Oxford Textbook of
Oncology

Free personal online access for 12 months

Individual purchasers of this book are also entitled to free personal access to the online edition for 12 months on Oxford Medicine Online (<http://oxfordmedicine.com/>). Please refer to the access token card for instructions on token redemption and access.

Online ancillary materials, where available, are noted at the end of the respective chapters in this book. Additionally, Oxford Medicine Online allows you to print, save, cite, email, and share content; download high-resolution figures as PowerPoint® slides; save often-used books, chapters, or searches; annotate; and quickly jump to other chapters or related material on a mobile-optimized platform.

We encourage you to take advantage of these features. If you are interested in ongoing access after the 12-month gift period, please consider an individual subscription or consult with your librarian.

Oxford Textbook of
Oncology

THIRD EDITION

Edited by

David J. Kerr

Daniel G. Haller

Cornelis J.H. van de Velde

Michael Baumann

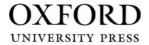

OXFORD
UNIVERSITY PRESS

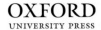

Great Clarendon Street, Oxford, OX2 6DP,
United Kingdom

Oxford University Press is a department of the University of Oxford.
It furthers the University's objective of excellence in research, scholarship,
and education by publishing worldwide. Oxford is a registered trade mark of
Oxford University Press in the UK and in certain other countries

First Edition © Oxford University Press, 1995
Second Edition © Oxford University Press, 2002
Third Edition © Oxford University Press, 2016
Chapter 10 © Baccelli, I. and Trumpp, A., 2012

The moral rights of the authors have been asserted

First Edition published in 1995
Second Edition published in 2002
Third Edition published in 2016

Impression: 1

Published in the United States of America by Oxford University Press
198 Madison Avenue, New York, NY 10016, United States of America

British Library Cataloguing in Publication Data
Data available

Library of Congress Control Number: 2015955657

ISBN 978–0–19–965610–3

Printed and bound in Great Britain by
Bell & Bain Ltd, Glasgow

Preface

The opportunity to compile a third edition of the *Oxford Textbook of Oncology* (after a gap of over ten years) represented a chance to deliver a definitive and comprehensive text detailing the evolution, evidence base, and current best practice in multidisciplinary cancer care. The first half of the textbook opens with introductory chapters covering the basic science that underpins our understanding of how cancer cells grow and function. These are then followed by sections looking specifically at the aetiology of cancer and the general principles governing modern approaches to oncology treatments. The first half of the book ends with a look at the unique challenges presented by treatment of cancer on a larger scale within population groups, and conversely the importance of recognizing and supporting the needs of individual patients both during and after treatment.

Our aim for the second half of the textbook was to provide a series of disease-based chapters written by expert teams from across the globe. Each chapter takes a multidisciplinary approach to the diagnosis and management of cancer, with sections covering the epidemiology, biology and pathology, radiotherapy, medical and surgical management of specific disease types.

When looking at the contents list for the new edition, you may notice that we have not included a chapter on childhood cancers. We felt that any discussion of paediatric oncology that was limited to only one chapter would inevitably be too superficial to cover even the most central aspects of this important discipline. Instead, readers will find that the focus of this volume is on the treatment and management of adult patients. For special paediatric considerations, we refer readers to *Cancer in Children: Clinical Management* (eds Michael C.G. Stevens and Hubert N. Caron, Oxford University Press, 2011). Now in its sixth edition, this book provides an excellent guide to the management of common childhood cancers.

One of the most important innovations in the third edition of the *Oxford Textbook of Oncology* is that it is available both in print, ebook, and online formats. One of the negatives of preparing a major textbook is that it may be out of date by the time of publication. We seek to overcome this with regular online updates when change in knowledge demands. Purchasers of the print book will receive a free 12-month access to the online version of the book. The online version contains all the material from the printed book, as well as extensive reference linking via PubMed. Over the lifetime of the book, additional case studies, figures, and other reference material will be made available as part of a series of regular updates that will be made to the online edition.

We would like to thank Beth Womack, Nicola Wilson, Caroline Smith, and the rest of the OUP team and the many international experts who contributed time, knowledge, and wisdom in writing this book.

This is a time of extraordinary advancement in oncology, with improvements seen in each of the major therapeutic areas, underpinned by basic and translational science leading to an increasingly personalized approach for many cancer patients. Drawing on the combined experience of an extensive list of internationally renowned contributors, we believe that this updated and revitalized third edition provides an essential resource for oncologists in all fields.

David J. Kerr
Daniel G. Haller
Cornelis J.H. van de Velde
Michael Baumann

Contents

List of abbreviations *xi*

List of contributors *xxi*

SECTION 1
Hallmarks of cancer

1 **The hallmarks of cancer: perspectives for cancer medicine** *3*
Douglas Hanahan and Robert A. Weinberg

2 **Growth factors and uncontrolled proliferation** *11*
Shujuan Liu and Ahmed Ashour Ahmed

3 **Cell signalling pathways** *23*
Stefan Knapp

4 **Cell cycle control** *31*
Simon M. Carr and Nicholas B. La Thangue

5 **Cancer cell death** *42*
Amanda S. Coutts, Sandra Maniam, and Nicholas B. La Thangue

6 **Angiogenesis** *49*
Yull E. Arriaga and Arthur E. Frankel

7 **Invasion and metastasis** *61*
Andrew P. Mazar, Andrey Ugolkov, Jack Henkin, Richard W. Ahn, and Thomas V. O'Halloran

8 **Genetic instability** *72*
Jennifer Wilding and Walter Bodmer

9 **DNA repair after oncological therapy (radiotherapy and chemotherapy)** *82*
Ekkehard Dikomey, Kerstin Borgmann, Malte Kriegs, Wael Y. Mansour, Cordula Petersen, and Thorsten Rieckmann

10 **Biology of cancer and metastasis stem cells** *86*
Andreas Trumpp and Irène Baccelli

11 **Biomarker identification and clinical validation** *98*
Richard D. Kennedy, Manuel Salto-Tellez, D. Paul Harkin, and Patrick G. Johnston

12 **Cancer, immunity, and inflammation** *109*
Campbell S.D. Roxburgh and Donald C. McMillan

13 **Cancer and metabolism** *119*
Cameron Snell, Kevin C. Gatter, Adrian L. Harris, and Francesco Pezzella

SECTION 2
Aetiology and epidemiology of cancer

14 **Smoking and cancer** *127*
Jonathan M. Samet

15 **Viruses** *136*
Chris Boshoff

16 **Chemical carcinogens** *142*
Paula A. Oliveira

17 **Radiation-induced cancer** *150*
Klaus R. Trott

18 **Aetiology and progression of cancer: role of body fatness, physical activity, diet, and other lifestyle factors** *155*
Fränzel J.B. van Duijnhoven and Ellen Kampman

SECTION 3
Principles of oncology

19 **Practice points for surgical oncology** *163*
Petra G. Boelens, C.B.M. van den Broek, and Cornelis J.H. van de Velde

20 Practice points for radiation oncology *173*
Annekatrin Seidlitz, Stephanie E. Combs,
Jürgen Debus, and Michael Baumann

21 Principles of chemotherapy *186*
David J. Kerr, Daniel G. Haller, and Jaap Verweij

22 Multidisciplinary cancer care *196*
David N. Church, Rachel Kerr, and David J. Kerr

**23 Principles of clinical
pharmacology: introduction to
pharmacokinetics
and pharmacodynamics** *209*
Michael Ong and Udai Banerji

24 Design and analysis of clinical trials *220*
Daniel J. Sargent and Qian Shi

25 Medical ethics in oncology *229*
Eric A. Singer

**26 Health economic assessment
of cancer therapy** *236*
Jeffrey Peppercorn

SECTION 4
Population health

27 Cancer control planning *245*
Massoud Samiei

28 Cancer prevention: vaccination *256*
Sarah E.B. Goltz and Julian Lob-Levyt

29 Cancer chemoprevention *262*
Hans-Joerg Senn, Nadir Arber, and Dirk Schrijvers

30 Population cancer screening *267*
Andrew Evans, C. Simon Herrington,
and Robert J.C. Steele

**31 Familial cancer syndromes and
genetic counselling** *276*
Henry T. Lynch, Carrie L. Snyder, and Jane F. Lynch

SECTION 5
Support for the cancer patient

32 Supportive and palliative care *293*
David Hui and Eduardo Bruera

33 Quality of life *302*
Neil K. Aaronson and Peter M. Fayers

34 Cancer survivorship and rehabilitation *312*
Rachel L. Yung and Ann H. Partridge

SECTION 6
Disease orientated chapters

35 Head and neck cancer *329*
Christine H. Chung, Andreas Dietz, Vincent Gregoire,
Marco Guzzo, Marc Hamoir, C. René Leemans, Jean-Louis
Lefebvre, Lisa Licitra, Adel K. El-Naggar, Brian O'Sullivan,
I. Bing Tan, Vincent Vandecaveye, Vincent Vander
Poorten, Jan B. Vermorken, and Michelle D. Williams

36 Oesophageal cancer *365*
Piet Dirix, Karin Haustermans, Eric Van Cutsem,
Xavier Sagaert, Christophe M. Deroose, Philippe
Nafteux, Hans Prenen, and Toni Lerut

37 Gastric cancer *388*
Hideaki Bando, Takahiro Kinoshita, Yasutoshi Kuboki,
Atsushi Ohtsu, and Kohei Shitara

**38 Rectal cancer and systemic therapy
of colorectal cancer** *408*
Regina Beets-Tan, Bengt Glimelius, and Lars Påhlman

39 Colorectal cancer *444*
Alex Boussioutas, Stephen B. Fox, Iris Nagtegaal,
Alexander Heriot, Jonathan Knowles, Michael Michael,
Sam Ngan, Kathryn Field, and John Zalcberg

40 Pancreatic cancer *478*
Jürgen Weitz, Markus W. Büchler, Paul D. Sykes,
John P. Neoptolemos, Eithne Costello, Christopher
M. Halloran, Frank Bergmann, Peter Schirmacher,
Ulrich Bork, Stefan Fritz, Jens Werner, Thomas B.
Brunner, Elizabeth Smyth, David Cunningham,
Brian R. Untch, and Peter J. Allen

41 Hepatobiliary cancers *508*
Graeme J. Poston, Nicholas Stern, Jonathan Evans,
Priya Healey, Daniel Palmer, and Mohandas K. Mallath

42 Peritoneal mesothelioma *533*
H. Richard Alexander, Jr., Dario Baratti, Terence C. Chua,
Marcello Deraco, Raffit Hassan, Marzia Pennati,
Federica Perrone, Paul H. Sugarbaker, Anish Thomas,
Keli Turner, Tristan D. Yan, and Nadia Zaffaroni

43 Cancer of the breast *546*
Martine Piccart, Toral Gathani, Dimitrios Zardavas, Hatem
A. Azim, Jr., Christos Sotiriou, Giuseppe Viale, Emiel J.T.
Rutgers, Mechthild Krause, Monica Arnedos, Suzette
Delaloge, Fabrice Andre, and Felipe Ades Moraes

44 Gynaecological cancers *576*
Richard Pötter, Shujuan Liu, Bolin Liu, Sebastien Gouy,
Sigurd Lax, Eric Leblanc, Philippe Morice, Fabrice Narducci,
Alexander Reinthaller, Maximilian Paul Schmid,
Catherine Uzan, and Pauline Wimberger

45 Genitourinary cancers *602*
John Fitzpatrick, Asif Muneer, Jean de la Rosette,
and Thomas Powles

46 Lung cancer *628*
Rafał Dziadziuszko, Michael Baumann,
Tetsuya Mitsudomi, Keith M. Kerr, Solange Peters,
and Stefan Zimmermann

47 Neoplasms of the thymus *655*
Rebecca Bütof, Axel Denz, Gustavo Baretton,
Jan Stöhlmacher-Williams, and Michael Baumann

48 Pleural mesothelioma *659*
Andrea S. Wolf, Assunta de Rienzo, Raphael Bueno,
Lucian R. Chirieac, Joseph M. Corson, Elizabeth H. Baldini,
David Jackman, Ritu Gill, Walter Weder, Isabelle Opitz,
Ann S. Adams, and David J. Sugarbaker

49 Skin cancer: melanoma *674*
John F. Thompson, Richard A. Scolyer,
and Richard F. Kefford

50 Skin cancer: non-melanoma *690*
Diona L. Damian, Richard A. Scolyer, Graham Stevens,
Alexander M. Menzies, and John F. Thompson

51 Acute leukaemias *699*
Adele K. Fielding, Charles G. Mullighan, Dieter Hoelzer,
Eytan M. Stein, Ghada Zakout, Martin S. Tallman,
Yishai Ofran, Jacob M. Rowe, and Ross L. Levine

52 Chronic leukaemias *754*
Hemant Malhotra, Lalit Kumar, Pankaj Malhotra,
Devendra Hiwase, and Ravi Bhatia

53 Myeloma *782*
Charlotte Pawlyn, Faith Davies,
and Gareth Morgan

54 Malignant lymphomas *808*
Frank Kroschinsky, Friedrich Stölzel, Stefano A. Pileri,
Björn Chapuy, Rainer Ordemann, Christian Gisselbrecht,
Tim Illidge, David C. Hodgson, Mary K. Gospodarowicz,
Christina Schütze, and Gerald G. Wulf

**55 Sarcomas of soft tissues
and bone** *844*
Alessandro Gronchi, Angelo P. Dei Tos,
and Paolo G. Casali

56 Craniospinal malignancies *867*
Puneet Plaha, Allyson Parry, Pieter Pretorius,
Michael Brada, Olaf Ansorge, and Claire Blesing

57 Tumours of the eye and orbit *904*
Daniel G. Ezra, Geoffrey E. Rose, Jacob Pe'er,
Sarah E. Coupland, Stefan Seregard, G.P.M. Luyten,
and Annette C. Moll

58 Endocrine cancers *918*
Andrew Weaver, Anthony P. Weetman,
Oliver Gimm, Ashley Grossman, Petra Sulentic,
Bertram Wiedenmann, Ursula Plöckinger,
Ulrich-Frank Pape, John Wass, Angela Rogers,
and Wouter de Herder

59 Cancer of unknown primary site *965*
Nicholas Pavlidis and George Pentheroudakis

Index *975*

List of abbreviations

2D-CRT	two-dimensional conformal treatment		ALA	aminolaevulinic acid
2GTKI	second generation TKI therapy		ALCL	anaplastic large-cell lymphoma
2-HG	2-hydroxyglutarate		ALFA	Acute Leukemia French Association
3DCRT	3D conformal radiotherapy		ALK	activin-receptor-like kinases; anaplastic lymphoma receptor tyrosine kinase
5-FU	5-fluorouracil			
5-FU/FA	5-fluorouracil and folinic acid (leucovorin)		ALL	acute lymphocytic leukaemia; acute lymphoblastic leukaemia
5-HIAA	5-hydroxy-indole acetic acid			
5-hmC	5-hydroxymethylcytosine		ALT	alternative lengthening of telomeres; atypical lipomatous tumour
5-mC	5-methylcytosine			
5'-TOP	5'-terminal oligopolypyrimidine		allo-HSCT	allogeneic-haematopoietic stem cell transplantation
^{18}F-FDG	^{18}F-fluoro-deoxyglucose			
			allo-SCT	allogeneic-stem cell transplantation
AA	African American; anaplastic astrocytomas		ALT	alternative lengthening of telomeres
AAH	atypical adenomatous hyperplasia		AMC	Advanced Market Commitment
aaIPI	age-adjusted IPI		AML	acute myelogenous leukaemia; acute myeloid leukaemia
ABC	advanced biliary cancer; activated B-cell			
ABVD	Adriamycin® (doxorubicin), bleomycin, vinblastine, and dacarbazine		AMPK	adenosine monophosphate-activated protein kinase
			AO	anaplastic oligoastrocytoma
AC	adrenal carcinoma		AOA	anaplastic oligoastrocytoma
ACA	additional cytogenetic abnormalities		AP	accelerated phase
ACC	adenoid cystic carcinoma		APA	aldosterone-producing adenoma
ACF	aberrant crypt foci		Apaf-1	apoptotic protease activating factor 1
ACS	American Cancer Society		APBD	anomalous pancreatic biliary duct
ACTH	adrenocorticotrophic hormone		APC	adenomatous polyposis coli
aCGH	array Comparative Genomic Hybridization		APC	anaphase promoting complex
ADC	antibody drug conjugate; apparent diffusion coefficient		APL	acute promyelocytic leukaemia
			array-CGH	array-based comparative genomic hybridization
ADCC	antibody-dependent cellular cytotoxicity		ARF	alternative reading frame
ADH	antidiuretic hormone		ARHG	AP29 RHOA GTPase-activating protein 29
ADME	absorption, distribution, metabolism, and excretion		ASCO	American Society of Clinical Oncology
ADOC	cyclophosphamide, Adriamycin® (doxorubicin), vincristine, and cisplatin		ASCT	autologous stem cell transplant
			ASOC	advanced stage ovarian cancer
AF	accelerated radiotherapy		ASR	age standardized rates
AFAP	attenuated FAP		Atg	autophagy-related gene
AFP	alpha-feto protein		ATL	adult T-cell leukaemia
AfrOx	Africa Oxford Cancer Foundation		ATM	ataxia telangiectasia mutated
AFX	atypical fibroxanthoma		ATO	arsenic trioxide
AICR	American Institute for Cancer Research		ATP	adenosine triphosphate
AIF	apoptosis inducing factor		ATRA	all-trans retinoic acid
AIS	adenocarcinoma in situ		Auto-SCT	autologous stem cell transplantation
AITL	angioimmunoblastic T-cell lymphoma		AUC	area under the curve
AJCC	American Joint Committee on Cancer		AVC	angiogenic vascular cells
AK	actinic keratosis		AYA	adolescents and young adults

β₂M β₂	microglobulin		CEUS	ultrasound contrast bubbles
β-TRCP	b-transducin repeat-containing protein		CF	conventional fractionation
BAD	BCL-2 antagonist of cell death		CGH	comparative genomic hybridization
BAFF	B-cell activating factor		CGIN	cervical glandular intraepithelial neoplasia
B-ALL	B-cell acute lymphocytic leukaemia		CHCC	combined hepatocellular and cholangiocarcinoma
BAO	basal acid output		CHD	carcinoid heart disease
BC	blast crisis		CHF	congestive heart failure
B-CLL	B-cell lymphocytic leukaemia		CHL	classic Hodgkin lymphoma
BBB	blood-brain barrier		CHOP	cyclophosphamide, doxorubicin, vincristine, and prednisone
BC	breast cancer; bladder cancer			
BCC	basal cell carcinomas; breast cancer cells		CHR	complete haematological response
BCG	Bacillus Calmette-Guérin		CI	confidence interval
Bcl-2	B-cell lymphoma 2		CIN	cervical intraepithelial neoplasia; chromosome instability
BCLC	Barcelona Clinic for Liver Cancer			
BCT	breast-conserving therapy		CIMP	CpG island methylator phenotype
BDWG	Biomarkers Definitions Working Group		CIS	carcinoma in situ
BEAM	BCNU, etoposide, cytarabine, and melphalan		CK	cytokeratin
BEP	cisplatin, etoposide, and bleomycin		CK-7	cytokeratin-7
BER	base excision repair		CKI	CDK inhibitor
BH	Bcl-2 homology		CLC	cardiotrophin-like cytokine
BHDS	Birt-Hogg-Dube syndrome		CLND	completion lymph node dissection
BL	Burkitt's lymphoma		CLL	chronic lymphocytic leukaemia
BM	bone marrow		CML	chronic myeloid leukaemia
BMD	bone mineral density		CMML	chronic myelomonocytic leukaemia
BMP	bone morphogenetic proteins		C-MIN	conjunctival melanocytic intraepithelial neoplasia
BOD	biologically optimal dose			
BP	blastic phase		CMR	complete molecular response
BRCP	breast cancer resistance protein		CMS	Centers for Medicare and Medicaid Services
BRPC	borderline resectable pancreatic cancer		CMV	cytomegalovirus
BRRM	bilateral risk reducing mastectomy		CNA	copy number alterations
BRT	bioradiotherapy		CNS	central nervous system
BSC	best supportive care		CNSL	central nervous system lymphoma
BTK	Bruton's tyrosine kinase		CNTF	ciliar neurotrophic factor
			CoC	Commission on Cancer
CA	cryoablation		COG	Children's Oncology Group
CAE	cyclophosphamide, Adriamycin® (doxorubicin), and etoposide		COO	cell-of-origin
			COPD	chronic obstructive pulmonary disease
CAF	cancer-associated fibroblast		CP	chronic phase
CAG	chronic atrophic gastritis		CR	complete remission
CAK	CDK activating kinase		CRAB	calcium, renal, anaemia, and bone abnormalities
CAIX	carbonic anhydrase IX		CRC	colorectal carcinoma
CALGB	Cancer and Leukemia Group B		CRKL	CRK-like protein
CARES	Cancer Rehabilitation Evaluation System		CRM	circumferential resection margin; continual reassessment method
CAT	computer-adaptive testing			
CAV	cyclophosphamide, doxorubicin, and vincristine		CRPC	castrate-resistant prostate cancer
CAVE	cyclophosphamide, doxorubicin, vincristine, and etoposide		CRRM	contralateral risk-reducing mastectomy
			CRS	cytoreductive surgery
CBE	complete blood count examination		CRT	chemoradiotherapy
CBR	clinical benefit rate		(C)RT	radiotherapy alone or with chemotherapy
CBV	cyclophosphamide, BCNU, etoposide		CS	carcinoid syndrome
cCR	clinical complete remission		CSA	cranio-spinal axis
CCRCC	clear cell renal cell carcinoma		CSC	cancer stem cell
CCRT	concurrent/concomitant chemoradiation therapy		CSF	cerebrospinal fluid
CCS	cancer control strategy		CSR	class switch recombination
CD	coeliac disease		CT	computed tomography
CDC	complement-dependent cytotoxicity		CT1	cardiotrophin
CDK	cyclin-dependent kinase		CTC	circulating tumour cell
CEA	carcino-embryonic antigen		CTL	cytotoxic T-lymphocyte
CED	convection-enhanced delivery		CTV	clinical target volume
CEP	circulating endothelial progenitors		CUP	cancer of unknown primary

CVA	cerebrovascular accidents	EGFR	epidermal growth factor receptor
CVD	cyclophosphamide, vincristine, and dacarbazine	EHCC	extrahepatocellular carcinoma
		eIF4E	eukaryotic translation initiation factor 4E
DAG	diacylglycerol	ELND	elective lymph node dissection
DAPK	death-associated protein kinase	EM	electron microscopy
DC	dendritic cell	EMA	endoscopic mucosal ablation
DCC	deleted in colon cancer	EMR	endoscopic mucosal resection
DCE	dynamic contrast enhanced	EMT	epithelial mesenchymal transformation/ transition
DCE-MRI	dynamic contrast-enhanced magnetic resonance imaging	EMZL	extranodal marginal zone B-cell lymphomas
DCIS	ductal carcinoma in situ	ENB	esthesioneuroblastomas
DD	death domain	ENETS	European Neuroendocrine Tumor Society
DEB	drug-eluting beads	EORTC	European Organization for Research and Treatment of Cancer
DEPTOR	DEP domain-containing mTOR-interacting protein	EORTC QLQ-C30	European Organization for Research and Treatment of Cancer Core QoL Questionnaire
DEXA	dual-energy X-ray absorptiometry		
DFCI	Dana Farber Cancer Institute		
DFS	disease-free survival	EPC	endothelial progenitor cells
DFSP	dermatofibrosarcoma protuberans	EPO	erythropoietin
DHAP	dexamethasone/high-dose ara-C/cisplatin	EPP	extrapleural pneumonectomy
DHFR	dihydrofolate reductase	EPT	electron-photon therapy
DIC	disseminated intravascular coagulation	EPT	endocrine pancreatic tumour
DFS	disease-free survival	EQ	erythroplasia of Queyrat
DFSP	dermatofibrosarcoma protuberans	ER	endoplasmatic reticulum
DIN	ductal intraepithelial neoplasia	ERAS	enhanced recovery after surgery
DISC	death-inducing signalling complex	ERCP	endoscopic retrograde cholangio-pancreatography
DKK	Dickkopfs	ERR	excess relevant risk; oestrogen related receptors
DLBCL	diffuse large B-cell lymphoma	ERUS	endorectal ultrasonography
DLL4	Delta-like ligand 4	ES	effect size
DLT	dose-limiting toxicity	ESAS	Edmonton Symptom Assessment Scale
DM	distant metastases	ESD	endoscopic submucosal dissection
DMPM	diffuse malignant peritoneal mesothelioma	ESMO	European Society of Medical Oncology
DOR	duration of response	ESS	Edmonton Staging System
DPD	dihydropyrimidine dehydrogenase	ESSO	European Society of Surgical Oncology
DRE	digital rectal examination	ET	essential thombocythaemia
DSB	double strand break	ETP	early T-cell precursor
DTC	direct-to-consumer; disseminated tumour cells	EUNICE	European Network for Indicators on Cancer
DTI	diffusion tensor tractography	EURECCA	European Registration of Cancer Care
Dvl	intracellular Dishevelled	EUS	endoscopic ultrasound
DWI	diffusion-weighted imaging	EUS-FNA	endoscopic ultrasound-guided fine needle aspiration
EAP	Expanded Access Programs	EUSOMA	European Society of Mastology
EATL	enteropathy-associated T-cell lymphoma		
EB	epidermolysis bullosa	FA	fluorescein angiography
EBMT	European Group for Blood and Marrow Transplantation	FACS	fluorescence-activated cell sorting
		FACT-G	Functional Assessment of Cancer Therapy
EBRT	external beam radiotherapy	FADD	Fas-associated DD
EBUS	endobronchial ultrasound	FAMM	facial artery musculo-mucosal; familial atypical multiple mole/melanoma
EBUS-FNA	endobronchial ultrasound-guided fine needle aspiration		
EBV	Epstein–Barr virus	FAMMM	familial atypical multiple mole/melanoma
EC	endometrial cancer	FAP	familial adenomatous polyposis
ECCO	European CanCer Organisation	FCTC	Framework Convention on Tobacco Control
ECF	epirubicin, cisplatin, and infusional 5-fluorouracil	FDA	Food and Drug Administration
ECM	extracellular matrix	FDG	fluorodeoxyglucose
ECOG	Eastern Cooperative Oncology Group	FDG-PET	18-fludeoxyglucose positron emission tomography
ECT	electrochemotherapy		
EEA	extended endoscopic approaches	FFCD	Fédération Francophone de Cancérologie Digestive
EFS	event-free survival rates		
EGF	epidermal growth factor	FFPE	formalin-fixed and paraffin-embedded
EGRF	epidermal growth factor receptor	FGF	fibroblast growth factor

FGFR	fibroblast growth factor receptor
FIT	faecal immunochemical testing
FISH	fluorescence in situ hybridization
FKHR	forkhead transcription factor
FLIC	Functional Living Index—Cancer
FN	fibronectin
FNA	fine needle aspiration
FNAC	fine needle aspiration cytology
FNR	false-negative rate
FL	follicular lymphoma
FLL	focal liver lesions
FLR	future liver remnant
FOB	fibreoptic bronchoscopy
FOLFOX	5-FU, leucovorin and oxaliplatin
FOXO	forkhead box O
FRO	familial renal oncocytoma
FRS2	FGFR substrate 2s
FS	flexible sigmoidoscopy
FTH	follicular T-helper
GAB1	GRB2-associated binding protein 1
GAP	GTPase activating protein
GARFT	glycinamide ribonucleotide formyltransferase
GASTRIC	Global Advanced/Adjuvant Stomach Tumour Research International Collaboration
GBC	gall bladder cancer; germinal centre B-cell
GBM	glioblastoma multiforme
GC	gemcitabine and carboplatin
GC	germinal centre
GCP	good clinical practice
GCSF	granulocyte colony stimulating factor
GDA	gastroduodenal artery
GDF	growth and differentiation factor
GDP	gemcitabine, dexamethasone, and cisplatin; guanosine diphosphate
GEF	guanine nucleotide exchange factor
GHRH	growth hormone-releasing hormone
GEJ	gastro-oesophageal junction
GEMM	genetically engineered mouse models
GEP	gastroenteropancreatic
GEP	gene expression profiling
GF	growth factor
GGR	global genome repair
GH	growth hormone
GINA	Genetic Information Nondiscrimination Act
GIST	gastrointestinal stromal tumour
GITSG	Gastrointestinal Tumour Study Group
GLUT4	glucose transporter type 4
GMALL	German Multicenter Study Group for Adult Acute Lymphoblastic Leukemia
GMP	good manufacturing procedure; granulocyte/macrophage progenitor
GM-CSF	granulocyte-macrophage colony-stimulating factor
GO	gemtuzumab ozogamicin
GPS	Glasgow Prognostic Score
GRA	glucocorticoid-remediable aldosteronism
GRB2	proteins growth-factor-receptor bound-2
GSK3	glycogen synthase kinase 3
GSK3-b	glycogen synthase kinase 3b

GTP	guanosine triphosphate
GTV	gross tumour volume
GvHD	graft-versus-host disease
GvL	graft-versus-leukaemia
GWAS	genome-wide association studies
HAART	highly active antiretroviral therapy
HAT	histone acetyl-transferase
HB	hepatobiliary
HBeAg	hepatitis B e antigen
HBsAg	hepatitis B surface antigen
HBOC	hereditary breast-ovarian cancer
HBV	hepatitis B virus
HCC	hepatocellular carcinoma
HCL	hairy cell leukaemia
HCL-v	hairy cell leukaemia-variant
HCT	haematopoietic cell transplantation
HCV	hepatitis C virus
HDAC	histone deacetylase
HDR	high dose rate
HDT	high-dose therapy
HDV	hepatitis delta virus
H&E	haematoxylin and eosin
Hep Par 1	hepatocyte paraffin 1 monoclonal antibody
HF	hyperfractionated radiotherapy
HGF	hepatocyte growth factor
HGFA	HGF activator
Hh	Hedgehog
HIDAC	high-doses cytarabine
HIF	hypoxia inducible factor; hypoxia inhibitory factor
HIFU	high intensity focused ultrasound
HICC	heated intracavity chemotherapy
HIPEC	hyperthermic perioperative chemotherapy
HLA	humoral leukocyte antigen
HNPCC	hereditary non-polyposis colorectal cancer
HNPGL	head and neck parasympathetic paraganglioma
HNSCC	head and neck squamous cell carcinoma
HPC	haemangiopericytoma
HPF	high power fields
HPRC	hereditary papillary renal carcinoma
HPV	human papilloma virus
HR	hazard ratio; homologous recombination
HRC	hereditary renal carcinoma
HRE	hypoxic response elements
HSC	haematopoietic stem cell
HSP90	heat shock protein 90
HT	hypertension
HTLV-1	Human T-cell leukaemia virus 1
IAP	inhibitor of apoptosis protein
IARC	International Agency for Research on Cancer
IASLC	International Association for the Study of Lung Cancer
IBI	International Breast Cancer Intervention Study
ICE	ifosfamide, carboplatin, etoposide
ICER	incremental cost-effectiveness ratio
ICL	interstrand cross-link
ICRP	International Commission on Radiation Protection

ICRU	International Commission on Radiation Units and Measurements
ICT	induction chemotherapy
IDC	NOS invasive ductal carcinoma not otherwise specified
IFFIm	International Finance Facility for Immunisation
IFL	irinotecan/bolus 5-FU, leucovorin
IFN	interferon
IFP	interstitial fluid pressure
IFRT	involved-field radiotherapy
IGABT	image-guided adaptive brachytherapy
IGF	insulin growth factor
IGF1	insulin growth factor 1
IGF2	insulin growth factor 2
IGFBP	IGF binding proteins
IGLC	International Gastric Cancer Linkage Consortium
IGRT	image-guided radiotherapy
IHA	idiopathic hyperaldosteronism
IHC	immunohistochemistry
IHCC	intrahepatic cholangiocarcinoma
IIC	infiltrating immune cell
IJCN	inflamed juvenile conjunctival naevi
IKK	IκB kinase
IKKB	IkB kinase b
IL	interleukin
IL1R	interleukin 1 receptor
IL6	Interleukin 6
ILC	invasive lobular carcinoma
ILND	inguinal lymph node dissection
ILP	isolated limb perfusion
iMR	intraoperative MR
IMRT	intensity-modulated radiation therapy
IMWG	International Myeloma Working Group
INCTR	International Network for Cancer Treatment
iNOS	inducible nitric oxide synthase
INRT	involved-node radiotherapy
Ins(1,4,5)P3	inositol-1,4,5- trisphosphate
IOM	Institute of Medicine
IORT	intraoperative radiotherapy
IOUS	intraoperative ultrasound
IP	intraperitoneal
IPAA	total proctocolectomy and ileoanal pouch
IPD	individual patient data
IPI	International Prognostic Index
IPMN	intraductal papillary mucinous neoplasms
iPS	induced pluripotent stem cells
IR	insulin receptor; ionizing radiation
IRA	ileorectal anastomosis
IRS	insulin receptor substrates
IRT	item response theory
ISGPF	International Study Group on Pancreatic Fistula Definition
ISGPS	International Study Group of Pancreatic Surgery
ITMIG	International Thymic Malignancy Interest Group
ITT	intention to treat
ITV	internal target volume
JAK	Janus kinase
JCOG	Japan Clinical Oncology Group

JGCA	Japanese Gastric Cancer Association
KA	keratoacanthoma
KPS	Karnofsky performance status
KS	Kaposi's sarcoma
KSHV	Kaposi's sarcoma-associated herpesvirus
KSR	kinase suppressor of Ras
LAPC	locally advanced pancreatic cancer
LAR	long-acting repeatable
LCC	large cell carcinoma
LCIS	lobular carcinoma in situ
LCL	lymphoblastoid cell line
LCNEC	large cell neuroendocrine carcinoma
LDDST	low-dose dexamethasone suppression test
LDH	lactate dehydrogenase
LDHA	lactate dehydrogenase A
LDR	low dose rate
LEF	lymphoid enhancer factor
LEF1	lymphoid enhancer-binding factor 1
LFS	leukaemia-free survival
LETZ	loop excision of the transformation zone
LIF	leukaemia inhibitory factor
LIN	lobular intraepithelial neoplasia
LMICs	low- and middle-income countries
LMP-1	latent membrane protein-1
LOH	loss of heterozygosity
LP	lymphocyte predominant
LPL	lymphoplasmacytic lymphoma
LRR	local and/or regional recurrences
LS	Lynch syndrome
LSC	leukaemic stem cell
LUTS	lower urinary tract symptoms
LVSI	lymphovascular space invasion
MAA	macro-aggregated albumin
mAb	monoclonal antibodies
MACs	microsatellite and chromosome stable
MAC-NPC	meta-analysis of chemotherapy in NPC
MALT	lymphoma mucosa-associated lymphatic tissue lymphoma
MAP3K	MAP kinase kinase kinases
MAPK	mitogen-activated protein kinases
MAP	MUTYH-associated polyposis
MBL	monoclonal B-cell lymphocytosis
mBL	molecular BL
MC	mitotic count
MCC	Merkel cell carcinoma
MCD	Multicentric Castleman's Disease
MCL	mantle cell lymphoma
MCN	mucinous cystic neoplasm
MCP-1	monocyte chemotactic protein
MCPM	multicystic peritoneal mesothelioma
MCR	macroscopic complete resection; molecular complete response
MCRC	metastatic colorectal cancer
MCV	Merkel cell polyomavirus
MDCT	multidetector computed tomography
MDR	multidrug resistant

MDRT	moderate-dose radiation therapy	NBOCAP	National Bowel Cancer Audit Programme
MDS	myelodysplastic syndromes	NCCN	National Comprehensive Cancer Network
MDSC	myeloid derived suppressor cells	NCCS	National Coalition for Cancer Survivorship
MDT	multidisciplinary team	NCD	non-communicable disease
MEC	mucoepidermoid carcinoma	NCI	National Cancer Institute
MELD	model of end-stage liver disease	NEC	neuroendocrine carcinoma
MelTUMP	melanocytic tumour of uncertain malignant potential	NEN	neuroendocrine neoplasia
MEN	multiple endocrine neoplasia	NER	nucleotide excision repair
MET	mesenchymal-to-epithelial transition	NET	neuroendocrine tumour
MFH	malignant fibrous histiocytoma	NETZ	needle excision of the transformation zone
MGUS	monoclonal gammopathy of undetermined significance	NGS	next-generation sequencing
		NHEJ	non-homologous end joining
		NHL	Non-Hodgkin lymphoma
MIBC	muscle invasive bladder carcinoma	NHSCSP	National Health Service Cervical Screening Programme
MIC	metastasis-initiating cells; microinvasive carcinoma	NICD	Notch intracellular domain
MIE	minimally invasive oesophagectomy	NLPHL	nodular lymphocyte-predominant Hodgkin lymphoma
MIF	Müllerian inhibitory factor	NLR	neutrophil:lymphocyte ratio
MIBG	metaiodobenzylguanidine	NMIBC	non-muscle invasive bladder carcinoma
MiSG	minor salivary glands	NMSC	non-melanoma skin cancer
MITF	micropthalmia transcription factor	NNK	N-nitrosamines
Miz1	Myc interacting zinc-finger protein		4-(methylnitrosamino)-1-(3-pyridyl)-1-butanone
MLC	multileaf collimators	NNN	N'-nitrosonornicenotine
MM	multiple myeloma	NOS2	nitric oxide synthase-2
MMMT	Mixed malignant Müllerian tumours	NOTES	natural orifice transluminal endoscopic surgery
MMP	matrix metalloproteinase	NPC	nasopharyngeal carcinoma
MMP-9	matrix metalloprotease-9	NPM	nucleophosmin gene
MMR	mismatch repair	NPV	negative predictive value
MNGGCT	malignant non-germinoma germ cell tumour	NRM	non-relapse mortality
MoAb	monoclonal antibody	NSABP	National Surgical Breast and Bowel Project
MOMP	mitochondrial outer membrane permeabilization	NSAID	non-steroidal anti-inflammatory drug
MOPP	mechlorethamine, vincristine, procarbazine, prednisone	NSE	neuron-specific enolase
		NSGCT	non-seminoma germ cell tumours
mOS	median overall survival	NSCLC	non-small-cell carcinoma; non-small-cell lung cancer
MPA	medroxyprogesterone acetate		
MPD	myeloproliferative diseases	NTCP	normal tissue complication probability
MPM	malignant peritoneal mesothelioma		
MPN	myeloproliferative neoplasms	OAR	organs at risk
MR	minimal response	OC	ovarian cancer
MRA	magnetic resonance angiography	OCA	other chromosomal abnormality
MRC	Medical Research Council	ONB	olfactory neuroblastoma
MRCP	magnetic resonance cholangiopancreatography	OPC	oropharyngeal cancer
MRD	minimal residual disease	ORR	overall response rate
MRF	mesorectal fascia	OS	overall survival
MRI	magnetic resonance imaging	OSCC	oral cavity squamous cell carcinoma; oropharyngeal squamous cell carcinoma
MRP	multidrug resistance-associated protein		
MSI	microsatellite instability		
MSI-H	high microsatellite instability	OSM	oncostatin M
MSI-L	low microsatellite instability	OSSN	ocular surface squamous neoplasia
MSKCC	Memorial Sloan Kettering Cancer Center		
MSS	microsatellite stable/stability	P13K	phosphoinositide 3 kinase
MTC	medullary thyroid carcinoma	PAC	cyclophosphamide, doxorubicin, and cisplatin
MTD	maximum tolerated dose	PAH	polycyclic aromatic hydrocarbon; primary adrenal hyperplasia
mTOR	mammalian target of rapamycin		
MZL	marginal zone lymphoma	PAM	primary acquired melanosis
		PanIN	pancreatic intraepithelial neoplasia
NAC	nipple areolar complex	PAR3	partitioning defective 3
NAMPT	nicotinamide phosphoribosyltransferase	PARP	poly(ADP-ribose)polymerase
NASH	non-alcoholic steatohepatitis	PBF	peripheral blood film
NBCC	nodular BCC		

PBMNC	peripheral blood mononuclear cell
PBPC	peripheral blood progenitor cells
PBT	proton beam therapy
PCD	programmed cell death
PCI	prophylactic cranial irradiation; peritoneal cancer index
PCL	plasma cell leukaemia
PCM	plasma cell myeloma
pCR	pathological complete remission
P/D	pleurectomy/decortication
PDGF	platelet-derived growth factor
PDGFR-α	platelet-derived growth factor receptor α
PDGFR-β	platelet-derived growth factor receptor β
PDK1	phosphoinositide-dependent kinase 1
PDT	photodynamic therapy
PE	phosphatidylethanolamine
PET	positron emission tomography
PF	cisplatin and fluorouracil
PFE	platinum/5-FU/Erbitux® (cetuximab)
PFS	progression-free survival
PG	paraganglioma
PGP	P170 membrane glycoprotein
PH	pleckstrin homology
PHC	primary health care
PHD	prolyl hydroxylase domain protein
PI3K	phosphoinositide-3-kinase
PI3P	phosphatidylinositol g3-phosphate
PIAS	PIAS protein inhibitor of active STAT
PIKK	PI3K-related protein kinase
PIN	point mutation instability
PKB	protein kinase B
PKD1	protein kinase D1
PLC	phospholipase C
PLGA	polymorphous low-grade adenocarcinoma
PlGF	placental growth factor
Plk	polo-like kinases
PLL	prolymphocytic leukaemia
PMBL	primary mediastinal large B-cell lymphoma
PMF	primary myelofibrosis
PMLBCL	primary mediastinal large B-cell lymphomas
PNET	primitive neuro-ectodermal tumours
PODXL	podocalyxin
POPF	post-operative pancreatic fistula
PPH	postpancreatectomy haemorrhage
PPI	proton-pump inhibitor
PPPD	pylorus-preserving pancreaticoduodenectomy
PPT	pineal parenchymal tumours
PPV	positive predictive value
pre-RC	pre-replicative complex
pRb	retinoblastoma protein
PROCARisE	Project on Cancer of the Rectum
PROMIS	Patient-Reported Outcome Measurement Information System
PRP	platelet-rich plasma
PRRT	peptide receptor-mediated radionuclide therapy
PRV	planning organ-at-risk volume
PSA	prostate-specific antigen
PSC	pancreatic stem cells; primary sclerosing cholangitis
PSOGI	Peritoneal Surface Oncology Group International

PTC	percutaneous transhepatic cholangiography
PTCL	peripheral T-cell lymphomas
PTCL-NOS	peripheral T-cell lymphomas not otherwise specified
PTE	proportion of treatment effect
PTH-rp	parathyroid hormone-related protein
PTLD	post-transplant lymphoproliferative disorders
PTV	planning target volume
PUNLMP	papillary urothelial neoplasm of low malignant potential
PUVA	psoralens and UVA
PV	polycythaemia vera
PVC	primary vaginal cancer
QALY	quality-adjusted life years
RARECARE	Surveillance of Rare Cancers in Europe
RASIP1	RAS-interacting protein 1
Rb	retinoblastoma
RBE	relative biological effectiveness
RCC	renal cell carcinoma
RECIST	Response Evaluation Criteria in Solid Tumours
rESS	revised Edmonton Staging System
RFA	radiofrequency ablation
RFR	relapse-free rate
RFS	relapse-free survival
RHEB	RAS homologue enriched in brain
RIC	reduced-intensity conditioning
RIC-allo-SCT	reduced-intensity conditioned allogeneic-stem cell transplantation
RILD	radiation induced lung disease
RIP	receptor-interacting protein
RIT	radioimmunotherapy
RKIP	RAF kinase inhibitor protein
R/M	recurrent/metastatic
ROLL	radio-guided occult lesion localization
ROS	reactive oxygen species
ROTI	myeloma-related organ and tissue impairment
RPE	retinal pigment epithelium
RPLS	reversible posterior leukoencephalopathy syndrome
RPS	retroperitoneal sarcomas
RR	response rate
RRSO	risk-reducing bilateral salpingo-oophorectomy
RS	recurrence score
RSCL	Rotterdam Symptom Checklist
RT	radiation therapy
RTK	receptor tyrosine kinase
RTOG	Radiation Therapy Oncology Group
RT-PCR	reverse transcriptase-polymerase chain reaction
RQ-PCR	real-time quantitative polymerase chain reaction
S1P	sphingosine-1-phosphate
SAP	serum amyloid P
SBCC	superficial BCC
SBRT	stereotactic body radiotherapy
SCC	squamous cell carcinoma
SCCHN	squamous cell carcinoma of the head and neck
SCLC	small-cell lung carcinoma

sCR	stringent complete response		STIC	serous tubal intraepithelial carcinoma
SDF-1	stromal derived factor-1		SUV	standardized uptake value
SDH	succinate dehydrogenase		SV40-T	simian virus large T antigen
SDPP	stroma-derived prognostic predictor		SVCS	superior vena cava syndrome
SEER	Surveillance, Epidemiology and End results		SWETZ	straight wire excision of the transformation zone
SEIC	serous endometrial intraepithelial carcinoma			
SEMS	self-expanding metallic stents		TA	telomerase activity
SERM	selective estrogen receptor modulators		TACE	transarterial chemoembolization
SET	sensitivity to endocrine therapy		TAM	tumour-associated macrophages
SES	socio-economic status		TBI	total-body irradiation
SFLC	serum free light-chains		TCD	T-cell depletion
SFRP	secreted frizzled-related protein		TCF	docetaxel, cisplatin, infusional 5-fluorouracil; T-cell factor
SGC	salivary gland cancer			
SGCT	seminoma germ cell tumour		TCP	tumor control probability
SH2	Src homology 2		TCR	transcription-coupled repair
SH3	Src homology 3		TEM	transanal endoscopic microsurgery
SHIP	SH2-domain-containing inositol-5-phosphatase		TG	total glansectomy
SHM	somatic hypermutation		TGF	transforming growth factor
SHS	secondhand smoke		TGFβ, TGF-b	transforming growth factor beta
SIB	simultaneous integrated boost		TGR	total glans resurfacing
SIGN	Scottish Intercollegiate Guidelines Network		TIEG1	TGFβ-inducible early-response gene
SIL	squamous intraepithelial lesion; single incision laparoscopy		TIGAR	TP-53-induced glycolysis and apoptosis regulator
sIL-2R	soluble interleukin-2 receptor		TIL	tumour-infiltrating lymphocytes
SIN3	squamous intraepithelial neoplasia 3		TK	tyrosine kinase
SIRT	selective internal radiation treatment		TKI	tyrosine kinase inhibitor
SLAM	signalling lymphocytic activation molecule		TLS	tumour lysis syndrome
SLNB	sentinel lymph node biopsy		TME	total mesorectal excision; tumour microenvironment
SMA	superior mesenteric artery		TNBC	triple-negative breast cancer
SMAC	second mitochondria derived activator		TNFR	tumour necrosis factor receptor
smCC	small-cell cancer		TNFR1	TNF receptor 1
SMM	smouldering myeloma		TNM	tumour node metastasis
SMV	superior mesenteric vein		TORS	transoral robotic surgery
SN	sentinel node		TOS	TOR signalling
SNP	single nuclear polymorphisms		T-PLL	T-cell prolymphocytic leukaemia
SNEC	sinonasal neuroendocrine		TPF	docetaxel, cisplatin, and 5-fluorouracil; Taxotere®, cisplatin, and fluorouracil
SNUC	sinonasal undifferentiated carcinoma			
SOCS	suppressor of cytokine signalling		TPMT	thiopurine methyltransferase
SOS	Son of Sevenless		TPS	treatment planning systems
SPARC	secreted protein acidic and rich in cysteine		TRADD	TNFR1-associated DD
SPB	solitary plasmacytoma of bone		TRAF	TNF receptor associated factor
SPEP	serum electrophoresis		TRAIL	TNF-related apoptosis inducing ligand
SPH	serine proteinase homology		TRAIL-R1	TRAIL receptor 1
SPT	secondary primary tumour		TRAIL-R2	TRAIL receptor2
SRE	skeletal-related event		TRM	treatment-related mortality
SREBP	sterol regulatory element binding proteins		TRU	terminal respiratory unit
SRM	standardized response mean		TRUS	transrectal ultrasonography
SRS	somatostatin-receptor scintigraphy		TS	thymidylate synthase; treatment score
SRS	stereotaxic radiosurgery		TSC2	tuberous sclerosis 2
SSA	single-strand annealing		TSG	tumour suppressor gene
SSA	somatostatin analogue		TSH	thyroid-stimulating hormone
SSB	single-strand break		TTF	time-to-treatment failure
SSCP	single strand conformational polymorphism		TTF1	thyroid transcription factor 1
SSRI	selective serotonin reuptake inhibitors		TTP	time-to-progression
SSS	superior sagittal sinus		TURT	transurethral resection of the tumour
STAT3	transcription 3			
STE	surrogate threshold effect		UFC	urinary free cortisol
STS	soft tissue sarcomas		UFT	uracil/tegafur
STAT5	signal transducer and activator of transcription-5		UGT	UDP-glucuronosyltransferase

UICC	Union for International Cancer Control
UKELD	United Kingdom end-stage liver disease score
uPAR	urokinase plasminogen activator receptor
UPEP	urine electrophoresis
UPR	unfolded protein response
US	ultrasound
USPIO	ultrasmall superparamagnetic particles of iron oxide
UTUC	upper tract urothelial cancer
UV	ultraviolet
VAIN	vaginal intraepithelial neoplasia
VATS	video-assisted thoracic surgery
VC	vaginal cancer; verrucous carcinoma
VDA	vascular disrupting agent
VEGF	vascular endothelial growth factor
VEGFR	vascular endothelial growth factor receptor
VEGF	MKI vascular endothelial growth factor multikinase inhibitors
VHL	von Hippel-Lindau
VIN	vulvar intraepithelial neoplasia
VIP	vasoactive intestinal polypeptide

WART	whole abdominal radiotherapy
WBC	white blood cell count
WBD	whole body dose
WBI	whole breast irradiation
WBRT	whole brain radiotherapy
WCRF	World Cancer Research Fund
WDLPS	well-differentiated liposarcoma
WDPPM	well-differentiated papillary peritoneal mesothelioma
WGS	Whole Genome Shotgun
WHEL	Women's Healthy Eating and Living
WIF1	Wnt inhibitory factor 1
WINS	Women's Intervention Nutrition Study
WLE	wide local excision
WM	Waldenström macroglobulinemia
XP	capecitabine plus cisplatin; xeroderma pigmentosum
ZES	Zollinger–Ellison syndrome
ZO1	zonula occludens 1

UICC	Union for International Cancer Control	
UKELD	United Kingdom end-stage liver disease score	
uPAR	urokinase plasminogen activator receptor	
UPEP	urine electrophoresis	
UPR	unfolded protein response	
US	ultrasound	
USPIO	ultrasmall superparamagnetic particles of iron oxide	
UTUC	upper tract urothelial cancer	
UV	ultraviolet	
VAIN	vaginal intraepithelial neoplasia	
VATS	video-assisted thoracic surgery	
VC	vaginal cancer verrucous carcinoma	
VEGF	vascular endothelial growth factor	
VEGFR	vascular endothelial growth factor receptor	
VEGF/VM	vasculo vascular endothelial growth factor multikinase inhibitors	
VHL	von Hippel-Lindau	
VIN	vulvar intraepithelial neoplasia	
VIP	vasoactive intestinal polypeptide	

WART	whole abdominal radiotherapy	
WBC	white blood cell count	
WBD	whole body dose	
WBI	whole breast irradiation	
WBR	whole brain radiotherapy	
WCRF	World Cancer Research Fund	
WDL	well differentiated liposarcoma	
WDPM	well differentiated papillary peritoneal mesothelioma	
WGS	Whole Genome Sequencing	
WHEL	Women's Healthy Eating and Living	
WHI	Women's Health Initiative	
WINS	Women's Intervention Nutrition Study	
WM	Waldenström macroglobulinemia	
XR	capecitabine plus Capecitabine xeloderma	
ZES	Zollinger-Ellison syndrome	
ZOL	zoledronic acid	

List of contributors

Neil K. Aaronson, The Netherlands Cancer Institute, Division of Psychosocial Research and Epidemiology, Amsterdam, The Netherlands

Ann S. Adams, Massachusetts General Hospital, Department of Surgery, Boston, MA, USA

Felipe Ades Moraes, Hospital Albert Einstein, São Paulo, Brazil

Ahmed Ashour Ahmed, Nuffield Department of Obstetrics and Gynaecology, University of Oxford, Oxford, UK

Richard W. Ahn, Northwestern University, Department of Chemistry, Evanston, IL, USA

H. Richard Alexander, Jr., University of Maryland School of Medicine, Baltimore, MD, USA

Peter J. Allen, David M. Rubenstein Center for Pancreatic Cancer Research, Memorial Sloan Kettering Cancer Centre, New York, NY, USA

Fabrice Andre, INSERM (Institut National des Sciences et de la Recherche Médicale); Institut Gustave Roussy, Villejuif, France

Olaf Ansorge, Nuffield Department of Clinical Neurosciences, University of Oxford, Oxford, UK

Nadir Arber, Integrated Cancer Prevention Center (ICPC), The Tel Aviv Sourasky Medical Center, Tel Aviv University, Tel Aviv, Israel

Monica Arnedos, Department Of Medical Oncology, Institut Gustave Roussy, Villejuif, France

Yull E. Arriaga, University of Texas Southwestern Medical Center, Dallas, TX, USA

Hatem A. Azim, Jr., Breast Cancer Translational Research Laboratory, Institut Jules Bordet, Université Libre de Bruxelles, Brussels, Belgium

Irène Baccelli, Institute for Research in Immunology and Cancer, Université de Montréal, Montreal, Canada

Elizabeth H. Baldini, Department of Radiation Oncology, DanaFarber; Cancer Institute and Brigham and Women's Hospital, Harvard Medical School, Boston, MA, USA

Hideaki Bando, Department of Gastroenterology and Gastrointestinal Oncology, National Cancer Center Hospital East, Chiba, Japan

Udai Banerji, The Institute of Cancer Research and The Royal Marsden, Drug Development Unit, London, UK

Dario Baratti, Department of Surgery, Fondazione IRCCS Istituto Nazionale Tumori, Milano, Italy

Gustavo Baretton, Institute of Pathology, Faculty of Medicine and University Hospital Carl Gustav Carus, Technische Universität Dresden, Dresden, Germany

Michael Baumann, Department of Radiation Oncology, OncoRay—National Center for Radiation Research in Oncology, Faculty of Medicine and University Hospital Carl Gustav Carus, Technische Universität Dresden, Dresden; Helmholtz-Zentrum Dresden—Rossendorf; Institute of Radiooncology German Cancer Consortium (DKTK), Dresden and German Cancer Research Center (DKFZ), Heidelberg, Germany

Regina Beets-Tan, Department of Radiology, The Netherlands Cancer Institute, Amsterdam, The Netherlands

Frank Bergmann, Institute of Pathology, University Hospital, Heidelberg, Germany

Ravi Bhatia, Director, Division of Hematology and Oncology, and Professor, Department of Medicine, University of Alabama Birmingham, Birmingham, AL, USA

Claire Blesing, Department of Oncology, Oxford Cancer Centre, Churchill Hospital, Oxford, UK

Walter Bodmer, Weatherall Institute of Molecular Medicine and Department of Oncology, University of Oxford, John Radcliffe Hospital, Oxford, UK

Petra G. Boelens, Department of Surgery, Leiden University Medical Center, Leiden, The Netherlands

Kerstin Borgmann, Laboratory of Radiobiology & Experimental Radiooncology, University Medical Center Hamburg Eppendorf, Hamburg, Germany

Ulrich Bork, Department of General, Visceral and Transplant Surgery, University of Heidelberg, Heidelberg, Germany

Chris Boshoff, Early Development, Translational and Immuno-Oncology, Pfizer Inc., La Jolla, CA, USA

Alex Boussioutas, Research Training, Dentistry and Health Sciences, The University of Melbourne; Peter MacCallum Cancer Centre and Royal Melbourne Hospital, Melbourne, Australia

Michael Brada, The Clatterbridge Cancer Centre, Liverpool, and the Department of Molecular and Clinical Cancer Medicine, University of Liverpool, Liverpool, UK

C.B.M. van den Broek, Leiden University Medical Center, Department of Surgery, Leiden, The Netherlands

Eduardo Bruera, Department of Palliative Care and Rehabilitation Medicine, The University of Texas MD Anderson Cancer Center, Houston, TX, USA

Thomas B. Brunner, Department of Radiation Oncology, University Hospitals Freiburg, Freiburg im Breisgau, Germany

Markus W. Büchler, Department of General, Visceral and Transplant Surgery, University of Heidelberg, Heidelberg, Germany

Raphael Bueno, Division of Thoracic Surgery, Brigham and Women's Hospital, and Professor of Surgery, Harvard Medical School, Boston, MA, USA

Rebecca Bütof, Department of Radiation Oncology, OncoRay—National Center for Radiation Research in Oncology, Faculty of Medicine and University Hospital Carl Gustav Carus, Technische Universität Dresden, Helmholtz-Zentrum Dresden–Rossendorf, Germany

Simon M. Carr, Laboratory of Cancer Biology, Department of Oncology, University of Oxford, Oxford, UK

Paolo G. Casali, Department of Cancer Medicine, Fondazione IRCCS Istituto Nazionale dei Tumori, Milano, Italy

Björn Chapuy, Deparment of Medical Oncology, Dana-Farber Cancer Institute, Harvard Medical School, Boston, MA, USA

Lucian R. Chirieac, Department of Pathology, Brigham and Women's Hospital, Harvard Medical School, Boston, MA, USA

Terence C. Chua, Ryde Hospital, Syndey, NSW, Australia

Christine H. Chung, Department of Oncology, Johns Hopkins University, Baltimore, MD, USA

David N. Church, Wellcome Trust Centre for Human Genetics, University of Oxford, Oxford, UK

Stephanie E. Combs, Department of Radiation Oncology, University Hospital of Heidelberg, Heidelberg, Germany

Joseph M. Corson, Department of Pathology, Harvard Medical School, Brigham and Women's Hospital, Boston, MA, USA

Eithne Costello, The Clatterbridge Cancer Centre, Liverpool, and the Department of Molecular and Clinical Cancer Medicine, University of Liverpool, Liverpool, UK

Sarah E. Coupland, Pathology, Department of Molecular and Clinical Cancer Medicine, University of Liverpool, Liverpool, UK

Amanda S. Coutts, Department of Oncology, University of Oxford, Oxford, UK

David Cunningham, Department of Medicine, Royal Marsden NHS Foundation Trust, Sutton, UK

Eric Van Cutsem, Digestive Oncology, University Hospitals Leuven and KULeuven, Leuven, Belgium

Diona L. Damian, Dermatology, University of Sydney and Melanoma Institute Australia, Sydney, NSW, Australia

Faith Davies, Myeloma Institute, University of Arkansas for Medical Sciences, Little Rock, AR, USA

Wouter de Herder, Erasmus MC, Department of Internal Medicine, Section of Endocrinology, Rotterdam, The Netherlands

Jean de la Rosette, Department of Urology, AMC University Hospital, Amsterdam, The Netherlands

Assunta De Rienzo, Division of Thoracic Surgery, Brigham and Women's Hospital, and Instructor in Surgery, Harvard Medical School, Boston, MA, USA

Jürgen Debus, Heidelberg Institute Radiation Oncology (HIRO), and German Consortium Translational Oncology (DKTK), Heidelberg, Germany

Angelo P. Dei Tos, General Hospital of Treviso, Department of Pathology, Treviso, Italy

Suzette Delaloge, Centre de Lutte Contre le Cancer (CLCC), Institut Gustave Roussy, Villejuif, France

Axel Denz, Department of Visceral, Thoracic and Vascular Surgery, Faculty of Medicine and University Hospital Carl Gustav Carus, Technische Universität Dresden, Dresden, Germany

Marcello Deraco, Fondazione IRCCS Istituto Nazionale dei Tumori, Milan, Italy

Christophe M. Deroose, Nuclear Medicine, University Hospitals Leuven, and Department of Imaging & Pathology, KU Leuven, Belgium

Andreas Dietz, ENT Department, University Hospital of Leipzig, Leipzig, Germany

Ekkehard Dikomey, Laboratory of Radiobiology & Experimental Radiooncology, University Medical Center Hamburg Eppendorf, Hamburg, Germany

Piet Dirix, Iridium Cancer Network, GZA St Augustinus Hospital, Department of Radiation Oncology, Antwerpen, Belgium

Fränzel J.B. van Duijnhoven, Division of Human Nutrition, Wageningen University, Wageningen, The Netherlands

Rafał Dziadziuszko, Department of Oncology and Radiotherapy, Medical University of Gdask, Gdask, Poland

Adel K. El-Naggar, The University of Texas M.D. Anderson Cancer Center, Houston, TX, USA

Andrew Evans, Dundee University, Dundee, UK

Jonathan Evans, Department of Radiology, The Royal Liverpool University Hospital, Liverpool, UK

Daniel G. Ezra, Adnexal Service, Moorfields Eye Hospital, Moorfields; NIHR Biomedical Research Centre, UCL Institute of Ophthalmology, London, UK

Peter M. Fayers, Institute of Applied Health Sciences, University of Aberdeen, UK and Norwegian University of Science and Technology (NTNU), Department of Cancer Research and Molecular Medicine, Trondheim, Norway

Kathryn Field, Royal Melbourne Hospital, and Clinical Research Fellow, Ludwig Institute Cancer Research, Melbourne, VIC, Australia

Adele K. Fielding, UCL Cancer Institute, London, UK

John Fitzpatrick (deceased), Irish Cancer Society, Dublin, Republic of Ireland

Stephen B. Fox, Peter MacCallum Cancer Centre, Melbourne, and Department of Pathology, University of Melbourne, Parkville, VIC, Australia

Arthur E. Frankel, University of Texas Southwestern Medical Center, Dallas, TX, USA

Stefan Fritz, Department of General, Visceral and Transplantation Surgery, University of Heidelberg, Heidelberg, Germany

Toral Gathani, Cancer Epidemiology Unit, Nuffield Department of Population Health, University of Oxford, Oxford, UK

Kevin C. Gatter, Nuffield Division of Clinical Laboratory Sciences, Radcliffe Department of Medicine, Oxford, UK

Ritu Gill, Department of Radiology, Harvard Medical School, and Associate Radiologist, Thoracic Radiology, Brigham and Women's Hospital, Boston, MA, USA

Oliver Gimm, Department of Clinical and Experimental Medicine, Division of Clinical Sciences, Linköping University, Linköping, Sweden

Christian Gisselbrecht, Institut d'Hématologie, Hôpital Saint Louis, Paris, France

Bengt Glimelius, Oncology Section, Department of Immunology, Genetics and Pathology, Uppsala University, Uppsala, Sweden

Sarah E.B. Goltz, Principal, Sage Innovation, Brooklyn, NY, USA

Mary K. Gospodarowicz, Princess Margaret Cancer Centre, University Health Network, University of Toronto, Toronto, ON, Canada

Sebastien Gouy, Gustave Roussy, Villejuif, France

Vincent Gregoire, Department of Radiation Oncology, UCL St Luc University Hospital, Catholic University of Louvain, Brussels, Belgium

Alessandro Gronchi, Department of Surgery, Fondazione IRCCS Istituto Nazionale dei Tumori, Milan, Italy

Ashley Grossman, Professor of Endocrinology, Oxford Centre for Diabetes, Endocrinology and Metabolism, University of Oxford, Oxford, UK

Marco Guzzo, Fondazione IRCCS Istituto Nazionale dei Tumori, Milan, Italy

Daniel G. Haller, Perelman School of Medicine, University of Pennsylvania, Philadelphia, PA, USA

Christopher M. Halloran, NIHR Pancreas Biomedical Research Unit, University of Liverpool, Liverpool, UK

Marc Hamoir, Cancer Center Cliniques universitaires SaintLuc, Brussels, Belgium

Douglas Hanahan, Swiss Institute for Experimental Cancer Research (ISREC), School of Life Sciences, Swiss Federal Institute of Technology Lausanne (EPFL), Lausanne, Switzerland

D. Paul Harkin, School of Medicine, Dentistry and Biomedical Sciences, and Centre for Cancer Research and Cell Biology, Queen's University, Belfast, UK

Adrian L. Harris, Molecular Oncology Laboratories, Oxford University Department of Oncology, Weatherall Institute of Molecular Medicine, Oxford, UK

Raffit Hassan, Thoracic and GI Oncology Branch, Center for Cancer Research, National Cancer Institute, Bethesda, MD, USA

Karin Haustermans, Department of Radiation Oncology, University Hospitals Leuven, Department of Oncology, KU Leuven, Leuven, Belgium

Priya Healey, Royal Liverpool and Broadgreen University Hospital, Liverpool, UK

Jack Henkin, Northwestern University, Center for Developmental Therapeutics, Evanston, IL, USA

Alexander Heriot, Department of Surgical Oncology, Peter MacCallum Cancer Centre, Melbourne, VIC, Australia

C. Simon Herrington, University of Edinburgh Division of Pathology, Edinburgh Cancer Research Centre, Institute of Genetics and Molecular Medicine, Edinburgh, UK

Devendra Hiwase, Haematology Department, Institute of Medical and Veterinary Science, Adelaide, SA, Australia

David C. Hodgson, Department of Radiation Oncology, University of Toronto, Toronto, ON, Canada

Dieter Hoelzer, ONKOLOGIKUM Frankfurt, am Museumsufer, Frankfurt, Germany

David Hui, University of Texas MD Anderson Cancer Center, Houston, TX, USA

Tim Illidge, Institute of Cancer Sciences, University of Manchester, Manchester Academic Health Science Centre, Manchester, UK

David Jackman, Harvard Medical School; Clinical Pathways, Dana-Farber Cancer Institute, Boston, MA, USA

Patrick G. Johnston, President and Vice Chancellor, Queen's University Belfast, Belfast, UK

Ellen Kampman, Division of Human Nutrition, Wageningen University, Wageningen, The Netherlands

Richard F. Kefford, Faculty of Medicine, Macquarie University, and Melanoma Institute Australia, Sydney, NSW, Australia

Richard D. Kennedy, Centre for Cancer Research and Cell Biology, Queen's University of Belfast, Belfast, and Vice President and Head of Research, Almac Diagnostics, UK

Rachel Kerr, Department of Oncology, University of Oxford, Oxford, UK

David J. Kerr, Nuffield Division of Clinical Laboratory Sciences, Nuffield Department of Medicine, University of Oxford, Oxford, UK

Keith M. Kerr, Department of Pathology, Aberdeen University Medical School, Aberdeen Royal Infirmary, Foresterhill, Aberdeen, UK

Takahiro Kinoshita, National Cancer Center, Tokyo, Japan

Stefan Knapp, Johann Wolfgang Goethe-University, Institute for Pharmaceutical Chemistry, Frankfurt am Main, Germany

Jonathan Knowles, Royal Free London, NHS Foundation Trust, London, UK

Mechthild Krause, Department of Radiation Oncology and OncoRay—National Center for Radiation Research in Oncology, Faculty of Medicine and University Hospital Carl Gustav, Technische Universität Dresden, Helmholtz-Zentrum Dresden—Rossendorf, Institute of Radiooncology, German Cancer Consortium (DKTK) Dresden and German Cancer Research Center (DKFZ) Heidelberg, Germany

Malte Kriegs, Laboratory of Radiobiology & Experimental Radiooncology, University Medical Center Hamburg Eppendorf, Hamburg, Germany

Frank Kroschinsky, Department of Internal Medicine I, University Hospital Carl Gustav Carus Dresden, Dresden, Germany

Yasutoshi Kuboki, Japanese Foundation for Cancer Research, Tokyo, Japan

Lalit Kumar, Department of Medical Oncology, All India Institute of Medical Sciences, New Delhi, India

Nicholas B. La Thangue, Department of Oncology, University of Oxford, Oxford, UK

Sigurd Lax, Institute for Pathology, General Hospital Graz West, Graz, Austria

Eric Leblanc, Lille Cancer Center, Centre Oscar Lambert (COL), Lille, France

C. René Leemans, Department of Otolaryngology/Head and Neck Surgery, VU University Medical Center, Amsterdam, The Netherlands

Jean-Louis Lefebvre, Lille Cancer Center, Centre Oscar Lambert (COL), Lille, France

Toni Lerut, Department of Thoracic Surgery, University Hospital Gasthuisberg, KU Leuven, Belgium

Ross L. Levine, Memorial Sloan Kettering Cancer Center, New York, NY, USA

Lisa Licitra, Istituto Nazionale dei Tumori, Milan, Italy

Bolin Liu, Department of Neurosurgery, Xijing Institute of Clinical Neuroscience, Xijing Hospital, Fourth Military Medical University, Xi'an, China

Shujuan Liu, Weatherall Institute of Molecular Medicine and Nuffield Department of Obstetrics and Gynaecology, University of Oxford, UK, and Department of Obstetrics and Gynaecology, Xijing Hospital, Fourth Military Medical University, Xi'an, China

Julian Lob-Levyt, Malaria Consortium; Formerly Gavi, the Vaccine Alliance

G.P.M. Luyten, Leiden University Medical Center, Leiden, The Netherlands

Henry T. Lynch, Department of Preventive Medicine, Creighton University, Omaha, NE, USA

Jane F. Lynch (deceased), Formerly of the Department of Preventive Medicine, Creighton University, Omaha, NE, USA

Hemant Malhotra, Division of Medical Oncology, RK Birla Cancer Center, SMS Medical College Hospital, Jaipur, India

Pankaj Malhotra, Department of Internal Medicine, Postgraduate Institute of Medical Education & Research, Chandigarh, India

Mohandas K. Mallath, Department of Digestive Diseases, Tata Medical Centre, Kolkata, West Bengal, India

Sandra Maniam, Pharmacology Unit, Department of Human Anatomy, Faculty of Medicine and Health Sciences, University Putra Malaysia, Serdang, Malaysia

Wael Y. Mansour, Laboratory of Radiobiology & Experimental Radiooncology, University Medical Center Hamburg Eppendorf, Hamburg, Germany

Andrew P. Mazar, Department of Pharmacology, Feinberg School of Medicine, Northwestern University, Chicago, IL, USA

Donald C. McMillan, Academic Unit of Surgery, School of Medicine, College of Medical, Veterinary and Life Sciences, University of Glasgow, Glasgow Royal Infirmary, Glasgow, UK

Alexander M. Menzies, Melanoma Institute Australia, University of Sydney, Sydney, NSW, Australia

Michael Michael, Peter MacCallum Cancer Centre, Division of Cancer Medicine, Colorectal Tumour Stream, Melbourne, VIC, Australia

Tetsuya Mitsudomi, Department of Surgery, Division of Thoracic Surgery, Faculty of Medicine, Kinki University, OsakaSayama, Japan

Annette C. Moll, VU University Medical Center, Amsterdam, The Netherlands

Gareth Morgan, Myeloma Institute, University of Arkansas for Medical Sciences, Little Rock, AR, USA

Philippe Morice, Gustave Roussy, Universite Paris XI, Villejuif, France

Charles G. Mullighan, Department of Pathology, St Jude Children's Research Hospital, Memphis, TN, USA

Asif Muneer, Department of Urology, University College Hospital, London, UK

Philippe Nafteux, Department of Thoracic Surgery, University Hospitals Leuven, Leuven, Belgium

Iris Nagtegaal, Department of Pathology, Radboud umc, Nijmegen, The Netherlands

Fabrice Narducci, Lille Cancer Center, Centre Oscar Lambert (COL), Lille, France

John P. Neoptolemos, Department of Molecular and Clinical Cancer Medicine at the University of Liverpool, Royal Liverpool and Broadgreen University Hospitals NHS Trust, Liverpool, UK

Sam Ngan, Division of Radiation Oncology, Peter MacCallum Cancer Centre, Melbourne, VIC, Australia

Brian O'Sullivan, Princess Margaret Cancer Centre, Department of Radiation Oncology, University of Toronto, Toronto, ON, Canada

Yishai Ofran, Hematology Department, Rambam Health Care Campus, Haifa, Israel

Thomas V. O'Halloran, Charles E. and Emma H. Morrison Professor of Chemistry, Professor of Molecular Biosciences, and Founding Director, Chemistry of Life Processes Institute and Department of Chemistry, Northwestern University, Evanston, IL, USA

Atsushi Ohtsu, National Cancer Center Hospital East, Kashiwa, Japan

Paula A. Oliveira, CITAB, Department of Veterinary Sciences, University of TrásosMontes, and Alto Douro, Vila Real, Portugal, Vila Real, Portugal

Michael Ong, Division of Medical Oncology, University of Ottawa, Faculty of Medicine, Ottawa, ON, Canada

Isabelle Opitz, Division of Thoracic Surgery, University Hospital Zurich, Zurich, Switzerland

Rainer Ordemann, University Hospital Carl Gustav Carus, Technical University Dresden, Dresden, Germany

Lars Påhlman, Department of Surgery, University Hospital Uppsala, Uppsala, Sweden

Daniel Palmer, Department of Molecular and Clinical Cancer Medicine, University of Liverpool, Liverpool, UK

Ulrich-Frank Pape, Charité University Medicine Berlin, Department of Hepatology and Gastroenterology, Berlin, Germany

Allyson Parry, John Radcliffe Hospital, Oxford, UK

Ann H. Partridge, DanaFarber Cancer Institute, Harvard Medical School, Boston, MA, USA

Nicholas Pavlidis, Medical School, University of Ioannina, Ioannina, Greece

Charlotte Pawlyn, The Institute of Cancer Research and The Royal Marsden NHS Foundation Trust, London, UK

Jacob Pe'er, Department of Ophthalmology, Hadassah Hebrew University Medical Center, Jerusalem, Israel

Marzia Pennati, Molecular Pharmacology Unit, Department of Experimental Oncology and Molecular Medicine, Fondazione IRCCS Istituto Nazionale dei Tumori, Milano, Italy

George Pentheroudakis, Medical School, University of Ioannina, Ioannina, Greece

Jeffrey Peppercorn, Massachusetts General Hospital, Cancer Center, Harvard Medical School, Boston, MA, USA

Federica Perrone, Laboratory of Experimental Molecular Pathology, Department of Pathology, Fondazione IRCCS Istituto Nazionale dei Tumori, Milan, Italy

Solange Peters, Medical Oncology, Oncology Department, CHUV, Lausanne, Switzerland

Cordula Petersen, Clinic of Radiotherapy and Radiooncology, University Medical Center Hamburg Eppendorf, Hamburg, Germany

Francesco Pezzella, Radcliffe Department of Medicine, John Radcliffe Hospital, University of Oxford, Oxford, UK

Martine Piccart, Department of Medicine, Institut Jules Bordet, Université Libre de Bruxelles, Brussels, Belgium

Stefano A. Pileri, Bologna University, European Institute of Oncology, Milan, Italy

Puneet Plaha, John Radcliffe Hospital, Oxford University Hospital NHS Trust, Oxford, UK

Ursula Plöckinger, Charité—Universitätsmedizin Berlin (CVK), Berlin, Germany

Vincent Vander Poorten, Department of Oncology, Section Head and Neck Oncology, KU Leuven, Otorhinolaryngology, Head and Neck Surgery, University Hospitals Leuven, Leuven Cancer Institute, Leuven, Belgium

Graeme J. Poston, School of Translational Studies, University of Liverpool, UK; Consultant Surgeon, Aintree University Hospital, UK

Richard Pötter, Department of Radiation Oncology, Comprehensive Cancer Center, Medical University of Vienna, Wien, Austria

Thomas Powles, Experimental Cancer Medicine, Barts Cancer Institute, Barts and The London School of Medicine and Dentistry, London, UK

Hans Prenen, Department of Oncology, University Hospitals Leuven, Catholic University, Leuven, Belgium

Pieter Pretorius, Department of Neuroradiology, The John Radcliffe Hospital, Oxford University Hospitals NHS Trust, Oxford, UK

Alexander Reinthaller, Medical University of Vienna, Wien, Austria

Thorsten Rieckmann, Laboratory of Radiobiology and Experimental Radiooncology, University Medical Center Hamburg, Eppendorf, Germany

Angela Rogers, Oxford Centre for Diabetes, Endocrinology and Metabolism, Radcliffe Department of Medicine, University of Oxford, Oxford, UK

Geoffrey E. Rose, Adnexal Service, Moorfields Eye Hospital , Moorfields; NIHR Biomedical Research Centre, UCL Institute of Ophthalmology; City University London, London, UK

Jacob M. Rowe, Rambam Health Care Campus and Technion, Israel Institute of Technology, Haifa, Israel

Campbell S.D. Roxburgh, School of Medicine, College of Medical Veterinary and Life Sciences, University of Glasgow, Glasgow, UK

Emiel J.T. Rutgers, Netherlands Cancer Institute, Amsterdam, The Netherlands

Xavier Sagaert, University Hospitals Leuven, Leuven, Belgium

Manuel Salto-Tellez, Northern Ireland Molecular Pathology Laboratory, Centre for Cancer Research and Cell Biology, Queens University Belfast & Belfast Health Trust, Belfast, UK

Jonathan M. Samet, Department of Preventive Medicine, Keck School of Medicine, Institute for Global Health, University of Southern California, Los Angeles, CA, USA

Massoud Samiei, International Atomic Energy Agency, Programme of Action for Cancer Therapy (PACT), Vienna, Austria

Daniel J. Sargent, Division of Biomedical Statistics and Informatics, Mayo Clinic, Rochester, MN, USA

Peter Schirmacher, Institute of Pathology, University Hospital, Heidelberg, Germany

Maximilian Paul Schmid, Department of Radiation Oncology, Medical University of Vienna, Wien, Austria

Dirk Schrijvers, Ziekenhuisnetwerk Antwerpen Middelheim, Antwerp, Belgium

Christina Schütze, Department of Radiation Oncology, OncoRay—National Center for Radiation Research in Oncology, Faculty of Medicine and University Hospital Carl Gustav Carus, Technische Universität Dresden, Helmholtz-Zentrum Dresden—Rossendorf, Germany

Richard A. Scolyer, Royal Prince Alfred Hospital; Sydney Medical School, The University of Sydney; Melanoma Institute, Sydney, NSW, Australia

Annekatrin Seidlitz, Department of Radiation Oncology, OncoRay—National Center for Radiation Research in Oncology, Faculty of Medicine and University Hospital Carl Gustav Carus, Technische Universität Dresden, Dresden; Helmholtz-Zentrum Dresden—Rossendorf; Institute of Radiooncology German Cancer Consortium (DKTK), Dresden; and German Cancer Research Center (DKFZ), Heidelberg, Germany

Hans-Joerg Senn, Tumor and Breast Center ZeTuP, St.Gallen, Switzerland

Stefan Seregard, St Erik Eye Hospital, Karolinska Institutet, Stockholm, Sweden

Qian Shi, Division of Biomedical Statistics and Informatics, Mayo Clinic, Rochester, MN, USA

Kohei Shitara, Department of Experimental Therapeutics (and Gastrointestinal Oncology), National Cancer Center Hospital East, Kashiwa, Japan

Eric A. Singer, Section of Urologic Oncology, Rutgers Cancer Institute of New Jersey, and Rutgers Robert Wood Johnson Medical School, New Brunswick, NJ, USA

Elizabeth Smyth, Department of Medicine, Royal Marsden NHS Foundation Trust, Sutton, UK

Cameron Snell, Nuffield Division of Clinical Laboratory Sciences, Radcliffe Department of Medicine, University of Oxford, Oxford, UK

Carrie L. Snyder, Department of Preventive Medicine, Creighton University, Omaha, NE, USA

Christos Sotiriou, Breast Cancer Translational Research Laboratory, Institut Jules Bordet, Université Libre de Bruxelles, Brussels, Belgium

Robert J.C. Steele, Division of Cancer, Medical Research Institute, School of Medicine, University of Dundee, Dundee, UK

Eytan M. Stein, Leukemia Service, Memorial Sloan-Kettering Cancer Center, New York, NY, USA

Nicholas Stern, Digestive Diseases Unit, Aintree University Hospital NHS Foundation Trust, Liverpool, UK

Graham Stevens, Department of Radiation Oncology, Orange Hospital, Orange, NSW, Australia

Jan Stöhlmacher-Williams, Medical Clinic and Policlinic I, Faculty of Medicine and University, Hospital Carl Gustav Carus, Technische Universität Dresden, Dresden, Germany

Friedrich Stölzel, Department of Internal Medicine I, University Hospital Carl Gustav Carus Dresden, Dresden, Germany

David J. Sugarbaker, Lung Institute, Baylor College of Medicine, Houston, TX, USA

Paul H. Sugarbaker, Center for Gastrointestinal Malignancies, MedStar Washington Hospital Center, Washington, DC, USA

Petra Sulentic, Department for Endocrinology and Diabetes, KBC "Sisters of Mercy", University of Zagreb, Zagreb, Croatia

Paul D. Sykes, Institute of Translational Medicine, University of Liverpool, Liverpool, UK

Martin S. Tallman, Memorial Sloan Kettering Cancer Center, New York, NY, USA

I. Bing Tan, Department of Head and Neck Oncology and Surgery, The Netherlands Cancer Institute, Amsterdam, The Netherlands

Anish Thomas, National Cancer Institute, National Institutes of Health, Bethesda, MD, USA

John F. Thompson, Melanoma Institute Australia, and Sydney Medical School, The University of Sydney, Sydney, NSW, Australia

Klaus R. Trott, Department of Radiation Oncology, Technical University of Munich, Munich, Germany

Andreas Trumpp, Division of Stem Cells and Cancer, German Cancer Research Center (DKFZ) and Heidelberg Institute of Stem Cell Technology and Experimental Medicine (HISTEM), Heidelberg, Germany

Keli Turner, Vanderbilt University School of Medicine, Nashville, TN, USA

Andrey Ugolkov, Center for Developmental Therapeutics, Northwestern University, Evanston, IL, USA

Brian R. Untch, Department of Surgery, Gastric and Mixed Tumor Service, Memorial Sloan Kettering Cancer Center, New York, NY, USA

Catherine Uzan, Gustave Roussy, Villejuif, France

Vincent Vandecaveye, Department of Radiology, University Hospitals Leuven, Department of Imaging and Pathology, Catholic University of Leuven, Leuven, Belgium

Cornelis J.H. van de Velde, Leiden University Medical Center, The Netherlands

Jan B. Vermorken, Antwerp University Hospital, Edegem, Belgium

Jaap Verweij, Erasmus MC Cancer Institute, Rotterdam, The Netherlands

Giuseppe Viale, Department of Pathology, European Institute of Oncology, University of Milan School of Medicine, Milan, Italy

John Wass, Royal College of Physicians, and Oxford University Hospitals NHS Trust, Oxford, UK

Andrew Weaver, Department of Oncology, Oxford University Hospitals NHS Trust, Oxford, UK

Walter Weder, Faculty of Medicine, University of Zurich, Zurich, Switzerland

Anthony P. Weetman, Faculty of Medicine, Dentistry and Health, University of Sheffield, Sheffield, UK

Robert A. Weinberg, Whitehead Institute for Biomedical Research, Ludwig/MIT Center for Molecular Oncology, MIT Department of Biology, Cambridge, MA, USA

Jürgen Weitz, Department of Visceral, Thoracic and Vascular Surgery, University Hospital Carl Gustav Carus, Technische Universität Dresden, Dresden, Germany

Jens Werner, Department of General Surgery, University of Heidelberg, Heidelberg, Germany

Bertram Wiedenmann, Charité University of Medicine, Berlin, Germany

Jennifer Wilding, Weatherall Institute of Molecular Medicine and Department of Oncology, University of Oxford, John Radcliffe Hospital, Oxford, UK

Michelle D. Williams, Department of Pathology, University of Texas, MD Anderson Cancer Center, Houston, TX, USA

Pauline Wimberger, Department of Gynecology and Obstetrics, TU Dresden, Dresden, Germany

Andrea S. Wolf, Department of Thoracic Surgery, The Icahn School of Medicine at Mount Sinai, The Mount Sinai Medical Center, New York, NY, USA

Gerald G. Wulf, Section Hematopoietic Stem Cell Transplantation, Haematology and Medical Oncology, Goettingen, Germany

Tristan D. Yan, Royal Prince Alfred Hospital, Sydney, NSW, Australia

Rachel L. Yung, Medical Oncology, DanaFarber Cancer Institute, Harvard Medical School, Boston, MA, USA

Nadia Zaffaroni, Molecular Pharmacology Unit, Department of Experimental Oncology and Molecular Medicine, Fondazione IRCCS Istituto Nazionale dei Tumori, Milano, Italy

Ghada Zakout, University College London Cancer Institute, London, UK

John Zalcberg, School of Public Health and Preventive Medicine, Faculty of Medicine, Nursing and Health Sciences, Monash University, Melbourne, VIC, Australia

Dimitrios Zardavas, Breast International Group, Brussels, Belgium

Stefan Zimmermann, Oncology Department, HFR Fribourg Hôpital Cantonal, Fribourg, Switzerland

SECTION 1

Hallmarks of cancer

1 **The hallmarks of cancer: perspectives for cancer medicine** 3
Douglas Hanahan and Robert A. Weinberg

2 **Growth factors and uncontrolled proliferation** 11
Shujuan Liu and Ahmed Ashour Ahmed

3 **Cell signalling pathways** 23
Stefan Knapp

4 **Cell cycle control** 31
Simon M. Carr and Nicholas B. La Thangue

5 **Cancer cell death** 42
Amanda S. Coutts, Sandra Maniam, and Nicholas B. La Thangue

6 **Angiogenesis** 49
Yull E. Arriaga and Arthur E. Frankel

7 **Invasion and metastasis** 61
Andrew P. Mazar, Andrey Ugolkov, Jack Henkin, Richard W. Ahn, and Thomas V. O'Halloran

8 **Genetic instability** 72
Jennifer Wilding and Walter Bodmer

9 **DNA repair after oncological therapy (radiotherapy and chemotherapy)** 82
Ekkehard Dikomey, Kerstin Borgmann, Malte Kriegs, Wael Y. Mansour, Cordula Petersen, and Thorsten Rieckmann

10 **Biology of cancer and metastasis stem cells** 86
Andreas Trumpp and Irène Baccelli

11 **Biomarker identification and clinical validation** 98
Richard D. Kennedy, Manuel Salto-Tellez, D. Paul Harkin, and Patrick G. Johnston

12 **Cancer, immunity, and inflammation** 109
Campbell S.D. Roxburgh and Donald C. McMillan

13 **Cancer and metabolism** 119
Cameron Snell, Kevin C. Gatter, Adrian L. Harris, and Francesco Pezzella

CHAPTER 1

The hallmarks of cancer
Perspectives for cancer medicine

Douglas Hanahan and Robert A. Weinberg

Introduction: a conceptual organizing principle

This textbook elaborates the landscape of a disease characterized by extraordinary complexity across the spectrum of organ sites and cell types. The growths that are grouped together under the rubric of cancer exhibit scrambled and mutated cell genomes, diverse histopathologies, highly variable timelines of pathogenesis and progression to symptomatic and metastatic disease, and a plethora of pathological effects. The simple premise in proposing a generic set of cancer hallmarks came from our belief that the bewildering complexity of cancer could be rationalized in terms of an underlying principle.

We envisaged these hallmarks as a set of acquired functional capabilities that act in combination to produce most forms of cancer, despite genetic and pathologic differences that might otherwise suggest a lack of mechanistic commonality. We imagined that each of these capabilities could be acquired by developing cancers through several alternative means, representing different solutions to the common challenges facing all incipient neoplasias. This concept, first presented in 2000 [1] and refined in 2011 [2], has proven to be a useful heuristic tool for distilling the underlying foundations of this disease.

The following sections provide a concise synopsis of this scheme, with a brief perspective on clinical applications in the last section. The reader is referred to the primary publications [1, 2], as well as to another perspective that expands on the roles of stromal cells in enabling the hallmarks of cancer [3]. A textbook on the biology of cancer [4] may provide additional detail on many of the mechanisms of cancer pathogenesis described in outline in this chapter.

The hallmarks of cancer: necessary functional capabilities

In the current conceptualization, there are eight hallmarks—acquired capabilities—that are common to many forms of human cancer (Figure 1.1). Each capability serves a distinct role in supporting the development, progression, and persistence of tumours and their constituent cells, as briefly explained below.

Hallmark 1: sustaining proliferative signalling

The essence of the disease is a deregulated programme that instructs cancer cells to grow and divide, doing so at inappropriate times and places, chronically. Many so-called 'driver mutations' that convert normal cellular genes into oncogenes (by mutational alteration of gene function or amplification in expression) serve to stimulate and sustain progression of cells through their growth-and-division cycles. They act by perturbing multiple nodes in the signal transduction circuits that normally transmit growth signals from the extracellular milieu into the cell nucleus. Many of these mutations alter regulatory circuits involving secreted growth-stimulatory proteins that bind as ligands to activate their cognate cell-surface receptors. Signal transduction into the cell nucleus is accomplished by cascades of protein–protein associations and protein phosphorylations, the most prominent of these signalling channels being growth-promoting signals transmitted through the RAS-RAF-MEK-MAPK pathway. Signal-sustaining mutational alterations of genes in this pathway are commonly observed in a wide variety of human cancers, illustrating its importance in enabling acquisition of this hallmark capability. We note, however, that activation in cancer cells of this central mitogenic pathway does not invariably depend on genetic changes acquired during the course of tumour progression. In certain instances, epigenetic deregulation of autocrine (auto-stimulatory) and paracrine (cell-to-cell) signalling circuits can also provide cancer cells with chronic growth-promoting signals, doing so in the apparent absence of underlying somatic mutations.

Hallmark 2: evading growth suppressors

The essential complement to proliferative signals in normal cells are braking mechanisms that serve either to overrule the initiation of, or to subsequently turn off, cell division stimulated by such signals. These countervailing regulatory mechanisms often involve the tissue microenvironments in which normal cells reside, ensuring that cell proliferation is not an entirely cell-autonomous process. The most prominent brakes are the direct regulators of the cell division cycle, embodied in the retinoblastoma protein (pRb) and several 'cyclin-dependent' kinase inhibitors that block progression of an individual cell through its growth-and-division cycle. The activity of this molecular braking system is regulated in part by extracellular pro- and anti-growth signals transduced by receptors on the cell surface in order to permit transitory proliferation, thereby ensuring normal tissue homeostasis.

In addition to the brakes that respond to extracellular growth-modulatory signals, an intracellular monitoring system, centred upon the p53 protein, serves to ensure that cells advance only through their growth-and-division cycles when the

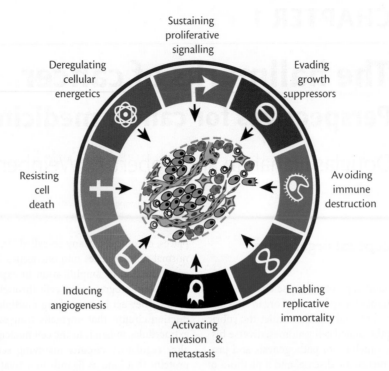

Fig. 1.1 The hallmarks of cancer. Eight distinctive functional capabilities—the hallmarks of cancer—are thought to be necessarily acquired during the multistep pathogenesis pathways leading to most forms of human cancer. Certain forms of cancer may be less dependent on one hallmark or another. Thus, adenomatous tumours evidently lack the capability for invasion and metastasis. Leukaemias may not require angiogenesis or invasive capabilities, although progression to lymphoma almost certainly requires both. And, the necessity for metabolic reprogramming or evading tumour immunity may be less pronounced in certain cancers.

Reprinted from *Cancer Cell*, Volume 21, Issue 3, Hanahan D, and Coussens LM, Accessories to the crime: functions of cells recruited to the tumor microenvironment, pp. 309–322, Copyright © 2012, with permission from Elsevier, http://www.sciencedirect.com/science/journal/15356108

physiologic state of the cell is appropriate. Thus, p53 serves to sense unrepaired damage to a cell's genome as well as other unresolved physiologic imbalances, and responds by shutting off the cell division cycle. In cases of severe genomic damage or physiological abnormalities, the p53 pathway can induce programmed cell death (see below), an extreme form of putting on the brakes to cell proliferation.

A number of component genes in both braking mechanisms—of the Rb and p53 pathways—are classified as tumour suppressors (TSGs) by virtue of their frequent loss-of-function via inactivating genetic mutations. Alternatively, the functions of TSGs can be lost by shutting down the expression of these genes through epigenetic mechanisms, notably those involving DNA and histone methylation. For example, while the p53 gene itself is mutated in ~40% of all human cancers, many other tumours carry genetic lesions that compromise p53 signalling in other ways. In sum, elimination or evasion of growth suppressors is clearly necessary to ensure that the chronic cell proliferation of cancer cells is not halted by braking mechanisms that, under normal conditions, would succeed in constraining cell proliferation.

Hallmark 3: resisting cell death

The second, qualitatively distinctive barrier to aberrant cell proliferation involves intrinsic mechanisms that can induce programmed cell death, a more drastic means to counteract inappropriate increases in cell number. The most prominent of these programmes is apoptosis, which helps to maintain tissue homoeostasis by inducing the suicide of aberrant cells, including ones that

are inappropriately proliferating. The apoptotic programme can be triggered by cell-intrinsic as well as non-cell-autonomous signals that detect different forms of cellular abnormality.

The apoptotic cell death programme involves the directed degradation of critical cellular organelles, the shrivelling of the cell, and its engulfment, either by their neighbours or by tissue-monitoring phagocytes, notably macrophages. All this transpires in less than an hour in mammalian tissues, explaining why apoptotic cells are usually relatively rare, even in a population of cells that is actively undergoing apoptosis, such as the cancer cells in tumours being subjected to cytotoxic chemotherapy. The rapid engulfment of apoptotic cell bodies ensures that their death does not release subcellular components that could inadvertently provoke an immune response; the resulting absence of responding immune cells contrasts with the programme of necrosis, which may be activated by various conditions, including oxygen and energy deprivation. Cells that are dying by necrosis rupture, releasing their contents and leaving their carcasses as debris; the relics of living cells incite an inflammatory response that, as discussed below, can have both tumour-promoting and tumour-antagonizing effects.

A third programme, termed autophagy, serves as a recycling system for cellular organelles that normally helps cells respond to conditions of nutrient deprivation; by degrading cellular organelles, autophagy generates the metabolites and nutrients that cells are unable to acquire from their surroundings. While normally operating as a survival system, extreme nutrient deprivation can lead to hyper-activation of autophagy that results in autophagic cell death when stressed cancer cells have cannibalized so many of their own organelles that they are inviable.

These three quite distinct mechanisms of programmed cell death must be circumvented or attenuated by cancer cells if they and their descendants are to continue their proliferative expansion in number and their evolution to states of heightened malignancy.

Hallmark 4: enabling replicative immortality

A third intrinsic barrier to chronic proliferation is integral to the linear structure of mammalian chromosomes: the telomeres at the ends of chromosomes record—by progressive reduction of their length during each cell division cycle—the number of successive cell generations through which a cell lineage has passed. The telomeres are composed of thousands of tandem copies of a specific hexanucleotide sequence. When the number of telomere repeats is reduced below a certain threshold, a tripwire is triggered, causing p53-dependent cell cycle arrest or apoptosis, the latter historically being termed 'crisis'. Circumventing these p53-induced anti-proliferative responses (e.g., by mutationally inactivating the p53 gene) does not on its own enable the cancer cell to avoid eventual elimination. Instead, continuing telomere erosion produces unstable chromosomes whose ends are no longer protected by telomeres, which can result in chromosomal translocations and rearrangements. If unchecked, these changes lead to mitotic catastrophe and consequent cell death.

Most cancer cells circumvent the barriers erected by the telomere replication clock by activating a mechanism of telomere maintenance used to preserve the replicative capacity of normal embryonic and tissue stem cells. This mechanism depends on upregulating the expression of the telomere-extending enzyme telomerase. Less frequently, they engage an alternative inter-chromosomal recombination-based mechanism for preserving telomere length. Thus, through one strategy or another, cancer cells acquire the capability to maintain their telomeres at healthy lengths, doing so indefinitely. By avoiding the barrier created by overly eroded telomeres, these cells acquire the unlimited replicative potential—termed cellular immortality—that is required to spawn large tumour masses.

Hallmark 5: inducing angiogenesis

Angiogenesis—the growth of new blood vessels—is critical for most neoplastic growths. Like normal organs, tumours require a steady supply of oxygen, glucose, and other nutrients, as well as a means to evacuate metabolic waste to sustain cell viability and proliferation; the vasculature serves these purposes. The deleterious effect that ischaemia has in normal tissue is well established clinically and experimentally: cells die, via one form of programmed cell death or another, causing tissue and organ degradation and dysfunction. Similarly, the growth of developing nests of cancer cells halts when their ability to acquire blood-borne nutrients becomes inadequate, typically when the nearest capillary is more than 200 microns away.

Cells at the diffusion limit from the nearest capillary activate various stress response systems, of which the most prominent involves the hypoxia-inducible transcription factor (HIF) system, which regulates hundreds of genes, including ones that directly or indirectly induce angiogenesis and other stress-adaptive capabilities. Much like cells in ischaemic tissues, cancer cells beyond the diffusion limit for oxygen and glucose will typically die, doing so

by necrosis, apoptosis, or autophagy. This explains why most vigorously growing tumours are well vascularized with evidence of ongoing active angiogenesis.

Of note, the tumour-associated neovasculature is usually aberrant, both morphologically and functionally. Tumour blood vessels are torturous, dilated, and leaky, with erratic flow patterns and 'dead zones' in which no blood flow is detectable, in marked contrast to the seamless blood flow operating in the normal microvasculature. Moreover, the degree of vascularity varies widely from one tumour type to another, ranging from intensely vascularized renal carcinomas to poorly vascularized pancreatic ductal adenocarcinomas.

Finally, we note that while chronic angiogenesis is a hallmark of the great majority of solid tumours, some may devise an alternative means to acquire access to the vasculature: in certain cases, cancers evidently co-opt normal tissue vasculature by employing the hallmark capability of invasion (see below). Thus, particular types of cancer cells can proliferate and grow along normal tissue capillaries, creating sleeves around the vessels. While vascular co-option is evident in certain cases (e.g., in glioblastoma) and in some tumours treated with potent angiogenesis inhibitors, most tumours rely to a considerable extent on chronic angiogenesis to support their expansive growth.

Hallmark 6: activating invasion and metastasis

The five hallmarks detailed above stand as logical necessities for the chronic proliferative programmes of cancer cells. The sixth is less intuitive: high-grade cancer cells become invasive and migratory. These interrelated programmes enable cancer cells to invade into adjacent tissue, and into both blood and lymphatic vessels (intravasation). Using these vessels as highways for dissemination, cancer cells can reach microvessels in other organs and extravasate across the walls of these vessels into new tissue parenchyma. Having entered the unfamiliar tissue microenvironments, seeded micrometastases generally die or lay dormant. However, on rare occasion, they may adapt to survival in such ectopic tissue locations and develop proliferative programs in these microenvironments, allowing them generate macroscopic metastases—the process termed 'colonization'.

The regulation of the intertwined capabilities for invasion and metastasis is extraordinarily complex, involving both cell-intrinsic programmes and assistance from accessory cells in the tissue microenvironment. Prominent amongst the cancer cell intrinsic regulatory mechanisms is the activation of a developmental programme termed the epithelial-mesenchymal transition (EMT) [2, 4], which is associated with cell migrations and tissue invasions during embryogenesis and organogenesis. A second overlapping regulatory programme engaged by some invasive and metastatic cancer cells is the aforementioned hypoxia response system, which triggers the activation of the hypoxia-inducible transcription factors HIF1a and HIF2a, consequently altering expression of hundreds of genes [5, 6]. Both transcriptional programmes control genes that can facilitate invasive migration as well as survival in the blood and lymphatic systems and in ectopic tissue locations.

Notably, the acquisition of this hallmark capability can occur at various points along the pathways of multistep tumour development that lead incrementally from normal cells of origin to those found in aggressive malignancies. In some cases, this capability for invasion and metastasis is acquired early, such that cancer cells in an ostensibly benign tumour may be capable of dissemination long before this growth exhibits the overt histopathological phenotypes associated with high-grade malignancy. More often than not, however, the capability arises late, reflecting the accumulated mutational and epigenetic changes that render a tumour overtly malignant and thus its constituent cells capable of disseminating in large numbers to distant sites in the body. Moreover, there are clear indications that in the case of carcinomas, the EMT programme may become transiently active and functionally important for driving dissemination and seeding, thereafter being switched off in macrometastatic colonies [7]. It remains unclear whether the acquired traits of invasion and metastasis are beneficial and hence actively selected during the evolution of primary tumours or, alternatively, represent incidental byproducts of activating global regulatory networks (e.g. EMT, HIF) that facilitate primary tumour formation via functional contributions to the other five hallmarks.

Hallmark 7: deregulating cellular energetics and metabolism

The concept that cancer cells alter their utilization of energy sources—notably glucose—to support their proliferation was introduced almost 90 years ago by Otto Warburg, who observed that certain cultured cancer cells exhibited enhanced uptake of glucose, which was then largely metabolized by glycolysis. This limited breakdown of glucose occurred even in the presence of oxygen levels that normally would favour the oxidative phosphorylation pathway operative in the mitochondria. The result was counterintuitive, since glycolysis is far less efficient than 'OxPhos' at producing ATP, the primary currency of intracellular energy. We now appreciate that the 'aerobic' glycolysis described by Warburg produces, in addition to ATP, many of the building blocks for the cellular macromolecules that are required for cell growth and division. Indeed, the metabolism of cancer cells resembles that of actively dividing normal cells rather than being a novel invention of neoplasia. Moreover, it is important to appreciate that there is not a bimodal switch from mitochondrial Ox-Phos to aerobic cytosolic glycolysis in cancer cells. Instead, cancer cells continue to utilize in different proportions the Krebs/citric acid cycle-associated Ox-Phos and glycolysis pathways, the balance of which may well be required for optimal growth by cancer cells in different tumour microenvironments.

Although glucose is the primary fuel source used by most cancer cells, glutamine is also emerging as another key blood-borne source of energy and a precursor of lipids and amino acids. In most cases, glutamine likely supplements and enhances glucose in supplying energy and biomaterials for growth and proliferation of cancer cells, although in some cases of glucose insufficiency, glutamine may be able to compensate [8].

A third player in metabolic fuelling is lactate. While long considered to be toxic waste that is secreted by cells undergoing aerobic and anaerobic glycolysis, lactate is now appreciated to have diverse tumour-promoting capabilities [9]. In certain cancer cells, particularly those suffering glucose deprivation, extracellular lactose can be imported via specific transporters and used as fuel for generation of ATP and biomaterials. Similarly, some cancer-associated fibroblasts (CAF) can utilize lactate. Hence, metabolic symbioses can be envisaged within some tumours, between glucose-importing/lactose-exporting cells and lactose-importing cells [9].

Finally, we note a still-unresolved question about this hallmark: Is it significantly independent of the six cited earlier in terms of its regulatory mechanisms, or is it controlled by one of these other hallmark traits and in this sense hardly an independently standing hallmark on its own? Thus, certain mutant cancer genes, such as *Kras, cMyc,* and *p53,* have been found able to reprogramme the energy metabolism of cancer cells. Given this ambiguity, we termed the reprogramming of cellular energetics and metabolism as as an 'emerging hallmark' [2]. Irrespective of this qualification, it is clearly a crucial hallmark component of the neoplastic cell phenotype [10].

Hallmark 8: avoiding immune destruction

The eighth hallmark has been apparent on the horizon for decades. As originally proposed, incipient neoplasias must find ways to circumvent active surveillance by the immune system that would otherwise eliminate aberrantly proliferating pre-malignant cells. While clearly demonstrable in highly antigenic tumours in mouse models, and implicated in virus-induced human cancers, the generality of immune surveillance of cancer cells as a barrier to neoplastic progression and subsequent tumour formation is unresolved. One factor militating against this notion is the phenomenon of immune tolerance: because a normally functioning immune system develops a tolerance toward self-antigens, a tumour may pass under the radar and evade recognition and attack, as it expresses only these normal tissue antigens. Exceptions evidently arise, however, if cancer cells come to express embryonic antigens toward which immune self-tolerance was never established, or express fully novel non-self antigens created by gene mutation or by an infectious agent.

In fact, the immune response to the ~20% of virus-induced human tumours is clear: oncogenic viruses express foreign antigens to which the immune system is not tolerant, resulting in humoural and cellular immune responses that can kill virus-infected cells and thus eradicate incipient neoplasias. The fact that virus-transformed cells can nevertheless succeed in evading immune elimination to produce cancer testifies to immune-evasive capabilities evolved by such tumour viruses or developed by these cells during the course of tumour progression.

Although the incidence of non-virus-induced human cancers is not markedly increased in the context of immunodeficiency, suggesting a lack of immune surveillance of incipient neoplasias in the other 80% of human cancers, various lines of evidence suggest that some tumour types must indeed deal with immune recognition and attack during later stages of tumour progression and, in response, acquire immune-evasive strategies. Here, histopathological and epidemiological analyses have shed light on the potential role of immune attack and immune evasion. For example, among patients with surgically resected colorectal carcinomas, those whose tumours contained dense infiltrates of cytotoxic T-lymphocytes (CTLs) had a better prognosis than patients with tumours of similar grade and size that had comparatively few infiltrating CTLs. Such data implicate the actions of the immune system as a significant obstacle to the progressive growth and dissemination of cancer cells, one that is necessarily circumvented in some aggressive tumour types [11]. Indeed, immune phenotyping of tumours, including their associated stroma, is being evaluated as a new metric in the prognosis of certain tumour types that may enable, when combined with traditional criteria, more accurate predictions of prognosis and more effective treatment decisions [12].

For these reasons, we view anti-tumour immune responses as a significant barrier to be circumvented during the lengthy multistage development of many forms of human cancer. However, rules of immune engagement remain ambiguous across the spectrum of human cancers. Thus, it is generally unclear when during organ-specific tumour development the attention of the immune system is attracted (or not), and what the characteristics and efficacy of resultant immune responses are. Nor is it evident how polymorphic genetic constitutions of patients and the tumours that they harbour may affect anti-tumour immunity. Nevertheless, evading immune destruction seems increasingly to be an important mandate for developing tumours and thus an evident (if still emerging) hallmark of cancer.

Taken together, we view these capabilities acquired by most forms of human cancer to constitute a set of eight distinct hallmarks (Figure 1.1). Importantly, one cannot ignore the complex underlying mechanistic realities: different tumours acquire these hallmarks by diverse mechanisms, co-opting distinct homoeostatic and developmental functions in order to achieve them.

Genomic instability and inflammation: facilitators of hallmark capabilities

The lengthy process of tumour development and malignant progression, long appreciated to involve a succession of rate-limiting steps, reflects the need of evolving cancer cells to acquire the eight hallmark capabilities enumerated above. How then are these functional capabilities acquired? Currently, there are two clearly established means by which the hallmarks are acquired: genome instability and the resulting mutation of hallmark-enabling genes, and inflammation by cells of the immune system that help provide such capabilities.

Genome instability and the consequent mutation of hallmark-enabling genes is the primary means of acquiring hallmark capabilities. The cell genome is subject to routine DNA damage inflicted by a variety of chemically reactive by-products of normal metabolism, by environmental insults, and by errors in DNA replication during cell division. The resulting defects, if left unrepaired, can become cell-heritable mutations, explaining the need for an elaborate array of proteins that continuously monitor DNA integrity and, in response to damage, undertake repair. Irreparable genome damage provokes the elimination of cells, a task orchestrated by the p53 tumour suppressor gene, which has therefore been dubbed the 'guardian of the genome'.

The elevated rates and persistence of ongoing proliferation of cells in neoplastic lesions creates cell lineages that have undergone far more successive growth-and-division cycles than is typical of normal tissues, accentuating the potential for mutation-generating replication errors. Moreover, critically shortened telomeres can catalyse chromosomal rearrangements and fusions; if advantageous, hallmark-enabling mutations result, and if telomerase is subsequently activated to stabilize the mutated genome before the telomere crisis become lethal, then mutant clones of cancer cells can selectively expand.

The fundamental association of genome instability and mutation with cancer has been strengthened by numerous demonstrations that many cancer cells carry identifiable defects in the complex machinery designed to monitor and repair genomic damage. Most

apparent are the frequently documented mutant alleles of p53 that have been found in perhaps 40% of all cancers; without p53 on duty, damaged DNA can persist unrepaired and mutant cells can survive and pass their damaged genomes on to their progeny. Other specialized DNA repair enzymes are also found in defective form in many tumours, and inherited familial defects in DNA repair can lead to elevated risk of cancer development, again by enabling the acquisition of tumour-promoting mutations.

The critical roles of somatic mutations in cancer pathogenesis are being further substantiated by the development of high-throughput DNA sequencing technologies and the associated ability to systematically analyse large numbers of independently arising cancer cell genomes. Complemented by other methods for genome scanning, such as comparative genomic hybridization to identify copy number variations, and 'chromosome painting' to detect karyotypic abnormalities such as translocations, the derangements of the cancer cell genome are being revealed in unprecedented detail [13–16].

The observations enabled by these various technologies substantiate the fact that almost every form of human cancer involves cancer cells whose genomes have been rearranged and mutated. The density of genetic alterations varies from one tumour type to another over many orders-of-magnitude, from very low numbers detected in certain paediatric cancers to the blizzards of mutations present in the genomes of UV-induced melanomas and tobacco-induced lung cancers. Thus, the aberrations can range from dozens of point mutations to hundreds of thousands per cancer cell genome, and from quasi-diploid chromosomal karyotypes to widespread aneuploidy, translocations, and multiple large-scale amplifications and deletions.

The data generated by these increasingly high-throughput genomic technologies presents a major challenge to determine which of the myriad mutational alterations actually contribute substantively to hallmark capabilities? The numbers that are being catalogued in many cancer cells greatly exceed those that are likely to be important in reshaping cell phenotype. The recurrence of specific mutations or mutated genes in multiple independently arising tumours of the same cancer type or subtype presents one compelling line of evidence concerning the functional importance of the involved gene. Yet other mutations may simply occur as consequences of the rampant stochastic mutations that accumulate in patients' tumours and, being non-recurrent, can be dismissed as 'passenger mutations' having little likelihood of contributing to tumour development; thus, such mutations would not seem to afford selective advantage and clonal expansion during tumour growth and progression. These phenomena have led to the emerging concept that cancer cells contain two classes of mutations: 'drivers' and 'passengers', the former being functionally important in driving tumour progression forward, while the latter are not. Identifying the important drivers becomes increasingly important as the effort to find potential therapeutic targets within cancer cells accelerates. An added dimension of complexity comes from the observations that certain hallmark traits may be conferred by driver mutations in some tumours, while in others comparable phenotypic advantage may be acquired by changes in the epigenome—the spectrum of heritable changes in chromatin that are not reflected by alterations in nucleotide sequence [17]. The field of cancer genetics is poised for an extraordinary decade during which tens of thousands of cancer cell genomes will be comprehensively analysed for multiple parameters (DNA sequence and copy number, gene transcription, and histone and DNA methylation). The challenge and the opportunity will be to distill the contributions of specific genomic alterations to hallmark-enabling functions from the mammoth datasets that are being generated, and to exploit such knowledge for improved detection, evaluation, and informed treatment of human cancers.

Tumour-promoting immune infiltration (inflammation) is the second important means by which developing cancers can acquire hallmark capabilities. Above we discussed the mandate of developing tumours to avoid immunological destruction by cells of the adaptive immune system, often by blocking or pacifying infiltrating cytotoxic T cells. At the same time, it is clear that most tumours are nevertheless infiltrated by other cells of the immune system (so-called infiltrating immune cells, or IICs [3]) that are often components of the innate arm of this system and function as mediators of inflammation. In principle, such inflammation by IICs might reasonably be thought to represent failed attempts by the immune system to eradicate tumours. However, the evidence now clearly shows a quite different role: IICs help in the acquisition of multiple hallmark capabilities, encompassing six of the eight hallmarks [3]. Many of these functions reflect the roles that IICs play in the processes of wound healing and associated transient inflammation. Thus IICs can variously supply proliferative and survival signals, pro-angiogenic factors, and facilitate local invasion and blood-borne metastasis. In addition, some of these IICs (T-regulatory and myeloid-derived suppressor cells) can actively suppress the cytotoxic T lymphocytes that have been dispatched by the immune system to eradicate cancer cells.

The identities of the recruiting signals that bring IICs into tumours—including an ensemble of chemokine and cytokine signalling factors—are still incompletely understood. In some cases, the nature of the neoplastic lesion may trigger tissue abnormality signals that attract IICs; in particular, innate immune cells and possibly also B and T lymphocytes of the adaptive arm of the immune system. In other cases, oncogenic signalling, by activating transcriptional networks, induces expression of cytokines and chemokines that recruit IICs. In early stage lesions, the recruited IIC can help incipient cancer cells to proliferate, survive, evade anti-growth controls, or activate angiogenesis. At later stages of progression, IICs at the margins of tumours can facilitate invasiveness. Some experiments reveal that IICs can pair with cancer cells as they migrate through the circulation and become established in distant locations [18]. Additionally, certain IICs, such as macrophages, can subject cancer cells to DNA-damaging reactive oxygen species, thereby contributing to the mutational alteration of the cancer cell genome.

Most types of solid tumours are associated with tumour-promoting immune infiltrations that range from histologically subtle to the obvious inflammatory responses recognized by pathologists. In addition, the long-appreciated epidemiologic association between chronic inflammation and carcinogenesis supports the proposition that pre-existing inflammatory conditions create fertile breeding grounds for the inception and progression of certain forms of cancer. Moreover, chronically inflamed tissues share features with wound healing; both involve induction of angiogenesis and stimulation of cell survival, proliferation and migration/invasion, involving the inflammatory IIC and other cell types (e.g., myofibroblasts) that they activate in the affected tissue. These multiple processes stimulated by inflammatory cells are of course hallmark capabilities, explaining why inflammation represents an important enabler of many types of cancer.

The tumour microenvironment (TME)

Historically, the simplistic description of the stroma posited that endothelial cells, through the process of angiogenesis, provided oxygen and nutrients, while carcinoma-associated fibroblasts (CAFs) provided structural support, and the IICs, discussed above, represented ineffectual anti-tumoural immune responses. We now appreciate the fact that the diverse cells forming the tumour-associated stroma can contribute to acquisition by cancer cells of seven of the eight hallmarks [3]. These three classes of stromal cell—angiogenic vascular cells (AVC), consisting of endothelial cells and pericytes; cancer-associated fibroblasts (CAF); and infiltrating immune (inflammatory) cells (IIC)—remain the most important actors within the TME in terms of their ability to facilitate tumour progression [3]. In fact, there are a number of distinct subtypes of mesenchymal cells within the stroma that have, in the past, been labeled simply as CAFs. The three most prevalent of these originate from alpha-smooth muscle actin-expressing myofibroblasts, mesenchymal stem cells, or connective tissue fibroblasts. These subtypes of CAFs are evidently generated by epigenetic reprogramming of their respective normal cells of origin by paracrine signals produced in the TME, reflecting similar signals that are responsible for orchestrating the complex process of wound healing.

The IIC cells described earlier are now known to be more diverse than previously appreciated. The list of tumour-promoting IICs includes various forms of macrophages, neutrophils, partially differentiated myeloid progenitors, and in some cases specialized B and T lymphocyte subtypes. The endothelial cells and pericytes of the tumour-associated vasculature are, superficially at least, relatively simple by comparison. However, both epitope and gene expression profiling have revealed tissue- and tumour-type-specific features of the endothelial cells, likely with subtle functional implications in terms of their ability to contribute to acquisition of hallmark phenotypes by nearby cancer cells.

This recent and more nuanced view of stromal cells elevates their importance in understanding the disease, by virtue of their hallmark-enabling functional contributions [2, 3]. CAFs, as an example not discussed above, can in different neoplastic contexts secrete proteases and signalling ligands that can, in turn, liberate epithelial cells from the growth-suppressive effects imposed by normal tissue architecture. Alternatively, CAFs may foster tumour-promoting inflammation, facilitate both local invasion and metastatic seeding, and even provide cancer cells with metabolic fuel. CAFs can also induce angiogenesis and, remarkably, act in an immune-suppressive fashion to blunt the attacks of tumoricidal CTLs.

Looking to the future, an important goal will be to continue mapping the multidimensional landscape of stromal cell types and subtypes operating within different tumour types and at different stages of progression, annotating the means of their recruitment and programming, and their respective functional contributions to hallmark capabilities and tumour phenotypes.

Finally, we note an additional dimension of intra-tumoral complexity revealed by findings indicating that most cancers contain distinct subpopulations of cancer cells with a greatly elevated ability to seed new tumours. Such tumour-initiating cells (TICs), often termed cancer stem cells (CSCs), contrast with the bulk of cells in most tumours, which lack tumour-initiating ability. CSCs typically proliferate relatively slowly and often express the distinctive cell-surface markers of tissue stem cells [7, 19]. The initial concept was that CSC spawned cancer cells much like normal tissue stem cells spawn differentiated progenitors, and indeed there are such cases. For example, the CSCs in squamous cell carcinomas of the skin, which produce partially differentiated cancer cells much as normal skin stem cells produce the squamous epithelium. But in other cases, there appears to a dynamic bidirectional relationship between CSCs and cancer cells, in that cancer cells can be converted into CSCs, and vice versa; in some such cases, the EMT appears to switch on the CSC phenotype in cancer cells, while its converse (the mesenchymal-to-epithelial transition, MET) does the opposite to CSCs [7, 19]. Independent of this interconvertibility, there are indications that more slowly proliferating CSCs are often more resistant to existing anti-cancer drugs, enabling their persistence after initial treatment, laying the foundation for the regrowth of tumours that leads to clinical relapse. As such, therapeutic targeting of CSCs may be crucial to achieving enduring cancer therapies.

Applications to cancer medicine?

What then are the applications to translational and clinical oncology research of this conceptualization that common principles underlie the diversity of human cancer? The most apparent is in helping elucidate the molecular and cellular mechanisms by which particular forms of human cancer develop and progress to malignancy. A wealth of data is being generated by multiplatform analyses of cancer cells and neoplastic lesions in different tumour types (see, for example, [20]). Moreover, there will be other extrapolations of such analytic technologies, including the comparison of the cells present in multiple stages in tumorigenesis and tumour progression including metastatic growths, as well as comparisons of tumours and metastases during the response and relapse phases. The hope is to distill these complex datasets into insights that enable the development of novel mechanism-targeted therapies. The challenges are indicated by a number of formidable problems, including developing computational strategies that will make it possible to integrate all of this information in order to reveal the key determinants of particular tumorigenic pathways, to identify new therapeutic targets within cancer cells, to identify modes of

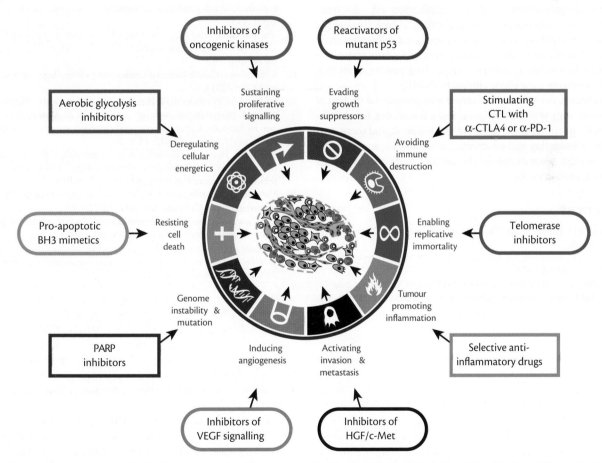

Fig. 1.2 Therapeutic targeting of the hallmarks of cancer. Drugs have been developed that disrupt or interfere with all eight of the hallmark capabilities, and with the two enabling facilitators (genome instability and tumour-promoting inflammation). Some of these hallmark-targeting drugs are approved for clinical use, while others are being tested in late-stage clinical trials; moreover, there is a pipeline full of new hallmark-targeting drugs that are in development and preclinical evaluation. Recognizing that eventual adaptive resistance during therapeutic treatment is apparent for virtually all of these hallmark-targeting drugs, a hypothesis has emerged: perhaps, by co-targeting multiple independent hallmarks, it will be possible to limit or even prevent the emergence of simultaneous adaptive resistance to independent hallmark-targeting drugs; clinical and preclinical trials are beginning to assess the possibilities.

Reprinted from *Cell*, Volume 144, Issue 5, Hanahan D, Weinberg RA, Hallmarks of cancer: the next generation, pp. 646–674, Copyright © 2011, with permission from Elsevier, http://www.sciencedirect.com/science/journal/00928674

adaptive resistance to therapy, and to use all of these data for diagnosis, prognosis, and treatment decisions. It is plausible, albeit still unproven, that conceptualizing these problems in terms of cancer's hallmarks will prove useful in this integration and distillation.

The hallmarks concept may prove useful in a second way. Thus, there are either approved drugs or drugs in late-stage clinical trials that target each of the eight hallmark capabilities and both of the enabling characteristics (Figure 1.2). For most of the ten, there are multiple drugs targeting a small set of mechanistic effectors. Unfortunately to date, such mechanism-based therapies targeting individual hallmarks have not proven to be been transformative for the treatment of late-stage, aggressive forms of human cancer. Typically, after a period of clinical response by tumours, adaptive resistance mechanisms kick in, enabling the surviving cancer cells (and CSCs) to resume progressive growth.

While different solutions can be proffered, one strategy involves applying the concept of the hallmarks as independent (or quasi-independent) and necessary components of a malignant cancer: by concomitantly targeting multiple hallmarks, it may be more difficult for cancer cells to concurrently develop multiple resistance mechanisms, allowing improvements in both initial efficacy and duration of clinical responses. As is always the case with multi-drug treatments, a major complication will arise from the toxicities that often accompany application of such therapeutic protocols. Anticipating such complications, genetically engineered mouse models of cancer and patient-derived xenografts may prove highly useful in reducing the numbers of drug combinations that should be tested in early phase clinical trials [21].

In conclusion, the hallmarks of cancer may provide the student of modern oncology with a foundation and a framework for absorbing the subsequent topical chapters of this textbook, and more generally for investigating and interpreting mechanisms, and applying such knowledge towards the development of more effective treatments for human cancers.

References

1. Hanahan D, Weinberg RA. The hallmarks of cancer. Cell 2000; 100: 57–70.
2. Hanahan D, Weinberg RA. Hallmarks of cancer: the next generation. Cell 2011; 144: 646–674.
3. Hanahan D, Coussens LM. Accessories to the crime: functions of cells recruited to the tumor microenvironment. Cancer Cell 2012; 21: 309–322.
4. Weinberg RA. The Biology of Cancer. New York: Garland Press, 2013.
5. Keith B, Johnson RS, Simon MC. HIF1α and HIF2α: sibling rivalry in hypoxic tumour growth and progression. Nature Reviews Cancer 2011; 12(1): 9–22.
6. Semenza GL. Hypoxia-inducible factors: mediators of cancer progression and targets for cancer therapy. Trends in Pharmacological Sciences 2012; 33: 207–214.
7. Baccelli I, Trumpp A. The evolving concept of cancer and metastasis stem cells. Journal of Cell Biology 2012; 198: 281–293.
8. Daye D, Wellen KE. Metabolic reprogramming in cancer: unraveling the role of glutamine in tumorigenesis. Seminars in Cell & Developmental Biology 2012; 23: 362–369.
9. Dhup S, Dadhich RK, Porporato PE, Sonveaux P. Multiple biological activities of lactic acid in cancer: influences on tumor growth, angiogenesis and metastasis. Current Pharmaceutical Design 2012; 18: 1319–1330.
10. Ward PS, Thompson CB. Metabolic reprogramming: a cancer hallmark even Warburg did not anticipate. Cancer Cell 2012; 21: 297–308.
11. Fridman WH, Pagès F, Sautès-Fridman C, Galon J. The immune contexture in human tumours: impact on clinical outcome. Nature Reviews Cancer 2012; 12: 298–306.
12. Galon J, Franck P, Marincola FM, Angell HK, Thurin M et al. Cancer classification using the Immunoscore: a worldwide task force. Journal of Translational Medicine 2012; 10(1): 205.
13. National Institute of Cancer, TCGA Data Portal Overview, <https://tcga-data.nci.nih.gov/tcga/tcgaHome2.jsp>, accessed on 14 April 2015.
14. The Wellcome Trust Sanger Institute's Cancer Genome Project 2013, <http://www.sanger.ac.uk/research/projects/cancergenome/>, accessed on 14 April 2015.
15. International Cancer Genome Consortium, <http://icgc.org/>, accessed on 14 April 2015.
16. NCI and NCBI's SKY/M-FISH and CGH Database 2001, <http://www.ncbi.nlm.nih.gov/sky/skyweb.cgi>, accessed on 20 April 2015.
17. You JS, Jones PA. Cancer genetics and epigenetics: two sides of the same coin? Cancer Cell 2012; 22: 9–20.
18. Labelle M, Hynes RO. The initial hours of metastasis: the importance of cooperative host-tumor cell interactions during hematogenous dissemination. Cancer Discovery 2012; 2: 1091–1099.
19. Visvader JE, Lindeman GJ. Cancer stem cells: current status and evolving complexities. Cell Stem Cell 2012; 10: 717–728.
20. The Cancer Genome Atlas Network. Comprehensive molecular portraits of human breast tumours. Nature 2012; 490: 61–70.
21. De Palma M, Hanahan D. The biology of personalized cancer medicine: facing individual complexities underlying hallmark capabilities. Molecular Oncology 2012; 6: 111–127.

CHAPTER 2

Growth factors and uncontrolled proliferation

Shujuan Liu and Ahmed Ashour Ahmed

Introduction to growth factors and uncontrolled proliferation

In spite of the significant diversity in their protein structures, growth factors have a remarkably similar overall mechanism of relaying signals (Figure 2.1). In general, ligand binding to receptors induces dimer formation (Figure 2.2) and autophosphorylation followed by recruitment of docking proteins and the activation of downstream signalling pathways that eventually modulate transcription. The specificity of growth factor signalling is governed by tissue-specific expression of pathway receptors, modulators, adaptors, and signalling molecules. The orderly regulation of components of growth factor pathways is governed by feedback loops that modulate the intensity and duration of a particular signal. A central feature of the majority of known cancers is the deregulation of one or more components of such feedback loops. Therefore, growth factor signalling pathways have attracted extensive drug discovery and drug development efforts that led to the introduction of many successful targeted therapies in cancer management. In general, these therapies have targeted the inactivation or blockage of ligands, receptors, or downstream signalling pathways (Figure 2.3). Here we outline the mechanisms involved in the regulation of some of the major growth factor signalling pathways, their deregulation in cancer and current approaches for growth factor targeted therapies.

Hepatocyte growth factor

Hepatocyte growth factor (HGF) was originally identified as a growth factor produced by platelets that stimulated DNA production in rat hepatocytes in primary culture that was biochemically distinct from platelet derived growth factor [1]. Subsequently, HGF and its ligand, the MET receptor tyrosine kinase [2] were implicated in various physiological and pathological processes.

HGF belongs to the plasminogen family of proteins and is transcribed and secreted in its inactive form as a single polypeptide, pro-HGF [3]. Subsequent site-specific proteolysis results in the formation of a dimer and this process is required for the biological activity of HGF [4]. This proteolytic step is mediated by a thrombin-like soluble enzyme called HGF activator (HGFA) or by the membrane bound proteolytic enzymes matriptase and hepsin [5, 6]. The activation of HGF is inhibited by proteolytic inhibitors HAI1 and HAI2 [7, 8].

Once HGF is activated, its serine proteinase homology (SPH) domain binds to the semaphorin (Sema) transmembrane domain of its receptor MET at the surface of cells. This binding results in the dimerization of the receptor and subsequent autophosphorylation of multiple tyrosine residues in its kinase domain. This results in subsequent activation and autophosphorylation of the substrate recognition site of the kinase and the adaptor proteins growth factor receptor-bound protein 2 (GRB2) and the GRB2-associated binding protein 1 (GAB1). It is important to note that the dimerization of the receptor is followed by internalization by endocytosis through clathrin-mediated coated pits and vesicles. Internalized receptor retains activity and there is recent evidence to suggest that certain MET mutations result in cytoplasmic localization of the receptor [9]. Once phosphorylated, MET, GBR2, and GAB1 act as docking sites for multiple substrates such as phosphoinositide 3 kinase (PI3K), CRK-like (CRKL) protein, and the protein tyrosine phosphatase SHP2 (also called PTPN11). Cytoplasmic MET becomes either degraded or recycled back to the membrane. Through docking these proteins, the HGF-MET pathway regulates several biological processes such as metabolism (PI3K signalling), proliferation (RAS/MAPK and PI3K signalling), epithelial mesenchymal transformation (EMT) and migration (RAC1/CDC42) [10]. Through modulating these signaling pathways, the HGF-MET pathway regulates important processes such as regeneration after skin [11, 12] or liver damage [13, 14] and EMT of myogenic progenitor cells in development [15].

The physiological regulation of HGF and MET is lost in cancers through multiple mechanisms including transcriptional deregulation, inadequate degradation, receptor crosstalk or synergies in downstream signalling pathways [2, 10, 16]. Induction of germ-line mutations of the HGF pathway in mice results in the generation of a variety of malignancies such as carcinomas, lymphomas, and sarcomas [17]. In addition, conditional activation of MET in the mammary gland results in the formation of basal-like carcinomas [18] and overexpression of MET is observed in a variety of tumours such as lung and renal carcinomas [19]. The activation of this pathway results in persistent activation of the RAS/MAPK pathway and the PI3K/AKT pathway that in turn results in increased proliferation, growth, and resistance to apoptosis. HGF/MET signalling is also a potent inducer of endothelial cell growth and angiogenesis [20–22]. Activation of MET results in increased VEGFA production and inhibition of thrombospondin production and this leads to enhanced angiogenesis [23]. MET also plays an important role in promoting metastasis of cancer cells through its role in regulating the RAS/MAPK [24] and RAC1/CDC42 regulation of the cytoskeleton [25].

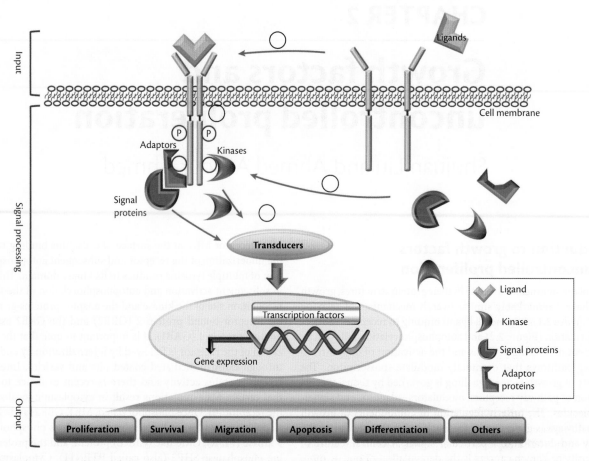

Fig. 2.1 General perspective of growth factor signal transduction. The basic mechanism of activation of growth factor signalling pathway starts by: (1) binding followed by (2) ligand-induced receptor dimerization, activation of intrinsic kinase activity and autophosphorylation at specific tyrosine residues or serine/threonine residues (in the case of TGFβ), then (3) the phosphorylated receptors act as docking sites for adaptor proteins or could directly bind to a wide range of molecules that could (4) activate downstream signalling pathways which, ultimately, regulate a variety of cellular processes. Most of these signalling pathways relay signals from the membrane through the cytoplasm to the nucleus, except for IL-6 which via STATs transmit signals directly from the membrane to the nucleus.

Because of its established role in transformation, tumour growth, metastasis, and angiogenesis, the HGF-MET pathway has been established as a target for therapy in many tumour types [19]. So far, there are several strategies targeting the HGF/MET pathway, including inhibitor of HGF/SF activators, anti-HGF humanized antibodies, MET decoy receptors as well as MET extracellular domain monoclonal antibodies. In addition, several selective and non-selective MET kinase inhibitors are under evaluation in clinical trials. In addition, several combinations of targeted therapies are ongoing in Phase II and Phase III studies [10, 19]. Promising results were obtained from a clinical trial of a MET antibody (METMab®) in combination with an EGFR inhibitor (erlotinib) to treat patients

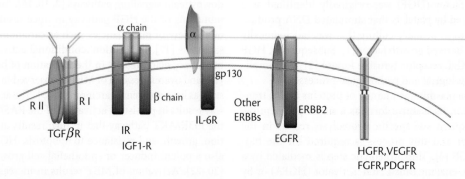

Fig. 2.2 Ligand binding could induce different types of receptor dimer formation depending on both the structural characteristics of the receptors. The most common form of dimerization is the formation of homodimers as is the case with HGF, VEGF, FGF, and PDGF receptors. EGF receptors form heterodimer complexes as not all of them can interact with ligands (e.g., ERBB2) or possess kinase activity (e.g., ERBB3). The TGFβ and IL-6 receptors usually form heteroterametric complexes (sometime hexamerization for IL-6) composed of two different isoforms of the receptor (for TGFβ, they are type I and type II TGFR. For IL-6, they are IL-6Rα and gp130). The IR and IGF1R isoforms are 'half' receptors that comprise a predominately extracellular α-chain and an intracellular β-chain. When actived, two half receptors form a holoreceptor for downstream signalling.

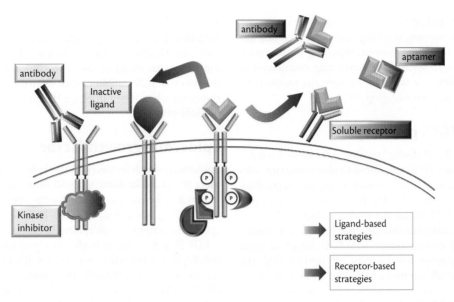

Fig. 2.3 Principles of pharmacological inhibition of growth factor signalling in cancer therapy. In general, the strategies targeting growth factor signalling pathways are divided into two major groups: (1) approaches for blocking the ligand or (2) blocking the receptor. The ligand can be blocked by neutralizing antibodies, dimeric soluble receptor extracellular domains, aptamers (stabilized oligonucleotides which could bind ligand proteins with high specific) or antisense oligonucleotides that target the ligand mRNA. Among the blocking receptor approaches, the receptor kinase inhibitors are the most widely developed pharmacological agents in cancer therapy. In addition, neutralizing antibodies targeting receptors and receptor kinase inhibitors are the most efficient and widely developed pharmacological approaches in cancer therapy.

with non small cell lung carcinoma (NSCLC). The combination treatment increased the progression-free survival (PFS) in cancers with high c-MET expression when compared with the group receiving erlotinib alone. Cancers with low or no c-MET expression showed no response to METMab® and patients had worse overall survival [10].

Insulin growth factor

Insulin is secreted from the β cells of the pancreas and functions as a classic hormone by influencing glucose uptake and carbohydrate metabolism in target cells that are distant from the pancreas. Insulin signals through insulin receptors (IR) that are formed of two αβ glycosylated polypeptides that together form a holoreceptor. The α chain of the receptor is predominantly localized at the surface while the β chain is transmembranous and harbours the kinase domain of the receptor [26]. Binding of insulin to the α chain of the receptor results in its activation and increased glucose uptake and downstream induction of glycolysis. This basic physiological process is crucial for the regulation of circulating glucose levels. IGFs have characteristics of both hormones and tissue growth factors. Similar to insulin, insulin-like growth factor 1 (IGF1) and IGF2 signal through a specific receptor, IGF1R, to regulate glucose metabolism, signal transduction, and a variety of physiological processes. Unlike insulin, IGF1 and IGF2 are widely expressed by many cell types and function in autocrine, endocrine, and paracrine fashions [27]. These ligands and their receptors have been implicated in driving the growth of many tumours [28, 29]. IRs exist in two splice variant isoforms: IRA and IRB, but the IGF1 receptor only has one isoform. IRB recognizes only insulin while IRA, which is most commonly expressed in tumours, recognizes both insulin and IGF2.

IGF1R shares 70% homology with IR (84% homology with its kinase domain [30]) and is a holoreceptor that is formed of αβ chains and together they form part of the transmembrane receptor tyrosine kinase superfamily. IGF1R acts as a receptor for both IGF1 and IGF2. Upon ligand activation, IGF1R undergoes conformational changes that result in binding of ATP to residue Lys1003 and activation of the kinase by autophosphorylation at tyrosine residues 1131, 1135, and 1136 [31] and subsequent binding and activation of docking substrate proteins such as insulin receptor substrates (IRS1-4). IRS tyrosine phosphorylation increases its affinity to the PI3K complex that results in translocation of PI3K to the membrane and its subsequent activation. IGF1R-mediated activation of PI3K as well as RAS/RAF/MAPK represent the key pathways through which IGF regulates cell proliferation and metabolism [27, 32].

There are several lines of regulation of IGF signalling. In general, IGF binding proteins (IGFBPs) have high affinity to insulin growth factors and limit their bioavailability to bind to IGFR1 [33]. IGFBPs expression is induced by p53, as well as many growth inhibitors such as vitamin D, anti-estrogens, retinoids, and transforming growth factor β [28]. Decreased expression of IGFBPs or mutations in TP53 result in increased IGF signalling and increased tumour proliferation [34]. Another line of regulation is through allelic dosing by imprinting and silencing of the maternal-derived allele of IGF2. Loss of imprinting carries a fivefold increased risk of colorectal neoplasia [35]. In addition, IGF2R, which specifically binds IGF2, lacks the kinase activity of IGF1. Therefore, IGF2R binding to IGF2 is thought to be a mechanism of inhibition of the pathway, and loss of function mutations of IGF2R have been found in a variety of tumours [36]. There is strong evidence that IGF signalling is either required for or facilitates the transforming signals of oncogenes. In vivo models demonstrated that loss of IGF2 reduced tumour development following TP53 or PTEN deletions in mice [37, 38].

Because of the strong evidence that the IGF signalling pathway is involved in driving tumour growth [28, 39, 40], it has been intensively investigated as a possible target for therapy. Several strategies have been evaluated including targeting the ligands or decreasing their bioavailability, developing blocking antibodies targeting the IGF receptors or blocking of downstream signalling via activation of the AMPK pathway. In spite of the continuing enthusiasm in evaluating IGF signalling as a target for therapy, the results from clinical trials have not been encouraging [29].

The IL6/JAK/STAT3 pathway

Initially identified as a T-cell-derived regulating factor in B cell differentiation, Interleukin 6 (IL6) was found to play important roles in a wide range of biological activities such as immune regulation, haematopoiesis, and oncogenesis [41]. IL6 belongs to a group of cytokines that include IL11, leukaemia inhibitory factor (LIF), cardiotrophin (CT1), cardiotrophin-like cytokine (CLC), ciliar neurotrophic factor (CNTF), and oncostatin M (OSM), which all share a common receptor: glycoprotein receptor 130 (gp130) [42]. IL6 binds to its receptor IL6R (composed of ILRα and gp130) leading to its tetramerization/hexamerization, which in turn leads to activation of JAK1/JAK2/TYK2 kinases [42–44]. Activated JAK1/JAK2/TYK2 leads to tyrosine phosphorylation of the cytoplasmic domain of the IL6R leading predominantly to recruitment of signal transducer and activator of transcription 3 (STAT3) via its SH2 domain and its subsequent phosphorylation by JAK1/JAK2/TYK2. Once phosphorylated, STAT3 dissociates from the receptor and forms active dimers in which a phosphorylated SH2 domain of one molecule of STAT3 binds to the phospho-tyrosine 705 of the other molecule. Unlike many other signalling pathways that relay signals from the membrane through the cytoplasm to the nucleus, STATs offer a direct route of signalling from the membrane to the nucleus. STAT3 activation leads to the transcription of pro-survival proteins such as the anti-apoptotic protein BcL-xl, the cell cycle promoter cyclin D1, MCL-1, XIAP, Fas, and the oncogene c-Myc, as well as angiogenic factors [45, 46]. The regulation of the IL6/JAK/STAT3 pathway is mediated by the SOCS (suppressor of cytokine signalling) feedback inhibitors and PIAS (protein inhibitor of active Stat) proteins [41]. In addition to activation of STAT3, IL6 also activates Ras, MAPK, Cox-2, Wnt and PI3K/AKT pathways [47].

Overexpression of IL6 and activation of IL6 pathway are reported in many tumour types such as ovarian cancer, breast cancer, prostate cancer, endometrial cancer, lung cancer, renal cell carcinoma, oral squamous cell carcinoma, and colon cancer [41]. IL6 and STAT3 have also been associated with cancer drug resistance in breast, prostatic, and ovarian cancer. Treatment targeting IL6 or STAT3 could sensitize ovarian cancer to paclitaxel [48–50]. In addition, serum IL6 has been found to correlate with patient survival and could be an independent prognostic factor for cancers [51]. Mutations of IL6 downstream kinases such as the JAK2 V617F have been identified in most myeloproliferative neoplasms [52].

Current therapeutic strategies targeting IL6 mainly focus on monoclonal antibodies against IL6 and IL6R. Several types of chimeric antibodies, such as CNTO 328 (siltuximab) and BE-8, and humanized monoclonal antibodies, such as CNTO 136 and ALD518, are undergoing clinical trials [41, 53]. In addition, strategies have been employed for targeting STAT3 signalling that can be broadly divided into rationalized inhibitor design and screening. Peptides, peptidomimetics, and small molecule derivatives have been developed to interrupt STAT3 dimerization by targeting the SH2 domain or by inhibiting the interaction between STAT3 dimers and DNA [54]. In addition, high throughput cell-based screening identified quinolines as possible inhibitors of STAT3 phosphorylation [55]. Despite intense research for discovering potent STAT3 inhibitors that could be tested in clinical trials, such agents still do not exist. JAK inhibitors such as ruxolitinib elicited significant responses when tested in phase III clinical trials for patients with myelofibrosis [56].

Epidermal growth factor

Epidermal growth factors (EGF) include 13 polypeptide ligands that share the EGF-like domain, a ~50 amino acid sequence characterized by a consensus six cysteine residue peptide and a β-sheet structure. EGF ligands include EGF, HB-EGF, neuregulins (1 through 6), epiregulin, amphiregulin, epigen, betacellulin, and TGFα. [57–59]

EGF ligands signal through a group of receptor tyrosine kinases called epidermal growth factor receptors (EGFRs, also called the ERBB receptors). The ERBB family of receptor tyrosine kinases includes ERBB1, ERBB2, ERBB3, and ERBB4 and share similar structural features. Broadly, they are formed of an extracellular ligand-binding domain, a transmembrane domain, a juxtamembrane domain, a kinase domain and a c-terminal tail that acts as a docking site for signalling proteins. In general, ligand binding results in homo- or heterodimerization, in which ERBB2-containing heterodimers are formed preferentially, and autophosphorylation on tyrosine residues. The latter provides docking sites for various adaptors or enzymes that initiate many signalling cascades [60]. In spite of broad similarities, ERBB receptors have distinct characteristics. For example, ERBB1, once bound to its ligands, undergoes conformational changes and autophosphorylation followed by binding to multiple docking proteins such as growth factor receptor bound 2 (GRB2) and members of the MAPK family of proteins but not PI3K [61]. Mouse knockouts of ERBB1 are fatal because of brain defects [62]. ERBB2, however, is thought to be a non-autonomous receptor tyrosine kinase that is incapable of binding to ligands but is capable of binding to a wide variety of substrates including the formation of heterodimers with other ERBB receptors and is, therefore, responsible for signal amplification in the EGF pathway [63]. ERBB3, while able to bind to ligands, is also thought to be non-autonomous as it lacks tyrosine kinase activity, albeit similar to the IGFR2 [64]. It does, however, form heterodimers with other ERBB receptors and is capable of binding to PI3K resulting in its relocation to the membrane followed by activation. ERBB4 is an autonomous tyrosine kinase that is capable of binding to ligands such as betacellulin, heparin-binding ligand, HB-EGF and epiregulin. Upon activation it is capable of recruiting GRB2, Shc, STAT5, and PI3K.

ERBB receptors are regulated via positive and negative feedback mechanisms. For example, ERBB receptor activation has been shown to induce TGFα and HB-EGF transcription [65]. Negative feedback loops either pre-exist, or are newly synthesized following stimulation of ERBBs by their respective ligands. The former primarily control receptors dephosphorylation and degradation. The latter, which is transcriptional up-regulated, may affect the ERBBs in multiple processes. For example, EGF stimulation results in the increased expression of the suppressor of cytokine signalling 5 (SOC5) that in turn promotes ERBB degradation through recruitment of E3 ubiquitin ligase [66]. In addition, the transmembrane leucine-rich repeat and immunoglobulin-like domains 1 protein (LRIG1) have been shown to inhibit EGF-mediated transformation of NIH3T3 fibroblast possibly through promoting ERBB receptor degradation [67].

Several mechanisms of deregulation of the EGF pathway have been described in cancer, which include overproduction of ligands, overproduction of receptors, or constitutive activation of receptors. In lung cancer, frequent mutations of ERBB1 at the ATP-binding cleft of the kinase domain have been described [68]. Such mutations are capable of activating downstream signalling pathways and increase the ability of ERBB1 to form heterodimers with other ERBB family members. Further, deletions of exon 2 to 7 of EGFR to form the oncogenic EGFRvIII mutant are commonly observed in glioblastoma [69]. In addition, genomic amplification of ERBB1 has been observed in lung, ovary, pancreas, breast, and head and neck cancers [70–72]. ERBB2 amplification and overexpression is frequently observed in breast cancer [73] and results in poor overall prognosis and resistance to taxane chemotherapy [74]. Overexpression results in EGFR-dependent pathway activation through delayed ligand induced degradation.

EGF targeting has been one of the most successful targeted therapy strategies for cancer treatment. Most efforts have concentrated on ERBB2 and ERBB1 owing to their increased expression in certain tumours, as mentioned before. Therapeutic approaches could be divided into immunological strategies (humanized antibody or naked monoclonal antibody), low molecular weight inhibitors (such as inhibitor of Hsp90), tyrosine kinase inhibitors and drug combinations. For example, trastuzumab, a monoclonal antibody against ERBB2, significantly improves survival in breast cancers that overexpress ERBB2 [75]. Similar results have been obtained with the EGFR monoclonal antibody cetuximab in EGF-expressing colorectal cancers that do not possess RAS mutations [76]. Tyrosine kinase inhibitors gefitinib (Iressa®) and erlotinib (Tarceva®) are also indicated in non-small-cell lung cancer [68]. Lapatinib is an ERBB1 and ERBB2 inhibitor that improves survival in ERBB2 positive metastatic breast cancer [77].

Fibroblast growth factors

Fibroblast growth factors (FGFs) [78] play many important physiological roles in regulating angiogenesis, wound repair, cell survival, and proliferation and differentiation. The FGF family includes 18 ligands and four transmembrane receptor tyrosine kinases (FGFR 1 through 4). FGFs are formed of glycoproteins that are secreted to the extracellular matrix and cell surface and are released from the matrix by the action of heparinases, proteases, or specific FGF-binding proteins that enable them to bind and activate their receptors. The specificity of the FGF–FGFR interaction is established by receptor paralogues, alternative splicing of FGFR, and the tissue-specific expression of ligands and receptors [79].

In general, the released FGFs bind to cell surface heparan sulphate proteoglycans (HPSGs) that stabilize the ligand–receptor interaction. FGF's binding to its receptors results in receptor dimerization, and subsequent formation of a ternary complex that comprises two receptor molecules, two FGFs, and one HSPG chain. The FGF signal leads to a conformational change of receptor structure that induces kinase domain activation and tyrosine phosphorylation of both the kinase domain and the receptor tail. This results in docking of a variety of signalling proteins of which the FGFR substrate 2 (FRS2) appears to be a key adaptor largely specific to FGFR. FGFRs phosphorylate FRS2 on several sites, and active FRS2 allows the recruitment of adaptor proteins, growth factor receptor bound 2 (GRB2) and Son of Sevenless 1 (SOS1) protein to promote guanine nucleotide exchange and activation of the RAS/RAF/MAPK pathway [80] and PI3K [81]. FGFRs are also capable of binding to other receptor tyrosine kinases such as anaplastic lymphoma receptor tyrosine kinase (ALK) [82]. Independently of FRS2 binding, the FGFRs could also bind to the SH2 domain of phospholipase Cγ (PLCγ) via its phosphotyrosin residue at the carboxyl terminus [83] and signals through the PKC/Ref/MAPK pathway. Several other pathways are also activated by FGFRs, such as p38 MAPK, Jun N-terminal kinase pathway, STAT signalling pathway [84], and ribosomal protein S6 kinase 2 (RSK2) [85]. The physiological functions of the FGF family are context dependent subject to cell-type specific expression pattern and cross-talk with other pathways. FGFRs play a key role in differentiation. For example, mutations in FGFR2 result in premature activation in development and premature closure of skull sutures resulting in a syndrome called craniosynostosis.

Important negative feedback mechanisms exist to suppress FGF signalling. For example, activation of the pathway has been shown to activate CBL-mediated monoubiquitylation and degradation of FGFRs [86]. MAPK activation downstream of FGFR results in induction of FRS2 expression which competes for and inhibits the binding of GRB2 to FGFR [82]. Further, FGFR signalling activates the MAPK phosphatase 3 (MKP3) which results in dephosphorylation and inactivation of ERK1 and ERK2 and, therefore, limiting MAPK signalling [87]. In addition, ERK1 and ERK2 signalling results in increased expression of Sprouty which either competes with SOS1 for binding to GRB2 and limits FGF-induced RAS activation, or directly binds to RAF to block the subsequent MAPK signalling [88, 89]. Similarly, the transmembrane form of interleukin 17 receptor D (IL17RD, also known as SEF) can directly bind to FGFRs [90] and inhibit ERK phosphorylation [91].

In cancer, several mechanisms of deregulation of the FGF pathway have been described including genomic FGFR alterations that drive ligand-independent receptor signalling such as gene amplifications, mutations, and translocations and alternation that result in ligand-dependent activation [79]. In a screen of more than 1000 somatic mutations found in the coding exons of 518 protein kinase genes from 210 different human cancers, the non-synonymous mutations of FGF signalling pathways were the most commonly identified mutations [92]. Most notably, mutations in the extracellular domain of FGFR3 that result in constitutive dimer formation have been described in 50% of bladder cancers [93]. Similar mutations have been observed in cervix cancer [94], prostate cancer [95] and multiple myeloma [96]. Mutations of FGFR2 occur in 12% of endometrial cancers [97]. Gene amplifications of FGFR2 are frequently observed in cancers such as being amplified in 10% of gastric cancers [98]. Similarly, amplification of the FGFR1-containing locus occurs in 10% of breast cancers [99]. Translocations that result in constitutive activation have also been observed in multiple myelomas where t(4;14) results in an FGFR3 to immunoglobulin H3 fusion which facilitates ligand-independent binding [100, 101]. In addition to FGFR deregulation, ligand-dependent mechanisms have also been observed in cancers through either autocrine production of ligand in cancer cells or paracrine overproduction of ligand from stromal cells that may be expressed physiologically or in response to cancer cells in a "paracrine loop" [79]. For example, antisense-mediated inhibition of FGFR1 or FGF2 regressed the growth of human melanoma xenografts, indicating that an FGF2–FGFR1 autocrine loop promotes the development of some melanoma [102]. FGF1 overexpression, which functions in a paracrine manner to promote angiogenesis, has been shown to correlate with poor survival in ovarian cancer [103].

Several mechanisms mediate the oncogenic potential of FGF deregulation. FGF signalling could affect cell proliferation, cell survival, migration, invasion, and angiogenesis in different tumour types. For example, activation of the pathway results in enhanced cancer cell survival and proliferation via activation of the PI3K–Akt pathway [104–106]. In addition, overexpression of FGF2 results in upregulation of the anti-apoptotic proteins BCL2, BCLx, XIAP, and IAP1 through the S6 kinase-mediated pathway, therefore promoting resistance to chemotherapy [107, 108, 109]. FGFR1 activation could result in increased MMP3-dependent invasion [110]. Importantly, endothelial blood vessels express high levels of FGFR1 and FGFR2, and FGF stimulation is known to have a potent angiogenic effect [111, 112].

In spite of the known oncogenic potential of FGF signalling, studies have shown that it has tumour suppressive functions in a context-dependent manner. For example, in a mouse model of developing endochondral and membranous bone, the FGFR3 and FGFR2 can negatively regulate proliferation and positively drive differentiation [113, 114]. Several studies of human tumours and cancer cell lines potentially support a tumour protective effect of FGFR2 signalling. For example, the expression of FGFR2-IIIb in FGFR2-IIIb negative bladder tumour cell lines blocks cell proliferation [115]. Given that in some circumstances FGFR2 signalling is clearly oncogenic, it is recognized that context-dependent differences in signalling can lead to either tumour promotion or senescence in response to active FGF signalling [79].

Several therapies targeting the FGF pathway are currently under investigation. FGFR tyrosine kinase inhibitors such as BIBF1120 [116], TK1258 [117], and TSU-68 [118] are in clinical trials. Such inhibitors have the advantage of targeting multiple pro-angiogenic growth factors (such as VEGF, PDGF, and FGF) but lack of specificity increases the potential side effects and limits the ability to deliver drugs at doses required for FGFR inhibition. Specific antibodies against mutant FGFR3 have been shown to be successful in bladder cancer and t(4;14) myeloma [119]. A third approach for targeting is the development of ligand traps. A fusion protein between the extracellular portion of FGFR1-IIIC and the Fc domain of IgG1 targets multiple FGF receptors by preventing ligand binding and has been shown to have anti-proliferative and anti-angiogenic effects [79]. Finally, recombinant FGF7 to stimulate FGFRs are used in treatment of mucositis induced by myelotoxic therapy requiring haematopoietic stem cell support [120].

Transforming growth factor beta

The transforming growth factor beta (TGFβ) pathway plays important roles in many physiological processes such as adhesion, migration, differentiation, apoptosis, and the determination of cell fate [121, 122]. In embryogenesis it plays an important role in germ line specification and patterning. The transforming growth factor family of ligands includes three TGFβ isoforms, four activin β chains, the protein nodal, ten bone morphogenic proteins (BMPs), and 11 growth and differentiation factors (GDFs) [123].

The basic mechanism of ligand-receptor activation includes dimerization of the pre-ligand protein followed by cleavage to generate an active ligand, followed by receptor binding. TGFβ receptors are formed of an extracellular cysteine-rich domain, a transmembrane domain, and a serine-threonine kinase domain

that distinguish this family of receptors from other transmembrane receptor tyrosine kinases [124]. TGFβ receptors are classified into two families: type I and type II. Type I family includes activin-like receptors (ALK 1 through 7). Type II includes receptors such as TGFRII, ACTRII, ACTRIIB, BMPRII, and AMHRII. Type II receptors are thought to phosphorylate type I receptors upon ligand activation. Phosphorylated type I receptors consequently recruit and phosphorylate the receptor-regulated TGFβ transducers SMAD proteins 1, 2, 3, 5, and 8 (R-SMADs). These SMADs consequently bind to SMAD4 and are translocated to the nucleus where they regulate transcription through regulating chromatin remodelling and histone modification [124]. In addition to the SMAD-dependent functions of the TGFβ pathway, TGFBRII has been shown to modulate disassembly of tight junctions through PAR6 [125].

Negative regulatory pathways exist to regulate the TGFβ pathway. For example, the inhibitory SMADs (I-SMADs), SMAD6 and SMAD7, are thought to inhibit other SMADs and terminate TGFβ-driven signal transduction [126]. TGFβ and BMP signalling and stimulation of R-SMADs results in the increase of transcription of SMAD6 and SMAD7 which compete with R-SMADs for binding to type I receptors and, therefore, limit signal transduction [127]. In addition, E3 ubiquitin ligases play a central role in regulating TGFβ signalling through the degradation of SMADs. Homologous to the E6-accessory protein C-terminus (HECT) E3 ubiquitin ligases, SMAD ubiquitin regulatory factor 1 (SMURF1) and SMURF2 are examples of key ubiquitin ligases involved in this process [128]. SMAD7 mediates the binding of SMURF1/2 to R-SMADs and their consequent degradation [129, 130]. In contrast, the RING-type E3 ubiquitin ligase Arkadia induces ubiquitination and degradation of SMAD7 and, therefore, augments TGFβ signalling [128]. SMAD6 may specifically compete with SMAD4 for binding to BMPR-activated SMAD1 by forming an inactive SMAD1/SMAD6 complex in the cytoplasm [131]. In addition, cross-talk between the TGFβ and the MAPK pathway (which includes ERK1/2, JNK and p38 pathways) is thought to induce positive and negative regulation of TGFβ signalling [132, 133]. For example, JNK, ERK, and p38 phosphorylate SMAD2/3 independent of TGFβ signalling [134–136]. There is also evidence that SMADs act upstream of MAPKs and mediate their activation. For instance, SMAD signalling plays an important role in promoting the invasive phenotype of human head and neck squamous carcinoma cells by p38-mediated upregulating collagenase expression [137]

The dual role of the TGFβ signalling pathway has recently become clearer [138, 139]. In early tumour formation, TGFβ induces a durable anti-proliferative effect by its cytostatic and apoptotic functions [140]. The cytostatic mechanism is thought to involve the upregulation of p21 and p15 and the consequent inhibition of CDK phosphorylation of retinoblastoma protein, halting the cell cycle [141]. In addition, TGFβ downregulates the transcription of c-Myc in a SMAD3-dependent manner. The apoptotic mechanism of TGFβ has important relationship with some pro-apoptotic target genes, which are controlled by SMAD transcriptional complexes such as the TGFβ-inducible early-response gene (TIEG1), the death-associated protein kinase (DAPK), and the SH2-domain-containing inositol-5-phosphatase (SHIP) [140]. Loss of this tumour suppressive function of TGFβ is thought to be a major step towards cancer progression. However, in established tumours, TGFβ signalling is thought to be overexpressed to create a local immunosuppressive environment that fosters tumour growth and exacerbates the pro-invasive and metastatic behaviour of tumour cells [140]. TGFβ induces the expression of several matrix metalloproteinases (MMPs) that lead to the degradation of the extracellular matrix and facilitate invasion. TGFβ also acts as a potent inducer of angiogenesis through a direct effect on VEGF expression and indirectly through inducing monocytes to release angiogenic cytokines [141]. In vivo models of breast cancer metastasis revealed that TGFβ signalling plays an important role in bone metastasis [142]. In addition, several signalling pathways have been implicated in TGFβ-induced epithelial-mesenchymal transition (EMT), such as SMADs, PI3K/Akt, RHOA, and p38 MAPK [140].

Therapeutic options targeting the TGFβ pathway in tumours have been developed [143, 144]. The most advanced TGFβ signalling antagonists in clinical development are large molecules including monoclonal antibodies and antisense oligonucleotides. For example, DNA oligonucleotides targeting TGFβ2 mRNA has been developed (trabedersen, AP12009, Antisense Pharma) for targeting high-grade gliomas, pancreatic cancer, and malignant melanomas [145]. Similarly, AP11014 is an antisense oligonucleotide against TGFβ1 that has also been developed for targeting non-small-cell lung cancer, colorectal cancer, and prostate cancer [146]. In addition, small-molecular TGFβ type I receptor kinase inhibitors have been the focus of drug discovery efforts, such as the ALK inhibitors SB431542 [147] and SB525334 [148]. Given the dual function of TGFβ signalling and the limitation of these therapeutic molecules, future studies may focus on exploring the potential clinical benefit of large and small molecule combination therapies and on determining the appropriate patient subpopulations for TGFβ therapies [143].

Platelet derived growth factors

Platelet derived growth factors [149, 150] are dimers of disulfide-linked polypeptide chains [151]. They are characterized by growth factor core domains with a conserved set of cysteine residues [152, 153]. The PDGF family consists of PDGFA, PDGFB, PDGFC, and PDGFD. The protein products of the genes form homodimers but PDGF-AB heterodimers have also been described. This family of growth factors is linked structurally and functionally to the VEGF family of proteins. PDGF receptors include PDGFRα and PDGFRβ. The receptors contain five extracellular immunoglobulin loops and a tyrosine kinase intracellular domain. They have structural similarities to FMS, c-Kit, and FLT3 which are the receptors for the CSF1, SCF, and FLT3 ligands, respectively. In vivo evidence confirmed that PDGF-AA and PDGF-CC dimers bind to PDGFRα while PDGF-BB binds to PDGFR-β [152, 154] PDGF expression in cultured cells is induced by several factors including hypoxia, thrombin, cytokines and growth factors including PDGF itself. PDGFA and PDGFC are predominantly expressed in epithelial cells, muscles, and neuronal progenitor cells. PDGFB is expressed in endothelial cells, megakaryocytes, and neurons while PDGFD is expressed in fibroblasts. PDGFR expression is generally low in mesenchymal cells but is increased following inflammation, TGFβ stimulation, estrogen, interleukin 1α, FGF2, and TNFα [151].

Similar to many other receptor tyrosine kinases, ligand binding of PDGF to its receptors induces dimer formation, autophosphorylation of the kinase domain and kinase activation. Phosphorylated sites act as docking sites for downstream signal transduction molecules and activate the RAS/MAPK pathway, the PI3K pathway, and PLC-γ.

GRB2 binds via its SH2 domain to phosphorylated PDGFR and via its SH3 domain to SOS1, which in turn activates RAS which signals to the RAF1 and MAPK pathway [155]. PI3K via its SH2 domain of regulatory subunit binds to PDGFR and actives a wide range of cell processes [156]. PLC-γ activation results in mobilization of intracellular calcium ions and the activation of PKC and downstream effects on cell growth and mobility [154]. In addition, PDGFR activation results in activation of the Src family of kinases promoting Myc transcription and mitogenic responses [157] and the FER/FES tyrosine kinases which induce cytoskeletal remodeling and differentiation.

PDGF signalling is controlled by the balance between the stimulatory signals mentioned above and negative feedback loops. SHP2 tyrosine phosphatase binds to PDGFR through the SH2 domain and dephosphorylates the receptor [158]. In addition, RAS-GAP binds to PDGFR-β and inactivates RAS [159]. Ligand-receptor interaction induces endocytotic receptor internalization and lysosomal degradation [160]. In addition, the adapter protein Alix binds to PDGFRB resulting in its increased ubiquitination and degradation via the CBl RING finger E3 ubiquitin ligase [161]. Phosphatase TC-PTP may also act as a negative regulator of PDGFR-β phosphorylation [162].

Many physiological functions have been attributed to the PDGF family. PDGF signalling plays a role in gastrulation and formation of cranial and cardiac neural crest. PDGFA and PDGFR-α null mice have severe impairment of early mesenchymal derivatives. PDGFR-α knockout mice and PDGFA/PDGFC double knockout mice have defective vertebral arch formation. PDGFs also have a conserved morphogenic function in guiding cell migration through the formation of growth factor gradients in the extracellular space. In addition, PDGF plays a key role in the development of several organs and tissue types such as being required for villous morphogenesis in the bowel tract, alveolar septum development, palate formation, glomerular formation in the kidney, hair follicles, and spermatogenesis. PDGFs are also involved in glial cell development and neuroprotection, and in the development of cardiovascular system, axial skeleton, and teeth [152].

PDGF signalling may be involved in modulating tumour behaviour through both autocrine and paracrine routes. Autocrine PDGF signalling has been implicated in glioblastoma, soft tissue sarcomas, and breast cancer, and contributes to proliferation, survival, invasion, and metastasis. A variety of tumours express high levels of PDGFA, PDGFC, and PDFGR-α. Such increased expression may be secondary to stimulation by other growth factors such as TGF-β in the case of some gliomas. Gene amplification has also been described in glioblastoma and esophageal squamous cell carcinoma. In addition to increased expression, activating mutations and chromosomal rearrangements also lead to autocrine PDGF signalling. For example, gastrointestinal stromal tumours that do not possess mutations in KIT frequently possess gain of function mutations in PDGFR-α. Several myeloid disorders and leukaemia have translocations that involve the PDGF receptors such as the ETV6-PDGFRB fusion that result in constitutive activation of the receptor. In addition, dermatofibrosarcoma protuberans (DFSP), a rare mesenchymal neoplasm of the dermis is characterized by a translocation that repositions the collagen type 1α1 promoter adjacent to the PDGF gene resulting in its overexpression and constitutive activation of PDGFR-β. Imatinib, a tyrosine kinase inhibitor that targets several kinases including PDGFR-β elicits up to 50% responses in this tumour [163]. PDGF signalling was found to be upregulated during TGFβ-induced EMT in breast cancer and promote metastasis in mouse mammary carcinomas. Paracrine PDGF signalling may play a role in malignant transformation by recruiting different types of stromal cells, such as endothelial cells, pericytes, and fibroblasts, to the tumour mass. Through its effect on these non-neoplastic stromal cells, PDGF signalling may directly and indirectly promote tumour growth, blood perfusion, metastatic dissemination, and drug resistance [164]. For example, in mouse fibrosarcoma, paracrine PDGF/PDGFR-β signalling enhances pericyte recruitment to the tumour vasculature, thereby promoting tumour cell growth, survival, and vessel stabilization [165]. PDGFR-β signalling could regulate interstitial fluid pressure (IFP) in normal tissue, and inhibition of PDGFR could reduce tumour IFP and enhance the uptake into tumours [166, 167]. Therefore, the PDGF signalling may be implicated causally in at least three cancer cell traits: self-sufficient growth, angiogenesis and metastasis, as well as in resistance to cytotoxic therapy [152].

Given the important role of PDGF signalling in tumours, several strategies have been tested for targeting this signalling pathway. Strategies include blocking PDGF and inhibiting PDGFR function. Neutralizing antibodies, recombinant dimeric soluble PDGF extracellular domain and nucleic acids (aptamers) have been employed to target PDGF. PDGFR function could be blocked by antibodies, dominant-negative ligands, and kinase inhibitors. Imatinib (ST1571, Gleevec®) is an oral tyrosine kinase inhibitor that inhibits PDGFR-α and PDGFR-β, as well as BCR-ABL fusion protein, c-Kit, and Flt3. Imatininb has been approved by the Food and Drug Administration for the treatment of patients with Philadelphia chromosome positive chronic myelogenous leukaemia and gastrointestinal stromal tumours. Most of the available PDGFR kinase inhibitors available are not completely specific and act on other tyrosine kinase such as c-Kit and Flt3; thus, it is difficult to determine how much of the response to these agents is actually due to the PDGF blockade [168].

Conclusion

While the general mechanisms of activation of growth-factor-dependent signalling are highly similar across multiple pathways, they serve distinct regulatory roles. The selectivity of growth factor function is largely driven by tissue specific expression of regulatory proteins. Deregulation of regulatory elements result in the development of tissue-specific diseases including tumours. The understanding of these pathways is essential for the development of growth factor targeted therapies. The successful development of many such therapies over the past two decades have already contributed to the control of many cancer types. However, major challenges to theses therapies such as tumour heterogeneity, the inevitable development of drug resistance, and the difficulties in achieving therapeutic selectivity are likely to be the focus of future research directions in this field.

Further reading

Blobe GC, Schiemann WP, Lodish HF. Role of transforming growth factor beta in human disease. New England Journal of Medicine 2000; 342(18): 1350–1358.

Bottaro DP, Rubin JS, Faletto DL, Chan AM, Kmiecik TE, et al. Identification of the hepatocyte growth factor receptor as the c-met proto-oncogene product. Science 1991; 251(4995): 802–804.

Chan JM, Stampfer MJ, Giovannucci E, Gann PH, Ma J, et al. Plasma insulin-like growth factor-I and prostate cancer risk: a prospective study. Science 1998; 279(5350): 563–566.

Cohen S. Epidermal Growth Factor. In Nobel Lectures, Singapore: World Scientific Publishing Co., 1993.

Gospodarowicz D. Localisation of a fibroblast growth factor and its effect alone and with hydrocortisone on 3T3 cell growth. Nature 1974; 249(453): 123–127.

Greenman C, Stephens P, Smith R, Dalgliesh GL, Hunter C, et al. Patterns of somatic mutation in human cancer genomes. Nature 2007; 446(7132): 153–158.

Heinrich C, Behrmann I, Müller-Newen G, Schaper F, Graeve L. Interleukin-6-type cytokine signalling through the gp130/Jak/STAT pathway. Biochemical Journal 1998; 334(Pt 2): 297–314.

Heldin CH. Structural and functional studies on platelet-derived growth factor. EMBO Journa, 1992; 11(12): 4251–4259.

Massague J, Blain SW, Lo RS, TGFbeta signaling in growth control, cancer, and heritable disorders. Cell 2000; 103(2): 295–309.

Rong S, Bodescot M, Blair D, Dunn J, Nakamura T, et al. Tumorigenicity of the met proto-oncogene and the gene for hepatocyte growth factor. Molecular and Cell Biology 1992; 12(11): 5152–5158.

Ross, R, Glomset J, Kariya B, Harker L. A platelet-dependent serum factor that stimulates the proliferation of arterial smooth muscle cells in vitro. Proceedings of the National Academy of Sciences USA 1974; 71(4): 1207–1210.

Ullrich A, Bell JR, Chen EY, Herrera R, Petruzzelli LM, et al. Human insulin receptor and its relationship to the tyrosine kinase family of oncogenes. Nature 1985; 313(6005): 756–761.

References

1. Nakamura T, Teramoto H, Ichihara A Purification and characterization of a growth factor from rat platelets for mature parenchymal hepatocytes in primary cultures. Proceedings of the National Academy of Sciences USA 1986; 83(17): 6489–6493.

2. Bottaro DP, Rubin JS, Faletto DL, Chan AM, Kmiecik TE et al. Identification of the hepatocyte growth factor receptor as the c-met proto-oncogene product. Science 1991; 251(4995): 802–804.

3. Gak E, Taylor WG, Chan AM, Rubin JS. Processing of hepatocyte growth factor to the heterodimeric form is required for biological activity. FEBS Letters 1992; 311(1): 17–21.

4. Parr C, Sanders AJ, Jiang WG, Hepatocyte growth factor activation inhibitors—therapeutic potential in cancer. Anti-Cancer Agents in Medicinal Chemistry 2010; 10(1): 47–57.

5. Miyazawa K, Shimomura T, Kitamura A, Kondo J, Morimoto Y, Kitamura N. Molecular cloning and sequence analysis of the cDNA for a human serine protease reponsible for activation of hepatocyte growth factor. Structural similarity of the protease precursor to blood coagulation factor XII. Journal of Biological Chemistry 1993; 268(14): 10024–10028.

6. Kataoka H, Miyata S, Uchinokura S, Itoh H. Roles of hepatocyte growth factor (HGF) activator and HGF activator inhibitor in the pericellular activation of HGF/scatter factor. Cancer Metastasis Review 2003; 22(2–3): 223–236.

7. Shimomura T, Denda K, Kitamura A, Kawaguchi T, Kito M, et al. Hepatocyte growth factor activator inhibitor, a novel Kunitz-type serine protease inhibitor. Journal of Biological Chemistry 1997; 272(10): 6370–6376.

8. Kawaguchi T, Qin L, Shimomura T, Kondo J, Matsumoto K et al. Purification and cloning of hepatocyte growth factor activator inhibitor type 2, a Kunitz-type serine protease inhibitor. Journal of Biological Chemistry 1997; 272(44): 27558–27564.

9. Joffre C, Barrow R, Ménard L, Calleja V, Hart IR, et al. A direct role for Met endocytosis in tumorigenesis. Natural Cell Biology 2011; 13(7): 827–837.

10. Gherardi E, Birchmeier W, Birchmeier C, Vande Woude G. Targeting MET in cancer: rationale and progress. Nature Reviews Cancer 2012; 12(2): 89–103.

11. Huelsken J, Vogel R, Erdmann B, Cotsarelis G, Birchmeier W. beta-Catenin controls hair follicle morphogenesis and stem cell differentiation in the skin. Cell 2001; 105(4): 533–545.

12. Chmielowiec J, Borowiak M, Morkel M, Stradal T, Munz B et al. c-Met is essential for wound healing in the skin. Journal of Cell Biology 2007; 177(1): 151–62.

13. Michalopoulos GK, DeFrances MC. Liver regeneration. Science 1997; 276(5309): 60–66.

14. Huh CG, Factor VM, Sánchez A, Uchida K, Conner EA et al. Hepatocyte growth factor/c-met signaling pathway is required for efficient liver regeneration and repair. Proceedings of the National Academy of Sciences USA 2004; 101(13): 4477–4482.

15. Bladt F, Riethmacher D, Isenmann S, Aguzzi A, Birchmeier C Essential role for the c-met receptor in the migration of myogenic precursor cells into the limb bud. Nature 1995; 376(6543): 768–771.

16. Rong S, Bodescot M, Blair D, Dunn J, Nakamura T et al. Tumorigenicity of the met proto-oncogene and the gene for hepatocyte growth factor. Molecular and Cell Biology 1992; 12(11): 5152–8.

17. Graveel C, Su Y, Koeman J, Wang LM, Tessarollo L, et al. Activating Met mutations produce unique tumor profiles in mice with selective duplication of the mutant allele. Proceedings of the National Academy of Sciences USA 2004; 101(49): 17198–17203.

18. Ponzo MG, Lesurf R, Petkiewicz S, O'Malley FP, Pinnaduwage D et al. Met induces mammary tumors with diverse histologies and is associated with poor outcome and human basal breast cancer. Proceedings of the National Academy of Sciences USA 2009; 106(31): 12903–12908.

19. Peters S, Adjei AA. MET: a promising anticancer therapeutic target. Nature Reviews Clinical Oncology 2012; 9(6): 314–326.

20. Abounader R, Laterra J Scatter factor/hepatocyte growth factor in brain tumor growth and angiogenesis. Neuro-Oncology 2005; 7(4): 436–451.

21. Bussolino F, Di Renzo MF, Ziche M, Bocchietto E, Olivero M et al. Hepatocyte growth factor is a potent angiogenic factor which stimulates endothelial cell motility and growth. Journal of Cell Biology 1992; 119(3): 629–41.

22. Grant DS, Kleinman HK, Goldberg ID, Bhargava MM, Nickoloff BJ et al. Scatter factor induces blood vessel formation in vivo. Proceedings of the National Academy of Sciences USA 1993; 90(5): 1937–41.

23. Zhang YW, Su Y, Volpert OV, Vande Woude GF. Hepatocyte growth factor/scatter factor mediates angiogenesis through positive VEGF and negative thrombospondin 1 regulation. Proceedings of the National Academy of Sciences USA 2003; 100(22): 12718–12723.

24. Webb CP, Taylor GA, Jeffers M, Fiscella M, Oskarsson M et al. Evidence for a role of Met-HGF/SF during Ras-mediated tumorigenesis/metastasis. Oncogene 1998; 17(16): 2019–2025.

25. Ridley AJ, Comoglio PM, Hall A Regulation of scatter factor/hepatocyte growth factor responses by Ras, Rac, and Rho in MDCK cells. Molecular and Cell Biology 1995; 15(2): 1110–1122.

26. De Meyts P Insulin and its receptor: structure, function and evolution. Bioessays 2004; 26(12): 1351–1362.

27. Pollak MN, Schernhammer ES, Hankinson SE. Insulin-like growth factors and neoplasia. Nature Reviews Cancer 2004; 4(7): 505–518.

28. Pollak M. Insulin and insulin-like growth factor signalling in neoplasia. Nature Reviews Cancer 2008; 8(12): 915–928.

29. Pollak M The insulin and insulin-like growth factor receptor family in neoplasia: an update. Nature Reviews Cancer 2012; 12(3): 159–169.

30. Sachdev D, Yee D Disrupting insulin-like growth factor signaling as a potential cancer therapy. Molecular Cancer Therapeutics 2007; 6(1): 1–12.

31. Kato H, Faria TN, Stannard B, Roberts CT Jr, LeRoith D. Essential role of tyrosine residues 1131 1135, and 1136 of the insulin-like growth factor-I (IGF-I) receptor in IGF-I action. Molecular Endocrinology 1994; 8(1): 40–50.

32. LeRoith D Insulin-like growth factor I receptor signaling: overlapping or redundant pathways? Endocrinology 2000; 141(4): 1287–1288.

33. Firth SM, Baxter RC. Cellular actions of the insulin-like growth factor binding proteins. Endocrine Reviews 2002; 23(6): 824–854.

34. Buckbinder L, Talbott R, Velasco-Miguel S, Takenaka I, Faha B et al. Induction of the growth inhibitor IGF-binding protein 3 by p53. Nature 1995; 377(6550): 646–649.

35. Kaneda A, Wang CJ, Cheong R, Timp W, Onyango P et al. Enhanced sensitivity to IGF-II signaling links loss of imprinting of IGF2 to increased cell proliferation and tumor risk. Proceedings of the National Academy of Sciences USA 2007; 104(52): 20926–20931.

36. De Souza AT, Hankins GR, Washington MK, Orton TC, Jirtle RL et al. M6P/IGF2R gene is mutated in human hepatocellular carcinomas with loss of heterozygosity. Nature Genetics 1995; 11(4): 447–449.

37. Church DN, Phillips BR, Stuckey DJ, Barnes DJ, Buffa FM et al. Igf2 ligand dependency of Pten(+/−) developmental and tumour phenotypes in the mouse. Oncogene 2012; 31(31): 3635–3646.

38. Haley VL, Barnes DJ, Sandovici I, Constancia M, Graham CF et al. Igf2 pathway dependency of the Trp53 developmental and tumour phenotypes. EMBO Molecular Medicine 2012; 4(8): 705–718.

39. Ullrich A, Bell JR, Chen EY, Herrera L, Petruzzelli LM, et al. Human insulin receptor and its relationship to the tyrosine kinase family of oncogenes. Nature 1985; 313(6005): 756–761.

40. Chan JM, Stampfer MJ, Giovannucci E, Gann PH, Ma J et al. Plasma insulin-like growth factor-I and prostate cancer risk: a prospective study. Science 1998; 279(5350): 563–566.

41. Guo Y, Xu F, Lu T, Duan Z, Zhang Z. Interleukin-6 signaling pathway in targeted therapy for cancer. Cancer Treatment Reviews 2012; 38(7): 904–910.

42. Heinrich PC, Behrmann I, Müller-Newen G, Schaper F, Graeve L. Interleukin-6-type cytokine signalling through the gp130/Jak/STAT pathway. Biochemical Journal 1998; 334(Pt 2): 297–314.

43. Lutticken C, Wegenka UM, Yuan J, Buschmann J, Schindler C, et al. Association of transcription factor APRF and protein kinase Jak1 with the interleukin-6 signal transducer gp130. Science 1994; 263(5143): 89–92.

44. Stahl N, Boulton TG, Farruggella T, Ip NY, Davis S, et al. Association and activation of Jak-Tyk kinases by CNTF-LIF-OSM-IL-6 beta receptor components. Science 1994; 263(5143): 92–95.

45. Imada K, Leonard WJ. The Jak-STAT pathway. Molecular Immunology 2000; 37(1–2): 1–11.

46. Bromberg J. Stat proteins and oncogenesis. Journal of Clinical Investigation 2002; 109(9): 1139–1142.

47. Weidle UH, Klostermann S, Eggle D, Krüger A. Interleukin 6/interleukin 6 receptor interaction and its role as a therapeutic target for treatment of cachexia and cancer. Cancer Genomics Proteomics 2010; 7(6): 287–302.

48. Dijkgraaf EM, Welters MJ, Nortier JW, van der Burg SH, Kroep JR et al. Interleukin-6/interleukin-6 receptor pathway as a new therapy target in epithelial ovarian cancer. Current Pharmaceutical Design 2012; 18(25): 3816–27.

49. Duan Z, Foster R, Bell DA, Mahoney J, Wolak K et al. Signal transducers and activators of transcription 3 pathway activation in drug-resistant ovarian cancer. Clinical Cancer Research 2006; 12(17): 5055–5063.

50. Wang Y, Niu XL, Qu Y, Wu J, Zhu YQ et al. Autocrine production of interleukin-6 confers cisplatin and paclitaxel resistance in ovarian cancer cells. Cancer Letters 2010; 295(1): 110–123.

51. Lauta VM. Interleukin-6 and the network of several cytokines in multiple myeloma: an overview of clinical and experimental data. Cytokine 2001; 16(3): 79–86.

52. LaFave LM, Levine RL. JAK2 the future: therapeutic strategies for JAK-dependent malignancies. Trends in Pharmacological Sciences 2012; 33(11): 574–582.

53. Trikha M, Corringham R, Klein B, Rossi JF. Targeted anti-interleukin-6 monoclonal antibody therapy for cancer: a review of the rationale and clinical evidence. Clinical Cancer Research 2003; 9(13): 4653–4665.

54. Kupferman ME, Jayakumar A, Zhou G, Xie T, Dakak-Yazici Y et al. Therapeutic suppression of constitutive and inducible JAK/STAT activation in head and neck squamous cell carcinoma. Journal of Experimental Therapeutics and Oncology 2009; 8(2): 117–127.

55. Xu J, Cole DC, Chang CP, Ayyad R, Asselin M et al. Inhibition of the signal transducer and activator of transcription-3 (STAT3) signaling pathway by 4-oxo-1-phenyl-1,4-dihydroquinoline-3-carboxylic acid esters. Journal of Medicinal Chemistry 2008; 51(14): 4115–4121.

56. Verstovsek S, Mesa RA, Gotlib J, Levy RS, Gupta V et al. A double-blind, placebo-controlled trial of ruxolitinib for myelofibrosis. New England Journal of Medicine 2012; 366(9): 799–807.

57. Olayioye MA, Neve RM, Lane HA, Hynes NE. The ErbB signaling network: receptor heterodimerization in development and cancer. EMBO Journal 2000; 19(13): 3159–3167.

58. Citri A, Yarden Y EGF-ERBB signalling: towards the systems level. Nature Reviews Molecular and Cell Biology 2006; 7(7): 505–516.

59. Cohen S Epidermal growth factor. In Nobel Lectures. Singapore: World Scientific Publishing, 1993.

60. Olayioye MA, Graus-Porta D, Beerli RR, Rohrer J, Gay B, Hynes NE. ErbB-1 and ErbB-2 acquire distinct signaling properties dependent upon their dimerization partner. Molecular and Cell Biology 1998; 18(9): 5042–5051.

61. Schulze WX, Deng L, Mann M. Phosphotyrosine interactome of the ErbB-receptor kinase family. Molecular Systems Biology 2005; 1: 2005 0008.

62. Sibilia M, Steinbach JP, Stingl L, Aguzzi A, Wagner EF. A strain-independent postnatal neurodegeneration in mice lacking the EGF receptor. EMBO Journal 1998; 17(3): 719–731.

63. Klapper LN, Glathe S, Vaisman N, Hynes NE, Andrews GC et al. The ErbB-2/HER2 oncoprotein of human carcinomas may function solely as a shared coreceptor for multiple stroma-derived growth factors. Proceedings of the National Academy of Sciences USA 1999; 96(9): 4995–5000.

64. Guy PM, Platko JV, Cantley LC, Cerione RA, Carraway KL 3rd. Insect cell-expressed p180erbB3 possesses an impaired tyrosine kinase activity. Proceedings of the National Academy of Sciences USA 1994; 91(17): 8132–8136.

65. Schulze A, Lehmann K, Jefferies HB, McMahon M, Downward J. Analysis of the transcriptional program induced by Raf in epithelial cells. Genes & Development 2001; 15(8): 981–994.

66. Nicholson SE, Metcalf D, Sprigg NS, Columbus R, Walker F et al. Suppressor of cytokine signaling (SOCS)-5 is a potential negative regulator of epidermal growth factor signaling. Proceedings of the National Academy of Sciences USA 2005; 102(7): 2328–33.

67. Laederich MB, Funes-Duran M, Yen L, Ingalla E, Wu X, Carraway KL 3rd et al. The leucine-rich repeat protein LRIG1 is a negative regulator of ErbB family receptor tyrosine kinases. Journal of Biological Chemistry 2004; 279(45): 47050–47056.

68. Lynch TJ, Bell DW, Sordella R, Gurubhagavatula S, Okimoto RA et al. Activating mutations in the epidermal growth factor receptor underlying responsiveness of non-small-cell lung cancer to gefitinib. New England Journal of Medicine 2004; 350(21): 2129–2139.

69. Stutz MA, Shattuck DL, Laederich MB, Carraway KL 3rd, Sweeney C et al. LRIG1 negatively regulates the oncogenic EGF receptor mutant EGFRvIII. Oncogene 2008; 27(43): 5741–52.

70. Moscatello DK, Holgado-Madruga M, Godwin AK, Ramirez G, Gunn G et al. Frequent expression of a mutant epidermal growth factor receptor in multiple human tumors. Cancer Research 1995; 55(23): 5536–9.

71. Nicholson RI, Gee JM, Harper ME. EGFR and cancer prognosis. European Journal of Cancer 2001; 37(Suppl. 4): S9–S15.

72. Ford AC, Grandis JR. Targeting epidermal growth factor receptor in head and neck cancer. Head & Neck 2003; 25(1): 67–73.

73. Ross JS, Fletcher JA, Linette GP, Stec J, Clark E et al. The Her-2/neu gene and protein in breast cancer 2003: biomarker and target of therapy. Oncologist 2003; 8(4): 307–25.

74. Slamon DJ, Godolphin W, Jones LA, Holt JA, Wong SG et al. Studies of the HER-2/neu proto-oncogene in human breast and ovarian cancer. Science 1989; 244(4905): 707–712.

75. Spiridon CI, Ghetie MA, Uhr J, Marches R, Li JL, Shen GL et al. Targeting multiple Her-2 epitopes with monoclonal antibodies results in improved antigrowth activity of a human breast cancer cell line in vitro and in vivo. Clinical Cancer Research 2002; 8(6): 1720–1730.

76. Cetuximab: new drug. Metastatic colorectal cancer: an inappropriate evaluation. Prescrire International 2005; 14(80): 215–217.

77. Gajria D, Gonzalez J, Feigin K, Patil S, Chen C, Theodoulou M et al. Phase II trial of a novel capecitabine dosing schedule in combination with lapatinib for the treatment of patients with HER2-positive metastatic breast cancer. Breast Cancer Research Treat 2012; 131(1): 111–116.

78. Gospodarowicz D. Localisation of a fibroblast growth factor and its effect alone and with hydrocortisone on 3T3 cell growth. Nature 1974; 249(453): 123–127.

79. Turner N, Grose R. Fibroblast growth factor signalling: from development to cancer. Nature Reviews Cancer 2010; 10(2): 116–129.

80. Eswarakumar VP, Lax I, Schlessinger J. Cellular signaling by fibroblast growth factor receptors. Cytokine Growth Factor Review 2005; 16(2): 139–149.

81. Altomare DA, Testa JR. Perturbations of the AKT signaling pathway in human cancer. Oncogene 2005; 24(50): 7455–7464.

82. Gotoh N. Regulation of growth factor signaling by FRS2 family docking/scaffold adaptor proteins. Cancer Science 2008; 99(7): 1319–1325.

83. Peters KG, Marie J, Wilson E, Ives HE, Escobedo J et al. Point mutation of an FGF receptor abolishes phosphatidylinositol turnover and Ca2+ flux but not mitogenesis. Nature 1992; 358(6388): 678–681.

84. Hart KC, Robertson SC, Kanemitsu MY, Meyer AN, Tynan JA et al. Transformation and Stat activation by derivatives of FGFR1, FGFR3, and FGFR4. Oncogene 2000; 19(29): 3309–3320.

85. Kang S, Elf S, Dong S, Hitosugi T, Lythgoe K et al. Fibroblast growth factor receptor 3 associates with and tyrosine phosphorylates p90 RSK2, leading to RSK2 activation that mediates hematopoietic transformation. Molecular and Cell Biology 2009; 29(8): 2105–2117.

86. Thien CB, Langdon WY. Cbl: many adaptations to regulate protein tyrosine kinases. Nature Reviews Molecular and Cell Biology 2001; 2(4): 294–307.

87. Zhao Y, Zhang ZY. The mechanism of dephosphorylation of extracellular signal-regulated kinase 2 by mitogen-activated protein kinase phosphatase 3. Journal of Biological Chemistry 2001; 276(34): 32382–32391.

88. Casci T, Vinos J, Freeman M. Sprouty, an intracellular inhibitor of Ras signaling. Cell 1999; 96(5): 655–665.

89. Hacohen N, Kramer S, Sutherland D, Hiromi Y, Krasnow MA. Sprouty encodes a novel antagonist of FGF signaling that patterns apical branching of the Drosophila airways. Cell 1998; 92(2): 253–263.

90. Tsang M, Friesel R, Kudoh T, Dawid IB. Identification of Sef, a novel modulator of FGF signalling. Natural Cell Biology 2002; 4(2): 165–169.

91. Tsang M, Dawid IB. Promotion and attenuation of FGF signaling through the Ras-MAPK pathway. Science's STKE 2004; 2004(228): pe17.

92. Greenman C, Stephens P, Smith R, Dalgliesh GL, Hunter C et al. Patterns of somatic mutation in human cancer genomes. Nature 2007; 446(7132): 153–158.

93. Cappellen D, De Oliveira C, Ricol D, de Medina S, Bourdin J et al. Frequent activating mutations of FGFR3 in human bladder and cervix carcinomas. Nature Genetics 1999; 23(1): 18–20.

94. Rosty C, Aubriot M-E., Cappellen D, Bourdin J, Cartier I et al. Clinical and biological characteristics of cervical neoplasias with FGFR3 mutation. Molecular Cancer 2005; 4(1): 15.

95. Hernández S, de Muga S, Agell L, Juanpere N, Esgueva R et al. FGFR3 mutations in prostate cancer: association with low-grade tumors. 8Modern Pathology 2009; 22(6): 848–56.

96. Onwuazor ON, Wen XY, Wang DY, Zhuang L, Masih-Khan E et al. Mutation, SNP, and isoform analysis of fibroblast growth factor receptor 3 (FGFR3) in 150 newly diagnosed multiple myeloma patients. Blood 2003; 102(2): 772–773.

97. Dutt A, Salvesen HB, Chen TH, Ramos AH, Onofrio RC et al. Drug-sensitive FGFR2 mutations in endometrial carcinoma. Proceedings of the National Academy of Sciences USA 2008; 105(25): 8713–8717.

98. Kunii K, Davis L, Gorenstein J, Hatch H, Yashiro M et al. FGFR2-amplified gastric cancer cell lines require FGFR2 and Erbb3 signaling for growth and survival. Cancer Research 2008; 68(7): 2340–2348.

99. Courjal F, Cuny M, Simony-Lafontaine J, Louason G, Speiser P et al. Mapping of DNA amplifications at 15 chromosomal localizations in 1875 breast tumors: definition of phenotypic groups. Cancer Research 1997; 57(19): 4360–4367.

100. Avet-Loiseau H, Li JY, Facon T, Brigaudeau C, Morineau N et al. High incidence of translocations t(11;14)(q13;q32) and t(4;14)(p16;q32) in patients with plasma cell malignancies. Cancer Research 1998; 58(24): 5640–5645.

101. Chesi M, Nardini E, Brents LA, Schröck E, Ried T et al. Frequent translocation t(4;14)(p16.3;q32.3) in multiple myeloma is associated with increased expression and activating mutations of fibroblast growth factor receptor 3. Nature Genetics 1997; 16(3): 260–264.

102. Wang Y, Becker D. Antisense targeting of basic fibroblast growth factor and fibroblast growth factor receptor-1 in human melanomas blocks intratumoral angiogenesis and tumor growth. Nature Medicine 1997; 3(8): 887–893.

103. Birrer MJ, Johnson ME, Hao K, Wong KK, Park DC et al. Whole genome oligonucleotide-based array comparative genomic hybridization analysis identified fibroblast growth factor 1 as a prognostic marker for advanced-stage serous ovarian adenocarcinomas. Journal of Clinical Oncology 2007; 25(16): 2281–2287.

104. Maeda T, Yagasaki F, Ishikawa M, Takahashi N, Bessho M. Transforming property of TEL-FGFR3 mediated through PI3-K in a T-cell lymphoma that subsequently progressed to AML. Blood 2005; 105(5): 2115–2123.

105. Memarzadeh S, Xin L, Mulholland DJ, Mansukhani A, Wu H et al. Enhanced paracrine FGF10 expression promotes formation of multifocal prostate adenocarcinoma and an increase in epithelial androgen receptor. Cancer Cell 2007; 12(6): 572–585.

106. Zhong C, Saribekyan G, Liao CP, Cohen MB, Roy-Burman P. Cooperation between FGF8b overexpression and PTEN deficiency in prostate tumorigenesis. Cancer Research 2006; 66(4): 2188–2194.

107. Pardo OE, Arcaro A, Salerno G, Raguz S, Downward J et al. Fibroblast growth factor-2 induces translational regulation of Bcl-XL and Bcl-2 via a MEK-dependent pathway: correlation with resistance to etoposide-induced apoptosis. Journal of Biological Chemistry 2002; 277(14): 12040–12046.

108. Pardo OE, Lesay A, Arcaro A, Lopes R, Ng BL et al. Fibroblast growth factor 2-mediated translational control of IAPs blocks mitochondrial release of Smac/DIABLO and apoptosis in small cell lung cancer cells. Molecular and Cell Biology 2003; 23(21): 7600–7610.

109. Pardo OE, Wellbrock C, Khanzada UK, Aubert M, Arozarena I et al. FGF-2 protects small cell lung cancer cells from apoptosis through a complex involving PKCepsilon, B-Raf and S6K2. EMBO Journal 2006; 25(13): 3078–3088.

110. Xian W, Schwertfeger KL, Vargo-Gogola T, Rosen JM. Pleiotropic effects of FGFR1 on cell proliferation, survival, and migration in a 3D mammary epithelial cell model. Journal of Cell Biology 2005; 171(4): 663–673.

111. Presta M, Dell'Era P, Mitola S, Moroni E, Ronca R et al. Fibroblast growth factor/fibroblast growth factor receptor system in angiogenesis. Cytokine Growth Factor Review 2005; 16(2): 159–178.

112. Kandel J, Bossy-Wetzel E, Radvanyi F, Klagsbrun M, Folkman J et al. Neovascularization is associated with a switch to the export of bFGF in the multistep development of fibrosarcoma. Cell 1991; 66(6): 1095–1104.

113. Yu K, Xu J, Liu Z, Sosic D, Shao J et al. Conditional inactivation of FGF receptor 2 reveals an essential role for FGF signaling in the regulation of osteoblast function and bone growth. Development 2003; 130(13): 3063–3074.

114. Colvin JS, Bohne BA, Harding GW, McEwen DG, Ornitz DM. Skeletal overgrowth and deafness in mice lacking fibroblast growth factor receptor 3. Nature Genetics 1996; 12(4): 390–397.

115. Ricol D, Cappellen D, El Marjou A, Gil-Diez-de-Medina S, Girault JM et al. Tumour suppressive properties of fibroblast growth factor receptor 2-IIIb in human bladder cancer. Oncogene 1999; 18(51): 7234–7243.

116. Hilberg F, Roth GJ, Krssak M, Kautschitsch S, Sommergruber W et al. BIBF 1120: triple angiokinase inhibitor with sustained receptor blockade and good antitumor efficacy. Cancer Research 2008; 68(12): 4774–4782.

117. Sarker D, Molife R, Evans TR, Hardie M, Marriott C et al. A phase I pharmacokinetic and pharmacodynamic study of TKI258, an oral, multitargeted receptor tyrosine kinase inhibitor in patients with advanced solid tumors. Clinical Cancer Research 2008; 14(7): 2075–2081.

118. Machida S, Saga Y, Takei Y, Mizuno I, Takayama T et al. Inhibition of peritoneal dissemination of ovarian cancer by tyrosine kinase receptor inhibitor SU6668 (TSU-68). International Journal of Cancer 2005; 114(2): 224–229.

119. Qing J, Du X, Chen Y, Chan P, Li H et al. Antibody-based targeting of FGFR3 in bladder carcinoma and t(4;14)-positive multiple myeloma in mice. Journal of Clinical Investigation 2009; 119(5): 1216–1229.

120. Spielberger R, Stiff P, Bensinger W, Gentile T, Weisdorf D et al. Palifermin for oral mucositis after intensive therapy for hematologic cancers. New England Journal of Medicine 2004; 351(25): 2590–2598.

121. Blobe GC, Schiemann W, Lodish HF. Role of transforming growth factor beta in human disease. New England Journal of Medicine 2000; 342(18): 1350–1358.

122. Massague J, Blain SW, Lo RS. TGFbeta signaling in growth control, cancer, and heritable disorders. Cell 2000; 103(2): 295–309.

123. Schmierer B, Hill CS. TGFbeta-SMAD signal transduction: molecular specificity and functional flexibility. Nature Reviews Molecular and Cell Biology 2007; 8(12): 970–982.

124. Shi Y, Massague J. Mechanisms of TGF-beta signaling from cell membrane to the nucleus. Cell 2003; 113(6): 685–700.

125. Ozdamar B, Bose R, Barrios-Rodiles M, Wang HR, Zhang Y et al. Regulation of the polarity protein Par6 by TGFbeta receptors controls epithelial cell plasticity. Science 2005; 307(5715): 1603–1609.

126. Itoh S, ten Dijke P. Negative regulation of TGF-beta receptor/Smad signal transduction. Current Opinion in Cell Biology 2007; 19(2): 176–184.

127. Hayashi H, Abdollah S, Qiu Y, Cai J, Xu YY et al. The MAD-related protein Smad7 associates with the TGFbeta receptor and functions as an antagonist of TGFbeta signaling. Cell 1997; 89(7): 1165–1173.

128. Inoue Y, Imamura T. Regulation of TGF-beta family signaling by E3 ubiquitin ligases. Cancer Science 2008; 99(11): 2107–2112.

129. Kavsak P, Rasmussen RK, Causing CG, Bonni S, Zhu H et al. Smad7 binds to Smurf2 to form an E3 ubiquitin ligase that targets the TGF beta receptor for degradation. Molecular Cell 2000; 6(6): 1365–1375.

130. Ebisawa T, Fukuchi M, Murakami G, Chiba T, Tanaka K et al. Smurf1 interacts with transforming growth factor-beta type I receptor through Smad7 and induces receptor degradation. Journal of Biological Chemistry 2001; 276(16): 12477–12480.

131. Hata A, Lagna G, Massagué J, Hemmati-Brivanlou A. Smad6 inhibits BMP/Smad1 signaling by specifically competing with the Smad4 tumor suppressor. Genes & Development 1998; 12(2): 186–197.

132. Javelaud D, Mauviel A. Crosstalk mechanisms between the mitogen-activated protein kinase pathways and Smad signaling downstream of TGF-beta: implications for carcinogenesis. Oncogene 2005; 24(37): 5742–5750.

133. Kretzschmar M, Doody J, Timokhina I, Massagué J. A mechanism of repression of TGFbeta/ Smad signaling by oncogenic Ras. Genes & Development 1999; 13(7): 804–816.

134. Brown JD, DiChiara MR, Anderson KR, Gimbrone MA Jr, Topper JN. MEKK-1, a component of the stress (stress-activated protein kinase/c-Jun N-terminal kinase) pathway, can selectively activate Smad2-mediated transcriptional activation in endothelial cells. Journal of Biological Chemistry 1999; 274(13): 8797–8805.

135. Engel ME, McDonnell MA, Law BK, Moses HL. Interdependent SMAD and JNK signaling in transforming growth factor-beta-mediated transcription. Journal of Biological Chemistry 1999; 274(52): 37413–37420.

136. Hayes SA, Huang X, Kambhampati S, Platanias LC, Bergan RC. p38 MAP kinase modulates Smad-dependent changes in human prostate cell adhesion. Oncogene 2003; 22(31): 4841–4850.

137. Leivonen SK, Ala-Aho R, Koli K, Grénman R, Peltonen J et al. Activation of Smad signaling enhances collagenase-3 (MMP-13) expression and invasion of head and neck squamous carcinoma cells. Oncogene 2006; 25(18): 2588–2600.

138. Akhurst RJ, Derynck R. TGF-beta signaling in cancer: a double-edged sword. Trends in Cellular Biology 2001; 11(11): S44–51.

139. Connolly EC, Akhurst RJ. The complexities of TGF-beta action during mammary and squamous cell carcinogenesis. Current Pharmaceutical Biotechnology 2011; 12(12): 2138–49.

140. Siegel PM, Massague J. Cytostatic and apoptotic actions of TGF-beta in homeostasis and cancer. Nature Reviews Cancer 2003; 3(11): 807–821.

141. Derynck R, Akhurst RJ, Balmain A. TGF-beta signaling in tumor suppression and cancer progression. Nature Genetics 2001; 29(2): 117–129.

142. Yin JJ, Selander K, Chirgwin JM, Dallas M, Grubbs BG et al. TGF-beta signaling blockade inhibits PTHrP secretion by breast cancer cells and bone metastases development. Journal of Clinical Investigation 1999; 103(2): 197–206.

143. Yingling JM, Blanchard KL, Sawyer JS. Development of TGF-beta signalling inhibitors for cancer therapy. Nature Reviews Drug Discovery 2004; 3(12): 1011–1022.

144. Akhurst RJ. Large- and small-molecule inhibitors of transforming growth factor-beta signaling. Current Opinion in Investigational Drugs 2006; 7(6): 513–521.

145. Jaschinski F, Rothhammer T, Jachimczak P, Seitz C, Schneider A et al. The antisense oligonucleotide trabedersen (AP 12009) for the targeted inhibition of TGF-beta2. Current Pharmaceutical Biotechnology 2011; 12(12): 2203–2213.

146. Leivonen SK, Kahari VM. Transforming growth factor-beta signaling in cancer invasion and metastasis. International Journal of Cancer 2007; 121(10): 2119–2124.

147. Halder SK, Beauchamp RD, Datta PK. A specific inhibitor of TGF-beta receptor kinase, SB-431542, as a potent antitumor agent for human cancers. Neoplasia 2005; 7(5): 509–521.

148. Kim YJ, Hwang JS, Hong YB, Bae I, Seong YS. Transforming growth factor beta receptor I inhibitor sensitizes drug-resistant pancreatic cancer cells to gemcitabine. AntiCancer Research 2012; 32(3): 799–806.

149. Ross R, Glomset J, Kariya B, Harker L. A platelet-dependent serum factor that stimulates the proliferation of arterial smooth muscle cells in vitro. Proceedings of the National Academy of Sciences USA 1974; 71(4): 1207–1210.

150. Heldin CH. Structural and functional studies on platelet-derived growth factor. EMBO Journal 1992; 11(12): 4251–4259.

151. Heldin CH, Westermark B. Mechanism of action and in vivo role of platelet-derived growth factor. Physiological Reviews 1999; 79(4): 1283–1316.

152. Andrae J, Gallini R, Betsholtz C. Role of platelet-derived growth factors in physiology and medicine. Genes & Development 2008; 22(10): 1276–1312.

153. McDonald NQ, Hendrickson WA. A structural superfamily of growth factors containing a cystine knot motif. Cell 1993; 73(3): 421–424.

154. Tallquist M, Kazlauskas A. PDGF signaling in cells and mice. Cytokine Growth Factor Review 2004; 15(4): 205–213.

155. Seger R, Krebs EG. The MAPK signaling cascade. FASEB Journal 1995; 9(9): 726–735.

156. Liu P, Cheng H, Roberts TM, Zhao JJ. Targeting the phosphoinositide 3-kinase pathway in cancer. Nature Reviews Drug Discovery 2009; 8(8): 627–644.

157. Erpel T, Courtneidge SA. Src family protein tyrosine kinases and cellular signal transduction pathways. Current Opinion in Cell Biology 1995; 7(2): 176–182.

158. Lechleider RJ, Sugimoto S, Bennett AM, Kashishian AS, Cooper JA et al. Activation of the SH2-containing phosphotyrosine phosphatase SH-PTP2 by its binding site, phosphotyrosine 1009, on the human platelet-derived growth factor receptor. Journal of Biological Chemistry 1993; 268(29): 21478–21481.

159. Fantl WJ, Escobedo JA, Martin GA, Turck CW, del Rosario M et al. Distinct phosphotyrosines on a growth factor receptor bind to specific molecules that mediate different signaling pathways. Cell 1992; 69(3): 413–423.

160. Heldin CH, Wasteson A, Westermark B. Interaction of platelet-derived growth factor with its fibroblast receptor. Demonstration of ligand degradation and receptor modulation. Journal of Biological Chemistry 1982; 257(8): 4216–4221.

161. Lennartsson J, Wardega P, Engström U, Hellman U, Heldin CH et al. Alix facilitates the interaction between c-Cbl and platelet-derived growth factor beta-receptor and thereby modulates receptor down-regulation. Journal of Biological Chemistry 2006; 281(51): 39152–39158.

162. Karlsson S, Kowanetz K, Sandin A, Persson C, Ostman A et al. Loss of T-cell protein tyrosine phosphatase induces recycling of the platelet-derived growth factor (PDGF) beta-receptor but not the PDGF alpha-receptor. Molecular Biology of the Cell 2006; 17(11): 4846–4855.

163. Malhotra B, Schuetze SM. Dermatofibrosarcoma protruberans treatment with platelet-derived growth factor receptor inhibitor: a review of clinical trial results. Current Opinion in Oncology 2012; 24(4): 419–424.

164. Liu KW, Hu B, Cheng SY. Platelet-derived growth factor signaling in human malignancies. Chinese Journal of Cancer 2011; 30(9): 581–4.

165. Abramsson A, Lindblom P, Betsholtz C. Endothelial and nonendothelial sources of PDGF-B regulate pericyte recruitment and influence vascular pattern formation in tumors. Journal of Clinical Investigation 2003; 112(8): 1142–1151.

166. Pietras K, Stumm M, Hubert M, Buchdunger E, Rubin K et al. STI571 enhances the therapeutic index of epothilone B by a tumor-selective increase of drug uptake. Clinical Cancer Research 2003; 9(10 Pt 1): 3779–3787.

167. Heldin CH, Rubin K, Pietras K, Ostman A. High interstitial fluid pressure—an obstacle in cancer therapy. Nature Reviews Cancer 2004; 4(10): 806–813.

168. Homsi J, Daud AI. Spectrum of activity and mechanism of action of VEGF/PDGF inhibitors. Cancer Control 2007; 14(3): 285–294.

CHAPTER 3

Cell signalling pathways

Stefan Knapp

Introduction to cell signalling pathways

Cellular functions are regulated by highly complex signalling networks containing thousands of interconnected nodes that tightly control cellular growth, migration, metabolism, differentiation, and cell death. However, these regulatory networks are far too complex to serve as predictive model systems for our understanding of cell signalling processes, forcing us to adhere to easier directional pathways that describe the main signalling avenues that transmit environmental cues from the plasma membrane to the nucleus. In most cancer types several key regulators in signalling pathways are perturbed, and each of these perturbations provides the cancer cell with a small survival and growth advantage. The advent of large-scale sequencing revealed that there are on average 80 mutations that alter amino acid residues in signalling proteins in a typical cancer biopsy. These mutations are composed of few commonly mutated genes but the majority of mutations occur with low frequency resulting in a complex picture of the cancer genome landscape. Analysis of these mutations by statistical methods predicts that most of the detected mutations have probably little or no functional consequences. However, it has been estimated that nevertheless around 15 mutations contribute either to the initiation, progression, or maintenance of a tumour. In late-stage metastatic cancer, multiple distinct and spatially separated inactivating mutations of tumour-suppressor genes have been identified within a single tumour leading to a considerable degree of intra-tumour heterogeneity, further complicating molecular mechanisms that lead to deregulation of signalling in cancer and consequently the rational design of new therapeutic strategies that target signal transduction pathways.

However, all cancers need to acquire a set of capabilities that are tightly controlled in normal cells. These hallmark capabilities lead to alterations in signalling that sustain growth factor-independent proliferation, evade growth suppression, suppress apoptotic mechanism and detection of cancer cells by the immune system, overcome the limited replication potential of somatic cells, guarantee sufficient nutrition supply by generating new blood vessel formation and by changing the cellular energy supply. These lead finally to the spread of the tumour in the body by inducing cell migration and metastasis. Here I review the principal regulatory mechanisms that control the main signalling pathways, with a particular focus on pathways that have been successfully targeted in cancer therapy.

Receptor tyrosine kinases and growth factor signalling

Tissue homoeostasis is tightly controlled by extracellular signalling molecules such as growth factors that bind to cell surface receptors located in the plasma membrane. Receptors of extracellular growth factors (GFs) are often receptor tyrosine kinases (RTKs) or receptors that tightly associate with RTKs. GF receptors share a number of characteristic regulatory features that allow efficient transmission of extracellular mitotic signals through the plasma membrane and the activation of downstream signalling pathways that transmit signals to the nucleus where they trigger activation of transcriptional programmes. Dysfunction of growth factor signalling is a hallmark of cancer and involves usually GF independent activation of growth-promoting signalling events. Due to the large diversity of GF receptors the description here is limited to three main receptor systems that play a central role in cancer and that are also current targets of drug development efforts.

Insulin and insulin growth factor signalling

The Insulin and insulin-like growth factor 1 (IGF1) signalling pathway has a pivotal role in regulating cellular proliferation and survival. This pathway evolved very early in evolution to regulate growth, body size, and longevity as a response to nutrient supply. The more specific role in regulation of carbohydrate metabolism evolved much later and is a specialized function of insulin and the insulin receptor (IR). IGF1 is mainly expressed in liver where expression of this growth factor is stimulated by growth hormone (GH). The IGF2 isoform is more widely expressed and is not regulated by GH. Free plasma levels of IGF1 and IGF2 are regulated by IGF binding proteins (IGFBPs). It has been estimated that more than 90% of circulating IGF is bound to IGFBPs which inactivate IGFs by competing with receptor binding. However, IGFBs also stabilize IGFs by prolonging their plasma half-life and may have IGF independent growth-inhibitory and pro-apoptotic functions.

The IRs, IGF1, and IGF2 are tetrameric and are composed of so-called half-receptors consisting of an extracellular binding domain (α-chain) and a transmembrane and cytoplasmic RTK (β-chain). The IR is expressed as two splice isoforms. The isoform 'IRB' recognizes exclusively insulin, but the 'IRA' isoform, which is also overexpressed in tumours, recognizes both insulin and IGF2. Two diverse receptors also exist for IGF (IGF1R and IGF2R). IGF2R has no catalytic domain and functions as a sink for free IGF2 and has therefore tumour-suppressor properties. Depending on their relative abundance IGF1R and IR half-receptors may associate into hybrid receptors. The direct downstream targets of IGF1R and IR are the insulin receptor substrates (IRS proteins) that trigger activation of a number of pathways including phosphatidylinositol 3-kinase, AKT, mammalian target of rapamycin (mTOR), and mitogen-activated protein kinases (MAPKs), which will be

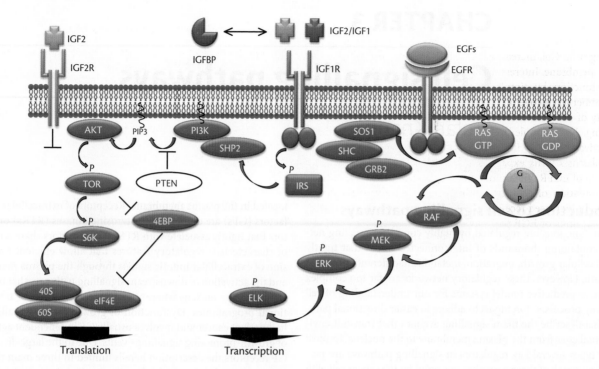

Fig. 3.1 Example of a receptor tyrosine kinase signalling pathway. Kinases are highlighted in blue, receptor tyrosine kinases and their substrates in green, phosphatases in white, GTPases in olive and adaptor and substrate proteins in red.

discussed later in this chapter. A graphical representation of the IGFR signalling pathway is shown in Figure 3.1.

Epidermal growth factor (EGF) signalling

Another group of growth factors comprise epidermal growth factor (EGF)-like proteins and neuregulins which activate members of the EGF receptor (EGFR) family of RTKs and consists of four members (EGFR/ErbB-1, HER2/ErbB2, HER3/ErbB3, and HER4/ErbB4). These RTKs have been originally named ERB because of their homology to the erythroblastoma viral gene product, *v-erbB*. More than 15 diverse ligands have been identified that contain a conserved EGF domain, creating a highly complex signalling network. However, knockout studies of specific EGFR ligands suggested a significant functional redundancy between EGF growth factors. For instance, knockout mice of EGF and the keratinocyte growth factor amphiregulin showed no significant phenotype. In contrast, deletion of the ErbB1 receptor revealed a non-redundant function of this receptor RTK which has a key role in epithelial cell development in many organs. Depending on the mouse strain used, ErbB1$^{-/-}$ mice die at mid-gestation or shortly after birth.

Similar to IR/IGFR receptors, receptor heterodimers, which may also involve receptors that have either a catalytically inactive kinase domain (HER3) or that lack the capacity binding growth factors (ErbB2), add additional layers of regulation to this complex signalling network. EGF receptors consist of a single polypeptide with an extracellular ligand binding domain as well as a cytoplasmic RTK domain which is activated by ligand induced dimerization. Interestingly, the dimerization of the cytoplasmic kinase domain is asymmetric in such a way that one kinase domain serves as an activator of the second catalytic domain through a docking interaction

reminiscent of the activation of cyclin dependent kinases (CDKs) by cyclins. As for other RTKs, kinase activation as well as cross-talk with other receptors and cytoplasmic kinases generates docking sites for adaptor proteins that stimulate signalling. A key adaptor molecule of EGF1R signalling is GRB2 (proteins growth-factor-receptor bound-2) which is responsible for recruitment of RAS and activation of the MAPK pathway. Another direct substrate of EGF1R is STAT5 (signal transducer and activator of transcription-5), which dimerizes upon phosphorylation resulting in nuclear import and increased transcription of a number of growth-promoting target genes. The survival pathway PI3K–AKT is also activated by EGF signalling—not directly but via activation of RAS and signalling through RAS-MAPK and RAS-PI3K pathways.

Inactivation of EGFR signalling occurs primarily through a process called endocytosis which either leads to receptor degradation or to recycling of the receptor to the cell surface. Endosomal trafficking is a key regulatory mechanism controlling receptor turnover. Several internalization mechanisms of membrane receptors have been identified. The best studied one is mediated by clathrin-coated vesicles. Once internalized, the clathrin-coated vesicles containing the receptor fuse with intracellular organelles known as the endosomes. In these early endosomes, which are characterized by low pH and the presence of GTPase proteins, the targeted receptor may be either subjected to a recycling pathway transporting the receptor back to the plasma membrane, or it is ubiquitinylated leading to proteosomal degradation in lysosomes. EGFR degradation is mediated by the ubiquitin ligase Cbl, which is recruited to the receptor by phosphorylation of a single tyrosine residue (Tyr1045). However, it is the stability of the activated ligand–receptor complex in the mildly acidic endosomal environment that determines the level of receptor recycling. For instance, EGFR homodimers are stable and remain bound to Cbl, resulting in increased receptor degradation, whereas the less stable EGFR–HER2 heterodimers escape lysosomal degradation by dissociating from Cbl, increasing the rate of receptor recycling to the plasma membrane. Interestingly, the oncogenic activity of viral Cbl (v-Cbl) functions by stimulating the receptor recycling pathway.

A number of oncogenic viruses harness EGFR signalling using a variety of different mechanisms that all lead to increased EGF signalling. For example, the hepatitis B virus and Epstein–Barr virus activate EGFR by increasing its expression, whereas the avian erythoblastosis virus expresses a truncated constitutively active viral form of EGFR. The human papilloma virus protein E5 blocks the degradation of EGFR by inhibiting an endosomal ATPase resulting in increased receptor recycling to the plasma membrane. The direct links of EGF pathway dysfunction to cancer development highlight the key role of the EGF pathway in maintaining tissue homoeostasis and offer therapeutic opportunities that have already been successfully explored by the development of HER2/ErbB2 inhibitors and therapeutic antibodies.

Janus Kinases (JAK) and STAT signalling

Janus Kinases (JAK1–3 and TYK2) play an essential role regulating haematopoiesis and proliferation of blood cells. A key discovery in this signalling field was the identification of the point mutation $JAK2^{V617F}$ that leads to activation of the JAK/STAT signalling pathways and development of myeloproliferative diseases (MPD) such as polycythaemia vera (PV), essential thombocythaemia (ET), and primary myelofibrosis (PMF). $JAK2^{V617F}$ is a somatic mutation, which means that it is present only in the haematopoietic cell compartment but not in germline DNA. This mutation has been identified in most MPD patients defining a common genetic mechanism for this disease.

JAKs contain no transmembrane domain and are therefore not receptor tyrosine kinases. They interact with specific cytokine receptors which lacks intrinsic kinase activity. However, much as in RTKs, ligand binding to the cytokine receptor results in JAK activation by autophosphorylation and phosphorylation of the cytokine receptor itself and the recruitment of members of the signal transducer and activator of the transcription (STAT) family. Cytokine receptors have different specificity for one of the JAK kinases, resulting in different signalling outcomes. For instance, genetic ablation of JAK2 blocks erythropoiesis, a result of deficient signalling through the erythropoietin (EPO) receptor that specifically binds JAK2. JAK family members contain seven homology domains (JH1-7) which include the tyrosine kinase domain (JH1), an inactive (pseudo)kinase domain (JH2), and several docking and protein interaction modules (JH3-7). Interestingly, the $JAK2^{V617F}$ point mutation is located in the pseudokinase domain which has an autoinhibitory function. It has been speculated that V617F releases this autoinhibitory block resulting in a constitutively active JAK2 kinase. Indeed, expression of $JAK2^{V617F}$ leads to cytokine hypersensitivity and cytokine-independent growth, a typical feature of haematopoietic colonies grown from PV patients. JAK activity is negatively regulated by binding of SOCS (suppressor of cytokine signalling) ubiquitine ligases which interact with phosphorylations sites on JAK, leading to degradation. JAK also activates the MAPK and PI3K signalling pathway, resulting in increased proliferation and survival of cells harbouring the $JAK2^{V617F}$ mutation.

Signalling downstream of GFRs

A number of protein interaction modules contributed critically to our understanding of the complex molecular events that mediate signalling downstream GFRs. Phosphorylation sites created by activated RTK activity lead to the recruitment of SH2 (Src homology 2) domain containing adapter proteins. The SH2 domain, first identified in the cytoplasmic tyrosine kinase Src, is a small phosphotyrosine specific binding. A second Src homology domain (SH3) is crucial for recruiting further binding partners by interacting with proline rich sequences in target molecules. One of these adaptor molecules is GRB2, which contains one SH2 and two SH3 domains. GRB2 links the activated phosphorylated GFR with the guanine nucleotide exchange factor SOS (Son of Sevenless), named after the Drosophila gene whose inactivation leads to lack of expression of the seventh, central photoreceptor (R7). Interaction with GRB2 stimulates SOS leading to the GDP/GTP exchange and activation of the RAS family of small GTPases. Active GTP-bound RAS activates members of the serine/threonine kinase RAF and consequently the MAPK pathway. Finally the discovery of phospholipid binding pleckstrin homology (PH) domains explained how phospholipid effector molecules can specifically activate protein kinases such as the Ser/Thr kinase AKT also known as protein kinase B (PKB), PKD1 (Protein kinase D1), as well as lipid kinases (PI(3)Ks).

The RAS/RAF/MAPK pathway

The name RAS refers to the discovery of the viral oncogene v-RAS (Rat Sarcoma). Mutations in members of the RAS family of small GTPase (H-Ras, N-Ras, and K-Ras) have been detected in 20–30% of all human tumours, highlighting the central role of these proteins in the regulation of cellular proliferation. Indeed, expression of oncogenic H-RAS is sufficient for driving G0 arrested cells into the cell cycle in the absence of mitotic signals. RAS family members share homology with the G_α subunit of heterotrimeric G proteins (large GTPases). GTPases cycle between a GDP bound-off state and a GTP bound-on state. The exchange of the nucleotide is catalysed by guanine nucleotide exchange factors (GEFs) and GTPase activating proteins (GAPs). RAS by itself has GTPase activity. However, hydrolysis of GTP is very slow in the absence of a GAP, which contributes additional catalytic residues leading ultimately to the inactive GDP-bound state. Inactivation of RAS activity by GAPs is a frequent target of somatic mutations found in oncogenic RAS variants. RAS is reactivated by GEFs such as SOS that facilitate reloading of GTP by a nucleotide exchange mechanism. GTP-bound RAS has high binding affinity for a number of effector molecules including the lipid kinase PI3K. RAS is recruited to the plasma membrane by covalent linkage to lipids (prenylation or palmitoylation). This multistep process involves several enzymes. The C-terminal peptide motif "CaaX box" is first farnesylated at the CaaX cysteine residue, loosely inserting RAS into the membrane of the endoplasmatic reticulum (ER) and other cellular membranes. The C-terminal tripeptide "aaX" is subsequently cleaved by a prenyl-protein specific endoprotease and the new C-terminus is methylated by a methyltransferase completing the insertion cycle.

The GTP-bound form of RAS has high affinity for the serine/threonine kinase c-RAF (RAF1), the proto-oncogene homologue to the viral v-RAF oncogene. There are two additional RAF kinases (A-RAF and B-RAF) encoded in humans and mutations in B-RAF have been found in several tumours. RAFs are MAP kinase kinase kinases (MAP3Ks) that function as the entry point for the MAPK pathway, a major signalling path that transmits membrane receptor signals to nuclear transcription factors.

RAF kinases harbour an N-terminal regulatory RAS binding domain and a C-terminal kinase domain. Oncogenic v-RAF lacks the regulatory domain and is constitutively active. However, activation of c-RAF is a multistep process. RAS binding exposes an inhibitory phosphorylation site (S259) that locks c-RAF in an inactive state to phosphatases such as PP2A, resulting in pS259 dephosphorylation. Several other kinases target c-RAF, introducing phosphorylation at several sites that modulate c-RAF activity but that are on their own insufficient for activation. Activated c-RAF phosphorylates the dual specificity kinase MEK which in turn phosphorylates and activates ERK. Several regulatory and scaffolding proteins guarantee tight control of this signalling pathway. For instance, the pseudokinase KSR (kinase suppressor of Ras) binds to MEK in quiescent cells but interacts with c-RAF and ERK in stimulated cells, whereas RKIP (RAF kinase inhibitor protein) disrupts the interaction between RAF and MEK. ERK has a large number of substrates, including transcription factors such as ELK1 necessary for activation of the proto-oncogene c-fos and Myc. Transcription factors regulated by MAPKs are of particular importance for the expression of proteins that regulate the cell cycle.

The PI(3)K/AKT pathway

Phosphatidylinositol (PtdIns) is a phospholipid located in membranes that can be phosphorylated at the 3, 4, and 5 positions of the inositol ring to generate seven diverse combinations of phosphoinositides. Phosphorylation of these messenger molecules is regulated by PI3K family members and the antagonizing activity of lipid phosphatases such as PTEN. The lipid kinase PI(3)K is recruited to receptor or IRS phosphotyrosine sites by means of SH2 domains located in its non-catalytic alpha subunit. PI(3)K can also be recruited to the cell membrane by means of Ras. Phospholipase C (PLC) hydrolyses PtdIns to generate two so-called second messengers: diacylglycerol (DAG) and inositol-1,4,5- trisphosphate (Ins(1,4,5)P3). Phosphoinositides stimulate phosphorylation dependent signalling by interaction with PH domains. In the protein kinase AKT (PKB), PtdIns(3,4)P2 binds to the PH domain of AKT, thereby releasing an autoinhibitory conformation resulting in partial kinase activation by the kinase PDK1 (phosphoinositide-dependent kinase 1). Full activation of AKT is accomplished by a second phosphorylation event carried out by mTORC2, the mammalian target of rapamycin complex 2, but other kinases have also been identified as secondary activators of AKT.

AKT was originally identified as an oncogene (v-AKT) of the transforming retrovirus AKT8. Three isoforms (AKT1–3) are expressed in mammals. Knockout of AKT1 in mice results in growth deficiency of the animals but normal glucose homoeostasis. AKT2-deficient mice have only mild growth defects but are diabetic, pointing to a pivotal role of this isozyme in signalling downstream of the insulin receptor. One of the main regulators of AKT is the tumour suppressor PTEN, a phosphatase that dephosphorylates PtdIns(3,4,5)P3 to PtdIns(4,5)P2, which removes AKT from the plasma membrane and significantly decreases the rate of AKT activation, leading to insensitivity to insulin and IGF1 growth signals.

AKT is a key regulator for a number of diverse cellular functions including inhibition of apoptotic pathways, regulation of protein synthesis and glucose metabolism as well as regulation of gene transcription and cell migration. In accordance with these diverse functions more than a hundred AKT substrates have been identified comprising, for instance, forkhead box O (FOXO) transcription factors, glycogen synthase kinase 3 (GSK3) in the insulin signalling pathway as well as the RAB GAP that regulates insulin-stimulated exocytosis of glucose transporter type 4 (GLUT4), the tuberous sclerosis 2 (TSC2) tumour suppressor, the pro-apoptotic protein BCL-2 antagonist of cell death (BAD), and the cell cycle regulators p21 and p27. A graphical representation of AKT activation and some downstream signalling partners is shown in Figure 3.2.

The mTOR pathway controls cellular growth and energy metabolism

Cellular systems have developed complex regulatory networks that allow them to transition between anabolic and catabolic states and which also determine if cells will survive, grow, or break down cellular organelles for the recycling of nutrients as a response to nutrient availability. The serine/threonine PI3K-related protein kinase (PIKK) mTOR (the mammalian target of rapamycin) plays a central role in the regulation of these processes. Dysfunction of mTOR has been linked to many diverse diseases and has stimulated a large number of drug development efforts on this signalling pathway. mTOR signalling is mediated by the two large protein complexes mTORC1 and mTORC2 which share the central mTOR kinase subunit. mTORC1 consists of mTOR, the activating subunits Raptor and mLST8, as well as two negative regulators, PRAS40 and DEPTOR. The scaffolding protein Raptor is regulated by phosphorylation and it facilitates substrate recruitment. The mTORC2 complex is not sensitive to rapamycin and, due to the lack of specific inhibitors, this complex is much less studied. Apart from the mTORC1 components mTOR, DEPTOR, and mLST8, mTORC2 also contains the subunits Rictor, mSIN1, Protor (protein observed with rictor-1), and Hsp70. The mSIN1 subunit is important for recruitment and activation of AKT. mTORC2 is activated by growth factors, stimulates AKT signalling, and regulates GTPases of the Rac and Rho family stimulating cell motility and survival.

mTORC1 is regulated by a large diversity of signalling pathways, as for instance insulin and IGF1, which stimulate the PI3K and Ras pathways. A common feature of effector kinases of these pathways (protein kinase B (AKT/PKB), extracellular-signal-regulated kinase 1/2 (ERK1/2), and ribosomal S6 kinase (RSK1)) is that they all phosphorylate and inactivate the tuberous sclerosis TSC1/TSC2 complex, an inhibitor of mTORC1. TSC1/TSC2 functions as a GAP RHEB (RAS homologue enriched in brain), converting it to its inactive GDP-bound form. Since GTP-bound RHEB strongly stimulates mTORC1 activity by binding to the complex, the GAP activity of TSC1/TSC2 leads to mTORC1 inactivation. To date no GEF for RHEB has been identified that would lead to mTORC1 reactivation. AKT additionally activates mTORC1 by phosphorylation of the mTORC1 inhibitor PRAS40, resulting in its dissociation from the mTORC1 complex.

Similarly, mTORC1 can be activated by TSC1/TSC2 phosphorylation by IkB kinase b (IKKb) as a response to inflammatory stimuli such as TNFα or through the Wnt pathway effector glycogen

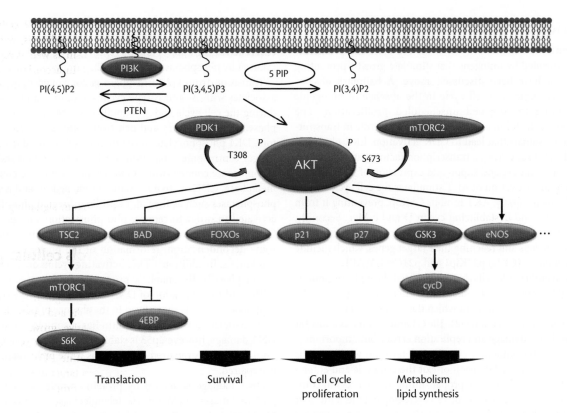

Fig. 3.2 Activation of AKT and main downstream signalling partners. Colours codes are as in Figure 3.1.

synthase kinase 3b (GSK3-β). Sensing of low nutrient levels or oxidative stress also acts at least in part through regulation of the TSC1/ TCC2 complex. For instance, adenosine monophosphate-activated protein kinase (AMPK) phosphorylates TSC2 and increases its GAP activity towards Rheb in response to hypoxia or low energy states, but, similarly to AKT, AMPK also directly regulates mTORC1 by phosphorylation of raptor leading to inhibition of mTORC1.

Regulation of protein synthesis by mTORC1 has been extensively studied. mTORC1 phosphorylates 4EBP1, a binding protein of the translational regulators eukaryotic translation initiation factor 4E (eIF4E). Phosphorylation inhibits the binding of 4EBP1 to the cap-binding protein eIF4E, preventing formation of the eIF4E/ eIF4F complex which is required for the initiation of cap-dependent translation. mTORC1 also directly phosphorylates and activates S6 kinase 1 (p70S6K1) stimulating mRNA biogenesis as well as translational initiation and elongation by phosphorylating the 40S ribosomal protein S6. S6 phosphorylation particularly enhances the translation of mRNAs containing a 5'-terminal oligopolypyrimidine (5'-TOP). Interestingly, 4EBP1 and p70S6K1 are specifically recruited to mTORC1 via the TOR signalling (TOS) motif, a conserved five-amino-acid sequence that interacts with the mTORC1 subunit Raptor. mTORC1 activity is also regulated by amino acid levels. Low amino acid levels in the growth medium lead to rapid dephosphorylation of the mTORC1 substrates 4EBP1 and p70S6K1. This effect is quickly reversed when amino acids are resupplied. The pathway regulating this effect is largely unknown but recent reports suggested that MAP4K3 senses amino acid levels and stimulates mTORC1. Several studies identified a negative feedback regulation by p70S6K1 to the upstream insulin/insulin growth factor effector IRS1 which is regulated transcriptionally by mTORC1 as well as

by direct phosphorylation by p70S6K1, preventing IRS1 binding to RTKs leading to down-regulation of PI3K and MAPK signalling.

mTORC1 also regulates another important catabolic process: autophagy, an evolutionary highly conserved process that leads to the degradation of cytoplasmic organelles, toxic protein aggregates, and intracellular pathogens in lysosomes. The autophagic programme allows cells to recycle catabolites by organelle breakdown, which can be used for essential biosynthetic and metabolic processes promoting survival during starvation. During autophagy intracellular vesicles named autophagosomes engulf cellular organelles and fuse them with lysosomes. Nutrient deprivation or specific inhibition of mTORC1 by rapamycin induces this survival programme. Autophagy has been extensively studied in yeast where TOR phosphorylates the protein kinase Atg1 (autophagy-related gene 1) which interacts with Atg13. These studies revealed that TOS motif-dependent phosphorylation of Atg1 by TOR inhibits Atg13/Atg1 complex formation, repressing autophagy. The mammalian Atg1 homologue is a family of four kinases (ULK1-4, UNC-51-like kinase) in which ULK1–3 seem to play a role in autophagy and ULK1–2 have been shown to be directly phosphorylated by mTORC1. The role of autophagy in tumour development and progression is controversial. On the one hand, repressing autophagy may impair tumorigenesis by reducing the ability of cancer cells to survive under energy-poor conditions. On the other hand, studies have shown that mice lacking essential components of the autophagy machinery have an increased rate of spontaneous tumour development, an effect that has been attributed to higher rates of DNA damage induced by reactive oxygen species that accumulate in cells with damaged mitochondria.

Regulation of the cell cycle and mitosis

The decision as to whether cells enter the cell cycle and proliferate is tightly controlled by mitogens that stimulate growth-promoting pathways that have been discussed above. A hallmark of cancer is that cells enter the cell cycle in the absence of mitogenic signals, leading to so-called unscheduled proliferation. The Ras–RAF-MEK–ERK kinase cascade plays a a key role in transmitting mitogenic signals that lead to CDK activation. ERK phosphorylates and stabilizes c-Myc, a transcription factor that induces the expression of cyclin D1 and suppresses expression of CDK inhibitors. Further, the activation of AKT stimulates the cell cycle by two main mechanisms: firstly, AKT inhibits GSK3β, preventing it from phosphorylating and destabilizing cyclin D and c-Myc. Secondly, AKT inhibits FOXO transcription factors, preventing them from entering the nucleus and reaching their target genes, which include the CDK inhibitors (CKIs) p27Kip1 and p21Cip1/WAF1.

Apart from embryonic cells that can proceed through continuous cycles of DNA replication (S phase) and division (M phase), the cell cycle contains four phases in which the S and M phase is interspersed by gap phases (G1 and G2). The G1 and G2 phases allow for the repair of DNA damage and replication errors, but, importantly, also interpret environmental cues that determine whether cells enter a new round of cell division or exit the cell cycle and enter a quiescent state (G0). To ensure proper timing and successful completion of each step, the eukaryotic cell cycle implements a number of checkpoints that includes the restriction point—a point of no return that commits cells to complete a division cycle even if mitogenic signals drop or, failing that, enter an apoptotic programme.

CDKs are the key regulators of the cell cycle. They require the binding of activating cyclin cofactors, which stabilizes the active state of these kinases. However, due to their central role in controlling the cell cycle, CDKs are regulated on several additional levels by activating and inactivating phosphorylation events as well as by interaction with CDK inhibitors (CKIs). Cyclin levels are tightly controlled during the different phases of the cell cycle, regulating CDK activity in a timely manner. In mammals the activity of three interphase CDKs (CDK2, CDK4, and CDK6), a mitotic CDK (CDK1, also known as cell division control protein 2 (CDC2)), and ten cyclins belonging to four diverse families (A-, B-, D-, and E-type cyclins) is orchestrated in a highly dynamic manner during the cell cycle. D-type cyclins are expressed during the initial phase of G1. Cyclin D bind and activate mainly CDK4 and CDK6, resulting in the partial inactivation of the retinoblastoma (RB) tumour suppressor by phosphorylation which imposes the first checkpoint. The partial inactivation of RB leads to the expression of E2F transcription factors and the expression of E-type cyclins which interact with and activate CDK2, resulting in the complete inactivation of RB by CDK2/cyclin E phosphorylation in late G1. From this point onwards the cell cycle progresses independently of mitogenic stimulation (restriction point) into S-phase.

Premature entry into S-phase is prevented by a number of CDK inhibitors comprising p27Kip1 and others, such as p15Ink4b, p16Ink4a, p21Cip1/WAF1, and p57Kip2, that rapidly inactivate CDK catalytic activity by blocking the ATP binding site. A number of mitogenic stimuli release CDK by suppressing p27Kip1 transcription and translation. Once activated, CDK2 rapidly inactivates p27Kip1 by phosphorylation that targets this inhibitor for polyubiquitination mediated by an SCF (Skp1/Cul1/F-box

protein)-ubiquitin-ligase complex and degradation by the proteasome system. CDK2 activation is completed by activation by CAK (CDK activating kinase) and by removal of an inhibitory phosphorylation by phosphatase of the CDC25 family.

Transition from G2 to M-phase is controlled by CDK1 which associates with A- and B-type cyclins. Cyclin A and B accumulate during the cell cycle and are rapidly degraded at the onset of anaphase, mediating entry and exit from mitosis. The master regulator CDK1 phosphorylates more than 70 substrates during G2/M to trigger centrosome separation, nuclear envelope breakdown, and chromosome condensation. Once chromosomes are condensed in metaphase, CDK1 activity is rapidly switched off and a number of phosphatases such as the Cdc14 proline-directed phosphatases are activated in order to remove phosphorylation sites generated by CDK1 activity. Elimination of these sites is required for chromosome decondensation, reformation of the nuclear envelope, and cytokinesis. In addition, CDK1 activating cyclins are degraded during anaphase by the anaphase promoting complex (APC).

The faithful replication of DNA is controlled by the p53 tumour suppressor which is short-lived in the absence of DNA damage due to its association with the ubiquitin ligase complex. In response to DNA damage, however, p53 is stabilized and causes cell cycle arrest until the DNA is repaired or apoptosis if the DNA damage cannot be repaired.

DNA damage is sensed by protein complexes containing the protein kinases ATM (ataxia telangiectasia mutated) and ATR (ATM-related). ATM and ATR activate the checkpoint kinases CHK2 and CHK1, which leads to inhibition of CDC25 phosphatases prompting the accumulation of inhibitory phosphorylation of CDKs. Cell cycle arrest is mediated at least in part by activation of the CDK inhibitor p21*waf/cip*, which inhibits cyclin E/CDK2 complexes, whereas apoptosis is induced by p53 activation of the expression of the pro-apoptotic proteins BAX and PUMA. Stability of p53 is increased by ARF which blocks the interaction between p53 and Mdm2. The acronym ARF stands for 'alternative reading frame' since ARF is encoded by the same locus as the CDK inhibitor p16ink4 but it is transcribed from a different promoter using a different reading frame. Interestingly, transcription of ARF is regulated by E2F transcription factors that are controlled by the RB tumour suppressor, suggesting that the loss of this locus in some cancers eliminates two tumour suppressors that control RB as well as p53 function.

The well established model of cell cycle regulation by CDKs has recently been challenged by genetic knockout studies in mice that surprisingly revealed a non-essential function of CDK2, CDK4, and CDK6. Instead, deletion in the mouse germline of each of the three interphase CDKs resulted only in developmental defects in highly specialized cell types. Moreover, deletion of multiple interphase CDKs only led to developmental defects in certain tissue types but had no effect on the cell cycle in general. Only deletion of CDK1 led to cell cycle arrest, preventing embryos from developing beyond the two-cell stage. This surprising observation suggests that CDK1 alone is needed to drive the cell cycle in most tissues and that the mammalian cell cycle is still quite similar to the cell cycle in yeast which expresses only a single CDK1 homologue. However, defects in cell cycle regulators such as overexpression of cyclin D or CDK2, and loss of the tumour suppressors RB and CDK inhibitors (p27Kip1, ARF, p16) are among the most frequent genetic alterations observed in tumours. In addition, c-Myc, is frequently overexpressed in cancer and has a key role in regulating the cell cycle.

All Myc isoforms (c-Myc, L-Myc, and N-Myc) strongly induce the expression of D-type cyclins and in complex with Miz1 (Myc interacting zinc-finger protein), c-Myc inhibits the expression of CDK inhibitors p21Cip1 and p15Ink4b.

Wnt signalling

Canonical Wnt signalling plays an important role in development, tissue homoeostasis, and dysfunction of this pathway has been implicated in the development of a cancer. The Wnt pathway has been discovered by the identification of the Int1 locus (Wnt1) as the factor required for mouse mammary tumour virus-driven tumorigenesis and by mutants in *Drosophila melanogaster* lacking wings (*Wingless* (*Wg*)).

The canonical Wnt pathway is initiated at the plasma membrane by binding for Wnt proteins (there are 19 identified Wnt genes in humans) to Frizzled receptors and their LRP5–LRP6 co-receptors. As for other receptor signalling pathways, there are several inhibitors of this pathways that antagonize Wnt function including secreted Frizzled-related proteins (SFRPs) that sequester Wnt ligands, Dickkopfs (DKKs), and Wnt inhibitory factor 1 (WIF1). The key event of the binding of Wnt ligands to the Frizzled receptor is the stabilization of β-catenin in the cytoplasm followed by translocation of β-catenin into the nucleus where it forms complexes with LEF (lymphoid enhancer factor) and TCF (T-cell factor) transcription factors. Genes activated by the β-catenin complexes with LEF and TGF transcription factors including c-MYC, Cyclin D, VEGF (vascular endothelial growth factor), and FGF4 (vascular endothelial growth factor). The discovery that Wnt signalling increases expression of c-MYC, and indirectly Cyclin D, has linked Wnt signalling with G1-phase progression and cell proliferation. In the absence of Wnt signalling, β-catenin is rapidly degraded by complex formation with APC (adenomatous polyposis coli) and axins as well as by phosphorylation by the serine kinases GSK3β and CK1α. Phosphorylated β–catenin is recruited to the E3 ubiquitin ligase subunit β-TRCP (β-transducin repeat-containing protein) and rapidly degraded by the ubiquitin system. In addition, LEF and TCF transcription factors are inactivated in the nucleus by interaction with proteins of the Groucho family.

Mutations in genes that control β–catenin stability, such as those that encode members of the destruction complex (APC or axins), or β–catenin itself, have been associated with tumorigenesis. Most notable are mutations or truncations in APC that lead to familial adenomatous polyposis (FAP). FAP patients develop large numbers of adenomatous polyps in the colon early in their lives that subsequently develop into malignant carcinomas. Sporadic mutations of the APC gene have also been detected in a large number of colon cancers. A general feature of mutations in the APC, AXIN1/2, and β-catenin locus is the inappropriate accumulation of β-catenin in the absence of Wnt signalling leading to aberrant Wnt pathway activation.

TGF-β signalling

The TGF-β family comprises 33 extracellular signalling molecules that play a key role in embryonic development, stem cell differentiation, immune response, and wound healing. The TGF-β family contains three TGF-β isoforms, the bone morphogenetic proteins (BMPs), growth and differentiation factors (GDFs), and Müllerian inhibitory factor (MIF) as well as activins or inhibins. TGF-β binds to heterodimeric cell surface receptors containing one type I and one type II receptor (TGFβRI and TGFβRII), each containing a cytoplasmic serine/threonine kinase domain. Seven type I receptors, also named activin-receptor-like kinases (ALKs), and five different type II receptors are expressed in humans. Two type III co-receptors (endoglin and betaglycan) have been described that however do not play an active role in signalling but may regulate ligand access to type I and type II receptors. TGF-β binds to the extracellular domains of type I and type II receptors leading to the formation of heterotetrameric active receptor complexes. TGFβRII are constitutively active and phosphorylate a glycine/serine-rich domain in the type I receptor, triggering the recruitment and phosphorylation of downstream effectors of the SMAD family of transcription factors.

The SMAD family is grouped into three classes of effector proteins depending on their function in signalling. The receptor-associated SMADs (R-SMADs) are directly phosphorylated by TGFβRIs leading to R-SMAD activation. R-SMADs are transcriptionally inactive and are retained in the cytoplasm by interaction with retention proteins. The R-SMAD family comprises five members—SMAD1, SMAD2, SMAD3, SMAD5, and SMAD8–which have specificity for different receptor families. After phosphorylation R-SMADs form a complex with the co-SMAD SMAD4. This complex translocates into the nucleus where it interacts with a number of transcription factors and co-activators regulating the expression of a large diversity of target genes. SMAD transcriptional activity is antagonized by inhibitory SMADs (I-SMADs) (SMAD6 and SMAD7) which disrupt the SMAD/Co-SMAD complex, providing a negative feedback loop for this pathway.

TGF-β1 was originally discovered as a factor stimulating growth of cultured rat fibroblasts in soft agar. However, the effect of receptor stimulation by TGF1β binding is highly context dependent. During early embryogenesis and in some adult mesenchymal cells TGF1β signalling promotes growth. In contrast, most adult tissues respond to TGF1β with cytostasis or even by induction of apoptosis. Activation of TGFβ signalling inhibits cell cycle progression in the G1 phase due to transcriptional up-regulation of CDK inhibitors, in particular InK4B and p21, and the inhibitor of protein translation 4EBP, as well as repression of Myc expression. The expression of cell cycle inhibitors such as p21 is transactivated by the SMAD/FOXO complexes. As discussed above, Forkhead transcription factors play a central role in regulating development, metabolism, and longevity under caloric restriction and are linked to the TORC1 pathway by interaction with AKT, which inactivates FOXO. In cancer, the growth-limiting antimitotic signals of the TGFβ pathway are often inhibited by inactivating mutations of the TGFβRs that are common in colon cancer. Other aspects of TGFβ signalling may however promote tumorigenesis.

One of these aspects that may lead to cancer progression is linked to the observation that TGFβ signalling can induce epithelial mesenchymal transition (EMT), a cellular programme that leads to loss of epithelial traits such as loss of cell adhesion by transcriptional repression of E-cadherins, a family of calcium-dependent adhesion proteins that mediate proper cell contacts. Loss of cadherin function results in increased cell mobility, a characteristic feature of mesenchymal cells. Several growth-promoting pathways have been shown to take part in this transformation including Wnt/β-catenin and Ras-MAPK signaling, which leads to activation of two transcription factors: Snail and Slug. Both proteins repress E-cadherin expression leading to destruction of desmosomal function and as a consequence increased cell spreading. Snail and Slug also regulate expression of p63, a transcription factor of the p53 family required for development of epithelial structures and proper cell polarity. TGFβ has been shown to down-regulate a number of proteins essential for the functions of tight junctions and R-SMAD can directly interact with Snail, resulting in transcriptional complexes that promote expression of EMT associated genes. The precise mechanistic contribution of TGFβ signalling to EMT has still to be clarified, but it is clear that this pathway plays an essential role in the initiation and completion of EMT in development as well as during tumour progression.

Further reading

Citri A, Yarden Y. EGF-ERBB signalling: towards the systems level. Nature reviews Molecular Cell Biology 2006; 7: 505–516.

Fedorov O, Muller S, Knapp S. (2010). The (un)targeted cancer kinome. Nature Chemical Biology 2010; 6: 166–169.

Gerlinger M, Rowan AJ, Horswell S, Larkin J, Endesfelder D et al. Intratumor heterogeneity and branched evolution revealed by multiregion sequencing. New England Journal of Medicine 2012; 366: 883–892.

Hanahan D, Weinberg RA. Hallmarks of cancer: the next generation. Cell 2011; 144: 646–674.

Ikushima H, Miyazono K. (2010). TGFbeta signalling: a complex web in cancer progression. Nature reviews cancer 2010; 10: 415–424.

Klaus A, Birchmeier W. Wnt signalling and its impact on development and cancer. Nature Reviews Cancer 2008; 8: 387–398.

Laplante M, Sabatini DM. mTOR signaling in growth control and disease. Cell 2012; 149: 274–293.

Levine RL, Pardanani A, Tefferi A, Gilliland DG. Role of JAK2 in the pathogenesis and therapy of myeloproliferative disorders. Nature Reviews Cancer 2007; 7: 673–683.

Malumbres M, Barbacid M. Cell cycle, CDKs and cancer: a changing paradigm. Nature Reviews Cancer 2009; 9: 153–166.

Pollak MN, Schernhammer ES, Hankinson SE. Insulin-like growth factors and neoplasia. Nature Reviews Cancer 2004; 4: 505–518.

Vanhaesebroeck B, Stephens L, Hawkins P. PI3K signalling: the path to discovery and understanding. Nature Reviews Molecular Cell Biology 2012; 13: 195–203.

Wood, LD, Parsons DW, Jones S, Lin J, Sjoblom T et al. The genomic landscapes of human breast and colorectal cancers. Science 2007; 318: 1108–1113.

CHAPTER 4

Cell cycle control

Simon M. Carr and Nicholas B. La Thangue

Introduction to cell cycle control

All cells arise by the division of existing cells. This process involves duplication of the cell contents, followed by the equal distribution of these contents into two daughter cells. Collectively, this highly regulated series of events is known as the cell cycle. Whilst duplication of cellular contents such as organelles and membranes occurs throughout all stages of the cell cycle, chromosomal DNA is replicated only once at a discrete stage known as S phase. Once DNA replication is complete, distribution of chromosomes and other cellular components occurs during the final stage of the cell cycle, known as M phase, or mitosis. The passage of a cell through the cell cycle is therefore regulated in a temporal fashion, so that entry into subsequent cell cycle stages only occurs once the previous stage has been efficiently completed. The cell has a number of signalling mechanisms at its disposal with which to monitor the integrity of cell cycle progression, and if problems are detected, later cell cycle stages can be delayed whilst these errors are corrected. This chapter aims to give an overview of the major control mechanisms that the cell utilizes to regulate cell cycle progression, and how these checkpoints are circumvented during the onset of cancer.

The cell cycle

The cell cycle can be divided into a number of discrete phases, based on the cellular activities which occur during each distinct stage [1, 2]. Duplication of chromosomal DNA, for example, is an early cell cycle event which occurs during S phase (Figure 4.1). The timing and coordination of DNA replication is tightly regulated, so that the genetic material within the cell is copied once and only once [1, 2]. Chromosome duplication itself requires the activity of a large number of proteins and enzymes which must be synthesized in the cell prior to the onset of DNA replication [3, 4]. A number of these proteins are involved in maintaining a tight association between the newly synthesized chromosomes, a step which is essential to ensure efficient segregation of the genetic material to daughter cells in a later cell cycle stage known as M phase (Figure 4.1) [1, 2]. At the midpoint of M phase, these linked chromosome pairs, known as sister chromatids, disassociate and migrate to opposite poles of the cell, where they are enveloped into two new daughter nuclei. This process is mediated by the attachment of sister chromatids to an array of microtubules called the mitotic spindle, which pull sister chromatids to opposite poles of the cell [1, 2]. Following chromosomal segregation, the cell pinches in two as a new plasma membrane forms between the daughter nuclei [1, 2].

S and M phases themselves are separated by two additional phases, known as the gap phases G1 and G2 (Figure 4.1). These gap phases provide additional time in which protein synthesis and cell growth can occur, since these processes are coordinated with cell division in most cell types [1, 2]. The gap phases also represent a time in which the cell can monitor extracellular and intracellular signals to ensure conditions are appropriate for it to progress to the next stage of the cell cycle. During G1, for example, cells become committed to cell division unless conditions are unfavourable, in which case they can pause in G1 or enter a prolonged, non-dividing state [5]. During G2, the integrity of DNA replication is assessed to ensure that sister chromatid segregation only occurs once chromosomal duplication is complete [6].

Cell cycle checkpoints

The function of the cellular machinery that carries out DNA replication and cell division is strictly regulated by a complex signalling network known as the cell cycle control system. This central control network is responsible for driving progression of the cell cycle through a number of restriction points known as checkpoints [1, 2]. When conditions are appropriate for cell proliferation, the cell cycle control system will drive the cell through its first checkpoint at the transition between G1 and S phase [5] (Figure 4.1). DNA replication is initiated, and new proteins are synthesized which drive early cell cycle events. The second checkpoint occurs at the entry to mitosis (the 'G2/M checkpoint'; Figure 4.1), where the assembly of the mitotic spindle is tightly controlled [6]. By the midpoint of mitosis (metaphase), sister chromatids are attached to microtubules originating from the cell poles and they are prepared for separation in the next stage of mitosis known as anaphase. This is where the third major checkpoint occurs (the 'metaphase to anaphase transition'; Figure 4.1), which commits the cell to chromatid separation and the completion of mitosis [6]. Progression through all of these checkpoints relies not only on the completion of previous cell cycle events, but also on receiving appropriate signals from the extracellular and intracellular environment.

The cell cycle control system

Whilst numerous proteins are involved in cell cycle control, the central components are a group of enzymes known as cyclin-dependent kinases (CDKs) [7]. These enzymes catalyse the addition of phosphate groups onto a plethora of target substrates involved in processes such as DNA replication, protein synthesis, and cell division. These phosphorylation events can promote or inhibit the activity of the receiving substrate, and can mediate or ablate additional protein–protein interactions. As such, the enzymatic activity of CDKs can be used to fine-tune the function of many cell

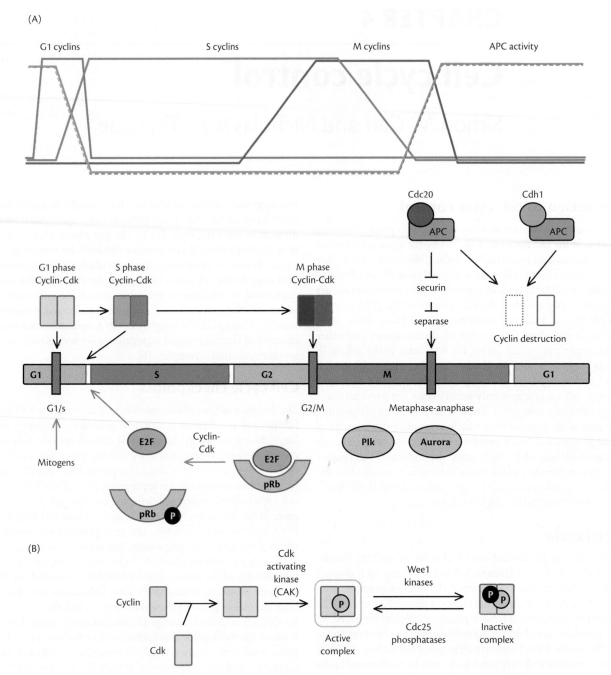

Fig. 4.1 Overview of cell cycle control. (A) The oscillating expression levels of specific cyclins involved in driving the main transitions between cell cycle phases is simplified in graphical format at the top of this figure. CDK levels generally remain constant throughout the cell cycle, so discrete cyclin–CDK complexes form in parallel with rises and falls in cyclin levels. G1-phase cyclin–CDK complexes commit the cell to cell cycle entry at the G1/S transition by targeting phosphorylation events onto the pocket proteins (i.e. pRb), which induces the release of E2F transcriptional activity and the expression of genes required for S-phase progression. M-phase cyclin–CDK complex activity begins to rise after completion of S phase and drives cells through the G2/M checkpoint by inducing chromosome condensation, nuclear envelope disassembly, and formation of the mitotic spindle. It also results in the activation of APC, which induces the loss of sister chromatid cohesion and triggers chromosome segregation at the metaphase-to-anaphase transition. Completion of mitosis also depends on the activity of the Plk and Aurora mitotic kinases, and on the destruction of S- and M-phase cyclins by APC activity. The main cell cycle checkpoints are indicated by vertical red bars. (B) CDK activity is not simply regulated by the formation of a complex between the CDK and its cyclin partner. Complete activation of CDKs requires a phosphorylation event mediated by CAK. Fully active cyclin–CDK complexes can be inhibited by further phosphorylation events mediated by the Wee1 family of kinases, and reactivated by removal of this phosphate group by Cdc25 family phosphatases. (Activatory phosphorylation events are displayed in yellow whilst inhibitory phosphorylation events are shown in black.)

regulatory proteins, as will be discussed in more detail in later sections of this chapter.

Many different CDK enzymes exist within the cell, and each possesses its own set of substrates, though there can be some overlap in target preference between family members [7]. The activity of each

CDK enzyme must therefore be controlled in a cell-cycle-dependent fashion so that substrates are only phosphorylated in an appropriate temporal way. This control is achieved primarily via the binding of regulatory subunits known as the cyclins [7], whose protein levels oscillate throughout the cell cycle (Figure 4.1A). Different cyclins are produced at discrete cell cycle stages, resulting in the formation of distinct cyclin–CDK complexes [8, 9]. This leads directly to cyclical changes in the phosphorylation of cell cycle machinery components. For example, at the transition between G1 and S phase, active cyclin–CDK complexes phosphorylate proteins involved in cell cycle entry and DNA replication [5, 10, 11]. During M phase, however, different cyclin–CDK complexes are involved in driving cells through the G2/M checkpoint by phosphorylating substrates involved in microtubule spindle assembly. CDK activity also needs to be switched off as the cell progresses from one cell cycle stage to another, and this is achieved via the degradation of the cyclin subunits themselves. This method of cyclin destruction is particularly prevalent at the end of mitosis, when all CDK activity declines whilst the cell prepares itself for a subsequent round of cell division (Figure 4.1A).

CDK activity is regulated by a variety of mechanisms

Whilst CDK activity requires the binding of a cyclin partner, this alone is not sufficient to fully activate CDKs. The creation and removal of phosphorylation events on the CDK itself are also important determinants of enzyme activity. For example, a phosphorylation event mediated by enzymes known as CDK-activating kinases (CAKs) is required for full CDK activity [7], whilst inhibitory phosphorylation events also occur and are particularly important in preventing the inappropriate activity of CDKs. These inhibitory events are mediated by the Wee1 family of protein kinases (Figure 4.1B).

CDK activity is also kept in check by a number of inhibitor proteins known as the CKIs (CDK inhibitors) that bind to and inactivate cyclin–CDK complexes [12]. These CKIs are expressed in response to cellular stress, and are important in triggering cell cycle arrest when unfavourable conditions, such as DNA damage, exist (discussed in 'The DNA damage response' below). They fall into two families with distinct methods of action, though the function of all is to inhibit those CDKs that drive the initial steps of the cell cycle when commitment to cell division is determined [12].

As discussed previously, destruction of cyclin subunits is another mechanism by which CDK activity can be regulated [13]. These proteins are targeted for destruction by a process known as ubiquitination, which involves the addition of multiple copies of the small protein ubiquitin to the cyclin. This leads to the generation of a ubiquitin chain, which functions to target the cyclin to a large protein complex known as the proteasome, which mediates the subsequent destruction of unwanted proteins in the cell. Ubiquitin is added to cyclins primarily by a multi-subunit enzyme known as the anaphase promoting complex, or APC [13]. Its ability to ubiquitinate substrates is controlled by a number of activator subunits, which vary during different stages of the cell cycle and function to target APC activity towards discrete subsets of cyclin–CDK complexes [13, 14].

The transition from G1 to S phase

E2F transcription factors and their regulation by the pocket proteins

Progression into the cell cycle requires the expression of a host of genes that are involved in cell cycle entry and DNA replication. As discussed above, the expression of a number of cyclin genes is also important to promote CDK activity during this stage. The majority of these genes are regulated by a family of transcription factors known as the E2Fs, of which eight members have been described to date [15–17]. These E2F members can be subdivided into two groups, based on whether they act to promote or inhibit the transcription of their target genes. The E2F 1, 2, and 3 proteins can generally be regarded as the 'activator' E2Fs, whilst E2Fs 4 through 8 are transcriptional repressors that bind to G1/S-phase regulated genes and inhibit gene expression. These two subgroups of E2F therefore work antagonistically towards each other, and the balance of activity between the activator and repressor E2Fs is important for reliable G1/S checkpoint control. Loss of activator E2Fs is often associated with tissue-specific defects in cell proliferation, whilst loss of repressor E2Fs can cause defects in cell cycle exit while cells begin to specialize in function [15–18]. It is also important to note that some E2F target genes function in other stages of the cell cycle too, such as during mitosis or in response to DNA damage, so E2F activity is not just restricted to the transition of cells from G1 to S phase.

The E2F transcription factors themselves are also highly regulated, to ensure that expression of genes required for S phase entry only occurs in proliferating cells. This regulation is primarily mediated by an interaction between E2Fs and the 'pocket' proteins (pRb, p107, and p130) [10, 19–21]. In mammalian cells, the activator E2Fs are bound and inactivated by pRb, whilst p107 and p130 act as co-repressors for E2F4–6 in non-proliferating cells [10, 19–21]. The pocket proteins inhibit E2F-dependent gene expression by binding directly to the domain of E2F involved in mediating its transcriptional activity, and thereby directly block its action. Cells lacking pocket proteins have severe defects in their ability to exit the cell cycle in response to stimuli such as DNA damage, and mutations affecting pRb-pathways are incredibly common in almost all human cancers described [21].

Regulation of E2F activity via post-translational modifications

Before entry into S phase, E2F-dependent gene expression is inhibited by the concerted action of the repressor E2Fs and the p107 and p130 pocket proteins [10, 19–21]. Activator E2Fs are present at very low levels, and their activity is suppressed by interactions with the pRb protein [10, 19–21]. As cells progress into the cell cycle, the pocket proteins dissociate from their E2F partners, causing a switch from a generally repressive environment to one that can promote transcription of genes. The protein levels of the activator E2Fs also increase at this time, favouring their association with promoters and the stimulation of gene expression [15–17]. The genes encoding the activator E2Fs are also E2F-responsive, ensuring a positive feedback loop that enhances further G1/S-phase-regulated gene expression.

The dissociation of pocket proteins from the E2Fs is regulated primarily by phosphorylation events catalysed by cyclin–CDK complexes [10] (Figure 4.1). The initial phosphorylation events are mediated by cyclin–CDK complexes that exist in early G1 [10, 22, 23]. However, this activity alone results in only partial pRb phosphorylation, and complete activation of E2F requires subsequent phosphorylation events mediated in late G1 by additional cyclin–CDK complexes [10, 24, 25]. S-phase cyclin–CDK complexes are also thought to be important for maintaining pRb phosphorylation levels throughout S phase and into mitosis [10], ensuring that E2F activity remains high as cells transition through the cell cycle. The ability of cyclin–CDK complexes to phosphorylate pRb can also be influenced by additional post-translational modifications [26, 27]. For example, acetylation and methylation of pRb are known to occur during processes such as cellular differentiation [26], or in response to signals mediated by DNA damage [27, 28]. In both scenarios the cell will not wish to begin cell division, so E2F activity must be held in check. This outcome is achieved since acetylation and methylation events act to block the recognition of pRb by cyclin–CDK complexes, effectively preventing its phosphorylation [26, 28].

Regulation of CDK activity in G1 by mitogenic signalling

In multicellular organisms, entry of a cell into a new cell cycle occurs only in response to appropriate extracellular signals mediated by mitogens. Mitogens are usually soluble peptides or small proteins that are secreted by neighbouring cells, and control the rate of division of several cell types in the body. They do this by binding to receptors located on the outer surface of the cell's plasma membrane, which then mediate a signalling cascade within the cell by promoting phosphorylation events. Whilst these signalling events involve a host of additional proteins and are complex in nature, a few key players are known to play an essential role in driving cell proliferation, and are often targeted by mutations in cancer (discussed in detail in Chapter 3). Mitogenic signalling activates a number of transcription factors which drive the expression of cyclin and CDK genes, and other genes involved in regulating cell growth [29, 30]. These signalling events therefore promote the accumulation of active cyclin–CDK complexes, which in turn enhances their ability to target proteins such as pRb and drive cell cycle progression. Signalling pathways involving anti-mitogenic signals are also important in cell cycle control, and these function to arrest the cell and prevent entry into the cell cycle whilst inappropriate environmental conditions exist. Such anti-mitogenic signalling usually leads to an increase in expression levels of the CKIs, which act to repress cyclin-CDK activity.

The degradation of CKIs

The G1/S-transition is driven primarily by the concerted activity of cyclin–CDK complexes, which promote an irreversible commitment to cell cycle entry and S phase [5, 7]. As described above, this depends in part on the ability of cyclin–CDK complexes to initiate E2F-dependent transcription [15–17]. However, the activity of cyclin–CDK complexes is held in check by CKIs during G1 [12], and these CDK inhibitor proteins need to be deactivated before the cell can enter S phase. This inactivation involves the targeted destruction of CKIs mediated by ubiquitin-conjugating enzymes found both in the nucleus and the cytoplasm [31, 32].

The control of DNA synthesis

Once the duplication of DNA begins, it usually proceeds to completion, and does not occur again in the same cell cycle. This ensures that each daughter cell inherits the precise amount of genetic material from the parental cell, a step which is essential to avoid abnormal loss or gain of genetic information which could cause aberrant function of the cell and lead to diseases such as cancer. This intricate level of DNA replication control is achieved by tightly regulating the initiation process in a temporal fashion that follows the cell cycle stages. In early G1, a complex of initiation proteins called the pre-replicative complex (pre-RC) forms at specific sites on the DNA and primes them for replication [4, 11, 33]. In early S phase, this complex is converted to the pre-initiation complex, which unwinds the DNA and loads the DNA replication machinery [4]. Once DNA replication has been triggered, the pre-RC breaks down, and its reassembly is inhibited until the next G1 [4, 11, 33].

In animal cells, the formation of the pre-RC is regulated by the activity of a number of inhibitor proteins, which are expressed during most stages of the cell cycle and help to prevent the formation of the pre-RC [11, 33]. This inhibition continues to exist until the G1 phase, when these inhibitor proteins are degraded and inactivated [34]. With the inhibitors removed, pre-RC components can be loaded onto the DNA in preparation for DNA replication. Once the machinery required for DNA synthesis has been expressed, the pre-RC is then converted to the pre-initiation complex, and finally, DNA replication itself is triggered by the combined activity of cyclin–CDK complexes and another kinase known as Cdc7 [35]. Once replication has begun, the levels of inhibitor proteins once again climb, resulting in the prevention of further rounds of pre-RC formation [4, 11, 33]. This ensures that re-replication of DNA does not occur during the later cell cycle phases, and that the genetic information in the cell is copied once and only once.

In addition to these inhibitor proteins, cyclin–CDK complexes also play an important role in regulating pre-RC formation, as they can directly phosphorylate pre-RC components and promote their destruction [36]. Since cyclin–CDK complex activity remains high throughout most cell cycle phases, and only begins to decline upon completion of M phase (Figure 4.1A), re-formation of the pre-RC complex is directly inhibited until all CDK activities decline at the end of the cell cycle.

Regulation of early mitotic events

During the approach to mitosis, the cell will confirm that DNA replication has proceeded in an efficient and accurate manner. If this is the case, the cell will then divide into two daughter cells, each containing one copy of the original cell's genetic material. This division process is again highly regulated and involves several steps, including the condensation and organization of chromosomes, breakdown of the membrane surrounding the nucleus, segregation of genetic material to opposite poles of the cell, and the formation of a new cell membrane between the poles to generate the two daughter cells. The following section of this chapter will focus on some of the initial events involved in mitosis, namely how chromosome organization is controlled, and the mechanism by which the genetic material is segregated to the poles of the cell. Once again, the activity of a number of kinases, including cyclin–CDK complexes, represents the main driving force for cell cycle progression, and will be outlined in further detail below.

Control of mitotic cyclin-CDK activity

In multicellular organisms, mitotic entry is regulated primarily by two cyclins and their CDK partners. The first cyclin–CDK complex has already been active during S phase, but will be degraded as mitosis progresses. It is involved in regulating early mitotic events such as chromosome condensation [6, 37]. The second and perhaps the most important cyclin–CDK complex for driving mitotic events consists of cyclin B and CDK1, and forms as cells progress through G2. This complex has a number of important roles throughout mitosis, and as such its activity is tightly regulated [6, 37].

The activity of CDK1, like most CDKs, is regulated by the binding of its cyclin partner. However, cyclin B-CDK1 complexes initially remain inactive as an enzyme due to an inhibitory phosphorylation event that exists on the CDK1 subunit (see 'CDK activity is regulated by a variety of mechanisms' 4 and Figure 4.1B) [7, 37]. As cells progress into mitosis, this inhibitory mark is removed by members of the Cdc25 phosphatase family, whose protein levels and activity rise markedly at this time. This control mechanism ensures that cyclin B-CDK1 activity is not triggered prematurely, which could result in inefficient segregation of the cell's genetic material.

The cellular localization of cyclin B and its CDK partner are also regulated throughout the cell cycle [6, 37, 38]. As cyclin B levels rise in G2, it is localized exclusively in the cytoplasm, but as mitosis progresses, cyclin B-CDK1 is rapidly relocated to the nucleus, where it is involved in promoting nuclear envelope breakdown [6, 37, 38]. This change in cyclin B-CDK1 localization is governed by the relative rates of the protein's nuclear import and export, and this balance is skewed towards import during early mitosis. Again, this results from phosphorylation events—only this time they occur on the cyclin subunit rather than the CDK itself [39, 40].

Involvement of other mitotic kinases

Several other kinases in addition to CDKs are activated at the onset of mitosis and help coordinate early mitotic events. The most important of these are two families of kinases known as the Polo-like kinases (Plk) and the Aurora kinases (Figure 4.1A). Plk protein levels rise in early mitosis as a result of increased gene expression and remain elevated till the end of mitosis, when the APC complex becomes active and targets Plk for degradation [40, 41]. Plk has a wide range of functions during M phase, being involved in activities such as chromatid separation and the formation of daughter cells [40, 41] (discussed later). Like Plk, Aurora kinase protein levels also rise during mitosis, and they function in regulating many mitotic processes such as chromosome condensation [41, 42].

Chromosome condensation

After DNA replication, chromosomes exists as two tightly associated sister chromatids. These sisters are held together not only by extensive intertwining of their DNA, but also by a protein complex known as cohesin, which links the duplicated DNA molecules together [1, 43]. This helps the cell to organize its replicated genetic material, since without a certain degree of housekeeping the cell would simply contain an unordered mass of DNA. Nevertheless, attempting to separate the sister chromatids in this tangled state would likely lead to extensive DNA breakage. To remedy this situation the sister chromatids are compacted in a process known as chromosome condensation, and this is mediated by a large protein complex called condensin [44]. At the same time, the majority of the cohesin complex holding sister chromatids together is removed, which will permit the separation of sisters at a later stage of mitosis. Condensin activity and cohesin removal are both regulated by the combined activity of several enzymes, including cyclin–CDK complexes, Plk, and Aurora kinases [40, 42–44].

Assembly of the mitotic spindle

At the midpoint of M phase, known as metaphase, the condensed chromosome pairs will be aligned in an ordered fashion across the centre of the cell. Once this step is complete, the sister chromatids can then be separated and pulled to opposite poles of the cell, where they will subsequently be enveloped into two new daughter nuclei. This process requires the creation of an important structure within the cell, known as the mitotic spindle, and the attachment of sister chromatids to this spindle. Without this structure, the correct alignment of chromosomes will not take place, and sister chromatids cannot be segregated to opposite poles of the cell [1, 2]. While the spindle apparatus consists of hundreds of proteins, the fundamental machinery is the spindle microtubules, which are capable of attaching to chromatids and causing their transit through the cell. The mitotic spindle is assembled in early mitosis whilst chromosome condensation occurs, and mitotic spindles are bipolar in nature, each spindle pole being focused at a large multi-protein organelle known as the centrosome [45]. In G1, cells possess a single centrosome, but as they enter the cell cycle this structure becomes duplicated to form two tightly associated centrosomes [46]. Upon entry into mitosis, the centrosomes migrate to opposite poles of the cell and mediate formation of the bipolar mitotic spindle [45, 47] onto which the sister chromatids are eventually attached. Once again, all of these processes are regulated via phosphorylation events, mediated by a number of cyclin–CDK complexes and the Aurora and Polo-like kinases [45–47]. Once sister chromatid separation is complete and the cell has divided, each daughter cell will once again possesses a single centrosome.

Breakdown of the nuclear envelope

In animal cells the nuclear envelope must be removed to allow the mitotic spindle, which exists in the cytoplasm, to gain access to the sister chromatids, which exist in the nucleus. Breakdown of the nuclear envelope requires the disassembly of a number of large protein complexes, which exist both within and attached to the surfaces of the nuclear membranes. This process again likely involves the activity of cyclin B–CDK1, since phosphorylation of the subunits of many structural membrane complexes causes their disassembly from the nuclear envelope [48]. This dismantling process results in a loss of overall nuclear envelope structure, and eventually the nuclear membrane will disperse completely. After mitosis is complete, nuclear membrane proteins are resorted into membranes to reform the nuclear envelope around the segregated chromosomes, a process that is thought to involve the reversal of cyclin B–CDK1 phosphorylation events [48].

Regulation of late mitotic events

After chromosomes have been compacted and attached to the mitotic spindle, they are arranged at the centre of the cell by forces pulling through the microtubules. The cell is now at metaphase, and late mitotic events will lead to the separation and segregation of the sister chromatids. During anaphase, sister chromatid cohesion is destroyed and the sisters separate until finally, in telophase, the mitotic spindle is disassembled and segregated chromosomes are repackaged into daughter nuclei. The metaphase-to-anaphase transition is one of the major cell cycle checkpoints in the cell and is initiated by a process that involves the destruction of several regulatory proteins by the APC. The dephosphorylation of CDK targets is also an important step in driving the late events of mitosis [49, 50], and together, these two processes help reset the cell cycle control system to its original G1 state.

The activation of APC is essential for anaphase

The APC is a large complex of subunit proteins whose main function in the cell is to trigger the transition from metaphase to anaphase, by tagging specific proteins for degradation via the process of ubiquitination (see 'CDK activity is regulated by a variety of mechanisms'). The activity of APC is regulated by the association of specific activator subunits, which target the APC to specific sets of substrates at different times in the cell cycle. During mitosis, the activator Cdc20 associates with APC, and this complex has numerous targets that function to regulate the completion of M phase. The proteins of most importance to get targeted for degradation by APC are the S- and M-phase cyclins, and a protein known as securin [14]. Securin is a protein which binds to and inhibits a protease known as separase, which in turn is responsible for promoting separation of sister chromatids during mitosis. The destruction of securin by the APC therefore enables chromatid cohesion to be disrupted and permits efficient segregation of sisters at anaphase [43] (Figure 4.1A). In addition to securin, the APC also targets the mitotic cyclins themselves. By promoting cyclin destruction, APC activity effectively inactivates CDK enzymes, which require their cyclin partners to function [14]. The loss of CDK activity subsequently permits the dephosphorylation of CDK targets [50], and this step is an important requirement for many late mitotic events, such as breakdown of the mitotic spindle and nuclear envelope reassembly.

Another APC activator subunit, known as Cdh1, also plays an important role during late M phase, when it functions to target APC activity towards proteins such as the Aurora and Polo-like kinases, which are not targets for Cdc20-containing APC. Destruction of these additional mitotic kinases at the end of M phase helps the cell to reset its cell cycle control machinery to a state that is found in G1 [14].

The spindle checkpoint

Accurate sister chromatid segregation requires that all sister pairs be correctly attached to microtubules originating from both poles of the mitotic spindle before they are separated. This requirement is monitored by the spindle checkpoint system, which only permits anaphase to occur once bi-orientation is attained. In this way, it acts to prevent the mis-segregation of genetic material to daughter cells that would result if the mitotic spindle attempted to separate inappropriately attached sister chromatids. The spindle checkpoint functions by preventing the activation of the APC, and whilst APC activity is held in check, the protein securin can continue to inhibit sister chromatid segregation [51]. However, once microtubules from each pole have successfully attached to the sister chromatids, the 'stop' signal generated by the spindle checkpoint system is silenced, and APC activity will drive the cell into anaphase.

Dephosphorylation of CDK targets is required for completion of anaphase and telophase

Although disruption of sister chromatid cohesion is required for chromosome segregation, normal chromosome movement towards each cell pole during anaphase requires regulated changes to microtubule behaviour (i.e. they need to be instructed to 'pull'). The activity of proteins involved in these processes is controlled in a cell-cycle-dependent fashion by their CDK-dependent phosphorylation in early mitosis and their subsequent dephosphorylation in anaphase once mitotic cyclins have been destroyed [49, 50]. After sister chromatids have been segregated to opposite poles of the cell, they need to be packaged into new daughter nuclei. The mitotic spindle is also disassembled at this time, and compacted chromosomes begin to decondense. Once again, the main driving force of these changes is dephosphorylation of CDK targets resulting from the degradation of cyclins and the inactivation of CDKs, particularly CDK1 [49, 50].

The DNA damage response

Every cell in the body is equipped to respond to the harmful effects of DNA damage, which can occur in a variety of ways in response to factors such as chemical changes or exposure to radiation. This DNA damage can result in gene mutations that impact on essential cellular processes and alter the cell's behaviour in a way that threatens the survival of the organism. The damage received by DNA can take many forms, ranging from small changes in base composition to breaks in both strands of the double helix [1, 52]. Such damage is recognized by sensor proteins that can recruit other enzymes to repair the DNA [52–54]. If the damage is extensive these sensors can also trigger the DNA damage response, which transmits signals to a number of effector proteins involved in transcription of genes involved in DNA repair. Alternatively, these effectors can lead to the activation of cell cycle checkpoints that cause cell cycle arrest [53, 55]. If the damage is subsequently repaired, the cell is permitted to re-enter the cell cycle. In multicellular organisms, however, extensive DNA damage results in a permanent cell cycle arrest or removal of the cell by apoptosis [53, 55].

In all eukaryotes, two protein kinases called ATM and ATR play a central role in the response to DNA damage. These proteins bind chromosomes at the damage site in combination with a number of other sensor proteins that assemble a platform upon which DNA repair complexes can be recruited [56–58]. Association of ATM and ATR with damaged DNA switches on their kinase activity and results in the phosphorylation of downstream targets (Figure 4.2). These initiate a number of signalling pathways that inhibit cell cycle progression and stimulate the expression of genes involved in DNA repair. For example, ATM and ATR activate E2F family members and the tumour-suppressor protein p53, which together trigger the expression of many genes involved in apoptosis or cell cycle arrest [59–61]. Mutations in DNA-damage-responsive components such as ATM, ATR, and p53 generally result in an increase in the accumulation of damaged DNA in cells, which leads to an increased risk of developing diseases such as cancer [54].

The regulation of p53 and E2F-1 activity

In a multicellular organism, a cell with severely damaged DNA can represent a threat to the survival of the organism as a whole. It is therefore important to prevent badly damaged cells from proliferating by arresting them permanently or removing them via apoptosis. The p53 protein plays an integral role in this response

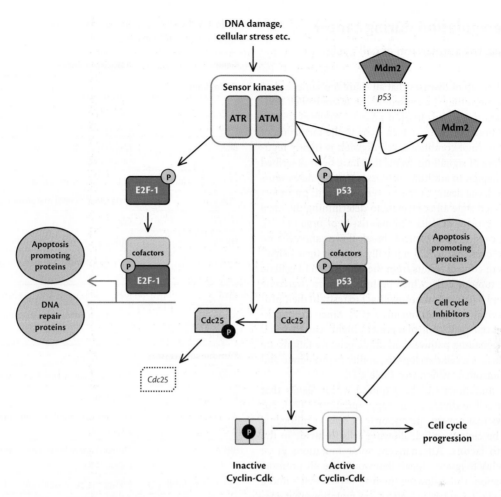

Fig. 4.2 The DNA damage response. DNA damage received throughout the cell cycle leads to the activation of the sensor kinases ATM and ATR. These kinases have a number of cellular targets including the Cdc25 family of phosphatases. Cyclin–CDK activity is therefore blocked, since inhibitory phosphorylation events on the CDK are not removed, and this prevents cell cycle progression. ATM and ATR are also capable of activating and stabilizing p53, by disrupting the Mdm2-p53 interaction. This promotes p53 activity, which is to drive the expression of genes involved in cell cycle arrest and apoptosis. Damage responsive kinases can also target the E2F-1 transcription factor, promoting its interaction with proteins that enhance E2F transcriptional activity. E2F-1 regulates the expression of several genes involved in cell death and DNA repair. (Activatory phosphorylation [P] events are displayed in yellow, whilst inhibitory phosphorylation events are shown in black.)

to DNA damage, illustrated by the fact that the p53 protein is inactivated in at least half of all cancers described. In the absence of functional p53, the DNA damage response is compromised, resulting in the accumulation of gene mutations that enhance the likelihood that cancer will develop [54, 62]. p53 is activated in response to several forms of DNA damage or cellular stress, and its function is tightly regulated by a number of modifications which result in its increased concentration and transcriptional activity [60, 63].

The major regulator of p53 is a protein known as Mdm2, which can tag p53 with ubiquitin and target the protein for destruction [63, 64]. In the absence of DNA damage, Mdm2 binds to p53 and keeps its concentration and activity low in cells (Figure 4.2). However, when DNA damage occurs, the activity of Mdm2 is reduced, which permits the stabilization of p53 protein levels and helps drive transcription of DNA-damage-responsive genes [63, 64]. p53 acetylation also helps to stabilize p53 protein levels after damage [65–67], and phosphorylation of p53 by kinases such as ATM helps to promote interactions with cofactors that drive transcription of DNA-damage-responsive genes [68, 69].

Like p53, a number of E2F family members are also known to be responsive to events that damage DNA. E2F-1, in particular, seems to be activated in response to stress, and once again, modifications of the protein seem to be important for driving its activity [70–75]. For example, ATM and ATR are both known to target E2F-1 directly (Figure 4.2) [70, 72], and as with p53, these modifications stabilize E2F-1 protein levels and promote interactions with other transcriptional cofactors that drive expression of genes involved in apoptosis and DNA repair [73, 76].

The DNA damage response and cell cycle arrest

Whilst DNA damage can be sustained at any point during the cell cycle, the outcome to this damage is usually the same: the cell either arrests during its current cell cycle stage to halt proliferation whilst the damage is repaired, or if the damage is extensive, the cell will be removed from the organism by apoptosis. These events are triggered by the activation of DNA-damage sensing kinases such as ATM and ATR, which initiate a number of signalling events that enforce cell cycle checkpoints (Figure 4.2).

Cell cycle deregulation during cancer

Mutations cause the subversion of cell cycle checkpoints

Cancer is a broad group of diseases that all share the same underlying property: namely, they are caused by the uncontrolled division of cells. This unregulated division process produces a mass of cells within an organ or tissue, which leads to the formation of a tumour. Under normal conditions, cell division is tightly regulated by the plethora of signalling events that have been described throughout this chapter. In addition, processes that regulate events such as cell survival, cell death, or the conversion of cells into a terminally differentiated state all contribute to determining the ideal number, size, and growth of cells within a tissue or organ [1, 2]. However, during cancer, such controls break down, and cells no longer respond to cues that would normally regulate their behavior [77]. This loss of control results from the acquisition of genetic mutations within tumour cells, which permits them to overcome the checkpoints and barriers that normally act to restrain their proliferation and survival within an organism [77]. Since the checkpoints that govern cell cycle control represent highly complex and often redundant signalling pathways, multiple gene mutations are usually required before a cell develops the ability to proliferate and spread in an uncontrolled fashion (see Table 4.1).

Initially, these mutations will be acquired within genes that enable the cancer cell to divide at an inappropriate rate [77]. For example, pathways that govern the response of cells to mitogenic signalling might be circumvented, allowing cells to divide in the absence of growth factors. Alternatively, some mutations grant cancer cells an ability to ignore signals that would usually promote cellular differentiation, thus allowing them to bypass entry into a non-dividing state [77]. Cancer cells also carry mutations that enable them to survive in conditions that would usually trigger cell death [77, 78], such as in response to DNA damage, meaning that they can escape the normal controls that act to remove potentially damaging cells from the body. Loss of p53 function, for example, is an incredibly common feature found in almost all tumour cells, and this event can impact on cell death since many p53 responsive genes are involved in cell cycle arrest and apoptosis [62, 79].

Mutations, therefore, play a key role in tumour evolution. Whilst a small fraction of these cancer-promoting mutations are inherited and associated with familial disease, most are acquired spontaneously as a result of natural errors during the replication, segregation or repair of DNA [1, 2]. These errors usually occur at a very low frequency, but mutation rates can be accelerated in response to environmental triggers that damage DNA, or in cells that have acquired mutations in genes that regulate the cell cycle control machinery [77, 80, 81] (see Chapter 8 on 'Genetic Instability').

Mutations in oncogenes and tumour suppressors

Throughout this chapter a large number of proteins have been highlighted, and their roles in cell cycle control described. Most of these proteins will fall into two groups: those that positively regulate entry and progression through the cell cycle, and those that function to halt it. The genes that encode these proteins are known as proto-oncogenes and tumour suppressor genes respectively, and both are frequently mutated in many forms of cancer [1, 2].

Proto-oncogenes can be converted to their cancer-promoting oncogenic form by a variety of mechanisms, but all lead to the

Table 4.1 Examples of oncogenes and tumour suppressor genes frequently mutated in cancer

Gene	Associated disease
Oncogenes	
ABL	CML, ALL
AKT	Ovarian, pancreatic cancers
BRAF	Melanoma, colorectal, thyroid, borderline ovarian cancers, NSCLC
CCND1 (Cyclin D1)	CLL, B-ALL, breast cancer
CDK4	Melanoma, familial malignant melanoma
EGFR	Glioma
HRAS	Infrequent sarcomas, rare other types
KRAS	Pancreatic, colorectal, lung, thyroid cancers, AML, others
MYC	Burkitt lymphoma, B-CLL, others
NRAS	Melanoma, MM, AML, thyroid cancer
PDGFR	GIST, AML, CML
Tumour suppressors	
ATM	T-PLL, leukaemia, lymphoma, ataxia telangiectasia
BCL2	NHL, CLL
BLM	Leukaemia, lymphoma, skin squamous cell, Bloom syndrome
BRCA1	Ovarian cancer, breast cancer, inherited ovarian and breast cancer
CDKN2A (p16INK4A)	Melanoma, pancreatic cancer, multiple other
NBS1	Glioma, medulloblastoma, Nijmegen breakage syndrome
PTEN	Glioma, prostatic, endometrial cancers, Cowden syndrome
RB1 (pRb)	Retinoblastoma, sarcoma, breast, small-cell lung cancer
TP53 (p53)	Breast, colorectal, lung, adrenocortical cancer, glioma, sarcoma, many others, Li–Fraumeni syndrome

ALL, acute lymphocytic leukaemia; AML, acute myelogenous leukaemia; B-ALL, B-cell acute lymphocytic leukaemia; B-CLL, B-cell lymphocytic leukaemia; CLL, chronic lymphocytic leukaemia; CML, chronic myeloid leukaemia; GIST, gastrointestinal stromal tumour; MM, multiple myeloma; NHL, non-Hodgkin lymphoma; NSCLC, non-small-cell lung cancer; T-PLL, T-cell prolymphocytic leukaemia.

overproduction or hyperactivity of the protein in question [1, 2]. Errors in DNA replication or DNA repair, for example, can lead to the acquisition of point mutations that lock cell signalling proteins in their active states, or promote the enzymatic activity of kinases. Alternatively, amplification of entire genes can lead to the production of a normal cellular protein at abnormal levels [1, 2]. This amplification could result from chromosomal segregation defects or errors in events that take place during DNA repair [81]. Chromosomal rearrangements such as this can also lead to a situation where the coding sequence of one gene comes under the control of another gene's promoter. A perfect example of this occurs with Burkitt lymphoma, where a chromosome translocation leads to the overproduction of a transcription factor that functions to drive the uncontrolled proliferation of lymphoid cells [82].

Mutations in tumour suppressor genes usually cause a loss of function; quite often, both alleles of the gene will need to be ablated [1, 2]. Again, this can occur by single point mutations, but often involves large deletions of the tumour suppressor genes themselves, resulting in the loss of large regions of the proteins they encode. For example, the loss of chromosomal regions containing genes encoding for CKIs such as p16 are common mutations found in many cancers [83]. In some cases, mutations in one allele of a tumour suppressor gene can be inherited, meaning an individual is more prone to develop a particular familial cancer disease [84]. Inherited mutations in one allele of the RB gene, for example, make individuals more prone to develop retinoblastoma, since complete loss of gene function now only requires the loss of the remaining normal allele [79, 84].

Conclusion

In every cell there is a complex combination of cell signalling pathways and checkpoint controls, which together constitute the highly conserved network of events that we collectively identify as the cell cycle control machinery. Progression of cells through the cell cycle involves the activity of a plethora of proteins that either permit or restrain advancement to the next stage, and it is this ordered set of events that culminates in the coordination observed between cell growth and division. Many of these cell cycle regulators become mutated in tumours, resulting in a breakdown of cell cycle control which permits cells to proliferate in an uncontrolled fashion—arguably the most fundamental hallmark of cancer.

Acknowledgements

Work in our laboratory is supported by CRUK, MRC, LRF, AICR, EU, and the Oxford NIHR Musculoskeletal Biomedical Research Unit.

Further reading

Bell SP, Dutta A. DNA replication in eukaryotic cells. Annual Review of Biochemistry. 2002; 71: 333–374.

DeGregori J, Johnson DG. Distinct and overlapping roles for E2F family members in transcription, proliferation and apoptosis. Current Molecular Medicine 2006, 6: 739–748.

Giacinti C, Giordano A. RB and cell cycle progression. Oncogene 2006; 25: 5220–5227.

Hanahan D, Weinberg RA. Hallmarks of cancer: The next generation. Cell 2011; 144: 646–674.

Jackson SP, Bartek J. The DNA-damage response in human biology and disease. Nature 2009, 461: 1071–1078.

Lindqvist A, Rodríguez-Bravo V, Medema R. The decision to enter mitosis: feedback and redundancy in the mitotic entry network. Journal of Cell Biology 2009; 185: 193–202.

Malumbres M, Barbacid M. Mammalian cyclin-dependent kinases. Trends in Biochemical Sciences 2005; 30: 630–641.

Neganova I, Lako M. G1 to S phase cell cycle transition in somatic and embryonic stem cells. Journal of Anatomy 2008; 213: 30–44.

Rieder CL. Mitosis in vertebrates: the G2/M and M/A transitions and their associated checkpoints. Chromosome Research 2011; 19: 291–306.

Sullivan M, Morgan DO. Finishing mitosis, one step at a time. Nature Reviews Molecular Cell Biology 2007; 8: 894–903.

References

1. Morgan DO. The Cell Cycle: Principles of Control. London: New Science Press, 2007.
2. Weinberg RA. The Biology of Cancer. New York: Garland Science, 2006.
3. Bell SP, Dutta A. DNA replication in eukaryotic cells. Annual Review of Biochemistry 2002; 71: 333–374.
4. Diffley JF. Regulation of early events in chromosome replication. Current Biology 2004; 14: R778–786.
5. Neganova I, Lako M. G1 to S phase cell cycle transition in somatic and embryonic stem cells. Journal of Anatomy 2008; 213: 30–44.
6. Rieder CL. Mitosis in vertebrates: the G2/M and M/A transitions and their associated checkpoints. Chromosome Research 2011; 19: 291–306.
7. Malumbres M, Barbacid M. Mammalian cyclin-dependent kinases. Trends in Biochemical Sciences 2005; 30: 630–641.
8. Brown NR, Noble ME, Endicott JA, Johnson LN. The structural basis for specificity of substrate and recruitment peptides for cyclin-dependent kinases. Nature Cell Biology 1999; 1: 438–443.
9. Loog M. and Morgan D.O. Cyclin specificity in the phosphorylation of cyclin-dependent kinase substrates. Nature 2005, 434: 104–108
10. Giacinti C, Giordano A. RB and cell cycle progression. Oncogene 2006; 25: 5220–5227.
11. Tanaka S and Araki H. Regulation of the initiation step of DNA replication by cyclin-dependent kinases. Chromosoma 2010; 119: 565–574.
12. Vidal A. and Koff A. Cell-cycle inhibitors: three families united by a common cause. Gene 2000; 247: 1–15.
13. Nakayama KL and Nakayama K. Ubiquitin ligases: cell-cycle control and cancer. Nature Reviews Cancer 2006; 6: 369–381.
14. Castro A, Bernis C, Vigneron S, Labbé JC, Lorca T. The anaphase-promoting complex: a key factor in the regulation of cell cycle. Oncogene 2005; 24: 314–325.
15. Dimova DK, Dyson NJ. The E2F transcriptional network: old acquaintances with new faces. Oncogene 2005; 24: 2810–2826.
16. DeGregori J, Johnson DG. Distinct and overlapping roles for E2F family members in transcription, proliferation and apoptosis. Current Molecular Medicine 2006; 6: 739–748.
17. Polager S, Ginsberg D. E2F—at the crossroads of life and death. Trends in Cell Biology 2008; 18: 528–535.
18. Chen HZ, Tsai SY, Leone G. Emerging roles of E2Fs in cancer: an exit from cell cycle control. Nature Reviews Cancer 2009; 9: 785–797.
19. Macaluso M, Montanari M, Giordano A. Rb family proteins as modulators of gene expression and new aspects regarding the interaction with chromatin remodeling enzymes. Oncogene 2006; 25: 5263–5267.
20. Genovese C, Trani D, Caputi M, Claudio PP. Cell cycle control and beyond: emerging roles for the retinoblastoma gene family. Oncogene 2006; 25: 5201–5209.
21. Burkhart DL, Sage J. Cellular mechanisms of tumour suppression by the retinoblastoma gene. Nature Reviews Cancer 2008; 8: 671–682.
22. Connell-Crowley L, Harper JW, Goodrich DW. Cyclin D1/Cdk4 regulates retinoblastoma protein-mediated cell cycle arrest by site-specific phosphorylation. Molecular Biology of the Cell 1997; 8: 287–301.
23. Takaki T, Fukasawa K, Suzuki-Takahashi I, Semba K, Kitagawa M et al. Preferences for phosphorylation sites in the retinoblastoma protein of D-type cyclin-dependent kinases, Cdk4 and Cdk6, in vitro. Journal of Biochemistry 2005; 137: 381–386.
24. Ezhevsky SA, Ho A, Becker-Hapak M, Davis PK, Dowdy SF. Differential regulation of retinoblastoma tumor suppressor protein by G(1) cyclin-dependent kinase complexes in vivo. Molecular and Cellular Biology 2001; 21: 4773–4784.

25. Kitagawa M, Higashi H, Jung HK, Suzuki-Takahashi I, Ikeda M et al. The consensus motif for phosphorylation by cyclin D1-Cdk4 is different from that for phosphorylation by cyclin A/E-Cdk2. EMBO Journal 1996; 15: 7060–7069.

26. Chan HM, Krstic-Demonacos M, Smith L, Demonacos C, La Thangue NB. Acetylation control of the retinoblastoma tumour-suppressor protein. Nature Cell Biology 2001; 3: 667–674.

27. Carr SM, Munro S, Kessler B, Oppermann U, La Thangue NB. Interplay between lysine methylation and Cdk phosphorylation in growth control by the retinoblastoma protein. EMBO Journal 2011; 30: 317–327.

28. Markham D, Munro S, Soloway J, O'Connor DP, La Thangue NB. DNA-damage-responsive acetylation of pRb regulates binding to E2F-1. EMBO Report 2006; 7: 192–198.

29. Adhikary S, Eilers M. Transcriptional regulation and transformation by Myc proteins. Nature Reviews Molecular Cell Biology 2005; 6: 635–645.

30. Shaulian E, Karin M. AP-1 as a regulator of cell life and death. Nature Cell Biology 2002; 4: E131-E136.

31. Kamura T, Hara T, Matsumoto M, Ishida N, Okumura F. Cytoplasmic ubiquitin ligase KPC regulates proteolysis of p27^{Kip1} at G1 phase. Nature Cell Biology 2004; 6: 1229–1235.

32. Hao B, Zheng N, Schulman BA, Wu G, Miller JJ et al. Structural basis of the Cks1-dependent recognition of p27^{Kip1} by the SCF^{Skp2} ubiquitin ligase. Molecular Cell 2005; 20: 9–19.

33. Arias EE, Walter JC. Strength in numbers: preventing rereplication via multiple mechanisms in eukaryotic cells. Genes & Development 2007; 21: 497–518.

34. Li A, Blow JJ. Non-proteolytic inactivation of geminin requires CDK-dependent ubiquitination. Nature Cell Biology 2004; 6: 260–267.

35. Labib K. How do Cdc7 and cyclin-dependent kinases trigger the initiation of chromosome replication in eukaryotic cells? Genes & Development 2010; 24: 1208–1219.

36. Nguyen VQ, Co C, Li JJ. Cyclin-dependent kinases prevent DNA re-replication through multiple mechanisms. Nature 2001; 411: 1068–1073.

37. Lindqvist A, Rodríguez-Bravo V, Medema R. The decision to enter mitosis: feedback and redundancy in the mitotic entry network. Journal of Cell Biology 2009; 185: 193–202.

38. Takizawa CG, Morgan DO. Control of mitosis by changes in the sub-cellular location of cyclin-B1-Cdk1 and Cdc25C. Current Opinion in Cell Biology 2000; 12: 658–665.

39. Toyoshima-Morimoto F, Taniguchi E, Shinya N, Iwamatsu A, Nishida E. Polo-like kinase 1 phosphorylates cyclin B1 and targets it to the nucleus during prophase. Nature 2001; 410: 215–220.

40. Archambault V, Glover DM. Polo-like kinases: conservation and divergence in their functions and regulation. Nature Reviews Molecular Cell Biology 2009; 10: 265–275.

41. Malumbres M. Physiological relevance of cell cycle kinases. Physiological Reviews 2011; 91: 973–1007.

42. Vader G, Lens SM. The Aurora kinase family in cell division and cancer. Biochimica et Biophysica Acta 2008; 1786: 60–72.

43. Nasmyth K, Haering CH. Cohesin: its roles and mechanisms. Annual Review of Genetics 2009; 43: 525–558.

44. Hirano T. Condensins: organizing and segregating the genome. Current Biology 2005; 15: R265-R275.

45. Walczak CE, Heald R. Mechanisms of mitotic spindle assembly and function. International Review of Cytology 2008; 265: 111–158.

46. Tsou M-FB, Stearns T. Controlling centrosome number: licenses and blocks. Current Opinion in Cell Biology 2006; 18: 74–78.

47. Tanenbaum ME, Medema RH. Mechanisms of centrosome separation and bipolar spindle assembly. Developmental Cell 2010; 19: 797–806.

48. Burke B, Ellenberg J. Remodelling the walls of the nucleus. Nature Reviews Molecular Cell Biology 2002; 3: 487–497.

49. Sullivan M, Morgan DO. Finishing mitosis, one step at a time. Nature Reviews Molecular Cell Biology 2007; 8: 894–903.

50. Bollen M, Gerlich DW, Lesage B. Mitotic phosphatases: from entry guards to exit guides. Trends in Cell Biology 2009; 19: 531–541.

51. Musacchio A, Salmon ED. The spindle-assembly checkpoint in space and time. Nature Reviews Molecular Cell Biology 2007; 8: 379–393.

52. Ciccia A, Elledge SJ. The DNA damage response: making it safe to play with knives. Molecular Cell 2010; 40: 179–204.

53. Su TT. Cellular responses to DNA damage: one signal, multiple choices. Annual Review of Genetics 2006; 40: 187–208.

54. Jackson SP, Bartek J. The DNA-damage response in human biology and disease. Nature 2009; 461: 1071–1078.

55. Clarke PR, Allan LA. Cell-cycle control in the face of damage—a matter of life or death. Trends in Cell Biology 2009; 19: 89–98.

56. Smith J, Tho LM, Xu N, Gillespie DA. The ATM-Chk2 and ATR-Chk1 pathway in DNA damage signaling and cancer. Advances in Cancer Research. 2010; 108: 73–112.

57. Bhatti S, Kozlov S, Farooqi AA, Naqi A, Lavin M et al. ATM protein kinase: the linchpin of cellular defences to stress. Cellular and Molecular Life Sciences 2011; 68: 2977–3006.

58. Cimprich KA, Cortez D. ATR: an essential regulator of genome integrity. Nature Reviews Molecular Cell Biology 2008; 9: 616–627.

59. Polager S, Ginsberg D. p53 and E2F: partners in life and death. Nature Reviews Cancer 2009; 9: 738–748.

60. Harris SL, and Levine AJ. The p53 pathway: positive and negative feedback loops. Oncogene 2005; 24: 2899–2908.

61. Meek DW. Tumour suppression by p53: a role for the DNA damage response? Nature Reviews Cancer 2009; 9: 714–723.

62. Rivlin N, Brosh R, Oren M, Rotter V. Mutations in the p53 tumor suppressor gene: important milestones at the various steps of tumorigenesis. Genes Cancer 2011; 2: 466–474.

63. Dai C, Gu W. p53 post-translational modification: deregulated in tumorigenesis. Trends in Molecular Medicine 2010; 16: 528–536.

64. Fuchs SY, Adler V, Buschmann T, Wu X, Ronai Z. Mdm2 association with p53 targets its ubiquitination. Oncogene 1998; 17: 2543–2547.

65. Gu W, Roeder RG. Activation of p53 sequence-specific DNA binding by acetylation of the p53 C-terminal domain. Cell 1997; 90: 595–606.

66. Liu L, Scolnick DM, Trievel RC, Zhang HB, Marmorstein R, et al. p53 sites acetylated in vitro by PCAF and p300 are acetylated in vivo in response to DNA damage. Molecular and Cellular Biology 1999; 19: 1202–1209.

67. Li M, Luo J, Brooks CL, Gu W. Acetylation of p53 inhibits its ubiquitination by Mdm2. Journal of Biological Chemistry 2002; 277: 50607–50611.

68. Lambert PF, et al. Phosphorylation of p53 serine 15 increases interaction with CBP. Journal of Biological Chemistry 1998; 273: 33048–33053.

69. Hirao A. et al. DNA damage-induced activation of p53 by the checkpoint kinase Chk2. Science 2000; 287: 1824–1827.

70. Lin WC, Kashanchi F, Radonovich MF, Shiekhattar R, Brady JN. Selective induction of E2F1 in response to DNA damage, mediated by ATM-dependent phosphorylation. Genes & Development 2001; 15: 1833–1844.

71. Stevens C, Smith L, La Thangue NB. Chk2 activates E2F-1 in response to DNA damage. Nature Cell Biology 2003; 5: 401–409.

72. Blattner C, Sparks A, Lane D. Transcription factor E2F-1 is upregulated in response to DNA damage in a manner analogous to that of p53. Molecular Cell Biology 1999; 19: 3704–3713.

73. Biswas AK, Johnson DG. Transcriptional and nontranscriptional functions of E2F1 in response to DNA damage. Cancer Research 2012; 72: 13–17.

74. Cho EC, Zheng S, Munro S, Liu G, Carr SM et al. Arginine methylation controls growth regulation by E2F-1. EMBO Journal 2012; 31: 1785–1797.

75. Kontaki H, Talianidis I. Lysine methylation regulates E2F1-induced cell death. Molecular Cell; 2010; 39: 152–160.

76. Milton AH, Khaire N, Ingram L, O'Donnell AJ, La Thangue NB. 14-3-3 proteins integrate E2F activity with the DNA damage response. EMBO Journal 2006; 25: 1046–1057.

77. Hanahan D, Weinberg RA. Hallmarks of cancer: The next generation. Cell 2011; 144: 646–674.

78. Kelly G, Strasser A. The essential role of evasion from cell death in cancer. Advances in Cancer Research 2011; 111: 39–96.

79. Sherr CJ, McCormick F. The RB and p53 pathways in cancer. Cancer Cell 2002; 2: 103–112.

80. Negrini S, Gorgoulis VG, Halazonetis TD. Genomic instability—an evolving hallmark of cancer. Nature Reviews Molecular Cell Biology 2010; 11: 220–228.

81. Gordon DJ, Resio B, Pellman D. Causes and consequences of aneuploidy in cancer. Nature Reviews Genetics 2012; 13: 189–203.

82. Janz S. Myc translocations in B cell and plasma cell neoplasms. DNA Repair 2006; 5: 1213–1224.

83. Kim WY, Sharpless NE. The regulation of INK4/ARF in cancer and aging. Cell 2006; 127: 265–275.

84. Garber JE, Offit K. Hereditary cancer predisposition syndromes. Journal of Clinical Oncology 2005; 23: 276–292.

CHAPTER 5

Cancer cell death

Amanda S. Coutts, Sandra Maniam, and Nicholas B. La Thangue

Introduction to cancer cell death

A defining feature of cancer cells is their uncontrolled proliferation and ability to overcome cell death mechanisms [1]. As most cancer treatments rely on the induction of cell death pathways, understanding how cancer cells circumvent these pathways is important in the development of novel therapeutic agents. Morphologically and biochemically, at least three types of cell death have been defined: apoptosis (type I), autophagy (type II), and necrosis (type III). This chapter will outline these three types of programmed cancer cell death and detail some of the specific pathways involved, highlighting the clinical relevance where appropriate.

Apoptosis

Apoptosis is a ubiquitous, energy-consuming form of cell suicide triggered and orchestrated by a defined set of molecular events. The term apoptosis was first used in 1972 by Kerr, Currie, and Wyllie, who described the main morphological features [2]. Thirty years later, Brenner, Horvitz, and Sulston received the Nobel Prize in Physiology and Medicine for unravelling some of the fundamental aspects of the biology of apoptosis using the nematode *Caenorhabditis elegans* as a model system [3]. Apoptosis can be triggered by either mitochondrial-dependent mechanisms or by ligand binding to cell surface death receptors (Figure 5.1). As such, apoptosis can be stimulated by a variety of internal and external stimuli and can be divided into the intrinsic and extrinsic pathways [4].

Caspases

Caspases are a family of cysteine proteases which orchestrate apoptotic execution pathways through proteolytic cleavage of target proteins. Caspases are initially synthesized as inactive precursors (procaspases) that are rapidly converted to active proteases upon induction of apoptosis. The caspases can be divided into two groups: initiators (caspase-8, -9, and -10) and effectors (also known as executioners; caspase-3, -6, -7). The caspases activate each other via cleavage leading to amplification of the signalling cascade. Of note, caspase-8 is essential for the extrinsic apoptosis pathway, while caspase-9 is necessary for the intrinsic signalling pathway. Both of these pathways converge on caspase-3 which is the predominant effector caspase involved in the cleavage of signalling components that effect the morphologic changes associated with apoptosis [5].

Hallmarks of apoptosis

Caspases cleave a number of cytoplasmic and nuclear substrates resulting in many of the morphological features associated with apoptosis. Proteolysis of cytoskeletal and nuclear proteins results in cell and nuclear shrinkage, leading to membrane blebbing as a consequence of a weakened cytoskeleton. One of the first biochemical hallmarks of apoptosis to be identified was the degradation of genomic DNA into ladder fragments as a result of endonuclease-mediated chromatin cleavage. Other classic hallmarks of apoptosis are condensed chromatin and nuclear fragmentation [6]. The cells eventually fragment into apoptotic bodies which are consumed by phagocytes with a minimal production of pro-inflammatory cytokines [6].

Intrinsic apoptosis

The intrinsic apoptosis pathway is tightly regulated by the Bcl-2 (B-cell lymphoma 2) family of proteins and is mainly activated by internal stimuli emanating from cellular damage sensors or physicochemical alterations produced by stressed cells (e.g., reactive oxygen species (ROS) or DNA damage; Figure 5.1). Mitochondria play a fundamental role in the intrinsic pathway of apoptosis by releasing key effector proteins such as cytochrome c and SMAC (second mitochondria derived activator). The release of effector proteins is a consequence of compromised integrity of the mitochondrial outer membrane by a process known as mitochondrial outer membrane permeabilization (MOMP). This release initiates caspase activation in the cytosol leading to caspase-mediated proteolysis of target proteins [6].

The Bcl-2 family members are grouped into two classes (Figure 5.1); the anti-apoptotic (e.g., Bcl-2, Bcl-xL, Bcl-w, and Mcl-1) and the pro-apoptotic (e.g., Bax, Bak, PUMA) proteins. The two pro-apoptotic family members Bax and Bak have been shown to be required for activation of the intrinsic apoptotic pathway [7]. Upon activation, Bax and Bak oligomerize within the outer mitochondrial membrane. The oligomers form pores in the mitochondrial outer membrane leading to MOMP [8]. Anti-apoptotic members bind to and inhibit Bax and Bak. Additional pro-apoptotic members, (BH3 only proteins such as PUMA, Bid, and Bad; Figure 5.1), can promote MOMP by binding to and activating Bax and Bak or by inhibiting the anti-apoptotic members.

Thus, key control of MOMP occurs through interactions between pro- and anti-apoptotic Bcl-2 family members to control

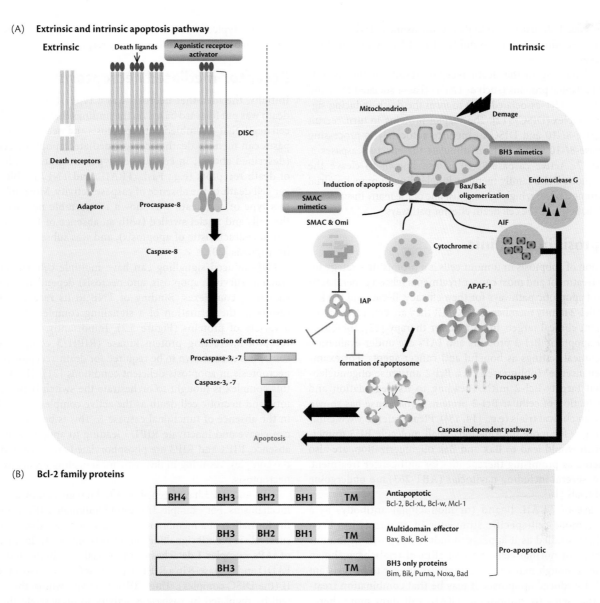

(A) **Extrinsic and intrinsic apoptosis pathway**

Extrinsic

Death ligands

Agonistic receptor activator

Intrinsic

Mitochondrion

Demage

DISC

Death receptors

BH3 mimetics

Adaptor

Procaspase-8

Induction of apoptosis

SMAC mimetics

Bax/Bak oligomerization

Endonuclease G

SMAC & Omi

AIF

Caspase-8

Cytochrome c

IAP

APAF-1

Activation of effector caspases

Procaspase-3, -7

formation of apoptosome

Caspase-3, -7

Procaspase-9

Apoptosis

Caspase independent pathway

(B) **Bcl-2 family proteins**

| BH4 | BH3 | BH2 | BH1 | TM | **Antiapoptotic** Bcl-2, Bcl-xL, Bcl-w, Mcl-1 |

| | BH3 | BH2 | BH1 | TM | **Multidomain effector** Bax, Bak, Bok |

| | BH3 | | | TM | **BH3 only proteins** Bim, Bik, Puma, Noxa, Bad |

Pro-apoptotic

Fig. 5.1 Apoptosis pathways. (A) Extrinsic and Intrinsic apoptosis. The extrinsic pathway is initiated by binding of ligands to death receptors, leading to the recruitment of adaptor proteins and caspase-8; This results in dimerization of caspase-8 which cleaves and activates the effector caspases. Intrinsic apoptosis stimuli activate Bcl-2 pro-apoptotic proteins such as Bax and Bak which promote MOMP. Following MOMP, soluble (blue circle) and insoluble (black circle) proteins are released to the cytosol. Cytochrome c binds to Apaf-1, inducing formation of the apoptosome which recruits procaspase-9; activated caspase-9 cleaves and activates executioner caspases leading to apoptosis. SMAC and OMI neutralize the inhibitory effect of IAP. AIF and endonuclease G translocate to the nucleus where they promote DNA fragmentation in a caspase-independent fashion. Promising clinical targets are labelled in green boxes. (B) Bcl-2 family proteins. The Bcl-2 family is comprised of anti-apoptotic and pro-apoptotic proteins that contain conserved functional Bcl-2 homology (BH) domains. The pro-apoptotic proteins can be subdivided into multi-domain and BH3-only proteins.

Bax and Bak oligomers leading to MOMP and release of proteins, like cytochrome c, into the cytosol. Once released into the cytosol, cytochrome c forms a complex referred to as the apoptosome which also contains caspase-9 and Apaf-1 (apoptotic protease activating factor 1). Caspase-9 is activated within the apoptosome, leading to cleavage and activation of the so-called executioner (or effector) caspases-3, -6, and -7 (Figure 5.1).

During apoptosis SMAC is also released from the mitochondria where it can activate apoptosis by relieving IAP (inhibitor of apoptosis protein) mediated inhibition of caspases [9]. MOMP also releases caspase-independent effectors such as apoptosis inducing factor (AIF) and endonuclease G. These proteins translocate to the

nuclear compartment where they promote DNA fragmentation and chromatin condensation [7].

Extrinsic apoptosis

The extrinsic pathway is activated via the binding of extracellular ligands to transmembrane death receptors and is mediated by members of the tumour necrosis factor (TNF) receptor superfamily (Figure 5.1; [10]). There are a number of well-characterized death receptors known to mediate apoptotic signalling including TNFR1 (TNF receptor 1), Fas, and TNF-related apoptosis inducing ligand (TRAIL) receptor 1 and 2 (TRAIL-R1/2) [11]. The death receptors contain a death domain (DD) in their cytoplasmic tail which facilitates the recruitment and assembly of multi-protein signalling complexes.

Ligand binding to the death receptor results in the recruitment of adaptor proteins (such as FADD (Fas-associated DD) and TRADD (TNFR1-associated DD) to form the death-inducing signalling complex (DISC) [12]. The adaptor proteins, in turn, recruit procaspase-8/-10 and DISC to mediate autocatalytic processing of caspase-8/-10 which in turn stimulate the effector caspases-3, -6, and -7. Active caspase-8/-10 is also known to cleave the pro-apoptotic Bcl-2 family member Bid, leading to mitochondrial cytochrome c release, highlighting just one of the many instances of cross-talk between the cell death effector pathways.

Apoptosis in the clinic

Activation of apoptosis in tumour cells is a promising strategy for cancer treatment and most cancer treatments rely on general activation of apoptotic pathways for their efficacy. Because of the key role of Bcl-2 family members in MOMP, they are considered to be important clinical targets in anti-cancer therapy [13]. Inhibitors of anti-apoptotic Bcl-2 proteins and IAPs are under evaluation in preclinical settings as hopeful anti-cancer agents. For example, Genansense® (oblimersen) is a Bcl-2 antisense oligonucleotide that targets Bcl-2 mRNA leading to its degradation and thus reduction of cellular Bcl-2 protein. Genansense has shown promise in clinical trials (e.g., [14, 15]). Please refer to www.clinicaltrials.gov for more information. Small molecule BH3 mimetics, which would lead to Bax and Bak oligomerization, are also considered as promising therapeutics for anti-cancer treatment. To date, several including navitoclax (ABT-263) are undergoing clinical trials [16].

The use of TRAIL ligand (or monoclonal antibody) as a potent tumour cell-specific stimulator of apoptosis has been intensively studied as it appears to induce apoptosis in tumour cells, but not normal cells. Several clinical trials have shown promise, although many human tumours appear to be resistant to TRAIL-induced apoptosis. It may be that combination treatments that sensitize tumours to TRAIL will show more therapeutic potential [17, 18].

Necrosis

Necrosis is a well-characterized form of cell death and was until recently thought to be largely accidental. While necrotic cell death is often associated with injury and trauma, such as ischaemia or exposure to toxins, it is also becoming increasingly clear that programmed necrosis (referred to hereafter as necroptosis) is an important cell death mechanism. Increasing evidence suggests that necroptosis relies on the induction of a variety of specific genes and signalling pathways (for example, see [19]).

Features of necrosis

Unlike apoptotic cells, necrotic cells do not fragment into discrete bodies. Instead, the induction of necrosis is associated with cell rounding, organelle and cell swelling, and a lack of chromatin condensation. This leads to an eventual increase in cell volume and rupture of the plasma membrane. In contrast to apoptosis, necrotic cell death typically proceeds in the absence of caspase activation and often promotes an inflammatory response.

Receptor-mediated necroptosis

Initially, the idea that necrosis was a type of programmed cell death was put forward based on the findings that TNF could cause cell death that resembled both apoptosis and necrosis. While caspases can mediate death-receptor-mediated apoptotic cell death (described above), in certain cell types treatment with ligands of death receptors (e.g., FasL, TRAIL, and TNF) is able to trigger cell death in the absence of caspase activity. Morphologically, this type of cell death was shown to resemble necrosis in that the cells and nuclei swelled (with an absence of DNA fragmentation characteristic of apoptosis), and was subsequently named necroptosis [20].

TNF-induced signalling can have multiple cellular outcomes (such as survival, apoptosis, and necrosis) dependent on distinct signalling complexes. Binding of TNF to its receptor, TNFR1, results in the formation of a signalling complex that contains a variety of proteins (Figure 5.2). Importantly, formation of a receptor-interacting protein kinase (RIP)1/3 complex (necrosome) has been shown to be required for death-receptor-mediated necroptosis in apoptosis-deficient conditions [21]. The activity of this complex is thought to orchestrate the switch between apoptotic and necrotic cell death as the active complex can only form in the absence of functional caspase-8. This is because caspase-8 can cleave and inactivate RIP1/3 leading to apoptosis; but in its absence, RIP1 and RIP3 are phosphorylated and activated within the complex, resulting in downstream signalling events to execute necroptosis.

RIP1 and RIP3 have been shown to be regulated by a variety of mechanisms. For example, IAP can ubiquitinate RIP1, resulting in the formation of a membrane-associated complex that favours cell survival via NF-κB signalling pathways (complex I). In the absence of IAPs, complex I detaches from the cell membrane and recruits FADD and caspase-8 in a RIP1-dependent fashion to form complex II (the DISC complex). Thus, RIP1/3 activity within this complex will be regulated by caspase-8 activity to orchestrate the switch between apoptosis or necroptosis.

Mediators of necrosis

Various agents such as pathogens, oxidative stress, ionizing radiation, DNA damage, and calcium overload can trigger necrotic cell death [22]. While in some cases the importance of RIP1/3 in this process is clear, precisely how necroptosis is executed downstream of RIP1/3 activation remains unclear.

Energy metabolism has been linked with necroptosis. Adenosine triphosphate (ATP) levels are an important determinant of whether cell death occurs via necrosis or apoptosis. This is because apoptosis demands energy in the form of ATP (which is immediately targeted by caspases), while necrosis can result from (and is thought to result in) ATP depletion. Activation of RIP3 can also result in the recruitment of metabolic enzymes to the RIP1/3 complex, leading to increased glycolysis and production of ROS. This suggests that ROS signalling may be involved in mediating necroptosis, and studies have shown that inhibition of ROS production can limit necroptotic cell death [23, 24].

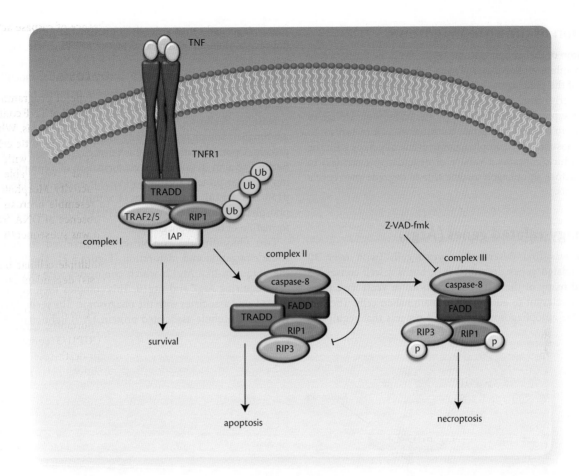

Fig. 5.2 TNF-induced necroptosis. TNFR1 activation results in recruitment of a TRADD containing complex I. IAP within this complex ubiquitinates (Ub) RIP1 leading to NF-κB signalling and cell survival. In the cytosolic complex II, FADD recruits and activates caspase-8 leading to cleavage of RIP1/3 and activation of apoptosis. In the absence of caspase-8 activity (e.g., Z-VAD-fmk), RIP1/3 are phosphorylated (p) and activated leading to necroptosis.

More recently, a complex containing RIP1 that is distinct from the TNF-induced complex, called the ripoptosome [25, 26], has been identified. This complex contains RIP1, FADD, and caspase-8, and, depending on the cell context, can promote apoptotic or necroptotic cell death. Interestingly, these studies suggest that this complex forms primarily in transformed cells, highlighting its potential importance in tumour cell death.

Necroptosis and cancer

Necrosis is commonly observed in human tumours and is also associated with chemotherapies and radiotherapies [21]. Importantly, the presence of necrotic cells can be a byproduct of other types of cell death and may not necessarily reflect the presence of programmed necrotic cell death. Currently there are no clear biomarkers for necroptosis, and in general necrotic cell death is identified by the absence of markers of apoptosis or autophagy. Several studies have examined necroptosis in the absence of apoptosis to identify signalling pathways that can impact on necroptosis [20, 27]. Interestingly, SMAC can inhibit IAPs, leading to the activation of RIP1, and small molecule mimetics of SMAC have been shown to prime apoptosis-resistant cells for necroptotic cell death in vitro [28]. It is likely that similar molecules may have clinical potential and could be exploited to target human cancers. As researchers gain a better understanding of the signalling molecules involved in programmed necrosis, this will no doubt open up therapeutic options and allow the development of compounds that effectively modulate necroptosis in a therapeutically beneficial manner.

Autophagy

Autophagy ('self-eating') is a catabolic process whereby cytosolic components and organelles are degraded in order to recycle key cellular materials. Autophagy is a constitutive process required for proper tissue homoeostasis but can be rapidly regulated by a variety of stimuli (e.g., nutrient starvation, pathogens, DNA damage, and hypoxia). Under normal conditions, cells undergo a basal level of autophagy, allowing the breakdown and recycling of long-lived or aggregated proteins, and damaged organelles. During times of metabolic stress and nutrient depletion, autophagy is an important mechanism by which cellular material is recycled to provide the biomaterials necessary for survival. For this reason autophagy is often thought of as a mechanism of tumour cell growth and survival, but unrestrained autophagy has been suggested to be an effective cell death inducer. At least three forms of autophagy have been described: macroautophagy, microautophagy, and chaperone-mediated autophagy, but in this chapter we will hereafter be using autophagy to relate primarily to macroautophagy.

Formation of the autophagosome

The formation of the autophagosome begins with the formation of a double membrane phagosome (Figure 5.3). In mammalian cells the origin of the phagosome is not entirely clear, but studies suggest it may derive from the endoplasmic reticulum, mitochondria, golgi, and the plasma membrane [29]. The phagosome elongates and encloses to engulf cytoplasmic constituents as it matures into the autophagosome. The autophagosome eventually fuses with the lysosome (which contains a variety of degradative enzymes) to become a mature autophagolysosome able to degrade and recycle its components.

Autophagy-related genes (Atgs)

Autophagy was first described in yeast cells (with over 30 autophagy-related genes described [6]), but is a well conserved process and many of the initial observations in yeast have been shown to be relevant to autophagy in mammalian cells. The formation of the autophagosome is a rapid process that requires a tightly regulated set of at least 18 mammalian proteins comprising several different complexes (Figure 5.3; [30, 31]). Signals feed into autophagosome formation via the ULK complex (unc-51-like kinases) which, along with Atg9, is recruited independently to the autophagosome formation site. These are required for the recruitment of the class III phosphatidylinositol-3-kinase (PI3K) complex containing Beclin 1 (Atg6). Beclin 1 is an important initiator of mammalian autophagy, originally identified as a Bcl-2 interacting protein. Upon starvation, Bcl-2 is released from Beclin 1, allowing Beclin 1 to activate autophagy via formation of a complex containing vacuolar protein sorting 34 (Vps34; a class III PI3K), Vps15/p150 and Atg14L (Barkor). Vps34 within this complex generates phosphatidylinositol 3-phosphate (PI3P) which is important for formation of the autophagosome.

Two ubiquitin-like complexes are involved in autophagosome elongation and maturation (Figure 5.3). The first involves the ubiquitin-like Atg12, which conjugates with Atg5 in a process requiring Atg7 and Atg10. This complex then interacts with Atg16L and associates with the phagosome. The second is the LC3 (Atg8/microtubule-associated protein 1A/B light chain 3; LC3-I)

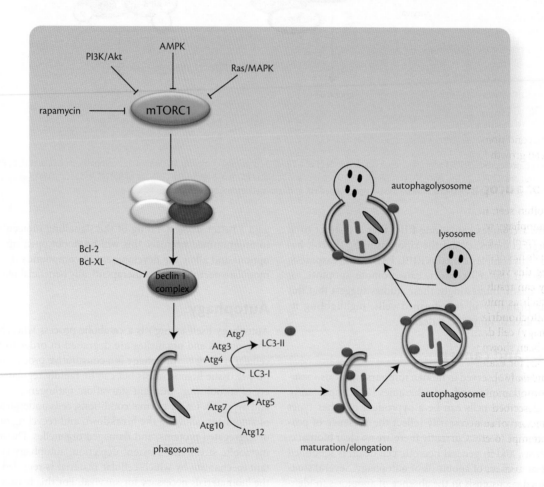

Fig. 5.3 Autophagy regulation and autophagosome formation. Numerous stresses activate autophagy signalling, leading to alterations in mTOR activity within the mTORC1 complex. Inhibition of mTOR under nutrient-replete conditions leads to activation of the ULK-containing complex and the Beclin 1 complex, both of which are required for phagosome formation. The phagosome elongates and matures, steps requiring the Atg12-5 and LC3 complexes. Atg12 is conjugated to Atg5, which requires Atg7 and Atg10; this complex interacts with Atg16L and associates with the phagophore. LC3-I is cleaved by Atg4 and lipidated to form LC3-II, which associates with the autophagosome. Closure of the phagophore resuts in the formation of the double-membrane autophagosome which can fuse with the lysosome, leading to degradation of cellular cargo.

family complex. Atg4 cleaves LC3-I which is then conjugated to phosphatidylethanolamine (PE) to form (LC3-II), allowing its association with the autophagosome. LC3-II remains bound to the autophagosome until it is recycled during lysosomal degradation and is thus considered one of the most reliable markers of autophagy.

Control of autophagy

mTOR

A variety of stimuli have been demonstrated to result in autophagy, including hypoxia, nutrient depletion, endoplasmic reticulum stress, and DNA damage. The most important regulator of autophagy is the serine-threonine kinase mTOR (mammalian target of rapamycin) pathway (Figure 5.3). Under normal growth conditions, when nutrients are replete, mTOR is active and acts to suppress autophagy. Rapamycin, for example, targets and inhibits mTOR, leading to induction of autophagy.

mTOR forms two complexes in cells (mTORC1 and 2) and it is only mTORC1 that is sensitive to inhibition by rapamycin. Numerous signalling pathways converge on mTORC1, including the PI3K/Akt, Ras proto-oncogene/mitogen activated protein kinase (MAPK), and AMPK (adenosine monophosphate protein kinase) signalling pathways (Figure 5.3). These pathways act upstream of mTORC1 to control its activation state. Active mTORC1 binds to the Atgs ULK1/2 within the ULK complex, leading to their phosphorylation and inhibition of autophagy (Figure 5.3). When nutrient levels are depleted, for example, AMPK is activated and will inhibit mTORC1 to result in enhanced autophagy. Conversely, in nutrient-replete conditions, active mTORC1 will stimulate protein synthesis and cell growth [32].

Dual role of autophagy in cancer

Autophagy is often seen in dying cells, which has led to the supposition that autophagy was responsible for the cell death, but how this occurs is currently unclear. In experimental systems, long-term starvation of cells has demonstrated that autophagy can lead to cell survival, calling this view into question. It has also been proposed that autophagy can result in the digestion of organelles necessary for survival, such as mitochondria. Indeed, when large enough numbers of mitochondria are removed by autophagy (a process termed mitophagy) cell death ensues. Certainly in a few situations autophagy has been shown to be directly responsible for the induction of apoptosis, for example during development of the salivary gland in *Drosophila* [33].

Although non-apoptotic cell death accompanied by autophagy has been well described in human cancer cells, it has been suggested that detection of autophagy in dying cells is the result of an unsuccessful attempt to cope with stress, rather than a bona fide death mechanism [27]. Indeed, the role of autophagy in cancer is currently unclear and autophagy is thought to play a paradoxical role in cancer, acting as both a survival and a death mechanism [21]. The tumour-suppressive nature of autophagy was first demonstrated by the finding that monoallelic loss of the autophagy regulator Beclin 1 could promote tumorigenesis in mice [34]. In human cancers monoallelic loss of Beclin 1 has also been observed. For example, roughly 75% of ovarian cancers and 50% of breast cancers are thought to be Beclin 1 haploinsufficient [21].

Conversely, autophagy can provide a survival advantage for tumour cells due to their high energy demand [35, 36]. Moreover, inhibition of autophagy can synergize with chemotherapy, supporting the notion that autophagy can play a protective role in cancer cell survival [35]. It may be that the genetic background and/or stage of the cancer plays a role in whether autophagy can promote or inhibit tumour cell death [37]. Moreover the situation is further complicated by the fact that there is substantial cross-talk between autophagy and apoptosis (e.g., the anti-apoptotic protein Bcl-2 can bind and inhibit Beclin 1).

mTOR hyperactivation has been found in several human cancers. Rapamycin is a natural inhibitor of mTOR, but rapamycin and several of its analogues have had limited clinical success [38]. This had led to attempts to develop more effective mTOR inhibitors (e.g., dual PI3K/Akt and mTOR inhibitors) but their clinical efficacy has yet to be demonstrated. The late-stage autophagy inhibitors chloroquine and hydrochloroquine have been evaluated in humans as they are commonly used anti-malaria drugs. Autophagy inhibitors in combination with other therapies could provide a more effective means to target human tumours [37]. Indeed, clinical trials evaluating hydrochloroquine along with other cytotoxic agents are currently underway (<www.clinicaltrials.gov>).

Conclusion

Given that the fundamental goal of cancer treatment is selective tumour cell killing, understanding the mechanisms responsible for tumour cell death is of primary clinical significance. It has been 40 years since the initial characterization of apoptosis, long assumed to be the only mechanism of programmed cell death. In the last decade it has become apparent that non-apoptotic programmed cell death mechanisms play vital roles in normal physiology as well as in disease states [9]. Moreover, as researchers further characterize the mechanisms and effectors involved in these pathways, it is becoming increasingly clear that there is extensive cross-talk between these pathways. Unravelling the complexities behind cell death will allow refinements in treatments tailored to specific tumour types, taking into account the genetic pathways and the primary modes of cell death involved.

Therapies aimed at inducing apoptosis in cancer cells have been clinically exploited as have biomarkers that can be used to predict the efficacy of such therapies. A long-standing issue with cancer therapy is the development of resistance to treatment. There are a plethora of genetic and epigenetic changes in tumour cells that can circumvent apoptotic pathways; as such, understanding and developing therapies that can target other death-signalling pathways could have great clinical significance. Indeed, as necroptosis seems to function in the absence of apoptosis, it may be an important target in apoptosis-deficient cancer cells. Therapies that can block the growth-favouring aspects of autophagy while enhancing apoptotic and necrotic death may also be of benefit. Further, the double-edged nature of autophagy requires a more comprehensive understanding of its outcome in human cancers. Indeed, much research is aimed at identifying autophagy response biomarkers but a clearer understanding of the outcome of autophagy in human tumours must be gained.

Given the complexity involved in the variety of cell death mechanisms, the challenge in oncology is how to harness these different modes of cell death in order to effectively eliminate cancer cells.

Acknowledgements

We thank the MRC and CRUK for their generous support. The authors apologize to those whose work could not be cited due to space limitations.

Further reading

Aggarwal BB. Signalling pathways of the TNF superfamily: a double-edged sword. Nature Reviews Immunology 2003; 3(9): 745–756.

Choi AM, Ryter SW, Levine B. Autophagy in human health and disease. New England Journal of Medicine 2013; 368(7): 651–662.

Hanahan D, Weinberg RA. Hallmarks of cancer: the next generation. Cell 2011; 144(5): 646–674.

Kreuzaler P, Watson CJ. Killing a cancer: what are the alternatives? Nature Reviews Cancer 2012; 12(6): 411–424.

Long JS, Ryan KM. New frontiers in promoting tumour cell death: targeting apoptosis, necroptosis and autophagy. Oncogene 2012; 31(49): 5045–5060.

Taylor RC, Cullen SP, Martin SJ. Apoptosis: controlled demolition at the cellular level. Nature Reviews Molecular Cell Biology 2008; 9(3): 231–241.

Tenev T, Bianchi K, Darding M, Broemer M, Langlais C et al. The Ripoptosome, a signaling platform that assembles in response to genotoxic stress and loss of IAPs. Molecular Cell 2011; 43(3): 432–448.

White E. Deconvoluting the context-dependent role for autophagy in cancer. Nature Reviews Cancer 2012; 12(6): 401–410.

References

1. Hanahan D, Weinberg RA. Hallmarks of cancer: the next generation. Cell 2011; 144(5): 646–674.

2. Kerr JF, Wyllie AH, Currie AR. Apoptosis: a basic biological phenomenon with wide-ranging implications in tissue kinetics. British Journal of Cancer 1972; 26(4): 239–257.

3. Horvitz HR. Nobel lecture. Worms, life and death. Bioscience Reports 2003; 23(5–6): 239–303.

4. Cotter TG, Apoptosis and cancer: the genesis of a research field. Nature Reviews Cancer 2009; 9(7): 501–507.

5. MacKenzie SH, Clark AC. Death by caspase dimerization. Advances in Experimental Medicine and Biology 2012; 747: 55–73.

6. Taylor RC, Cullen SP, Martin SJ. Apoptosis: controlled demolition at the cellular level. Nature Reviews Molecular Cell Biology 2008; 9(3): 231–241.

7. Kilbride, SM, Prehn JH. Central roles of apoptotic proteins in mitochondrial function. Oncogene 2012; 32(22): 2703–2711.

8. Chipuk JE, Green DR. How do BCL-2 proteins induce mitochondrial outer membrane permeabilization? Trends in Cell Biology 2008; 18(4): 157–164.

9. Shiozaki, EN, Shi Y. Caspases, IAPs and Smac/DIABLO: mechanisms from structural biology. Trends in Biochemical Sciences 2004; 29(9): 486–494.

10. Aggarwal BB. Signalling pathways of the TNF superfamily: a double-edged sword. Nature Reviews Immunology 2003; 3(9): 745–756.

11. Jain MV, Paczulla AM, Klonisch T, Dimgba FN, Rao SB et al. Interconnections between apoptotic, autophagic and necrotic pathways: implications for cancer therapy development. Journal of Cellular and Molecular Medicine 2013; 17(1): 12–29.

12. Wilson NS, Dixit V, Ashkenazi A. Death receptor signal transducers: nodes of coordination in immune signaling networks. Nature Immunology 2009; 10(4): 348–355.

13. Kale J, Liu Q, Leber B, Andrews DW. Shedding light on apoptosis at subcellular membranes. Cell 2012; 151(6): 1179–1184.

14. Ott A, Chang J, Madden K, Kannan R, Muren C et al. Oblimersen in combination with temozolomide and albumin-bound paclitaxel in patients with advanced melanoma: a phase I trial. Cancer Chemotherapy and Pharmacology 2013; 71(1): 183–191.

15. Galatin S, Advani RH, Fisher GA, Francisco B, Julian T et al. Phase I trial of oblimersen (Genasense®) and gemcitabine in refractory and advanced malignancies. Investigational New Drugs 2011; 29(5): 971–977.

16. Liu Q, Wang HG. Anti-cancer drug discovery and development: Bcl-2 family small molecule inhibitors. Communicative & Integrative Biology 2012; 5(6): 557–565.

17. Kruyt FA. TRAIL and cancer therapy. Cancer Letters 2008; 263(1): 14–25.

18. Holoch A, Griffith TS. TNF-related apoptosis-inducing ligand (TRAIL): a new path to anti-cancer therapies. European Journal of Pharmacology 2009; 625(1–3): 63–72.

19. Hitomi J, Christofferson DE, Ng A, Yao J, Degterev A et al. Identification of a molecular signaling network that regulates a cellular necrotic cell death pathway. Cell 2008; 135(7): 1311–1323.

20. Degterev A, Huang Z, Boyce M, Li Y, Jagtap P et al. Chemical inhibitor of nonapoptotic cell death with therapeutic potential for ischemic brain injury. Nature Chemical Biology 2005; 1(2): 112–119.

21. Kreuzaler P, Watson CJ. Killing a cancer: what are the alternatives? Nature Reviews Cancer 2012; 12(6): 411–424.

22. Vanlangenakker N, Vanden Berghe T, Vandenabeele P. Many stimuli pull the necrotic trigger, an overview. Cell Death Differentiation 2012; 19(1): 75–86.

23. Vanlangenakker N, Vanden Berghe T, Bogaert P, Laukens B, Zobel K et al. cIAP1 and TAK1 protect cells from TNF-induced necrosis by preventing RIP1/RIP3-dependent reactive oxygen species production. Cell Death Differentiation 2011; 18(4): 656–665.

24. Zhang DW, Shao J, Lin J, Zhang N, Lu BJ et al. RIP3, an energy metabolism regulator that switches TNF-induced cell death from apoptosis to necrosis. Science 2009; 325(5938): 332–336.

25. Feoktistova M, Geserick P, Kellert B, Dimitrova DP, Langlais C et al. cIAPs block Ripoptosome formation, a RIP1/caspase-8 containing intracellular cell death complex differentially regulated by cFLIP isoforms. Molecular Cell 2011; 43(3): 449–463.

26. Tenev T, Bianchi K, Darding M, Broemer M, Langlais C et al. The Ripoptosome, a signaling platform that assembles in response to genotoxic stress and loss of IAPs. Molecular Cell 2011; 43(3): 432–448.

27. Kepp O, Galluzzi L, Lipinski M, Yuan J, Kroemer G. Cell death assays for drug discovery. Nature Reviews Drug Discovery 2011; 10(3): 221–237.

28. Laukens B, Jennewein C, Schenk B, Vanlangenakker N, Schier A et al., Smac mimetic bypasses apoptosis resistance in FADD- or caspase-8-deficient cells by priming for tumor necrosis factor alpha-induced necroptosis. Neoplasia 2011; 13(10): 971–979.

29. Mari M, Tooze SA, Reggiori F. The puzzling origin of the autophagosomal membrane. F1000 Biology Reports 2011; 3: 25.

30. Dall'Armi C, Devereaux KA, Di Paolo G. The role of lipids in the control of autophagy. Curr Biology 2013; 23(1): R33–R45.

31. Lamb CA, Dooley HC, Tooze SA. Endocytosis and autophagy: shared machinery for degradation. Bioessays 2013; 35(1): 34–45.

32. Janku F, McConkey DJ, Hong DS, Kurzrock R. Autophagy as a target for anticancer therapy. Nature Reviews Clinical Oncology 2011; 8(9): 528–539.

33. Berry DL, Baehrecke EH. Growth arrest and autophagy are required for salivary gland cell degradation in Drosophila. Cell 2007; 131(6): 1137–1148.

34. Yue Z, Jin S, Yang C, Levine AJ, Heintz N. Beclin 1, an autophagy gene essential for early embryonic development, is a haploinsufficient tumor suppressor. Proceedings of the National Academy of Sciences USA 2003; 100(25): 15077–15082.

35. Choi AM, Ryter SW, Levine B. Autophagy in human health and disease. New England Journal of Medicine 2013. 368(7): 651–662.

36. White E. Deconvoluting the context-dependent role for autophagy in cancer. Nature Reviews Cancer 2012; 12(6): 401–410.

37. Long JS, Ryan KM. New frontiers in promoting tumour cell death: targeting apoptosis, necroptosis and autophagy. Oncogene 2012; 31(49): 5045–5060.

38. Rodon J, Dienstmann R, Serra V, Tabernero J. Development of PI3K inhibitors: lessons learned from early clinical trials. Nature Reviews Clinical Oncology 2013; 10(3): 143–153.

CHAPTER 6

Angiogenesis

Yull E. Arriaga and Arthur E. Frankel

Introduction to angiogenesis

Blood vessels arose in vertebrates to improve supply of oxygen, nutrients, and immune defence cells to different tissues and organs [1]. The initial vascular architecture is assembled in a process called 'vasculogenesis'. The process employs deposition of embryonal angioblasts next to each other to create the initial capillary network. Subsequently, angiogenesis is used to expand the vascular network within growing organs. Different organs provide organ-specific signals and markers to the endothelium [2]. Angiogenesis is critical both in vertebrate vegetative functions and immune defence and employs unique tissue-specific pathways to meet organ needs. Not surprisingly, such an important system is regulated by many cell and molecular components. Co-option of the angiogenesis process by tumours is critical for their survival and pathology since uncontrolled growth alone fails without nutrients and a permissive extracellular environment. The discovery of the role of angiogenesis in cancer growth began with microscopic histology in the nineteenth century followed by the discovery of pro-angiogenic molecules and their receptors with molecular biology tools at the end of the twentieth century. Ultimately, protein and small molecular weight inhibitors of one of the pro-angiogenic factors were used to successfully palliate patients with a number of metastatic cancers.

History

Virchow and other German pathologists noted exuberant vessel proliferation in tumours in the 1880s [3]. In the 1920s, Lewis observed markedly different vascular patterns among different tumour types [4]. Ide and Algire reported tumour hypervascularity in the 1930s and 1940s [5, 6]. Several decades later, Ehrmann and Greenblatt identified a filterable molecule produced by tumours that triggered endothelial proliferation [7, 8]. Based on this work, Folkman hypothesized in 1971 that inhibitors to pro-angiogenic factors would 'starve' tumours and be a new class of targeted cancer therapeutics [9]. In the following decade, Folkman's lab optimized microvascular endothelial culture conditions that permitted an in vitro assay for the search for endothelial growth factors. Subsequently, numerous investigators evaluated fibroblast growth factor and tumour growth factor beta and other molecules, but none met the rigorous requirements for induction of endothelial growth in its presence and loss of endothelial growth in its absence. Finally, in the late 1980s, the endothelial mitogen, vascular endothelial growth factor (VEGF), was purified and characterized by Ferrara and colleagues from pituitary follicular cell conditioned media [10]. VEGF met Koch's postulates—its presence enhanced angiogenesis and its absence by genetic or immunologic means inhibited angiogenesis. Ferrara's group then synthesized blocking monoclonal antibodies [11]. Other groups established the VEGF receptors (VEGFRs) as a family of tyrosine kinases and developed small molecular weight tyrosine kinase inhibitors (TKIs) [12]. Clinical studies in the last decade were associated with US Food & Drug Administration approval of the anti-VEGF antibody, bevacizumab, for metastatic colorectal carcinoma (CRC), metastatic non-small-cell lung carcinoma (NSCLC), metastatic renal cell carcinoma (RCC), and glioblastoma and approval of the VEGFR TKIs—sunitinib, sorafenib, pazopanib, and axitinib for metastatic renal carcinoma. Sunitinib and sorafenib were also approved for gastrointestinal stromal tumours (GIST) and hepatocellular carcinoma (HCC), respectively [13]. Regorafenib was approved for metastatic colorectal carcinoma (CRC) and for GIST. While encouraging, these VEGF-VEGFR targeted agents have produced modest several-month improvements in disease-free survival and overall survival. Currently, there are several hundred clinical trials of novel anti-angiogenesis compounds and new predictive biomarkers based on an improved understanding of the biology. Hence, a deeper understanding of angiogenesis should be fruitful to cancer scientists, pharmacologists, and physicians.

Biology

Angiogenesis is an orchestrated, elegantly controlled series of steps as diagrammed simplistically in Figure 6.1. The steps are listed temporally and include (a) tumour cell release of pro-angiogenic factors and attraction of stromal fibroblasts and macrophages, (b) endothelial tip cell selection with extension of filipodia, loosening of the endothelial cell junctions, degradation of the extracellular matrix, migration towards the tumour, pericyte detachment from vessel wall, and increased permeability of the endothelial cell layer with deposition of a provisional extracellular matrix-ECM scaffold, (c) endothelial stalk cell proliferation with intercellular junctions, (d) lumen formation, (e) tip cell fusion, (f) blood flow, and (g) phalanx cell quiescence with production of basement membrane and coverage by pericytes.

The molecular machinery for the changes in the endothelium, stromal cells and extracellular matrix employs multiple reactions influenced by time and space. Because of the inherent lack of organization in the tumour microenvironment, the resulting vascular network is only partially functional, generating the disparate vascular patterns found in different tumour types and incompletely handling the nutritional needs, waste removal, and immune cell repair of normal tissue wounds. The tumour vessels are dilated,

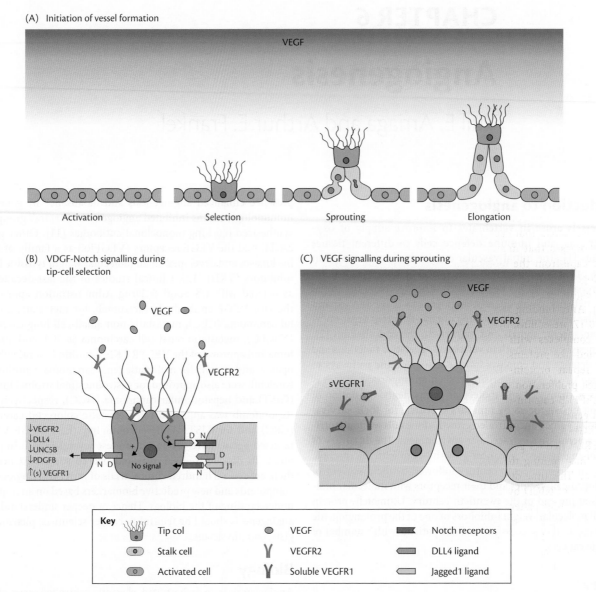

Fig. 6.1 Sprout induction. (A) The initiation of blood vessel formation. The presence of VEGF (blue gradient) activates the endothelium (yellow cells) of existing blood vessels. A VEGF/notch-dependent regulatory mechanism ensures the selection of a limited number of tip cells (green) by blocking tip cell formation in the immediate neighbours (via lateral inhibition). Tip cells sprout towards the VEGF gradient, and the adjacent stalk cells follow the guiding tip cell and proliferate to support sprout elongation. (B) VEGF/notch regulatory feedback during tip cell selection. The activation of VEGFR2 (pink) by VEGF (blue circles) induces the expression of the notch ligand DLL4 (D; blue). The subsequent activation of notch (N; red) by DLL4 in contacting cells reduces their expression of VEGFR2 and DLL4, thereby making them less sensitive to VEGF-mediated activation and limiting their ability to activate notch signalling in neighbouring cells. The expression of other tip cell enriched genes, such as UNC5B and PDGFB is reduced in stalk cells, whereas the expression of the non-signalling VEGF decoy receptors VEGFR1 and soluble (s) VEGFR1 is increased, further reducing the likelihood of VEGFR2 activation in these cells. Furthermore, jagged1 (J1; yellow), which is selectively expressed in stalk cells, competes with DLL4 in cis for binding to notch receptors on tip cells. Jagged1 binds, but does not activate the notch receptor, thereby preventing notch activation in the tip cells. (C) VEGF signalling during sprouting. Soluble VEGFR1 (sVEGFR1; brown) produced by the cells immediately next to the outgrowing vessel branch sequesters VEGF molecules, thereby creating a corridor of higher VEGF levels perpendicular to the parent vessel. This corridor might act to optimize spreading of the vascular network and to avoid contact with nearby emerging sprouts.

Reproduced with permission from Geudens I, Gerhardt H, Coordinating cell behaviour during blood vessel formation, *Development*, Volume 138, pp. 569–583, Copyright © 2011. Published by The Company of Biologists Ltd, doi:10.1242/dev.062323

tortuous, hyperpermeable, and show heterogeneity within the tumour bed [14]. Despite the complexity, some of the major chemical pathways have been identified [15, 16].

Tumour tissues—tumour cells and stromal cells—over-express VEGF-A proteins including splice variants VEGF121, VEGF165, VEGF189, and VEGF206 [17]. VEGF transcription is induced by local hypoxia or VHL mutation with stabilization of HIF1α [18],

local inflammation with stabilization of NFκB [19], and/or as a product of multiple activated oncogenes [20]. A VEGF gradient develops in the tumour tissue with soluble and heparan sulfate matrix bound VEGF molecules. In addition, both tumour and stromal cells (fibroblasts and macrophages) from the hypoxic and inflammatory tumour microenvironment produce other pro-angiogenic peptides including VEGF-C, placental growth factor (PlGF), fibroblast growth factor (FGF), Bv8/PK2—a homologue of endocrine-derived VEGF, IL-8, SDF-1, and PDGF-C [21–27].

The endothelial VEGF receptor VEGFR-2 is composed of extracellular immunoglobulin repeats and intracellular tyrosine kinase domains [28]. After VEGF-A binds VEFGR-2, the receptor homodimerizes, autophosphorylates at tyrosines 951, 1054, 1059, 1175, and 1214, and activates downstream FAK, Src, PLCγ, AKT, and p38 MAK kinase [29]. The endothelial cell converts to a 'tip cell' with filipodia, enhanced migration, decreased intercellular adhesions, increased vascular permeability, induction of Delta-like ligand 4 (DLL4), and Fringe glycosyltransferase [29]. Neuropilins NRP1 and NRP2 act as VEGF co-receptors. The tip cell Notch receptor becomes glycosylated by Fringe. Tip cells release ANG2 that causes pericyte release, express matrix metalloproteases that degrade the basement membrane, and permit escape from the bloodstream of proteins facilitating a pro-angiogenic ECM.

The neighbour 'stalk' endothelial cell has Notch receptors [28]. After binding the tip cell DLL4, Notch is cleaved by ADAM10/17/presenilins; the released Notch intracellular domain (NICD) complexes with transcription factor FBPj/CBF1 and Mastermind-like proteins; transcription occurs of Notch-related ankyrin repeat protein-NRARP. NRARP triggers transcription of cell proliferation genes, lymphoid enhancer-binding factor 1 (LEF1)/β-catenin-dependent Wnt-mediated intercellular adhesion genes, Jagged1 inhibitory Notch ligand gene, VEGFR1 decoy VEGF-A receptor gene and downregulates transcription of VEGFR2/VEGFR3 genes. NRARP also promotes NICD degradation thus limiting the time duration of the 'stalk' and 'tip' phenotypes. This time duration is fine-tuned by acetylation and deacetylation of NICD by SIRT1. These temporal controls determine the branching pattern of the vessels.

Blood vessel lumen formation occurs by different processes in different tissues [30]. In cases of large capillaries with constant perfusion, stalk cells retain the apical-basal polarity when they bud from the larger vessel. In other cases, lumen formation requires a series of discrete steps [28, 31]. Stalk multicellular rods first establish basal surface β1-integrin binding to ECM collagen/fibrin. This causes RAS-interacting protein 1 (RASIP1), RHOA GTPase-activating protein 29 (ARHGAP29), and partitioning defective 3 (PAR3) to transfer to the basal area and trigger basal redistribution of junctional proteins including zonula occludens 1 (ZO1), claudin 5, VE-cadherin and CD99. CD34 and podocalyxin (PODXL) move to the apical surface where their sialic acid negatively charged electrostatic repulsion generates a lumen. Protein kinase C-PKC phosphorylates moesin and binds filamentous actin-F-actin to PODXL. RHO-associated coiled-coil kinase-ROCK links non-muscle myosin II to the apical F-actin, and actomyosin contraction occurs, which expands the lumen. In addition, exocytic vacuole trafficking to the apical surface aids lumen expansion. Tip cells fuse by VE-cadherin formation of adhesion junctions first at filipodia and then throughout the cell interface [30]. Macrophages can assist in the process.

Once the capillary sprouts with lumens have fused, blood flow ensues. Blood flow activates the shear stress-responsive transcription factor Kruppel-like factor 2 (KLF2), which transcribes miR-126 [15, 28]. miR-126 represses SPRED1 and PIK3R2, which are MAPK and PI3K inhibitors, respectively. The signal pathway activation promotes vessel integrity.

Finally, the new vessel matures and quiescent 'phalanx' cells produce basement membrane and recruit and interact with pericytes [15]. Molecularly, phalanx cell TGFβ binds pericyte TGFBR2/endoglin/Alk-1 to enhance pericyte proliferation and differentiation. Phalanx cell PDGFB binds pericyte PDGFRβ for cell recruitment. Phalanx sphingosine-1-phosphate (S1P) reacts with pericyte and phalanx S1PR and triggers N-cadherin-containing phalanx-pericyte junctions. Phalanx DLL4 binds pericyte Notch3 and enhances mural and endothelium maturation. Pericyte ANG1 binds phalanx TIE-2 and prevents phalanx cell VE-cadherin internalization. Phalanx nitric oxide synthetase and thrombomodulin maintain vessel patency. Phalanx VE-cadherin dephosphorylates VEGFR2 maintaining quiescence. Phalanx intracrine VEGF prevents cell apoptosis. Pericyte FGF binds phalanx FGFR and preserves adherens and tight junctions. Phalanx cells also produce PAI-1 and TIMPs to preserve the basement membrane. Further, phalanx prolyl hydroxylase domain proteins (PHDs) respond to tissue oxygen to adjust cell shape via HIF2α signalling.

Clinical applications

Efficacy

Only a few anti-angiogenesis compounds have been FDA approved for use in cancer as shown in Table 6.1 and previously reviewed [32]. The humanized anti-VEGF-A antibody bevacizumab in combination with chemotherapy is used for metastatic colorectal carcinoma (CRC) and non-small-cell lung carcinoma (NSCLC), in combination with interferon-2α for metastatic renal cell carcinoma (RCC) and as monotherapy for recurrent glioblastoma multiforme (GBM). Food and Drug Administration (FDA) approved indications of bevacizumab in cancer therapy are shown in Table 6.2.

The VEGFR TKI sunitinib is used as a single agent for metastatic RCC, pancreatic neuroendocrine tumours, and imatinib-refractory GIST. The VEGFR TKI sorafenib is given for metastatic RCC and HCC. The VEGFR TKI pazopanib is used for metastatic RCC. The VEGFR TKI axitinib is given for metastatic RCC. The VEGFR TKI regorafenib is used as a single agent for chemotherapy refractory metastatic CRC and as third-line therapy for metastatic GIST.

Sunitinib monotherapy improved median PFS and OS by 6 and 4.6 months, respectively, versus interferon-α in the metastatic RCC NCT00083889 trial [33]. Similarly, sunitinib improved median PFS versus placebo by 5.5 months in the imatinib refractory GIST SUN1112 study [34]. OS data is not mature. Finally, sunitinib improved median PFS versus best supportive care by 5.9 months in the pancreatic neuroendocrine tumour NCT00428597 trial [35]. Again, OS data is not available but the sunitinib death hazard ratio was 0.41.

Sorafenib monotherapy for metastatic RCC yielded an improvement in median PFS and OS of 2.7 months and 3.5 months, respectively, versus placebo after censoring for placebo crossovers in the TARGET trial [36]. Sorafenib monotherapy versus placebo for HCC showed an improved median PFS based on radiologic progression and OS of 2.7 months and 2.8 months, respectively, in the SHARP trial [37].

Pazopanib achieved an improvement in median PFS improvement of 5 months versus placebo in metastatic RCC patients in the VEG105192 trial [38]. OS data were not mature.

Table 6.1 US FDA-approved anti-angiogenesis agents

Agent	Disease	Rr (%)	Pfs improvement (Mo)	Os Improvement (Mo)	References
Bevacizumab	CRC	ND	1.4, 2.6, 4.2	1.4, 2.6, 4.7	[82]
					[83]
					[84]
	NSCLC	ND	1.7	2	[85]
	RCC	ND	4.8	2, 0.9	[86]
					[87]
	GBM	23	4	ND	[88]
Sunitinib	RCC	ND	6	4.6	[33]
	GIST	ND	5.5	ND	[34]
	NET	ND	5.9	ND	[35]
Sorafenib	RCC	ND	2.7	3.5	[36]
	HCC	ND	2.7	2.8	[37]
Pazopanib	RCC	ND	5	ND	[38]
Axitinib	RCC	ND	2	ND	[39]

Axitinib compared to sorafenib as second-line therapy for metastatic RCC produced a two-month improvement in median PFS in the AXIS study [39]. Again, OS data were not available.

Anti-VEGF/VEGFR therapies are not completely cross-resistant. Patients may respond to a second TKI after progression on the first TKI [40, 41].

Lack of efficacy of bevacizumab as adjuvant therapy for micrometastatic disease

The National Surgical Breast and Bowel Project (NSABP) C-08 study was a prospective randomized open label multi-institutional phase III clinical trial which evaluated the safety and benefit of adding bevacizumab for 12 months to adjuvant chemotherapy with infusional 5 fluorouracil (5-FU), leucovorin and oxaliplatin (FOLFOX) after complete resection of the primary tumour in patients with high-risk stage II and stage III colon cancer [42]. In this study, patients who received adjuvant bevacizumab plus FOLFOX for treatment of micrometastases had a significant but transient improvement in disease-free survival (DFS) after the first 15 months of follow-up (hazard ratio: 0.62; p <.001). The early improvement in DFS in patients who received bevacizumab plus FOLFOX was lost with longer follow-up. At a median follow-up of 35.6 months there was no statistically significant difference in DFS in patients who received bevacizumab plus FOLFOX compared to those who received adjuvant FOLFOX without bevacizumab. Another prospective randomized study, the AVANT clinical trial, evaluated the safety and efficacy of adjuvant bevacizumab for 12 months added to adjuvant FOLFOX or to adjuvant capecitabine plus oxaliplatin (XELOX) in patients with resected high-risk stage II or stage III colon cancer [43]. Like the NSABP-C08 study, the goal of the AVANT clinical trial was to evaluate the role of adjuvant bevacizumab in the treatment of micrometastatic disease. The AVANT study did not show a significant improvement in DFS in patients who received adjuvant bevacizumab plus FOLFOX or XELOX. The lack of DFS and overall survival (OS) benefit of adjuvant bevacizumab added to standard chemotherapy in patients with high-risk stage II and stage III colon cancer after complete resection of the primary tumour is in contrast with the significant improvements in DFS and OS seen in patients with metastatic CRC, metastatic NSCLC, and GBM treated with bevacizumab plus chemotherapy.

To date, results from prospective randomized clinical trials in patients with solid tumours without gross metastases do not support the use of adjuvant bevacizumab for the treatment of micrometastases after complete resection of the primary tumour. The underlying molecular mechanisms explaining the lack of benefit of adjuvant bevacizumab for the treatment of micrometastatic disease are unknown. Angiogenesis signalling pathways might be different in the primary tumour, micrometastases, and macrometastatic lesions. Effects of bevacizumab on the primary tumour and on gross metastatic lesions include:

- inhibition of neoplastic blood vessel formation
- inhibition of vessel co-option
- decreased intratumoural vascular density
- normalization of intratumoral pressure

Table 6.2 Approved indications of bevacizumab for metastatic malignancies

Malignancy	Clinical benefit
Colorectal cancer (CRC)	Improvement in median overall survival-OS and median PFS: • Bevacizumab plus irinotecan/bolus 5-flourouracil-5FU/leucovorin-IFL, AVF2107 trial [82] • Bevacizumab plus infusional 5FU/leucovorin/oxaliplatin-FOLFOX, N016966 trial [83] • Bevacizumab plus infusional 5FU/leucovorin/oxaliplatin-FOLFOX4 in patients previously treated with a fluoropyrimidine and irinotecan. E3200 trial [84]
Non-small-cell lung cancer (NSCLC)	Improvement in median overall survival-OS and median PFS: • Bevacizumab plus carboplatin/paclitaxel, E4599 trial [85]
Renal cell carcinoma- RCC	Improvement in median overall survival-OS and median PFS: • Bevacizumab plus interferon-2α, AVOREN trial [86]; CALGB90206 trial [87]
Glioblastoma Multiforme-GBM	Improvement in median PFS: • Single agent bevacizumab (monotherapy), AVF3708 study [88]

♦ normalization of abnormal neoplastic blood vessel

♦ enhanced delivery of cytotoxic chemotherapy to cancer cells

♦ enhanced sensitivity of tumour endothelial cells to the cytotoxic effects of chemotherapeutic agents

♦ direct cytostatic effects in tumour cells.

The effects of adjuvant bevacizumab on micrometastases may be different when compared to the anti-angiogenic effects of bevacizumab demonstrated in primary tumours and in macrometastatic lesions.

Toxicities

The VEGFR inhibitors have distinct side effects compared to cytotoxic chemotherapy and require different management. The antibody and small molecule TKIs show slightly different side effect patterns.

Bevacizumab produces haemorrhage, wound healing complications, gastrointestinal perforation, arterial thromboembolism, bleeding, congestive heart failure (CHF), hypertension (HT), proteinuria/nephritic syndrome, infusion reactions, and reversible posterior leukoencephalopathy syndrome (RPLS) [44]. Bevacizumab avoidance in patients with haemotypsis, squamous NSCLC, or full anticoagulation will reduce bleeding events; bevacizumab avoidance 60 days before until 30 days after surgery will reduce wound healing complications; cautious bevacizumab use in patients with active intra-abdominal inflammation, large tumours, or prior abdominopelvic irradiation will reduce GI perforations; guarded bevacizumab use in patients >65 years old or with a history of arterial thromboembolism reduces arterial thromboses; vigilant bevacizumab use in CHF/prior anthracycline/chest wall irradiation patients should impact the frequency of CHF; bevacizumab use with blood pressure monitoring and addition of antihypertensive therapy will impact HT toxicity; bevacizumab use with urine protein regular measurements will avoid severe proteinuria/nephrotic syndrome; and finally, attention to rare infusion reactions or RPLS with appropriate intervention will avoid these life-threatening side effects.

The spectra of VEGF TKI toxicities are similar but show different frequencies of events for the different molecules [45]. Sorafenib most often produces hypertension, hand-foot syndrome, rash, anaemia, fatigue, diarrhoea, arterial thromboembolism, nausea, hepatotoxicity, hypocalcaemia, haemorrhage, elevated lipase, hypophosphatemia, and alopecia. Sunitinib also produces hypertension, hand-foot syndrome, rash, anaemia, fatigue, diarrhoea, arterial thromboembolism, nausea, hepatotoxicity, and a greater incidence of CHF, prolonged QT, myelosuppression, mucositis, asthenia, vomiting, and hypothyroidism. Pazopanib has a significant rate of proteinuria, hepatotoxicity, hypothyroidism, hyperglycaemia, and wound healing complications. Axitinib has commonly hypertension, fatigue, nausea, vomiting, hypothyroidism, proteinuria, diarrhoea, anorexia, and hand-foot syndrome. Rare complications of VEGFR TKIs are RPLS, intracranial haemorrhage, renal thrombotic microangiopathy, and mesenteric vein thrombosis [46]. Patient management includes monitoring of blood pressure, urine protein, TSH, liver functions, blood sugar, calcium, phosphate, ECG, and cardiac ejection fraction with dose adjustments and medications as needed. Palliative treatments are given including topical care for hand-foot syndrome, topical lidocaine for mucositis, hydrocortisone cream for rash, loperamide for diarrhoea, and ondansetron for nausea.

Economics

A six-month course of bevacizumab, sorafenib, sunitinib, pazopanib, and axitinib cost US pharmacies $54K, $51K, $54K, $39K, and $54K, respectively. These calculations do not include pharmacy markups, clinic visits, and monitoring laboratory tests [47].

Predictive tests/biomarkers

It is questionable that improvements in PFS and OS derived from the use of small molecule anti-angiogenic multikinase inhibitors in cancer therapy result from their anti-angiogenic effects. Blockade of the VEGF pathway or other angiogenesis signalling pathways by multikinase inhibitors may not result in tumour shrinkage [48]. The clinical benefit of anti-angiogenic multikinase inhibitors is modest. Fundamentally, these agents have a cytostatic effect in cancer cells and their anti-neoplastic effects may be indirect. These agents induce tumour endothelial cell apoptosis which in turn may result in tumour cell apoptosis, inhibition of tumour cell proliferation, and inhibition of distant metastatic spread. Their systemic effects on trafficking and function of haematopoietic progenitor cells and effector immune cells may result in tumour regression or growth [49, 50]. Patient selection with pre-treatment or early post-treatment predictive assays would improve benefit, reduce unnecessary exposure to toxicities, and reduce societal and patient costs. Patients with post-treatment grade 3 or 4 toxicities—HT, hypothyroidism, hand-foot syndrome—have the highest response rate, PFS, and OS [51–53]. Pilot, unconfirmed predictors of improved response/PFS/OS include pre-treatment low plasma IL-8 and SDF-1α, post-therapy decreased forward volume transfer constant-K^{trans}, and reverse reflux rate constant-K_{ep} using dynamic contrast enhanced (DCE) MRI, and post-therapy high plasma PlGF, IL-8, and low plasma MMP-2, bFGF, sTIE2, sVEGFR1, IL6, and SDF-1α [54–56]. In additional preliminary studies, in RCC elevated tissue carbonic anhydrase IX and in metastatic breast cancer (MBC) elevated tissue CD31 and PDGFRβ predict higher response rates to sorafenib and bevacizumab, respectively [57–58]. Genotype VEGF-2578AA/1154AA and IL8-251A TT are associated with MBC and ovarian cancer response to paclitaxel plus bevacizumab and cyclophosphamide plus bevacizumab, respectively [59–60]. All these potential biomarkers require confirmatory studies.

Anti-VEGFR agents in development

Current clinical trials of anti-angiogenesis and anti-tumour vascular drugs in cancer include at least four categories of studies. First, approved anti-VEGFR agents are tested in new indications and in association with biomarkers. Second, second-generation anti-VEGFR agents are being tested in phase III clinical trials.

Bevacizumab: additional indications

Bevacizumab produced improvements in PFS and OS in subsets of ovarian cancer and MBC patients. Addition of bevacizumab to carboplatin plus paclitaxel in high-risk ovarian cancer patients—FIGO stage IV or FIGO stage III with >1cm residual disease after debulking—yielded five-month and eight-month improvements in PFS and OS, respectively, in two studies [61, 62]. Neoadjuvant chemotherapy with the addition of bevacizumab for triple negative MBC yielded a higher rate of pathologic complete response than neoadjuvant therapy lacking bevacizumab [63, 64]. Bevacizumab plus chemotherapy given to gastric, breast, and pancreas cancer patients with elevated plasma soluble low molecular weight iso-forms of VEGF-A yielded improvements in PFS and OS compared to treatment without bevacizumab [65]. These disease states are excellent candidates for further phase III clinical trials leading to US FDA approval.

Approved VEGFR TKI additional indications

Pazopanib showed clinical efficacy in HCC with 73% of patients showing PR or stable disease [66]. A phase III randomized placebo controlled trial of pazopanib in patients with angiogenesis-naïve non-adipocytic soft tissue sarcomas showed an improvement in PFS of 3 months compared to placebo [67]. Sunitinib plus irra-diation produced a partial remission in a chondrosarcoma patient [68]. These VEGFR TKIs may obtain additional approvals for these disease states after confirmation of safety and efficacy in phase III clinical trials.

Second-generation VEGFR TKIs

AEE788, brivanib, motesanib, OSI-930, tandutinib, vatalanib, BIBF1120, tivozanib, and cediranib have shown sufficient activity to merit randomized phase II/III studies in different malignancies. AEE788 is a HER1/2 and VEGFR TKI in clinical testing in solid tumours—NCT100118456 and GBM-00116376 [69]. Brivanib is a FGFR and VEGFR TKI with activity in sorafenib-refractory HCC evidenced by a disease control rate of 46%, a median PFS of 2.7 months, and a median OS of 9.8 months [70]. Motesanib is a VEGFR and PDGFR TKI tested in NSCLC with carbopl-atin and paclitaxel [71]. OSI-930 is a KIT and VEGFR TKI in a phase I evaluation—NCT100513851 [69]. Tandutinib is a FLT3 and VEGFR TKI with activity in prostate cancer and AML [72]. Vatalanib is a PDGFR and VEGFR TKI with activity in GIST and high serum LDH colorectal cancers [73]. BIBF1120 is a PDGFR, FGFR, and VEGFR TKI undergoing clinical testing in ovarian cancer and NSLCL [74, 75]. Tivozanib is a VEGFR TKI active in RCC [76]. Cediranib is a VEGFR and PDGFR TKI with activ-ity in RCC [77]. Several other TKI cross-react with VEGFR, but their predominant and clinically important inhibition is likely for other receptors—vandetanib for RET and cabozantinib for MET [69]. Many of these compounds will be approved in differ-ent subsets of cancer patients enhancing 'personalized or preci-sion medicine'.

Protein anti-VEGF/VEGFR agents

Two proteins modify VEGF signalling and are in late stage clini-cal trials. Aflibercept is composed of the second immunoglobu-lin domain of VEGFR-1, the third immunoglobulin domain of VEGFR-2, and the constant region of human IgG1 antibody. Aflibercept binds VEGF-A, VEGF-B, and PlGF. When combined with FOLFIRI, the combination extended PFS by 2.2 months and OS by 1.5 months in CRC compared to FOLFIRI alone in the VELOUR trial [78]. Aflibercept combined with docetaxel yielded seven partial remissions and 32 stable disease among 54 advanced solid tumour patients for an overall disease control rate of 72% [79]. Epistaxis, proteinuria, dysphonia, and HT occurred in >50% of patients. Ramucirumab is a human antibody reac-tive with VEGFR-2. Fifteen of 37 advanced solid tumour patients showed a partial remission or stable disease lasting >6 months on ramucirumab [80].

Novel anti-angiogenesis agents in clinical studies

As described above, there are additional critical signalling pathways that modulate angiogenesis. These have recently become targets for clinical tests of new anti-angiogenesis treatments. These targets include PlGF, PDGFR, VEGFR1, NRP-1, DLL4, ANG1/2, and S1P. Anti-angiogenesis agents that are not VEGFR directed are in phase I and phase II trials. A summary of anti-angiogenesis monoclonal antibodies and recombinant peptide proteins in clinical trials are presented in Table 6.3.

Small molecule vascular disrupting agents (VDAs) in clinical development

The modest results with anti-angiogenesis compounds may be due to several reasons including multiple pro-angiogenic hormones, pathways, and participating cells, unacceptable toxicities to nor-mal blood vessels, promotion of metastases by slight increases in tumour tissue hypoxia, and reduced potency on established tumour vessels. An alternative approach is to target mature tumour blood vessels with a vascular disrupting agent (VDA). VDAs depend upon differences in intracellular or surface molecules between tumour and normal vessels. A small molecule VDA modifies intra-cellular tumour vessel functions leading to cell death or endothelial dysfunction. A number of small-molecule VDAs have reached the clinic and some are in various stages of testing in solid tumours. A summary of small-molecule VDAs in clinical trials are presented in Table 6.4.

In summary, a few small-molecule VDAs are continuing in development. The class appears to have modest efficacy, but, in selected cases, may be combined with cytotoxic chemotherapy or other therapies due to non-overlapping toxicities.

Ligand-directed VDAs in clinical development

Ligand-directed VDAs contain a peptide ligand which binds cell surface tumour endothelial antigens and an effector domain which produce vessel injury or thrombosis [80]. The ligand improves the tumour endothelial specificity of the VDA. Ligands include cyclic peptide mimetics and monoclonal antibodies. Effector domains include Fc fragments, radionuclides, or cytokines. Different tumours employ different angiogenesis pathways, and hence dif-ferent ligands and targets may be optimal for different patient tumours. A summary of ligand-directed VDAs in clinical trials are presented in Table 6.5.

Table 6.3 Anti-angiogenesis monoclonal antibodies and recombinant peptide proteins in clinical trials

Agent	Class	Target	Effects and clinical trials
TB-403	Humanized antibody	PlGF	◆ Interruption of PlGF signalling to VEGFR1 ◆ Expected activity in tumours over-expressing PlGF and unresponsive to VEGF inhibition ◆ Phase I study in advanced solid tumours [89]
MEDI-575	Fully human antibody	PDGFR	◆ Expected activity in tumours unresponsive to VEGF inhibition ◆ Two phase I studies in advanced solid tumours ◆ Ongoing studies in NSCLC and GBM [90]
Icrucumab or IMC-18F1	Fully human antibody	VEGFR1	◆ Effects on tumour cell, endothelial cell, circulating haematopoietic cell, macrophage, and stromal cell VEGFR1 ◆ Safe at pharmacologically active dose levels in advanced solid tumours [91] ◆ Ongoing phase II studies in breast and bladder cancer
MRNP1685A	Fully human antibody	NRP1	◆ Safe in inter-patient dose escalation study [92, 93] ◆ Phase IB study in combination with bevacizumab plus paclitaxel in NSCLC [94]
OMP-21M18	Humanized antibody	DLL4	◆ Induces hyperproliferation of non-functional tumour vasculature leading to tumour ischaemia ◆ Study as single agent in advanced solid tumours [95] ◆ Ongoing studies in combination with carboplatin plus pemetrexed in NSCLC and with gemcitabine in pancreas cancer
Sonepcizumab	Humanized antibody	S1P	◆ Inhibition of SIP binding to S1PRs inhibits endothelial cell communication with pericytes ◆ Phase I study in advanced solid tumours [96]
REGN910	Fully human antibody	ANG2	◆ Ongoing phase I study in advanced solid tumours [97]
AMG 386	Recombinant peptide-Fc fusion protein	ANG1/2	◆ Binding of ANG1/2 blocks interaction with TIE2 [98] ◆ twenty-two ongoing clinical trials as single agent or in combination with chemotherapy, bevacizumab, or small-molecule TKIs: GBM, CRC, gastric/oesophageal adenocarcinoma, RCC, HCC, ovarian carcinoma, triple negative breast cancer

Table 6.4 Small molecule vascular disrupting agents (VDAs) in clinical trials

Agent	Effect	Clinical studies
Vadimezan, DMXAA or ASA404	Induces tumour endothelial cell apoptosis	◆ Flavonoid vascular disrupting agent [99] ◆ Increases intratumoral TNF-α concentrations ◆ Ongoing study with carboplatin plus paclitaxel in SCLC
Fosbretabulin or combretastatin A-4 disodium	Binds tubulin	◆ Inhibits microtubule assembly, destabilizes cytoskeleton, disrupts adherens junction complexes, increases tumour vessel permeability, blocks tumour blood flow [100] ◆ Single-agent studies in advanced solid tumours [101] ◆ Phase II study of carboplatin/paclitaxel/bevacizumab +/−ß fosbretabulin in NSCLC [102] ◆ Ongoing study of bevacizumab +/− fosbretabulin in ovarian cancer
OXi4503 or combretastatin A1 diphosphate	Binds tubulin	◆ More potent than fosbretabulin ◆ Phase I studies in advanced solid tumours [103]
Ombrabulin and crolibulin	Microtubule-directed agent	◆ Ongoing studies in sarcoma-ombrabulin and anaplastic thyroid cancer-crolibulin
ABT-751	Binds tubulin	◆ Sulphonamide vascular disrupting agent ◆ Phase I and phase II single-agent studies in advanced solid tumours [104, 105]
Plinabulin	Binds tubulin	◆ Depolimerizes microtubules ◆ Phase I studies with and without chemotherapy in advanced solid tumours [106, 107]
Solblidotin or TZT-1027	Binds tubulin	◆ Cytotoxic dolastatin-10 analog ◆ Inhibits microtubule assembly ◆ Three phase I studies in advanced solid tumours and NSCLC [108–110]
ADH-1	Vascular disrupting agent	◆ Cyclic pentapeptide N-cadherin antagonist ◆ Two phase I studies in advanced solid tumours [111, 112]

Table 6.5 Ligand-directed VDAs in clinical trials

Agent	Class	Clinical studies
Bavituximab	Anti-β2-glycoprotein 1 mouse-human chimeric antibody	◆ Single-agent study in advanced solid tumours [113] ◆ Four studies in combination with chemotherapy showed efficacy: ◆ With docetaxel, second line—MBC [114] ◆ With carboplatin/paclitaxel, first line—MBC [47] ◆ With carboplatin/paclitaxel—NSCLC [115, 116] ◆ Ongoing studies: in combination with cabazitaxel-castration resistant prostate cancer-CRPC, with paclitaxel—triple negative MBC, with sorafenib—HCC, with gemcitabine-pancreas cancer
Cilengitide	Cyclic RGD-containing pentapeptide. Blocks αvβ3/αvβ5-ECM interaction	◆ Study in recurrent GBM [117] ◆ Study in combination with temozolomide+radiotherapy, first line for GBM [118] ◆ Randomized phase III trials +/– chemotherapy: GBM—CENTRIC trial, H&N carcinoma—ADVANTAGE trial ◆ Ongoing NSCLC—CERTO trial
Intetumumab	Fully human anti-αv monoclonal antibody	Three studies: melanoma, angiosarcoma, and castration-resistant prostate cancer [119, 121]
PF 04605412	Fully human anti- αvβ3/α5β1 monoclonal antibody	Ongoing phase I study in advanced solid tumours
GLPG 0187	Anti- α5β1 peptidomimetic	Ongoing phase I study in refractory solid tumours
E7820	Sulphonamide derivative-α2 integrin inhibitor	Ongoing randomized study in combination with irinotecan in CRC
TRC105	Anti-endoglin human/murine chimeric IgG1 monoclonal antibody	◆ Studies in advanced solid tumours [122, 123] ◆ Dramatic responses in CRC, ovarian cancer and endometrial cancer ◆ Ongoing studies in combination with chemotherapy: MBC, HCC, CRPC, and other solid tumours
J591	Anti-PSMA murine monoclonal antibody conjugated to different radionuclides	◆ Conjugated to ^{111}In: ◆ Study in advanced solid tumours [124, 125] ◆ Tumour vasculature selectively and safely targeted ◆ Conjugated to ^{177}Lu: ◆ Remissions reported in CRC [126] ◆ Ongoing study in non-prostate metastatic solid tumours
^{131}I-L19SIP	L19 anti-ED-B FN human antibody Fv fused to CH4 and radiolabeled with ^{131}I	◆ Two phase I studies [127, 128] ◆ Ongoing studies in combination with radiotherapy or chemoradiotherapy for brain metastases and NSCLC
L19IL2	L19 anti-ED-B FN human antibody Fv fused to IL2	◆ Studies in RCC [129] and other solid tumours ◆ Study in combination with dacarbazine-melanoma [130] ◆ Ongoing studies in combination with dacarbazine-melanoma and with gemcitabine-pancreas cancer
NGR-hTNF	NGR peptide coupled with human tumour necrosis factor α	◆ NGR selectively binds CD13 on tumour endothelial cells ◆ Studies in advanced solid tumours, mesothelioma, CRC, and HCC [131–134] ◆ Randomized phase II study evaluating combinations with chemotherapies—NSCLC [135] ◆ Studies in combination with doxorubicin-refractory solid tumours, SCLC, and ovarian cancer [136–138] ◆ Studies in combination with capecitabine/oxaliplatin-refractory CRC and with cisplatin-solid tumours [139, 140] ◆ Ongoing studies in combination with doxorubicin for platinum-resistant ovarian cancer, study in soft tissue sarcoma and randomized phase II study in combination with standard chemotherapy—NSCLC ◆ Ongoing randomized phase II study-relapsed mesothelioma and maintenance therapy—mesothelioma

Conclusion

Angiogenesis consists of an orchestrated series of steps leading from vessel sprouting, tube and lumen formation, vessel fusion, and, finally, quiescence. How these steps and their associated molecular components relate to non-physiologic, tumour angiogenesis is still being defined. Several anti-angiogenic drugs have reached the clinic. They all target the VEGF/VEGFR signalling pathway. They provide modest clinical benefit, but at a cost of significant and sometimes life-threatening toxicities. Progress is occurring with application of new predictive biomarkers to extend anti-VEGF-A/VEGFR approved drugs to new indications and more appropriate patient subsets. New, more selective VEGFR TKIs and novel protein drugs modifying VEGF–VEGFR interactions are likely to be approved soon for routine cancer care. Other components of tumour angiogenesis have been targeted, including ANG1/2 and S1P, and led to disease control. Ligand-directed VDAs—particularly antibodies to PS-β2 glycoprotein, endoglin [81], and CD13—have shown safety and excellent clinical activity. With enhanced understanding of vascular biology and advances in targeted therapy design, medical oncology practice will see an expanding role for tumour endothelial directed therapies.

Further reading

Carmeliet P, Jain RK. Molecular mechanisms and clinical applications of angiogenesis. Nature 2011; 473: 298–307.

Crawford Y, Ferrara N. Tumor and stromal pathways mediating refractoriness/resistance to anti-angiogenic therapies. Trends in Pharmacological Sciences 2009; 30: 624–630.

Ferrera N. Pathways mediating VEGF-independent tumor angiogenesis. Cytokine & Growth Factor Reviews 2010; 21: 21–26.

Ivy SP, Wick JY, Kaufman, BM. An overview of small-molecule inhibitors of VEGFR signaling. Nature Reviews Clinical Oncology 2009; 6: 569–579.

Jayson G C, Hicklin DJ, Ellis LM. Antiangiogenic therapy—evolving view based on clinical trial results. Nature Reviews Clinical Oncology 2012; 9(5): 297–303.

Kerbel RS. Tumor angiogenesis. New England Journal of Medicine 2008; 358: 2039–2049.

Munoz-Chapuli R. Evolution of angiogenesis. International Journal of Developmental Biology 2011; 55: 345–351.

Potente M, Gerhardt H, Carmeliet P. Basic and therapeutic aspects of angiogenesis. Cell 2011; 146: 873–887.

Sato Y. Persistent vascular normalization as an alternative goal of anti-angiogenic cancer therapy. Cancer Science 2011; 102: 1253–1256.

Semenza GL. Hypoxia-inducible factor in physiology and medicine. Cell 2012; 148: 399–408.

References

1. Munoz-Chapuli R. Evolution of angiogenesis. International Journal of Developmental Biology 2011; 55: 345–351.

2. Rocha SF, Adams RH. Molecular differentiation and specialization of vascular beds. Angiogenesis 2009; 12: 139–147.

3. Ferrara N. VEGF and the quest for tumour angiogenesis factors. Nature Reviews Cancer 2002; 2: 795–803.

4. Lewis WH. The vascular pattern of tumors. Johns Hopkins Hospital Bulletin 1927; 41: 156–162.

5. Ide AG, Baker NH, Warren SL. Vascularization of the Brown–Pearce rabbit epithelioma transplant as seen in the transparent ear chamber. American Journal of Roentgenology 1939; 42: 891–899.

6. Agire GH, Chalkley HW. Vascular reactions of normal and malignant tissues in vivo. I Vascular reactions of mice to wounds and to normal and neoplastic transplants. Journal of the National Cancer Institute 1945; 6: 73–85.

7. Ehrmann RL, Knoth M Choriocarcinoma: transfilter stimulation of vasoproliferation in the hamster cheek pouch studied by light and electron microscopy. Journal of the National Cancer Institute 1968; 41: 1329–1341.

8. Greenblatt M, Shubik P (1968). Tumor angiogenesis: transfilter diffusion studies in the hamster by the transparent chamber technique. Journal of the National Cancer Institute 1968; 41: 111–124.

9. Folkman J Tumor angiogenesis: therapeutic implications. New England Journal of Medicine 1971; 285: 1182–1186.

10. Leung DW, Cachianes G, Kuang WJ, Goeddel DV, Ferrara N Vascular endothelial growth factor is a secreted angiogenic mitogen. Science 1989; 246: 1306–1309.

11. Ferrara N Vascular endothelial growth factor and the regulation of angiogenesis. Recent Progress in Hormone Research 2000; 55: 15–35.

12. Ivy SP, Wick JY, Kaufman, BM. An overview of small-molecule inhibitors of VEGFR signaling. Nature Reviews Clinical Oncology 2009; 6: 569–579.

13. Sato Y Persistent vascular normalization as an alternative goal of anti-angiogenic cancer therapy. Cancer Science 2011; 102: 1253–1256.

14. Goel S, Duda DG, Xu L, Munn LL, Boucher Y et al. (2011). Normalization of the vasculature for treatment of cancer and other diseases. Physiological Reviews 2011; 91: 1071–1121.

15. Potente M, Gerhardt H, Carmeliet P. Basic and therapeutic aspects of angiogenesis. Cell 2011; 146: 873–887.

16. Carmeliet P, Jain RK. Molecular mechanisms and clinical applications of angiogenesis. Nature 2011; 473: 298–307.

17. Ferrera N. Pathways mediating VEGF-independent tumor angiogenesis. Cytokine & Growth Factor Reviews 2010; 21: 21–26.

18. Semenza GL. Hypoxia-inducible factor in physiology and medicine. Cell 2012; 148: 399–408.

19. Wang S, Liu Z, Wang L, Zhang X. NF-kappa B signaling pathway, inflammation and colorectal cancer. Cell Molecular Immunology 2009; 6: 327–334.

20. Mukhopadhyay P, Datta K. Multiple regulatory pathways of vascular permeability factor/vascular endothelial growth factor (VPF/VEGF) expression in tumors. Seminars in Cancer Biology, 2004; 14: 123–130.

21. Tammela T, Zarkada G, Nurmi H, Jakobsson L, Heinolainen K et al. VEGFR-3 controls tip to stalk conversion at vessel fusion sites by reinforcing Notch signaling. Nature Cell Biology, 2011; 13: 1202–1213.

22. Salgado R, Benoy I, Vermevlen P, Van Dam P, Van Marck P et al. Circulating basic fibroblast growth factor is partly derived from the tumour in patients with colon, cervical and ovarian cancer. Angiogenesis 2004; 7: 29–32.

23. Cheng SJ, Lee JJ, Cheng SL, Chen HM, Chang HH et al. Increased serum placental growth factor level is significantly associated with progression, recurrence and poor prognosis of oral squamous cell carcinoma. Oral Oncology, 2012; 48(5): 424–428.

24. Shojaei F, Wu X, Zhong C, Yu L, Liang XH et al. Bv8 regulates myeloid cell-dependent tumour angiogenesis. Nature 450: 825–831.

25. Pavlakovic H, Havers W, Schweigerer L. Multiple angiogenesis stimulation in a single malignancy: implications for anti-angiogenic tumour therapy. Angiogenesis 2001; 4: 259–262.

26. Orimo A, Gupta PB, Sgroi DC, Aranzana-Seisdedes F, Delaunay T et al. Stromal fibroblasts present in invasive human breast carcinomas promote tumor growth and angiogenesis through elevated SDF/CXCRL12 secretion. Cell 2005; 121: 335–348.

27. Crawford Y, Ferrara N. Tumor and stromal pathways mediating refractoriness/resistance to anti-angiogenic therapies. Trends in Pharmacological Sciences 2009; 30: 624–630.

28. Herbert SP, Stainier DYR. (2011). Molecular control of endothelial cell behaviour during blood vessel morphogenesis. Nature Reviews Molecular Cell Biology 2011; 12: 551–564.

29. Patel-Hett S, D'Amore PA. Signal transduction in vasculogenesis and developmental angiogenesis. International Journal of Developmental Biology 2011; 55: 353–363.

30. Geudens I, Gerhardt H. Coordinating cell behaviour during blood vessel formation. Development 2011; 138: 4569–4583.

31. Wacker A, Gerhardt H. Endothelial development taking shape. Current Opinion in Cell Biology 2011; 23: 676–685.

32. Ebos JM, Kerbel RS. Antiangiogenic therapy: impact on invasion, disease progression, and metastasis. Nat Reviews Clinical Oncology 2011; 8: 210–221.

33. Motzer RJ, Hutson TE, Tomczak P, Michaelson MD, Bukowski RM et al. Overall survival and updated results for sunitinib compared with interferon alpha in patients with metastatic renal cell carcinoma. Journal of Clinical Oncology 2009; 27: 3584–3590.

34. Goodman VL, Rock EP, Dagher R, Ramchandani RP, Abraham S. Approval summary: sunitinib for the treatment of imatinib refractory or intolerant gastrointestinal stromal tumors and advanced renal cell carcinoma. Clinical Cancer Research 2007; 13: 1367–1373.

35. Raymond E, Dahan, L, Raoul JL, Bang YJ, Borbath I et al. Sunitinib malate for the treatment of pancreatic neuroendocrine tumors. New England Journal of Medicine 2011 364: 501–513.

36. Escudier B, Eisen T, Stadler WM, Szczylik C, Staehler M et al. Sorafenib for treatment of renal cell carcinoma: final efficacy and safety results of the phase III treatment approaches in renal cancer global evaluation trial. Journal of Clinical Oncology 2009; 27: 3312–3318.

37. Llovet JM, Ricci S, Mazzaferro V, Hilgard P, Gane E et al. (2008) Sorafenib in advanced hepatocellular carcinoma. New England Journal of Medicine 2008; 359: 378–390.

38. Sternberg CN, Davis ID, Mardiak J, Szczylik C, Lee E et al. (2010). Pazopanib in locally advanced or metastatic renal cell carcinoma: results of a randomized phase III trial. Journal of Clinical Oncology 28: 1061–1068.

39. Rini BI, Escudier B, Tomczak P, Kaprin A, Szczylik C, et al. Comparative effectiveness versus sorafenib in advanced renal cell carcinoma (AXIS): a randomised phase 3 trial. Lancet 2011; 378: 1931–1939.

40. Oudard S, Elaidi RT. Sequential therapy with targeted agents in patients with advanced renal cell carcinoma: optimizing patient benefit. 2012 38(8): 981–987.

41. Zimmerman K, Schmittel A, Steiner U, Asemissen AM, Knoedler M et al. Sunitinib treatment for patients with advanced clear-cell renal-cell carcinoma after progression on sorafenib. Oncology 2009; 76: 350–354.

42. Allegra CJ, Yothers G, O'Connell MJ, Sharif S, et al. (2011). Phase III trial assessing bevacizumab in stages II and III carcinoma of the colon: results of NSABP protocol C-08. Journal of Clinical Oncology 2011; 29: 11–16.

43. de Gramont A, Van Cutsem E, Schmoll HJ, Tabernero J, et al. (2012). Bevacizumab plus oxaliplatin-based chemotherapy as adjuvant treatment for colon cancer (AVANT): a phase 3 randomised controlled trial. Lancet Oncol., 12: 1225–1233

44. Gressett SM, Shah SR. Intricacies of bevacizumab-induced toxicities and their management. Annals of Pharmacotherapy, 2009; 43: 490–501.

45. Cohen RB, Oudard S. Antiangiogenic therapy for advanced renal cell carcinoma: management of treatment-related toxicities. Investigational New Drugs 2012; 30(5): 2066–2079.

46. Keefe D, Bowen J, Gibson R, Tan T, Okera M et al. Noncardiac vascular toxicities of vascular endothelial growth factor inhibition in advanced cancer: a review. Oncologist 2011; 16: 432–444.

47. Jain M, Raizada N, Kuttan R, Shan J, Digumarti R et al. Phase II study of bavituximab plus paclitaxel and carboplatin in locally advanced or metastatic breast cancer: interim results. Journal of Clinical Oncology 2010; 28 Suppl: 15s.

48. Hamzah J, Jugold M, Kiessling F, Rigby P, Manzur M et al. Vascular normalization in Rgs5-deficient tumours promotes immune destruction. Nature 2008; 453: 410–414.

49. Kerbel RS. Tumor angiogenesis. New England Journal of Medicine 2008; 358: 2039–2049.

50. Yuasa T, Takahashi S, Hatake K, Yonese J, Fukui I. Biomarkers to predict response to sunitinib therapy and prognosis in metastatic renal cell cancer. Cancer Science 2011; 102: 1949–1957.

51. Di Fiore F, Rigal O, Menager C, Michel P, Pfister C et al. Severe clinical toxicities are correlated with survival in patients with advanced renal cell carcinoma treated with sunitinib and sorafenib. British Journal of Cancer 2011; 105: 1811–1813.

52. Li XS, Wu X, Zhao PJ, Huang LH, Song Y et al. Efficacy and safety of sunitinib in the treatment of metastatic renal cell carcinoma. Chinese Medical Journal 2011; 124: 2920–2924.

53. Zhu AX, Sahani DV, Duda DG, di Tomaso E, Ancukiewicz M et al. Efficacy, safety, and potential biomarkers of sunitinib monotherapy in advanced hepatocellular carcinoma: a phase II study. Journal of Clinical Oncology 27: 3027–3035.

54. Xu L, Duda DG, di Tomaso E, Ancukiewicz M, Chung DC et al. Direct evidence that bevacizumab, an anti-VEGF antibody, up-regulates SDF1α, CXCR4, CXCL6, and neuropilin 1 in tumors from patients with rectal cancer. Cancer Research 2009; 69: 7905–7910.

55. Batchelor TT, Duda DG, di Tomaso E, Ancukiewicz M, Plotkin SR et al. Phase II study of cediranib, an oral pan-vascular endothelial growth factor receptor tyrosine kinase inhibitor, in patients with recurrent glioblastoma. Journal of Clinical Oncology 2010; 28: 2817–2823.

56. Choueiri TK, Regan MM, Rosenberg JE, Oh WK, Clement J et al. Carbonic anhydrase IX and pathologic features as predictors of outcome in patients with metastatic clear-cell renal cell carcinoma receiving vascular endothelial growth factor-targeted therapy. BJU International 2010; 106: 772–778.

57. Yang SX, Steinberg SM, Nguyen D, Modrusan Z et al. Gene expression profile and angiogenic marker correlates with response to neoadjuvant bevacizumab followed by bevacizumab plus chemotherapy in breast cancer. Clinical Cancer Research 2008; 14: 5893–5899.

58. Schneider BP, Wang M, Radovich M, Sledge GW, Badve S et al. Association of vascular endothelial growth factor and vascular endothelial growth factor receptor-2 genetic polymorphisms with outcome in a trial of paclitaxel compared with paclitaxel plus bevacizumab in advanced breast cancer. Journal of Clinical Oncology 2008; 26: 4672–4678.

59. Schultheis AM, Lurje G, Rhodes KE, Zhang W, Yang D et al. Polymorphisms and clinical outcome in recurrent ovarian cancer treated with cyclophosphamide and bevacizumab. Clinical Cancer Research 2008; 14: 7554–7563.

60. Perren TJ, Swart AM, Pfisterer J, Ledermann JA, Pujade-Lauraine E et al. A phase 3 trial of bevacizumab in ovarian cancer. New England Journal of Medicine 2011; 365: 2484–2496.

61. Burger RA, Brady MF, Bookman MA, Fleming GF, Monk BJ et al. Incorporation of bevacizumab in the primary treatment of ovarian cancer. New England Journal of Medicine 2011; 365: 2473–2483.

62. Bear HD, Tang G, Rastogi P, Geyer CE, Robidoux A et al. Bevacizumab added to neoadjuvant chemotherapy for breast cancer. New England Journal of Medicine 2012; 366, 310–320.

63. Von Minckwitz G, Eidtmann H, Rezai M, Fasching PA, Tesch H et al. Neoadjuvant chemotherapy and bevacizumab for HER2-negative breast cancer. New England Journal of Medicine 2012; 366, 299–309.

64. Jayson G C, Hicklin DJ, Ellis LM. Antiangiogenic therapy—evolving view based on clinical trial results. Nature Reviews Clinical Oncology 2012; 9(5): 297–303.

65. Yau T, Chen PJ, Chan P, Curtis CM, Murphy PS, et al. Phase I dose-finding study of pazopanib in hepatocellular carcinoma: evaluation of early efficacy, pharmacokinetics, and pharmacodynamics. Clinical Cancer Research 2011; 17: 6914–6923.

66. Van der Graaft WT, Blay JY, Chawla SP, Kim DW et al. Pazopanib for metastatic soft tissue sarcoma (PALETTE): a randomized double-blind, placebo controlled phase 3 trial. Lancet 2012; 379: 1879–1886.

67. Dallas J, Imanirad I, Rajani R, Dagan R et al. Response to sunitinib in combination with proton beam radiation in a patient with chondrosarcoma: a case report. Journal of Medical Case Reports 2012, 6: 41.

68. Ribatti D, Djonov V. Angiogenesis in development and cancer today. International Journal of Developmental Biology 2011; 55: 343–344.

69. Finn RS, Kang YK, Mulcahy M, Polite BN, Lim HY et al. Phase II, open-label study of brivanib as second-line therapy in patients with advanced hepatocellular carcinoma. Clinical Cancer Research 2012; 18(7): 2090–2098.

70. Blumenschein GR, Kabbinavar F, Menon H, Moks TS, Stephenson J et al. A phase II, multicenter, open-label randomized study of motesanib or bevacizumab in combination with paclitaxel and carboplatin for advanced nonsquamous non-small-cell lung cancer. Annals of Oncology 2011; 22: 2057–2067.

71. DeAngelo DJ, Stone RM, Heaney ML, Nimer SD, Paquette RL et al. Phase 1 clinical results with tandutinib (MLN518), a novel FLT3 antagonist, in patients with acute myelogenous leukemia or high-risk myelodysplastic syndrome: safety, pharmacokinetics, and pharmacodynamics. Blood 2006; 108: 3674–3681.

72. Joensuu H, De Braud F, Grignagni G, De Pas T, Spitalieri G et al. Vatalanib for metastatic gastroinstinal stromal tumour (GIST) resistant to imatinib: final results of a phase II study. British Journal of Cancer 2011; 104: 1686–1690.

73. Ledermann JA, Hackshaw A, Kaye S, Jayson G, Gabra H et al. Randomized phase II placebo-controlled trial of maintenance therapy using the oral triple angiokinase inhibitor BIBF1120 after chemotherapy for relapsed ovarian cancer. Journal of Clinical Oncology 2011; 29: 3798–3804.

74. Reck M, Kaiser R, Eschbach C, Stefanic M, Love J et al. A phase II double-blind study to investigate efficacy and safety of two doses of the triple angiokinase inhibitor BIBF1120 in patients with relapsed advanced non-small-cell lung cancer. Annals of Oncology 22: 1374–1381.

75. Eskens FA, de Jonge MJ, Bhargava P, Isoe T, Cotroe MM et al. Biological and clinical activity of tivozanib (AV-951, KRN-951), a selective inhibitor of VEGF receptor-1, -2, and -3 tyrosine kinases, in a 4-week-on, 2-week-off schedule in patients with advanced solid tumors. Clinical Cancer Research 2011; 17: 7156–7163.

76. Mulders P, Hawkins R, Nathan P, de Jong I, Osanto S et al. Cediranib monotherapy in patients with advanced renal cell carcinoma: results of a randomised phase II study. European Journal of Cancer 2012; 48: 527–537.

77. Gaya A, Tse V. A preclinical and clinical review of aflibercept for the management of cancer. Cancer Treatment Reviews 2012; 38(5): 484–493.

78. Isambert N, Freyer G, Zanetta S, You B, Fumoleau P et al. (2012). Phase I dose-escalation study of intravenous aflibercept in combination with docetaxel in patients with advanced solid tumors. Clinical Cancer Research 2012; 18(6): 1743–50.

79. Spratlin JL, Cohen RB, Eadens M, Gore L, Camdige DR et al. Phase I pharmacologic and biologic study of ramucirumab (IMC-1121B), a fully human immunoglobulin G1 monoclonal antibody targeting the vascular endothelial growth factor receptor-2. Journal of Clinical Oncology 2010; 28: 780–787.

80. Alghisi, G.C., Ponsonnet, L., Ponsonnet, L., Ruegg, C. (2009). The integrin antagonist cilengitide activates αvβ3, disrupts VE-cadherin localization at cell junctions and enhances permeability in endothelial cells. PLoSONE, 4: e4449.

81. Nassiri F, Cusimano MD, Scheithauer BW, Rotondo F, et al. (2011). Endoglin (CD105): a review of its role in angiogenesis and tumor diagnosis, progression and therapy. Anticancer Res., 31: 2283–2290.

82. Hurwitz H, Fehrenbacher L, Novotny W, Cartwright T, Hainsworth J et al. Bevacizumab plus irinotecan and leucovorin for metastatic colorectal cancer. New England Journal of Medicine 2004; 350(23): 2335–2342.

83. Saltz LB, Clarke S, Diaz-Rubio E, Scheithauer W, Figer A et al. Bevacizumab in combination with oxaliplatin-based chemotherapy as first-line therapy in metastatic colorectal cancer: a randomized phase III. Journal of Clinical Oncology 2008; 26(12): 2013–2019.

84. Giantonio BJ, Catalano PJ, Meropol NJ, O'Dwyer PJ, Mitchell EP et al. Bevacizumab in combination with oxaliplatin, fluorouracil, and leucovorin (FOLFOX4) for previously treated metastatic colorectal cancer: results from the Eastern Cooperative Oncology Group Study E3200.Journal of Clinical Oncology 2007; 25(12): 1539–1544.

85. Sandler A, Gray R, Perry MC, Brahmer J, Schiller JH et al. Paclitaxel-carboplatin alone or with bevacizumab for nonsmall lung cancer. New England Journal of Medicine 2006; 355(24): 2542–2550.

86. Escudier B, Bellmunt J, Negrier S, Bajetta E, Melichar B et al. Phase III trial of bevacizumab plus interferon alfa-2b in patients with metastatic renal cell carcinoma (AVOREN): final analysis of overall survival. Journal of Clinical Oncology 2010; 28(13): 2144–2150.

87. Rini BI, Halabi S, Rosenberg JE, Stadler WM, Vaena DA et al. Phase III trial of bevacizumab plus interferon alfa versus interferon alfa monotherapy in patients with metastatic renal cell carcinoma: final results of CALGB 90206. Journal of Clinical Oncology 2010; 28(13): 2137–2143.

88. Cohen MH, Shen YL, Keegan P, Pazdur R. FDA drug approval summary: bevacizumab (Avastin) as treatment for recurrent glioblastoma multiforme. Oncologist 2009; 14(11): 1131–1138.

89. Lassen U, Nielsen DL, Sorensen M, Winstedt L, Niskanen T et al. A phase I, dose-escalation study of TB-403, a monoclonal antibody directed against PlGF, in patients with advanced solid tumours. British Journal of Cancer 2012; 106: 678–684.

90. Teicher BA. Antiangiogenic agents and targets: a perspective. Biochemical Pharmacology 2011; 81: 6–12.

91. Schwartz JD, Rowinsky EK, Youssoufian H, Pytowski B, et al. Vascular endothelial growth factor receptor-1 in human cancer. Cancer 2010; 116(Suppl 4): 1027–1032.

92. Xin Y, Xiang H, Dresser M, Brachmann R, et al. (2010). Characterization of MNRP1685A (Anti-NRP1) clinical pharmacokinetics in the first-in-human phase I study. AAPS Journal; 12(Suppl 1): 363.

93. Xin Y, Li J, Wu J, Kinard R, Weekes CD et al. Pharmacokinetic and pharmacodynamic analysis of circulating biomarkers of anti-NRP1, a novel antiangiogenesis agent, in two phase I trials in patients with advanced solid tumours. Clinical Cancer Research 2012; 18: 6040-6048.

94. Weekes CD, LoRusso P, Ramakrishnan V, Shih LM, Darbonne WC et al. A phase Ib study for MNRP1685A (anti-NRP1) administered intravenously with bevacizumab with or without paclitaxel to patients with advanced solid tumors. Journal of Clinical Oncology 2011; 29 Suppl: 3050.

95. Yan M. Therapeutic promise and challenges of targeting DLL4/NOTCH1. Vascular Cell 2011; 3: 17.

96. Sabbadini RA. Sphingosine-1-phosphate antibodies as potential agents in the treatment of cancer and age-related macular degeneration. British Journal of Pharmacology 2011; 162: 1225–1238.

97. Papadopoulos KP, Chau NG, Patnaik A, Adriaens L, Lalani C et al. A phase I first-in-human study of REGN910, a fully human and selective angiopoietin-2 monoclonal antibody, in patients with advanced solid tumor malignancies. Journal of Clinical Oncology 2011; 29 Suppl: TPS159.

98. Mita AC, Takimoto CH, Mita M, Tolcher A, Sankhala K et al. Phase 1 study of AMG386, a selective angiopoietin1/2-neutralizing peptibody, in combination with chemotherapy in adults with advanced solid tumors. Clinical Cancer Research 2010; 16: 3044–3056.

99. Lara PN, Douillard JY, Nakagawa K, von Pawel J, et al. (2011). Randomized phase III placebo-controlled trial of carboplatin and paclitaxel with or without the vascular disrupting agent vadimezan (ASA404) in advanced non-small cell lung cancer. Journal of Clinical Oncology 29: 2965–2971.

100. Nagaiah G, Remick SC. Combretastatin A4 phosphate: a novel vascular disrupting agent. Future Oncology 2010; 6: 1219–1228.

101. Siemann DW, Chaplin DJ, Walicke PA. A review and update of the current status of the vasculature-disrupting agent combretastatin-A4 phosphate (CA4P). Expert Opinion on Investigational Drugs 2009; 18: 189–197.

102. McKeage MJ. Clinical trials of vascular disrupting agents in advanced non-small cell lung cancer. Clinical Lung Cancer 2011; 12: 143–147.

103. Patterson DM, Zweifel M, Middleton MR, Price PM, Folkes LK et al. Phase I clinical and pharmacokinetic evaluation of the vascular disrupting agent OXi4503 in patients with advanced solid tumors. Clinical Cancer Research 2012; E18(5): 1415–1425.

104. Hande KR, Hagey A, Berlin J, Cai Y, Meek K et al. The pharmacokinetics and safety of ABT-751, a novel orally bioavailable sulfonamide antimitotic agent: results of a phase I study. Clinical Cancer Research 2006; 12: 2834–2840.

105. Mauer AM, Cohen EE, Ma PC, Kozloff MF, Schwartzerg L et al. A phase II study of ABT-751 in patients with advanced non-small cell lung cancer. Journal of Thoracic Oncology 2008; 3: 631–636.

106. Mita MM, Spear MA, Yee LK, Mita AC, Heath EI et al. Phase 1 first-in-human trial of the vascular disrupting agent plinabulin (NPI-2358) in patients with solid tumors or lymphomas. Clinical Cancer Research 2010; 16: 5892–5899.

107. Millward M, Mainwaring P, Mita A, Federico K, Lloyd GK et al. Phase 1 study of the novel vascular disrupting agent plinabulin (NPI-2358) and docetaxel. Investigational New Drugs 2011; 30(3): 1065–1070.

108. Horti J, Juhasz E, Monostori Z, Maeda K, Eckhardt S et al. (2008). Phase I study of TZT-1027, a novel synthetic dolastatin 10 derivative, for the treatment of patients with non-small cell lung cancer. Cancer, Chemotherapy and Pharmacology 2008; 62: 173–180.

109. Yamamoto N, Andoh M, Kawahara M, Fukuoka M, Niitani H. Phase I study of TZT-1027, a novel synthetic dolastatin 10 derivative and inhibitor of tubulin polymerization, given weekly to advanced solid tumor patients for 3 weeks. Cancer Science 2009; 100: 316–321.

110. Tamura K, Nakagawa K, Kurata T, Satoh T, et al. Phase I study of TZT-1027, a novel synthetic dolastatin 10 derivative and inhibitor of tubulin polymerization, which was administered to patients with advanced solid tumors on day 1 and 8 in 3-week courses. Cancer, Chemotherapy and Pharmacology 2007 July; 60: 285–293.

111. Perotti A, Sessa C, Mancuso A, Noberasco C, Cresta S et al. Clinical and pharmacological phase I evaluation of Exherin (ADH-1), a selective anti-N-cadherin peptide in patients with N-cadherin-expressing solid tumours. Annals of Oncology 2009; 20: 741–745.

112. Yarom N, Stewart D, Malik R, Wells J, Avruch L et al. Phase I clinical trial of Exherin (ADH-1) in patients with advanced solid tumors. Currents in Clinical Pharmacology 2015; 10(4).

113. Gerber DE, Stopeck AT, Wong L, Rosen LS, Thorpe PE et al. Phase I safety and pharmacokinetic study of bavituximab, a chimeric phosphatidylserine-targeting monoclonal antibody, in patients with advanced solid tumors. Clinical Cancer Research 2011; 17: 6888–6896.

114. Tabagari D, Nemsadze G, Janjalia M, Jincharadze M, Shan J et al. Phase II study of bavituximab plus docetaxel in locally Advanced or metastatic breast cancer. Journal of Clinical Oncology 2010; 28 Suppl: 15s.

115. Digumarti R, Suresh AV, Bhattacharyya GS, Dasappa L, Shan J et al. Phase II study of bavituximab plus paclitaxel and carboplatin in untreated locally advanced or metastatic non-small cell lung cancer: interim results. Journal of Clinical Oncology 2010; 28 Suppl: 15s.

116. Thorpe PE. Targeting anionic phospholipids on tumor blood vessels and tumor cells. Thrombosis Research 2010; 125 Suppl 2: S134–S137.

117. Reardon DA, Fink KL, Mikkelsen T, Cloughesy TF, O'Neill A et al. Randomized phase II study of cilengitide, an integrin-targeting arginine-glycine-aspartic acid peptide, in recurrent glioblastoma multiforme. Journal of Clinical Oncology 2008; 26: 5610–5617.

118. Stupp R, Hegi ME, Neyns B, Goldbrunner R, Schlegel U et al. Phase I/IIa study of cilengitide and temozolomide with concomitant radiotherapy followed by cilengitide and temozolomide maintenance therapy in patients with newly diagnosed glioblastoma. Journal of Clinical Oncology 2010; 28: 2712–2718.

119. O'Day SJ, Pavlick AC, Albertinni MR, Hamid O, Schalch H et al. Clinical and pharmacologic evaluation of two dose levels of intetumumab (CNTO 95) in patients with melanoma or angiosarcoma. Investigational New Drugs 2011; 30(3): 1074–1081.

120. Chu FM, Picus J, Fracasso PM, Dreicer R, Lang Z et al. A phase 1, multicenter, open-label study of the safety of two dose levels of a human monoclonal antibody to human α(v) integrins, intetumumab, in combination with docetaxel and prednisone in patients with castrate-resistant metastatic prostate cancer. Investigational New Drugs 2011; 29: 674–679.

121. O'Day S, Pavlick A, Loquai C, Lawson D, Gutzmer R et al. A randomized, phase II study of intetumumab, an anti-αv-integrin mAb, alone and with dacarbazine in stage IV melanoma. British Journal of Cancer 2011; 105: 346–352.

122. Adelberg D, Apolo AB, Madan RA, Gulley JL, Adelberg DE et al. A phase I study of TRC105 (anti-CD105 monoclonal antibody) in metastatic castration-resistant prostate cancer (mCRPC). Journal of Clinical Oncology 2011; 29(Suppl): 171.

123. Goldman JW, Gordon MS, Hurwitz H, Pili R, Mendelson BJ et al. A phase I study of TRC105 (anti-CD105 antibody) in patients with advanced solid tumors. Journal of Clinical Oncology 2011; 29(Suppl): 3073.

124. Milowsky MI, Nanus DM, Kostakoglu L, Sheehan CE, Vallabhajosoula S et al. Vascular targeted therapy with anti-prostate-specific membrane antigen monoclonal antibody J591 in advanced solid tumors. Journal of Clinical Oncology 2007; 25: 540–547.

125. Morris MJ, Pandit-Taskar N, Divgi CR, Bender S, O'Donoghue JA et al. Phase I evaluation of J591 as a vascular targeting agent in progressive solid tumors. Clinical Cancer Research 2007; 13: 2707–2713.

126. Tagawa ST, Beltran H, Vallabhajosula S, Goldsmith SJ, Osborne J et al. Anti-prostate-specific membrane antigen-based radioimmunotherapy for prostate cancer. Cancer 2010; 116(Suppl 4): 1075–1083.

127. Sauer S, Erba PA, Petrini M, Menrad A, Giovannoni L et al. Expression of the oncofetal ED-B-containing fibronectin isoform in hematologic tumors enables ED-B-targeted 131I-L19SIP radioimmunotherapy in Hodgkin lymphoma patients. Blood 2009; 113: 2265–2274.

128. Del Conte G, Tosi D, Fasolo A, Chiesa C, et al. A phase I trial of anti-fibronectin 131I-L19-small immunoprotein (L19-SIP) in solid tumors and lymphoproliferative disease. Journal of Clinical Oncology 2008; 26(Suppl): 2575.

129. Johannsen M, Spitaleri G, Curigliano G, Roigas J, Weikert S et al. The tumour-targeting human L19-IL2 immunocytokine: preclinical safety studies, phase I clinical trial in patients with solid tumours and expansion into patients with advanced renal cell carcinoma. European Journal of Cancer 2010; 46: 2926–2935.

130. Eigentler TK, Weide B, Spitaleri G, De Braud FG, Romanini A et al. A dose confirmation and signal-generating study of the immunocytokine L19-IL2 in combination with dacarbazine in patients with metastatic melanoma. Journal of Clinical Oncology 2011; 29(Suppl): 2531.

131. Van Laarhoven HWM, Fiedler W, Desar IME, van Asten JJA, Marréaud S et al. Phase I clinical and magnetic resonance imaging study of the vascular agent NGR-hTNF in patients with advanced cancers (EORTC Study 16041). Clinical Cancer Research 2010; 16: 1315–1323.

132. Gregorc V, Zucali PA, Santoro A, Ceresoli GL, Citterio G et al. Phase II study of asparagine-glycine-arginine-human tumor necrosis factor alpha, a selective vascular targeting agent, in previously treated patients with malignant pleural mesothelioma. Journal of Clinical Oncology 2010; 28: 2604–2611.

133. Santoro A, Rimassa L, Sobrero AF, Citterio G, Sclafani F et al. Phase II study of NGF-hTNF, a selective vascular targeting agent, in patients with metastatic colorectal cancer after failure of standard therapy. European Journal of Cancer 2010; 46: 2746–2752.

134. Santoro A, Pressiani T, Citterio G, Rossoni G, Donadoni G et al. Activity and safety of NGR-hTNF, a selective vascular-targeting agent, in previously treated patients with advanced hepatocellular carcinoma. British Journal of Cancer 2010; 103: 837–844.

135. Gregorc V, Zilembo N, Grossi F, Rossoni G, Pietrantonio E et al. Randomized, phase II trial of NGR-hTNF and chemotherapy in chemotherapy-naïve patients with non-small cell lung cancer (NSCLC): preliminary results. Journal of Clinical Oncology 2011; 29 Suppl: 7568.

136. Gregorc V, Santoro A, Bennicelli E, Punt CJA, Citterio G et al. Phase Ib study of NGR-hTNF, a selective vascular targeting agent, administered at low doses in combination with doxorubicin to patients with advanced solid tumours. British Journal of Cancer 2009; 101: 219–224.

137. Vigano MG, Cavina R, Novello S, Grossi F, Santoro A et al. Phase II trial of NGR-hTNF and doxorubicin in relapsed small cell lung cancer (SCLC). Journal of Clinical Oncology 2011; 29 Suppl: 7077.

138. Scanbia G, Lorusso D, Amadio G, Trivellizzi N, et al. Phase II study of NGR-hTNF plus doxorubicin in relapsed ovarian cancer (OC). Journal of Clinical Oncology 2011; 29 Suppl: 5022.

139. Mammoliti S, Andretta V, Bennicelli E, Caprioni F, Comandini D et al. Two doses of NGR-hTNF in combination with capecitabine plus oxaliplatin in colorectal cancer patients failing standard therapies. Annals of Oncology 2011; 22: 973–978.

140. Gregorc V, De Braud FG, De Pas TM, Scalamogna R, Citterio G et al. Phase I study of NGR-hTNF, a selective vascular targeting agent, in combination with cisplatin in refractory solid tumors. Clinical Cancer Research 2011b; 17: 1964–1972.

CHAPTER 7

Invasion and metastasis

Andrew P. Mazar, Andrey Ugolkov, Jack Henkin, Richard W. Ahn, and Thomas V. O'Halloran

Introduction to invasion and metastasis

Malignant (from Latin *malignus* = born to be bad) cancer has three characteristic features: anaplasia, invasiveness and the capacity to metastasize. Invasion involves the capacity of malignant cells to escape the primary tumour and to access a means of dissemination such as the lymphatics or the circulation (intravasation). Metastasis (from Greek *meta* = beyond; *stasis* = a standing still) is defined as dissemination of cancer cells from a primary malignant tumour to another part (or organ) of the human body followed by growth of the disseminated tumour in another organ site distant from the primary tumour. Benign tumours are not capable of invasion or metastasis [1]. Although most malignant tumours can metastasize, there are two exceptions: glioma (malignant tumours of the glial cells in the brain) and basal cell carcinoma (malignant tumours of the skin) [1]. Glioma and basal cell carcinoma are highly invasive tumours and can become locally advanced but they rarely form metastases [1].

Cancer invasion

Malignant tumours grow by progressive invasion and destruction of adjacent benign tissue. Proteases that are expressed or recruited by cancer cells such as matrix metalloproteinases (MMPs), cathepsins, plasmin, and urokinase plasminogen activator can break down extracellular matrix (ECM) adjacent to tumour cells as well as basement membrane that surrounds blood vessels to promote invasion [2, 3]. In addition, the transformed metabolism of cancer cells supports destruction of adjacent normal cells, further facilitating the invasive process [4, 5]. In contrast to normal cells, many malignant cells rely on anaerobic glycolysis even in the presence of abundant oxygen (Warburg effect) [6, 7]. Because anaerobic metabolism is energy inefficient, it is compensated by increased glucose uptake by cancer cells [8]. This high consumption of glucose by cancer cells (up to 50 times higher than normal cells) [6, 7] was used as a basis to establish the positron emission tomography (PET) imaging technique to detect primary and metastatic cancer [9], which utilizes the positron-emitting radionuclide glucose analogue fluorodeoxyglucose (^{18}FdG). This inefficiency in ATP production might be thought to represent a significant competitive disadvantage for cancer cell survival. However, mathematical modelling of the tumour–host interface proposes that anaerobic glycolysis actually supports tumour cell invasion [10]. In cancer cells, glycolysis leads to increased excretion of protons that decreases the extracellular pH around the tumour leading to p53

mediated apoptosis of normal cells that are adjacent to cancer cells, impaired immune cell response, and loss of intercellular gap junctions. Cancer cells survive this low pH milieu because they are p53-mutant or p53-null.

The molecular mechanisms of cancer cell invasion through benign tissue and into lymphatic and blood vessels are still poorly understood. Can cancer cells migrate and invade independently within benign human tissue? Despite many years of investigation into cancer cell invasion and metastasis, this simple but critical question remains to be addressed. In vitro migration and invasion assays (e.g. Matrigel®, wound healing) indirectly support the theory of cancer cell migration and epithelial mesenchymal transition (EMT) [11, 12]. However, these in vitro systems are extremely artificial in that they do not recapitulate the tumour microenvironment faithfully. As investigators set up more complex systems that take into consideration the various cell–cell and cell–ECM interactions that occur within a tumour, many of the conclusions drawn based on older migration and invasion results are being called into question. For example, EMT is defined as a process of cell transdifferentiation from an epithelial to a mesenchymal phenotype characterized by loss of cell adhesion and repression of E-cadherin (a tumour suppressor) expression [12]. The concept of EMT is based on the developmental phenomenon in embryogenesis although none of the cells are defined as epithelial or mesenchymal at embryogenesis, and thus the extrapolation of what is observed during embryogenesis to tumour invasion is tenuous at best [13]. The reversibility of EMT has been proposed based on the obvious similarity in the E-cadherin expression pattern in primary and metastatic tumours although reversibility has not been demonstrated experimentally [14, 15]. The major mechanistic support for EMT occurring in the first place is based on microscopic images of 2D tumour section that provide the impression that small separated clumps of 'migrating' E-cadherin-negative cancer cells invade surrounding benign tissue (Figure 7.1). However, recent experimental results using more sophisticated systems that reconstruct a tumour in 3D (rather than just looking at a tumour section in a single plane) indicate that all cancer cells within a tumour specimen are interconnected, forming a 3D network of cancer cell invading roots resembling a 'hair ball' in which the space between microscopic invading roots of cancer cells is filled with benign cells (Figure 7.1). These observations suggest that cancer cell proliferation rather than EMT-mediated migration is a primary driving force of cancer invasion. Three-dimensional modelling of tumour

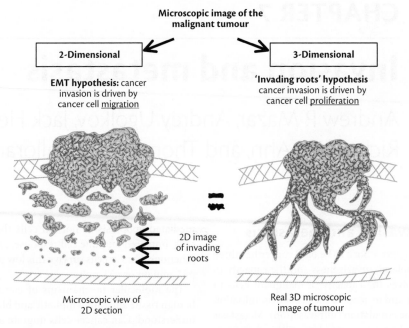

Fig. 7.1 The schematic presentation of EMT and 'invading roots' hypotheses in human cancer.

sections suggests that invading roots might penetrate venules at multiple points, budding and releasing proliferating cancer cells into the blood circulation, leading to metastasis. Thus, cancer cell invasion and seeding into blood circulation (metastasis) may be driven by continuous proliferation of cancer cells. This hypothesis is further supported by the fact that most proliferating cancer cells are typically located at the invasive front of a tumour (Figure 7.1). This 'invading roots' hypothesis can explain the clonal selection of metastatic cancer cells (located at invasive ends of roots). These metastatic cells, selected by their capacity to survive and proliferate in this harsh environment, would have evolved over thousands of generations of proliferation from the originating cancer cells.

Cancer metastasis

Cancer cell dissemination and formation of metastasis occurs in several ways: (1) lymphatic (lymphogenous) dissemination; (2) haematogenous dissemination; (3) direct dissemination to cavities and surfaces of the human body.

Lymphatic metastasis

The most common route of cancer cell dissemination for many carcinomas is the lymphatics [1]. Lymph node metastasis follows the routes of lymphatic drainage. In many types of cancer, regional lymph nodes represent barriers to further spread of cancer cells. There are numerous interconnections between the lymphatic and vascular systems suggesting the possible involvement of lymphatic spreading in haematogenous metastasis as well [1].

Haematogenous metastasis

Common sites of distant haematogenous metastasis are the liver, lungs, and bones (Table 7.1) [1]. Haematogenous spreading of cancer cells is typical for sarcomas but is also observed in certain carcinomas such as renal cell [1]. Cancer cells detach from the primary

tumour and intravasate into venous flow. These disseminated cells are then delivered to target organs to form metastases (Figure 7.2). There are two hypotheses to explain the process of haematogenous metastasis: 'mechanistic' (blood flow) and 'seed and soil' (organ microenvironment) originally proposed by Paget [16, 17]. These hypotheses complement each other to explain how metastasis develops. Mechanistically, the prevalence of certain metastatic sites depends on where the primary tumour is localized in the body. For example, the liver is the first organ through which venous blood flow from colon, gastric, and pancreatic cancer passes, so these types of cancer frequently metastasize to the liver (Table 7.1). Metastatic breast cancer cells are delivered by venous flow to the right heart, which delivers blood to the lungs. Metastasis to brain and bone is formed by cancer cells delivered with arterial blood. In this case, metastatic cancer cells (from the primary tumour) pass

Table 7.1 Common metastatic sites of human cancer

Type of cancer	Metastatic site
Breast	Lungs, liver, bones, brain
Prostate	Bones, lungs, liver
Colon	Liver, peritoneum, lungs
Lungs	Adrenal gland, liver, brain
Melanoma	Lungs, liver, brain
Pancreas	Liver, lungs, peritoneum
Kidney	Lungs, liver, bones
Ovary	Peritoneum, liver, lungs
Stomach	Liver, lungs, bones
Bladder	Bone, lungs, peritoneum
Endometrial	Lungs, liver

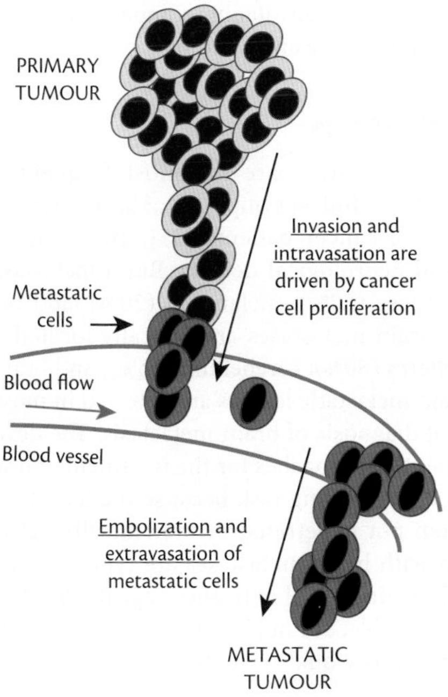
PRIMARY
TUMOUR
Invasion and
intravasation are
driven by cancer
cell proliferation
Metastatic
cells
Blood flow
Blood vessel
Embolization and
extravasation of
metastatic cells
METASTATIC
TUMOUR

Fig. 7.2 Schematic illustration of sequential steps in the process of haematogenous metastasis.

through the pulmonary vascular system, or lung metastatic lesions release cancer cells to seed secondary metastasis in brain and bone as seen for breast and lung cancer.

The 'seed and soil' hypothesis suggests that seeding and growth of cancer cells is regulated by the biologically specific microenvironment of the target organ (soil) [16]. Indeed, it has been demonstrated in vivo that certain kinds of cancer prefer to metastasize to specific organs regardless of blood flow or vascular anatomy [16]. However, the 'seed and soil' hypothesis is also compatible with the mechanistic hypothesis of metastasis because tumour cells must reach target organs by flow and be trapped there, at which time the 'soil' determines whether those trapped cells will progress to true metastases. Wood et al. [17] were the first to demonstrate the development of haematogenous metastasis in vivo. V2 carcinoma cells (rabbit carcinoma) were injected into small arteries in the rabbit's ear, into which a chamber was inserted to observe the ear capillary network. V2 cancer cells were rapidly trapped in the capillaries and a thrombus formed within 30 minutes of tumour cell injection. Division of cancer cells started in 24 hours with subsequent invasion through the endothelium (extravasation) which became obvious by 48 hours after injection. A metastatic lesion was established 72 hours post injection. This study was the first to illustrate that the process of haematogenous metastasis consisted of a series of sequential steps (Figure 7.2). This was also the first study to suggest that metastasis is an inefficient process, later confirmed by Fidler and co-workers [18] and others, since the vast majority (99.9%) of circulating cancer cells were destroyed quickly. Since potential metastatic cells are detached from the ECM and are essentially anchorage-independent until they seed, many of these cells likely undergo anoikis, a form of programmed cell death, upon detachment at this stage of metastasis [19]. A variety of host factors (e.g. blood viscosity and turbulence, platelets, T-cells, natural killer cells, and macrophages) also contribute to the rapid death of circulating cancer cells [20]. Moreover, the passage of disseminated tumour cells through capillaries leads to cancer cell lysis by shear forces [20]. Because only a few cancer cells end up seeding a metastatic site, a recent hypothesis that micrometastases (defined as metastatic tumours that are not clinically detectable) arise from cancer stem cells has been proposed [19, 21]. This hypothesis is currently under investigation in a variety of laboratories looking at many different tumour types. One of the challenges to studying metastasis is the lack of good animal models that completely recapitulate the metastatic process. However, this is changing as investigators develop new approaches that utilize genetically engineered mouse models (GEMM) and patient-derived xenografts (which use fresh patient tumours implanted directly into mice) to study the metastatic process [22, 23].

Direct dissemination to body cavities and surfaces

Direct dissemination of cancer cells into body cavities occurs when cancer grows through the target organ and into a body cavity; for example, the penetration of the colonic serosal layer by colon carcinoma leads to peritoneal dissemination. Pleural effusions and peritoneal dissemination are the most common metastases to represent direct ways in which cancer cells spread into a body cavity [1], and peritoneal dissemination is a common feature of ovarian cancer.

Molecular pathways involved in invasion and metastasis

A detailed discussion of the molecular pathways implicated in metastasis is beyond the scope of this chapter. However, a representative list of these molecules and pathways is provided in Table 7.2 along with references that discuss them in detail.

Clinical implication of metastasis

The kinetics of metastasis development varies in different tumours. For example, breast cancer metastasis can arise 10 to 15 years after primary tumour resection [24], leading some investigators to hypothesize that metastatic cells in breast cancer lie dormant (see below). In contrast, pancreatic cancer often demonstrates a very short time (<1 year) between primary tumour detection and clinical manifestation of metastasis. In general, tumour size, depth of cancer cell invasion, and, in some cancer types, necrosis (which correlates with tumour size) are considered to be valuable clinical predictors of increased risk for metastasis. The larger and more invasive the primary malignancy, the greater the probability of metastasis. For example, gastric carcinomas with progressively more invasion to mucosal, submucosal, muscle, and serosal layers have an increasing incidence of lymph node metastasis (5%, 23%, 52%, and 82%, respectively) [25–27].

Malignant primary tumours in human vital organs (brain, lung, liver) can lead to patient death because of primary tumour growth; however, the majority of cancer deaths (>90%) occur in patients with metastatic disease [28]. Many of these patients do not die from their tumour burden but rather from complications associated with metastatic disease. For example, approximately 30% of cancer deaths are caused by cachexia [29], a wasting syndrome, which develops in advanced stages of cancer and is therefore associated with metastasis. Cachexia is characterized by anorexia, progressive

Table 7.2 A representative listing of molecules and pathways involved in metastasis

Adhesion molecules [92–95]				
Cadherins	Selectins	CD44/ hyaluronate	integrins	ECM and basement membrane
uPAR	thronbospondin			
Proteolytic pathways [2–4]				
uPA and uPAR	MMPs/TIMPs	Cathepsins	Maspin	Plasmin
Cell signalling [96–99]				
TGFβ and Smads	Chemokines/ Chemokine receptors	IGF	HGF/c-Met	Endocrine pathways
RankL/CD95	RTK's	Notch	Ras	MEK
RAF	ERK	mTOR	PI3K	
Transcription factors [100–107]				
p53	Myc	NF-κB	Hormone receptors	various micro RNA
HIF	STATs	Fos/Jun	Drg-1	Sp/KLF family
Epigenetic factors [108–111]				
HDAC	Histone demethylases	GSK-3		

loss of body fat and muscles, weakness and anaemia [30]. Patients with cachexia have decreased survival due to a loss of total body protein, leading to significant impairment in respiratory and heart muscle function [30]. In contrast to starvation, providing extra calories does not reverse the loss of fat and muscle in cancer patients with cachexia; the mechanism of cachexia is not well understood. In other cases, metastasis leads to cancer-related death due to the failure of organs affected by progressive metastatic disease (lungs, liver, and brain).

Lung metastasis

Metastasis to the lung is common in different types of carcinoma (Table 7.1). Sarcoma metastasizes almost exclusively to the lungs [1] and the incidence of lymphoma metastasis to the lung is increasing as these patients live longer due to improvements in therapy [31]. In many cases, there are no lung-related symptoms when lung metastases are detected. However, the symptoms of lung metastases can include chest pain, bloody sputum, cough, and shortness of breath. Complications of lung metastases include pneumonia, bleeding, respiratory failure, collapsed lung, and formation of effusions.

Liver metastasis

The colonization of cancer cells in the liver leads to progressive liver damage. Liver metastases can block bile ducts, leading to jaundice and intoxication. Liver metastasis is generally not curable [32] although surgery and local and systemic treatment of metastatic lesions has led to improved clinical outcomes with five-year survival now approaching 25–40% when surgery and chemotherapy

are combined [33]. Life-threatening complications of liver metastasis include hepatic failure and bleeding.

Brain metastasis

Metastases in the brain are the most frequent intracranial tumours [34, 35]. Clinical symptoms of brain metastasis develop in up to 10% of cancer patients [35]. These include seizures, headache, and neurological deficits. Brain metastases originate from lung cancer (50%), melanoma (20%), and breast cancer (25%) [35]. Brain metastases are typically located in the cerebral hemispheres (80%), cerebellum (15%), and brainstem (5%). Multiple brain metastatic lesions are detected in most of patients at the time of diagnosis of brain metastasis. The development of novel therapeutic approaches for the treatment of brain metastases remains a challenging task because the blood–brain barrier (BBB) is often not penetrated by systemically delivered drugs, and patients with brain metastases are typically excluded from clinical trials testing novel anticancer agents. Most brain metastases are not curable, although palliation with radiation therapy is utilized to improve quality of life.

Bone metastasis

Bone metastases are detectable in over 50% of patients who die of cancer [36]. There are two types of bone metastases: osteoclastic (breast cancer, lung cancer, multiple myeloma, some prostate cancer) and osteoblastic (prostate cancer). Reciprocal interactions are observed between tumour and bone cells in osteoclastic (osteolytic) lesions where cancer cells secrete factors that activate osteoclasts leading to degradation of the bone matrix, which releases growth factors to stimulate cancer cells to secrete more of these factors [19]. Osteoblastic metastases activate osteoblasts, leading to abnormal bone formation. Clinical signs of bone metastasis include severe pain, bone fractures, anaemia, affected mobility, and spinal cord compression. Osteolytic metastasis can also lead to life-threatening hypercalcaemia.

Peritoneal dissemination (carcinomatosis)

The peritoneum is a common site for surface metastasis in ovarian and gastrointestinal cancers with median survival of <6 months once they occur [37, 38]. Peritoneal dissemination may not produce any unusual symptoms in its early stages. Ascites is a typical feature of progressing peritoneal dissemination and may cause abdominal pain, breathing problems, loss of appetite, nausea, and constipation. Cytological analysis of ascitic fluid is performed to confirm peritoneal dissemination.

Metastatic dormancy and outgrowth

Following complete remission or maximum apparent shrinkage of tumours post-treatment, micrometastases can already be expected to be established at various distant sites, and a fraction of these are in microenvironments which are or will become permissive for outgrowth. These micrometastases contain live tumour cells that have survived chemotherapy, and may remain dormant through the course of treatment and for prolonged periods thereafter. Even in patients who undergo curative resections of early-stage disease, some will have recurrent metastatic disease suggesting that micrometastatic disease was already present at the time of surgery [39]. Since metastatic outgrowth is the major cause of cancer death, the mechanisms by which these cancer cells persist over long periods of time in ectopic sites is of great importance, because the characteristics which allow these cells to survive also enable their outgrowth as new conditions evolve, often with enhanced malignancy and resistance to treatment that is associated with relapse [40, 41]. Dormant tumour cells may have been refractory to treatment because they are not dividing or they may express active drug resistance mechanisms which protect them from therapy. Thus, a deeper understanding of the mechanisms underlying dormancy presents an unmet therapeutic opportunity. This would also allow development of probes which home to dormant cells to detect their specific locations in patients who harbour them.

Three categories of molecules may be classified according to their contribution to metastasis and some of these are summarized in Table 7.2: (1) molecules which initiate metastasis through imparting an advantage in cell escape and invasiveness; (2) molecules providing an advantage in survival at the ectopic microenvironment; and (3) molecules promoting progression at those sites ('soil') by enhancing angiogenesis, stromal contributions to metastatic progression, or immune evasion [42]. Metastases that arise soon after primary tumour ablation likely derive from disseminated tumour cells (DTC) which have spread recently from an advanced tumour, then progress linearly at their new location. Micrometastases that remain dormant for long periods may be recent DTCs which are halted in their new setting or they may have originated from an early stage of the tumour, and then progressed in parallel. Owing to selection pressure and genetic instability, parallel progression of the DTC predicts independent disparate accumulation of genetic and epigenetic changes. These would vary among DTC according to their times of original dissemination and according to the niche in which they land, leading to heterogeneity. Genetic diversity, growth rate, and death rate in the examination of patients and their metastatic samples in relation to primary tumour stage are consistent with the parallel progression hypothesis in cases of long-term dormancy [43]. In the period of dormancy where micrometastases are present but are not clinically apparent, the mechanisms responsible for tumour cell dormancy and ultimate outgrowth are not well understood. However, based on both experimental and clinical information, two general mechanisms have been postulated. In the first case, tumour cells are thought to exist in a quiescent solitary state that is resistant to therapies directed against rapidly dividing cells [44]. Thus, in the case of adjuvant treatment, these cells would survive. The conversion of quiescent solitary cells into progressive disease may depend on the rate of accumulation of genetic changes. In the second case, small tumour cell clusters do proliferate but are balanced by a rate of apoptosis that gives no net increase in tumour size. These may remain in a state of zero net growth for long periods of time. Dormant tumours that begin to progress may experience outgrowth that occurs more rapidly and can be attributed only to new additional genetic changes [45]. This suggests that other mechanisms contribute to metastatic progression once dormant tumour cells are activated, such as the regulation of dormancy through the interaction of micrometastatic tumour cells with their microenvironment ('soil').

Tumour microenvironment and metastasis

DTCs interact with ECM, and their survival and ultimate progression to metastatic disease may be influenced by cross-talk with stromal cells, endothelial cells (EC), and endothelial progenitor cells (EPC) during angiogenesis, and interactions (or suppression of interactions) with immune system cells. It is likely that all of these contribute to the escape of a micrometastasis from dormancy, and each probably represents new opportunities for therapeutic targeting. For example, in the microenvironment invasion model, the genetic alterations in a tumour cell initiate transient changes in stromal gene expression [46] through epigenetic or phenotypic changes, and these could contribute to the progression of metastasis. Conversely, the failure of tumour cells to engage their environment may lead to their quiescence. New 3D cell culture systems comprised of basement membranes depleted of growth factors have been used to recapitulate transitions to or from dormancy, showing how ECM components can first impose signals inhibiting growth. In these model systems, dormant metastatic tumour cells show a unique cytoskeletal organization with minimal adhesive interactions with the ECM, but the switch to proliferation is accompanied by internal cytoskeletal rearrangements in the tumour cell and new interactions with ECM associated with the formation of actin stress fibres. In this switch to proliferation, actin stress fibres are formed through β1 integrin signalling that leads to myosin light chain phosphorylation. This requires fibronectin (FN) secretion by the tumour cells, which then mediates the interaction to the α5β1 integrin [47], inducing the switch from quiescence to malignant growth. In fact, dormant cell lines in this model system could be induced to aggressive behaviour by the simple addition of FN to the 3D milieu. In another study looking at dormancy in a model of head and neck cancer, increased urokinase plasminogen activator receptor (uPAR) and its binding to α5β1 integrin led to increased fibronectin fibril formation and tumour cell proliferation, whereas down-regulation of uPAR led to reduced signalling via α5β1 integrin and induced dormancy. Assembly of fibronectin fibrils via the uPAR-α5β1integrin interaction activates the Ras/ERK pathway and abrogates growth arrest [48].

In general, normal tissue architecture, intact ECM components, and protease inhibitors are suppressive of cancer cell outgrowth. Myoepithelial cells, fibroblasts, and immune system cells such as macrophages likewise initially resist tumour progression. However, these cells exhibit plasticity and. under the influence of cross-talk with cancer cell signals in the complex stromal milieu described above, can become significantly altered to create a tumour-permissive or enhancing environment.

Premetastatic niche

For many years, tumour stromal cells were thought to be mere observers in cancer progression, with tumour cells being the major driver in cancer progression. An abundance of evidence now indicates that tumours are complex systems with cancer-associated fibroblasts (CAFs), endothelial cells, and immune cells acting in concert to promote cancer progression and metastasis [49]. Two distinct populations of cells contribute to the progression of metastatic disease: the first is comprised of resident stromal cells and includes fibroblasts and endothelial cells; the second is derived from bone marrow precursors and includes macrophage, neutrophils, mast cells, myeloid derived suppressor cells (MDSC), and progenitor cells [50]. In many tumours, the microenvironment is characterized by a chronic inflammatory state with prominent infiltration of bone marrow derived cells, including neutrophils, lymphocytes, and macrophages. Over time, this chronic inflammatory state undergoes cross-talk with the tumour cells to promote the transformation of normal stromal cells to tumour-associated cells that further contribute to metastatic progression [51]. Many of the molecules and pathways listed in Table 7.2 are implicated in this pathway including chemokines, proteases, cell-surface adhesive proteins, and the tumour ECM.

The immune system has a dual role in the development of cancer and metastasis [52]. Under normal conditions, most immune cells are tumour suppressive. In the tumour microenvironment, immune cells can be recruited and co-opted by the tumour to promote local invasion, angiogenesis, and metastasis. Tumour-associated macrophages (TAM) are a key player in this process and a growing body of evidence supports the role of TAM in tumour invasion, tumour growth, tumour angiogenesis, and metastasis by producing chemokines and growth factors, secreting proteases, and directly interacting with other tumour cells [53]. Further, the role of TAM may depend on its local environment, with individual subpopulations of TAMs promoting angiogenesis or invasion [54]. TAMs are attracted to a tumour by colony-stimulating factor CSF-1 and their increased infiltration into a tumour correlates with poor survival. While class M1 macrophages may initially resist tumour expansion, recruited M2-type TAMs enhance progression, as they secrete matrix metalloprotease-9 (MMP-9), which releases matrix-bound VEGF-A to promote angiogenesis. Identification of unique TAM genes in M2 (not found in MI types) may provide targets for maintaining dormancy. Mast cells, another type of immune cell, are attracted to tumour by monocyte chemotactic protein (MCP-1) and are also associated with poor prognosis. Mast cells are an abundant source of VEGF, bFGF, and TNFα [55], which can drive angiogenesis.

Immune suppression has a principal role in the development of metastasis. Particularly important to this immunosuppression are myeloid derived suppressor cells (MDSC), which are present in tumours, peripheral blood, the lymph nodes, and bone marrow of cancer patients and preclinical cancer models [56]. MDSC are CD11b+ immature bone marrow derived cells that suppress CD4+ and CD8+ T-cells, increase regulatory T-cell levels, and inhibit natural killer cells. Since MDSC are a heterogeneous population of cells, eliciting their exact role has been challenging. Peripheral blood MDSC have been identified in many solid tumours, and increased peripheral blood MDSC is associated with advanced stage and certain chemotherapy regimens [57]. The combination of permissive stromal microenvironment and the recruitment of MDSC to this microenvironment generates a premetastatic niche that is favourable to the outgrowth of metastases. This premetastatic niche is characterized by the presence of the CD11b+MDSC that allows metastatic tumour cells to seed and proliferate through the suppression of the immune system.

In addition to TAM and MDSC, other critical intermediaries that regulate tumour progression include various bone marrow derived progenitor cells. Bone marrow (BM) is a rich reservoir of haematopoietic and other types of progenitor cells stem cells that are anchored to the endosteal surface. Once the premetastatic niche is seeded by tumour cells and metastatic outgrowth begins, these tumours begin to secrete soluble growth factors which promote the mobilization of progenitor cells into the circulation, which are then recruited to the tumour via chemo-attractant gradients. Stress from tissue injury (e.g., surgical resection of tumour) or remodeling, such as occurs when tumour cells seed a niche, leads to release of angiogenic factors, including VEGF, which mobilize these stem cells to the circulation. VEGF interacts with its receptors, expressed on endothelial stem cells, and thereby promotes recruitment of these endothelial precursor cells (EPC), also called circulating endothelial progenitors (CEP) to neo-angiogenic sites [58]. It has been proposed that these EPC are initiators of tumour angiogenesis and required for metastatic outgrowth [59]. EPC are thought to merge with the wall of growing blood vessels and then differentiate into EC. EPC are key contributors to the growth of small tumours but appear less critical for angiogenesis once tumour vessels are more established [60]. In a direct study of full thickness skin wounds in mice, EPC were found to peak at day 3 following wound creation [61]. Thus, in patients undergoing surgical or radiation ablation of tumour, the trauma effect on EPC mobilization may lead to a period of days or weeks with enhanced angiogenic sensitivity to drive small-tumour outgrowth. This implies that brief anti-angiogenic treatment may be a reasonable anti-metastatic strategy following surgical cancer resection [62]. In addition, typical cancer treatment with cycles of chemotherapy delivered at the maximum tolerated dose (MTD), followed by rest periods for recuperation of damaged tissues, has actually been found to induce increased levels of circulating EPC and mobilization during these necessary pauses, mimicking the rebound of neutrophils after their ablation by chemotherapy. EPC arrival and integration at sites of minimal residual disease stimulates local angiogenesis and can facilitate tumour repopulation, and may also stimulate otherwise dormant tumours to grow. In lymphoma xenografts, MTD dosing of cyclophosphamide with 21-day rest cycles was compared with lower doses delivered more frequently and not including recovery periods. The latter 'metronomic' regimen gave a more durable tumour response with consistent reduction in EPC while the MTD regimen showed robust increases in EPC after the end of each treatment cycle, and rapid development of tumour resistance [63]. In a review of many similar model studies, it was concluded that anti-VEGF agents given before the post-chemotherapy EPC spike can effectively blunt the surge of EPC observed in the rest cycle and may therefore limit metastatic outgrowth at its earliest stages. Additional evidence to this effect comes from studies of paclitaxel, which induces EPC mobilization via release of CXCR4 stores from platelets. Tumour response to paclitaxel therapy was demonstrated to be superior in Id mutant mice, which can make all normal BM cells but lack EPC mobilization, compared to wild-type mice, consistent with EPC enhancement of malignancy [64]. Since MTD cyclic dosing of at least some chemotherapeutic drugs seems to create tumour rebound driven at least in part by a pro-angiogenic surge, several strategies are being examined to counter this clinically. One is to include anti-angiogenic therapy during rest cycles of chemotherapy [65], and metronomic dosing has already proven to be superior to MTD dosing in several cases [66]. Another is to include metronomic dosing in combination with an antiangiogenic agent (e.g., pazopanib), although such strategies may be most pragmatic when both agents are orally available since they will be taken daily [67, 68].

In addition to co-opting immune cells and recruiting BM-derived cells to promote metastatic progression, tumour cells alter the gene expression of fibroblasts in their microenvironment, which reciprocate in turn. Fibroblasts are highly abundant in the stroma of tumours. Xenograft studies indicate that about one-third of cancer-associated fibroblasts (CAFs) originate from recruited precursors from bone marrow. Secretion of TGFβ also 'educates' resident fibroblasts to become CAFs, and many of these show epigenetic changes that are significantly mediated by microRNAs (miRs). MiRs with 19 to 25 nucleotides regulate gene expression post-transcriptionally by hybridizing to complementary sites in untranslated regions of target genes, leading to inhibition of transcription, or increased mRNA instability, leading to more rapid mRNA degradation. These miRs may function as oncogenes or tumour suppressors. MiRs can also be shed in exosomes of the plasma membrane and taken up by neighbouring cells, a key method of cell–cell cross-talk. Different miRs are dysregulated in CAF derived from a variety of cancers. Thus, it is likely that CAF and tumour cells reciprocally influence each other via exchange of miRs in addition to signals mediated via adhesion, junctional contact, and proteases, as discussed above. Breast cancer cells (BCC) which have metastasized to the BM can be very aggressive and resistant to treatment, with poor prognosis, although BCC can remain dormant for many years before undergoing metastatic progression. However, this suggests that their coexistence with BM stroma is thus important. At least four miRs have been identified which are delivered to these cells from BM stroma and target the stimulatory chemokine CXCL12 (aka SDF-1, stromal derived factor-1). The miRs move from stroma to BCC with the aid of gap junction proteins like connexin 43 to down-regulate expression of the growth stimulatory chemokine to maintain quiescence. When these miRs eventually fail to be secreted, BCC can grow. Exogenous delivery of the most potent of these, miR-197, might represent a future approach to restoring lost dormancy as a maintenance strategy in the treatment of metastatic breast cancer [69].

Circulating tumour cells

Circulating tumour cells (CTCs) were first described in a report dating from 1869 [70] and have been extensively studied because of their presumed role in the dissemination metastatic disease. To date, circulating tumour cells have been identified in many tumour types including breast [71], prostate [72], colorectal [73], and others [74]. The presence of circulating tumour cells has been correlated with disease progression and decreased survival in breast, colorectal, and prostate cancers. The number of CTCs increases with disease progression and CTCs have been identified early in the course of disease, prior to the detection of metastatic disease, but not all patients with CTCs have metastatic disease. This suggests that the sub-population of CTCs that can establish metastasis is a fraction of the total isolated CTCs and that some CTC may simply be shed cells with no metastatic potential. The recent advent of single cell profiling of CTCs has demonstrated heterogeneity of CTCs in several metastatic cancer types including breast cancer and castrate-resistant prostate cancer [75, 76], which supports the hypothesis that not all CTCs are metastatic. A commercial assay (CellSearch®, Veridex®) for the isolation and quantitation of CTCs is FDA approved for metastatic prostate, breast, and colorectal cancer patients. However, routine evaluation of CTC burden (liquid

biopsy) is not yet recommended in NCCN or ASCO guidelines. Nevertheless, being able to study CTCs at the single cell level is expected to yield new insights into metastatic disease in the future.

Treatment of metastatic disease

Despite years of progress in cancer therapy, curative treatments are not available for the majority of patients with metastatic solid tumours. Curative therapies have only been identified in a few metastatic cancer types including testicular cancer, choriocarcinoma, and papillary thyroid cancer [77]. Reports of successful treatment of diffuse metastatic disease date back to the 1950s [78]. Choriocarcinoma, which occurs most commonly after a molar pregnancy, was the first tumour to be cured with a combination of chemotherapy, radiation, and surgery. Testicular germ cell tumours are the most common solid tumour in young men (ages 15–35) [79]. Combinations of cisplatin-based chemotherapy, surgery, and radiation therapy have drastically improved the prognosis of these tumours. Several subtypes of thyroid cancer that avidly uptake radioactive iodine are also curable after metastasis [80]. Treatment with radioiodine relies on the unique physiology of the thyroid follicular cell and is not beneficial for the treatment of other tumour types. The early success in treating the tumour types described above led to the hypothesis that other chemosensitive tumours would be curable after identification of an appropriate chemotherapeutic regimen, a prediction that unfortunately has not come to fruition [81].

Despite the limited progress towards the cure of patients with metastatic solid tumours, notable progress has been made in the treatment of subsets of patients with metastatic breast, colorectal, and prostate cancers. Newly developed molecularly targeted chemotherapy, aggressive surgical management of liver metastasis, and the development of new local-regional cancer therapies have all contributed to this end. These management strategies are described in detail elsewhere in this volume.

The development of molecularly directed breast cancer therapies has improved the prognosis of most breast cancer patients, including tumours that over-express the estrogen, progesterone, and HER2/neu receptors. HER2/neu overexpression was considered to be a poor prognostic factor for the 20–30% of patients where it is over-expressed. The development of trastuzumab (Herceptin®, Genentech), a humanized monoclonal antibody against the HER2/neu antigen (member of the ErbB/EGFR family) drastically improved the prognosis of this disease. Treatment with trastuzumab as a single agent results in complete or partial response in about 25% of patients with HER2 positive metastatic metastatic breast cancer [82], while combination therapy of docetaxel and trastuzumab increases the complete or partial response to 72% [83]. Despite this impressive efficacy, most patients eventually progress on trastuzumab therapy, though a minority (9% in a recent report) has a durable complete response of greater than five years [84]. This subset of patients suggests that further gains in the treatment of HER2-positive cancers are possible and include: the development of antibodies against additional EGFR family members with synergistic activity with trastuzumab; the development of a trastuzumab drug conjugate; and the development of HER2-targeted nanoliposomes containing doxorubicin.

The first site of metastasis is the liver for a majority of patients with colorectal cancer. Patients with metastatic colorectal cancer (MCRC) are treated with combinations of 5-fluorouracil and oxaliplatin (FOLFOX) or irinotecan (FOLFIRI) [85]. More recently, monoclonal antibodies against VEGF and EGFR have been added to these regimens with increased progression-free survival. While many patients initially respond to chemotherapy, and patients may even achieve a complete clinical response from chemotherapy, recurrence and eventual disease progression is likely. Surgical resection of colorectal metastasis can be attempted if there is complete resection with adequate liver reserve and survival for these patients ranges at 30–50% at five years, though not all patients are surgical candidates [86]. Neoadjuvant chemotherapy can also be utilized to reduce disease burden prior to surgery. More recently, techniques have also been utilized to reduce metastatic disease burden prior to surgery and for palliation. These include transarterial chemoembolization or Y-90 brachytherapy [87].

While the prognosis of some cancer patients has improved, other solid tumours remain refractory to curative therapy. These include pancreatic, ovarian, lung, and many others. Many factors contribute to the dearth of effective treatment options for these therapies including poor drug delivery to metastatic tumour sites, development of resistance, and progressive immune dysfunction [88]. Pancreatic adenocarcinomas are difficult to treat because of their hypovascular and fibrotic nature [89]. This relatively low vascularity impairs drug delivery to pancreatic cancers, which is thought to contribute to the poor prognosis. Moreover, pancreatic tumours are often asymptomatic and patients are frequently inoperable because of invasion of local structures and liver metastasis by the time they present and their disease is diagnosed. However, even with optimal surgical management, the overall survival of pancreatic patients remains dismal.

Most newly diagnosed ovarian cancer and small-cell lung cancer patients respond to cisplatin-based therapies, but these tumours rapidly acquire resistance to these therapies [90]. These include increased expression of glutathione, increased activity of DNA-repair pathways, increased drug efflux through export proteins, mutations in target enzymes, and loss of apoptosis pathways and other mechanisms, all of which contribute to metastasis of these cancer types. Another factor that contributes to the failure of therapy is the late diagnosis of both small-cell lung cancer and ovarian cancer, given that both are asymptomatic until late in progression and no screening tests are available [91].

Evidence that adjuvant chemotherapy and adjuvant radiotherapy can prevent the development of metastatic disease supports the hypothesis that drugs are most effective at treating micrometastasis. The American College of Surgeons Oncology Group Z0011 trial demonstrated equivalent survival in early-stage breast cancer patients with positive lymph nodes who undergo lumpectomy with whole breast radiation and systemic therapy at the discretion of their physician combined with either complete axillary lymph node dissection or no further treatment [53]. This study suggests that micrometastatic disease in the setting of the breast can be successfully treated using the combination of radiation and chemotherapy.

There is substantial effort ongoing in both academia and industry to discover and develop new drugs to treat metastatic disease that are based on the explosion of new knowledge of the molecular pathways that drive metastatic progression. These include agents targeted at a variety of kinase targets and signalling pathways, epigenetic signalling, oncogenes, targeted chemotherapy, and novel cytotoxic agents. Some of these new drugs used in mid- and late-stage clinical trials are summarized in Table 7.3 (not intended to be all-inclusive but merely representative) with a brief description of their mechanism of action.

Table 7.3 A sampling of new drugs in development for metastatic cancer

Type of drug	Name	Target or mechanism of action	Indication
Kinase inhibitors	regorafenib	VEGFR, FGFR, RET, PDGFR	mCRC
	selumetinib	MEK	melanoma
	vandetanib	EGFR	NSCLC
	pazopanib	VEGFR-1, -2, -3, PDGFR	RCC
	ibrutinib	Bruton's tyrosine kinase	Mantle cell lymphoma
Epigenetic modulators	panobinostat	HDAC	various
	belinostat	HDAC	various
	SB939	HDAC	Prostate cancer
Targeted chemotherapy (ADC)	T-DM1	HER2 targeted cytotoxic agent	Breast cancer
Other targeted agents	Brentuximab vedotin	CD30	Various lymphomas
	ASG-5ME	SLC44A4	Pancreatic, gastric
	Lorvotuzumab mertansine	CD56	SCLC
	rilotumumab	c-Met	Gastric cancer
	figitumumab	IGF-1R	various
Novel cytotoxics	epothilones	Microtubule targeting agents	various
	ARW501	DNA damage check point inhibitor	pancreatic
	S1	DPD inhibitor	various

Further reading

Aguirre-Ghiso JA. Models, mechanisms and clinical evidence for cancer dormancy. Nature Reviews Cancer 2007; 11: 834–846.

de Visser KE, Eichten A, Coussens, LM. ****Paradoxical roles of the immune system during cancer development. Nature Reviews Cancer 2006; 6: 24–37.

Fidler I. The pathogenesis of cancer metastasis: the 'seed and soil' hypothesis revisited. Nature Reviews Cancer 2003; 3: 453–458.

Gao D, Mittal V. The role of bone-marrow-derived cells in tumor growth, metastasis initiation and progression. Trends in Molecular Medicine 2009; 15: 333–343.

Gottfried E, Kreutz M, Mackensen A. Tumor metabolism as modulator of immune response and tumor progression. Seminars in Cancer Biology 2012; 22: 335–341.

Lee JM, Dedhar S, Kalluri R, Thompson EW. The epithelial-mesenchymal transition: new insights in signaling, development, and disease. Journal of Cell Biology 2006; 172: 973–981.

Liotta LA, Kohn, EC. The microenvironment of the tumour-host interface. Nature 2001; 411: 375–379.

Shaked Y, Henke E, Roodhart JM, Mancuso P, Langenberg MH et al. Rapid chemotherapy-induced acute endothelial progenitor cell mobilization: implications for antiangiogenic drugs as chemosensitizing agents. Cancer Cell. 2008; 14: 263–273.

Steeg PS. Tumor metastasis: mechanistic insights and clinical challenges. Nature Medicine 2006; 12: 895–904.

Tarin D. The fallacy of epithelial mesenchymal transition in neoplasia. Cancer Research 2005; 65: 5996–6000.

References

1. Cotran RS, Kumar V, Robbins SL. Robbins Pathologic Basis of Disease, 8th ed. Philadelphia, PA: W.B. Saunders Company, 2009.

2. Yue J, Zhang K, Chen J. Role of integrins in regulating proteases to mediate extracellular matrix remodeling. Cancer Microenvironment 2012; 5: 275–283.

3. Mason SD, Joyce JA. Proteolytic networks in cancer. Trends in Cell Biology 2011; 21: 228–237.

4. McCawley LJ, Matrisian LM. Matrix metalloproteinases: multifunctional contributors to tumor progression. Molecular Medicine Today 2000; 6: 149.

5. Gatenby RA, Gawlinski ET. The glycolytic phenotype in carcinogenesis and tumor invasion: insights through mathematical models. Cancer Research 2003; 63: 3847–3854.

6. Warburg O. The metabolism of tumors. London: Constable Press, 1930.

7. Warburg O. On the origin of cancer cells. Science 1956; 123: 309–314.

8. Garber K. Energy boost: the Warburg effect returns in a new theory of cancer. Journal of the National Cancer Institute 2004; 96: 1805–1806.

9. Czernin J, Phelps ME. Positron emission tomography scanning: current and future applications. Annual Review of Medicine 2002; 53: 89–112.

10. Gottfried E, Kreutz M, Mackensen A. Tumor metabolism as modulator of immune response and tumor progression. Seminars in Cancer Biology 2012; 22: 335–341.

11. Crnic I, Christofori G. Novel technologies and recent advances in metastasis research. International Journal of Developmental Biology 2004; 48: 573–581.

12. Lee JM, Dedhar S, Kalluri R, Thompson EW. The epithelial-mesenchymal transition: new insights in signaling, development, and disease. Journal of Cell Biology 2006; 172: 973–981.

13. Tarin D. The fallacy of epithelial mesenchymal transition in neoplasia. Cancer Research 2005; 65: 5996–6000.

14. Thompson EW, Newgreen DF. Carcinoma invasion and metastasis: a role for epithelial-mesenchymal transition? Cancer Research 2005; 65: 5991–5995.

15. Christiansen JJ, Rajasekaran AK. Reassessing epithelial to mesenchymal transition as a prerequisite for carcinoma invasion and metastasis. Cancer Research 2006; 66: 8319–8326.

16. Fidler I. The pathogenesis of cancer metastasis: the 'seed and soil' hypothesis revisited. Nature Reviews Cancer. 2003; 3: 453–458.

17. Wood S Jr, Robinson RR, and Marzocchi B. Factors influencing the spread of cancer: Locomotion of normal and malignant cells in vivo. In Wissler RW, Dao TL, Wood S Jr, eds, Endogenous Factors Influencing Host–Tumor Balance. Chicago: University of Chicago Press, 1967, 223–237.

18. Fidler IJ. Metastasis: quantitative analysis of distribution and fate of tumor emboli labeled with 125 I-5-iodo-2'-deoxyuridine. Journal of the National Cancer Institute 1970; 45: 773–782.

19. Steeg PS. Tumor metastasis: mechanistic insights and clinical challenges. Nature Medicine 2006; 12: 895–904.

20. Wirtz D, Konstantopoulos K, Searson PC. The physics of cancer: the role of physical interactions and mechanical forces in metastasis. Nature Reviews Cancer 2011; 11: 512–522.

21. Diehn M, Majeti R. Metastatic cancer stem cells: an opportunity for improving cancer treatment? Cell Stem Cell 2010; 6: 502–503.

22. Politi K, Pao W. How genetically engineered mouse tumor models provide insights into human cancers. Journal of Clinical Oncology 2011; 29: 2273–2281.

23. Tentler JJ, Tan AC, Weekes CD, Jimeno A, Leong S, et al. Patient-derived tumour xenografts as models for oncology drug development. Nature Reviews Clinical Oncology 2012; 9: 338–350.

24. Karrison TG, Ferguson DJ, Meier P. Dormancy of mammary carcinoma after mastectomy. Journal of the National Cancer Institute 1999; 91: 80–85.

25. Roviello F, Rossi S, Marrelli D, Pedrazzani C, Corso G, et al. Number of LN metastases and its prognostic significance in early gastric cancer: A multicenter Italian study. Journal of Surgical Oncology 2006; 94: 275–280.

26. Nakajima T, Ota K, Ishihara S, Oyama S, Nishi, M. Indication for the lymph node dissection of gastric cancer based on the pattern analysis small of lymphatic spread (in Japanese). Gan to Kagaku Ryoho 1994; 21: 1751–1755.

27. Akagi T, Kitano S. Lymph node metastasis of gastric cancer. Cancers 2011; 3: 2141–2159.

28. Lu DY, Lu TR, Cao S. Cancer metastases and clinical therapies. Cell & Developmental Biology 2012; 1: 1–3.

29. Barton BE. IL-6-like cytokines and cancer cachexia: consequences of chronic inflammation. Immunol Research 2001; 23: 41–58.

30. Tisdale MJ. Biology of cachexia. Journal of the National Cancer Institute 1997; 89: 1763–1773.

31. Vargas HA, Hampson FA, Babar JL, Shaw AS. Imaging the lungs in patients treated for lymphoma. Clinical Radiology 2009; 64: 1048–1055.

32. Lygidakis NJ, Pearl A. Metastatic liver disease: a review. Hepatogastroenterology 1997; 44: 1484–1487.

33. Ismaili N. Treatment of colorectal liver metastases. World Journal of Surgical Oncology 2011; 9: 154.

34. Koay E, Sulman EP. Management of brain metastasis: past lessons, modern management, and future considerations. Current Oncology Reports 2012; 14: 70–78.

35. Eichler AF, Chung E, Kodack DP, Loeffler JS, Fukumura D et al. The biology of brain metastases: translation to new therapies. Nature Reviews Clinical Oncology 2011; 8: 344–356.

36. Mundy GR. Metastasis to bone: causes, consequences and therapeutic opportunities. Nature Reviews Cancer 2002; 2: 584–593.

37. Nissan A, Stojadinovic A, Garofalo A, Esquivel J, Piso P. Evidence-based medicine in the treatment of peritoneal carcinomatosis: past, present, and future. Journal of Surgical Oncology 2009; 100: 335–344.

38. Raptopoulos V, Gourtsoyiannis N. Peritoneal carcinomatosis. European Radiology 2001; 11: 2195–2206.

39. Wikman H, Vessella R, Pantel K. Cancer micrometastasis and tumour dormancy. APMIS 2008; 116: 754–770.

40. Aguirre-Ghiso JA. Models, mechanisms and clinical evidence for cancer dormancy. Nature Reviews Cancer 2007; 11: 834–846.

41. Barkan D, Green JE, Chambers AF. Extracellular matrix: a gatekeeper in the transition from dormancy to metastatic growth. European Journal of Cancer 2010 ; 46: 1181–1188.

42. Sleeman JP, Christofori G, Fodde R, Collard JG, Berx G. Concepts of metastasis in flux: the stromal progression model. Seminars in Cancer Biology 2012; 22: 174–186.

43. Klein CA. Parallel progression of primary tumours and metastases. Nature Reviews Cancer 2009; 9: 302–312.

44. Naumov GN, Townson JL, MacDonald IC, Wilson SM, Bramwell VH. Ineffectiveness of doxorubicin treatment on solitary dormant mammary carcinoma cells or late-developing metastases. Breast Cancer Research and Treatment 2003; 82: 199–206.

45. Klein CA, Hölzel D. Systemic cancer progression and tumor dormancy: mathematical models meet single cell genomics. Cell Cycle 2006; 5: 1788–1798.

46. Reddy BY, Lim PK, Silverio K, Patel SA, Won BW et al. The microenvironmental effect in the progression, metastasis, and dormancy of breast cancer: a model system within bone marrow. International Journal of Breast Cancer 2012; 2012: 721659.

47. Barkan D, Kleinman H, Simmons JL, Asmussen H, Kamaraju AK et al. Inhibition of metastatic outgrowth from single dormant tumor cells by targeting the cytoskeleton. Cancer Research 2008; 68: 6241–6250.

48. Allgayer H, Aguirre-Ghiso JA. The urokinase receptor (u-PAR): a link between tumor cell dormancy and minimal residual disease in bone marrow? APMIS 2008; 116: 602–614.

49. Liotta LA, Kohn, EC. The microenvironment of the tumour–host interface. Nature 2001; 411: 375–379.

50. Gao D, Mittal V. The role of bone-marrow-derived cells in tumor growth, metastasis initiation and progression. Trends in Molecular Medicine 2009; 15: 333–343.

51. Mantovani A, Allavena P, Sica A, Balkwill F. Cancer-related inflammation. Nature 2008; 454: 436–444.

52. de Visser KE, Eichten A, Coussens, LM. Paradoxical roles of the immune system during cancer development. Nature Reviews Cancer 2006; 6: 24–37.

53. Giuliano AE, Hunt KK, Ballman KV, Beitsch PD, Whitworth PW, Blumencranz PW, Leitch AM, Saha S, McCall LM, Morrow M. Axillary dissection vs no axillary dissection in women with invasive breast cancer and sentinel node metastasis: a randomized clinical trial. JAMA 2011; 305: 569–575.

54. Joyce JA, Pollard JW. Microenvironmental regulation of metastasis. Nature Reviews Cancer 2009; 9: 239–252.

55. Ch'ng S, Wallis RA, Yuan L, Davis PF, Tan ST. Mast cells and cutaneous malignancies. Modern Pathology 2006; 19: 149–159.

56. Ostrand-Rosenberg S, Sinha P. Myeloid-derived suppressor cells: linking inflammation and cancer. Journal of Immunology 2009; 182: 4499–4506.

57. Diaz-Montero CM, Salem ML, Nishimura MI, Garrett-Mayer E, Cole DJ et al. Increased circulating myeloid-derived suppressor cells correlate with clinical cancer stage, metastatic tumor burden, and doxorubicin-cyclophosphamide chemotherapy. Cancer Immunology, Immunotherapy 2009; 58: 49–59.

58. Rabbany SY, Heissig B, Hattori K, Rafii S. Molecular pathways regulating mobilization of marrow-derived stem cells for tissue revascularization. Trends in Molecular Medicine 2003; 9: 109–117.

59. Mancuso P, Calleri A, Bertolini, F. Circulating endothelial cells and circulating endothelial progenitors. Recent Results Cancer Research 2012; 195: 163–170.

60. Bertolini F, Mancuso P, Benayoun L, Gingis-Velitski S, Shaked Y. Evaluation of circulating endothelial precursor cells in cancer patients. Methods in Molecular Biology 2012; 904: 165–172.

61. Morris LM, Klanke CA, Lang SA, Pokall S, Maldonado AR et al. Characterization of endothelial progenitor cells mobilization following cutaneous wounding. Wound Repair and Regeneration 2010; 18: 383–390.

62. Retsky MW, Hrushesky WJ, Gukas ID. Hypothesis: primary antiangiogenic method proposed to treat early stage breast cancer. BMC Cancer 2009; 9: 7.

63. Bertolini F, Paul S, Mancuso P, Monestiroli S, Gobbi A et al. Maximum tolerable dose and low-dose metronomic chemotherapy have opposite effects on the mobilization and viability of circulating endothelial progenitor cells. Cancer Research 2003; 63: 4342–4346.

64. Shaked Y, Henke E, Roodhart JM, Mancuso P, Langenberg MH et al. Rapid chemotherapy-induced acute endothelial progenitor cell mobilization: implications for antiangiogenic drugs as chemosensitizing agents. Cancer Cell 2008 14: 263–273.

65. Shaked Y, Kerbel RS. Antiangiogenic strategies on defense: on the possibility of blocking rebounds by the tumor vasculature after chemotherapy. Cancer Research 2007; 67: 7055–7058.

66. André N, Abed S, Orbach D, Alla CA, Padovani L. Pilot study of a pediatric metronomic 4-drug regimen. Oncotarget 2011; 2: 960–965.

67. Hashimoto K, Man S, Xu P, Cruz-Munoz W, Tang T et al. Potent preclinical impact of metronomic low-dose oral topotecan combined with the antiangiogenic drug pazopanib for the treatment of ovarian cancer. Molecular Cancer Therapeutics 2010; 9: 996–1006.

68. Eichbaum M, Mayer C, Eickhoff R, Bischofs E, Gebauer G et al. The PACOVAR-trial: a phase I/II study of pazopanib (GW786034) and cyclophosphamide in patients with platinum-resistant recurrent, pretreated ovarian cancer. BMC Cancer 2011; 11: 453.

69. Lim PK, Bliss SA, Patel SA, Taborga M, Dave MA et al. Gap junction-mediated import of microRNA from bone marrow stromal cells can elicit cell cycle quiescence in breast cancer cells. Cancer Research 2011; 71: 1550–1560.

70. Ashworth T. A case of cancer in which cells similar to those in the tumours were seen in the blood after death. Australasian Medical Journal 1869; 14: 146–149.

71. Cristofanilli M, Budd GT, Ellis MJ, Stopeck A, Matera J. Circulating tumor cells, disease progression, and survival in metastatic breast cancer. New England Journal of Medicine 2004; 351: 781–791.

72. Moreno JG, Miller MC, Gross S, Allard WJ, Gomella LG et al. Circulating tumor cells predict survival in patients with metastatic prostate cancer. Urology 2005; 65: 713–718.

73. Cohen SJ, Punt CJ, Iannotti N, Saidman BH, Sabbath KD. Relationship of circulating tumor cells to tumor response, progression-free survival, and overall survival in patients with metastatic colorectal cancer. Journal of Clinical Oncology 2008; 26: 3213–3221.

74. Allard WJ, Matera J, Miller MC, Repollet M, Connelly MC et al. Tumor cells circulate in the peripheral blood of all major carcinomas but not in healthy subjects or patients with nonmalignant diseases. Clinical Cancer Research 2004; 10: 6897–6904.

75. Powell AA, Talasaz AH, Zhang H, Coram MA, Reddy A et al. Single cell profiling of circulating tumor cells: transcriptional heterogeneity and diversity from breast cancer cell lines. PLoS One 2012; 7:e33788.

76. Miyamoto DT, Lee RJ, Stott SL, Ting DT, Wittner BS et al. Androgen receptor signaling in circulating tumor cells as a marker of hormonally responsive prostate cancer. Cancer Discovery 2012; 2: 995–1003.

77. Lurain, JR. Gestational trophoblastic disease I: epidemiology, pathology, clinical presentation and diagnosis of gestational trophoblastic disease, and management of hydatidiform mole. American Journal of Obstetrics & Gynecology 2010; 203: 531–539.

78. Li MC, Hertz R, Bergenstal DM. Therapy of choriocarcinoma and related trophoblastic tumors with folic acid and purine antagonists. New England Journal of Medicine 1958; 259: 66–74.

79. Einhorn LH. Curing metastatic testicular cancer. Proceedings of the National Academy of Sciences of the USA 2002; 99: 4592–4595.

80. Mazzaferri EL, Kloos RT. Current approaches to primary therapy for papillary and follicular thyroid cancer. Journal of Clinical Endocrinology & Metabolism 2001; 86: 1447–1463.

81. Einhorn LH. Testicular cancer as a model for a curable neoplasm: the Richard and Hinda Rosenthal Foundation Award Lecture. Cancer Research 1981; 41: 3275–3280.

82. Vogel CL, Cobleigh MA, Tripathy D, Gutheil JC, Harris LN et al. Efficacy and safety of trastuzumab as a single agent in first-line treatment of HER2-overexpressing metastatic breast cancer. Journal of Clinical Oncology 2002; 20: 719–726.

83. Valero V, Forbes J, Pegram MD, Pienkowski T, Eiermann W et al. Multicenter phase III randomized trial comparing docetaxel and trastuzumab with docetaxel, carboplatin, and trastuzumab as first-line chemotherapy for patients with HER2-gene-amplified metastatic breast cancer (BCIRG 007 study): two highly active therapeutic regimens. Journal of Clinical Oncology 2011; 29: 149–156.

84. Gullo G, Zuradelli M, Sclafani F, Santoro A, Crown J. Durable complete response following chemotherapy and trastuzumab for metastatic HER2-positive breast cancer. Annals of Oncology 2012; 23: 2204–2205.

85. Gallagher DJ, Kemeny N. Metastatic colorectal cancer: from improved survival to potential cure. Oncology 2010; 78: 237–248.

86. Kopetz S, Chang GJ, Overman MJ, Eng C, Sargent DJ et al. Improved survival in metastatic colorectal cancer is associated with adoption of hepatic resection and improved chemotherapy. Journal of Clinical Oncology 2009; 27: 3677–3683.

87. Mulcahy MF, Lewandowski RJ, Ibrahim SM, Sato KT, Ryu RK et al. Radioembolization of colorectal hepatic metastases using yttrium‐90 microspheres. Cancer 2009; 115: 1849–1858.

88. Nguyen DX, Bos PD, Massague J. Metastasis: from dissemination to organ-specific colonization. Nature Reviews Cancer 2009; 9: 274–284.

89. Komar G, Kauhanen S, Liukko K, Seppänen M, Kajander S et al. Decreased blood flow with increased metabolic activity: a novel sign of pancreatic tumor aggressiveness. Clinical Cancer Research 2009; 15: 5511–5517.

90. van Moorsel CJ, Pinedo HM, Veerman G, Bergman AM, Kuiper CM et al. Mechanisms of synergism between cisplatin and gemcitabine in ovarian and non-small-cell lung cancer cell lines. British Journal of Cancer 1999; 80: 981–990.

91. Cannistra SA. Cancer of the ovary. New England Journal of Medicine 2004; 351: 2519–2529.

92. Li J, King MR. Adhesion receptors as therapeutic targets for circulating tumor cells. Frontiers in Oncology 2012; 2: 79.

93. Zhong X, Rescorla FJ. Cell surface adhesion molecules and adhesion-initiated signaling: understanding of anoikis resistance mechanisms and therapeutic opportunities. Cell Signal 2012; 24: 393–401.

94. Makrilia N, Kollias A, Manolopoulos L, Syrigos K. Cell adhesion molecules: role and clinical significance in cancer. Cancer Investigation 2009; 27: 1023–1037.

95. Mousa SA. Cell adhesion molecules: potential therapeutic & diagnostic implications. Molecular Biotechnology 2008; 38: 33–40.

96. Torsvik A, Bjerkvig R. Mesenchymal stem cell signaling in cancer progression. Cancer Treatment Review 2012; Apr 9. doi:http://dx.doi.org/10.1016/j.ctrv.2012.03.005.

97. Spano D, Heck C, De Antonellis P, Christofori G, Zollo M. Molecular networks that regulate cancer metastasis. Seminars in Cancer Biology 2012; 22: 234–249.

98. Weis SM, Cheresh DA. Tumor angiogenesis: molecular pathways and therapeutic targets. Nature Medicine 2011; 17: 1359–1370.

99. Valastyan S, Weinberg RA. Tumor metastasis: molecular insights and evolving paradigms. Cell 2011; 147: 275–292.

100. Semenza GL. Hypoxia-inducible factors: mediators of cancer progression and targets for cancer therapy. Trends in Pharmacological Sciences 2012; 33: 207–214.

101. Reshmi G, Sona C, Pillai MR. Comprehensive patterns in microRNA regulation of transcription factors during tumor metastasis. Journal of Cellular Biochemistry 2011; 112: 2210–2217.

102. Braeuer RR, Zigler M, Villares GJ, Dobroff AS, Bar-Eli M. Transcriptional control of melanoma metastasis: the importance of the tumor microenvironment. Seminars in Cancer Biology 2011; 21: 83–88.

103. Schneider G, Krämer OH. NFκB/p53 crosstalk-a promising new therapeutic target. Biochimica et Biophysica Acta 2011; 1815: 90–103.

104. Pratap J, Lian JB, Stein GS. Metastatic bone disease: role of transcription factors and future targets. Bone 2011; 48: 30–36.

105. O'Malley BW, Kumar R. Nuclear receptor coregulators in cancer biology. Cancer Research 2009; 69: 8217–8222.

106. Devarajan E, Huang S. STAT3 as a central regulator of tumor metastases. Current Molecular Medicine 2009; 9: 626–633.

107. Mees C, Nemunaitis J, Senzer N. Transcription factors: their potential as targets for an individualized therapeutic approach to cancer. Cancer Gene Therapy 2009; 16: 103–112.

108. Huynh KT, Hoon DS. Epigenetics of regional lymph node metastasis in solid tumors. Clinical & Experimental Metastasis 2012; 29: 747–756.

109. Deb M, Sengupta D, Patra SK. Integrin-epigenetics: a system with imperative impact on cancer. Cancer Metastasis Rev. 2012; 31: 221–234.

110. Kasinski AL, Slack FJ. Epigenetics and genetics. MicroRNAs en route to the clinic: progress in validating and targeting microRNAs for cancer therapy. Nature Reviews Cancer 2011; 11: 849–864.

111. Chik F, Szyf M, Rabbani SA. Role of epigenetics in cancer initiation and progression. Advances in Experimental Medicine and Biology 2011; 720: 91–104.

CHAPTER 8

Genetic instability

Jennifer Wilding and Walter Bodmer

Introduction to genetic instability

DNA integrity is constantly under threat from both exogenous and endogenous DNA-damaging agents as well as from errors that occur during DNA replication and the distribution of chromosomes between daughter cells during cell division. Complex mechanisms have evolved to identify and repair damaged or incorrectly copied DNA, and it is the disruption of these mechanisms that can lead to genetic instability and, ultimately, cancer.

Normal cells are estimated to make errors approximately once every 10^4 to 10^5 nucleotides, but the vast majority of these are corrected through proofreading and mismatch repair (MMR) mechanisms, resulting in a mutation rate of approximately 10^{-8} per base per cell division [1, 2]. In addition to errors during DNA replication, changes such as deamination, depurination, alkylation, oxidation, and DNA breaks induced by reactive oxygen species (ROS) can also result in errors in the DNA sequence (reviewed in [3]). Exogenous factors, such as UV light, ionizing radiation (IR), and chemical exposure add to the burden of DNA damage with which cells must cope. Repair pathways that specialize in the repair of DNA lesions or base pair mismatches include:

- nucleotide excision repair (NER)
- base excision repair (BER)
- mismatch repair (MMR).

Repair of double-strand DNA breaks is accomplished via recombinatorial repair pathways involving:

- homologous recombination (HR)
- interstrand cross-link (ICL) repair
- non-homologous end joining (NHEJ).

In addition to the repair of small-scale DNA damage, chromosomal integrity and ploidy are protected by pathways that regulate chromosome segregation and centrosome duplication during cell division.

This chapter will give a very brief summary of the main features of the major DNA damage response and repair pathways and the nature of the different types of genetic instability that have been observed in human cancers (Figure 8.1). We will discuss the difference between genetic instability arising in germline predisposition syndromes compared to genetic instability in sporadic cancers, and the meaning of these distinctions with regard to the ongoing debate over the necessity (or lack thereof) of genetic instability for the development and progression of all cancers. Finally, we offer an overview of some of the possible mechanisms through which sporadic cancers may become genetically unstable.

It is widely quoted that most cancers exhibit some form of genetic instability at either the nucleotide or chromosome level. Genetic instability at the nucleotide level includes microsatellite instability (MIN/MSI+/RER+) in addition to the comparatively seldom cited and poorly understood phenomenon of point mutation instability (PIN). Genetic instability at the level of the chromosomes is referred to as chromosome instability (CIN) and is characterized by the accumulation of structural chromosome changes. Aneuploidy describes changes in chromosome number, but the term CIN is often used to encompass a wider range of changes in chromosome number and/or structure.

Germline mutations in DNA repair genes commonly confer a much higher than normal risk of development of cancer in an affected individual (but only when they are homozygous). Given that germline mutations in DNA damage response genes give rise to cancers that are genetically unstable, and that most sporadic cancers are also perceived to exhibit genetic instability, it is tempting to speculate that genetic instability is a driving force for the development and progression of all cancers because it accelerates the accumulation of potentially oncogenic mutations. There has been much debate as to whether it is absolutely required for cancer development or whether the genetic instability is simply a byproduct/bystander effect of selection for some other crucial mechanism such as escape from apoptosis [4, 5].

We can gain crucial insight into the nature of genetic instability by comparing its perturbation in inherited and sporadic cancers. Most heritable cancer predisposition syndromes are recessive, meaning that both copies of the DNA repair gene are mutated in every cell in these patients (Figure 8.2). No further event is needed to cause genetic instability in the cancer: the defect is present in all cells, hugely increasing the chance of developing the cancer through selectively advantageous mutations. However, it is important to note that heterozygote germline carriers for recessive cancer predisposing syndromes are not generally at any higher risk than the normal population of developing cancer. This is despite the fact that, in these cases, every cell harbours a mutation in one of the DNA repair genes and therefore has a theoretically much higher potential for genetic instability (through a single further somatic mutation in any cell). For genetic instability to arise through similar gene inactivation in a sporadic cancer requires two sequential inactivating mutations in a given DNA damage response or mismatch repair pathway gene in the same individual somatic cell. The crucial difference between the two is that while genetically unstable cancers arising in germline cancer predisposing conditions can be explained through mutation of DNA repair genes, these genes are rarely mutated in the sporadic cancers that exhibit similar modes of genetic instability [6–9].

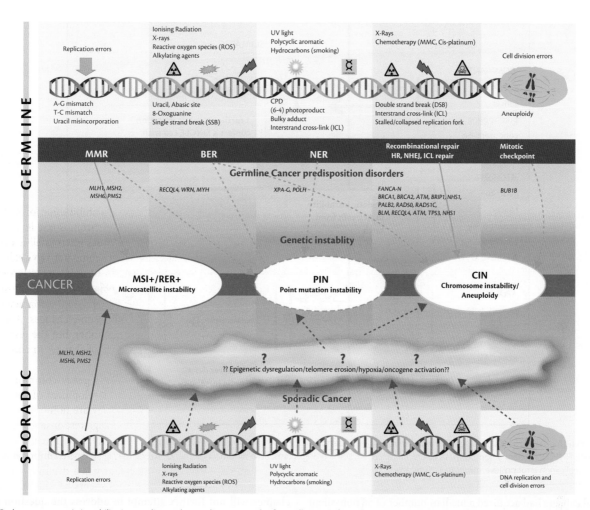

Fig. 8.1 Pathways to genetic instability in germline and sporadic cancers. The figure illustrates from the top-down, the origin of DNA damage, the repair pathway affected, and the nature of resulting genetic instability arising through inactivation of respective pathways in germline cancer predisposing syndromes. The parallel mechanisms leading to sporadic cancers are illustrated from the bottom up. Whilst germline and sporadic cancers are subject to the same errors of replication and sources of DNA damage, with activation of the same damage response pathways and similar features of genetic instability, the genetic nature of the perturbation of the respective pathways is well characterized in germline cancers, but remains elusive in sporadic cancers. DNA repair mechanisms are differentially activated depending on the nature and location of the DNA damage. Solid lines linking affected DNA repair pathways to specific types of genetic instability indicate clearly defined and well characterized mechanisms, whereas dashed lines indicate an inferred mechanism through which the observed instability is achieved. Dashed outline for PIN indicates a less well-defined form of genetic instability.

Abbreviations: MMR, mismatch repair; BER, base excision repair; NER, nucleotide excision repair; HR, homologous recombination; NHEJ, non homologous end joining; ICL, interstrand cross link; UV, ultraviolet; MMC, mitomycin; CCPD, cyclobutane pyrimidine dimers; HNPCC, hereditary non-polyposis colorectal cancer; MAP, MYH associated polyposis; MSI+, microsatellite instability; RER+, replication error positive.

Perhaps we need to question whether or not it is fair to claim that most sporadic cancers display some form of genetic instability. It is important to point out that genetic instability is defined by an increase in *rate* (compared to normal) of generation and accumulation of mutations or changes in chromosome number or structure. The presence of large numbers of mutations or structural/numeric chromosomal changes provides no information regarding the rate at which they were generated nor whether they reflect a current state of genetic instability.

Is it really the case that cancers nearly always exhibit features of *instability*, or is the number of mutations/CIN/aneuploidy observed in any particular cancer more or less what could be expected simply from Darwinian selection of mutations that have occurred at no higher a rate than normal? The incidence of certain mutations that are selected for is necessarily much higher than would be predicted from the mutation rate alone. It is only the incidence of 'neutral' or

bystander mutations that should give some estimate of the mutation rate. Additionally, somatic mutation rates are not at all well defined. These are mostly based on mutations identified from a mixture of uncloned cells, where only mutations common to the majority of cells are detected (in contrast to the tumour, which is clonal) and so do not give valid estimates of the mutation rate [4]. There is, in fact, evidence that a sizeable proportion of at least some cancers do not display any form of genetic instability. For example, a subset of colorectal cancers termed MACs (microsatellite and chromosome stable) has been identified and accounts for up to one-third of all sporadic colorectal cancers [10–13]. This, in itself, argues strongly against a genetic requirement of instability for the development of cancer.

Results from recent whole-genome and -exome sequencing of individual cancers provide some further insight. For example, the recent TCGA study determined that more than 80% of 224

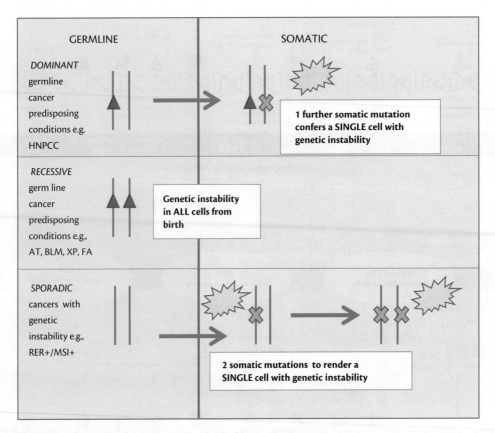

Fig. 8.2 Genetic mechansims leading to genetic instability in germline and sporadic cancers.
Abbreviations: HNPCC, hereditary non-polyposis colorectal cancer; AT, ataxia telangiectasia; BLM, Bloom syndrome; XP, xeroderma pigmentosum; FA, Fanconi anaemia; RER+/MSI+, replication error positive/microsatellite unstable.

colorectal cancers had acquired a median number of 58 non-silent mutations [14]. Does that number reflect a background of genetic instability? Without knowing the length of time each of those cancers has taken to manifest, it is hard to approximate a rate of mutation necessary to account for the observed numbers of mutations in any particular cancer. Further arguments against the requirement of genetic instability are supported by mathematical models, which show that genetic instability is not necessary for accumulation of the requisite number of mutations for a cancer to develop [15]. For example, lack of an increase in mutation rate (up to 1000 times higher in genetically unstable tumours) can be compensated for by a similar-fold increase in cell number such that the overall likelihood of accumulating each new mutation would be similar in a genetically stable tumour that has undergone clonal expansion [5]. In addition, the basic role of natural selection in the evolution of a cancer is often overlooked: the selective advantage conferred to the cell which acquires the initial inactivating mutation in one of the components of a DNA repair pathway cannot feasibly be related to the increase in mutation rate in subsequent progeny. Rather, there must be an advantage, such as escape from apoptosis, from which the initiating cell derives a selective advantage. It may well be that a basic requirement of all cancers is that in the early stages they overcome apoptotic signals, and that the simplest mechanism through which this can be achieved is via inactivation of DNA repair signalling pathways. Thus, even if genetic instability is present in a sporadic cancer, this may simply be a byproduct of the requirement for escape from apoptosis. Although the issue is key to understanding the role of genetic instability in cancer, this

chapter will not further attempt to address the question of how common true genetic instability is in sporadic cancers, but rather to give an overview of the types of genetic instability that may occur, and the mechanisms that might give rise to them in both sporadic cancers and those arising as a result of germline mutations in key genes.

Genetic instability at the nucleotide level

Mismatch repair pathway and microsatellite instability

The most clearly understood form of genetic instability at the nucleotide level in human cancer arises through inactivation of the MMR pathway. It is significant that it is the only form of genetic instability seen in a range of both germline and sporadic cancers that can be explained through the inactivation of the key genes in the relevant pathway.

MMR plays a crucial role in maintaining the fidelity of the genome by repairing DNA replication errors such as base–base mismatches and insertion/deletion loops that can occur during DNA synthesis. The MMR process is reported to improve the fidelity of DNA replication by 100- to 1000-fold and to reduce the replication error rate to one per 10^{10} bases [16]. The MMR system is comprised of several subunits including *MSH2* (mutS homolog 2) on chromosome 2p16, *MLH1* (mutL homolog 1) on chromosome 3p21, *MSH6* (mutS homolog 6) on chromosome 2p16, and *PMS2* (postmeiotic segregation 2) on chromosome 7p22. These assemble to form two heterodimeric complexes: MSH2-MSH3 (MutSβ), which preferentially recognizes and binds to larger insertion/deletion loops, and MSH2-MSH6 (MutSα), which recognizes smaller insertion deletion loops as well as single base-pair mismatches [17–20]. MLH1 and PMS2 then heterodimerize and interact with the MSH2-containing heterodimers and recruit other proteins (including PCNA) required for the repair process.

Hereditary non-polyposis colorectal cancer (HNPCC), also known as Lynch Syndrome, is an autosomal dominant condition characterized by germline mutations in one of the DNA MMR genes. DNA repair is not impaired in the heterozygous state, but somatic alteration of the remaining copy of the normal gene results in the increased rate of accumulation of mutations in mono-, di-, and trinucleotide repeats throughout the genome.

Patients have an estimated 80% lifetime risk of developing colorectal cancer and an increased risk of developing a wide range of other malignancies including ovarian, gastric, brain, pancreatic, endometrial, biliary, small bowel, and urinary tract cancers [21]. Approximately 70% of germline mutations in HNPCC patients occur in either MSH2 or MLH1, whereas mutations in MSH6 are usually associated with an increased risk of endometrial cancer.

Loss of MMR function typically occurs through a combination of epigenetic silencing (promoter methylation) or mutation, coupled with loss of heterozygosity (LOH), of MLH1 and less frequently MSH2 or MSH6 [22, 23]. As a result, such tumours are replication error positive (RER+), which leads to the accumulation of insertion/deletion mutations in mono-, di-, tri-, and tetranucleotide repeats throughout the genome. The altered length of these microsatellite repeats is the 'phenotypic' manifestation of an inactive MMR, and is referred to as microsatellite instability (MSI+). This form of genetic instability in sporadic cancers has been described best in colorectal cancer and is found in up to 15% of sporadic colorectal tumours [23]. Crucially, MSI+ colorectal cancers tend not to exhibit genetic instability at the chromosome level (i.e. CIN) and often have diploid or pseudodiploid karyotypes. Most cancers that are MSI+ also show minimal evidence of widespread LOH (reviewed in [24]), whereas cancers with CIN show numerical chromosome alterations in addition to LOH and copy neutral LOH (LOH followed by reduplication such that while heterozygosity is lost, copy numbered is retained).

The underlying genetic instability in RER+ tumors (whether from sporadic or germline mutation derived cancers) results in a genetic profile that is distinct from RER– tumors and is characterized by mutation of 'susceptible' genes containing repeat sequences within their protein coding regions. In addition, studies in colorectal cancer have shown that deletions in regulatory, non-protein coding 3'UTR mononucleotide repeat sequences account for much of the mRNA expression profile differences seen between MMR proficient (MSI–/RER–) vs MMR deficient (MSI+/RER+) tumours [25].

This type of genetic instability is unique in that the genetic or epigenetic mechanisms involved in MMR inactivation are common to both sporadic cancers as well as cancers from patients harbouring germline mutations in one of the MMR genes. Thus MSI+ cancers always arise through inactivation of both alleles of one of the MMR genes.

Nucleotide excision repair (NER)

The NER pathway consists of 20 to 30 proteins that repair DNA damage caused by UV light as well as chemically-induced cross-links and bulky adducts. As with all DNA repair pathways, NER involves recognition of the damage, excision of the damaged nucleotides, and repair of the DNA strand. The NER pathway repairs complex lesions through the removal of approximately 30 bases. Exposure to UV causes two common mutagenic lesions, cyclobutane pyrimidine dimers (CPD) and pyrimidine (6-4) pyrimidone photoproducts (6-4PPs). If the lesion is in the transcribed strand of an active gene, it is repaired by the transcription-coupled repair (TCR) sub-pathway [26]. If the lesion falls within a transcriptionally inactive part of the genome, it is repaired by global genome repair (GGR) sub-pathway [27]. The two pathways differ in the mechanism by which damage is recognized but involve the same proteins for excision and resynthesis.

The first DNA repair disorder ever identified, xeroderma pigmentosum (XP), is an autosomal recessive disorder, which arises through inactivation of both copies of one of the XP genes active in the NER pathway. Diminished levels of the affected protein component of the NER pathway in these patients can reduce the level of DNA repair to 5% of normal. Individuals with XP are extremely sensitive to UV-induced cancers in addition to exhibiting neurological, ocular, and developmental abnormalities (reviewed [28]). The cells of XP patients are defective in their capacity to excise DNA cross-links and bulky adducts, and the persistence of these UV-induced lesions renders the genome vulnerable to their mutagenic effects. Skin cancers in these patients are characterized by high mutation rates at pyrimidine dimers and whilst they are genetically unstable at the nucleotide level and have been described as NER unstable (NIN), they tend not to exhibit gross changes in chromosome number (CIN) [29]. It is noteworthy that XP heterozygotes are not at an increased risk of developing cancer.

Base excision repair (BER)

The BER mechanism repairs DNA damage induced by metabolic processes such as methylation, deamination, reactive oxygen species (ROS) and hydrolysis [30]. Generally speaking, this pathway serves to repair and replace nucleotides with small chemical alterations. There are two BER pathways known as 'short patch' and 'long patch' depending upon the number of nucleotides replaced during repair. Both pathways are initiated by a specific glycosylase that recognizes the damaged nucleotide and releases it from the DNA leaving an apurinic or apyrimidinic (AP) site. An AP endonuclease or an AP lyase then nicks the DNA, and a DNA polymerase processes the nick and fills in the resulting gap. Finally, a DNA ligase completes the repair process by joining the newly synthesized 'patch' to the preexisting DNA strand.

At least 11 different human glycosylases have been discovered. Germline mutations in one of these, the *MutY* homolog *MUTYH*, lead to a cancer-predisposing syndrome called *MUTYH*-associated polyposis (MAP). Impaired function of MUTYH leads to the inability to repair G:A mismatches in DNA, leading to an increase of G:C to T:A transversions. MAP is an autosomal recessive disorder (the common variants are Tyr165Cys and Gly382Asp [31]), characterized by colorectal adenomatous polyps and a very high risk of the development of colorectal cancer in addition to a moderate risk for several extra-intestinal cancers.

The form of genetic instability in cancers from these patients is not, however, clearly defined, with reports of both aneuploidy as well as near diploid karyotypes.

Mouse models deficient for components of NER, BER, and MMR pathways provide important evidence for the roles of these genes in cancer. Mice deficient for individual components of both the NER and BER pathways do not generally result in spontaneous cancer phenotypes. In contrast, MMR deficient mouse models cause spontaneous cancers with nearly complete penetrance. Similarly, patients heterozygous for MMR gene mutations are tumour prone, whilst heterozygotes for BER gene mutations (and many other recessive cancer prone repair mutations) are not.

Point mutation instability (PIN)

This form of genetic instability has been described but is generally not widely accepted, perhaps because unlike MSI and CIN, there is no easy and standardized way to confirm the presence of PIN. Cancers with aneuploid karyotypes are easily identified as having CIN, whilst MSI can be inferred from the identification of a mutation or promoter methylation of one of the MMR genes, or confirmed by measuring changes in the repeat length of several widely used microsatellite loci. An increased rate in the accumulation of point mutations outside microsatellite repeats, diagnostic of PIN, would be difficult to confirm. This is especially true for sporadic cancers, where the genetic mechanisms underlying PIN are largely unknown. Cancer predisposition syndromes with germline mutations in genes affecting the NER and BER pathways lead to cancers that may be chromosome and microsatellite stable, but may accumulate mutations at the nucleotide level at an accelerated rate, and as such, could be considered to exhibit PIN. However, recent data from exome-capture DNA sequencing of 224 sporadic colorectal and rectal cancers identified cancers with two clear levels of mutation: the majority of cancers fell into a group with a median of 58 mutations versus a second group (13%) with a median of 728 mutations, which the authors designated as hypermutated cancers [14]. All but one of the 'hypermutated' cancers were mutated or epigenetically silenced at one of the MMR genes and 13 of them had an additional mutation in *POLE*, a DNA polymerase that together with another polymerase *POLD1*, has recently been found to predispose individuals carrying germline mutations within the proofreading domains to colorectal cancer [32]. However, only one of the hypermutated cancers had a *POLE* mutation where no concomitant mutation in an MMR gene was found. Using the standard definition of MSI+, which only tests for accumulation of mutations in five mono- or di- nucleotide repeat sequences, some of the hypermutated cancers with a mutant MMR gene other than *MLH1* were classified as microsatellite stable. It is possible that since most of these were mutant for MMR genes other than *MLH1* and that some also carried POLE mutations, the profile of accumulated mutations could be different in these cancers, and the genetic instability conferred by these genes would not be detected efficiently using the standard panel of five microsatellites. In fact, evidence from mouse models shows that the mutation spectrum arising from inactivation of *MSH3* is different from that in *mlh1* deficient mice, with around 40% of the frameshift mutations occurring outside of repetitive sequences [33]. If PIN existed as a separate entity from MSI+, high throughput sequencing studies should have revealed a group of cancers with no evidence of mutation in MMR genes, but with evidence of a higher than normal burden of point mutations. Thus, these two bodies of evidence [14] call into question the existence of a form of point mutation genetic instability distinct from that generated by inactive MMR in sporadic cancers.

DNA damage response (DDR) pathway

This is a signal transduction pathway that recognizes DNA damage and replication stress (accumulation and collapse of stalled DNA replication forks). It encompasses the recombinational repair of double strand breaks (DSBs), single strand breaks (SSBs), and interstrand cross-links (ICLs).

Almost all forms of replication-independent DNA damage require unwinding of double stranded DNA by helicases, cleavage of the DNA strand, and repair of the DNA by polymerases. In humans, DNA DSBs are repaired preferentially by a process called non-homologous end joining (NHEJ), which joins the broken DNA strands. Less commonly, homologous recombination (HR) uses genetic exchange with the homologous sister chromatid to repair the break, and this process involves a complex of proteins including BRCA1, BRCA2, and RAD51. During G0, most DSBs are repaired by one of two NHEJ pathways: the Ku-mediated and the more precise ataxia telangiectasia-mutated (ATM)-mediated.

The XRCC5/XRCC6 heterodimer (also known as KU) constitutes the DNA recognition component, which together with the catalytic subunit, DNA-PKcs, forms the DNA-dependent protein kinase (DNA–PK) complex required for repair of DSBs.

Epigenetic inactivation through promoter methylation of XRCC5 has been shown in approximately 20% of sporadic non-small cell lung cancers (NSCLCs).

Germline mutations in a range of genes involved in repair of DNA DSBs or DNA ICLs cause predisposition to a number of cancers including breast, ovarian, and leukaemia/lymphoma. These genes include: breast cancer susceptibility 1 (*BRCA1*), *BRCA2*, partner and localizer of *BRCA2* (*PALB2*), *BRCA1*-interacting protein 1 (*BRIP1*), *RAD50*, Nijmegen breakage syndrome protein 1 (*NBS1*), Werner syndrome helicase (*WRN*), Bloom syndrome helicase (*BLM*), RecQ protein-like 4 (*RECQLA4*) and the Fanconi anaemia (*FA*) genes [34–36]. Many of these proteins are components of the ataxia telangiectasia mutated (ATM) and ataxia telangiectasia and RAD3-related (ATR) signalling pathways. ATR responds to stalled replication forks and SSBs, whereas ATM is activated by DSBs. Both ATM and ATR signal through activation of the cell cycle checkpoint kinases CHK1 and CHK2, which phosphorylate chromatin-bound factors and promote fork stability and restart collapsed or stalled replication forks. This process is also dependent on several other factors including DNA helicases and translocases such as BLM, WRN and FANCM.

BRCA1 acts during the S and G2 phases of the cell cycle when it co-localizes with RAD51 at sites of DNA DSBs, and it is required for HR mediated repair of DSBs. There is also evidence that it is involved in other DNA repair processes, including transcription-coupled repair, NEJM and NER (reviewed in [37]).

Germline mutations in the FA genes (all but 2% of which are recessive) predispose affected individuals to a range of conditions, and the majority of patients develop haematological abnormalities, bone marrow failure, and eventually, acute myelogenous leukaemia. There are 15 genes in the FA family and they play a key role in the recognition and repair of ICLs and DSBs. Cells from people with FA are defective in their ability to repair ICLs and are thus sensitive to drugs such as mitomycin-C, which treat cancer by causing DNA cross-links.

Poly(ADP-ribose)polymerase (PARP) proteins localize to sites of single (and double) strand breaks, where they recruit XRCC1 and induce structural changes in local chromatin that lead to the recruitment of other DNA repair proteins. The role of PARPs is particularly crucial in patients with *BRCA* mutations, where the repair of DSBs has already been compromised. Treating these patients with PARP inhibitors results in an effect called synthetic lethality, which arises when the combined inhibition of complementary pathways (one through homozygous inactivation of the *BRCA* gene in the cancer and the other through drug inhibition of another component of the DSB repair pathway) results in lethality not seen through inhibition of either pathway alone. Crucially, all non-cancerous cells within patients with germline mutations of *BRCA* genes retain one functional copy of the *BRCA* gene and are able to survive. Treatment of patients with *BRCA* mutations with PARP inhibitors has provided a substantial improvement to the outcome of these patients.

Genetic instability at the chromosome level

CIN and aneuploidy

Boveri proposed more than 100 years ago that cancer was caused by abnormal chromosome segregation [38]. Structural chromosome changes leading to CIN are generated most commonly through errors in the recombinational repair of DSBs and include translocations, inversions, deletions, and duplications. Numerical changes can occur as a result of errors within mitotic control pathways regulating chromosome segregation and centrosome duplication.

The factors underlying aneuploidy in sporadic cancers are poorly understood but several genes, including *MAD2* (*MXI1*), *BUB1B*, *BUB3*, and *CENPE* [39, 40], involved in the alignment and segregation of chromosomes during mitosis (reviewed in [41]), have been suggested to play a role in the formation of aneuploidy. *APC* [42], which is mutated in about 85% of colorectal cancers, has also been implicated in the genesis of aneuploidy in colorectal cancer. However, the fact that *APC* is also mutated in a large number of MMR deficient colorectal cancers where aneuploidy is not present suggests it is unlikely that *APC* plays a major role in the development of aneuploidy in colorectal cancer.

In yeast, more than 100 genes that can cause genetic instability at the level of the chromosome have been identified [43]. That disruption of these genes *can* generate a CIN or aneuploidy phenotype in model organisms does not necessarily mean that they are the cause of CIN or aneuploidy in human cancers. There have been reports of mutations in some of these genes in cancers, but the numbers are modest at best and can in no way account for the incidence of CIN or aneuploidy in human cancers. That these genes behave as typical tumour suppressor genes, requiring somatic inactivation of both copies of the relevant gene in sporadic cancers, may account for the low incidence of observed mutations in genes within these pathways in sporadic cancers. It may well be that genetic instability in sporadic cancers arises through some other mechanism with fewer steps and that, once again, CIN/aneuploidy is possibly just a side effect of selection for escape from one of the many tumour suppressive mechanisms employed by the cell.

Clearly, the lack of mutations identified in nearly all candidate genes studied to date indicates that the genetic and/or epigenetic factors that lead to CIN and aneuploidy in the majority of sporadic human malignancies have yet to be uncovered.

Mechanisms implicated in the development of genetic instability in sporadic cancers

If we accept that genetic instability is common in both sporadic cancers as well as those arising in patients carrying germline mutations for DNA repair pathways, we must also note that that the genetic instability in sporadic cancers clearly arises through a mechanism other than genetic or epigenetic inactivation of those genes associated with heritable cancer risk. There are only two possible explanations for this difference: genetic instability is required for development of cancer in general, but sporadic and germline-derived cancers reach this end through different mechanisms, or while genetic instability clearly occurs through genetic inactivation of key genes in DNA repair pathways in germline cancer predisposing conditions, the genetic instability seen in sporadic cancers is incidental and secondary to some other process. The mechanisms discussed below have all been implicated in the development of CIN in sporadic cancers. While it is clear that each of these plays a role in the development and progression of sporadic cancers, their causative role in the development of genetic instability in sporadic cancers remains unproven. They are therefore listed here to give a more complete overview of the currently held views that might explain genetic instability in sporadic human cancers. The assumption for each of these is that, if they provide a mechanism through which the rate at which genetic, epigenetic, or chromosomal changes could be generated (albeit transiently in some circumstances), they could be considered as mechanisms contributing to genetic instability.

Epigenetic alterations

Epigenetic alterations in cancer typically involve DNA hypermethylation of CpG dinucleotides (clustered into regions called CpG islands in the promoters of genes), which mostly result in the transcriptional inactivation of the associated genes [44]. Almost half of all genes are predicted to contain a CpG rich region that fulfils the criteria of being a CpG island [45]. Promoter methylation is a 'metastable' change affecting gene expression and may undergo selective pressure in tumorigenesis in just the same way as mutations. Thus, disruption of the epigenetic signature in cancer represents a theoretical alternative to genetic instability in providing a similar, heritable mechanism involved in the progression of cancer. This has been explored in the greatest depth in colorectal cancer, where the concept of a CpG island methylator phenotype (CIMP) was first described [46]; reviewed in [47].

The term refers to cancer-related aberrant methylation of CpG islands in the promoters of a range of genes, termed CIMP markers. Methylation of CIMP markers is broadly interpreted to indicate the presence of a disrupted methylation maintenance system and may be associated with more targeted methylation of tumour suppressor genes.

Telomeres

Telomeres protect the ends of chromosomes and stop them from being recognized by the DNA damage response machinery as DSBs.

Embryonic stem cells and adult tissue stem cells in humans express both the ribonucleoprotein (hTERC/hTR) as well as the catalytic component (hTERT) of the protein complex telomerase, which acts to maintain telomere length and protect cells from a type of cell cycle arrest known as replicative cell senescence (see [48, 49] for recent reviews). Most other somatic cells only express one ribonucleoprotein subunit, and lack hTERT expression. Consequently, they are unable to maintain telomere length during replication and eventually undergo replicative cell senescence. Cells with shortened telomeres which have become resistant to senescence have been shown to undergo chromosome fusion and develop CIN [50]. It has been shown that about 85–90% of human cancers express active telomerase [51]. It is unclear whether this is due to reactivation via re-expression of the catalytic subunit, or whether the cancers arose from a stem cell or early progenitor cell in which telomerase was already active. However, there is evidence that some early cancers and pre-cancerous cells undergo telomere loss-induced crisis and end-to-end chromosomal fusions, which can generate unstable dicentric chromosomes and potentially lead to CIN [52].

Hypoxia

Hypoxia is a common feature of developing cancers as they outgrow existing blood supply and before angiogenic stimuli lead to new vasculature. There is emerging evidence that hypoxia and cyclical hypoxia and re-oxygenation result in the induction of genetic instability and increased mutation frequencies [53, 54] through transcriptional repression of MMR genes including *MLH1*, *MSH2*, and *MSH6* [55, 56]. Hypoxic conditions have also been reported to result in oxidative base damage [57, 58], gene amplification [59], and DNA over-replication [60].

Recent studies have suggested a mechanism involving DNA replication stress which may account for the genetic instability (most commonly in the form of CIN) seen in sporadic cancers [61, 62]. Unresolved DNA replication forks, also known as DNA replication stress, can arise through any mechanism that interferes with the normal progression of DNA replication forks, including changes in the levels of dNTPs or proteins involved in dNTP synthesis, DNA synthesis, or damage to the DNA itself. If unresolved, stalled replication forks can lead to DSBs and complex chromosomal rearrangements (CIN) (reviewed in [3, 62, 63]).

Oncogene-induced DNA replication stress model

The oncogene-induced DNA replication stress model arose from the observation that early precancerous lesions tend to have an increase in the number of DNA DSBs thought to be caused by stalled DNA replication forks, in addition to constitutive activation of the ATM-CHK2 DNA damage response pathway [64, 65]. Importantly, this occurs in the absence of mutation of any of the DNA damage repair pathway genes such as *TP53*.

It was subsequently shown that activating mutations in several oncogenes including *RAS*, *MYC*, *CCNE1* (cyclin E), *CDC25A*, and *E2F1* are capable of inducing DSBs, LOH, and genetic instability in various animal model systems ranging from human to mouse and even yeast [64, 66–69]. Thus, the oncogene-induced DNA replication stress model argues that *RAS* and other oncogenes cause collapse of DNA replication forks and DSBs in early and precancerous

cells, which then provides selective pressure for the loss of DNA checkpoint genes like *TP53* in order to escape apoptosis.

Although there is some evidence for oncogene induction of this mechanism, and although the model would provide an explanation for why nearly all sporadic cancers are thought to have genetic instability in the absence of mutations in DNA repair pathway genes, there is currently no understanding of the mechanism by which the presence of activated oncogenes might cause DNA replication stress. There are also clear examples where precancerous lesions, such as colorectal adenomas, are not commonly aneuploid.

Conclusion

It is now undisputed that cancer arises as a result of the sequential accumulation of genetic and epigenetic changes, each of which is selected for in a Darwinian evolutionary process because they provide a selective advantage to the developing cancer. It is also clear that disruptions of the mechanisms that have evolved to maintain the fidelity of the genome result in increased rates of mutation and can accelerate tumorigenesis. It is widely accepted that many if not most cancers harbour some form of genetic instability, either manifested through CIN and aneuploidy, or via inactivation of MMR with resultant MSI. These observations have led some to hypothesize the existence of a mutator phenotype. The mutator hypothesis argues that genetic instability is present in precancerous lesions and drives tumour development by increasing the spontaneous mutation rate [70]. The key assumption with this argument is that spontaneous mutation rates are not high enough to give rise to the mutations that are selected for in the outgrowth of a cancer. The counter-argument is that mutation rates are large enough if selection is properly taken into account [4]. In hereditary cancers, genetic instability facilitates the accumulation of critical mutations in oncogenes and tumour suppressor genes, and these cancers almost certainly fulfil the requirements of the mutator hypothesis in that genetic instability occurs early in the development of the cancer and results in an increased rate of accumulation of spontaneous mutation. However, the germline cancer predisposition syndromes are almost always autosomal recessive and do not, in the heterozygous state, affect genome stability. If genetic instability were selected for in cancer, one might expect that individuals who are heterozygotes for mutations in repair genes associated with diseases like AT, BLM, XP, and FA would carry a much higher risk of developing cancers (through the single further step of somatic inactivation of the second allele) in the same way that individuals heterozygous for mutations in MMR genes have a 100% risk of developing colorectal cancer. But this is not found to be the case, strongly suggesting that the selective advantage conferred by MMR deficiency is not due to the increased mutation rate per se, but rather due to the acquisition of some phenotype directly related to growth and survival, such as resistance to apoptosis.

The key issue with genetic and epigenetic changes that increase genetic instability is whether their selective advantage is due solely to their effect on mutation rate, or whether it is due to a more direct effect, and that the increase in mutation rate is a bystander effect. The rationale for the argument against the mutator hypothesis rests on the fundamentals of natural selection; any selective advantage must be conferred in the first change that does not yet increase the mutation rate. Exhaustive studies of sporadic cancers have failed to identify common mutations in DNA repair and mitotic checkpoint genes in a wide range of cancers (reviewed in [63]; [14, 71]). The low frequency of these mutations in sporadic cancers has confounded expectations and argues against the mutator hypothesis for sporadic cancers [4, 14].

DNA repair mechanisms generally result in activation of apoptotic pathways once a critical level of damage accumulates [72, 73]. This protective mechanism allows the cell to attempt repair, but in the event that the damage cannot be repaired, activation of apoptosis ensures that fidelity is retained. It then stands to reason that part of the role of the protein complexes involved in recognition and repair of damaged DNA is simultaneously to recruit and activate apoptotic pathways. Thus, inactivation of one or more of the components of DNA repair is likely also to affect the ability to escape apoptotic signals resulting from accumulation of excessive levels of damage. This escape from apoptosis would provide the most likely selective advantage conferred to a cell in which somatic inactivation of a DNA damage repair gene occurred.

It has yet to be determined whether transient telomere deficiency, epigenetic dysregulation, cycles of hypoxia and re-oxygenation, the oncogene-induced DNA-damage model, or some combinations thereof are responsible for CIN in sporadic human cancers. Similarly, there is no clear answer to the question of whether genetic instability in sporadic cancers is simply a common byproduct of, for example, the selective pressures against apoptotic signals that arise from activation of repair pathways in the face of DNA damage. Experimental and theoretical evidence do not support the concept of genetic instability as a universal and required driving force for all cancers, but where it is evident in sporadic cancers, we still have some way to go before we fully understand the underlying mechanisms.

Further reading

Bodmer W, Bielas JH, Beckman RA. Genetic instability is not a requirement for tumor development. Cancer Research 2008; 68(10):3558–3560; discussion 60–61.

Ciccia A, Elledge SJ. The DNA damage response: making it safe to play with knives. Molecular Cell 2010; 40(2): 179–204.

Comprehensive molecular characterization of human colon and rectal cancer. Nature 2012; 487(7407): 330–337.

Dereli-Oz A, Versini G, Halazonetis TD. Studies of genomic copy number changes in human cancers reveal signatures of DNA replication stress. Molecular Oncology 2011; 5(4): 308–314.

Fousteri M, Mullenders LH. Transcription-coupled nucleotide excision repair in mammalian cells: molecular mechanisms and biological effects. Cell Research 2008; 18(1): 73–84.

Garber K. At loose ends: telomere theories of aging and cancer begin to converge. Journal of the National Cancer Institute 2012; 104(11): 803–806.

Gordon DJ, Resio B, Pellman D. Causes and consequences of aneuploidy in cancer. Nature Review Genetics 2012; 13(3): 189–203.

Hassen S, Ali N, Chowdhury P. Molecular signaling mechanisms of apoptosis in hereditary non-polyposis colorectal cancer. World Journal of Gastrointestinal Pathophysiology 2012; 3(3): 71–79.

Lynch M. Rate, molecular spectrum, and consequences of human mutation. Proceedings of the National Academy of Sciences USA 2010; 107(3): 961–968.

Sieber OM, Heinimann K, Tomlinson IP. Genomic instability: the engine of tumorigenesis? Nature Reviews Cancer 2003; 3(9): 701–708.

Tomlinson I, Sasieni P, Bodmer W. How many mutations in a cancer? The American Journal of Pathology 2002; 160(3): 755–758.

References

1. Lynch M. Rate, molecular spectrum, and consequences of human mutation. Proceedings of the National Academy of Sciences USA 2010; 107(3): 961–968.
2. Roach JC, Glusman G, Smit AF, Huff CD, Hubley R et al. Analysis of genetic inheritance in a family quartet by whole-genome sequencing. Science 2010; 328(5978): 636–639.
3. Ciccia A, Elledge SJ. The DNA damage response: making it safe to play with knives. Molecular Cell 2010; 40(2): 179–204.
4. Bodmer W, Bielas JH, Beckman RA. Genetic instability is not a requirement for tumor development. Cancer Research 2008; 68(10): 3558–3560; discussion 60–1.
5. Sieber OM, Heinimann K, Tomlinson IP. Genomic instability: the engine of tumorigenesis? Nature Reviews Cancer 2003; 3(9): 701–708.
6. Cahill DP, da Costa LT, Carson-Walter EB, Kinzler KW, Vogelstein B et al. Characterization of MAD2B and other mitotic spindle checkpoint genes. Genomics 1999; 58(2): 181–187.
7. Cahill DP, Lengauer C, Yu J, Riggins GJ, Willson JK et al. Mutations of mitotic checkpoint genes in human cancers. Nature 1998; 392(6673): 300–303.
8. Rajagopalan H, Lengauer C. Aneuploidy and cancer. Nature 2004; 432(7015): 338–341.
9. Wang Z, Cummins JM, Shen D, Cahill DP, Jallepalli PV et al. Three classes of genes mutated in colorectal cancers with chromosomal instability. Cancer Research 2004; 64(9): 2998–23001.
10. Silver A, Sengupta N, Propper D, Wilson P, Hagemann T et al. A distinct DNA methylation profile associated with microsatellite and chromosomal stable sporadic colorectal cancers. International Journal of Cancer 2012; 130(5): 1082–1092.
11. Cai G, Xu Y, Lu H, Shi Y, Lian P et al. Clinicopathologic and molecular features of sporadic microsatellite- and chromosomal-stable colorectal cancers. International Journal of Colorectal Disease 2008; 23(4): 365–373.
12. Tang R, Changchien CR, Wu MC, Fan CW, Liu KW et al. Colorectal cancer without high microsatellite instability and chromosomal instability: an alternative genetic pathway to human colorectal cancer. Carcinogenesis 2004; 25(5): 841–846.
13. Hawkins NJ, Tomlinson I, Meagher A, Ward RL. Microsatellite-stable diploid carcinoma: a biologically distinct and aggressive subset of sporadic colorectal cancer. British Journal of Cancer 2001; 84(2): 232–236.
14. Comprehensive molecular characterization of human colon and rectal cancer. Nature 2012; 487(7407): 330–337.
15. Tomlinson I, Sasieni P, Bodmer W. How many mutations in a cancer? The American Journal of Pathology 2002; 160(3): 755–758.
16. Modrich P, Lahue R. Mismatch repair in replication fidelity, genetic recombination, and cancer biology. Annual Review of Biochemistry 1996; 65: 101–133.
17. Acharya S, Wilson T, Gradia S, Kane MF, Guerrette S et al. hMSH2 forms specific mispair-binding complexes with hMSH3 and hMSH6. Proceedings of the National Academy of Sciences USA 1996; 93(24): 13629–13634.
18. Alani E. The Saccharomyces cerevisiae Msh2 and Msh6 proteins form a complex that specifically binds to duplex oligonucleotides containing mismatched DNA base pairs. Molecular Cell Biology 1996; 16(10): 5604–5615.
19. Genschel J, Littman SJ, Drummond JT, Modrich P. Isolation of MutSbeta from human cells and comparison of the mismatch repair specificities of MutSbeta and MutSalpha. Journal of Biological Chemistry 1998; 273(31): 19895–19901.
20. Marsischky GT, Kolodner RD. Biochemical characterization of the interaction between the Saccharomyces cerevisiae MSH2-MSH6 complex and mispaired bases in DNA. Journal of Biological Chemistry 1999; 274(38): 26668–26682.
21. Jasperson KW, Tuohy TM, Neklason DW, Burt RW. Hereditary and familial colon cancer. Gastroenterology 2010; 138(6): 2044–2058.

22. Giacomini CP, Leung SY, Chen X, Yuen ST, Kim YH et al. A gene expression signature of genetic instability in colon cancer. Cancer Research 2005; 65(20): 9200–9205.

23. Peltomaki P. Role of DNA mismatch repair defects in the pathogenesis of human cancer. Journal of Clinical Oncology 2003; 21(6): 1174–1179.

24. Vilar E, Gruber SB. Microsatellite instability in colorectal cancer: the stable evidence. Nature Reviews Clinical Oncology 2010; 7(3): 153–162.

25. Wilding JL, McGowan S, Liu Y, Bodmer WF. Replication error deficient and proficient colorectal cancer gene expression differences caused by 3'UTR polyT sequence deletions. Proceedings of the National Academy of Sciences USA 2010; 107(49): 21058–21063.

26. Fousteri M, Mullenders LH. Transcription-coupled nucleotide excision repair in mammalian cells: molecular mechanisms and biological effects. Cell Research 2008; 18(1): 73–84.

27. Sugasawa K, Okamoto T, Shimizu Y, Masutani C, Iwai S et al. A multistep damage recognition mechanism for global genomic nucleotide excision repair. Genes & Development 2001; 15(5): 507–521.

28. Dworaczek H, Xiao W. Xeroderma pigmentosum: a glimpse into nucleotide excision repair, genetic instability, and cancer. Critical Reviews in Oncogenesis 2007; 13(2): 159–177.

29. Heim S, Mitelman F eds. Cancer Cytogenetics. New York: Wiley-Liss, 1995.

30. Wood RD, Mitchell M, Sgouros J, Lindahl T. Human DNA repair genes. Science. 2001; 291(5507): 1284–1289.

31. Al-Tassan N, Chmiel NH, Maynard J, Fleming N, Livingston AL et al. Inherited variants of MYH associated with somatic G:C–>T:A mutations in colorectal tumors. Nature Genetics 2002; 30(2): 227–232.

32. Palles C, Cazier JB, Howarth KM, Domingo E, Jones AM et al. Germline mutations affecting the proofreading domains of POLE and POLD1 predispose to colorectal adenomas and carcinomas. Nature Genetics 2012.

33. Chen PC, Kuraguchi M, Velasquez J, Wang Y, Yang K et al. Novel roles for MLH3 deficiency and TLE6-like amplification in DNA mismatch repair-deficient gastrointestinal tumorigenesis and progression. PLoS Genetics 2008; 4(6): e1000092.

34. Bachrati CZ, Hickson ID. RecQ helicases: suppressors of tumorigenesis and premature aging. Biochemical Journal 2003; 374(Pt 3): 577–606.

35. Kennedy RD, D'Andrea AD. DNA repair pathways in clinical practice: lessons from pediatric cancer susceptibility syndromes. Journal of Clinical Oncology 2006; 24(23): 3799–3808.

36. Ripperger T, Gadzicki D, Meindl A, Schlegelberger B. Breast cancer susceptibility: current knowledge and implications for genetic counselling. European Journal of Human Genetics 2009; 17(6): 722–731.

37. Aly A, Ganesan S. BRCA1, PARP, and 53BP1: conditional synthetic lethality and synthetic viability. Journal of Molecular Cell Biology 2011; 3(1): 66–74.

38. Boveri T. Über mehrpolige Mitosen als Mittel zur Analzyse des Zellkerns. Verhandlungen der physicalisch-medizinischen Gesselschaft zu Würzburg. 1902; 35: 67–90.

39. Grady WM. Genomic instability and colon cancer. Cancer Metastasis Review 2004; 23(1–2): 11–27.

40. Barber TD, McManus K, Yuen KW, Reis M, Parmigiani G et al. Chromatid cohesion defects may underlie chromosome instability in human colorectal cancers. Proceedings of the National Academy of Sciences USA 2008; 105(9): 3443–3448.

41. Gordon DJ, Resio B, Pellman D. Causes and consequences of aneuploidy in cancer. Nature Review Genetics 2012; 13(3): 189–203.

42. Alberici P, Fodde R. The role of the APC tumor suppressor in chromosomal instability. Genome Dynamics 2006; 1: 149–170.

43. Yuen KW, Warren CD, Chen O, Kwok T, Hieter P. Systematic genome instability screens in yeast and their potential relevance to cancer. Proceedings of the National Academy of Sciences USA 2007; 104(10): 3925–3930.

44. Herman JG, Baylin SB. Gene silencing in cancer in association with promoter hypermethylation. New England Journal of Medicine 2003; 349(21): 2042–2054.

45. Antequera F, Bird A. Number of CpG islands and genes in human and mouse. Proceedings of the National Academy of Sciences USA 1993; 90(24): 11995–11999.

46. Toyota M, Ahuja N, Ohe-Toyota M, Herman JG, Baylin SB et al. CpG island methylator phenotype in colorectal cancer. Proceedings of the National Academy of Sciences USA 1999; 96(15): 8681–8686.

47. Curtin K, Slattery ML, Samowitz WS. CpG island methylation in colorectal cancer: past, present and future. Pathology Research International 2011; 2011: 902674.

48. Allen ND, Baird DM. Telomere length maintenance in stem cell populations. Biochimica et Biophysica Acta 2009; 1792(4): 324–328.

49. Garber K. At loose ends: telomere theories of aging and cancer begin to converge. Journal of the National Cancer Institute 2012; 104(11): 803–806.

50. Counter CM, Avilion AA, LeFeuvre CE, Stewart NG, Greider CW et al. Telomere shortening associated with chromosome instability is arrested in immortal cells which express telomerase activity. EMBO Journal 1992; 11(5): 1921–1929.

51. Jefford CE, Irminger-Finger I. Mechanisms of chromosome instability in cancers. Critical Reviews in Oncology/Hematology 2006; 59(1): 1–14.

52. Raynaud CM, Hernandez J, Llorca FP, Nuciforo P, Mathieu MC et al. DNA damage repair and telomere length in normal breast, preneoplastic lesions, and invasive cancer. American Journal of Clinical Oncology 2010; 33(4): 341–345.

53. Reynolds TY, Rockwell S, Glazer PM. Genetic instability induced by the tumor microenvironment. Cancer Research 1996; 56(24): 5754–5757.

54. Papp-Szabo E, Josephy PD, Coomber BL. Microenvironmental influences on mutagenesis in mammary epithelial cells. International Journal of Cancer 2005; 116(5): 679–685.

55. Mihaylova VT, Bindra RS, Yuan J, Campisi D, Narayanan L et al. Decreased expression of the DNA mismatch repair gene Mlh1 under hypoxic stress in mammalian cells. Molecular Cell Biology 2003; 23(9): 3265–3273.

56. Koshiji M, To KK, Hammer S, Kumamoto K, Harris AL et al. HIF-1alpha induces genetic instability by transcriptionally downregulating MutSalpha expression. Molecular Cell 2005; 17(6): 793–803.

57. Hammond EM, Green SL, Giaccia AJ. Comparison of hypoxia-induced replication arrest with hydroxyurea and aphidicolin-induced arrest. Mutation Research 2003; 532(1–2): 205–213.

58. Lindahl T. Instability and decay of the primary structure of DNA. Nature 1993; 362(6422): 709–715.

59. Coquelle A, Toledo F, Stern S, Bieth A, Debatisse M. A new role for hypoxia in tumor progression: induction of fragile site triggering genomic rearrangements and formation of complex DMs and HSRs. Molecular Cell 1998; 2(2): 259–265.

60. Young SD, Marshall RS, Hill RP. Hypoxia induces DNA over-replication and enhances metastatic potential of murine tumor cells. Proceedings of the National Academy of Sciences USA 1988; 85(24): 9533–9537.

61. Dereli-Oz A, Versini G, Halazonetis TD. Studies of genomic copy number changes in human cancers reveal signatures of DNA replication stress. Molecular Oncology 2011; 5(4): 308–314.

62. Burhans WC, Weinberger M. DNA replication stress, genome instability and aging. Nucleic Acids Research 2007; 35(22): 7545–7556.

63. Negrini S, Gorgoulis VG, Halazonetis TD. Genomic instability: an evolving hallmark of cancer. Nature Reviews Molecular Cell Biology 2010; 11(3): 220–228.

64. Bartkova J, Horejsi Z, Koed K, Kramer A, Tort F et al. DNA damage response as a candidate anti-cancer barrier in early human tumorigenesis. Nature 2005; 434(7035): 864–870.

65. Gorgoulis VG, Vassiliou LV, Karakaidos P, Zacharatos P, Kotsinas A et al. Activation of the DNA damage checkpoint and genomic instability in human precancerous lesions. Nature 2005; 434(7035): 907–913.

66. Bartkova J, Rezaei N, Liontos M, Karakaidos P, Kletsas D et al. Oncogene-induced senescence is part of the tumorigenesis barrier imposed by DNA damage checkpoints. Nature 2006; 444(7119): 633–637.

67. Denko NC, Giaccia AJ, Stringer JR, Stambrook PJ. The human Ha-ras oncogene induces genomic instability in murine fibroblasts within one cell cycle. Proceedings of the National Academy of Sciences USA 1994; 91(11): 5124–5128.

68. Di Micco R, Fumagalli M, Cicalese A, Piccinin S, Gasparini P et al. Oncogene-induced senescence is a DNA damage response triggered by DNA hyper-replication. Nature 2006; 444(7119): 638–642.

69. Tsantoulis PK, Kotsinas A, Sfikakis PP, Evangelou K, Sideridou M et al. Oncogene-induced replication stress preferentially targets common fragile sites in preneoplastic lesions. A genome-wide study. Oncogene 2008; 27(23): 3256–3264.

70. Loeb LA. Mutator phenotype may be required for multistage carcinogenesis. Cancer Research 1991; 51(12): 3075–3079.

71. Barbieri CE, Baca SC, Lawrence MS, Demichelis F, Blattner M et al. Exome sequencing identifies recurrent SPOP, FOXA1 and MED12 mutations in prostate cancer. Nature Genetics 2012; 44(6): 685–689.

72. O'Brien V, Brown R. Signalling cell cycle arrest and cell death through the MMR System. Carcinogenesis 2006; 27(4): 682–692.

73. Hassen S, Ali N, Chowdhury P. Molecular signaling mechanisms of apoptosis in hereditary non-polyposis colorectal cancer. World Journal of Gastrointestinal Pathophysiology 2012; 3(3): 71–79.

CHAPTER 9

DNA repair after oncological therapy (radiotherapy and chemotherapy)

Ekkehard Dikomey, Kerstin Borgmann, Malte Kriegs,
Wael Y. Mansour, Cordula Petersen,
and Thorsten Rieckmann

Introduction to DNA repair

Normally, tumours are treated by combined modalities among which radiotherapy is of great importance. To achieve maximal tumour control, all malignant cells need to be killed. With ionizing irradiation, this is mostly achieved via non- and mis-repaired DNA double-strand breaks (DSBs) finally resulting in lethal chromosome aberrations.

Induction and repair of DNA damage

Induction and repair of double-strand breaks

Exposure to ionizing irradiation leads to numerous types of DNA lesions with about 30 DSBs per diploid cell per 1 Gy X-ray. In tumour cells this number may vary by a factor of two with substantial impact on the cellular radiosensitivity.

The repair kinetics of X-ray-induced DSBs are characterized by a biphasic curve finally approaching a constant plateau (Figure 9.1). There is a fast exponential component with a half-time ranging between 5 and 30 minutes, mostly associated with the repair in euchromatin, and a slow component with a half-time of 2–5 hours representing repair in heterochromatin. The final plateau represents the number of non-misrepaired and probably also misrepaired DSBs [1, 2]. Differences in the repair kinetics, especially in the final plateau, indicate defects either in damage response, chromatin organization, repair pathways, or repair regulation.

Initial DNA damage response

Upon induction of DNA damage, cells react with a complex DNA damage response (DDR). DSBs will be detected, marked and processed for repair. As a part of DDR, cell proliferation will be regulated to give more time for repair before entering highly sensitive cell cycle phases such as S phase and mitosis [3]. ATM kinase and MRN complex (Mre11, Rad50, Nibrin) play a critical role in the recognition of DSBs initiating phosphorylation of the histone 2AX for up to one to two megabase pairs. This phosphorylated histone, generally termed as γH2AX, recruits MDC1, which serves as a platform that stimulates the recruitment of other repair proteins forming so-called repair foci which can easily be detected via immunofluorescence.

Mechanisms of DSB repair

DSBs can be repaired by several distinct pathways that differ not only in the underlying mechanism and proteins involved but also in the preferred DNA structure needed (Figure 9.1). Mammalian cells have evolved three main DSB repair pathways: non-homologous end joining (NHEJ), homologous recombination (HR), and single-strand annealing (SSA). NHEJ is the central pathway, which requires no sequence homology and, hence, can act on DSB with different structures and also in all cell cycle phases [4]. The central unit of NHEJ is the DNA PK complex composed of the heterodimer Ku70/80 and the catalytic subunit PKcs, which keeps the two DSB ends together. Final ligation is then performed by Artemis and Pol μ together with XRCC4, LigIV and XLF [5].

HR is active only in late S and G2 phase [6], where the sister chromatid (the most appropriate homology sequence) is available (Figure 9.1). Rad51 as the central HR player forms a nucloprotein filament, which invades the sister chromatid and searches for homology. HR is specifically required for repairing one-ended DSBs which are generated when single-strand breaks run into the replication fork. Repair of such lesions by HR prevent their dissociation and thereby strongly guarantee genomic stability of the DNA [6].

When NHEJ is defective, mammalian cells may rejoin DSB via an alternative end-joining mechanism (Alt-NHEJ) which requires PARP1, XRCC1, and LigIII. Alt-NHEJ is error-prone and is characterized by slow kinetics. Interestingly, Alt-NHEJ has also been shown to mediate both intra-chromosomal joining for class switch recombination (CSR) and inter-chromosomal translocation junctions, and may therefore strongly contribute to an oncogenic transformation.

SSA is stimulated when a DSB is generated between two repetitive sequences of 20 to 50 base pairs. An extensive resection of the DSB ends is required for SSA before homologous sequences are identified by Rad52 (the central SSA player) followed by the removal of the overhanging ends [7].

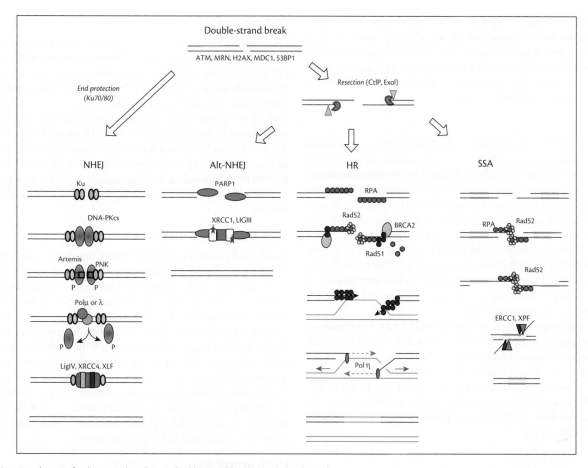

Fig. 9.1 Repair pathways of radiation-induced DNA double-strand breaks in mammalian cells.
Abbreviations: NHEJ, non-homologous end joining; Alt-NHEJ, alternative non-homologous end joining; HR, homologous recombination; SSA, single-strand annealing.
Adapted from Springer Verlag, *The Impact of Tumor Biology on Cancer Treatment and Multidisciplinary Strategies*, 2009, pp. 251–271, DNA repair and cell cycle regulation after ionizing irradiation, Iliakis G, Dahm-Daphi J, and Dikomey E, Copyright © 2009. With kind permission of Springer Science+Business Media

A functional hierarchy has recently been reported to exist between these three repair pathways to ensure fast and accurate repair of a DSB by canonical/classical NHEJ, which dominates over the other two pathways [8]. However, in many tumours this hierarchy is disturbed so that these two pathways are more active.

Targeting DSB repair

To enhance tumour radiosensitivity aiming to increase tumour cure, DSB repair is considered to be an optimal target, because it is the main determinant of the cellular radiosensitivity.

Radiochemotherapy

Radiochemotherapy is a main regimen for many tumors. Radiotherapy is combined with chemotherapy in an adjuvant or neo-adjuvant regimen but also may be given simultaneously. However, for most of the conventional drugs used there is rarely a synergistic effect observed but mostly only an additive effect, even for the often applied combination of radiation and cisplatin.

Molecular targeting

The great knowledge about the DSB repair mechanisms and their regulation achieved in the last years has paved the way in developing new specific targets to inhibit DSB repair in tumour cells to increase cellular radiosensitivity.

Epidermal growth factor receptor

The epidermal growth factor receptor (EGFR) is often over-expressed in tumours, and is known to regulate DSB repair. This receptor can be targeted either by specific antibodies (AB) such as cetuximab or tyrosine kinase inhibitors (TKI) such as erlotinib or gefitinib. A first clinical study with advanced head and neck tumours has demonstrated that at least cetuximab can be used in combination with radiotherapy (RT) to improve local tumour control [9]. Surprisingly, no such increase was seen when RT was combined with a TKI.

The mechanisms leading to this cetuximab-mediated improved tumour control are not yet fully understood. Cetuximab was found to suppress DSB repair by blocking both NHEJ and HR. However, an even stronger effect was seen for erlotinib, for which no cellular radiosensitization was seen. These data might indicate that the inhibition of DSB is only transient and might not result in an increased cell inactivation, because EGFR inhibition also blocks cell proliferation. Probably these cell cycle effects leading to premature senescence are more important for EGFR targeting [10].

Recent research focuses on downstream targets of EGFR such as the MAPK signalling pathways, which are known to regulate DSB repair. Probably, targeting of these two signalling pathways is more effective, because it cannot be compensated by other signalling cascades.

Due to its abundant expression in tumours, the EGFR may also be used for immunotherapy by applying radio-labelled AB. This approach specifically induces DSBs in tumours heavily over-expressing EGFR which are known to be highly resistant [11]. When combined with external irradiation, tumour control is already achieved with fairly low doses.

PARP-1

The poly (ADP ribose) polymerase 1 (PARP-1) plays an essential role in base excision repair (BER). As a consequence, upon suppression of PARP-1 by specific inhibitors more single-strand breaks or base damage will collide with replication fork leading to the formation of one-ended DSB (see "Mechanisms of DSB repair"). In cells with normal HR activity, these lesions are still repaired efficiently. However, in tumours with deficiency in HR, these lesions are not repaired. Therefore, targeting of PARP-1 will then lead to grossly increased lethality in HR-deficient tumours [12]. This concept, also termed as 'synthetic lethality', is considered to be a very promising tool specifically to inactivate tumour cells, because an HR defect is often seen in malignant cells [13].

PARP-1 is also involved in the Alt-NHEJ (see "Mechanisms of DSB repair"), which is known to be active in tumour cells. Therefore, when tumour cells using Alt-NHEJ are damaged either by radiation or specific chemicals such as cisplatin, inhibition of PARP-1 would lead to an enhanced cell killing. To apply this approach successfully in cancer therapy, biomarkers need to be established to allow identification of tumours which use Alt-NHEJ or are defective in HR.

HPV

Recent data indicate that in addition to cervix carcinoma, other types of tumour are also induced by a high-risk human papilloma virus (HPV) such as oropharyngeal squamous cell carcinoma (OSCC). Surprisingly, this tumour reacts much better to RT and RCT, when compared to HPV-negative head and neck tumours [14]. This higher local control was shown to be mediated by an extensive G2 block and an elevated level of residual DSBs [15]. When this G2 block is suppressed by specific inhibitors, a radiosensitization is seen in most HPV-negative OSCC, but not in normal human fibroblasts.

Chk1 und Chk2

In most tumours, the G1/S checkpoint is not active because p53 is mutated. As a consequence, these tumours especially rely on intra-S-phase as well as the G2 checkpoint, to prevent cell proliferation and to provide more time for efficient DSB repair. Both intra-S-phase and G2 checkpoints are initiated either by ATM or ATR, depending on the type of damage induced, which will then activate Chk1 and Chk2. There are several inhibitors available targeting either or both of these kinases which are already used in the clinics. These inhibitors are known to suppress DSB repair and with that specifically enhance tumour cell radio- as well as chemo-sensitivity [16, 17].

Prediction by DSB repair

Given its central role in cellular radiosensitivity, DSB repair may also be used to predict tumour response. Several tools are available reporting either directly or indirectly specific DSB repair capacity.

DSB repair foci

DSB repair foci, as measured by immunofluorescence, are considered an optimal parameter to determine specific repair capacity. For most tumour cell lines, an excellent correlation was reported between the residual number of DSB repair foci measured 24 hours after irradiation and cellular radiosensitivity [18]. It should, however, be noted that a difference in repair capacity of 1% has already been shown to have a strong effect on cell survival [19]. This technique may also be applied for tumour tissue slides irradiated both *in situ* or ex-vivo [18, 20]. However, there are still numerous problems to be solved such as hypoxic regions as well as contamination by normal tissue before this technique can be used in a daily clinical routine.

Immunohistochemistry

Beside many other factors, DSB repair capacity is also determined by the expression level of key repair proteins. Substantial variations in the amount of repair proteins have been reported in tumours both intra- and inter-individually. Among several proteins studied, the broadest variation has been reported for the heterodimer Ku protein, which is involved in NHEJ. For this protein, a clear and highly significant association was seen with an elevated expression leading to a high DSB repair capacity resulting in a poor prognosis after radiotherapy [21]. Such an analysis via immunohistochemistry may also include other proteins showing only an indirect effect on DSB repair such as EGFR and survivin [22, 23]. It should, however, be considered that this technique only allows determination of the relative amount of the protein present.

Gene expression

DSB repair capacity may also be estimated by gene expression analysis. This can be done either by a whole genome analysis or by specifically derived DSB repair tools. There are several studies showing an excellent correlation between a specific gene expression profile and tumour radiosensitivity [24, 25]. Surprisingly, however, these profiles did not include DSB repair genes.

Conclusion

There has been great improvement of our understanding about DSB repair and its regulation both in normal tissue as well as in tumours. These data revealed that tumours deviate in many aspects of DSB repair: the DNA damage response, the expression of DNA repair proteins, its hierarchy as well as its regulation. These deviations will allow us to establish new targets to specifically block DSB repair in tumours. One of the main objectives to achieve in the next few years is to establish tools allowing determination for each tumour its specific DSB repair defect, which can then be targeted by a specific therapy either in combination with RT or RCT.

Further reading

Begg AC, Stewart FA, Vens C. Strategies to improve radiotherapy with targeted drugs. Nature Reviews Cancer 2011; 11: 239–253.

Fong PC, Boss DS, Yap TA, et al. Inhibition of poly(ADP-ribose) polymerase in tumors from BRCA mutation carriers. New England Journal of Medicine 2009; 361: 123–134.

Helleday T, Lo J, van Gent DC, Engelward BP. DNA double-strand break repair: from mechanistic understanding to cancer treatment. DNA Repair (Amst) 2007; 6: 923–935.

Jackson SP, Bartek J. The DNA-damage response in human biology and disease. Nature 2009; 461: 1071–1078.

Mansour WY, Schumacher S, Rosskopf R, Rhein T, Schmidt-Petersen F et al. Hierarchy of nonhomologous end-joining, single-strand annealing and gene conversion at site-directed DNA double-strand breaks. Nucleic Acids Research 2008; 36: 4088–4098.

Moeller BJ, Yordy JS, Williams MD, Giri U, Raju U et al. DNA repair biomarker profiling of head and neck cancer: Ku80 expression predicts locoregional failure and death following radiotherapy. Clinical Cancer Research 2011; 17: 2035–2043.

Rothkamm K, Lobrich M. Evidence for a lack of DNA double-strand break repair in human cells exposed to very low x-ray doses. Proceedings of the National Academy of Sciences USA 2003; 100: 5057–5062.

References

1. Dahm-Daphi J, Dikomey E. Rejoining of DNA double-strand breaks in X-irradiated CHO cells studied by constant- and graded-field gel electrophoresis. International Journal of Radiation Biology 1996; 69: 615–621.

2. Rothkamm K, Lobrich M. Evidence for a lack of DNA double-strand break repair in human cells exposed to very low x-ray doses. Proceedings of the National Academy of Sciences USA 2003; 100: 5057–5062.

3. Jackson SP, Bartek J. The DNA-damage response in human biology and disease. Nature 2009; 461: 1071–1078.

4. Roth DB, Porter TN, Wilson JH. Mechanisms of nonhomologous recombination in mammalian cells. Molecular Cell Biology 1985; 5: 2599–2607.

5. Weterings E, Chen DJ. The endless tale of non-homologous end-joining. Cell Research 2008; 18: 114–124.

6. Helleday T, Lo J, van Gent DC, Engelward BP. DNA double-strand break repair: from mechanistic understanding to cancer treatment. DNA Repair (Amst) 2007; 6: 923–935.

7. Shinohara A, Shinohara M, Ohta T, Matsuda S, Ogawa T. Rad52 forms ring structures and co-operates with RPA in single-strand DNA annealing. Genes to Cells 1998; 3: 145–156.

8. Mansour WY, Schumacher S, Rosskopf R, Rhein T, Schmidt-Petersen F et al. Hierarchy of nonhomologous end-joining, single-strand annealing and gene conversion at site-directed DNA double-strand breaks. Nucleic Acids Research 2008; 36: 4088–4098.

9. Bonner JA, Harari PM, Giralt J, Azarnia N, Shin DM et al. Radiotherapy plus cetuximab for squamous-cell carcinoma of the head and neck. New England Journal of Medicine 2006; 354: 567–578.

10. Wang M, Morsbach F, Sander D, Gheorghiu L, Nanda A et al. EGF receptor inhibition radiosensitizes NSCLC cells by inducing senescence in cells sustaining DNA double-strand breaks. Cancer Research 2011; 71: 6261–6269.

11. Saker J, Kriegs M, Zenker M, Heldt JM, Eke I, Pietzsch HJ et al. Inactivation of HNSCC cells by 90Y-labeled cetuximab strictly depends on the number of induced DNA double-strand breaks. Journal of Nuclear Medicine 2013; 54: 416–423.

12. Fong PC, Boss DS, Yap TA, et al. Inhibition of poly(ADP-ribose) polymerase in tumors from BRCA mutation carriers. New England Journal of Medicine 2009; 361: 123–134.

13. Mason KA, Raju U, Buchholz TA, Wang L, Milas ZL et al. (ADP-ribose) Polymerase Inhibitors in Cancer Treatment. American Journal of Clinical Oncology 2012; 46(1): 9–20.

14. Lassen P, Eriksen JG, Hamilton-Dutoit S, Tramm T, Alsner J et al. Effect of HPV-associated p16INK4A expression on response to radiotherapy and survival in squamous cell carcinoma of the head and neck. Journal of Clinical Oncology 2009; 27: 1992–1998.

15. Rieckmann T, Tribius S, Grob TJ, et al. HNSCC cell lines positive for HPV and p16 possess higher cellular radiosensitivity due to an impaired DSB repair capacity. Radiotherapy & Oncology 2013; 107: 242–246.

16. O'Connor MJ, Martin NM, Smith GC. Targeted cancer therapies based on the inhibition of DNA strand break repair. Oncogen. 2007; 26: 7816–7824.

17. Begg AC, Stewart FA, Vens C. Strategies to improve radiotherapy with targeted drugs. Nature Reviews Cancer 2011; 11: 239–253.

18. Olive PL. Retention of gammaH2AX foci as an indication of lethal DNA damage. Radiotherapy and Oncology 2011; 101: 18–23.

19. Kasten-Pisula U, Tastan H, Dikomey E. Huge differences in cellular radiosensitivity due to only very small variations in double-strand break repair capacity. International Journal of Radiation Biology 2005; 81: 409–419.

20. Menegakis A, Eicheler W, Yaromina A, Thames HD, Krause M et al. Residual DNA double strand breaks in perfused but not in unperfused areas determine different radiosensitivity of tumours. Radiotherapy & Oncology 2011; 100: 137–144.

21. Moeller BJ, Yordy JS, Williams MD, Giri U, Raju U et al. DNA repair biomarker profiling of head and neck cancer: Ku80 expression predicts locoregional failure and death following radiotherapy. Clinical Cancer Research 2011; 17: 2035–2043.

22. Ang KK, Andratschke NH, Milas L. Epidermal growth factor receptor and response of head-and-neck carcinoma to therapy. International Journal of Radiation Oncology Biology Physics 2004; 58: 959–965.

23. Rödel F, Reichert S, Sprenger T, Gaipl US, Mirsch J et al. The role of survivin for radiation oncology: moving beyond apoptosis inhibition. Current Medicinal Chemistry 2010; 18: 191–199.

24. Pramana J, Van den Brekel MW, van Velthuysen ML, Wessels LF, Nuyten DS et al. Gene expression profiling to predict outcome after chemoradiation in head and neck cancer. International Journal of Radiation Oncology Biology Physics 2007; 69: 1544–1552.

25. Spitzner M, Emons G, Kramer F, Gaedcke J, Rave-Fränk M et al. A gene expression signature for chemoradiosensitivity of colorectal cancer cells. International Journal of Radiation Oncology Biology Physics 2010; 78: 1184–1192.

26. Iliakis G, Dahm-Daphi J, Dikomey E. DNA repair and cell cycle regulation after ionizing irradiation. In Molls M, Vaupel P, Nieder C, Anscher MS eds, The Impact of Tumor Biology on Cancer Treatment and Multidisciplinary Strategies. Berlin Heidelberg: Springer Verlag, 2009, 251–271.

CHAPTER 10

Biology of cancer and metastasis stem cells

Andreas Trumpp and Irène Baccelli

Introduction to biology of cancer and metastasis stem cells

Over the past 20 years, the concept of the cancer stem cell (CSC) has emerged after identification and characterization of CSC-enriched populations in several distinct cancer entities (Table 10.1) [1–3]. Although the concept remains controversial [4–6], new observations from clinical studies and basic research including transplantation experiments, in vivo lineage tracing experiments as well as clonal analysis of tumours have led to a more comprehensive CSC model of tumorigenesis, disease recurrence, and metastasis formation. The CSC concept is expected to contribute to the development of better therapeutic approaches to target residual disease, and break chemotherapy resistance and metastasis. The chapter is an updated and extended version of our recent review [7].

Historical background

Paget's landmark review on cancer in 1889 proposes that cancer might not be initiated by an accumulation of black bile produced by the stomach and the spleen (as initially proposed by Hippocrates and Galen), but rather by the encounter of a 'seed' (cancer cell) with an appropriate 'soil' (microenvironment). Indeed, as early as 1937, Furth and Kahn could demonstrate that one single mouse leukaemic cell is able to seed and form a new tumour in a healthy recipient mouse. The clonality of human cancers assessed by genetic markers was also demonstrated later on, confirming that cancers can arise from one transformed initiating cellular clone [8].

A clonal evolution model or multistep carcinogenesis model has subsequently been proposed to explain cancer development [9]. This model proposes that cells acquire tumorigenicity by accumulating mutations or genetic alterations, which occur stochastically in all neoplastic cells. This ultimately leads to the development of tumours, from benign to highly aggressive, depending on the type and number of newly acquired genetic alterations. For instance, this model has been thoroughly described for colon carcinoma [9].

However, accumulating evidence indicates that neoplastic cells do not always acquire tumorigenicity stochastically. Instead, tumours are often hierarchically organized, as are adult tissues [2, 10]. This was first demonstrated in mouse squamous cell carcinoma, where, by DNA lineage tracking, Pierce and colleagues could document the hierarchy between non-differentiated cells giving rise to well differentiated cells. The differentiated progeny was no longer able to form tumours in secondary recipients, contrary to non-differentiated cells. This observation, among many others, marked the beginning of the CSC research field [2, 10].

The classical concept of cancer stem cells

Adult regenerating tissues (such as the skin, the gastrointestinal mucosa or the haematopoietic system) are hierarchically organized [11–13]. At the top of the cellular organization, normal adult stem cells maintain tissues during homoeostasis and facilitate their regeneration, for example in response to infection or to cell loss due to injury or chemotherapy. These physiological stem cells are defined by their functional properties: they have the life-long capacity to self-renew (ability to give rise to a new stem cell following cell division), are multipotent, and can reversibly enter quiescent or even dormant states and resist cytotoxic drugs [11, 13–15]. Similar to regenerative tissues, many tumours follow a hierarchical organization and, like physiological stem cells, CSCs are defined by a series of functional traits [2, 10, 16] (Figure 10.1).

Universal CSC functional traits

At the helm of tumour hierarchy

First, CSCs can generate all cell types present in a tumour. Located at the top of the tumour hierarchy, CSCs can self-renew and also generate non-CSC progeny, which form the tumour bulk (differentiated progeny). Hierarchical organization of tumours, governed by CSCs, have been reported for many tumour types including germ cell cancers, leukaemia, breast cancer, brain cancer, colon cancer, pancreatic cancer, melanoma, and several others [7] (Table 10.1).

Unlimited self-renewal potential

In striking contrast with their differentiated progeny, CSCs can undergo unlimited self-renewing divisions. Typically, the presence of human CSCs within a cell population is experimentally addressed by serial transplantation of tumour cells into immunocompromised mice or rats (Table 10.1). Although considered state of the art, this assay has limitations and only imperfectly recapitulates the in vivo situation found in patients. Indeed, the immunocompromised mouse models lack an adaptive immune system (neither mouse nor human) and express cytokines/chemokines and other environmental components of mouse origin, such as the tumour vasculature. Furthermore, the detection and enumeration of functional CSCs by these methods remains highly assay-dependent, as several different immunocompromised mouse strains and many methods of tumour dissociation and implantation exist [34, 38, 39]. Nevertheless, human CSCs cannot be simply reduced to technical artefacts due to their detection in xenografts. Indeed, mouse CSCs have also been

Table 10.1 Identification of human primary tumour CSC biomarkers using in vivo assays. Studies reporting the existence of enriched human CSC populations are listed. In the first five columns, the main parameters influencing the efficiency of tumour engraftment are listed. *From left to right*: the tumour entity, the type of immunocompromised mouse strain used, the route of transplantation of human tumour cells, preconditioning of the recipient mice, treatment of mice during the assay, and whether the tumour cells were mixed with matrigel upon transplantation. In the next four columns, the main results of these studies are summarized. *From left to right*: the frequency of the identified CSC-enriched population observed in the given tumour entity, the biomarkers identified for this CSC-enriched population, the minimal number of tumour cells expressing these biomarkers able to give rise to a human tumour, as well as the reference of the corresponding study [7]

Cancer	Animal	Type of injection	Treatment of recipient mice	Injection with matrigel	% of csc-enriched population in tumour	Biomarkers	Minimal # of biomarker + cells to obtain a tumour	Reference
ALL (B-ALL)	NOD/SCID/IL2rγc⁻/⁻ newborns	intravenous	sub-lethal irradiation	no	82.50%	CD34+/CD19+	$2–6.10^4$	[17]
AML	NOD/SCID	intravenous	sub-lethal irradiation	no	0.75%	CD34+/CD38-	2.10^5	[1]
AML	NOD/SCID, NOD/SCID/β₂m⁻/⁻ and NOD/SCID/IL2rγc⁻/⁻	intravenous and intra-bone	IVIG of CD122 pre-treatment and sub-lethal irradiation	no	0.076 % (*)	CD34+/CD38- (*) or CD34+/CD38+ (**) (in samples with lowest CD34+/CD38- fraction)	$7.5\ 10^3$ (*) or 10^6 (**)	[18]
AML	NOD/SCID	intra-femoral	IVIG of CD122 pretreatment and sub-lethal irradiation	no	0.06% to 0.00009% of bulk	NA	NA	[19]
Bladder	Rag2γcDKO	intra-dermal	NA	yes	3–36.3%	CD44	100	[20]
Breast	NOD/SCID	mammary fat pad	VP–16, oestrogen pellets	no	11–35%	ESA+/CD44^high/CD24^low-neg	200	[21]
Breast	NOD/SCID	humanized mammary fat pad	oestrogen pellets	yes	3–10%	ALDH1+	500	[22]
BREAST ctcs	NOD/SCID/IL2rγc⁻/⁻	intra-femoral	oestrogen pellets	yes	1%–44%	CD44+/MET+/CD47+	1000 blood CTCs	[23]
Brain	NOD/SCID	intracranial	NA	no	6–29%	CD133+	100	[24]
Colorectal	NOD/SCID	renal capsule	sub-lethal irradiation	yes	1.8–24.5%	CD133+	100	[25]
Colorectal	NOD/SCID	subcutaneous	NA	no	2.60%	ESA^high/CD44+	200	[26]
Colorectal	NOD/SCID	subcutaneous	NA	yes	3.50%	ALDH1+	25 serially passaged	[27]
Head and neck squamous cell carcinoma	NOD/SCID and Rag2γcDKO	subcutaneous	NA	yes	10–12%	CD44+	5000	[28]
Liver	SCID	intra-hepatic	NA	no	2.50%	CD45-/CD90+	10^3	[29]
Lung	SCID and NUDE	subcutaneous, after in vitro expansion	NA	yes	0.4–1.5%	CD133+	10^4	[30]
Lung	NOD/SCID/IL2rγc⁻/⁻	subcutaneous	NA	yes	median 15%	lin-/CD166+	≤500	[31]
Melanoma	NOD/SCID	subcutaneous	NA	no	1.6–20.4%	ABCB5+	10^5	[32]
Melanoma	Rag2γcDKO	intra-dermal	NA	yes	2.5–41%	CD271+	100	[33]
Melanoma	NOD/SCID/IL2rγc⁻/⁻	subcutaneous	NA	yes	NA	NA	1 (in 28% of cases)	[5]
Melanoma	NUDE, (NOD/SCID, NOD/SCID/IL2rγc⁻/⁻)	subcutaneous	NA	yes	8–11%	CD271+	1000	[34]

(Continued)

Table 10.1 Continued

Cancer	Animal	Type of injection	Treatment of recipient mice	Injection with matrigel	% of csc-enriched population in tumour	Biomarkers	Minimal # of biomarker + cells to obtain a tumour	Reference
Ovarian	NUDE	subcutaneous	NA	yes	0.20%	CD44+cKIT-CD117+	100	[31]
Ovarian	NOD/SCID	subcutaneous	NA	yes	0.5% - >70%	CD133+	100–500	[35]
Pancreatic	NOD/SCID	subcutaneous and intra-pancreatic	NA	yes	0.2–0.8%	ESA+/CD44+/ CD24+	100	[36]
Pancreatic	NUDE	intra-pancreatic	NA	no	3.6 cells per high power field	ESA+/CD133+	500	[37]

Abbreviation: CTC, circulating tumour cells isolated from the blood of patients.

© Baccelli, I. and Trumpp, A., 2012. Reproduced with permission from *The Journal of Cell Biology*, The evolving concept of cancer and metastasis stem cells, Volume 198, Issue 3, pp. 281–93, DOI: 10.1083/Jcb.201202014

reported in syngeneic mouse models of leukaemia, breast cancer, and skin cancer, providing strong evidence that CSCs govern many tumour types [7].

In addition to transplantation experiments, in vivo lineage tracing methods have been developed and used in syngeneic mouse tumour models and lentivirally marked human tumour xenografts to assess the fate of individual CSCs as well as the clonal composition within tumours (reviewed in [40]). For example, clonal analysis of human colon cancer xenografts revealed long-term transient as well as dormant clones. The latter ones only appeared in secondary and tertiary transplants suggesting that there is a significant fluctuation during the progression of tumour growth over time. Interestingly, slow-cycling dormant clones showed the highest resistance to chemotherapy showing that the clones that drive initial tumour growth might be distinct from the ones that reinitiate growth and relapse after therapy. Importantly, these data demonstrate that tumour heterogeneity is not exclusively the consequence of genetic heterogeneity, but also caused by epigenetically distinct tumour cells following the cancer stem cell model [15, 41].

Other CSC functional traits

Quiescence or slow-cycling states

Although cellular quiescence does not seem to be a universal feature, some CSCs have been reported to shuttle between quiescent, slow-cycling, and active states, in a way similar to the behaviour of many adult stem cell types [14, 42–45]. For example, the presence of quiescent leukaemic stem cells (LSCs) has been reported in a mouse model for acute myeloid leukaemia (AML) [46]. Moreover, using clonal tracking techniques, delayed-contributing CSC clones were identified both in AML and in colon carcinoma, suggesting the existence of long-term quiescent/dormant pools of human CSCs [15, 41]. In line with these findings, a report showed a strong correlation between the number of slow-cycling breast cancer cells, as measured by retention of the membrane dye PKH26 in mammosphere cultures and the frequency of CSCs, assessed by tumorigenicity assay in mice. Of major importance, quiescence or slow-cycling states might render CSCs less likely to be responsive to conventional chemotherapy, which mainly targets cycling cells.

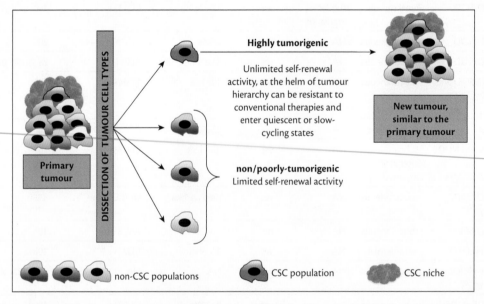

Fig. 10.1 The classical 'cancer stem cell' (CSC) concept. Tumours are heterogeneous and hierarchically organized entities. Upon dissociation and transplantation into an immunocompromised animal, human CSCs can be functionally distinguished from non/poorly tumorigenic cell populations by their ability to reinitiate and grow a similar heterogeneous tumour in vivo.

© Baccelli I, Trumpp A, 2012. Reproduced with permission from *The Journal of Cell Biology*, The evolving concept of cancer and metastasis stem cells, Volume 198, Issue 3, pp. 281–293, doi: 10.1083/Jcb.201202014

Moreover, quiescent normal stem cells can re-enter the cell cycle after injury in order to repair a tissue [14, 42, 46]. In agreement with this stem cell feature, it has been hypothesized that potential reactivation of quiescent CSCs might induce tumour relapse, which sometimes occurs decades after completion of therapy [47].

Increased resistance to conventional therapies

Similar to physiological stem cells, some CSCs were reported to exhibit remarkable resistance to chemotherapies. For instance, breast CSCs were found to accumulate in women with locally advanced tumours after cytotoxic chemotherapy had eliminated the bulk of the tumour cells [48]. Similarly, in chronic myeloid leukaemia (CML), BCR-ABL-driven LSCs are resistant to tyrosine kinase inhibitors (TKIs) such as imatinib, whereas these compounds eliminate the rest of the leukaemic cells, often even achieving a complete molecular response (undetectable levels of BCR-ABL mRNA by RT-PCR) [49, 50]. Accordingly, during STOP trials, in which TKI treatments are discontinued, tumour relapse was observed in the majority of patients. This was most likely caused by new tumour cell production by resistant CML-LSCs, as the relapsed 'non-LSC' leukaemic cells remained sensitive to the initially used TKI [51, 52]. Another case of resistant CSCs was reported for myelodysplasia carrying a 5q deletion. While the majority of tumour cells were efficiently targeted by treatment with the immunomodulator lenalidomide, leading to a complete clinical and cytogenetic remission, most patients relapsed due to the outgrowth of remaining resistant CSCs [53].

CSC resistance might first of all be caused by increased drug efflux capacities, mediated by expression of multidrug resistance (MDR) transporters [54]. Indeed, cancer cells named 'side population', due to their ability to efflux the fluorescent dye Hoechst, have been reported to be highly enriched for both normal and cancer stem cells [55]. Second, aldehyde dehydrogenase-1 (ALDH-1), a cytosolic enzyme involved in the catalysis of aldehyde oxidation, was reported to be specifically active in several CSCs [56]. In a retrospective study, ALDH-1 activity was significantly higher in breast cancer metastatic cells, which developed resistance to cyclophosphamide, compared to sensitive cells [57]. This suggests that ALDH-1 might also play a role in cytotoxic drug resistance. Third, genotoxic treatments like ionizing radiation might be evaded by CSCs due to increased DNA damage check point response and DNA repair capacities, as observed in CD133-expressing glioblastoma CSC-enriched populations compared to CD133-negative populations [58]. Last, CSCs might counterbalance the radiation-induced reactive oxygen species (ROS) production by increased expression of free radical scavengers, as reported for murine and human breast CSCs [59]. This ability might selectively protect CSCs from ROS-mediated DNA damage and hence explain their resistance to irradiation. Importantly, in vitro studies of drug-sensitive tumour cell lines suggest that cancer cells might transiently and reversibly acquire drug resistance, indicating that drug resistance might not always be a stable trait [60].

The CSC niche

The tumour microenvironment is composed of diverse immune cells, stromal cells, as well as extracellular components [61, 62]. CSC functional traits might be sustained by this microenvironment, termed 'niche' [63]. For instance, vascular endothelial cells maintained self-renewal and promoted tumorigenicity of glioma CSCs in a mouse xenograft model [64]. Hypoxia, notably via the hypoxia-inducible factor 2-alpha (HIF2α) increased glioma CSC self-renewal and

tumorigenic capacities [65]. Moreover, inflammatory cells and molecules such as interleukin 6, secreted by infiltrating immune cells in the tumour, enhanced the proliferation of colitis-associated CSCs [66].

The CSC niche might not only regulate CSC traits but might also directly provide CSC features to non-CSCs. For instance, tumour-associated myofibroblasts enhanced self-renewal of colorectal CSCs via HGF production but also strongly enhanced the in vivo tumorigenicity of non-CSCs through their secreted factors [67]. Extracellular matrix proteins such as periostin and Tenascin-C are critical for the outgrowth of breast cancer metastatic cells in the lung, possibly by coordinating the interaction with neighbouring cells and by enhancing signalling mediated by growth-promoting signalling factors [63].

In leukaemia and in prostate carcinoma cancer, cells could hijack existing physiological stem cell niches. Although physiological stem cell niches are known to play important roles for quiescence maintenance and resistance to stress-inducing treatments [68, 69], the influence of the tumour niche on CSC function at the cellular and molecular levels still remains to be elucidated.

Origin of CSCs

Importantly, the CSC concept has to be separated from the 'cell of origin' question: as outlined above, CSCs are defined by a series of functional tumour-propagating traits. However, the tumour 'cell of origin' defines the cell type from which the disease is derived, meaning the cell type first hit by an oncogenic mutation. However, this 'cell of origin' does not necessarily immediately acquire a CSC phenotype [70]. Having said this, CSCs might indeed originate from stem cells, as they are already capable of almost limitless self-renewal. For instance, embryonic stem cells can form teratomas when transplanted subcutaneously in recipient mice.

Nevertheless, CSCs can also originate from more differentiated progenitors that acquire stemness traits by accumulation of genetic or epigenetic abnormalities. For instance, progenitors derived from stem cells that already carry initiating genetic mutations acquire further mutations during differentiation that will finally lead to transformation. This would mean that the 'cell of origin' for the first mutation is a stem cell, but that the CSC that drives the tumorigenic clone would be a more differentiated progenitor. Such a scenario has been reported for chronic myeloid leukaemia (CML). Although the BCR–ABL fusion protein is the first event and is present in haematopoietic stem cell (HSC)-like CML cells (suggesting that the 'cell of origin' of the disease is a normal HSC), advanced-stage LSCs during blast crisis were found to be in a state similar to granulocyte/macrophage progenitors (GMPs) [71]. Similarly, in AML, the AML–ETO fusion protein is present in HSCs ('cell of origin' of the disease) but the functional leukaemic stem cells were detected in a Thy1-progenitor cell state. However, in acute promyelocytic leukaemia (APL), the MLL–AF9 fusion protein was not detected in HSCs, but when introduced in mouse GMPs, it could induce leukaemia, indicating that both the 'cell of origin' and the leukaemic stem cells were found in progenitors rather than in HSCs [72].

Recent work on induced pluripotent stem cells (iPS) has demonstrated that contrary to all expectations, the acquisition of self-renewal and pluripotency starting from any cell type can be achieved by activation of as little as four transcription factors [73]. Importantly, this reprogramming process requires the transient repression of p53 and INK4a, two of the most frequently mutated tumour suppressor loci in human cancers [74]. Similarly, loss of the same tumour suppressors causes an activation of a self-renewal programme in normally non-self-renewing haematopoietic progenitors; consequently, these cells start to behave as haematopoietic stem cells in vivo despite maintaining a progenitor phenotype. Thus, these cells do not de-differentiate, but rather acquire self-renewal potential after loss of tumour suppressors [75]. These data raise the possibility that the accumulation of mutations in certain oncogenes and tumour suppressors may lead to a process that may be described as a partial reprogramming, with the acquisition of self-renewal activity paralleling the development of CSC activity. Indeed, in vitro reprogramming of human skin fibroblasts by stable expression of hTERT, H-RasV12 and SV40 LT and ST antigens leads to the generation of cells with CSC properties, able to form hierarchically organized tumours in mice [76]. Similarly, experimentally induced expression of the depolarization-inducing transcription co-activator TAZ [77] as well as experimentally induced expression of epithelial to mesenchymal transition (EMT)-inducing transcription factors TWIST or SNAIL [78] was reported to provide CSC-like properties to non-CSC cells.

Identification of cancer stem cell biomarkers

The cancer stem cell concept proposes that one of the major parameters to evaluate therapy efficacy is the quantification of remnant CSCs within minimal residual disease and not of gross measurement of tumour regression, as is typically used in clinical drug trials. Therefore, one major aim in the field is to identify reliable and specific CSC biomarkers for each tumour type.

Bonnet and Dick identified LSCs in AML by limiting dilution transplantations in non-obese diabetic/severe combined immunodeficient (NOD/SCID) mice as CD34+/CD38- leukaemic cells, closely resembling normal HSCs [1]. However, in the meantime, examination of a large set of AML patients revealed that functional CSC clones reside within several distinct immunophenotypically defined cellular compartments, showing significant inter-patient heterogeneity [19].

For solid tumours, a first leap forward was achieved in 2003, when Michael Clarke and colleagues reported the identification of breast CSCs within the EPCAM+/CD44+/CD24low-neg population of mammary pleural effusion and tumour samples. As few as a hundred EPCAM+/CD44+/CD24low-neg cells were able to reinitiate the original tumour in NOD/SCID mice, while 10,000 cells with an alternate phenotype were not [21]. Subsequently, breast cancer metastasis-initiating cells (MICs) were identified in the blood of hormone receptor-expressing luminal breast cancer patients. These EPCAM+/CD44+/MET+/CD47+ cells had the potential to initiate new metastasis after transplantation into immunocompromised mice, directly demonstrating that an often small proportion of circulating tumour cells had MIC activity [23].

Following these landmark publications, CSCs were identified in many more solid and haematopoietic human tumours as summarized in Table 10.1. Importantly, several reports indicate the existence of CSC-enriched populations displaying different, sometimes non-overlapping, sets of markers for the same tumour type. For example, only 1% of breast cancer cells simultaneously express both reported CSC phenotypes EPCAM+/CD44+/CD24low-neg and ALDH-1+. This discrepancy might be due to several different reasons. First, differences in methods could be responsible for these differences [34, 38]. Second, several CSC clones may co-exist within primary tumours [19] and the research groups may have detected different CSC populations. Third, functional CSC clones might reside within several immunophenotypically defined

cellular compartments [19, 79]. Last but not least, cancer entities are rarely uniform. For instance, during the last few years, various genome-wide gene expression profiling efforts combined with biomarker and clinical approaches have led to the sub-classification of breast cancers into increasing numbers of molecular subtypes [80, 81]. The mutational patterns vary between the different subtypes and this genetic heterogeneity is likely paralleled by a heterogeneous CSC complexity. Different CSC phenotypes might thus be associated with genetically diverse cancer-subtypes.

Therapeutic targeting of cancer stem cells

Studies on AML show that the signature of functionally validated LSCs is a good predictor for poor patient survival independent of any biomarker [19]. These data strongly suggest that therapeutic targeting of CSCs should be relevant for patients. However, many technical hurdles still need to be overcome.

Targeting CSC biomarkers

CD44, a transmembrane glycoprotein involved in cell–cell and cell–matrix adhesion is expressed on many tumour CSCs (Table 10.1). Altering CD44 function by a specific antibody inhibited AML-LSC proliferation in xenograft studies probably by inhibiting LSC-niche interactions [82]. However, universal targeting of CD44, which is also expressed by many adult stem cells, might be deleterious for patients. Undesirable effects might be evaded by targeting different isoforms of CD44 specifically expressed by tumour cells, such as CD44v6 [83]. However, severe skin toxicity has been reported in a phase I clinical trial of bevatuzumab (an anti-CD44v6 antibody) in the case of head and neck squamous cell carcinoma [84]. Nevertheless combination of the immunoconjugate bevatuzumab–mertansine with external beam radiotherapy provided improved local tumour control with possible targeting of CSCs [85].

More recently, successful eradication of AML-LSC was described by targeting of CD123 (interleukin-3 (IL3) receptor alpha chain), using a blocking antibody in xenografted mice. However, since CD123 is also expressed by normal HSCs, there is a risk of severe side effects. Targeting ABC transporters expressed by CSCs has also been explored [86] but was put on hold after realizing that these transporters play pivotal roles in blood-brain-barrier maintenance as well as in adult stem cell maintenance.

Targeting CSC molecular pathways

Based on the hypothesis that cancer cells might be more dependent on the activation of oncogenic pathways than their normal counterparts, a phenomenon termed 'oncogene addiction' [87], pharmaceutical companies have applied major efforts to target signalling pathways activated in CSCs and cancer cells in general. For instance, the NFκB pathway has been successful targeted and allowed selective eradication of AML and final phase (blast crisis) CML-LSCs. Guzman and colleagues treated in vitro leukaemic cells with parthenolide, a drug known to directly bind IκB kinase (IKK) as well as to modify p50 and p65 subunits. This pretreatment induced higher levels of ROS, which lead to a decrease of CD34+CD38- leukaemic populations and an impaired capacity of leukaemic cells to engraft in NOD/SCID mice, suggesting that mainly LSCs were targeted [88]. Similarly, inhibition of NOTCH signalling using gamma-secretase inhibitors in CD133 expressing medulloblastoma CSCs led to the diminution of CD133+ cells and correlated with impaired tumour engraftment in vivo [89]. Last, but not least, inhibition of the TGFβ pathway by bone morphogenetic proteins (BMPs) was reported to lead to the differentiation of brain CSCs and successive cure of the disease in a xenograft model, providing a first proof of principle for the possible efficacy of a 'differentiation therapy'.

Sensitization to therapy

A number of studies have aimed to sensitize CSCs to therapy. For instance, in colon cancer IL4 blockade successfully primed CSCs to chemotherapy. In glioblastoma, a CHK kinase inhibitor increased the radiosensitivity of CSCs [58]. In addition, recent reports showing that dormant and chemotherapy-resistant normal stem cells can be activated and simultaneously sensitized to chemotherapy-mediated killing might provide a strategy to target dormant CSCs [42, 46]. Here a sequential treatment scheme would be used in which dormant CSCs would first be 'primed' and activated, followed by chemotherapy leading to complete elimination of the tumour including the initially dormant and resistant CSCs. Such a strategy was successfully applied in mouse models of AML and CML [46]. However, activation of dormant cancer stem cells may harbour the risk of disease progression and requires a highly efficient therapeutic option for the second phase, such as tyrosine kinase inhibitors in case of BCR-ABL driven CML. Finally, in a mouse model of APL, LSCs expressing PML-RARα (promyelocytic leukaemia-retinoic acid receptor alpha) could be forced out of self-renewal into differentiation by cooperative treatment of arsenic, cyclic AMP, and retinoic acid, leading to LSC clearance and impressive remission in patients [90].

Novel strategies to target CSCs

Some new hope might arise from the development of bi-specific or tri-specific antibodies that are able to specifically target cell populations. For instance, T-cell recognition via an anti-CD3 antibody can be combined with cancer cell recognition via an additional antigen-binding site such as EPCAM (catumaxomab) or HER2 (ertumaxomab) [91, 92].

In addition, high-throughput screening of drugs selectively inhibiting CSCs, rather than other tumour cells, has been successfully used to uncover compounds such as salinomycin. This antibiotic drug targets putative breast CSCs (grown as mammospheres in culture), as well as CLL LSCs, probably via inhibition of the Wnt pathway [93]. However, the toxicity of this molecule on physiological stem cells remains unexplored.

Last, but not least, recent discoveries concerning specific CSC biological properties might lead to the development of novel targeting strategies: for instance, glioma stem cells were found to be mechanistically distinct from their less tumorigenic counterparts regarding production of nitric oxide via nitric oxide synthase-2 (NOS2). NOS2 inhibition successfully slowed down tumour growth in a xenograft glioma model [94]. Similarly, glycine decarboxylase activity was found to be critical for non-small-cell lung CSCs suggesting that glycine metabolism might be a novel anti-CSC target [31]. However, in both cases, general toxicity of such treatments has not yet been thoroughly investigated.

In summary, therapeutic applications deriving from CSC studies are less straightforward than was initially anticipated, notably due to the large overlap in molecules expressed by CSCs and their respective normal stem cells that has so far hampered their use in the clinic due to collateral toxicity [95]. Nevertheless, without the efficient eradication of CSCs, a long-term cure for many cancer patients appears unreachable. Innovative efforts will therefore be required from the field to achieve this goal in the not too distant future.

Dynamic model of CSCs

Given the pace of research in the field and the diverse nature of the results, the classical view of CSCs needs to be updated. In this section, we introduce a more dynamic model for CSCs and integrate recent results into this model.

Multiple genetic CSC clones within one tumour

Recent studies in which several subregions of the primary tumour and metastases of pancreatic and kidney cancers were sequenced revealed an unexpected degree of intra-tumour heterogeneity [96–98]. This often highly underestimated heterogeneity may result from the fact that CSCs are genetically unstable. Indeed, in colon cancer such genetic instability was reported, leading to the formation of new CSC clones deriving from an initial 'parental' CSC clone [99]. In addition, two landmark studies in human ALL studied the genetic architecture of LSCs over time and following successive transplantations in xenografted mice. Both studies showed that several LSC clones co-exist within single patients. During disease progression, after therapy, and following serial xeno-transplantation, different LSC clones can take over and initiate new tumours [100, 101]. This might explain, at least partially, the observed 'acquired resistance' to targeted therapy observed in some patients. That is, after successfully targeting sensitive CSC clones, already present resistant clones may take over, mimicking an acquisition of resistance to the applied treatment. As a consequence, tumours might not be faithfully represented by single-headed hierarchical structures bur rather might resemble more oligarchic structures, displaying multiple heads: if one head, i.e. a CSC clone, is cut off (by targeted therapy, for instance), another one might take over, repopulating the tumour. Thus, dynamic hierarchies might exist within a single CSC clone and its progeny (intra-CSC clone hierarchy), but also between different genetically diverse CSC clones that compete with each other (inter-CSC clone hierarchy) (Figure 10.2A).

CSCs need not be rare

CSCs do not need to be rare, as shown by Kelly and colleagues using leukaemia and lymphoma genetic mouse models [4]. Indeed, CSC-enriched populations have been reported to represent extremely variable proportions of bulk tumour cells, ranging from 0.2% to 82.5% (Table 10.1). Moreover, the frequency of CSCs might increase during tumour progression, as recently shown by in vivo limiting dilution assays of grade 1 and grade 3 breast tumours [102].

During the last few years, the idea that CSCs must be rare, which is based on our knowledge of physiological stem cells, has often led to a questioning of the CSC hypothesis. For instance, it was reported that melanoma stage III to IV tumorigenic cells are very abundant, representing up to 30% of the tumour bulk. Moreover, the screening of a very high number of cell surface markers failed to distinguish these tumorigenic cells from other tumour cells [5]. From these results it was proposed that melanoma does not follow a CSC model but rather a stochastic model, where tumorigenicity is a random feature distributed among all tumour cells [103].

Although this is certainly possible, there are also alternative explanations to these observations. The difficulty of finding any relevant biomarkers for stage III to IV tumorigenic melanoma cells might be technically explained by the temporary loss of surface proteins due to the use of trypsin. Without using this enzyme, CD271 could be identified as a melanoma CSC marker by two other groups [33, 34].

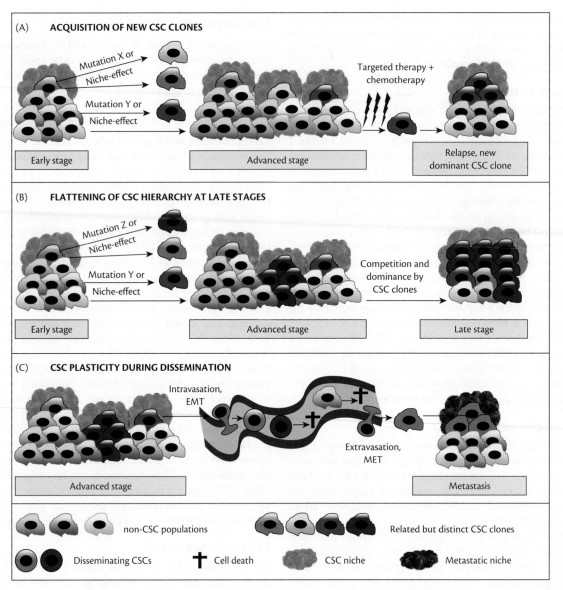

Fig. 10.2 The dynamic CSC concept. (A) Although early-stage tumours might be governed by a single CSC clone, advanced-stage tumours might contain several distinct but related clones, either arising from the initial CSC clone or from its differentiated progeny via mutations or via induction by the CSC niche. Targeted therapy and/or chemotherapy eliminate(s) the tumour mass including possibly some of the CSCs. At least one resistant CSC clone is then responsible (possibly after acquiring additional mutations) for tumour relapse. (B) Advanced-stage tumours contain several distinct but related CSC clones. Some acquire enhanced self-renewal capabilities with simultaneously decreased differentiation. During tumour progression, the CSC clones compete with each other, leading to the dominance of at least one CSC clone with the subsequent loss of differentiated tumour progeny. Over time, this leads to a flattening of the hierarchical structure and to a selection of the most aggressive CSCs. Late-stage tumours may thus be comprised almost exclusively of aggressive, multiresistant CSCs, a situation similar to the one proposed by the stochastic model. (C) Carcinoma CSCs display a dynamic phenotype during systemic dissemination: they are able to at least partially lose epithelial traits through epithelial to mesenchymal transition (EMT). Probably only a subset of such disseminating CSCs is able to survive in the systemic circulation, extravasate, reacquiring epithelial features (MET), to seed in a new microenvironment and to initiate metastasis. All three scenarios illustrated in (A), (B), and (C) occur in parallel and/or during different phases of tumour progression.

© Baccelli I, Trumpp A, 2012. Reproduced with permission from *The Journal of Cell Biology*, The evolving concept of cancer and metastasis stem cells, Volume 198, Issue 3, pp. 281–293, doi: 10.1083/Jcb.201202014

Alternatively, late-stage melanoma might consist of several distinct CSC clones displaying different cell surface biomarkers that are all highly malignant. These CSC clones might even differ from patient to patient, as described for ALL [100, 101]. Moreover, a likely scenario is a high selection and enrichment of CSC clones, which have retained little or no differentiation capacity. In this scenario, the initial hierarchy in the tumour is steadily decreased and flattened, leading to late-stage tumours composed almost exclusively of heterogeneous CSC clones (Figure 10.2B).

Plasticity of CSC phenotype

In recent years, the EMT process, in which epithelial polarized adherent cells are converted into mesenchymal-like depolarized migratory tumour cells, has been linked to the CSC phenotype and function in breast, pancreatic, and colorectal tumours. CSCs were found to express EMT-inducing transcription factors such as TWIST, SNAIL, and SLUG and, vice versa, EMT-undergoing cells were found enriched for CSC activities compared with cells not undergoing EMT [104]. The process can be controlled by a ZEB1/mir200 feedback loop mechanism (maintaining stemness), itself controlled by p53 [105]. Overall, these findings suggest that epithelial markers might be down-regulated in carcinoma CSCs and would therefore be missed in typical screens, which generally exclude cells lacking epithelial markers such as EPCAM. Furthermore, they underline the fact that epithelial CSCs might strongly modulate their phenotype during tumour progression: for example, a CSC detected in an early-stage primary tumour might have a completely different phenotype from the one of a CSC circulating in the blood (Figure 10.2C). As a consequence of this plasticity, some of the reported CSC biomarkers might be relevant in some stages of tumour progression but obsolete in others.

Generating a dynamic concept of CSCs

These recent data and others suggest a more complex and dynamic CSC model integrating the three main additional features.

First, tumours are by definition genetically unstable entities. Therefore, the cellular composition of a tumour in an early-stage disease, at relapse, or at late stages may display significant genetic differences including genetic heterogeneity. The available data suggest that in early neoplasms only a single or very few CSC clones drive tumour growth. During disease progression, new CSC clones can arise either from existing CSC clones or from the differentiated progeny via mutation-mediated partial reprogramming. After eradication of the majority of tumour cells by chemotherapy and/or targeted approaches, one or a few CSC clones may survive and expand, leading to a change in the clonal and cellular composition of the relapsing cancer (Figure 10.2A).

Second, the different genetically distinct CSC clones may also compete with each other, leading to the selection of CSC clones with high self-renewing activity and simultaneous loss of differentiation capacity. This would provide an explanation for the observed flattening of the cellular hierarchy within advanced-stage tumours, which creates a situation similar to what is proposed by the stochastic model (Figure 10.2B). Third, CSC biomarkers can be unstable, as indicated by studies on EMT in solid tumours (Figure 10.2C). Thus, reported CSC biomarkers might only be relevant for a given tumour stage and therefore need to be validated for each case in conjunction with functional analyses.

Importantly, this dynamic CSC model suggests that only complex combinatorial treatments are likely to be efficacious to target late-stage tumours or metastasis. First, mutations that are commonly present in all clones have to be identified, for instance, by whole-genome sequencing of various regions within a single tumour mass [96, 106]. The associated deregulated pathways of these common mutations present in all subregions (likely including the various tumour subclones) need then to be targeted by pathway-specific strategies. Second, these strategies need to be complemented by therapies targeting additional CSC-specific features (see above) to eliminate not only the non-CSC parts of each tumour clone, but also the various CSCs present in advanced-stage tumours or metastasis.

CSCs and metastasis-initiating clones (MICs)

Metastasis might be initiated by a subset of CSC clones

Systemic dissemination and metastasis is responsible for most cancer-related deaths. To date, human MICs have not yet been prospectively identified. However, several lines of evidence indicate that MICs might be found within subpopulations of CSCs. First of all, carcinoma CSCs possess tumour-initiating capacity, which is a mandatory trait for the establishment of secondary tumours in distant organs. Second, they express EMT markers [105], suggesting that they are able to migrate, as well as making them likely candidates for metastasis-initiating activities.

More specifically, several reports suggest that MICs might be comprised within CSC populations: CD44+ breast cancer cells (comprising a breast CSC phenotype) were proposed to have enriched metastatic activities in xenograft studies [21, 23]. Similarly, CD44+CXCR4+ cells, a subfraction of the putative pancreatic CSCs present at the invasive front of cell-line-induced pancreatic tumours, were reported to be enriched for metastatic capabilities [37]. Along the same lines, CD26, in combination with the CSC marker CD133 has been proposed as a marker for colorectal MIC-enriched tumour populations in primary tumour xenograft experiments [40].

MICs might be late-stage disseminating CSC clones

MICs might disseminate at an early stage during tumour progression or might derive from late-stage disseminating CSC clones [107]. Through mapping of the genetic evolution of both pancreatic primary tumours and metastases by next-generation sequencing, two recent studies identified the genealogy of metastatic clones [96]. Both studies suggest that even if both primary tumours and metastases consist of heterogeneous clones, additional driver mutations are present in the metastasis-initiating clones compared to the clones present in the primary tumours. In addition, metastatic clones were evaluated to be arising rather late within primary pancreatic tumours [96], even if the dissemination process itself might start rather early [108], suggesting that functional MICs are typically disseminating from advanced-stage tumours rather than from early-stage primary tumours.

MICs must be found among disseminating tumour cells

Since metastasis results from the successful dissemination of primary tumour cells into a distant organ, MICs should be found among disseminating tumour cells. These include circulating tumour cells (CTCs) as well as disseminated tumour cells (DTCs), found, respectively, in the blood or in the bone marrow of carcinoma patients. In the case of many carcinomas and in particular for breast cancer, the presence and/or number of DTCs or CTCs are linked to poor clinical outcome [109, 110]. Interestingly, variable proportions of CTCs and DTCs have been reported to display CSC phenotypes by immunocytochemistry or flow cytometry [23, 110]. However, the detection methods for carcinoma CTCs remain controversial. This is due to the use of EPCAM and cytokeratins (CKs) as positive selection markers, as they are not specific to tumour cells, but rather detect epithelial cells. Moreover, these epithelial proteins might be down-regulated during EMT-mediated dissemination. Indeed, in breast cancer CTCs simultaneously express mesenchymal and epithelial markers. Moreover, during disease progression and in response to therapies, reversible shifts between these cell fates have been observed, suggesting that EPCAM-based detection methods may miss many CTCs in breast cancer patients [111]. In a mouse model for pancreatic ductal adenocarcinomas, less than 40% of genetically YFP-labeled CTCs expressed CK19 or EPCAM, suggesting that a large proportion of CTCs undergo EMT and lose expression of epithelial markers. Further, more than 40% of the detected YFP-labelled CTCs expressed the previously reported pancreatic CSC markers (CD44+/CD24+) and showed high clonogenicity in vitro, suggesting that at least some of the detected CTCs have self-renewing potential [108].

Functional in vivo analyses of different subfractions of human CTCs or DTCs using xenograft assays are required to test whether phenotypic disseminating CSCs are indeed functionally involved in metastasis initiation. Recently, it could be demonstrated that primary CTCs isolated from metastatic hormone receptor positive breast cancer patients can initiate new bone, liver, and lung metastasis after transplantation into immunocompromised mice [23]. These MICs expressed cell surface receptors previously implicated in tumour and metastasis, including CD44, the receptor tyrosine kinase and HGF receptor MET, as well as CD47, an inhibitor of macrophage activity. Presence of these MICs correlated with poor clinical outcome, suggesting that these cells are causatively involved in metastasis formation. These cell surface receptors may serve as biomarkers and may offer new possibilities for the detection and targeting of MICs [23].

The metastasis-initiating cell model

MICs likely arise from subpopulations of late-stage CSC clones, hence the relevance for characterizing CSCs, even in late-stage tumours. In addition to the functional capacities of CSCs, MICs have to display metastatic capacities, meaning that they must disseminate, survive in the systemic circulation, extravasate at the metastatic site and seed and grow in the new environment. Several metastatic clones might co-exist during dissemination, exhibiting different site-specific migration and seeding capacities (Figure 10.3). Indeed, Massagué and colleagues have proposed that, in the context of breast cancer, different metastatic populations can be distinguished according to their capacity to metastasize to the bone, the lung, or the brain in patients with systemic disease [112]. This appears to be related to their capacity to directly or indirectly generate a metastatic niche [63].

Summary

CSCs are a specific subset of transformed cells that are able to sustain primary tumour growth following a hierarchical pattern. Strong evidence for the existence of such cells exists in many cancer types, although the model may not be appropriate for all cancer types and/or all stages. Like any model, the CSC concept needs to be constantly adapted to the currently available data and is thus steadily evolving. Recent findings uncovering high intra-tumour genetic heterogeneity have led to the observation that several CSC-controlled clones can co-exist and compete with each other within a tumour. Furthermore, CSCs may have unstable phenotypes and genotypes,

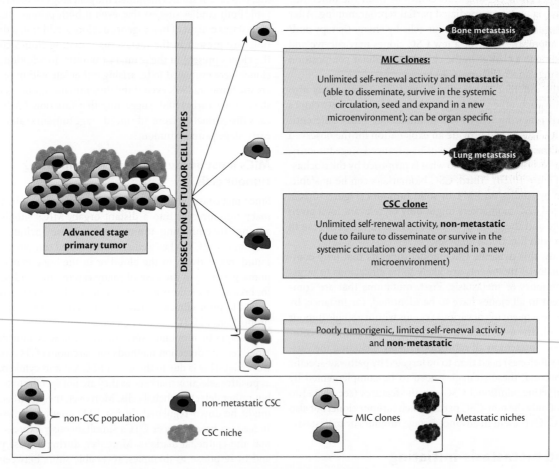

Fig. 10.3 The 'metastasis-initiating cell' (MIC) concept. Advanced-stage primary tumours are heterogeneous and multihierarchical structures. Upon dissociation and transplantation in immunocompromised hosts, MICs can be functionally distinguished from CSC clones by their metastatic ability in vivo (dissemination, survival in the systemic circulation, extravasation, seeding, and expansion in a new microenvironment, termed 'metastatic niche'). MICs are adapted descendants and therefore subpopulations of CSCs with metastatic capacity and possibly organ specificity.

© Baccelli I, Trumpp A, 2012. Reproduced with permission from *The Journal of Cell Biology*, The evolving concept of cancer and metastasis stem cells, Volume 198, Issue 3, pp. 281–293, doi: 10.1083/Jcb.201202014

which makes it difficult to identify reliable and robust biomarkers and develop associated targeted therapies. In addition, cell-extrinsic factors provided by the CSC niche might provide yet another dimension to the complexity of CSC regulation. Importantly, most cancer-related deaths are a consequence of metastasis development rather than due to growth of the primary tumour. Therefore the better characterization of MICs will become pivotal in the future, in order to prevent and target so far insufficiently treatable metastatic disease. Importantly, the identification of CSCs is also therapeutically relevant for late-stage tumours since MICs in the blood or in distant tissues are likely a subset of CSCs. Evolving the CSC concept will help to focus research towards developing improved therapies by lowering the risk of tumour recurrence and allow the development of targeting strategies for fatal late-stage cancers.

Acknowledgement

Chapter © Baccelli, I. and Trumpp, A., 2012. Adapted with permission from *The Journal of Cell Biology*, The evolving concept of cancer and metastasis stem cells, Volume 198, Issue 3, pp. 281–93, DOI: 10.1083/Jcb.201202014.

Further reading

Al-Hajj M, Wicha MS, Benito-Hernandez A, Morrison SJ, Clarke MF. Prospective identification of tumorigenic breast cancer cells. Proceedings of the National Academy of Sciences of the USA 2003; 100(7): 3983–3988.

Baccelli I, Schneeweiss A, Riethdorf S, Stenzinger A, Schillert A et al. Identification of a population of blood circulating tumor cells from breast cancer patients that initiates metastasis in a xenograft assay. Nature Biotechnology 2013; 31(6): 539–544.

Dick JE. Stem cell concepts renew cancer research. *Blood* 2008; 112: 4793–4807.

Magee JA, Piskounova E, Morrison SJ. Cancer stem cells: impact, heterogeneity, and uncertainty. Cancer Cell 2012; 21(3): 283–296.

Mani SA, Guo W, Liao MJ, Eaton EN, Ayyanan A et al. The epithelial-mesenchymal transition generates cells with properties of stem cells. Cell 2008; 133(4): 704–715.

Marmé F, Sinn HP, Pantel K, Weichert W, Trumpp A. Identification of a population of blood circulating tumor cells from breast cancer patients that initiates metastasis in a xenograft assay. Nat Biotechnology 2013; 31(6): 539–544.

Martinez N, Matthews A, Stewart P, Tarpey I, Varela B et al. Intratumor heterogeneity and branched evolution revealed by multiregion sequencing. New England Journal of Medicine 2012; 366:883–892.

Notta F, Mulligan CG, Wang JC, Poeppl A, Doulatov S et al. Evolution of human BCR-ABL1 lymphoblastic leukaemia-initiating cells. Nature 2011; 469(7330): 362–367.

Pantel K, Alix-Panabieres A, Riethdorf S. 2009. Cancer micrometastases. Proceedings of the National Academy of Sciences of the USA 2009; 100:3983–3988.

Reya T, Morrison SJ, Clarke MF, Weissman IL. Stem cells, cancer, and cancer stem cells. Nature 2001; 414(6859): 105–111.

Trumpp A, Wiestler OD. Mechanisms of disease: cancer stem cells—targeting the evil twin. Nature Clinical Practice Oncology 2008; 5(6): 337–347.

References

1. Bonnet D, Dick JE. Human acute myeloid leukemia is organized as a hierarchy that originates from a primitive hematopoietic cell. Nature Medicine 1997; 3(7): 730–737.

2. Reya T, Morrison SJ, Clarke MF, Weissman IL. Stem cells, cancer, and cancer stem cells. Nature 2001; 414(6859): 105–111.

3. Trumpp A, Wiestler OD. Mechanisms of disease: cancer stem cells—targeting the evil twin. Nature Clinical Practice Oncology 2008; 5(6): 337–347.

4. Kelly PN, Dakic A, Adams JM, Nutt SL, Strasser A. Tumor growth need not be driven by rare cancer stem cells. Science 2007; 317(5836): 337.

5. Quintana E, Shackleton M, Foster HR, Fullen DR, Sabel MS, et al. Phenotypic heterogeneity among tumorigenic melanoma cells from patients that is reversible and not hierarchically organized. Cancer Cell 2010; 18(5): 510–523.

6. Magee JA, Piskounova E, Morrison SJ. Cancer stem cells: impact, heterogeneity, and uncertainty. Cancer Cell 2012; 21(3): 283–296.

7. Baccelli I, Trumpp A. The evolving concept of cancer and metastasis stem cells. Journal of Cell Biology 2012; 198(3): 281–293.

8. Fialkow PJ. The origin and development of human tumors studied with cell markers. New England Journal of Medicine 1974; 291(1): 26–35.

9. Fearon ER, Vogelstein B. A genetic model for colorectal tumorigenesis. Cell 1990; 61(5): 759–767.

10. Dick JE. Stem cell concepts renew cancer research. Blood 2008; 112(13): 4793–4807.

11. Fuchs E, Nowak JA. Building epithelial tissues from skin stem cells. Cold Spring Harbour Symposia on Quantitive Biology 2008; 73: 333–350.

12. Murphy MJ, Wilson A, Trumpp A. More than just proliferation: Myc function in stem cells. Trends in Cellular Biology 2005; 15(3): 128–137.

13. Clevers H. Stem cells: A unifying theory for the crypt. Nature 2013; 495(7439): 53–54.

14. Wilson A, Laurenti E, Oser G, van der Wath RC, Blanco-Bose W et al. Hematopoietic stem cells reversibly switch from dormancy to self-renewal during homeostasis and repair. Cell 2008; 135(6): 1118–1129.

15. Kreso A, O'Brien CA, van Galen P, Gan OI, Notta F et al. Variable clonal repopulation dynamics influence chemotherapy response in colorectal cancer. Science 2013; 339(6119): 543–548.

16. Nguyen LV, Vanner R, Dirks P, Eaves CJ. Cancer stem cells: an evolving concept. Nature Reviews Cancer 2012; 12(2): 133–143.

17. Kong Y, Yoshida S, Saito Y, Doi T, Nagatoshi Y, Fukata M, Saito N, Yang SM, Iwamoto C, Okamura J et al. CD34+CD38+CD19+ as well as CD34+CD38-CD19+ cells are leukemia-initiating cells with self-renewal capacity in human B-precursor ALL. Leukemia 2008; 22:1207–1213.

18. Taussig DC, Pearce DJ, Simpson C, Rohatiner AZ, Lister TA, Kelly G, Luongo JL, Danet-Desnoyers GA, and Bonnet D. Hematopoietic stem cells express multiple myeloid markers: implications for the origin and targeted therapy of acute myeloid leukemia. Blood 2005; 106:4086–4092.

19. Eppert K, Takenaka K, Lechman ER, Waldron L, Nilsson B et al. Stem cell gene expression programs influence clinical outcome in human leukemia. Nature Medicine 2011; 17(9): 1086–1093.

20. Chan KS, Espinosa I, Chao M, Wong D, Ailles L, Diehn M, Gill H, Presti J Jr., Chang HY, Rijn M van de et al. Identification, molecular characterization, clinical prognosis, and therapeutic targeting of human bladder tumor-initiating cells. Proc. Natl. Acad. Sci. USA 2009; 106:14016–14021.

21. Al-Hajj M, Wicha MS, Benito-Hernandez A, Morrison SJ, Clarke MF. Prospective identification of tumorigenic breast cancer cells. Proceedings of the National Academy of Sciences of the United States of America. 2003; 100(7): 3983–3988.

22. Ginestier C, Hur MH, Charafe-Jauffret E, Monville F, Dutcher J, Brown M, Jacquemier J, Viens P, Kleer CG, Liu S et al. ALDH1 is a marker of normal and malignant human mammary stem cells and a predictor of poor clinical outcome. Cell Stem Cell 2007; 1:555–567.

23. Baccelli I, Schneeweiss A, Riethdorf S, Stenzinger A, Schillert A et al. Identification of a population of blood circulating tumor cells from breast cancer patients that initiates metastasis in a xenograft assay. Nature Biotechnology 2013; 31(6): 539–544.

24. Singh SK, Hawkins C, Clarke ID, Squire JA, Bayani J, Hide T, Henkelman RM, Cusimano MD and Dirks PB. Identification of human brain tumour initiating cells. Nature 2004; 432:396–401.

25. O'Brien CA, Pollett A, Gallinger S and Dick JE. A human colon cancer cell capable of initiating tumour growth in immunodeficient mice. Nature 2007; 445:106–110.

26. Dalerba P, Dylla SJ, Park IK, Liu R, Wang X, Cho RW, Hoey T, Gurney A, Huang EH, Simeone DM et al. Phenotypic character- izationof-humancolorectalcancerstemcells. Proc.Natl.Acad.Sci.USA 2007; 104:10158–10163.

27. Huang EH, Hynes MJ, Zhang T, Ginestier C, Dontu G, Appelman H, Fields JZ, Wicha MS and Boman BM. Aldehyde dehydrogenase 1 is a marker for normal and malignant human colonic stem cells (SC) and tracks SC overpopulation during colon tumorigenesis. Cancer Res 2009; 69:3382–3389.

28. Prince ME, Sivanandan R, Kaczorowski A, Wolf GT, Kaplan MJ, Dalerba P, Weissman IL, Clarke MF and Ailles LE. Identification of a subpopula- tion of cells with cancer stem cell properties in head and neck squamous cell carcinoma. Proc. Natl. Acad. Sci. USA 2007; 104:973–978.

29. Yang ZF, Ho DW, Ng MN, Lau CK, Yu WC, Ngai P, Chu PW, Lam CT, Poon RT and Fan ST. Significance of CD90+ cancer stem cells in human liver cancer. Cancer Cell 2008; 13:153–166.

30. Eramo A, Lotti F, Sette G, Pilozzi E, Biffoni M, Di Virgilio A, Conticello C, Ruco L, Peschle C and De Maria R. Identification and expansion of the tumorigenic lung cancer stem cell population. Cell Death Differ 2008; 15:504–514.

31. Zhang WC, Shyh-Chang N, Yang H, Rai A, Umashankar S et al. Glycine decarboxylase activity drives non-small cell lung cancer tumor-initiating cells and tumorigenesis. Cell 2012; 148(1–2): 259–272.

32. Schatton T., Murphy GF, Frank NY, Yamaura K, Waaga-Gasser AM, Gasser M, Zhan Q, Jordan S, Duncan LM, Weishaupt C, et al. Identification of cells initiating human melanomas. Nature 2008; 451:345–349.

33. Boiko AD, Razorenova OV, van de Rijn M, Swetter SM, Johnson DL et al. Human melanoma-initiating cells express neural crest nerve growth factor receptor CD271. Nature 2010; 466(7302): 133–137.

34. Civenni G, Walter A, Kobert N, Mihic-Probst D, Zipser M et al. Human CD271-positive melanoma stem cells associated with metas- tasis establish tumor heterogeneity and long-term growth. Cancer Research 2011; 71(8): 3098–3109.

35. Curley MD, Therrien VA, Cummings CL, Sergent PA, Koulouris CR, Friel AM, Roberts DJ, Seiden MV, Scadden DT, Rueda BR, Foster R. CD133 expression defines a tumor initiating cell population in primary human ovarian cancer. Stem Cells. 2009 Dec; 27(12):2875–83. doi: 10.1002/stem.236.

36. Li C, Heidt DG, Dalerba P, Burant CF, Zhang L, Adsay V, Wicha M, Clarke MF and Simeone DM. Identification of pancreatic cancer stem cells. Cancer Res 2007; 67:1030–1037.

37. Hermann PC, Huber SL, Herrler T, Aicher A, Ellwart JW et al. Distinct populations of cancer stem cells determine tumor growth and metastatic activity in human pancreatic cancer. Cell Stem Cell 2007; 1(3): 313–323.

38. Quintana E, Shackleton M, Sabel MS, Fullen DR, Johnson TM et al. Efficient tumour formation by single human melanoma cells. Nature 2008; 456(7222): 593–598.

39. Ishizawa K, Rasheed ZA, Karisch R, Wang Q, Kowalski J et al. Tumor- initiating cells are rare in many human tumors. Cell stem Cell 2010; 7(3): 279–282.

40. Beck B, Blanpain C. Unravelling cancer stem cell potential. Nature Reviews Cancer 2013; 13(10): 727–738.

41. Dieter SM, Ball CR, Hoffmann CM, Nowrouzi A, Herbst F et al. Distinct types of tumor-initiating cells form human colon cancer tumors and metastases. Cell Stem Cell 2011; 9(4): 357–365.

42. Essers MA, Offner S, Blanco-Bose WE, Waibler Z, Kalinke U et al. IFNalpha activates dormant haematopoietic stem cells in vivo. Nature 2009; 458(7240): 904–908.

43. Fuchs E. The tortoise and the hair: slow-cycling cells in the stem cell race. Cell 2009; 137(5): 811–819.

44. Goff DJ, Recart AC, Sadarangani A, Chun HJ, Barrett CL et al. A Pan-BCL2 inhibitor renders bone-marrow-resident human leukemia stem cells sensitive to tyrosine kinase inhibition. Cell Stem Cell 2013; 12(3): 316–328.

45. Chen J, Li Y, Yu TS, McKay RM, Burns DK et al. A restricted cell population propagates glioblastoma growth after chemotherapy. Nature 2012; 488(7412): 522–526.

46. Trumpp A, Essers M, Wilson A. Awakening dormant haematopoietic stem cells. Nature Reviews Immunology 2010; 10(3): 201–209.

47. Aguirre-Ghiso JA. Models, mechanisms and clinical evidence for can- cer dormancy. Nature Reviews Cancer 2007; 7(11): 834–846.

48. Li X, Lewis MT, Huang J, Gutierrez C, Osborne CK et al. Intrinsic resistance of tumorigenic breast cancer cells to chemotherapy. Journal of the National Cancer Institute 2008; 100(9): 672–679.

49. Goldman JM. Chronic myeloid leukemia: a historical perspective. Seminars in Hematology 2010; 47(4): 302–311.

50. Perrotti D, Jamieson C, Goldman J, Skorski T. Chronic myeloid leukemia: mechanisms of blastic transformation. Journal of Clinical Investigation 2010; 120(7): 2254–2264.

51. Druker BJ, Guilhot F, O'Brien SG, Gathmann I, Kantarjian H et al. Five-year follow-up of patients receiving imatinib for chronic myeloid leukemia. New England Journal of Medicine 2006; 355(23): 2408–2417.

52. Ross DM, Hughes TP, Melo JV. Do we have to kill the last CML cell? Leukemia 2011; 25(2): 193–200. Epub 2010/09/17.

53. Tehranchi R, Woll PS, Anderson K, Buza-Vidas N, Mizukami T et al. Persistent malignant stem cells in del(5q) myelodysplasia in remission. New England Journal of Medicine 2010; 363(11): 1025–1037.

54. Dean M, Fojo T, Bates S. Tumour stem cells and drug resistance. Nature Reviews Cancer 2005; 5(4): 275–284.

55. Wulf GG, Wang RY, Kuehnle I, Weidner D, Marini F et al. A leukemic stem cell with intrinsic drug efflux capacity in acute myeloid leukemia. Blood 2001; 98(4): 1166–1173.

56. Ran D, Schubert M, Taubert I, Eckstein V, Bellos F et al. Heterogeneity of leukemia stem cell candidates at diagnosis of acute myeloid leuke- mia and their clinical significance. Experimental Hematology 2012; 40(2): 155–165 e1.

57. Douville J, Beaulieu R, Balicki D. ALDH1 as a functional marker of cancer stem and progenitor cells. Stem Cells Development 2009; 18(1): 17–25.

58. Bao S, Wu Q, McLendon RE, Hao Y, Shi Q et al. Glioma stem cells promote radioresistance by preferential activation of the DNA damage response. Nature 2006; 444(7120): 756–760.

59. Diehn M, Cho RW, Lobo NA, Kalisky T, Dorie MJ et al. Association of reactive oxygen species levels and radioresistance in cancer stem cells. Nature 2009; 458(7239): 780–783.

60. Sharma SV, Lee DY, Li B, Quinlan MP, Takahashi F et al. A chromatin-mediated reversible drug-tolerant state in cancer cell subpopulations. Cell 2010; 141(1): 69–80.

61. Bissell MJ, Hines WC. Why don't we get more cancer? A proposed role of the microenvironment in restraining cancer progression. Nature Medicine 2011; 17(3): 320–329.

62. Hanahan D, Coussens LM. Accessories to the crime: functions of cells recruited to the tumor microenvironment. Cancer Cell 2012; 21(3): 309–322.

63. Oskarsson T, Massague J. Extracellular matrix players in metastatic niches. EMBO Journal 2012; 31(2): 254–256.

64. Calabrese C, Poppleton H, Kocak M, Hogg TL, Fuller C et al. A perivascular niche for brain tumor stem cells. Cancer Cell 2007; 11(1): 69–82.

65. Li Z, Bao S, Wu Q, Wang H, Eyler C et al. Hypoxia-inducible factors regulate tumorigenic capacity of glioma stem cells. Cancer Cell 2009; 15(6): 501–513.

66. Grivennikov S, Karin E, Terzic J, Mucida D, Yu GY et al. IL-6 and Stat3 are required for survival of intestinal epithelial cells and development of colitis-associated cancer. Cancer Cell 2009; 15(2): 103–113.

67. Vermeulen L, De Sousa EMF, van der Heijden M, Cameron K, de Jong JH et al. Wnt activity defines colon cancer stem cells and is regulated by the microenvironment. Nature Cell Biology 2010; 12(5): 468–476.

68. Ehninger A, Trumpp A. The bone marrow stem cell niche grows up: mesenchymal stem cells and macrophages move in. Journal of Experimental Medicine 2011; 208(3): 421–428.

69. Park D, Sykes DB, Scadden DT. The hematopoietic stem cell niche. Frontiers in Bioscience 2012; 17: 30–39.

70. Visvader JE. Cells of origin in cancer. Nature 2011; 469(7330): 314–322.

71. Jamieson CH, Ailles LE, Dylla SJ, Muijtjens M, Jones C et al. Granulocyte-macrophage progenitors as candidate leukemic stem cells in blast-crisis CML. New England Journal of Medicine 2004; 351(7): 657–667.

72. Krivtsov AV, Twomey D, Feng Z, Stubbs MC, Wang Y et al. Transformation from committed progenitor to leukaemia stem cell initiated by MLL-AF9. Nature 2006; 442(7104): 818–822.

73. Takahashi K, Tanabe K, Ohnuki M, Narita M, Ichisaka T et al. Induction of pluripotent stem cells from adult human fibroblasts by defined factors. Cell 2007; 131(5): 861–872.

74. Utikal J, Polo JM, Stadtfeld M, Maherali N, Kulalert W et al. Immortalization eliminates a roadblock during cellular reprogramming into iPS cells. Nature 2009; 460(7259): 1145–1148.

75. Akala OO, Park IK, Qian D, Pihalja M, Becker MW et al. Long-term haematopoietic reconstitution by Trp53-/-p16Ink4a-/-p19Arf-/- multi-potent progenitors. Nature 2008; 453(7192): 228–232.

76. Scaffidi P, Misteli T. In vitro generation of human cells with cancer stem cell properties. Nature Cell Biology 2011; 13(9): 1051–1061.

77. Cordenonsi M, Zanconato F, Azzolin L, Forcato M, Rosato A et al. The Hippo transducer TAZ confers cancer stem cell-related traits on breast cancer cells. Cell 2011; 147(4): 759–772.

78. Mani SA, Guo W, Liao MJ, Eaton EN, Ayyanan A et al. The epithelial-mesenchymal transition generates cells with properties of stem cells. Cell 2008; 133(4): 704–715.

79. Gibbs KD Jr, Jager A, Crespo O, Goltsev Y, Trejo A et al. Decoupling of Tumor-Initiating Activity from Stable Immunophenotype in HoxA9-Meis1-Driven AML. Cell stem Cell 2012; 10(2): 210–217.

80. Herschkowitz JI, Simin K, Weigman VJ, Mikaelian I, Usary J et al. Identification of conserved gene expression features between murine mammary carcinoma models and human breast tumors. Genome Biol. 2007; 8(5): R76.

81. Curtis C, Shah SP, Chin SF, Turashvili G, Rueda OM et al. The genomic and transcriptomic architecture of 2,000 breast tumours reveals novel subgroups. Nature 2012.

82. Jin L, Hope KJ, Zhai Q, Smadja-Joffe F, Dick JE. Targeting of CD44 eradicates human acute myeloid leukemic stem cells. Nature Medicine 2006; 12(10): 1167–1174.

83. Orian-Rousseau V. CD44, a therapeutic target for metastasising tumours. European Journal of Cancer 2010; 46(7): 1271–1277.

84. Riechelmann H, Sauter A, Golze W, Hanft G, Schroen C et al. Phase I trial with the CD44v6-targeting immunoconjugate bivatuzumab mertansine in head and neck squamous cell carcinoma. Oral Oncology 2008; 44(9): 823–829.

85. Gurtner K, Hessel F, Eicheler W, Dorfler A, Zips D et al. Combined treatment of the immunoconjugate bivatuzumab mertansine and fractionated irradiation improves local tumour control in vivo. Radiotherapy & Oncology 2012; 102(3): 444–449.

86. Lou H, Dean M. Targeted therapy for cancer stem cells: the patched pathway and ABC transporters. Oncogene 2007; 26(9): 1357–1360.

87. Weinstein IB. Cancer. Addiction to oncogenes—the Achilles heal of cancer. Science 2002; 297(5578): 63–64.

88. Guzman ML, Rossi RM, Karnischky L, Li X, Peterson DR et al. The sesquiterpene lactone parthenolide induces apoptosis of human acute myelogenous leukemia stem and progenitor cells. Blood 2005; 105(11): 4163–4169.

89. Fan X, Matsui W, Khaki L, Stearns D, Chun J et al. Notch pathway inhibition depletes stem-like cells and blocks engraftment in embryonal brain tumors. Cancer Research 2006; 66(15): 7445–7452.

90. de The H, Chen Z. Acute promyelocytic leukaemia: novel insights into the mechanisms of cure. Nature Reviews Cancer 2010; 10(11): 775–783.

91. Hess J, Ruf P, Lindhofer H. Cancer therapy with trifunctional antibodies: linking innate and adaptive immunity. Future Oncology 2012; 8(1): 73–85.

92. Shen J, Zhu Z. Catumaxomab, a rat/murine hybrid bispecific monoclonal antibody for the treatment of cancer. Current Opinion in Molecular Therapy 2008; 10(3): 273–284.

93. Lu D, Choi MY, Yu J, Castro JE, Kipps TJ et al. Salinomycin inhibits Wnt signaling and selectively induces apoptosis in chronic lympho-cytic leukemia cells. Proceedings of the National Academy of Sciences of the United States of America. 2011; 108(32): 13253–13257.

94. Eyler CE, Wu Q, Yan K, MacSwords JM, Chandler-Militello D et al. Glioma stem cell proliferation and tumor growth are promoted by nitric oxide synthase-2. Cell 2011; 146(1): 53–66.

95. Deonarain MP, Kousparou CA, Epenetos AA. Antibodies targeting cancer stem cells: a new paradigm in immunotherapy? MAbs. 2009; 1(1): 12–25.

96. Yachida S, Jones S, Bozic I, Antal T, Leary R et al. Distant metastasis occurs late during the genetic evolution of pancreatic cancer. Nature 2010; 467(7319): 1114–1117.

97. Fisher R, Pusztai L, Swanton C. Cancer heterogeneity: implications for targeted therapeutics. British journal of cancer. 2013; 108(3): 479–485.

98. Koboldt DC, Steinberg KM, Larson DE, Wilson RK, Mardis ER. The next-generation sequencing revolution and its impact on genomics. Cell 2013; 155(1): 27–38.

99. Odoux C, Fohrer H, Hoppo T, Guzik L, Stolz DB et al. A stochastic model for cancer stem cell origin in metastatic colon cancer. Cancer research. 2008; 68(17): 6932–6941.

100. Notta F, Mullighan CG, Wang JC, Poeppl A, Doulatov S et al. Evolution of human BCR-ABL1 lymphoblastic leukaemia-initiating cells. Nature 2011; 469(7330): 362–367.

101. Anderson K, Lutz C, van Delft FW, Bateman CM, Guo Y et al. Genetic variegation of clonal architecture and propagating cells in leukaemia. Nature 2011; 469(7330): 356–361.

102. Pece S, Tosoni D, Confalonieri S, Mazzarol G, Vecchi M et al. Biological and molecular heterogeneity of breast cancers correlates with their cancer stem cell content. Cell 2010; 140(1): 62–73.

103. Gupta PB, Fillmore CM, Jiang G, Shapira SD, Tao K et al. Stochastic state transitions give rise to phenotypic equilibrium in populations of cancer cells. Cell 2011; 146(4): 633–644.

104. Scheel C, Weinberg RA. Cancer stem cells and epithelial-mesenchy-mal transition: concepts and molecular links. Seminars in Cancer Biology 2012; 22(5-6): 396–403.

105. Brabletz T. EMT and MET in metastasis: where are the cancer stem cells? Cancer Cell 2012; 22(6): 699–701.

106. Gerlinger M, Rowan AJ, Horswell S, Larkin J, Endesfelder D et al. Intratumor heterogeneity and branched evolution revealed by multiregion sequencing. New England Journal of Medicine 2012; 366(10): 883–892.

107. Klein CA. Parallel progression of primary tumours and metastases. Nature Reviews Cancer 2009; 9(4): 302–312.

108. Rhim AD, Mirek ET, Aiello NM, Maitra A, Bailey JM et al. EMT and Dissemination Precede Pancreatic Tumor Formation. Cell 2012; 148(1-2): 349–361.

109. Cristofanilli M, Hayes DF, Budd GT, Ellis MJ, Stopeck A et al. Circulating tumor cells: a novel prognostic factor for newly diagnosed metastatic breast cancer. J Clin Oncol. 2005; 23(7): 1420–1430.

110. Kang Y, Pantel K. Tumor cell dissemination: emerging biological insights from animal models and cancer patients. Cancer Cell 2013; 23(5): 573–581.

111. Yu M, Bardia A, Wittner BS, Stott SL, Smas ME et al. Circulating breast tumor cells exhibit dynamic changes in epithelial and mesen-chymal composition. Science 2013; 339(6119): 580–584.

112. Vanharanta S, Massague J. Origins of metastatic traits. Cancer Cell 2013; 24(4): 410–421.

CHAPTER 11

Biomarker identification and clinical validation

Richard D. Kennedy, Manuel Salto-Tellez,
D. Paul Harkin, and Patrick G. Johnston

Introduction to biomarker identification and clinical validation

With a few notable exceptions, most cancer therapy is given in a 'one size fits all' manner depending on the anatomical site involved and basic histopathology. In addition, drug dosage has been calculated from clinical trials using toxicity as an endpoint. Although these approaches have been quite successful in the past, an improved understanding of cancer at a molecular level has questioned how we develop novel drugs and how we select appropriate patients in the clinic.

Studies in solid and haematological cancers have demonstrated that cancers originating from a single anatomical site can represent complex diseases with several molecular subtypes. For example, breast cancer comprises at least five distinct diseases, which have different clinical outcomes and respond to therapies differently. This heterogeneity in diseases may explain why single-agent chemotherapy drugs rarely exceed 30% response rates and why the attrition rate in clinical trials remains high in cancer medicine.

A better knowledge of cancer biology has also led to therapies that target specific molecular pathways. These drugs are highly unlikely to work in the context of an unselected patient population and are also often very expensive. It is clear that some strategy will be required to select appropriate patients for these therapeutic approaches. In addition, these drugs do not result in the toxicities associated with conventional cytotoxic agents, such as bone marrow suppression, making the endpoints in dose escalation studies more challenging.

Biomarkers that allow personalization of treatment to a patient's specific disease offer a solution to these issues. The USA National Institute of Health defines a biomarker as: 'a characteristic that is objectively measured and evaluated as an indicator of normal biologic processes, pathogenic processes, or pharmacologic responses to a therapeutic intervention' [1]. There are many cancer-related biomarkers that have been published in peer-reviewed articles; however, very few have made an impact on patient care. This is largely due to a failure to demonstrate clinical validity. In this chapter we aim to explain the process of biomarker discovery and delivery with a view to helping the practising physician and translational researcher appreciate what constitutes a valid biomarker suitable for clinical use.

Types of biomarker used in cancer management

The biomarkers used in cancer management can be categorized into seven major groups that cover the spectrum through from identification of patients at risk to treatment decisions (Figure 11.1). Each of these is discussed in more detail below.

Biomarkers of cancer risk

These are typically inherited somatic mutations in tumour suppressor genes that can be detected by sequencing or sequence-specific PCR approaches using normal cells (often white blood cells). They predict a high risk of developing cancer within an individual's lifetime. Examples are mutations within the BRCA1 or BRCA2 gene that predict increased risk of breast and ovarian cancer [2, 3], mutations in the mismatch repair genes MSH2, MSH6, and MLH1 that predict increased risk of colorectal cancer, ovarian cancer, and endometrial cancer (hereditary non-polyposis coli [4]) and mutations in the p53 gene that predict increased risk of breast, connective tissue and brain tumours (Li-Fraumeni syndrome [5]). These markers are used to inform primary screening approaches such as regular mammography, ultrasonography, or colonoscopy as well as surgical prophylaxis.

Tumour markers

These biomarkers help the clinician to estimate the amount of viable tumour in a patient either as an adjunct to imaging approaches or as a sensitive test for small levels of disease below radiological detection. They can also, in some circumstances, be used as diagnostic tests, although most are relatively non-specific and should not be used alone. Typically, they are glycoproteins that are expressed from tumour sites and can be measured by ELISA assays. Examples are CA-125 for ovarian cancer, carcinoembryonic antigen (CEA) for colorectal cancer, prostatic specific antigen (PSA) for prostate cancer, CA19-9 for pancreatic cancer, beta-2 microglobulin for lymphoproliferative diseases, paraproteins for multiple myeloma, alpha-fetoprotein (AFP) for hepatoma, beta-human chorionic gonadotrophin (beta-HCG) for choriocarcinoma and beta-HCG/alpha-fetoprotein for germ cell tumours. Recently, technology has been developed that can isolate and

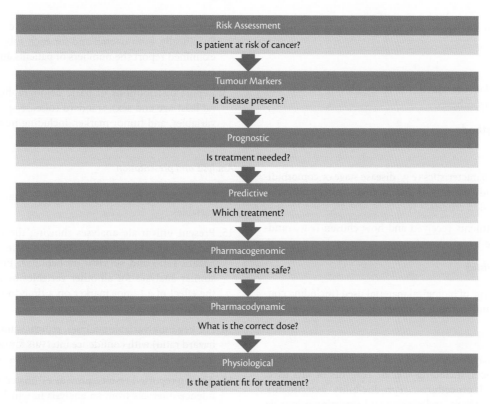

Fig. 11.1 Biomarkers in clinical practice.

quantitate circulating tumour cells in patients with solid tumours. This technique promises to be a further approach to estimating tumour response in the future [6].

Prognostic biomarkers

These biomarkers are used to estimate the outcome for a patient, usually in terms of disease-free, progression-free, or overall survival in the absence of a specific treatment. For example, high tumour grade is a prognostic factor associated with a higher chance of disease relapse in many cancer types. The presence of meta-static disease in the regional lymph nodes in breast or colorectal cancer patients has been a useful prognostic biomarker and has guided treatment towards adjuvant chemotherapy after surgery. More recently, the multigene OncotypeDx® breast cancer test has been shown to estimate the likelihood of disease recurrence following surgery in early oestrogen receptor positive breast cancer in the absence of adjuvant cytotoxic chemotherapy [7]. Those at high risk of recurrence have been shown to benefit from the addition of chemotherapy. Similarly, it has recently been reported that the presence of microsatellite instability in stage II colon cancer may indicate a biomarker of good prognosis and therefore indicate no requirement for adjuvant chemotherapy [8]. The National Cancer Institute–European Organization for Research and Treatment of Cancer working group on cancer diagnostics have published Reporting recommendations for tumor marker prognostic studies (REMARK criteria, Box 11.1) [9].

Predictive biomarkers

These estimate the likelihood of a patient benefiting from a specific therapy either in terms of an objective response or in terms

of disease-free or overall survival. A number are already used in the clinic to guide treatment (Table 11.1). Predictive markers can be used to improve drug development in two major ways. First, in early first-in-man studies, predictive biomarkers can be used to select patients thought likely to benefit. This is often referred to as a 'trial enrichment strategy'. The development of drugs that show no activity in these enriched populations may be halted in favour of more active compounds. An example was the selection of BRCA1 and BRCA2 mutant patients for first-in-man studies with single-agent olaparib, a PARP inhibitor [10].

The second application is the selection of patients that show superior outcomes to conventional therapy in drug registration studies (usually phase III). In this context the biomarker effectively becomes part of the treatment as it is required prior to administering the drug (referred to as 'on-label') and its validation falls under the appropriate regulatory authority such as the EMA or FDA. An example would be the on-label use of FDA-approved HER2 tests for patients receiving trastuzumab.

Pharmacogenomic markers

Although the response to cancer treatment often depends on tumour-specific molecular factors, naturally occurring genetic variations in normal somatic cells can also influence outcome. Single nuclear polymorphisms (SNPs) are base variations in genetic sequences, which occur in over 1% of the population. They can lead to altered metabolism of cancer drugs that increase or decrease their activity, and can therefore have important clinical consequences. Examples of SNPs that result in decreased metabolism are those in dihydropyrimidine dehydrogenase (DPD) which increase toxicity with 5 fluorouracil [11], in UDP-glucuronosyltransferase

Box 11.1 REMARK criteria

Introduction

1. State the marker examined, the study objectives, and any pre-specified hypotheses.

Materials and methods

Patients

2. Describe the characteristics (e.g., disease stage or comorbidities) of the study patients, including their source and inclusion and exclusion criteria.

3. Describe treatments received and how chosen (e.g., randomized or rule-based).

Specimen characteristics

4. Describe the type of biological material used (including control samples) and methods of preservation and storage.

Assay methods

5. Specify the assay method used and provide (or reference) a detailed protocol, including specific reagents or kits used, quality control procedures, reproducibility assessments, quantitation methods, and scoring and reporting protocols. Specify whether and how assays were performed blinded to the study end point.

Study design

6. State the method of case selection, including whether the study design was prospective or retrospective and whether stratification or matching (e.g., by stage of disease or age) was used. Specify the time period from which cases were taken, the end of the follow-up period, and the median follow-up time.

7. Precisely define all clinical endpoints examined.

8. List all candidate variables initially examined or considered for inclusion in models.

9. Give rationale for sample size; if the study was designed to detect a specified effect size, give the target power and effect size.

Statistical analysis methods

10. Specify all statistical methods, including details of any variable selection procedures and other model-building issues, how model assumptions were verified, and how missing data were handled.

11. Clarify how marker values were handled in the analyses; if relevant, describe methods used for cutpoint determination.

Results

Data

12. Describe the flow of patients through the study, including the number of patients included in each stage of the analysis (a diagram may be helpful) and reasons for dropout. Specifically, both overall and for each subgroup extensively examined report the numbers of patients and the number of events.

13. Report distributions of basic demographic characteristics (at least age and sex), standard (disease-specific) prognostic variables, and tumor marker, including numbers of missing values.

Analysis and presentation

14. Show the relation of the marker to standard prognostic variables.

15. Present univariate analyses showing the relation between the marker and outcome, with the estimated effect (e.g., hazard ratio and survival probability). Preferably provide similar analyses for all other variables being analyzed. For the effect of a tumor marker on a time-to-event outcome, a Kaplan–Meier plot is recommended.

16. For key multivariable analyses, report estimated effects (e.g., hazard ratio) with confidence intervals for the marker and, at least for the final model, all other variables in the model.

17. Among reported results, provide estimated effects with confidence intervals from an analysis in which the marker and standard prognostic variables are included, regardless of their statistical significance.

18. If done, report results of further investigations, such as checking assumptions, sensitivity analyses, and internal validation.

Discussion

19. Interpret the results in the context of the pre-specified hypotheses and other relevant studies; include a discussion of limitations of the study.

20. Discuss implications for future research and clinical value.

Reprinted by permission from Macmillan Publishers Ltd: *Nature Reviews Clinical Oncology*, McShane LM, et al., Reporting recommendations for tumor marker prognostic studies (REMARK), Volume 2, Number 8, p. 419, Copyright © 2005, doi:10.1038/ncponc0252

(UGT) which result in toxicity with irinotecan [12] or in thiopurine s-methyltransferase (TPMT) that predisposes to severe toxicity with 6-mercaptopurine [13]. SNPs may also result in decreased drug activation leading to loss of drug efficacy such as those affecting CYP2D6 that decrease the activity of tamoxifen [14].

Pharmacodynamic biomarkers

These biomarkers are used to measure the effect of a drug on its specific target and are used in dose optimization studies. This approach has become increasingly important as modern therapies that are targeted to specific molecular pathways are unlikely to have the same toxic effects observed for conventional DNA-targeted treatments. This can mean that traditional dose escalation to grade 3–4 toxicity may result in a drug dosage far

Table 11.1 Examples of predictive biomarkers used in routine clinical practice

Biomarker	Technology	Disease	Drug	References
BCR-ABL translocation	FISH	Chronic myeloid leukaemia	Imatinib	[25]
BRCA 1/2 mutation	Sequencing	Breast and ovarian cancer	Olaparib	[26]
BRAF mutation	PCR/sequencing	Melanoma	Vemurafenib	[27]
CD20 expression	Immunohistochemistry	B Cell lymphoma	Rituximab	[28]
C-kit mutation	PCR/Sequencing	Gastrointestinal stromal tumour	Imatinib	[29]
EGFR mutation	PCR/sequencing	Non-small-cell lung cancer	Gefitinib	[30]
EML4-ALK translocation	PCR/FISH	Lung adenocarcinoma	Crizotinib	[31]
HER2 amplification	Immunohistochemistry/in-situ hybridization	Breast Cancer	Trastuzumab	[32]
KRAS mutation	PCR/sequencing	Colorectal cancer	Cetuximab, panitumumab	[33, 34]
Oestrogen receptor Expression	Immunohistochemistry	Breast cancer	Tamoxifen, anastrozole	[35]

in excess of that required for complete inhibition of the pathway of interest. Pharmacodynamic (PD) markers allow investigators to find an appropriate biologically active drug dosage that may be well below toxic levels. This can make the treatment more tolerable to patients, save on the amount of drug administered with economical benefits, and reduce the likelihood of additive toxicity if the drug is combined with other more conventional cytotoxic therapies.

Ideally, the PD marker is measured in the tissue of interest and is directly related to the drug's mechanism of action, such as dephosphorylation of tumour PRAS40 for AKT inhibitors [15]. Alternatively, markers of proliferation such as tumour expression of Ki67 can be used to demonstrate drug activity as has been reported for aromatase inhibitors in breast cancer treatment [16]. In some studies, peripheral tissue has been used to demonstrate drug activity such as eyelash bulb H2AX expression for PARP inhibitors [10] or peripheral blood white cells for histone deacetylase activity following administration of HDAC inhibitors [17].

Radiological approaches are also being investigated as PD markers in cancer drug development. For example, dynamic contrast enhanced MRI and contrast-enhanced ultrasound have been used to measure tumour blood vessel response to anti-angiogenic agents [18, 19].

Biomarkers of physiological processes

The measurement of physiological processes such as renal function, liver function, and bone marrow function by electrolyte, metabolite, and blood cell and platelet counts is an important biomarker in cancer patient management. The clinician can potentially give or withhold treatment based on these measurements so it is essential they are measured with the same quality and their limitations understood as much as in the case of other cancer biomarkers.

Biomarker discovery

Biomarker discovery can either be hypothesis driven, where an investigator knows the likely molecular pathway that influences

patient outcome, or investigational, where a biomarker is discovered in an unbiased fashion. An example of a hypothesis-driven approach would be where a drug is known to target a specific molecular pathway that can be affected by a cancer-related mutation. Examples are the use of activating BRAF mutations as predictive biomarkers for BRAF inhibitors or activating EGFR mutations as predictive biomarkers for EGFR-targeted therapies. A pure investigational approach may be taken where it is unclear which pathways are responsible for patient outcome such as the DNA-microarray-based discovery of a 70-gene prognostic test for early breast cancer (Mammaprint®) [20].

Biomarker discovery study designs

Biomarker discovery can be performed using three main approaches.

Preclinical model systems

Human cell lines and animal model systems can be used in the laboratory to model how a tumour may behave and respond to treatment in specific molecular contexts. This has the advantage that very specific questions around the biological relevance of a biomarker can be asked using single agent drugs. Preclinical systems, however, can also be misleading, as cancer behaviour can often be influenced by the immune system and tumour–stromal interactions. For example, human cell lines may demonstrate overexpression of genes that are unique to the artificial Petri dish environment and xenograft models for anti-angiogenic agents may not adequately model the biological pathways active in human tumours.

Retrospective archived tissue analysis

In this approach, archived material is analysed for biomarker discovery. This may be particularly useful in the case of prognostic biomarkers as the clinical follow-up and outcome data for a specific patient may be available. In addition, with the standard approach to tumour archiving there may be large numbers of samples available among clinical centres, particularly if formalin-fixed paraffin-embedded tissues are used. In the case of predictive markers for novel therapies, however, it is unlikely that archived material will be available. Archived tumour material may also demonstrate degradation over time, introducing 'noise' to the analysis [21].

Prospective biomarker discovery

This may be the most appropriate approach when discovering a biomarker for a novel drug agent as material from responding and non-responding patients can be analysed to look for differences at a molecular level. One difficulty, however, may be the adequate powering of the study. Considering the heterogeneity that can occur in cancer, it is likely that at least 20 to 30 samples each from responding and non-responding patients will be required. If a drug agent has an expected response rate of 10% in a general population, 300 patients would need to be recruited to get 30 tissue samples from responders, which may be impractical. Novel adaptive trial designs may help to deal with this issue (Figure 11.2). Another problem is that novel agents are often combined with conventional drugs as part of a clinical trial. This makes it very difficult to identify biomarkers that are specific to the agent in question rather than for the combination of agents.

Given the importance of retrospective and prospective tissue collections in biomarker discovery and validation (see below), it is essential that those centres involved in such activities pay special attention to the quality of their retrospective and prospective biological collections. This is done through the establishment of institutional biobanks, which are tailored to provide samples for biomarker discovery and/or validation of the best possible quality and following the strictest ethical frameworks. In many instances, the quality of an institution's biobank is an indicator of the quality of its biomarker discovery programme.

Important issues with biomarker study design

Balancing for confounding factors

In the process of identifying a biomarker, samples from two populations with different outcomes are compared for molecular differences. These populations must be properly balanced for factors that may result in molecular differences independent from outcome or due to known prognostic or predictive factors. For example, if there is an over-representation of female patients in one of the sample sets then the biomarker may predict gender rather than outcome. If one sample set is predominantly comprised of high-grade tumours whereas the comparator is comprised of low-grade tumours, it is likely the resultant biomarker will predict outcome but this will have no clinical utility above standard histopathological examination. Examples of other factors to be considered for balancing between datasets are age, ethnicity, tumour stage, type of surgery, and concomitant medication.

Reagent effects

Many laboratory reagents are manufactured for research use only. They do not have the quality standards applied that would be expected for diagnostic tests and therefore demonstrate considerable variation between batches. This can result in considerable variation in biomarker results depending on which batch of reagent is used. For example, two batches of antibody may vary in concentration resulting in different immunohistochemical staining for the same sample. Ideally, this issue is dealt with by using GMP (good manufacturing procedure) grade reagents. Alternatively, the laboratory may choose to test every batch of new reagents to ensure correct performance or pool several batches of reagent to average out any batch-specific effects.

Population effects

When developing a biomarker it is important to ensure that it applies to the population in which it will be used. For example, a biomarker of response to androgen ablation in prostate cancer in a Caucasian population may not apply to an Afro-Caribbean population due to differences in prostate cancer biology between the groups.

Centre effects

A biomarker that is discovered using tumour material from one clinical centre may not work for patients from other centres. Factors such as centre-specific approaches to surgery, specific tumour fixation protocols, physician-specific chemotherapy regimens, and user biases on the assessment of tumour response may lead to a biomarker that only works in a centre-specific context. Ideally, biomarkers should be developed using tumour material and clinical data collected from multiple centres. In addition, each centre should provide samples representing the two populations of interest such as responders and non-responders.

Laboratory operator effects

Biomarkers that are discovered by a single laboratory operator risk validating only in the hands of the same individual. Biomarkers should be developed using defined standard laboratory operating procedures and, as much as possible, automated laboratory systems to prevent user-specific variation in protocols. In addition, samples for biomarker discovery should be randomized between several operators to remove the influences of any one individual.

Biomarker substrates

With the exception of radiological biomarkers, most cancer biomarkers are measured using biological materials. Examples are listed in Table 11.2. To date, many biomarkers have been measured using tumour material but this can raise some practical issues. First, tumour material may be difficult to biopsy. Patients with liver or lung metastases may require a surgical procedure that could be potentially harmful and is likely to reduce recruitment to biomarker-focused clinical studies. Alternatively, tumour material from an original diagnostic resection may be used but this may not be representative of the current disease in patients who have undergone tumour-cell selection by multiple courses of chemotherapy. Less invasive approaches to biomarker measurement, such as using circulating tumour cells, free plasma DNA/RNA/miRNA, urine, saliva, or faeces are being developed to try to circumvent these issues.

Important practical considerations for biomarker discovery

Sample practicality

Although a technology may be very successful in discovering a potential biomarker in the research laboratory it may not be

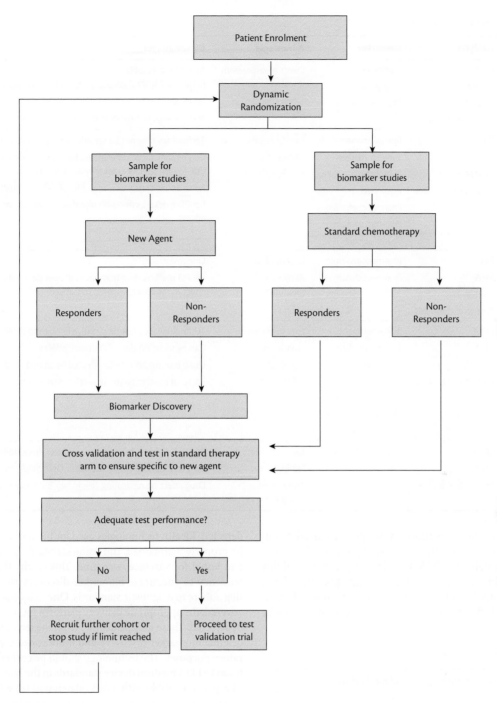

Fig. 11.2 An example of an adaptive trial design for biomarker discovery.

practical for every day use in the clinic. For example, a requirement for fresh frozen tumour tissue will necessitate a change in clinical practice, as the surgeon will need to have liquid nitrogen available in the operating theatre for every tumour. Similarly, DNA-damage-induced repair foci detected by immunohistochemistry in irradiated fresh tumour biopsies are a good measure of DNA damage response and may guide the use of DNA damaging chemotherapy or PARP inhibitor treatment [22]. It is unlikely, however, that a process could be put in place where every tumour is harvested at the time of surgery and irradiated. Certain technologies such as mass spectrometry or full genome sequencing may

also be excellent for biomarker discovery but are at this moment too laborious and time consuming for use in a regular diagnostic lab.

In addition, a biomarker strategy that requires invasive sampling techniques that could result in significant patient morbidity or mortality is unlikely to succeed as a diagnostic in routine clinical practice.

Technology

A list of potential technologies for biomarker discovery and delivery are given in Table 11.3. Some technologies may be excellent for research purposes but may not be suitable for biomarker discovery.

Table 11.2 Biomarker sample sources

Source	Analytes	Biomarker	Advantages	Disadvantages
Tumour	DNA mRNA miRNA Protein metabolites	Predictive Prognostic Pharmacodynamics	Direct measure from disease of interest Often collected in diagnostic process	May be inaccessible Biopsy may not be representative of whole tumour due to heterogeneity May be large normal or stromal cell component
Blood	DNA mRNA miRNA Protein metabolites	Risk assessment Tumour markers Prognostic Predictive Pharmacogenomic Pharmacodynamic Physiological	Easy to obtain Allows serial measurements	Technology may not be sensitive enough to detect analyte Can be difficult to differentiate tumour-specific analytes from those due to non-specific disease-related effects Renal and liver function may affect levels of some biomarkers For PD markers, effects on blood cells may not represent tumour effects
Mucosa/Skin biopsy	DNA RNA miRNA Protein metabolites	Pharmacogenomic Pharmacodynamic	Easy to obtain Allows serial measurements	Uncomfortable For PD markers drug may have different penetration or biological effect in mucosa compared to tumour
Excreted/ Secreted Urine/Faeces/ Saliva	DNA RNA miRNA Protein metabolites	Risk assessment Tumour markers Prognostic Predictive Pharmacogenomic Pharmacodynamic Physiological	Easy to obtain Non-invasive Allows serial measurements	Technology may not be sensitive enough to detect analyte Can be variation due to dilutional effects Urine biomarkers may be affected by altered renal function Bacterial contamination may affect some assays
Eye lash/hair bulb	DNA RNA Protein metabolite	Pharmacodynamic	Easy to obtain No-invasive Allow serial measurements	Best suited for Immunohistochemistry/ Immunofluorescence Very small amounts of material for DNA/RNA/metabolite analysis. Drug effect on replicating cells in hair bulb may not represent tumour

Problems can arise where a platform is not properly quality controlled, leading to variable results and a loss of precision. For example, a poorly maintained q-PCR machine may generate highly variable results, which are discordant from a high-quality platform. These issues may not be immediately apparent in a research environment where a drift in biomarker results over time would not be detected. Ideally, technologies used for biomarker discovery should be properly maintained, run using standard operating procedures, and tested for variance over time. This is why there is currently a tendency to encourage biomarker discovery work in laboratories that adhere to diagnostic standards. Once a biomarker has been discovered, the appropriate delivery platform for the clinic will need to be selected. These may be distinct from the technologies used in the original biomarker discovery and more suited for diagnostic laboratory purposes. The technology should be cost effective, manufactured to FDA medical device standards in the USA or CE marked in Europe, compatible with a fast turnaround time (preferably under one week), and easy to use in a general hospital laboratory setting. Examples of these technologies are ELISA, Immunohistochemistry, and q-PCR. Occasionally more complex biomarker technologies such as DNA microarrays or DNA sequencing can be delivered from a central laboratory as a service, providing the test is not cost prohibitive, can be delivered in a realistic timescale, and fulfils the regulatory quality standards.

Table 11.3 Biomarker technologies

Analyte	Discovery technology	Clinical delivery
DNA	DNA microarray Sequencing (Sanger/Next Generation)	Polymerase Chain Reaction (PCR) Sequencing In-Situ hybridization
RNA	cDNA microarray Sequencing	Reverse transcriptase PCR (RT-PCR)
Protein	2D Gels Mass spectometry Protein Microarray	Immunohistochemistry Enzyme-linked immunosorbent assay (ELISA)
Metabolites	Mass spectrometry Nuclear magnetic resonance (NMR) Spectroscopy	ELISA Chemical/colourmetric assays

Expense

A biomarker with excellent performance characteristics that is discovered using an expensive technology but cannot be moved to a less expensive platform may not be successful. A cost versus patient benefit analysis will need to be adequately compelling to encourage reimbursement from national health or insurance schemes.

Cancer biomarker validation

It is an absolute necessity that a cancer biomarker is adequately validated prior to being used in patient management. Depending on the risks associated with its use there are various levels of validation expected under guidance from the EMA in Europe, and the FDA and CLIA legislation in the USA. These requirements are complex and evolving and readers seeking more detailed guidance are advised to contact these authorities. Some attempts are now being made to standardize these requirements globally due to the complexity of running international biomarker-focused clinical trials.

There are, however, some underlying basic principles in the validation of all biomarkers. These can be described as analytical validation, clinical validation, and evidence of clinical utility.

Analytical validation

The analytical characteristics of a biomarker must be known. These can be described as follows.

Precision

This is a measure of the repeatability of a biomarker result. Obviously an assay that gives differing results each time it is used for the same sample will be of limited use to a clinician. Specific factors that can cause low precision are inadequate operator training, variability in reagent batches due to poor supplier quality control, choice of a technology with inherent variable results such as phosphoantibody analysis on IHC, or poor maintenance of laboratory equipment. Another factor that may affect precision that is somewhat unique to cancer biomarkers delivered from tumour tissue is the effects of stroma and normal tissue on the result. Some tumour samples can have large amounts of fibrous tissue that may give a different biomarker signal to the malignant cell content. This effect can be reduced by macrodissection or microdissection of tumour material to standardize malignant cell content.

Accuracy

This is a measure of how close the assay result is to the known truth. In many cases the truth may be the results from a reference laboratory or as reported using the gold standard technology. Factors that may affect accuracy are improper sample handling prior to analysis, or a suboptimal operating procedure or technology. Another issue that can affect accuracy is the timing of tumour biopsy. A biomarker result measured from an original diagnostic tumour sample may be very different from the result from the same patient's tumour that has undergone selective pressure from chemotherapy or radiotherapy. Ideally, for predictive biomarkers, the assay should be performed immediately prior to starting the agent in question.

Detection limits

This is a measure of the amount of material that is needed in order to give an accurate result. For example, in the case of tumour material at least 20% of the specimen needs to be viable malignant cells in order to detect a mutation by conventional sequencing [23].

Reportable range

This is a measure of the expected normal population distribution of the assay result. This may be important when the target population for a drug is defined on a population basis such as the top quartile of patients expressing the highest level of a specific gene or protein. It also allows the laboratory to detect outlying results that could be due to the wrong sample type being submitted, sample handling errors, or diagnostic laboratory error.

Reference range

Most biomarkers have a predefined cutoff of what constitutes a positive or negative result. In the case of mutations this is straightforward, but for biomarkers with a continuous numerical result it can be more complicated. Most cutoffs in continually variable assays are set at the optimal sensitivity and specificity for the assay as defined from clinical trials. For multivariate assays, such as q-PCR or DNA-microarray measurement of several mRNA transcripts, the cutoff is usually a score from a computational algorithm. The software that is used for this calculation must also be validated and demonstrated to be consistent.

Internal controls

Appropriate internal positive and negative control samples must be developed for biomarker assays. These allow the laboratory to know if a technical problem has developed with the assay. This could be a simple operator mistake causing a sudden failure of control results or could be a reagent or equipment problem that could result in a gradual drift in results. To detect the latter, diagnostic laboratories will typically record and plot control results over time and apply statistical algorithms, such as the Westgard rules, to alert operators to an issue [24].

Clinical validation

For a biomarker to be useful it must have adequate clinical performance. The performance for a biomarker that dichotomizes a population into two groups, such as into predicted responder or non-responder or into predicted recurrence or non-recurrence at a defined time point, can be described in the terms of sensitivity, specificity, negative predictive value, and positive predictive value. Sensitivity is a measure of how well the assay detects true positive patients whereas specificity measures how well it excludes true negative patients. Negative and positive predictive values are dependent on the distribution of true positive and negative patients in a patient population and measure the proportion of subjects with a positive or negative test result respectively who are correctly diagnosed.

Some biomarkers predict a particular outcome on a time-to-event basis, such as disease-free or overall survival. This may be appropriate where there is no logical time point to act as a cutoff for a dichotomized approach. An example is early-stage oestrogen receptor positive stage breast cancer where recurrence events can continue beyond ten years. In such cases the biomarker performance may be best measured in terms of a hazard ratio with confidence limits.

It is absolutely essential that biomarker performance metrics be validated on a patient cohort completely independent from those used for assay discovery. This is to prevent 'over-fitting', where artificially high performance characteristics are observed for an assay applied to the same population used to discover it.

The appropriate design for biomarker validation studies is a subject of much debate, as some require large numbers of patients and are consequently very expensive. Most designs, however, can be classified as a prospective treatment interaction design, a prospective treatment stratified design, or a retrospective validation design (Figure 11.3). Prospective designs are usually required for the

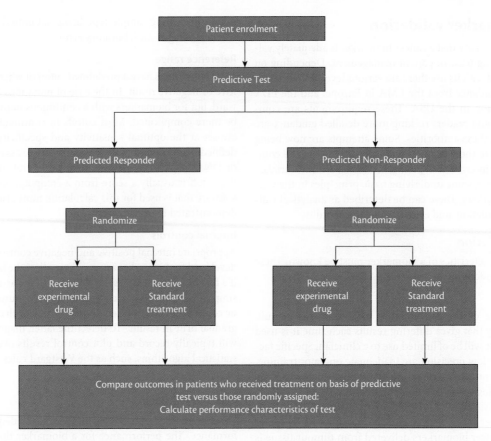

Fig. 11.3 A treatment interaction biomarker validation study design.

validation of predictive biomarkers for novel therapeutic agents as no archived tissue is available. Retrospective validation can be performed on archived tissue where this is available and this approach may be particularly useful for prognostic tests where patient outcomes are known. It is important, however, that the material has been collected in a standardized manner consistent with how it will be collected in clinical use.

Clinical utility

An important consideration for a cancer biomarker before implementation is how it is likely to alter patient management. For example, it could be argued that for a cancer with a poor prognosis and few treatment options, a predictive biomarker would have to be extremely specific before a clinician would elect not to offer treatment. Assuming that the biomarker is not a regulatory prerequisite for offering a drug (on-label), a clinician may simply decide to offer chemotherapy to a patient with measurable disease and reassess after a few weeks rather than pay for an expensive predictive test. Obviously, in the case of adjuvant chemotherapy, this approach would not work, and a predictive test may be more important.

For the pharmaceutical industry, an important consideration will be how well a novel drug performs in the context of a biomarker when compared to the standard treatment arm in a registration study. If the combination of biomarker and drug demonstrates an improved outcome, the test will become 'on-label' and effectively become part of the drug therapy. In this case clinicians will be expected to perform the assay before offering the novel drug.

Quality control of biomarkers

Once a biomarker has been validated and entered clinical practice there must be system for quality control to protect patients from erroneous results. Unfortunately, this is often overlooked when biomarkers are measured in an academic environment. Quality control can take the form of internal and external activities. Internally, control sample results can be measured to ensure there is no drift in results. A random selection of samples should be rerun every few months to ensure consistency in reporting. Operators must all have demonstrable training and adhere to standard operating procedures. Equipment must be maintained to high standards and reagents must be batch tested to ensure no changes in specification. These activities are part of the core review of agencies to certify a laboratory adequate for diagnostics. Indeed, the quality of the laboratory's internal quality control scheme is a measure of its overall quality, although it can increase substantially the cost of the final laboratory test.

External quality control takes the form of formalized comparisons of results to reference laboratories and audits from approved bodies such as UKAS and the College of Pathologists.

Conclusion

With the development of targeted therapies, it is inevitable that oncology will be an increasingly biomarker-dependent discipline. The adoption of biomarkers is likely to benefit patients who will receive treatments that are more likely to work and are less likely to result in needless toxicity. Health care providers will also benefit, as limited resources will be better targeted towards successful outcomes. Similarly, health insurance companies and national health services will be better able to pay for expensive new therapies, as fewer patients will be considered eligible for them. Finally, the appropriate use of pharmacodynamic, predictive, and prognostic biomarkers in clinical trials will identify ineffective therapies earlier in the development process and will improve the likelihood of successful agents reaching the clinic.

There are, however, challenges to the adoption of biomarkers in the clinic. First, it is unclear who should pay for their development. As discussed earlier, the validation process can require large clinical studies. To date these have been paid for by pharmaceutical and diagnostic companies. It could be argued that insurance companies and health services would benefit from adoption of these approaches and should become engaged in their development. In addition, there can be a perception in some pharmaceutical companies that biomarkers may limit the market for some drugs by selecting patient subgroups. Although this may be true, a non-biomarker-driven approach opens the possibility that a competitor may capture the market with an on-label predictive test, which may restrict the patient numbers but also demonstrates superior therapeutic responses.

In the next few years it is likely these issues will be resolved and the use of biomarkers will become increasingly commonplace in everyday clinical practice. When this occurs it will be the responsibility of every oncologist to ensure that these assays are properly validated and have the appropriate level of quality control so that patients gain the maximum benefit.

Further reading

Biomarkers Definitions Working Group. Biomarkers and surrogate endpoints: preferred definitions and conceptual framework. Clinical Pharmacology & Therapeutics 2001; 69(3): 89–95.

Friedman LS, Ostermeyer EA, Szabo CI, Dowd P, Lynch ED et al. Confirmation of BRCA1 by analysis of germline mutations linked to breast and ovarian cancer in ten families. Nature Genetics 1994; 8(4): 399–404.

Lynch HT, Watson P, Shaw TG, Lynch JF, Harty AE et al. Clinical impact of molecular genetic diagnosis, genetic counseling, and management of hereditary cancer. Part II: Hereditary nonpolyposis colorectal carcinoma as a model. Cancer 1999; 86(11 Suppl): 2457–2463.

McShane LM, Altman DG, Sauerbrei W, Taube SE, Gion M et al. Reporting recommendations for tumor marker prognostic studies (REMARK). Journal of the National Cancer Institute 2005; 97(16): 1180–1184.

Westgard. Westgard Rules and Multirules. Available from: https://www.westgard.com/westgard-rules.htm, last accessed on 11 May 2015.

References

1. Biomarkers Definitions Working Group. Biomarkers and surrogate endpoints: preferred definitions and conceptual framework. Clinical Pharmacology & Therapeutics 2001; 69(3): 89–95.
2. Friedman LS, Ostermeyer EA, Szabo CI, Dowd P, Lynch ED et al. Confirmation of BRCA1 by analysis of germline mutations linked to breast and ovarian cancer in ten families. Nature Genetics 1994; 8(4): 399–404.
3. Wooster R, Neuhausen SL, Mangion J, Quirk Y, Ford D et al. Localization of a breast cancer susceptibility gene, BRCA2, to chromosome 13q12-13. Science 1994; 265(5181): 2088–2090.
4. Lynch HT, Watson P, Shaw TG, Lynch JF, Harty AE et al. Clinical impact of molecular genetic diagnosis, genetic counseling, and management of hereditary cancer. Part II: Hereditary nonpolyposis colorectal carcinoma as a model. Cancer 1999; 86(11 Suppl): 2457–2463.
5. Varley JM. Germline TP53 mutations and Li-Fraumeni syndrome. Human Mutation 2003; 21(3), 313–320.
6. de Bono JS, Scher HI, Montgomery RB, Parker C, Miller MC et al. Circulating tumor cells predict survival benefit from treatment in metastatic castration-resistant prostate cancer. Clinical Cancer Research 2008; 14(19): 6302–6309.
7. Paik S, Shak S, Tang G, Kim C, Baker J et al. A multigene assay to predict recurrence of tamoxifen-treated, node-negative breast cancer. New England Journal of Medicine 2004; 351(27): 2817–2826.
8. Sinicrope FA, Foster NR, Thibodeau SN, Marsoni S, Monges G et al. DNA mismatch repair status and colon cancer recurrence and survival in clinical trials of 5-fluorouracil-based adjuvant therapy. Journal of the National Cancer Institute 2011; 103(11): 863–875.
9. McShane LM, Altman DG, Sauerbrei W, Taube SE, Gion M et al. Reporting recommendations for tumor marker prognostic studies (REMARK). Journal of the National Cancer Institute 2005; 97(16): 1180–1184.
10. Tutt A, Robson M, Garber JE, Domchek SM, Audeh MW et al. Oral poly(ADP-ribose) polymerase inhibitor olaparib in patients with BRCA1 or BRCA2 mutations and advanced breast cancer: a proof-of-concept trial. Lancet 2010; 376(9737): 235–244.
11. Diasio RB, Beavers TL, Carpenter JT. Familial deficiency of dihydropyrimidine dehydrogenase. Biochemical basis for familial pyrimidinemia and severe 5-fluorouracil-induced toxicity. Journal of Clinical Investigation 1988; 81(1): 47–51.
12. Iyer L, King CD, Whitington PF, Green MD, Roy SK et al. Genetic predisposition to the metabolism of irinotecan (CPT-11). Role of uridine diphosphate glucuronosyltransferase isoform 1A1 in the glucuronidation of its active metabolite (SN-38) in human liver microsomes. Journal of Clinical Investigation 1998; 101(4): 847–854.
13. Krynetski EY, Tai HL, Yates CR, Fessing MY, Loennechen T et al. Genetic polymorphism of thiopurine S-methyltransferase: clinical importance and molecular mechanisms. Pharmacogenetics 1996; 6 (4): 279–290.
14. Schroth W, Goetz MP, Hamann U, Fasching PA, Schmidt M et al. Association between CYP2D6 polymorphisms and outcomes among women with early stage breast cancer treated with tamoxifen. Journal of the American Medical Association 2009; 302(13): 1429–1436.
15. Yap TA, Yan L, Patnaik A, Fearen I, Olmos D et al. First-in-man clinical trial of the oral pan-AKT inhibitor MK-2206 in patients with advanced solid tumors. Journal of Clinical Oncology 2011; 29(35): 4688–4695.
16. Dowsett M, Smith IE, Ebbs SR, Dixon JM, Skene A et al. Prognostic value of Ki67 expression after short-term presurgical endocrine therapy for primary breast cancer. Journal of the National Cancer Institute 2007; 99(2): 167–170.
17. Bonfils C, Kalita A, Dubay M, Siu LL, Carducci MA et al. Evaluation of the pharmacodynamic effects of MGCD0103 from preclinical models to human using a novel HDAC enzyme assay. Clinical Cancer Research 2008; 14(11): 3441–3449.
18. Forsberg F. Can the effect of antiangiogenic treatments be monitored and quantified noninvasively by using contrast-enhanced US? Radiology 2010; 254(2): 317–318.
19. Hahn OM, Yang C, Medved M, Karczmar G, Kistner E et al. Dynamic contrast-enhanced magnetic resonance imaging pharmacodynamic biomarker study of sorafenib in metastatic renal carcinoma. Journal of Clinical Oncology 2008; 26(28): 4572–4578.
20. van de Vijver MJ, He YD, van't Veer LJ, Dai H, Hart AA et al. A gene-expression signature as a predictor of survival in breast cancer. New England Journal of Medicine 2002; 347(25): 1999–2009.
21. Farragher SM, Tanney A, Kennedy RD, Paul Harkin D. RNA expression analysis from formalin fixed paraffin embedded tissues. Histochemistry and Cell Biology 2008; 130(3): 435–445.

22. Kennedy RD, D'Andrea AD. DNA repair pathways in clinical practice: lessons from pediatric cancer susceptibility syndromes. Journal of Clinical Oncology 2006; 24(23): 3799–3808.

23. Chin TM, Anuar D, Soo R, Salto-Tellez M, Li WQ et al. Detection of epidermal growth factor receptor variations by partially denaturing HPLC. Clinical Chemistry 2007; 53(1): 62–70.

24. Westgard. Westgard Rules and Multirules. Available from: https://www.westgard.com/westgard-rules.htm, last accessed on 11 May 2015.

25. Druker BJ, Talpaz M, Resta DJ, Peng B, Buchdunger E et al. Efficacy and safety of a specific inhibitor of the BCR-ABL tyrosine kinase in chronic myeloid leukemia. New England Journal of Medicine 2001; 344(14): 1031–1037.

26. Audeh MW, Carmichael J, Penson RT, Friedlander M, Powell B et al. Oral poly(ADP-ribose) polymerase inhibitor olaparib in patients with BRCA1 or BRCA2 mutations and recurrent ovarian cancer: a proof-of-concept trial. Lancet 2010; 376 (9737): 245–251.

27. Sosman JA, Kim KB, Schuchter L, Gonzalez R, Pavlick AC et al. Survival in BRAF V600-mutant advanced melanoma treated with vemurafenib. New England Journal of Medicine 2012; 366(8): 707–714.

28. Maloney DG, Grillo-López AJ, White CA, Bodkin D, Schilder RJ et al. IDEC-C2B8 (Rituximab) anti-CD20 monoclonal antibody therapy in patients with relapsed low-grade non-Hodgkin's lymphoma. *Blood* 1997; 90(6): 2188–2195.

29. Joensuu H, Dimitrijevic S. Tyrosine kinase inhibitor imatinib (STI571) as an anticancer agent for solid tumours. Annals of Medicine 2001; 33(7): 451–455.

30. Lynch TJ, Bell DW, Sordella R, Gurubhagavatula S, Okimoto RA et al. Activating mutations in the epidermal growth factor receptor underlying responsiveness of non-small-cell lung cancer to gefitinib. New England Journal of Medicine 2004; 350(21): 2129–2139.

31. Koivunen JP, Mermel C, Zejnullahu K, Murphy C, Lifshits E et al. EML4-ALK fusion gene and efficacy of an ALK kinase inhibitor in lung cancer. Clinical Cancer Research 2008; 14(13): 4275–4283.

32. Vogel CL, Cobleigh MA, Tripathy D, Gutheil JC, Harris LN et al. Efficacy and safety of trastuzumab as a single agent in first-line treatment of HER2-overexpressing metastatic breast cancer. Journal of Clinical Oncology 2002; 20(3): 719–726.

33. Amado RG, Wolf M, Peeters M, Van Cutsem E, Siena S et al. Wild-type KRAS is required for panitumumab efficacy in patients with metastatic colorectal cancer. Journal of Clinical Oncology 2008; 26(10); 1626–1634.

34. Van Cutsem E, Köhne CH, Hitre E, Zaluski J, Chang Chien CR et al. (2009). Cetuximab and chemotherapy as initial treatment for metastatic colorectal cancer. New England Journal of Medicine 2009; 360(14): 1408–1417.

35. Fisher B, Redmond C, Brown A, Wickerham DL, Wolmark N et al. Influence of tumor estrogen and progesterone receptor levels on the response to tamoxifen and chemotherapy in primary breast cancer. Journal of Clinical Oncology 1983; 1(4): 227–241.

CHAPTER 12

Cancer, immunity, and inflammation

Campbell S.D. Roxburgh and Donald C. McMillan

Introduction to cancer, immunity, and inflammation

In recent years, the failure of the somatic mutation hypothesis of cancer progression to provide meaningful improvements in outcome in non-hereditary cancers has given way to a more complex paradigm in which host inflammatory responses are central. There is also now persuasive evidence that inflammation is key to tumourigenesis (reviewed in [1]) via DNA damage, stimulation of angiogenesis and proliferation, and inhibition of apoptosis. Indeed, inflammation is now considered a key hallmark of cancer [2]. However, the present chapter will focus on the role of immunity and inflammation in established cancer.

Work carried out in a number of common solid tumours including breast, gastrointestinal, urological, and lung cancer have been important in the current understanding of the importance of immunity and inflammation in tumour growth and progression, and it is clear that such findings are likely to be of importance in most sporadic cancers.

There have long been suspicions that dysregulated immune and inflammatory responses promote the progression and dissemination of established cancers [3]. For example, Dvorak [4] proposed that a 'tumour is a wound which does not heal'. Further, in patients with gastrointestinal tumours there have been repeated clinical observations that patients presenting as emergencies (with blood loss, obstruction, or perforation) or who develop an anastomotic leak following surgery have poorer cancer survival compared with those who did not, independent of tumour staging (e.g., [5–7]).

Cancer-associated alterations in patient immune and inflammatory responses are complex but are clearly linked. To examine such associations some arbitrary divisions have been made to differentiate various aspects of these responses. One rational approach would be to consider local responses in the tumour microenvironment and systemic responses in tissues distant from the tumour. Within these divisions it is then reasonable to consider innate, humoral, and adaptive responses (see Figure 12.1). By examining these responses and the mediators that link local and systemic immune/inflammatory responses it is possible to identify key mediators that can be targeted in future work. Finally, it is possible to comment on whether the up-regulation or attenuation of these responses may be important for disease progression and survival in patients with colorectal cancer.

Local immune and inflammatory responses

It is increasingly apparent that tumour progression is not a tumour-cell autonomous process [8]. There are a multitude of complex interactions between the host immune response and the tumour that dictate oncological outcome. As tumour cells proliferate and neoplasms grow in size, up to 90% of the tumour can consist of stroma and inflammatory cells [9]. In addition, tumour microsatellite instability status, CpG island methylator phenotype, and intra-tumoural HLA expression appear to be associated with tumour inflammatory cell infiltrate. This is consistent with a pronounced inflammatory cell infiltrate being more common in early-stage disease, degrading with increasing tumour size or T stage presumably reflective of tumour escape. Therefore, the tumour microenvironment plays a crucial role in determining disease progression, representative of the host–tumour interface where immune cells interact with each other and tumour cells.

With reference to the local immune and inflammatory response, more than 100 studies over the last 40 years have reported that immune cells in the immediate tumour microenvironment play an important role in determining survival in a number of common solid tumours [10, 11]. Recent work confirms that a pronounced tumour inflammatory infiltrate predicts good outcome and it has been proposed this may be used routinely to predict survival.

Klintrup and co-workers determined that, through a simple routine assessment of the entire immune/inflammatory reaction at both the invasive margin and in the central part of the tumour, a high-grade infiltrate was associated with improved recurrence-free and cancer-specific survival in colorectal cancer [12]. When the components of this inflammatory cell infiltrate were examined, a high-grade infiltrate was mainly composed of macrophages, lymphocytes, neutrophils, and plasma cells whereas a low-grade inflammatory cell infiltrate was almost exclusively composed of macrophages such that the macrophage count was similar in both high- and low-grade Klintrup scores [13]. Similar results have been reported in primary operable breast cancer [14].

Therefore, in general, where present an effective anti-cancer adaptive immune response is associated with improved outcome and where absent, other forms of innate myeloid derived cellular immune responses predominate and appear to be associated with poorer outcome. However, it is also increasingly clear that there is

Cancer immunity and inflammation

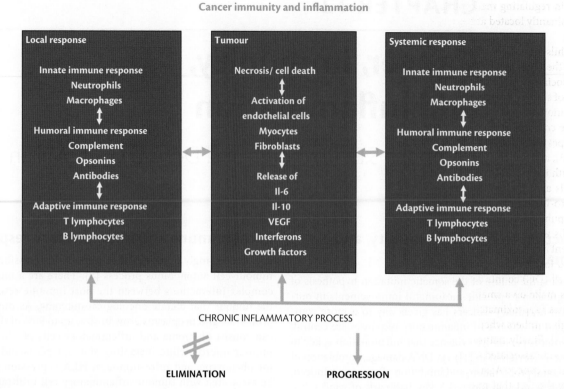

Fig. 12.1 Cancer immunity and inflammation.

significant plasticity of these myeloid and lymphoid-derived cells exerting different pro- and anti-tumour effects as a result of signals from the tumour microenvironment. As a consequence, depending on the tumour, microenvironment (including stroma, immune cell type, and polarization and humoral immune responses) can act to attenuate or to promote tumour growth and spread. In particular, pro-tumour stromal responses are varied but can contribute to the production of factors that create an inflammatory microenvironment resulting in prolonged tumour cell survival, tissue remodelling, angiogenesis, increased proliferation, and increased metastatic potential [15, 16]. This area is currently the subject of intensive investigation.

Local innate immune and inflammatory response

The innate immune response comprises the immediate or front-line response to tissue injury or pathogens. Myeloid cells, including granulocytes, macrophages, mast cells, dendritic cells, and natural killer cells are known to be important in this response. It is generally non-specific and through chemokine and cytokine release acting on stromal cells, including fibroblasts, results in wound healing and tissue repair. In the acute setting, dendritic cells also act as antigen-presenting cells responsible for lymphocyte recruitment generating the adaptive component of the immune response. However, within the tumour microenvironment, host and tumour factors can act chronically to activate the innate response and there is a failure of resolution. The key cell types that are known to be involved include macrophages/monocytes, granulocytes, and mast cells, all of which are involved in tissue repair and can produce growth factors that act directly on

cancer cells or confer mitogenic capabilities (EGF, TGFβ, TNFα, interleukins, and chemokines).

With reference to cancer-associated inflammation, macrophages appear to be an important innate cell type. Higher relative densities of tumour-associated macrophages (TAMs) are associated with poorer prognosis in a variety of common solid tumours and targeting them has recently been associated with improved chemotherapeutic outcomes [17, 18]. There are two main subsets of macrophages; those exposed to pro-inflammatory Type 1 cytokines including IFNγ, IL6, IL12, iNOS, and TNFα are classically activated or M1 polarized and demonstrate anti-tumour activity. In contrast, macrophages exposed to IL4 and prostaglandins are termed alternatively activated or M2-polarized macrophages. These M2 phenotypes appear to make up the majority of TAMs and play a role in angiogenesis and metastasis. For example, M2 TAMs specifically produce chemokines including CCL17 and CCL27 that recruit non-cytotoxic T-cells (Th2 and T regulatory cells T_{regs}). Furthermore, M2 cells can produce CCL18 capable of attracting naïve T-cells. A tumour microenvironment composed of M2 macrophages, T_{regs} and naïve T-cells is likely to create lymphocytic anergy with ineffective anti-tumour responses compounding pro-tumour effects of M2 polarized cells [19].

However, the published literature on the association between tumour macrophage infiltration and cancer outcomes is inconsistent and high TAMs have been reported to be associated with both improved and poorer outcomes [10–20]. These results may reflect heterogeneity of macrophage function, including M1/M2 subtypes, and this has not been specifically examined in the majority of studies. Nevertheless, recent studies including M1 and M2 markers have related high M2 density to improved outcome (e.g., [21]). Therefore, it may be that the tumour microenvironment plays a key role in regulating macrophage function since macrophages are predominantly located at the invasive margin and around areas of necrosis.

Neutrophils have been reported to contribute approximately 15–20% of the inflammatory cell infiltrate in colorectal cancer and are also associated with increasing tumour necrosis (e.g., [13, 22]). A number of studies have reported that increasing tumour neutrophil infiltration was associated with improved survival. However, this may be confounded by the observation that many inflammatory cell types increase together and are associated with improved survival [23], and therefore any association of a particular immune cell type with improved survival is not necessarily causal.

Mast cells are other innate immune cells capable of degranulation of pro-inflammatory mediators. For example, in six out of the seven published studies in colorectal cancer, high numbers of mast cells were associated with improved survival particularly when present at the invasive margin. Similarly, four out of six studies reported lower recurrence and improved survival with higher dendritic cell (DC) counts or densities [11]. In addition, although eosinophils make up a small proportion of tumour inflammatory cell infiltrates (approximately 2%), based on five of six published studies, high numbers when present are associated with improved outcome [11]. Finally, natural killer cells when present in increasing numbers are associated with an improved prognosis in patients with colorectal cancer. Again, the above relationships may be confounded by the fact that many inflammatory cell types increase together [23].

Local humoral immune and inflammatory response

Despite the current intense interest in immune and inflammatory responses in the tumour microenvironment there has been little work to investigate the importance of the components of the humoral immune and inflammatory response in patients with cancer. The humoral response can be considered to include the complement pathways, opsonins, and antibodies, and these are intimately linked to promote tumour cell lysis and phagocytosis. Indeed, there is good evidence from animal models to indicate their importance in determining innate and adaptive immune responses in the tumour microenvironment and the likelihood of tumour progression (e.g., [24–26]). Therefore, there is a considerable and pressing need to translate such findings from animal work into patient investigation of the tumour microenvironment.

Tumour stroma and local immune and inflammatory response

Given the increasing recognition of the tumour microenvironment in determining immune cell and inflammatory responses (see above) there is increasing interest in the role of the stroma in determining tumour growth and spread. De Wever and Mareel [27] proposed that changes in the stroma drive the key hallmarks of cancer, invasion and metastases. In particular, the appearance of myofibroblasts, cells sharing characteristics of smooth muscle cells and fibroblasts, was associated with increased cancer cell invasion. Indeed, they proposed that induction of apoptosis in these cancer-associated myofibroblasts may be a useful therapeutic target since the tumour microenvironment is similar to that of wound

healing, including the presence of myofibroblasts. Furthermore, consistent with the concept that 'tumour is a wound that does not heal', myofibroblasts do not disappear by apoptosis as in wound healing. More recently, this insight has been applied to the prediction of outcome in patients undergoing surgery for colorectal cancer. Higher numbers of stromal myofibroblasts, identified using specific staining, have been reported to be associated with shorter disease-free survival, independent of tumour stage [28]. Similar associations, independent of tumour stage, have been reported using routine H&E slides and calculating the proportion of tumour cells to stroma [29]. However, the relationship between the proportion of stroma and nature of the inflammatory cell infiltrate is not, as yet, clear.

Local adaptive immune and inflammatory response

The adaptive immune cells infiltrating the tumour are largely composed of T and B lymphocytes (TILs). Indeed, the association between a pronounced lymphocytic infiltrate and improved survival within breast and gastrointestinal tumours has been appreciated for more than 30 years [10, 11]. More recently, there has been interest in identifying subsets of TILs within tumours with CD3+, CD8+, CD45RO+, and FOXP3+ and to establish their prognostic value. Polarization of helper T lymphocytes (CD4+) towards a Th1 or Th2 type response appears to be key to determining the relationship between adaptive immune response and the tumour [30]. Generally, an effector cytotoxic T-cell (CD8+) or Th1 CD4+-type response is associated with a good outcome in many common solid tumours, and conversely infiltrates of T-regulatory lymphocytes (FOXP+) and a Th2 CD4+ response are associated with poorer outcome.

Th1-type responses appear to be driven mainly by CD4+T lymphocyte secretion of IFNγ, TNFα, IL2, and IL12. Th1 responses improve immune surveillance by the up-regulation of antigen presentation on MHC I and II molecules of antigen-presenting cells. In addition to recruiting CD8+ cytotoxic T lymphocytes, Th1 CD4+ lymphocytes also have cytotoxic capabilities through release of cytokines and cytolytic granules [30]. The primary effector cell of the Th1 adaptive immune response is the CD8+ cytotoxic T lymphocyte that recognizes antigens after exposure associated with humoral leukocyte antigen (HLA) class I proteins. After exposure to tumour antigen/HLA complexes, CD8+ cells clonally expand and have strong cytotoxic capacity, releasing cytolytic granules (perforin and granzyme B).

In contrast, Th2 CD4+ lymphocytes appear to release mediators including IL4, IL5, and IL10 that act to inhibit cytotoxic T-lymphocyte responses inducing T-lymphocyte anergy or unresponsiveness. The main role of the Th2 (CD4+) polarization appears to be the clonal expansion of B lymphocytes and the consequent production of antibodies. B lymphocytes have a role in mediating and regulating immune responses and also act as antigen-presenting cells to stimulate T-lymphocyte responses. However, their role in cancer is not as well established as that of T lymphocytes. Indeed, there remains ongoing controversy given that they may have pro and anti-T-lymphocyte effects effects in differing tumour microenvironments. For example, in a study examining the constituent cell types of the generalized lymphocytic/inflammatory cell infiltrate in colorectal tumours (Klintrup–Makinen Score), B lymphocytes (assessed as plasma cells on H&E) were found to comprise 10% of all cell types and were significantly related to improved survival [13].

Another adaptive cell type of increasing interest is the T regulatory (CD4+ CD25+ Foxp3+) lymphocytes. T-regulatory lymphocytes are known to suppress the activity of CD8+, natural killer cells, and dendritic cells [31] through mechanisms including increasing immunosuppressive cytokines including IL10 and IFN-γ and direct cytolytic activity [32, 33]. A higher density of tumour T-regulatory-lymphocyte infiltrate has been associated with poorer survival in a variety of common solid tumours. However, for example in colorectal cancer, several studies have described contradictory results with higher density of FOXP3+ associated with improved survival in several studies [11]. The paradoxical role of FOXP3+T-cells in colorectal cancer has been hypothesized to relate to the possibility that T-regulatory lymphocytes also play an anti-microbial role in dampening pro-tumour inflammation due to bacterial translocation across the gut mucosal barrier [34]. Again, these reports may simply reflect that many inflammatory cell types increase together, and the independence of such an association with improved outcome requires further investigation.

A recently described subset of helper T lymphocytes is the Th17 group which is also capable of exerting pro- and anti-tumour activity based on surrounding mediators and site [35]. They exert their effects through secretion of IL17, IL21, and IL22. Pro-tumour effects may include stimulation of angiogenesis and recruitment of myeloid cells.

The concept of suppressor cells that undermine cytotoxic T-lymphocyte responses was developed in the 1980s by Schreiber and co-workers. A group of cells expressing CD11b and Gr-1 are now known as myeloid derived suppressor cells (MDSCs). MDSCs lack markers of mature myeloid cells (e.g., F4/80) and have high potential to suppress immune responses in common with M2 macrophages [36]. The two subsets of MDSCs are polymorphonuclear or monocytic MDSCs. MDSCs can suppress CD8+T lymphocytes through MHC dependent and independent mechanisms inhibiting IFNγ release. MDSCs and M2 macrophages foster an immunosuppressive microenvironment, coordinating recruitment of CD4+/FOXP3+ T_{regs} targeting CD8+ T lymphocyte apoptosis in addition to increasing metastatic potential [37]. In colorectal cancer, few studies have examined the prognostic value of MDSCs; however, increasing intra-tumoral MDSCs have been related to advancing disease stage and as a result have been hypothesized to be associated with disease progression.

Clearly, if such work is to have clinical relevance there is a need to have routine assessment tools that can be simply reported and understood. However, the routine assessment of the tumour inflammatory cell infiltrates and their use to predict outcome in patients with cancer is in its infancy and such tools are in rapid development. A relatively simple but subjective assessment of the tumour cell infiltrate was introduced as part of the Jass classification in the mid-1980s [38]. However, the reproducibility of the assessment was repeatedly questioned and the assessment was not incorporated into routine practice. More recently, an H&E based assessment of peri-tumoral inflammation (Klintrup–Makinen score, 12) has also consistently demonstrated tumour stage-independent prognostic value with lymphocytes as the predominant cell type [10–12]. In addition, over the last decade, many adaptive immune cell markers have been studied using immunohistochemistry. The evidence is strongest for CD3+, CD45RO, and CD8+T lymphocytes. In particular, a high CD8+ density at the invasive margin and within colorectal tumours has been consistently reported to predict improved oncological outcome in over 30 clinical studies [10, 11]. This knowledge has led to the development of several CD8+T lymphocyte-based prognostic scores including the Immune Score described by Galon and Pages based on CD8+and CD45RO+(memory T-cell), recently superseded by the immunoscore based on CD3+ (generic T-cell marker) and CD8+ [39].

It may be that tumour necrosis, as a result of a tumour outgrowing its blood supply, becoming relatively hypoxic and inducing the up-regulation of cellular stress genes in the tumour and the inflammatory cell infiltrate, is important in the induction of immune and inflammatory responses. Indeed, it has been postulated that the combination of inflammation and necrosis provides an environment in which the epigenetic regulation of genes, cell death, cell proliferation, and mutagenesis occurs [3]. At sites of chronic inflammation, cells are continuously dying as a consequence of hypoxic stress, an event in turn promoting growth and proliferation of the local epithelium. The apoptotic to necrotic conversion that is associated with unscheduled cell death and the subsequent release of necrotic mediators is recognized not to be a 'clean' death, but instead stimulates inflammatory pathways [3, 40]. These inflammatory pathways are now recognized to be important for angiogenesis, stromagenesis, and the promotion of epithelial proliferation, all of which are required for tumour growth.

In summary, most innate and adaptive immune cell types have been reported to play a role in tumour immune responses. Taken together the evidence suggests that a strong coordinated cytotoxic T-cell (adaptive) response is associated with improved cancer survival. However, when such a response is absent, other immune cell types, in particular M2 macrophages, MDSCs, Th2 CD4+cells, and FOXP3+T-cells, are associated with poorer cancer survival. As the tumour increases in size and disseminates there is a degradation of lymphocytic anti-tumour responses and development of T-cell suppressor responses (M2 macrophages and MDSCs). Therefore, a pronounced tumour inflammatory cell infiltrate appears to primarily reflect a down-regulation and up-regulation of the innate and adaptive immune systems, respectively, in the tumour microenvironment. In order that the above information is consolidated into the routine assessment of patients with cancer, standardized measurements of the tumour inflammatory cell infiltrate are required.

Systemic immune and inflammatory response

With reference to the systemic inflammatory response, more than 100 studies have reported the prognostic value of the systemic inflammatory response using blood biochemical or haematological markers, such as elevated C-reactive protein concentrations, hypoalbuminaemia or increased white cell, neutrophil, lymphocyte, and platelet counts or their combinations, such as the Glasgow Prognostic Score and the neutrophil:lymphocyte ratio (NLR), in patients with cancer [41–43]. For example, since the initial work a decade ago that the combination of C-reactive protein and albumin, the Glasgow Prognostic Score (GPS), had independent prognostic value in patients with cancer, there have been more than 60 studies (>30,000 patients) that have examined and validated the use of the GPS or the modified GPS (mGPS) in a variety of cancer scenarios [42]. Similarly, over 60 studies (>37,000 patients) to date have examined the clinical utility of the NLR to predict patient outcomes in a variety of cancers [43].

Consistent with this is that there are significant associations between these systemic inflammatory response markers [44]. There is also robust evidence of their prognostic value in other gastrointestinal cancers and lung cancer. It is becoming clear what the optimal thresholds for these systemic inflammatory response markers are and the optimal combination of these markers for the prediction of survival [45]. Due to the simplicity and reliability of these markers, this is an area currently subject to intensive investigation and consolidation. It is, therefore, of interest to consider what these markers of the systemic inflammatory response might reflect in terms of the tumour–host responses.

Systemic innate immune and inflammatory response

The circulating innate immune cells, according to number, include neutrophils, monocytes/macrophages, mast cells, dendritic cells, basophils and eosinophils, and natural killer cells. Increased numbers of these circulating cells are associated with a non-specific response to infection or cell injury.

Accounting for the majority of circulating white cells, elevated numbers of circulating neutrophils are associated with increasing tumour stage and poorer survival in a variety of common solid tumours including colorectal cancer (e.g., [44, 45]). Furthermore, the role of neutrophils in effectively stratifying patient response to treatment is becoming clearer [46]. For example, circulating neutrophils above the upper limit of normal were independently associated with poorer outcome in patients with metastatic colorectal cancer treated with FOLFIRI or XELOX plus anti-VEGF. Further, in similar patients receiving palliative chemotherapy, a neutrophil/lymphocyte ratio >5 was independently associated with poorer survival [43]. Therefore, an elevated pretreatment neutrophil count appears to be a strong independent predictor of poor outcome in patients with cancer [46, 45]. Moreover, it would appear that neutrophils, similar to other inflammatory cells, are capable of polarization of N1 and N2 phenotypes, a matter that is currently the subject of investigation [46].

In addition, although they are less numerous, elevated numbers of circulating monocytes have been reported to be associated with increasing tumour stage and poorer survival in colorectal cancer [44]. Unlike tumour cell infiltration, little work has been carried out to examine the relationship between the phenotype of such circulating monocytes and cancer outcome. However, it is clear from work in other disease states that monocytes leave the bloodstream and migrate into tissues where, following conditioning by the local inflammatory milieu, they differentiate into macrophage or dendritic cell populations. Although passage of monocytes is essential for effective control of infections, such monocytes also contribute to the pathogenesis of inflammatory disease states [47] and possibly cancer.

Few studies have examined the associations between circulating mast cells, dendritic cells, basophils and eosinophils, and natural killer cells and survival. The acute phase proteins, including the prototypical C-reactive protein, rise during a period of infection, tissue injury, or necrosis. In response to such stimulus, circulating

C-reactive protein concentrations may rise up to 50,000-fold. The increase in circulating concentrations is principally due to factors released by macrophages such as IL6. As its half-life is constantly circulating, concentrations of C-reactive protein are mainly determined by the rate of production in the liver. C-reactive protein is considered to be part of the innate immune response since it is thought to assist in complement binding to foreign and damaged cells and enhances phagocytosis by macrophages (opsonin-mediated phagocytosis). Indeed, there is evidence that neutrophils and macrophages have Fcγ receptors that can be activated by C-reactive protein. In addition, some tumours types stain for C-reactive protein [48]. Furthermore, Yang and co-workers [49] reported that, in myeloma cells, C-reactive protein can activate membrane-bound Fcγ receptors and in turn activate PI3K/Akt, ERK, and NF-kB pathways and inhibit caspase cascade activation resulting in increased tumour cell proliferation and inhibition of apoptosis. It is also of interest that circulating C-reactive protein concentrations were directly associated with tumour size and necrosis [50]. Therefore, it may be that C-reactive protein plays both an indirect and a direct role in tumour progression that ultimately leads to its strong association with poorer cancer-specific survival in patients with cancer.

Systemic humoral immune and inflammatory response

It is of interest that circulating concentrations of a number of the molecules that are associated with the activation of the components of the humoral immune and inflammatory response in patients with cancer have been reported to have prognostic value independent of tumour-based factors. These include the pattern-recognition molecules, complement C3a (e.g., [51, 52]), C-reactive protein (see above), mannose-binding lectin and complexes MASP-2 [53, 54], and antibodies [55–57].

Given that the function of the humoral immune and inflammatory mediators is to connect local and systemic response, these are ideally suited to sense tumour immune surveillance. It is therefore surprising that these molecules have not been subject to more investigation and exploited as prognostic and therapeutic markers. Again, there is a considerable and pressing need to extend and consolidate such findings into routine investigation of patients with cancer.

Mediators linking local and systemic immune and inflammatory responses

There are a number of plausible mediators linking local and systemic inflammatory responses. For example, Kantola and colleagues [58] have reported the pattern of alterations of 13 serum cytokine concentrations between >80 normal controls and patients newly diagnosed with colorectal cancer. Compared with controls, the presence of colorectal cancer was associated with a significant increase in IL6, IL7, IL8, IL12, IFN-gamma, MCP-1, and PDGF-BB. Sex, tumour site, and N stage had little association with the serum cytokine alterations reported. Furthermore, increasing T stage was only associated with a significant increase in IL6, IL8, and MCP-1; increasing grade was only associated with a significant increase in IL6 and IL8; while the presence of metastasis was associated with a significant increase in IL4, IL6, IL7, IL8, MCP-1, and PDGF-BB. In contrast, the presence of a systemic inflammatory response, as evidenced by the modified Glasgow Prognostic Score (mGPS), was significantly associated with IL-1ra, IL6, IL7, IL8, IL9, IL12, IFN-gamma, IP-10, MCP-1, MIP-1B, and PDGF-BB. Taken together, these results would suggest that circulating IL6 and IL8 concentrations may link the tumour with the systemic inflammatory response. With reference to the inflammatory cell type, few inflammatory cells, with the exception of monocytes/macrophages, can produce such a spectrum of cytokines and growth factors, in particular IL6. These findings are consistent with the hypothesis that tumour necrosis (which increases with T stage) plays an important in both linking local and systemic inflammatory responses in patients with colorectal cancer [50].

It has long been recognized that tumour-associated macrophages localize to hypoxic regions of the tumour microenvironment. Therefore, it is plausible that the relative density of macrophages (perhaps M2) determined by the tumour microenvironments is important in the local and systemic production of IL6 and the nature of local and systemic immune and inflammatory responses [59]. Alternatively, recent work has suggested that an accumulation of myeloid-derived suppressor cells in the tumour microenvironment may be important in these observations.

Systemic adaptive immune and inflammatory response

The circulating adaptive immune cells, according to number, primarily include T and B lymphocytes. Increased numbers of T lymphocytes, in particular CD4+ and CD8+ subpopulations, are associated with a specific response to an antigen. Therefore, it is somewhat surprising that little in vivo work has been carried out to examine the relationship between circulating T lymphocyte subsets and outcome in patients with cancer, particularly since blood measurements are more readily available to assess and to monitor patient response to treatment.

Small studies have shown that in addition to increased circulating neutrophil counts there is a significant reduction in the percentage of CD3 T lymphocytes and in the numbers of CD4+ T lymphocytes but no difference in CD8 T lymphocytes in those patients who have colorectal cancer compared with controls and subsequently develop recurrence following curative surgery [60, 61]. More recently, small studies examining peripheral blood regulatory T lymphocytes (CD4+CD25+Foxp3+) in patients with colorectal cancer have reported that increased numbers of these immunosuppressive cells [62] are associated with increasing tumour stage and inflammatory cell infiltration, and are not normalized on resection of the tumour [63]. Therefore, an alteration of circulating T-lymphocyte subpopulations appears to be a feature of common solid tumours and is consistent with impaired immune function at the systemic level. However, further work is clearly required in this area.

In summary, work on routinely available markers of the systemic inflammatory response is now being consolidated in the form of systemic-inflammation-based prognostic scores such as the GPS and the NLR, primarily reflecting activation of the innate immune and inflammatory response. However, to date little work has been carried out to characterize the phenotype of circulating innate and adaptive immune cells. Nevertheless, the systemic inflammatory response appears primarily to reflect an up-regulation and down-regulation of the circulating innate and adaptive immune processes, respectively.

Therapeutic intervention in immune and inflammatory responses

There is great interest in potential strategies to manipulate immune and inflammatory responses in cancer for therapeutic gain. Generally speaking, this will involve restoration of a targeted anti-tumour-cell mediated immune response. Potential strategies that may improve oncological outcome include targeting both local and systemic innate and adaptive immune responses: for example, at a local level, repolarization of tumour-associated neutrophils and macrophages towards N1 and M1 phenotypes, respectively, and inhibition of myeloid-derived suppressor cell activity, as well as repolarization towards Th1 anti-tumour cytotoxic T-cell responses and suppressing T-regulatory cell activity. Other promising future strategies may include specific immune cell depletion or inactivation, and, at a systemic level, maintaining cell-mediated adaptive immune responses and suppressing development of non-specific innate cellular responses such that the host systemic inflammatory response and its associated detrimental effects on body composition and quality of life and survival are abrogated. Such therapeutic goals may be achieved using non-selective anti-inflammatory agents or using highly selective agents subtly to attenuate targeted mediators or pathways of the immune and inflammatory responses to cancer.

Non-selective agents

Aspirin and non-steroidal anti-inflammatory drugs including cyclooxygenase-2 inhibitors have been described as potential chemotherapeutic agents, most commonly in colorectal cancer. There is consistent evidence of a chemo-preventative reduction in colorectal cancer incidence and mortality, based on epidemiological studies [64].

With reference to advanced cancer, NSAIDs have been shown to attenuate the systemic inflammatory response and moderate cachexia [65]. In contrast, it is only relatively recently that a potential benefit in patients with early-stage colorectal cancer has been realized, with NSAID users less likely to present with recurrence. Indeed, emerging evidence of as much as a 40% reduction in recurrence and mortality in patients undergoing curative surgery for colorectal cancer makes the concept of the use of NSAIDs as adjuvant treatment in high-risk disease more compelling [66, 67]. Several prospective randomized trials are under way to determine the role of aspirin/NSAIDs as adjuvant therapy in colorectal cancer [67].

Several mechanistic pathways, including a myriad of COX-dependent and independent pathways, have been implicated in the direct and indirect effects of aspirin/NSAIDSs on tumour cells, the tumour microenvironment, and innate and adaptive immune responses: for example, the inhibition of several signal transduction pathways including Wnt/β-catenin and nuclear factor-kappa B (NF-κB). Recently, in the context of randomized trial data, patients with mutated *PIK3* in their tumours where shown to have increased survival compared with the non-mutated form [68], and a reduced risk of cancer with NSAIDs in patients with mutations within the NF-κB pathway [69]. In addition, there is good evidence of their effect on platelet function and some evidence that NSAIDs may play a role in enhancing cytotoxic T-cell activity preventing cancer-associated immune suppression [70].

Nevertheless, for those patients likely to benefit from NSAIDs there is a clear need to identify treatment markers of immune and inflammatory response.

The 3-hydroxy-3-methylglutaryl coenzyme A (HMG-CoA) reductase inhibitors, commonly known as statins, are primarily used in the treatment of hypercholesterolaemia and atherosclerotic cardiovascular disease. However, they are known to have a number of pleiotropic effects on cell proliferation, angiogenesis, inflammation, and endothelial cell function. A number of epidemiological studies have reported a reduction in risk of colorectal cancer with statin use[71]. In particular, there is evidence from clinical trials of a 90% reduction in risk of inflammatory bowel-disease-related colorectal cancer [72].

Statins have a variety of actions that may potentially alter immune and inflammatory responses in cancer. For example, in cardiovascular disease prevention trials there are clearly identified anti-inflammatory effects, with down-regulation of pro-inflammatory cytokines and increased cardiovascular risk reduction in patients with elevated serum inflammatory markers [73]. Furthermore, favourable effects on organ rejection following heart and renal transplant suggest a potent immunomodulatory effect, potentially through a direct effect on MHC class II expression and subsequent T-cell activation [74].

Selective agents

With the increasing knowledge of the immune and inflammatory dysfunction in patients with cancer, specific and selective immunomodulatory agents are having an emerging role in oncological practice. In general, these include targeted agents aiming at specific manipulation of cytokines/chemokines or blocking cellular responses to encourage a rebalancing of immune and inflammatory responses. Novel methods of achieving this goal include the development of cancer vaccines and adoptive cell transfer.

The lead for such work has come from the newer treatments of chronic inflammatory diseases in non-cancer conditions. There have been therapeutic successes in targeting pro-inflammatory cytokines such as IL6 and TNF-α. To date, anti-IL6 immunotherapies (siltuximab) have been employed in phase II trials for ovarian and renal cancer with some promising results including stabilization of disease and attenuation of systemic inflammatory responses.

Further, monoclonal antibodies with specific effects on host–tumour immunity encouraging cytotoxicity include ipilimumab (anti-CTL-4), an immunostimulatory antibody that has been shown to enhance anti-tumour immunity and also counter the immunosuppressive inflammatory response created by the tumour in melanoma. The trial of ipilimumab in melanoma patients published in 2010 was the first ever positive randomized phase III drug trial in melanoma. Other monoclonal antibodies which encourage antibody-dependent cellular cytotoxicity include rituximab, a CD20 antibody which has been used in lymphoma leading to B-cell depletion, and catumaxomab, an anti-CD3 EpCAM chimeric antibody which has been used in the treatment of malignant ascites.

A recent promising strategy is to manipulate adaptive T-cell function. Programmed cell death 1 (PD-1) protein is a T-cell receptor mediating T-cell inhibition and along with its ligands (PD-L1 and PD-L2) plays an important role in regulating T-cell responses. Blocking interactions between PD-1 and PD-L1 with anti-PD-L1 antibody has been shown in phase I studies of breast, ovarian, melanoma, lung, and colorectal cancer patients to improve anti-tumour T-cell activity with encouraging clinical results [75].

Finally, there has been recent interest in the use of autologous dendritic cell pulsed with tumour peptides and injected as a vaccine directly into tumour tissue. This technique has been observed in early human studies to provoke potential anti-tumour adaptive immune responses with increased CD4+ and CD8+ T-cells [76]. Sipuleucel-T is a novel dendritic-cell-based vaccine that has been employed successfully in castration-resistant metastatic prostate cancer. Autologous peripheral blood mononuclear cells and antigen-presenting cells are extracted from the patient, activated ex vivo with a recombinant fusion protein (PA2024) which consists of prostatic acid phosphatase, a common prostatic cancer antigen linked to granulocyte-macrophage colony-stimulating factor (GM-SF). This cancer vaccine is then delivered back into the patient resulting in stimulation of host CD4+ and CD8+T-cell responses targeting prostate cancer cells. To date, three phase III trials have reported positive improvements in survival with infusions of Sipuleucel-T [77].

In summary, along with the now widespread appreciation of the pivotal role of the immune/inflammatory responses in dictating human cancer outcome, there has been a recent rapid expansion of therapies aimed at manipulation of these responses. Broad-spectrum anti-inflammatory drugs have long been appreciated as playing a role in oncological progression; however, stratification using more accurate immune/inflammatory or molecular profiling may help to identify those patients who may derive greatest therapeutic benefit. Recently, there have been impressive results observed in melanoma and renal cell cancer. It remains to be determined whether the use of such immunotherapies will apply to most tumour types.

Conclusion

It is clear that immune and inflammatory responses, both local and systemic, are intimately linked and impact on cancer survival. However, the mechanisms by which these inflammatory responses are activated, maintained, and interact are not clear. An interesting concept is that a cell-signalling mediator such as IL6 or pattern recognition molecules may have a key role. It also may be, at least in non-hereditary disease, that inflammation becomes the key hallmark on which all the other hallmarks of cancer are dependent. Therapeutic intervention using non-selective anti-inflammatory agents is widely advocated and likely to become part of routine clinical practice in the near future. Selective therapeutic intervention directed at the immune and inflammatory responses in cancer is in its infancy.

Further reading

Bonovas S, Filioussi K, Flordellis CS, Sitaras NM. Statins and the risk of colorectal cancer: a meta-analysis of 18 studies involving more than 1.5 million patients. Journal of Clinical Oncology 2007; 25: 3462–3468.

Coussens LM, Zitvogel L, Palucka AK. Neutralizing tumor-promoting chronic inflammation: a magic bullet? Science 2013; 339(6117): 286–291.

De Wever O, Mareel M. Role of tissue stroma in cancer cell invasion. Journal of Pathology 2003; 200: 429–447.

Galon J, Pagès F, Marincola FM, Angell HK, Thurin M et al. Cancer classification using the Immunoscore: a worldwide task force. Journal of Translational Medicine 2012; 10: 205.

Germano G, Mantovani A, Allavena P. Targeting of the innate immunity/inflammation as complementary anti-tumor therapies. Annals of Medicine 2011; 43: 581–593.

Liao X, Lochhead P, Nishihara R, Morikawa T, Kuchiba A et al. Aspirin use, tumor PIK3CA mutation, and colorectal-cancer survival. New England Journal of Medicine 2012; 367(17): 1596–1606.

Qian BZ, Pollard JW. Macrophage diversity enhances tumor progression and metastasis. Cell 2010; 141(1): 39–51.

Roxburgh CS, McMillan DC. Role of systemic inflammatory response in predicting survival in patients with primary operable cancer. Future Oncology 2010; 6(1): 149–163.

Roxburgh CS, McMillan DC. The role of the in situ local inflammatory response in predicting recurrence and survival in patients with primary operable colorectal cancer. Cancer Treatment Review 2012; 38: 451–466.

Vakkila J, Lotze MT. Inflammation and necrosis promote tumour growth. Nature Reviews Immunology 2004; 4(8): 641–648.

References

1. Grivennikov SI, Greten FR, Karin M. Immunity, inflammation, and cancer. Cell 2010; 140(6): 883–899.

2. Hanahan D, Weinberg RA. Hallmarks of cancer: the next generation. Cell 2011; 144: 646–674.

3. Vakkila J, Lotze MT. Inflammation and necrosis promote tumour growth. Nature Reviews Immunology 2004; 4(8): 641–648.

4. Dvorak HF. Tumors: wounds that do not heal. Similarities between tumor stroma generation and wound healing. New England Journal of Medicine 1986; 315(26): 1650–1659.

5. McArdle CS, McMillan DC, Hole DJ. Impact of anastomotic leakage on long-term survival of patients undergoing curative resection for colorectal cancer. British Journal of Surgery 2005; 92: 1150–1154.

6. Lagarde SM, de Boer JD, ten Kate FJ, Busch OR, Obertop H et al. Postoperative complications after esophagectomy for adenocarcinoma of the esophagus are related to timing of death due to recurrence. Annals of Surgery 2008; 247: 71–76.

7. Mirnezami A, Mirnezami R, Chandrakumaran K, Sasapu K, Sagar P et al. Increased local recurrence and reduced survival from colorectal cancer following anastomotic leak: systematic review and meta-analysis. Annals of Surgery 2011; 253: 890–899.

8. Ogino S, Galon J, Fuchs CS, Dranoff G. Cancer immunology: analysis of host and tumor factors for personalized medicine. Nature Reviews Clinical Oncology 2011; 8: 711–719.

9. Mesker WE, Junggeburt JM, Szuhai K, de Heer P, Morreau H et al. The carcinoma-stromal ratio of colon carcinoma is an independent factor for survival compared to lymph node status and tumor stage. Cell Oncology 2007; 29: 387–398.

10. Mohammed ZM, Going JJ, Edwards J, McMillan DC. The role of the tumour inflammatory cell infiltrate in predicting recurrence and survival in patients with primary operable breast cancer. Cancer Treatment Review 2012; 38: 943–955.

11. Roxburgh CS, McMillan DC. The role of the in situ local inflammatory response in predicting recurrence and survival in patients with primary operable colorectal cancer. Cancer Treatment Review 2012; 38: 451–466.

12. Klintrup K, Mäkinen JM, Kauppila S, Väre PO, Melkko J et al. Inflammation and prognosis in colorectal cancer. European Journal of Cancer 2005; 41: 2645–2654.

13. Richards CH, Flegg KM, Roxburgh CS, Going JJ, Mohammed Z. The relationships between cellular components of the peritumoural inflammatory response, clinicopathological characteristics and survival in patients with primary operable colorectal cancer. British Journal of Cancer 2012; 106: 2010–2015.

14. Mohammed ZM, Going JJ, Edwards J, Elsberger B, Doughty JC. The relationship between components of tumour inflammatory cell infiltrate and clinicopathological factors and survival in patients with primary operable invasive ductal breast cancer. British Journal of Cancer 2012; 107: 864–873.

15. Mantovani A, Romero P, Palucka AK, Marincola FM. Tumour immunity: effector response to tumour and role of the microenvironment. Lancet 2008; 371(9614): 771–783.

16. DeNardo DG, Johansson M, Coussens LM. Immune cells as mediators of solid tumor metastasis. Cancer Metastasis Review 2008; 27: 11–18.

17. Germano G, Mantovani A, Allavena P. Targeting of the innate immunity/inflammation as complementary anti-tumor therapies. Annals of Medicine 2011; 43: 581–593.

18. Mitchem JB, Brennan DJ, Knolhoff BL, Belt BA, Zhu Y et al. Targeting tumor-infiltrating macrophages decreases tumor-initiating cells, relieves immunosuppression, and improves chemotherapeutic responses. Cancer Research 2013; 73: 1128–1141.

19. Qian BZ, Pollard JW. Macrophage diversity enhances tumor progression and metastasis. Cell 2010; 141(1): 39–51.

20. Zhang QW, Liu L, Gong CY, Shi HS, Zeng YH. Prognostic significance of tumor-associated macrophages in solid tumor: a meta-analysis of the literature. PLoS One 2012; 7(12):e50946.

21. Edin S, Wikberg ML, Dahlin AM, Rutegård J, Öberg Å et al. The distribution of macrophages with a M1 or M2 phenotype in relation to prognosis and the molecular characteristics of colorectal cancer. PLoS One 2012; 7(10):e47045.

22. Salama P, Platell C. Host response to colorectal cancer. ANZ Journal of Surgery 2008; 78(9): 745–753.

23. Nielsen HJ, Hansen U, Christensen IJ, Reimert CM, Brünner N et al. Independent prognostic value of eosinophil and mast cell infiltration in colorectal cancer tissue. Journal of Pathology 1999; 189(4): 487–495.

24. Rozanov DV, Savinov AY, Golubkov VS, Postnova TI, Remacle A et al. Cellular membrane type-1 matrix metalloproteinase (MT1-MMP) cleaves C3b, an essential component of the complement system. Journal of Biological Chemistry 2004; 279(45): 46551–46557.

25. Imai M, Ohta R, Varela JC, Song H, Tomlinson S. Enhancement of antibody-dependent mechanisms of tumor cell lysis by a targeted activator of complement. Cancer Research 2007; 67(19): 9535–9541.

26. Varela JC, Imai M, Atkinson C, Ohta R, Rapisardo M et al. Modulation of protective T cell immunity by complement inhibitor expression on tumor cells. Cancer Research 2008; 68(16): 6734–6742.

27. De Wever O, Mareel M. Role of tissue stroma in cancer cell invasion. Journal of Pathology 2003; 200: 429–447.

28. Tsujino T, Seshimo I, Yamamoto H, Ngan CY, Ezumi K et al. Stromal myofibroblasts predict disease recurrence for colorectal cancer. Clin Cancer Research 2007; 13: 2082–2090.

29. Huijbers A, Tollenaar RA, v Pelt GW, Zeestraten EC, Dutton S et al. The proportion of tumor-stroma as a strong prognosticator for stage II and III colon cancer patients: validation in the VICTOR trial. Annals of Oncology 2013; 24: 179–185.

30. DeNardo DG, Andreu P, Coussens LM. Interactions between lymphocytes and myeloid cells regulate pro- versus anti-tumor immunity. Cancer Metastasis Review 2010; 29(2): 309–316.

31. Strauss L, Bergmann C, Whiteside TL. Functional and phenotypic-characteristics of CD4+CD25highFoxp3+ Treg clones obtained from peripheral blood of patients with cancer. International Journal of Cancer 2007; 121: 2473–2483.

32. Feuerer M, Hill JA, Mathis D, Benoist C. Foxp3+ regulatory T cells: differentiation, specification, subphenotypes. Nature Immunology 2009; 10: 689–695.

33. Cao X, Cai SF, Fehniger TA, Song J, Collins LI, et al. Granzyme B and perforin are important for regulatory T cell-mediated suppression of tumor clearance. Immunity 2007; 27: 635–646.

34. Ladoire S, Martin F, Ghiringhelli F. Prognostic role of FOXP3+ regulatory T cells infiltrating human carcinomas: the paradox of colorectal cancer. Cancer Immunology, Immunotherapy 2011; 60(7): 909–918

35. Coussens LM, Zitvogel L, Palucka AK. Neutralizing tumor-promoting chronic inflammation: a magic bullet? Science 2013; 339(6117): 286–291.

36. Gabrilovich DI, Nagaraj S. Myeloid-derived suppressor cells as regulators of the immune system. Nature Reviews Immunology 2009; 9(3): 162–174.

37. Mantovani A, Sica A. Macrophages, innate immunity and cancer: balance, tolerance, and diversity. Current Opinion in Immunology 2010; 22(2): 231–237.

38. Jass JR, Love SB, Northover JM. A new prognostic classification of rectal cancer. Lancet 1987; 1(8545): 1303–1306.

40. Harris AL. Hypoxia: a key regulatory factor in tumour growth. Nature Reviews Cancer 2002; 2(1): 38–47.

39. Galon J, Pagès F, Marincola FM, Angell HK, Thurin M et al. Cancer classification using the Immunoscore: a worldwide task force. Journal of Translational Medicine 2012; 10: 205.

41. Roxburgh CS, McMillan DC. Role of systemic inflammatory response in predicting survival in patients with primary operable cancer. Future Oncology 2010; 6(1): 149–163.

42. McMillan DC. The systemic inflammation-based Glasgow Prognostic Score: A decade of experience in patients with cancer. Cancer Treatment Review 2013; 39(5): 534–540.

43. Guthrie, GJK, Charles KA, Roxburgh CSD, Horgan PG, McMillan DC et al. The systemic inflammation-based neutrophil–lymphocyte ratio: experience in patients with cancer. Critical Reviews in Oncology/Haematology 2013; 88(1): 219–230.

44. Leitch EF, Chakrabarti M, Crozier JE, McKee RF, Anderson JH et al. Comparison of the prognostic value of selected markers of the systemic inflammatory response in patients with colorectal cancer. British Journal of Cancer 2007; 97(9): 1266–1270.

45. Proctor MJ, Horgan PG, Talwar D, Fletcher CD, Morrison DS et al. Optimization of the systemic inflammation-based Glasgow Prognostic Score: A Glasgow Inflammation Outcome Study. Cancer 2013; 119(12): 2325–2332.

46. Donskov F. Immunomonitoring and prognostic relevance of neutrophils in clinical trials. Seminars in Cancer Biology 2013; 23(3): 200–207.

47. Shi C, Pamer EG. Monocyte recruitment during infection and inflammation. Nature Reviews Immunology 2011; 11(11): 762–774.

48. McCall P, Catlow J, McArdle PA, McMillan DC, Edwards J. Tumoral C-reactive protein and nuclear factor kappa-B expression are associated with clinical outcome in patients with prostate cancer. Cancer Biomarkers 2011–2012; 10(2): 91–99.

49. Yang J, Wezeman M, Zhang X, Lin P, Wang M et al. Human C-reactive protein binds activating Fcgamma receptors and protects myeloma tumor cells from apoptosis. Cancer Cell 2007; 12(3): 252–265.

50. Richards CH, Roxburgh CS, Anderson JH, McKee RF, Foulis AK et al. Prognostic value of tumour necrosis and host inflammatory responses in colorectal cancer. British Journal of Surgery 2012; 99: 287–294.

51. Habermann JK, Roblick UJ, Luke BT, Prieto DA, Finlay WJ et al. Increased serum levels of complement C3a anaphylatoxin indicate the presence of colorectal tumors. Gastroenterology 2006; 131(4): 1020–1029

52. Solassol J, Rouanet P, Lamy PJ, Allal C, Favre G et al. Serum protein signature may improve detection of ductal carcinoma in situ of the breast. Oncogene 2010; 29(4): 550–560.

53. Ytting H, Christensen IJ, Jensenius JC, Thiel S, Nielsen HJ. Preoperative mannan-binding lectin pathway and prognosis in colorectal cancer. Cancer Immunology, Immunotherapy 2005; 54(3): 265–272.

54. Ytting H, Christensen IJ, Thiel S, Jensenius JC, Nielsen HJ. Serum mannan-binding lectin-associated serine protease 2 levels in colorectal cancer: relation to recurrence and mortality. Clinical Cancer Research 2005; 11(4): 1441–1446.

55. Tan EM, Zhang J. Autoantibodies to tumor-associated antigens: reporters from the immune system. Immunology Review 2008; 222: 328–340.

56. Ramoner R, Rahm A, Falkensammer CE, Leonhartsberger N, Thurnher M. Serum IgG against Candida predict survival in patients with metastatic renal cell carcinoma. Cancer Immunology, Immunotherapy 2010; 59(8): 1141–1147.

57. Heegaard NH, West-Nørager M, Tanassi JT, Houen G, Nedergaard L et al. Circulating antinuclear antibodies in patients with pelvic masses are associated with malignancy and decreased survival. PLoS One 2012; 7(2):e30997.

58. Kantola T, Klintrup K, Väyrynen JP, Vornanen J, Bloigu R et al. Stage-dependent alterations of the serum cytokine pattern in colorectal carcinoma. British Journal of Cancer 2012; 107: 1729–1736.

59. Guthrie GJ, Roxburgh CS, Horgan PG, McMillan DC. Does interleukin-6 link explain the link between tumour necrosis, local and systemic inflammatory responses and outcome in patients with colorectal cancer? Cancer Treatment Review 2013; 39: 89–96.

60. McMillan DC, Fyffe GD, Wotherspoon HA, Cooke TG, McArdle CS. Prospective study of circulating T-lymphocyte subpopulations and disease progression in colorectal cancer. Diseases of the Colon & Rectum 1997; 40: 1068–1071.

61. Attallah AM, Tabll AA, El-Sadany M, Ibrahim TA, El-Dosoky I. Dysregulation of blood lymphocyte subsets and natural killer cells in schistosomal liver cirrhosis and hepatocellular carcinoma. Clinical and Experimental Medicine 2003; 3: 181–185.

62. Campbell DJ, Koch MA. Phenotypical and functional specialization of FOXP3+ regulatory T cells. Nature Reviews Immunology 2011; 11: 119–130.

63. Ling KL, Pratap SE, Bates GJ, Singh B, Mortensen NJ et al. Increased frequency of regulatory T cells in peripheral blood and tumour infiltrating lymphocytes in colorectal cancer patients. Cancer Immunity 2007; 7: 7.

64. Chan AT, Detering E. An emerging role for anti-inflammatory agents for chemoprevention. Recent Results Cancer Research 2013; 191: 1–5.

65. Solheim TS, Fearon KC, Blum D, Kaasa S. Non-steroidal anti-inflammatory treatment in cancer cachexia: a systematic literature review. Acta Oncologica 2013; 52(1): 6–17.

66. Rothwell PM, Wilson M, Price JF, Belch JF, Meade TW et al. Effect of daily aspirin on risk of cancer metastasis: a study of incident cancers during randomised controlled trials. Lancet 2012; 379(9826): 1591–1601.

67. Chia WK, Ali R, Toh HC. Aspirin as adjuvant therapy for colorectal cancer--reinterpreting paradigms. Nature Reviews Clinical Oncology 2012 Oct; 9(10): 561–570.

68. Liao X, Lochhead P, Nishihara R, Morikawa T, Kuchiba A et al. Aspirin use, tumor PIK3CA mutation, and colorectal-cancer survival. New England Journal of Medicine 2012; 367(17): 1596–1606.

69. Seufert BL, Poole EM, Whitton J, Xiao L, Makar KW et al. IκBKβ and NFκB1, NSAID use and risk of colorectal cancer in the Colon Cancer Family Registry. Carcinogenesis 2013; 34: 79–85.

70. Lönnroth C, Andersson M, Arvidsson A, Nordgren S, Brevinge H et al. Preoperative treatment with a non-steroidal anti-inflammatory drug (NSAID) increases tumor tissue infiltration of seemingly activated immune cells in colorectal cancer. Cancer Immunity 2008; 8: 5.

71. Bonovas S, Filioussi K, Flordellis CS, Sitaras NM. Statins and the risk of colorectal cancer: a meta-analysis of 18 studies involving more than 1.5 million patients. Journal of Clinical Oncology 2007; 25: 3462–3468.

72. Samadder NJ, Mukherjee B, Huang SC, Ahn J, Rennert HS et al. Risk of colorectal cancer in self-reported inflammatory bowel disease and modification of risk by statin and NSAID use. Cancer 2011; 117(8): 1640–1648.

73. Jain MK, Ridker PM. Anti-inflammatory effects of statins: clinical evidence and basic mechanisms. Nature Reviews Drug Discovery 2005; 4(12): 977–987.

74. Kwak B, Mulhaupt F, Myit S, Mach F. Statins as a newly recognized type of immunomodulator. Nature Medicine 2000; 6(12): 1399–1402.

75. Brahmer JR, Tykodi SS, Chow LQ, Hwu WJ, Topalian SL et al. Safety and activity of anti-PD-L1 antibody in patients with advanced cancer. New England Journal of Medicine 2012; 366(26): 2455–2465.

76. Aarntzen EH, De Vries IJ, Lesterhuis WJ, Schuurhuis D, Jacobs JF et al. Targeting CD4(+) T-helper cells improves the induction of antitumor responses in dendritic cell-based vaccination. Cancer Research 2013; 73: 19–29.

77. Karan D, Holzbeierlein JM, Van Veldhuizen P, Thrasher JB. Cancer immunotherapy: a paradigm shift for prostate cancer treatment. Nature Reviews Urology 2012; 9(7): 376–385.

CHAPTER 13

Cancer and metabolism

Cameron Snell, Kevin C. Gatter,
Adrian L. Harris, and Francesco Pezzella

Introduction to cancer and metabolism

It was recognized in the mid-twentieth century that tumour cells exhibited characteristic changes in metabolism, in particular the use of glucose for glycolysis rather than for oxidative phosphorylation in the presence of adequate oxygen. This metabolic switch, named after Otto Warburg, who first made this observation (the Warburg effect) [1] was originally hypothesized to be causative in the development of cancer. Tumour development is now known to be driven by the activation of cancer oncogenes and loss of tumour suppressors. However, we now recognize that mutations in some metabolic enzymes can indeed cause cancer and intermediate products of metabolism may be able to promote tumour progression.

Proliferating cancer cells have a high energy requirement, to maintain homoeostatic cellular processes in the setting of a neoplastic microenvironment. The shift in energy production to aerobic glycolysis, whilst being much more rapid, yields far less energy than oxidative phosphorylation (2 net molecules of ATP per glucose molecule for glycolysis compared to 36 for aerobic glycolysis) [2]. An increased demand for glucose by tumour cells is potentiated by hypoxia and Akt signalling, and is the basis for positron emission tomography (PET) positivity by increased uptake of the glucose analogue 2-fluorodeoxy-D-glucose (^{18}F-FDG).

There is some debate about the selective advantage that glycolysis affords tumour cells. Initially, it was thought that mitochondria were intrinsically defective in tumours, although more recently it has been recognized that mitochondria retain the capacity for oxidative phosphorylation and consume oxygen at similar rates to normal tissues [3]. The increased rate of energy production possible with aerobic glycolysis has also been proposed as a selection advantage. Alternatively, high rates of glycolysis may be co-selected with factors that promote the increased expression of hypoxia-related genes (such as those required for angiogenesis) as an oxygen-independent energy source. Finally, increased intermediate products of glycolysis can be shunted into biosynthetic pathways required for serine and nucleotide synthesis and lipid synthesis [4] (Figure 13.1).

A more complex picture of metabolic transformation in tumours, beyond the switch to aerobic glycolysis, has emerged over the last decade and is increasingly linked to specific disturbances in cell-signalling pathways [5]. Additionally, tumours with the same genetic perturbations develop different metabolic adaptations depending on the host-tissue in which they arise, suggesting the stromal environment plays a role in shaping the metabolic profile [6]. The increased growth and metabolic requirements of tumours also require a corresponding increase in the production of NADPH as a reducing agent in anabolic reactions and to maintain cellular redox balance.

Supporting tumour growth: from angiogenesis to metabolic reprogramming

Warburg raised two important questions regarding how tumour cells are supplied by glucose and by oxygen [1]. Folkman's work addressed the latter issue and answered the question of how cancer cells are supplied by oxygen by raising the hypothesis that 'tumour growth is angiogenesis-dependent' [7]. Subsequent work led to the recognition of angiogenesis as one of the hallmarks of cancer [8].

Lack of angiogenesis and metabolic reprogramming

Although robust evidence has been reached that angiogenesis is crucial in cancer, this is not always the case, and some tumours can grow in the absence of angiogenesis by co-opting pre-existing vessels [9].

Non-angiogenic growth was first identified histologically in lung cancer as neoplastic cells fill the alveolar spaces co-opting the pre-existing capillary network and producing a characteristic 'chicken-wire' appearance [9]. A gene expression signature for non-angiogenic non-small cell lung cancer (NSCLC) was published in 2005, derived by comparing the expression of mRNA transcripts by microarray in 12 non-angiogenic and 30 angiogenic tumours [10]. Sixty-two genes were found to separate the two types of tumour, 40 of which were more highly expressed in non-angiogenic tumours. Surprisingly, rather than classic angiogenesis-related genes, the differentially expressed genes were involved in mitochondrial metabolism, transcription, protein synthesis, and the cell cycle. This result suggests that response to hypoxia does not necessarily trigger neo-angiogenesis but could, according to the genetic background of the neoplastic cells, lead to metabolic reprogramming [10].

Sustained signalling promotes metabolic reprogramming

Cancer cells are driven by constant activation of growth signals, which are integrated into cellular adaptive responses in metabolism including increased glucose uptake, lipid, protein, and nucleic acid

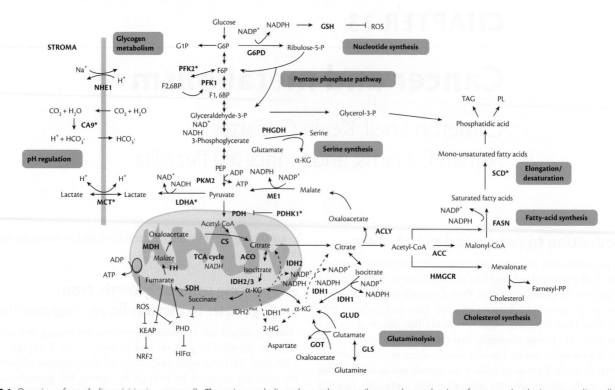

Fig. 13.1 Overview of metabolic activities in cancer cells. The main metabolic pathways that contribute to the production of macromolecules in mammalian cells are nucleotide synthesis, the pentose phosphate pathway, serine synthesis, glutaminolysis, cholesterol synthesis, fatty-acid synthesis, and elongation desaturation. Glycogen synthesis and pH regulation contribute to cellular bioenergetics. The enzymes involved in these pathways are shown in bold, those induced in response to hypoxia are marked with an asterisk. Metabolic enzymes in the TCA cycle, fumarate hydratase (FH) and succinate dehydrogenase (SDH), can act as tumour suppressors. 2-hydroxyglutarate (2-HG) is produced from α-ketoglutarate (α-KG) by the mutant forms of isocitrate dehydrogenase 1 (IDH1) and IDH2 enzymes that are found in cancer (grey dashed arrow). Reductive carboxylation of α-KG by IDH1 and IDH2 produces citrate for lipid synthesis in hypoxic cells (black dashed arrow). Abbreviations: ACC, acetyl-CoA carboxylase; ACLY, ATP citrate lyase; ACO, aconitase; CA9, carbonic anhydrase 9; CoA, coenzyme A; CS, citrate synthase; FASN, fatty-acid synthase; F1,6BP, fructose-1,6- bisphosphate; F2,6BP, fructose-2,6-bisphosphate; F6P, fructose-6-phosphate; GLS, glutaminase; GLUD, glutamate dehydrogenase 1; GOT, glutamic- oxaloacetic transaminase; GSH, glutathione; G1P, glucose-1-phosphate; G6P, glucose-6-phosphate; G6PD, G6P dehydrogenase; HIF, hypoxia inducible factor; HMGCR, 3-hydroxy-3-methylglutaryl-CoA reductase; KEAP, kelch-like ECH-associated protein 1; LDHA, lactate dehydrogenase A; MCT, monocarboxylate transporters; MDH, malate dehydrogenase; ME1, malic enzyme 1; NHE1, Na+/H+exchange protein 1; NRF2, nuclear factor (erythroid-derived 2)-like 2; PDH, pyruvate dehydrogenase; PDHK1, pyruvate dehydrogenase kinase; PEP, phosphoenolpyruvate; PFK, phosphofructokinase; PHD, prolyl hydroxylases; PHGDH, phosphoglycerate dehydrogenase; PKM2, pyruvate kinase M2; PL, phospholipids; ROS, reactive oxygen species; SCD, stearoyl-CoA desaturase; TAG, triacylglycerides.

Reprinted by permission from Macmillan Publishers Ltd: *Nature*, 2012; Volume 491, Issue, 7424, pp. 364–373, Schulze A, Harris AL, How cancer metabolism is tuned for proliferation and vulnerable to disruption, Copyright © 2012, doi:10.1038/nature11706

synthesis. Increased glutamine uptake and glutaminolysis are also characteristic of malignancies, and this serves to replenish TCA cycle intermediates used in biosynthetic reactions (Figure 13.2).

PI3K pathway

Growth factors usually activate receptor tyrosine kinases (RTKs) which then promote signalling through two pathways, the phosphatidylinositol 3-kinase (PI3K) and the Ras-Raf-MAP kinase (ERK) pathway. The PI3K is one of the most commonly mutated and activated pathways in tumour cells, often following inactivation of the tumour suppressor PTEN. Activation of downstream AKT integrates growth signals with increased metabolic requirements leading to higher glucose uptake by glucose transporters; it follows increases the activity of hexokinase and glycolytic flux. AKT1 signalling also strongly stimulates mTOR function by phosphorylating and inhibiting the negative regulator tuberous sclerosis 2 (TSC2) [11].

mTOR

Growth factors can promote the activation of mTOR beside the PI3K pathway. ERK signalling also phosphorylates TSC2 to inhibit

it and promote mTOR activity. The convergence of multiple growth factor pathways, as well as the ability to sense free amino acids, supports mTOR as a key signal integrator and effector of metabolic control: its activation in cancer drives anabolism, energy storage, and consumption. It also activates translation, cell mass increase, and lipogenesis while inhibiting autophagy. There is mounting evidence that inhibition of autophagy promotes tumorigenesis, as mice deficient for the autophagy genes beclin and ATG4C are prone to developing tumours. mTOR is also able to promote the activity of hypoxia inhibitory factor (HIF), even under normoxic conditions [12].

AMPK

AMP-activated protein kinase (AMPK) is a crucial sensor of cellular energetic status, opposes the effect of AKT1, and is a potent inhibitor of mTOR signalling [13]. During periods of energy depletion or stress, AMPK is activated in response to increased AMP/ATP ratio, promoting oxidative phosphorylation and inhibiting cellular proliferation. In this way, exogenous growth signalling pathways must overcome the checkpoint role of AMPK activation in order to proliferate under conditions that are less energetically favourable (such as in hypoxia). Many tumours, therefore, decouple

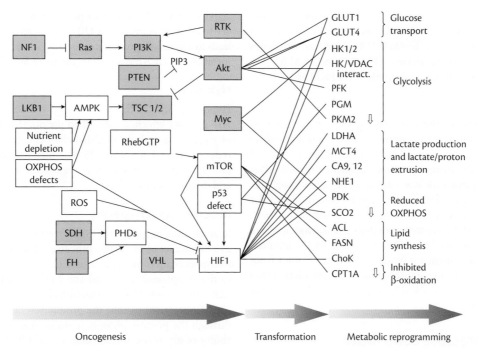

Fig. 13.2 Molecular mechanisms of cancer-specific metabolic reprogramming. As a result of oncogenic gain-of-function events (pink) or the loss of tumor suppressors (green) affecting the PI3K/Akt/mTOR/HIF axis and/or inactivation of the p53 system, a stereotyped pattern of metabolic changes is induced, leading to cancer-associated alterations in metabolism. Note that arrows connecting different proteins do not necessarily indicate direct interactions.
Abbreviations: ACL, ATP citrate lyase; AMPK, AMP-activated kinase; CA9 and CA12, carbonic anhydrases 9 and 12; ChoK, choline kinase; CPT, carnitine palmitoyltransferase; FH, fumarate hydratase; GLUT, glucose transporter; HIF, hypoxia-inducible factor; HK, hexokinase; OXPHOS, oxidative phosphorylation; LAT1, L-type amino acid transporter 1; LDHA, lactate dehydrogenase isoform A; MCT, monocarboxylate transporter; mTOR, mammalian target of rapamycin; NF, neurofibromin; PDK, pyruvate dehydrogenase kinase; PFK, phosphofructokinase; PI3K, phosphatidylinositol 3-kinase; PIP3, phosphatidylinositol triphosphate; PGM, phosphoglycerate mutase; PHD, prolyl hydroxylase; PKM2, pyruvate kinase isoform M2; SCO2, synthesis of cytochrome c oxidase 2; SDH, succinate dehydrogenase; TSC, tuberous sclerosis complex; VDAC, voltage-dependent anion channel; VHL, von Hippel-Lindau ubiquitin ligase.

Reprinted from *Cancer Cell*, Volume 13, Issue 6, Kroemer G, Pouyssegur J, Tumor cell metabolism: cancer's Achilles' heel, pp. 472–482., Copyright © 2008, with permission from Elsevier, http://www.sciencedirect.com/science/journal/15356108

the activity of AMPK from growth signals, including by mutations in liver kinase B1 (LKB1), which is required for AMPK activity. The loss of LKB1, mutated in Peutz–Jeghers syndrome and sporadically in several other tumours [14], leads to increased mTOR and HIF1 activity and promotes the shift to glycolytic metabolism.

Oestrogen-related receptors

Oestrogen-related receptors (ERRs) have unique functions distinct from oestrogen receptors (ERs) although they share significant homology. There are three ERRs (ERRα, ERRβ and ERRγ), which do not associate with a known steroid hormone, and they are highly expressed in normal tissues with high-energy demands and many cancers. In breast cancer the expression of ERα is inversely related to the expression of ERRα. A high level of ERRα can promote glycolytic metabolic reprogramming, whereas ERRγ can sustain oxidative phosphorylation. ERR signalling is modulated by mitogenic signalling, and ERRα activity is promoted by EGFR and ERRB2 (HER2) signalling. ERRs are not affected by current hormonal therapies used in breast cancer [15].

Transcription factors orchestrate the metabolic switch

Hypoxia-inducible factors (HIFs)

A heterodimer of an unstable alpha subunit (in normoxia) and a constitutively present and stable beta subunit, HIF binds to DNA at specific locations called hypoxic response elements (HREs) and elicits a transcriptional up-regulation of genes required to respond appropriately to hypoxia. HIF1, the ubiquitously expressed isoform, promotes the transcription of genes encoding glucose transporters and most glycolytic enzymes increasing the capacity to perform glycolysis. HIF1 also prevents the entry of pyruvate into the TCA cycle by inducing the expression of pyruvate dehydrogenase kinase 1 (PDK1), altering the expressed isoforms of cytochrome c oxidase (from isoform 1 to 2) and inhibiting mitochondrial biogenesis. This causes reduced levels of oxygen consumption and a shift away from oxidative phosphorylation. HIF1 can be activated under normoxic conditions in tumours by oncogenic pathways such as PI3K and by mutations in VHL, succinate dehydrogenase, and fumarate hydratase [16].

MYC

High expression of the oncogene c-Myc is capable of immortalizing cells in vitro and it is overexpressed and amplified in approximately 30% of human cancers. Myc is a transcription factor capable of influencing expression of about 15% of all proteins, including a higher than expected presence of mitochondrial proteins. Oncogenic levels of Myc increase glutaminolysis leading to glutamine addiction of Myc-transformed cells [17]. In collaboration with HIF1, Myc can promote expression of several glycolytic enzymes and glucose transporters as well as lactate dehydrogenase A (LDHA) and PDK1 [18]. The relationship between HIF1 and Myc is complicated, and there is evidence that the two can regulate each other's activity. One example is that HIF-1 can inhibit c-Myc activity, and thus inhibit mitochondrial biogenesis and respiration in hypoxia [19]. Myc also promotes the alternative splicing of the pyruvate kinase gene PKM leading to enhanced expression of the embryonic form PKM2 [20].

PKM2

Pyruvate kinase catalyses the rate-limiting step of glycolysis in which phosphoenolpyruvate is converted to pyruvate, producing ATP. The M2 isoform, up-regulated in many different types of tumour and highly proliferating tissues, can switch from a tetrameric to a dimeric form with lower activity [21]. This lower efficiency allows the accumulation of glycolytic intermediates for use in biosynthetic pathways, including the hexosamine pathway, glycerol synthesis, and the pentose phosphate shunt. High levels of Myc cause the expression of the M2 isoform and PKM2 interacts directly with HIF-1α, enhancing binding and transcription from HREs [22]. By increasing the transcription of proglycolytic genes such as *LDHA* and *SLC2A1*, PKM2 can promote a shift towards anaerobic metabolism.

Tumour suppressors contribute to increased glycolysis

Tumour suppressors also regulate glycolytic metabolism, and the loss of p53 can result in the Warburg effect, consequent to its role in maintaining expression of mitochondrial cytochrome c oxidase 2. P53 normally controls glycolysis through the TP-53-induced glycolysis and apoptosis regulator (TIGAR), increased expression of which inhibits glycolysis and increases the availability of glucose-6-phosphate [23]. P53 can also increase the amount of glucose-6-phosphate by inducing the expression of hexokinase II [24]. This metabolite is used in the pentose phosphate pathway and promotes the synthesis of nucleotides as part of the DNA damage response.

   From the limited description of the metabolic consequences of high-frequency mutations in a wide variety of tumours as described, it is clear that metabolic derangements in cancer provide the conditions to support a high proliferative rate. This is not only through energetic supply, but also by promoting the accumulation of biosynthetic precursors for fatty acid, nucleotide, and protein synthesis. As a consequence of the ensuing cancer environment, tumour cells must adapt to survive in conditions of reduced oxygen and altered acid-base and redox balance.

Metabolic changes that support uncontrolled proliferation

Lactate and pH

The increased rate of glycolysis and conversion to lactate produces an acidic intracellular compartment and high concentrations of lactate. Regulation of intracellular pH is maintained in tumour cells by the Na^+/H^+ exchanger protein NHE1, required for tumour cell proliferation [25]. Carbonic anhydrase 9 (CA9), a target gene of HIF1, catalyses the conversion of carbon dioxide into bicarbonate at the extracellular aspect of the plasma membrane, promoting the removal of excess protons from the cell [26]. Lactate transport out of tumour cells is facilitated by the monocarboxylate transporters MCT1 and MCT4 which require the ancillary protein CD147 (basigin) for their

activity. Renal-cell tumours are particularly reliant on MCT4, secondary to aberrant activation of HIF1 by inactivation of VHL [27]. This leads to a pseudohypoxic state, resulting in a predominant glyocolytic metabolism which has a high requirement for efficient lactate export.

Hypoxia

Hypoxia promotes the stability and transcription activity of the HIF proteins which, as described previously, are efficient inducers of glycolytic metabolism. Other than effects on HIF, hypoxia also reduces the activity of mTOR and may reactivate autophagy and promote survival under stress, angiogenesis, metastasis, glycolysis and drug resistance.

Reactive oxygen species

Reactive oxygen species (ROS) are a set of radical species produced as a byproduct of metabolic processes. The mitochondrial electron transport chain is the main source of ROS and these can contribute to the cytoplasmic pool and affect cell signalling. Mitochondrial ROS can promote HIF stabilization [28], and inhibit PKM2 activity [29]. Consequent to this, the production of NADPH is increased through the pentose phosphate shunt, due to the increased availability of glycolytic intermediates. NADPH is required to maintain the activity of antioxidant systems including glutathione and thioredoxin. High levels of ROS are deleterious to the cell, causing macromolecular damage (including DNA), senescence, and apoptosis.

Metabolic genes with oncogenic or tumour suppressor activity

In addition to the contribution that alterations of oncogenes and tumour suppressor genes make towards driving metabolic transformation, it has been recognized that metabolic derangements can also actively participate in the transformation process.

Oncogenic mutation of metabolic enzymes

Mutations in IDH1 and IDH2 are commonly found in glioblastoma and always cause a single amino acid change (Arg132 in IDH1, Arg172 in IDH2). These characteristic changes lead to neomorphic enzyme properties promoting the conversion of alpha-ketoglutarate to 2-hydroxyglutarate [2-HG] [30]. 2-HG can modulate gene expression in tumours by inhibiting the DNA demethylase TET2 [31], leading to increased genome-wide CpG island methylation and repression of differentiation in astrocytes. Consequently, this metabolite can promote the development of poorly differentiated tumours by directing gene expression. These properties have led it to be named an 'oncometabolite'.

Mitochondrial enzyme tumour suppressor genes

Inherited mutations in the nuclear genes encoding mitochondrial proteins succinate dehydrogenase (SDHB, SDHC, SDHD) and fumarate hydratase (FH) lead to familial cancer syndromes and have implicated these genes as tumour suppressors [32]. Mutations in succinate dehydrogenase lead to accumulation in succinate, which inhibits the activity of HIF prolyl hydroxylases. The HIF prolyl hydroxylases hydroxylate HIF-α subunits in an oxygen-dependent manner, labelling it for VHL-mediated ubiquitination [33]. In effect, higher levels of succinate and fumarate lead to higher levels of HIF signalling by inhibiting its degradation. This may provide the metabolic conditions conducive to oncogenic transformation.

Lipid biosynthesis is up-regulated in cancer

In order to support increased proliferation, tumour cells increase their rate of de novo fatty-acid synthesis. The expression of enzymes involved in lipogenesis is largely controlled by the sterol regulatory element binding proteins (SREBPs). The activity of SREBPs is regulated by AKT and is dependent on mTOR [34]. Increased lipid synthesis is required for the generation of structural lipids that are required for building biological membranes. Other lipids, such as triacylglycerols are used as an energy source, whilst others such as monoacylglycerol lipase may be a signalling molecule-inducing gene expression promoting invasion and metastasis [35]. The precise contribution of increased lipogenesis in tumours is not yet clear; however, SREBP1 expression correlates with breast cancer progression [36].

An increased rate of fatty acid synthesis in prostate cancer can occur in the absence of significant glucose uptake, making the staging of the disease problematic using ^{18}F-FDG PET. Increased fatty acid synthesis can be imaged using ^{11}C-acetate PET, enhancing patient management, and may also potentially be used to predict response to novel anti-fatty acid synthase inhibitors [37].

Glycogen synthesis in cancer

Despite the increased rate of glycolysis in tumours, many tumours and cell lines have been shown to accumulate glycogen. Glycogen accumulation performs a critical role, as inhibiting the breakdown by small molecule inhibition leads to apoptosis in pancreatic tumour cells. On the other hand, reducing the levels of glycogen phosphorylase, which leads to glycogen accumulation, leads to premature senescence of tumour cells and impairs tumour growth [38]. Tumoural glycogen maintains levels of NADPH and ROS, and potentially allows for regulation of substrate entry into the glycolytic pathway.

Potential strategies for targeting metabolic transformation

Metabolic reprogramming provides the opportunity for targeted drugs to selectively exert toxic effects on tumour cells. This may require tumour phenotyping to select patients who are most likely to benefit from therapies that target tumour metabolism [5]. As we have described, functional targeting of oncogenic pathways such as *PI3K* and *KRAS*, may reduce the downstream pathways that promote metabolic transformation as well as reducing growth of the tumour.

Metformin is an antidiabetic drug that is in widespread use and inhibits mitochondrial ATP production, causing activation of AMPK. This reduces the anabolic function of mTOR signalling and triggers autophagy. P53 loss sensitizes cells to the effects of metformin [39] and trials are currently underway evaluating whether metformin may be able to alter tumour metabolism in patients.

ERRα represents a new therapeutic target which may be able to reverse the global metabolic programming that occurs in tumours [15]. Drugs that reduce HIF signalling are also likely to be particularly efficacious given its central role in mediating increased glycolysis, angiogenesis, and metastasis.

One of the most convincing ways of targeting metabolism to produce anticancer effects is synthetic lethality. Lactate dehydrogenase A (LDHA) catalyses the conversion of pyruvate to lactate-producing NAD+, which itself is required for glycolysis. NAD+ can also be recycled from nicotinamide through the salvage pathway using the enzyme nicotinamide phosphoribosyltransferase (NAMPT). NAMPT inhibitors potentiate the effect of LDHA inhibitors [40]. In addition, NAMPT combined with genotoxic chemotherapy and radiotherapy may produce significant effect.

Conclusions

Although many tumours show a stereotypical altered metabolic phenotype with regard to enhanced glucose uptake, it is clear that a variety of metabolic pathways can produce this effect. Many of the metabolic pathways show commonality with hypoxic-induced changes. The changes are adaptive, allowing for strict ROS balance and biosynthetic function, and therapeutic strategies that interrupt these homoeostatic mechanisms may form the basis for future anti-metabolic treatments in cancer.

Acknowledgements

The authors would like to thanks Professor Tom Donnem for critically reading the manuscript.

Further reading

Favaro E, Bensaad K, Chong MG, Tennant DA, Ferguson DJ et al. Glucose utilization via glycogen phosphorylase sustains proliferation and prevents premature senescence in cancer cells. Cell Metabolism 2012; 16(6): 751–764.

Gatenby RA, Gillies RJ. Why do cancers have high aerobic glycolysis? Nature Reviews Cancer 2004; 4(11): 891–899.

Gottlieb E, Tomlinson IP. Mitochondrial tumour suppressors: a genetic and biochemical update. Nature Reviews Cancer 2005; 5(11): 857–866.

Hanahan D, Weinberg RA. Hallmarks of cancer: the next generation. Cell 2011; 144(5): 646–674.

Hu J, Bianchi F, Ferguson M, Cesario A, Margaritora S et al. Gene expression signature for angiogenic and nonangiogenic non-small-cell lung cancer. Oncogene 2005; 24(7): 1212–1219.

Kroemer G, Pouyssegur J. Tumor cell metabolism: cancer's Achilles' heel. Cancer Cell 2008; 13(6): 472–482.

Pezzella F, Pastorino U, Tagliabue E, Andreola S, Sozzi G et al. Non-small-cell lung carcinoma tumor growth without morphological evidence of neo-angiogenesis. American Journal of Pathology 1997; 151(5): 1417–1423.

Schulze A, Harris AL. How cancer metabolism is tuned for proliferation and vulnerable to disruption. Nature 2012; 491(7424): 364–373.

Vander Heiden MG, Cantley LC, Thompson CB. Understanding the Warburg effect: the metabolic requirements of cell proliferation. Science 2009; 324(5930): 1029–1033.

Warburg O. The metabolism of tumours in the body. Journal of General Physiology 1927; 8: 519–530.

References

1. Warburg O. The metabolism of tumours in the body. Journal of General Physiology 1927; 8: 519–530.
2. Gatenby RA, Gillies RJ. Why do cancers have high aerobic glycolysis? Nature Reviews Cancer 2004; 4(11): 891–899.

3. Frezza C, Gottlieb E. Mitochondria in cancer: not just innocent bystanders. Seminars in Cancer Biology 2009; 19(1): 4–11.

4. Vander Heiden MG, Cantley LC, Thompson CB. Understanding the Warburg effect: the metabolic requirements of cell proliferation. Science 2009; 324(5930): 1029–1033.

5. Schulze A, Harris AL. How cancer metabolism is tuned for proliferation and vulnerable to disruption. Nature 2012; 491(7424): 364–373.

6. Yuneva MO, Fan TW, Allen TD, Higashi RM, Ferraris DV et al. The metabolic profile of tumors depends on both the responsible genetic lesion and tissue type. Cell metabolism 2012; 15(2): 157–170.

7. Folkman J. Tumor angiogenesis: therapeutic implications. New England Journal of Medicine 1971; 285(21): 1182–1186.

8. Hanahan D, Weinberg RA. Hallmarks of cancer: the next generation. Cell 2011; 144(5): 646–674.

9. Pezzella F, Pastorino U, Tagliabue E, Andreola S, Sozzi G et al. Non-small-cell lung carcinoma tumor growth without morphological evidence of neo-angiogenesis. American Journal of Pathology 1997; 151(5): 1417–1423.

10. Hu J, Bianchi F, Ferguson M, Cesario A, Margaritora S et al. Gene expression signature for angiogenic and nonangiogenic non-small-cell lung cancer. Oncogene 2005; 24(7): 1212–1219.

11. Wong KK, Engelman JA, Cantley LC. Targeting the PI3K signaling pathway in cancer. Current Opinion in Genetics & Development 2010; 20(1): 87–90.

12. Zoncu R, Efeyan A, Sabatini DM. mTOR: from growth signal integration to cancer, diabetes and ageing. Nature Reviews Molecular Cell Biology 2011; 12(1): 21–35.

13. Shackelford DB, Shaw RJ. The LKB1-AMPK pathway: metabolism and growth control in tumour suppression. Nature Reviews Cancer 2009; 9(8): 563–575.

14. Jenne DE, Reimann H, Nezu J, Friedel W, Loff S et al. Peutz–Jeghers syndrome is caused by mutations in a novel serine threonine kinase. Nature Genetics 1998; 18(1): 38–43.

15. Deblois G, Giguere V. Oestrogen-related receptors in breast cancer: control of cellular metabolism and beyond. *Nature Reviews Cancer* 2013; 13(1): 27–36.

16. Denko NC. Hypoxia, HIF1 and glucose metabolism in the solid tumour. Nature Reviews Cancer 2008; 8(9): 705–713.

17. Wise DR, DeBerardinis RJ, Mancuso A, Sayed N, Zhang XY et al. Myc regulates a transcriptional program that stimulates mitochondrial glutaminolysis and leads to glutamine addiction. Proceedings of the National Academy of Sciences of the United States of America 2008; 105(48): 18782–18787.

18. Dang CV, Kim J-w, Gao P, Yustein J. The interplay between MYC and HIF in cancer. Nature Reviews Cancer 2008; 8(1): 51–56.

19. Fukuda R, Zhang H, Kim J-w, Shimoda L, Dang CV et al. HIF-1 regulates cytochrome oxidase subunits to optimize efficiency of respiration in hypoxic cells. Cell 2007; 129(1): 111–122.

20. David CJ, Chen M, Assanah M, Canoll P, Manley JL. HnRNP proteins controlled by c-Myc deregulate pyruvate kinase mRNA splicing in cancer. Nature 2010; 463(7279): 364–368.

21. Sun Q, Chen X, Ma J, Peng H, Wang F et al. Mammalian target of rapamycin up-regulation of pyruvate kinase isoenzyme type M2 is critical for aerobic glycolysis and tumor growth. Proceedings of the National Academy of Sciences of the United States of America 2011; 108(10): 4129–4134.

22. Luo W, Hu H, Chang R, Zhong J, Knabel M et al. Pyruvate kinase M2 is a PHD3-stimulated coactivator for hypoxia-inducible factor 1. Cell 2011; 145(5): 732–744.

23. Bensaad K, Tsuruta A, Selak MA, Vidal MNC, Nakano K et al. TIGAR, a p53-inducible regulator of glycolysis and apoptosis. Cell 2006; 126(1): 107–120.

24. Mathupala SP, Heese C, Pedersen PL. Glucose catabolism in cancer cells: The type II hexokinase promoter contains functionally active response elements for the tumor suppressor p53. Journal of Biological Chemistry 1997; 272(36): 22776–22780.

25. Chiche J, Brahimi-Horn MC, Pouyssegur J. Tumour hypoxia induces a metabolic shift causing acidosis: a common feature in cancer. Journal of Cellular and Molecular Medicine 2010; 14(4): 771–794.

26. McIntyre A, Patiar S, Wigfield S, Li J-L, Ledaki I et al. Carbonic anhydrase IX promotes tumor growth and necrosis in vivo and inhibition enhances anti-VEGF therapy. Clinical Cancer Research 2012; 18(11): 3100–3111.

27. Gerlinger M, Santos CR, Spencer-Dene B, Martinez P, Endesfelder D et al. Genome-wide RNA interference analysis of renal carcinoma survival regulators identifies MCT4 as a Warburg effect metabolic target. Journal of Pathology 2012; 227(2): 146–156.

28. Klimova T, Chandel NS. Mitochondrial complex III regulates hypoxic activation of HIF. Cell Death and Differentiation 2008; 15(4): 660–666.

29. Anastasiou D, Poulogiannis G, Asara JM, Boxer MB, Jiang JK et al. Inhibition of pyruvate kinase M2 by reactive oxygen species contributes to cellular antioxidant responses. Science 2011; 334(6060): 1278–1283.

30. Dang L, White DW, Gross S, Bennett BD, Bittinger MA et al. Cancer-associated IDH1 mutations produce 2-hydroxyglutarate. Nature 2010; 465(7300): 966.

31. Figueroa ME, Abdel-Wahab O, Lu C, Ward PS, Patel J et al. Leukemic IDH1 and IDH2 mutations result in a hypermethylation phenotype, disrupt TET2 function, and impair hematopoietic differentiation. Cancer Cell 2010; 18(6): 553–567.

32. Gottlieb E, Tomlinson IP. Mitochondrial tumour suppressors: a genetic and biochemical update. Nature Reviews Cancer 2005; 5(11): 857–866.

33. Kaelin WG, Ratcliffe PJ. Oxygen sensing by metazoans: the central role of the HIF hydroxylase pathway. Molecular Cell 2008; 30(4): 393–402.

34. Porstmann T, Santos CR, Griffiths B, Cully M, Wu M et al. SREBP activity is regulated by mTORC1 and contributes to Akt-dependent cell growth. Cell Metabolism 2008; 8(3): 224–236.

35. Nomura DK, Long JZ, Niessen S, Hoover HS, Ng SW et al. Monoacylglycerol lipase regulates a fatty acid network that promotes cancer pathogenesis. Cell 2010; 140(1): 49–61.

36. Hilvo M, Denkert C, Lehtinen L, Muller B, Brockmoller S et al. Novel theranostic opportunities offered by characterization of altered membrane lipid metabolism in breast cancer progression. Cancer Research 2011; 71(9): 3236–3245.

37. Haseebuddin M, Dehdashti F, Siegel BA, Liu J, Roth EB et al. 11C-Acetate PET/CT before radical prostatectomy: nodal staging and treatment failure prediction. Journal of Nuclear Medicine 2013; 54(5): 699–706.

38. Favaro E, Bensaad K, Chong MG, Tennant DA, Ferguson DJ et al. Glucose utilization via glycogen phosphorylase sustains proliferation and prevents premature senescence in cancer cells. Cell Metabolism 2012; 16(6): 751–764.

39. Buzzai M, Jones RG, Amaravadi RK, Lum JJ, DeBerardinis RJ et al. Systemic treatment with the antidiabetic drug metformin selectively impairs p53-deficient tumor cell growth. Cancer Research 2007; 67(14): 6745–6752.

40. Le A, Cooper CR, Gouw AM, Dinavahi R, Maitra A et al. Inhibition of lactate dehydrogenase A induces oxidative stress and inhibits tumor progression. Proceedings of the National Academy of Sciences USA 2010; 107(5): 2037–2042.

Aetiology and epidemiology of cancer

14 Smoking and cancer *127*
Jonathan M. Samet

15 Viruses *136*
Chris Boshoff

16 Chemical carcinogens *142*
Paula A. Oliveira

17 Radiation-induced cancer *150*
Klaus R. Trott

18 Aetiology and progression of cancer: role of body fatness, physical activity, diet, and other lifestyle factors *155*
Fränzel J.B. van Duijnhoven and Ellen Kampman

Aetiology and epidemiology of cancer

CHAPTER 14

Smoking and cancer

Jonathan M. Samet

Introduction to smoking and cancer

Historical perspective

The global impact of tobacco use on health is staggering. Worldwide, there are more than one billion users of tobacco products, including about 750,000 people who smoke cigarettes regularly [1]. The resulting burden of premature mortality, about 6 million deaths in 2011, makes tobacco use the world's leading cause of avoidable premature mortality [2]. Of the six million deaths, an estimated 2.12 million (33%) are from cancer [3]. This chapter provides a perspective on tobacco smoking as a cause of cancer, summarizing the evidence from epidemiological studies and reviewing a now extensive literature on how tobacco smoke causes cancer. It also covers the topic of tobacco control. In-depth reviews are available on these topics, such as Monographs 83 and 100E of the World Health Organization's International Agency for Research on Cancer (IARC), volumes 11 through 14 of the IARC Handbooks of Cancer Prevention, and the 2004, 2006, 2010, and 2014 reports of the United States Surgeon General.

Cancer has figured prominently in the identification of tobacco use as a major cause of disease worldwide. Although there were writings on the dangers of tobacco use for health centuries ago, the body of evidence that constitutes the foundation of understanding of tobacco as a cause of disease dates to approximately the mid-twentieth century. Even earlier, clinical case reports and case series had called attention to the likely role of smoking and chewing tobacco as a cause of cancer. The rise of diseases that had once been uncommon, such as lung cancer (Figure 14.1), was noticed early in the twentieth century and motivated studies to determine if the increases were 'real' or an artefact of changing detection. By mid-century, there was certainty that the increases were real and continuing, and the focus of research shifted to finding the causes of the new epidemics of 'chronic diseases' with an emphasis initially on lung cancer and coronary heart disease.

The rise of smoking had antedated the rise of lung cancer (Figure 14.1) and consequently smoking was among the postulated causes of the increase, but other factors were also considered. In initiating their pioneering case-control study of lung cancer in the late 1940s, Doll and Hill, the British epidemiologists, gave equal weight to smoking and to air pollution as possible causes of lung cancer. The key initial observations were made in epidemiologic studies of smoking and lung cancer with the earliest carried out in the late 1920s and 1930s [4]. Consistent results were reported from five case-control studies reported in 1950, all showing a strong association of cigarette smoking with lung cancer in men [5–9]. The case-control results were soon followed by confirmatory findings from cohort (longitudinal studies) including the landmark study of British physicians carried out by Doll and Hill [10, 11].

These initial observations sparked complementary laboratory studies on the mechanisms by which tobacco smoking causes disease. By the early 1950s cigarette smoke was known to contain benzo(a)pyrene, a recognized carcinogen, and in 1953, Wynder and colleagues reported that painting the shaved skin of mice with cigarette smoke condensate caused tumours [12]. The mounting evidence received formal review and evaluation by government committees, leading to conclusions that smoking caused lung cancer in the late 1950s and early 1960s, including the landmark reports from the Royal College of Physicians and the Advisory Committee to the US Surgeon General [13, 14]. Subsequent reports have led to a progressively lengthier list of cancers caused by smoking (Table 14.1). Even 40 years after the first Surgeon General's report, the 2004 report found the evidence for a number of malignancies sufficient to classify the associations as causal, including cervical cancer and acute myelogenous leukaemia [15], and IARC's Monograph 83 found the relationship to be causal for liver cancer [16]. The 2014 report of the US Surgeon General added colorectal cancer as causally associated with smoking [17]. These causal conclusions have long been critical in motivating aggressive tobacco control.

The issue of passive smoking and cancer has a briefer history. The 1972 report of the Surgeon General was the first to call attention to passive smoking in a chapter titled 'Public exposure to air pollution from tobacco smoke' [18]. The first major studies on passive smoking and lung cancer in non-smokers were reported in 1981, including the cohort study of Japanese women carried out by Hirayama which showed high lung cancer mortality among non-smoking women married to smokers compared with those married to non-smokers [19], and by 1986 the evidence supported the conclusion that passive smoking was a cause of lung cancer in non-smokers, a conclusion reached by the IARC, the US Surgeon General, and the US National Research Council. This conclusion has had widespread public health impact, serving as a key driver for smoke-free indoor environments including public places and workplaces. Research continues on passive smoking and other cancers, particularly for breast cancer—a still controversial topic [20].

Mechanisms of carcinogenesis

Tobacco smoke components

Tobacco smoke is a rich mixture of particles sufficiently small to reach the bronchioles and alveoli and of gases. Fresh tobacco

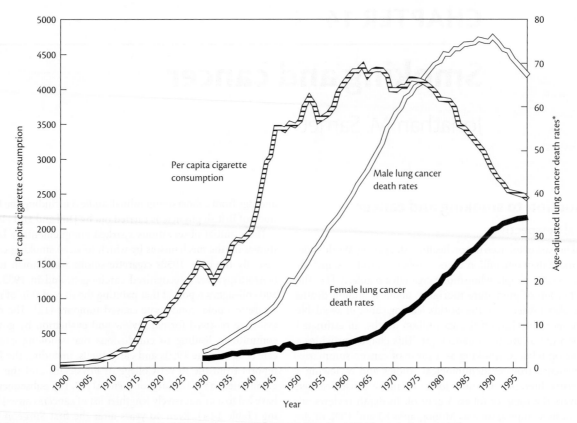

Fig. 14.1 Tobacco use and lung cancer mortality, US, 1900–1997 (per 100,000 and age-adjusted to 1970 US standard population).
Reproduced with permission from Hecht SS and Samet JM, Cigarette Smoking, pp. 1521–1551, in Rom WM (Ed.), *Environmental and Occupational Medicine*, Fourth Edition, Wolters Kluwer/Lippincott Williams & Wilkins, Philadelphia, USA, Copyright © 2007

smoke is reported as containing about 7000 distinct chemicals, including numerous known carcinogens, such as benzo(a)pyrene, tobacco-specific nitrosamines, benzene, polonium, and toxins [21]. These components contribute directly and indirectly to carcinogenesis. Tobacco smoke has high oxidative potential and causes inflammation in the lung and systemically. Tobacco smoke components move from the lungs into the circulation and reach throughout the body, thus leading to tissue doses of carcinogens, not only at the site of absorption, but to most organs of the body. The liver is a site of carcinogen metabolism and activation and the kidneys and bladder are involved in the excretion of carcinogens.

Tobacco smoke contains numerous known carcinogens, including many that have been evaluated for carcinogenicity by IARC [16, 22]. Broad classes of carcinogens include polycyclic aromatic hydrocarbons (PAHs), N-nitrosamines, aromatic amines, volatile aldehydes, and phenolic amines. The PAHs result from incomplete combustion and include benzo(a)pyrene, one of the first carcinogens identified in tobacco smoke. They act locally and bind to DNA. *N*-nitrosamines are a large class of carcinogens that includes the tobacco-specific nitrosamines *N*-nitrosamines 4-(methylnitrosamino)-1-(3-pyridyl)-1-butanone (NNK) and *N'*-nitrosonornicotine (NNN). The N-nitrosamines are potent systemic carcinogens and NNK causes lung and other tumours in animal models. Aromatic amines, also combustion products, include recognized human bladder carcinogens in occupational settings, 2-naphthylamine and 4-aminobiphenyl. Some other carcinogens in tobacco smoke are formaldehyde, catechol, and 1,3 butadiene,

and the leukemogen benzene. Diverse metals and the radionuclide ^{210}Po are also present in cigarette smoke.

The doses of carcinogens and other tobacco smoke components received can be assessed using biomarkers. Cotinine, a major nicotine metabolite, is a widely used biomarker for active and passive smoking that can be measured in blood, urine, saliva, and hair [16]. The doses of cigarette smoke carcinogens resulting from inhalation of tobacco smoke are reflected in levels of these carcinogens or their metabolites in the blood and urine of smokers. Certain biomarkers are associated with exposure to specific cigarette smoke carcinogens, such as urinary metabolites of the tobacco-specific nitrosamine NNK and haemoglobin adducts of aromatic amines. Levels of these biomarkers can be used as highly specific indicators of exposure to tobacco smoke carcinogens, while nicotine or its metabolites (particularly cotinine) are used as indicators of exposure to tobacco smoke generally, both for active and passive smoking. For example, the NNK metabolite, NNAL, can be measured in the urine of active smokers and of passive smokers [23].

Tobacco smoke and carcinogenesis

Figure 14.2 provides a general schema for the causation of cancer by the carcinogens in tobacco smoke. There are both specific and non-specific pathways by which smoking is thought to cause cancer. The figure begins with initiation of cigarette smoking and addiction; it is the maintained contact with tobacco smoke carcinogens consequent to addiction that leads to the very high risk of cancer in those who smoke daily throughout their lives, the general pattern of the addicted smoker. However, the sustained, but

Table 14.1 Cancers caused by active smoking, as identified by the United States Surgeon General or by the World Health Organization's International Agency for Research on Cancer (IARC)

Cancer type	Highest level conclusion available for active smoking	
	US Surgeon General	**IARC**
Bladder and ureter	Causal	Causal
Brain (adults only)	Suggestive of no causal relationship	–
Breast (women only)	Suggestive but not sufficient to infer causal relationship [17]	Positive association
Cervical	Causal	Causal
Colorectal	Causal [17]	Causal
Endometrial	Reduced risk in postmenopausal women	Evidence suggesting lack of carcinogenicity (postmenopausal)
Oesophageal	Causal	Causal
Kidney	Causal	Causal
Laryngeal	Causal	Causal
Leukaemia	Causal	Causal
Liver	Causal	Causal
Lung	Causal	Causal
Oral and pharyngeal	Causal	Causal
Ovarian	Inadequate to infer presence or absence of causal relationship	Causal (mucinous)
Pancreatic	Causal	Causal
Prostate	Suggestive of no causal relationship	–
Sinonasal	–	Causal
Stomach	Causal	Causal
Thyroid	–	Evidence suggesting lack of carcinogenicity

Source: data from US Department of Health and Human Services, *The Health Consequences of smoking: A Report of the Surgeon General*, US Department of Health and Human Services, Atlanta, Georgia, USA, 2004; International Agency for Research on Cancer (IARC), *Tobacco Smoke and Involuntary Smoking*, IARC Monograph 83, International Agency for Research on Cancer, Lyon, France, Copyright © 2004 and International Agency for Research on Cancer (IARC), *A Review of Human Carcinogens, Part E: Personal Habits and Indoor Combustions*, Monograph 100E, International Agency for Research on Cancer, Lyon, France, Copyright © 2012.

lower-level exposures of passive smokers are also sufficient to cause cancer. The figure highlights the multiple processes that lead to uncontrolled cell growth and malignancy and the multiple points in these processes at which tobacco smoke components contribute to carcinogenesis. Emphasis has been given to DNA binding and mutations but research also shows that tobacco smoke contributes to increased cancer risk through epigenetic mechanisms.

For many tobacco smoke carcinogens, metabolic activation is needed and genetic determinants of rates of activation may modify the risk of cancer in smokers [21]. The metabolic activation of cigarette smoke carcinogens by cytochrome P-450 enzymes has a direct effect on the formation of DNA adducts. There is consistent evidence that a combination of polymorphisms in the CYP1A1 and GSTM1 genes of the cytochrome P-450 system leads to higher DNA adduct levels in smokers and higher relative risks for lung cancer than in smokers without this genetic profile. Tobacco-specific carcinogens form adducts and lead to mutations in oncogenes and tumour suppressor genes. Smoking has been found specifically to increase the frequency of DNA adducts of cigarette smoke carcinogens such as benzo(a)pyrene and tobacco-specific nitrosamines in

the lung and other organs, and to cause DNA damage and mutations in key oncogenes and tumour suppressor genes, including *TP53* and *KRAS*. There is also evidence showing that smoking leads to the presence of promoter methylation of key tumour suppressor genes such as *P16* in lung cancer and other smoking-caused cancers. More recent research is more specifically characterizing the pathways by which smoking causes cancer. For example, the 2010 report of the Surgeon General found that smoke constituents, such as nicotine and NNK, can activate signal transduction pathways directly through receptor-mediated events, allowing the survival of damaged epithelial cells that would normally die.

Epidemiology of smoking and cancer
Overview

Smoking causally increases risk for multiple cancer sites (Table 14.1). Table 14.2 provides relative risk estimates for cancer death for major sites in the two cohort studies of the American Cancer Society, Cancer Prevention Study (CPS) I (1959–1965) and CPS II (1982–1988) [15]. Several general findings are notable: (1) the

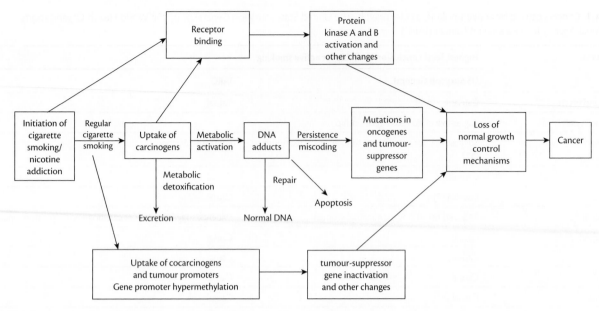

Fig. 14.2 Link between cigarette smoking and cancer through carcinogens in tobacco smoke.
Reproduced from US Department of Health and Human Services, *How Tobacco Smoke Causes Disease: The Biology and Behavioral Basis for Smoking-Attributable Disease: A Report of the Surgeon General*, US Department of Health and Human Services, Atlanta, Georgia, USA, 2010.

relative risks for current and former smokers compared to never smokers are remarkably high for some sites, such as lung and laryngeal cancer; (2) former smokers uniformly have decreased relative risks in comparison with current smokers; (3) relative risks have tended to be lower in females than in males; and (4) relative risks tended to increase for females over the two decades between the two studies. Findings of more recent studies suggest that relative risks have continued to rise as more recent cohorts of women have started to smoke at a similarly young age as men and smoked with the same intensity.

Lung and laryngeal cancers

The impact of smoking on lung cancer in the twentieth century in the US can be seen in Figure 14.1. Cigarette smoking was rare in the early part of the twentieth century, as was lung cancer. Smoking increased due to mass production of cigarettes, increased advertising, pervasive availability of cigarettes by military personnel during World War I, and increased use by women at the time of World War II. Cigarette smoking peaked in the 50s and 60s, and began to decline after the wave of studies documenting its risks appeared and the publication of the first Surgeon General's Report in 1964. Mortality due to lung cancer in men can be seen to follow the curve for smoking prevalence by about 30 years, beginning to decrease in the mid-1990s. Lung cancer became the most common cause of cancer death in US women, surpassing breast cancer in 1988, and only now has the overall lung cancer death rate reached a plateau.

Lung cancer was the first cancer causally associated with cigarette smoking and the epidemiological data for lung cancer illustrate the power of smoking as a cause of cancer, the variation in risk with duration and amount of smoking, and the beneficial consequences of smoking cessation. Recent studies show about a 20-fold increase in risk of lung cancer in current smokers, compared with non-smokers and the relative risks are now comparable in male and female smokers in western countries. The strongest

determinant of lung cancer in smokers is duration of smoking, and risk also increases with the number of cigarettes smoked, but not so steeply as for duration of smoking. Thus, earlier age of initiation of smoking greatly increases lung cancer risk. Cessation of smoking at any age avoids the further increase in risk of lung cancer caused by continued smoking, but the risk of ex-smokers for lung cancer remains elevated for years after cessation, compared to the risk of never smokers, and even with long-term successful quitting it does not return to the risk of the never smoker (Table 14.2).

Smoking increases the risk of all major histologic types of lung cancer [16]. Initially, the association of smoking with adenocarcinoma of the lung was weak, but in more recent decades that association has become stronger. In fact, changes in cigarette design are postulated as causing the shift in histological types of lung cancer over recent decades with adenocarcinoma replacing squamous cell carcinoma as the most common type of lung cancer caused by smoking in the US and elsewhere. The design changes are postulated to have led to deeper inhalation of smoke and greater doses of tobacco-specific nitrosamines which are linked to adenocarcinoma.

Lung cancer has multiple causes other than cigarette smoking but in populations with early age of initiation and average consumption of about 20 cigarettes per day, approximately 90% of lung cancer cases are due to cigarette smoking. For some occupational and environmental causes of lung cancer, such as asbestos and radon, synergistic interactions are well documented [16].

The general patterns are also similar for laryngeal cancer (Table 14.2). However, for laryngeal cancer, smoking interacts synergistically with alcohol consumption, greatly increasing risk for those who both smoke and drink alcohol heavily [16]. Risk patterns and synergism with alcohol are similar for cancers of the oropharynx and oesophagus as well and the comparable epidemiological patterns for these upper airway and digestive sites have led to the introduction of the concept of 'aerodigestive tumours'.

Table 14.2 Age-adjusted relative risks of death from smoking-related cancers from the Cancer Prevention Study (CPS) I and CPS-II

Disease category (ICD-9 code)	CPS-I (1959–1965)				CPS-II (1982–1988)			
	Males		Females		Males		Females	
	CS	FS	CS	FS	CS	FS	CS	FS
Lip, oral cavity, pharynx (140–149)	6.3	2.7	2.0	1.9	10.9	3.4	5.1	2.3
Oesophagus (150)	3.6	1.3	1.9	2.2	6.8	4.5	7.8	2.8
Stomach (151)	1.8	1.7	1.0	1.0	2.0	1.5	1.4	1.3
Pancreas (157)	2.3	1.3	1.4	1.4	2.3	1.2	2.3	1.6
Larynx (161)	10.0	8.6	3.8	3.1	14.6	6.3	13.0	5.2
Trachea, bronchus, lung (162)	11.4	5.0	2.7	2.6	23.3	8.7	12.7	4.5
Cervix uteri (180)	NA	NA	1.1	1.3	NA	NA	1.6	1.1
Urinary bladder (188)	2.9	1.8	2.9	2.3	3.3	2.1	2.2	1.9
Kidney, other urinary (189)	1.8	1.8	1.4	1.5	2.7	1.7	1.3	1.1
Acute myeloid leukaemia (204–208)	1.6	1.6	1.0	1.0	1.9	1.3	1.1	1.4

ICD-9 = International Classification of Diseases, 9th Revision

CS = Current smokers

FS = Former smokers

Results presented for persons ≥35 years of age unless otherwise indicated

Source: data from US Department of Health and Human Services, *The Health Consequences of Smoking: A Report of the Surgeon General*, US Department of Health and Human Services, Atlanta, Georgia, USA, 2004.

Other cancers

Cigarette smoking is causally associated with diverse other cancers (Tables 14.1 and 14.2). Similar to lung cancer, for these sites risk increases with smoking duration and number of cigarettes smoked, and cessation avoids further increases in risk. However, the magnitudes of the relative risks are substantially lower than for lung cancer (Table 14.2). For some sites, the evidence has long been sufficient to support a causal association, including cancers of the oral cavity, oesophagus, and urinary bladder. The evidence has also become sufficiently strong to causally link smoking to cancers of the stomach, pancreas, and kidney. For some of these sites, there has been careful attention to other factors and aetiological research has controlled for such factors, for example alcohol and carcinoma of the oesophagus, and explored the combined effects of smoking with these other factors [16].

For several sites, there are other strong causal agents, for example hepatitis B virus infection and hepatocellular carcinoma, and smoking has been causally linked to their aetiology only after epidemiological research fully clarified the role of smoking in the context of these other factors. The IARC identified smoking as a cause of hepatocellular carcinoma after summarizing epidemiological studies showing that the association with smoking was not arising from confounding by the other causal agents, particularly alcohol consumption. Additionally, there was a positive relationship with indicators of dose and a decline of risk after cessation. Similarly, cigarette smoking is a cause of cervical squamous cell carcinoma, accelerating the development of cervical malignancy in women with human papilloma virus, the apparent cause of most cases of cervical cancer. Myeloid leukaemia in adults is also causally related to cigarette smoking. Cigarette smoke contains benzene, a known leukomogen. The 2014 report of the US Surgeon General found the relationship of smoking with colorectal cancer to be causal [17].

For some cancer sites, the evidence is suggestive of a causal association but not yet judged conclusive. The most controversial findings relate to breast cancer for which the overall association with active smoking has been previously null. The breast tissue of smokers is exposed to tobacco smoke carcinogens, but smoking alters estrogen metabolism to a profile that may lower breast cancer risk [15]. Epidemiological studies have explored whether particular subgroups of smokers may be at increased risk, as defined by clinical characteristics, genotype for carcinogen metabolism, or risk factor profile. The evidence remains mixed. However, several groups have classified active smoking as a cause of breast cancer [24, 25]. The 2014 Surgeon General's report, based on an exhaustive evaluation of the literature and meta-analysis found the evidence to be suggestive of a causal relationship [17]. For prostate cancer, mortality, but not incidence, is increased in cigarette smokers [15].

Other types of tobacco use

Cigar and/or pipe smoking are strongly related to cancers of the oral cavity, oropharynx, hypopharynx, larynx, and oesophagus, with the risk being similar to that of cigarette smoking [26]. Dose-response relationships have been documented. Cigar and/or pipe smoking are causally associated with lung cancer and possibly with cancers of the pancreas, stomach, and urinary bladder [27].

Bidis, smoked by millions in India, Bangladesh, and other countries in Asia, are comprised of flakes of tobacco rolled within a leaf and held together by a string [1, 28]. Typically, they are made at the local level, but distributed widely. Toxicological and biomarker studies document a profile that indicates a potential for risks comparable to those in smokers of cigarettes. Although the evidence is limited, epidemiological studies show increased risk for aerodigestive cancers in bidi smokers.

Passive smoking and cancer

Secondhand smoke (SHS) inhaled by never smokers has also been causally linked to lung cancer. Secondhand tobacco smoke is a mixture, mainly of the smoke generated between puffs, called side-stream smoke, and a minor portion of mainstream smoke constituents exhaled by a smoker. Although the levels of certain carcinogens in sidestream tobacco smoke are greater than in mainstream smoke per gram tobacco burned, SHS is diluted by air and the carcinogen dose received by a nonsmoker exposed to SHS is substantially less than that received by an active smoker.

Epidemiologic studies of secondhand tobacco smoke and lung cancer have typically found relative risks between 1 and 2. Over the decades since the first studies, meta-analyses have been repeatedly carried out. The 2002 evaluation by IARC compiled more than 50 studies of involuntary smoking and lung cancer risk in non-smokers. The IARC Monograph 83 concluded that there is a significant and consistent association between lung cancer risk in spouses of smokers and secondhand tobacco smoke exposure, with the excess risk being about 20% in women and 30% in men. Workplace exposures to SHS also increased lung cancer risk in non-smokers, by 12–19%. The findings of subsequent meta-analyses have been similar; a 2007 report based on 22 studies found that workplace exposure was associated with a 24% increase in risk [29].

The literature on SHS exposure and breast cancer is mixed and controversial, in part because of the inconsistent findings on active smoking, unlike lung cancer. The association of SHS exposure with breast cancer risk is strongest in case-control studies of premenopausal breast cancer, but less clear in cohort studies and for postmenopausal breast cancer. As for active smoking, several groups have concluded that passive smoking is a cause of breast cancer [24, 25], but neither IARC nor the US Surgeon General have yet reached this conclusion (Table 14.1).

Global burden of smoking-caused cancer

The global burden of smoking-attributable premature death is over six million annually, of which 2.1 million, or one-third of the total burden, are from malignancy. Not surprisingly, the number is greatest for lung cancer at 1.1 million [3]. Other leading sites include the oropharynx, oesophagus, stomach, and liver. In high-income countries, about half of the cancer burden is attributable to smoking; that percentage is currently lower in less developed countries, but anticipated to rise, absent effective tobacco control [30]. For passive smoking, 603,000 premature deaths are attributable to SHS exposure worldwide [31].

Tobacco control

Tobacco control has had a lengthy evolution that has been closely linked to the increasing evidence on the health effects of active and passive smoking and on what tobacco control modalities are efficacious [32, 33]. Historically, the initial findings on lung cancer and smoking were followed by efforts to educate the public about the risks of smoking with the expectation that they would stop. Since then, we have learned that tobacco control requires far more complex approaches that acknowledge the hierarchy of factors that determine the use of tobacco and the interplay of these factors across the lifecourse, as health is damaged by smoking from conception on. At each age, the emphasis of tobacco control shifts, moving from ending maternal smoking during pregnancy and SHS exposure during childhood, to preventing initiation, and then to promoting successful cessation. Additionally, tobacco control efforts need to be dynamic in time, changing as the tobacco industry attempts to counter any tobacco control measures.

Figure 14.3 provides a hierarchical model that is useful for framing tobacco control [34]. At the lowest level, emerging evidence shows that genetic factors figure in determining liability to addiction and risk for disease in smokers. Intermediate levels are also relevant: the roles of family and peers in initiation are well established. The broader neighbourhood, municipal and state and national levels are also critical in establishing both positive and negative pressures for tobacco use and in setting the critical 'cultural norm' around smoking. The cultural norm may be that smoking is acceptable as in present-day China where cigarettes have well-established roles in social interactions, or unacceptable as in much of the US today, where workplaces and public places are generally smoke-free. Advertising bans, pack warnings, and taxation rates—potentially determined at multiple governmental levels—also affect the environment for smoking and tobacco control. The global level is ever more relevant as the tobacco industry has consolidated into a limited number of multinational companies, including Philip Morris International, British American Tobacco, Japan Tobacco International, and Imperial Tobacco/Altadis [2]. The largest producer is China National Tobacco Corporation, a state monopoly that manufactures more than 90% of cigarettes consumed by China's 300 million smokers.

The industry has a critical role, as the 'root cause' of the tobacco epidemic. Considered in the classic epidemiological triangle of agent, vector, and host, the tobacco industry is the vector that conveys tobacco to people, the host. It also contributes to setting the environment by advertising and promoting its addicting product. We have learned that the industry also attempted to affect the environment around smoking by paying for placement of smoking in movies [35]. Viewing of smoking in movies has been causally linked to increased tobacco use [35]. Notably, the industry is an 'adaptive' vector that changes strategies in a dynamic way to target by host characteristics (age, gender, and race) and to counter efforts at tobacco control. The need to address the industry broadly is reflected in control measures that directly address its activities, including regulation, litigation, and the World Health Organization's Framework Convention on Tobacco Control (FCTC) [36].

Over time, approaches to tobacco control have evolved such that they incorporate a package of interventions. This evolution reflects the expanding understanding of the impact of various tobacco control strategies. For example, the finding that passive smoking caused lung cancer motivated the implementation of smoking bans in public places and workplaces and initiated a change in social norms around smoking that moved smoking from being viewed as acceptable to unacceptable. As noted by Surgeon General Koop in the preface to his 1986 report, 'The right of smokers to smoke ends where their behaviour affects the health and well-being of others' [37]. Approaches to smoking cessation became more effective when nicotine was identified as addicting, nicotine replacement therapy and other pharmacological approaches were introduced,

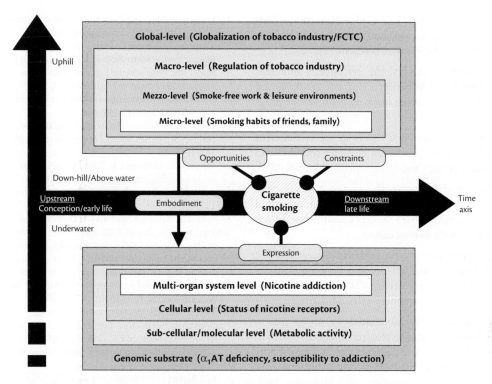

Fig. 14.3 Axes of time and nested hierarchical structures for tobacco control.

Adapted from *Social Science Medicine*, Volume 62, Issue 7, Glass TA and McAtee MJ, Behavioral science at the crossroads in public health: extending horizons, envisioning the future, pp. 1650–1671, Copyright © 2005, with permission from Elsevier, http://www.sciencedirect.com/science/journal/02779536

and stronger behavioural approaches were introduced. Research and experience also documented the need to raise taxes, to use aggressive counter-marketing to denormalize smoking, and to protect children from the reach of the tobacco industry. Most importantly, decades of evidence shows that a multicomponent strategy is needed that targets non-smokers to keep them from smoking and that encourages and supports smokers to quit. Recent experience in New York City, for example, shows that an aggressive, multifaceted programme can have rapid impact. Following implementation of a smoking ban, tax increases, hard-hitting anti-smoking campaigns, and an active cessation programme, smoking prevalence fell from 21.6% to 19.2% between 2002 and 2003, signifying a reduction of approximately 140,000 smokers during this period [38].

Many nations have implemented tobacco control programs. Most importantly, there is now the FCTC, ratified and in force for most nations of the world, although not for the US and Indonesia. Many universal elements of national tobacco control policy are core provisions of the FCTC. Key provisions include a comprehensive ban on tobacco advertising, promotion, and sponsorship; a ban on misleading descriptors such as 'light'; and a mandate to place rotating warnings that cover at least 30% of tobacco packaging and encouragement for even larger, graphic warnings. The FCTC also urges countries to implement smoke-free workplace laws, address tobacco smuggling, and increase tobacco taxes. The FCTC has now been in place for more than five years and progress is slowly being made in implementing its components [39].

Building on the FCTC process, the WHO released its first 'Report on Control of the Tobacco Epidemic' entitled 'MPOWER' in 2008 [40]. MPOWER is a comprehensive tobacco control strategy intended to provide a programmatic counterpart to the FCTC. MPOWER includes six key tobacco control measures including

Monitoring the epidemic, Protecting non-smokers from exposure to SHS, Warning smokers of the health effects of smoking with strong, effective health warnings, Enforcing advertising bans, and Raising the price of tobacco products. The WHO is tracking implementation of MPOWER and coverage of the world's population by its provisions. To date, its reach is still limited, although increasing coverage of the world's population by its elements can be anticipated [41]. Fortunately, global tobacco control has benefited greatly from funding from the Bloomberg Family Foundation and the Bill and Melinda Gates Foundation, first made available in 2007 and now slated to continue through 2016. These funds have supported capacity building in tobacco control, policy advocacy, regulation, and surveillance.

Cancer, smoking, and oncology

This brief review highlights the role of tobacco smoking as the leading cause of avoidable death from lung cancer. As for all health professionals, oncologists should be actively supportive of tobacco control at all levels—from local to global. In providing patient care, they need actively to promote cessation for those patients who smoke after diagnosis. These individuals are at high risk for a second malignancy, particularly at a site of smoking-caused cancer, and smoking has unfavourable consequences for outcome (see [42], for example, with regard to early-stage lung cancer). In a study of people treated for cancer at Roswell Park Cancer Institute, continued smoking after diagnosis increased both overall mortality and disease-specific mortality [43]. Unfortunately, smoking status has received little attention in cancer clinical trials and survey data for the US show that about 15% of adult cancer survivors are current smokers [44, 45].

The 2014 report of the US Surgeon General includes a comprehensive review of the evidence on smoking and cancer outcomes. Four notable conclusions for oncologists were reached [17]:

1. In cancer patients and survivors, the evidence is sufficient to infer a causal relationship between cigarette smoking and adverse health outcomes. Quitting smoking improves the prognosis of cancer patients.

2. In cancer patients and survivors, the evidence is sufficient to infer a causal relationship between cigarette smoking and increased all-cause mortality and cancer-specific mortality.

3. In cancer patients and survivors, the evidence is sufficient to infer a causal relationship between cigarette smoking and increased risk for second primary cancers known to be caused by cigarette smoking, such as lung cancer.

4. In cancer patients and survivors, the evidence is suggestive but not sufficient to infer a causal relationship between cigarette smoking and (1) the risk of recurrence, (2) poorer response to treatment, and (3) increased treatment-related toxicity.

These conclusions provide a powerful rationale for oncologists to address smoking by their patients. Oncologists should have skills in smoking cessation and monitor and address smoking cessation by their patients. They see them during multiple 'teachable moments' and they should be prepared to intervene with strategies, both pharmacologic and non-pharmacologic, of proven efficacy [46].

Summary

Tobacco smoking, as well as its use in other products, is the leading cause of avoidable premature mortality, including from cancer, worldwide. For some sites, such as lung cancer, risks are remarkably high in cigarette smokers and smoking has been linked to malignancy of most organs. Thus, tobacco control provides a tremendous opportunity for cancer prevention. A global public health treaty, the World Health Organization's FCTC, calls for the ratifying nations, now numbering 176, to implement a set of effective tobacco control policies [36]. The FCTC has now been in force for more than five years, creating a global tobacco control movement.

For oncologists, emerging evidence points to clinical implications of smoking with regard to therapy and outcomes in cancer. As for all clinical encounters, smoking needs to be assessed routinely and cessation counseled vigorously for cancer patients who are smoking. The American Society for Clinical Oncology advocates engagement of oncologists in smoking cessation as well as tobacco control generally [47]. The literature suggests that smoking cessation after the diagnosis of cancer improves prognosis.

Further reading

Hecht SS, Samet JM. Cigarette smoking. In Rom WM, ed., Environmental and Occupational Medicine, 4th ed. Philadelphia: Wolters Kluwer/ Lippincott Williams & Wilkins, 2007, 1521–1551.

Glass TA, McAtee MJ. Behavioral science at the crossroads in public health: extending horizons, envisioning the future. Social Science & Medicine 2006; 62(7): 1650–1671.

References

1. Giovino GA, Mirza SA, Samet JM, Gupta PC, Jarvis MJ et al. Tobacco use in 16 countries with 4 billion population: the GATS collaborative group. Lancet 2012; 380(9842): 668–679.

2. Eriksen M, Mackay J, Ross H. The Tobacco Atlas, 4th ed. Atlanta: American Cancer Society, World Lung Foundation, 2012.

3. Mathers CD, Loncar D. Projections of global mortality and burden of disease from 2002 to 2030. PLoS Med 2006; 3(11): e442.

4. Samet JM. What was the first epidemiological study of smoking and lung cancer? Peventive Medicine 2012; 55(3): 178–180.

5. Doll R, Hill AB. Smoking and carcinoma of the lung. British Medical Journal 1950; 2(4681): 739–748.

6. Levin ML, Goldstein H, Gerhardt PR. Cancer and tobacco smoking: a preliminary report. Journal of the American Medical Association 1950; 143: 336–338.

7. Wynder EL, Graham EA. Tobacco smoking as a possible etiologic factor in bronchiogenic carcinoma: a study of six hundred and eighty-four proved cases. Journal of the American Medical Association 1950; 143(4): 329–336.

8. Schrek R, Baker LA, Ballard GP, Dolgoff S. Tobacco smoking as an etiologic factor in dieases I. Cancer. Cancer Research 1950; 10 (1): 49–58.

9. Mills CA, Porter MM. Tobacco smoking habits and cancer of the mouth and respiratory system. Cancer Research 1950; 10(9): 539–542.

10. Doll R, Hill AB. Lung cancer and other causes of death in relation to smoking: a second report on the mortality of British doctors. British Medical Journal 1956(5001): 1071–1081.

11. Doll R, Hill AB. Mortality in relation to smoking: ten years' observations of British doctors. British Medical Journal 1964; 1: 1399–1410.

12. Wynder EL, Graham EA, Croninger AB. Experimental production of carcinoma with cigarette tar. Cancer Research 1953; 13: 855–864.

13. Royal College of Physicians of London. Smoking and Health. Summary of a Report of the Royal College of Physicians of London on Smoking in Relation to Cancer of the Lung and Other Diseases. London: Pitman Medical Publishing Co., Ltd, 1962.

14. US Department of Health Education and Welfare. Smoking and Health. Report of the Advisory Committee to the Surgeon General. Washington, DC: U.S. Government Printing Office, 1964 DHEW Publication No. [PHS] 1103.

15. US Department of Health and Human Services. The Health Consequences of Smoking. A Report of the Surgeon General. Atlanta, GA: U.S. Department of Health and Human Services, Centers for Disease Control and Prevention, National Center for Chronic Disease Prevention and Health Promotion, Office on Smoking and Health, 2004.

16. International Agency for Research on Cancer. Tobacco Smoke and Involuntary Smoking. IARC monograph 83. Lyon, France: International Agency for Research on Cancer, 2004.

17. US Department of Health and Human Services. The Health Consequences of Smoking–50 years of Progress: A Report of the Surgeon General. Atlanta–GA: US Department of Health and Human Services, Centers for Disease Control and Prevention, National Center for Chronic Disease Prevention and Health Promotion, Office on Smoking and Health, 2014.

18. US Department of Health Education Welfare. The Health Consequences of Smoking. A Report of the Surgeon General. Atlanta, GA: US Government Printing Office, 1972.

19. Hirayama T. Non-smoking wives of heavy smokers have a higher risk of lung cancer: A study from Japan. British Medical Journal (Clinical Research Ed) 1981; 282(6259): 183–185.

20. Institute of Medicine. Breast Cancer and the Environment: A Life Course Approach. Washington, DC: National Academies Press, 2012.

21. US Department of Health and Human Services. How Tobacco Smoke Causes Disease: The Biology and Behavioral Basis for Smoking-Attributable Disease. A report of the Surgeon General. Atlanta, GA: US Department of Health and Human Services, Centers for Disease Control and Prevention, National Center for Chronic Disease Prevention and Health Promotion, Office on Smoking and Health, 2010.

22. International Agency for Research on Cancer. A Review of Human Carcinogens. Part E: Personal Habits and Indoor Combustions. Monograph 100E. Lyon, France: International Agency for Research on Cancer, 2012.

23. Hecht SS, Carmella SG, Murphy SE, Akerkar S, Brunneman KD et al. A tobacco-specific lung carcinogen in the urine of men exposed to cigarette smoke. New England Journal of Medicine 1993; 329(21): 1543–1546.

24. Cal/EPA. Carcinogenic effects, 7.4.1. Breast cancer. In Proposed Identification of Environmental Tobacco Smoke as a Toxic Air Contaminant. Part B: Health Effects. Final Report. Sacramento, CA: California Environmental Protection Agency, Office of Environmental Health Hazard Assessment, California Air Resources Board, 2005.

25. Collishaw NE, Boyd NF, Cantor KP, Hammond SK, Johnson KC et al. Canadian Expert Panel on Tobacco Smoke and Breast Cancer Risk. Toronto, Canada: Ontario Tobacco Research Unit, 2009.

26. US Department of Health and Human Services. The Health Consequences of Smoking: Cancer. A Report of the Surgeon General. Washington, DC: US Department of Health and Human Services, Public Health Service, Office on Smoking and Health, 1982 -32676. Report No.: DHHS Publication No. (PHS) 82-50179.

27. National Cancer Institute. Cigars: Health Effects and Trends. Smoking and Tobacco Control Monograph 9. Bethesda, MD: National Institutes of Health, 1998.

28. Asma S, Gupta PC, eds. Bidi Smoking and Public Health. Mumbai: India Ministry of Health, 2008.

29. Stayner L, Bena J, Sasco AJ, Smith R, Steenland K et al. Lung cancer risk and workplace exposure to environmental tobacco smoke. American Journal of Public Health 2007; 97(3): 545–551.

30. Jha P. Avoidable global cancer deaths and total deaths from smoking. Nature reviews Cancer 2009; 9(9): 655–664.

31. Oberg M, Jaakkola MS, Woodward A, Peruga A, Pruss-Ustun A. Worldwide burden of disease from exposure to second-hand smoke: a retrospective analysis of data from 192 countries. Lancet 2011; 377(9760): 139–146.

32. US Department of Health and Human Services. Reducing Tobacco Use: A Report of the Surgeon General. Atlanta, GA: U.S. Department of Health and Human Services, Centers for Disease Control and Prevention, National Center for Chronic Disease Prevention and Health Promotion, Office on Smoking and Health, 2000 S/N 017-001-00544-4.

33. Wipfli H, Samet JM. Global economic and health benefits of tobacco control: part 2. Clinical Pharmacology & Therapeutics 2009; 86(3): 272–280.

34. Samet JM, Wipfli HL. Ending the tobacco epidemic: from the genetic to the global level. In Sommer M, Parker R, eds. Structural Approaches in Public Health. New York: Routledge, 2013.

35. National Cancer Institute. The Role of the Media in Promoting and Reducing Tobacco Use. Smoking and Tobacco Control Monograph no. 19. Bethesda, MD: US Department of Health and Human Services, National Institutes of Health, National Cancer Institute, 2008.

36. World Health Organization. WHO Framework Convention on Tobacco Control (FCTC) (cited 28 August 2012). Available from: http://www.who.int/fctc/en/index.html, accessed 11 May 2015.

37. US Department of Health and Human Services. The Health Consequences of Involuntary Smoking. A Report of the Surgeon General. Washington, DC: US Department of Health and Human Services, Public Health Service, Office on Smoking and Health, 1986 -32676. Report No.: DHHS Publication No. (CDC) 87-8398.

38. Frieden TR, Mostashari F, Kerker BD, Miller N, Hajat A et al. Adult tobacco use levels after intensive tobacco control measures: New York City, 2002–2003. American Journal of Public Health 2005; 95(6): 1016–1023.

39. Samet JM, Wipfli HL. Globe still in grip of addiction. Nature 2010; 463(7284): 1020–1021.

40. World Health Organization. WHO Report on the Global Tobacco Epidemic, 2008: The MPOWER package. Geneva: World Health Organization, 2008.

41. World Health Organization. WHO Report on the Global Tobacco Epidemic, 2011: Warning about the Dangers of Tobacco. Geneva: World Health Organization, 2011.

42. Parsons A, Daley A, Begh R, Aveyard P. Influence of smoking cessation after diagnosis of early stage lung cancer on prognosis: systematic review of observational studies with meta-analysis. British Medical Journal 2010; 340: b5569.

43. Warren GW, Kasza KA, Reid ME, Cummings KM, Marshall JR. Smoking at diagnosis and survival in cancer patients. International Journal of Cancer 2012; 132(2): 401–410.

44. Peters EN, Torres E, Toll BA, Cummings KM, Gritz ER et al. Tobacco assessment in actively accruing national cancer institute cooperative group program clinical trials. Journal of Clinical Oncology 2012; 30(23): 2869–2875.

45. Underwood JM, Townsend JS, Stewart SL, Buchannan N, Ekwueme DU et al. Surveillance of demographic characteristics and health behaviors among adult cancer survivors: Behavioral Risk Factor Surveillance System, United States, 2009. MMWR Surveillance Summary 2012; 61(1): 1–23.

46. US Preventive Services Task Force. Counseling and Interventions to Prevent Tobacco Use and Tobacco-Caused Disease in Adults and Pregnant Women: Reaffirmation Recommendation Statement. Rockville: Agency for Healthcare Research and Quality; April 2009. Available from: http://www.uspreventiveservicestaskforce.org/uspstf09/tobacco/tobaccors2.htm, accessed 11 May 2015.

47. Zon RT, Goss E, Vogel VG, Chlebowski RT, Jatoi I et al. American Society of Clinical Oncology policy statement: the role of the oncologist in cancer prevention and risk assessment. Journal of Clinical Oncology 2009; 27(6): 986–993.

CHAPTER 15

Viruses

Chris Boshoff

Introduction to viruses

Viral infection accounts for 15% of all human cancers. Seven viruses are known to be implicated in human malignancy (Table 15.1). The immune system is crucial in controlling oncogenic virus-infected cells, as is exemplified by the increased incidence of virus-induced cancers in immunosuppressed individuals. Oncogenesis is a multifactorial process and only a fraction of infected individuals will develop a tumour, particularly in the absence of immunosuppression. Tumour viruses establish long-term persistent infections in humans, with malignancy an accidental side effect of viral replication.

Animal and human oncogenic viruses have played crucial roles in our understanding of cancer biology. In particular, the discoveries of both oncogenes and tumour suppressor genes were made possible by studying animal oncogenic viruses. The discovery of the Rous sarcoma virus in 1911, an avian retrovirus, and other animal oncoviruses led to the eventual discovery of viral oncogenes (e.g. src, ras, and myc), and subsequently a plethora of human proto-oncogenes. The tumour suppressor protein p53 was discovered by studying the oncogenic functions of simian virus large T antigen (SV40-T). SV40-T interacts and abrogates the activity of p53, resulting in uncontrolled cellular proliferation.

Herpesviruses

Over 100 herpesviruses have been identified. Herpesviruses share a common virion architecture and become latent and persist for life in their hosts. They are large (100–140 kbp) DNA viruses with circular, double-stranded genomes. Latent viral genomes take the form of circular episomes.

Epstein Barr virus (EBV)

EBV is the prototype of gammaherpesviruses. In vitro, EBV infection of primary B lymphocytes induces transformation into permanent cell lines (lymphoblastoid cell lines, LCLs).

EBV-infected B lymphocytes are highly immunogenic and elicit powerful cytotoxic T-lymphocyte (CTL) responses. EBV-specific CTLs target human leukocyte antigen (HLA) class 1-associated peptides derived from the EBV latent proteins.

Although EBV is a highly transforming virus, only a small number of EBV-infected individuals develop an EBV-driven neoplasm, and despite the targeting of EBV-infected B cells by CD8+T-lymphocytes, EBV persists in B-lymphocytes. These two apparent paradoxes are explained by the down-regulation of all growth-promoting viral proteins, which include those known to elicit CTL responses in persistently infected B-lymphocytes. Only EBNA-1 (EBV nuclear antigen 1) is expressed in these cells. EBNA-1 is essential to maintain the stability of the viral episome, does not evoke an immune response, and does not induce cell proliferation.

Burkitt's lymphoma (BL)

The recognition of BL and of its associations with malaria and EBV infection is one of the great achievements of twentieth-century medicine. Post-World War II, the Irish surgeon Denis Burkitt studied a peculiar lymphoma common in African children, with a specific geographical distribution. His lecture tours brought him into contact with Anthony Epstein who suspected an infective agent was the culprit. Epstein used electron microscopy to discover EBV.

Only EBNA-1 is expressed in BL cells. These cells thus represent the resting persistently infected B cells in the circulation. However, BL cells are in cell cycle and rapidly proliferating due to the universally present translocation of the c-myc gene. This translocation brings c-myc under the control of an immunoglobulin enhancer. This translocation induces resting EBNA-1-expressing B cells to proliferate.

Nasopharyngeal carcinoma (NPC)

EBV enters epithelial cells from permissively infected lymphocytes trafficking through lymphoid-rich epithelium. The establishment of infection in epithelial cells could be the trigger for NPC development. EBV latent membrane protein-1 (LMP-1) is expressed in NPC and induces NF-κB, and consequently cell proliferation. Epidemiological data indicate that consumption of large quantities of salted fish (e.g., in South East China) is a co-factor.

Hodgkin disease (HD)

The finding of clonal EBV genomes in Reed–Sternberg cells and the restricted pattern of latent viral gene expression in nearly 30–50% of all HD cases suggest that EBV is not simply a passenger in HD. A positive association between a history of infectious mononucleosis and subsequent HD further supports a causal role.

Post-transplant lymphoproliferative disorder (PTLD)

PTLD represents one of the most common complications of immunosuppression following organ transplantation. Predisposing factors include primary EBV infection at or postdating transplantation, and high cumulative doses of immunosuppressive drugs.

Table 15.1 Infection and human cancer

Year when association with cancer was first established, or pathogen discovered	Discoverer/s	Agent	Viral Transcript involved in oncogenesis/ mechanism of oncogenesis	Neoplasm
1964	Epstein, Achong, Barr	Epstein–Barr virus	EBNA1-6 Latent membrane proteins (LMPs) Viral microRNAs	Burkitt's lymphoma, Hodgkin's disease, HIV-related lymphoma, Post-transplant lymphoproliferative disease, Nasopharyngeal carcinoma, *Leiomyosarcoma
1967–1968	**Blumberg, Okochi, Prince, Vierrucci	Hepatitis B virus	Hepatocyte regeneration	Hepatocellular carcinoma
1980	Gallo	Human T-cell leukaemia virus 1	Tax	T-cell leukaemia/lymphoma
1983	Zur Hausen	Human papillomavirus	E6, E7	Cervical and vulvar carcinoma, Anal carcinoma, Penile carcinoma, Oropharyngeal carcinoma
1989	Houghton	Hepatitis C virus	Hepatocyte regeneration	Hepatocellular carcinoma
1994	Chang and Moore	Kaposi's sarcoma-associated herpesvirus	viral cyclin LANA viral FLIP viral microRNAs	Kaposi's sarcoma, Multicentric Castleman's disease, Primary effusion lymphoma
2008	Chang and Moore	Merkel cell polyomavirus	Large T, Small T	Merkel cell carcinoma

*HIV-infected children with EBV positive leiomyosarcoma have been described.

**Between 1967-1968, Blumberg, Okochi, Prince, and Vierrucci reported that the Australian antigen is involved in the development of hepatitis B.

EBV+ lymphoproliferative disorders also occur in congenital immunodeficiencies, for example X-linked lymphoproliferative syndrome. Phenotypically, PTLD resembles in vitro transformed B lymphocytes, i.e. LCLs, where the tumour cells express all the latent viral proteins. Tumour cells are able to proliferate due to a lack of CTL responses in the immunocompromised host.

CD20 is frequently expressed on the tumour cells and immunotherapy against this antigen (e.g., anti-CD20 antibody rituximab) is an effective treatment option. Treatment also includes the infusion of EBV-specific CTLs.

AIDS-associated lymphomas

Up to 50% of HIV-related systemic lymphomas and 100% of brain lymphomas contain EBV DNA. PCR detection of EBV in the cerebrospinal fluid helps in the differential diagnosis of CNS lesions in HIV-infected individuals.

Kaposi's sarcoma-associated herpesvirus (KSHV)

For over 100 years, Kaposi's sarcoma (KS) remained a rare curiosity, until it emerged as a defining feature of the acquired immunodeficiency syndrome (AIDS). In 1872, the Hungarian dermatologist Moriz Kaposi published case histories of male patients in Vienna with *idiopathic multiple pigmented sarcomas* of the skin. *Classic KS* occurs predominantly in elderly male patients of Southern and East European ancestry. In some equatorial African countries, KS existed prior to HIV (*endemic KS*).

KS can develop after organ transplantation (*post-transplant or iatrogenic KS*). In 1981, two rare diseases in young men, KS and *Pneumocystis carinii* pneumonia, heralded the AIDS pandemic and *AIDS-KS* is today the most common form of KS.

Chang and colleagues [1] employed molecular techniques to identify sequences of a new herpesvirus (KSHV, or human herpesvirus-8 (HHV-8)) in AIDS-KS biopsies.

Kaposi's sarcoma (KS)

KSHV DNA is present in all four epidemiological forms of KS. Seroepidemiological surveys show that general populations at risk of developing KS have a higher prevalence of KSHV infection (Figure 15.1).

KSHV infects endothelial cells, and KSHV-encoded proteins provide a growth advantage to these cells and facilitate their escape from host immune responses. KSHV induces cytokines and other inflammatory molecules in the tumour microenvironment, promoting cell proliferation and angiogenesis.

The introduction of anti-HIV therapy has led to a decline in the incidence of AIDS-KS and also in the resolution of KS in those

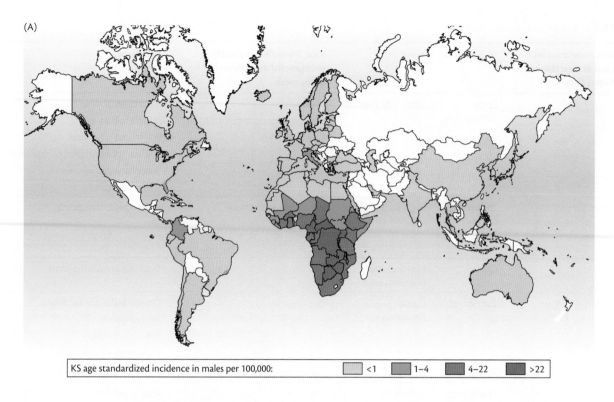

KS age standardized incidence in males per 100,000: □ <1 □ 1–4 □ 4–22 □ >22

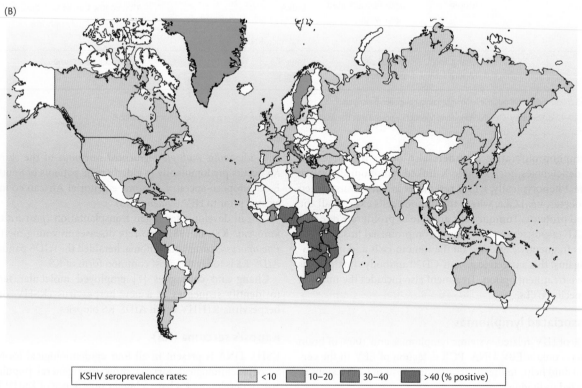

KSHV seroprevalence rates: □ <10 □ 10–20 □ 30–40 □ >40 (% positive)

Fig. 15.1 Geographical prevalence of KS and seroprevalence of KSHV. (A) The standardized incidence of Kaposi's sarcoma (KS) is depicted for males. (B) KSHV seroprevalence rates were compiled from multiple studies.

Reprinted by permission from Macmillan Publishers Ltd: *Nature Reviews Cancer*, Volume 10, Issue 10, pp. 707–719, EA Mesri, E Cesarman, C Boshoff, Kaposi's sarcoma and its associated herpesvirus, Copyright © 2010.

already affected. This indicates that cellular immune responses are important in the control of KSHV infection and in KS pathogenesis. Post-transplant KS also regresses when immunosuppression is discontinued.

Multicentric Castleman's Disease (MCD)

MCD is a lymphoproliferative disorder associated with multiple organ involvement, especially spleen and lymph nodes with weight loss and fever. MCD is mostly diagnosed in HIV-infected individuals and is associated with increased circulating IL6 levels. KSHV DNA is found in up to 50% of MCD cases. Treatment includes cytotoxics, anti-CD20, or anti-IL6 antibody therapies.

Papillomaviruses (HPV)

The papillomaviruses are small (~8 kbp) DNA viruses with circular, double-stranded genomes. Over 100 distinct HPVs have been identified to date. The majority of infections result in a benign tumours (warts). Cells are usually infected at the terminal stages of epithelial cell differentiation and lysed, so virus-induced proliferation is self-limiting and does not progress to transformation. However, a number of HPV types (oncogenic subtypes) can induce cancer.

An infectious aetiology for cervical cancer was suggested by the observation that the most important risk factor is the number of sexual partners. Zur Hausen first hypothesized that this malignancy is caused by HPV, and in 1983 he and colleagues identified HPV sequences in this tumour. HPV-16 is found in nearly 60% and HPV-18 in 20% of cervical cancers. Other HPV types are also associated with cervical cancer.

A key step in cervical cancer progression is the accidental integration of viral DNA sequences into the genome of cells in the basal layer, i.e. the cells in which papillomaviruses normally persist. As a result, as the cells move upwards from the basal layer to the surface, replication to new virions can no longer occur, and progress of the virus infectious cycle has been interrupted. Integrated viral DNA retains the capacity to express HPV early genes (E6 and E7) which directly drive cellular proliferation. Secondary somatic genetic changes occurring in these latently infected cells give rise to malignancy.

Some HPV types (e.g., 16, 18, 31, and 33) are termed high risk because they are found in lesions that progress to malignancy. Other types, such as 6 and 11, are termed low risk, only rarely giving rise to tumours. E6 and E7 abrogate the activities of the tumour suppressor proteins P53 and pRb, respectively. Cells from a particular aggressive cervical cancer removed in 1951 (named HeLa cells after the patient **H**enrietta **La**cks) became a common source of human cancer cells. After decades of HeLa cells growing in laboratories, these cells remain dependent on HPV-18 E6 and E7 expression (i.e. oncogene addiction).

The implementation of a successful vaccine against the high-risk HPV types is poised to transform the incidence of cervical cancer and also the increasing incidence of HPV-associated oral cancer.

Human T-cell leukaemia virus 1 (HTLV-1)

In 1977 it was reported that a range of certain T-cell leukaemias in Japanese patients can be described as one syndrome: adult T-cell leukaemia (ATL)/lymphoma. Gallo and colleagues [2] discovered a virus with reverse transcriptase activity from a T-cell lymphoma cell line. This was the first isolated human retrovirus and therefore termed HTLV-1. Hinuma (1982) and colleagues demonstrated that retrovirus particles from an ATL cell line are identical to HTLV-1. Epidemiological studies showed that HTLV-1 and ATL co-localize in Japan, coastal regions of central Africa, in the Caribbean basin and in Taiwan.

HTLV-1 is transmitted from mother to child, either via infected maternal T lymphocytes across the placenta or via breast milk. HTLV-1 is also transmitted sexually or through blood products. Up to 6% of those infected develop ATL. The incubation period between infection and malignancy is 20–40 years, indicating that additional secondary somatic mutations are required. In vitro, HTLV-1 immortalizes and transforms primary human T lymphocytes.

HTLV-1 is a typical retrovirus: two copies of an RNA genome of 9000 nucleotides encode the *gag*, *pol*, and *env* genes surrounded by short terminal repeat sequences. One region of the HTLV-1 provirus encodes two additional genes expressing the proteins Tax and Rex. Tax is a transcriptional activator, promoting the transcription of viral and cellular proteins involved in cell proliferation including IL2 and IL2 receptor, both of which are required to initiate T-cell division, PDGF, and NF-κB. Tax is the principle oncogene involved in oncogenesis.

Adult T-cell leukaemia (ATL) is a malignant proliferation of CD4+T cells with high expression of the IL2 receptor. Circulating antibodies to HTLV-1 are present in >90% of patients and their spouses. Skin involvement, lymphadenopathy, hepatosplenomegaly, hypercalcaemia and lytic bone lesions are frequent. Few patients survive >6 months.

HTLV-1-infected tumour cells are clonal and each cell in the transformed lymphocyte clone contains virus integrated into the same site; however, this site varies from patient to patient. This indicates that HTLV-1 does not initiate malignancy by insertional mutagenesis.

There is currently no vaccine against HTLV-1.

Hepatitis B virus (HBV)

HBV belongs to the hepadnavirus group, which includes viruses of woodchucks and squirrels. These agents contain a DNA genome that is partially double-stranded and partially a single strand. The virion core enzymes convert the partially single-stranded DNA to a complete, double-stranded DNA helix. The entire genome is then transcribed, producing an RNA that is a full-length copy of the viral DNA. The longest RNA transcript acts as a template for a reverse transcriptase that is also the DNA polymerase. Reverse transcriptase copies the RNA template into a complementary DNA strand. This viral enzyme is blocked by reverse transcriptase inhibitors, which are currently being used to treat HBV infection.

Today, the most important routes of transmission in the West are through needle sharing among drug users and by sexual transmission. The responses in individuals undergoing a primary infection with HBV vary significantly: mild or subclinical infections being the most common. Up to 10% of adults with HBV infection do not clear the virus, but continue to synthesize viral antigens, developing chronic hepatitis.

Hepatocellular carcinoma (HCC)

The incidence of HCC correlates with the worldwide prevalence of HBV and persistence. The risk of developing liver cancer is 100 to 200 times greater for HBsAg carriers than for non-carriers.

Chronic HBV infection leads to the continuous production of viral antigens and attack of infected cells by the immune system with subsequent liver cell regeneration, and repeated immune attack of newly infected cells. Continuing hepatocyte division leads to an increased risk of mutations. Epidemiological studies indicate that the consumption of food contaminated with the fungus aflatoxin might act synergistically with HBV infection to induce HCC.

A successful recombinant vaccine against HBV was developed in the 1980s. In countries with effective universal vaccination programmes, for example Taiwan, the incidence of HCC has been dramatically reduced.

Hepatitis C virus (HCV)

HCV was first described in 1989. It is estimated that over 170 million people are globally infected. The 2–3% seroprevalence in the UK and USA is towards the lower seropositivity incidence. HCV is a single-strand RNA virus of 9400 bases, associated with acute and chronic hepatitis and liver cirrhosis. Virus replication is dependent on a viral-encoded RNA polymerase, which does not have proofreading capability, resulting in numerous genetic variations of the virus within an infected individual. This impacts both on viral replicative fitness, as well as on the selection of virus resistance to mechanism-based antivirals.

Most patients with haemophilia who were treated with blood products prior to the use of virus-inactivation procedures were infected with HCV. HCV infection is also more common among intravenous drug users.

Hepatocellular carcinoma (HCC)

Compared with HBV or HCV mono-infections, co-infections are associated with a higher risk of HCC. In HBV and HCV low-endemic areas (e.g., Sweden), these viruses play a minor role in the pathogenesis of HCC, compared to alcohol-related cirrhosis. The incubation period between infection and cancer is up to four decades. The high turnover of hepatocytes due to the ongoing cycle of liver injury and regeneration associated with cirrhosis predisposes to somatic mutations and eventual malignancy.

Current therapy for HCV infection includes pegylated interferon, usually co-administered with ribavirin, a nucleoside analogue. More recently, protease inhibitors have been developed, which may cure selected patients. Two viral enzymes, the NS3/4A serine protease and the NS5B RNA-dependent RNA polymerase, are being targeted with small molecules to develop mechanism-based therapeutics. An HCV vaccine is not yet available and may be difficult to develop because of the high variability of viral proteins.

Therapy for HCC includes surgical resection, radiofrequency ablation, transarterial chemoembolization, molecular targeted therapy (e.g., sorafenib), and chemotherapy. Orthotopic liver transplantation offers an effective treatment strategy for HCC, even in the setting of HCV or HBV cirrhosis. HCC recurrence is uncommon after transplant in properly selected patients and disease-specific long-term survival approaches 90%.

Merkel cell polyomavirus (MCV)

Polyomaviruses are small (~5400 base pair), non-enveloped, double-stranded DNA viruses. MCV is genetically related to the African green monkey lymphotropic polyomavirus. MCV encodes characteristic polyomavirus genes including the large T antigen and small T antigen. MCV T antigens have similar features to the T antigens of other polyomaviruses, known oncoproteins, and is expressed in human tumours.

Although MCV is a ubiquitous human virus, its mode of transmission is unclear. In human cancer, Merkel cell carcinoma (MCC), the virus is unable to replicate, because the viral T antigen is mutated, leaving the T antigen unable to initiate the DNA replication needed to propagate the virus. Therefore, MCC can be considered a 'dead-end host' for MCV.

Merkel cell carcinoma (MCC)

This aggressive skin tumour was originally described in 1972. It presents as a painless nodule on the skin, often in the head or neck region, and metastasizes early. Eighty per cent of MCC cases have MCV integrated in a monoclonal pattern, inferring that infection is present in a precursor cell prior to clonal expansion. The tumour usually develops on sun-exposed skin and ultraviolet light could be a co-factor. MCC development is modified by the immune system, as the incidence is increased significantly in immunosuppressed individuals. As with other virus-induced cancers, it is likely that additional somatic mutations act in concert with the viral T antigens to precipitate MCC.

Summary

- Up to 15% of all human cancers are caused by viruses.

- The incubation period between infection and malignancy can be decades.

- Virus-driven malignancies often require co-factors.

- Virus-driven cancers are more common in immunosuppressed individuals.

- Viruses may be either direct (e.g., HPV, EBV, HTLV-1), or indirect (e.g., HCV, HBV) oncogenic agents.

- Patients with cirrhosis resulting from any cause, including HBV or HCV, have a greater risk of developing liver cancer (hepatocellular carcinoma).

- Cervical cancer is one of the most common cancers in sub-Saharan Africa.

- Universal vaccination against HPV and HBV will have a major global impact on cancer incidence.

Glossary

Episomenon: Integrated viral or bacterial circular DNA; DNA element that is not incorporated into the genome.

Insertional mutagenesis: Mutagenesis of DNA by the insertion of one or more bases of DNA (virus or other), e.g., integrating a provirus near a normal cellular proto-oncogene, resulting in activation of the proto-oncogene and cellular transformation.

Latency: Life-long persistence of virus, where only of fraction of viral proteins are expressed; ability of a virus to remain dormant or *latent* within a cell.

Orthotopic: Relating to a tissue transplant grafted into its normal place in the body.

Plasmablast: Pre-terminally differentiated B-cell; precursor of a plasma cell.

Proto-oncogene: Cellular gene that has the ability to induce cellular proliferation and transformation; normal gene that can become an oncogene due to mutations or over-expression.

Reverse transcriptase (or RNA-dependent DNA polymerase): An enzyme (DNA polymerase) that converts or transcribes an RNA template into a complementary DNA strand. For example, the RNA genome of HIV is converted by the HIV-encoded *reverse transcriptase* into virus DNA that integrates into the host genome.

Somatic mutation: DNA alteration or mutation that occurs in the host genome after conception (therefore not a germline mutation).

Transcriptional activator: Protein that binds to DNA and stimulates the activation of nearby genes.

Transform/transformation: Process by which normal cells become malignant or acquire the properties of cancer.

Tumour suppressor protein (or anti-oncogene): A protein that can block cellular transformation, and therefore prevent cancer; loss or mutation of a tumour suppressor protein (e.g., p53) can predispose to cellular transformation.

Virion: Virus particle; virus structure.

Further reading

Beral V, Peterman TA, Berkelman RL, Jaffe, HW. Kaposi's sarcoma among persons with AIDS: a sexually transmitted infection? Lancet 1990; 335: 123–128.

Burkitt DP. A sarcoma involving the jaws in African children. British Journal of Surgery 1958; 197: 218–223.

Castleman B, Iverson L, Menendez VP. Localized mediastinal lymph-node hyperplasia resembling thymoma. Cancer 1956; 9: 822–830.

Chang Y, Cesarman E, Pessin MS, Lee F, Culpepper J et al. Identification of herpesvirus-like DNA sequences in AIDS-associated Kaposi's sarcoma. Science 1994; 266, 1865–1869.

Choo QL, Kuo G, Weiner AJ, Overby LR, Bradley DW et al. Isolation of a cDNA clone derived from a blood-borne non-A, non-B viral hepatitis genome. Science 1989; 244: 359–362.

Epstein M, Achong B, Barr Y. Virus particles in cultured lymphoblasts from Burkitt's lymphoma. Lancet 1964; 1: 702–703.

Feng H, Shuda M, Chang Y, Moore PS. Clonal integration of a polyomavirus in human Merkel cell carcinoma. Science 2008; 319:s 1096–1100.

Frizzera G, Massarelli G, Banks PM, Rosai J. A systemic lymphoproliferative disorder with morphologic features of Castleman's disease. American Journal of Surgical Pathology 1983; 7: 211–231.

Gissmann L, Wolnik L, Ikenberg H, Koldovsky U, Schnürch HG. Human papillomavirus types 6 and 11 DNA sequences in genital and laryngeal papillomas and in some cervical cancers. Proceedings of the National Academy of Sciences USA 1983; 80: 560–563.

Goedert JJ, Cote TR, Virgo P, Scoppa SM, Kingma DW et al. Spectrum of AIDS-associated malignant disorders. The Lancet 1998; 351: 1833–1839.

Heslop HE, Rooney CM. Adoptive cellular immunotherapy for EBV lymphoproliferative diseases. Immunological Reviews 1997; 157: 217–222.

Kaposi, M. Idiopathisches multiples pigmentsarcom der haut. Archiv für Dermatologie und Syphilis 1872; 4: 265–273.

Klein, G. Epstein–Barr virus strategy in normal and neoplastic B cells. Cell 1994; 77, 791–793.

Kuehnle I, Huls MH, Liu Z, Semmelmann K, Krance RA et al. CD20 monoclonal antibody (rituximab) for therapy of Epstein–Barr virus lymphoma after hemapoietic stem-cell transplantation. Blood 2000; 95: 1502–1505.

Lane DP, Crawford LV. T antigen is bound to a host protein in SV40-transformed cells. Nature 1979; 278: 261–263.

Linzer DIH, Levine AJ. Characterization of a 54K dalton cellular SV40 tumor antigen present in SV40-transformed cells and uninfected embryonal carcinoma cells. Cell 1979; 17: 43–52

Manolov G, Manolova Y. Marker band in one chromosome 14 from Burkitt lymphoma. Nature 1972; 237: 33–34.

Mesri EA, Cesarman E, Boshoff C. Kaposi's sarcoma and its associated herpesvirus. Nature Reviews Cancer 2010; 10, 707–719

Poiesz BJ, Ruscetti FW, Gazdar AF, Bunn PA, Minna JD et al. Detection and isolation of type C retrovirus particles from fresh and cultured lymphocytes of a patient with cutaneous T-cell lymphoma. Proceedings of the National Academy of Sciences USA 1980; 77, 7415–7419.

Rickinson AB, Moss DJ. Human cytotoxic T lymphocyte responses to Epstein–Barr virus infection. Annual Review of Immunology 1997; 15: 405–431.

Rosenberg N, Jolicoeur P. Retroviral pathogenesis. In Coffin JM, Hughes SH, Varmus HE, eds. Retroviruses. Cold Spring Harbor, NY: Cold Spring Harbor Laboratory Press, 1997, 475–585.

Service PH. Kaposi's sarcoma and pneumocystis pneumonia among homosexual men in New York City and California. MMWR 1981; 30: 305–308.

Sitas F, Carrara H, Beral V, Newton R, Reeves G et al. Antibodies against human herpesvirus-8 in black South African patients with cancer. New England Journal of Medicine 1999; 340: 1863–1871.

Soulier J, Grollet L, Oksenhendler E, Cacoub P, Cazals Hatem D et al. Kaposi's sarcoma-associated herpesvirus-like DNA sequences in multicentric Castleman's disease. Blood 1995; 86: 1276–1280.

Yates JL, Warren N, Sugden B. Stable replication of plasmids derived from Epstein–Barr virus in various mammalian cells. Nature 1985; 313: 812–815.

Yoshida M, Miyoshi I, Hinuma Y. A retrovirus from human leukemia cell lines: its isolation, characterization, and implication in human adult T-cell leukemia (ATL). Princess Takamatsu Symposium 1982; 12: 285–294.

Yu MC, Huang TB, Henderson BE. Diet and nasopharyngeal carcinoma: a case control study in Guangzhou, China. International Journal of Cancer 1989; 43: 1088–1094.

References

1. Chang Y, Cesarman E, Pessin MS, Lee F, Culpepper J et al. Identification of herpesvirus-like DNA sequences in AIDS-associated Kaposi's sarcoma. Science 1994; 266, 1865–1869.
2. Poiesz BJ, Ruscetti FW, Gazdar AF, Bunn PA, Minna JD et al. Detection and isolation of type C retrovirus particles from fresh and cultured lymphocytes of a patient with cutaneous T-cell lymphoma. Proceedings of the National Academy of Sciences USA 1980; 77, 7415–7419.

CHAPTER 16

Chemical carcinogens

Paula A. Oliveira

Introduction to chemical carcinogens

The word carcinogenic was initially defined as the ability of a compound to unchain the process of cancer development in man and animals under suitable conditions, by acting on one or several organs or tissues [1]. With the discovery of the diverse mechanisms implicated in carcinogenesis, this description is now incomplete [2]. From an experimental point of view, a chemical compound is considered carcinogenic when its administration to laboratory animals induces a statistically significant increase in the incidence of one or more histological types of neoplasia, compared with the animals in the control group which were not exposed to the compound [3]. Humans can be exposed to chemical carcinogens when they are present in food, air, water, their workplace, etc. Chemical carcinogens can be classified as natural chemicals, synthetic compounds, or mixtures of both that are synthesized or used for industrial, agricultural, or commercial purposes. According to Irigaray and Belpomme [4] chemical carcinogens should be classed as either chemicals of endogenous origin, i.e. chemicals that result from human/animal natural metabolic intermediates, or exogenous chemicals. These authors also consider exogenous chemicals to be more prone to causing cancer than endogenous natural molecules. Only exogenous chemicals will be considered in this chapter, since exogenous chemical carcinogens may be the major contributors to human cancer.

Exogenous chemical carcinogenesis is a very complex multifactorial process throughout which gene–environment interactions involving exposure to chemical carcinogens and polymorphisms of cancer-susceptibility genes add further complexity. There are currently hundreds of individual chemical compounds shown to induce cancer and many thousands of additional chemical compounds are suspected carcinogens. Despite the fact that many lists of human chemical carcinogens have been published, they differ widely because of the strength of the accepted evidence provided. The problem behind their identification in humans is due to the lengthy latent periods involved (potentially over 20 years) between exposure to these agents and the first appearance of cancer. This chapter is concerned with main types of exogenous chemical carcinogens, how they are classified and their mode of action, absorption and metabolism, as well as the principal tests available for evaluating their carcinogenicity.

A historical perspective on the identification of chemical carcinogens

The history of the identification of chemical carcinogens is based on epidemiologic observations and animal experiments that identified cancer-causing chemicals. Chemical carcinogenesis was first suggested by clinicians some 200 years ago. According to Hayes [5], it was the English surgeon Percivall Pott who in 1775 first documented the causal association between contact to chemical substances and neoplastic development. This author described the incidence of neoplasias in the skin of the scrotum of London chimney sweeps as a result of repeated localized contamination with soot. Also in the eighteenth century, John Hill observed a high percentage of cancerous alterations in the nasal mucosa of snuff users and related it to the localized long-term exposure to snuff. In 1895, Rehn reported a high incidence of urinary bladder cancer in workers in the European dye industry. More recently, observations were made concerning the induction of angiosarcomas in patients exposed to contrast material use for radiological imaging studies [1, 6–10].

Based on these observations, in the early twentieth century several researchers conducted the first experimental studies on chemical carcinogenesis using laboratory animals. The primary investigational work was carried out in 1915 by Katsusaburo Yamagiwa and Koichi Ichikawa [11]. They rubbed rabbits' ears with coal tar and latter observed the development of malignant tumours at the site. These results were used to confirm epidemiologic observations of scrotal and nasal mucosa tumours by Pott and Hil,l respectively. In the meantime, other researchers evaluated the effects of several chemical carcinogens on the urinary bladder, liver, kidneys, pancreas, and lungs using laboratory animals. Later, Beremblum and Shubik [12] studied carcinogenesis on the skin of mice. By applying polycyclic aromatic hydrocarbons and croton oil, they described two phases in cancer development: initiation and promotion. For the first time, chemical carcinogens were being classified as initiators and promoters according to their involvement in each phase. In 1954, Foulds [13] individualized a third stage, termed progression, to account for all post-initiation events that occur during carcinogenesis after promotion. The overview of DNA as genetic material by Avery, MacLeod, and McCarthy [14] and the description of the structure of DNA by Watson and Crick [15] showed that DNA was the cellular target for chemical carcinogens and that mutation was the key to understanding mechanisms of cancer development.

The above described experimental studies, allied with epidemiological studies, have shown an apparent relationship between the induction of cancer in humans and rodents and exposure to chemical compounds. However, human life is led under very different circumstances from experimental procedures. While the process of carcinogenesis is analogous between man and animals in experimental situations, the various chemical compounds to which humans are exposed during their lives can modify the speed of cancer development and the occurrence of mutations, the speed of cell growth and the phenotypical expression of the mutated genes. On the other hand, the individual's relative levels of vulnerability and protection mechanisms have their own part to play, which modifies each of the neoplastic stages.

Carcinogenic classification and their mode of action

Carcinogenic classification is by no means consensual [2, 16] and is in most cases based on the carcinogen's mode of action. Since chemical carcinogenesis comprises the three sequential and successive steps—initiation, promotion, and progression—according to the involvement of carcinogenic chemicals in each of the steps, several authors classify chemical carcinogens as initiators, promoters and progressors [17, 18].

Tumour initiators are those carcinogenic compounds capable of inducing an initial driving DNA mutation, using numerous mechanisms, in a dividing cell, via direct or indirect mutagenesis, so that an initial clone of mutated cells can emerge [4]. Initiators are chemicals that are DNA reactive, either directly or following metabolic activation. They can induce DNA changes such as interruptions of the DNA chain, errors in DNA repair, or elimination of a base repair. Examples of carcinogenic initiators include alkylating agents, polycyclic aromatic hydrocarbons, aromatic amines, metals (cadmium, chromium and nickel), aflatoxins, and nitrosamines.

Chemical carcinogens classified as promoters accelerate or promote the transformation process when applied repeatedly after initiators. Promoters can also act as initiators at the same time, though promoters are usually not initiators when used in isolation at the same dosage at which they promote. The promoter has to be present for weeks, months, and years in order to be effective and its effectiveness depends on its concentration in the target tissue [19]. Some promoter agents are specific to a particular tissue, but others can act on several tissues at the same time [20, 21]. Promoter compounds do not interact directly with DNA and unchain biological effects without being metabolically activated [19, 20, 22, 23]. They may induce some alterations in initiated cells, such as the alteration of cell-surface sensitivity to various growth factors, alteration of cell-surface glycoproteins and glycolipids, alteration of cell morphology, increased phospholipid and glucose metabolism, stimulation of DNA synthesis and cell proliferation, increased production of free oxygen radicals, the induction of disproportionate DNA replication within one cell cycle via gene amplification, and preventing apoptosis [4, 18]. Initiators require the application of promoters to induce cancer development in experimental models. However, in studies of chemical carcinogenesis with prolonged exposure and using high doses, almost all promoter agents induced neoplasias without the prior application of initiators [3, 24]. Examples of this are exposure to phenobarbital, benzene, and asbestos, which, even without the previous use of initiator agents, lead to neoplastic development [25, 26]. The following are some examples of chemical carcinogens classified as promoters: diethylstilbesterol, cyclamates, phorbol 12-myristate 13-acetate, and saccharin.

Chemical carcinogens can also be classified as progressors. These agents are chemical compounds that move mutated cells on from the promotion to progression phase, i.e. they enable premalignant mutated cells irreversibly to obtain the phenotype of fully malignant cells. Progressor agents include alkylating agents, arsenic salts, asbestos, and benzene [4, 17]. Complete carcinogens are capable of triggering all three stages of carcinogenesis.

Other authors classify chemical carcinogens according to the function of their mechanisms of action, and according to their involvement with DNA as being genotoxic and non-genotoxic (mitogenic and cytogenic) [7, 19, 23, 27, 28]. Genotoxic carcinogens are chemicals, or their metabolites, that have the capacity to directly react, or interact with DNA or genetic material to generate DNA adducts and subsequently mutations, chromosomal aberrations, and/or changes in chromosome number [29, 30]. They exhibit a direct analogy among their structure and activity, are mutagenic in in vitro assays, are active in high doses, and could affect various animal species and injure diverse organs [3, 28, 31]. DNA adducts are covalent bonds established with macromolecules, and if not removed prior to DNA replication, these adducts can result in mutations. If such mutations occur in critical oncogenes or the tumour suppressor genes that control cell proliferation, cancer development may follow [32]. Adduct repair is coordinated by numerous enzymes and is controlled by different genes. It can be done via the excision of bases, or nucleotides, recombined repair or mismatched repair and direct-damage reversal [33–36]. The detection of adducts suggests that chemical carcinogens were absorbed, metabolized, and distributed by tissues, thus fleeing from the body's detoxification and repair mechanisms [8, 37, 38]. Adduct detection can be done by techniques such as immunohistochemistry, immunoassays with ^{32}P, gaseous chromatography associated with mass spectrometry, and HPLC associated with fluorescent spectroscopy [39].

Non-genotoxic carcinogens have been shown to act as promoters and do not require metabolic activation. Little is known about this group of carcinogens but evidence from known non-genotoxic carcinogens suggests that in a high proportion multiple pathways need to be changed for cancer induction to occur [40]. As their name implies, they do not react directly with DNA, do not raise adducts, and are negative on mutagenicity tests carried out in in vivo and in in vitro studies, while genotoxic events may occur but are secondary to another biological activity [19, 28, 23, 30, 41]. Non-genotoxic carcinogens have a huge diversity of mechanisms of cancer induction including receptor-mediated endocrine modulation, non-receptor mediated endocrine modulation, tumour promotion, induction of tissue-specific toxicity and inflammatory responses, immunosuppressants, and gap-junction intercellular communication inhibitors. The diversity of modes of action for each non-genotoxic carcinogen, their tissue specificity, and their lack of genotoxicity makes their detection and description very difficult [40]. Non-genotoxic compounds potentiate the effects of genotoxic compounds, do not demonstrate a direct association among structure and activity, and their action is conditioned by their concentration. They are tissue- and species-specific [2, 25, 28, 33, 42]. Non-genotoxic carcinogens are classified as mitogenic and cytotoxic in regard to whether their activity is mediated by a receptor or not [2, 43, 44]. Mitogenic compounds induce cell proliferation in target tissues through interaction with a precise cellular receptor [44]. Cytotoxic carcinogens cause cell death in vulnerable tissues followed by compensatory hyperplasia [19, 28, 45]. The more nearby cells augment the number of cell divisions through regenerative events, the more likely it is that they will end up being prematurely recruited for the cell cycle and that the time available for DNA repair will be inferior—this increases the probability of mutations occurring [25, 43]. On the other hand, necrotized cells are destroyed by the immune system and endogenous chemicals such as reactive oxygen species (ROS), reactive nitrogen species (RNS), and proteolytic enzymes are produced [18, 46, 47]. When production of these ROS and RNS exceeds the cellular anti-oxidant capacity, it may cause lipid peroxidation, oxidative DNA damage, oxidative damage to RNA, oxidative damage to proteins, and DNA mutations [18]. Mitogenic compounds should be present in adequate concentrations in order to promote their action. In contrast, the action of cytotoxic compounds is independent of their concentrations [2, 19].

In 2004, Bolt et al. [16] suggested the separation of genotoxic compounds into two groups: those which react with DNA, and those which are genotoxic at a chromosomal level. Compounds which react with DNA are subdivided into three different groups: initiators (with unlimited doses), borderline, and weak genotoxic (they act via a secondary mechanisms). In 2006, Butterworth [29] classified chemical compounds that can act on chromosomal structure and induce aneuploidy and changes in chromosome number as clastogenic. Since then, DNA damage at the chromosome level is being studied as an essential part of chemical carcinogenesis [48]. In 2011, Cohen and Arnold [49] suggested a refinement of chemical carcinogen classification into those chemicals that increase the risk of cancer that are non-DNA reactive and do so by increasing the number of DNA replications in the target cell population (increased cell proliferation) and those chemicals that are DNA reactive. According to these authors, this classification allows us to make the distinction between classes of chemicals based on their ability to generate DNA reactivity. To this day, this is the basis for the classification of chemical carcinogens and forms the basis for the distinction of potential risks to humans in regulatory decision-making.

According to their chemical structure chemical carcinogens can be classified as polycyclic aromatic hydrocarbons, alkylating agents, aromatic amines/amides, aminoazo dyes, carbamates, halogenated compounds, natural carcinogens, metalloids and hormones. In Table 16.1 they are brought together under the following headings: group, compound, mechanism of action, and affected organs/cancer type.

Table 16.1 Chemical carcinogenic agents

Group	Compounds	Major origins	Mechanism of action	Affected organs/ Cancer type
Polycyclic aromatic hydrocarbons	Benzo[a]pyrene [50]	Charcoal broiled foods Cigarette smoke	DNA adducts	Skin, lungs, stomach
	Dimethylbenz[a]anthracene [31]	Diesel exhaust Residential heating	DNA adducts	Liver, skin
Alkylating agents	Nitrosamides (N-ethyl-N-nitrosurea; N-methyl-N-nitrosurea; N-methyl-N-nitro-N-nitrosoguanidine) [51]	Chemical solvents	DNA adducts, methylation and ethylation reactions	Liver, lungs, kidneys, brain
	Nitrogen mustards (chlorambucil, cyclophosphamide) [31]	Cancer chemotherapy	DNA adducts, DNA strand breaks, DNA alkylation	Leukaemia Nasal tumors
	Ethylene oxide; propylene oxide vinyl chloride [52]		DNA adducts	Liver tumours, lung tumours, tumours from the hematopoetic system
Aromatic amines/amides	Aniline dyes, 2-naphthylamine, benzidine, 2-acetylaminofluorene [53]	Oil refining, synthetic polymers, dyes, adhesives and rubbers, pharmaceuticals, pesticides, explosives, cigarette smoke, hair dyes, diesel exhaust, burning/pyrolysis of protein-rich vegetable matter	DNA adducts	Liver, urinary bladder
	4-Aminobiphenyl [31]	Industrial exposition, cigarette smoke	DNA adducts	Urinary bladder
Aminoazo dyes	o-Aminoazotoluene; N,N-dimethyl-4-aminoazobenzene [54]	Dyes and pigments	Adducts with DNA and haemoglobin	Liver, lungs, urinary bladder Lungs, liver
Carbamates	N-methylcarbamate esters: propoxur [55]	Insecticides	Chromosome aberration, gene mutation, cell transformation	Experimental results showed liver, kidneys and testes degeneration
Halogenated compounds	Trichloroethylene, methylene chloride, chloroform, chloroisoprene, trichlorobenzene [56]	Industry involved in the production of polymers, pesticides, and fire retardants	Somatic mutations, modification of cell cycle pathways	Experimental results showed kidney, liver and lung cancer

(continued)

Table 16.1 Continued

Group	Compounds	Major origins	Mechanism of action	Affected organs/Cancer type
Natural carcinogens	Aflatoxin B1 [57]	Food contamination (grains, nuts, peanut butter) by *Aspergillus flavus*	Forms adducts with guanine, react with RNA and proteins	Liver cancer
	Asbestos [31]	Environmental media (air, water and soil); human activities (product manufacture, construction activities and transport)	Mutagenecity	Mesothelioma, lung cancer
	Ptaquiloside [58]	*Pteridium aquilinum*	DNA adducts	Urinary bladder
Metals	Arsenic [59, 60]	Natural and anthropogenic sources (drinking water, gold mining activities, etc.)	Cell cycle checkpoint dysregulation, DNA damage response, abnormal chromosomal segregation, defects in cell cycle checkpoints, disabled apoptosis, telomere dysfunction, altered chromatin structure	Skin, lungs, liver, lungs, prostate, kidneys, urinary bladder
	Cadmium [59]	Burning of coal and tobacco	Interferes with antioxidant defence mechanisms, inhibit apoptosis	Lungs, nasal cavity, breast
	Nickel [59, 61]	Industrial processes	Oxidative stress, recombination and repair of DNA	Respiratory cancer
	Chromium [62]	Industrial processes	DNA adducts, oxidative DNA damage	Lungs and nasal cavity
Hormones	Ethinyl estradiol [63]	Medicinal exposure	Cell cycle	Uterus and prostate
	Estradiol [64]	Medicinal exposure	Cell cycle	Breast
	Tamoxifen [65]	Medicinal exposure	Cell cycle arrest	Breast
	Estrogen [66]	Medicinal exposure	Cellcycle	Breast cancer, endometrial cancer, ovarian cancer

Absorption and metabolism of chemical carcinogens

Following exposure, chemical carcinogens may be absorbed in a number of ways (ingestion, inhalation, skin absorption, injection, or other possible contamination routes) and distributed across several tissues (Figure 16.1). Absorption depends on the physicochemical properties of the substance. Substances absorbed orally pass through the liver and only then they are distributed in the body; those absorbed in the lungs are distributed by the blood prior to reaching the liver at a later stage [67, 68]. Those chemical carcinogenic compounds classified as direct act directly on DNA, causing mutations and forming DNA adducts without being metabolized. These chemicals are also defined as activation-independent carcinogens and ultimate carcinogens. It has been estimated that approximately 25% of all carcinogens are direct carcinogens [4]. The relative carcinogenic strength of direct-acting carcinogens depends in part on the relative rates of interaction between the chemical and genomic DNA, as well as competing reactions with the chemical and other cellular nucleophiles. The relative carcinogenic activity of direct-acting carcinogens is dependent upon such competing reactions and also on detoxification reactions. Chemical stability, transport, and membrane permeability determine the chemical's carcinogenic activity. Direct carcinogens are typically carcinogenic at multiple sites and in all species examined [69].

On the other hand, most chemical carcinogens, approximately 75% of them, require metabolic activation to be carcinogenic and are labelled as indirect, procarcinogens or indirect-acting genotoxic carcinogens [31, 70]. The terms procarcinogen, proximate carcinogen, and ultimate carcinogen have been coined to classify the parent compound (procarcinogen) and its metabolite form as well as the intermediate (proximate carcinogen) or final form (ultimate carcinogen) that reacts with DNA. The final form of the carcinogen is most likely to be the chemical species that results in mutation and neoplastic transformation. Indirect-acting genotoxic carcinogens usually produce their neoplastic effects, not at the site of exposure (as seen with direct-acting genotoxic carcinogens) but at the target tissue where their metabolic activation occurs. Metabolic activation occurs mainly in the liver at the plain endoplasmic reticulum, where the cytochrome P450 is abundant, and/or in other enzymes located in urothelium, skin, gastrointestinal system, oesophagus, kidneys, and lungs. The final product is an electrophilic compound that directly interacts with proteins, RNA, and DNA to form adducts [71]. The P450 system not only activates chemical carcinogens but also other drugs. Although some of these metabolic processes lead to activation in reactive electrophiles, many actually lead to inactivation of the chemicals by increasing aqueous solubility and leading to their increased excretion either in urine or in faeces [49]. Thus, exposure to any chemical initiates competing metabolic pathways for activation versus inactivation [49, 72]. The

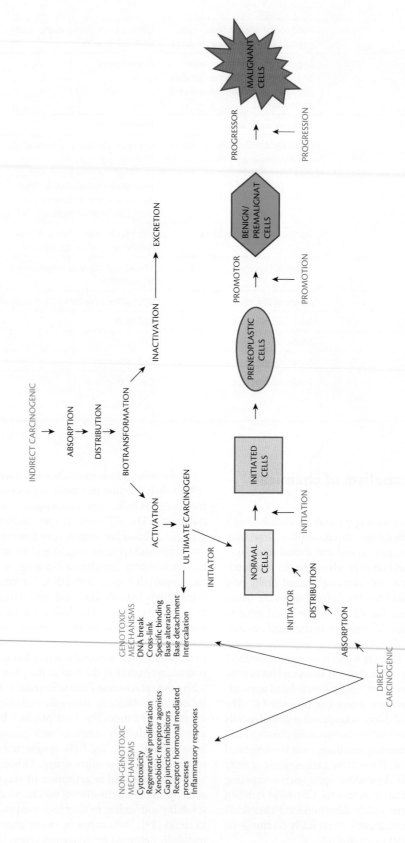

Fig. 16.1 Absorption and metabolism of chemical carcinogens.

specificity of the activation systems of diverse tissues is dependent on genetic polymorphisms, which control the expression and distribution of the P450 enzyme, and the resulting susceptibility to cancer development. Metabolic pathways are equally important for both humans and animals, although qualitative and quantitative differences among them do exist. These have led to incorrect interpretations when animal models are used in the research and analysis of carcinogenic properties of chemical compounds [38, 41, 73].

Testing for carcinogenicity

Experimental assays with animal models and in vitro assays as well as epidemiological studies allow the recognition of carcinogenic chemical compounds and the analysis of many aspects of chemical carcinogenesis.

Animal models

Animal models should reflect the exposure to carcinogens or the genetic predisposition that is present in at-risk humans. In addition, pathological lesions should reflect the molecular changes and histological characteristics seen in human cancers [74]. The standard approach to carcinogenicity testing is to conduct two-year bioassays in small laboratory rodents (rats and/or mice). However, this kind of assay uses large numbers of animals, is time-consuming and expensive and is also fraught with sources of controversy regarding the relevance of the mode of action to humans or the dose used in the study compared with human exposure levels [49, 75]. The uncertainty in the extrapolation of results is particularly high for non-genotoxic carcinogens. This is because non-genotoxic carcinogens are likely to have a dose-response curve that is not linear and that includes a threshold. Furthermore, they could induce cancer in animals via a mechanism that is not applicable to humans. Achieving a positive result in a conventional assay only indicates that there is a potential hazard. Its significance for human health will depend on other factors, several of which need additional studies [76].

In vitro assays

In vitro models can be used to identify and to study chemical carcinogens. In vitro assays use prokaryotic, human, and animal cells, mimic some key stages of in vivo multistep carcinogenesis, measure induction of phenotypical alterations, have differing levels of complexity, and can overcome the ethical aspects related to animal experiments, as well as being faster, more cost-efficient and reduced reliance on animals. In vitro models have been shown to have a good concordance with rodent bioassay results, detecting both genotoxic and non-genotoxic carcinogens [77]. However, we do not have appropriate cell lines available which appropriately mimic the in vivo response, all the metabolic activation and inactivation processes are not maintained in vitro, and current in vitro approaches are unable to address the frequent occurrence of organ interactions that are implicated in many toxic end points. The first test described to evaluate the carcinogenic properties of chemical compounds in vitro was the malignant transformation of Syrian hamster embryo cells [78]. In 1970 the Ames test emerged. This test semi-quantitatively analyses a chemical's capacity to induce mutations in *Salmonella typhimurium* in a culture medium improved by using microsomatic enzymes [79]. Between 70% and 90% of

identified chemical carcinogens showed positive results on the Ames test. Due to the high correlation that exists between mutagenicity and carcinogenicity, the Ames test is currently still used to assess the carcinogenic potential of chemicals.

Epidemiological studies

Global epidemiological studies have identified environmental and occupational chemicals as potential carcinogens. Epidemiological studies are retrospective and unless a big number of individuals are studied their levels of sensitivity is low [80, 81]. Epidemiological advances in the identification of chemical carcinogens are limited for two main reasons. First, only relatively high risks can be detected and, second, epidemiological surveys are based on observations of the effects resulting as a consequence of exposure that took place many years before.

Other methods

Computational approaches for genotoxicity prediction have existed for over two decades. The carcinogenic capacity of a chemical substance can be given using software that thoroughly reproduces man's physiological and metabolic procedures and relates them to the molecular configuration of the substance being evaluated [82, 83]. These chemical characteristics are correlated to the molecular structure of chemical, physical, and toxicological properties [84, 85].

Statistical learning methods have been explored as a new advance in genotoxicity prediction without any restrictions on the features of structures or types of molecules. As an alternative to focusing on specific structural characters or a particular group of related molecules, these methods classify molecules into genotoxic positive or non-genotoxic agents, based on their general structural and physicochemical properties, regardless of their structural and chemical types [86].

Further reading

Bertram JS. The molecular biology of cancer. Molecular Aspects of Medicine 2001, 21: 167–223.

Bolt HM, Foth H, Hengstler JG, Degen GH. Carcinogenicity categorization of chemicals-new aspects to be considered in a European perspective. Toxicology Letters 2004, 151: 29–41.

Butterworth BE, Popp JA, Conolly RB, Goldsworthy TL. Chemically induced cell proliferation in carcinogenesis. IARC Scientific Publications 1992, 116: 279–305.

Butterworth BE. A classification framework and practical guidance for establishing a mode of action for chemical carcinogens. Regulatory Toxicology and Pharmacology 2006, 45: 9–23.

Cohen SM, Arnold LL. Chemical carcinogenesis. Toxicological Sciiences 2011; 120(Suppl. 1): S76–S92.

Hanahan D, Weinberg RA. The hallmarks of cancer. Cell 2000, 100: 57–70.

Irigaray P, Belpomme D. Basic properties and molecular mechanisms of exogenous chemical carcinogens. Carcinogenesis 2010; 31: 135–148.

Klaunig JE, Kamendulis LM, Xu Y. Epigenetic mechanisms of chemical carcinogenesis. Human and Experimental Toxicology 2000, 19: 543–555.

Oliveira PA, Colaço A, Chaves R, Guedes-Pinto H, De la Cruz LF et al. Chemical carcinogenesis. Anais da Academia Brasileira de Ciências 2007; 79: 593–616.

Pogribny IP, Beland FA. DNA methylome alterations in chemical carcinogenesis. Cancer Lett. 2012, doi:pii: S0304–3835[12]00559-9 10.1016/j.canlet.2012.09.010.

References

1. Huff J. Chemicals associated with tumours of the kidney, urinary bladder and thyroid gland in laboratory rodents from 2000 US National Toxicology Program/National Cancer Institute bioassays for carcinogenicity. IARC Scientific Publications 1999; 147: 211–225.

2. Butterworth BE, Bogdanffy MS. A comprehensive approach for integration of toxicity and cancer risk assessments. Regulatory Toxicology and Pharmacology 1999; 29: 23–36.

3. Gutiérrez JB, Salsamendi ALC. Fundamentos de ciencia toxicológica. Madrid: Diaz de Santos, 2001, 155–177.

4. Irigaray P, Belpomme D. Basic properties and molecular mechanisms of exogenous chemical carcinogens. Carcinogenesis 2010; 31: 135–148.

5. Hayes RB. Genetic susceptibility and occupational cancer. Medicina del Lavoro 1995; 86: 206–213.

6. Vajdic CM, McDonald SP, McCredie MR van, Leeuwen MT, Stewart JH et al. Radiation-induced primary liver tumors in 'Thorotrast patients'. Recent Results Cancer Research 1986; 100: 16–22.

7. Cohen SM, Ellwein LB. Genetic errors, cell proliferation, and carcinogenesis. Cancer Research 1991; 51: 6493–6505.

8. Garner RC. The role of DNA adducts in chemical carcinogenesis. Mutation Research 1998; 402: 67–75.

9. Dybdahl M, Frentz G, Vogel U, Wallin H, Nexo BA. Low DNA repair is a risk factor in skin carcinogenesis: a study of basal cell carcinoma in psoriasis patients. Mutation Research 1999; 433: 15–22.

10. Bertram JS. The molecular biology of cancer. Molecular Aspects of Medicine 2001; 21: 167–223.

11. Yamagiwa K, Ichikawa K. Experimental study of the pathogenesis of carcinoma. Journal of Cancer Research 1918; 3: 1–29.

12. Beremblum I, Shubik P. The role of croton oil applications, associated with a single painting of a carcinogen, in tumor induction of the mouse's skin. British Journal of Cancer 1947; 1: 379–382.

13. Foulds L. The experimental study of tumor progression: a review. Cancer Research 1954; 14: 327–339.

14. Avery OT, MacLeod CM, McCarty M. Studies on the chemical nature of the substance inducing transformation of pneumococcal types. Inductions of transformation by a desoxyribonucleic acid fraction isolated from pneumococcus type III. Journal of Experimental Medicine 1979; 149: 297–326.

15. Watson JD, Crick FH. The structure of DNA. Cold Spring Harbor Symposia on Quantitative Biology 1953; 18: 123–131.

16. Bolt HM, Foth H, Hengstler JG, Degen GH. Carcinogenicity categorization of chemicals-new aspects to be considered in a European perspective. Toxicology Letters 2004; 151: 29–41.

17. Hanahan D, Weinberg RA. The hallmarks of cancer. Cell 2000; 100: 57–70.

18. Klaunig JE, Wang Z, Pu X, Zhou S. Oxidative stress and oxidative damage in chemical carcinogenesis. Toxicology and Applied Pharmacology 2011; 254: 86–99.

19. Butterworth BE, Popp JA, Conolly RB, Goldsworthy TL. Chemically induced cell proliferation in carcinogenesis. IARC Scientific Publications 1992; 116: 279–305.

20. Yuspa SH, Hennings H, Lichti U, Kulesz-Martin M. Organ specificity and tumor promotion. Basic Life Sciences 1983; 24: 157–171.

21. Yuspa SH, Poirier MC. Chemical carcinogenesis: from animal models to molecular models in one decade. Advances in Cancer Research 1988; 50: 25–70.

22. Weisburger JH. Worldwide prevention of cancer and other chronic diseases based on knowledge of mechanisms. Mutation Research 1998; 402: 331–337.

23. Williams GM. Mechanisms of chemical carcinogenesis and application to human cancer risk assessment. Toxicology 2001; 161: 3–10.

24. Pitot HC, Dragan YP. Facts and theories concerning the mechanisms of carcinogenesis. FASEB Journal 1991; 5: 2280–2286.

25. Melnick RL, Kohn MC, Portier CJ. Implications for risk assessment of suggested non-genotoxic mechanisms of chemical carcinogenesis. Environmental Health Perspectives 1996; 104: 123–134.

26. Trosko JE. Commentary: is the concept of 'tumor promotion' a useful paradigm? Molecular Carcinogenesis 2001; 30: 131–137.

27. Nguyen-Ba G, Vasseur P. Epigenetic events during the process of cell transformation induced by carcinogens (review). Oncology Reports 1999; 6: 925–932.

28. Klaunig JE, Kamendulis LM, Xu Y. Epigenetic mechanisms of chemical carcinogenesis. Human and Experimental Toxicology 2000; 19: 543–555.

29. Butterworth BE. A classification framework and practical guidance for establishing a mode of action for chemical carcinogens. Regulatory Toxicology and Pharmacology 2006; 45: 9–23.

30. Pogribny IP, Beland FA. DNA methylome alterations in chemical carcinogenesis. Cancer Letters 2012; 334(1): 39–45.

31. Luch A. Nature and nurture: lessons from chemical carcinogenesis. Nature Reviews Cancer 2005; 5: 113–125.

32. Spencer WA, Lehmler HJ, Robertson LW, Gupta RC. Oxidative DNA adducts after Cu(2+)-mediated activation of dihydroxy PCBs: role of reactive oxygen species. Free Radical Biology and Medicine 2009; 46: 1346–1352.

33. Farmer PB. Carcinogen adducts: use in diagnosis and risk assessment. Clinical Chemistry 1994; 40: 1438–1443.

34. Moustacchi E. Molecular mechanisms of carcinogenesis: the role of systems of DNA repair. Bulletin de l'Academie nationale de medecine 1998; 182: 33–46.

35. Miller MC, Mohrenweiser HW, Bell DA. Genetic variability in susceptibility and response to toxicants. Toxicology Letters 2001; 120: 269–280.

36. Hanawalt PC, Ford JM, Lloyd DR. Functional characterization of global genomic DNA repair and its implications for cancer. Mutation Research 2003; 544: 107–114.

37. Airoldi L, Pastorelli R, Magagnotti C, Fanelli R. Carcinogen–DNA adducts as tools in risk assessment. Advances in Experimental Medicine and Biology 1999; 472: 231–240.

38. Guengerich FP. Metabolism of chemical carcinogens. Carcinogenesis 2000; 21: 345–351.

39. Santella RM, Gammon M, Terry M, Senie R, Shen J et al. DNA adducts, DNA repair genotype/phenotype and cancer risk. Mutation Research 2005; 592: 29–35.

40. Hernández LG, van Steeg H, Luijten M, van Benthem J. Mechanisms of non-genotoxic carcinogens and importance of a weight of evidence approach. Mutation Research 2009; 682: 94–109.

41. Gonzalez FJ. The use of gene knockout mice to unravel the mechanisms of toxicity and chemical carcinogenesis. Toxicology Letters 2001; 120: 199–208.

42. Gomes-Carneiro MR, Ribeiro-Pinto LF, Paumgartten FJ. Environmental risk factors for gastric cancer: the toxicologist's standpoint. Cadernos de Saúde Pública 1997; 13(Suppl): 27–38.

43. Cohen SM. Analysis of modifying factors in chemical carcinogenesis. Progress in Experimental Tumor Research 1991; 33: 21–40.

44. Cohen SM, Garland EM, Ellwein LB. Cancer enhancement by cell proliferation. Progress in Clinical and Biological Research 1992; 374: 213–229.

45. Cohen SM, Purtilo DT, Ellwein LB. Ideas in pathology. Pivotal role of increased cell proliferation in human carcinogenesis. Modern Pathology 1991; 4: 371–382.

46. Lutz WK. Dose-response relationships in chemical carcinogenesis: superposition of different mechanisms of action, resulting in linear-nonlinear curves, practical thresholds, J-shapes. Mutation Research 1998; 405: 117–124.

47. Ohshima H, Tazawa H, Sylla BS, Sawa T. Prevention of human cancer by modulation of chronic inflammatory processes. Mutation Research 2005; 591: 110–122.

48. Fenech M. The micronucleus assay determination of chromosomal level DNA damage. Methods in Molecular Biology 2008; 410:185–216.

49. Cohen SM, Arnold LL. Chemical carcinogenesis. Toxicological Sciiences 2011; 120(Suppl. 1): S76–S92.

50. Baan R, Grosse Y, Straif K, Secretan B, El Ghissassi F et al. WHO International Agency for Research on Cancer Monograph Working Group. A review of human carcinogens. Part F: chemical agents and related occupations. Lancet Oncology 2009; 10: 1143–1144.

51. Dietrich M, Block G, Pogoda JM, Buffler P, Hecht S et al. A review: dietary and endogenously formed N-nitroso compounds and risk of childhood brain tumors. Cancer Causes and Control 2005; 16(6): 619–635.

52. Guha N, Loomis D, Grosse Y, Lauby-Secretan B, El Ghissassi F. International Agency for Research on Cancer Monograph Working Group. Carcinogenicity of trichloroethylene, tetrachloroethylene, some other chlorinated solvents, and their metabolites. Lancet Oncology 2012;13:1192–1193.

53. Pinheiro HM, Touraudb E, Thomas O. Aromatic amines from azo dye reduction: status review with emphasis on direct UV spectrophotometric detection in textile industry wastewaters Dyes and Pigments 2004; 61: 121–139.

54. Golka K, Kopps S, Myslak ZW. Carcinogenicity of azo colorants: influence of solubility and bioavailability. Toxicology Letters 2004; 151: 203–210.

55. Wang TC, Chiou CM, Chang YL. Genetic toxicity of N-methylcarbamate insecticides and their N-nitroso derivatives. Mutagenesis 1998; 13: 405–408.

56. Lock EA, Reed CJ, McMillan JM, Oatis JE Jr, Schnellmann RG. Lack of formic acid production in rat hepatocytes and human renal proximal tubule cells exposed to chloral hydrate or trichloroacetic acid. Toxicology 2007; 230: 234–243.

57. Wild CP, Garner RC, Montesano R, Tursi F. Aflatoxin B1 binding to plasma albumin and liver DNA upon chronic administration to rats. Carcinogenesis 1986; 7: 853–858.

58. Gil da Costa R, Bastos M, Oliveira P, Lopes C. Bracken-associated human and animal health hazards: chemical, biological and pathological evidence. Journal of Hazardous Materials 2012; 5(203–204): 1–12.

59. Schmitz-Spanke S, Rettenmeier AW. Protein expression profiling in chemical carcinogenesis: a proteomic-based approach. Proteomics 2011; 11: 644–656.

60. Bhattacharjee P, Banerjee M, Giri AK. Role of genomic instability in arsenic-induced carcinogenicity. A review. Environment International 2013; 53: 29–40.

61. Goodman JE, Prueitt RL, Thakali S, Oller AR. The nickel ion bioavailability model of the carcinogenic potential of nickel-containing substances in the lung. Critical Reviews in Toxicology 2011; 41: 142–174.

62. Nickens KP, Patierno SR, Ceryak S. Chromium genotoxicity: A double-edged sword. Chemico-Biological Interactions 2010; 188: 276–288.

63. Hyder SM, Chiappetta C, Stancel GM. Synthetic estrogen 17alpha-ethinyl estradiol induces pattern of uterine gene expression similar to endogenous estrogen 17beta-estradiol. Journal of Pharmacology and Experimental Therapeutics 1999; 290: 740–747.

64. Russo J, Fernandez SV, Russo PA, Fernbaugh R, Sheriff FS et al. 17-Beta-estradiol induces transformation and tumorigenesis in human breast epithelial cells. FASEB Journal 2006; 20: 1622–1634.

65. King CM. Tamoxifen and the induction of cancer. Carcinogenesis 1995; 16:1449–1454.

66. Singh B, Bhat NK, Bhat HK. Induction of NAD(P)H-quinone oxidoreductase 1 by antioxidants in female ACI rats is associated with decrease in oxidative DNA damage and inhibition of estrogen-induced breast cancer. Carcinogenesis 2012; 33: 156–163.

67. King C, Wang C, Gorelick N, Frederick C. Genotoxicity in the rodent urinary bladder. Food and Chemical Toxicology 1995; 33: 757–769.

68. van Leeuwen IM, Zonneveld C. From exposure to effect: a comparison of modeling approaches to chemical carcinogenesis. Mutation Research 2001; 489:17–45.

69. Klaunig JE and Kamendulis LM. Chemical carcinogens. In Klaassen CD, ed. Toxicology: The Basic Science of Poisons, 7th ed. Columbus, OH: McGraw-Hill 2008, 329–380.

70. Poirier MC, Santella RM, Weston A. Carcinogen macromolecular adducts and their measurement. Carcinogenesis 2000; 21: 353–359.

71. Oda Y. Analysis of the involvement of human N-acetyltransferase 1 in the genotoxic activation of bladder carcinogenic arylamines using a SOS/umu assay system. Mutation Research 2004; 554: 399–406.

72. Park BK, Kitteringham NR, Maggs JL, Pirmohamed M, Williams DP. The role of metabolic activation in drug-induced hepatotoxicity. Annual Review of Pharmacology and Toxicology 2005; 45: 177–202.

73. Gonzalez FJ, Kimura S. Understanding the role of xenobiotic-metabolism in chemical carcinogenesis using gene knock-out mice. Mutation Research 2001; 477: 79–87.

74. Oliveira PA, Colaço A, Chaves R, Guedes-Pinto H, De la Cruz LF et al. Chemical carcinogenesis. Anais da Academia Brasileira de Ciências 2007; 79: 593–616.

75. Huff J. Chemical toxicity and chemical carcinogenesis. Is there a causal connection? A comparative morphological evaluation of 1500 experiments. IARC Scientific Publications 1992; 116: 437–475.

76. Maronpot RR, Boorman GA. The contribution of the mouse in hazard identification studies. Toxicologic Pathology 1996; 24: 726–731.

77. OECD. Detailed review paper on cell transformation assays for detection of chemical carcinogens. OECD Environment, Health and Safety Publications, Series on Testing and Assessment 2007, No. 3: 11–164.

78. Berwald Y, Sachs L. In vitro transformation of normal cells to tumor cells by carcinogenic hydrocarbons. Journal of the National Cancer Institute 1965; 35: 641–661.

79. Ames BN. The detection of environmental mutagens and potential carcinogens. Cancer 1984; 53: 2034–2040.

80. Weinstein IB. Strategies for inhibiting multistage carcinogenesis based on signal transduction pathways. Mutation Research 1988; 202: 413–420.

81. Tennant RW. Evaluation and validation issues in the development of transgenic mouse carcinogenicity bioassays. Environmental Health Perspectives 1998; 106: 473–476.

82. Loew GH, Poulsen M, Kirkjian E, Ferrell J, Sudhindra BS et al. Computer-assisted mechanistic structure-activity studies: application to diverse classes of chemical carcinogens. Environmental Health Perspectives 1985; 61: 69–96.

83. Naven RT, Greene N, Williams RV. Latest advances in computational genotoxicity prediction. Expert Opinion on Drug Metabolism and Toxicology 2012; 8(12): 1579–1587.

84. Barratt MD, Rodford RA. The computational prediction of toxicity. Current Opinion in Chemical Biology 2001; 5: 383–388.

85. Feng J, Lurati L, Ouyang H, Robinson T, Wang Y et al. Predictive toxicology: benchmarking molecular descriptors and statistical methods. Journal of Chemical Information and Computer Sciences 2003; 43: 1463–1470.

86. Li H, Ung CY, Yap CW, Xue Y, Li ZR et al. Prediction of genotoxicity of chemical compounds by statistical learning methods. Chemical Research in Toxicology 2005; 18: 1071–1080.

CHAPTER 17

Radiation-induced cancer

Klaus R. Trott

Introduction to radiation-induced cancer

The first case of a radiation-induced cancer in a radiology technologist who suffered from severe atrophic skin damage (roentgenoderm) was demonstrated in 1904. Since then, ionizing radiations have been established as one possible cause of cancer. Numerous radiologists in the first three decades of the twentieth century developed radiation-induced malignancies: either skin cancers as a consequence of late skin damage or leukaemia. The full extent of the risk of radiation carcinogenesis and its dependence on dose and exposed organ was only assessed after the long-term follow-up studies of the survivors of the A-bombs in Hiroshima and Nagasaki were established.

Molecular mechanisms of radiation carcinogenesis

Radiation-induced DNA damage preferentially causes deletions. Therefore, it is generally assumed that the inactivating mutation of tumour suppressor genes is the most probable mechanism of the induction of cancer by low radiation doses and that a single radiation track traversing the nucleus has a finite probability, albeit very low, of generating the specific DNA damage that results in cancer growth. This hypothesis supports the assumption that cancer risk increases proportionally with radiation dose without threshold [1]. Yet, the conclusion that this mechanism excludes the possibility of a dose threshold has been debated very controversially. Other biological mechanisms such as low-dose hypersensitivity which may specifically eliminate cells harbouring DNA damage, and non-targeted radiation effects such as radiation-induced genomic instability, bystander effects, and immunological surveillance mechanisms may modify the consequences of direct radiation-induced transforming mutations. The complex mechanisms elicited by initial processes continue to be the subject of radiobiological research [2].

The A-bomb survivor lifespan study, cancer mortality, and cancer incidence

The dramatic experience of the people of Hiroshima and Nagasaki in 1945 initiated a programme for life-long follow-up of all A-bomb survivors. This is arguably the largest, most comprehensive, and most detailed epidemiological study ever performed. The results of this study are the main data source on which rules and regulations of radiation protection are based.

The Life Span Study (LLS) comprises 120,321 people, including about 54,000 atomic bomb survivors who were within 2.5 km of the hypocentre at the time of the explosion. Of the study population 52% was still alive in 1999, including >85% of the nearly 50,000 individuals who were children or adolescents in August 1945.

For >90% of the total study population, detailed information was collected by Japanese interviewers on their exact location at the moment of explosion. The dose assessment (called the DS 86) is based on Monte Carlo calculations of track passage from the source in the exploding bomb through the air and the buildings to the body of the individual, calculating mean organ doses for different critical organs.

The most significant long-term health damage observed in the LSS is a dose-dependent increased mortality from cancer [3]. Among the 44,771 deceased members of the LLS cohort with dosimetric information, there were 9335 deaths from cancer and 582 deaths from leukaemia. By analysing the relationship with radiation exposure, it was concluded that until 1997, 440 cancer deaths (4%) and nearly 100 leukaemia deaths (15%) have been attributable to the radiation exposure. Significant dose relationships were found for death from leukaemia and carcinoma of the stomach, colon, lung, breast, oesophagus, bladder, ovary, and liver. Since, at the time of the last analysis nearly 50% of the cohort was still alive, it is not possible to make well-founded statements on the life-time risk of dying for people who were young at the time of exposure.

The publication of cancer incidence data 1958 to 1998 [4] is the most comprehensive and detailed analysis of the late carcinogenic effects of radiation. Of the 17,448 cancer cases observed in this study, 7851 occurred in individuals who had received a dose of >0.005 Gy and thus were considered exposed. Of these 853, i.e. 11%, were attributable to the radiation exposure. For a person aged 70 exposed to 1 Gy at the age of 30, the excess relative risk (ERR) was 0.47 for all cancers combined (0.58 for females and 0.35 for males).

The Chernobyl accident

The Chernobyl accident in 1986 was the most severe accident in the civil use of nuclear energy, so far. In the aftermath, many thousands of rescue workers, called liquidators, who were spread all over the former Soviet Union, were concerned about possible health damage from the radiation they had been exposed to during and after the accident. It was impossible to set up a comprehensive research programme such as after the Hiroshima and Nagasaki bomb explosions which covered all affected people. However, several epidemiological studies have been initiated and continue to provide important information on health consequences which complement the information gathered from the bomb survivors [5]. The liquidator studies as well as studies of populations living in areas of radioactive contamination from accidents and bomb tests will provide important comparisons of radiation risks in people with different background cancer rates and from low dose rate radiation exposure with those in Japanese bomb survivors.

The most important findings in the populations exposed by the Chernobyl accident relate to the massive epidemic of thyroid cancer among the young which, until 2002, has affected nearly 5000 people who were under 17 in 1986. The data could be well fitted to a no-threshold linear dose response relationship with an eightfold increase of risk after 1 Gy thyroid dose. The highest risk was in children under 4 years at exposure. In young adults, the risk was much lower. The Chernobyl thyroid cancer cases provide a unique opportunity for studying specific molecular alterations caused by radiation since >90% of cancers occurring in those born between 1980 and 1986 are radiation-induced, whereas <10% of those occurring in those born after 1987 are radiation-induced. So far, few of the patients have died from thyroid cancer or treatment-related complications; the overall prognosis appears good [5].

Patients treated for benign diseases

Up to the 1960s, more patients were treated with radiotherapy for non-cancer diseases than for cancer. Although the number of indications has been reduced, it is still employed in the treatment of a variety of painful degenerative joint disorders. Doses are less than 10% of those given to treat cancer; results are usually fast and persistent. Some of these treatments are regarded as obsolete today; for example, for conditions such as ankylosing spondylitis pharmacological treatment options are available which are more convenient to doctor and patient. Moreover, some treatments used in the past were associated with a significantly increased risk of leukaemia and cancer [6, 7] analysed the mortality of 14,554 patients irradiated for ankylosing spondylitis between 1935 and 1954. Among the 1582 recorded deaths, the most striking finding was a tenfold increase in fatal leukaemia: 52 patients, compared to five expected. Post-partum mastitis was a very successful indication for low-dose radiotherapy. If irradiated early, one or two 0.5 Gy fractions will abolish the inflammation within a day or two, no abscess develops, no antibiotics or surgery are required, and breast feeding can be resumed quickly. Yet in most countries, this indication for radiotherapy has been abandoned as the extraordinary radiosensitivity of the breast of young women with regard to cancer induction became apparent. Shore et al. [8] studied 601 American women who had been irradiated between 1940 and 1957 for acute post-partum mastitis with a median dose of 3.5 Gy. After a mean follow-up of 30 years, they observed 56 women with breast cancer, whereas according to observation of the patients' sisters, only 32 would have been expected.

These observations led to the recommendation that indication, planning, and performance of radiotherapy for selected non-malignant diseases should be made with the same care as definitive radiotherapy for cancer, limiting field sizes, avoiding critical organs, and reducing radiation to the lowest effective dose.

Radon exposure of hard rock miners or in homes

The publication of a report in 1879 on lung diseases among the miners in Schneeberg (Saxony, Germany) is a milestone in the history of occupational medicine. Härting and Hesse [9] proved that miners working underground died from lung cancer, usually after about 20 years working underground. By cleaning the air by forced ventilation and the introduction of wet drilling, the cancer rate was significantly reduced within ten years. Lung cancer was caused by the exposure of the miners to the radioactive decay products of radon gas which attach to aerosols in the air, and are inhaled and deposited on the bronchial epithelial, irradiating the epithelial stem cells with α-particles.

Several large cohort studies of uranium miners confirmed the early findings. All types of lung cancer are increased in the uranium miners. There is a supra-additive interaction between exposure to radon and cigarette smoking, with silica dust in the mines also contributing to the cancer risk. The results of these studies suggest the possibility that exposure to radon in houses may cause lung cancer in the general population. Radon concentrations in houses vary by orders of magnitude and in some regions with special geological features they can reach values which cause concern. In several European countries and in China large case control studies on the contribution of radon exposure to the lung cancer risk have been performed. In the German study [10], nearly 3000 cases of lung cancer and 4200 controls were investigated. In addition to a comprehensive interrogation, radon concentration measurements were performed in current and previous homes. As expected, the most important risk factor for lung cancer was cigarette smoking. Despite this strong influence of smoking, a clear dependence of relative risk on radon concentration in homes was observed, as was also the case in studies in Finland, Sweden, and the UK. The overall excess lung cancer risk at a radon concentration of 100 Bq/m^3 was 10%. The excess risk from radon was found to exist for smokers as well as for non-smokers, with the risks interacting in a multiplicative way. Up to 10% of all lung cancers may be caused by radon in homes.

Second cancers after cancer therapy

During the typical follow-up period of a patient treated for cancer with radical radiotherapy, many patients will present with a second cancer. The frequency varies between <1% and >10%, depending on age and sex. Results of epidemiological studies demonstrate that after radiotherapy, the increased lifespan of cured patients, and not direct radiation effects, is the most important underlying cause leading to second cancers.

The International Commission on Radiation Protection (ICRP) developed a method to estimate the risk of radiation-induced cancer from the occupational and environmental exposure of workers and the general population which has been also widely used in estimating risk of second cancers after radiotherapy of first cancers. Yet the ICRP [1] strongly advised against using this method to estimate the risks of radiation-induced cancer after radiotherapy since the dose distributions within and between organs are completely different. Second cancer risks estimated this way are orders of magnitude higher than those derived directly from epidemiological investigations on radiotherapy patients. The risk of radiation-induced second cancers should be estimated by the comparison of second cancer rates in patient cohorts who were cured from their first cancer by either radiotherapy or by surgery. This method avoids the influence of competing risks from underlying genetics and lifestyle which may differ between cancer patients and members of the general population. However, important information can also be derived from studies on the topographical relationship of primary and second cancer in symmetrical organs, in particular in patients with a primary breast cancer and a secondary lung cancer. Moreover, studies on second cancers after radiotherapy of young people and their comparison with age-matched healthy populations provide information after very long follow-up, but interpretation is difficult because of strong genetic susceptibility factors influencing risks. A comprehensive review by the National Council of Radiation Protection of the USA has been summarized by Travis et al. [11].

Carcinoma of the prostate

The results of the large cohort study on more than 120,000 prostate cancer patients registered in the SEER program who either had surgery or radiotherapy [12] demonstrate the extent of the problem for clinical radiotherapy well.

Of the approximately 17,000 prostate cancer patients who survived more than five years after radical radiotherapy, 1185 (7%) developed a second cancer. More than 1000 of those second cancers (>85%) are due to the increased lifespan after cure from the first cancer. Just about 120 to 150 of those second cancers among 51,584 prostate cancer patients (0.3%) are related to radiotherapy, in particular:

* approximately 50 cases of bladder cancer;
* approximately 15 cases of cancer of the rectum;
* approximately 50 cases of lung cancer;
* approximately 12 cases of leukaemia.

The most important message of the prostate cancer study is that half of all radiation-induced second cancers occur in the high-dose organs (bladder, rectum) and the other half in the organs exposed to low doses (lung). It is likely that different mechanisms are involved in the high- and low-dose organs. The mechanisms of low-dose radiation carcinogenesis have been explored in radiation protection research [13]. On the other hand, high radiation doses may lead to chronic radiation injury characterized by microvascular damage, parenchymal atrophy and chronic inflammation, a typical pre-cancerous lesion.

Breast cancer

Patients treated with post-operative radiotherapy for breast cancer receive significant radiation doses of more than 5% of the target dose to the contralateral breast. Since second cancers in the contralateral breast occur more frequently than expected and comprise nearly half of all second cancers in women with breast cancer, a causal relationship with the radiation exposure from the treatment of the first cancer was suggested. A case control study by Stovall et al. [14] embedded into the WECARE Study with 708 women with asynchronous bilateral breast cancer and 1399 women with unilateral breast cancer (controls) demonstrated that women <40 years of age who received >1Gy to the specific quadrant of the contralateral breast had a 2.5-fold greater risk for contralateral breast cancer than unexposed women. No excess was observed in women >40 years of age. It is particularly in young breast cancer patients that the dose to the contralateral breast should be carefully controlled.

Patients treated with post-operative radiotherapy for breast cancer receive very different doses to the ipsilateral compared to the contralateral lungs. Darby et al. [15] reported that among 115,165 women treated for breast cancer using radiotherapy 482 women died from lung cancer for which the affected side was clearly defined in the records. Of the cases, 283 (59%) were ipsilateral and 199 (41%) were contralateral. From these findings an absolute risk of 0.6% of radiation-induced lung cancer was estimated. Grantzau et al. [16] analysed the long-term risk of second primary solid non-breast cancers in the Danish national population-based cohort of more than 46,000 patients treated according to national guidelines of the Danish Breast Cancer Cooperative Group for early breast cancer between 1982 and 2007. About half received post-operative radiotherapy and were compared to those not receiving radiotherapy. Altogether, 2358 second cancers had occurred during the follow-up. The hazard ratio was not increased for sites distant from the treatment field; however, it progressively increased with duration of follow-up for sites in the thorax, in particular the lungs. The estimated attributable risk of developing a secondary cancer in the thorax (excluding contralateral breast) translates into one radiation-induced second cancer in every 200 women treated with radiotherapy.

Hodgkin lymphoma

Dores et al. [17] reported results of a large international study on 32,591 Hodgkin lymphoma patients with 2861 patients followed up for more than 20 years and 1111 patients for more than 25 years. Mean age at treatment was 37 years. Second malignancies developed in 2153 patients (7%) which, compared to the age- and sex-adjusted general population, was an increase of more than a factor of 2. The risk of late-developing solid cancers was particularly increased after radiotherapy while second leukaemias were mostly related to chemotherapy. The highest absolute excess second cancer risk was for cancers of the lung and breast. The authors calculated a 25-year cumulative risk of treatment-induced second cancers of 11.7%, most of which was related to radiotherapy.

In their review of late effects after treatment for Hodgkin lymphoma, Swerdlow and van Leeuwen [18] concluded that the substantial increase in solid tumour risk with time since diagnosis necessitated careful, lifelong medical surveillance of all patients. In particular, women treated with mantle field irradiation before the age of 30 are at greatly increased risk of breast cancer and follow-up of these women should include yearly mammography; however, the efficacy of these measures has not yet been demonstrated.

Paediatric malignancies

The chances of children with cancer being cured and having a near normal life-expectancy have reached a level unimaginable 30 years ago. But the price for this progress has been high. Neglia et al. [19] investigated a cohort of 13,581 children from the Childhood Cancer Survivor Study register in the USA who survived at least five years. After a mean latency of 12 years, 298 second malignancies were observed. Whereas the risk of secondary leukaemia (altogether 24 cases) increased to a peak after five to nine years, the risk of solid second cancers, in particular breast, thyroid, and CNS was significantly elevated during the entire follow-up period of up to 30 years. The study of de Vathaire et al. [20] specifically looked at the impact of radiotherapy on childhood solid malignancies on the risk of second cancers. They analysed the second cancer risk in 4400 three-year survivors treated in France and the UK, 3109 (71%) of whom received radiotherapy. For 2831 (91%) of these children, individual radiation doses at 151 points of the body were determined, based on the individual treatment plans using a computer phantom. Of these, 113 patients (4%) developed a solid second malignant tumour. Twenty-five years after treatment of the primary malignancy, the cumulative risk was 5%; five years later it approached 8%. In 543 patients who had already attained an age >30 years, 16 second cancers were diagnosed while only 3.3 were expected, a fivefold increase. Diallo et al. [21] analysed the anatomical relationship between the location of fatal second cancers and the anatomy of the planning target volume (PTV) for sarcomas, brain tumours, breast cancer, and thyroid cancer. Of fatal second cancers, 50% were sarcomas, nearly 90% developed in or close to the PTV while the majority of central nervous system tumours occurred at a distance from the PTV. Tukenova et al. [22] reported that sarcomas occurred earlier than carcinomas but stayed constant after 20 years while the rate of carcinomas continued to increase steadily with increasing follow-up time.

In a study on 102 second cancers among 930 children treated for Hodgkin disease, Constine et al. [23] reported a threefold higher risk for female children treated for Hodgkin disease than for males of developing second cancers. This is mainly due to the high rate of cancers of the breast, but also of thyroid carcinomas and of sarcomas in females. These three cancer types comprise three-quarters of all second cancers in female Hodgkin survivors. Second cancers after childhood cancer radiotherapy are a particularly serious problem in female patients.

Conclusion

In a comprehensive analysis of data stored in the US Surveillance, Epidemiology and End Results Cancer Registries, Berrington de Gonzalez et al. [24] determined the proportion of second cancers which are attributable to radiotherapy treatments in 647,672 adults who survived their first cancer for more than five years and were followed up for another seven years. Of these 60,271 (9%) developed a second solid cancer between five and 12 years after treatment of the first cancer. The relative risk of second cancer and the proportion of cancers attributable to radiotherapy were calculated by comparing cancer rates for patients receiving radiotherapy versus patients not receiving radiotherapy in the definitive treatment of 15 types of first malignancy. In total, an estimated 3266 excess solid cancers could be related to radiotherapy in these five-year survivors, i.e. 8% of the total second cancers diagnosed in the cancer survivors who had received radiotherapy. The authors estimated that for every 1000 patients treated with radiotherapy there were an estimated three excess cancers by ten years after first cancer diagnosis which increased to five excess cases by 15 years. Over half of the excess cases occurred in organs likely to have received >5 Gy. The risk of radiation-induced second cancers is much greater in young and very young cancer patients. Increased cancer rates may persist lifelong.

All estimates of treatment-related second cancers made above are inevitably based on retrospective analyses of results from treating patients many years ago, yet the situation has changed dramatically in radiation oncology during the last two decades. Today, patients rarely receive radiotherapy alone. In particular, studies in patients treated as children with chemotherapy plus radiotherapy demonstrated that both treatment modalities increase the risk of secondary malignancy in cured patients, both regarding leukaemias and solid cancers. Therefore, the risk of cancer induced by the combination of chemotherapy, radiotherapy, and novel molecular agents cannot be predicted from the results of these studies on past patients, and the combinatory effects need to be closely watched in future.

Further reading

Berrington de Gonzalez A, Curtis RE, Kry SF, Gilbert E, Lamart S et al. The proportion of second cancers attributable to radiotherapy treatment in adults: a prospective cohort study in the US SEER cancer registries. Lancet Oncology 2011; 12: 353–360.

Brenner DJ, Curtis RE, Hall EJ, Ron E. Second malignancies in prostate carcinoma patients after radiotherapy compared with surgery. Cancer 2000; 88: 398–406.

Preston DL, Ron E, Tokuoka S, Nishi N, Soda M et al. Solid cancer incidence in atomic bomb survivors: 1958–1996. Radiation Research 2007; 168: 1–64.

Travis LB, Ng AK, Allan JM, Pui CH, Kennedy AR et al. Second malignant neoplasms and cardiovascular disease following radiotherapy. Journal of the National Cancer Institute 2012; 104: 357–370.

UNSCEAR. Annex A: Epidemiological studies of radiation and cancer. In Sources and Biological Effects of Ionizing Radiation. Report to the General Assembly, United Nations, 2006.

References

1. ICRP. The 2007 Recommendations of the International Commission on Radiological Protection. ICRP publication 103. Annals of the ICRP 297; 37: 1–332.

2. Tubiana M. Dose-effect relationships and estimation of the carcinogenic effects of low doses of ionising radiation. The joint report of the Académie des Sciences (Paris) and of the Académie Nationale de Médecine. International Journal of Radiation Oncology* Biology* Physics 2005; 63(2): 317–319.

3. Preston DL, Shimizu Y, Pierce A, Suyama A, Mabuchi K. Studies of mortality of atomic bomb survivors. Report 13: solid cancer and non-cancer disease mortality. Radiation Research 2003; 160: 31–407.

4. Preston DL, Ron E, Tokuoka S, Nishi N, Soda M et al. Solid cancer incidence in atomic bomb survivors: 1958–1996. Radiation Research 2007; 168: 1–64.

5. World Health Organization. Health Effects of the Chernobyl Accident and Special Health Care Programmes. Bennet B, Repacholi M, Carr Z eds. Geneva: WHO, 2006.

6. Trott KR, Kamprad F. Side effects and long-term risks from radiotherapy of non-malignant diseases. In Seegenschmiedt MH, Makoski HB, Trott KR, Brady LW eds, Radiotherapy for non-malignant diseases. Heidelberg: Springer, 2008.

7. Court-Brown WM, Doll R. Mortality from cancer and other causes after radiotherapy for ankylosing spondylitis. British Medical Journal 1965; 1327–1332.

8. Shore RE, Hildreth N, Woodard E, Dvoretsky P, Hempelmann L et al. Breast cancer among women given X-ray therapy for acute posst-partum mastitis. Journal of the National Cancer Institute 1986; 77: 689–696.

9. FM, Hesse W. Der Lungenkrebs, die Bergkrankheit in den Schneeberger Gruben. Vierteljahreszeitschrift für Gerichtliche Medizin 1879; 30: 296-309, 31: 102.132, 31: 312-337.

10. Wichmann HE, Schaffrath Rosario A, Heid IM, Kreuzer M, Heinrich J et al. Increased lung cancer risk due to residential radon in a pooled and extended analysis of studies in Germany. Health Physics 2005; 88: 71–79.

11. Travis LB, Ng AK, Allan JM, Pui CH, Kennedy AR et al. Second malignant neoplasms and cardiovascular disease following radiotherapy. Journal of the National Cancer Institute 2012; 104: 357–370.

12. Brenner DJ, Curtis RE, Hall EJ, Ron E. Second malignancies in prostate carcinoma patients after radiotherapy compared with surgery. Cancer 2000; 88: 398–406.

13. UNSCEAR. Annex A: Epidemiological studies of radiation and cancer. In Sources and Biological Effects of Ionizing Radiation. Report to the General Assembly, United Nations, 2006.

14. Stovall M, Smith SA, Langholz BM, Boice JD Jr, Shore RE et al. Dose to the contralateral breast from radiotherapy and risk of second primary breast cancer in the WECARE study. International Journal of Radiation Oncology* Biology* Physics 2008; 71: 1021–1030.

15. Darby SC, McGale P, Taylor CW, Peto R. Long-term mortality from heart disease and lung cancer after radiotherapy for early breast cancer: prospective cohort study of about 300,000 women in US SEER cancer registries. Lancet Oncology 2005; 6: 557–565.

16. Grantzau T, Mellemkjär L, Overgaard J. Second primary cancers after adjuvant radiotherapy in early breast cancer patients: A national population based study under the Danish Breast Cancer Cooperative Group. Radiotherapy & Oncology 2013; 106: 42–49.

17. Dores GM, Metayer C, Curtis RE, Lynch CF, Clarke EA et al. Second malignant neoplasms among long-term survivors of Hodgkin's disease: a population-based evaluation over 25 years. Journal of Clinical Oncology 2002; 20: 3484–3494.

18. Swerdlow AJ, van Leeuwen FE. Late effects after treatment for Hodgkin's lymphoma. In Dembo AJ, Linch DC, Lowenberg B eds, Textbook of Malignant Hematology. Abingdon: Taylor & Francis, 2005, 758–768.

19. Neglia JP, Friedman DL, Yasui Y, Mertens AC, Hammond S et al. Second malignant neoplasms in five-year survivors of childhood cancer: childhood cancer survivor study. Journal of the National Cancer Institute 2001; 93: 618–629.

20. de Vathaire F, Hawkins M, Campbell S. Second malignant neoplasms after a first cancer in childhood: temporal pattern of risk according to type of treatment. British Journal of Cancer 1999; 79: 1884–1893.

21. Diallo I, Haddy N, Adjadi E, Samand A, Quiniou E et al. Frequency distribution of second solid cancer locations in relation to the irradiatred volume among 115 patients treated for childhood cancer. International Journal of Radiation Oncology* Biology* Physics 2009; 74: 876–883.

22. Tukenova M, Guibout C, Hawkins M, Quiniou E, Mousannif A et al. Radiation therapy and late mortality from second sarcoma, carcinoma and hematological malignancies after a solid cancer in childhood. International Journal of Radiation Oncology * Biology * Physics 2011; 80: 339–346.

23. Constine L, Tarbell N, Hudson MM. Subsequent malignancies in children treated for Hodgkin's disease: association with gender and radiation dose. International Journal of Radiation Oncology * Biology * Physics 2008 72: 24–33.

24. Berrington de Gonzalez A, Curtis RE, Kry SF, Gilbert E, Lamart S et al. The proportion of second cancers attributable to radiotherapy treatment in adults: a prospective cohort study in the US SEER cancer registries. Lancet Oncology 2011; 12: 353–360.

CHAPTER 18

Aetiology and progression of cancer
Role of body fatness, physical activity, diet, and other lifestyle factors

Fränzel J.B. van Duijnhoven and Ellen Kampman

Introduction to aetiology and progression of cancer

The occurrence of cancer varies across the world. Among men in more developed regions, prostate cancer is most common, followed by lung and colorectal cancer [1]. Among men in less developed regions, lung cancer is most prominent, followed by stomach and liver cancer. Among women, breast cancer is the most frequently occurring form of cancer in developed regions of the world, followed by cancer of the colorectum and the lung. In less developed regions, breast cancer is also the most common type of cancer among women, followed by cervix uteri, lung, and stomach cancer. Migrant studies, in which people moved from one part of the world to another, have shown that cancer rates among these populations change rapidly over generations and become comparable to the cancer rates of the host country [2–6]. These observations indicate that in addition to genes, lifestyle, including diet and physical activity, is important in the aetiology of cancer.

In 1981, Doll and Peto estimated that about 35% of all cancer deaths are attributable to dietary habits [7]. A similar conclusion is drawn in the policy report of the World Cancer Research Fund (WCRF) in collaboration with the American Institute for Cancer Research (AICR) which appeared in 2009: about a quarter to a third of all cancers in higher-income countries and about a fifth to a quarter in lower-income countries could be prevented through eating healthily, being physically active, and maintaining a healthy weight [8]. This report was built on evidence from their second expert report *Food, Nutrition, Physical Activity and the Prevention of Cancer: A Global Perspective* [9]. In addition to the influence of lifestyle factors on the occurrence of cancer later in life, the second expert report also acknowledged that research on lifestyle factors during and after cancer is important, because the number of people that are diagnosed with cancer as well as those who survive cancer is increasing.

This chapter describes the evidence on the role of body fatness, physical activity, diet, and other lifestyle factors[1] in the aetiology as well as the progression of cancer, it discusses what proportion of cancer cases is attributable to these factors, and it provides evidence-based recommendations for the general public.

Development of cancer

Body fatness

As greater body fatness strongly and consistently increases the risk of many types of cancer, it is one of the most important risk factors for cancer as a whole. The evidence that it causes cancer of the breast (after menopause), colorectum, pancreas, oesophagus (only adenocarcinomas), endometrium, and kidney is convincing, whereas it is probable for gallbladder cancer [9–11]. In contrast, greater body fatness probably protects against breast cancer before menopause.

It is not only the amount of fat tissue, but also the location of fat tissue within the body that is important in the development of cancer. Greater abdominal (central) fatness is convincingly associated with an increased risk of colorectal cancer and it probably also causes breast cancer (after menopause), pancreatic cancer, and endometrial cancer [9–11].

The mechanism behind these associations is thought to run via increased circulating concentrations of hormones and growth factors, such as sex hormones, insulin, and insulin-like growth factor, which are involved in carcinogenesis [12, 13]. In addition, body fatness is characterized by elevated levels of pro-inflammatory factors, which can promote cancer development [12, 13].

Although estimates of population attributable fractions vary between studies according to the methodology used, the number of cancer cases that are attributable to body fatness also differ by type of cancer and by population (Table 18.1; [9, 14]). For example, about 34–38% of endometrial cancers are estimated to be attributable to body fatness in the UK, which is regarded as a high-income country, whereas it is about 18% in China, which is considered to be a low-income country. For colorectal cancer, 7–13% is estimated to be attributable to body fatness in the UK and 3% in China.

Given the high impact of body fatness, WCRF/AICR as well as the American Cancer Society (ACS) recommend individuals to achieve and maintain a healthy weight throughout life [9, 15]. A healthy weight is best achieved by choosing diets based on foods with low-energy density, avoiding sugary drinks, and being physically active throughout life.

Table 18.1 Estimates of population attributable fractions of body fatness, physical activity, and dietary factors for 12 cancer sites [8, 14]

	Population attributable fraction (%)		
	Parkin et al. 2011 [14]	WCRF/AICR 2009 [8]	WCRF/AICR 2009 [8]
	UK	UK	China
Mouth, pharynx, and larynx			
Non-starchy vegetables	53	34	12
Fruits		17	30
Alcoholic drinks	29	41	10
Total estimate	67	67	44
Oesophagus			
Non-starchy vegetables	46	21	11
Fruits		5	16
Alcoholic drinks	21	51	11
Body fatness	22	31	17
Total estimate	67	75	44
Stomach			
Non-starchy vegetables	36	21	10
Fruits		18	26
Salt	24	14	*
Total estimate	51	45	33
Colon—Rectum			
Foods containing fibre	12	12	*
Red meat	21	5	7
Processed meat		10	1
Alcoholic drinks	12	7	1
Physical activity	3	12	7
Body fatness	13	7	3
Total estimate	48	43	17
Liver			
Alcoholic drinks	9	17	6
Gallbladder			
Body fatness	18	16	6
Pancreas			
Foods containing folate	*	23	*
Body fatness	12	24	14
Total estimate	12	45	14
Lung			
Fruits	9	33	38
Breast			
Alcoholic drinks	6	22	1
Physical activity	3	12	8

(continued)

Table 18.1 Continued

	Population attributable fraction (%)		
	Parkin et al. 2011 [14]	WCRF/AICR 2009 [8]	WCRF/AICR 2009 [8]
Body fatness	9	16	12
Total estimate	17	42	20
Endometrium			
Physical activity	4	30	20
Body fatness	34	38	18
Total estimate	36	56	34
Prostate			
Foods containing lycopene	*	20	*
Kidney			
Body fatness	24	19	8
12 Cancers combined	*	39	27
All cancers	18	26	20

*Not evaluated

Adapted with permission from Parkin et al., The fraction of cancer attributable to lifestyle and environmental factors in the UK in 2010, *British Journal of Cancer*, Volume 105, S77–81, Copyright © 2011 Cancer Research UK and World Cancer Research Fund/American Institute for Cancer Research, Policy and Action for Cancer Prevention, *Food, Nutrition, and Physical Activity: A Global Perspective*, Washington DC: AICR, Copyright © 2009.

Physical activity

Physical activity consistently reduces the risk of colon cancer and probably also protects against postmenopausal breast cancer and endometrial cancer. In addition to the beneficial effect of physical activity on body fatness, this may be due to its favourable influence on endogenous steroid hormone metabolism and immune function [16].

Around 3–12% of colorectal cancer cases are estimated to be preventable by being physically active on a regular basis in the UK, while it is around 7% in China (Table 18.1). It is advised to adopt a physically active lifestyle [9, 15]. This means building regular moderate, and some vigorous physical activity into everyday life, and diminishing the time spent sitting.

Diet

Plant foods

In general, plant foods are assumed to protect against cancer, as most diets that decrease the risk of cancer mainly contain foods of plant origin. The observed inverse associations between plant foods separately and the development of cancer, however, are relatively weak and are still debated [17].

The evidence that has currently been established is the following: a relatively high consumption of non-starchy vegetables, which includes green, leafy vegetables, cruciferous vegetables, and allium vegetables, probably protects against cancer of the upper-gastrointestinal tract (mouth, pharynx, larynx, oesophagus, and stomach) [9]. Allium vegetables alone probably also protect against stomach cancer, whereas garlic specifically has been shown to decrease the risk of colorectal cancer [9, 11]. The consumption of fruits probably decreases the risk of cancer of the mouth, pharynx, larynx, oesophagus, lung, and stomach.

Foods containing dietary fibre, which also includes vegetables and fruits, is convincingly protective against colorectal cancer [11, 18].

In addition to dietary fibre, the beneficial effects of vegetables and fruits may be due to specific vitamins or other bioactive compounds, such as carotenoids including beta-carotene and lycopene (coloured vegetables), folates (green leafy vegetables and brassica), glucosinolates (brassica), and allyl sulphides (garlic and onions). Non-starchy vegetables and fruits are also typically low in energy density; thus a diet high in these products probably also protects against weight gain.

For cancers of the mouth, pharynx, and larynx, around 34% and 17% in the UK and 12% and 30% in China are estimated to be attributable to non-starchy vegetables and fruit, respectively (Table 18.1). Consuming an adequate amount of fibre is thought to prevent around 12% of colorectal cancer cases in the UK (Table 18.1).

The consumption of plant foods is encouraged by both the WCRF/AICR and ACS [9, 15]. WCRF recommends eating at least five portions/servings (at least 400 g or 14 oz) and ACS advises at least 2.5 cups of vegetables and fruits each day. In addition, they both promote the consumption of unprocessed cereals (whole grains) and limit the consumption of refined grain products.

Animal foods

Animal foods typically include meat, poultry, fish, eggs, as well as milk and other dairy products. The evidence for most of these foods in relation to the development of cancer is limited, with the exception of meat and milk.

Red meat, which includes beef, pork, lamb, and goat, as well as processed meat, meaning meats that are preserved by smoking, curing, salting, or the addition of chemical preservatives (e.g., ham, bacon, pastrami, salami, and sausages), are convincingly associated with an increased risk of colon as well as rectal cancer [11].

The exact mechanism by which red and processed meat increases colorectal cancer risk is unclear [11]. Factors that may play a role in colorectal carcinogenesis are specific mutagens, such as heterocyclic amines and polycyclic aromatic hydrocarbons, which are formed when meat is cooked well done at a very high temperature or over a direct flame (e.g., grilling, frying, or barbecuing). A specific component in red meat that may also be involved in the carcinogenic process is heme iron. This compound, which gives meat its red colour, may act through two different pathways: (1) it catalyses the peroxidation of fat in the gastrointestinal tract, which produces cytotoxic and mutagenic alkenals; (2) it induces the production of carcinogenic N-nitroso-compounds in the gastrointestinal tract. These latter N-nitroso-compounds can also be formed when nitrates and nitrites are added as preservatives to processed meats during the curing process.

Around 5% and 10% of colorectal cancers in the UK and 7% and 1% in China are estimated to be attributable to red and processed meats, respectively (Table 18.1). The guidelines to prevent cancer emphasize diminishing the consumption of red meat [15] (less than 500 g a week according to WCRF/AICR [9]) and limiting [15] or even avoiding [9] the consumption of processed meat.

Although the evidence on milk and the development of cancer is not limited, it is conflicting [9]. On the one hand, the consumption of milk probably protects against cancer of the colon and rectum, which is thought to occur at least in part due to a higher consumption of dietary calcium. On the other hand, diets high in calcium are probably associated with an increased risk of prostate cancer.

Based on these findings, it may be hypothesized that calcium both has an inhibiting as well as a promoting role in the carcinogenic process, which may differ by cell type.

Calcium may reduce colorectal carcinogenesis by binding to secondary bile acids and fatty acids, which prevents them from exerting their proliferative effects on colonic epithelial cells. In addition, calcium may directly influence the colorectal carcinogenic process by inducing differentiation in normal cells and apoptosis in transformed cells [9]. The mechanism of calcium in prostate carcinogenesis is proposed to involve vitamin D. A high intake of calcium down-regulates the formation of 1,25 dihydroxyvitamin D, which may result in increased cell proliferation in the prostate [9].

Due to these conflicting results, the proportion of cancers that can be prevented by drinking or not drinking milk cannot be determined and no recommendations are provided.

Alcohol

Alcoholic beverages cause several types of cancer. A high consumption of alcoholic drinks is convincingly associated with cancer of the mouth, pharynx, larynx, oesophagus, and breast (before and after menopause). It is also convincingly a cause of colorectal cancer in men, whereas it is probably a cause for colorectal cancer in women, and for liver cancer [9].

It is not the type of alcohol drink that is consumed that is important but the total intake of ethanol. The primary metabolite of ethanol, acetaldehyde, as well as other reactive metabolites, may be carcinogenic. In addition, alcohol may influence the production of prostaglandins, lipid peroxidation, and the generation of free-radical oxygen species. It also may act as a solvent, thereby enhancing penetration of carcinogens into cells, and it may change folate metabolism, with unfavourable effects on DNA-synthesis and DNA-methylation [9, 15, 19].

In the UK, 21–51% of oesophageal cancer is estimated to be attributable to alcohol consumption, whereas it is 11% in China (Table 18.1). If only the evidence on cancer was taken into account, all amounts of alcohol should be avoided. However, as low to moderate intake of alcoholic drinks is associated with a reduced risk of coronary heart disease, both the WCRF and the ACS recommend consuming no more than one drink for women and two drinks for men, per day, when alcohol is consumed [9, 15].

Preservation, processing, and preparation of foods

Some methods of food preservation, processing, and preparation may affect cancer risk. The strongest evidence exists for processed meat (described under 'Animal foods'), for salt and salt-preserved foods, and for foods that are contaminated with aflatoxins, such as cereals (grains) and pulses (legumes) [9].

It is the overall amount of salt that is consumed in itself and with salt-preserved foods that probably causes stomach cancer. Aflatoxins are produced by some moulds when the above-mentioned foods are stored too long in warm temperatures. These aflatoxin-contaminated foods cause liver cancer.

In the UK, 14–24% of stomach cancers are estimated to be attributable to salt intake, while there are no estimates for the impact of aflatoxin-contaminated foods on the total number of liver cancer cases (Table 18.1). WCRF/AICR recommends avoiding salt-preserved, salted, or salty foods to ensure an intake of less than 6 g (2.4 g sodium) a day. In addition, they suggest not eating mouldy grains and legumes.

Other lifestyle factors

Dietary supplements

The findings for dietary supplements in the development of cancer are inconsistent [9]. Some studies have observed decreased risks for certain types of cancer, while others did not find any association or even reported an increased risk for particular forms of cancer. These results are based on specific populations which received specific doses of supplements. More research is needed to determine the role of high as well as low doses and natural as well as synthetic forms of supplements. In addition, combinations of different vitamins, minerals, or other compounds may be relevant when investigating supplements. For now, the use of supplements for the general population to prevent cancer is not recommended. The consumption of foods instead of dietary supplements is advocated as the best source of nutrients [9, 15]. However, in specific groups and in specific situations, the use of dietary supplements may be advisable. An example is the use of vitamin D for people who are not exposed to enough sunlight or those who are not able to synthesize a sufficient amount of vitamin D from sunlight [9].

Breastfeeding

There is strong and consistent evidence that lactation, breastfeeding by the mother, protects the mother against breast cancer at all ages thereafter [10]. This may be due to the fact that the lifetime exposure to menstrual cycles is shortened, which influences hormone levels and thereby influences breast cancer risk [9]. In addition, cells with potential initial DNA damage may be removed because of the strong exfoliation of breast tissue during lactation and the immense epithelial apoptosis at the end of breastfeeding, which may reduce breast cancer risk. For women with babies it is therefore recommended to breastfeed for at least six months after the baby is born [9].

Progression of cancer

In contrast to the enormous amount of original research studies that have been performed on the role of body fatness, physical activity, dietary and other lifestyle factors in the development of cancer, relatively few well-designed investigations have focused on the influence of these lifestyle factors on survival from cancer [9]. This new area of research, however, is now expanding. Most studies have focused on outcomes in breast, colorectal, and prostate cancer patients, as these are most prevalent in high-income countries. In addition to the fact that these are specific populations, these investigations are limited because there is a lot of heterogeneity in the type of exposure and especially the timing of exposure. Body fatness, physical activity, diet, and other lifestyle factors may have a different impact when patients receive treatment than when patients have finished their treatment. To make sure that changing these lifestyle factors is not harmful for patients at any time, the influence of lifestyle factors should first be evaluated in observational studies before feasible and effective intervention trials can be planned and conducted among cancer survivors.

The major challenge in conducting studies among cancer patients in combination with the lack of homogeneous studies in this field makes it difficult to draw firm conclusions for the cancer population at large [20, 21]. Since there is hardly any consistent scientific evidence available, the current recommendation for patients who have finished treatment is to aim to follow the guidelines to prevent cancer [9]: achieve and maintain a healthy weight, engage in regular physical activity, and adopt a healthy diet [9, 22].

Conclusion

The important involvement of body fatness, physical activity, diet, and other lifestyle factors in the development of cancer has been established and evidence-based recommendations for the general public have been set. The focus of investigations on lifestyle factors in the development of cancer will now be directed towards refining this knowledge: for instance, by unravelling the underlying mechanism and identifying the most relevant bio-active compounds, specific dietary patterns, or susceptible subgroups. The current recommendations to maintain a healthy weight, to adopt a physically active lifestyle, and to consume a healthy diet should help to reduce the number of persons that will be diagnosed with cancer worldwide. For the people who are diagnosed with cancer, however, evidence-based guidelines to improve their progression and quality of life still need to be determined. To define these guidelines, future research will be devoted to the role of body fatness, physical activity, diet, and other lifestyle factors in cancer progression.

Note

1 Given the overwhelming body of evidence on smoking in relation to cancer and other diseases, the importance of not smoking and avoiding exposure to tobacco smoke is now generally acknowledged and is, therefore, not part of this section. See Chapter 14 'Smoking and cancer'.

Further reading

Kushi LH, Doyle C, McCullough M, Rock CL, Demark-Wahnefried W et al. American Cancer Society Guidelines on nutrition and physical activity for cancer prevention: reducing the risk of cancer with healthy food choices and physical activity.CA: A Cancer Journal for Clinicians 2012; 62(1): 30–67.

Parkin DM, Boyd L, Walker LC. The fraction of cancer attributable to lifestyle and environmental factors in the UK in 2010. British Journal of Cancer 2011; 105(Suppl. 2): S77–S81.

Rock CL, Doyle C, Demark-Wahnefried W, Meyerhardt J, Courneya KS et al. Nutrition and physical activity guidelines for cancer survivors. CA: A Cancer Journal for Clinicians 2012; 62(4): 242–274.

World Cancer Research Fund/ American Institute for Cancer Research. Food, Nutrition, Physical Activity, and the Prevention of Cancer: A Global Perspective. Washington, DC: AICR, 2007.

World Cancer Research Fund/ American Institute for Cancer Research. Policy and Action for Cancer Prevention. Food, Nutrition, and Physical Activity: A Global Perspective. Washington, DC: AICR, 2009.

References

1. GLOBOCAN 2008 v1.2, Cancer Incidence and Mortality Worldwide: IARC CancerBase No 10 [Internet]. Lyon, France: International Agency for Research on Cancer, 2010. Available from: http://globocan.iarc.fr, accessed on 26 April 2012.
2. Flood DM, Weiss NS, Cook LS, Emerson JC, Schwartz SM et al. Colorectal cancer incidence in Asian migrants to the United States and their descendants. Cancer Causes Control 2000; 11(5): 403–411.
3. Hemminki K, Li X. Cancer risks in second-generation immigrants to Sweden. International Journal of Cancer 2002; 99(2): 229–237.

4. Hemminki K, Li X, Czene K. Cancer risks in first-generation immigrants to Sweden. International Journal of Cancer 2002; 10; 99(2): 218–228.

5. McMichael AJ, Giles GG. Cancer in migrants to Australia: extending the descriptive epidemiological data. Cancer Research 1988; 48(3): 751–756.

6. McMichael AJ, McCall MG, Hartshorne JM, Woodings TL. Patterns of gastro-intestinal cancer in European migrants to Australia: the role of dietary change. International Journal of Cancer 1980; 25(4): 431–437.

7. Doll R, Peto R. The causes of cancer: quantitative estimates of avoidable risks of cancer in the United States today. Journal of the National Cancer Institute 1981; 66(6): 1191–1308.

8. World Cancer Research Fund/ American Institute for Cancer Research. Policy and Action for Cancer Prevention. Food, Nutrition, and Physical Activity: A Global Perspective. Washington, DC: AICR, 2009.

9. World Cancer Research Fund/ American Institute for Cancer Research. Food, Nutrition, Physical Activity, and the Prevention of Cancer: A Global Perspective. Washington, DC: AICR, 2007.

10. World Cancer Research Fund/ American Institute for Cancer Research. Continuous Update Project Report: The Associations between Food, Nutrition and Physical Activity and the Risk of Breast Cancer. Washington DC: AICR, 2010.

11. World Cancer Research Fund/ American Institute for Cancer Research. Continuous Update Project Report: The Associations between Food, Nutrition and Physical Activity and the Risk of Colorectal Cancer, Washington DC: AICR, 2011.

12. Calle EE, Kaaks R. Overweight, obesity and cancer: epidemiological evidence and proposed mechanisms. Nature Reviews Cancer 2004; 4(8): 579–591.

13. Pischon T, Nothlings U, Boeing H. Obesity and cancer. Proceedings of the Nutrition Society 2008; 67(2): 128–145.

14. Parkin DM, Boyd L, Walker LC. The fraction of cancer attributable to lifestyle and environmental factors in the UK in 2010. British Journal of Cancer 2011; 105(Suppl. 2): S77–S81.

15. Kushi LH, Doyle C, McCullough M, Rock CL, Demark-Wahnefried W et al. American Cancer Society Guidelines on nutrition and physical activity for cancer prevention: reducing the risk of cancer with healthy food choices and physical activity.CA: A Cancer Journal for Clinicians 2012; 62(1): 30–67.

16. McTiernan A. Mechanisms linking physical activity with cancer. Nature Reviews Cancer 2008; 8(3): 205–211.

17. Key TJ. Fruit and vegetables and cancer risk. British Journal of Cancer 2011; 104(1): 6–11.

18. Aune D, Chan DS, Lau R, Vieira R, Greenwood DC et al. Dietary fibre, whole grains, and risk of colorectal cancer: systematic review and dose-response meta-analysis of prospective studies. British Medical Journal 2011; 343:d6617.

19. Boffetta P, Hashibe M. Alcohol and cancer. Lancet Oncology 2006; 7(2): 149–156.

20. Kampman E, Vrieling A, van Duijnhoven FJ, Winkels RM. Impact of diet, body mass index, and physical activity on cancer survival. Current Nutrition Reports 2011; 1(1): 30–36.

21. Vrieling A, Kampman E. The role of body mass index, physical activity, and diet in colorectal cancer recurrence and survival: a review of the literature. American Journal of Clinical Nutrition 2010; 92(3): 471–490.

22. Rock CL, Doyle C, Demark-Wahnefried W, Meyerhardt J, Courneya KS et al. Nutrition and physical activity guidelines for cancer survivors. CA: A Cancer Journal for Clinicians 2012; 62(4): 242–274.

SECTION 3

Principles of oncology

19 **Practice points
for surgical oncology** *163*
Petra G. Boelens, C.B.M. van den Broek,
and Cornelis J.H. van de Velde

20 **Practice points for radiation oncology** *173*
Annekatrin Seidlitz, Stephanie E. Combs,
Jürgen Debus, and Michael Baumann

21 **Principles of chemotherapy** *186*
David J. Kerr, Daniel G. Haller, and Jaap Verweij

22 **Multidisciplinary cancer care** *196*
David N. Church, Rachel Kerr, and David J. Kerr

23 **Principles of clinical pharmacology:
introduction to pharmacokinetics
and pharmacodynamics** *209*
Michael Ong and Udai Banerji

24 **Design and analysis of clinical trials** *220*
Daniel J. Sargent and Qian Shi

25 **Medical ethics in oncology** *229*
Eric A. Singer

26 **Health economic assessment
of cancer therapy** *236*
Jeffrey Peppercorn

CHAPTER 19

Practice points for surgical oncology

Petra G. Boelens, C.B.M. van den Broek, and Cornelis J.H. van de Velde

Introduction to surgical oncology

Surgical oncology remains the cornerstone of curative oncology treatment for most solid cancers. Historically, surgery was the only cure for cancer for a long time. If a tumour was mobile, thus movable by the surgeon on palpation, it could be taken out. With respect to modern surgical oncology, it has become far more innovative and complex. Nevertheless, surgical removal of solid cancer still offers the best chance of long-term survival over all other treatment modalities for most cancers.

Precision diagnosis using high-tech imaging techniques such as ultrasound, MRI and CT-scanning, and sometimes PET/CT, can personalize the surgical approach. Cancer surgery especially has benefited from advances in imaging. Cancers are nowadays clinically staged as either resectable or potentially resectable or unresectable, depending on patient characteristics such as fitness and comorbidity, preferences, TNM stage, and appearance on imaging. As expected, enhanced pre-operative staging has implications for treatment options. For example, MR-based staging of rectal cancer is very accurate in T-staging and definition of mesorectal fascia (MRF) involvement [1], separating good prognosis patients from poor prognosis, and determining who should receive upfront treatment with radiation and/or chemoradiation therapy. MR-based restaging in rectal cancer after primary treatment with radiation or chemoradiation defines response and definitive surgery.

Minimal invasive surgery such as laparoscopic techniques in colorectal surgery were introduced and showed to be safe with respect to long-term oncological outcomes [2–4]. For the direct post-operative period, benefits of laparoscopic surgery are lower risk of mortality and morbidity and shorter hospital stay. In the field of breast cancer, breast-conserving surgery in combination with post-operative radiation therapy versus mastectomy is similar in long-term survival in numerous randomized trials [5, 6]. Some studies also describe significant benefit in body image and satisfaction with breast-conserving therapy in comparison to mastectomy, although decreasing in time due to late effects of radiation therapy; others have seen that body image problems did not differ at two years after any type of surgery. Shared decision-making between the surgeon and patient has a role in achieving long-term satisfaction by the treatment choice that fits the patient the best according to her preferences. Decision aids, web-based or digital, assist in this aim.

In some fields, a more extensive surgical resection results in better outcome such as the Dutch D1D2 trial: the standardized extended (D2) lymphadenectomy leads to better results than standardized limited (D1) lymphadenectomy in patients with resectable primary adenocarcinoma of the stomach. After a median follow-up of 15 years, D2 lymphadenectomy had lower locoregional recurrence and gastric-cancer-related death rates than D1 surgery. Of note, the D2 procedure was associated with more post-operative mortality, morbidity, and reoperation rates. Because a safer, spleen-preserving D2 resection technique is currently available in high-volume centres, this modified D2 lymphadenectomy is the recommended surgical approach for patients with resectable (curable) gastric cancer [7].

Perioperative care has become better over time; therefore, surgeons are less hindered by age, stage, comorbidity and advanced disease for deciding on surgical management. In case of resectable liver metastases of colorectal cancer, the sequence and timing to treat the primary or metastases with surgery or systemic therapy play a role in treatment [8]. Chemotherapy and radiofrequency ablation (RFA) may be options to consider in borderline resectable disease.

Cancer care now involves a wide spectrum of systemic therapies with pre- or post-operative, induction, and/or palliative treatment(s). Specifics about these are elaborated in other chapters of this textbook. Consequently, managing cancer is increasingly a multidisciplinary alliance. Dedicated health care professionals from all different disciplines should discuss all the possible options of treatment at several decision points in time before sharing this with the patient. Presentation of a patient with cancer in a multidisciplinary team (MDT) is the preferred approach.

History of surgical oncology

The earliest surgical operations in human history were carried out in prehistoric times (2000 BC) in several parts of the world—in Europe, in Asia and particularly in Peru, where well-preserved mummies endure. Many of these mummies have a hole in the skull which is the product of trepanning (also known as trephining or trephination) which was thought to be helpful in releasing evil spirits. Surgery in the old days was obviously a risky business.

With regards to surgical oncology, in the Greek and Roman empires people such as Hippocrates started to recognize and treat cancers. The introduction of general anaesthesia (nitric oxide and ether to start with), antisepsis (principles discovered by Lister, Semmelweis, and Pasteur), and many surgical pioneers (such as Moore and Halsted for introducing radical breast surgery, Kocher for the approach in thyroid surgery, and Miles for the abdominoperineal resection for rectal cancer) were at the base of modern surgical oncology. In the last decades, many advances have been made toward better surgical oncological outcome and better quality of life.

Cancer surgery and resectability

Although it sounds very logical that resectability means that a tumour can be resected, it is a bit more complex than that. Final determination of resectability requires a multifaceted evaluation of tumour anatomy by imaging, existence of local and/or distant disease, age, comorbidities, functional status, and sometimes results of laboratory tests to determine the risk–benefit profile of surgery. This evaluation may take more than one outpatient visit to complete for the patient and at least one MDT discussion to decide on treatment strategies. Moreover, if upfront non-surgical treatment is considered; restaging might reveal additional surgical options.

Now, with diverse types of high-tech imaging techniques within reach, the definition of resectability is far more complicated. For example, what is resectable pancreatic cancer? According to the cancer staging systems this would be cancer not associated with disease outside the pancreas. The anatomic extent of the primary cancer is pre-operatively and primarily determined by CT scan; this means there should not be tumour extension into the major blood vessels (such as branches from the celiac trunk, common hepatic artery, superior mesenteric vein or artery, or portal vein) or adjacent organs. Until recently, tumours that appeared to involve any of the major abdominal blood vessels were considered unresectable because survival following surgical procedures that required resection and reconstruction of these vessels was poor. In some centres, however, pancreatic tumours are resected with the involvement of major blood vessels, with good long-term outcome. It should be recognised that this can only be done in expert centres.

In cancer surgery, outcome is generally measured by comparing survival and disease-specific outcomes. It has become more accepted to implement other measures of quality such as quality of life, infectious complications, body image, or cosmetic outcome as outcome measures. The preferences of the patient in these processes are important to sustain long-term satisfaction with the choices that were made.

Age and comorbidity

In Western countries, the fastest growing part of the population is people aged 65 years or older, and the highest incidence of colorectal cancer is among those aged between 70 and 80 years old. In recent years, the focus on elderly colorectal cancer patients has increased. It is important to realize that the elderly population forms a very heterogeneous group of patients. Not only can calendar age be very different from biological age, but the definition of elderly also varies widely from ≥65 years to ≥80 years in different studies. Calendar age alone is, therefore, not the primary influence on outcome; rather, the combination of comorbidities and decreased physical reserve to recover from adverse events that may occur may determine the outcome for elderly patients. This is also

referred to as biological age. Hence, calendar age itself should not be a contraindication for more aggressive or adjuvant treatment. Comorbidities, on the other hand, are of critical importance in the care of a patient.

However, comorbid conditions do not alone determine post-operative outcome in elderly patients; fitness or frailty must also be taken into account. Unfortunately, there is scarce information available on pre-operative conditions of fitness at advanced age, including factors such as 'frailty', age-related muscle loss (sarcopenia), and malnutrition. These factors indicate which elderly individual is more vulnerable in encountering adverse outcome. Hence, identifying 'frail' octogenarians is of utmost importance to acquire a realistic prognosis of cancer surgery. Currently, instruments developed for this are unfortunately both time-consuming and rather impractical.

Malnutrition is highly prevalent in elderly populations; approximately one-third to one-half of hospitalized patients are malnourished at the time of admission, which leads to higher post-operative morbidity rates. This suggests that consideration of the perioperative nutritional status is especially important in elderly patients.

Staging and restaging

Staging cancer is the process of establishing the anatomical location, size, and depth of the tumour growth, the locoregional extent in adjacent organs, and the spread of cancer either to lymph nodes or distant organs. Staging is important in planning a surgical approach (if possible) and to gather information about prognosis. Usually, a higher stage is associated with worse outcome and has varying potentials for treatment. It is important that staging is discussed in a multidisciplinary board, because all treatments are based on anatomy and stage.

The TNM classification is one of the most commonly used staging systems. This system has been accepted by the International Union Against Cancer (UICC) and the American Joint Committee on Cancer (AJCC). Most medical facilities use the TNM system as their leading classification for cancer reporting. MDTs are encouraged to discuss clinical TNM stage and pathology TNM as pre-operative and post-operative bases for treatment regimes.

The TNM system gives information about the extent of the tumour (T), the extent of spread to the lymph nodes (N), and the presence of distant metastasis (M). For example, the T stage of the primary tumour will be described as TX when the primary tumour cannot be evaluated or is unknown and T0 if there is no evidence of a primary tumour. If the primary tumour is an in situ carcinoma, it is called Tis (pre-invasive cancer), and the following are sequential in size T1, T2, T3. T4 indicates growth into an adjacent organ, including the skin. Regional lymph nodes (N) are classified according to the same method: NX—regional lymph nodes cannot be evaluated; N0—no regional lymph node involvement; and N1, N2, N3—involvement of regional lymph nodes in ascending numbers (number of lymph nodes and/or extent of spread). For distant metastasis (M), the methodology is similar and describes as: MX–distant metastasis cannot be or are not evaluated; M0—no distant metastases are present; and M1—distant metastases are present.

With the development of pre-operative therapies—radiation therapy, chemotherapy or biologics—the initial staging will be part of the comparison of the restaging after induction or pre-operative treatments on therapeutic effects or response and give information about final surgical outcome and prognosis. Restaging is usually less accurate because of biological changes to the tissue such as fibrosis which makes pathology difficult to interpret. MRI, for example, is the standard restaging modality for rectal cancer and breast cancer. In some fields—pancreatic cancer, ovarian cancer, and hepatic malignancies—PET-CT could assist in monitoring therapy for staging and restaging.

Anatomical surgery

The best option on long-term survival and reduced local recurrence is precise surgery if possible; the tumour needs to be confined to a resectable organ or organ part or en bloc with draining lymph nodes.

Some sites in the body have very delicate and clear surgical landmarks of the tissue to be resected (thyroid cancer, rectal cancer, pancreatic cancer) while other areas are less clearly defined anatomically such as breast tissue or liver parenchyma.

The aim of oncological surgical resections is a clear margin around the tumour. If there is extension of the tumour in the surrounding tissue, this is called locally advanced disease, which requires a different surgical approach. Locally advanced disease does not always adhere to anatomical landmarks. It is imperative for surgeons to know the anatomy of the tumour at hand. Nerves, vessels, and adjacent organs should be respected if not involved in the tumour process.

A clear margin of one millimetre equals complete resection in most cancers, although a larger margin reduces the risk of local recurrence. For instance, in breast cancer, Halsted introduced the radical mastectomy (surgical removal of the breast, pectoralis major, and minor muscles en bloc with a full axillary lymph node dissection). In 1983, Maddox et al. compared the Halsted radical mastectomy to the modified radical mastectomy (not resecting the muscles) and had similar results on ten-year survival, although local recurrence was lower after radical mastectomy [9]. In the same period, breast preservation (wide local excision of the breast mass with locoregional irradiation) was studied, and nowadays it is very well established that breast preservation can result in equal long-term outcome when compared to mastectomy. With local treatment, pathological exam of the surgical margins became important. Before the 1990s, only margins where tumour tissue was suspected when checked macroscopically were investigated microscopically. From 1990 and beyond, margins were evaluated more intensively, but evaluations were not standardized.

A 2 mm free margin is regarded sufficient in breast cancer. Proximal and distal margin are terms used, for example, in colon cancer, which depend on the vascular supply of the segment of the colon that needs to be resected.

In rectal cancer, the border surrounding the mesorectum (the fatty tissue around the serosal layer of the rectal wall harbouring the locoregional draining lymph nodes), the mesorectal fascia (MRF), is best described by a pre-operative MRI, measured in millimetres towards the tumour. This is the clinical differentiation between clinical T3 and T4 disease and will give the best prediction of whether a negative circumferential resection margin (CRM) will be possible. A CRM >1 mm is associated with better survival and a lower incidence of local recurrence [1, 10].

Prophylactic surgery in hereditary cancer CRC

About 3–5% of colorectal cancers are of hereditary origin. If there is clinical suspicion of polyposis or Lynch syndrome, the patient should be referred to a specialist in human genetics for genetic testing. Clinical suspicion is based on clinical criteria or on molecular screening in the context of a suggestive personal or family history.

Lynch syndrome (LS/hereditary non-polyposis colorectal cancer [HNPCC]) is the most common hereditary colorectal cancer syndrome and is estimated to account for 3–5% of all CRC cases. LS is caused by mutations in DNA mismatch repair (MMR) genes which are inherited in an autosomal dominant pattern and are associated with accelerated development of cancers. Life-time risk for colorectal and endometrial cancers approaches 70–80% and 40–60%, respectively. At-risk family members who undergo screening colonoscopy have a reduced risk of developing HNPCC-related cancers and lower mortality. It is recommended that colonoscopies with polypectomies and endometrial biopsies with transvaginal ultrasonography are repeated frequently in Lynch syndrome. With surveillance intervals of one to two years, members of families with Lynch syndrome have a lower risk of developing CRC than with surveillance intervals of two to three years.

Familial adenomatous polyposis (FAP), which is caused by mutations in the adenomatous polyposis coli (APC) gene, is characterized by the development of multiple adenomas in the rectum and colon starting during the second decade of life. Individuals with FAP carry a 100% life-time risk of CRC. Cancer prevention—including prophylactic colectomy-- and maintaining a good quality of life are the main goals of management, and regular and systematic follow-up and supportive care should be offered to all patients.

Important topics in hereditary colorectal cancer syndromes that are open for discussion are which patient must be treated earlier, ideal timing for surgery, and the extent of surgery. In FAP patients, by the late teens or early twenties, colorectal cancer prophylactic surgery is advocated. The recommended options are total proctocolectomy and ileoanal pouch (IPAA) or ileorectal anastomosis (IRA) for attenuated FAP.

Desmoid tumors are rare non-metastasizing fibromatoses that can occur in association with familial adenomatous polyposis. Desmoids have a prevalence of 10–26% in FAP and are usually a major source of morbidity and one of the most common causes of death in these patients. An interaction between female gender and early (<18 years) colectomy of patients developing desmoids has been investigated, with a hazard ratio (HR) of 2.5.

Breast and ovarian cancer

Although a family history of breast and/or ovarian cancer is common in women diagnosed with breast or ovarian cancer, less than 10% of all breast cancers and less than 15% of ovarian cancers are associated with inherited genetic mutations. The majority of hereditary breast and ovarian cancers are associated with mutations in two genes, breast cancer type 1 and 2 susceptibility genes (BRCA1 and BRCA2). Less commonly, breast cancer is due to other hereditary cancer syndromes, such as Li-Fraumeni and Cowden syndromes, which are related to mutations in the TP53 and PTEN genes, respectively.

Women with BRCA1 and BRCA2 have markedly elevated risks of breast cancer and ovarian cancer, with a lifetime risk of breast cancer of 50 to 85% and a 15 to 40% chance of developing ovarian cancer. There is also an increased risk of a second breast cancer diagnosis. Men with BRCA1 and BRCA2 also have an increased risk of breast cancer and prostate cancer. Whereas the increased lifetime risk for men with BRCA1 of breast cancer and prostate cancer is undefined, the lifetime risk of breast cancer of men with BRCA2 appears to be under 10%, and the lifetime risk of prostate cancer is elevated five- to sevenfold. Besides breast, ovarian, and prostate cancer, patients with mutations in the BRCA2 gene have elevated risks of other cancer types, such as pancreatic cancer.

Patients with hereditary breast and ovarian cancer are counselled to initiate screening considerably earlier than average risk patients due to the early age of diagnosis. Expert recommendations include clinical breast examination two to four times annually beginning at age 25, with annual MRI and mammography screening from the age of 30. Twice per year, screening for ovarian cancer using transvaginal ultrasound and serum CA-125 levels should begin at age 35. Besides prophylactic mastectomy, bilateral salpingo-oophorectomy should be offered at completion of childbearing. For men, clinical breast examination semi-annually is advised, as well as a baseline mammogram and appropriate prostate cancer screening.

Other hereditary disorders

MEN1 is a rare heritable disorder classically characterized by a predisposition to tumours of the parathyroid glands, anterior pituitary, and pancreatic islet cells. In patients with MEN1, known MEN1 carriers, and family members whose risk has not been eliminated by DNA testing, clinical vigilance should be maintained for symptoms or signs that could be due to MEN1-associated tumours. These include symptoms of nephrolithiasis, amenorrhoea, galactorrhoea, erectile dysfunction, peptic ulcer disease, diarrhoea, and neuroglycopenic or sympathoadrenal symptoms from hypoglycaemia. We typically measure serum calcium annually to detect asymptomatic hyperparathyroidism, which may be treated surgically.

CDKN2A mutations, also known as FAMMM syndrome (familial atypical multiple mole/melanoma syndrome), is an autosomal dominant genodermatosis characterized by multiple melanocytic nevi, usually more than 50, and a family history of melanoma. This syndrome is associated with a wide variety of other tumour types and may be among the most common mutations in human cancer. Besides melanoma, families with CDKN2A mutations appear to have an increased risk of exocrine pancreatic cancer. This is more specifically in families with CDKN2A mutations that impaired the function of p16. Screening for melanoma in those susceptible to FAMMM should begin at age 10 with a baseline total body skin examination including scalp, oral mucosa, genital area, and nails, as family members may develop melanoma in their early teens.

There are currently no successful screening methods to detect early, operable pancreatic carcinoma. The anatomic location of the pancreas and late-presenting, often non-specific, initial symptoms of pancreatic cancer hinder the ability to detect masses at an early, resectable stage. However, promising results have been seen with the use of endoscopic ultrasound (EUS) and endoscopic retrograde cholangiopancreatography (ERCP) in clinical trials evaluating high-risk families. These tests are not currently considered standard of care, and patients and families at high risk for a pancreatic cancer, such as those with FAMMM syndrome, should be referred for consideration of clinical research screening programs.

Minimal invasive surgery

Laparoscopy

Laparoscopic surgery is a minimal invasive surgical modality that has increased its acceptance in oncological surgery in the last decades in some surgical fields. It is a keyhole technique that requires small incisions and the use of a laparoscope. To work with the laparoscope, a pneumoperitoneum is necessary to elevate the abdominal wall to create viewing and working space; to obtain this, carbon dioxide is insufflated intra-abdominally. In 1902, the first laparoscopic procedure was reported in dogs and in 1910 in humans. Prior to 1990, the only specialty performing laparoscopy regularly was gynaecology. In general surgery the laparoscopic cholecystectomy was the first accepted procedure. Conceptually, the laparoscopic approach is intended to minimize post-operative pain and reduce recovery times, while maintaining an enhanced visual field for surgeons. Disadvantages are loss of tactility, range of motion, poor depth perception, and a longer learning curve and operation time. Late conversion to open surgery is mostly due to complications such as bleeding or perforation and can bring the patient into a worse position than open surgery. From the societies (e.g., EAES) strict recommendations have been made to train professionals in laparoscopic techniques in order to optimize surgical quality. Due to improved patient outcomes in the last two decades, laparoscopic surgery has been adopted by various surgical subspecialties including gastrointestinal surgery, gynaecologic surgery, and urology. Based on numerous prospective randomized controlled trials, the approach has proven to be beneficial in reducing post-operative morbidities such as wound infections and incisional hernias, and is now deemed safe when applied to surgery for cancers such as cancer of the colon. Moreover, it renders similar outcomes with respect to overall survival and disease-specific survival. It should be taken into account that patient selection remains crucial; obesity, tumour extension to other organs or vessels, and previous abdominal surgeries increase the complexity or impossibility of laparoscopy [2–4].

Laparoscopic and/or thoracoscopic techniques have been developed for oesophageal cancer surgery, colon cancer, lung cancer surgery, rectal cancer surgery (confined to the rectal wall T2–T3 a/b), liver surgery, pancreas resection, adrenalectomy, nephrectomy, and even for breast cancer and small thyroid cancers.

Newer techniques include single incision laparoscopy (SIL) only using one port to execute the surgical procedure. Robotic approaches are used for prostatectomy and pelvic lymphadenectomy in expert centres and are ergonomically friendly for the surgeon but are still costly. Natural orifice transluminal endoscopic surgery (NOTES) is an experimental surgical technique whereby 'scarless' abdominal operations can be performed with an endoscope passed through a natural orifice (mouth, urethra, anus, etc.), then through an internal incision in the stomach, vagina, bladder, or colon, thus avoiding any external incisions or scars. This is not in widespread use yet.

Local treatments

There are many local treatments for early or palliative for advanced and borderline resectable cancer, usually at a risk of being less safe or not treating micrometastases in locoregional lymph nodes. Many techniques are still experimental and there is little hard evidence to promote them; expert centres could be consulted for advice.

TEM rectal cancer

A minimally invasive procedure called transanal endoscopic microsurgery (TEM) is indicated for removal of benign or premalignant rectal tumours and early-stage rectal cancers (T1). A full thickness excision is performed from the rectal wall and the mesorectum with the draining lymph nodes left in situ. Of course, there are many benefits of minimizing rectal cancer surgery, such as no abdominal scars, better sexual and urinary function, and less surgical complications.

However, it should always be noted that unknown lymph node metastasis (in pT1 approximately 8%) are not treated; TME surgery is recommended when the pathology report reveals high-risk features such as lymphovascular invasion, tumour stage more than T1sm2, poor differentiation grade, or incomplete resection. Follow-up is recommended frequently with endoscopy, CEA, and additional imaging and/or biopsies in case of symptoms.

Polypectomy, ESD, EMR, and EMA in colon cancer

For early colon cancers, advanced techniques such as endoscopic mucosal resection (EMR), endoscopic submucosal dissection (ESD), or even endoscopic mucosal ablation (EMA) are available. However, there are no data currently available showing long-term safety and equivalence with regards to oncologic outcomes. The main hesitation in using these endoscopic techniques for early colon cancer is that submucosal cancer invasion and/or lymph node involvement cannot be endoscopically recognized. Early colon cancer is defined as cancer that has progressed in the mucosa and/or submucosa, with or without lymph node involvement. Early colon cancer generally has a very good five-year prognosis and is traditionally treated surgically. Assessing the risk of lymph node metastasis should include a pathology exam with description of histological features such as moderate/poor differentiation, lymphatic invasion, positive margins, and depth of submucosal invasion. In contrast to their advice on surgical resection, expert groups are debating that surgery for early colon cancer without lymph node metastasis is unnecessary with respect to post-operative risks.

RFA in liver surgery

Local treatment in liver surgery has been developed to avoid large resections with its accompanying morbidity for borderline or unresectable disease. Of course, not all tumours or patients are suitable for these approaches. Because cryosurgery, using liquid nitrogen, or a probe that is very cold, to freeze and kill cancer cells is not being widely performed, this section will focus on RFA. RFA can be carried out percutaneously or during laparotomy. In RFA, a needle is inserted into the liver, usually under the guidance of ultrasonography or CT. Once it has been placed within the tumour, a rapidly alternating current (radiofrequency energy) is produced that destroys the tumour. It cannot be used for very large lesions or lesions that are on top of blood vessels. It can potentially leave small islands of remaining tumour cells, and is therefore regarded as a second-best choice after primary resection.

Laser surgery

Laser surgery uses a powerful beam of light, which can be directed at specific parts of the body, without making a large incision, to destroy cancer. For example, in the digestive system, a laser is often used to remove colon polyps (e.g., EMA). Laser surgery has been used to treat abnormal tissue, carcinoma in situ, and early cancer of the cervix, vagina, and vulva, to name a few.

Hyperthermic Intraperitoneal Chemotherapy (HIPEC)

Isolated peritoneal carcinomatosis in advanced colorectal cancer represents a special biologic entity with poor prognosis with systemic chemotherapy alone or with no intervention. Current data, including one randomized controlled trial and numerous prospective and retrospective studies, suggest a role for colorectal surgery and HIPEC in a multimodal treatment regimen that may improve PFS as well as OS for selected patients with peritoneal carcinomatosis. In the randomized trial, after a median follow-up of 21.6 months, the median survival was longer in the experimental arm than in the control arm (22.4 months versus 12.6 months, hazard ratio 0.55, 95% CI 0.32–0.95). The mortality rate was 8% in the HIPEC group, and the most severe toxicity was due to small intestinal leakage and sepsis.

HIPEC can be performed with acceptable morbidity and low mortality in specialized centres. Nevertheless, pre-operative patient selection is crucial for the success of the combined treatment concept. Main selection criteria are good general health status, limited intraperitoneal tumour dissemination (peritoneal cancer index, PCI < 20), limited small bowel disease, and no extra-abdominal metastasis [11].

Perioperative care

Fast track surgery

Fast track protocols in surgery were designed to minimize surgical complications by providing a multimodal approach, implementing as far as possible evidence-based tools to achieve early recovery after major surgery [12, 13]. This was first carried out for patients undergoing colectomy. ERAS (enhanced recovery after surgery) focuses on the following elements: improving patient education, reducing pain, reducing nausea and vomiting, stimulating normal diet, and getting the patient out of bed as soon as possible. Implementation of ERAS has resulted in a large reduction in length of hospital stay (see http://www.erassociety.org/). It takes teamwork from the patient, surgeon, anaesthesiologist, general practitioner, and nurses to make such a protocol work.

Surgical checklists and safety

Perioperative surgical checklists are mandated by many hospitals, as determined by the reduction in morbidity and mortality seen as a result of the use of the World Health Organization's Surgical Safety Checklist. Implementation of checklists has been associated with a reduction in surgical complications and mortality in hospitals with a high standard of care [14, 15].

Curative and palliative surgery

Curative surgery

Surgery gives the best chance to cure cancer; this means that all tumours should be removed during surgery. Curative surgeries remove partial or total organs of origin and in some cases the draining lymph nodes that might contain (micro)metastases.

Palliative surgery

The aim of palliative surgery is mainly to reduce pain or symptoms for the patient. The surgery may not necessarily aim to eradicate any or all cancer tissue in the patient. In fact, palliative surgery is often deemed to be worthwhile and feasible by cancer specialists when the disease is not responsive to any type of curative treatment. A successful palliative surgery may not only make the patient's life more comfortable, but may in some cases also prolong the patient's life. Palliative surgery which removes cancer tissue is recorded as cancer-directed surgery. Palliative surgery, such as a nerve block procedure to interrupt pain signals in the nervous system, or a stent placement to alleviate obstruction, etc., which does not remove cancer tissue is recorded as non-cancer-directed surgery. Deviating stoma formation can be done through a small incision to decompress an ileus due to obstructing colon or rectal carcinoma. A double bypass is an example of a palliative procedure ensuring the passage of food while a pancreatic cancer or duodenal cancer is obstructing the proximal intestines.

Locally advanced disease

In locally advanced disease, it is always advisable to ensure that a patient is sent to the appropriate referral centre for this specific cancer. The opportunities to be cured by surgery are higher in expert high-volume centres. In expert centres, experimental studies might offer the up-front non-surgical therapies to downsize the tumour and result in as much organ-sparing surgery as possible.

Local relapse and salvage treatment

In breast cancer, local recurrences can be operated by excision, salvage mastectomy, or salvage axillary clearance. Recurrent rectal cancer can be operated by wide excision and stoma formation, which can be very large resections with concomitant blood loss and post-operative recovery, yet still offering the best possibility for secondary cure. If a peri-anastomotic recurrence happens in colon cancer, this has a relative better prognosis than, for instance, peritoneal metastases. Salvage treatment should always be discussed in multidisciplinary teams and/or referral centres should be consulted to obtain the best treatment strategy.

Timing of Surgery

Upfront Surgery vs up-front systemic therapy vs up-front radiation or CRT therapy

Over the past decades, additional treatments for cancer have been introduced. Overall, surgery remains the cornerstone of cancer treatment in most cases. The addition of radiotherapy, chemotherapy, and the combination of radiotherapy and chemotherapy, has been investigated in many cancer types. The timing of these additional treatments has been under discussion.

In case of non-metastatic rectal cancer, patients could receive pre-operative radiotherapy or pre-operative chemoradiation, depending on the size and location of the tumour, whether the circumferential margin is threatened, and the possible malignant lymph nodes found on imaging. Pre-operative radiotherapy or chemoradiation is preferred over post-operative treatment, since the toxicity, local control, and compliance are better when pre-operative treatment is given. When pre-operative radiotherapy is chosen, the timing of the surgery to follow it is investigated at this point. In the Dutch TME trial, pre-operative radiotherapy is followed by surgery within ten days of the first fraction of radiotherapy [16, 17]. Several studies have suggested that an interval of more than three days between radiotherapy and surgery could lead to worse survival. The ongoing Stockholm III trial is investigating whether delayed surgery, with an interval of four to eight weeks between radiotherapy and surgery, is feasible, safe, and introduces downstaging of the tumour [18]. Pre-operative chemoradiation is preferred when downstaging of the tumour is needed. The timing between pre-operative chemoradiation and surgery is still under discussion, as it seems that the longer the interval, the more downstaging is achieved. In certain cases, this could lead to pathological complete responses, which are associated with excellent long-term outcome.

In breast cancer, adjuvant therapies for patients with a higher risk of recurrence are chemotherapy, hormonal therapy, or targeted drugs like trastuzumab. Tumour grade, stage, hormone receptor status, Her2 status, and lymph node status are factors involved in the decision for additional therapies. Many randomized trials report equivalent outcomes of neoadjuvant systemic therapies in comparison with adjuvant [19, 20]. The main benefit is to downsize the tumour and make it possible to discuss breast-conserving therapy (wide local excision combined with radiation therapy).

Specific procedures in surgical oncology

Sentinel node

In breast cancer, it has been established that the sentinel node (SN) procedure is very relevant for lymph node staging in clinically non-metastasized patients and plays a crucial role in the decision tree for initiation of adjuvant therapy. Even in patients with a biopsy of DCIS (ductal carcinoma in situ), a sentinel node is advised in the following situations: indication of mastectomy due to the large size of the DCIS, a small DCIS with risks of harbouring an invasive part such as in patients younger than 55 years of age, solid lesion on mammogram, or moderate or poor differentiated DCIS in the biopsy.

A sentinel node in melanoma is recommended for nodal staging of patients without clinical apparent metastases and in melanoma thicker than 1 mm. The recommendations are derived from studies showing no clinical relevance if there are already metastases because of a median survival of seven months, and in thin melanoma a very low incidence of lymph node metastases. From Dutch studies, five-year survival appears to be about 90% if the sentinel node is negative, in contrast to 65% when it is positive in clinically non-metastasized patients. It has a clear relevance in nodal staging in clinically non-metastasized melanoma. The evidence for additional lymph node dissection when the SN (sentinel node) is positive is still under investigation; no or weak differences in survival or disease-specific survival are currently described.

Two recent meta-analyses have acknowledged that a sentinel node procedure in patients undergoing resection for colorectal cancer has low sensitivity and little clinical relevance.

Role of the Multidisciplinary Teams (MDT)

Due to the difficult biology of cancer and the many specialties involved in the treatment, potentially suboptimal care could be given quite easily. In an ideal situation, patients would receive optimal treatment from an expert specialist, coordinated by one case officer. Over the past two decades, there has been growing recognition that shared decision-making was needed for optimal cancer care. Therefore, multidisciplinary care has become an integral part of cancer care in many Western countries. MDT meetings were established to ensure that care delivery is consistent with the best available evidence. The presence of different specialists means that consideration of the full range of therapeutic modalities is available for each patient. There is clear evidence that MDT meeting result in changes in patient management. And although limited, evidence indicates that MDTs are associated with improved patient outcomes for many cancer types, probably due to influencing various aspects of patient care. These factors include adherence to guidelines, nurse education, increased surgical volume and experience, and improved interdisciplinary working. Although multidisciplinary care is considered standard practice in many countries, access to such care still varies among countries and hospitals. The importance of good communication cannot be overstated, and is likely to become more rather than less important as cancer is determined to be a greater number of biomarker-determined disease subtypes. Both the European CanCer Organisation (ECCO) and the European Society of Surgical Oncology (ESSO) have as part of their mission the encouragement of true multidisciplinary cancer care.

Cancer management in Europe

Reflecting on cancer management in Europe, the EUROCARE-4 (EUROpean CAncer REgistry-based study on survival and CARE of cancer patients; http://www.eurocare.it/) analysis showed improved survival for all cancers and for all major cancer sites [21]. To collect good data on cancer management is demanding and time-consuming; however, these data are imperative to generate information on the quality of care. To give insight on variation between hospitals or countries, it is important to define best practices to learn from and to study subgroups of patients, such as the elderly, who are excluded from or underrepresented in randomized controlled trials. Large epidemiological research has been providing us with crude annual incidences and outcome comparisons of almost all cancers in Europe. The limitations of these studies are that they rely on completeness and quality of data from the available sources, mostly national cancer registries, and that not all countries have a national coverage of registry of patients with cancer.

Striving for multidisciplinary care is the vision of ECCO and ESSO. This means integrating the expertise and insights of the different professions and stakeholders that constitute the oncology community to achieve the best possible patient outcomes—taking into consideration the trends that impact on cancer, the complexity of the disease, and the specificity of each cancer patient.

A lot has changed in quality assurance in surgical oncology in many European countries as a result of introducing quality-control indicators and delivering voluntary or obligatory registries and audit structures. The improvements in cancer care have been spectacular. The next part of the chapter is dedicated to European surgical registries and audits and their results.

A history of cancer registries

Since the beginning of the twentieth century, cancer registries have provided population-based, comparative survival statistics for cancer patients. The task of the first population-based registry in Denmark, which started in 1943, was outlined as the collection of data in order to serve as a basis for individual follow-up of patients. The goal was to obtain reliable morbidity statistics with a view to an accurate estimate of therapeutic results and variations in the incidence of malignant neoplasms. From the mid-1940s, cancer registries were started up in a number of countries.

In 1989, EUROCARE was funded, based on collaboration between the Istituto Nazionale Tumori (Milan, Italy), the Istituto Superiore di Sanità (Rome, Italy) and a large number of population-based cancer registries from 12 European countries. EUROCARE is a cancer epidemiology research project on the incidence and survival of European cancer patients. It aims to describe any differences between populations, and if so, how large they are, how they evolve and how reliable the survival estimates are [22]. This project was the first to compare cancer survival rates among populations.

A comparison of the survival of patients diagnosed with cancer among different populations may be profoundly difficult to interpret, as longer survival may depend on either later death or earlier diagnosis (adding 'lead time'). In order to compare survival rates among different registries, it is necessary to have standardized information on disease stage at diagnosis, on the actual diagnostic procedures used for staging, and on treatment. These items are usually not available from population-based cancer registries.

Quality assurance in surgical oncology

Currently, quality assurance is a hot topic, although it is relatively new in surgical oncology. Audits have achieved excellent results at the national level, but differences between countries remain and cannot be easily explained. To reduce those differences by identifying and spreading best practice, ECCO and ESSO have initiated an international, multidisciplinary, outcome-based quality improvement programme, the European Registration of Cancer Care (EURECCA). EURECCA was founded in 2007 for rectal cancer; now, there are subgroups for colon and rectal cancer, breast cancer, oesophago-gastric cancer, and hepato-pancreatico-biliary cancer.

Surgical outcome showed large variation among centres. Surgery is steadily shifting from being a craft to becoming a transparent and well-defined skill. Training, specialization, knowledge, teamwork, and continuous quality improvement are considered mandatory for surgeons of the twenty-first century.

Since the beginning of the 1990s, several surgical audits have been set up in Europe. Initially, most of the audits were for rectal cancer, because of its poor outcome and variation both among hospitals and individual surgeons. Using audits, the Nordic countries were able to improve outcome in rectal cancer patients and showed that this process reduces healthcare-related costs.

Registries and audits of cancer in Europe

In the last two decades, there have been several European surgical audits. An audit is a quality instrument that collects detailed clinical data from different healthcare providers, which can be adjusted for baseline risk and subsequently fed back to individual hospitals or surgeons. In this way, 'best practices' can be identified, communicated, and broadly adopted.

Rectal cancer surgical audits

Most audits were initially set up for rectal cancer, as mentioned above, because of poor outcome and remarkable variation among hospitals and individual surgeons. Later, most rectal cancer audits expanded with the registry of the outcomes of colon cancer. Between 1993 and 2009, eight surgical (colo)rectal audits were performed in Europe. The oldest is the Norwegian Rectal Cancer Project started in 1993. Outstanding results were achieved after four years: the proportion of applied TME surgery increased from 78% to 92% and the local recurrence rate dropped from 28% to 7%. Moreover, they proved to be very cost effective. Currently, the audit is called the Norwegian Colorectal Cancer Project because colon cancer has also been incorporated. After the excellent results of the Norwegian Rectal Cancer Project, several other countries initiated audits on (colo)rectal cancer, including the Swedish Rectal Cancer Registry, the Danish Colorectal Cancer Database, the National Bowel Cancer Audit Programme (NBOCAP) from the UK, the International Quality Assurance in Colorectal Carcinoma from Germany, Poland, Italy, and Lithuania, the Project on Cancer of the Rectum (PROCARE) from Belgium, the Spanish TME project, and the Dutch Surgical Colorectal Audit.

EURECCA colorectal aims to improve care for patients with colorectal cancer in Europe by forming a European platform for sharing the data of registries and audits in order to be able to learn from them, and to form a core dataset in Europe. More information can be found at www.canceraudit.eu.

Breast cancer audits

Several projects have shown that the quality of breast cancer care can be improved by auditing as well. To illustrate, EUSOMA (the European Society of Mastology) is the organization representing breast cancer specialists in all disciplines in Europe. It promotes dedicated breast units by accreditation/certification, covering all aspects of breast cancer care, and developing guidelines and recommendations in order to form a basis for auditing [23].

Volume of procedures and outcome

It has been suggested that preventable surgical deaths may have been related to inadequate experience with the surgical procedures involved [24]. In the absence of better information or criteria that describe surgical quality, task forces aiming to improve surgical safety and surgical quality have embraced the volume norm. High-risk elective procedures in high-volume centres should reduce the risk of operative death [25].

An inverse relationship between volumes of surgical procedures per hospital and surgical outcome is at present relevant to many surgical cancer treatments. Hospitals are divided between high and low volume depending on the procedure. The surgeon and procedural volume have an effect on post-operative mortality and long-term survival.

Ever since the manuscript of Birkmeyer et al. [25] was published, a large number of studies on the effect of hospital volume on outcomes after gastrectomy have been published. Nowadays, centralization of gastric cancer surgery is implemented in the UK, Sweden, Finland, Denmark, Sweden, and the Netherlands. As in the Netherlands, oesophagectomies had already been centralized before; there will be also be upper gastrointestinal (GI) centres in other countries. This enables the formation of dedicated upper GI MDTs. Beside upper GI cancers, many other cancer surgery types are currently being centralized, such as pancreatic cancer surgery, hepatic surgery, breast cancer surgery, and colon and rectal cancer surgery.

Using hospital volume as the sole basis for referral to improve outcome has been criticized. Low-volume hospitals can have excellent outcomes, and vice versa. Studies on the surgeon's volume have been performed, but sometimes with contradictory results. It has been suggested that centralization combined with auditing is more effective in comparison with centralization alone. With auditing, providers of care are being monitored, and their performance is being benchmarked against others.

Shared decision-making

In cancer management, it is important that all steps are carefully discussed with the patient and that the physician listens and takes notice of the patient's preferences in the treatment. In 'shared decision-making' (SDM) clinicians and patients make decisions together using the best available evidence. This sounds logical, but not all surgeons have been trained to elucidate patients' preferences in the same session that diagnosis and treatment are discussed or even when the operation is scheduled. It has been postulated that physicians do not always choose according to the patient's preferences but substitute their own views [26]. In a study of 150 patients with prostate cancer facing radiation therapy, physicians were asked to judge which patient would choose which dosage if given the possibility of choosing between two dosages of radiation. Patients were provided with a decision aid (DA), clearly showing all the benefits and risks of each dosage scheme. Physicians proposed the preference that the patient would choose and then the actual patient preferences were compared. Physicians tended to underestimate the patients' decision-making preferences and made the assumption that patients would choose the less toxic treatment [26]. It might not just be the patient who needs counselling but also the physician who needs to be modernized in information flow to and from the patient.

In order to illustrate this important issue, given that we know that breast conserving therapy and mastectomy result in similar long-term outcomes, we raise the question as to whether patients diagnosed with early breast cancer, given the choice of breast-conserving or mastectomy, would make a high-quality choice [5]. Women diagnosed with breast cancer were given up-to-date, complete information about the risks and benefits of breast-conserving surgery and mastectomy in a controlled, supportive setting. After going through DA, the women completed exercises in explicit values clarification. Women were afterwards seen by a surgeon who endorsed a shared and informed decision-making process. Collins reported high knowledge scores, significant associations between patient values and treatment choice, and low decisional conflict [27]. In this study, a third of the women chose mastectomy, the more radical and potentially mutilating procedure [27]. Self-possession and peace of mind as a result of breast removal and having avoided radiation were rated significantly higher by participants choosing mastectomy. Other features and outcomes, such as avoiding local recurrence, did not differ between those choosing mastectomy over breast-conserving surgery.

A recent Cochrane meta-analysis concluded that using DAs improves the knowledge of patients about the intervention options relating to their disease and reduces decisional conflict [28]. Implementation of a web-based DA for breast cancer surgery increased patients' readiness to make a decision about their surgery, and was reinforced by having the surgery option at hand [29]. For an example of a website with a DA relating to surgery of the breast in breast cancer, see www.bresdex.com.

Further reading

Birkmeyer JD, Siewers AE, Finlayson EV, Stukel TA, Lucas FL et al. Hospital volume and surgical mortality in the United States. New England Journal of Medicine 2002 Apr 11; 346(15): 1128–1137.

Cardoso F, Loibl S, Pagani O, Graziottin A, Panizza P et al. The European Society of Breast Cancer Specialists recommendations for the management of young women with breast cancer. European journal of Cancer 2012; 48(18): 3355–3377.

de Cuba EM, Kwakman R, Knol DL, Bonjer HJ, Meijer GA et al. Cytoreductive surgery and HIPEC for peritoneal metastases combined with curative treatment of colorectal liver metastases: Systematic review of all literature and meta-analysis of observational studies. Cancer Treatment Review 2013; 39(4): 321–327.

Kapiteijn E, Marijnen CA, Nagtegaal ID, Putter H, Steup WH et al. Preoperative radiotherapy combined with total mesorectal excision for resectable rectal cancer. New England Journal of Medicine 2001; 345(9): 638–646.

Kehlet H. Multimodal approach to control postoperative pathophysiology and rehabilitation. British Journal of Anaesthesia 1997; 78(5): 606–617.

Nagtegaal ID, Quirke P. What is the role for the circumferential margin in the modern treatment of rectal cancer? Journal of Clinical Oncology 2008; 26(2): 303–312.

Nordlinger B, Sorbye H, Glimelius B, et al. Perioperative chemotherapy with FOLFOX4 and surgery versus surgery alone for resectable liver metastases from colorectal cancer (EORTC Intergroup trial 40983): a randomised controlled trial. Lancet 2008; 371(9617): 1007–1016.

Songun I, Putter H, Kranenbarg EM, Sasako M, van de Velde CJ. Surgical treatment of gastric cancer: 15-year follow-up results of the randomised nationwide Dutch D1D2 trial. Lancet Oncology 2010; 11(5): 439–449.

van der Hage JA, van de Velde CJ, Julien JP, Tubiana-Hulin M, Vandervelden C et al. Preoperative chemotherapy in primary operable breast cancer: results from the European Organization for Research and Treatment of Cancer trial 10902. Journal of Clinical Oncology 2001; 19(22): 4224–4237.

References

1. Glimelius B, Beets-Tan R, Blomqvist L, et al. Mesorectal fascia instead of circumferential resection margin in preoperative staging of rectal cancer. Journal of Clinical Oncology 2011; 29(16): 2142–2143.

2. Clinical Outcomes of Surgical Therapy Study Group. A comparison of laparoscopically assisted and open colectomy for colon cancer. New England Journal of Medicine 2004; 350(20): 2050–2059.

3. Kuhry E, Schwenk WF, Gaupset R, Romild U, Bonjer HJ. Long-term results of laparoscopic colorectal cancer resection. Cochrane Database System Review 2008(2): CD003432.

4. Lee JK, Delaney CP, Lipman JM. Current state of the art in laparoscopic colorectal surgery for cancer: Update on the multi-centric international trials. Annals of Surgical Innovation and Research 2012; 6(1): 5.

5. Litiere S, Werutsky G, Fentiman IS, Rutgers E, Christiaens MR et al. Breast conserving therapy versus mastectomy for stage I-II breast cancer: 20 year follow-up of the EORTC 10801 phase 3 randomised trial. Lancet Oncology 2012; 13(4): 412–419.

6. Simone NL, Dan T, Shih J, et al. Twenty-five year results of the national cancer institute randomized breast conservation trial. Breast Cancer Research and Treatment 2012; 132(1): 197–203.

7. Songun I, Putter H, Kranenbarg EM, Sasako M, van de Velde CJ. Surgical treatment of gastric cancer: 15-year follow-up results of the randomised nationwide Dutch D1D2 trial. Lancet Oncology 2010; 11(5): 439–449.

8. Nordlinger B, Sorbye H, Glimelius B, et al. Perioperative chemotherapy with FOLFOX4 and surgery versus surgery alone for resectable liver metastases from colorectal cancer (EORTC Intergroup trial 40983): a randomised controlled trial. Lancet 2008; 371(9617): 1007–1016.

9. Maddox WA, Carpenter JT Jr, Laws HT, Soong SJ, Cloud G et al. Does radical mastectomy still have a place in the treatment of primary operable breast cancer? Archives of Surgery 1987; 122(11): 1317–1320.

10. Nagtegaal ID, Quirke P. What is the role for the circumferential margin in the modern treatment of rectal cancer? Journal of Clinical Oncology 2008; 26(2): 303–312.

11. de Cuba EM, Kwakman R, Knol DL, Bonjer HJ, Meijer GA et al. Cytoreductive surgery and HIPEC for peritoneal metastases combined with curative treatment of colorectal liver metastases: Systematic review of all literature and meta-analysis of observational studies. Cancer Treatment Review 2013; 39(4): 321–327.

12. Kehlet H. Multimodal approach to control postoperative pathophysiology and rehabilitation. British Journal of Anaesthesia 1997; 78(5): 606–617.

13. Kehlet H, Slim K. The future of fast-track surgery. British Journal of Surgery 2012; 99(8): 1025–1026.

14. de Vries EN, Prins HA, Crolla RM, den Outer AJ, van Andel G et al. Effect of a comprehensive surgical safety system on patient outcomes. New England Journal of Medicine 2010; 363(20): 1928–1937.

15. de Vries EN, Eikens-Jansen MP, Hamersma AM, Smorenburg SM, Gouma DJ et al. Prevention of surgical malpractice claims by use of a surgical safety checklist. Annals of Surgery 2011; 253(3): 624–628.

16. Kapiteijn E, Marijnen CA, Nagtegaal ID, Putter H, Steup WH et al. Preoperative radiotherapy combined with total mesorectal excision for resectable rectal cancer. New England Journal of Medicine 2001; 345(9): 638–646.

17. van Gijn GW, Marijnen CA, Nagtegaal ID, Kranenbarg EM, Putter H et al. Preoperative radiotherapy combined with total mesorectal excision for resectable rectal cancer: 12-year follow-up of the multicentre, randomised controlled TME trial. Lancet Oncology 2011; 12(6): 575–582.

18. Pettersson D, Cedermark B, Holm T, Radu C, Påhlman L et al. Interim analysis of the Stockholm III trial of preoperative radiotherapy regimens for rectal cancer. British Journal of Surgery 2010; 97(4): 580–587.

19. Mauri D, Pavlidis N, Ioannidis JP. Neoadjuvant versus adjuvant systemic treatment in breast cancer: a meta-analysis. Journal of the National Cancer Institute 2005; 97(3): 188–194.

20. van der Hage JA, van de Velde CJ, Julien JP, Tubiana-Hulin M, Vandervelden C et al. Preoperative chemotherapy in primary operable breast cancer: results from the European Organization for Research and Treatment of Cancer trial 10902. Journal of Clinical Oncology 2001; 19(22): 4224–4237.

21. Verdecchia A, Francisci S, Brenner H, Gatta G, Micheli A et al. Recent cancer survival in Europe: a 2000-02 period analysis of EUROCARE-4 data. Lancet Oncology 2007; 8(9): 784–796.

22. Berrino F. The EUROCARE Study: strengths, limitations and perspectives of population-based, comparative survival studies. Annals of Oncology 2003; 14(Suppl. 5): v9–13.

23. Cardoso F, Loibl S, Pagani O, Graziottin A, Panizza P et al. The European Society of Breast Cancer Specialists recommendations for the management of young women with breast cancer. European Journal of Cancer 2012; 48(18): 3355–3377.

24. Dudley RA, Johansen KL, Brand R, Rennie DJ, Milstein A. Selective referral to high-volume hospitals: estimating potentially avoidable deaths. Journal of the American Medical Association 2000; 283(9): 1159–1166.

25. Birkmeyer JD, Siewers AE, Finlayson EV, Stukel TA, Lucas FL et al. Hospital volume and surgical mortality in the United States. New England Journal of Medicine 2002 Apr 11; 346(15): 1128–1137.

26. Stalmeier PF, van Tol-Geerdink JJ, van Lin EN, Schimmel E, Huizenga H et al. Doctors' and patients' preferences for participation and treatment in curative prostate cancer radiotherapy. Journal of Clinical Oncology 2007; 25(21): 3096–3100.

27. Collins ED, Moore CP, Clay KF, Kearing SA, O'Connor AM et al. Can women with early-stage breast cancer make an informed decision for mastectomy? Journal of Clinical Oncology 2009; 27(4): 519–525.

28. Stacey D, Bennett CL, Barry MJ, Col NF, Eden KB et al. Decision aids for people facing health treatment or screening decisions. Cochrane Database System Review 2011(10): CD001431.

29. Sivell S, Edwards A, Manstead AS, Reed MW, Caldon L et al. Increasing readiness to decide and strengthening behavioral intentions: evaluating the impact of a web-based patient decision aid for breast cancer treatment options (BresDex: www.bresdex.com). Patient Education and Counselling 2012; 88(2): 209–217.

CHAPTER 20

Practice points for radiation oncology

Annekatrin Seidlitz, Stephanie E. Combs,
Jürgen Debus, and Michael Baumann

Introduction to radiation oncology

Radiotherapy is an indispensable treatment modality in modern oncology with curative potential in a wide spectrum of malignancies. About half of all cancer patients today receive radiotherapy during the course of their disease either with curative or palliative intent. The proportion of cancer patients treated by radiotherapy is steadily increasing as a consequence of outcomes which are equivalent to surgical approaches in several tumours, increased use of function-preserving approaches in oncology, better access to radiotherapy, and other factors. Radiotherapy is often combined with surgery or cytostatic drugs; increasingly, combinations with molecular targeted drugs are being introduced in clinical practice. In contrast to systemic treatment approaches, curative radiation therapy aims to obtain permanent local or locoregional tumour control by eradicating all macroscopic or microscopic tumour in the irradiated volume. Because of the spatial distribution of dose, radiotherapy is highly dependent on imaging information. Throughout its history radiotherapy has been an interprofessional approach integrating clinical oncology, medical physics and technology, and radiation biology. Progress in all of these fields has contributed to today's high efficacy of radiotherapy [1]. Technological developments in treatment machines, imaging, and information technology for rapid treatment planning allow delivery of highly conformal radiation dose distributions which cover the tumour and spare surrounding normal tissues. These technologies have been rapidly translated into clinical practice. Radiotherapy regularly uses model-based approaches to individualize treatment based on imaging information and radiobiological data on tumour control (TCP) and normal tissue complication (NTCP) probabilities. This personalized radiation treatment is expected to be enhanced in the coming years beyond anatomical and clinical data by relevant biomarkers, particularly bioimage-based information.

The scope of this brief chapter cannot be to give a comprehensive overview of the foundations and practice of radiooncology; excellent textbooks are available for this [2–5]. Rather, we focus on some important basic principles, practice points, and developmental strategies which are of relevance to the non-radiation oncologist which might be of use for discussions in the multidisciplinary setting.

Aim of radiotherapy and therapeutic window

The aim of radiotherapy is to achieve uncomplicated local or locoregional tumour control by permanently inactivating all cancer cells in the irradiated volume without inducing severe normal tissue reactions. This concept was laid out by H. Holthusen in the 1930s [6]. After variable threshold doses, steep and usually sigmoid-shaped increases of TCP and NTCP are observed. If, for a given radiation treatment technique and schedule the TCP curve is located left of the NCTP curve, uncomplicated local tumour control initially increases, with the effect on the tumour reaching a maximum before it falls again when the NTCP also increases. The therapeutic window depends therefore on the relative position of the TCP and NTCP curves as they reflect the overall radiosensitivity of a given tumour versus the surrounding normal tissue. The aim of clinical radiotherapy is to prescribe for an individual patient a dose close to the maximum of uncomplicated local tumour control. This almost always means that some risk of severe normal tissue reactions has to be accepted, which has important implications for informed consent discussions and for follow-up of patients after treatment. The aim of research in radiation oncology is to broaden the therapeutic window by either increasing the radiosensitivity of tumours or by making normal tissues more radioresistant or, optimally, both.

Radiation effects on tumours

Radiotherapy given alone or in combination with drugs is highly effective in permanently inactivating cancer stem cells (CSC). CSCs are defined functionally as cells that have the ability to expand and form a recurrent tumour after high dose irradiation [7]. Cancer cells as well as normal cells can be radiation-inactivated through several mechanisms. Generally speaking, unrepaired or not correctly repaired DNA damage is underlying radiobiological radiation-induced cell kill. Of particular importance is the presence of oxygen directly at the time of irradiation, as free oxygen may fix DNA damage which otherwise is scavenged. Thus, cells irradiated in the presence of oxygen are more sensitive than cells irradiated under hypoxic conditions (oxygen effect) by a factor of approximately three. This effect is clinically highly relevant as many tumours contain a large proportion of hypoxic cells [8]. As DNA damage frequently occurs in every cell of the body, different efficient repair mechanisms have evolved during evolution (see Chapter 9 'DNA Repair after Oncological Therapy' in this volume). Unrepaired DNA double-strand breaks or clusters of such damage are considered to be the most important DNA damage leading to cell death after radiotherapy. The leading mode of radiation-induced cell death is mitotic cell death (or mitotic catastrophe) caused by severe chromosome damage which results in the inability of the cell to divide correctly in the next (or one of the next) M-phase of the cell cycle. Autophagy as well as direct radiation-induced cell necrosis play a minor role in the inactivation of non-haematological tumour cells. Direct cellular necrosis does not significantly contribute to radiation-induced cell kill, but may play a role as an unregulated process of cell destruction due to ischaemia and inflammation. Apoptotic cell death plays a major role after irradiation of haematopoietic and lymphatic neoplasm and some normal tissues but only a minor role in the majority of solid tumours. Radiation-induced senescence is one of the central mechanisms in normal tissue reactions like fibrosis, as will be explained later.

Permanent local control after radiotherapy is only achieved if all CSCs are inactivated by radiation or killed by the host (e.g., immune reactivity) or if surviving CSCs are remaining in a permanent dormant state [9]. If one or more CSCs survive irradiation and escape inactivation by the host, recurrence will occur. Radiobiological studies indicate that inactivation of CSC is an exponential function of dose and that after the high radiation doses typically applied in curative radiotherapy on average only few CSCs survive (see Figure 20.1A). This has important implications, as drugs which often have only relatively weak effects on CSCs may show significant anti-tumour effects when combined with radiation.

Selected key points of general importance for multidisciplinary oncology which can be derived from the radiation dose-effects on CSC include the following:

Geographic miss needs to be avoided

As a single surviving CSC may cause a recurrence and radiation dose response relationships in general are steep, it is of the utmost importance to ensure that all tumour cells are covered by the prescribed dose. While this may sound trivial, it certainly is not, given the severe limitations of imaging technologies to define small tumour extensions and microscopic disease, the motion of tumours and normal tissues during the treatment series and individual fractions, and changing anatomy during treatment (e.g., weight loss related decrease of fatty and soft tissues, tumour growth or regression). Much of the

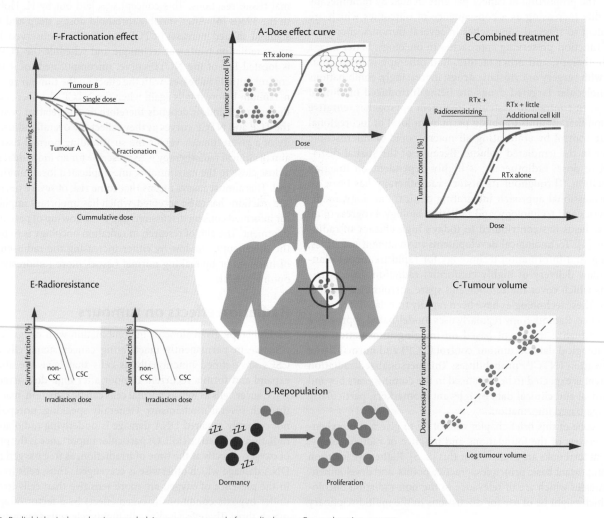

Fig. 20.1 Radiobiological mechanisms underlying tumour control after radiotherapy. For explanation see text.

Adapted from *Radiotherapy and Oncology: Journal of the European Society for Therapeutic Radiology and Oncology*, Volume 108, Issue 3, Butof R et al., Clinical perspectives of cancer stem cell research in radiation oncology, pp. 388–396, Copyright © 2013 with permission from Elsevier, http://www.sciencedirect.com/science/journal/aip/01678140

recent technological advances in image-guided radiotherapy, with increasing use of in-room imaging equipment, are aimed at minimizing these problems. It is also important to understand that scientific evaluation of local tumour control after radiotherapy requires detailed knowledge of the site of recurrence and the dose applied to this site (Figure 20.2). Only from such data can information on, for example, the radiosensitivity of a given tumour be derived.

The dose necessary for permanent local eradication of a tumour increases with the logarithm of the number of CSCs present in the tumour

In a given tumour site and histology, tumour volume is a clinically valid approximation of CSC number [9, 10]. Frequently, lower doses are therefore prescribed to areas with low tumour burden, such as subclinical or microscopic residual disease, compared with macroscopic tumours of different volumes. Because of exponential radiation cell kill, the dose levels needed to eradicate tumours of different volumes do not increase linearly but on a logarithmic basis (Figure 20.1C). This leads in clinical practice to relatively small differences in prescribed dose which, for example on tumour boards, are often found counterintuitive by oncologists not trained in radiobiological principles. A clinically particularly important example is macroscopic incomplete resection of tumour ('removal of bulk'). Even if 90% of the tumour is resected, the radiation oncologist has to apply almost or exactly the same dose to the residual tumour, as if it has not been resected, because logarithmic cell kill 90% removal corresponds generally to about 2 fractions of 2 Gy. Thus, while the effect of macroscopic incomplete resection is small or nil, there may be added unwarranted treatment effects on normal tissues from surgery and radiotherapy. Notable exceptions include situations where due to (incomplete) resection, the radiation volume can be importantly reduced or critical normal tissues, such as the optic nerve, can be excluded altogether from the treatment volume. It is obvious that such approaches require detailed interdisciplinary discussion and treatment planning before administering therapy. On the other hand, because of the steep dose-response relationships, relatively small escalations in total dose to macroscopic tumours may lead to significant increase of local tumour control rates. This is one of the reasons underlying the enthusiasm of radiation oncologists toward highly conformal precision techniques because these may allow escalation of the total dose without exceeding (volume-dependent, see below) normal tissue tolerance.

Regression of tumours after chemotherapy may not allow significant reduction of total radiation dose

Another important clinical practice point originating from the exponential cell kill of radiation is that partial regression of tumours after drug treatment, even if impressive, usually does not allow a significant reduction in the radiation dose to the tumour. In addition, regression after induction treatment may importantly disturb the relationship of volume and CSC number if the drugs applied are mainly effective on non-CSCs [7]. As there are currently no clinically suitable tests for CSC survival after induction treatment,

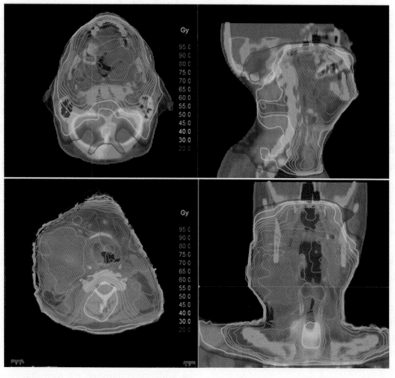

Fig. 20.2 Individual and scientific evaluation of treatment outcome after radiotherapy requires detailed knowledge of the site of recurrence and the dose applied to this site. 18Fluor-deoxyglucose uptake in recurrent tumours detected by PET-CT in two patients treated with identical radiochemotherapy for advanced head and neck cancer was superimposed to the original treatment plans. (*Upper panels*) 36 m after end of treatment of a T4 N2 carcinoma of the tongue a recurrence was detected within the former high-dose region. (*Lower panels*) 6 m after treatment recurrence was diagnosed in a region formerly spared from radiation for normal tissue protection in a patient with T2 N3 carcinoma of the piriform sinus. While the tumour in the upper panels was resistant to the treatment, no statement on resistance is possible for the second tumour.

reduction of radiation doses based on regression after drug treatment may potentially jeopardize local control and should therefore be reserved for the clinical research setting. However, one potential advantage of induction chemotherapy is that the radiation target volume may be reduced after response to the drugs.

The dose necessary for local control of tumours of equal size depends on the density and radiosensitivity of CSC

It is well recognized that the radiosensitivity of different tumour entities differs widely. While lymphomas and germ cell tumours are often exquisitely radiosensitive, sarcomas and high-grade gliomas are usually highly radioresistant. The most frequent tumour entities, squamous cell or adenocarcinomas, range between these extremes [11]. In addition to these differences of radiosensitivity among tumour entities there is also vast heterogeneity of radiosensitivity between tumours of the same histology and size in different patients (intertumoral heterogeneity). Recent research indicates that even different subvolumes of the same tumour in the same patient may differ in radiosensitivity (intratumoral heterogeneity). It is obvious that knowledge of the radiosensitivity of individual tumours obtained from predictive tests before the start of treatment would provide an opportunity to better tailor the treatment to individual patients. Currently several such tests are under preclinical and clinical investigation. Radiobiological mechanisms that may underlie differences in radiosensitivity of tumours of equal volume include:

- CSC density/total CSC number to inactivate
- intrinsic cellular radiosensitivity of CSC and repair capacity of CSC during fractionated radiotherapy. Radiosensitivity of some CSC may differ from non CSC (Figure 20.1E–F)
- repopulation of CSC during treatment (Figure 20.1D)
- hypoxia and other microenvironmental factors may increase radioresistance of CSC.

Combination of irradiation with drugs will increase local tumour control only if the drugs kill additional CSCs or if they radiosensitize CSCs

Figure 20.1B illustrates that combination with radiosensitizing substances or drugs which directly kill CSC can shift the dose-response curve for local tumour control to the left, i.e. may achieve a higher curative potential for the same radiation dose. This can be clinically very important if the radiation doses applied cannot be further escalated because of risk of normal tissue complications and if at the same time no (or little) overlapping toxicities exist between the drugs and radiation for the dose-limiting normal tissue [12]. A large number of clinical trials have corroborated this strategy in the past decades, and simultaneous drug plus radiation treatment is today more the rule than the exception. Different mechanisms have been shown to underlie the improvement through combined modality treatment, most importantly independent kill of CSCs. However, direct cellular radiosensitization or more indirect mechanisms such as reduction of repopulation or the improved oxygenation status of CSCs may improve local control after combining radiotherapy with drugs. Further exploitable mechanisms of combined radiochemotherapy include spatial cooperation (i.e.

radiation to kill the macroscopic tumour bulk and chemotherapy to destroy micrometastases) or modification of treatment volumes in sequential approaches [13]. It should be noted, however, that particularly in the field of molecular targeted drugs many combinations with radiation have shown more pronounced tumour regression and longer growth delay but no impact on local tumour control. Such drugs obviously are effective on the bulk of non-CSCs in the tumour but ineffective at killing CSCs in the context of radiotherapy (Figure 20.1B). As it has been shown that novel drugs might also modulate the radiation response of normal tissues in both directions, it will be important carefully to investigate if the therapeutic window can be broadened by new approaches.

Radiation effects on normal tissues

The radiosensitivity of organs at risk depends on the types of tissue of which they are composed, their structure, function, pre-existing defects, and remaining potential for compensation. In addition, the different parameters of radiotherapy, including beam quality, total dose, dose per fraction, time interval between fractions, dose per week, overall treatment time, volume irradiation, and spatial dose-distribution, have significant impact on radiation effects in normal tissues (as well as in tumours). The challenge of radiation treatment planning is to minimize the risk of normal tissue damage while fully covering the tumour. To facilitate this complex and dynamic process the radiation oncologist utilizes data derived from detailed long-term observation of irradiated patients. Through the use of appropriate radiobiological and biostatistical methodology, data with high spatial resolution on normal tissue effects are correlated with dose-volume-fractionation parameters under consideration of clinical parameters, for example on pre-existing damage. From these data NTCP-curves are established that will then be used in a model-based approach in the radiation treatment planning of future patients. Although considerable inter-patient heterogeneity exists in the risk of a given normal tissue reaction after the same treatment, NTCP curves tend to be significantly steeper than TCP curves due to more extensive intertumoral heterogeneity. In general, it is useful to differentiate between two broad classes of normal tissue effects in radiotherapy, i.e. early and late effects.

Early radiation-induced normal tissue reactions

Early (or acute) normal tissue reactions occur during radiotherapy and usually resolve within weeks or a few months after treatment. The underlying radiobiological mechanism is the kill of stem or precursor cells with subsequent cell depletion in tissues with high turnover. Typical examples include haematological effects, mucositis, dermatitis, or hair loss. Incidence and severity and to some extent time of onset of early radiation-induced normal tissue reactions increase with:

- increasing total dose
- increased dose-intensity (weekly dose), i.e. short overall treatment times
- increased volume
- additional damage, e.g. simultaneous cytotoxic therapy

Early side effects cannot only importantly compromise the patients' wellbeing but may also cause treatment interruptions or dose limitation, thereby potentially decreasing the chance of local tumour control.

Intermediate late reactions

Radiogenic pneumonitis and demyelination disorders of the central nervous system such as Lhermitte's syndrome are examples of intermediate late side effects of radiotherapy. Radiobiological parameters are neither typical for early or late reactions. For example, the risk of pneumonitis increases after both short overall treatment times and high doses per fraction.

Consequential late effects

Consequential late effects are defined as late effects occurring after particularly severe early normal tissue reactions and, while follow the radiobiology of early normal tissue reactions, show the typical time course and morphology of late normal tissue reactions.

Late radiation-induced normal tissue reactions

In contrast to early effects, late normal tissue reactions occur months or even years after completion of radiotherapy, and are usually irreversible and often even progressive. Typical examples include subcutaneous or lung fibrosis, telangiectasia, necrosis, vascular stenosis, or damage of nerves and radionecrosis of CNS tissue. Fibrosis, for example, is often already fully expressed after one or few years, while coronary stenosis is an example of a late damage often occurring a decade or later after end of treatment. For a long time it has been assumed that, much as early normal tissue damage, late effects are caused by cellular depletion. Long turnover times of target cells were assumed to be the cause of clinical delay of damage. While this radiobiological mechanism remains part of the explanation of the clinical time course, it is now known that molecular events in cells, tissue and potentially even the whole organism cascade over long time intervals and contribute to the development of subclinical and overt late damage. Incidence and severity of late radiation-induced normal tissue reactions increase with:

+ increasing total dose
+ increased dose per fraction
+ short time intervals between fractions
+ increased volume
+ additional damage, e.g. simultaneous cytotoxic therapy, trauma, or infection to irradiated tissue.

Today the radiation dose applied to the tumour is usually limited by the risk of late normal tissue reactions. Late NTCP can only be considered during prescription and treatment planning, which relies on continuous evaluation of detailed clinical data of patients treated in the past [14, 15].

Secondary malignancies

Ionizing radiation is well recognized as a potential cause of secondary malignancies. This issue is reviewed in detail by K. Trott in Chapter 17 'Radiation' in this volume.

Management of radiation-induced normal tissue effects

The management of side effects requires a high level of expertise. Early reactions need intense supportive care during radiation treatment to prevent treatment interruption or other unwarranted modifications of treatment. Patients with early normal tissue reactions should always be seen by their radiation oncologists who needs to review whether these are expected based on the treatment plan or, if unexpected, will re-review the parameters of radiotherapy. The radiation oncologist also recommends supportive measures to ameliorate the symptoms as well as for skin care, nutrition, and pain control during treatment. Suspected late normal tissue damage also needs to be evaluated by the radiation oncologist because such damage occurs only in irradiated volumes and usually follows closely the biological effective radiation dose distribution. Not infrequently, radiation damage is assumed by other healthcare professionals to underlie a new lesion or symptom in a patient previously treated by radiotherapy, while this is judged to be extremely unlikely after expert review, necessitating further diagnostic evaluation. Last but not least, the radiation oncologist should be involved in cases of further treatment such as surgery (or even surgical dental care) when this affects pre-irradiated tissues. This enhances the pre-therapeutic assessment of the risk of complications, and frequently allows modification of the procedure. Even on histopathological exam it is not possible to determine if a tumour has been induced by radiation. Therefore, suspected radiation-induced tumours should be reported to the radiation oncologist. As late normal tissue reactions are the main dose-limiting factor in modern radiotherapy, detailed follow-up of patients with analysis of outcome is the only option for the radiation oncologists to further refine model-based radiation treatment planning. Therefore, long-term follow-up of patients is established good clinical practice in radiotherapy, and in some countries even mandatory by law.

Utilizing radiobiological knowledge: dose per fraction, overall treatment time, volume

Fractionation in curative treatment is aimed at broadening the therapeutic window

Early in the twentieth century, both radiation treatment with a high-dose single irradiation or few fractions (German school) and treatments with a large number of fractions (French school) were in use in radiotherapy [1, 16]. Fractionated radiotherapy with 2 Gy per fraction and five fractions per week to different total doses (dependent on tumour entity, size and location) over several weeks became an international standard for many decades (so-called conventional fractionation, CF) and probably continues to be the most often applied fractionation schedule [17, 18]. Some centres, particularly in the UK and in Canada, applied somewhat higher doses per fraction to lower total doses in a shorter overall treatment time on a routine basis. Such schedules would be categorized as moderately hypofractionated and accelerated radiotherapy. Treatment with single doses or few fractions were reintroduced to curative clinical radiotherapy in the context of modern stereotactic ablative radiotherapy approaches. From a radiobiological point of view, fractionated radiotherapy has the following main advantages compared to single-dose treatments or radiotherapy with few fractions [19, 20]:

+ Early normal tissue damage depends significantly on overall treatment time, that is on dose-intensity (dose per week). Thus, fractionated treatments over longer treatment periods lead to less early normal tissue reactions and are better tolerated by the patients. The downside is that CSC may repopulate the tumours during treatment which decreases the change of permanent local tumour control. Such repopulation has been demonstrated for a variety of tumours, most notably squamous cell carcinoma of the head and neck, lung, and other sites but at a lower magnitude for prostate cancer, for example.

- ◆ Late normal tissue damage increases with increasing dose per fraction, while this is not the case for many tumours. Thus, application of higher number of low-dose fractions widens the therapeutic window between tumours and late-responding normal tissues, given that the time interval between the fractions is long enough (usually six to eight hours; for some tissues even more). The downside here is that there are notable exceptions among tumours. For example, the probability of locally controlling breast cancer and likely prostate cancer at the same total dose increases with dose per fraction; however, there might be significant intertumoral heterogeneity.

- ◆ Tumours often contain large proportions of hypoxic radioresistant CSCs while there is little or no hypoxia in surrounding normal tissues. Radiation first kills the sensitive cells but, dependent on dose and the proportion of hypoxic cells, these will dominate the overall effect. During fractionated radiotherapy, hypoxic tumour cells may reoxygenate, which would enhance the therapeutic effect.

Over the past decades modified fractionation schedules have been developed based on the following radiobiological principles.

Accelerated radiotherapy (AF)

AF entails application of the total dose in shorter overall treatment time. AF that counteracts CSC repopulation has been shown in a number of randomized trials (HNSCC and lung cancer) to increase locoregional control at the same total dose as used for CF, or to result in equivalent local tumour control at decreased total radiation doses. With AF, early normal tissue reactions are increased, while late normal tissue reactions are either constant or slightly increased. The latter may be the consequence of too short time intervals between fractions or very intense normal tissue reactions leading to consequential late effects. A very important lesson learned from AF clinical trials is that overall treatment times in curative radiotherapy should not be prolonged beyond prescription [21, 22]. Evidence is emerging that for concurrent radiochemotherapy the impact of overall treatment time on local tumour control is less than for radiotherapy given alone.

Hyperfractionated radiotherapy (HF)

HF is the application of doses per fraction less than 2 Gy (usually 1.1–1.3 Gy, two fractions per day). HF intends to decrease late normal tissue damage, thereby allowing an increase in the total dose to the tumour. This finds support in randomized trials on HNSCC; however, late normal tissue damage was usually not reduced to the anticipated extent. HF is often combined with AF, allowing an increase in total dose or a decrease in late normal tissue reactions and at the same time counteracting repopulation.

Moderate hypofractionation

In tumours with potentially high repair capacity, such as breast cancer, moderate hypofractionation, with, for example, 3 Gy per fraction, can achieve the same local tumour control at lower total dose, that is at a lower number of fraction. Whether this approach widens the therapeutic ratio is still under debate. Notably, moderate hypofractionation is usually also accelerated and thereby might

also counteract repopulation of CSC. Moderate hypofractionation has, among techniques, an emerging role in particle therapy.

Single-dose treatment or hypofractionation

Single-dose treatment of hypofractionation doses per fractions of 3 Gy or more is regularly used for palliative treatments where total doses are low (e.g., 10 x 3 Gy, 4 x 5 Gy, 1-2 x 8 Gy) and life expectancy is usually short. It also is used clinically on a routine basis for high-precision stereotactic radiotherapy to small tumours using high, so-called ablative doses.

High-precision conformal radiotherapy

As outlined above, all CSCs have to be inactivated to achieve local tumour control. For this the gross tumour volume (GTV) has to be identified and delineated in the treatment plan ([23, 24], see Figure 20.5D). The tumour position often changes during a single fraction (e.g., respiratory motion in lung cancer) or between fractions. This can today be taken into account by image-guided daily set-up, by motion control, or by 4D CT based treatment planning (iGTV). Furthermore, there are microscopic tumour extensions or microscopic deposits of tumour cells which cannot be depicted by imaging but need to be defined by statistical experience (e.g., from resection specimens) in the so-called CTV (clinical target volume: [23, 24], see Figure 20.5D). Further margins need to be added, for example, for physical beam characteristics and remaining geometrical and motion uncertainties (planning target volume, PTV: [23, 24], see Figure 20.5D). In earlier times, generous margins were applied to account for all these uncertainties. However, both early and late NTCP increases with increasing high-dose volume (and to some extent also with low-dose volume). Thus, high-precision radiotherapy, which conforms the dose to the tumour and spares as much sensitive normal tissue as possible, reduces the risk of normal tissue damage substantially and widens the therapeutic window as long as all tumour tissue is covered. Conformal radiotherapy has also allowed substantial escalation of the doses applied over the past decades, thereby significantly improving local tumour control rates.

Essentials of physics and technology in radiotherapy

Most radiation treatments are given as external beam radiotherapy (EBRT) using megavoltage photons. These are applied either using cobalt 60 units or, much more frequently today, linear electron accelerators (linacs). In linacs, high-energy electrons are stopped at a target, thereby generating X-rays with maximum photon energies typically from 4 to 20 MV. Particle therapy with protons, carbon ions, or other ions is emerging as a new clinical treatment modality, but currently is available at only a few centres worldwide. Figure 20.3 compares the depth dose distribution of different beam qualities. Electrons have an energy-dependent finite range in tissue and are therefore mainly suitable for treatment of superficial tumours where they can spare underlying deeper normal tissues. Megavoltage X-rays of different energies show an energy-dependent build-up region at the entrance surface before they reach their dose maximum at the depth of a few centimetres. This build-up reflects the energy transfer onto secondary electrons which is of great clinical importance for sparing skin

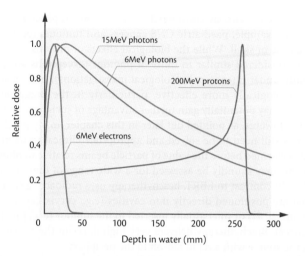

Fig. 20.3 Depth dose distribution of different beam qualities. For further explanation see text.

Source: data for proton curve drawn from Richter C, *Dosimetrische Charakterisierung laserbeschleunigter Teilchenstrahlen für in vitro Zellbestrahlungen*, Dissertation, Technische Universität Dresden, Germany, Copyright © 2013.

and superficial structures. Introduction of megavoltage beams into clinical radiotherapy between the 1950s and 1970s because of their depth-dose characteristics has been a major technological breakthrough compared to lower energy X-rays used before.

These orthovoltage X-rays did not have skin-sparing effects and therefore frequently resulted in dose-limiting skin reactions. For photon beams there is an energy-dependent decrease of dose behind the dose maximum. In contrast, protons and heavier ions have a lower entrance channel dose. At the end of the range, a large portion of their energy is deposited over a very small distance, resulting in the so called Bragg peak. The range of the particles in tissue and thereby the depth of the Bragg peak depends on the beam energy. Thus, compared to photon beams, particle beams show an inverted dose distribution which can be utilized for improved protection of normal tissues. For treatment with photons, normal tissues before and behind the tumour will always be irradiated to relatively high doses (Figure 20.4); this is not true for particle beams where dose to normal tissues behind the tumour can be effectively avoided. To spare dose to normal tissues while achieving relatively homogeneous dose distribution in the tumour, photon beams in clinical practice are almost always applied using several fields from different directions (Figure 20.4). This concentrates the high-dose region to the tumour (crossfire irradiation), but at the cost of smearing lower doses to larger volumes of normal tissues. Arc treatments extend this concept to an extreme by delivering the radiation practically through an infinite number of fields. Stereotactic body or brain radiotherapy also uses this concept, utilizing either arcs or a high number of fields to treat small tumours with very steep fall-off of dose to the periphery. To

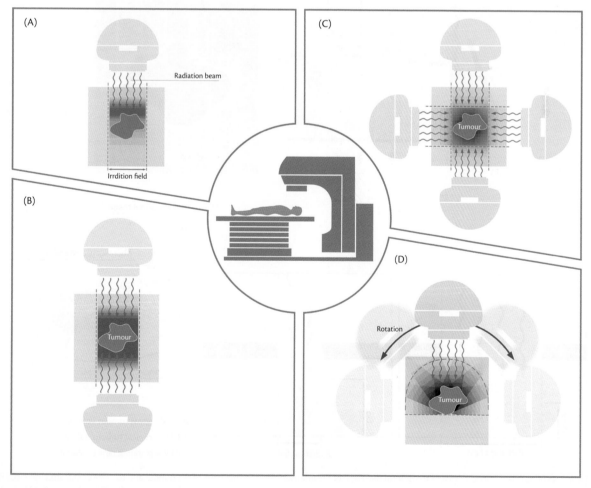

Fig. 20.4 Dose distributions for different beam arrangements. With increasing number of treatment fields the conformality of the high-dose region to the tumour increases, while low doses are smeared to larger volumes.

achieve conformality while blocking tissue that is not intended to be irradiated from that direction, radiation fields are shaped by individual customized metal blocks or, today, by motorized multileaf collimators (MLC) which may assume essentially each shaping geometry (Figure 20.5A and 20.5B). As the leaves of MLC can be moved during treatment, it is also possible to modify the dose in the different segments of each field, which is utilized in intensity-modulated radiotherapy (IMRT), showing further improved conformality of photon beams (Figure 20.5C). Particle beams may be conformed to the target volume by passive scattering using scatter foils, collimating-apertures, range shifter and compensators to shape the field and spread out the Bragg peak. Alternatively, the Bragg peak may be actively scanned over the tumour volume allowing for intensity-modulated proton therapy. With usually only few fields, particle beams may achieve in several clinical situations advantageous dose distributions compared to even optimal photon therapy (Figure 20.6). In particular, the irradiated volume which receives low or intermediate radiation doses may often be significantly reduced and some structures may be spared altogether. This advantage explains the enthusiasm to introduce these beams more widely in clinical practice where they

are currently already considered to be superior to photon beams in, for example, paediatric CNS cancers and tumours located at the base of skull. While the biological effects of protons are usually considered similar to those of photons (exceptions are currently under intense radiobiological investigations), heavier ions are biologically more effective, particularly in the Bragg peak, which may potentially gain further advantage of such beam qualities. However, as pointed out later in this chapter, many practical issues still need to be solved and appropriate clinical trials must be performed before the value of particle beams relative to photon beams may soundly be assessed for a wide range of tumour sites [25]. In contrast to EBRT, brachytherapy uses radioactive sources that are positioned directly into cavities (e.g., cervix cancer, see Figure 20.7]) or interstitially inserted in the tumour (e.g., prostate cancer). Brachytherapy delivers very high doses in the proximity of the source with a rapid fall-off to the periphery.

Treatment planning today is performed using fast computerized treatment planning systems (TPS). Target volumes and normal tissues at risk are usually defined on the basis of CT images in treatment position for conformal planning in three dimensions of the appropriate beam number, beam direction, beam quality,

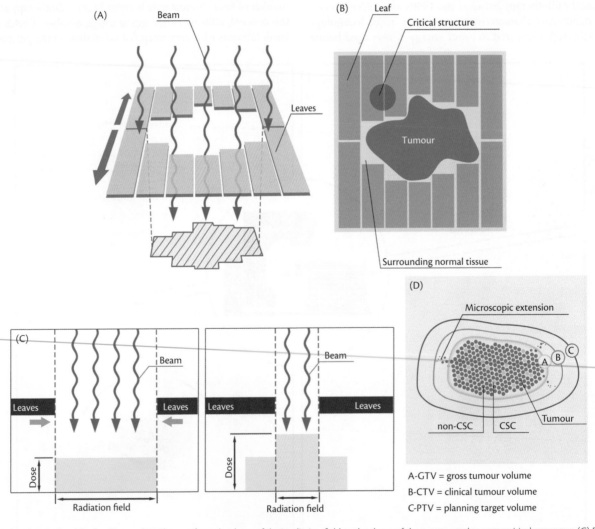

Fig. 20.5 (A, B) Use of multileaf collimator (MLC) to conform the shape of the irradiation field to the shape of the tumour and to spare critical structures. (C) By motorized movement of leaves during irradiation, inhomogeneous doses within each field for intensity-modulated radiotherapy (IMRT) can be generated. (D) Target volume terminology according to the International Commission on Radiation Units and Measurements ICRU [23, 24].

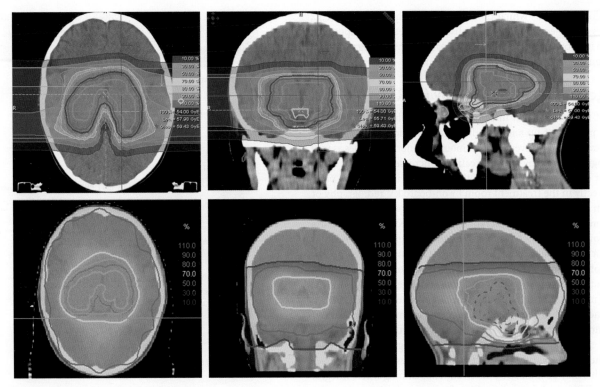

Fig. 20.6 Comparison of the dose distribution of proton therapy with two entrance fields (*upper panels*) to intensity-modulated photon radiotherapy (IMRT) with seven entrance fields (*lower panels*) in a 5-year-old girl with brain stem glioma. Considerably larger volumes of normal brain are irradiated to lower doses with photon therapy than with proton therapy.

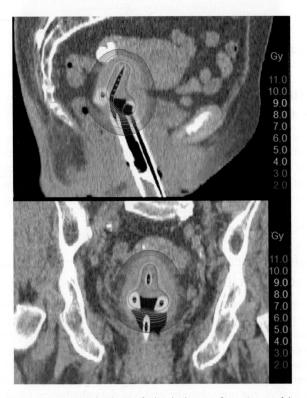

Fig. 20.7 Radiation dose distribution for brachytherapy of a carcinoma of the cervix. Note the steep dose gradient to the periphery.

and energy. Vast advances have been seen over the past decades in developing very fast algorithms which allow the optimal dose distribution for each patient to be defined with great precision. Two-dimensional treatment planning or standard radiographic simulation can still be reasonable, especially in the palliative set-up.

Advanced treatment techniques of particular importance for current clinical practice include the following:

Intensity-modulated radiation therapy (IMRT)

Usually optimized by means of so-called inverse dose planning, IMRT may significantly enhance conformation of the dose to the target volume compared to standard forward-planned 3D conformal radiotherapy (3DCRT). It is particularly beneficial in tumours with complex irregular shapes, for example concave tumours located around critical normal tissues. IMRT is widely considered an established standard for cancers of the prostate, head, and neck or lung, for example. However, while the distribution of high doses is more conformal for IMRT, greater volumes of normal tissues are irradiated to lower doses compared to 3DCRT. Application of IMRT is therefore not generally advantageous to 3DCRT, and the optimal planning approach for specific sites and for the individual patient's anatomy needs expert assessment.

Simultaneous integrated boost (SIB)

IMRT allows the application of a SIB (higher dose to the GTV or suspected areas of radioresistance) in parallel to the application of lower doses to areas which do not require such high doses (e.g., volumes of suspected microscopic disease). Whether this approach leads to improved clinical outcome (in particular with regard to late radiation damage) needs to be explored further.

Image-guided radiotherapy (IGRT)

State-of-the-art in-room imaging equipment allows higher precision of patient set-up and of radiotherapy application [27]. Inter- and intrafractional movement of tumours and normal tissues as well as changes in anatomy during treatment increase the risk of missing part of the target. Control of the geometric in-treatment position directly in the treatment room by on-board kV radiography or in-room CT and, very recently, also MRI significantly enhances the precision with which radiotherapy may be applied, allowing the use of narrower margins. Advanced radiotherapy approaches such as IMRT or SBRT require combination with IGRT to meet their potential. Motion control, for example by breath holding techniques, abdominal compression, jet ventilation under general anaesthesia, gating (turning the beam off when the target volume moves out of a predefined window setting) or tracking (the beam follows the moving tumour) may be used to further decrease margins in specific clinical settings. Four-dimensional CT may register images over time, thereby providing an exact time–space resolution of movement. This may be utilized by 4D treatment planning where integral GTV or CTV are defined as the basis for beam selection.

Stereotactic brain or body radiotherapy (SBRT)

Because of the steep dose gradient that can be achieved using SBRT techniques, small tumours or metastases may be treated to very high biological doses (ablative doses) in a single session or using few fractions. For ablative single-dose irradiation the term radio-surgery is also used. Usually the use of EBRT for SBRT is limited to a few small tumours or metastases. SBRT to ablative doses has been shown to be a valid alternative to surgical procedures, for example in early lung cancer or lung metastases. An emerging role for SBRT is treatment of oligometastases with locally curative doses.

Workflow of radiotherapy

Today radiotherapy is usually an integral part of an overall multidisciplinary workflow in oncology, with the radiation oncologist being involved at several steps. This is because Multidisciplinary Teams (MDTs) give superior clinical results. A simplified workflow is outlined in Figure 20.8.

Clinical assessment of the patient and steering of diagnostic procedures

It is the opinion of the authors of this chapter that each oncologist who treats patients, independently of discipline, should be educated expertly to steer basic workup and staging of patients, and that institutional guidelines or multidisciplinary clinics should ensure that this is performed to the same standards for all patients. Basic evaluation needs to be supplemented by specialist assessment, for example in making decisions on the applicability of radiotherapy or specific radiotherapy techniques.

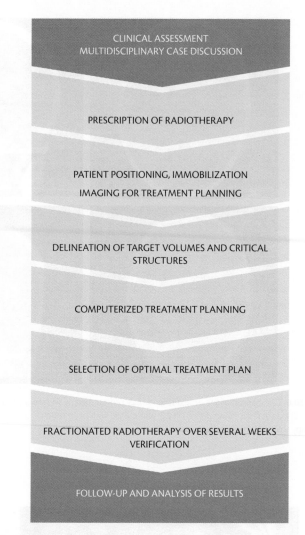

Fig. 20.8 Synopsis of the standard workflow in radiation oncology.

Multidisciplinary case discussion in tumour boards

Discussions should be performed as soon as all necessary information on patient characteristic and tumour histology, localization, and stage is available and certainly before treatment is initiated. Further multidisciplinary discussions are frequently necessary after completion of individual treatment steps in the multidisciplinary workflow, for example after completion of neoadjuvant radiochemotherapy before surgery.

Informed consent discussion and prescription of radiotherapy

Before start of treatment planning, the radiation oncologist informs the patient in detail about the recommended radiotherapy procedure, its goal, and relevant early and late normal tissue reactions. Alternative treatment options should also be covered and, if appropriate, discussions with specialists from other disciplines should be offered. As the basis for the treatment planning process, the radiation oncologist prescribes the details of the radiotherapy schedule to the target volume (e.g., total dose, dose per fraction, overall treatment time, beam quality) and specifies constraints of dose to critical normal tissues.

Patient set-up and imaging in treatment position

The patients need to be positioned for radiotherapy precisely, reproducibly, and as convenient as possible. The choice of the optimal treatment portals must anticipate later treatment planning and application, and endeavour not to compromise them. Various individual customized materials are used for positioning, such as thermoplastic masks for fixing the head, and body casts for immobilization of the trunk or extremities. Skin marking with robust stain or tattoos is essential to match the patient's position within the therapy room via a laser alignment system. CT imaging in treatment positions is performed.

Delineation of target volume and normal tissues at risk

Treatment planning is today usually performed based on CT in which the Hounsfield units represent the electron density of the tissue which is directly related to absorption of the beam in the tissues of the individual patient. For complex delineations, for example, requiring high contrast of soft tissues planning CT can be matched with MRI. Matching with PET images may provide important information on metabolic activity, allowing improved definition of tumour versus normal tissues. Once all pre-planning imaging has been done, the radiation oncologist delineates the target volumes ([23, 24], see Figure 20.5D: GTV, CTV, PTV) and normal tissues at risk of radiation damage in the planning CT images.

Generation of treatment plans

Treatment plans are usually generated by the dosimetrist or by the medical physicist, using sophisticated treatment planning software. Often alternative plans for comparative analysis are provided. Although algorithms for radiation treatment planning have become significantly faster over the last few years, generation of an optimal treatment plan may still need several days, in particular in complex clinical situations or when very advanced radiotherapy techniques are being used. Treatment plans have to be reviewed for tumour coverage and sparing of normal tissues as well as robustness to possible deviations, and must be signed off by the radiation oncologist and the medical physicist, who have to work closely together for optimal results. Quantitative analyzing tools supporting the evaluation, such as dose-volume histograms for all delineated structures, are implemented in all modern treatment planning systems. However, particularly when several critical normal tissues need to be considered, the decision for the optimal treatment plan may be extremely difficult. At this stage it may also be necessary to adapt the prescribed dose or the intended target volume or, infrequently, to re-start the process accounting for different patient positioning or a change of treatment strategy. When the final treatment plan has been decided upon, further quality assurance by the medical physicist is required as well as the production of auxiliary materials. In many instances, the application of the treatment plan is simulated before treatment using kV radiographic equipment with the geometry of the treatment machine, a dedicated CT simulator, or at the treatment machine itself using onboard imaging equipment.

Irradiation is delivered over weeks requiring periodically verification

Radiotherapists (or radiotherapy technologists or radiotherapy assistants) treat the patient under supervision of the radiation oncologist and medical physicist at the treatment machine. In many instances, treatments are given daily over several weeks. Because of this long duration, ongoing treatment monitoring and set-up verification is necessary. There are many sources of uncertainty during treatment. These may be patient-related (e.g., weight loss, variable filling of bowel or bladder) or attributed to the treatment application. The latter include incorrect positioning, variations in field or rotational settings, deviations in isocentre position, errors in collimator alignment or shape of blocks, varieties of treatment couches between simulator and accelerator, deviations in the in-room alignment system, light beam incongruence. Systematic errors usually have more severe consequences (e.g., if the tumour is partly missed) while random errors may wash out during the treatment. However, in settings requiring the highest precision these random errors may also have significant consequences. A number of monitoring and verification procedures are used during the course of radiotherapy to detect inaccuracies and errors during treatment and correct for them. Adaptive radiotherapy techniques (often requiring re-planning) are also being increasingly implemented to correct for changes in patients' anatomy. In addition, patients are closely monitored during treatment by the radiation oncologist for side effects of radiotherapy on normal tissues, which often require supportive measures and sometimes modification of the treatment.

Follow-up after radiotherapy

After the end of treatment patients need to be followed up for tumour control as well as for evaluation of normal tissue reactions, and data should be included in registers for quality assurance and for scientific evaluations. Follow-up is frequently integrated in multidisciplinary clinics, but evaluation of normal tissue effects requires special expertise and detailed comparison with dose distributions, necessitating the participation of the radiation oncologist in follow-up.

Workflow for oncological emergencies

Oncological emergencies including neurological deficits caused by metastases in the vertebrae or superior vena cava syndrome need consultation of the MDT, including a radiation oncologist, within hours. Diagnostic procedures and the start of treatment must be performed without delay. When the decision is made for radiotherapy, simple techniques are often applied in such situations, at least for the initial treatments.

Emerging directions

Particle therapy and other very high-precision (bio-) image guided technologies

As outlined above, these technologies can apply high doses at lower normal tissue toxicity, which may significantly further improve outcome in those tumours that still recur frequently. They may potentially also allow for a reduction in the number of radiation fractions, which may decrease the time for the patient at the treatment centre and may spare resources. While protons are considered to be associated with a comparable relative biological effectiveness (RBE) as photons, heavier charged particles such as carbon ions have the potential to modulate the biological effect of radiotherapy due to the higher RBE produced by the specific and severe radiation damage of high-LET beams. This RBE can vary depending on several factors, but mostly ranges between 2 and 5 [26]. It must be noted, however, that the potential of very high precision beams can only be exploited if the whole chain of radiotherapy is optimized: most importantly, pre-therapeutic imaging, treatment planning, and in-room monitoring, in particular accounting for additional range uncertainties compared to photon beam treatment. Continuously adapted radiotherapy which considers tumour size, location, and movement as well as the position of normal tissues at each treatment day is another promising strategy to increase the therapeutic window of radiotherapy but requires substantial further technological improvements such as ultra-fast recalculation of treatment plans, enhanced in-room imaging, and automated fast non-rigid registration technologies. Emerging integrated imaging-therapeutic facilities include among others, MR-Linac hybrids.

Large databases and automated clinical decision-support systems

Because the spatial distribution of dose is an important determinant of radiation response in tumours and normal tissues, and because the exact distribution of dose may be highly variable even for patients with well-matched anatomy and tumours, large-scale databases (including imaging information, dose plans, and spatially resoluted follow-up information) are powerful tools for developing prediction models for radiotherapy. Clinical decision-support systems based on the predictive and prognostic data of several sources can be utilized substantially to enhance a variety of steps in radiotherapy planning and application, including prescription, delineation, or treatment plan optimization. Overall, this requires the implementation of intense multi-institutional networks to generate databases of the necessary size and quality as well as powerful analysis tools [28].

Biological individualization in radiation oncology

Today radiotherapy is a highly individualized treatment modality for cancer, with dose-volume prescriptions based on individual anatomy and utilization of model-based parameters for TCP and NTCP on an individual patient basis. Dose distribution is a powerful surrogate marker for radiation effects in both tumours and normal tissue. Technological advances over the past few decades, together with careful clinical studies and clinical-radiobiological analysis have been the basis for these achievements. Further advances in individualized radiotherapy are expected from integration of this technology with modern biology. A number of putative predictive biomarkers for radiosensitivity of tumours are currently under preclinical and clinical evaluation. Examples include determination of residual DNA double-stand breaks after irradiation by measurement of γH2AX foci which closely correlate with cellular radiosensitivity, determination of the extent of tumour hypoxia, and re-oxygenation by bio-imaging using PET and hypoxia-specific tracers such as 18F-misonidazole, or high-throughput methodologies such as whole exon sequencing which may provide a broader spectrum of markers indicating radioresistance. Only one predictive biomarker for radiosensitivity would add significantly

to the stratification and individualization already established in radiotherapy today. Because of the spatial distribution of dose, predictive bio-imaging methodology is widely being considered as particularly relevant for radiotherapy. Further considerable promise for individualized approaches in radiation oncology bears the combination with specific drugs which either overcome radiobiological mechanisms of radioresistance (e.g. hypoxic cell sensitizers in hypoxic tumours or DNA repair inhibitors in tumours with high capacity for repair of radiation induced double-strand breaks). Such treatment combinations require application according to predictive biomarkers for development of individualized approaches. Monoclonal antibodies against the epidermal growth factor receptor (EGFR) have been the prime example of successful radiosensitization by targeting a specific molecule in combination with radiotherapy; however, to date no reliable biomarker is available for this approach, excluding a biological-driven individualized application.

Novel study design

A challenge for oncology in general is to develop study designs which can cope with individualized treatment approaches, i.e. an increasing number of treatment strata of patients with a decreasing number of eligible patients for such studies per centre. This is further complicated by the fact that the number of potential treatments rapidly increases and that frequently (though sometimes unintentionally) different parameters are variable in the same trial (e.g., in a study testing a new drug combined with radiotherapy, dose distribution may be very heterogeneous; see Figure 20.2). These trends necessitate formation of large study networks (for prospective as well as retrospective data) as well as substantial investments in quality control and new biostatistical assessment techniques.

Further reading

Baumann M, Krause M, Hill R. Exploring the role of cancer stem cells in radioresistance. Nature Reviews Cancer 2008; 8(7): 545–554.

Bentzen SM, Trotti A. Evaluation of early and late toxicities in chemoradiation trials. Journal of Clinical Oncology 2007; 25(26): 4096–4103.

Bentzen SM, Harari PM, Bernier J. Exploitable mechanisms for combining drugs with radiation: concepts, achievements and future directions. Nature Clinical Practice Oncology 2007; 4(3): 172–180.

Bernier J, Hall EJ, Giaccia A. Radiation oncology: a century of achievements. Nature reviews. Cancer 2004; 4(9): 737–747.

Combs SE, Bohl J, Elsasser T, Weber Kj, Schulz-Ertner D et al. Radiobiological evaluation and correlation with the local effect model (LEM) of carbon ion radiation therapy and temozolomide in glioblastoma cell lines. International Journal of Radiation Biology 2009; 85(2): 126–137.

Holthusen H. Erfahrungen über die Verträglichkeitsgrenze für Röntgenstrahlen und deren Nutzanwendung zur Verhütung von Schäden. Strahlentherapie 1936; 57: 254–268.

Horsman MR, Mortensen LS, Petersen JB, Busk M, Overgaard J. Imaging hypoxia to improve radiotherapy outcome. Nature Reviews Clinical Oncology 2012; 9(12): 674–687.

Lambin P, van Stiphout RG, Starmans MH, Rios-Velazquez E, Nalbantov G et al. Predicting outcomes in radiation oncology—multifactorial decision support systems. Nature Reviews Clinical Oncology 2013; 10(1): 27–40.

Verellen D, De Ridder M, Linthout N, Tournel K, Soete G et al. 2007. Innovations in image-guided radiotherapy. Nature Reviews Cancer, 7(12): 949–960.

References

1. Bernier J, Hall EJ, Giaccia A. Radiation oncology: a century of achievements. Nature reviews. Cancer 2004; 4(9): 737–747.

2. Hall EJ, Giaccia AJ. Radiobiology for the Radiologist. Seventh Edition, 7th ed. Philadelphia, PA: Lippincott Williams & Wilkins, 2012.

3. Halperin EC, Perez CA. Perez & Brady's Principles and Practice of Radiation Oncology. 6th ed. Philadelphia, PA: Lippincott Williams & Wilkins, 2013.

4. Joiner M and van der Kogel A. Basic Clinical Radiobiology. 4th ed. London: Hodder Education.

5. Thames HD, Hendry JH. Fractionation in Radiotherapy. 1st ed. London, New York: Taylor & Francis, 1987

6. Holthusen H. Erfahrungen über die Verträglichkeitsgrenze für Röntgenstrahlen und deren Nutzanwendung zur Verhütung von Schäden. Strahlentherapie 1936; 57: 254–268.

7. Baumann M, Krause M, Hill R. Exploring the role of cancer stem cells in radioresistance. Nature Reviews Cancer 2008; 8(7): 545–554.

8. Horsman MR, Mortensen LS, Petersen JB, Busk M, Overgaard J. Imaging hypoxia to improve radiotherapy outcome. Nature Reviews Clinical Oncology 2012; 9(12): 674–687.

9. Butof R, Dubrovska A, Baumann M. Clinical perspectives of cancer stem cell research in radiation oncology. Radiotherapy and Oncology 2013; 108(3): 388–396.

10. Dubben HH, Thames HD, Beck-Bornholdt HP. Tumor volume: a basic and specific response predictor in radiotherapy. Radiotherapy and Oncology 1998; 47(2): 167–174.

11. Ang KK, Baumann M, Bentzen SM, Brammer I, Budach W et al. 1993. Medical radiology. In Beck-Bornholdt HP ed., Diagnostic imaging and radiation oncology. Berlin: Springer-Verlag, 1993, 87.

12. Bentzen SM, Trotti A. Evaluation of early and late toxicities in chemoradiation trials. Journal of Clinical Oncology 2007; 25(26): 4096–4103.

13. Bentzen SM, Harari PM, Bernier J. Exploitable mechanisms for combining drugs with radiation: concepts, achievements and future directions. Nature Clinical Practice Oncology 2007; 4(3): 172–180.

14. Emami B, Lyman J, Brown A, Coia L, Goitein M et al. 1991. Tolerance of normal tissue to therapeutic irradiation. International Journal of Radiation Oncology Biology Physics 1991; 21(1): 109–122.

15. Bentzen Sm, Constine Ls, Deasy Jo, Eisbruch A, Jackson A et al. 2010. Quantitative analyses of normal tissue effects in the clinic (QUANTEC): an introduction to the scientific issues. International Journal of Radiation Oncology Biology Physics 2010; 76(Suppl. 3): S3–S9.

16. Thames HD, Bentzen SM, Turesson I, Overgaard M, van den Bogaert W. Fractionation parameters for human tissues and tumors. International Journal of Radiation Biology 1989; 56(5): 701–710.

17. Fowler JF. Heavy particles in radiotherapy. In Steel GG, Adams GE, Peckham MT eds, The biological basis of radiotherapy. Amsterdam: Elsevier, 1983, 181–194.

18. Good JS, Harrington KJ. The hallmarks of cancer and the radiation oncologist: updating the 5Rs of radiobiology. Clinical Oncology 2013; (10): 569–577.

19. Fletcher GH. Textbook of Radiotherapy, 3rd ed. Philadelphia: Lea & Febiger, 1980.

20. Wang CC. Clinical Radiation Oncology: Indications, Techniques, and Results. Massachusetts, MA: PSG Publishing Company, Inc., 1988.

21. Bentzen SM, Thames HD. Clinical evidence for tumor clonogen regeneration: interpretations of the data. Radiotherapy and Oncology 1991; 22(3): 161–166.

22. Butof R, Baumann M. 2013. Time in radiation oncology—keep it short! Radiotherapy and Oncology 2013; 106 (3): 271–275.

23. International Commission on Radiation Units and Measurements (ICRU). Prescribing, Recording, and Reporting Photon Beam Therapy ICRU Report 50, 1993.

24. International Commission on Radiation Units and Measurements (ICRU). Prescribing, Recording, and Reporting Photon Beam Therapy ICRU Report 62 (Supplement to ICRU report 50), 1999.

25. Allen AM, Pawlicki T, Dong L, Fourkal E, Buyyounouski M et al. 2012. An evidence based review of proton beam therapy: the report of ASTRO's emerging technology committee. Radiotherapy and Oncology 2012; 103(1): 8–11.

26. Combs SE, Bohl J, Elsasser T, Weber Kj, Schulz-Ertner D et al. Radiobiological evaluation and correlation with the local effect model (LEM) of carbon ion radiation therapy and temozolomide in glioblastoma cell lines. International Journal of Radiation Biology 2009; 85(2): 126–137.

27. Verellen D, De Ridder M, Linthout N, Tournel K, Soete G et al. 2007. Innovations in image-guided radiotherapy. Nature Reviews Cancer, 7(12): 949–960.

28. Lambin P, van Stiphout RG, Starmans MH, Rios-Velazquez E, Nalbantov G et al. Predicting outcomes in radiation oncology—multifactorial decision support systems. Nature Reviews Clinical Oncology 2013; 10(1): 27–40.

29. Richter C. Dosimetrische Charakterisierung laserbeschleunigter Teilchenstrahlen für in vitro Zellbestrahlungen. Dissertation, Technische Universität Dresden, 2013.

CHAPTER 21

Principles of chemotherapy

David J. Kerr, Daniel G. Haller, and Jaap Verweij

Introduction to principles of chemotherapy

The treatment of cancer is one of the best settings for a multidisciplinary approach to treatment in medicine. Surgery and radiotherapy are frequently still the primary choice of treatment for patients with malignant tumours. However, since 60–70% of patients with cancer will develop metastatic disease during their lifetime despite local control of their cancer, for most patients cancer may be considered a systemic disease, requiring systemic treatment. In addition, along with radiation and surgery, systemic therapy is frequently given as part of primary treatments with curative intent. The development of systemic therapy over the last few decades has therefore created an important role for medical oncologists in the care of patients with cancer. One of the dominant reasons for the emergence of medical oncology as a subspecialty was the significance of the toxicity associated with conventional cytotoxic drugs. Classically, these agents have steep dose response curves and narrow therapeutic ratios, and therefore a small increment in dose can lead to a large increase in toxicity. Famously, the French philosopher René Descartes declared, 'Cogito ergo sum,' (I think, therefore I am), and we may be able to modify this statement to justify the emergence of medical oncology in the early days to 'Veneno, ergo sum,' (I poison, therefore I am). The types of systemic treatment available to the medical oncologist are continually expanding with newly emerging pharmacological and biological therapies that have clinical activity. We can predict that the role of medical oncology will become increasingly important in the near future.

Every medical oncologist must be aware of the scientific rationale for choosing specific drugs, combinations of drugs, or combinations of different types of treatment. This chapter summarizes the basis of chemotherapy, and addresses important issues in the development of new approaches using molecular targets in a more sophisticated way to try to obtain tumour cell kill, dormancy, or enhanced immune rejection of the cancer.

Principles of chemotherapy

In the majority of patients with cancer, chemotherapy will be considered for use at some time during the course of their illness, aiming either at cure, prolongation of life, or palliation, depending on tumour type, stage, and the relative fitness of the patient.

In an ideal world, the design of chemotherapy regimens should be based on specific knowledge about cell cycle kinetics, pharmacokinetics, biochemical–pharmacological factors, and bioinformatic analysis of the consequences of inhibition of signal transduction pathways. However, this is often still trumped by empirical knowledge of the responsiveness of specific tumours to specific drugs, and a more traditional disease-oriented approach to anticancer drug development. Although much has been made of the remarkable insights that cell and molecular biology has given the oncology community and a belief that it would be possible to treat cell targets and pathways rather than specific tumour types, it has become clear that a 'driver mutation' in, for example, lung cancer may not operate in the same way in colorectal or breast cancer, given the differing mutational landscape in these diverse tumour types. This lends greater weight to the computational statisticians' attempts to model what the consequences of inhibition of pathway X are on pathway Y, and how different resistance escape mechanisms might operate depending on the constellation of background mutations.

Mechanism of action of commonly available drugs

Anthracyclines

Anthracyclines (doxorubicin, daunomycin, epirubicin, daunorubicin) are anti-tumour antibiotics used in cancer chemotherapy derived from the Streptomyces bacteria and have three mechanisms of action:

◆ inhibits DNA and RNA synthesis by intercalating between base pairs of the DNA/RNA strand, thus preventing the replication of rapidly-growing cancer cells

◆ inhibits topoisomerase II enzyme, preventing the relaxing of super-coiled DNA and thus blocking DNA transcription and replication

◆ creates iron-mediated free oxygen radicals that damage the DNA and the lipid domain of cell membranes.

Vinca alkaloids

Vinca alkaloids (vincristine, vinorelbine, vinblastine, vindesine) are antimitotic and antimicrotubule agents that were originally derived from the periwinkle plant Catharanthus roseus. The principal mechanisms of cytotoxicity relate to their interactions with tubulin and disruption of microtubule function, particularly of microtubules comprising the mitotic spindle apparatus, leading to metaphase arrest.

Taxanes

Taxanes (docetaxel, paclitaxel, nab-paclitaxel) are diterpenes produced by the plants of the genus Taxus (yews). The principal mechanism of action of the taxane class of drugs is the disruption of microtubule function. Microtubules are essential to cell division, and taxanes stabilize GDP-bound tubulin in the microtubule, thereby inhibiting the process of cell division—a 'frozen mitosis'. Thus, in essence, taxanes are mitotic inhibitors. In contrast to the taxanes, the vinca alkaloids destroy mitotic spindles. Both taxanes and vinca alkaloids are together named spindle poisons.

Alkylating agents

Alkylating agents (nitrogen mustards—cyclophosphamide, ifosfamide, melphalan, chlorambucil; nitrosoureas—carmustine, lomustine, streptozocin; alkyl sulphonate—busulfan). Their principal mechanism of action is to allkylate the N7 residue of the guanine which can crosslink nucleobases in DNA double-helix strands. This makes the strands unable to uncoil and separate, leading ultimately to apoptotic cell death. The anti-tumour antibiotic, mitomycin, isolated from Streptomyces caespitosus can also be considered an alkylating agent as it is activated to produce a species which crosslinks guanine residues in the sequence 5'-CpG-3'.

Bleomycin

Bleomycin is a glycopeptide antibiotic produced by the bacterium Streptomyces verticillus which induces DNA strand breaks by generating superoxide free radicals.

Platinum-based agents

These include cisplatin, carboplatin, and oxaliplatin. Platinum-based agents also bind N7 guanine and can cause intra- and interstrand DNA crosslinks, inhibiting DNA synthesis and inducing programmed cell death.

Antimetabolites

Antimetabolites (purines, pyrimidines, anti-folates) are chemicals that inhibit the use of a naturally occurring metabolite that is essential for the cell's normal economy; for example, DNA and protein synthesis. Such drugs are often similar in structure to the metabolite with which they interfere. Purine analogues (mercaptopurine, thioguanine, fludarabine, pentostatin, and cladribine) are antimetabolites that mimic the structure of metabolic purines and that therefore inhibit DNA synthesis. Pyrimidine analogues (5-fluorouracil, gemcitabine, floxuridine, cytosine arabinoside) are antimetabolites that mimic the structure of metabolic pyrimidines and that inhibit DNA and RNA synthesis. Antifolate analogues (methotrexate, pemetrexed) are drugs that impair the function of folic acids. A well-known example is methotrexate. This is a folic acid analogue, which, owing to structural similarity with it, binds and inhibits the enzyme dihydrofolate reductase (DHFR), and thus prevents the formation of tetrahydrofolate. Because tetrahydrofolate is essential for purine and pyrimidine synthesis, methotrexate inhibits production of DNA, RNA, and proteins (as tetrahydrofolate is also involved in the synthesis of amino acids serine and methionine).

Topoisomerase inhibitors

Topoisomerase inhibitors (topo 1—irinotecan, topotecan; topo 2—etoposide, amsacrine, teniposide), inhibit the two enzymes that regulate the overwinding or underwinding of DNA and lead to single and double-strand DNA breaks that can induce apoptosis.

Hormonal agents

Hormonal therapy involves the manipulation of the endocrine system through exogenous administration of specific hormones, particularly steroid hormones, or drugs which inhibit the production or activity of such hormones (hormone antagonists). Because steroid hormones are powerful drivers of gene expression in certain cancer cells, changing the levels or activity of certain hormones can cause cytostasis, or cell death.

Aromatase inhibitors

At menopause, oestrogen production in the ovaries ceases, but other tissues continue to produce oestrogen through the action of the enzyme aromatase on androgens produced by the adrenal glands. Aromatase blockade reduces oestrogen levels in postmenopausal women, causing growth arrest and/or apoptosis of hormone-responsive cancer cells. Letrozole and anastrozole are aromatase inhibitors which have been shown to be superior to tamoxifen for the first-line treatment of breast cancer in postmenopausal women, and exemestane is an irreversible 'aromatase inactivator' which is superior to megestrol for treatment of tamoxifen-refractory metastatic breast cancer. Analogues of gonadotropin-releasing hormone (GnRH) can induce chemical castration, complete suppression of the production of oestrogen, progesterone and testosterone from the reproductive organs via the negative feedback effect of continuous stimulation of the pituitary gland by these hormones. Leuprolide and goserelin are GnRH analogs which are used primarily for the treatment of hormone-responsive prostate cancer.

Oestrogen receptor antagonists (SERM)

Tamoxifen is a partial agonist, which can actually increase oestrogen receptor signalling in some tissues, such as the endometrium. Raloxifene is another partial agonist SERM which does not seem to promote endometrial cancer, and is used primarily for chemoprevention of breast cancer in high-risk individuals. Toremifene and fulvestrant are SERMs with little or no agonist activity.

Antiandrogens

Antiandrogens are a class of drug which bind and inhibit the androgen receptor, blocking the growth- and survival-promoting effects of testosterone on certain prostate cancers. There are steroidal antiandrogens and 'pure' antiandrogens. The steroidal antiandrogens include megestrol. The 'pure' or nonsteroidal antiandrogens include bicalutamide, flutamide, and nilutamide.

Cell signalling inhibitors

This broad classification underpins the remarkable insights that cell and molecular biology have yielded over the past two decades that have resulted in druggable targets, several of which are used as biomarkers to select chemosensitive patient subpopulations.

Anti-angiogenic inhibitors (bevacizumab, aflibercept, sorafenib, sunitinib, pazopanib and everolimus)

Angiogenesis requires the binding of signalling molecules, such as vascular endothelial growth factor (VEGF), to receptors on the surface of normal endothelial cells. When VEGF and other endothelial growth factors bind to their receptors on endothelial cells, signals within these cells are initiated that promote the growth and survival of new blood vessels. Angiogenesis inhibitors interfere with various steps in this process; for example, bevacizumab is a monoclonal antibody that specifically recognizes and binds to VEGF, preventing it from activating its receptor. Other angiogenesis inhibitors, including sorafenib, regorafenib, and sunitinib, bind to receptors on the surface of endothelial cells or to other proteins in the downstream signalling pathways, blocking their activities. Ramucirumab is a fully human monoclonal antibody (IgG1) being developed for the treatment of solid tumors. It is directed against the vascular endothelial growth factor receptor 2 (VEGFR2). By binding to VEGFR2, it works as a receptor antagonist blocking the binding of vascular endothelial growth factor (VEGF) to VEGFR2. VEGFR2 is known to mediate the majority of the downstream effects of VEGF in angiogenesis.

Growth factor receptor inhibitors

Aberrant expression of the epidermal growth factor receptor (EGFR) system has been reported in a wide range of epithelial cancers. In some studies, this has also been associated with a poor prognosis and resistance to the conventional forms of therapies. These discoveries have led to the strategic development of several kinds of EGFR inhibitors, which comprise the anti-EGFR monoclonal antibodies cetuximab and panitumumab, and the small molecule EGFR tyrosine kinase inhibitors gefitinib and erlotinib. Human epidermal growth factor receptor 2 (HER2) is the target of the monoclonal antibody trastuzumab, which is effective only in cancers where HER2 is over-expressed.

One of the difficulties in classifying signal transduction inhibitors is that they often have multiple targets and it may be impossible to be precise about the dominant mode of action. Some of the main pharmacologic types are:

- multitargeted tyrosine kinase inhibitors which include erlotinib, imatinib, gefitinib, dasatinib, sunitinib, nilotinib, lapatinib, sorafenib, crizotinib, regorafenib
- proteasome inhibitors, such as bortezomib
- mTOR inhibitors, such as temsirolimus, everolimus
- histone deacetylase inhibitors, such as vorinostat (SAHA)
- hedgehog pathway inhibitors, such as vismodegib.

Cellular principles of chemotherapy

For cytotoxic treatment, the following characteristics of tumour growth are important in determining outcome:

- cell cycle time
- tumour doubling time
- growth fraction
- tumour size, or the number of cells in the population.

Decades ago, Skipper et al. [1] found that the doubling time of proliferating murine cancer cells is constant, forming a straight line on a semilog plot. Death of the animals resulted when the malignant cells reached a critical fraction of body weight. Since other experiments [2] had shown that a single surviving cell leads to treatment failure, and there is still no evidence that normal levels of host defence are capable of eliminating a few remaining tumour cells, for a given amount of chemotherapy survival was related to tumour size at the time of diagnosis (Figure 21.1).

These studies were performed in model systems, often using murine leukaemic cell lines, showing logarithmic (exponential) growth. All of the cells were in cycle and dividing, with no cells in a resting phase, and the cell number doubling at a tumour-specific rate. While knowledge based on these model characteristics is important, the rules only apply to the cells in the proliferation compartment. Unfortunately, only a few human cancers have a large proportion of such responsive proliferating cells. In most tumours there is a large non-proliferating compartment; therefore, these model systems, though important in their time, are not truly representative of the kinetics of human solid tumours [3].

Most human tumours are diagnosed when they are relatively large and kinetically and genetically heterogeneous. Due to a variety of factors such as poor vascularity, hypoxia [4], and competition for nutrients, they exhibit decelerating growth at this stage. Larger tumours contain a high fraction of slowly or non-dividing cells (termed G0 cells) and as a consequence the growth fraction is low. Therefore, in treating human tumours, the fractional cell kill hypothesis probably does not apply as well as in animal tumour models. Non-proliferating cells are less sensitive to antineoplastic agents, particularly because they have time to repair the damaged DNA. As many antineoplastic agents are most effective against rapidly dividing cells, the cell-kinetic situation at tumour diagnosis is unfavourable for treatment with most drugs.

Unlike the tumour models used by Skipper, and related to the fact that the proliferating cell population is distinct from the non-proliferating population, human tumours are thought to follow a different growth pattern. Attempts have been undertaken to describe human tumour growth by mathematical models. Two available models are the so-called Gompertzian growth model and the exponential growth model. The primary distinction between the two models is that in Gompertzian growth kinetics

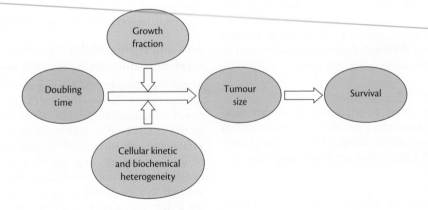

Fig. 21.1 Cancer dynamics.

the growth fraction of the tumour is not constant but decreases exponentially with time. Exponential growth implies that the time taken for a tumour to double its volume is constant. A significant problem is that most tumours only become clinically manifest by approximately 10^9 tumour cells (equating approximately to a size of 1 cm^3, representing the last part of the tumour's growth curve). Thus, estimating growth curves of human primary tumours based on multiple time points of tumour volume appeared to be difficult, if not impossible. Overall, the available data suggest that the Gompertzian growth model (sigmoid in shape on a log scale) is the most probable model (it is interesting to reflect that Gompertz was an economist and developed his models around how industrialized economies behaved).

Apart from cell-kinetic heterogeneity, genetic and biochemical heterogeneity of human tumours may also reduce the likelihood of cure. Although most human tumours evolve from a single clone of malignant cells [5], more recent studies have shown that this homogeneity does not persist during further stages of tumour growth, presumably as a result of further somatic mutations of the original tumour line. When non-homogeneous tumour cells are exposed to drugs, sensitive tumour cells will be destroyed while resistant cells will survive and proliferate [6]. As a result, tumour cell kill tends to decrease with subsequent courses of treatment, as resistant cells are selected. Paradoxically, normal tissues never change their level of sensitivity to chemotherapy, emphasizing an important difference in relative genetic stability.

Pharmacological principles of chemotherapy

The scheduling of drug treatments is based on both practical and theoretical considerations. Intermittent cycles of treatment are used to allow periods of recovery of normal tissues. This strategy aims at re-treatment with full therapeutic doses as frequently as possible, in keeping with the fractional cell kill hypothesis, but also allowing the normal tissues to recover from the unintended effects of cytotoxic treatment. The outcome of chemotherapy will obviously largely depend on the overall intrinsic sensitivity of the treated tumour.

Fractional cell kill means that a given drug concentration applied for a defined time period will kill a constant fraction of the total cell population, independent of the absolute number of cells. In other words, each treatment cycle kills a specific fraction (percentage) of the remaining cells. Since this fraction is never 100%, a single drug administration will never be sufficient to eradicate a tumour completely. Therefore, treatment results will also be a direct function of the drug concentration and exposure time and the frequency of repeating treatment. Drug concentration and exposure time will be dependent on pharmacokinetic (PK) factors such as drug absorption, metabolism, and elimination (Figure 21.2). These will have to be considered in general in determining the dose, schedule, and route of drug administration. In addition, inter-patient variations in PK parameters are usually large and this may be one reason for the inconsistency in responses of 'sensitive' tumours.

The bioavailability of a drug describes the proportion of a dose of a drug that enters the systemic circulation (e.g., for intravenous 5-FU this would be 100% compared to 10–25% for oral 5-FU). For drugs taken orally that are intended for systemic action, a significant proportion of a given dose may not even enter the systemic circulation. This may be due to poor absorption from the gastrointestinal (GI) tract, or metabolism in the gut wall or liver (called first-pass metabolism).

Various processes are involved in drug elimination, although hepatic and renal processes are the most important. The liver is the main organ of drug metabolism. There are generally two types of reaction (Phase I and Phase II) that have two important effects:

- Make the drug more water soluble—to aid excretion by the kidneys.

- Inactivate the drug—in most cases, the metabolite is less active than the parent drug, although in some cases the metabolite can be as active, or more so, than the parent (e.g., irinotecan, tamoxifen).

Phase I metabolism involves oxidation, reduction, or hydrolysis reactions. Oxidation reactions are most common and are catalysed by cytochrome P450 isoenzymes located primarily in the liver. Phase II metabolism involves conjugation reactions, such as glucuronidation (such as UGT1a1) or sulphation, which produce more water-soluble compounds, enabling rapid elimination.

The main route of excretion of drugs is the kidney. Renal elimination is dependent on multiple factors that include:

- glomerular filtration rate (GFR)

- active tubular secretion (may involve P-gp)

- passive tubular secretion.

If a drug is metabolized mainly to inactive compounds (e.g., 5-flourouracil), renal function will not greatly affect the elimination.

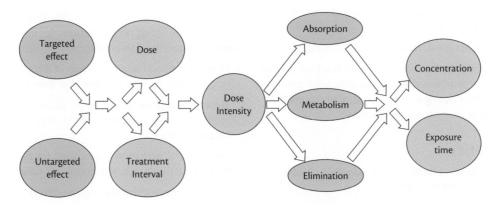

Fig. 21.2 Pharmacodynamics in cancer chemotherapy.

If, however, the drug is excreted largely unchanged (e.g., carboplatin), or an active metabolite is excreted via the kidney (e.g., morphine), changes in renal function will influence the elimination, and dose adjustments may be necessary.

Effect of hepatic and renal impairment

Impaired liver function can affect the pharmacokinetics and pharmacodynamics of many anticancer drugs (e.g., anthracyclines, taxanes, vinca alkaloids, and 5-FU). Reduction in hepatic blood flow and a potential fall in the number and the activity of hepatocytes can alter liver function and impact on drug clearance. A reduced synthesis of albumin can result in reduced drug–protein binding, thereby affecting the volume of distribution. Cholestasis can affect the biliary excretion of drugs and metabolites. Patients with impaired hepatic function may also develop a degree of renal impairment due to decreased renal plasma flow and GFR. Unlike impaired renal function, there is no simple test that can determine the impact of liver disease on drug handling. A combination of factors needs to be considered before such impact can be assessed, which include liver function tests (LFTs), diagnosis, and physical symptoms.

In general, the metabolism of drugs is unlikely to be affected unless the patient has severe liver disease. Most problems are seen in patients with jaundice, ascites, and hepatic encephalopathy. As such, doses of drugs should be reviewed in the following situations:

- hepatically metabolized drug with narrow therapeutic index
- there is a significant involvement of the cytochrome P450 system (CYP3A4/5 is highly susceptible to liver disease, while CYP2D6 appears relatively refractory)
- international normalized ratio (INR) >1.2.
- bilirubin >100micromol/L
- albumin <30g/L
- signs of ascites and/or encephalopathy.

The elimination of several cytotoxic drugs and their metabolites is dependent upon renal function (capecitabine, carboplatin, cisplatin, methtrexate). Impaired renal function, coupled with rising urea plasma concentrations, induces changes in drug pharmacokinetics and pharmacodynamics. Implications for drug therapy include:

- increased risk of undesirable effects and toxicity through reduced excretion of the drug and/or metabolite(s)
- increased sensitivity to drug effects, irrespective of route of elimination, (e.g., antipsychotics)
- increased risk of further renal impairment (e.g., NSAIDs).

Many of these problems can be avoided by simple adjustment of daily dose or frequency of administration. The dose nomogram for carboplatin is an excellent example of this. In other situations, however, an alternative drug may need to be chosen.

Pharmacogenetics

If it were not for the great variability among individuals, medicine might as well be a science and not an art.

William Osler

Pharmacogenetics is the study of how variation in an individual gene affects the response to drugs which can lead to adverse drug reactions, drug toxicity, therapeutic failure, and drug interactions. Genetic variability can affect an individual's response to drug treatment by influencing pharmacokinetic and pharmacodynamic processes (e.g., variations in genes that encode cytochrome P450 isoenzymes, drug receptors, or transport proteins can determine clinical response). Pharmacogenetics can aid in the optimization of drug therapy through the identification of individuals who are likely to respond to treatment, or those who are most likely at risk of an adverse drug reaction. For example, with tamoxifen the active metabolite, endoxifen, is produced by a reaction involving CYP2D6. Patients with a PM phenotype are at risk of therapeutic failure with tamoxifen. Drugs that inhibit CYP2D6 will also mimic the PM phenotype and should be avoided. Warfarin bleeding effects are more common with CYP2D9 polymorphisms; patients with mutations in UGT1a1 reduce metabolism of irinotecan and are associated with more toxicity.

Dose intensity

Most cancer chemotherapeutic agents in vitro and in vivo exhibit a steep dose-response curve. Consequently, it is considered desirable to administer them in humans at the highest possible dose-intensity, since in theory even small reductions in dose would lead to substantial reductions of tumour cell kill. The importance of dose intensity in tumour responsiveness in humans was first suggested in heavily criticized retrospective analyses performed by Levin and Hryniuk [8] and others [9]. These investigators suggested dose response correlations for 5-fluorouracil in colon cancer, cisplatin in ovarian cancer, doxorubicinin in breast cancer, and vincristine in Hodgkin's disease. Subsequently, for some of these, prospective randomized trials of a relatively small sample size have supported or refuted the concept.

It is generally accepted that the most important measure of drug exposure would be the area under the curve in a plot of local tumour drug concentration against time.

Obviously, there is a hierarchy ranging from simple plasma levels of unbound and activated drug (where appropriate) to activated drug concentrations within the target tumour cell. Unfortunately, there are scarcely any data from humans to suggest that plasma drug levels do correlate with tumour levels and response.

Locoregional drug administration

Regional perfusion with antineoplastic drugs can generate higher than expected drug concentrations in the body compartment which harbours the dominant tumour burden.

1. Direct intrathecal administration of drugs such as methotrexate or cytarabine enables a higher local dose in a sanctuary site.

2. Hepatic artery or portal vein infusion in theory allows an increased drug concentration to liver primary or secondary tumours [10].

3. Intra-arterial perfusion can be used for metastatic and primary liver cancer, limb melanomas and soft tissue sarcomas.

4. Intraperitoneal chemotherapy is effective for ovarian cancer [11–13].

Dose intensification using local administration in uncontrolled studies has suggested improved response rates. However, with the exception of intrathecal therapy in acute lymphocytic leukaemia, hepatic arterial infusion for metastatic colorectal cancer, and intra-peritoneal therapy for ovarian cancer, none of the regional methods has been reported in randomized trials to produce a longer survival than conventional systemic methods of drug administration.

An increase of the dose per administration

The dose per administration can be increased without changing the intervals between administrations. One such method to increase tumour cell kill is to use doses of chemotherapy that cause pro-longed bone marrow suppression and to rescue the host either with autologous bone marrow harvested before treatment or with allogenic marrow from a histocompatible donor.

With the use of high-dose chemotherapy, new dose-limiting tox-icities to organs other than bone marrow emerge, such as nitrosou-rea toxicity to lung, kidneys, or liver [14]. For this reason, its use is still limited to certain classes of drugs. To date, marrow-ablative chemotherapy in humans has only been shown effective in leukae-mias and lymphomas, tumour types with high growth fractions and intrinsic sensitivity to chemotherapy.

Shortening treatment intervals

This method has been used, especially in solid tumours, as another way of increasing dose intensity. The introduction of drugs such as the 5-hydroxytryptamine-3 antagonist anti-emetics and the haematopoietic growth factors has greatly facilitated this approach. Although weekly [15] or biweekly administration of relatively high doses of drugs previously given at three- to four-week intervals seems feasible and yields interesting results in uncontrolled trials, it is too early to conclude if the resulting increases in dose intensity produce an increase in cure rate (an exception may be in the use of dose-dense adjuvant chemotherapy for breast cancer).

Principles of combination chemotherapy

As a consequence of somatic mutations, tumour cell kill tends to decrease with subsequent courses of treatment, as genetically resistant cell types are selected out.

For this reason, single-agent treatment is rarely curative. Therefore, and for a variety of other reasons discussed here, cancer chemotherapy is most frequently given as a combination of differ-ent drugs. Favourable and unfavourable interactions between drugs must be considered in developing such combination regimens. These interactions may be pharmacokinetic, cytokinetic, or bio-chemical, and may influence the effectiveness of the components of the combination. The theoretical and sometimes proven superi-ority of combination chemotherapy over single-agent treatment is derived from the principles listed in Box 21.1.

When any drugs are administered in combination, three out-comes are possible: additive, subtractive, or synergistic effects. With additive effects, the drugs act completely independently of each other, presumably through non-overlapping biochemical pathways, and have no pharmacokinetic interactions which alter the quantum of drug reaching its active site. For subtractive or negative syner-gistic effects, one drug interferes with the other to reduce efficacy. This could be competition at the active site, altered pharmacokinet-ics inducing one of the enzyme systems responsible for the other

> **Box 21.1** Principles of combination chemotherapy
>
> Use drugs active as a single agent
>
> Use drugs with different mechanisms of action
>
> Use drugs with different mechanisms of resistance
>
> Use drugs with different side effects
>
> Beware of drug-drug interactions

drug's metabolism, or the unexpected consequence that inhibition of a biochemical pathway might have on up-/down-regulation of the target kinase of the companion drug. Synergy is defined as an interaction between drugs where the effects are stronger than their mere sum and may be driven by both pharmacokinetic and pharmacodynamic interactions. The best way of demonstrating true synergy is to use the Chou–Talalay method for drug combina-tion. This is based on the median-effect equation, derived from the mass-action law principle, which is the unified theory that provides the common link between single entity and multiple entities, and first-order and higher-order dynamics. It is possible, therefore, to apply stringent equations in the preclinical setting, both in vitro and in vivo to empirical cytotoxic drug combinations to determine whether true synergy can be documented and therefore used as a piece of supporting evidence to take specific anticancer drug com-binations into the clinic.

Activity as a single agent

Drugs with at least activity as a single agent should be selected. Because of primary resistance (see later), which is frequent for any single agent even in the most responsive tumours, complete response rates of single agents rarely exceed 20%.

Different mechanisms of action

Drugs with different mechanisms of action (and toxicity profiles) should be combined. The various anticancer agent classes have different targets in the cell. Thus, even if a certain target cannot be exploited in a given tumour cell, another target might. Even if tumours are initially sensitive, they usually rapidly acquire resist-ance after drug exposure. This is probably due to selection of pre-existing resistant tumour cells in the biochemically heteroge-neous tumour cell population. In other words, the chemotherapy destroys the sensitive cell population, but is less effective against the non-sensitive population of cells that is subsequently able to con-tinue expanding. In addition, cytotoxic drugs themselves appear to increase the rate of mutation to resistance, at least in tumour mod-els [16]. The use of multiple agents with different mechanisms of action enables independent cell killing by each agent. Cells that are resistant to one agent might still be sensitive to the other drug(s) in the regimen, and might thus still be killed. Known patterns of cross-resistance must be taken into consideration in the design of drug combinations.

Different mechanisms of resistance

Drugs with different mechanisms of resistance should be com-bined. Resistance to many agents may be the result of mutational changes unique to those agents. However, in other circumstances a single mutational change may lead to resistance to a variety of

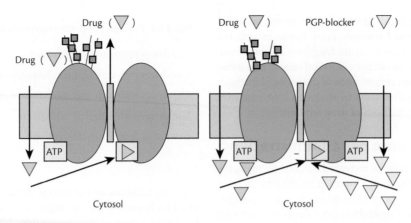

Fig. 21.3 P-glycoprotein: action and inhibition. The blocking agent binds to the cytoplasmic binding site of the drug, inhibiting its efflux.

different drugs. The number of potential mechanisms of resistance is continually increasing and is partly drug dependent.

The most investigated form of multidrug resistance is the one mediated by increased expression of the P170 membrane glycoprotein (PGP). Primary (intrinsic) over-expression of this protein has been identified in tumours derived from healthy tissues in which the protein also occurs [17]. Secondary (acquired) over-expression has also been found following chemotherapy in various diseases. PGP mediates the efflux of drugs such as anthracyclines, vinca alkaloids, epipodophyllotoxins, and various others, all derived from natural resources. PGP-mediated active efflux results in decreased intracellular drug levels, resulting in decreased cell kill. Agents that compete for the protein such as calcium-channel blockers, cyclosporin, and various synthetically produced drugs can, at least in models, reverse the effect of PGP (Figure 21.3). The clinical relevance of this type of resistance and its reversal is still unclear.

For several of the classic alkylating agents (cisplatin, cyclophosphamide, melphalan) resistance appears to be related to enhanced repair of drug-induced DNA damage.

There are many other mechanisms of resistance, including alterations in target proteins (e.g., dihydrofolate reductase with altered affinity for methotrexate) and carrier-mediated drug uptake (e.g., reduced folate). In the heterogeneous human tumours, there are frequently various mechanisms of resistance that play a role. Reversing only one of these is unlikely to yield a major impact. Resistance reversal is therefore pursued in only limited numbers of tumours. Because of the presence of drug-resistant mutants at the time of clinical diagnosis, the earliest possible use of drugs that are not cross-resistant is recommended to avoid the selection of double mutants by sequential chemotherapy. Adequate cytotoxic doses of drugs have to be administered as frequently as possible to achieve maximal kill of both sensitive and moderately resistant cells. Less desirable alternatives are the use of different regimens in alternating cycles of therapy or the use of multiple cycles of one regimen given to the point of maximal response, followed by a second regimen.

Different dose-limiting toxicities

If possible, drugs with different dose-limiting toxicities should be combined. In the case of non-overlapping toxicity it is more likely that each of the drugs can be used at full dose and thus the effectiveness of each agent will be maintained in the combination. Unfortunately, for many cytotoxic agents the side effects frequently involve myelosuppression. If there is overlapping myelotoxicity,

arbitrary scales of dose adjustment according to bone marrow toxicity can be used, or haematopoietic growth factors can be added to reduce the risk related to myelosuppression. Clearly, drugs that have low bone marrow toxicity, such as vincristine, cisplatin, and bleomycin, are favoured to combine with myelosuppressive agents. Drugs with renal or hepatic side effects in theory can alter the elimination of other agents through these routes and therefore must be used with caution in combinations. For example, cisplatin causes renal toxicity and is known to alter the pharmacokinetics of other agents (such as methotrexate or bleomycin) that depend on renal elimination as their primary mechanism of excretion.

Cell cycle-related and biochemical interactions

Cell cycle-related and biochemical interactions between drugs can also be used to design combinations. Examples of drug interactions are listed in Box 21.2.

Provided that the drugs used are active in a particular disease, knowledge of cell kinetics can be used to consider initiation of therapy with agents that are not specific for cell cycle (the alkylating

---

Box 21.2 Drug interactions in combination chemotherapy

Antagonism of anti-tumour effect

L-Asparaginase prior to methotrexate

5-Fluorouracil prior to methotrexate

Enhancement of anti-tumour effect

Nitroimidazoles enhance alkylating agent activity

Leucovorin increases 5-flourouracil inhibition of thymidylate synthase

Inhibitors of pyrimidine synthesis enhance 5-flourouracil incorporation into RNA

Reversal of drug resistance

Calcium-channel blocker inhibits efflux by P-glycoprotein

Prevention or reversal of toxicity

Allopurinol blocks 5-flourouracil activation by normal tissues

Leucovorin prevents methotrexate toxicity

Deoxycytidine prevents toxicity of cytarabine

agents and nitrosoureas), first to reduce tumour bulk and second to recruit slowly dividing cells into active DNA synthesis. Once the latter is achieved, therapy can be continued within the same cycle of treatment with agents specific for cell cycle phase (such as methotrexate or the fluoropyrimidines) that mainly affect cells during periods of DNA synthesis. Further, repeated courses with S-phase-specific drugs, such as cytosine arabinoside and methotrexate, that block cells during the period of DNA synthesis, are most effective if they are administered during the rebound rapid recovery of DNA synthesis that follows the period of suppression of DNA synthesis [18]. For cytosine arabinoside, for instance, this occurs approximately ten days after the first treatment with this agent.

An example of biochemical interaction suggesting a rational combination of drugs is shown by the example of leucovorin (5-formyltetrahydrofolate) enhancing 5-fluorouracil, by ternary stabilization of its metabolite (fluorodeoxyuridine monophosphate) with thymidylate synthase [19].

Adjuvant and neoadjuvant systemic therapy

Drug therapy is also used to benefit patients who exhibit no evidence of residual disease after initial therapy, but are at high risk of relapse (adjuvant therapy), or those with bulky primary disease to reduce this bulk preceding local therapy (neoadjuvant therapy).

Adjuvant therapy

There are two major reasons why adjuvant chemotherapy might be considered: (1) the high rate of recurrence after surgery for some, apparently localized tumours and (2) the failure of systemic therapy or combined modality treatment to cure patients with clinically apparent metastatic disease. These issues may in turn be related to the following three points. First, once the tumour bulk is reduced to clinically undetectable levels with local therapy, the number of cells yet to be destroyed by subsequent chemotherapy is relatively small, in contrast to the large numbers of cells in the case of clinical metastatic disease. According to the principles of log cell kill in the first situation, the likelihood of completely eradicating the remaining tumour cells is much higher than in the latter (Figure 21.4).

Second, as mentioned earlier, there is evidence from tumour models that supports the hypothesis that tumours are most sensitive to chemotherapy at their earliest stages of growth. This is thought to be related to their high growth fraction (most cells are in active progression through the cell cycle), shorter cell cycle times, and therefore greater fractional cell kill for a given dose of drug [20]. Once tumours progress to clinical detectability, their growth fraction falls, the cell cycle time lengthens, and they become much less sensitive to treatment.

Third, there is a relationship between tumour bulk and tumour cell resistance. The probability of the occurrence of resistant cells in a tumour population is a function of the total number of cells present and mutation rates. Therefore, subclinical (occult) tumours rather than clinically detectable tumours are more likely to be cured by chemotherapy.

On the other hand, there are obviously potential disadvantages of adjuvant chemotherapy that have to be taken into account. They relate to immediate, short-, and long-term side effects of such treatment. Since a significant fraction of patients receiving adjuvant treatment is already cured by the primary surgical procedure they would therefore experience needless toxicity and risks if treated with adjuvant therapy. The immediate side effects obviously relate to potentially lethal infectious complications from neutropenia, bleeding, and less hazardous—but very inconvenient—side effects such as alopecia and nausea and vomiting.

Late complications such as carcinogenicity and permanent sterility assume greater importance, but neither risk has been adequately quantified for all drugs and combinations. The risks of other late effects such as bone marrow hypoplasia from alkylating agents and nitrosoureas, the cardiotoxicity of doxorubicin, neurotoxocity of platins and taxanes, and pulmonary toxicity of bleomycin and the nitrosoureas should obviously not outweigh the potential benefits. In balancing these risks with the outcome as far as tumour eradication is concerned, adjuvant chemotherapy has become a standard of care in many cancers of childhood, the breast, the colon, and the ovary.

Neoadjuvant therapy

If chemotherapy is used as initial treatment, preceding a form of local therapy, it is called 'neoadjuvant therapy' or 'induction therapy'. Such neoadjuvant chemotherapy has attracted increasing attention in the treatment of some adult solid tumours. Factors

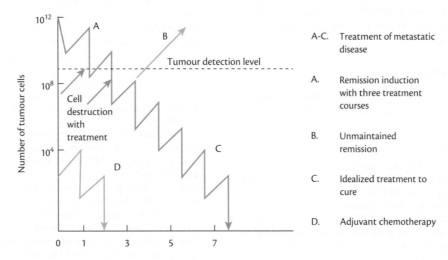

Fig. 21.4 The principle of adjuvant chemotherapy as opposed to treatment of measurable disease.

related to the response to neoadjuvant chemotherapy are similar to those that may affect adjuvant chemotherapy, namely growth rate, presence of drug resistance, and tumour mass. The potential benefits of neoadjuvant chemotherapy involve the control of the primary tumour as well as of potential micrometastases.

There are several potential advantages for control of the primary tumour [21, 22]. First, local reduction of the tumour may facilitate the use of more conservative surgery and/or radiotherapy. Second, administering chemotherapy prior to the local therapy avoids the potential of poor distribution and penetration of drug at the tumour site due to the compromised vascularity that may result from surgery and/or radiation therapy. Third, cytotoxic drugs can be combined concurrently with radiation therapy to increase the local control rate. Fourth, post-chemotherapy surgery offers a unique opportunity to assess the correlation between clinical tumour response measurements and actual pathological changes. Fifth, the response of the primary tumour to chemotherapy may reflect the response of micrometastases and therefore influence further patient management.

The disadvantages of neoadjuvant chemotherapy are similar to those mentioned for adjuvant chemotherapy. Additional disadvantages may be:

1. Selection of drug-resistant clones

2. An increase in toxicity from subsequent therapies

3. A failure of cytotoxic agents to reduce the primary tumour significantly, thereby possibly allowing further subclinical progression of disease

4. A loss of the advantage of attacking micrometastases after surgical resection of the primary tumour mass, when they may exhibit more favourable cell kinetics.

Conclusion

Despite the insights in tumour biology gained by modern molecular genetics, the broad principles governing medical oncology and the delivery of systemic anticancer therapy have remained intact over the past few decades. It is all about delivering sufficient quantities of the drug to its site of action and a molecular target which is differentially or uniquely expressed relative to normal tissue. We can respond to but not control the genetic background of the tumour, utilizing predictive and prognostic biomarkers [23, 24] but we can control drug dose and this must remain the cornerstone of effective medical oncology.

Acknowledgements

The authors would like to acknowledge the contributions made by Kees Nooter and Gerrit Stoter to previous editions of this chapter.

Further Reading

Fojo AT, Ueda K, Slamon DJ, Poplack DG, Gottesman MM et al. Expression of a multidrug-resistance gene in human tumors and tissues. Proceedings of the National Academy of Sciences USA 1987; 84: 265–269.

Folkman J. Tumor angiogenesis. In Mendelsohn J, Israel MA, Liotta LA eds, The Molecular Basis of Cancer. Philadelphia: WB Saunders, 1995, 206–232.

Goldie JH, Coldman AJ. A mathematic model for relating the drug sensitivity of tumors to their spontaneous mutation rate. Cancer Treatment Reports 1979; 63: 1727–1733.

Hill RP, Chambers AF, Ling V. Dynamic heterogeneity: rapid generation of metastatic variants in mouse B16 melanoma cells. Science 1984; 224: 998–1000.

Howell SB. Intraperitoneal chemotherapy for ovarian carcinoma. Journal of Clinical Oncology 1988; 6: 1673–1675.

La Thangue NB, Kerr DJ. Predictive biomarkers: a shift towards personalised cancer medicine. Nature Reviews Clinical Oncology 2011; 8: 587–596.

Skipper HE. Historic milestones in cancer biology: a few that are important to cancer treatment (revisited). Seminars in Oncology 1979; 6: 506–514.

References

1. Skipper HE. Historic milestones in cancer biology: a few that are important to cancer treatment (revisited). Seminars in Oncology 1979; 6: 506–514.
2. Furth J, Kahn MC. The transmission of leukemia of mice with a single cell. American Journal of Cancer 1937; 31: 276–282.
3. Mendelsohn ML. The growth fraction: a new concept applied to tumors. Science 1960; 132: 1496.
4. Tannock IF. The relationship between proliferation and the vascular system in a transplanted mouse mammary tumor. British Journal of Cancer 1968; 22: 258–273.
5. Fialkow PJ. Clonal origin of human tumors. Biochimica et Biophysica Acta 1976; 458: 283–321.
6. Curt GA, Chabner BA. Gene amplification in drug resistance: of mice and men. Journal of Clinical Oncology 1984; 2: 62–64.
7. Osler W. The Principles and Practice of Medicine. New York: D. Appleton and Co., 1892.
8. Levin L, Hryniuk WM. Dose intensity analysis of chemotherapy regimens in ovarian carcinoma. Journal of Clinical Oncology 1987; 5: 756–767.
9. Longo DL, et al. Twenty years of MOPP therapy for Hodgkin's disease. Journal of Clinical Oncology 1986; 4: 1295–1306.
10. Alberts DS, Peng YM, Chen HS, Struck RF. Effect of phenobarbital on plasma levels of cyclophosphamide and its metabolites in the mouse. British Journal of Cancer 1978; 38: 316–324.
11. Kemeny N, Schneider A. Regional treatment of hepatic metastases and hepatocellular carcinoma. Current Problems in Cancer 1989; 13: 197–284.
12. Howell SB. Intraperitoneal chemotherapy for ovarian carcinoma. Journal of Clinical Oncology 1988; 6: 1673–1675.
13. Alberts DS, et al. Phase III study of intraperitoneal cisplatin (CDDP)/intravenous cyclophosphamide (CPA) vs i.v. CDDP/i.v. CPA in patients with optimal disease stage III ovarian cancer: a SWOG-GOG-ECOG Intergroup study. Proceedings of the American Society of Clinical Oncology 1995; 14: 273.
14. Tchekmedyian NS, et al. High-dose chemotherapy without autologous bone marrow transplantation in melanoma. Journal of Clinical Oncology 1986; 4: 1811–1818.
15. Philips GL, et al. Intensive 1.3-bis(2-chloroethyl)-1 nitrosourea (BCNU) (NSC-4366650) and cryopreserved autologous marrow transplantation for refractory cancer. A phase I–II study. Cancer 1983; 52: 1792–1802.
16. Planting ASTh, Van der Burg MEL, De Boer-Dennert M, Stoter G, Verweij J. Phase I/II study of a short course of weekly cisplatin in patients with advanced solid tumors. British Journal of Cancer 1993; 68: 789–792.
17. Rice GC, Hoy C, Schimke RT. Transient hypoxia enhances the frequency of DHFR gene amplification in Chinese hamster ovary cells. Proceedings of the National Academy of Sciences USA 1986; 83: 5978–5982.
18. Deffie AM, Batra JK, Goldenberg GJ. Direct correlation between topoisomerase II activity and cytotoxicity in adriamycin-sensitive and -resistant P388 leukemia cell lines. Cancer Research 1989; 49: 58–62.
19. Cadman E, Heimer R, Davis L. Enhanced 5-fluorouracil nucleotide formation after methotrexate administration: explanation for drug synergism. Science 1979; 205: 1135–1137.

20. Grem JL, Hoth DF, Hamilton JM, King SA et al. Overview of the current status and future directions of clinical trials with fluorouracil and folinic acid. Cancer Treatment Reports 1987; 71: 1249–1264.

21. Goldie JH, Coldman AJ. A mathematic model for relating the drug sensitivity of tumors to their spontaneous mutation rate. Cancer Treatment Reports 1979; 63: 1727–1733.

22. De Boer-Dennert M, de Wit R, Schmitz PI, Djontono J, v Beurden V et al. Patient perception of the side-effects of chemotherapy: the influence of 5HT3 antagonists. British Journal of Cancer 1997; 76: 1055–1061.

23. Domingo E, Church DN, Sieber O, Ramamoorthy R, Yanagisawa Y et al. Evaluation of PIK3CA mutation as a predictor of benefit from nonsteroidal anti-inflammatory drug therapy in colorectal cancer. Journal of Clinical Oncology 2013, published online before print. doi: 10.1200/JCO.2013.50.0322.

24. La Thangue NB, Kerr DJ. Predictive biomarkers: a shift towards personalised cancer medicine. Nature Reviews Clinical Oncology 2011; 8: 587–596.

CHAPTER 22

Multidisciplinary cancer care

David N. Church, Rachel Kerr, and David J. Kerr

Introduction to multidisciplinary cancer care

Given the complex biology of the disease and the many different medical specialties required to deliver a cancer management plan in keeping with current best practice, it is not surprising that cancer care has the real potential to become fragmented, arbitrary, and suboptimal. The ideal scenario would be one in which the patient moved seamlessly along the care pathway, receiving appropriate interventions from expert specialists as tumour type and stage demanded. This 'journey' would be coordinated by a case officer managing the various interfaces and streamlining communication so that the patient felt supported, informed and confident that each element was part of a cohesive whole. It might be worth pause for reflection now so that the reader might consider the situation in their own hospital, centre, or clinic and how far from or close to this ideal their own practice may be.

Certainly in the UK ten to 15 years ago there was a growing recognition, driven initially by the compartmentalization of cancer care, the length of waiting times for operations or access to radiotherapy, and the fact that the UK's cancer outcomes fell short of the major European nations and the USA that changes in the delivery of care were much needed [1, 2]. A major policy decision taken at that time was to promote multidisciplinary working as a key element in service improvement. The definition of multidisciplinary cancer care is variable [3–6], and may include multidisciplinary clinics [7–9], multidisciplinary protocols for diagnosis and treatment [10], and multidisciplinary team (MDT) meetings [11]. However, it is undoubtedly the last category that has had the greatest impact on working practices, as MDT discussion has become mandated for all new incident cases of cancer in the UK over the last two decades. The MDT is typically defined as a group of doctors and other health professionals with expertise in a specific cancer, who discuss each case before tailoring a personalized management plan. The specific composition of any MDT depends on the tumour type cared for, but most teams will involve one or several surgeons, radiologists, histopathologists, medical oncologistsand clinical radiation oncologists, palliative care physicians and clinical nurse specialists. Other health professionals, including clinical geneticists, physiotherapists, occupational therapists, psychologists, dieticians, speech therapists, and pharmacists, may also be involved.

Since their inception, MDTs have become progressively more site specialised, and although initially this was manifested predominantly as surgeons focusing their attention on particular tumour types in order to increase and refine their caseloads, over time there has been a shift to a tumour-specific focus for all team members. Clearly this raises issues for staffing and time commitments, and

begs the question as to whether there is sufficient capacity to support this degree of specialization. Irrespective of their composition, however, the importance of MDTs in many healthcare systems has increased substantially over recent years. In the UK, the proportion of cancer cases managed by an MDT has increased from less than 20% to greater than 80% over the last two decades [12], and multidisciplinary care is mandated by healthcare organizations in the UK, mainland Europe, the USA, and Australia [4, 13–15]. In addition to improved coordination and delivery of care, many other benefits of MDTs working for patients and healthcare professionals have been suggested. However, the organization of MDT care requires substantial time and cost commitments, and the cost-effectiveness of MDTs is difficult to ascertain. Furthermore, high-quality evidence of benefit of MDTs working on patient outcomes is at best scanty, for reasons discussed below. Nevertheless, the UK NHS cancer plan regards MDTs as an essential part of the management of common cancers, and has recommended the extension of multidisciplinary care to rare tumours.

Organization and delivery of multidisciplinary cancer care

The purpose of the MDT is to collate sufficient clinical, pathological, and radiological data to enable the team to make a consensus recommendation for the optimum modality and sequence of treatment. In general, the patient history is presented by either the clinician who made primary contact or the clinical nurse specialist who has been appointed the 'key worker' for the patient; the histopathologist reports the tumour characteristics (ideally using a nationally agreed proforma designed to capture validated prognostic factors in addition to conventional TNM staging); and the radiologist delineates the primary tumour and annotates the presence/absence of distant metastases (Figure 22.1). The MDT may request further information (e.g., MRI scan of liver if there is doubt on the CT scan about presence of hepatic metastases), but if there are sufficient data, a treatment plan is formulated and a referral to initiate treatment made to the primary clinician, who could be a surgeon, radiotherapist, medical oncologist, or palliative care specialist, depending on clinical circumstance. Coordination is essential as often the patient will have to meet new clinical teams situated in different areas of the hospital or even in a completely different centre. The roles of the MDT coordinator and the clinical nurse specialists are pivotal as, for the MDT to function effectively, the results of the discussions need to be disseminated to the relevant healthcare professionals, and to the patients themselves, accurately and expeditiously.

As mentioned, in response to the unacceptable delays in treatment for cancer of a decade ago, the NHS in the UK has mandated

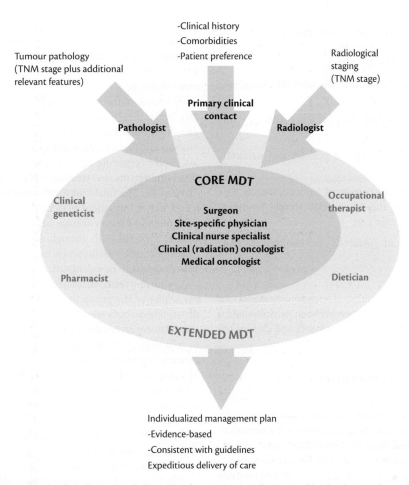

Fig. 22.1 Organization of MDT meetings. The clinical history and other salient features are typically presented by the clinician who made primary contact with the patient, or the clinical nurse specialist (CNS). The tumour pathology is summarized by the histopathologist and the imaging findings presented by the radiologist. The MDT then discusses the case and a tailored management plan is formulated. This should be both evidence-based and consistent with national and international guidelines. By collecting many specialists together, the MDT should expedite delivery of care when compared with sequential referrals between specialists.

that all new cancer patients should be discussed by an MDT, and that this is subject to audit as a quality surrogate in an ongoing national programme. The frequency of MDT meetings varies with caseload and tumour prevalence, though MDTs for the common solid tumours (lung, breast, colorectal, and urogenital) tend to meet weekly. The implementation of MDT working has helped to reduce waiting times to more internationally acceptable figures and has also improved the patient experience of the cancer journey.

Potential benefits of multidisciplinary care

By pooling the expertise of healthcare professionals from various clinical specialities, MDTs aim to provide a personalized and optimum management plan for each case discussed. As a result, patients should benefit from expert diagnosis and staging, with secondary review of imaging and pathology resulting in improved diagnostic accuracy, particularly in uncommon cancers [16, 17]. The presence of different specialists should mean that consideration is given to the full range of therapeutic modalities available for each patient, rather than the preferred therapy of the primary physician or surgeon [18, 19]. This is of particular importance for complex cases, for patients with comorbidities and for cases where combined modality therapy—such as chemoradiotherapy—is indicated. For more

straightforward situations, MDT teamwork may facilitate closer adherence to evidence-based guidelines [20, 21]. In addition, MDT discussion should prevent inappropriate referrals and expedite care delivery compared with the traditional model of sequential consultations with different specialists.

More generally, the structure of MDT meetings is consistent with the application of peer review, and the teamworking required may help promote initiatives for service improvement [22]. The MDT provides an ideal forum at which to identify patients who may be eligible for clinical trials, and the presence of a research nurse at the MDT may help ensure that the option of study participation is available to all eligible. Improved data collection as a result of MDTs should facilitate audit and research. In response to a survey of MDTs in the UK in 2009, characteristics of effective MDTs have been published to serve as a model for MDT improvement [23, 24]. Intended benefits for patients from having their case managed by an MDT are summarized in Box 22.1.

In addition to directly improving patient care, participating healthcare professionals may also benefit from working in a MDT. Communication between different team members is also often better where they have a formal working relationship but within the structure of regular discourse and mutual support. For challenging cases, the reassurance of corporate decision-making may

Box 22.1. Benefits of multidisciplinary cancer care

- Greater accuracy of diagnosis and staging
- Selection from a choice of treatments decided by a group of experts, rather than by one doctor
- Better coordination and continuity of care through all disease stages
- Treatment in line with locally agreed policies and national guidelines
- Provision of appropriate and consistent information, as the healthcare provider giving the information should be more aware of the team's strategy for care
- Greater consideration of patient's psychological and social needs.

be beneficial, although the legal position of such recommendations is unclear [25]. The open communication between professionals is also conducive to learning about novel treatments and clinical trials [26, 27].

Challenges for multidisciplinary care

A typical MDT meeting involves ten to 20 healthcare professionals, lasts between one and three hours, and may require substantial preparation for participants—particularly radiologists and pathologists who may have to review 20 to 30 cases beforehand. The average clinician may attend between one and three such meetings a week, and even the most cursory of calculations will demonstrate the significant time commitments that MDT working demands from members. Consequently, it is perhaps unsurprising that a common contributor to suboptimal MDT effectiveness is lack of attendance at meetings [28–30]. A study of breast cancer MDTs showed that while surgeons and clinical nurse specialists were present for the entire meeting 95% of the time, and pathologists and radiologists in 90–95% of cases, the proportion of clinical oncologists who attended the entire meeting was 70%, and medical oncologists were present throughout in only 44.1% of cases. Medical oncologists were more likely to attend the whole MDT meeting if it was held in a protected session (71% versus 54%), though only 28% of MDT meetings were in protected time. A subsequent study of breast cancer MDTs reported similar findings, and lack of attendance of core members has also been noted in colorectal and head and neck cancer MDTs [29–31]. Time pressures may also lead to challenges in ensuring each case is discussed in sufficient detail to permit the formulation of a detailed management plan. As a representative example, the Oxford colorectal cancer MDT comprises 12 to 15 consultants, four to six specialist nurses and two MDT coordinators, and discusses an average of 30 to 40 new patients each week in a 1–1.5-hour slot. The team is absolutely committed to joint working, but feels that the need to spend more time discussing more complex or difficult cases means that a 'tick-box' mentality is sometimes applied to straightforward cases.

The logistics of conducting an MDT meeting is in itself a substantial undertaking. Meeting rooms require information technology support to permit projection of imaging and histopathology, and in many cases to enable videoconferencing with other hospitals. The MDT coordinator plays a pivotal role in ensuring that correct meeting facilities are booked, that the necessary patient information is available, and that the result of discussions is accurately recorded and expeditiously disseminated to all those involved in the patient's care [18, 30, 32].

As a result of the staff and support costs, MDT working requires substantial investment, and it has been shown that funding strategies often underestimate the true costs of MDT service. A recent analysis collated all salary and support costs of breast MDTs in one UK cancer centre during 2009. During this period the MDT met 53 times and formulated treatment plans for 1315 patients from 2343 discussions. The total cost for the year was £114,948, translating to a cost per management plan of £87.41—similar to the NHS estimate of £85.62 for an average MDT decision. Staff costs comprised 86% of the total [33]. Though this likely represents a worthwhile investment, such evaluation is essential if the true value of MDTs to patient care is to be calculated.

As with any team, successful MDT working is also dependent on the ability of the group to perform well together, a characteristic dependent on both team composition and size [33]. The MDT chair should foster an environment in which all members are encouraged to contribute, with mutual respect for opinions that may differ, and constructive feedback provided on previous decisions [18, 34–37]. This aspect of MDT working is potentially at odds with the historical role of the clinician as largely autonomous care provider, and teams do not typically function well without guidance and training for members [20, 38]. To address this common deficiency, in the UK an MDT self-assessment programme, MDT-FIT ('feedback for improving team-working') is under development with the aim of improving MDT performance [39].

A further potential Achilles heel of MDT working is that central decision-making may be perfectly coordinated but delivery of the treatment plan may be fragmented. Although the ideal of patients moving smoothly along the care pathway from one specialty to another is entirely achievable, the many transitions along the route have the potential to lead to a rather disjointed and daunting experience for the patient at a time of maximum vulnerability. This risk is significantly reduced by the availability of a clinical nurse specialist or key care worker able to accompany the patient when they attend for primary and subsequent treatments in order to maintain continuity and ensure that patients do not get lost in the system. Although many clinical nurse specialists perform this function excellently, again, time pressures prevent them from providing this level of care and support as routine and in every case.

Evidence of benefit from the MDT approach

There are relatively few studies evaluating the effect of MDT working in any form, and those focusing on its effect on cancer outcomes are even less common. The logistics of organizing a randomized controlled trial comparing MDT working with non-MDT working would be challenging to say the least, and as MDT working is both common, and in many cases mandated, internationally such a study is highly unlikely to be performed. Consequently, most data are retrospective, with many before-and-after studies that run substantial risk of confounding due to improvements in care outwith the MDT during the study period. A systematic review of MDT effectiveness published in 2010 [6] identified two systematic reviews [40, 41], one abstract, and 18 original studies [42–58] analysing the effects of MDT working on cancer survival. Of these, 12 studies (one prospective [57]) and six retrospective cohort studies [42–44, 46, 54, 58], five before-and-after series [47, 50–52, 56] reported statistically significant associations between multidisciplinary care and patient survival. However, significant methodological limitations, including heterogeneity of the definition of multidisciplinary care and a lack of comparison with control groups were common. Thus, it was possible that some of the benefit of MDT working was in fact due to confounding factors including biases in patient selection and improved survival secondary to improved treatments during the study period [6, 40]. Consequently, although the collective weight of evidence to date suggests that multidisciplinary care improves cancer survival, this cannot be authoritatively asserted at present. More controversial still is the evaluation of whether the costs of MDT working justify clinical benefits. Studies evaluating the effects of MDT working on treatment and outcomes for common cancers are discussed below and summarized in Table 22.1.

Breast cancer

MDT management of breast cancer is now standard in the UK and much of the developed world. However, despite early studies reporting that breast MDT cancer care was associated with frequent alteration of patient management plans [11, 59], shorter time to treatment, and greater patient satisfaction [7], a systematic review in 2006 found no evidence that MDTs were associated with improved survival for patients with breast cancer [40]. The authors concluded that while MDT care should in theory be associated with improvement in survival, there was a lack of high-quality evidence to support this.

An important recent report by Kesson and colleagues from Scotland has gone some way to correcting this apparently anomalous situation [60]. In 1995 MDT care was introduced in the Greater Glasgow health board area as part of an initiative to improve the quality of care, but not in areas managed by other health boards in the west of Scotland. Following this introduction, care in the intervention area applied common principles of MDT care—regular meetings, application of evidence-based guidelines and audit—while care in the non-intervention area remained organized along traditional lines, with surgeons unilaterally responsible for making decisions on surgery and adjuvant therapy. Following publication of national guidance on cancer care in 1999, the non-intervention areas also adopted MDT care, and the discrepancy ceased to exist. By comparing outcomes between areas before the introduction of MDT care (analysed time period January 1990 to September 1995) and during the intervention period (time period October 1995 to December 2000), the authors were able to address many of the limitations of previous studies, by defining the composition of an MDT at the outset, observing the effect of care where no other model was available, and including a contemporaneous comparison population to adjust for temporal improvements in survival. Before the introduction of MDTs, breast cancer mortality was 11% higher in the intervention area than in the non-intervention area (hazard ratio adjusted for year of incidence, age at diagnosis, and deprivation = 1.11; 95% confidence interval 1.00 to 1.20). After multidisciplinary care was introduced, breast cancer mortality was 18% lower in the intervention area than in the non-intervention area (0.82, 0.74–0.91). All cause mortality did not differ significantly between populations in the earlier period, but was 11% lower in the intervention area than in the non-intervention area in the later period (HR 0.89, CI 0.82–0.97). Interrupted time series analyses showed a significant improvement in breast cancer survival in the intervention area in 1996, compared with the expected survival in the same year had the pre-intervention trend continued (P = 0.004). This improvement was maintained after the intervention was introduced. It would appear therefore, that multidisciplinary care was associated with improved survival and reduced variation in survival among hospitals. These results provide the most convincing evidence of benefit for patients with any tumour type from MDT care to date.

Lung cancer

The diagnostic workup for suspected lung cancers often requires multiple investigations, including imaging studies such as ^{18}FDG-PET, bronchoscopy, endobronchial ultrasound (EBUS), mediastinoscopy, and thoracoscopy, many of which are performed by different specialists. In addition, management is frequently multimodal and both the type and scheduling of treatment vary substantially depending on tumour histology and stage. Intuitively, MDTs would be expected to have substantial impact in this tumour type.

In an early effort to assess the effectiveness of MDT working in lung cancer, a pilot study to assess the feasibility and efficacy of referral to a central multidisciplinary diagnostic clinic for diagnostic workup compared with conventional investigation was conducted by investigators at the Royal Marsden Hospital in London. Reported in 2003, this showed that MDT review was associated with shorter time to initiation of treatment though on follow-up no difference in survival between groups was detected. Although the investigators confirmed the feasibility of the pilot, they noted that expanding the study to a size powered to detect survival change would require substantial commitment from patients and physicians [45]. Another study evaluated treatment and survival of patients with non-small-cell lung cancer (NSCLC) before and after the implementation of MDT care in a single centre in Scotland [50]. The pre- and post-cohorts were well matched for baseline variables. Adoption of MDT care was associated with significant increases in the proportion of patients treated with chemotherapy (23% versus 7%; P < 0.001) and in overall survival (6.6 months versus 3.2 months; P < 0.001). However, the before-and-after nature of this study might mean that improvements in systemic therapy and supportive care during the study period may have contributed to the results.

Both of these studies were included in a systematic review of the effect of MDT working on lung cancer outcomes published in 2008. Sixteen studies met the authors' inclusion criteria, including several in which the primary focus was not MDT care per se. Statistical pooling was not possible due to a clinical heterogeneity; however, only two publications, including the study by Forrest, reported improved survival [41]. Both were potentially confounded by the before-and-after design and the authors concluded that although MDT review may be associated with improved survival in lung cancer, the published evidence did not provide conclusive support for this at present. In an attempt to address these deficiencies by minimizing confounding due to temporal changes in management, Boxer and co-workers compared outcomes for 988 patients diagnosed with NSCLC between 2005 and 2008 in Southwestern Australia according to whether or not their cases were discussed

Table 22.1 Summary of studies evaluating the effects of MDT working

Tumour type	Intervention evaluated	Comparison group used	Study design	Sample size	Effect of MDT care on patient management	Effect of MDT care on patient survival	Notes	Reference
Breast cancer	Effect of introduction of MDT care in health board areas (intervention area)	Adjacent health board areas without introduction of MDT care (non-intervention area)	Temporally matched comparison before and after introduction of MDTs	N = 14, 358	Not reported	18% reduction in breast cancer mortality (HR 0.82, 0.74–0.91) and 11% reduction in all cause mortality (0.89, 0.82–0.97) in intervention area compared to compared to non-intervention area	Highest quality evidence of benefit of MDT care on cancer survival. Screen-detected cancers excluded to avoid bias. Survival improvement persisted after adjustment for confounders	[60]
	Receipt of multimodality treatment/high surgical caseload (> 30 cases/year)	Patients not treated with multimodality therapy/low surgical caseload	Population-based retrospective cohort study (1979–1988)	N = 12,861	Patients treated by surgeons with high caseload more likely to receive adjuvant chemotherapy and hormone therapy	Receipt of multimodality therapy associated with improved survival	High surgical caseload likely to be associated with MDT working	[43]
	Receipt of multimodality treatment/high surgical caseload (> 30 cases/year)	Patients not treated with multimodality therapy/low surgical caseload	Population-based retrospective cohort study (1989–1994)	N = 11,329	Patients treated by surgeons with high caseload more likely to receive chemotherapy	Management by surgeon with high caseload associated with five-year survival of 68% versus 60% for cases managed by surgeons with lowest caseload	High surgical caseload likely to be associated with MDT working	[46]
	Impact of Calman–Hine recommendations, including MDTs	Cases managed by surgeons with less adoption of MDT working	Population-based, retrospective cohort study	N = 12,961	Increased adherence of teams to manual of cancer service standards associated with greater use of postoperative radiotherapy following breast-conserving surgery (OR = 1.22, P = 0.05)	Trend towards improved survival with increasing surgical site specialization (HR = 0.93, 95% P = 0.1)	Study noted variable implementation of Calman–Hine recommendations	[53]
	Introduction of one-stop multidisciplinary clinic	Cases managed prior to introduction of multidisciplinary clinic	Single centre, before–after study	N₁ = 162 N₂ = 177	Significant decrease in time to initiation of treatment with MDT clinic (29.6 days versus 42.2 days; P = 0.0008). Improved patient satisfaction	Not reported	Authors note pivotal role of nursing coordinator in multidisciplinary care delivery	[7]
	Effect of MDT review on diagnosis/ management plan	Nil	Single centre, retrospective review of during six-month period	N = 75	MDT revised treatment plans in 32 cases (43%)	Not reported		[11]
	Effect of MDT review on diagnosis/ management plan	Nil	Single centre, retrospective review during one-year period	N = 149	Change in interpretation of imaging in 67 cases (45%) and to interpretation of pathology in 43 patients (29%). Alteration of management plans in 77 cases (52%)	Not reported		[59]

<small>N₁ = 162 N₂ = 177 should read:</small>

	Intervention	Study design	N	Process findings	Survival findings	Notes	Ref
Lung cancer	MDT case discussion	Retrospective study of all patients with lung cancer diagnosed between 2005 and 2008	988	MDT case discussion associated with increased use of chemotherapy (46% versus 29%; P < 0.01), radiotherapy (66% versus 33%; P < 0.01) and palliative care (66% versus 53%; P < 0.01)	No change in survival	Greater number of patients >80 years age in non-MDT group (25% versus 13%)	[61]
	Introduction of MDT meetings for non-small cell lung cancer	Single centre, before-after study comparing two one-year periods (N_1: 1997, N_2: 2001)	$N_1 = 117$ $N_2 = 126$	Implementation of MDT working associated with increased use of chemotherapy (23% versus 7%; P < 0.001)	MDT care associated with improved survival: 6.6 versus 3.2 months (P<0.001)	MDT meetings contained respiratory physicians, medical and clinical oncologists, palliative care physician, radiologist and lung CNS	[50]
	Implementation of MDT meetings and appointment of specialist thoracic surgeon	Before-after series	$N_1 = 65$ $N_2 = 175$	Significant increase in overall resection rate (23.4% versus 12.2%; P < .001) and operations in the elderly (18% versus 4%; P = 0.02)	No change in five-year survival (31% versus 32%)		[49]
	Central multidisciplinary two-stop clinic for patients with suspected lung cancer	Randomized, controlled pilot study	N = 88	Time to initiation of treatment significantly less in MDT group (three weeks versus seven weeks; P < 0.0025)	No difference in survival at two years	Authors noted that definitive trial would require substantial commitment for patients and clinicians	[45]
Gastrointestinal cancer	Impact of Calman–Hine recommendations, including MDTs for colorectal cancer	Population-based, retrospective cohort study	N = 12, 358	Increased use of preoperative radiotherapy for rectal cancer with increase in team specialization (HR = 1.43, P < 0.04)	3% decrease in relative risk of death per 25% increase in team score (HR = 0.97, 95% CI 0.94–0.99)	Team score reflected implementation of Calman–Hine recommendations, including MDT care	[54]
	Impact of introduction of colorectal cancer MDT	Before-after study (N_1: 1997–2002, N_2: 2002 to 2005)	$N_1 = 176$ $N_2 = 134$	Increased use of adjuvant chemotherapy after introduction of MDT care (31% versus 13%; P < 0.01)	Increased three-year overall survival for patients with stage III disease following MDT implementation (66% versus 58%; P–0.023)		[56]
	Impact of introduction of dedicated MDT with liver surgeon for metastatic colorectal cancer	Prospective cohort study	N = 331	Frequency of preoperative chemotherapy not reported	Five-year survival greater for patients referred via specialist MDT (49.9% versus 43.3%; P = 0.0001)		[57]
	Impact of MDT on outcome for patients with oesophageal cancer	Before-after study (N_1: 1991–1997, N_2: 1998 to 2003)	$N_1 = 77$ $N_2 = 67$	Greater use of radical radiotherapy (P = 0.001) and palliative chemotherapy and radiotherapy (P<0.0001) following adoption of MDT working	Five-year survival in group managed by MDT 52% versus 10% for historical controls (P<0.001)	MDT comprised specialist surgeons, oncologist, radiologists, pathologist, gastroenterologists, CNS	[52]

(continued)

Table 22.1 Continued

Tumour type	Intervention evaluated	Comparison group used	Study design	Sample size	Effect of MDT care on patient management	Effect of MDT care on survival	Notes	Reference
	Impact of tertiary centre MDT review for pancreatic cancer	Nil	Prospective study of 203 cases in one-year period		Revision to radiological staging in 38 cases (18.7%), to pathological interpretation in 7 cases (3.4%). Alteration of management plan in 48 patients (23.6%)	Not reported		[62]
Urological cancer	Introduction of concurrent multidisciplinary clinic for low risk prostate cancer	Sequential specialist consultations	Retrospective multicentre study during one-year period	N = 701	Higher proportion of patients in MDT cohort managed with active surveillance (43% versus 22%; P<0.001)	Not reported	High rate of patient satisfaction from MDT clinic	[66]
	Effect of MDT meetings on patient management for urological cancers	Nil	Prospective single-centre study during six-month period	N = 124	Major change to diagnosis/staging* in 2 cases (1.6%), minor change in 5 cases (4.0%)	Not reported	Prior to MDT referring clinicians documented proposed management plans and comparison was made with MDT recommendation	[67]
	Central MDT discussion of selected urologic cancers	Local MDT discussion	Retrospective review of 87 cases during one-year period	N = 87	Change in management from local MDT plan recommended in 0/67 prostate, 4/19 (21.0%) bladder, and 1/1 renal cancer cases	Not reported	Referral to central MDT based on pre-defined criteria	[67]
Gynaecologic cancer	Management of ovarian cancer at multidisciplinary clinic	Patients not managed at joint clinic during same period	Population-based retrospective cohort (one-year period)	N = 533	Patients twice as likely to receive platinum-based chemotherapy (P < 0.001)	Five-year survival 35.3% versus 19.2% (P < 0.001)	130 patients of 479 assessable during study period seen at joint clinic. Improved survival unlikely to be due solely to chemotherapy use	[42]
	Management of ovarian cancer by multidisciplinary team at cancer centre	Patients treated at peripheral units	Retrospective cohort study	N = 287	Higher proportion of patients managed by MDT in cancer centre treated with postoperative platinum-based chemotherapy (98% versus 86%; P = 0.008)	Survival in cases managed in peripheral units significantly less than in those managed by MDT (HR 1.79; P = 0.02)	Service evaluation prior to introduction of management guidelines for ovarian cancer	[58]
	Tumour board discussion of gynaecologic cancers	Nil	Retrospective review during 3-year period (391 new cases, 68 recurrences)	N = 459	Major revision to diagnosis/ staging* in 23 cases (5.0%), minor change in 9 cases (2.0%)	Not reported	Authors concluded tumour board review affects patient care	[71]

Tumour type	Intervention	Study design	Control	N	Result	Survival	Conclusion	Ref
	MDT discussion of gynaecologic cancers	Retrospective review during one-year period	Nil	N = 509	Major revision to diagnosis/staging* in 30 patients (5.9%) and minor discrepancies in 16 cases (3.1%) Commonest alterations were recommendations for chemotherapy and surgery	Not reported	Authors concluded tumour board review affects patient care	[69]
	Tumour board discussion of gynaecologic cancers	Prospective analysis over one-year period	Nil	N=153	Major revision to diagnosis/staging resulting in change in management in 8.5% and minor change in 26.1%	Not reported		[80]
	Discussion of cases of uterine sarcoma at MDT meeting	Population-based retrospective cohort study	Cases not discussed at MDT	N = 87	Less use of adjuvant chemotherapy in patients discussed by MDT	No impact of MDT discussion on survival apparent		[30]
Head and neck squamous cell carcinoma (HNSCC)	Multidisciplinary clinic with surgeons and oncologists	Retrospective audit—before-after (1: 1996–1997, 2: 1999–2000)	Cases prior to adoption of MDT working	$N_1 = 566$, $N_2 = 727$	Not reported	MDT management associated with trend to improved two-year survival in first audit (P = 0.1) and significant improvement in second audit (P = 0.02)	Greater use of MDT working following publication of Calman-Hine report	[47]
Miscellaneous tumour types	Adoption of weekly MDT meetings as part of creating of dedicated cancer centre	Before-after series	Patients managed before MDT implementation, SEER data	$N_1 = 5,487$, $N_2 = 10,548$	Decrease in proportion of cases managed with surgery alone (36.9% to 31.0%; P<0.0001). Increase in proportion of patients treated with systemic therapy (24.6% to 42.1%; P<0.0001)	Increase in five-year actuarial survival for all tumour types (52% to 58%; P<0.0001]. Significantly improved survival for cancers of breast, lung, prostate, stomach, pancreas, oral cavity	Authors conclude multiple advantages to multidisciplinary team approach	[51]

Notes: * resulted in change in patient management.

in an MDT. Cases discussed at MDT had better documentation of disease stage and performance status, and these patients were also more likely to receive chemotherapy, radiotherapy, and palliative care referrals that patients whose cases were not discussed (P < 0.001 all comparisons). Despite this, no effect of MDT discussion on patient survival was evident [61].

Consequently, although MDT working clearly impacts on patient management in lung cancer, current data do not conclusively prove its benefit in improving patient outcome.

Gastrointestinal cancer

Several studies have examined the effect of MDT working on gastrointestinal malignancies. In an early study, Stephens and colleagues compared outcomes for 67 consecutive patients with oesophageal cancer treated after the adoption of MDT working in 1997 with 77 consecutive historical controls managed by individual surgeons previously [52]. Five-year survival was dramatically higher in the group managed by MDT (52% versus 10%, P<0.0001). Patients managed by MDT were significantly more likely to receive palliative chemotherapy and radiotherapy, though the proportion of patients treated with preoperative chemotherapy was not documented. Though it is likely that the improvement in outcome resulted from multiple factors, many of these are likely to have been secondary to the adoption of MDT working. The effect of MDT care on management of pancreatic cancer was examined in 203 patients treated at a tertiary centre multidisciplinary clinic between 2006 and 2007. MDT review of imaging led to a change in disease stage in 38 cases (18.7%), and in pathological interpretation in seven cases (3.4%). The treatment recommendation of the MDT differed from that previously planned for the patient in 48 cases [62]. Survival outcomes were not reported in this study.

In common with the examples cited above in breast and lung cancer, a multidisciplinary approach to colorectal cancer management can result in alteration in management [63]. A study performed by Burton and co-workers demonstrated that MDT discussion of staging MRI for rectal cancer cases reduced positive circumferential resection margins through improved preoperative treatment [64], and MDT management was associated with increased use of neo-adjuvant therapy in a US study [63]. A large study examining the effect of the Calman–Hine recommendations on colorectal cancer care in Yorkshire in the UK ranked colorectal cancer teams according to how closely they adhered to the ideal MDT published in the UK manual of cancer standards, with increasing team score indicating closer adherence. The investigators found no significant link between increase in team score and the frequency of chemotherapy overall, or of preoperative radiotherapy for rectal cancers. However, for every 25% increase in team score a statistically significant 3% reduction in risk of death for all colorectal cancer patients was observed (HR = 0.97, 95% CI = 0.94–0.99) [54]. Although the large size of this study (12,358 patients) and its population-based nature strengthen these conclusions when compared to single-centre studies, the possibility that the improvements in survival may have resulted from factors other than MDT working remains. The multimodality management of liver metastases from colorectal cancer is a notable success of contemporary cancer medicine, and multidisciplinary care has been an integral component in this. However, specialist radiology and surgical review are required to identify cases suitable for curative resection and absence of these may result in patients being denied radical treatment inappropriately.

Therefore, in most large centres discussion of such patients at a specialist hepatobiliary MDT is recommended. A recent study retrospectively identified patients with colorectal liver metastases treated with palliative chemotherapy by oncologists without specialist hepatobiliary MDT review. Imaging prior to chemotherapy was reviewed by liver surgeons blinded to patient management [65]. Of 52 patients with liver-only disease, 33 (63%) were considered potentially resectable by the expert panel. Although this decision was based on purely radiological grounds, it is unlikely that all of these patients would have been unfit for surgery.

Urological cancer

Prostate cancer is a heterogeneous malignancy, the optimum management of which varies from active surveillance to radical prostatectomy or radical radiotherapy. Treatment recommendations for patients may vary according to care providers' biases, and a noteworthy recent study provides an interesting insight into the effects of multidisciplinary working on this. In this large retrospective study of men with low-risk prostate cancer, review at a concurrent multidisciplinary clinic (including a urologist, radiotherapist, and medical oncologist) was associated with a higher proportion of men selected for active surveillance and lower rates of treatment with radical prostatectomy or radiation than in patients seen by practitioners sequentially [66]. This difference was not due to temporal change in practice as all patients were treated in 2009, and the authors conclude that these results may have significant clinical implications. In contrast to these data, Acher and colleagues examined the frequency with which MDT review changed management plans for urology patients in a single centre over a six-month period. Prior to each meeting, referring surgeons completed a form for patients stating their proposed management plan, and this was then compared with the team decision made at the meeting. There was concordance between the two in over 98% of cases, and the authors concluded that it may be possible to reserve MDT discussion for challenging cases without compromising patient care [67]. Similarly, in a report analysing the importance of central MDT review (based on defined criteria) for urological malignancies, management was not changed in any cases of prostate cancer, while for bladder malignancies 4 out of 19 cases (21.0%) had a change in management [68].

Gynaecologic cancer

Several studies report that MDT review of gynaecological malignancies frequently results in change in diagnosis and staging [69–71]. Cohen and co-workers investigated the frequency with which pathological and radiological findings were altered by discussion at a specialist gynaecology MDT in New Zealand [69]. Discrepancies were classified as major if they resulted in a change in patient management, and minor if they did not. From 509 cases discussed during the one-year period analysed, 46 deviations were found (9%), with 30 major (5.9%) and 16 minor (3.1%) discrepancies. The most frequent changes to patient management were recommendations for chemotherapy and surgery. Similar findings were noted in an early study of the effects of multidisciplinary working for all cases of ovarian cancer diagnosed in Scotland in 1997, in which MDT management was associated with increased use of platinum-based chemotherapy. Notably in this study, MDT care was also associated with improved survival, with an effect beyond that explicable by the greater use of platinum-based treatment in this group [42].

Head and neck squamous cell carcinoma

Birchall audited cases of head and neck cancer in the southwest of England before and after the publication of the Calman–Hine report, which promoted MDT working (periods examined 1996/1997 and 1999/2000). Although two-year overall survival was unchanged between the two periods, in both audits MDT management was significantly associated with improved survival [47]. The proportion of patients treated with surgery, radiotherapy, and chemotherapy did not alter between the first and second audits; however, whether use of these treatment modalities was more common in cases managed by MDT is not reported.

Other evidence for effectiveness of MDT care

Although as discussed above, MDTs should improve communication and enhance coordination of treatment, few studies have addressed this. One audit of head and neck cancer found that although referral pathways appeared satisfactory, delays occurred due to waits for investigations, beds, and specialist treatments, particularly radiotherapy [29]. A further concern was that MDTs were frequently understaffed. Another questionnaire-based survey published in 2003 found that 62% of lead clinicians of colorectal MDTs stated that there were difficulties in running the MDT, with 32% lacking a dedicated MDT coordinator. The authors emphasized the essential role of MDT coordinators, and stressed the importance of mapping the patient care pathway to identify bottlenecks where delays occurred [30]. A study of breast cancer teams found that clinical performance was improved by the number of breast care nurses, and positively correlated with the workload of the MDT. This study also demonstrated that teams with a number of leaders were associated with greater effectiveness, while a single, clear leader negatively predicted innovation and effectiveness in audit and research. Interestingly, levels of psychiatric morbidity were lower for MDT members than those reported for other health teams and the NHS workforce in general [35], a finding mirrored by another report which found less psychiatric morbidity overall in MDT members than previously published rates for UK clinicians. However, this average is perhaps an oversimplification as the researchers found substantial variation within teams and high rates of emotional exhaustion in MDT leaders [72]. Although commonly postulated as an advantage of MDT working, evidence for an impact of MDT working on clinical trial recruitment is limited, though published data are consistent with increased frequency of clinical trial participation in patients identified as eligible by MDTs [26, 73, 74].

The future of multidisciplinary cancer care

Cancer is largely a disease of ageing, and the increasing proportion of the elderly who suffer malignant disease poses a particular challenge of MDT working. Although meetings are generally excellent at recording disease stage and pathological factors, documentation of other patient factors such as performance status and comorbidities is frequently variable and occasionally absent. A study of patients with upper gastrointestinal cancers discussed at MDTs found that in 15.1% of cases the MDT recommendation was not implemented. In 43.9% of these cases the discordance was due to comorbidity and in 34.2% to patient choice. The authors concluded that more information on comorbid disease was required for MDTs to make informed recommendations on patient care [75]. Other studies have reported that MDT treatment plans for patients were not actioned in 10–24% cases of colorectal cancer, and 4.4% of lung cancer cases [76] due mainly to a combination of comorbidities and patient refusal [21, 77]. Although validated scales such as the Charlson comorbidity index provide prognostic information for patients with cancer [78] they are not commonly used outside clinical trials. Incorporation of such indices into MDT discussion would substantially strengthen recommendations for the elderly, and is increasingly straightforward using the computer-based applications available. At the very least, a minimum dataset comprising performance status and concurrent illnesses should be available for each patient discussed.

Given the general acceptance that MDT meetings are integral to current best practice in oncology, attention is likely to focus on the refinement, standardization, and streamlining of MDT function. The application of modern information technology (IT) methodology promises significant improvements in all areas. The current MDT model of discussion of each case by core MDT members followed by formulation of an optimum management plan is typically accompanied by limited, if any, documentation of the factors decisions are based upon and little context between one patient and the next. To the external observer, particularly those from backgrounds in engineering and decision science, MDT meetings are in large part art and in small part science. Though the development of evidence-based checklists to structure MDT meetings [39] is a step in the right direction, it is possible to develop integrative software tools to record, display, and report the decision-making process and its outcome in a structured way. Such a system, MATE (Multidisciplinary meeting Assistant and Treatment sElector), developed at the Royal Free Hospital in London was designed to capture patient data including pathology and imaging results, identify patients eligible for clinical trials, and suggest evidence-based treatment recommendations. The developers performed a prospective evaluation through 2008 and 2009 during which MDT patient data was entered onto MATE, though the MDT were unaware of the treatment recommendations generated by the software. On analysis, the recommendations made by MATE displayed better concordance with clinical practice guidelines than MDT recommendations (97% versus 93.2%); in addition, the software identified 61% more patients eligible for clinical trials than the MDT [79].

It is likely that in the next few years MATE, and similar software, will be sufficiently adaptable to contain multifactorial analysis based on genomic data in addition to traditional prognostic factors in order to take advantage of the revolution in genomics which underpins personalized cancer medicine. The logical endpoint of this development will be a suite of software for the management of cancer patients, not only combining current patient data, but also able to display it within the context of a database of previous patients with annotated outcomes, and links to national cancer treatment guidelines and expert disease management systems. This will propel the MDT into an era in which clinical outcomes become the gold standard used to compare the quality of teams and hospitals and, when made publicly available, allow citizens better to choose the centres to which they would prefer referral.

Conclusions

There is clear evidence that MDT working results in change in patient management, and, though limited, outcome data are consistent with a benefit for patients with cancer from MDT care. As discussed previously, the widespread adoption of MDT working internationally means that such a randomized controlled trial of MDT care is unlikely to take place, although prospective audits should help to confirm that the benefits of MDT working are being realized in practice.

Multidisciplinary care probably improves patient outcomes by influencing various aspects of care. These factors include adherence to guidelines and nurse education, increased surgical volume and experience, and improved interdisciplinary working. Although multidisciplinary care is considered standard practice in many countries, access to such care still varies. However, these results support the universal provision of cancer care by specialist, multidisciplinary teams. The importance of good communication cannot be overstated, and is likely to become more rather than less important as cancer is resolved into a greater number of biomarker-determined disease subtypes. While it is likely that MDTs will remain site-based for the foreseeable future, there will be increasing specializations around targeted molecular pathways as the application of high-throughput sequencing technologies to clinical samples becomes routine. Further work should address other cancer types, tease out which are the most important contributory elements of team-delivered cancer care, and address the issue of cost-effectiveness.

Further reading

Birchall M, Bailey D, King P, South West Cancer Intelligence Service Head and Neck Tumour Panel. Effect of process standards on survival of patients with head and neck cancer in the south and west of England. British Journal of Cancer 2004; 91(8): 1477–1481.

Blazeby JM, Wilson L, Metcalfe C, Nicklin J, English R et al. Analysis of clinical decision-making in multi-disciplinary cancer teams. Annals of Oncology 2006; 17(3): 457–460.

Boxer MM, Vinod SK, Shafiq J, Duggan KJ. Do multidisciplinary team meetings make a difference in the management of lung cancer? Cancer 2011; 117(22): 5112–5120.

Catt S, Fallowfield L, Jenkins V, Langridge C, Cox A. The informational roles and psychological health of members of 10 oncology multidisciplinary teams in the UK. British Journal of Cancer 2005; 93(10): 1092–1097.

Coory M, Gkolia P, Yang IA, Bowman RV, Fong KM. Systematic review of multidisciplinary teams in the management of lung cancer. Lung Cancer 2008; 60(1): 14–21.

Fennell ML, Das IP, Clauser S, Petrelli N, Salner A. The organization of multidisciplinary care teams: modeling internal and external influences on cancer care quality. Journal of the National Cancer Institute Monographs 2010; 2010(40): 72–80.

Fleissig A, Jenkins V, Catt S, Fallowfield L. Multidisciplinary teams in cancer care: are they effective in the UK? Lancet Oncology 2006; 7(11): 935–943.

Forrest LM, McMillan DC, McArdle CS, Dunlop DJ. An evaluation of the impact of a multidisciplinary team, in a single centre, on treatment and survival in patients with inoperable non-small-cell lung cancer. British Journal of Cancer 2005; 93(9): 977–978.

Gabel M, Hilton NE, Nathanson SD. Multidisciplinary breast cancer clinics. Do they work? Cancer 1997; 79(12): 2380–2384.

Gillis CR, Hole DJ. Survival outcome of care by specialist surgeons in breast cancer: a study of 3786 patients in the west of Scotland. British Medical Journal 1996; 312(7024): 145–148.

Haward R, Amir Z, Borrill C, Dawson J, Scully J et al. Breast cancer teams: the impact of constitution, new cancer workload, and methods of operation on their effectiveness. British Journal of Cancer 2003; 89(1): 15–22.

Hong NJL, Wright FC, Gagliardi AR, Paszat LF. Examining the potential relationship between multidisciplinary cancer care and patient survival: an international literature review. Journal of Surgical Oncology 2010; 102(2): 125–134.

Houssami N, Sainsbury R. Breast cancer: multidisciplinary care and clinical outcomes. European Journal of Cancer 2006; 42(15): 2480–2491.

Jones RP, Vauthey J-N, Adam R, Rees M, Berry D et al. Effect of specialist decision-making on treatment strategies for colorectal liver metastases. British Journal of Surgery 2012; 99(9): 1263–1269.

Junor EJ, Hole DJ, Gillis CR. Management of ovarian cancer: referral to a multidisciplinary team matters. British Journal of Cancer 1994; 70(2): 363–370.

Kesson EM, Allardice GM, George WD, Burns HJG, Morrison DS. Effects of multidisciplinary team working on breast cancer survival: retrospective, comparative, interventional cohort study of 13 722 women. British Medical Journal 2012; 344:e2718.

Lamb BW, Sevdalis N, Vincent C, Green JSA. Development and evaluation of a checklist to support decision making in cancer multidisciplinary team meetings: MDT-QuIC. Annals of Surgical Oncology 2012; 19(6): 1759–1765.

Lordan JT, Karanjia ND, Quiney N, Fawcett WJ, Worthington TR. A 10-year study of outcome following hepatic resection for colorectal liver metastases: the effect of evaluation in a multidisciplinary team setting. European Journal of Surgical Oncology 2009; 35(3): 302–306.

Morris E, Haward RA, Gilthorpe MS, Craigs C, Forman D. The impact of the Calman–Hine report on the processes and outcomes of care for Yorkshire's colorectal cancer patients. British Journal of Cancer 2006; 95(8): 979–985.

Morris E, Haward RA, Gilthorpe MS, Craigs C, Forman D. The impact of the Calman–Hine report on the processes and outcomes of care for Yorkshire's breast cancer patients. Annals of Oncology 2008; 19(2): 284–291.

Murray PV, O'Brien MER, Sayer R, Cooke N, Knowles G et al. The pathway study: results of a pilot feasibility study in patients suspected of having lung carcinoma investigated in a conventional chest clinic setting compared to a centralised two-stop pathway. Lung Cancer 2003; 42(3): 283–290.

Patkar V, Acosta D, Davidson T, Jones A, Fox J et al. Using computerised decision support to improve compliance of cancer multidisciplinary meetings with evidence-based guidance. British Medical Journal Open 2012; 2(3).

Ruhstaller T, Roe H, Thürlimann B, Nicoll JJ. The multidisciplinary meeting: an indispensable aid to communication between different specialities. European Journal of Cancer 2006; 42(15): 2459–2462.

Sainsbury R, Haward B, Rider L, Johnston C, Round C. Influence of clinician workload and patterns of treatment on survival from breast cancer. Lancet 1995; 345(8960): 1265–1270.

Simcock R, Heaford A. Costs of multidisciplinary teams in cancer are small in relation to benefits. British Medical Journal 2012; 344: e3700.

Tattersall MHN. Multidisciplinary team meetings: where is the value? Lancet Oncology 2006; 7(11): 886–888.

Twelves CJ, Thomson CS, Young J, Gould A. Entry into clinical trials in breast cancer: the importance of specialist teams. Scottish Breast Cancer Focus Group and Scottish Cancer Therapy Network. European Journal of Cancer 1998; 34(7): 1004–1007.

References

1. Department of Health. A Policy Framework for Commissioning Cancer Services: A Report by the Expert Advisory Group on Cancer to the Chief Medical Officers of England and Wales. London: Department of Heath, 1995.
2. Haward RA. The Calman–Hine report: a personal retrospective on the UK's first comprehensive policy on cancer services. Lancet Oncology 2006; 7(4): 336–346.
3. Tripathy D. Multidisciplinary care for breast cancer: barriers and solutions. Breast Journal 2003; 9(1): 60–63.
4. Fleissig A, Jenkins V, Catt S, Fallowfield L. Multidisciplinary teams in cancer care: are they effective in the UK? Lancet Oncology 2006; 7(11): 935–943.

5. Zorbas H, Barraclough B, Rainbird K, Luxford K, Redman S. Multidisciplinary care for women with early breast cancer in the Australian context: what does it mean? Medical Journal of Australia 2003; 179(10): 528–531.

6. Hong NJL, Wright FC, Gagliardi AR, Paszat LF. Examining the potential relationship between multidisciplinary cancer care and patient survival: an international literature review. Journal of Surgical Oncology 2010; 102(2): 125–134.

7. Gabel M, Hilton NE, Nathanson SD. Multidisciplinary breast cancer clinics. Do they work? Cancer 1997; 79(12): 2380–2384.

8. Frost MH, Arvizu RD, Jayakumar S, Schoonover A, Novotny P et al. A multidisciplinary healthcare delivery model for women with breast cancer: patient satisfaction and physical and psychosocial adjustment. Oncology Nursing Forum 1999; 26(10): 1673–1680.

9. Kanbour-Shakir A, Harris KM, Johnson RR, Kanbour AI. Breast care consultation center: role of the pathologist in a multidisciplinary center. Diagnostic Cytopathology 1997; 17(3): 191–196.

10. Kovner F, Spigel S, Rider I, Otremsky I, Ron I et al. Radiation therapy of metastatic spinal cord compression. Multidisciplinary team diagnosis and treatment. Journal of Neurooncology 1999; 42(1): 85–92.

11. Chang JH, Vines E, Bertsch H, Fraker DL, Czerniecki BJ et al. The impact of a multidisciplinary breast cancer center on recommendations for patient management: the University of Pennsylvania experience. Cancer 2001; 91(7): 1231–1237.

12. Griffith C, Turner J. United Kingdom National Health Service, Cancer Services Collaborative 'Improvement Partnership,' Redesign of Cancer Services: A National Approach. Eur Journal of Surgical Oncology 2004; 30(Suppl. 1): 1–86.

13. Anderson BO, Carlson RW, Kaufman CS, Kiel KD. Ensuring optimal interdisciplinary breast care in the United States. Breast Journal 2009; 15(6): 569–570.

14. Van Belle S. How to implement the multidisciplinary approach in prostate cancer management: the Belgian model. BJU International 2008 Mar.; 101 Suppl 2: 2–4.

15. Lehmann K, Guller U, Bugnon S, Zuber M. Interdisciplinary tumour boards in Switzerland: quo vadis? Swiss Med Wkly 2008; 138(9–10): 123–127.

16. Delaney RJ, Sayers CD, Walker MA, Mead GM, Theaker JM. The continued value of central histopathological review of testicular tumours. Histopathology 2005; 47(2): 166–169.

17. Khalifa MA, Dodge J, Covens A, Osborne R, Ackerman I. Slide review in gynecologic oncology ensures completeness of reporting and diagnostic accuracy. Gynecologic Oncology 2003; 90(2): 425–430.

18. Ruhstaller T, Roe H, Thürlimann B, Nicoll JJ. The multidisciplinary meeting: an indispensable aid to communication between different specialities. European Journal of Cancer 2006; 42(15): 2459–2462.

19. Rougier P, Neoptolemos JP. The need for a multidisciplinary approach in the treatment of advanced colorectal cancer: a critical review from a medical oncologist and surgeon. European Journal of Surgical Oncology 1997; 23(5): 385–396.

20. Carter S, Garside P, Black A. Multidisciplinary team working, clinical networks, and chambers; opportunities to work differently in the NHS. Quality and Safety in Health Care 2003; 12(Suppl. 1): i25–28.

21. Kurtz J-E, Heitz D, Serra S, Brigand C, Juif V et al. Adjuvant chemotherapy in elderly patients with colorectal cancer. A retrospective analysis of the implementation of tumor board recommendations in a single institution. Critical Reviews in Oncology/Hematology 2010; 74(3): 211–217.

22. Nicholls S, Cullen R, O'Neill S, Halligan A. Clinical governance: its origins and its foundations. Clinical Performance and Quality Healthcare 2000; 8(3): 172–178.

23. National Cancer Action Team (NACT). The Characteristics of an Effective Multidisciplinary Team (MDT). London: NHS, 2010.

24. Action Team (NACT). The Characteristics of an Effective Multidisciplinary Team (MDT). February 2010: NHS. Available from: <http://www.ncin.org.uk/cancer_type_and_topic_specific_work/multidisciplinary_teams/mdt_development>, accessed 18 July 2015.

25. Tattersall MHN. Multidisciplinary team meetings: where is the value? Lancet Oncology 2006; 7(11): 886–888.

26. Magee LR, Laroche CM, Gilligan D. Clinical trials in lung cancer: evidence that a programmed investigation unit and a multidisciplinary clinic may improve recruitment. Clinical Oncology 2001; 13(4): 310–311.

27. Twelves CJ, Thomson CS, Young J, Gould A. Entry into clinical trials in breast cancer: the importance of specialist teams. Scottish Breast Cancer Focus Group and Scottish Cancer Therapy Network. European Journal of Cancer 1998; 34(7): 1004–1007.

28. Kee F, Owen T, Leathem R. Decision making in a multidisciplinary cancer team: does team discussion result in better quality decisions? Medical Decision Making 2004; 24(6): 602–613.

29. Bradley PJ, Zutshi B, Nutting CM. An audit of clinical resources available for the care of head and neck cancer patients in England. Clinical Oncology 2005; 17(8): 604–609.

30. Kelly MJ, Lloyd TDR, Marshall D, Garcea G, Sutton CD et al. A snapshot of MDT working and patient mapping in the UK colorectal cancer centres in 2002. Colorectal Disease 2003; 5(6): 577–581.

31. Whelan JM, Griffith CDM, Archer T. Breast cancer multi-disciplinary teams in England: much achieved but still more to be done. Breast 2006; 15(1): 119–122.

32. Douek M, Taylor I. Good practice and quality assurance in surgical oncology. Lancet Oncology 2003; 4(10): 626–630.

33. Simcock R, Heaford A. Costs of multidisciplinary teams in cancer are small in relation to benefits. British Medical Journal 2012; 344: e3700.

34. Fennell ML, Das IP, Clauser S, Petrelli N, Salner A. The organization of multidisciplinary care teams: modeling internal and external influences on cancer care quality. Journal of the National Cancer Institute Monographs 2010; 2010(40): 72–80.

35. Haward R, Amir Z, Borrill C, Dawson J, Scully J et al. Breast cancer teams: the impact of constitution, new cancer workload, and methods of operation on their effectiveness. British Journal of Cancer 2003; 89(1): 15–22.

36. Madge S, Khair K. Multidisciplinary teams in the United Kingdom: problems and solutions. Journal of Pediatric Nursing 2000; 15(2): 131–134.

37. Lamb B, Payne H, Vincent C, Sevdalis N, Green JSA. The role of oncologists in multidisciplinary cancer teams in the UK: an untapped resource for team leadership? Journal of Evaluation in Clinical Practice 2011; 17(6): 1200–1206.

38. Barr O. Interdisciplinary teamwork: consideration of the challenges. British Journal of Nursing 1997; 6(17): 1005–1010.

39. Lamb BW, Sevdalis N, Vincent C, Green JSA. Development and evaluation of a checklist to support decision making in cancer multidisciplinary team meetings: MDT-QuIC. Annals of Surgical Oncology 2012; 19(6): 1759–1765.

40. Houssami N, Sainsbury R. Breast cancer: multidisciplinary care and clinical outcomes. European Journal of Cancer 2006; 42(15): 2480–2491.

41. Coory M, Gkolia P, Yang IA, Bowman RV, Fong KM. Systematic review of multidisciplinary teams in the management of lung cancer. Lung Cancer 2008; 60(1): 14–21.

42. Junor EJ, Hole DJ, Gillis CR. Management of ovarian cancer: referral to a multidisciplinary team matters. British Journal of Cancer 1994; 70(2): 363–370.

43. Sainsbury R, Haward B, Rider L, Johnston C, Round C. Influence of clinician workload and patterns of treatment on survival from breast cancer. Lancet 1995; 345(8960): 1265–1270.

44. Gillis CR, Hole DJ. Survival outcome of care by specialist surgeons in breast cancer: a study of 3786 patients in the west of Scotland. British Medical Journal 1996; 312(7024): 145–148.

45. Murray PV, O'Brien MER, Sayer R, Cooke N, Knowles G et al. The pathway study: results of a pilot feasibility study in patients suspected of having lung carcinoma investigated in a conventional chest clinic setting compared to a centralised two-stop pathway. Lung Cancer 2003; 42(3): 283–290.

46. Stefoski Mikeljevic J, Haward RA, Johnston C, Sainsbury R, Forman D. Surgeon workload and survival from breast cancer. British Journal of Cancer 2003; 89(3): 487–491.

47. Birchall M, Bailey D, King P, South West Cancer Intelligence Service Head and Neck Tumour Panel. Effect of process standards on survival of patients with head and neck cancer in the south and west of England. British Journal of Cancer 2004; 91(8): 1477–1481.

48. Wong S, Rosenthal MA, deBoer R, Green MD, Fox RM. Five years managing metastatic non-small cell lung cancer: experience at a teaching hospital. Internal Medicine Journal 2004; 34(8): 458–463.

49. Martin-Ucar AE, Waller DA, Atkins JL, Swinson D, O'Byrne KJ et al. The beneficial effects of specialist thoracic surgery on the resection rate for non-small-cell lung cancer. Lung Cancer 2004; 46(2): 227–232.

50. Forrest LM, McMillan DC, McArdle CS, Dunlop DJ. An evaluation of the impact of a multidisciplinary team, in a single centre, on treatment and survival in patients with inoperable non-small-cell lung cancer. British Journal of Cancer 2005; 93(9): 977–978.

51. Dillman RO, Chico SD. Cancer patient survival improvement is correlated with the opening of a community cancer center: comparisons with intramural and extramural benchmarks. Journal of Oncology Practice 2005; 1(3): 84–92.

52. Stephens MR, Lewis WG, Brewster AE, Lord I, Blackshaw GRJC et al. Multidisciplinary team management is associated with improved outcomes after surgery for esophageal cancer. Diseases of the Esophagus 2006; 19(3): 164–171.

53. Morris E, Haward RA, Gilthorpe MS, Craigs C, Forman D. The impact of the Calman–Hine report on the processes and outcomes of care for Yorkshire's breast cancer patients. Annals of Oncology 2008; 19(2): 284–291.

54. Morris E, Haward RA, Gilthorpe MS, Craigs C, Forman D. The impact of the Calman–Hine report on the processes and outcomes of care for Yorkshire's colorectal cancer patients. British Journal of Cancer 2006; 95(8): 979–985.

55. Downing A, Mikeljevic JS, Haward B, Forman D. Variation in the treatment of cervical cancer patients and the effect of consultant workload on survival: a population-based study. European Journal of Cancer 2007; 43(2): 363–370.

56. MacDermid E, Hooton G, MacDonald M, McKay G, Grose D et al. Improving patient survival with the colorectal cancer multi-disciplinary team. Colorectal Disease 2009; 11(3): 291–295.

57. Lordan JT, Karanjia ND, Quiney N, Fawcett WJ, Worthington TR. A 10-year study of outcome following hepatic resection for colorectal liver metastases: the effect of evaluation in a multidisciplinary team setting. European Journal of Surgical Oncology 2009; 35(3): 302–306.

58. Shylasree TS, Howells REJ, Lim K, Jones PW, Fiander A et al. Survival in ovarian cancer in Wales: prior to introduction of all Wales guidelines. International Journal of Gynecological Cancer 2006; 16(5): 1770–1776.

59. Newman EA, Guest AB, Helvie MA, Roubidoux MA, Chang AE et al. Changes in surgical management resulting from case review at a breast cancer multidisciplinary tumor board. Cancer 2006; 107(10): 2346–2351.

60. Kesson EM, Allardice GM, George WD, Burns HJG, Morrison DS. Effects of multidisciplinary team working on breast cancer survival: retrospective, comparative, interventional cohort study of 13 722 women. British Medical Journal 2012; 344:e2718.

61. Boxer MM, Vinod SK, Shafiq J, Duggan KJ. Do multidisciplinary team meetings make a difference in the management of lung cancer? Cancer 2011; 117(22): 5112–5120.

62. Pawlik TM, Laheru D, Hruban RH, Coleman J, Wolfgang CL et al. Evaluating the impact of a single-day multidisciplinary clinic on the management of pancreatic cancer. Annals of Surgical Oncology 2008; 15(8): 2081–2088.

63. Levine RA, Chawla B, Bergeron S, Wasvary H. Multidisciplinary management of colorectal cancer enhances access to multimodal therapy

and compliance with National Comprehensive Cancer Network (NCCN) guidelines. International Journal of Colorectal Disease 2012; 27(11): 1531–1538.

64. Burton S, Brown G, Daniels IR, Norman AR, Mason B et al. MRI directed multidisciplinary team preoperative treatment strategy: the way to eliminate positive circumferential margins? British Journal of Cancer 2006; 94(3): 351–357.

65. Jones RP, Vauthey J-N, Adam R, Rees M, Berry D et al. Effect of specialist decision-making on treatment strategies for colorectal liver metastases. British Journal of Surgery 2012; 99(9): 1263–1269.

66. Aizer AA, Paly JJ, Zietman AL, Nguyen PL, Beard CJ et al. Multidisciplinary care and pursuit of active surveillance in low-risk prostate cancer. Journal of Clinical Oncology 2012; 30(25): 3071–3076.

67. Acher PL, Young AJ, Etherington-Foy R, McCahy PJ, Deane AM. Improving outcomes in urological cancers: the impact of 'multidisciplinary team meetings'. International Journal of Surgery 2005; 3(2): 121–123.

68. Sooriakumaran P, Dick JA, Thompson AC, Morley R. The central urology multidisciplinary team—is it time to change the referral criteria? An audit of practice in a district general hospital in London. Annals of the Royal College of Surgeons of England 2009; 91(8): 700–702.

69. Cohen P, Tan AL, Penman A. The multidisciplinary tumor conference in gynecologic oncology—does it alter management? International Journal of Gynecological Cancer 2009; 19(9): 1470–1472.

70. Croke JM, El-Sayed S. Multidisciplinary management of cancer patients: chasing a shadow or real value? An overview of the literature. Current Oncology 2012; 19(4): e232–e238.

71. Santoso JT, Schwertner B, Coleman RL, Hannigan EV. Tumor board in gynecologic oncology. International Journal of Gynecological Cancer 2004; 14(2): 206–209.

72. Catt S, Fallowfield L, Jenkins V, Langridge C, Cox A. The informational roles and psychological health of members of 10 oncology multidisciplinary teams in the UK. British Journal of Cancer 2005; 93(10): 1092–1097.

73. McNair AGK, Choh CTP, Metcalfe C, Littlejohns D, Barham CP et al. Maximising recruitment into randomised controlled trials: the role of multidisciplinary cancer teams. European Journal of Cancer 2008; 44(17): 2623–2626.

74. Kuroki L, Stuckey A, Hirway P, Raker CA, Bandera CA et al. Addressing clinical trials: can the multidisciplinary Tumor Board improve participation? A study from an academic women's cancer program. Gynecologic Oncology 2010; 116(3): 295–300.

75. Blazeby JM, Wilson L, Metcalfe C, Nicklin J, English R et al. Analysis of clinical decision-making in multi-disciplinary cancer teams. Annals of Oncology 2006; 17(3): 457–460.

76. Leo F, Venissac N, Poudenx M, Otto J, Mouroux J et al. Multidisciplinary management of lung cancer: how to test its efficacy? Journal of Thoracic Oncology 2007; 2(1): 69–72.

77. Wood JJ, Metcalfe C, Paes A, Sylvester P, Durdey P et al. An evaluation of treatment decisions at a colorectal cancer multi-disciplinary team. Colorectal Disease 2008; 10(8): 769–772.

78. Extermann M. Measuring comorbidity in older cancer patients. European Journal of Cancer 2000; 36(4): 453–471.

79. Patkar V, Acosta D, Davidson T, Jones A, Fox J et al. Using computerised decision support to improve compliance of cancer multidisciplinary meetings with evidence-based guidance. British Medical Journal Open 2012; 2(3).

80. Gatliffe TA, Coleman RL. Tumor board: more than treatment planning: a 1-year prospective survey. Journal of Cancer Education 2008; 23(4): 235–237.

CHAPTER 23

Principles of clinical pharmacology
Introduction to pharmacokinetics and pharmacodynamics

Michael Ong and Udai Banerji

Introduction to principles of clinical pharmacy

Pharmacology is the branch of medicine that studies the uses, effects, and modes of action of drugs. In oncology, principles of pharmacology have been critical in addressing the balance between therapeutic and toxic drug properties—a challenging matter considering that many anticancer drugs are dosed at or near their maximum tolerated dose (MTD) [1, 2]. Two major domains of pharmacology are pharmacokinetics—'what the human body does to a drug', and pharmacodynamics—'what the drug does to the body'. In this chapter, we give an overview of how studies of pharmacokinetics and pharmacodynamics have influenced and continue to guide the development of anticancer drugs in use today.

Pharmacokinetic analyses describe drug absorption, distribution, metabolism, and excretion (ADME) in the body. Pharmacokinetic studies aim to define a dose-response relationship for both therapeutic and toxic drug effects, and describe variation in drug exposure between individuals. A key pharmacokinetic concept is that drug response in individuals is related to drug concentration at the target site. Since intratumoural drug concentrations cannot be practically obtained in clinical practice [3], pharmacokinetic studies typically describe plasma drug concentrations over time as a surrogate measure of tumour exposure. Mathematical models can thereafter be formulated to describe and predict pharmacokinetic processes that take place following administration.

Drug pharmacokinetics are affected by both physicochemical drug characteristics [4] (cell membrane permeability, biotransformation, and protein binding) and physiological parameters [5] (body composition, gastrointestinal motility, organ blood perfusion, and urine flow). The array of influencing factors makes it unsurprising that most anticancer therapies carry substantial pharmacokinetic variability as high as tenfold between individuals [6]. This variability may be very significant since the majority of anticancer agents have narrow therapeutic indices—small differences between the minimum effective dose and the minimum toxic dose—potentially leading to suboptimal drug dosing in some patients or, conversely, toxic dosing in others [7].

Understanding of pharmacokinetics has a key influence on attempts to reduce the interpatient variability of drug exposure. Examples of important influences of pharmacokinetic studies on oncological practice include defining drug dosing by adjusting for patient body surface area [8–12] (e.g., paclitaxel) as drug clearance can increase as a function of body size; routine drainage of third-space fluids prior to administration of methotrexate to prevent drug-fluid distribution and increased late toxicity [13]; alkalinization of urine to promote renal excretion of high-dose methotrexate [14]; carboplatin dose calculation through estimation of renal function [15]; and understanding and reduction of drug–drug interactions as a result of cytochrome P450 activity [16] (see section on 'Absorption').

Pharmacodynamic analyses describe drug effects on the body and tumour, with key pharmacodynamic effects observed for anticancer drugs being host toxicity and tumour response. Host toxicity can be characterized using standardized criteria commonly utilized in clinical trials [17]. The severity of toxicity is important in defining the maximally tolerated dose of a drug. A common dose-limiting toxicity of conventional chemotherapy and, in particular, DNA-damaging and tubulin-binding agents has been myelosuppression [18]. It is possible to model myelosuppression in relation to pharmacokinetic parameters, clinical parameters, or pharmacodynamics biomarkers such as DNA adduct formation [19, 20].

However, pharmacodynamic assessments have evolved as advances in cancer biology have spurred the development of molecularly targeted drugs against the hallmark traits of cancer such as cell signalling and angiogenesis [21]. This paradigm shift towards targeted treatment has redefined the ways in which new anticancer drugs are developed and evaluated [22]. Sophisticated pharmacodynamic biomarkers in both normal and tumour tissues can be used to confirm an appropriate level and duration of target and pathway modulation [1]. Therefore, demonstration that a drug can modulate the biological target of interest and thereby invoke functional consequences represents an essential goal of pharmacodynamic assessments in modern clinical trials.

Pharmacodynamic biomarkers can assess drug effect at the target site (e.g., tumour) or at a surrogate site (e.g., platelet-rich plasma), and are broadly divided into 'proof-of-mechanism' biomarkers that demonstrate drug modulation of the intended target in the human

Table 23.1 Examples of types of biomarkers used to define doses and schedules of targeted agents

Type of PD Biomarker	Target	Biomarker	Drug
Proof-of-mechanism	ABL	p-CRKL	Imatinib
	m-TOR	p-S6	Everolimus
	HDAC	Acetylated histone	Vorinostat
Proof-of-concept	EGFR	Ki67	Gefitinib
	BRAF	FDG-PET	Vemurafenib
	VEGF	DCE-MRI	Bevacizumab

body; and 'proof of principle' biomarkers which demonstrate functional consequences of inhibiting a target (see Table 23.1). For example, the degree of p-ERK inhibition caused by the BRAF inhibitor, vemurafenib, is linked to its efficacy [23]. An increasingly important concept is that a biologically effective dose range exists that appropriately modulates the target and may be different than the maximally tolerated dose, as is the case for bevacizumab [24, 25].

Principles of pharmacokinetics and pharmacodynamics play crucial roles in the way drugs are developed and used as monotherapy or combination therapy. Integrating pharmacokinetic and pharmacodynamic information is challenging, but very informative, and aids in optimizing the dose and schedule of targeted anticancer agents. Understanding pharmacologic principles, combined with specific information regarding an individual drug and patient, underlies the individualized optimal use of anticancer drugs.

Pharmacokinetic parameters

Describing the time-course of a drug in an individual begins with serial sampling of plasma drug concentrations following drug administration. These concentrations are then serially plotted against time in a concentration-time profile, as shown in Figure 23.1. Pharmacokinetic parameters that can be directly derived from this profile include:

◆ **Cmax**: the peak drug concentration in plasma observed

◆ **Tmax**: the time to peak drug concentration

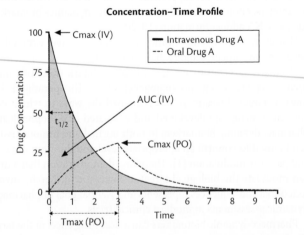

Concentration–Time Profile

Fig. 23.1 Examples of a pharmacokinetic profile of intravenous and oral drugs following linear pharmacokinetics.
IV, intravenous; PO, oral.

◆ **Half-life (t$_{1/2}$)**: the time it takes for half of the drug to be eliminated from the body;

◆ **Area under the curve (AUC)**: the mathematically integrated area under the concentration-time curve; expresses in a single value the person's overall exposure to drug.

These parameters are useful to describe the expected duration and extent of drug exposure, intrapatient and interpatient variation, and changes in drug exposure as a result of factors such as concomitant drug interactions or liver dysfunction. Half-life is useful to understand the rate of elimination or accumulation of a drug. A drug takes four to five half-lives after dosing to be 93–97% eliminated from the body. Conversely, if a drug is dosed regularly at intervals shorter than the half-life, concentrations will reach higher levels until a steady state is achieved, in which drug entry is equally balanced by drug elimination. Since drugs with a very long half-life (e.g., trastuzumab half-life is 6–16 days) may require a long time to reach steady state, a loading dose may be considered to achieve therapeutic levels faster [26]. Cmax and AUC are useful to describe drug exposure and may be associated with pharmacodynamic effects. For example, Cmax of pegylated liposomal doxorubicin is associated with stomatitis grade and leukocyte nadir [27]; a higher AUC of drugs such as cisplatin, docetaxel, and vinorelbine is associated with a higher response rate of solid tumours [7] and greater haematological toxicity [28, 29].

Absorption

Drug absorption is a key factor that affects the concentration time-course of a drug in the body. Traditional cytotoxic chemotherapies have been largely administered as intravenous agents, which achieve maximum plasma concentrations (Cmax) nearly instantaneously since absorption across membranes is not required. In contrast, many newer molecularly targeted anticancer agents are now developed in oral formulation [30]. Orally administered drugs undergo absorption through a dynamic transfer process from the gastrointestinal lumen, across the intestinal epithelium, and into portal blood. Cmax of orally administered drugs are not instantaneously achieved, may be lower than an equivalent intravenous dosage, and may take hours to peak (Figure 23.1).

A relevant concept for orally (and other non-intravenously) administered agents is bioavailability (F)—the fraction of the administered drug reaching the systemic circulation as intact drug compared with intravenous dosing:

$$\text{Bioavailability (\%)} = \frac{\text{AUC}_{\text{non-intravenous}}}{\text{AUC}_{\text{intravenous}}} \times 100$$

Absolute bioavailability compares exposure to drug in oral formulation compared to the same drug in intravenous formulation; relative bioavailability compares two products to each other, and is commonly used to show bioequivalence for a generic formulation to the original formulation. Typical bioavailability of commonly administered oral anticancer agents is depicted in Table 23.2.

Drug bioavailability may be affected by:

◆ **Drug physicochemical properties**: lower molecular weight, increased solubility, increased lipophilicity, and non-ionization favour good oral bioavailability [4]. These characteristics promote passive uptake of drug from the gastrointestinal lumen, a rate-limiting step for absorption of most oral drugs [31].

- **'First-pass metabolism' by intestinal/hepatic enzymes**: oral, but not intravenous, drugs are subject to 'first-pass metabolism', in which metabolizing enzymes within enterocytes inactivate drug prior to the drug reaching the systemic circulation (e.g., 5-fluorouracil). Intestinal metabolism occurs mainly via phase I metabolic reactions (described in the 'Metabolism' section) performed by cytochrome P450 (CYP) 3A monooxygenases within enterocytes. Interestingly, grapefruit juice contains furanocoumarins that directly downregulate and inhibit intestinal CYP3A4, leading to less CYP3A4-mediated first-pass metabolism and potentially greater drug exposure and effect of oral drugs [32, 33].

- **Patient factors, including food-effects**: interpatient variation in the amount of gut surface area, gut transit time, and gastric/intestinal pH can all affect absorption of orally administered agents. Concurrent ingestion of food also affects drug bioavailability by affecting drug solubility and gastrointestinal physiology. For example, lapatinib bioavailability is increased fourfold with a high-fat meal and erlotinib 1.6-fold [34].

- **Active drug efflux into bowel lumen**: efflux transporters situated on the apical/luminal membrane of the intestine can limit oral bioavailability of drugs (e.g., paclitaxel [35]) by pumping drug out into the bowel lumen. Key intestinal efflux transporters include P-glycoprotein (P-gp; *ABCB1*), members of the multidrug resistance-associated protein (MRP; *ABCC*) family, and the breast cancer resistance protein (BRCP; *ABCG*).

Because the need for drug absorption alters ADME significantly, orally administered agents have characteristically greater pharmacokinetic variability than intravenous agents; this must be carefully considered with agents such as etoposide which can be administered by either route [36, 37]. A non-intravenous route should be avoided if bioavailability is poor or variable, particularly for drugs with narrow therapeutic indices [38].

Distribution

Drug distribution into extravascular tissues can occur once drug is delivered intravenously or absorbed via the gut into the intravascular space. The apparent extent of distribution of drug out into the extravascular tissues and away from the intravascular space (plasma) can be described by the volume of distribution (Vd):

$$\text{Vd} = \text{Amount of drug in the body/concentration} \\ \text{of drug in plasma at equilibrium}$$

Vd theoretically relates the measured drug concentration in plasma to what volume would be required if the body was a uniform space in which drug was distributed. In general, larger Vd indicates greater diffusibility of the drug, but the numerical value of Vd does not relate to a specific physiological volume. Vd can be no less than that of the plasma volume (approximately 3 litres (L)/70 kilogram (kg) man), but can be far greater than that of the total body water volume (42 L/70 kg man). However, larger Vd does not necessarily equate to a higher degree of drug penetration into tumour

tissue; mitoxantrone, for example, has a high Vd because it is highly sequestered by DNA binding and entrapment in acid vesicles of normal cells, and has limited tumour tissue penetration [39]. Table 23.2 lists Vd for commonly administered anticancer agents.

Vd is affected by the following factors:

- **Drug physicochemical properties**: highly lipid-soluble, non-polar compounds are generally able to penetrate cell membranes and fatty tissues more easily with a greater drug distribution than more polar, water-soluble compounds [4]. Penetration beyond the blood–brain barrier (BBB) into the central nervous system (CNS) is largely determined by lipid solubility, and secondarily by molecular size [40]. Formulation can drastically affect drug distribution; pegylated liposomal doxorubicin has 600-fold lower Vd due to stable retention of drug encapsulated by liposomes in circulation [27].

- **Degree of protein binding**: generally, unbound (free) drug is considered to be 'active' and available to bind to receptors, undergo metabolism, and be eliminated from the body. Protein binding predominantly occurs with albumin and/or alpha1-acid glycoprotein. Theoretically, highly protein-bound drugs are susceptible to large increases in free drug fraction by drug-displacement interactions such as salicylates displacing protein-bound methotrexate [41].

- **Active drug efflux and 'pharmacokinetic sanctuaries'**: drug-efflux transporters can affect distribution by limiting transcellular drug entry at the BBB, blood–testis, and blood–ovarian interfaces. At the BBB, drug entry into the brain is limited by endothelial cell tight junctions blocking paracellular uptake, and luminal efflux transporters including P-gp that actively pump drug away from the CNS [42]. The BBB may be impaired in brain metastases, leading to better penetration of drugs traditionally thought to have poor CNS penetration such as paclitaxel and trastuzumab [43, 44]. Poor or suboptimal drug penetration into pharmacokinetic sanctuaries may require circumvention by alternative treatment modalities: intrathecal methotrexate or external beam radiotherapy in children's acute lymphoblastic leukaemia can prevent CNS relapse [45]; delayed orchiectomy is indicated for advanced germ-cell cancer initially treated with chemotherapy because of a relatively high incidence of residual germ-cell cancer or teratoma in the unresected testis [46, 47].

- **Third-space fluid distribution**: third-space fluid such as pleural effusions can influence drug kinetics, especially with drug properties such as methotrexate (MTX) where the Vd is relatively small (approximately 40 L) and protein binding is low (~50%) [13]; thus, drainage of effusions is recommended prior to administration because MTX may accumulate and exit slowly from third-space fluids, leading to prolonged half-life, drug exposure, and toxicity [48].

Metabolism

Drug metabolism is a critical step in the disposition of most drugs, and primarily occurs in the liver. However, enzymes involved in metabolism are also present in many tissues including the intestine and tumour. Drugs typically undergo enzymatic biotransformation by drug metabolizing enzymes into more water-soluble states to increase the rate of excretion through urine and bile. Usually these reactions transform drugs into inactive metabolites; in some cases parent drugs, such as capecitabine, are inactive (pro-drug) and

Table 23.2 Pharmacokinetic properties of commonly administered anticancer agents.

Class	Drug	Absorption			Distribution				Metabolism			Excretion		
		Admin route	Oral bioavailability	Food effect	Dose adjust	Approx. Vd (L)*	Protein bound**	Crosses CNS	Metabolic reaction	Metabolism	Active Metabolite	Approx. $t_{1/2}$ (hr)**	Excretion route	Dose adjust
Alkylating Agents	Carmustine	IV	-	-	BSA	250	80%	15-70%	-	L	Yes	0.33	U	R
	Cyclophosphamide	IV/PO	90%	No	BSA	40	No	Poor	CYP	L	Yes+	6.5	U	R, H
	Dacarbazine	IV	-	-	BSA	40	20%	Poor	CYP	L	Yes+	5	U	R
	Ifosfamide	IV	-	-	BSA	50	20%	Poor	CYP	L	Yes+	7	U	-
	Lomustine	PO	100%	-	BSA	-	50%	15-30%	CYP	L	Yes	72	U	R
	Procarbazine	PO	100%	-	BSA	-	-	Yes	CYP	L	Yes+	1	U	R, H
	Temozolomide	IV/PO	100%	↓9%	BSA	30	15%	9-29%	Hydrolysis	-	Yes	2	U	-
Antitumour Antibiotics	Bleomycin	IV/SC/IM	-	-	BSA	20	5%	No	Hydrolase	L,K	-	3	U	R
	Doxorubicin	IV	-	-	BSA	1800	75%	No	Reduction	L	Yes	36	F	H
	Lipo-Doxorubicin	IV	-	-	BSA	3	-	No	Reduction	L	Yes	74	F	H
	Epirubicin	IV	-	-	BSA	1800	80%	No	CYP	L	Yes	35	F	H
	Mitoxantrone	IV	-	-	BSA	1000	80%	No	CYP	L	-	75	F	H
Anti-metabolites	5-fluorouracil	IV	40-70%	-	BSA	15	10%	Yes	DPD	T	Yes+	0.25	U	H
	Capecitabine	PO	100%	↓	BSA	-	60%	-	CES, CDA, TP, DPD	L,T	Yes+	0.75	U	R, H
	Gemcitabine***	IV	-	-	BSA	90-600	5%	No	DCK; CDA	L,P,T	Yes+	1 to 7	U	-
	Methotrexate	IV/IM/PO	Good <25mg/m²	↓	BSA	40	50%	5-10%	FPGS	L	Yes+	10	U	R, H
	Mitomycin-C	IV	-	-	BSA	40	-	No	CYP, DTD	L,T	-	0.83	F	R
	Pemetrexed	IV	-	-	BSA	15	80%	-	FPGS	L	Yes+	20	U	R
Platinums	Carboplatin	IV	-	-	AUC	15	0%	Yes	Aquation	P,T	Yes+	144	F	R
	Cisplatin	IV	-	-	BSA	70	95%	No	Aquation	P,T	Yes+	0.5	U	R
	Oxaliplatin	IV	-	-	BSA	600	98%	-	Aquation	P,T	Yes+	240	U	R
Taxanes	Abraxane	IV	-	-	BSA	1100	95%	-	CYP	L	Yes	27	F	-
	Docetaxel	IV	-	-	BSA	110	95%	Poor	CYP	L	No	11	F	H
	Paclitaxel	IV	-	-	BSA	120	90%	No	CYP	L	No	20	F	H

Class	Drug	IV/PO	Bioavail.	Food effect	Dosing	Vd (L)	Protein binding	Extensive metabolism	Enzyme	Excretion	Active metabolite	t½ (h)	Excretion route	Clearance organ
Topoisomerase inhibitors	Etoposide	IV/PO	50%	No	BSA	20	95%	Poor	GLU	L	Yes	7	U	R, H
	Irinotecan	IV	-	-	BSA	300	45%	-	CES	L,PT	Yes+	9	F	H
	Topotecan	IV	-	-	BSA	130	25%	30%	Hydrolysis	P	Yes	3	U	R
Vinca alkaloids	Vinblastine	IV	-	-	BSA	1900	99%	Poor	CYP	L	Yes	25	F	H
	Vincristine	IV	-	-	BSA	200	75%	Poor	CYP	L	Yes	85	F	H
	Vinorelbine	IV/PO?	-	-	BSA	2200	80%	Yes	CYP	L	Yes	35	F	H
Targeted antibodies	Bevacizumab	IV	-	-	Weight	3	-	-	-	-	-	480	-	-
	Cetuximab	IV	-	-	Weight	3	-	-	-	L,T	No	150	-	-
	Panitumumab	IV	-	-	Weight	3	-	-	-	L,T	No	156	-	-
	Trastuzumab	IV	-	-	Weight	3	-	-	-	L	No	384	-	-
Hormone therapies	Anastrazole	PO	85%	→	Fixed	-	40%	-	Multiple	L	No	50	F	-
	Exemestane	PO	42%	↑	Fixed	-	90%	-	CYP, Reduction	L	No	24	F	H
	Fulvestrant	IM	-	-	Fixed	280	99%	-	CYP	L	Yes	-	F	-
	Letrozole	PO	100%	→	Fixed	130	5%	-	GLU	L	No	-	U	-
	Tamoxifen	PO	100%	↑	Fixed	1400	99%	Yes	CYP	L	Yes+	240	F	H
Targeted small molecules	Erlotinib	PO	60%	↑	Fixed	250	95%	Likely	CYP	L	Yes	36	F	H
	Everolimus	PO	30%	→	Fixed	-	75%	Yes	CYP	L	No	30	F	H
	Gefitinib	PO	60%	No	Fixed	1500	90%	-	CYP	L	No	35	F	H
	Imatinib	PO	98%	No	Fixed	300	95%	Poor	CYP	L	Yes	18	F	H
	Lapatinib	PO	Incomplete	↑	Fixed	-	99%	Yes	CYP	L	-	24	F	H
	Sorafenib	PO	45%	→	Fixed	-	99%	-	CYP, GLU	L	Yes	36	F	H
	Sunitinib	PO	100%	No	Fixed	2200	95%	Likely	CYP	L	Yes	50	F	H
	Temsirolimus	IV	-	-	Fixed	175	-	-	Hydrolysis, CYP	L	Yes	17	F	-

*Approximated by calculating Vd in a 70kg man, height 160cm, BSA = 1.73 mg/m²; **parent drug, not applicable to metabolites; ***longer length of infusion of gemcitabine beyond 70 minutes increases Vd and t$_{1/2}$(92).

IV, intravenous; IM, intramuscular; PO, orally; BSA, body surface area (mg/m²); CYP, cytochrome P450; CDA, cytidine deaminase; DPD, dihydropyridimine dehydrogenase; CES, carboxylesterases; FGPS, folylpolyglutamate synthetase; GLU, glucuronidation; DCK, deoxycydicine kinase; R, Renal; H, Hepatic; L, Liver; K, Kidney; U, Urine; F, Feces; T, Tumour; P, Plasma.

require metabolic activation [31]; while occasionally both parent drug and metabolites are active.

Drug metabolism reactions are broadly categorized into phase I reactions performed by cytochrome P450 (CYP) monooxygenases, and phase II reactions responsible for drug conjugation.

Phase I reactions non-synthetically form new or modify existing functional groups on a parent drug to improve water solubility and enhance reactivity for further metabolism or excretion. Phase I oxidation reactions are most commonly performed by CYP enzymes located in the hepatocyte endoplasmic reticulum. Over a hundred CYP enzymes are known, of which CYP3A4 and CYP2D6 have the greatest potential for drug metabolism. CYP3A4 alone accounts for 60% of all hepatic cytochromes, and is involved in the metabolism of many anticancer drugs [49]. Because CYP activity is dependent on concentration, degree of induction, and potentially functional genetic polymorphisms, substantial interpatient variability of CYP drug metabolism has been described [50].

A number of clinically significant drug interactions can occur on the basis of alteration of CYP function, and require careful consideration. For example, tamoxifen is converted into its active metabolites via CYP2D6, but antidepressants, beta-blockers and antipsychotic drugs can potentially inhibit CYP2D6 activity and thus tamoxifen bioactivation [51]. Warfarin is an oral anticoagulant whose more active enantiomer, S-warfarin, is metabolized almost exclusively by CYP2C9. A significant interaction occurs with concurrently administered capecitabine, resulting in exaggerated warfarin anticoagulant activity and the need for careful monitoring.

Non-CYP phase I enzymes may also catalyse drug oxidation, reduction, or hydrolysis and include ketoreductase, aldehyde dehydrogenase, carboxylesterases (CES), dihydropyrimidine dehydrogenase (DPD), and cytosine deaminase (CDA). A well-known, clinically relevant functional variant is DPD deficiency. DPD is the rate-limiting and most important enzyme in catabolism of 5-fluorouracil. Partial (3–5% of patients) or complete (0.1%) DPD deficiency may occur in unselected patients, potentially leading to myelosuppression, diarrhoea, mucositis, and neurotoxicity in those treated with 5-fluorouracil [52].

Phase II reactions predominantly occur in the hepatocyte cytoplasm, and are catalysed by the enzymes uridine diphosphate glucuronosyltransferases (UGT1 and UGT2), sulfotransferases, and glutathione S-transferases. Phase II reactions add large water-soluble polar groups to the parent drug or its oxidized metabolites to make compounds more hydrophilic and generally more inert. The reactions are synthetic in nature, and the polar groups that can be added include glucuronic acid, sulfate, acetate, glycine, glutathione, or methyl groups.

Phase II enzymes can be genetically polymorphic, with functional consequences. A well-known functional polymorphism is described for *UGT1A1*, the phase II metabolic enzyme responsible for glucuronidation of SN-38, the active metabolite of irinotecan. Patients with the *UGT1A1 7/7* genotype (10% in North America) have functional deficiency *UGT1A1*, leading to higher patient exposure to SN-38 and a higher risk of severe neutropenia and diarrhoea [53–55].

Excretion

Drugs and/or their metabolites are mainly eliminated from the body via the biliary tract or the kidneys.

Biliary excretion

Drugs may be secreted by hepatocytes into the bile via efflux transporters such as P-gp, MRPs, and BCRP. Generally, larger (>500 daltons), lipid-soluble, amphipathic, or acid-conjugated metabolites are secreted into the bile, whereas smaller compounds are excreted in the urine. Drugs with hepatic elimination may need dose adjustment in the setting of liver dysfunction as detailed in Table 23.2. Reabsorption of drugs via the enterohepatic circulation can occur, leading to prolonged drug exposure and pharmacological effect. For example, the active metabolite SN-38 undergoes enterohepatic recirculation as characterized by rebound increase in SN-38 levels after discontinuation of irinotecan infusion [56].

Renal excretion

Free, unbound drug may be filtered by the kidney glomerulus, actively secreted into the proximal tubule, or reabsorbed in the distal tubule of the kidney nephron; the net excretion rate by the kidney is the sum of these three processes. For example, methotrexate and pemetrexed are eliminated unchanged in the urine via glomerular filtration and active tubular secretion [57, 58]. Drugs with renal elimination may need dose adjustment in the setting of renal dysfunction as detailed in Table 23.2. Urine pH may alter the excretion of drug; for example, the excretion of methotrexate is improved by co-administration of sodium bicarbonate to alkalinize the urine [14]. Concurrent drugs may also affect renal excretion of drugs. Concurrent administration of ASA, NSAIDs, penicillins, cephalosporins, and probenecid appears to inhibit renal drug transporter functions [59], decreasing renal elimination of methotrexate and resulting in clinical toxicity [60]. Renal elimination of paclitaxel, etoposide, ifosfamide, methotrexate, and bleomycin may also be reduced by concurrent platinum chemotherapy [61].

Clearance (Cl) is a pharmacokinetic parameter that describes the efficiency of irreversible drug elimination from the body. A drug is considered to be eliminated by either metabolism or excretion of the parent drug. For example, a molecule that has undergone glucuronidation is described as having been cleared, even though the molecule itself may have not yet left the body. Clearance occurs mainly via the liver or kidneys, but drug may also be eliminated in expired air, sweat, or saliva.

In pharmacokinetic terms, Cl is expressed as the volume of blood from which a drug can be completely removed per unit of time (e.g., 100 mL/min):

$$Clearance = Dose/AUC \text{ (estimated by } [0.693 \times Vd]/t1/2)$$

Clearance can be especially useful in optimizing dosing of patients because it describes the efficiency of drug elimination from the body. Clinical factors such as age, gender, race, nutrition, and organ function may be predictive of drug clearance; for example, it has been described that patients over the age of 70 have an approximately 30% decrease in clearance related to CYP enzyme activity [62]. Clearance of a parent drug (e.g., temozolamide or dacarbazine) may still yield active metabolites and it is important to consider the further metabolism and elimination of such compounds [63].

Pharmacokinetic models

Animal models are used to test toxicity and efficacy of an anticancer drug before it is administered to humans. Regulatory requirements vary, but often a rodent and non-rodent species is tested. The first-in-human starting dose for evaluation in clinical trials is often calculated by allometric scaling [64]. Extensive pharmacokinetic-pharmacodynamic efficacy modelling is also conducted as a part of drug discovery for targeted agents to define a pharmacologically active dose range in these models. It is possible to relate findings in human trials to these animal models while making go/no-go decisions at the end of phase I studies.

Linear, one-compartment pharmacokinetic models treat the body as a 'well-stirred' single compartment in which drug distributes instantaneously. Drug metabolism/excretion occurs at a rate directly proportional to drug concentration: doubling of drug concentration will be met with doubling of drug metabolism/excretion. Functionally, this is relevant in the case where therapeutic drug concentrations only occupy a small proportion of the available metabolizing or transporting enzyme sites.

Multicompartment pharmacokinetic models account for the time of drug distribution between tissue and plasma by dividing the body up into compartments in which drug can distribute and/or eliminate. The pharmacokinetic behaviour of most drugs is best described using a two-compartment model, in which a central compartment (blood plus the extracellular spaces of well-perfused tissues) and a peripheral compartment (less well-perfused tissues into which the drug permeates more slowly) are defined. Notably in these models, an alpha phase will characterize the rate of distribution away from plasma, while a beta phase (terminal half-life) will characterize the rate of elimination from plasma [65].

Non-linear pharmacokinetics (zero-order kinetics) may occur because drug excretion, metabolism, or protein-binding processes become saturated at typical blood concentrations. In this situation, increases in drug are not met with increasing metabolism or transport. Drug concentrations in blood rise unexpectedly and potentially dangerously with increasing dosage. Paclitaxel has been described as following non-linear pharmacokinetics [66], likely resulting from an interaction with the Cremophor® excipient used to dissolve paclitaxel. Furthermore, doxorubicin given concomitantly with paclitaxel can exhibit non-linear pharmacokinetics as well, possibly as a result of saturation of biliary excretory mechanisms [67]. Drugs may exhibit linear pharmacokinetics at low doses but non-linear pharmacokinetics at high-doses, as is observed for cyclophosphamide [68].

Population pharmacokinetics is the study of the variability in plasma drug concentrations between individuals who receive standard dosage regimens and who represent the target patient population. Population pharmacokinetic models aim to account for observed inter-individual variation by quantification of covariates using specific patient parameters to determine the optimal dose for the individual.

Pharmacokinetic-pharmacodynamic (PK-PD) models can provide a means of exploring important pharmacological and toxicological properties of a drug by describing the time course of the pharmacological effect of a given dose. Three components are required for a PK-PD model: a pharmacokinetic model, characterizing the time-course of a drug and metabolite concentrations in plasma; a pharmacodynamic model, characterizing the relationship between concentration and effect(s); and a link model, which serves to account for the often observed delay of the effect relative to the plasma concentration.

Pharmacodynamic biomarkers

Proof-of-mechanism biomarkers

Biomarkers crucial to demonstrating the mechanism of action of an anticancer agent are considered to be 'proof-of-mechanism' biomarkers. The aims of such assays are to demonstrate that the drug is modulating its intended target in the human body. In the case of tyrosine kinase inhibitors, it could be measurement of activation of the downstream signal transduction pathway; for example, measurement of inhibition of ERK phosphorylation as a pharmacodynamic readout of the EGFR inhibitor, gefitinib [69], or the study of S6 phosphorylation as a readout of an m-TOR inhibitor such as everolimus [70]. While these markers often measure biomarkers downstream of the intended biological target, pharmacodynamic biomarkers could also include quantification of accumulation of an upstream biological protein; for example, the quantification of accumulation of corticosterone upstream of the intended CYP17 was used to help define the dose of the CYP17 inhibitor, abiraterone [71].

While proof-of-mechanism biomarkers may be used to tailor the dose and schedule of anticancer drugs in phase I studies, they are also crucial in go/no-go decisions to stop the development of a drug if toxicity-limiting dose escalation occurs at doses of drug which does not cause proof-of-mechanism biomarker modulation.

Proof-of-concept biomarkers

Proof-of-concept biomarkers study the functional consequences of inhibiting a target. An example of a proof-of-concept biomarker includes measuring volume transfer constant (Ktrans) via dynamic contrast-enhanced magnetic resonance imaging (DCE-MRI) to measure vascular permeability while evaluating an anti-angiogenic agent such as bevacizumab or axitinib [72]. As proof-of-concept biomarkers study downstream functional events on inhibiting a target, they are sometimes not specific to the target itself. For example, measurement of Ki67 to determine the reduction of proliferation could be used as a proof-of-concept biomarker for an EGFR inhibitor such as gefitinib [73] or the BRAF inhibitor, vemurafenib [74]. In some instances, a change in proof-of-concept biomarker can also be investigated for use as a predictive biomarker of response. For example, the use of 18-fludeoxyglucose positron emission tomography (FDG-PET) to study the pharmacodynamic effects of imatinib in gastrointestinal stromal tumours [75].

Tissues for pharmacodynamic biomarkers

The gold standard for performing pharmacodynamic biomarker assays remains cancer tissue. Depending on the tumour being studied or the platform being used to assess pharmacodynamic biomarkers, it is possible to perform multiple assessments of pharmacodynamic changes before and after treatment with an anticancer agent. Examples of instances where it is possible to study pharmacodynamic biomarkers in tumour serially include the study of phosphorylation of CRKL in circulating leukaemia cells after treatment with the tyrosine kinase inhibitor imatinib, or the study of Ktrans using DCE-MRI of tumour to assess the anti-angiogenic effects of a VEGFR inhibitor such as axitinib [72]. Limitations of pre- and post-tumour biopsies include (1) the fact that often only one pre- and one post-treatment samples are taken due to safety considerations and therefore a sampling error may occur in relation to the time at which pharmacodynamic changes occur; and (2) the area of tumour sampled may not contain the biologically relevant drivers due to intra-tumoral heterogeneity [76]. Tumour biopsies are often performed in the later stages of a phase I study when it has been demonstrated that the drug has reached pharmacologically relevant plasma concentrations, and if appropriate assays are present to demonstrate modulation of proof-of-mechanism biomarkers in normal tissue. An exception to this rule is if the drug target itself resides in normal tissue, as in the case of ipilimumab, which modulates cytotoxic T-cell activation [77].

As multiple repeat sampling of tumour tissue is often not possible, pharmacodynamic biomarkers are often also assessed in normal tissue. It is often possible to sample normal tissue on multiple occasions, from which pharmacodynamic information may help to decide on scheduling of a drug. Commonly used tissues include peripheral blood mononuclear cells (PBMNCs) or platelet-rich plasma (PRP) to measure a diverse set of biomarkers such as p-ERK [78], p-AKT [79], acetylated histone H3 [80–82], and HSP70 [83], which are useful to study a variety of drugs targeting MEK, AKT, histone deacetylase (HDAC), or heat shock protein 90 (HSP90). Disadvantages of using PBMNCs and PRP are that the tissue being sampled consists of terminally differentiated and non-proliferating tissue which may not have relevant genetic abnormalities such as mutations in BRAF or amplified HER2. Normal tissue such as skin and hair follicles has the potential advantage that it demonstrates pharmacodynamic activity in extravascular space [69, 79, 81].

Technical aspects of pharmacodynamic biomarkers and validation

Pharmacodynamic biomarkers must be quantifiable across a dynamic range, taking into account the degree of normal variability in the patient sample being studied. If studying normal tissue, it is possible to look at variation in normal volunteers [84]. If studying tumour tissue, fortunately, interpatient variability may be partially controlled by the patient acting as their own control, i.e. the post-treatment samples are compared to pre-treatment samples. However, studies in variation of pharmacodynamic biomarkers in tumour may require multiple pre-treatment biopsies, or can be investigated using serial imaging [85]. Attention to the degree of reproducibility of the assay, and the processing and stability of samples once stored are crucial to valid interpretation of pharmacodynamic data [85].

Pharmacogenomics

Pharmacogenomics is the study of how an individual's genetic inheritance (his/her genome) or tumour genetics may affect drug pharmacokinetics and pharmacodynamics. Due to rapid advances in DNA sequencing techniques, individualized analysis of inherited germline DNA and/or tumoural DNA has become feasible and potentially useful for individualizing drug dosing and selection. However, interpreting the functional consequences of genetic changes such as single-nucleotide polymorphisms is complex because gene phenotypes are commonly polygenic (determined by multiple genes), and the outcomes of interest such as drug toxicity of irinotecan may not rely solely on a single genetic change such as a *UGT1A1* gene polymorphism [53–55]. Nevertheless,

pharmacogenomics is an increasingly studied field in oncology and carries great potential to inform individualized drug dosing and selection [86].

Conclusions

Pharmacokinetic principles crucially underpin the safe prescription and effective administration of anticancer drugs. Practices such as dose adjustments based on body surface area, clinical factors, and organ function have evolved out of pharmacokinetic studies in an effort to reduce interpatient variability to drug exposure. Further attention to variability as a result of oral administration of drugs, concomitant medications, drug formulation, and syndromes of host metabolic deficiency are important to an oncologist's routine practice. Individualization of drug doses based on these factors and assays such as therapeutic drug monitoring and pharmacogenomics can potentially identify patient populations with a high likelihood of toxicity [87].

Pharmacodynamic principles have become increasingly important to the development of molecularly targeted agents as our knowledge of cancer biology has evolved. Both proof-of-mechanism and proof-of-concept biomarkers allow demonstration of anticancer activity at pharmacological doses different to the maximally tolerated dose. Information from pharmacodynamic biomarkers potentially allows us to define drug dosing with wider therapeutic indices, optimal scheduling, and favoured combinatorial approaches [88, 89]. As new therapies targeting the hallmark traits of cancer are developed and evaluated, pharmacological principles will continue to increase in importance for optimizing anticancer drug delivery and minimizing toxicity [1].

Further reading

Baker SD, van Schaik RHN, Rivory LP, Ten Tije AJ, Dinh K et al. Factors affecting cytochrome P-450 3A activity in cancer patients. Clinical Cancer Research 2004; 10(24): 8341–8345

Baselga J, Rischin D, Ranson M, Calvert H, Raymond E et al. Phase I safety, pharmacokinetic, and pharmacodynamic trial of ZD1839, a selective oral epidermal growth factor receptor tyrosine kinase inhibitor, in patients with five selected solid tumor types. Journal of Clinical Oncology 2002; 20(21): 4292–4302.

Bollag G, Hirth P, Tsai J, Zhang J, Ibrahim PN et al. Clinical efficacy of a RAF inhibitor needs broad target blockade in BRAF-mutant melanoma. Nature 2010; 467(7315): 596–599.

Calvert AH, Newell DR, Gumbrell LA, O'Reilly S, Burnell M et al. Carboplatin dosage: prospective evaluation of a simple formula based on renal function. Journal of Clinical Oncology 1989; 7(11): 1748–1756.

Evans WE, McLeod HL. Pharmacogenomics—drug disposition, drug targets, and side effects. New England Journal of Medicine 2003 Feb 6; 348(6): 538–549.

Gerlinger M, Rowan AJ, Horswell S, Larkin J, Endesfelder D et al. Intratumor heterogeneity and branched evolution revealed by multiregion sequencing. New England Journal of Medicine 2012; 366(10): 883–892.

Lipinski CA, Lombardo F, Dominy BW, Feeney PJ. Experimental and computational approaches to estimate solubility and permeability in drug discovery and development settings. Advanced Drug Delivery Reviews 2001; 46(1–3): 3–26.

Smorenburg CH, Sparreboom A, Bontenbal M, Stoter GK. Randomized cross-over evaluation of body-surface area-based dosing versus flat-fixed dosing of paclitaxel. Journal of Clinical Oncology 2003; 21(2): 197–202.

Undevia SD, Gomez-Abuin G, Ratain MJ. Pharmacokinetic variability of anticancer agents. Nature Reviews Cancer 2005; 5(6): 447–458.

Yap TA, Sandhu SK, Workman P, de Bono JS. Envisioning the future of early anticancer drug development. Nature Reviews Cancer 2010; 10(7): 514–523.

References

1. Yap TA, Sandhu SK, Workman P, de Bono JS. Envisioning the future of early anticancer drug development. Nature Reviews Cancer 2010; 10(7): 514–523.

2. LoRusso PM, Boerner SA, Seymour L. An overview of the optimal planning, design, and conduct of phase I studies of new therapeutics. Clinical Cancer Research 2010; 16(6): 1710–1718.

3. Elias D, Bonnay M, Puizillou JM, Antoun S, Demirdjian S et al. Heated intra-operative intraperitoneal oxaliplatin after complete resection of peritoneal carcinomatosis: pharmacokinetics and tissue distribution. Annals of Oncology 2012; 13(2): 267–272.

4. Lipinski CA, Lombardo F, Dominy BW, Feeney PJ. Experimental and computational approaches to estimate solubility and permeability in drug discovery and development settings. Advanced Drug Delivery Reviews 2001; 46(1–3): 3–26.

5. Prado CMM, Baracos VE, McCargar LJ, Reiman T, Mourtzakis M et al. Sarcopenia as a determinant of chemotherapy toxicity and time to tumor progression in metastatic breast cancer patients receiving capecitabine treatment. Clinical Cancer Research 2009; 15(8): 2920–2926.

6. Undevia SD, Gomez-Abuin G, Ratain MJ. Pharmacokinetic variability of anticancer agents. Nature Reviews Cancer 2005; 5(6): 447–458.

7. Schellens JHM, Ma J, Planting AST, vanderBurg MEL, vanMeerten E, deBoerDennert M et al. Relationship between the exposure to cisplatin, DNA-adduct formation in leucocytes and tumour response in patients with solid tumours. British Journal of Cancer 1996; 73(12): 1569–1575.

8. Sparreboom A, Wolff AC, Mathijssen RHJ, Chatelut E, Rowinsky EK et al. Evaluation of alternate size descriptors for dose calculation of anticancer drugs in the obese. Journal of Clinical Oncology 2007; 25(30): 4707–4713.

9. Smorenburg CH, Sparreboom A, Bontenbal M, Stoter GK. Randomized cross-over evaluation of body-surface area-based dosing versus flat-fixed dosing of paclitaxel. Journal of Clinical Oncology 2003; 21(2): 197–202.

10. Gurney H. Dose calculation of anticancer drugs: a review of the current practice and introduction of an alternative. Journal of Clinical Oncology 1996; 14(9): 2590–2611.

11. Gurney HP, Ackland S, Gebski V, Farrell G. Factors affecting epirubicin pharmacokinetics and toxicity: evidence against using body-surface area for dose calculation. Journal of Clinical Oncology 1998; 16(7): 2299–2304.

12. de Jongh FE, Verweij J, Loos WJ, de Wit R, de Jonge MJA et al. Body-surface area-based dosing does not increase accuracy of predicting cisplatin exposure. Journal of Clinical Oncology 2001; 19(17): 3733–3739.

13. Li J, Gwilt P. The effect of malignant effusions on methotrexate disposition. Cancer Chemotherapy and Pharmacology 2002; 50(5): 373–382.

14. Pitman SW, Frei E. Weekly methotrexate-calcium leucovorin rescue: effect of alkalinization on nephrotoxicity; pharmacokinetics in the CNS and use in CNS non-Hodgkin's lymphoma. Cancer Treatment Reports 1977; 61(4): 695–701.

15. Calvert AH, Newell DR, Gumbrell LA, O'Reilly S, Burnell M et al. Carboplatin dosage: prospective evaluation of a simple formula based on renal function. Journal of Clinical Oncology 1989; 7(11): 1748–1756.

16. Scripture CD, Figg WD, Sparreboom A. The role of drug-metabolising enzymes in clinical responses to chemotherapy. Expert Opinion on Drug Metabolism and Toxicology 2006; 2(1): 17–25.

17. Common Terminology Criteria for Adverse Events, National Cancer Institute, US National Institutes of Health. Available from: <http://ctep.cancer.gov/protocolDevelopment/electronic_applications/ctc.htm>.

18. Joerger M, Huitema ADR, Richel DJ, Dittrich C, Pavlidis N et al. Population pharmacokinetics and pharmacodynamics of paclitaxel and carboplatin in ovarian cancer patients: a study by the European Organization for Research and Treatment of Cancer-Pharmacology and Molecular Mechanisms Group and New Drug Development group. Clinical Cancer Research 2007; 13(21): 6410–6418.

19. Schmitt A, Gladieff L, Laffont CM, Evrard A, Boyer J-C et al. Factors for hematopoietic toxicity of carboplatin: refining the targeting of carboplatin systemic exposure. Journal of Clinical Oncology 2010; 28(30): 4568–4574.

20. Ratain MJ, Schilsky RL, Conley BA, Egorin MJ. Pharmacodynamics in cancer therapy. Journal of Clinical Oncology 1990; 8(10): 1739–1753.

21. Hanahan D, Weinberg RA. Hallmarks of cancer: the next generation. Cell 2011; 144(5): 646–674.

22. Collins I, Workman P. New approaches to molecular cancer therapeutics. Nature Chemical Biology 2006; 2(12): 689–700.

23. Bollag G, Hirth P, Tsai J, Zhang J, Ibrahim PN et al. Clinical efficacy of a RAF inhibitor needs broad target blockade in BRAF-mutant melanoma. Nature 2010; 467(7315): 596–599.

24. Wolf M, Swaisland H, Averbuch S. Development of the novel biologically targeted anticancer agent gefitinib: determining the optimum dose for clinical efficacy. Clinical Cancer Research 2004; 10(14): 4607–4613.

25. Bocci G, Man S, Green SK, Francia G, Ebos JML et al. Increased plasma vascular endothelial growth factor (VEGF) as a surrogate marker for optimal therapeutic dosing of VEGF receptor-2 monoclonal antibodies. Cancer Research 2004; 64(18): 6616–6625.

26. Leyland-Jones B, Gelmon K, Ayoub J-P, Arnold A, Verma S et al. Pharmacokinetics, safety, and efficacy of trastuzumab administered every three weeks in combination with paclitaxel. Journal of Clinical Oncology 2003; 21(21): 3965–3971.

27. Lyass O, Uziely B, Ben-Yosef R, Tzemach D, Heshing NI et al. Correlation of toxicity with pharmacokinetics of pegylated liposomal doxorubicin (Doxil) in metastatic breast carcinoma. Cancer 2000; 89(5): 1037–1047.

28. Marty M, Fumoleau P, Adenis A, Rousseau Y, Merrouche Y et al. Oral vinorelbine pharmacokinetics and absolute bioavailability study in patients with solid tumors. Annals of Oncology 2001; 12(11): 1643–1649.

29. Extra JM, Rousseau F, Bruno R, Clavel M, Lebail N et al. Phase I and pharmacokinetic study of taxotere (RP-56976, NSC-628503) given as a short intravenous infusion. Cancer Research 1993; 53(5): 1037–1042.

30. Burris H a, Taylor CW, Jones SF, Koch KM, Versola MJ et al. A phase I and pharmacokinetic study of oral lapatinib administered once or twice daily in patients with solid malignancies. Clinical Cancer Research 2009; 15(21): 6702–6708.

31. Blum JL, Dieras V, Lo Russo PM, Horton J, Rutman O et al. Multicenter, Phase II study of capecitabine in taxane-pretreated metastatic breast carcinoma patients. Cancer 2001; 92(7): 1759–1768.

32. Bailey DG, Malcolm J, Arnold O, Spence JD. Grapefruit juice-drug interactions. British Journal of Clinical Pharmacology 1998; 46(2): 101–110.

33. Lown KS, Bailey DG, Fontana RJ, Janardan SK, Adair CH et al. Grapefruit juice increases felodipine oral availability in humans by decreasing intestinal CYP3A protein expression. Journal of Clinical Investigation 1997; 99(10): 2545–2553.

34. Koch KM, Reddy NJ, Cohen RB, Lewis NL, Whitehead B et al. Effects of food on the relative bioavailability of lapatinib in cancer patients. Journal of Clinical Oncology: 2009; 27(8): 1191–1196.

35. Kruijtzer CMF, Beijnen JH, Schellens JHM. Improvement of oral drug treatment by temporary inhibition of drug transporters and/or cytochrome P450 in the gastrointestinal tract and liver: an overview. Oncologist 2002; 7(6): 516–530.

36. Clark PI, Slevin Ml, Joel SP, Osborne RJ, Talbot DI et al. A randomized trial of 2 etoposide schedules in small-cell lung-cancer—the influence of pharmacokinetics on efficacy and toxicity. Journal of Clinical Oncology 1994; 12(7): 1427–1435.

37. Miller AA, Herndon JE, Hollis DR, Ellerton J, Langleben A et al. Schedule dependency of 21-day oral versus 3-day intravenous etoposide in combination with intravenous cisplatin in extensive-stage small-cell lung-cancer—a randomized phase-III study of the Cancer and Leukemia Group-B. Journal of Clinical Oncology 1995; 13(8): 1871–1879.

38. Thomas VH, Bhattachar S, Hitchingham L, Zocharski P, Naath M et al. The road map to oral bioavailability: an industrial perspective. Expert Opinion on Drug Metabolism and Toxicology 2006; 2(4): 591–608.

39. Rentsch KM, Schwendener RA, Pestalozzi BC, Sauter C, Wunderli-Allenspach H. Pharmacokinetic studies of mitoxantrone and one of its metabolites in serum and urine in patients with advanced breast cancer. European Journal of Clinical Pharmacology 1998; 54(1): 83–89.

40. Muldoon LL, Soussain C, Jahnke K, Johanson C, Siegal T et al. Chemotherapy delivery issues in central nervous system malignancy: a reality check. Journal of Clinical Oncology 2007; 25(16): 2295–2305.

41. Rolan PE. Plasma protein binding displacement interactions: why are they still regarded as clinically important? British Journal of Clinical Pharmacology 1994; 37(2): 125–128.

42. Cordon-Cardo C, O'Brien JP, Casals D, Rittman-Grauer L, Biedler JL et al. Multidrug-resistance gene (P-glycoprotein) is expressed by endothelial cells at blood-brain barrier sites. Proceedings of the National Academy of Sciences USA 1989; 86(2): 695–698.

43. Stemmler H-J, Schmitt M, Willems A, Bernhard H, Harbeck N et al. Ratio of trastuzumab levels in serum and cerebrospinal fluid is altered in HER2-positive breast cancer patients with brain metastases and impairment of blood-brain barrier. Anti-Cancer Drugs 2007; 18(1): 23–28.

44. Fellner S, Bauer B, Miller DS, Schaffrik M, Fankhänel M et al. Transport of paclitaxel (Taxol) across the blood-brain barrier in vitro and in vivo. Journal of Clinical Investigation 2002; 110(9): 1309–1318.

45. Tubergen DG, Gilchrist GS, O'Brien RT, Coccia PF, Sather HN et al. Prevention of CNS disease in intermediate-risk acute lymphoblastic leukemia: comparison of cranial radiation and intrathecal methotrexate and the importance of systemic therapy: a Children's Cancer Group report. Journal of Clinical Oncology 1993; 11(3): 520–526.

46. Bart J, Hollema H, Groen HJM, de Vries EGE, Hendrikse NH et al. The distribution of drug-efflux pumps, P-gp, BCRP, MRP1 and MRP2, in the normal blood-testis barrier and in primary testicular tumours. European Journal of Cancer 1990; 40(14): 2064–2070.

47. James PP, Mead GM. Sanctuary site relapse in chemotherapy-treated testicular cancer. Annals of Oncology 1992; 3(1): 41–43.

48. Pauley JL, Panetta JC, Schmidt J, Kornegay N, Relling MV et al. Late-onset delayed excretion of methotrexate. Cancer Chemotherapy and Pharmacology 2004; 54(2): 146–152.

49. Thummel KE, Wilkinson GR. In vitro and in vivo drug interactions involving human CYP3A. Annual Review of Pharmacology and Toxicology 1998; 38: 389–430.

50. Baker SD, van Schaik RHN, Rivory LP, Ten Tije AJ, Dinh K et al. Factors affecting cytochrome P-450 3A activity in cancer patients. Clinical Cancer Research 2004; 10(24): 8341–8345.

51. Sideras K, Ingle JN, Ames MM, Loprinzi CL, Mrazek DP et al. Coprescription of tamoxifen and medications that inhibit CYP2D6. Journal of Clinical Oncology 2010; 28(16): 2768–2776.

52. Saif MW, Choma A, Salamone SJ, Chu E. Pharmacokinetically guided dose adjustment of 5-fluorouracil: a rational approach to improving therapeutic outcomes. Journal of the National Cancer Institute 2009; 101(22): 1543–1552.

53. Cecchin E, Innocenti F, D'Andrea M, Corona G, De Mattia E et al. Predictive role of the UGT1A1, UGT1A7, and UGT1A9 genetic variants and their haplotypes on the outcome of metastatic colorectal cancer patients treated with fluorouracil, leucovorin, and irinotecan. Journal of Clinical Oncology 2009; 27(15): 2457–2465.

54. Han JY, Lim HS, Shin ES, Yoo YK, Park YH et al. Comprehensive analysis of UGT1A polymorphisms predictive for pharmacokinetics and treatment outcome in patients with non-small-cell lung cancer treated with irinotecan and cisplatin. Journal of Clinical Oncology 2006; 24(15): 2237–2244.

55. Innocenti F, Kroetz DL, Schuetz E, Dolan ME, Ramírez J et al. Comprehensive pharmacogenetic analysis of irinotecan neutropenia and pharmacokinetics. Journal of Clinical Oncology 2009; 27(16): 2604–2614.

56. Chabot GG, Abigerges D, Catimel G, Culine S, Deforni R. Extra JM et al. Population pharmacokinetics and pharmacodynamics of irinotecan (CPT-11) and active metabolite SN-38 during phase-I trials. Annals of Oncology 1995; 6(2): 141–151.

57. Shen DD, Azarnoff DL. Clinical pharmacokinetics of methotrexate. Clinical Pharmacokinetics 1978; 3(1): 1–13.

58. Joerger M, Omlin A, Cerny T, Früh M. The role of pemetrexed in advanced non small-cell lung cancer: special focus on pharmacology and mechanism of action. Current Drug Targets 2010; 11(1): 37–47.

59. Lee W, Kim RB. Transporters and renal drug elimination. Annual Review of Pharmacology and Toxicology 2004; 44: 137–166.

60. Ellison NM, Servi RJ. Acute renal failure and death following sequential intermediate-dose methotrexate and 5-FU: a possible adverse effect due to concomitant indomethacin administration. Cancer Treatment Reports 1985; 69(3): 342–343.

61. Relling MV, McLeod HL, Bowman LC, Santana VM. Etoposide pharmacokinetics and pharmacodynamics after acute and chronic exposure to cisplatin. Clinical Pharmacology & Therapeutics 1994; 56(5): 503–511.

62. Sotaniemi EA, Arranto AJ, Pelkonen O, Pasanen M. Age and cytochrome P450-linked drug metabolism in humans: an analysis of 226 subjects with equal histopathologic conditions. Clinical Pharmacology & Therapeutics 1997; 61(3): 331–339.

63. Baker SD, Wirth M, Statkevich P, Reidenberg P, Alton K et al. Absorption, metabolism, and excretion of 14C-temozolomide following oral administration to patients with advanced cancer. Clinical Cancer Research 1999; 5(2): 309–317.

64. Reagan-Shaw S, Nihal M, Ahmad N. Dose translation from animal to human studies revisited. FASEB Journal 2008; 22(3): 659–661.

65. Bruno R, Washington CB, Lu JF, Lieberman G, Banken L et al. Population pharmacokinetics of trastuzumab in patients with HER2+ metastatic breast cancer. Cancer Chemotherapy and Pharmacology; 2005; 56(4): 361–369.

66. Gianni L, Kearns CM, Giani A, Capri G, Viganó L et al. Nonlinear pharmacokinetics and metabolism of paclitaxel and its pharmacokinetic/pharmacodynamic relationships in humans. Journal of Clinical Oncology 1995; 13(1): 180–190.

67. Gianni L, Viganò L, Locatelli A, Capri G, Giani A et al. Human pharmacokinetic characterization and in vitro study of the interaction between doxorubicin and paclitaxel in patients with breast cancer. Journal of Clinical Oncology 1997; 15(5): 1906–1915.

68. Chen TL, Passos-Coelho JL, Noe DA, Kennedy MJ, Black KC et al. Nonlinear pharmacokinetics of cyclophosphamide in patients with metastatic breast cancer receiving high-dose chemotherapy followed by autologous bone marrow transplantation. Cancer Research 1995; 55(4): 810–816.

69. Baselga J, Rischin D, Ranson M, Calvert H, Raymond E et al. Phase I safety, pharmacokinetic, and pharmacodynamic trial of ZD1839, a selective oral epidermal growth factor receptor tyrosine kinase inhibitor, in patients with five selected solid tumor types. Journal of Clinical Oncology 2002; 20(21): 4292–4302.

70. O'Donnell A, Faivre S, Burris HA, Rea D, Papadimitrakopoulou V et al. Phase I pharmacokinetic and pharmacodynamic study of the oral mammalian target of rapamycin inhibitor everolimus in patients with advanced solid tumors. Journal of Clinical Oncology 2008; 26(10): 1588–1595.

71. Reid AHM, Attard G, Danila DC, Oommen NB, Olmos D et al. Significant and sustained antitumor activity in post-docetaxel, castration-resistant prostate cancer with the CYP17 inhibitor abiraterone acetate. Journal of Clinical Oncology 2010; 28(9): 1489–1495.

72. O'Connor JPB, Jackson A, Parker GJM, Roberts C, Jayson GC. Dynamic contrast-enhanced MRI in clinical trials of antivascular therapies. Nature Reviews Clinical Oncology 2012; 9(3): 167–177.

73. Daneshmand M, Parolin DAE, Hirte HW, Major P, Goss G et al. A pharmacodynamic study of the epidermal growth factor receptor tyrosine kinase inhibitor ZD1839 in metastatic colorectal cancer patients. Clinical Cancer Research 2003; 9(7): 2457–2464.

74. Flaherty KTKT, Puzanov I, Kim KBKB, Ribas A, McArthur GA et al. Inhibition of mutated, activated BRAF in metastatic melanoma. New England Journal of Medicine 2010; 363(9): 809–819.

75. van Oosterom AT, Judson I, Verweij J, Stroobants S, Donato di Paola E et al. Safety and efficacy of imatinib (STI571) in metastatic gastrointestinal stromal tumours: a phase I study. Lancet 2001; 358(9291): 1421–1423.

76. Gerlinger M, Rowan AJ, Horswell S, Larkin J, Endesfelder D et al. Intratumor heterogeneity and branched evolution revealed by multiregion sequencing. New England Journal of Medicine 2012; 366(10): 883–892.

77. Kaehler KC, Piel S, Livingstone E, Schilling B, Hauschild A, Schadendorf D. Update on immunologic therapy with anti-CTLA-4 antibodies in melanoma: identification of clinical and biological response patterns, immune-related adverse events, and their management. Seminars in Oncology 2010; 37(5): 485–498.

78. Banerji U, Camidge DR, Verheul HMW, Agarwal R, Sarker D et al. The first-in-human study of the hydrogen sulfate (Hyd-sulfate) capsule of the MEK1/2 inhibitor AZD6244 (ARRY-142886): a phase I open-label multicenter trial in patients with advanced cancer. Clinical Cancer Research 2010; 16(5): 1613–1623.

79. Yap TA, Yan L, Patnaik A, Fearen I, Olmos D et al. First-in-man clinical trial of the oral pan-AKT inhibitor MK-2206 in patients with advanced solid tumors. Journal of Clinical Oncology: 2011; 29(35): 4688–4695.

80. Kelly WK, O'Connor OA, Krug LM, Chiao JH, Heaney M et al. Phase I study of an oral histone deacetylase inhibitor, suberoylanilide hydroxamic acid, in patients with advanced cancer. Journal of Clinical Oncology 2005; 23(17): 3923–3931.

81. Banerji U, van Doorn L, Papadatos-Pastos D, Kristeleit R, Debnam P et al. A phase I pharmacokinetic and pharmacodynamic study of CHR-3996, an oral class I selective histone deacetylase inhibitor in refractory solid tumors. Clinical Cancer Research 2012; 18(9): 2687–2694.

82. Banerji U, O'Donnell A, Scurr M, Pacey S, Stapleton S et al. Phase I pharmacokinetic and pharmacodynamic study of 17-allylamino, 17-demethoxygeldanamycin in patients with advanced malignancies. Journal of Clinical Oncology 2005; 23(18): 4152–4161.

83. Banerji U, Walton M, Raynaud F, Grimshaw R, Kelland L et al. Pharmacokinetic-pharmacodynamic relationships for the heat shock protein 90 molecular chaperone inhibitor 17-allylamino, 17-demethoxygeldanamycin in human ovarian cancer xenograft models. Clinical Cancer Research 2005; 11(19 Pt 1): 7023–7032.

84. Medved M, Karczmar G, Yang C, Dignam J, Gajewski TF et al. Semiquantitative analysis of dynamic contrast enhanced MRI in cancer patients: variability and changes in tumor tissue over time. Journal of Magnetic Resonance Imaging 2004; 20(1): 122–128.

85. Cummings J, Ward TH, Dive C. Fit-for-purpose biomarker method validation in anticancer drug development. Drug Discovery Today 2010; 15(19-20): 816–825.

86. Evans WE, McLeod HL. Pharmacogenomics—drug disposition, drug targets, and side effects. New England Journal of Medicine 2003 Feb 6; 348(6): 538–549.

87. Gao B, Yeap S, Clements A, Balakrishnar B, Wong M et al. Evidence for therapeutic drug monitoring of targeted anticancer therapies. Journal of Clinical Oncology 2012; 30(32): 4017–4025.

88. Al-Lazikani B, Banerji U, Workman P. Combinatorial drug therapy for cancer in the post-genomic era. Nature Biotechnology 2012; 30(7): 679–692.

89. Kola I, Landis J. Can the pharmaceutical industry reduce attrition rates? Nature Reviews Drug Discovery 2004; 3(8): 711–715.

CHAPTER 24

Design and analysis of clinical trials

Daniel J. Sargent and Qian Shi

Introduction to design and analysis of clinical trials

Overall mortality rates for cancer patients have maintained a declining rate of more than 1% per year for the past ten years, with substantial contributions to this decline from four major cancers sites: lung, colorectum, breast, and prostate [1]. Recent exciting advances in genomics, proteomics, and computational power empower scientists with new tools to understand the causes and prognoses of cancer at the molecular level. Innovative targeted compounds are being developed with great potential to battle the disease. In the face of these advances, the high failure rates of late-phase clinical trials in oncology [2] are of substantial concern. In this chapter, we aim to present general concepts and principles, as well as current innovations and issues and future directions of design and analysis of clinical trials in oncology from a statistical perspective, with an expectation that adherence to these principles will ultimately increase clinical trial quality and reduce the phase III trial failure rate.

The intended audience of this chapter is a wide range of professionals in oncology research, especially those involved in clinical trials. We will not devote attention to mathematical theories of statistical design and analysis methods, but rather will provide a high-level overview on the relevant topics. Several excellent texts provide comprehensive discussions of the development and applications of statistical methods in clinical trials; we cite several such references.

Scientifically sound study design and conduct are fundamental and essential to the success of any research. This is particularly true for oncology therapeutic development in this new era of emerging personalized medicine. Successful clinical design and analysis are never easy tasks, which involve, but are not limited to, framing the right question based on high-quality scientific evidence, identifying the targeted disease population, selecting well-defined and most relevant endpoints, determining the cost-effective sample size and sampling schema, carefully controlling the impact of unknown or non-measurable confounders, formulating decision rules based on comprehensive operating characteristics assessment, prespecifying subgroup analyses and correlative studies, and building in continuous patient safety and therapeutic efficacy review.

Design of clinical trials

It is increasingly recognized among oncology researchers that collaboration with statisticians in the early stage of planning a study is not only valuable but critical. This is especially true for oncology clinical trials, to prevent costly mistakes in both financial burden to society and devastating losses to patients and their families. These mistakes can be due to methodological errors, underpowered studies with severe adverse effects, or misinterpretation of collected data. Optimal clinical trial design can simplify subsequent analyses by defining data collection processes appropriately, reducing bias and variability, and minimizing the influence of complicating confounders. In this way, stronger or more convincing evidence can be revealed by simple statistical analysis methods with fewer assumptions [3].

The section presents the principles, methodologies, and several illustrative examples related to the design of oncology clinical trials. Traditional or so-called standard designs will be presented, followed by two key elements of designing a clinical trial: endpoint selection and sample size determination. For additional technical background regarding clinical trial design and analysis, we refer readers to other sources such as Armitage and Berry [4] and Marubini and Valsecchi [5].

Traditional designs

A *clinical trial* is an experiment testing the safety and efficacy of a treatment or a medical procedure on human subjects through a rigorously defined protocol. This includes application of treatment, ascertainment of outcome(s), safety monitoring, decision rules, analysis plans, and specimen collection [3]. Clinical trials are generally classified as phase I, II, and III according to their primary aims and the stage in the timeline of drug development.

Phase I studies

Phase I studies are generally aimed at identifying the optimal dose level and treatment schedules based on an assessment of a new regimen's toxicity. In recent phase I studies, an extended cohort may be added to confirm the optimal dose level identified during the trial, to allow the generation of preliminary efficacy data, and to further define the basic clinical pharmacology of the drug.

A traditional and commonly used phase I design in oncology is the cohort-of-three design. The fundamental assumption is that treatment benefit and the toxicity are both increasing in a monotone fashion as the dose increases (e.g., with cytotoxic agents). Under this assumption, the balance between maximizing the treatment response and protecting patients from severe toxicities can be achieved by identifying the maximum tolerated dose (MTD). The MTD is defined as the highest dose level at which the percent of patients experiencing dose-limiting toxicity (DLT) reaches the pre-specified acceptable limit. In the cohort-of-three design, the limit of this percent is set to be 1/3. In general, DLTs are defined as serious or fatal side effects of the new regimen.

Practical considerations require the study design to prespecify a small set of doses, optimally based on preclinical evidence, with patients treated adaptively according to the observed rate of toxicity at each of the previously studied dose levels. In the cohort-of-three design, three patients are treated at the starting dose level. If no DLT is observed, three patients will be treated at the next higher dose level. If more than one DLT is observed, three patients will be treated at the next lower dose level. If one DLT is observed, an additional three patients will be treated at the same dose level. The MTD will be considered as exceeded if two or more DLTs are observed out of three or six patients at a given dose level. The next lower dose level will be defined as the MTD as long as six patient have been evaluated on that level.

The cohort-of-three design has several appealing features: it is straightforward to conduct, decision-making of dose escalations is transparent, and there is no need for sophisticated computing programs. However, this design may require a long time and many patients to reach the MTD, with many patients treated at the suboptimal dose levels. For example, 56 patients were accrued during 38 months, and 13 dose levels were tested in a study assessing irinotecan for patients with advanced cancer [6]. In addition, multiple simulation studies have demonstrated that model-based approaches can more accurately determine the true MTD, perhaps with fewer patients [7]. In the modern era of therapeutic development of treating cancer, more than one-dimensional dose-finding strategies are needed for testing combinations of new standard compounds. Many novel therapies with cytostatic or targeted compounds do not share the same dose-response assumption of cytotoxic agents. Innovative designs which account for efficacy data in dose-finding decision-making may be more appropriate in many cases than traditional cohort-of-three phase I study design [8, 9].

Phase II studies

Phase II trials are aimed at quickly screening new treatments or regimens based on early evidence of their efficacy, as well as further characterizing the toxicity of a regimen. As opposed to phase I studies, a focused disease population (e.g., a particular tumour type with specific stage) is generally considered. Historically, single-arm designs were commonly used in this setting. As oncology research has advanced, a randomized design has become more frequent. Regardless of the design, these clinical trials are vital to determine if the new treatment should be tested in large-scale comparative (phase III) studies. In addition, the feasibility of the new treatment, including safety, administration, and cost, will be informed during this phase of development.

Single-arm phase II studies construct the design using two benchmarks of the underlying treatment effect based on historical data. For instance, if the response rate (RR) is used to measure the treatment effect, then the first benchmark is a clinically uninteresting rate, p_0. If the true RR of the new regimen is as low as p_0, then it is not worthwhile continuing evaluation. The second benchmark is the targeted rate, p_1 ($> p_0$). An RR which is as high as p_1 will

be considered to warrant a large-scale comparative trial. By pre-specifying acceptable type I and II error rates (explained in a later section), the required number of patients (i.e. sample size) and the number of responses (i.e. boundary of efficacy-decision rule) can be calculated.

For ethical considerations, it is desirable to minimize the number of patients treated with ineffective or inferior treatments. Stopping trials based on results of interim analyses is commonly applied. From a statistical perspective, there are two reasons for stopping a trial early—stop for superiority (i.e. efficacy) or stop for inferiority (i.e. futility). The first situation applies when there is overwhelming evidence that the experimental treatment is superior to historical control (or a concurrent control in a randomized two-arm study). Stopping for futility (i.e. lack of efficacy) implies that based on an interim analysis result it is highly unlikely that the trial will achieve the targeted treatment effect even if all patients are enrolled. Due to the small sample size of phase II trials, a substantially large treatment effect (usually beyond what is realistic) will need to be observed to meet the early stopping criteria for efficacy.

Simon's optimal two-stage design [10] is a widely used method for single-arm phase II trials in oncology. For a typical phase II study, for example, to test the null hypothesis that the RR of a regimen is at most 60% versus the alternative hypothesis that the RR is greater than 75%, Simon's design requires a maximum sample size of 71 patients to achieve 90% power at the significance level of 0.1. A planned interim analysis (i.e. the first stage) will be conducted when 34 patients are enrolled and the response data are available. If 21 or fewer responses are observed, the trial will be terminated early for futility. Otherwise, an additional 37 patients will be accrued. If the study proceeds to the second stage and more than 47 responses are observed, the new regimen may warrant further investigation. Other designs and further discussion can be found in many references [11–16].

One of the major drawbacks of the single-arm design is the lack of robust knowledge of historical success rates due to heterogeneity of study population, limitations of previous studies (poor design or data quality), or even lack of relevant studies. This has been considered to be one of the reasons that contribute to the high failure rate of subsequent phase III studies [17, 18]. An alternative to the single-arm design is randomized phase II studies. Randomized selection and screening designs have been proposed and used in oncology drug development. In a selection design, multiple experimental arms are tested. A 'winner' will be selected for a future phase III trial either based on the highest estimated success rate for the primary endpoint [19], or between multiple arms if the difference in treatment effect between the best arm and less optimal arm(s) is larger than a prespecified criterion [20]. In a screening design, the experimental regimen is compared to standard-of-care treatment in a head-to-head manner [21]. A screening phase II design is very similar to phase III randomized trial design, but with higher type II error rate and lower power.

Phase III studies

Phase III clinical trials are pivotal, designed to provide the definitive evidence to move a new regimen or modality into patient care, or to definitively refute the usefulness of the proposed new treatment. Under most circumstances, phase III clinical trials are designed to compare concurrent arms with randomized allocation of patients. Randomization continues to be considered as a simple and reliable tool to prevent bias in allocating treatments in comparative studies, includes biases due to treatment selection based on patients' prognostic factors, and known/unknown (measured/unmeasured) confounding factors. For more practice and theory associated with randomization, we refer readers to the discussions by Lachin [22, 23].

There are two classes of design for phase III trials: the superiority design and the non-inferiority/equivalence design. In a randomized clinical trial (RCT) with a superiority design, the primary aim of the study is to show whether the new therapy is superior to an established therapy or placebo. Alternatively, if the alternative treatment is easier to administrate, costs less, or is less toxic than standard of care, showing superiority is not necessary; a definitive demonstration of non-inferiority is all that would be required [24–27]. Non-inferiority or equivalence trials are designed to show the alternative therapy is not inferior to or equivalent to an established therapy, respectively. The different aims of these two types of design lead to significantly different design aspects from a statistical perspective, such as the planning, analysis, and reporting of an RCT. Figure 24.1 illustrates the difference in specifications of null and alternative hypotheses comparing these designs.

Randomization is one of the fundamental principles for RCTs. It balances known and unknown prognostic factors. However, within a particular trial (especially a trial with small sample size), random chance may lead to imbalances with respect to important prognostic factors [28, 29]. To prevent the potential failure of randomization, randomization procedures can be implemented within subpopulations defined by different levels of patient baseline characteristics which influence prognosis. This is called *stratification* of treatment assignments. The patient characteristics (i.e. prognostic factors) are referred to as *stratification factors*. In addition to the benefit of assurance that compared groups are similar with respect to known prognostic factors, stratified randomization also protects against type I error [30, 31], increases power [32, 33], reduces sample size (especially for equivalence trials) [34], and facilitates subgroup analyses [35]. Generally speaking, fewer strata are better. With fewer stratification factors, the trial is more likely to avoid incomplete fills of blocks (*over-stratification*) and to assure equal distribution of stratification factor among treatment groups [36].

In randomized studies, blinding (or 'masking'), when possible, is another critical method for reducing bias. Blinding is a procedure that withholds information from specific groups of individuals [37]. For instance, patients are blinded to what treatment arm (intervention versus control) they are receiving. This is aimed to reduce the response bias associated with the psychological impact of being treated with an intervention perceived as superior to a control treatment. Blinding the treatment allocation to patients also prevents the attrition bias (i.e. dropout from control arm), non-compliance and co-intervention bias (i.e. patients in control group may seek out alternative interventions or obtain experimental intervention) [38]. Other groups that are commonly blinded are healthcare providers and outcome assessors. The knowledge of the treatment assignment of a patient may induce differences in the quality of patient–provider interaction, for example selective decisions to cross over from the control to the experimental

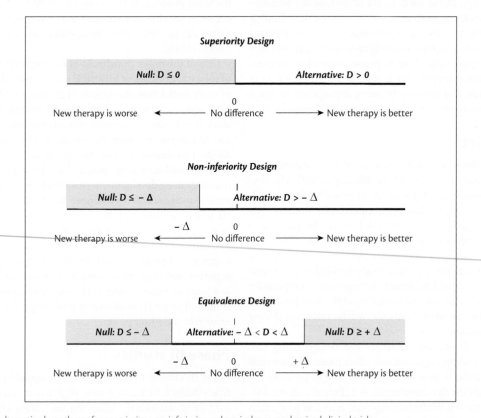

Fig. 24.1 The null and alternative hypotheses for superiority, non-inferiority and equivalence randomized clinical trials.

Note: D is the treatment effect (e.g. difference) between new therapy and control therapy. Δ is the non-inferiority and equivalence margin in non-inferiority and equivalence design, respectively.

intervention [37]. Blinding to outcome assessors helps prevent the tendency for evaluators to assess patients treated with the experimental intervention more favourably [39]. Using a placebo which is identical in appearance to the treatment drug is a common procedure for blinding in randomized trials [40, 41].

Endpoints

Types of endpoint

The primary endpoint(s) is one of the most critical elements in formulating the design, data collection, and statistical analyses plan of a clinical trial. It is a quantitative measurement implied or required by the primary objective(s) of a study, and will be determined in each study subject. The best endpoint is a clinical measurement reflecting the most relevant potential treatment effect of the new regimen that can be defined with rigorous mathematical and statistical properties. Many times, a clinical objective may imply more than one quantitative definition of an endpoint. For example, 'improve survival'—a common goal in oncology studies—might mean prolonged median survival, higher five-year survival rate, or a lower death rate specifically due to disease. These three quantitative definitions may require different methods or schedules of assessment, and need not yield the same sample size or analysis plan. In other instances, various study teams may define the same endpoint differently. For example, pre-operative morbidity could be defined as disease-specific, treatment-specific, or a composite; every primary endpoint must be clear and unambiguous.

The phase of clinical trials also affects the choice of endpoints. For example, the presence of a DLT during the first cycle of treatment is commonly used in phase I dose-finding trials. Short-term tumour-related measures (e.g., response status during treatment) may be a suitable primary endpoint for phase II screening trials. For confirmatory phase III oncology studies, overall survival, defined as time from randomization to death due to any cause, is a standard endpoint. From a statistical perspective, there are several types of endpoint that are likely to be used in various clinical trials. These include continuous endpoints (e.g., prostate-specific antigen level), dichotomous endpoints (e.g., response rate), or time-to-event endpoints (e.g., time to disease recurrence). Determining a proper endpoint that can be obtained reliably and repeatedly in a particular clinical trial is an essential task for the statistician and involves careful communication between the statistician and clinical investigators.

Surrogate endpoints

As mentioned in the previous section, overall survival (OS) is considered a standard clinical primary endpoint in phase III trials of life-threatening diseases, such as cancer. However, using OS as an endpoint frequently increases the duration or sample size of a clinical trial. For example, in early-stage cancer trials, sufficient power has to be achieved by extending patient follow-up or increasing the sample size due to a low death rate. This clearly hinders rapid development of effective therapies. To overcome this problem, using surrogate endpoints which are measured earlier, more frequently, more conveniently, or at less cost to replace the 'true' endpoint of OS seems to be an attractive solution.

There are various definitions of surrogate endpoints in the literature [42]. For example, the Biomarkers Definitions Working Group (BDWG) defines a surrogate endpoint as 'a biomarker that is intended to substitute for a clinical endpoint. A surrogate endpoint is expected to predict clinical benefit (or harm or lack of benefit or harm) based on epidemiologic, therapeutic, pathophysiologic, or other scientific evidence' [43]. A critical requirement of a valid surrogate endpoint is that the treatment effect observed on a surrogate endpoint should reliably predict the treatment effect on the clinical endpoint. This implies a stronger requirement for a surrogate endpoint than simply a significant correlation between it and the clinical endpoint.

There are two branches of statistical surrogate evaluation methodologies: a single-trial or a meta-analytic evaluation. In the single-trial approach, the 'proportion of treatment effect' (PTE) [44, 45] explained by the surrogate, has been the predominant approach. Recent innovative methods of evaluating surrogate endpoints using single-trial data have emerged, including the semi-competing risks paradigm [46] and the use of causal models [47]. On the other hand, work in the meta-analytic framework [48] and regression-based approaches [49, 50], based on multiple randomized trials, is frequently used to evaluate the potential time-to-event surrogate endpoints in oncology. Burzykowski et al. further developed the concept of a 'surrogate threshold effect' (STE) that estimates from existing trials the magnitude of a surrogate needed in a future trial to predict benefit on the true proposed endpoint [51]. Lassere has proposed [52] a biomarker surrogacy evaluation scheme to better enable integration of surrogacy into the clinical context.

In oncology studies, there has been a long history of utilizing surrogate endpoints. For example, tumour shrinkage or delayed tumour growth, improved levels of biomarkers, such as prostate-specific antigen (PSA) in prostate cancer, are considered as good prognostic factors for long-term clinical outcomes. Therefore, tumour response, time to progression or recurrence, and measures defined by certain forms of biomarkers over time are frequently used as primary outcomes in early phase clinical trials. Many times, these substitutes for the true clinical endpoint, such as OS, are used without any formal validation. However, as we gain a greater understanding of the validation conditions for surrogate endpoints, the process of formally evaluating a potential surrogate endpoint has been increasingly adopted. Shi and Sargent summarized recent applications of evaluating surrogate endpoints in oncology studies including colorectal, prostate, and breast cancer [42]. In the adjuvant colorectal cancer setting, Sargent et al. successfully validated three-year disease-free survival (DFS) as a surrogate endpoint for five-year OS [53]. In metastatic colorectal cancer, progression-free survival (PFS) has also demonstrated promising surrogacy [54], but such surrogacy was not established in advanced breast cancer [55]. No studies, to our knowledge, have successfully established strong surrogacy of tumour response for OS in any disease.

Power and sample size considerations

Errors and biases

In the statistical design of any clinical trial, control of possible error is a critical concept. Generally speaking, there are two types of error. One is random, which is purely due to chance. Another is systematic, known as bias, which describes errors that are not a consequence of chance alone [3].

We borrow Piantadosi's analogy to distinguish random errors and bias [3]: if the treatment effect in a clinical trial is the 'sound or signal' we aim to detect, then random errors can be considered to be the 'background noise', whereas bias is signal distortion. There are often a set of factors (well-known) that contribute to the possibility of bias. In many cases, these sources of bias can be understood well enough to be controlled. This is fundamentally different from random errors: pure random errors have no preferred direction. Clinically, averaging over a large number of observations or long enough time periods, the relative effect of random errors on treatment effect detection (hypothesis testing or parameter estimation) will be sufficiently small. However, bias cannot be reduced by averaging after repletion or taking additional observations. For controlling bias, randomization and stratification are two critical principles. Concurrent controls, objective assessments, active follow-up and endpoint ascertainment, and no post hoc exclusions are also critical considerations to reduce bias [3].

In a clinical context, although bias can arise in numerous ways, the critical ones are generally well understood and can usually be removed or reduced by good design and proper conduct of the clinical trial. However, due to sampling variability, subject heterogeneity, measurement error, and other sources of noise, the random error can never be completely eliminated. One aspect of the design of a clinical trial is to control and reduce the random error to an acceptably low level, while still maintaining the feasibility of conducting a trial ethically and financially. This goal is mainly achieved by the careful consideration of sample size calculations in respect of two types of error: false positive (type I) and false negative (type II) errors.

Significance level and power

Regardless of whether a design is based on hypothesis testing, significance testing, or confidence interval estimation, the statistical design of a clinical trial is centred on controlling type I and type II errors. A type I error is a 'false positive' result and occurs if there is no treatment effect or difference but investigators incorrectly conclude that there is. On the other hand, a type II error occurs when there is a treatment effect but investigators fail to detect it—a 'false negative' result. The significance level (frequently denoted as α) is the boundary of the acceptable type I error rate, i.e. the risk level the investigators are willing to accept that an observed significant treatment effect is not 'truthful' and instead due to chance. The significance level is usually set to be 0.05 in trials targeted to provide confirmatory results. For early phase studies (e.g., phase II), α can be as high as 0.2. The type II error rate usually is denoted by β. The value of $1-\beta$ is commonly known as power. The power of the study is the likelihood of concluding a treatment effect or difference exists when in fact it does.

For a particular design, the type I error rate and power depends on sample size, the null hypothesis regarding the treatment effect (e.g., no difference for a superiority design), the clinically meaningful effect size of the new treatment compared to standard care or placebo (alternative hypothesis), and the specific statistical model which depends heavily on the choice of the primary endpoint.

Study operating characteristics

When designing a clinical trial, the sample size and decision rules provide direct guidance for conducting the study. When a study is simple, for example without any interim looks, and a single primary endpoint, and a traditional design is considered, controlling type I and II error rates is straightforward. Many statistical software packages can perform the sample size/power calculations. If one or more interim looks are desired, then sample size calculations must be adjusted accordingly, as type I error rates are inflated due to multiple testing—multiple looks will increases the rate of positive findings purely by chance [3]. In some situations, the power will be also affected. Hence, a comprehensive evaluation of the proposed study design before launching the study is critical. From a statistical perspective, this consists of evaluating the study operating characteristics—calculations of probabilities of discovering the treatment effect and the likelihood of stopping the study early at interim looks under a range of assumptions of the true treatment effect. These assumptions usually range from no effect (null hypothesis) to the targeted clinical meaningful treatment difference (alternative hypothesis). In complex designs, simulation studies can be powerful tools to assess the study-operating characteristics. In these studies, the clinical outcomes can be generated based on design parameters under statistical models (the one chosen to determine the sample size and decision rules), and a designed study can be repeatedly 'conducted' and 'produce' the hypothetical outcome data a large amount of times (>1000]. It is not uncommon for existing statistical designs to be inadequate or for their underlying assumptions to be unfit for the situation in hand. In these circumstances, simulation studies provide a flexible tool to perform sample size and power calculations and define optimal decision rules.

Advanced designs

Phase I cancer therapies are shifting from cytotoxic compounds to cytostatic or targeted therapies. The shape of dose-response curves of these new regimens is usually unknown. It could be monotone non-decreasing, non-linear, or increasing with a plateau. The traditional cohort-of-three design is not appropriate in such cases. The continual reassessment method (CRM) [56] is a novel alternative design for phase I dose-finding studies. CRM phase I design uses the statistical model to update the estimated the DLT rate of each dose level, and determine the dose level for the next patient after observing each patient's DLT status at a given dose level, with all previous patients' data incorporated. As therapies become increasingly targeted, with reduced off-target effects (i.e. toxicity), the primary goal of many phase I trials is also changing towards defining a biologically optimal dose (BOD)—a dose that has maximal efficacy with acceptable toxicity. Modified CRM designs to identify the BOD, and other newer phase I designs have been proposed and developed [57–59].

It is well recognized that the long time period and high cost of conducting clinical trials is problematic. One appealing novel design is to combine phase II and III stages by conducting phase II/III studies. Theoretically, by streamlining the plan and conduct of the study, and allowing the inclusion of phase II patients into the phase III analysis, efficiency can be enhanced. Although the overall type I rate and power need special treatment, by adjusting the sample size and carefully formulating the decision rules in both phase II and III components, there are several flexible approaches to apply this design. Different designs can be used in the phase II portion, including single-arm efficacy analysis (e.g., a phase II/III study testing FOLFIRINOX versus gemcitabine in metastatic pancreatic cancer [60]), screening design (e.g., CALGB-80802 [61]),

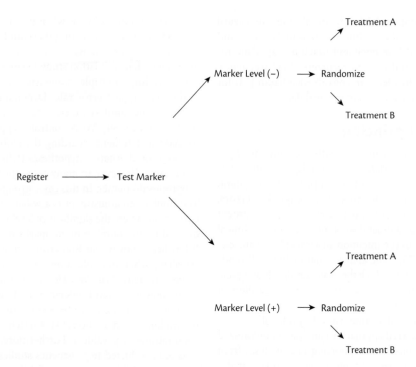

Fig. 24.2 Treatment-by-marker interaction designs as in [53].

Reproduced with permission from Sargent DJ, Conley BA, Allegra C, Collette L, Clinical trial designs for predictive marker validation in cancer treatment trials, *Journal of Clinical Oncology*, Volume 23, Issue 9, pp. 2020–2027, Copyright © 2005 American Society of Clinical Oncology.

and a selection design (CALGB-30610 [62]). Furthermore, different design aspects such as assessing multiple primary endpoints, mixtures of non-inferiority and superiority, or inclusion of multidimensional interim looks can be accommodated in this design (e.g., the Alliance intermediate risk rectal trial [63]).

To further streamline clinical trials, adaptive designs have been increasingly proposed. An important difference in adaptive design from traditional phase III randomized design is that this design can address more than one question through prespecified ongoing modification of the trial based on accumulating data [64]. Adaptations can include adding or dropping arms/doses, changing the proportion of patients randomized to each arm, adaptively defining an indication or responder population, and seamlessly transitioning between phases of clinical trials [65]. I-SPY2 [66, 67] is an example of an adaptive study aimed at prospectively identifying efficacious compounds in biomarker-defined patient populations. Multiple compounds from different drug companies and multiple biomarkers are being tested. Throughout the trial, the design algorithm continuously calculates the predictive probability of each regimen being successful in a 300-patient phase III confirmatory trial.

Based on the growing role of biomarkers in clinical trials, novel trial designs for validating prognostic and predictive biomarkers are in active development. The clinical utility of a predictive biomarker is to determine whether an individual patient will respond to a particular therapy or not, which can guide the individualized therapy [68]. Prospective designs include enrichment designs (only patients with biomarker-positive status will be studied) [69], treatment-by-marker interaction designs (patients with valid biomarker tests, both positive and negative, are randomized within each biomarker strata) [68, 70] (see Figure 24.2), marker-based strategy designs, and adaptive designs [68, 71].

Analysis of clinical trials

Among experiments in medical research, it is likely the case that clinical trials are the ones with the largest portion of effort expanded in the planning stage. A prospectively defined clinical trial protocol includes a carefully formulated statistical design, a well-planned assessment schedule and method for outcomes classification, well-established data monitoring and reporting programs, etc. As such, proper experimental design and execution tend to simplify the data analysis tasks, which in turn strengthen the evidence a clinical trial can deliver. Hence, analysis of clinical trial data can often follow basic and common statistical methods. For standard endpoints, depending on their nature, the commonly used statistical tests or regression techniques can be used to compare endpoints between groups and assess the associations between endpoints and other baseline factors, respectively. For example, the two sample t-test and chi-squared test are suitable to compare continuous and binary endpoints between treatment groups, respectively. Multivariate logistic regression is useful to assess the treatment effect on binary endpoints adjusting for confounders. When the primary endpoint is a time-to-event outcome (e.g. OS), log-rank and Cox proportional hazards models are used for simple comparison and association analysis, respectively. In addition, confidence intervals with a prespecified confidence level (e.g. 95% = (1–0.05) × 100%, where 0.05 is the significance level) are often used to give the interval estimate of the treatment effect. The length of the confidence interval provides an idea of the precision of the point estimate and strongly depends on sample size. The interpretation of a 95% confidence interval of a hazard ratio comparing overall survival times between two treatment groups is that, over the collection of all 95% confidence intervals that could be constructed from repeated random samples, 95% will contain the true hazard ratio. We refer readers for further technical details to Armitage and Berry [4], Everitt [72], and Campbell and Machin [73]. Time-to-event endpoints (e.g., OS and time to recurrence) are frequently used in oncology studies. Readers can consult Kleinbaum [74] for complete introduction to the analysis of survival data.

Intention-to-treat principle

The findings of a clinical trial can be sensitive to how investigators handle imperfections in data, for example non-adherence to protocol treatment, missing and incomplete measurement, non-protocol-specified treatment cross-overs, eligibility errors, follow-up dropouts, etc. Among these data imperfections, treatment non-adherence has received a great deal of attention in the clinical trial literatures. This leads to the intention-to-treat (ITT) principle, as stated by Fisher et al. [75]: 'The analysis that includes all randomized patients in the groups to which they were randomly assigned, regardless of their adherence with the entry criteria, regardless of the treatment they actually received, and regardless of subsequent withdrawal from treatment or deviation from the protocol.'

ITT has become the preferred approach to analysing randomized clinical trials based on a consensus supporting ITT analyses from statistical and clinical perspectives. An alternative to an ITT analysis is the per-protocol analysis, where patients are analysed according to the treatment actually received, even if the randomization called for something else. Per-protocol analysis has been shown to be potentially misleading and may confuse rather than help the interpretation of results, since there might be confounders which are associated with patients' adherence or non-adherence to the treatment [76] such as other treatments, disease status, lifestyle, or other unknown factors. For these reasons, the ITT analysis has been suggested as the standard analysis for a randomized clinical trial by several authors [77, 78]. Lagakos et al. [79] also showed that the size of an ITT analysis is not distorted by early treatment termination, although a loss of power can occur. From a clinical standpoint, the reasons for exclusion of patients due to non-adherence are frequently associated with prognosis or can affect the treatment groups differently. Although per-protocol analysis may be a better method in some circumstances, for example a non-inferiority design, or if required by a certain biological question, it should generally not be considered as the primary analysis of a randomized clinical trial.

Control for multiple comparisons

Within a clinical trial, besides the primary endpoint, several secondary endpoints are also generally prospectively specified to address questions beyond the primary objective. In addition, there might be one or more correlative studies which examine the prognostic value of genetic, pathological, or imaging biomarkers, for example. In this sense, clinical trial data often lend themselves to exploratory or hypothesis-generating analyses. Multiple endpoint analyses lead to multiple uses of the same data, i.e. multiple comparisons. The major problem associated with multiple comparisons is the inflation of type I (false positive) errors. If a nominal significance level is set to be 5%, two independent comparisons will increase the overall type I error rate of detecting at least one significant result to 9.8%, and three comparisons will increase it to 14.3%. Multiple comparisons also frequently arise when subgroup analyses are carried out. Hence, investigators must be aware

of these types of problems when performing exploratory analyses. A good practice in reporting these findings is to acknowledge the hypothesis-generating nature of the analysis and always carry out an independent validation study to confirm the results.

Controlling multiple comparisons refers to controlling the family-wise type I error rate. Depending on what inferences are intended, the family-wise error rate can be controlled in the *weak* or *strong* sense [80]. Weak control is appropriate only if one wants to make a statement regarding the global null hypothesis against any kind of alternative hypotheses (where the deviance lies is not important). However, in many cases, the specific differences among subgroups do matter. In this case, strong control should be applied. The Bonferroni adjustment is a widely used multiple comparisons correction, where the significance level is set to be the nominal level divided by the number of comparisons planned to be conducted. It has been shown that Bonferroni adjustment is too conservative, especially when multiple comparisons are correlated to each other. Improved methods include Holm [81] and Hommel [82] procedures (more powerful than Bonferroni method), fixed-sequential testing methods [83] (based on prespecified sequence of hypotheses), and resampling-based methods [84, 85] (which release the distributional assumptions of p-values). Furthermore, when a large number of tests are conducted (e.g., genetics studies), control of the false discovery rate [86] is a more powerful (i.e. more liberal) method.

Conclusions

In this chapter we addressed several key statistical issues associated with clinical trials. It should be recognized that a clinical trial is often a moving target. Decisions regarding modification and termination of a trial can (and will) be influenced by the advancing knowledge gained over the course of the study, both internally and externally. Communication and collaboration among the investigators and statisticians throughout the conduct of a trial are thus critical. Essential discussions between these experts involve the key questions to the practical planning and conduct of a study, including what the targeted disease population is, how 'success' is defined, what the clinical meaningful treatment effect is, and what the existing knowledge of the new regimen may be. With the discovery of genetic signatures and biological pathways, biomarker-directed therapy has an increasing role in oncology therapeutic research. Innovative clinical trial design is needed. By building an understanding of the principles and methods in clinical trial design with increasing experience with clinical trial principles, progress toward more effective therapeutic development can be accelerated.

Further reading

Berry DA. Adaptive clinical trials in oncology. Nature Reviews Clinical Oncology 2012; 9: 199–207.Campbell MJ, Machin D, editors. Medical Statistics. New York 1990.

Goulart BH, Clark JW, Pien HH, Roberts TG, Finkelstein SN et al. Trends in the use and role of biomarkers in phase I oncology trials. Clinical Cancer Research 2007; 13(22 Pt 1): 6719–6726.

Mandrekar SJ, Sargent DJ. Clinical trial designs for predictive biomarker validation: theoretical considerations and practical challenges. Journal of Clinical Oncology 2009; 27(24): 4027–4034.

Piantadosi S ed. Clinical Trials: A methodological perspective. New York: Wiley, 1997.

Ratain MJ, Sargent DJ. Optimising the design of phase II oncology trials: the importance of randomisation. European Journal of Cancer 2009; 45(2): 275–280.

Rogatko A, Schoeneck D, Jonas W, Tighiouart M, Khuri FR et al. Translation of innovative designs into phase I trials. Journal of Clinical Oncology 2007; 25(31): 4982–4986.

Rubin EH, Gilliland DG. Drug development and clinical trials: the path to an approved cancer drug. Nature Reviews Clinical Oncology 2012; 9(4): 215–222.

Sargent DJ, Goldberg RM. A flexible design for multiple armed screening trials. Statistics in Medicine 2001; 20(7): 1051–1060.

Shi Q, Sargent DJ. Meta-analysis for the evaluation of surrogate endpoints in cancer clinical trials. International Journal of Clinical Oncology 2009; 14(2): 102–111.

References

1. Siegel R, Naishadham D, Jemal A. Cancer statistics, 2012. CA: A Cancer Journal for Clinicians 2012; 62(1): 10–29.

2. Arrowsmith J. Trial watch: phase III and submission failures: 2007–2010. Nature Reviews Drug Discovery 2011; 10(2): 87.

3. Piantadosi S ed. Clinical Trials: A methodological perspective. New York: Wiley, 1997.

4. Armitage P, Berry G eds. Statistical methods in medical research. 3rd ed. Oxford: Blackwell, 1994.

5. Marubini E, Valsecchi MG eds. Analyzing survival data from clinical trials and observational studies: John Wiley & Sons, Inc.; 1995.

6. Goldberg RM, Kaufmann SH, Atherton P, Sloan JA, Adjei AA et al. A phase I study of sequential irinotecan and 5-fluorouracil/leucovorin. Annals of Oncology 2002; 13(10): 1674–1680.

7. Rogatko A, Schoeneck D, Jonas W, Tighiouart M, Khuri FR et al. Translation of innovative designs into phase I trials. Journal of Clinical Oncology 2007; 25(31): 4982–4986.

8. Rubin EH, Gilliland DG. Drug development and clinical trials: the path to an approved cancer drug. Nature Reviews Clinical Oncology 2012; 9(4): 215–222.

9. Goulart BH, Clark JW, Pien HH, Roberts TG, Finkelstein SN et al. Trends in the use and role of biomarkers in phase I oncology trials. Clinical Cancer Research 2007; 13(22 Pt 1): 6719–6726.

10. Simon R. Optimal two-stage designs for phase II clinical trials. Controlled Clinical Trials 1989; 10(1): 1–10.

11. Gehan EA. The determinatio of the number of patients required in a preliminary and a follow-up trial of a new chemotherapeutic agent. Journal of Chronic Diseases 1961; 13: 346–353.

12. Herson J. Predictive probability early termination plans for phase II clinical trials. Biometrics 1979; 35(4): 775–783.

13. Fleming TR. One-sample multiple testing procedure for phase II clinical trials. Biometrics 1982; 38(1): 143–151.

14. Chang MN, Therneau TM, Wieand HS, Cha SS. Designs for group sequential phase II clinical trials. Biometrics 1987; 43(4): 865–874.

15. Therneau TM, Wieand HS, Chang MN. Optimal designs for a grouped sequential binomial trial. Biometrics 1990; 46: 771–781.

16. Thall PF, Simon RM, Estey EH. Bayesian sequential monitoring designs for single-arm clinical trials with multiple outcomes. Statistics in Medicine 1995; 14(4): 357–379.

17. Tang H, Foster NR, Grothey A, Ansell SM, Goldberg RM et al. Comparison of error rates in single-arm versus randomized phase II cancer clinical trials. Journal of Clinical Oncology 2010; 28(11): 1936–1941.

18. Ratain MJ, Sargent DJ. Optimising the design of phase II oncology trials: the importance of randomisation. European Journal of Cancer 2009; 45(2): 275–280.

19. Simon R, Wittes RE, Ellenberg SS. Randomized phase II clinical trials. Cancer Treatment Reports 1985; 69(12): 1375–1381.

20. Sargent DJ, Goldberg RM. A flexible design for multiple armed screening trials. Statistics in Medicine 2001; 20(7): 1051–1060.

21. Rubinstein LV, Korn EL, Freidlin B, Hunsberger S, Ivy SP et al. Design issues of randomized phase II trials and a proposal for phase II screening trials. Journal of Clinical Oncology 2005; 23(28): 7199–7206.

22. Lachin JM. Properties of simple randomization in clinical trials. Controlled Clinical Trials 1988; 9(4): 312–326.

23. Lachin JM. Statistical properties of randomization in clinical trials. Controlled Clinical Trials 1988; 9(4): 289–311.

24. Garrett AD. Therapeutic equivalence: fallacies and falsification. Statistics in Medicine 2003; 22(5): 741–762.

25. Blackwelder WC. 'Proving the null hypothesis' in clinical trials. Controlled Clinical Trials 1982; 3(4): 345–353.

26. Greene WL, Concato J, Feinstein AR. Claims of equivalence in medical research: are they supported by the evidence? Annals of Internal Medicine 2000; 132(9): 715–722.

27. Costa LJ, Xavier AC, del Giglio A. Negative results in cancer clinical trials—equivalence or poor accrual? Controlled Clinical Trials 2004; 25(5): 525–533.

28. Zelen M. The randomization and stratification of patients to clinical trials. Journal of Chronic Diseases 1974; 27(7–8): 365–375.

29. Buyse M. Centralized treatment allocation in comparative clinical trials. Applied Clinical Trials 2000; 1: 32–37.

30. Feinstein AR, Landis JR. The role of prognostic stratification in preventing the bias permitted by random allocation of treatment. Journal of Chronic Diseases 1976; 29(4): 277–284.

31. Birkett NJ. Adaptive allocation in randomized controlled trials. Controlled Clinical Trials 1985; 6(2): 146–155.

32. Green SB, Byar DP. The effect of stratified randomization on size and power of statistical tests in clinical trials. Journal of Chronic Diseases 1978; 31(6–7): 445–454.

33. Lachin JM, Bautista OM. Stratified-adjusted versus unstratified assessment of sample size and power for analyses of proportions. Cancer Treat Research 1995; 75: 203–223.

34. Nam JM. Sample size determination in stratified trials to establish the equivalence of two treatments. Statistics in Medicine 1995; 14(18): 2037–2049.

35. Armitage P, Gehan EA. Statistical methods for the identification and use of prognostic factors. International Journal of Cancer 1974; 13(1): 16–36.

36. Makuch RW, Johnson MF eds. Biostatistical considerations for head and neck cancer research. Boston: tinus Jijhoff, 1985.

37. Psaty BM, Prentice RL. Minimizing bias in randomized trials: the importance of blinding. Journal of the American Medical Association 2010; 304(7): 793–794.

38. Hrobjartsson A, Gotzsche PC. Is the placebo powerless? An analysis of clinical trials comparing placebo with no treatment. New England Journal of Medicine 2001; 344(21): 1594–1602.

39. Guyatt GH, Pugsley SO, Sullivan MJ, Thompson PJ, Berman L et al. Effect of encouragement on walking test performance. Thorax 1984; 39(11): 818–822.

40. Boutron I, Estellat C, Guittet L, Dechartres A, Sackett DL et al. Methods of blinding in reports of randomized controlled trials assessing pharmacologic treatments: a systematic review. PLoS Medicine 2006; 3(10): e425.

41. Boutron I, Guittet L, Estellat C, Moher D, Hrobjartsson A et al. Reporting methods of blinding in randomized trials assessing nonpharmacological treatments. PLoS Medicine 2007; 4(2): e61.

42. Shi Q, Sargent DJ. Meta-analysis for the evaluation of surrogate endpoints in cancer clinical trials. International Journal of Clinical Oncology 2009; 14(2): 102–111.

43. Biomarkers and surrogate endpoints: preferred definitions and conceptual framework. Clinical Pharmacology & Therapeutics 2001; 69(3): 89–95.

44. Freedman LS, Graubard BI, Schatzkin A. Statistical validation of intermediate endpoints for chronic diseases. Statistics in Medicine 1992; 11(2): 167–178.

45. Lin DY, Fleming TR, De Gruttola V. Estimating the proportion of treatment effect explained by a surrogateker. Statistics in Medicine 1997; 16(13): 1515–1527.

46. Ghosh D. On assessing surrogacy in a single trial setting using a semicompeting risks paradigm. Biometrics 2009; 65(2): 521–529.

47. Frangakis CE, Rubin DB. Principal stratification in causal inference. Biometrics 2002; 58(1): 21–29.

48. Daniels MJ, Hughes MD. Meta-analysis for the evaluation of potential surrogatekers. Statistics in Medicine 1997; 16(17): 1965–1982.

49. Buyse M, Molenberghs G, Burzykowski T, Renard D, Geys H. The validation of surrogate endpoints in meta-analyses of randomized experiments. Biostatistics 2000; 1(1): 49–67.

50. Burzykowski T, Molenberghs G, Buyse M, Geys H, Renard D. Validation of surrogate end points in multiple randomized clinical trials with failure time end points. Applied Statistics 2001; 50(4): 405–422.

51. Burzykowski T, Buyse M. Surrogate threshold effect: an alternative measure for meta-analytic surrogate endpoint validation. Pharmaceutical Statistics 2006; 5(3): 173–186.

52. Lassere MN, Johnson KR, Boers M, Tugwell P, Brooks P et al. Definitions and validation criteria for biomarkers and surrogate endpoints: development and testing of a quantitative hierarchical levels of evidence schema. Journal of Rheumatology 2007; 34(3): 607–615.

53. Sargent DJ, Wieand HS, Haller DG, Gray R, Benedetti JK et al. Disease-free survival versus overall survival as a primary end point for adjuvant colon cancer studies: individual patient data from 20,898 patients on 18 randomized trials. Journal of Clinical Oncology 2005; 23(34): 8664–8670.

54. Buyse M, Burzykowski T, Carroll K, Michiels S, Sargent DJ et al. Progression-free survival is a surrogate for survival in advanced colorectal cancer. Journal of Clinical Oncology 2007; 25(33): 5218–5224.

55. Burzykowski T, Buyse M, Piccart-Gebhart MJ, Sledge G, Carmichael J et al. Evaluation of tumor response, disease control, progression-free survival, and time to progression as potential surrogate end points in metastatic breast cancer. Journal of Clinical Oncology 2008; 26(12): 1987–1992.

56. O'Quigley J, Pepe M, Fisher L. Continual reassessment method: a practical design for phase 1 clinical trials in cancer. Biometrics 1990; 46(1): 33–48.

57. Thall PF, Millikan RE, Mueller P, Lee SJ. Dose-finding with two agents in Phase I oncology trials. Biometrics 2003; 59(3): 487–496.

58. Zhang W, Sargent DJ, Mandrekar S. An adaptive dose-finding design incorporating both toxicity and efficacy. Statistics in Medicine 2006; 25(14): 2365–2383.

59. Braun TM, Wang S. A hierarchical Bayesian design for phase I trials ofel combinations of cancer therapeutic agents. Biometrics 2010; 66(3): 805–812.

60. Conroy T, Desseigne F, Ychou M, Bouche O, Guimbaud R et al. FOLFIRINOX versus gemcitabine for metastatic pancreatic cancer. New England Journal of Medicine 2011; 364(19): 1817–1825.

61. [CALGB-80802] US National Library of Medicine. ClinicalTrials.gov [online] Sorafenib tosylate with or without doxorubicin hydrochloride in treating patients with locally advanced or metastatic liver cancer, 2012. Available from: <http://clinicaltrials.gov/show/NCT01015833>, accessed on 15 May 2015.

62. [CALGB-30610] US National Library of Medicine. ClinicalTrials.gov [online] Three different radiation therapy regimens in treating patients with limited-stage small cell lung cancer receiving cisplatin and etoposide, 2012.

63. Chemotherapy alone or chemotherapy plus radiation therapy in treating patients with locally advanced rectal cancer undergoing surgery, 2012. Available from: <http://clinicaltrials.gov/show/NCT01515787>, accessed on 15 May 2015.

64. Berry DA. Adaptive clinical trials in oncology. Nature Reviews Clinical Oncology 2012; 9: 199–207.

65. Chang M ed. Adaptive desing theory and implementation using SAS and R. Boca Raton, FL: Chapman & Hall/CRC, 2008.

66. Medicine IUNLo. 2011. Available from: <http://clinicaltrials.gov/ct2/show/NCT01042379>, accessed on 15 May 2015.

67. Barker AD, Sigman CC, Kelloff GJ, Hylton NM, Berry DA et al. I-SPY 2: an adaptive breast cancer trial design in the setting of neoadjuvant chemotherapy. Clinical Pharmacology & Therapeutics 2009; 86(1): 97–100.

68. Sargent DJ, Conley BA, Allegra C, Collette L. Clinical trial designs for predictiveker validation in cancer treatment trials. Journal of Clinical Oncology 2005; 23(9): 2020–2027.

69. McShane LM, Hunsberger S, Adjei AA. Effective incorporation of biomarkers into phase II trials. Clinical Cancer Research 2009; 15(6): 1898–1905.

70. Mandrekar SJ, Sargent DJ. Clinical trial designs for predictive biomarker validation: theoretical considerations and practical challenges. Journal of Clinical Oncology 2009; 27(24): 4027–4034.

71. Sargent D, Allegra C. Issues in clinical trial design for tumorker studies. Seminars in Oncology 2002; 29(3): 222–230.

72. Everitt BS ed. Statistical methods for medical investigations. New York: Hodder Arnold, 1989.

73. Campbell MJ, Machin D eds. Medical Statistics. New York: Wiley, 1990.

74. Kleinbaum DG ed. Survival analysis: a self-learning text. New York: Springer, 1996.

75. Fisher LD, Dixon DO, Herson J, eds. Intention-to-treat in clinical trials. In Peace KE ed, Statistical Issues in Drug Research and Development. New York: Marcel Dekker, 1990, 331–350.

76. Influence of adherence to treatment and response of cholesterol on mortality in the coronary drug project. New England Journal of Medicine 1980; 303(18): 1038–1041.

77. Lee YJ, Ellenberg JH, Hirtz DG, Nelson KB. Analysis of clinical trials by treatment actually received: is it really an option? Statistics in Medicine 1991; 10(10): 1595–1605.

78. Peduzzi P, Wittes J, Detre K, Holford T. Analysis as-randomized and the problem of non-adherence: an example from the Veterans Affairs Randomized Trial of Coronary Artery Bypass Surgery. Statistics in Medicine 1993; 12(13): 1185–1195.

79. Lagakos SW, Lim LL, Robins JM. Adjusting for early treatment termination in comparative clinical trials. Statistics in Medicine 1990; 9(12): 1417–1424; discussion 33–37.

80. Westfull PH, Wolfinger RD. Closed multiple testing procedures and PROC MULTTEST. Observations: Technical Journal for SAS Software Users 23. Available from: <http://support.sas.com/documentation/periodical/obs/obswww232000>.

81. Holm S. A simple sequentially rejective multiple test procedure. Scandinavian Journal of Statistics 1979; 6: 65–70.

82. Hommel G. A stagewise rejective multiple procedure based on a modified Bonferroni test. Biometrika 1988; 75: 383–386.

83. Hsu JC, Berger RL. Stepwise confidence intervals without multiplicity adjustment for dose-response and toxicity studies. Journal of the American Statistical Association 1999; 94: 468–482.

84. Westfull PH, Young SS. P-value adjustment for multiple tests in multivariate binomial models. Journal of the American Statistical Association 1989; 84: 780–786.

85. Westfull PH, Tobias RD, Rom D, Tobias R eds. Multiple comparisons and multiple tests using the SAS system. Cary, NC: SAS Institute, 1999.

86. Benjamini Y, Hochberg Y. Controlling the false discovery rate: a new and powerful approach to multiple testing. Journal of the Royal Statistical Society, Series B 1995; 57: 1289–1300.

CHAPTER 25

Medical ethics in oncology

Eric A. Singer

Introduction to medical ethics

The ethical practice of medicine is often taken for granted by physicians, our colleagues, and our patients. It is assumed that as members of a learned profession, doctors instinctively understand how to dissect complex ethical dilemmas and fulfil the expressed and implied standards of the Hippocratic tradition [1]. This is assumed despite the remarkable advances in both diagnostic and therapeutic technology that would make contemporary medical practice seem unrecognizable to physicians of 100 years ago, let alone the fifth century BC. Fortunately, the ethical underpinnings of medicine remain unchanged: alleviating suffering, avoiding harm, and a healing relationship based on trust [2]. The aim of this chapter is to examine several areas of ethics that are of particular concern to oncologists.

Ethics in oncology

For most practitioners, ethics was taught in medical school or at university prior to the decision to pursue career specialization; we were not yet oncologists or urologists or paediatricians. The fundamentals to which we were exposed should still serve us well, but it can be helpful to explore subspecialty-specific dilemmas that occur with increased frequency. Given the central role that clinical trials play in oncology, this chapter will highlight some of issues involved with human subject research and the sequelae of advances in translational research and novel therapeutics. The reader will also gain valuable knowledge from several other chapters within this text that focus on complementary topics including clinical trial design, health care economics, cancer screening and prevention, and palliative care and supportive oncology (see Chapters 24, 26–30, and 33–35).

Research ethics

Ethics is more often about balancing competing principles or goods than simply choosing between right and wrong or good and bad. In the realm of clinical oncology research, the desire to generate knowledge and identify new or improved therapies is a compelling good. However, research involving human subjects includes a genuine risk of harm. To help establish a framework within which to examine conflicts in research ethics, one can turn to a collection of international statements that were written in response to severe ethical lapses with the goal of preventing future abuses.

The Nuremberg Code, written in 1947 in response to the atrocities performed by Nazi doctors during World War II, emphasizes the primacy of obtaining voluntary consent from all research participants and the importance of using human subjects only when the research results will benefit society and are not otherwise obtainable [3, 4]. The Declaration of Helsinki, adopted in 1964 and most recently updated by the World Medical Association in 2008, focuses on physicians performing research with patients and states that 'the well-being of the individual research subject must take precedence over all other interests' [5]. The seventh update of the Declaration of Helsinki was updated in 2013. Readers are encouraged to visit the World Medical Association's website at <www.wma.net> to review the latest iteration of this important document, which is published on the website of the Journal of American Medical Association (JAMA). In the United States, the Belmont Report, issued in 1979, emphasizes the principles of respect for persons, beneficence, and justice when evaluating the ethical nature of human subjects research [6]. Despite the guidance offered in these and other codes of research ethics, there has not been a widely acknowledged, comprehensive framework that is universal in its applicability [7].

Requirements for ethical research

Emanuel and colleagues describe seven requirements for the conduct of ethical clinical research in their seminal paper published in 2000 [7]. These central tenets include: (1) social or scientific value; (2) scientific validity; (3) fair subject selection; (4) favourable risk–benefit ratio; (5) independent review; (6) informed consent; and (7) respect for potential and enrolled subjects. Table 25.1 defines each of these seven requirements, lists the supporting ethical framework for their inclusion, and describes the skill set needed to evaluate whether each requirement has been met.

Some of the advantages of this rubric are that the seven requirements for ethical human subjects research are applicable to studies performed in economically developed as well as developing countries; that they are relevant to trials examining diagnosis, treatment, or prevention in both oncology and non-oncology domains; and that they encapsulate the values and priorities of multiple international statements on the ethical conduct of research without having been created in response to a specific crisis or incident [7]. Despite these benefits, questions about research ethics persist. Several contemporary concerns include clinical cancer research involving phase I trials, placebo-controlled trials, and the use of mandatory research biopsies.

Phase I trials

The primary endpoints for phase I oncology studies are to characterize the safety, tolerability, and side effects associated with novel therapies. Response to treatment, such as reduction in tumour size or number, improvement in disease symptoms, or prolonged

Table 25.1 Seven requirements for determining whether a research trial is ethical

Requirement	Explanation	Justifying ethical values	Expertise for evaluation
Social or scientific value	Evaluation of a treatment, intervention, or theory that will improve health and well-being or increase knowledge	Scarce resources and non-exploitation	Scientific knowledge; citizen's understanding of social priorities
Scientific validity	Use of accepted scientific principles and methods, including statistical techniques, to produce reliable and valid data	Scarce resources and non-exploitation	Scientific and statistical knowledge; knowledge of condition and population to assess feasibility
Fair subject selection	Selection of subjects so that stigmatized and vulnerable individuals are not targeted for risky research and the rich and socially powerful not favoured for potentially beneficial research	Justice	Scientific knowledge; ethical and legal knowledge
Favourable risk–benefit ratio	Minimization of risks; enhancement of potential benefits; risks to the subject	Non-maleficence, beneficence, and non-exploitation	Scientific knowledge; citizen's understanding of social values are proportionate to the benefits to the subject and society
Independent review	Review of the design of the research trial, its proposed subject population, and risk–benefit ratio by individuals unaffiliated with the research	Public accountability; minimizing influence of potential conflicts of interest	Intellectual, financial, and otherwise independent researchers; scientific and ethical knowledge
Informed consent	Provision of information to subjects about purpose of the research, its procedures, potential risks, benefits, and alternatives, so that the individual understands this information and can make a voluntary decision whether to enrol and continue to participate	Respect for subject autonomy	Scientific knowledge; ethical and legal knowledge
Respect for potential and enrolled subjects	Respect for subjects by 1. Permitting withdrawal from the research 2. Protecting privacy through confidentiality 3. Informing subjects of newly discovered risks or benefits 4. Informing subjects of results of clinical research 5. Maintaining welfare of subjects.	Respect for subject autonomy and welfare	Scientific knowledge; ethical and legal knowledge; knowledge of particular subject population

*Ethical requirements are listed in chronological order from conception of research to its formulation and implementation.

Reproduced with permission from Emanuel EJ, Wendler D, Grady C. What makes clinical research ethical?, *Journal of American Medical Association*, Volume 283, Issue 20, pp. 2701–2711, Epub 2000/05/20, Copyright © 2000 American Medical Association. All rights reserved.

survival may be assessed as secondary endpoints but they are not the driving factor behind phase I trials. Concerns regarding the ethics of phase I oncology trials have been debated for more than 30 years [8–14].

The fundamental issues in this debate centre on a potentially unfavourable risk–benefit ratio (limited likelihood of benefit despite a considerable risk of toxicity) and the adequacy of the informed consent process required prior to study participation [8]. Despite these ethical concerns, phase I trials continue to be a critical aspect of oncology drug development and many large cancer centres have dedicated phase I or developmental therapeutics teams whose primary goal is to engage in translational and early human cancer studies.

A favourable risk–benefit ratio is one of the seven requirements for ethical research [7]. While making such a determination is not always straightforward, allowing oncology patients, many of whom have advanced disease that has failed to respond to approved therapies, to consider participating in a phase I trial that is evaluating a drug that is supported by encouraging preclinical evidence is reasonable. The likelihood of direct personal benefit is small, but so is the expected benefit from using a third- or fourth-line

standard chemotherapy for most malignancies. Additionally, the level of evidence supporting extended-line therapies is often weak as agents may lack a specific indication and are used off label. Lastly, these extended-line treatments come with definite toxicities that are often very similar to those expected in phase I trials. In fact, the American Society of Clinical Oncology (ASCO) in its statement on individualized care for patients with advanced cancer suggests that patients consider enrolling in a clinical trial so that they may 'gain access to promising new interventions when standard therapy has little to offer and to do so in a highly regulated setting that offers a chance to contribute to improvement in outcomes for future patients' [15].

Since direct patient benefit is not the primary goal of phase I oncology protocols, some critics contend that only patients who don't fully grasp the purpose of early oncology trials would be willing to enrol in them. Patients must mistakenly believe that the purpose of a given study is to provide them with personalized and effective cancer care rather than to generate medical knowledge that might help future patients. This scenario, which was first described in psychiatric research, is referred to as the therapeutic misconception [16, 17].

Pentz and colleagues sought to understand the prevalence of the therapeutic misconception among subjects enrolled in phase I oncology studies at an academic medical centre during the first month of trial participation [18]. Among research subjects they interviewed and surveyed, 68.4% of respondents (65 of 95 subjects) could not correctly describe that the purpose of phase I research is to produce generalizable knowledge rather than direct personal benefit and that the treatments provided on the trial were set by the protocol rather than individualized by their treating physician. When examining demographic factors that were associated with therapeutic misconception, these researchers found that lower education and lower family income correlated with an increased risk. However, they also noted that having limited treatment options was not associated with an increased likelihood of therapeutic misconception, indicating that cancer patients were not more likely to confuse the purpose and design of clinical research with standard treatment because of the lack of therapeutic choices. While there are numerous limitations to this small single-centre study, it demonstrates that the therapeutic misconception continues to be a challenge to the proper conduct of phase I research.

Rather than claiming that cancer patients cannot participate in phase I clinical trials because of the possibility of not understanding the purpose and methods of research, Wendler proposes a slightly different approach to dealing with the therapeutic misconception. While ensuring that potential research subjects understand the differences between standard clinical care and clinical research is important, he suggests that investigators focus their efforts on confirming that subjects understand the *specific facts* about the *specific protocol* they are considering [19]. This 'task-specific' approach concerns itself less with the general differences between routine clinical care and a clinical trial and instead works to have the research subject appreciate how his/her treatment, testing, follow-up, and potential for benefit/harm will change if an investigative approach is chosen over standard therapy.

The therapeutic misconception is a genuine problem in the conduct of ethical clinical cancer research, but as Pentz and colleagues and Wendler have shown, the fact that some patients have difficulty understanding or articulating the differences between clinical research and standard clinical care is not an insurmountable problem and should not result in a moratorium on early-phase oncology research. Increased attention to clear, readable, culturally competent informed consent documents, the use of patient/subject advocates, and attention to the specific differences between routine and experimental treatment in a specific protocol can help ensure that research subjects are choosing to enrol in clinical trials with the necessary information and for the right reasons [20].

Use of placebos

Prospective, randomized clinical trials are the foundation of modern oncology. However, when designing such a study, considerable attention must be paid to the comparison arm as well as the experimental arm. Should the comparison arm be the 'standard of care' or a placebo? The use of inactive controls in trials enrolling subjects with cancer diagnoses remains controversial.

Emanuel and Miller describe the placebo-controlled trial debate as one that focuses on two opposing and unwavering camps [21]. Proponents of placebo-controlled trials emphasize the methodological purity attainable when there is no active comparison arm. Since the purpose of clinical research is to create generalizable information, placebo-controlled studies are appealing in that the statistical analysis is much more straightforward and accurate. However, opponents of placebo use believe that an active control must always be used whenever one is available as a way of minimizing the risks of forgoing treatment for research subjects. Supporters of active controls often cite the Declaration of Helsinki, which requires new therapies always be tested against the best current therapy available [5]. In setting up these opposing 'orthodoxies', Emanuel and Miller offer a compromise as the best way forward. This middle ground permits placebo-controlled studies when there are strong methodological reasons for omitting active controls (assuming the study meets all seven criteria for ethical research listed above), it is clear that subjects who receive placebo will not suffer serious harm, and that the research protocol has adequate safeguards to minimize any risks associated with subjects receiving placebo rather than a standard, active therapy [21].

Within the realm of oncology trials specifically, placebo-controlled studies are ethically justifiable when studying a condition that has a high placebo response rate; that fluctuates in the severity of its symptoms; that has an unpredictable course; for which existing treatments are of little benefit or highly toxic; or in relation to which there is no recognized standard therapy for a specific disease state [22]. If one or more of these conditions are met, and a placebo is to be used, additional safeguards are required to ensure that those subjects randomized to receive placebo are not at an increased risk of death, serious harm, or severe discomfort [22]. The research protocol and informed consent process must clearly explain these safeguards and the likelihood with which subjects will receive the placebo.

Best supportive care should be offered to all research participants regardless of the study arm to which they are randomized, and a detailed supportive care management plan should be stipulated in the research protocol. The reader is referred to Chapters 32–34 in this volume for additional details about supportive oncology and palliative care. Similarly, careful selection of the clinical trial design, such as with a randomized discontinuation design, can help reduce the number of subjects exposed to placebo and allow crossover to the study drug or other standard therapies upon progression [23]. Detailed information about study design and analysis is available in Chapter 24.

Mandatory research biopsies

The growing emphasis on 'personalized' or 'precision' medicine has led to the inclusion of research biopsies in clinical trials with increasing frequency [24–27]. The purpose of these biopsies is to facilitate correlative science, such as identifying predictors of treatment response or resistance, and might be required at multiple time points during the trial. Increasing our understanding of biomarkers and targetable pathways is crucial to enhancing treatment options, but the vast majority of these benefits are years from fruition and are unlikely to benefit the research subject [28–31]. Therefore, the incorporation of mandatory research biopsies raises several questions pertaining to subject autonomy/informed consent and minimizing risks while maximizing potential benefits for trial participants [32, 33].

In order to examine the issue of mandatory oncology research biopsies with greater granularity, Peppercorn and colleagues describe three different types of biopsy: clinical biopsy; research biopsy for correlative science; and research biopsy for an integral biomarker study [34]. A clinical biopsy is performed as part of the routine diagnosis of most malignancies and provides a direct benefit to the patient by helping to determine the type of treatment needed. Unused portions of a clinical biopsy can be used for correlative science with the patient's consent via a tumour bank or biorepository. A research biopsy performed to evaluate for an integral biomarker may or may not provide benefit to the research subject. In this scenario the utility of the integral biomarker is what is under investigation and the biopsy is necessary to determine if the biomarker is present in a tumour. The integral biomarker biopsy will determine the subject's eligibility to participate in a trial, which might provide a benefit. Lastly, a biopsy for correlative science provides an unclear benefit to the patient and will not be used to determine trial eligibility or to drive standard patient care. Correlative science biopsies may be exploratory or used to answer a specific hypothesis. The concern regarding mandatory correlative research biopsies arises from the requirement that subjects consent to future invasive procedures with potentially significant risks and no potential direct benefits in order to participate in a clinical trial now [35].

In order to further elucidate the risks associated with oncology research biopsies, Overman and colleagues examined the complication rates seen at their comprehensive cancer centre during a five-year period [36]. They identified 38 trials that required at least one mandatory research biopsy. Analysis of tumour tissue was a study endpoint in 95% of the trials. The primary reason for a research biopsy was for integral biomarker analysis or correlative science in 32% and 68% of the studies, respectively. In terms of complications from 745 biopsies, overall and major complication rates were 5.2% and 0.8%, respectively. However, among 211 thoracic or 189 abdominal/pelvic biopsies the complication rates increased to 17.1% and 1.6%, respectively. Overman and colleagues concluded by calling for improved informed consent documents that explicitly state the lack of benefit and investigative nature of non-integral biomarker biopsies and to provide organ or body-site-specific complication rates to help potential subjects understand the risks involved with research biopsies.

A recent position statement from ASCO provides five conditions that must be met in order ethically to justify the added risk associated with the inclusion of a mandatory research biopsy in a clinical trial [34]. These conditions include: (1) strong scientific rationale—a properly powered and independently reviewed protocol; (2) adequate informed consent—nature of the research, type of biopsy to be done, lack of direct benefit, and description of risk are clearly explained; (3) risk minimization—use of the least invasive technique targeting the safest site; (4) timing—combine research biopsies with other routine tests/procedures; (5) lack of other options—study cannot be performed without mandatory biopsies from all research subjects (e.g., analysing previously obtained tissue, using optional biopsies, or using another tissue source such as circulating tumour cells, etc.).

The need for correlative and translation science will continue to grow as the role of targeted therapies expands into new disease states. Likewise, clinical oncology research will continue to be possible because research subjects decide that the known risks and potential benefits of participating in cancer research have been minimized and maximized, respectively. Mandatory research biopsies are ethically permissible but must be considered the method of last resort and undertaken with great care so that research subjects are protected and empowered to make an informed decision.

Oncology drug shortages and the cost of cancer care

In addition to the myriad dilemmas pertaining to the ethical conduct of clinical oncology research, some of which are described above, there are two significant issues related to approved or standard of care oncology drugs that are occurring with greater frequency. The first is shortages of once readily available oncology medications and the second is the rapidly increasing cost of oncology treatments and technologies.

Managing oncology drug shortages

Becker and colleagues examined the incidence of oncology drug shortages at their urban, academic cancer centre from April to September 2010 and again in 2011 [37]. They found that 12 oncology drugs were in shortage in 2010 while the number increased to 22 in 2011. During the 2011 study period, nearly 10% of oncology patients had documented therapy changes due to the limited availability of chemotherapeutics compared to zero changes in 2010. In surveying their centre's oncologists, 30.4% felt these alternative regimens were less evidence-based and 34.8% believed they came with an increased risk of toxicity. While this is only an illustrative example, oncology drug shortages are a reality and a management plan should be developed in advance of an actual crisis [38].

Rosoff and colleagues logically state that the first step in dealing with an oncology drug shortage is to maximize efficiency and minimize waste [39, 40]. When this is inadequate to alleviate the shortage, they suggest using the 'accountability for reasonableness' process created by Daniels and Sabin to develop a rationing schema [41, 42]. Box 25.1 lists and defines the four ethical requirements of the accountability for reasonableness rationing system: (1) relevance, (2) transparency, (3) revision, and (4) enforcement.

Since the cause, duration, and scope of oncology drug shortages are constantly in flux, medical centres and oncologists should create their management strategies well in advance of an actual shortage. Table 25.2 describes factors that Valgus and colleagues believe should be considered when developing a response to oncology drug shortages. These factors include: (1) drug indication, (2) patient goals of care, (3) patient cycle of treatment, (4) presence of suitable alternative agents, (5) medical necessity, (6) informed consent, and (7) timing of the policy [43]. Rationing standard, conventional chemotherapeutics may seem jarring in the age of targeted therapies and novel biologics. However, failing to develop and implement a logical, just, prospective plan that includes the input of physicians, nurses, pharmacists, social workers, ethics committee members, and patient representatives is ill advised and could lead to suboptimal as well as unethical treatment decisions.

Cost of cancer care

In keeping with issues of access to cancer care, the costs of treatment are a significant barrier to many patients [44–47]. The proliferation of expensive targeted therapies, biologics, new radiation delivery methods, and robotic-assisted surgery has the potential to markedly increase the overall, as well as out-of-pocket, costs of cancer treatment. While this type of dilemma is largely dependent upon the type of healthcare system in which a patient finds him or herself, some of the ethical questions that arise have broad appeal. Namely, what should the role of the oncologist be in managing the

Table 25.2 Factors to consider when faced with an oncology drug shortage

Indication	**Approved indication versus off-label use**
	Patients being treated with a medication that has an approved indication for their condition should receive priority over off-label uses of a shortage drug.
	First-line versus subsequent-line
	Patients receiving first-line therapy should receive priority over patients getting second- and subsequent-line therapy.
Goals of care	**Curative intent versus palliation**
	Patients who may be cured of their disease should receive a shortage drug over those who are not curable or who are using the drug for palliation. Best supportive care should be offered to all patients regardless of goals of care, treatment indication, or line of therapy.
Cycle of treatment	**Ongoing regimen versus treatment plan being developed**
	Patients who have started a treatment regimen should receive a shortage drug over those who have not yet started therapy in order to avoid a situation where a patient receives the toxicity of therapy, and possibly that of another agent, but is not able to receive the potential benefit of a full course of the originally intended treatment.
Suitable alternatives	**Alternative approved and available versus not**
	Patients who may be treated with multiple regimens supported by high levels of medical evidence should be encouraged to choose the medication or combination of medications that avoids or uses the least amount of the shortage drug.
Ability to pay	Medical necessity should trump the patient's insurance status/financial resources when making allocation decisions. Drug hoarding, gray- or black-market purchases, price gouging, and bidding wars are unethical. Market forces certainly do affect healthcare and oncology, but they should not determine how healthcare providers handle oncology drug shortages.
Informed consent	Coping with a cancer diagnosis and treatment is extremely difficult when all recommended options are available. The stress, anxiety, and frustration our patients feel because of oncology drug shortages must be considered.
	In order for patients to make an informed treatment decision, oncologists must communicate:
	♦ what treatment is recommended
	♦ how a shortage will be managed
	♦ likely ramifications of a treatment disruption
	♦ whether alternative treatments, such as surgery, radiation, or another drug/regimen are available.
Policy timing	**Proactive versus reactive**
	Oncology drug shortages are a reality and will continue to challenge practitioners and patients alike. Congress and specialty societies are aware of the issue and working to lessen the likelihood of future events. However, each health system, medical centre, and practice must proactively develop plans for how to deal with oncology drug shortages.
	These plans, like those in place to manage a mass casualty incident, natural disaster, or a pandemic flu outbreak, should be informed by the best science available, be created with the input of diverse stakeholders (physicians, nurses, pharmacists, social workers, patient representatives, ethics committees, etc.), and be regularly reviewed and updated.

economic impact of a cancer diagnosis on the individual patient as well as the healthcare system as a whole?

ASCO's guidance statement on the cost of cancer care suggests a multifaceted approach to this problem [48]. It states that, on the individual patient level, oncologists must continue to strive to provide each patient with the best evidence-based care available. However, when competing therapies with similar efficacy and toxicity are available, it is reasonable to disclose this fact and allow cost to help inform treatment recommendations. Likewise, patients may reasonably decline a proven therapy, even one that might prolong their lives, because of the high associated out-of-pocket costs. As an oncology community, quality of life, cost-effectiveness, and survival metrics need to be incorporated into clinical trials whenever possible so that discussions about the cost of cancer care can be based on much more robust data than are presently available.

Oncology specialists may be asked to advise government health agencies, healthcare organizations, or insurance companies as these bodies set policy or make coverage determinations. Their recommendations should be based on the best science available,

transparent to all stakeholders, mindful of existing health disparities, and include a robust review/appeal mechanism. The previously described 'accountability for reasonableness' model can serve as a useful framework for this type of project as well [41–43] (Box 25.1).

Oncology ethics resources

Shuman and colleagues recently reviewed the ethics consultation databases of two comprehensive cancer centres [49]. They identified 207 adult oncology ethics consultations performed between 2007 and 2011 and found that the most common issues pertained to code status and advanced directives (25%), surrogate decision-making (17%), and medical futility (13%). Additionally, they identified communication problems and interpersonal conflicts in 41% and 51% of cases, respectively. Unfortunately, this chapter cannot address all of these topics in detail. However, additional resources are available.

Tenner and Helft have published an annotated bibliography of oncology ethics literature that will enhance the ability of novices

---

Box 25.1 Putting ethical priority setting into practice

Relevance

◆ Develop a rationale for each priority-setting decision.

◆ Use decision criteria based on your mission, vision, and values.

◆ Collect data/information related to each criterion.

◆ Consult with internal/external stakeholders to ensure relevance of decision criteria and to collect relevant information.

◆ Make decisions using a multidisciplinary group of informed stakeholders.

Transparency

◆ Communicate the decision and its rationale.

◆ Use an effective communication strategy to engage internal/external stakeholders around priority-setting goals, criteria, processes, and decisions.

Revision

◆ Incorporate opportunities for iterative decision review.

◆ Develop a formal decision-review process based on explicit decision-review criteria.

Enforcement

◆ Lead by example (i.e. ethical leadership).

◆ Evaluate and improve the priority-setting process.

---

and experts alike to handle the challenges of contemporary oncology practice [50]. Professional societies such as ASCO, the European Society of Medical Oncology, and the American Society for Bioethics and Humanities also have web-based content, position papers, and educational tracks at their annual meetings that can help augment practitioner knowledge and skill. Lastly, and perhaps most importantly, early ethics consultation can help address concerns or problems before they worsen and potentially place patients or research subjects at risk.

Conclusions

It is an exciting time to be an oncologist. However, despite the proliferation of novel treatments and the promise of precision medicine, conflicts between competing goods or obligations will continue to arise. This brief chapter has attempted to highlight several of the most common issues faced by oncology specialists in order to provide a framework for ethical reasoning. Readers are encouraged to examine the primary sources cited in this chapter so they may deepen their understanding of the ethical foundations of the practice of oncology.

Acknowledgements

I am indebted to Professors Raphael Catane and Nathan Cherny for their thoughtful review of this manuscript.

Further reading

Agrawal M, Emanuel EJ. Ethics of phase 1 oncology studies: reexamining the arguments and data. Journal of the American Medical Association 2003; 290(8): 1075–1082.

Daugherty CK, Ratain MJ, Siegler M. Pushing the envelope: informed consent in phase I trials. Annals of Oncology 1995; 6(4): 321–323.

Emanuel EJ, Wendler D, Grady C. What makes clinical research ethical? Journal of the American Medical Association 2000; 283(20): 2701–2711.

Meropol NJ, Schrag D, Smith TJ, Mulvey TM, Langdon RM, Jr. et al. American Society of Clinical Oncology guidance statement: the cost of cancer care. Journal of Clinical Oncology 2009; 27(23): 3868–3874.

Pellegrino ED. The internal morality of clinical medicine: a paradigm for the ethics of the helping and healing professions. Journal of Medicine and Philosophy 2001; 26(6): 559–579.

Pellegrino ED. The internal morality of clinical medicine: a paradigm for the ethics of the helping and healing professions. Journal of Medicine and Philosophy 2001; 26(6): 559–579.

Pellegrino ED. Professionalism, profession and the virtues of the good physician. Mount Sinai Journal of Medicine 2002; 69(6): 378–384.

Peppercorn J, Shapira I, Collyar D, Deshields T, Lin N et al. Ethics of mandatory research biopsy for correlative end points within clinical trials in oncology. Journal of Clinical Oncology 2010; 28(15): 2635–2640.

Tenner LL, Helft PR. Ethics in oncology: an annotated bibliography of important literature. Journal of Oncology Practice. 2013; ePub ahead of print. doi:10.1200/JOP.2012.000679

Valgus J, Singer EA, Berry SR, Rathmell WK. Ethical challenges: managing oncology drug shortages. Journal of Oncology Practice 2013; 9(2): e21–e23.

Wendler DS. Time to stop worrying about the therapeutic misconception. Journal of Clinical Ethics 2012; 23(3): 272–287.

References

1. Pellegrino ED. Professionalism, profession and the virtues of the good physician. Mount Sinai Journal of Medicine 2002; 69(6): 378–384.
2. Pellegrino ED. The internal morality of clinical medicine: a paradigm for the ethics of the helping and healing professions. Journal of Medicine and Philosophy 2001; 26(6): 559–579.
3. Shuster E. Fifty years later: the significance of the Nuremberg Code. New England Journal of Medicine 1997; 337(20): 1436–1440.
4. The Nuremberg Code. Journal of the American Medical Association 1996; 276(20): 1691.
5. Association WM. World Medical Association Declaration of Helsinki: Ethical Principles for Medical Research Involving Human Subjects 2008 (cited 2013 April 2); Available from: <http://www.wma.net/en/30publications/10policies/b3/>, accessed on 15 May 2015.
6. Research NCftPoHSoBaB. The Belmont Report. Washington, DC: US Government Printing Office, 1979.
7. Emanuel EJ, Wendler D, Grady C. What makes clinical research ethical? Journal of the American Medical Association 2000; 283(20): 2701–2711.
8. Agrawal M, Emanuel EJ. Ethics of phase 1 oncology studies: reexamining the arguments and data. Journal of the American Medical Association 2003; 290(8): 1075–1082.
9. Daugherty C, Ratain MJ, Grochowski E, Stocking C, Kodish E, Mick R, et al. Perceptions of cancer patients and their physicians involved in phase I trials. Journal of Clinical Oncology 1995; 13(5): 1062–1072.
10. Daugherty CK, Ratain MJ, Siegler M. Pushing the envelope: informed consent in phase I trials. Annals of Oncology 1995; 6(4): 321–323.

11. Emanuel EJ. A phase I trial on the ethics of phase I trials. Journal of Clinical Oncology 1995; 13(5): 1049–1051.

12. Joffe S, Miller FG. Rethinking risk–benefit assessment for phase I cancer trials. Journal of Clinical Oncology 2006; 24(19): 2987–2990.

13. Kodish E, Stocking C, Ratain MJ, Kohrman A, Siegler M. Ethical issues in phase I oncology research: a comparison of investigators and institutional review board chairpersons. Journal of Clinical Oncology 1992; 10(11): 1810–1816.

14. Penman DT, Holland JC, Bahna GF, Morrow G, Schmale AH et al. Informed consent for investigational chemotherapy: patients' and physicians' perceptions. Journal of Clinical Oncology 1984; 2(7): 849–855.

15. Peppercorn JM, Smith TJ, Helft PR, Debono DJ, Berry SR et al. American society of clinical oncology statement: toward individualized care for patients with advanced cancer. Journal of Clinical Oncology 2011; 29(6): 755–760.

16. Appelbaum PS, Roth LH, Lidz C. The therapeutic misconception: informed consent in psychiatric research. International Journal of Law and Psychiatry 1982; 5(3–4): 319–329.

17. Appelbaum PS, Roth LH, Lidz CW, Benson P, Winslade W. False hopes and best data: consent to research and the therapeutic misconception. Hastings Center Report 1987; 17(2): 20–4.

18. Pentz RD, White M, Harvey RD, Farmer ZL, Liu Y et al. Therapeutic misconception, misestimation, and optimism in participants enrolled in phase 1 trials. Cancer 2012; 118(18): 4571–4578.

19. Wendler DS. Time to stop worrying about the therapeutic misconception. Journal of Clinical Ethics 2012; 23(3): 272–287.

20. Emanuel EJ, Menikoff J. Reforming the regulations governing research with human subjects. New England Journal of Medicine 2011; 365(12): 1145–1150.

21. Emanuel EJ, Miller FG. The ethics of placebo-controlled trials: a middle ground. New England Journal of Medicine 2001; 345(12): 915–919.

22. Daugherty CK, Ratain MJ, Emanuel EJ, Farrell AT et al. Ethical, scientific, and regulatory perspectives regarding the use of placebos in cancer clinical trials. Journal of Clinical Oncology 2008; 26(8): 1371–1378.

23. Rosner GL, Stadler W, Ratain MJ. Randomized discontinuation design: application to cytostatic antineoplastic agents. Journal of Clinical Oncology 2002; 20(22): 4478–4484.

24. Banerji U, de Bono J, Judson I, Kaye S, Workman P. Biomarkers in early clinical trials: the committed and the skeptics. Clinical Cancer Research 2008; 14(8): 2512; author reply 3–4.

25. Cannistra SA. Performance of biopsies in clinical research. Journal of Clinical Oncology 2007; 25(11): 1454–1455.

26. Goulart BH, Clark JW, Pien HH, Roberts TG, Finkelstein SN et al. Trends in the use and role of biomarkers in phase I oncology trials. Clinical Cancer Research 2007; 13(22 Pt 1): 6719–6726.

27. Meric-Bernstam F, Farhangfar C, Mendelsohn J, Mills GB. Building a personalized medicine infrastructure at a major cancer center. Journal of Clinical Oncology 2013; 31(15): 1849–1857

28. Helft PR. Personalized medicine: medicine for the privileged? Oncology (Williston Park) 2012; 26(9): 814.

29. McGuire AL, McCullough LB, Evans JP. The indispensable role of professional judgment in genomic medicine. Journal of the American Medical Association 2013; 309(14): 1465–1466.

30. Tuckson RV, Newcomer L, De Sa JM. Accessing genomic medicine: affordability, diffusion, and disparities. Journal of the American Medical Association 2013; 309(14): 1469–1470.

31. Soden SE, Farrow EG, Saunders CJ, Lantos JD. Genomic medicine: evolving science, evolving ethics. Personalized Medicine 2012; 9(5): 523–528.

32. Kleiderman E, Avard D, Black L, Diaz Z, Rousseau C et al. Recruiting terminally ill patients into non-therapeutic oncology studies: views of health professionals. BMC Medical Ethics 2012; 13: 33.

33. Black L, Batist G, Avard D, Rousseau C, Diaz Z et al. Physician recruitment of patients to non-therapeutic oncology clinical trials: ethics revisited. Frontiers in Pharmacology 2013; 4: 25.

34. Peppercorn J, Shapira I, Collyar D, Deshields T, Lin N et al. Ethics of mandatory research biopsy for correlative end points within clinical trials in oncology. Journal of Clinical Oncology 2010; 28(15): 2635–2640.

35. Peppercorn J. Toward improved understanding of the ethical and clinical issues surrounding mandatory research biopsies. Journal of Clinical Oncology 2013; 31(1): 1–2.

36. Overman MJ, Modak J, Kopetz S, Murthy R, Yao JC et al. Use of research biopsies in clinical trials: are risks and benefits adequately discussed? Journal of Clinical Oncology 2013; 31(1): 17–22.

37. Becker DJ, Talwar S, Levy BP, Thorn M, Roitman J et al. Impact of oncology drug shortages on patient therapy: unplanned treatment changes. Journal of Oncology Practice 2013; 9(4): e122–e128.

38. Rochon PA, Gurwitz JH. Drug shortages and clinicians: no time for complacency. Archives of Internal Medicine 2012; 172(19): 1499–1500.

39. Rosoff PM. Unpredictable drug shortages: an ethical framework for short-term rationing in hospitals. American Journal of Bioethics 2012; 12(1): 1–9.

40. Rosoff PM, Patel KR, Scates A, Rhea G, Bush PW et al. Coping with critical drug shortages: an ethical approach for allocating scarce resources in hospitals. Archives of Internal Medicine 2012; 172(19): 1494–1499.

41. Daniels N, Sabin J. Limits to health care: fair procedures, democratic deliberation, and the legitimacy problem for insurers. Philosoph & Public Affairs 1997; 26(4): 303–350.

42. Daniels N, Sabin J. The ethics of accountability in managed care reform. Health Affairs 1998; 17(5): 50–64.

43. Valgus J, Singer EA, Berry SR, Rathmell WK. Ethical challenges: managing oncology drug shortages. Journal of Oncology Practice 2013; 9(2): e21–e23.

44. Brawley OW. The American Cancer Society and the American health care system. Oncologist 2011; 16(7): 920–925.

45. Fojo T, Grady C. How much is life worth: cetuximab, non-small cell lung cancer, and the $440 billion question. Journal of the National Cancer Institute 2009; 101(15): 1044–1048.

46. Kantarjian H, Experts C. The price of drugs for chronic myeloid leukemia (CML) is a reflection of the unsustainable prices of cancer drugs: from the perspective of a large group of CML experts. Blood 2013; 121(22): 4439–4442.

47. Zafar SY, Peppercorn JM, Schrag D, Taylor DH, Goetzinger AM et al. The financial toxicity of cancer treatment: a pilot study assessing out-of-pocket expenses and the insured cancer patient's experience. Oncologist 2013; 18(4): 381–390.

48. Meropol NJ, Schrag D, Smith TJ, Mulvey TM, Langdon RM, Jr. et al. American Society of Clinical Oncology guidance statement: the cost of cancer care. Journal of Clinical Oncology 2009; 27(23): 3868–3874.

49. Shuman AG, Montas SM, Barnosky AR, Smith LB, Kissane DW et al. Clinical Ethics Consultation in oncology. Journal of Clinical Oncology 2012; 30(15 Suppl.): 9121.

50. Tenner LL, Helft PR. Ethics in oncology: an annotated bibliography of important literature. Journal of Oncology Practice 2013; ePub ahead of print. doi:10.1200/JOP.2012.000679

CHAPTER 26

Health economic assessment of cancer therapy

Jeffrey Peppercorn

Introduction to health economic assessment of cancer therapy

Our ability to deliver high-quality cancer care is increasingly influenced by our ability to understand and manage the costs of care. Delivery of cancer therapy requires both an effective intervention and the ability to provide access to the intervention for patients in need. Much of the research of recent decades has been devoted, appropriately, to developing effective interventions in a variety of cancer settings. However, it is now clear that providing access to these interventions to patients in need is a global challenge requiring providers and policy makers to address the costs of cancer care both in the clinic for individual patients and at the level of the healthcare system.

At the level of national healthcare systems, the costs of healthcare in general, and the costs of cancer care in particular, are high. High costs are threatening to undermine or actively undermining the sustainability of national budgets. In the United States in 2011 it was estimated that total healthcare expenditures reached $2.7 trillion [1]. By the year 2020, it is projected that healthcare costs will account for roughly 20% of the US Gross Domestic Product (GDP) [2]. While the US leads other nations in healthcare spending as a percentage of GDP, rising costs threaten national budgets in nearly all developed countries [3]. Though there are considerable differences in the ways healthcare is financed and administered in different nations, there is a common need to deliver high-quality care at sustainable costs.

At the level of the individual patient, there is again considerable variation in the cost of care on the basis of their disease and setting. Both the total cost of care for a given patient and the percentage of that cost, if any, that will be paid out of pocket directly by the patient varies by national system and insurance coverage. However, costs for an individual patient impact care in virtually all settings whether due to direct financial hardship, uncertainty of access due to personal wealth or health insurance status (in the US) or due to national policy regarding access to care in countries with national healthcare systems (UK).

This chapter will review recent estimates of the aggregate costs of cancer care, discuss methods for determining cost-effectiveness or value in cancer care, provide a framework for understanding the components of cost at the societal and individual levels, and discuss efforts to control cost while preserving or improving quality and outcomes.

What does cancer care cost?: the societal perspective

The magnitude of costs of cancer care can be measured in terms of total spending, percentage of national GDP, or in terms of the cost to care for a single patient. In the US, total healthcare spending for 2013 is estimated at 2.98 trillion dollars, accounting for 17.6% of the GDP [2]. This amount of spending as a percentage of GDP exceeds that of other developed countries, with the closest being the Netherlands at 12% and France at 11.8% [4]. Estimating the component of total healthcare spending attributable to cancer can be difficult, particular in a fragmented healthcare system, but the US National Cancer Institute estimates that total cost of cancer care in the US was 124.5 billion dollars in 2010 [5]. This represents less than 5% of total healthcare spending and is generally consistent with the percentage of total spending attributable to cancer estimated for other developed countries [6]. For example, though total spending is lower in the UK, the National Health Service estimates that 5.4% of total healthcare spending for 2010/2011 was devoted to cancer care, compared to 11% of spending for mental healthcare, and 7.2% for cardiology-related care [7].

Total spending is a very crude way to estimate where and why money is being spent in cancer care. Many streams of spending contribute to total costs, including hospital fees, physician services, ancillary services (nursing, physical therapy), drug costs, surgical costs, radiation therapy, and durable medical goods. In the US, the Centers for Medicare and Medicaid Services (CMS) provide a breakdown of spending by services and funding source, but a comparable breakdown spending on components of cancer care is not currently available. At the level of total healthcare spending for major categories of medical services, the US spent 37% on hospital care, 24% on physician services, 12% on prescription drugs, 7% on nursing home care, 5% on dental care, and 3% on home healthcare in 2011 [1].

In addition to considering costs of cancer care by service or intervention, we can attempt to break down costs by individual cancer. In 2010, in the US it was estimated that total spending was 16.5 billion for breast cancer, 14.1 billion for colorectal cancer, 12.1 billion for lymphoma, 12.1 billion for lung cancer, and 11.9 billion for prostate cancer, with lesser amounts for other malignancies. Thus, we appear to be spending the most money on the most prevalent cancers, as would be expected. To truly understand costs at the public health level, however, we would need data on spending by intervention category or service for each of these diseases, and ultimately for each stage of disease. Obtaining data at this level of granularity is difficult, particularly in a healthcare system with multiple payers and limited public availability of data. However, this level of detail is needed to identify areas that may be experiencing higher than expected inflation, or where spending is not consistent with disease prevalence or clinical benefit. Effort to understand and control total spending without this level of detail should proceed with a large dose of caution.

Efforts to understand and control rising costs of care

Policy makers are concerned not just with the level of spending, but with the increase in spending, or what has been termed the 'cost curve'. A major objective in recent healthcare reform debates within the US, and indeed an objective worldwide, is to 'bend the cost curve' in a downward direction, or at least achieve a less steep upward slope over time to control the growth of spending. With projections that, by 2020, healthcare spending will to rise to 20% of GDP, or one-fifth of the entire US economy, there is legitimate concern about the impact this will have on other valued social goods such as education, housing, and even research to improve future delivery of healthcare. While oncology is only a small part of total healthcare spending by some estimates, there is concern that through a combination of higher incidence of disease, increased care delivery per patient, and rising costs for prescription drugs and other aspects of care that inflation in this area will contribute a disproportionate amount to increased healthcare spending and must be addressed now. Total oncology spending in the US is projected to grow from 27 billion in 1990 to 157 billion dollars by 2020, representing a staggering 600% increase in 30 years [8].

Identifying the factors and specific elements of spending that are responsible for the aggregate increases in cost can be challenging from available data. Using available data from the public system, Medicare, which covers care for older and disabled patients, Warren et al. found that between 1991 and 2002 the large increase in the spending for lung, colorectal, and breast cancer was driven by both utilization (the amount of care delivered) and charges for services and for hospital care. During this period, the percentage of patients with breast cancer receiving chemotherapy increased from 11% to 24% and the cost of chemotherapy increased from roughly $6,000 per patient to almost $13,000 [9]. In another study of Medicare spending, Dinan and colleagues found that PET scans and MRI utilization have increased across most types of cancer. Radiology may be a disproportionate driver of costs due both to innovation and relatively high margins on services. Between 1999 and 2006 the cost of imaging for cancer increased by 5.1% to 10.3% each year, while the cost of all cancer care increased by only 1.8% to 4.6% [10].

Rising aggregate costs of cancer care derive both from the cost of treating individual patients and from the number of patients who require treatment. Demographic, environmental, and behavioural factors that modify the risk of cancer in a population can have a large impact on societal costs of care. While cancer can strike at any age, it is predominantly a disease of older patients. Projected growth of the percentage of patients aged 50 years and older, and particularly an increase in the percentage of elderly patients in the population, are expected to translate into a dramatic increase in the number of patients with cancer unless there are countervailing advances in cancer prevention. Cancer is also rapidly becoming more common in developing countries as populations are living longer due to improvements in nutrition, successful treatment of infectious disease, reductions in infant mortality, and improvements in paediatric care [11]. In 1990, there were close to six million deaths from cancer estimated worldwide, but by 2010 roughly eight million cancer deaths occurred, a 38% increase [12]. In the US, due to a combination of changing demographics as well as success in management of cardiovascular disease, cancer has become the leading cause of death among those under age 85 [13].

Factors responsible for rising cancer incidence vary by nation. In China, dominant factors include chronic infection, including hepatitis B leading to liver cancer, and tobacco use [14]. In France, it is estimated that roughly 24% of cancer deaths are attributable to tobacco use, and obesity may contribute to 3% of cancer deaths [15]. There is concern worldwide, and particularly in the US, that rising levels of obesity will contribute to increases in cancer in addition to other adverse health consequences. In the US, more than one-third of the population is now characterized as obese. Among adult non-smokers in the US, close to 15% of cancers among men and nearly 20% of cancer among women are attributable to obesity [16]. From a policy perspective, prevention through modification of risk factors across a population may be one of the most effective means to control total societal costs without adverse impact on the quality of care for individuals diagnosed with cancer.

It should be noted that the societal costs of cancer care delivery are only a portion of the total economic consequences of cancer for society. The societal economic burden of cancer includes costs for care delivery, but also indirect costs caused by loss of economic productivity of individuals suffering the morbidity and mortality caused by cancer, as well as their family members who become caregivers. In Germany, for example, it was estimated that the direct cost of cancer care in 2004 was 12.1 billion euros [6]. The indirect cost, virtually all related to lost production due to cancer deaths, was estimated at 14.7 billion euros. In the US, a 2002 estimate listed direct costs of cancer care at $61 billion US dollars versus $110 billion in indirect costs [6]. Thus, in considering the costs of cancer care to society, we must consider not only the spending on care delivery but also the downstream impact of that spending. If spending on radiology leads to earlier diagnosis and improved treatment and outcomes, spending on a genomic predictor of recurrence leads to a decision to forgo systemic therapy, or spending on an expensive targeted adjuvant therapy improves cure rates, spending on some aspects of care may rise, but the overall economic impact may be favourable.

Impact of costs on individual patients

In addition to the impact of cancer care costs on societal budgets, the impact on individual patients can be considerable. In all settings, costs can impact the individual due to decisions made at the national level regarding coverage and access. In the majority of developed countries there is universal access to healthcare, but there are differing thresholds and mechanisms for determining what aspects of healthcare are provided and how it is allocated.

In the US, pending the full implementation of the Affordable Care Act of 2010, there is no guarantee of access to cancer care (or any other care other than emergency room services). In this context, the impact of costs of care to individual patients can be extraordinary. For example, a one-year course of adjuvant trastuzumab therapy for HER2 positive breast cancer costs approximately $50,000. This figure, already greater than the median family annual income in the US, does not include the provider costs, costs of other chemotherapy typically given with trastuzumab, costs for surgery, pathology, radiation therapy, lab work, hospitalization, and many other aspects of care. The newly approved drug TDM1 for the same disease in the metastatic setting costs approximately $98,000 for a one-year course of treatment, again on top of other healthcare expenses incurred during this time. Given these costs, only those with adequate insurance coverage can be sure to gain the benefits of these interventions. Cost presents a true barrier to care.

The impact of the high costs of cancer care in the US has been demonstrated in multiple studies. Patients with no health insurance or even inadequate insurance tend to present later in the course of illness and to experience worse cancer outcomes, including death, compared to patients with adequate health insurance [17]. Unfortunately, in some studies the public insurance system for poor people, Medicaid, qualifies as inadequate with outcomes similar to no insurance at all [17]. In addition to 52 million uninsured patients in the US, it is estimated that 29 million are 'underinsured', meaning coverage is inadequate to guarantee access to quality healthcare as of 2010 [18]. Underinsured patients may forgo non-cancer-related medical care, reduce expenditures on food, clothing, and shelter in order to cope with the costs of cancer medication [19]. Some patients also report discontinuation of cancer therapy due to cost [18].

Oncologists report that cost impacts cancer treatment decisions and that discussions of costs of cancer care with patients are deemed important. However, in a 2008 survey conducted by Neuman and colleagues, 58% of physicians reported inadequate knowledge to discuss costs of care with their patients [20].

Measuring the value of cancer care

Given the issues and concerns noted above there is a need to ensure that resources committed to cancer care are well spent. This is true if the spending is from the state budget, from an insurance provider, or from the patient's own pocket. We need to be able to identify not only the medical risks and benefit of any potential intervention, but to assess the relative benefit compared to the resources expended, or the 'value' of care. Developing an operational definition of value is complex.

In determining value, we need to be able to identify and, to some extent, quantify the medical benefits, toxicities, and risks of an intervention and the direct and indirect costs associated with its use. We must then determine what threshold of cost for a given net clinical benefit is reasonable or worthwhile. We are generally most concerned with financial evaluation of those interventions (a diagnostic test, drug, procedure, or any other aspect of care) where there is some marginal clinical benefit that may or may not, in the context of cost, offer good 'value'. If the harms outweigh the clinical

benefits or the cost is negligible (such as information on diet or exercise), we don't generally need to take a hard look at value.

Assigning value implies that we can define the overall worth of an intervention and make choices between options that take into account the totality of benefits, harms, and costs, and to some degree, alternatives. In truth, there is no ideal formula or even a broad consensus on how value should be assessed in cancer care or at what threshold of benefits and costs an intervention becomes 'high value'. However, there are well-validated methods of assessing relative clinical benefit and cost that move us in the direction of defining value.

All methods to evaluate clinical benefit relative to cost have at their core a goal of allowing us to assess value and make decisions about whether a given component of care should or should not be provided. Assigning value is not equivalent, per se, to rationing, which can be defined as a programme of distribution for scarce goods and services according to a rational prespecified framework. However, assigning value can be fairly seen as a necessary step in guiding medical decision that considers financial costs and that predictably will result in some level of constraints on care on the basis of factors other than clinical benefit alone. In a world of infinite resources, we might consider only clinical factors and provide all interventions in any setting with possible marginal benefit. In reality, resources are not infinite, so that a policy of considering marginal benefit only is unsustainable, and we need to be able to assess value to guide medical decisions.

It should be noted that efforts to define a rational basis to make healthcare allocation decisions date at least back to the days of triage in the army of Napoleon. In this early example, concern was not the cost of care, but given limited supplies and medics, inadequate available care to meet the needs of all soldiers injured in battle. The utility of care to the patient (as distinct from the severity of the illness) was made a primary consideration for allocation, or rationing, of care. In modern medicine, outside of the solid organ transplant setting, we are more often concerned with financial scarcity. However, drug shortages in oncology have recently become more common, resulting in further consideration of explicit rationing in oncology [21].

One of the most common methods of assessing value in oncology is to perform a cost-effectiveness analysis. As the name implies, the goal is to determine the cost of an intervention and weigh this against the effectiveness for the outcome of interest. If the objective is survival in metastatic pancreatic cancer, then to determine the cost-effectiveness of systemic therapy interventions for this disease we would need to know their cost for a course of treatment and their impact on improving survival. Any clinical goal can be considered, from survival to disease response rate to relief of pain, as long as it can be quantified as a measure of effectiveness and it is clearly defined.

Continuing with this example, if we consider three available interventions, gemcitabine, gemcitabine + erlotonib, or the FOLFIRINOX regimen (consisting of 5 FU, leucovorin, irinotecan, and oxaliplatin), we might calculate a ratio of the cost in dollars per increased weeks in expected survival compared to survival and costs with symptom management alone (or placebo). This would allow us to consider the cost-effectiveness of each intervention discretely and to make value-based comparisons between interventions.

In this example, one can quickly see why a basic calculation of cost and one measure of clinical effectiveness—weeks of survival—may be inadequate to fully assess value. What if a six-week extension in survival is at both a higher financial cost and at the cost of several months more of severe toxicity, such that the patient is alive but spending most of their time in bed feeling tired or nauseous? What if the cost of the intervention itself is modest but it requires expensive additional medications to treat side effects, or is likely to require prolonged hospitalization in a subset of patients? In addition, some distinguish the definition of 'efficacy', taken as the impact of an intervention of a clinical outcome in a near-idealized setting such as highly regulated randomized control trial versus 'effectiveness' defined as the impact of an intervention on the outcome of interest in a real-world broader population context. Either setting can be used in cost-effectiveness analysis, but it is important to be able to make the distinction and recognize that the 'effectiveness' of an intervention in practice is often somewhat less than its 'efficacy' in a clinical trial. Further complicating these issues, what if we wish to assess the cost effectiveness of first-line interventions for metastatic breast cancer or castrate-resistant prostate cancer in terms of impact on survival? How do we account for the impact of subsequent treatments or consider surrogate endpoints that may or may not correlate well with survival?

To address some of these challenges several steps have been taken to improve the methodology of cost-effectiveness assessment. First, one can try to define a meaningful outcome that considers not just longevity but also quality of life to facilitate meaningful comparisons in effectiveness among diverse interventions. Thus, instead of measuring survival alone in terms of weeks, months, or years, we can estimate gain in terms of quality-adjusted life years or 'QALYs'. What we gain in beginning to incorporate quality of life, however, we start to lose in the objectivity of our measurement because two individuals may have different definitions of what constitutes quality of life under different clinical scenarios. Because this calculation implies a measure not just of the intrinsic value of a clinical objective like survival time, but also of the subjective utility individuals assign to survival in differing conditions, calculation of cost-effectiveness involving QALYs is sometimes referred to as cost–utility analysis.

Often, one of the purposes of cost-effectiveness analysis is to compare the incremental benefit provided by a new expensive intervention to a standard less costly intervention. We want to ask if the marginal improvement in outcomes is 'worth it'. To do this, health economists use the incremental cost-effectiveness ratio or 'ICER'. The benefits of the interventions can be described in terms of QALYs or some other measure of outcome, the costs of a course of therapy identified, and the ratio of absolute difference in QALY over net increase in cost provides the ICER. To take a real-world published example, using the regimens for pancreatic cancer listed above, Tam and colleagues calculated the ICER for use of more effective but more expensive regimens. They determined utility of health states with pancreatic cancer by surveying physicians to calculate QALYs and used the pharmacy records from a Canadian cancer centre to determine cost. In Canadian dollars, the cost of a one-month course of gemcitabine was roughly $29,000 versus $41,000 with the addition of erlotinib versus $57,000 for FOLFIRINOX. Although gemcitabine plus erlotinib was cheaper, the ICER for this regimen was $153,631 per QALY versus $133,184 for FOLFIRINOX, suggesting that the latter, while more expensive in absolute terms, appears to provide better value [22].

In addition to the challenge of determining which outcome to use in measuring cost-effectiveness, determination of cost involves choices as well. First, cost can vary in some health systems depending on negotiations between payers and providers or manufacturers. It is important to distinguish between the charge for the intervention (the amount of money requested by the supplier) and the cost (the actual amount of money that changes hands). Second, one needs to consider whether to use the isolated cost of the intervention itself or the cost of the intervention and all associated ancillary care measures, such as drugs or hospitalizations, that might occur to treat symptoms or complications. Some studies use 'cost consequences' analysis to try to capture all associated costs with one plan of care over a longer timeframe to allow more financially realistic comparisons between two options. In such analyses, there remain questions over what time period should be used and what costs incurred during that period should be included.

As a 'consumer' of cost-effectiveness studies it is important for oncologists and policy makers to be aware of the many variables that can be considered in study design and the fact that such studies can be biased by these decisions. Some analyses of the field of cost-effectiveness research in medicine have found that there is bias among studies sponsored by the pharmaceutical industry, and more generally strong publication bias towards studies demonstrating favourable ICERs [23]. There has been a steep rise in the number of published cost-effectiveness studies over the past two decades, with variable quality [24]. The reader should carefully evaluate the underlying assumptions in the methodology, sources of data, and potential sources of bias.

Controlling costs

Determination of what constitutes good value in cancer care and how and whether cost control to ensure good value will be implemented differs by national healthcare system. A threshold of less than $50,000 per QALY gained is usually accepted as a clear measure of good value in most developed countries, although the exact threshold can vary [25]. Many cancer therapies that are used in the US do not meet this threshold and it has been suggested that a threshold of $100,000 per QALY or more may be more reasonable [21]. As might be expected, in nations where healthcare delivery, not just financing of healthcare, is a public service, there tends to be the greatest emphasis on ensuring that all care provided reaches a specified threshold of value, and the greatest means to enforce such care delivery.

In the UK, where the National Health Service is an example of both public financing and delivery of healthcare, the National Institute for Health and Clinical Excellence (NICE) explicitly evaluates both clinical effectives and cost-effectiveness of cancer care interventions. NICE provides the NHS with recommendations for which cancer therapy should or should not be provided on the basis of cost per QALY gained. In Canada, there is public funding for healthcare with universal access. Providers may be private or practice and government-funded hospitals. Many coverage decisions about healthcare resources are made at the level of the regional province. However, cancer therapy and other drugs are now subject to Common Drug Review by the Canadian Expert Drug Advisory Committee, which explicitly considers cost-effectiveness in its recommendations. Provinces are not required to follow the committee's recommendations but reportedly do so up to 90% of the time [26].

In Australia, there is universal healthcare with all citizens covered by one of 15 public insurance companies, with supplemental private health insurance available for a price. Diagnostic studies and cancer treatment, including chemotherapy, are covered without cost to the individual by the public system [27]. In the Australian system, decisions about cancer drugs availability are guided by the Pharmaceutical Benefits Advisory Committee, which explicitly considers both effectiveness and cost. A therapy will only become available if there is a favourable review by the committee [26].

In contrast, the US Food and Drug Administration by statute may not consider cost when determining approval for new drugs and the Centers for Medicaid and Medicare (which provide public financing of healthcare for elderly, poor, and disabled Americans) may not consider cost in benefits coverage decisions. These policies leave little leverage to promote high-value healthcare and control costs. Thus, the 2010 Patient Protection and Affordable Care Act, in addition to attempting to establish near universal access to care, established the Patient Centered Outcome Institute to support development of an evidence base to guide policy makers' decisions on coverage and access. However, unlike NICE, this new agency was still prohibited from establishing a cost–benefit threshold for healthcare and (like those of NICE) its recommendations are non-binding [28].

In the absence of an agency that determines value or cost-effectiveness for cancer care, in the US efforts to control costs while maintaining quality have fallen to private payers and to the profession. One mechanism seen as promising is the promotion of guidelines or pathways of care. With a defined guideline for a clinical scenario, evidence-based care can be promoted and costs can be better predicted, which allows insurance companies to attempt to match premiums to expenses. Data from an insurance provider-sponsored study of lung cancer care demonstrated that following guidelines resulted in equivalent outcomes but at substantially lower cost (35% reduction in total costs of care) compared to standard practice [29].

At the level of the profession, the American Society of Clinical Oncology joined 26 other medical specialties in participating in the 'choosing wisely campaign' in which several practices were identified that can be eliminated with no detriment (or possible improvement) in quality and resulting cost savings [30]. One does not have to agree on a definition of value to decide that an intervention without proven benefit (particularly when it has been well studied) should be eliminated. The first five practices identified were: (1) Don't use cancer-directed therapy among patients with very poor performance status and/or no proven benefit from further intervention in the patient's setting; (2) Don't perform staging studies for asymptomatic patients with early-stage low-risk prostate cancer; (3) Don't perform staging studies in asymptomatic patients with early-stage breast cancer; (4) Don't use serum biomarker or imaging studies as part of routine surveillance for asymptomatic patients with breast cancer after initial treatment; and (5) Don't use white cell growth factors for patients with low risk of febrile neutropenia [30].

Further work is underway to provide additional examples. At this time, the impact of this campaign is unknown and the cost savings depend primarily on physician behaviour and discretion. However, perhaps in part as a result of markedly increased attention to cost and to high-value practice in the US media, and the resulting impact on decision-making by physicians and patients, healthcare inflation has already started to decline, prior to full implementation of healthcare reform [31].

Clinical discretion in cost control

In any healthcare system, there is balance between allowing for physician discretion in medical decision-making and controlling quality and costs through regulation, access to interventions, and reimbursement policies. Physicians have an active role to play in ensuring that care delivered meets high standards of effectiveness and efficiency. In keeping with the goals of promoting high-quality care and preserving physician discretion to provide needed care to individual patients, cost-effectiveness must be considered in clinic.

While determination of value remains complex, a framework for identification of interventions that can be eliminated without negative impact on quality has been proposed [3]. By attempting to eliminate interventions that are not evidence based, those that are duplicative, and those that would not be pursued if the patient was offered the opportunity to make an informed choice, we can eliminate some costs of care while improving quality.

Two challenges to providing cost-effective care in oncology are constraints on the clinician's time with a patient and physician awareness of the costs of therapy [3]. When seeing patients with advanced cancer, it can be easier and faster to propose and review an intervention than to engage in a longer conversation to assess the patient's preferences and discuss the option of palliative care alone [32]. Similarly, when evaluating a new symptom, an oncologist may find it easier to simply order an expensive scan than to take a detailed history and physical to guide evaluation rationally [33, 34].

Oncologists may be up to date on the latest interventions, which are often featured in scientific and lay press, but less aware of evidence suggesting areas where care can be safely limited. For example, two large randomized trials have demonstrated that for asymptomatic patients with early-stage breast cancer there is no proven utility to obtaining tumour markers or routine staging studies for surveillance [35, 36]. Despite this decades-old evidence, use of these tests continues in some practices, necessitating identification of this issue by ASCO as one clear way to reduce costs without detriment to quality, as noted above [37]. It is worth noting that in the context of the medico-legal landscape in the US, 'defensive medicine', or practice based on fear of lawsuits, may guide some care decisions. While several studies show minimal financial impact of defensive medicine, clinicians continue to report that legal considerations impact decisions in some settings [38–40]. In addition, financial incentives in the US likely contribute to over-utilization.

In addition to clinical discretion, patient demand likely contributes to over-utilization of cancer care, or at least some of the ancillary aspects of cancer care to some degree. While it is doubtful that anyone requests more chemotherapy or surgery than they absolutely need, in the realm of diagnostic tests, provider visits, and in some cases pursuit of high-cost interventions with marginal to negligible proven benefit, patient preference and insensitivity to cost may play a role. This is the flipside of the economic burden and barriers to care imposed by cancer on many patients, particularly in the US. If patients do not bear any responsibility for costs of care, they are likely to be more indifferent to costs to society, or value of care, and to focus on marginal clinical benefits alone. This is described as 'moral hazard', where one party of a medical decision is shielded from the financial consequences. Surveys of patients suggest that they are open to considering both effectiveness and cost in medical decisions, and may be willing to pay more out of pocket for higher-value care [41]. Cost-sharing, in which patients pay a percentage of the costs of care through co-payments or deductibles, is increasingly seen in the US as a way to promote higher-value care. However, it is possible that cost-sharing indiscriminately reduces utilization of both low- and high-value care, requiring carefully analysis of the impact of cost-sharing when it is implemented.

Cancer care at the end of life

One aspect of cancer care that deserves special consideration in discussions of value is care at the end of life. Currently, many patients with cancer will ultimately die from their disease, and prevention of death is not an achievable goal. At some point, further disease-directed therapy becomes futile and, worse, potentially harmful to the patient. While we strive to define value in other aspects of cancer care, it is clear that resources devoted to disease-directed therapy past the point of potential for benefit are wasteful (as opposed to resources devoted to promoting quality of life and palliating symptoms). Unfortunately, studies suggest that a large portion of total spending for cancer care is for care delivered in the last weeks or days of life when this care may be both futile and inconsistent with the preferences of an informed patient [42–44]. This futile disease-directed care may have financial consequences for the patient's family and society and may compromise the patient's quality of life during the weeks prior to death as well as detract from a needed focus on palliative care [45].

Steps forward to understand and address the costs of cancer care

As outlined in this chapter, there is a need to consider the financial consequences of treatment decisions on our patients and for society. Regardless of the national healthcare system, there are constraints and tradeoffs in the resources that can be committed to healthcare and other societal goods, including cancer research itself. There may also be tradeoffs to consider among the care that can or should be provided to a single patient and our ability to provide care for all patients in need. Further research and public debate among interested and informed stakeholders is needed to guide rational policy and to promote quality care.

We need improve evaluation of the cost of cancer care in the clinic. We need to find efficient means to provide information on the direct and indirect financial impact of treatment decisions on patients and their families at the point of care. To the extent that we wish conversations over cost to enter the clinical encounter, we need to determine what the content and goals of these conversations should be, and what the impact will be on treatment decisions and on the patient's experience of cancer. It is clear that patients are interested in knowing how treatment decisions will affect them economically; it is less clear that they want conversations about the societal costs of care to enter the clinic or impact decisions.

At the policy level we need to strike the right balance between cost control, physician discretion, and allowing for patient autonomy where reasonable. In some areas of oncology, we have excellent evidence to guide practice. Support of guidelines through incentives, reimbursement, formulary policy, and other means can support quality care and control costs. In other areas, or in rare presentations of common cancers, evidence is limited and we may never have data from large randomized trials to guide practice. Patients in such settings require care that may not easily be reduced to a guideline or pathway, or best practices may be defined by rapidly evolving clinical literature that requires flexibility in the system to allow timely access to appropriate care. It is important for clinicians to be able to assess the clinical needs of individual patients and practice evidence-based medicine. It is also increasingly important to recognize that continued access to high-quality care and support for further innovation in oncology is now tightly linked to our collective ability to achieve sustainability in the healthcare system and promote high-value care.

Further reading

Clement FM, Harris A, Li JJ, Yong K, Lee KM et al. Using effectiveness and cost-effectiveness to make drug coverage decisions: a comparison of Britain, Australia, and Canada. Journal of the American Medical Association 2009; 302(13): 1437–1443.

Greenberg D, Earle C, Fang CH, Eldar-Lissai A, Neumann PJ. When is cancer care cost-effective? A systematic overview of cost-utility analyses in oncology. Journal of the National Cancer Institute 2010; 102(2): 82–88.

Mariotto AB, Yabroff KR, Shao Y, Feuer EJ, Brown ML. Projections of the cost of cancer care in the United States: 2010–2020. Journal of the National Cancer Institute 2011; 103(2): 117–128.

Peppercorn JM, Smith TJ, Helft PR, Debono DJ, Berry SR et al. American Society of Clinical Oncology statement: toward individualized care for patients with advanced cancer. Journal of Clinical Oncology 2011; 29(6): 755–760.

Schnipper LE, Smith TJ, Raghavan D, Blayney DW, Ganz PA et al. American Society of Clinical Oncology identifies five key opportunities to improve care and reduce costs: the top five list for oncology. Journal of Clinical Oncology 2012; 30(14): 1715–1724.

Sullivan R, Peppercorn J, Sikora K, Zalcberg J, Meropol NJ et al. Delivering affordable cancer care in high-income countries. Lancet Oncology 2011; 12(10): 933–980.

Yabroff KR, Lund J, Kepka D, Mariotto A. Economic burden of cancer in the United States: estimates, projections, and future research. Cancer Epidemiology, Biomarkers & Prevention 2011; 20(10): 2006–2014.

References

1. Hartman M, Martin AB, Benson J, Catlin A. National health spending in 2011: overall growth remains low, but some payers and services show signs of acceleration. Health Affairs 2013; 32(1): 87–99.
2. Keehan SP, Sisko AM, Truffer CJ, Poisal JA, Cuckler GA et al. National health spending projections through 2020: economic recovery and reform drive faster spending growth. Health Affairs 2011; 30(8): 1594–1605.
3. Sullivan R, Peppercorn J, Sikora K, Zalcberg J, Meropol NJ et al. Delivering affordable cancer care in high-income countries. Lancet Oncology 2011; 12(10): 933–980.
4. Squires DA. Explaining high health care spending in the United States: an international comparison of supply, utilization, prices, and quality. Commonwealth Fund pub. 1595 2012; 10.
5. Yabroff KR, Lund J, Kepka D, Mariotto A. Economic burden of cancer in the United States: estimates, projections, and future research. Cancer Epidemiology, Biomarkers & Prevention 2011; 20(10): 2006–2014.
6. Jönsson B, Wilking N. The burden and cost of cancer. Annals of Oncology 2007; 18(Suppl. 3): iii8–iii22.
7. Harker R. NHS funding and expenditure. Commons Briefing papers SN00724, 2012.
8. Mariotto AB, Yabroff KR, Shao Y, Feuer EJ, Brown ML. Projections of the cost of cancer care in the United States: 2010–2020. Journal of the National Cancer Institute 2011; 103(2): 117–128.

9. Warren JL, Yabroff KR, Meekins A, Topor M, Lamont EB, Brown ML. Evaluation of trends in the cost of initial cancer treatment. Journal of the National Cancer Institute 2008; 100(12): 888–897.

10. Dinan MA, Curtis LH, Hammill BG, Patz EF Jr, Abernethy AP et al. Changes in the use and costs of diagnostic imaging among Medicare beneficiaries with cancer, 1999–2006. Journal of the American Medical Association 2010; 303(16): 1625–1631.

11. Farmer P, Frenk J, Knaul FM, Shulman LN, Alleyne G et al. Expansion of cancer care and control in countries of low and middle income: a call to action. Lancet 2010; 376(9747): 1186–1193.

12. Lozano R, Naghavi M, Foreman K, Lim S, Shibuya K et al. Global and regional mortality from 235 causes of death for 20 age groups in 1990 and 2010: a systematic analysis for the Global Burden of Disease Study 2010. Lancet 2012; 380(9859): 2095–2128.

13. Jemal A, Siegel R, Xu J, Ward E. Cancer statistics, 2010. CA: A Cancer Journal for Clinicians 2010; 60(5): 277–300.

14. Wang JB, Jiang Y, Liang H, Li P, Xiao HJ et al. Attributable causes of cancer in China. Annals of Oncology 2012; 23(11): 2983–2989.

15. Boffetta P, Tubiana M, Hill C, Boniol M, Aurengo A et al. The causes of cancer in France. Annals of Oncology 2009; 20(3): 550–555.

16. Schottenfeld D, Beebe-Dimmer JL, Buffler PA, Omenn GS. Current perspective on the global and United States cancer burden attributable to lifestyle and environmental risk factors. Annual Review of Public Health 2013; 34: 97–117.

17. Halpern MT, Ward EM, Pavluck AL, Schrag NM, Bian J et al. Association of insurance status and ethnicity with cancer stage at diagnosis for 12 cancer sites: a retrospective analysis. Lancet Oncology 2008; 9(3): 222–231.

18. Schoen C, Doty MM, Robertson RH, Collins SR. Affordable Care Act reforms could reduce the number of underinsured US adults by 70 percent. Health Affairs 2011; 30(9): 1762–1771.

19. Zafar SY, Peppercorn JM, Schrag D, Taylor DH, Goetzinger AM et al. The financial toxicity of cancer treatment: a pilot study assessing out-of-pocket expenses and the insured cancer patient's experience. Oncologist 2013; 18(4): 381–390.

20. Neumann PJ, Palmer JA, Nadler E, Fang C, Ubel P. Cancer therapy costs influence treatment: a national survey of oncologists. Health Affairs 2010; 29(1): 196–202.

21. Peppercorn J, Armstrong A, Zaas DW, George D. Rationing in urologic oncology: lessons from sipuleucel-T for advanced prostate cancer. Urologic Oncology 2012; 31(7): 1079–1084.

22. Tam VC, Ko YJ, Mittmann N, Cheung MC, Kumar K et al. Cost-effectiveness of systemic therapies for metastatic pancreatic cancer. Current Oncology 2013; 20(2): e90–e106.

23. Bell CM, Urbach DR, Ray JG, Bayoumi A, Rosen AB et al. Bias in published cost effectiveness studies: systematic review. British Medical Journal 2006; 332(7543): 699–703.

24. Greenberg D, Earle C, Fang CH, Eldar-Lissai A, Neumann PJ. When is cancer care cost-effective? A systematic overview of cost-utility analyses in oncology. Journal of the National Cancer Institute 2010; 102(2): 82–88.

25. Pearson SD, Rawlins MD. Quality, innovation, and value for money: NICE and the British National Health Service. Journal of the American Medical Association 2005; 294(20): 2618–2622.

26. Clement FM, Harris A, Li JJ, Yong K, Lee KM et al. Using effectiveness and cost-effectiveness to make drug coverage decisions: a comparison of Britain, Australia, and Canada. Journal of the American Medical Association 2009; 302(13): 1437–1443.

27. Micheli A, Coebergh JW, Mugno E, Massimiliani E, Sant M et al. European health systems and cancer care. Annals of Oncology 2003; 14(Suppl. 5): v41–v60.

28. Clancy C, Collins FS. Patient-Centered Outcomes Research Institute: the intersection of science and health care. Science Translational Medicine 2010; 2(37): 37cm18.

29. Neubauer MA, Hoverman JR, Kolodziej M, Reisman L, Gruschkus SK et al. Cost effectiveness of evidence-based treatment guidelines for the treatment of non-small-cell lung cancer in the community setting. Journal of Oncology Practice 2010; 6(1): 12–18.

30. Schnipper LE, Smith TJ, Raghavan D, Blayney DW, Ganz PA et al. American Society of Clinical Oncology identifies five key opportunities to improve care and reduce costs: the top five list for oncology. Journal of Clinical Oncology 2012; 30(14): 1715–1724.

31. Lowery A. Slower growth of health costs eases budget deficit. New York Times, 11 February 2013.

32. Peppercorn JM, Smith TJ, Helft PR, Debono DJ, Berry SR et al. American Society of Clinical Oncology statement: toward individualized care for patients with advanced cancer. Journal of Clinical Oncology 2011; 29(6): 755–760.

33. Bishop TF, Federman AD, Keyhani S. Physicians' views on defensive medicine: a national survey. Archives of Internal Medicine 2010; 170(12): 1081–1083.

34. Goodman RL. Commentary: health care technology and medical education: putting physical diagnosis in its proper place. Academic Medicine 2010; 85(6): 945–946.

35. Rosselli Del Turco M, Palli D, Cariddi A, Ciatto S, Pacini P et al. Intensive diagnostic follow-up after treatment of primary breast cancer. A randomized trial. National Research Council Project on Breast Cancer follow-up. Journal of the American Medical Association 1994; 271(20): 1593–1597.

36. Impact of follow-up testing on survival and health-related quality of life in breast cancer patients. A multicenter randomized controlled trial. The GIVIO Investigators. Journal of the American Medical Association 1994; 271(20): 1587–1592.

37. Foster JA, Abdolrasulnia M, Doroodchi H, McClure J, Casebeer L. Practice patterns and guideline adherence of medical oncologists in managing patients with early breast cancer. Journal of the National Comprehensive Cancer Network 2009; 7(7): 697–706.

38. Mello MM, Chandra A, Gawande AA, Studdert DM. National costs of the medical liability system. Health Affairs 2010; 29(9): 1569–1577.

39. Hellinger FJ, Encinosa WE. The impact of state laws limiting malpractice damage awards on health care expenditures. American Journal of Public Health 2006; 96(8): 1375–1381.

40. Studdert DM, Mello MM, Sage WM, DesRoches CM, Peugh J et al. Defensive medicine among high-risk specialist physicians in a volatile malpractice environment. Journal of the American Medical Association 2005; 293(21): 2609–2617.

41. Wong YN, Hamilton O, Egleston B, Salador K, Murphy C et al. Understanding how out-of-pocket expenses, treatment value, and patient characteristics influence treatment choices. Oncologist 2010; 15(6): 566–576.

42. Mack JW, Weeks JC, Wright AA, Block SD, Prigerson HG. End-of-life discussions, goal attainment, and distress at the end of life: predictors and outcomes of receipt of care consistent with preferences. Journal of Clinical Oncology 2010; 28(7): 1203–1208.

43. Zhang B, Wright AA, Huskamp HA, Nilsson ME, Maciejewski ML et al. Health care costs in the last week of life: associations with end-of-life conversations. Archives of Internal Medicine 2009; 169(5): 480–488.

44. Earle CC, Landrum MB, Souza JM, Neville BA, Weeks JC et al. Aggressiveness of cancer care near the end of life: is it a quality-of-care issue? Journal of Clinical Oncology 2008; 26(23): 3860–3866.

45. Temel JS, Greer JA, Muzikansky A, Gallagher ER, Admane S et al. Early palliative care for patients with metastatic non-small-cell lung cancer. New England Journal of Medicine 2010; 363(8): 733–742.

SECTION 4

Population health

27 **Cancer control planning** *245*
   Massoud Samiei

28 **Cancer prevention: vaccination** *256*
   Sarah E.B. Goltz and Julian Lob-Levyt

29 **Cancer chemoprevention** *262*
   Hans-Joerg Senn, Nadir Arber, and Dirk Schrijvers

30 **Population cancer screening** *267*
   Andrew Evans, C. Simon Herrington, and Robert Steele

31 **Familial cancer syndromes and genetic counselling** *276*
   Henry T. Lynch, Carrie L. Snyder, and Jane F. Lynch

SECTION 4

Population health

27 Cancer control planning, 265
Mango O Samet

28 Cancer prevention vaccination, 256
Noah D. Cohen and Allan Hildesheim

29 Cancer chemoprevention, 269
Hans-Jörg Senn, Nadia Alber and Dirk Schrijvers

30 Population cancer screening, 263
Andrew Evans, Christa Horn and Robert Steele

31 Familial cancer syndromes and
genetic counseling, 272
Henry Lynch, Carrie Snyder and Jane F. Lynch

CHAPTER 27

Cancer control planning

Massoud Samiei

Background

Among the non-communicable diseases (NCDs), cancer is rapidly becoming a serious burden for the populations and health authorities in all low- and middle-income countries (LMICs). As the World Health Organization (WHO) stresses, there is no country in the world where cancer does not occur [1]. Despite all the progress made in cancer research and in the fight against cancer, it is a fact that the disease cannot be completely eradicated in the foreseeable future. A logical public health measure must therefore focus all efforts on preventing and confining the disease or, in other words, a systematic and coordinated approach is needed to reduce the impact of cancer on populations. Such an organized approach is called *cancer control*.

WHO places great emphasis on the rising impact of NCDs and cancer in LMICs, and the disproportionate suffering they cause in poor and disadvantaged populations [2]. The growing cancer epidemic in LMICs presents a major challenge to global public health. If present trends continue, more and more people will die prematurely and needlessly from cancer. Most countries are unable to cope with the current trends due to severely limited or non-existent resources and necessary medical infrastructure, which are needed to prevent, diagnose, and treat cancer. Even worse, few LMICs, if any, are prepared to deal with the increased cancer burden looming on the horizon. The cancer epidemic will certainly get worse with immense social and economic consequence unless more concrete and concerted actions are taken at global, regional, and country levels. In particular, with the rapid changes taking place in cancer risk and cancer burden in LMICs, there is an urgent need for governments to enact effective *cancer control policies* and *strategies* to facilitate the development of appropriate cancer control action plans [3]. Unfortunately, due to the absence of NCDs and cancer in the Millennium Development Goals, the international donor community still has difficulty considering cancer control a priority in LMICs; as a result, donor funding has been very limited for cancer control efforts.

The good news is that a clearer picture of the global issues of cancer is emerging and quite a number of evidence-based targets and cost-effective interventions for prevention and for reduction of morbidity and mortality can be identified for most common cancers [4]. It is for this reason that the establishment of a *national cancer control strategy* (or *policy*) to facilitate the planning and implementation of various activities to control cancer is strongly encouraged for all countries. More importantly, as some cancers are avoidable and others treatable when detected early, any systematic and organized measures to control cancer should be able to reduce cancer mortality and morbidity to improve the quality of life of cancer patients and their families. Even in low-resource countries, cancer control activities are necessary [1, 4].

As the resources are constrained everywhere and there are many competing healthcare priorities, effective plans with well-defined activities are needed to ensure that the limited resources are distributed in accordance with identified priority cancer control needs, and accessed equitably and sustainably. These actions should be systematic and form part of a holistic and coordinated approach, involving the public sector, non-governmental organizations (NGOs), academia, and the private sector. This should ensure that the selection and implementation of best practices in cancer prevention, early detection, treatment, and care are *resource-level appropriate* (that is, appropriate for the income level of the country) and are consistent with the country's prevailing social and cultural circumstances. Policy makers and cancer advocacy groups in LMICs should therefore consider *cancer control planning* and its financing and implementation a *public health necessity* and not an option [1].

The efforts described above are collectively referred to as a *national cancer control plan* or *programme* (NCCP). Other terminologies such as *cancer control strategy, comprehensive cancer control plan* or *population-based cancer control strategy/plan/programme* are also commonly used with the same meaning. Often, the words 'strategy', 'plan', and 'programme' are used interchangeably. In the context of cancer control, a *programme* is a collection of all national strategies and *plans* of action intended to reduce the impact of cancer in the *entire country and its population* relying on *all the resources* available during a determined period. An NCCP is described by the WHO as: 'a public health programme designed to reduce cancer incidence and mortality and improve quality of life of cancer patients, through the systematic and equitable implementation of evidence-based strategies for the prevention, early detection, diagnosis, treatment and palliation, making the best use of available resources' [5]. NCCPs provide a platform for the application of best evidence-based practices in cancer prevention and treatment. WHO emphasizes that the implementation of a carefully planned NCCP offers the most cost-effective means of achieving a tangible degree of cancer control, even where resources are limited [4]. The comprehensive cancer control approach also allows all stakeholders in a country to share with each other their skills, knowledge, and resources, so that the country can take advantage of all its potentials to more quickly and efficiently reduce the burden of cancer for all its population. Naturally, any intervention that is selected to be part of the NCCP must be economically feasible and, more importantly, culturally appropriate for the intended population and setting in mind.

Cancer control planning or NCD control planning?

It is important to take note of some recent developments concerning cancer and NCDs, which will have a bearing on future approaches to cancer control planning.

Although the growing burden of NCDs had been recognized since late 1980s, only in the past decade or so has there been increased attention to these diseases among health policy makers with growing concern about the severity and the magnitude of NCDs throughout the world. More significantly, health authorities worldwide have become aware about the increased prevalence of NCDs in LMICs and the cost of treating them, which has contributed to a widening of the healthcare gap between various sectors of society. As a result, the question of providing affordable means of treating the growing number of patients with cancer and other chronic diseases in LMICs, particularly in terms of medicine and health technology, has become increasingly prominent in the minds of policy makers and health authorities, in addition to concerns about the most feasible strategies for prevention and control. This has also become a priority for many United Nations (UN) agencies and active international organizations, but has been given a new emphasis following the comprehensive resolution approved by all UN member states in September 2011 on the prevention and control of non-communicable diseases [6], among which cancer is a leading cause of death. The matter has been given even higher urgency following the May 2012 World Health Assembly's decision to set *a global target of 25% reduction of premature mortality from NCDs by 2025* as a key target, amongst others, for the implementation of the UN resolution [7].

It is clear, therefore, that controlling cancer does not need to be at the expense of other diseases in LMICs or done in isolation. As a matter of fact, WHO underscores that 'National cancer control programmes evaluate the best ways to control and prevent cancer at country level. Governments who early on committed to address non-communicable diseases are already seeing progress in reducing cancer, diagnosing sooner and saving lives. Based on these successful examples, more countries should implement similar programme' [8]. The prevention and control of cancer should therefore be integrated into all major horizontal and vertical actions for other NCDs and all aspects of cancer control plans—from prevention to management of cancer and related research priorities—should be part of the national plans for strengthening the health system [9]. It is understood that strengthening health systems will make national efforts to reduce the burden of both communicable and non-communicable diseases more effective and sustainable. A recent WHO report on the global status of NCDs has put forward a series of interventions known to be effective, feasible, and affordable in any resource setting [10]. Primary healthcare (PHC) is identified as the best framework for implementing recommended interventions. The report highlights that NCCPs fit into the broader WHO framework to strengthen health systems with a major focus on PHC, and are part of the implementation of the *Action Plan of the Global Strategy for the Preventions and Control of NCDs*, which was endorsed by the World Health Assembly in May 2008 [2]. WHO has recently issued a new update of this Action Plan for 2013–2020 with the approval of its member states [11]. There are already a number of initiatives in various regions showing that this is the most feasible approach [9, 12, 13].

Elements of cancer control

Cancer control involves a number of key elements, which generally consist of four main components considered by WHO to be the cancer control priorities [1]: *prevention, early detection and screening, diagnosis and treatment*, and *palliative care*. Often, additional components are necessary which could be included in the NCCP, or within one of the above, especially where more resources are available. The most crucial among these are: a population-based cancer registry and surveillance system (to assess cancer burden, identify needs to support planning, monitor outcomes of all actions, and support cancer control evaluation); cancer advocacy and public education; survivorship and psychosocial support for patients and their families (more broadly called *cancer rehabilitation* aiming to help a person with cancer obtain the best physical, social, psychological, and work-related functioning during and after cancer treatment); and cancer research and clinical trials. Sometimes, other titles are used to describe the main components: for example, *primary prevention* (prevention), *secondary prevention* (early detection and screening), and *tertiary prevention, tertiary care*, or *cancer management* (diagnosis, treatment, and palliative care).

Whatever terminology is used, the important issue to note is that cancer control planning is about *all actions* that can reduce the impact of cancer and improve the quality of life for patients. Prevention, early detection and screening, diagnosis and treatment, palliative care, and psychosocial support are the components of cancer control that can reduce the burden of cancer. Advocacy and public education are essential prerequisites to inform and engage the population. Surveillance, research, monitoring, and evaluation are necessary to understand the causes of cancer, the effects of various interventions, and to analyse the country's cancer burden, as well as to measure progress for feedback into the cancer plan.

It is the responsibility of the health planners and policy makers to ensure that the NCCP planning process brings together all cancer stakeholders in the country to work on assessing strategic options and choosing those that are feasible, effective, and cost-effective bearing in mind the specific conditions of their country. Only then can they find the best combination of priorities and cost-effective interventions that will suit their resource setting and social and cultural boundaries to address cancer effectively within an overall national NCD strategy [10].

Naturally, very few countries will be able to have a comprehensive plan involving all cancer components right from the beginning. Experience from high-income countries suggests that cancer control capacity can develop in a step-by-step approach, starting with a few high-priority and implementable components (such as a focus on two to three common curable cancer sites, on risk factors such as tobacco control and banning public smoking, and on improved palliative care services). Later on, more components and interventions can be added as results are achieved and more resources become available. In most regions, perhaps the key indicator of progress would be a change of attitude and perception by the public about cancer as a non-preventable and non-curable disease, or that a cancer diagnosis is considered a death sentence [14, 15].

The planning process

The cancer control planning process can start when a country's national authorities decide to create a new cancer control plan or update an existing one. The development of a national cancer control plan and programme involves a number of logical and systematic steps similar to any other strategic planning process. Experience shows that it is vital to follow these steps to arrive at valid and workable strategies and plans. WHO has published managerial guidelines for cancer control [1], and a set of six modules entitled 'Cancer Control: Knowledge into Action' on how to develop and implement an effective cancer control plan to combat cancer effectively [4, 16]. The Union for International Cancer Control (UICC) has also very useful cancer control planning guidelines and toolkits for NGOs [17, 18]. WHO and the International Atomic Energy Agency (IAEA) jointly have developed a self-assessment tool that can help kick-start the planning process [19]. More planning guidelines, toolkits, and assessment models are also available from other organizations [20–23]. These are essential references for all planning stages.

Pre-planning prerequisites

In order to develop a successful NCCP, leadership and the relevant stakeholders need to be identified early on in the process to form a *cancer control* or *NCCP planning group* so that all partners can participate and take ownership and responsibility for the programme. The most important early first step for the initiator of the cancer control planning process is, therefore, to identify and invite and engage all governmental and non-governmental national stakeholders and service providers, including the private sector and patient organizations (where active). The process must involve all stakeholders from the beginning to the end. This systematic approach is the only manner in which a country's health authorities will be able to establish an effective programme to translate cancer control knowledge into appropriate actions in line with existing resources and available capacity [4]. To be effective and have enough authority, the NCCP planning group in LMICs needs to be established under the auspices of the Ministry of Health, and act as a *Steering Committee for Cancer Control* in the country, led by a *Programme Coordinator* who would oversee the entire process from planning to implementation and evaluation.

During pre-planning, all participants in the process would benefit from a review of existing cancer control strategies, plans or programmes, and discussion on possible opportunities, feasible interventions, lessons learned, and areas needing more attention such as quality health data and equitable access to cancer control [4, 24–26]. They should also review the different approaches adopted in similar countries for planning and delivery of population-based cancer control, and their accomplishments or failures, to decide how best to proceed in line with their aspirations, commitment, political will, local conditions, capacity, and resources [4, 27–29]. One option that has proven critical for many countries is that governments may seek external technical support (available from several organizations, particularly WHO, IAEA, UICC, IARC, INCTR, and AfrOx) to advise their Ministry of Health and the cancer control group on all issues related to NCCP planning.

Next, the NCCP planning group must familiarize themselves with the various dimensions of the cancer problem in the country with planning and implementation methodologies based on existing cancer control guidelines and tools from WHO, UICC, and other sources as indicated above. Every country should also adopt some *guiding principles* and a *set of values* to direct and

help its policy makers and participants in the NCCP planning processes to remain within a defined framework when analysing the situation, selecting cancer control interventions, making recommendations, or taking decisions for any action. A list of such principles and values based on experience in some 50 countries is presented here:

1. *Management and coordination*: cancer control leadership is expected to create clarity and unity of purpose; encourage team building; ensure broad participation, ownership of the process and mutual recognition of the efforts made; and involves everyone in continuous learning.

2. *Performance*: a strong focus on quality and the development of a culture of measurement and quality assurance.

3. *People*: a strong focus on rights and entitlements of patients, their families, and care providers. People's needs must come first.

4. *Collaboration*: a greater emphasis on partnership with community and voluntary sectors.

5. *Equity*: addressing health inequalities among different population groups.

6. *Accessibility*: an affordable, timely, and equitable access for all sectors of the population to a comprehensive range of health services regardless of ability to pay.

7. *Gender and culture*: recognition of and respect for gender sensitivity, cultural diversity, and ethical values of communities targeted.

8. *Evidence based*: a system of planning and evaluating policy and service delivery based on needs assessment, scientific evidence, and appropriate health technologies.

9. *Sustainability*: support long-term sustainability of the healthcare system by dealing effectively with and reducing the rise in the number of cancer cases.

10. *Efficiency*: use public resources wisely and promote the efficient use of these resources throughout the cancer system.

11. *Integration*: use available resources in a more efficient, balanced, and equitable manner by adopting cancer control strategies that are *integrated* within the *healthcare system* (linked to NCD strategy or linked to other existing services such as palliative care). In addition, recognize the common risk factors and opportunities for collaboration and integrated actions simultaneously to reduce the incidence of other chronic diseases.

12. *Stepwise approach*: follow WHO recommendations to adopt *primary healthcare* (PHC) and a stepwise approach to planning and implementing interventions, based on local considerations and needs. (See, for example, the definition of and a discussion on the stepwise approach to palliative care [29].)

In addition to the above, the planning group should bear in mind that although many specific objectives of an NCCP are achievable within five to ten years, its aims of reducing significantly the incidence of cancer and mortality, and maximizing cancer survival, will require more than 20 to 40 years to materialize. Thus, the final plan can only be successfully implemented if there is an equally long-term commitment on the part of government and partners (stakeholders) to carry out all its elements with close attention to realistic objectives, governance, resource allocation, financing issues, and regular monitoring and performance assessment.

Planning stages

Although WHO [4, 5, 19], the UICC [17, 18], the US Centers for Disease Control and Prevention (CDC) [20, 21], the IAEA [23, 31], and other organizations [32] have developed NCCP-related guidelines, toolkits, and needs assessment tools and models, as highlighted by a recent report from Imperial College London, there is no internationally agreed common format of an NCCP nor a commonly accepted framework to adapt them to local conditions [33]. In addition, no framework is available for NCCP evaluation or comparison, except for a few recent reviews where some criteria have been defined [33, 35]. As a result, a centrally maintained database on NCCPs and their performance worldwide does not exist, which would be ideal for measuring progress made in various regions. Additionally, there are significant differences across regions in the types of prevalent cancers, resources available for cancer control, organizational structure of healthcare system and service delivery, and existing cancer services, making it difficult to propose a single model for a cancer control plan and related interventions. As a result, the structure and framework of cancer plans will also vary; no single model will be suitable for all countries, although similarities in terms of goals, objectives, and planned actions are common among NCCPs.

The overall process can start following pre-planning consultations and the formalization of the planning group and its membership, and their familiarization with, and adherence to, the guiding principles outlined above as adapted in the country (which should preferably be issued by the Ministry of Health). The planning group must carefully review the country's epidemiological data, including data collected by cancer registries, where available, and then jointly set goals, objectives, strategies, and priorities for action considering the country's capacity and resources [4]. They should also work on mobilizing support for the implementation of the plan, and put in place an evaluation system to monitor implementation progress. Ideally, the planning group should be involved in implementation as well (and that is why it is essential for the planning group to be appointed formally by the Minister of Health as the *Steering Committee for Cancer Control* to have the overall responsibility for the entire process). The planning group might seek advice from others within the country or internationally in all stages of their work, but particularly in situation analysis [19, 23], and in comparative assessment of interventions and health technologies. This entire process might take as long as five to six years, a year or more to complete the plan, and normally a period of five years to implement each NCCP cycle. Time should also be allocated for evaluation of each plan and preparation of the next plan cycle.

Planning model

The model proposed here is a *hybrid* one, where the most relevant elements of models and cancer systems available [32, 33], and the actual experience in LMICs engaged in cancer control planning and implementation [31, 34] have been combined to present a more structured planning framework. To start with, the planning process can be summarized into ten major Steps, which are further divided in four set of activities as outlined in Figure 27.1.

As the planning moves forward, each set of Steps in Figure 27.1 represents a period of time and activities which can be considered as a response to two specific questions: one about cancer control status/situation, and the other about cancer control actions. These questions are outlined on the flowchart in Figure 27.2 for each set of Steps in similarly coloured boxes as in Figure 27.1 (the Steps corresponding to each *question* are also indicated in the boxes). It can easily be seen that the four *status/situation-oriented* questions (questions A to D) lead to the four *action-oriented* questions starting with a '*What*'. These four '*What*' questions form the basis for a planning model that was originally developed by a group of public health and cancer experts in the US and also adopted here [32].

Fundamentally, responses to questions A to D form the structure of an NCCP. During the preparatory stages of planning and drafting a consensus NCCP document, eight key questions in Figure 27.2 need to be answered by the Ministry of Health and the group assigned to the task. Arranging the original ten Steps into this set of questions somewhat simplifies the planning process for the planning group, although the responses will require extensive discussion. It is also clear from question D in Figure 27.2 that the process is not linear but cyclic and the process returns to question A once every few years (similar to *project life cycle* idea used in management [36]).

Based on the above analysis, cancer control planning and implementation can be looked at within a framework consisting of *four main* and *two intermediate stages*. The stages are linked in a cycle which can be presented graphically as depicted in Figure 27.3. The 'blue' boxes represent the main stages of the cycle from A to D (corresponding to boxes in Figure 27.2), and the 'orange' ones are intermediate stages highlighting the two key 'milestones' of the planning process; one after Stage C, the agreement on a 'Cancer Control Strategy', the completion of the NCCP formal document and the launching of the NCCP, and the other after Stage D, the evaluation report of NCCP and the revised NCCP for the next cycle. The central 'grey' box defines the vital prerequisites and the enabling conditions for the progress and success of the NCCP. This box is also the information centre for the NCCP, linking all cancer control data, inputs, activities, and outputs from all stages of the cycle.

Stage A: setting desired aims, goals, and objectives (What should be done?)

Here the NCCP planning group is established and a coordinator is nominated in partnership with stakeholders. To respond to the question 'Where does the country stand now in terms of cancer control?', they analyse all available cancer data to assess the magnitude of the cancer burden, the populations at risk, the risk factors, and any existing gaps in cancer control services. The minimum data needed is a reasonable estimate of all new cases per year, and reliable information on the proportion that may be curable after diagnosis. The top few cancers in the country for which effective prevention is available and those for which early diagnosis can be effective should be listed with estimates of number of people affected. Most LMICs will lack reliable data on cancer incidence, mortality, prevalence, and five-year survival from diagnosis, due to absence of population-based registries. (The only alternative is to rely on data published regularly by the IARC, which provides estimates of cancer incidence for most countries [37].) Special attention must be paid to cancer risk factors. Countries with a high percentage of young people (a triangular population pyramid with broad base) may not have a large cancer incidence but will have a significant prevalence of cancer risk factors [10]. A review of the common types of cancer can provide hints to what

1. Review of epidemiological data and prevailing cancers (if available from cancer registries or other sources), and country specific cancer risk factors

2. Assessment of existing infrastructure and services, and relevant gaps and needs

3. Setting measureable cancer control aims, goals and objectives

4. Agreement on possible strategies for cancer control, and *'resource-level-appropriate'* initial actions, activities, interventions, and related indicators (targets) for each objective

5. Estimation of timeline for achieving the specific objectives (5 years and beyond)

6. Agreement on 5-year priorities and the level and sources of financing

7. Development of implementation plan, and plans for raising additional funds

8. Selection of institutions responsible for delivering the NCCP components (and identification of potential partners)

9. Arrangements for management and implementation of the NCCP

10. Monitoring and evaluation of the results at the end of timeline, feedback to the management of NCCP, and revised NCCP for a new cycle (restart the Steps)

Fig. 27.1 The ten major Steps in cancer control planning.
Reproduced courtesy of Massoud Samiei.

the risks are (e.g., smoking and lung cancer, Hepatitis B infection and liver cancer) but a high-quality random population-based survey will usually be necessary to measure risk factor frequency and to help set priorities for prevention [27]. At the end of this Stage, the aims, goals, and optimal objectives of the NCCP are defined[1], which must be reviewed in the next two stages based on resource-level-appropriate strategies. The activities and outcomes of this stage are driven by *data*.

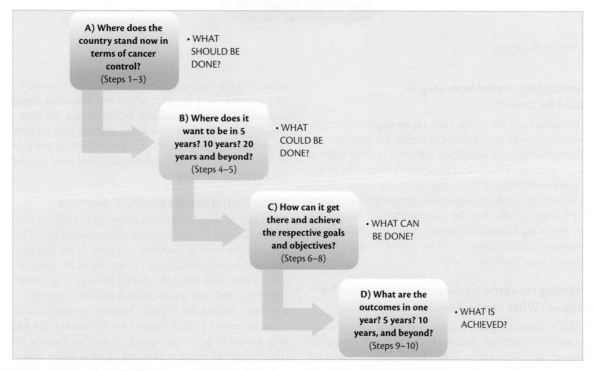

Fig. 27.2 The key questions driving the cancer control planning process.

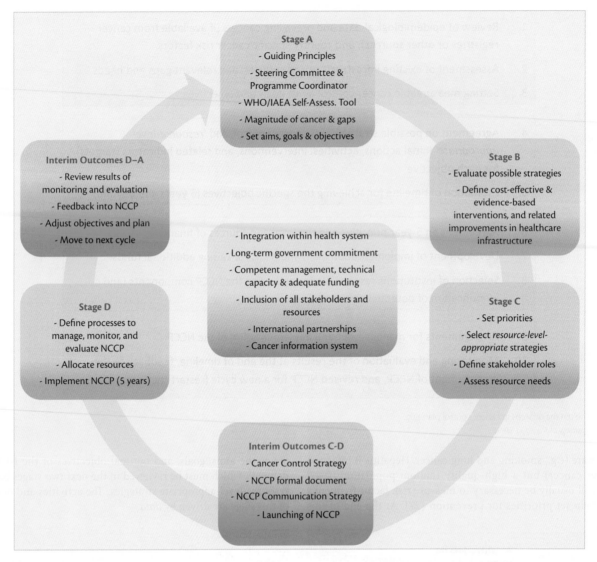

Fig. 27.3 Cancer control planning life cycle.

Stage B: evaluating available strategies (What could be done?)

Based on the objectives set above, relevant strategies are evaluated in consultation with stakeholders to define the interventions and related improvements in healthcare infrastructures in order to respond to the question 'Where does the country want to be in five years, ten years, and beyond?' This stage is mainly *science driven* as it relies on current evidence-based interventions to find those most effective (and cost-effective) for a given setting. If expertise is required for reviewing scientific information and the costs of various interventions, outside experts could be invited through WHO, or other relevant organizations, to help.

Stage C: setting resource-level-appropriate priorities and strategies (What can be done?)

Here the NCCP planning group needs to respond to the question 'How can the country get there and achieve the desired goals and objectives?' In coordination with stakeholders, they must choose amongst possible strategies from Stage B those that are implementable and acceptable locally, and correspond to the country's available and possible additional resources (funds, trained professionals, equipment, and facilities) and the type of cancers targeted (the effectiveness and the costs of intervention strategies for prevention, early detection, curative therapy, and palliative care of common cancers vary substantially and need careful technical review) [9, 24–27].

Cancer control strategy and NCCP document

At the end of Stage C, most countries opt to produce a formal document to present the findings and recommendations of the planning group in the form of a *strategy* or *policy*. Some countries prefer to call such formal documents, when issued by the government, a *policy paper*, and when developed through a partnership of governmental and non-governmental entities, a *strategy*. In general, a strategy defines the overall character, mission and direction of a cancer control plan. Strategies are formulated and implemented with a view to achieving specific goals, but they do not say specifically how to arrive at that end. That is where *policy* is needed to provide direction to all involved on how goals will be achieved.

While the development of possible and feasible strategies (Stages A, B, and C above) and the implementation plan (Stage D) are the responsibility of the Steering Committee for Cancer Control, policy is the responsibility of the government.

This document is then approved and signed by the Minister of Health (or higher authorities to ensure longer-term commitment and political support) and endorsed as a formal document of the government. A well-formulated cancer control strategy (CCS) provides a solid platform and guidelines for implementing and maintaining cancer control measures and for making cancer control an integral part of the nation's healthcare programme. According to WHO, such a document may be defined as 'an explicit commitment by the government and its partners that provides objectives for a balanced cancer control programme, specifies the relative priority of each objective and indicates the resources and measures required to attain the objectives' [1]. An excellent example of such a document is the 2010 Cancer Policy Framework of the Newfoundland and Labrador province in Canada [38]. This document outlines the provincial government's response to the burden of cancer in the province by providing key policy directions that will be used to guide cancer control efforts and specific action plans in the province in the coming years.

NCCP Document

The NCCP planning group and their coordinator must also produce a written version of the NCCP (that is the CCS and its implementation plan), and have it agreed as a consensus document by all concerned and ratified by the Minister of Health. This formal document is vital for further action by the government and the planning group, and is also needed to ensure an efficient and effective management of the NCCP and its continuity. Additionally, an *NCCP communication strategy* needs to be discussed and documented to ensure full public and media understanding and support for the plan and its actions. These documents will later be the main reference for officially adopting the NCCP, launching it, and managing its implementation.

Although the NCCP formulation will follow each country's specific situation and needs, the structure of the written document will be generally similar everywhere, i.e. an assessment of the cancer burden in the country; definition of aims, goals, and objectives; identification of the priority needs of the country; the cancer control strategies adopted; setting of realistic performance indicators (targets) and timeline, identifying those responsible for each; and review of resources available within the health system and sources of future funding (for examples of NCCPs see the 'Further reading' list at the end of this chapter).

Stage D: implementing and evaluating (What is achieved?)

The last stage provides a response to the question 'What has been achieved in one year, five years, ten years, and beyond?' It is basically an *outcome-driven* stage for implementing in cooperation with stakeholders the strategies reviewed during Stage B and selected during Stage C to meet the objectives defined during Stage A. The first action is to develop an implementation plan and define the processes to manage, monitor, and evaluate it (an implementation plan is needed whether a CCS has been formally approved at the end of Stage C or not).

Stage D is the longest period within the cycle and is normally set to five years. As it involves the management of NCCP's implementation processes, it requires adequate administrative, financial and technical capacity at national level [1, 4].

Evaluation report and revised NCCP

After the implementation period, there is a year of NCCP review and evaluation of results to provide feedback for the new cycle. Monitoring and evaluation are crucial to measure what various stakeholders and partners who have been given responsibility for the implementation of agreed interventions and actions have achieved. In addition, any shortcomings or failures must be addressed with recommendations for the next cycle. The results are reflected in a report and then utilized for feedback into NCCP to adjust objectives, intervention strategies, and activities as necessary, and to secure the resources for the next five-year cancer plan. A *new Stage A and NCCP cycle* with an enhanced cancer control status and programme in the country can then begin.

The success of this model, apart from being dependent on the efficient organization of the entire process, the long-term government commitment, the effectiveness of the planning group (Steering Committee and its Coordinator), resources available, and the collaboration of all partners involved, depends greatly on the availability and functionality of a pool of data and knowledge for decision-making in all its stages (the enabling condition presented in the 'grey' box in Figure 27.3). The data should ideally be centrally maintained or compiled, as part of the cancer surveillance and information system, using a computerized cancer information system with oversight of the Steering Committee.

Challenges facing planners

In this short overview of cancer control planning steps and processes, it is not possible to highlight all critical issues and challenges that are most relevant for LMICs. A recent WHO survey on national capacity for NCDs [10] in 185 countries revealed major gaps in cancer control planning and services. WHO reports that 'even if countries developed cancer plans or policies, many countries are struggling to move from commitment to action. Often these plans are not integrated into wider national health and development planning. In addition, many countries lack institutional capacity, as well as decisive leadership to ensure adequate national funding for cancer control' [39].

To guide the professionals interested in the topic, it suffices to stress that experience with operational NCCPs shows that those with more *realistic objectives and strategies*, corresponding to the *level of resources available*, have accomplished more [4, 24]. In such NCCPs, priority is given to effective (and cost-effective) interventions and programmes that are *resource-level-appropriate* and beneficial to the largest part of the population. Beyond resources, effective NCCPs are those that are *managed* well by a dedicated team and its leader, namely the *Steering Committee* and the *Programme Coordinator*, particularly in terms of continuous monitoring, evaluation, and periodical adjustments during implementation [25, 27].

Until quite recently, one area of concern for developing cancer plans in LMICs was the lack of sufficient or consolidated evidence and information in some fields relevant to low-resource settings. Despite the progress made, the experience in many LMICs shows that cancer control planning groups and policy makers often face more complicated questions, especially technical ones, related to planning Stages A, B, and C, for which there are not always readily available responses, either due to the lack of adequate scientific evidence relevant to their particular setting, or the lack of a clear or agreed definition of some of the terminology used in the cancer control literature. For example, to quote from an excellent reference on the subject [24]: 'What level of cancer incidence justifies a prevention or early detection programme? How do policy-makers know what specific approach or intervention is likely to succeed under their own circumstances? What is a comprehensive approach? What are necessary resources?' Alternatively, more specific ones as often discussed in cancer control conferences: What are the most appropriate screening approaches for common cancers? What are the right diagnostic and treatment technologies and infrastructure for the country? Or: How many professionals are needed to establish a reasonable cancer treatment service?

Fortunately, there have been a number of international initiatives and substantial scientific publications on cancer-control-related work and practice in the past decade, which are gradually shedding light on most of the 'What' and 'How' questions. For instance, the publication in 2006 of a set of guidelines by Breast Health Global Initiative intended to help policy makers and healthcare providers in LMICs adapt evidence-based, economically feasible and culturally appropriate practices, has strengthened efforts to improve breast healthcare and outcomes for women in LMICs through NCCPs [40]. Additional work has shed further light on *what's needed, what works*, and *how it should be done* [26, 29, 34, 41]. Further, there have been a few recent evaluations and reviews of existing NCCPs that are helpful in pinpointing some of the opportunities and key requirements for success [24, 33, 35, 42].

Finally, national efforts may be further enhanced or strengthened by being linked to global efforts spearheaded by international organizations (such as the HBV and HPV vaccination campaigns), in addition to seeking their assistance for situation analysis, NCCP planning, or certain plan implementation aspects (as mentioned above).

To learn more about best practices and cost-effective strategies in different settings, the most instructive approach is the review of existing NCCP documents of other countries and their reported experience. The online References and Additional resources provide an extensive list for further reference and reading. In addition to relevant material posted on the websites of organizations involved in cancer control as cited here, cancer control plans or strategies of a number of countries, including those of LMICs, can be found on the Internet, many of which can be instructive for anyone working on cancer control.

Note

1 The cancer control *aims, goals and objectives* need to be stated clearly in the NCCP document. As these terms could often be confusing in different languages, some examples are given below using WHO and other guidelines in the literature: Aims: (a) Reducing the overall incidence and mortality of selected cancers in the country, as well as improving overall survival and the quality of life of cancer patients and their families; Goals: (b) Preventing cancer and raising public awareness about the high priority cancers in the country and means of combating them; (c) Detecting cancers early and facilitating early access to treatment and follow-up; (d) Providing high quality cancer care for every patient diagnosed with cancer, with an emphasis on palliative care during the early stages of the plan; (e) Investing in expansion and improvement of existing

services to cover larger populations; (f) Ensuring adequate availability of workforce, and facilitating education and training in cancer control components; (g) Ensuring cancer services are gradually available and accessible across the country at affordable costs; Objectives: (Objectives are country, burden and resource dependent and can be general or more specific. For each goal, there can be a number of objectives – and often for each objective, more specific ones are defined): (h) Reducing incidence of cancers caused by tobacco; (i) Reducing tobacco smoking rates among health care professionals and patients attending primary care clinics.

References

1. WHO. National Cancer Control Programmes: Policies and Managerial Guidelines, 2nd ed. Geneva: WHO, 2002.

2. WHO. 2008–2013 Action Plan for the Global Strategy for the Prevention and Control of Non-Communicable Diseases. WHO: Geneva, 2008. Available from: http://www.who.int/nmh/publications/9789241597418/en/index.html, accessed on 20 October 2012.

3. Boyle P, Howell A. The globalisation of breast cancer, Breast Cancer 2010; Research 12(Suppl. 4): S7.

4. WHO. Cancer Control: Knowledge into Action. WHO Guide for Effective Programmes, Mod. 1: Planning. Geneva: WHO, 2006. Available from: <http://www.who.int/cancer/publications/cancer_control_planning/en/index.html>, accessed on 20 September 2012.

5. WHO. Cancer: National cancer control programmes. Geneva: WHO, 2012. Available from: <http://www.who.int/cancer/nccp/en/, accessed on 20 October 2012.

6. WHO. UN high-level meeting on non-communicable diseases prevention and control. Geneva: WHO, 19–20 September 2011, <http://www.who.int/nmh/events/un_ncd_summit2011/en/>, accessed on 24 February 2013.

7. WHO, Media centre, 65th World Health Assembly closes with new global health measures, 25 May 2012, <http://www.who.int/mediacentre/news/releases/2012/wha65_closes_20120526/en/index.html>, accessed on 24 February 2013.

8. WHO. Dr Oleg Chestnov, Assistant Director-General for Non-Communicable Diseases and Mental Health, WHO, at the 2012 UICC World Cancer Leaders' Summit, 27 August 2012, Montréal, Canada. Available from: <http://www.worldcancercongress.org/experts-warn-human-and-economic-cost-inaction-cancer>, accessed on 24 February 2013.

9. Sullivan R, Purushottham A. Towards an international cancer control plan: policy solutions for the global cancer epidemic. Network: The Magazine of the INCTR 2010; 9(4): 1–8.

10. WHO. Global Status Report On Non-Communicable Diseases. Geneva: WHO, 2010.

11. WHO. Global Action Plan for the Prevention and Control of Non-Communicable Diseases 2013–2020 (. WHO: Geneva, 2013. Available from < http://www.who.int/global-coordination-mechanism/publications/global-action-plan-ncds-eng.pdf >, accessed on 28 May 2015.

12. Narain JP. Integrating services for non-communicable diseases prevention and control: use of primary health care approach, Indian Journal of Community Medicine 2011; 36(Suppl. 1): 67–71.

13. Nishtar S. Prevention of non-communicable diseases in Pakistan: an integrated partnership-based model. Health Research Policy and Systems 2004; 2: 7.

14. Cancer as a disease, not a death sentence. New York Times, 17 June 2008. Available from: <http://www.nytimes.com/2008/06/17/health/17brody.html?_r=2&>, accessed on 24 February 2013.

15. Cancer is 'not a death sentence' anymore. Dominion Post, 19 April 2012. Available from: <http://www.stuff.co.nz/dominion-post/news/6764731/Cancer-is-not-a-death-sentence-anymore>, accessed on 25 Apr 2012.

16. WHO. Cancer Control: WHO Guide for Effective Programmes. Geneva: WHO, 2006. Available from: <http://www.who.int/cancer/modules/en/index.html>, accessed on 25 October 2012.

17. UICC. National Cancer Control Planning: Resources for Non-Governmental Organizations. Geneva: UICC, 2005. Available from <http://www.uicc.org/resources/national-cancer-control-planning-nccp>, accessed on 28 September 2012.

18. UICC. Supporting National Cancer Control Planning: A Toolkit for Civil Society Organisations. Geneva: UICC, 2012.

19. Sepulveda C, Samiei M. National cancer control programs capacity assessment: a joint WHO–IAEA initiative. Tumori 2009; 95: 573–574.

20. Centers for Disease Control and Prevention, USA (2002). Guidance for Comprehensive Cancer Control Planning, Volume 1: Guideline. Division of Cancer Prevention and Control, Centers for Disease Control and Prevention. Atlanta. Available from <http://www.cdc.gov/cancer/ncccp/pdf/Guidance-Guidelines.pdf>, accessed on 20 October 2012.

21. Centers for Disease Control and Prevention, USA (2002). Guidance for Comprehensive Cancer Control Planning, Volume 2: Toolkit. Atlanta: CDCP, 2002. Available from <http://www.cdc.gov/cancer/ncccp/pdf/Guidance-Toolkit.pdf>, accessed on 20 October 2012.

22. Edwards BK, Vinson CA, Stinchcomb DG. The Cancer Control PLANET (Plan, Link, Act, Network with Evidence-based Tools) online web portal—a widely used tool in North America for effective program planning, implementation, and evaluation, Tumori 2009 95: 572–573.

23. IAEA. Programme of Action for Cancer Therapy (PACT): Terms of Reference for imPACT (integrated missions of PACT). Vienna: IAEA, 2008. Available from: < http://www-naweb.iaea.org/pact/documents/impactTOR.pdf>, accessed on 28 May 2015.

24. Committee on Cancer Control in Low- and Middle-Income Countries. Cancer Control Opportunities in Low- and Middle-Income Countries, Sloan FA, Gelband H eds. Washington DC; National Academic Press, 2006. Available from <http://books.nap.edu/openbook.php?record_id=11797>, accessed on 12 November 2012.

25. Otter R, Qiao YL, Burton R, Samiei M, Parkin M et al. Organization of population-based cancer control programs: Europe and the World. Tumori 2009; 95: 623–636. Available from: <http://www.tumorionline.it/r.php?v=455&a=5377&l=5325&f=allegati/00455_2009_05/fulltext/06-Otter%20(623-636).pdf>, accessed on 26 September 2012.

26. Hanna TP, Kangolle ACT. Cancer control in developing countries: using health data and health services research to measure and improve access, quality and efficiency. BMC International Health and Human Rights 2010; 10: 24. Available from: <http://www.biomedcentral.com/1472-698X/10/24>, accessed on 4 November 2012.

27. Harford JB, Edwards BK, Nandakumar A, Ndom P, Capocaccia R et al. Cancer control-planning and monitoring population-based systems. Tumori 2009; 95: 568–578.

28. WHO. Overview: National Strategy for Cancer Control in Vietnam (2010–2020). Geneva: WHO, 2006. Available from: <http://www.who.int/cancer/modules/Viet%20Nam.pdf>, accessed on 4 November 2012.

29. Romero T. Changing the paradigm of cancer control in Cuba. MEDICC Review 2009; 11(3). Available from: <http://www.medicc.org/mediccreview/articles/mr_97.pdf>, accessed on 20 October 2012.

30. WHO. Cancer control: knowledge into action. WHO guide for effective programmes, mod. 5: Palliative Care. Geneva: WHO, 2007. Available from: <http://www.who.int/cancer/media/FINAL-Palliative%20Care%20Module.pdf>, accessed on 24 February 2013.

31. Samiei M. Building partnerships to stop the cancer epidemic in the developing world. UN Special 2008; 676, Sept. 2008. Available from: <http://www.unspecial.org/UNS676/t31.html>, accessed on 20 September 2012.

32. Abed J, Reilly B, Odell Butler M, Kean T, Wong F et al. Developing a framework for comprehensive cancer prevention and control in the United States, Journal of Public Health Management Practice 2000; 6(2): 67–78.

33. Atun R, Ogawa T, Martin-Moreno JM. Analysis of National Cancer Control Programmes in Europe, Imperial College Business School. London 2009. Available from <https://spiral.imperial.ac.uk/bitstream/10044/1/4204/1/Cancer%20Control%20vf2.pdf>, accessed on 20 February 2013.

34. Samiei M. Health systems strengthening for cancer control. In: Stewart BW, Wild CP, eds. World Cancer Report 2014. Geneva: International Agency for Research on Cancer. Available from: <http://apps.who.int/bookorders/anglais/detart1.jsp?codlan=1&codcol=80&codcch=275>, accessed on 28 May 2015.

35. Gorgojo L, Harris M, Garcia-Lopez E. National cancer control programmes: Analysis of primary data from questionnaires. European Partnership for Action Against Cancer, 2012. Available from: <http://www.epaac.eu/news/219-final-report-qnational-cancer-control-programmes-analysis-of-primary-data-from-questionnairesq-published>, accessed on 24 February 2013.

36. European Commission. Project Life Cycle Management Handbook. Freiburg: European Commission. Available from <http://www.sle-berlin.de/files/sletraining/PCM_Train_Handbook_EN-March2002.pdf>, accessed on 28 September 2012.

37. IARC. Cancer Incidence in Five Continents. IARC Scientific Publication No. 160. Lyon: IARC. Available from: <http://www.iarc.fr/en/publications/pdfs-online/epi/sp160/>, accessed on 15 May 2015. (More details on definition of terms available from: <http://globocan.iarc.fr>, accessed on 20 October 2012.)

38. Department of Health and Community Services, Newfoundland Labrador. Gaining Ground: A Provincial Cancer Control Policy Framework for Newfoundland and Labrador. ST Johns, NL: DHCS. Available from: <http://www.health.gov.nl.ca/health/publications/gaining_ground_provincial_cancer_control_policy.pdf>, accessed on 22 September 2012.

39. WHO, Media Centre. 1 in 2 countries unprepared to prevent and manage cancers, says WHO survey. Geneva: WHO, 2013. Available from: <http://www.who.int/mediacentre/news/notes/2013/world_cancer_day_20130201/en/index.html>, accessed on 24 February 2013)

40. BHGI. Guidelines for international breast health and cancer control implementation. Cancer 2008; 113 (Suppl. 8): i–ix, 2215–2371.

41. Pisani P. The cancer burden and cancer control in developing countries. Environmental Health 2011; 10(Suppl. 1): S2.

42. ECCO (European CanCer Organisation). Oncpolicy Forum 2011: National Cancer Plans. ECCO, 2011. Available from <http://www.ecco-org.eu/~/media/ECCO%20documents/ECCO%20sections/Public%20Affairs/Oncopolicy%20Forum/2011/Final%20Session%20Six.pdf>, accessed on 24 February 2013.

Additional resources

Organizations

1. World Health Organization (WHO), http://www.who.int/cancer/nccp/en/

2. Union for International Cancer Control (UICC), http://www.uicc.org/

3. International Agency for Research on Cancer (IARC), http://www.iarc.fr/

4. International Atomic Energy Agency/Programme of Action for Cancer Therapy (IAEA/PACT), http://cancer.iaea.org/whoarewe.asp

5. International Network for Cancer Treatment and Research (INCTR), http://cancer-control.wikidot.com/site-structure

6. American Cancer Society (ACS), http://www.cancer.org

7. African Organisation for Research and Training in Cancer (AORTIC), http://www.aortic-africa.org/index.php/about/about/

8. Breast Health Global Initiative (BHGI), http://portal.bhgi.org/Pages/Default.aspx

9. American Society of Clinical Oncology (ASCO), http://www.asco.org

10. European Society for Medical Oncology (ESMO), http://www.esmo.org/about-esmo.html

11. London School of Hygiene and Tropical Medicine, http://www.lshtm.ac.uk/pressoffice/press_releases/2008/cancersurvival.html

12. Africa Oxford Cancer Foundation (AfrOx), http://www.afrox.org/

13. Cancer Council of South Australia, http://www.cancersa.org.au/aspx/about_us.aspx
14. National Cancer Institute (INCA), Brazil, http://www.inca.gov.br/english/
15. Canadian Cancer Society, http://www.cancer.ca
16. Canadian Partnership against Cancer, http://www.partnershipagainst-cancer.ca
17. National Cancer Institute (NCI), Cairo University, Egypt, http://www.nci.cu.edu.eg
18. Institut National du Cancer (INCa), France, http://www.e-cancer.fr/en
19. Irish Cancer Society, http://www.cancer.ie
20. Instituto de Cancerología, México, http://www.incan.salud.gob.mx/contenido/acercade/english.html
21. Institut Català d'Oncologia, Spain, http://www20.gencat.cat/portal/site/salut/menuitem.d4e38b9cb651e7ec3bfd8a10b0c0e1a0/?vgnextoid=834f0225c538c210VgnVCM2000009b0c1e0aRCRD&vgnextchannel=834f0225c538c210VgnVCM2000009b0c1e0aRCRD&vgnextfmt=default&newLang=en_GB
22. National Cancer Institute (NCI), USA, http://www.cancer.gov
23. International Cancer Control Congress Association (ICCCA), http://www.icccassociation.com/index.html

National cancer strategies or plans

1. Albania, National Cancer Control Program 2011–2020, Ministry of Health, http://www.thewpca.org/EasysiteWeb/getresource.axd?AssetID=109009&type=Full&servicetype=Attachment
2. Australia, Cancer Australia Strategic Plan 2011–2014, http://canceraustralia.gov.au/publications-resources/cancer-australia-publications/strategic-plan-2011-2014
3. Bangladesh, National Cancer Control Strategy and Plan of Action 2009–2015, http://www.ban.searo.who.int/LinkFiles/Publication_Cancer_Strategy.pdf.pdf
4. Belgium, National Cancer Plan, 2008–2010, https://webgate.ec.europa.eu/sanco/heidi/images/2/27/Belgium_National_Cancer_Plan_2008-2010_English.pdf
5. Canada, 2012–2017 Strategic Cancer Plan: Sustaining Action Toward a Shared Vision, http://www.partnershipagainstcancer.ca/wp-content/uploads/Sustaining-Action-Toward-a-Shared-Vision-Full-Document.pdf
6. China, Programme of Cancer Control and Prevention in China, 2004–2010, http://www.chinacancernet.org.cn/links/english.html
7. Colombia, Plan Nacional para el Control del Cáncer 2010–2019 (Spanish), http://www.cancer.gov.co/contenido/contenido.aspx?conID=1061&catID=1
8. Estonia, National Cancer Strategy 2007–2015, https://webgate.ec.europa.eu/sanco/heidi/images/a/a5/Estonia_National_Cancer_Strategy_2007-2015_English.pdf
9. France, Institut National du Cancer: Plan Cancer 2003–2007: http://www.e-cancer.fr/Institut-national-Cancer/plan-cancer-2003-2007/op_1-it_112-la_1-ve_1.html
10. Hungary, National Cancer Control Programme, http://www.thewpca.org/EasysiteWeb/getresource.axd?AssetID=92889&type=Full&servicetype=Attachment
11. India, National Cancer Control Programme, http://www.nihfw.org/NDC/DocumentationServices/ NationalHealthProgramme/NATIONALCANCERCONTROLPROGRAMME.html
12. Ireland, A Cancer Control Strategy for Ireland, 2006, http://www.hse.ie/eng/services/Publications/HealthProtection/Public_Health_/National_Cancer_Control_Strategy.pdf
13. Kenya, National Cancer Control Strategy, 2011–2016, http://www.ipcrc.net/pdfs/Kenya-National-Cancer-Control-strategy.pdf
14. Rep of Korea, National Cancer Control Program in Korea, 2010, http://www.pitt.edu/~super4/41011-42001/41041-41051.pdf
15. Mauritius, National Cancer Control Programme: Action Plan 2010–2014, http://www.gov.mu/portal/goc/moh/file/cancer-ap.pdf
16. Mongolia, National Cancer Centre, Sub-Programme on Cancer Prevention and Control, 2009, http://eng.cancer-center.gov.mn/index.php?coid=31&cid=191
17. Morocco, Plan National de Prévention et de Contrôle du Cancer (French), http://www.contrelecancer.ma/site_media/uploaded_files/Synthese_PNPCC_2010-1019.pdf
18. Netherlands, National Comprehensive Cancer Control Programme 2005–2010, available from: http://www.NPKnet.nl
19. New Zealand, Cancer Control Strategy, 2003, Ministry of Health, http://www.cancernz.org.nz/assets/files/Resources_Auckland/Cancer%20Control%20Strategy.pdf
20. New Zealand, Cancer Control Strategy and Action Plan, 2005–2010, http://www.health.govt.nz/our-work/diseases-and-conditions/cancer-programme/cancer-control-strategy-and-action-plan
21. New Zealand, Capital & Coast District, Cancer Control Plan 2010–2015, http://www.ccdhb.org.nz/services/Cancer/CCP%202010-2015%20Section%201.pdf
22. Northern Ireland, Cancer Control Programme, 2010–2013, http://www.cancerni.net/cancerinni/cancerpolicytargets/cancercontrolprogramme
23. Ontario (Canada), Cancer Plan 2011–2015, http://ocp.cancercare.on.ca/common/pages/UserFile.aspx?fileId=84206
24. Qatar, National Cancer Strategy, http://www.nhsq.info/national-cancer-strategy
25. Spain, Estrategia en Cáncer del Sistema Nacional de Salud (Spanish), https://webgate.ec.europa.eu/sanco/heidi/images/4/40/Spain_National_Cancer_Strategy_Spanish.pdf
26. Sudan, Comprehensive National Cancer Control Programme, 2006, http://www.researchgate.net/publication/6983953_Cancer_initiatives_in_Sudan
27. Switzerland, National Cancer Programme for Switzerland, 2011–2015, http://www.thewpca.org/EasysiteWeb/getresource.axd?AssetID=93070&type=Full&servicetype=Attachment
28. Thailand, National Cancer Control Programme, http://www.senkyo.co.jp/apcc20th_abstract/pdf/apcc0009_Cancer%20Control_Dr.%20Khuhaprema.pdf
29. Turkey, National Cancer Control Program, 2011–2015, http://www.calameo.com/books/000713529dde4800f9572 (this is a public website that allows viewing of the full document only)
30. United Kingdom, Improving Outcomes: A Strategy for Cancer, 2011, http://www.dh.gov.uk/en/Publicationsandstatistics/Publications/PublicationsPolicyAndGuidance/DH_123371
31. United States, National Comprehensive Cancer Control Program, 1998 (last updated 2012), http://www.cdc.gov/cancer/ncccp/about.htm

Additional papers on cancer control

1. Pan American Health Organization. Regional Plan of Action for Cancer Prevention & Control, 2008. Available from: http://www.paho.org/english/ad/dpc/nc/pcc-stakeholders-mtg-June08-rpt.pdf, accessed on 24 October 2013.
2. WHO Regional Office for the Eastern Mediterranean. Towards a strategy for cancer control in the Eastern Mediterranean Region. WHO Regional Office for the Eastern Mediterranean, 2009. Available from: http://applications.emro.who.int/dsaf/dsa1002.pdf, accessed on 28 September 2012.
3. Cancer Control Council of New Zealand (2006). Evaluation and Monitoring Framework. Available from: http://cancercontrolnz.govt.nz/sites/default/files/ccc-evaluation-monitoring-framework.pdf, accessed on 24 February 2013.
4. Knaul, FM, Anderson, B, Bradley, C, Kerr, D. Access to Cancer Treatment in Low- and Middle-Income Countries: An Essential Part of Global Cancer Control, 2010. Submitted based on Working Paper by CanTreat International: Anderson B, Ballieu M, Bradley C, Elzawawy A, Cazap E et al. Access to Cancer Treatment in

Low- and Middle-Income Countries—An Essential Part of Global Cancer Control, 2010. Available from SSRN: http://ssrn.com/abstract=2055441, accessed on 4 November 2012.

5. Datta NR, Samiei M, Bodis S. Radiation therapy infrastructure and human resources in low- and middle-income countries: present status and projections for 2020. See comment in PubMed Commons below Int J Radiat Oncol Biol Phys. 2014 Jul 1;89(3):448-57. doi: 10.1016/j.ijrobp.2014.03.002. Epub 2014 Apr 18.

6. Datta NR, Samiei M, Bodis S. Radiotherapy infrastructure and human resources in Europe – Present status and its implications for 2020.

European Journal of Cancer, Volume 50, Issue 15, October 2014, Pages 2735–2743.

7. Samiei M. Challenges of making radiotherapy services accessible in developing countries in cancer control 2013: Global health dynamics in association with International Network for Cancer Treatment and Research (INCTR). Available at: http://globalhealthdynamics.co.uk/cc2013/wp-content/uploads/2013/04/83-96-Samiei-varian-tpage-incld-T-page_2012.pdf. Accessed 28 May 2015.

CHAPTER 28

Cancer prevention
Vaccination

Sarah E.B. Goltz and Julian Lob-Levyt

Introduction to cancer prevention vaccination

Since the development of the first successful vaccine—smallpox in 1796—vaccines have played a critical role in improving individual and public health globally. Few advances in medicine and science have had as substantial an impact on global morbidity and mortality as vaccines. Even in the lowest resource settings, vaccines have delivered important advances against disease. In the face of a growing global burden of cancer, the potential for vaccines to prevent, and possibly even to treat, cancers presents an important opportunity in cancer prevention, treatment, and control in all countries.

Over the past several decades, vaccine research and development have expanded greatly, resulting in an arsenal of powerful new vaccines that effectively protect against bacterial and viral causes of disease. Cutting-edge science has delivered new prophylactic vaccines that are unmatched in their safety and effective protection against disease. A new generation of highly effective prophylactic vaccines has been created through the novel use of adjuvants to boost immune response, and the development of conjugate vaccines that can provide high levels of individual protection and foster greater herd immunity.

The current growing interest and investment in cancer vaccines is particularly timely and important. The 2010 Global Burden of Disease Study revealed that a major epidemiological transition was well underway, particularly in low- and middle-income countries. This research illustrated a significant epidemiological shift that challenged assumptions that chronic diseases, including cancers, were limited to high-resource settings. This research showed a heavy burden of cancer and other chronic and non-communicable diseases in low- and middle-income countries [1]. Increases in smoking, dietary and lifestyle changes and toxic environmental exposure, together with longer life expectancy have contributed to the growing public health challenge of cancer worldwide. Increasingly, resource-poor health systems struggle to meet the need for cancer prevention, treatment, and control.

In the face of a growing global burden of cancer, vaccine solutions to prevent and possibly treat cancer are particularly relevant. Currently, there are three cancer vaccines. Two of these vaccines protect against cancer-causing viruses: hepatitis B virus (HBV) and the human papillomavirus (HPV). The third vaccine is a cancer treatment vaccine, which is an immunostimulant for late-stage prostate cancer. Other treatment vaccines are currently in development targeting other major cancers including bladder cancer, Hodgkin lymphoma, prostate cancer, and breast cancer. To date, these and others in development have yet to prove effective.

Current prophylactic cancer vaccines

Hepatitis B virus and liver cancer

Hepatitis B (HepB) is an infectious inflammatory illness of the liver caused by the HBV. Globally, more than two billion people are infected with HBV and more than 600,000 die each year from HepB [2, 3]. Transmitted sexually and through blood-to-blood contact, including mother-to-child transmission at birth, HBV is one of the most highly infectious viruses known today. HBV is 50 to 100 times more infectious than HIV [2].

HBV infection can cause both acute and chronic disease. Only chronic disease has been shown to cause cancer. Most individuals who are chronically infected with HBV are asymptomatic and remain unaware of their disease status. These individuals are particularly at risk both for spreading HBV and for suffering long-term health consequences, including cirrhosis of the liver and hepatocellular carcinoma (HCC). The likelihood of developing chronic infection—and thus, cancer risk—is directly related to the age at which an individual becomes infected with HBV [2].

In developing countries, perinatal transmission is a common route of infection often due to a lack of knowledge about the mother's status as a chronic carrier of the virus and poor management of mother-to-child transmission prevention protocols. If infected perinatally, infants are far less likely to develop acute illness than children over 5 years and adults. However, once infected, 90% of infants and 30–50% of children will develop chronic HepB disease [4]. Individuals with chronic HBV infection, often unaware of their HBV status, have a 15–25% risk of dying prematurely from HBV-related causes include hepatitis, liver cirrhosis, and HCC [5]. Research indicates that chronic HBV infection accounts for 75–80% of HCC in many parts of Asia [6], where as much as 66% of the total global burden of HCC exists [7].

Effective screening tests are available to diagnose HBV infection. Although no medical treatment is available for acute infection, chronic infection can be managed with medicines, where available and appropriate. Chronic HBV infection remains a leading cause of cancer in Asia, Amazonia, and Southern and Eastern Europe. In Asia, 8–10% of the adult population is chronically infected [8]. In Western Europe and North America, less than 1% of the adult population is chronically infected [2].

Hepatitis B vaccines

HepB vaccines are recommended in most countries for all infants, unvaccinated children under 19, and individuals at high risk for exposure, including health professionals, men who have sex with men, intravenous drug users, diabetics less than 60 years of age, and haemodialysis patients [9, 14]. As HepB is relatively rare in the UK, the National Health Service does not provide universal infant and childhood vaccination. Only children of HBV-positive mothers and high-risk individuals are routinely vaccinated in the UK. However, in over 110 countries where infection rates remain high, universal childhood vaccination is the norm [15].

Today, there are multiple formulations of the Hep B vaccine. HepB is often included in combination vaccines targeting multiple pathogens with a single vaccine administration. Only one formulation, the single antigen vaccine, is used to prevent vertical transmission and it must be administered within 24 hours of birth. These have been registered and are in use worldwide. HepB vaccination is among the vaccines prioritized and recommended by the World Health Organization (WHO) and national authorities globally. According to the WHO, over one billion doses of Hep B vaccine have been administered worldwide since 1982. The strong safety profile of the Hep B vaccine has been confirmed through continual global monitoring and expert reviews [8].

When delivered in complete series, Hep B vaccination is known to be 95% effective at preventing HBV infection and the resulting disease. According to the WHO, HepB vaccination imparts immune protection for 20 years [2]. As chronic disease is most often a consequence of infection early in life, immune protection afforded by early vaccination has been deemed sufficient to establish lifetime protection and no booster is recommended. Findings from a follow-up study of individuals vaccinated as infants through Taiwan's universal Hep B vaccination programme demonstrate the vaccine's protective effect and a statistically significant decrease in HCC twenty years post-vaccination [11]. Where HCC was present among vaccinated adults, it was directly linked to incomplete or unsuccessful HBV vaccination and poor prevention of mother-to-child transmission [11].

The Hep B vaccine offers an important case study for what can be done to make life-saving vaccines affordable and accessible globally. For nearly a decade, Hep B vaccine was beyond reach of most low- and middle-income countries. Galvanized by a 1992 World Health Assembly resolution to universally recommend Hep B vaccination, the WHO led an international effort to quickly scale up availability of HepB vaccine in low- and middle-income countries. Both Gavi, the Vaccine Alliance (focused on providing access to vaccines in the world's poorest countries) and the Pan American Health Organization (PAHO, focused on providing technical support and cooperation in Latin American countries) have stepped forward to provide valuable technical, vaccine pricing, and procurement support for many low- and middle-income countries. Both organizations have been instrumental in expediting widespread uptake and reducing the costs of vaccines, including Hep B, for countries where the burden of vaccine-preventable diseases is highest.

The impact of these efforts is significant. The price of the vaccine has dropped dramatically from US$100 per dose in the early 1980s [12] to just over US$0.17 in 2013 [13]. As a result of lower prices and greater international support, between 1992 and 2011, the number of countries that routinely vaccinated for HepB rose from 31 to 179 [2]. Among these countries, China has made unprecedented strides to implement a nationwide effort to prevent perinatal transmission of HepB. With catalytic Gavi support for initial pilots, first dose at birth vaccination has increased from 64% to over 90% in less than one decade. This increase in coverage—achieved even in China's most remote areas—was accomplished by expanding affordable access to the vaccine for the government, while increasing awareness and demand for hospital-based delivery of HepB vaccine among mothers. A recent study indicates that the partnership between the Government of China and Gavi prevented 3.82 million chronic infections and 685,000 future deaths in the areas jointly targeted between 2002 and 2011 [14]. According to Gavi, today less than 1% of children in China are chronic carriers of HBV [15]. Since routine vaccination began, other countries have reported similar drops in chronically infected children (Figure 28.1) [2].[25]

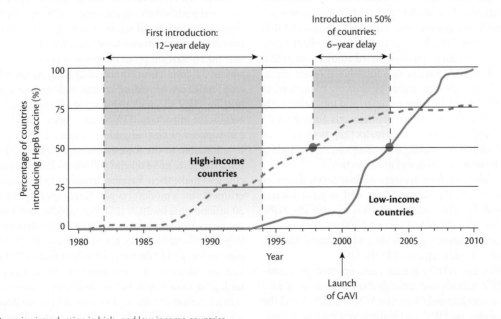

Fig. 28.1 Hepatitis B vaccine introduction in high- and low-income countries.

Human papillomavirus and cervical cancer

The HPV group contains over 150 viruses. Over 40 of these viruses are transmitted sexually and can cause cervical, vaginal, vulvar, anal, oral, and throat cancers. HPV can also cause tumours in the head, neck, urethra, and penis. Infection with HPV is common and usually cleared by an individual's immune system. Only persistent HPV infection can lead to cervical and other cancers. Cervical cancer is the largest cancer killer among women in most low-income countries. Each year, approximately 500,000 women develop cervical cancer and 275,000 women die from the disease [16].

In developed countries, high rates and frequency of cytology-based screening and early and effective treatment for pre-cancerous lesions has led to a significant drop in cervical cancer mortality. The limited or failed replication of an effective cytology-based cervical screening system—reliant on sufficient pathologists and follow-up treatment and referral systems—has caused cervical cancer screening to stagnate in developing countries. In 2006, only an estimated 5% of women in developing countries were screened for cervical pathology, compared to 75% of women in developed countries [17]. Over the past decade, a robust international effort has been underway to address this disparity and identify new screening and early treatment tools that could make cervical screening programmes viable in all resource settings. These efforts have been successful in identifying promising new tools, but have yet to be taken to scale in most resource-poor settings. As such, the swift rollout of the HPV vaccine is essential in order to reduce the overall burden of cervical cancer in the coming decades.

HPV vaccines

HPV vaccines became available in 2006. Currently, there are three HPV vaccines available—a bivalent (Cervarix®), a quadrivalent (Gardasil®), and a nine-valent (Gardasil 9®), which was approved in the US in late 2014. All three vaccines are non-infectious recombinant vaccines and protect against HPV 16 and 18, the two types of HPV responsible for 70% of cervical cancer cases globally and most HPV-induced genital, head and neck cancers. The quadrivalent vaccine also protects against HPV 6 and 11, which cause 90% of genital warts [18]. Manufacturers of the bivalent and quadrivalent claim some degree of cross-protection against other oncogenic strains of HPV, including HPV 45 and 31 [19]. Both vaccines have excellent safety profiles [19, 20, 21]. A recent population-based study in Australia, where the quadrivalent HPV vaccine was introduced nationally to girls since 2007, validated clinical studies by showing reductions in infections from HPV 16 and 18 among women and indicating early protective effects of the vaccine against genital warts among vaccinated women and herd immunity among males [22]. Both vaccines are safe and can be administered along with other vaccines including HepB, diphtheria, tetanus, pertussis and poliomyelitis.

The novel nine-valent vaccine protects against cervical cancer from HPV 16, 18, 31, 33, 45, 52, and 58, as well as genital warts causing HPV 6 and 11. This vaccine protects against the HPV types responsible for 90% of cervical cancer. Unlike Cervarix® and Gardasil®, which are registered worldwide and recommended by the WHO, Gardasil 9® is only registered in the US.

In December 2014, the WHO expanded and updated its recommendations for HPV vaccine use through the publication of new guidelines. In these recommendations, the WHO underscored the importance of introducing HPV vaccination as a part of a comprehensive cervical cancer control strategy where cervical cancer is a public health priority, would not compromise existing screening programmes for women, and is financially sustainable and cost-effective. As HPV exposure is common at sexual debut, HPV vaccination is recommended in early adolescence prior to first sexual contact. The WHO continued its recommendation that the vaccine be delivered to girls between the ages of 9-13 years of age. The dosing recommendations for girls vaccinated before the age of 15 was changed from a three-dose schedule to a two-dose schedule for both Cervarix® and Gardasil® at a six-month interval. Girls who were vaccinated with less than a six-month interval, or are immunocompromised, or are over the age of 15 should receive the three doses of the vaccine according to the original schedule of 0, 1–2, and 6 months. These guidelines do not incorporate any specific vaccination recommendations for the nine-valent vaccine, which has not yet been approved by the WHO.

While newly vaccinating countries exclusively targeting girls aged 9–12 can begin to focus on a two-dose schedule, the three-dose schedule will likely continue to be used in high-income countries where girls above the age of 15 are commonly vaccinated. In fact, many high-income countries have national HPV vaccine programmes that target girls up to the age of 26. In 2011 and 2012, several countries also expanded the registration of the quadrivalent vaccine to include protection for boys against genital warts and anal, oral, and throat cancers.

The UK, Australia, Canada, New Zealand, and the US were among the first countries to introduce HPV vaccine in 2007 and early 2008. Some countries initiated catch-up campaigns for girls and young women in order to maximize the potential benefit of the vaccine. These countries included Australia, Canada, Denmark, the Netherlands, New Zealand, and the UK [23]. In 2011 and 2012, several countries including Australia and the US included the vaccination of boys in their national HPV prevention efforts. In developing countries where adolescent health services are weak or non-existent, HPV vaccination programmes have the potential to act as a springboard for strengthened adolescent health programmes and services.

Unlike the HepB vaccine, which took several decades to scale in low- and middle-income countries, HPV vaccine has taken a much faster trajectory in all resource settings. As of September 2014, 73 countries and territories have included HPV vaccine in their routine immunization programmes and pilot programmes are underway in 37 countries (Figure 28.2) [24]. As with HepB, both Gavi and PAHO are providing critical technical and procurement support for HPV vaccine introduction. These organizations also had a significant impact on HPV vaccine price. Gavi has provided financial support to Gavi-eligible countries, allowing these vaccines to be affordable to the lowest-income countries. Gavi has secured a purchase price of $4.50 and will use its funds to purchase HPV vaccine and make these vaccines available to low-income country governments for a modest co-pay. Gavi expects to vaccinate more than 30 million girls by 2020 [25]. For middle- and low-middle-income countries in Latin America, PAHO's Revolving Fund has secured largely affordable prices for HPV vaccines. In 2013, these prices were as low as $13.08 for the bivalent and $13.79 for the quadrivalent for countries in Latin America. These vaccine prices are still far higher than HepB, but are following a similar trajectory over a shorter period of time and will need to come down further if they are to be truly affordable for the poorest and even middle-income countries [25].

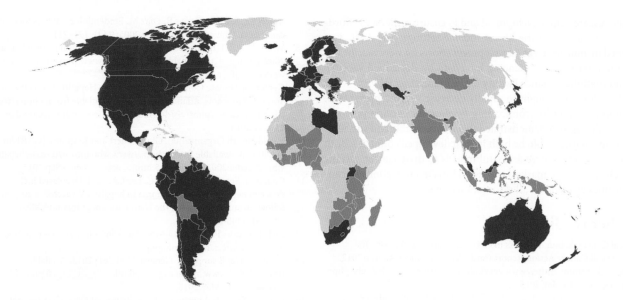

Fig. 28.2 Global Progress in HPV vaccine introduction: September 2014. Dark blue: countries with national HPV vaccination programmes Light blue: countries with HPV vaccine pilot programmes.
Reproduced with permission from Cervical Cancer Action, *Global Progress in HPV Vaccination,* Copyright © 2014 Cervical Cancer Action. All Rights Reserved. Available from http://www.cervicalcanceraction.org/comments/comments3.php

Several emerging issues could hasten the already rapid uptake of HPV vaccine in the coming years. First, the recent WHO recommendations for countries vaccinating girls under the age of 15 to switch to a two-dose schedule will have a considerable positive impact on the cost and challenges associated with the introduction of this vaccine. Second, the recent approval of the nine-valent introduces the possibility that in the future girls vaccinated with vaccine that covers such significant oncogenic HPV types might not require screening as adults. Finally, as HPV vaccination becomes more commonplace and affordable, the question of whether national programmes should vaccinate boys will likely get more attention. HPV vaccine could become an important strategy to protect males against other HPV-related cancers, as well as reduce the spread of HPV infection from males to females.

Cancer treatment and vaccines

The use of vaccines for cancer treatment is an exciting and evolving area of biomedical innovation. While the HepB and HPV vaccines offer protection against viruses that can cause cancer, cancer treatment vaccines mount a direct attack on a cancer that has already developed. Treatment vaccines are intended to delay cancer cell growth, cause shrinkage of existing tumours, prevent cancer recurrence, or eliminate cancerous cells that were not killed by other forms of treatment [26]. Treatment vaccines present a particularly difficult challenge as cancer cells often adapt quickly to changes in their environment and may have defence mechanisms that weaken anticancer immune responses [26]. Current tumour cell vaccines under development are made from harvested DNA or cells collected from the diseased person or tumour. These cells are then altered chemically or genetically. In theory, once altered, the modified DNA or cells are injected back into the diseased person in order to trigger an immune response that will directly alter cancer cells or increase the immune strength of a cancer patient.

Despite considerable research and interest in this area, only one cancer treatment vaccine is currently approved and available. Sipuleucel-T (Provenge®) is a treatment vaccine for prostate cancer. It is currently only approved for use in the US and is used in men with metastatic disease. This treatment vaccine is used to prolong survival, not to cure or reduce disease burden. The vaccine's impact on overall survival rate has been approximately four months [27]. Studies are underway to understand if the vaccine could be effectively used to increase survival time in less advanced cancer patients.

Sipuleucel-T is an autologous vaccine—created for each individual patient—making widespread commercialization and cost important barriers to widespread use. Immune cells from the diseased patient are collected through leukapheresis. These cells are then used to develop each patient's unique dose of Sipuleucel-T, which is then delivered to the patient intravenously 3 times over 2 week intervals [26]. This vaccine is currently in use exclusively in the US. Its current cost and reliance on sophisticated technology to develop the vaccine puts it far beyond reach of low- and middle-income countries.

Other cancer treatment vaccine trials are underway including pancreatic, brain, lung, and breast cancers as well as multiple myeloma, leukaemia, and melanoma.

Innovative strategies to drive cancer vaccine development and access

As cancer rates continue to grow globally, novel strategies are necessary to encourage and support scientific and biomedical efforts to develop new cancer prevention and treatment vaccines. Over the past several years, a number of notable innovative financing mechanisms were developed to encourage the creation or purchase of new vaccines for low-income countries. The Advanced Market Commitment (AMC) was created to frontload investment in vaccine research and development and to ensure earlier and affordable vaccine access in the lowest income settings. The AMC was designed to 'pull' or trigger development efforts for new vaccines by securing international financing for yet-to-be-developed vaccine. The International Finance Facility for Immunisation (IFFIm) was a broader effort that sought to rapidly decrease vaccine-preventable childhood diseases by frontloading funding for vaccine procurement. By doing so, it demonstrated that a large, viable and sustainable vaccine market could be built in least developed countries. Both mechanisms could serve as useful models to drive cancer vaccine research and secure markets that would make innovations in cancer vaccines available in all resources settings.

Further reading

Cervical Cancer Action. Progress in Cervical Cancer Prevention: The Cervical Cancer Action Report Card. Cervical Cancer Action, 2012. Available from: <http://www.cervicalcanceraction.org/pubs/pubs.php>, accessed on 15 May 2015.

Chang M, You S, Chen C, Liu, C, Lee CM et al. Decreased incidence of Hepatocellular carcinoma in Hepatitis V vaccine: a 20-year follow-up study. Journal of the National Cancer Institute 2009; 101(19): 1348–1355.

Hariri S, Markowitz L. Monitoring HPV vaccine impact: early results and ongoing challenges. Journal of Infectious Diseases 2012; advance publication. Available from: <http://jid.oxfordjournals.org/content/early/2012/10/17/infdis.jis593.full.pdf+html>, accessed on 15 May 2015.

Lozano R, Naghavi, N Forman K, Lim S, Shibuya, V et al. Global and regional mortality from 235 causes of death for 20 age groups in 1990 and 2010: a systematic analysis for the Global Burden of Disease Study 2010. Lancet 2012; 35: 2095–2127.

National Cancer Institute. Cancer vaccines. National Cancer Institute, 2011. Available from: <http://www.cancer.gov/cancertopics/factsheet/Therapy/cancer-vaccines>, accessed on 15 May 2015.

GAVI Alliance. Hepatitis B vaccine support. Geneva: GAVI Alliance, 2013. Available from: <http://www.gavialliance.org/support/nvs/Hepb/>, accessed on 15 May 2015.

World Health Organization. Hepatitis B Factsheet Number 204. Geneva: WHO, 2012. Available from: <http://www.who.int/mediacentre/factsheets/fs204/en/>, accessed on 15 May 2015.

References

1. Lozano R, Naghavi, N Forman K, Lim S, Shibuya, V et al. Global and regional mortality from 235 causes of death for 20 age groups in 1990 and 2010: a systematic analysis for the Global Burden of Disease Study 2010. Lancet 2012; 35: 2095–2127.
2. World Health Organization. Hepatitis B Factsheet Number 204. Geneva: WHO, 2012. Available from: <http://www.who.int/mediacentre/factsheets/fs204/en/>, accessed on 8 Sep 2015.
3. Goldstein ST, Zhou F, Hadler SC, Bell BP, Mast EE et al. A mathematical model to estimate global hepatitis B disease burden and vaccination impact. International Journal of Epidemiology 2005; 34: 1329–1339
4. Center for Disease Control and Prevention. Hepatitis B FAQs for the Public. Atlanta: Center for Disease Control, 2009. Available from <http://www.cdc.gov/hepatitis/B/bFAQ.htm#bFAQ38>, accessed on 15 May 2015.
5. World Health Organization. Hepatitis B. Geneva: WHO, 2012. Available from: <http://www.who.int/biologicals/vaccines/Hepatitis_B/en/index.html>, accessed on 15 May 2015.
6. Yuen, MF, Hou, JL, Chutaputti A. Hepatocellular carcinoma in the Asia pacific region. Journal of Gastroenterology and Hepatology 2009; 24(3): 346–353.
7. Bosch FX, Ribes J, Cleries R, Díaz M. Epidemiology of hepatocellular carcinoma. Clinical Liver Disease 2005; 9 (2): 191–211.
8. World Health Organization. Weekly epidemiological record: No. 40, 2009, 84, 405–420. Available from: <http://www.who.int/wer/2009/wer8440.pdf>, accessed on 15 May 2015.
9. Center for Disease Control and Prevention. Hepatitis B Vaccine. What You Need to Know. Atlanta: CDC, 2009. Available from: <http://www.cdc.gov/vaccines/pubs/vis/downloads/vis-hep-b.pdf>, accessed on 15 May 2015.
10. World Health Organization. Global Alert and Response (GAR) for Hepititis B. Available from: <http://www.who.int/csr/disease/hepatitis/whocdscsrlyo20022/en/index5.html>, accessed on 5 Sep 2015.
11. Chang M, You S, Chen C, Liu, C, Lee CM et al. Decreased incidence of hepatocellular carcinoma in hepatitis V vaccine: a 20-year follow-up study. Journal of the National Cancer Institute 2009; 101(19): 1348–1355.
12. PATH. Seattle: PATH, 2013 Available from: <http://www.path.org/vaccineresources/hep-b-info.php>.
13. UNICEF. HepB suppliers. Geneva. UNICEF; 2013. Available from: <http://www.unicef.org/supply/files/13_01_25_HepB.pdf>, accessed on 15 May 2015.
14. Chee G, Xie Z, Nakhimovsky S. Evaluation of Gavi–Government of China Hepatitis B vaccination programme. Abt Associates, 2012. Available from <http://www.Gavialliance.org/results/evaluations/evaluation-of-the-Gavi-government-of-china-hepatitis-b-vaccination-programme/>, accessed on 15 May 2015.
15. Gavi Alliance. China's dramatic fall in hepatitis B infections. Geneva: Gavi Alliance, 2010. Available from: <http://www.Gavialliance.org/library/news/roi/2010/china-s-dramatic-fall-in-hepatitis-b-infections/>, accessed on 15 May 2015.
16. Ferlay J, Shin HR, Bray F, Forman D, Mathers C, Parkin DM. GLOBOCAN 2008, Cancer incidence and mortality worldwide. IARC CancerBase No. 10. Lyon: International Agency for Research on Cancer, 2010.
17. Denny L, Quinn M, Sankaranarayanan R. Screening for cervical cancer in developing countries. Vaccine 2006; 24(S3): 71–77.
18. Villa LL, Costa RL, Petta CA, Andrade RP, Ault KA et al. Prophylactic quadrivalent human papillomavirus (types 6, 11, 16, and 18) L1 virus-like particle vaccine in young women: a randomised double-blind placebo-controlled multicentre phase II efficacy trial. Lancet Oncology 2005; 6(5): 271–278.
19. Harper D, Franco E, Wheeler C, Moscicki AB, Romanowski B et al. Sustained efficacy up to 4·5 years of a bivalent L1 virus-like particle vaccine against human papillomavirus types 16 and 18: follow-up from a randomised control trial. Lancet 367(9518): 1247–1255.
20. Gasparini R, Bonanni P, Levi M, Bechini A, Boccalini S et al. Safety and tolerability of bivalent HPV vaccine: an Italian post-licensure. Human Vaccine 2011(Suppl. 7): 136–146.
21. The Medicines and Healthcare Products Regulatory Agency (UK). Human papillomavirus immunisation programme: second year safety review. 2010. Available from: <http://www.mhra.gov.uk/Safetyinformation/DrugSafetyUpdate/CON096806>.
22. Hariri S, Markowitz L. Monitoring HPV vaccine impact: early results and ongoing challenges. Journal of Infectious Diseases 2012; advance publication. Available from: <http://jid.oxfordjournals.org/content/early/2012/10/17/infdis.jis593.full.pdf+html>, accessed on 15 May 2015.
23. Cervical Cancer Action. Progress in Cervical Cancer Prevention: The Cervical Cancer Action Report Card. Cervical Cancer Action, 2012. Available from: <http://www.cervicalcanceraction.org/pubs/pubs.php>, accessed on 15 May 2015.
24. Gavi Alliance. GAVI funds vaccines to protect girls against cervical cancer. Geneva: Gavi Alliance; 2013. Available from <http://www.Gavialliance.org/library/news/press-releases/2013/Gavi-funds-vaccines-to-protect-girls-against-cervical-cancer/>, accessed on 15 May 2015.

25. The World Bank. How we classify countries. Available from: <http://data.worldbank.org/about/country-classifications>, accessed on 15 May 2015.

26. National Cancer Institute. Cancer vaccines. National Cancer Institute, 2011. Available from: <http://www.cancer.gov/cancertopics/factsheet/Therapy/cancer-vaccines>, accessed on 15 May 2015.

27. National Institute of Health (United States). FDA Approval for Sipuleucel-T. National Institute of Health, 2013. Available from: <http://www.cancer.gov/cancertopics/druginfo/fda-sipuleucel-T>, accessed on 15 May 2015.

CHAPTER 29

Cancer chemoprevention

Hans-Joerg Senn, Nadir Arber, and Dirk Schrijvers

Introduction to cancer chemoprevention

Cancer chemoprevention is defined as the pharmacologic intervention by specific substances (drugs or nutrient-components) with the process of carcinogenesis, in order to prevent the development of overt, invasive malignant neoplasms [1]. This preventive attempt is particularly challenging in cancer types which have a long subclinical developmental phase, because of their low cellular proliferation rate and their slow preclinical evolution, until they become clinically detectable and therapeutically as well as prognostically relevant. Therefore, only certain specific cancer types are presently the focus of clinical chemoprevention, especially those with rather slow evolution such as adenocarcinomas. Additionally, such efforts are directed only those for which there exist relatively mild and tolerable ways of pharmacological intervention in otherwise (still) healthy individuals with only a statistically elevated risk of developing certain types of cancer on the basis of either their genetic background and family history or else their professional and personal exposure.

This means that the list of cancer types in which cancer chemoprevention presently constitutes a valuable primary preventive option is still short and actually confined to breast and colon cancer (see Table 29.1), with some candidate neoplasms such as prostate cancer at the doorstep of wider clinical interest [2]. In addition, another major limitation is operative in hormone-dependent tumours such as breast and prostate cancer: the anti-endocrine pathway of interaction with carcinogenesis is only effective in individuals developing target-oriented, receptor-positive disease.

Chemoprevention in (invasive and non-invasive) breast cancer

Epidemiology and the importance of the problem

Breast cancer is the most common cancer type of European women with 425,147 cases being diagnosed in 2008 and an overall incidence rate of 66.7/100,000 women and 128,737 dying from breast cancer, with a mortality rate of 16.9/100,000 women [3]. Despite remarkable progress in the primary curative treatment of early, localized disease, the overall mortality of breast cancer on a worldwide scene has been increasing during recent years due to the growth in the incidence of invasive breast cancer in heavily populated Asian countries, mainly due to changing living habits and significant increase of the lifespan of their populations [4]. In addition, it has become increasingly evident that the realistic gains of long-standing efforts of secondary breast cancer prevention (nationwide mammography screening) on ultimate survival figures in the Western hemisphere remain lower than previously anticipated [5]. For this reason, hitherto rather marginalized attempts to prevent breast cancer development 'at the roots', i.e. primary chemo- or pharmacological prevention, will become increasingly important in the future. These chemopreventive efforts have been greatly enhanced during the last two to three decades by the uncontested success of post-surgical adjuvant chemo- and endocrine therapy results obtained in multiple clinical trials by international groups, which clearly show decreased relapse and increased overall survival rates as a result of adjuvant chemotherapy and adjuvant antihormonal interventions [6, 7]. It is therefore logical to apply these successful attempts to prevent cancer relapse to the situation of primary cancer development and its potential prevention.

Chemoprevention by anti-oestrogens (SERM's) and aromatase inhibitors

In the last 15 years, innovative efforts by the National Surgical Adjuvant Breast and Bowel Project (NSABP) in the US and others such as the International Breast Cancer Intervention Study System (IBIS) have made it possible to test this concept of chemoprevention by anti-hormones (first tamoxifen, later also raloxifene and other SERMs) in a series of important clinico-preventive trials. These trials resulted nearly uniformly in a remarkable decrease in the development of overt, invasive breast cancer as well as localized precursors (DCIS and LCIS) in women with an increased chance of developing breast cancer on the basis of their risk profile [8]. The actual decrease of developing overt cancer over a latent period of presently around ten years is 35–50%, figures that have been confirmed—and even surpassed—by similar prevention trials with newer SERMs (arzoxifene, lozofoxifene) or aromatase inhibitors by other international trial groups such as the IBS-I trial with tamoxifen [9] and the exemestane trial [10]. More such breast cancer chemopreventive trials, including simple 'non-oncological' compounds such as daily low-dose aspirin and the anti-diabetic compound metformin, are currently in progress, usually involving five years of medication to selected female populations with increased breast cancer risk (Table 29.2).

Problems and obstacles related to the concept of chemoprevention in breast cancer

Despite these encouraging preventive results, there is still much resistance in health politics— on the part of the medical profession and the public itself—to transferring these positive trial results to clinical reality. This true even in the US, virtually the only country in which breast cancer chemoprevention by anti-hormones such as

Table 29.1 Mechanisms of action for chemopreventive drugs

Agent	Tumour type	Target	Mechanism of action	Pathway
Tamoxifen	Breast cancer	Cell membrane	Blocks peripheral action of oestrogen (SERM = selective oestrogen receptor modulator)	Oestrogen receptor
Raloxifene	Breast cancer	Cell membrane	Blocks peripheral action of oestrogen (SERM)	Oestrogen receptor
Anastrozole Exemestane	Breast cancer	Aromatase enzyme	Inhibits biosynthesis of oestrogen (e.g., conversion of androgens to oestrogens)	Oestrogen receptor
Aspirin	Colorectal cancer	COX-1 and COX-2	Open, diverse	Prostaglandin PG)-Synthesis, NF-kappa-B
Celecoxib Ofecoxib	Colorectal cancer	COX-2	Inhibition of proliferation, induction of apoptosis, immune modulating, COX-2 inhibitor (Rofecoxib = withdrawn)	PG synthesis, Leukotriens synthesis NF-kappa-B
Finasteride	Prostate Cancer	5α-reductase	Inhibition metabolism dihydrotestosterone to testosterone	Androgen receptor
Dutasteride	Prostate Cancer	5α-reductase	Inhibition metabolism dihydrotestosterone to testosterone	Androgen receptor

tamoxifen and raloxifene is already approved by the drug regulatory agency the US-FDA. The reasons are multifold: involved females at risk—still healthy and not afflicted by disease pressure—dislike the prospect of five years of drug-induced, variable anti-oestrogenic side effects; the doctors involved do not like the idea of being seen to be responsible for causing side effects and doing potential harm; and the industry is afraid of costly legal interaction and liability suits on the part of (still) healthy individuals at risk, possibly resulting in detriment to their normal way of life as a result of taking potentially unnecessary or ineffective cancer-preventive drugs.

Nevertheless, the potential means for successful, long-term primary (chemo-) prevention of invasive breast cancer and its localized precursors (DCIS, LCIS) are in our grasp should medicine and society accept them on a broader scale. Meanwhile, even potentially more appealing, non-oncological, and less toxic drugs, such as the anti-diabetic metformin, hold promise for breast cancer chemoprevention [11]. Whether these pharmacological preventive interventions will finally lower not only the incidence but also the mortality

of breast cancer remains to be shown with longer follow-up in the future.

Chemoprevention in colorectal cancers (CRC)

Epidemiology and importance of the problem

CRC is the second and third, most common cause of cancer death among men and women, relatively, aged 40 to 79 years. There were 229,219 (203,185) cases diagnosed in 2008 with an overall incidence of 13.5/100,000 individuals in both sexes and 110,059 (102,110 in women) dying from CRC with a mortality rate of 10.0 (10.6 in women) [3]. On a worldwide basis, there were more than 1,200,000 new cases in 2012, with more than 600,000 deaths. The progression of adenomatous polyps to overt invasive cancer spans over more than a decade; hence, CRC provides a window of opportunity actively to prevent the disease by drug intervention [12]. Screening

Table 29.2 Results of randomized major trials with different chemopreventive agents (anti-oestrogens) against breast cancer

Agent	Trial	Number individuals	MFU months	RR (ER+)	Comments
Tamoxifen (20mg/d)	NSABP P-1	13,388	>108	0.38	Significant decrease in the development of invasive and non-invasive breast cancer in TAM-treated risk-women
	IBIS-1	7139	>96	0.66	
	Royal Marsden	2471	>158	0.61	
	Italian trial	5408	>132	0.77	
Raloxifene (60mg/d)	MORE/CORE	7705/4011	>96	0.24	Breast cancer was sec. endpoint, but raloxifene active (RAL versus TAM!)
	RUTH	10,101	>69	0.45	
	STAR-trial	19,747	>93	1.24	
Lasofoxifene (0.25 vs 0.5 mg/d)	PEARL-trial	8556	>72	0.19	Higher dose more active
Arzoxifene (20mg/d)	Generations	9354	>60	0.30	Highly significant breast cancer preventive effect
Exemestane	MAP-3 trial	4560	>14	0.35	Exemestane reduces risk for invasive breast cancer significantly

Abbreviations: MFU, median follow up; RR, relative risk; TAM, tamoxifen; RAL, raloxifene.

Adapted with permission from Senn et al., The antihormonal preventive therapy of breast cancer and prostate cancer, *Hormone Molecular Biology and Clinical Investigation*, Volume 5, Issue 2, pp. 117–123, Copyright © 2011, DOI10.1515/hmbci.2010.079

colonoscopy would represent an attractive and effective prevention option, yet it is a relatively expensive procedure that carries some risk, require expertise, and whose acceptance rate by healthy individuals is rather low. As the emphasis of screening is shifting more towards real prevention, colonic adenomas, as the premalignant lesions, has become an attractive target for chemoprevention. This latter intervention is most useful in high-risk subjects, such as those with familial adenomatous polyposis or HNPCC [13].

General ways of pharmacologically preventing CRC

In average-risk populations the picture is less convincing, although chemopreventive strategies have been extensively studied to reduce the incidence and recurrence of adenomas and to delay their progression to CRC. There are many agents with some proven but minor efficacy (e.g., calcium, curcumin, vitamin D, fibre, etc.). But in most cases the effect is controversial, and in the best-case scenario the preventive effect is less than 20% [13].

CRC prevention by non-steroidal anti-inflammatory drugs (NSAIDs)

NSAIDs have been proven to be promising and most attractive candidates for chemoprevention of CRC. The preventive efficacy of these agents is supported by a multitude of randomized animal trials, and by 67 out of 69 epidemiological studies [14]. All of them clearly demonstrate that NSAID consumption prevents adenoma formation and decreases the incidence of and mortality from CRC. The attractiveness of these drugs partly stems from their ability to influence multiple mechanisms and components of the carcinogenesis pathway, from initiation to progression. The consumption of NSAIDs is not at all free of toxicity [13].

There are at least three isoforms of the cyclo-oxygenase (COX) enzymes. COX-1 is constitutively expressed in normal tissues and protects intestinal mucosal integrity. COX-2 is an early-response gene that is highly inducible by neoplastic and inflammatory stimuli. COX-3 is a variant form of COX-1. COX enzymes are probably the most common therapeutic drug targets in human history. Three international multicentre, randomized, placebo-controlled studies (PreSAP, APC, Approve) were launched at the beginning of the 21st century to evaluate the efficacy and safety of COX-2 inhibitors in preventing the recurrence of sporadic colorectal adenomas. The trials lasted five years: threes year on-drug with an additional two years of follow-up off-drug. In all these studies, the use of COX-2 inhibitors was clearly associated with a significant reduction in the risk of adenoma recurrence, particularly of advanced adenomas, which carry the highest risk for malignant transformation [14–16]. However, worldwide attention predominantly centred upon unexpected cardiovascular side effects [17]. Thus, cardiovascular toxicity caused the early termination of all COX-2 trials and the use of these agents in chemoprevention.

CRC prevention using aspirin (ASA)

Aspirin was first synthesized 120 years ago. There is vast experience with its cardiovascular protective effects, and strong evidence demonstrating that low-dose aspirin prevents adenoma recurrence, reduces the incidence of CRC, and is even associated with lower CRC mortality. The effect is mostly seen in COX-2-expressing tumours, in the right colon, and if taken for at least a decade [19]. The risk–benefit balance for cancer prevention should be weighed

up in conjunction with the benefits in prevention of the three major modern health catastrophes: other cancers, vascular illnesses, and Alzheimer's disease. ASA might be this 'magic bullet'. However, the ideal chemopreventive agent remains to be defined in the context of drug acceptance by the respective risk populations and of the principle of 'primum non nocere' (first: do no harm). Combinations of agents may be preferred, due to their potential of maximizing effectiveness, while limiting drug toxicity. Individualized approaches may emerge in the future, based on personal risk–benefit ratios by specific genetic profiles [20].

Chemoprevention in prostate cancer

Epidemiology and importance of the problem

Prostate cancer is the most common cancer type in European men with 370,733 being diagnosed in 2008, an incidence rate of 59.3/100,000 males, and 89,629 dying from prostate cancer, with a mortality rate of 12.0/100,000 [3]. Prostate cancer is a good candidate for chemoprevention due to its high prevalence, long latency, hormonal dependency, serum marker (PSA) for monitoring, and the existence of defined histological precursor lesions. Strategies for prevention include limiting accumulation of genetic damage with dietary antioxidants, anti-inflammatory agents, or hormonal manipulations. Several chemopreventive agents and strategies have been studied to decrease the incidence and development of this potentially lethal and invalidating disease.

Chemoprevention of prostate cancer by nutritional agents

Several nutritional treatments (selenium, vitamin E and D, lycopene, green tea, pomegranate, silymarin, phytoestrogens) have been studied in the prevention of prostate cancer. However, the interpretation of these studies has been hampered by their variable design and because their results were based on cohort, case-control, or only small randomized phase II studies [21]. Data from several randomized trials are available (Table 29.3), but so far none of these interventions have proven to be convincingly beneficial and ready for general use [22, 23], while vitamin E was even shown to increase the risk of prostate cancer [24].

Chemoprevention of prostate cancer by anti-inflammatory drugs

Inflammation is an important factor in the carcinogenesis of prostate cancer and several anti-inflammatory drugs have been tested as preventive agents [25]. However, studies were limited to cohort or prospective registry studies. No data of randomized phase III trials are available.

Chemoprevention by hormone-interfering drugs

Two phase III randomized trials with 5α-reductase inhibitors, finasteride in the Prostate Cancer Prevention Trail (PCPT) [26] and dutasteride in the REDUCE trial [27], in men aged above 50 years with a prostate-specific antigen (PSA) level within normal range and no suspicious prostate examination and/or a negative prostate biopsy, showed a decreased risk of prostate cancer development compared to placebo (a 24.8% relative reduction over a seven-year period in the PCPT and a 22.8% reduction in prevalence over a four-year period in the REDUCE) (Table 29.3). However, when

Table 29.3 Randomized chemopreventive phase III trials in prostate cancer

Author (year)	No. pts	Agent	Control	Outcome
Lippman (2008) Klein (2011)	35,533	Selenium; vitamin E; combination	Placebo	HR not different among groups; vitamin E significantly increased PC
Marshall (2011)	423	Selenium	Placebo	No difference in PC
Thompson (2003)	18,882	Finasteride	Placebo	24.8% reduction in prevalence over 7 years (P < 0.001); more high grade PC
Andriole (2010)	6,729	Dutasteride	Placebo	Relative risk reduction of 22.8% (P < 0.001) over 4 years; more high grade PC

Abbreviations: No, number; pts, patients; HR, hazard ratio; PC, prostate cancer.

prostate cancer was diagnosed, the median Gleason score (= differentiation grade) was higher in the treatment arm compared to the placebo arm, which might result in prostate cancer with a more aggressive behaviour. This should be discussed with men asking for primary prostate cancer prevention. Although much effort has gone into determining the role of primary chemoprevention in prostate cancer, it has not yet found its way into daily clinical practice in Europe, and only selectively in the US. Patients should be informed about the advantages and disadvantages of prostate cancer chemoprevention in order to make an informed personal decision [28].

Table 29.4 Selected chemopreventive trials in lung cancer

Setting	Phase	No. pts	Agents	Primary end point
Primary	**III**			
Smokers		29,133	BC/vitamin E	Harm/neutral
Smokers/asbestos		18,314	BC + retinol	Harm
Secondary	**II**			
Metaplasia		150	Etretinate	Neutral
Metaplasia		87	Isotretinoin	Neutral
Metaplasia		68	Fenretinide	Neutral
Sputum atypia		73	Vitamin B_{12} + folic acid	Neutral
Sputum atypia		755	BC + retinol	Neutral
Tertiary	**III (SPT)**			
NSCLC		307	RP	Neutral
NSCLC + HNC		2,592	NAC/RP	Neutral/neutral

Abbreviations: No, number; pts, patients; BC, beta-carotene; SPT, second primary tumour; NSCLC, non–small-cell lung cancer; HNC, head and neck cancer; NAC, N-acetylcysteine; RP, retinyl palmitate.

Source: data from Keith RL, Chemoprevention of lung cancer, *Proceedings of the American Thoracic Society*, Volume 6, Issue 2, pp. 187–193, Copyright © 2009.

Chemoprevention in lung cancer

Lung cancer is one of the most common cancers in Europe with an incidence of 391,000 new patients and 342,000 dying from lung cancer in 2008 [3]. Since smoking is involved in the majority of lung cancers, preventing people from starting smoking or helping them quit tobacco use is certainly the most effective method of prevention, although the realization of these aims at the political and personal levels is still difficult. In patient groups defined as 'high risk' due to a smoking history, cellular atypias in sputum, airflow obstruction, or a prior surgically cured non-small-cell lung cancer, several interventions have been tested [29]. But most trials have been negative, while some even showed the use of some chemopreventive agents caused harm, possibly due to the combination of smoking and the preventive agent itself (Table 29.4). At least at present, no chemopreventive measures are recommended in patients at high risk for the development of lung cancer.

References

1. Keloff GJ, Boone CW eds. Cancer chemopreventive agents. Drug development status and future prospects. Journal of Cellular Biochemistry 1994; Suppl. 20: 1–303.
2. Senn HJ, Morant R, Otto F. The antihormonal preventive therapy of breast cancer and prostate cancer. Hormone Molecular Biology and Clinical Investigation 2011; 5: 117–123.
3. Fast stats. Globocan 2008. Available from: <http://globocan.iarc.fr/factsheet.asp>.
4. Shin, HR, Joubert C, Boniol, Hery C, Ahn SH et al. Recent trends and patterns in breast cancer incidence among Eastern and Southeastern Asian women. Cancer Causes Control 2010; 21: 1777–1785.
5. Kalager M, Adami HO, Bretthauer M, Tamimi RM. Overdiagnosis of invasive breast cancer due to mammographic screening: Results from the Norwegian screening program. Annals of Internal Medicine 2012; 156: 491–496.
6. Goldhirsch A, Woods WC, Coates AC, Gelber RD, Thürlimann B et al. Strategies for subtypes—dealing with the diversity of breast cancer: highlights of the St. Gallen International Expert Consensus on the primary therapy of early breast cancer. Annals of Oncology 2011; 22: 1736–1747.
7. Peto R, Boreham J, Clarke M. et al. UK and USA breast cancer death rates down 25% in year 2000 at ages 20–69 years. Lancet 2000; 355: 1822–1826.
8. Fisher B, Costantino JP, Wickerham DL, Redmond CK, Kavanah M et al. Tamoxifen for the prevention of breast cancer: report of the NSABP- P-1 study. Journal of the National Cancer Institute 1998; 18: 1371–1388.
9. Cuzick J, Forbes JF, Sestak I, Cawthorn S, Hamed H et al. Long-term results of Tamoxifen prophylaxis for breast cancer: 96 months follow-up of the randomized IBIS-1 trial. Journal of the National Cancer Institute 2007; 99: 272–282.
10. Goss P, Ingle JN, Alés-Martinez JE, Cheung AM, Chlebowski RT et al. Exemestane for breast cancer prevention in postmenopausal women. New England Journal of Medicine 2011; 364: 2381–2391.
11. Chlebowski RT, McTiernan A, Wactawski-Wende, J, Manson JE, Aragaki AK et al. Diabetes, metformin and breast cancer in postmenopausal women. Journal of Clinical Oncology 2012; 30: 2845–2852.
12. Fearon ER, Vogelstein BA. A genetic model for colorectal tumorigenesis. Cell 1990; 61: 759–767.
13. Arber N, Levin B. Chemoprevention of colorectal neoplasia: the potential for personalized medicine. Gastroenterology 2008; 134: 1224–1237.
14. D'Avivi M, Moshkowitz E, Detering N, Arber N. The role of low-dose aspirin in the prevention of colorectal cancer. Expert Opinion on Therapeutic Targets 2012; 1:S51–S62.

15. Arber N, Eagle CJ, Spicak J, Rácz I, Dite P et al. Celecoxib for prevention of colorectal adenomas. New England Journal of Medicine 2006; 355: 885–895.

16. Bertagnolli MM, Eagle CJ, Zauber AG, Redston M, Solomon SD et al. Celecoxib for the prevention of sporadic colorectal adenomas. New England Journal of Medicine 2006; 355: 873–884.

17. Baron JA, Sandler RS, Bresalier RS, Quan H, Riddell R et al. A randomized trial of rofecoxib for the chemoprevention of colorectal adenomas. Gastroenterology 2006; 131: 1674–1682.

18. Solomon SD, Wittes J, Finn PV, Fowler R, Viner J et al. Cardiovascular risk of celecoxib in 6 randomized placebo-controlled trials: the cross trial safety analysis. Circulation 2008; 117: 2104–2113.

19. Chan AT, Arber N, Burn J, Chia WK, Elwood P et al. Aspirin in the chemoprevention of colorectal neoplasia: an overview. Cancer Prevention Research (Philadelphia) 2012; 5: 164–178.*

20. Martinez ME, O'Brien TG, Fultz KE, Babbar N, Yerushalmi N et al. Pronounced reduction in adenoma recurrence associated with aspirin use and a polymorphism in the ornithine decarboxylase gene. Proceeding of the National Academy of Sciences USA 2003; 100: 7859–7864.

21. Schmid HP, Fischer C, Engeler DS, Bendhack ML, Schmitz-Dräger BJ. Nutritional aspects of primary prostate cancer prevention. Recent Results in Cancer Research 2011; 188: 101–107.*

22. Lippman SM, Klein EA, Goodman PJ, Lucia MS, Thompson IM et al. Effect of selenium and vitamin E on risk of prostate cancer and other cancers: the Selenium and Vitamin E Cancer Prevention Trial (SELECT). Journal of the American Medical Association 2009; 301: 39–51.

23. Marshall JR, Tangen CM, Sakr WA, Wood DP Jr, Berry DL et al. Phase III trial of selenium to prevent prostate cancer in men with high-grade prostatic intraepithelial neoplasia: SWOG S9917. Cancer Prevention Research (Philadelphia) 2011; 4: 1761–1769.

24. Klein EA, Thompson IM Jr, Tangen CM, Crowley JJ, Lucia MS et al. (2011). Vitamin E and the risk of prostate cancer: the Selenium and Vitamin E Cancer Prevention Trial (SELECT). Journal of the American Medical Association 2011; 306: 1549–1556.

25. Hamid AR, Umbas R, Mochtar CA. Recent role of inflammation in prostate diseases: chemoprevention development opportunity. Acta Medica Indonesiana 2011; 43: 59–65.

26. Thompson IM, Goodman PJ, Tangen CM, Lucia MS, Miller GJ et al. The influence of finasteride on the development of prostate cancer. New England Journal of Medicine 2003; 349: 215–224

27. Andriole GL, Bostwick DG, Brawley OW, Gomella LG, Marberger M et al. (2010). REDUCE Study Group. Effect of dutasteride on the risk of prostate cancer. New England Journal of Medicine 2010; 362: 1192–202.

28. Ferlay J, Parkin DM, Steliarova-Foucher E. Estimates of cancer incidence and mortality in Europe in 2008. European Journal of Cancer 2010; 46: 765–781.

29. Keith, RL. Chemoprevention of Lung Cancer. Proceedings of the American Thoracic Society 2009; 6(2): 187–193.

CHAPTER 30

Population cancer screening

Andrew Evans, C. Simon Herrington, and Robert J.C. Steele

Introduction to population cancer screening

Screening is the process whereby theoretically asymptomatic individuals are tested to diagnose a disease at an early stage of its development with the aim of improving treatment outcome. In cancer, this includes not only detecting early invasive disease but also, where possible, the detection of premalignant disease so that the screening process may have an effect on disease incidence as well as outcome. It is important to be absolutely clear that the primary aim of population screening is to decrease the burden of disease on large groups so that the screening test must be affordable, acceptable, and associated with minimal risk.

The criteria for effective population screening were first established by Wilson and Jungner [1] and these are itemized in Box 30.1. Although the detection of early disease may seem to have obvious benefits, screening is associated with biases that have the effect of making screen-detected disease appear to have a better prognosis than symptomatic disease irrespective of whether or not the outcome has actually been affected by the screening process. The terms used to describe these biases are volunteer bias, length bias, and lead time bias. Volunteer bias results from invitations to be screened being taken up more readily by people who are health conscious. In other words, people who accept screening invitations are more likely to experience a better outcome from their disease anyway; for example, they may be more likely to take exercise and less likely to smoke. Length bias is a consequence of intermittent screening tests tending to pick up slow-growing disease that is more likely to be associated with a good prognosis than more aggressive, fast-growing disease that is likely to present between screening episodes. Finally, lead time bias is an inevitable consequence of early diagnosis; detecting disease at an early stage of its development inevitably leads to an observed improved duration of survival simply by virtue of shifting the point of diagnosis forward in time.

To prove that screening is effective, these biases must be eliminated, and to do this, population-based randomized controlled trials (RCTs) are required. In these trials, it is essential that the group randomized to be offered screening be analysed as a whole, including those who do not choose to participate in the process and those who are diagnosed with interval cancers (cancers that are diagnosed after a negative screening test in the interval until the next screening invitation). The disease-specific mortality in this group must then be compared with that seen in a randomly selected control group which is not offered screening, and only if a significant improvement is seen in the test group can screening be considered to be unequivocally beneficial.

In the UK and in many other countries, screening is available for breast, cervical, and colorectal cancer. For breast and colorectal disease population-based RCTs have been carried out; this is not the case for cervical cancer, but the observed benefits accrued from the programmes already in place make it impossible to perform such studies.

Breast cancer screening

Breast cancer incidence has risen worldwide for many decades and the disease is particularly common in the Western world. In the UK a woman's lifetime risk of developing breast cancer is 1 in 7 and it is now the commonest cancer in UK women, although lung cancer is now the commonest cause of cancer death. Breast cancer cannot currently be broadly prevented and the disease shows a strong size/outcome relationship making screening for breast cancer attractive. The recent decrease in breast cancer mortality in the UK appears to be due to a combination of earlier presentation of symptomatic cancer, better treatment, and the introduction of mammographic screening. Mammographic screening is now widespread throughout the developed world, and its introduction followed the results of a number of RCTs, the first of which was the HIP study from New York which took place during the 1960s.

Screening modalities

The only screening modality which has been shown to reduce population mortality from breast cancer is mammography. Screening using clinical examination and breast self-examination has not been shown to be effective in reducing breast cancer mortality. In recent years, ultrasound screening has been shown to increase the number of small node-negative cancers detected in women with mammographically dense breasts, but the impact of this increased cancer yield on mortality is unknown. However, ultrasound screening is time consuming and has poor specificity. MRI is now widely used to screen women at high risk of breast cancer, particularly women with BRCA1 and BRCA2 mutations. Again, the effect of such screening on breast cancer mortality is not known [2].

The screening process

In the UK, women are invited for screening appointments either at static screening units or on mobile vans where mammograms are performed by specially trained radiographers or assistant practitioners. The mammograms are then double read by radiologists or advanced radiographic practitioners. Non-concordant results are commonly resolved by arbitration. Between 3.8% and 8.6% of women are recalled for assessment; of these, about one in seven women will have cancer [3]. When women are recalled they are assessed by a multidisciplinary team which can carry out further mammography,

Box 30.1 Principles of screening

1. The condition should be an important health problem.

2. There should be an accepted treatment for patients with recognized disease.

3. Facilities for diagnosis and treatment should be available.

4. There should be a recognizable latent or early symptomatic stage.

5. There should be a suitable test or examination.

6. The test should be acceptable to the population.

7. The natural history of the condition, including development for latent to declared disease, should be adequately understood.

8. There should be an agreed policy on whom to treat as patients.

9. The cost of case-finding (including diagnosis and treatment of patients diagnosed) should be economically balanced in relation to possible expenditure on medical care as a whole.

10. Case finding should be a continuing process and not a 'once and for all' project.

Reproduced with permission from Wilson JM and Jungner F, Principles and practice of screening for disease, *Public Health Papers*, No. 34, pp. 26–27, WHO, Geneva, Switzerland, Copyright © 1968, available from http://whqlibdoc.who.int/php/WHO_PHP_34.pdf

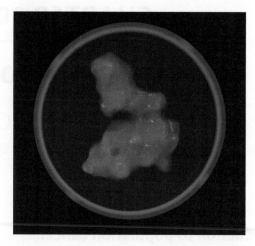

Fig. 30.1 Vacuum biopsy specimen X-ray of mammographic calcification.

Due to continuing criticisms of breast screening, which suggested that the overall mortality may be higher in those undergoing screening due to possible adverse effects of treatment, all-cause mortality was also assessed. This showed a relative risk of dying of any cause in the study arm of 0.98, which was of borderline statistical significance [5]. The precise mortality reduction attributable to screening is controversial as RCTs may underestimate the benefit of screening due to non-attendance and contamination (mammography occurring within the control group). Regular attendance for mammographic screening may result in a 63% reduction in breast cancer death for individual women [6].

Which age groups should be screened?

There is strong evidence from RCTs for a reduction in breast cancer mortality in women aged 55–69. Previous meta-analyses have supported the introduction of screening at age 50 but these data are based on ten-year age bands. Data analysis based on five-year age bands of screening women aged 50–55 has never shown a mortality benefit in this age group. The reasons for this are unclear but it has been suggested that this may be due to unusual behaviour of breast cancer in perimenopausal women.

There is no evidence from RCTs to support the screening of women over the age of 70, but the number of women over the age of 70 in these studies is small. Although the mammograms of older women are easy to read because of their low mammographic density and the incidence of cancer is high, there is an increased risk of over-diagnosis in this age group. A recent evaluation of service screening in northern Sweden showed significant mortality reductions for women aged 40–49 (RR 0.64 (0.43–0.97)) and women aged 50–69 (RR 0.70 (0.54–0.91)), but no mortality benefit was seen for women age 70–74 (RR 1.08 (0.58–2.03)) [7].

The most recent meta-analysis of RCTs screening women aged 39–49 at randomization has shown a statistically significant mortality reduction of 17% [8], and the Malmo [9] and Gothenburg [10] studies have both shown statistically significant mortality reductions in younger women. As breast cancer is only half as common in women in their forties compared with women in their fifties, some have suggested that presenting data in terms of percentage reduction in population mortality may be misleading. On the other hand, preventing breast cancer deaths in younger women will result in a larger number of life years gained and it has been shown that

ultrasound, clinical examination, and image-guided biopsy during a single appointment. Approximately 95% of invasive cancers and 90% of DCIS lesions are diagnosed preoperatively (Figure 30.1). Most benign lesions excised following screening are removed because of their uncertain malignant potential.

Quality assurance

For screening to be effective all the components have to be carried out to a very high level of performance. To ensure this, the performance of mammography, screen reading, non-operative diagnosis and treatment are subject to strict scrutiny against a set of national guidelines at both a unit and individual level. Performance of many of the components of screening has been shown to be related to volume. Therefore individuals involved in providing screening have to achieve minimum standards in terms of both quantity and quality [4].

The evidence for screening

Data from RCTs provide the strongest evidence of the efficacy of screening in reducing breast cancer mortality, and the most recent and highest quality RCTs of screening have been carried out in Sweden. The last overview of the Swedish trials included data from Malmo, Gothenburg, Stockholm, and the Ostergotland arm of the Two Counties study. Data from the Kopparberg arm of the Two Counties study was not included. Almost a quarter of a million women were included in these studies, with half being invited for screening and the other half making up the control group. The median trial time was 6.5 years and the median follow-up 15.8 years. The summated results indicated a 21% reduction in breast cancer mortality, with the largest reduction in women aged 60–69 (33%).

breast cancers arising in women in their forties account for 34% of life years lost to breast cancer.

The RCTs of screening were not originally designed to look at breast cancer mortality reductions in particular age groups and such subanalyses have been criticized. In particular, some of the screening episodes occurring in women aged 40–49 at randomization actually occurred when women were over 50. In addition, women in the control groups of these studies were not always screened at 50 or screened at all. Therefore, it is possible that part of the mortality benefit demonstrated in these women may be due to screening episodes over the age of 50. However, re-analysis based on age at diagnosis rather than randomization suggests that cancers detected by screening episodes before age 50 do impact on mortality. The UK Age Trial was the only RCT to perform all screening episodes before age 50 [11]. Participants aged 39–41 were randomly selected and were screened annually. The RR of breast cancer death in this study group was 0.83 (95% ci 0.66–1.04).

The low cancer incidence in women under the age of 50 results in the specificity of both recall and surgical biopsy being lower than that in older women. It has been said that there is reduced mammographic sensitivity in women in their forties; however, recent data suggest that the use of two views, high-film density and digital mammography [12], has substantially improved mammographic sensitivity in younger women. The most important obstacle to screening younger women is the short lead time of screening, the high frequency of screening required in younger women and the low incidence of breast cancer, which has led some to question the cost-effectiveness of screening in this age group. However, these disadvantages may be at least partly negated by the large number of life years gained per life saved.

Screening frequency

The lead time of screening is the time between mammographic detection and clinical presentation, and for screening to be effective the screening frequency has to be less than the lead time. The lead time achieved by mammographic screening is age dependent. For women under 50 the lead time of screening is just less than two years. The presence of this short lead time indicates the need to screen more frequently in women under the age of 50, so that the ideal screening interval is 12 months.

For women over 50 years the lead time of screening is between 3 and 4.5 years. Two-yearly screening should therefore be effective in this age group, as indicated by a recent analysis of pooled interval cancer data from six European countries. Interval cancer rates of 29% of the expected breast cancer incidence without screening in year 1 and 63% in year 2 [13] indicate that two yearly is the maximum screening interval that is appropriate. A recent analysis of interval cancer rates in the NHSBSP gave very similar results [14].

Over-diagnosis and over-treatment

Over-diagnosis and over-treatment imply the detection and treatment of cancers that would not become clinically apparent in the patient's lifetime or threaten life. Over-diagnosis probably occurs in about 10% of cancers detected when screening women aged 50–70 [15]. The rate is likely to be significantly higher when screening women aged over 70 years due to the decreased life expectancy and more indolent tumour profile in women of this age. Low-grade ductal carcinoma in situ (DCIS) and invasive tubular cancers are

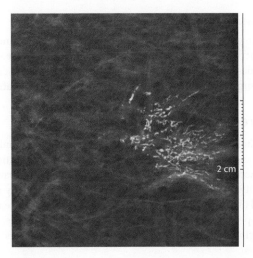

Fig. 30.2 Mammographic image of DCIS manifesting as impalpable calcification.

currently being over-treated. A number of studies are now addressing this issue by suggesting either less invasive treatment or a watch and wait policy for such lesions.

Ductal carcinoma in situ (DCIS)

About 25% of the cancers detected by screening are DCIS. Such lesions are usually diagnosed following the stereotactic sampling of impalpable mammographic calcification (Figure 30.2). Detection and treatment of high-grade DCIS is likely to beneficial by preventing the development of high-grade invasive cancer within a few years, but low-grade DCIS has a very indolent clinical course with many lesions not progressing to invasive disease after many years follow-up. The detection and treatment of such lesions almost certainly involves a degree of over-diagnosis and over-treatment [16]. About 70% of screen-detected DCIS is high grade, 15% intermediate grade, and 15% low grade.

Prognostic factors for screen-detected invasive cancers

The three classical breast cancer prognostic factors are size, histological grade, and lymph node stage. However, these factors were derived from symptomatic breast cancer series and they have been found to be of less value in predicting the behaviour of small screen-detected cancers. Histological grade is a prognostic factor for screen-detected cancers as a whole but not for cancers under 15 mm in size. Lymph node stage has been found to be a powerful prognostic factor for screen-detected cancers including small lesions; however, node positivity is present in less than half of the women with small screen-detected cancers who die of their disease. A number of studies have found that the presence of lymphovascular invasion in the resected specimen is an important prognostic factor, especially in node-negative women.

In recent years a number of studies have shown that the mammographic features of breast cancer contain important prognostic information. Tabar has shown that mammographic comedo calcification indicates a poor prognosis for small screen-detected lesions [17, 18]. Mammographic spiculation has been found to indicate a good prognosis for screen-detected breast cancer. This is probably a reflection of the fact that screen-detected cancers with a basal phenotype, which carry a poor prognosis, are rarely spiculated [19].

Conclusion: breast cancer screening

Mammographic screening can reduce breast cancer mortality in women aged 55–69 and probably in women from age 40. The downsides of mammographic screening are false positive screening recall/surgical interventions, over-diagnosis, and over-treatment.

Colorectal cancer screening

Colorectal cancer continues to be the fourth most commonly diagnosed cancer worldwide, and the most important prognostic factor in colorectal cancer is stage at diagnosis. As symptoms have poor sensitivity for colorectal cancer [20], screening is the only reliable method of early detection, and in this section, the evidence regarding the performance of currently available screening tests, factors influencing the uptake, and the potential adverse effects will be addressed.

Guaiac based faecal occult blood testing (gFOBT)

Until recently, detecting blood in faeces has relied on the guaiac test but this is an indirect measure of haemoglobin, relying on its ability to react with peroxidase. Within a screening context, the sensitivity of gFOBT for cancer is probably in the region of 50% owing to its low analytical sensitivity for blood and due to the fact that cancers bleed intermittently. On the other hand, the specificity (percentage of disease-free individuals with a negative test) is around 98%, which, although not perfect, makes gFOBT suitable for population screening.

Now that immunological tests for blood in faeces are available gFOBT is becoming obsolete, but the original population-based trials of colorectal cancer screening utilized gFOBT. As the results of these trials proved that screening for colorectal cancer is effective, they are worthy of consideration [21]. Three studies comparing biennial unrehydrated Haemoccult II® with uninvited controls took place in England, Denmark, and Sweden, but the first to report was carried out in the US. Here, volunteers were randomized into three groups, including annual and biennial screening with rehydrated Haemoccult II® in addition to a control group. A further study from France also studied biennial gFOBT, but was not strictly randomized, but compared different regions, some of which were offered screening.

The trials from England, Denmark, Sweden, and France all demonstrated reductions in colorectal-cancer-specific mortality of between 15% and 18% with a positivity rate of around 2%. The American study achieved better results, owing to the use of a rehydrated gFOBT which gives a higher positivity, and, indeed, around 30% of the population randomized to screening underwent colonoscopy.

These five studies are of the utmost importance as they are the only controlled studies of population screening compared to no intervention. The consistent reduction in disease-specific mortality indicates that early detection of colorectal cancer is truly beneficial and population screening by gFOBT can be estimated to reduce colorectal cancer mortality by 16%, increasing to 23% when adjusted for uptake [21].

In the UK, the National Screening Committee advised a demonstration pilot of biennial gFOBT screening to determine whether or not the results of the randomized trials could be reproduced within the UK National Health Service. This pilot was successfully carried out in two areas of the UK, one in Scotland and one in England

[22], and as a result, the UK Health Departments have now rolled out screening programmes. The initial outcomes indicate that the national programmes should produce the expected results [23, 24]. These programmes involve sending out test kits and invitations in the post, and the completed tests are returned for analysis at central 'hub' laboratory.

Faecal immunochemical testing

Faecal immunochemical testing for blood (FIT) is specific for human haemoglobin and there are now several manufacturers who produce quantitative FIT that provides a measure of the concentration of haemoglobin in faeces. Thus, FIT has significant advantages over gFOBT.

Qualitative FIT may be used in concert with gFOBT in order to reduce the false-positive rate created by the non-specific nature of the guaiac test and this approach has been introduced into the Scottish Bowel Screening Programme [25]. However, although it reduces the numbers of negative colonoscopies it does not address the issue of low clinical sensitivity seen with gFOBT. For this reason, there has been major interest in using *quantitative* FIT as the first-line screening test.

In two recent studies, a quantitative FIT has been compared with the Haemoccult II® gFOBT. In the first, from France, 10,677 individuals undergoing screening were offered both gFOBT and FIT [26]. Using a cut-off of 20 ng Hb/ml, the gain in sensitivity produced by the FIT was 50% for cancer and 256% for high-risk adenoma. This, however, was offset by a decrease in specificity. In the second study from the Netherlands, 20,623 individuals between 50 and 75 years of age were randomized to either a Haemoccult II gFOBT® or a quantitative FIT [27]. For the FIT, a cut-off of 100 ng Hb/ml was used to trigger colonoscopy. The positivity rate of the FIT was 5.5% compared with 2.4% for the gFOBT. However, the number needed to scope to find one cancer was the same between the two tests, and the detection rates for advanced adenomas and cancer were significantly higher for FIT than gFOBT.

From the relatively limited amount of information available, it would appear that a low cut-off for quantitative FIT in the region of 50 ng Hb/ml will detect most, although not all, cancers but will miss a substantial number of adenomas, particularly those of small size. Of course, the price for detecting a higher proportion of cancers and adenomas is a higher false-positive rate and a higher colonoscopy rate.

Flexible sigmoidoscopy

Given that 75% of cancers arise in the left colon, it was proposed that flexible sigmoidoscopy (FS), with removal of all adenomas, would provide effective screening that would reduce the mortality *and* incidence of colorectal cancer. This hypothesis has been tested in three multicentre randomized controlled trials, one from Italy (SCORE) [28] one from the UK (Flexiscope®) [29], and one from the US (PLCO) [30]. In all three studies, reductions in colorectal cancer mortality and incidence were observed, although the effects were largely restricted to left-sided cancers. The importance of these three studies is that they demonstrate beyond doubt that endoscopy and polypectomy can reduce the incidence of colorectal cancer and that FS is a credible candidate as a first-line screening test. Indeed, in England, 'once-only' FS is to be rolled out as a screening modality between the ages of 55 and 60, i.e. before FOBT screening starts.

However, uptake of FS screening poses a problem. Because the FS trials were performed in volunteers, the population uptake of FS could not be estimated. A Norwegian population-based randomized trial of FS achieved a participation rate of 67% [31], but a randomized study from the Netherlands comparing gFOBT, FIT, and FS achieved participation rates of 32.4% for FS compared with 49.5% and 61.5% for gFOBT and FIT [32]. On the other hand, a study from Italy found a similar participation rate for FIT and FS, although both were low at 32% of those invited [33]. It seems likely that both cultural issues and differences in level of deprivation are likely to be important in determining uptake of FS.

Colonoscopy

Colonoscopy would seem to be the ideal screening test; false positive results for neoplasia are not possible, the specificity is 100%, and the sensitivity is very high, albeit not 100%. In addition, colonoscopy is used widely for opportunistic screening and there is good epidemiological evidence that colonoscopy can reduce the incidence of colorectal cancer by means of polypectomy [34]. Despite this, the use of colonoscopy as a population-screening tool remains controversial, and although there are currently four randomized trials of colonoscopy screening worldwide, none of these have reported and there are relatively little data from which conclusions can be drawn.

It is interesting to note, however, that the effect of colonoscopy in reducing colorectal cancer mortality and incidence is less strong for the right side of the colon than the left [35]. This may reflect quality of colonoscopy; bowel preparation is often poorer in the right colon than the left colon and adenomas in the right colon are often flat and subtle when compared with the polypoid lesions seen on the left.

Radiology

There is increasing interest in CT colography as a screening tool. A recent randomized trial from the Netherlands which compared colonoscopy with CT colography found that uptake of CT colography (34%) was significantly better than with colonoscopy (22%), but that colonoscopy identified significantly more advanced neoplasia than was found on CT colography [36]. Interestingly, on an intention to screen basis, the diagnostic yield was similar for both strategies, but it should be noted that the uptake for both modalities was poor.

Uptake

Uptake is a crucial performance indicator for a screening programme. For gFOBT screening, population uptake generally ranges from 50% to 60% but, of course, the uptake required to produce a measurable reduction in incidence or mortality depends on the sensitivity of the test. As mentioned above, the type of test affects uptake, and most of the evidence indicates that gFOBT or FIT is more acceptable than flexible sigmoidoscopy which, in turn, is more acceptable than colonoscopy. Sociodemographic factors also have a profound influence on uptake. UK studies show that uptake of gFOBT screening falls with increasing deprivation and that women are consistently more likely to accept an invitation for colorectal cancer screening than men [37].

As uptake is central to the success of population screening, there has been great interest in interventions aimed at improving participation. Continuing to invite individuals for screening even if they do not accept the first invitation is the most obvious; a recent analysis of prevalence and incidence screening in Scotland demonstrated that the cumulative uptake of the first screening invitation rose from 53% to 63% over three biennial rounds [38]. Different forms of faecal testing also influence uptake; there is good evidence from randomized studies that the sampling method has an important effect as FIT seems to be more acceptable than gFOBT [39].

Endorsements by general practitioners and pre-notification have also been tested. Receiving the invitation from a family physician appears to be important [40], and comparisons of invitations with or without endorsement from a general practitioner have confirmed this [41]. Pre-notification is also effective as evidenced by randomized studies [42].

Adverse effects of screening

Any screening strategy is associated with false negative results leading to the development of interval cancers, defined as cancers that are diagnosed after a negative screening test in the interval before the next test date. It is held that a negative test result can falsely reassure people so that they ignore symptoms, creating a diagnostic delay—the 'certificate of health effect'.

A recent analysis of interval cancers in the Scottish gFOBT Programme found that interval cancers comprised about 50% of all cancers in the screened population in the first three rounds [43]. However, both overall and cancer-specific survival were significantly better for patients with interval cancers when compared to an equivalent population that had not been offered screening [43]. Thus, interval cancers have a relatively good prognosis when compared with cancers arising in the absence of screening, but it has to be accepted that, with gFOBT screening, high interval cancer rates occur.

This study raised two other concerns; namely that gFOBT screening tends to miss cancers in both the right side of the colon and the rectum and that it preferentially detects cancers in men when compared to women. The gender effect is almost certainly due to the fact that faecal occult blood testing is less sensitive for cancer in women than in men, and quantitative FIT testing has shown that faecal haemoglobin concentrations are higher in men than in women [44]. This suggests that differential cut-offs should be employed for male and female participants.

The issue of the effect of screening on 'all cause' mortality has created some controversy recently [45] and it has been suggested that screening programmes should be assessed on the basis of their effect on this parameter rather than on disease-specific mortality. It must be appreciated, however, that because colorectal cancer accounts for only 2% of all deaths, to demonstrate an effect on all-cause mortality would require a randomized trial that would be prohibitively large.

Conclusion: colorectal cancer screening

Currently, faecal testing for blood and lower gastrointestinal endoscopy are the only credible strategies for colorectal cancer screening, and there is good evidence from RCTs to support both strategies. Novel approaches, including faecal DNA markers, DNA methylation-specific RNAs, and specific protein panels are under investigation [46–48] and volatile compounds may also be useful [49]. None of these approaches have yet emerged as a practical solution, however, and refinement of the application of FIT and FS seems the most promising way forward at present.

Cervical cancer screening

Screening programmes aim to reduce mortality from invasive cancer by detecting and treating pre-invasive disease and/or early invasive tumours, but the purpose of screening is not to make a diagnosis; rather, it aims to reduce risk by identifying those who require further investigation to establish a definitive diagnosis, on the basis of which appropriate treatment can be undertaken. Cervical carcinoma, whether squamous cell carcinoma or adenocarcinoma, arises from well-defined pre-invasive (intraepithelial) lesions termed cervical intraepithelial neoplasia (CIN) or cervical glandular intraepithelial neoplasia (CGIN) respectively. These lesions, particularly CIN, can be sampled relatively easily as (1) they involve the surface of the cervix and (2) the cervix is easily accessible. These factors make cervical carcinoma particularly amenable to prevention through population screening. It is important to appreciate that cervical screening programmes are designed primarily to detect squamous epithelial disease and are less effective for the detection of glandular abnormalities, as these are both less consistently represented in cervical smears and more difficult to identify colposcopically. HPV testing may play a role in improving the detection of these glandular abnormalities.

The National Health Service Cervical Screening Programme (NHSCSP) was introduced in the UK in 1988. This programme is based on regular screening of women through a call-recall system, with subsequent investigation and management of women with abnormal smears using colposcopy and a range of treatment modalities. At the time of writing, the age range over which screening is provided in England and Northern Ireland is 25–64 years, with three-yearly screening from 25 to 49 and five-yearly screening from 50 to 64 [50, 51]. Over the age of 65, smears are only taken from women who have not been screened since the age of 50, or who have had abnormal smears that justify continued screening. In Scotland and Wales, screening commences at age 20, is undertaken at three-yearly intervals and finishes at 60 [52, 53]. In the Republic of Ireland, screening is offered to women aged 25 to 60: three-yearly from 25 to 44 and, if two consecutive results are negative, five-yearly from 45 to 60 [54]. Quality assurance of all elements, including cytology, colposcopy, and histopathology, against agreed auditable standards is important for the provision of a high-quality programme.

Cervical sampling and the investigation of abnormal cervical smears

Most cervical carcinomas, and pre-invasive cervical lesions, arise in the cervical transformation zone, where the native cervical columnar/glandular epithelium has been replaced, in response to cervical eversion after puberty, by metaplastic squamous epithelium. This zone can be sampled effectively by taking a cervical smear. Cervical smears can show a range of abnormalities that correlate with the nature and severity of the underlying lesion. Different terminologies are used to describe these abnormalities in different countries, although there is general agreement that there is a spectrum of abnormality ranging from the effects of human papillomavirus (HPV) infection through grades of cytological atypia to invasive carcinoma. In the UK, the term dyskaryosis is used to describe this atypia which is graded mild, moderate, and severe, terms that correlate broadly with the presence of CIN grades 1, 2, and 3, histologically. Glandular abnormalities are more difficult to detect but, when present, are referred to as glandular dyskaryosis, which may indicate a CGIN lesion. In general, women with smears showing moderate or severe squamous dyskaryosis, or glandular dyskaryosis, are referred for colposcopy and further management, whereas those with mild squamous dyskaryosis or more minor abnormalities (termed borderline changes) are recalled for repeat smears at shorter time intervals than is routine.

Colposcopic examination involves both direct inspection of the cervix at low magnification and assessment of the effect of the application of both acetic acid (which turns epithelium with a high nuclear content white) and iodine (which stains glycogenated epithelium); in general, abnormal squamous epithelium is acetowhite and iodine negative. The colposcopist can choose to take biopsies from abnormal areas to determine the histological diagnosis, or to treat the lesion directly. This can be performed using either ablative methods such as laser ablation or cold coagulation, in which case biopsies should be taken prior to treatment; or by excision using loop excision of the transformation zone (LETZ), straight wire excision of the transformation zone (SWETZ) or needle excision of the transformation zone (NETZ). These latter procedures not only treat the lesion but also produce a tissue specimen for histopathological analysis.

Tissue biopsies and other excision specimens are used to determine the nature and grade of any lesion present and to assess whether the lesion has been excised. Excisional methods of treatment therefore carry the advantage that a histological diagnosis is reached on the entire lesion and hence, in particular, early invasive lesions can be identified and managed appropriately. Subsequent management of CIN and CGIN is determined by the grade and extent of the lesion but may involve further excision. All patients with high-grade lesions (CIN 2, CIN 3, high-grade CGIN) are followed up with regular cervical smears according to the relevant screening programme guidelines. The management of patients with invasive lesions, whether squamous cell carcinoma or adenocarcinoma, is discussed at the gynaecological oncology multidisciplinary meeting and is dependent on stage and, to some extent, tumour type.

HPV testing and vaccination

The recognition that HPV infection is necessary (but not sufficient) for the development of cervical carcinoma [55], and the development of effective prophylactic HPV vaccines [56, 57], is beginning to have an impact on the cervical screening programmes in the UK. A UK-wide HPV vaccination programme started in 2008, offering a bivalent HPV vaccine against HPV 16 and HPV 18 to all 12–13-year-old and 17–18-year-old girls. Girls aged 13–18 y were offered the vaccine over the subsequent two years as part of a catch-up programme. An accelerated catch-up programme was implemented at the end of 2008 such that all girls born on or after 1 September 1990 could be protected before the end of the academic year 2009/2010. The effects of the HPV vaccination programme are not yet clear; as it is a prophylactic vaccine, its efficacy is due to prevention of infection and hence, given the long lead time to development of CIN/CGIN and invasive carcinoma, it will be some time before any effects on mortality from cervical carcinoma will be measurable. Moreover, the effects of preventing infection by HPV 16 and 18 on the prevalence of other HPV types that infect the lower genital tract [58, 59] are not yet clear. It is of note that the vaccine changed from September 2012 to a quadrivalent formulation that includes HPV 6 and HPV 11 in addition to HPV 16 and 18 [60]. This extends the efficacy of the vaccine to the prevention of genital warts, the majority of which are caused by infection with these two HPV types.

The strong link between HPV infection and cervical carcinoma has also prompted consideration of HPV testing as an adjunct to cytology in cervical screening, where it may have a particular role in the triage of women with mild cytological abnormalities and as a 'test of cure' on follow-up after treatment [61, 62]. Although HPV testing can lead to an increase in colposcopy rate, this is balanced by returning up to a third of women with mildly abnormal smears to routine recall, reducing the number of cervical smears being taken from this group of women. This relates to the high negative predictive value of HPV testing, which is also relevant to its use after treatment as most women with a negative HPV test in this setting can be returned to routine recall rather than being managed conventionally with more frequent cervical smears and, potentially, further colposcopy. By carrying out HPV testing using a centralized model, these two applications have been shown to be cost-effective [63].

Conclusion: cervical screening

It is clear that cervical screening has reduced mortality due to cervical carcinoma. However, the introduction of HPV vaccination and HPV testing is likely to improve the programme still further by prevention of HPV infection and by the optimization of management and follow-up strategies [64]. However, continuous audit and research are needed to assess the impact of these changes on the primary objective of the programme, i.e. mortality reduction.

Prostate and lung cancer screening

Two other common cancers that have attracted a lot of interest from a screening point of view are prostate and lung cancer. Prostate cancer screening has been based on detecting raised blood levels of prostate-specific antigen (PSA), and to date there have been five randomized trials of good quality. A recent Cochrane systematic review incorporating these trials has concluded that prostate cancer screening does not significantly reduce either all-cause or prostate-cancer-specific mortality [65]. In addition, PSA testing is associated with substantial risk of harm owing to high false-positive rates, over-diagnosis and adverse outcomes after both transrectal ultrasound biopsies and radical prostatectomy for screen-detected cancers. Currently, therefore, population screening for prostate cancer screening cannot be recommended.

Lung cancer screening has received a lot of attention following the publication of a randomized comparison of low-dose CT or single-view chest radiography which demonstrated a significant reduction in lung cancer mortality in the group allocated to CT [66]. This was not, however, a population-based trial of lung cancer screening, as only those who had agreed to participate were randomized, and there was no control 'no screening' arm. Until the results of population-based trials are available no recommendations can be made, and great care must be taken to avoid the use of lung cancer screening as an alternative to smoking cessation.

References

1. Wilson JM, Jungner F. Principles and practice of screening for disease. Public Health Papers No. 34. Geneva: WHO, 1968.
2. Rijnsburge A, Obdeijn I, Kaas R, Tilanus-Linthorst M, Boetes C, et al. BRCA1-associated breast cancers present differently from BRCA2-associated and familial cases: long-term follow-up of the Dutch MRISC Screening Study. Journal of Clinical Oncology 2010; 28: 5265–5273.
3. Bennett RL, Blanks RG, Patnick J, Moss SM. Results from the UK NHS Breast Screening Programme 2000–05. Journal of Medical Screening 2007; 14: 200–204.
4. National Health Service (NHS) Breast Screening Radiologists Quality Assurance Committee. Quality assurance guidelines for radiologists. NHSBSP publication No. 59. Sheffield: NHSBSP, 2005.
5. Nyström L, Andersson I, Bjurstam N, Frisell J, Nordenskjöld B et al. Long-term effects of mammographic screening: update overview of the Swedish randomised trials. Lancet 2002; 359: 909–919.
6. Tabar L, Vitak B, Chen HH, Yen MF, Duffy SW et al. Beyond randomized controlled trials: organized mammographic screening substantially reduces breast carcinoma mortality. Cancer 2001; 91: 1724–1731.
7. Jonsson H, Bordas P, Wallin H, Nyström L, Lenner P. Service screening with mammography in Northern Sweden: effects on breast cancer mortality: an update. Journal of Medical Screening 2007; 14: 87–93.
8. Magnus MC, Ping M, Shen MM, Bourgeois J, Magnus JH. Effectiveness of mammography screening in reducing breast cancer mortality in women aged 39–49 years: a meta-analysis. Journal of Women's Health 2011; 20(6): 845–852.
9. Andersson I, Janzon L. Reduced breast cancer mortality in women under age 50: updated results from the Malmo mammographic screening program. Journal of the National Cancer Institute Monographs 1997; 22: 63–68.
10. Bjurstam N, Bjorneld L, Duffy SW, Smith TC, Cahlin E et al. The Gothenburg breast screening trial: first results on mortality, incidence and mode of detection for women ages 39–49 years at randomization. Cancer 1997; 80: 2091–2099.
11. Moss SM, Cuckle H, Evans A, Johns L, Waller M et al. Effect of mammographic screening from age 40 years on breast cancer mortality at 10 years' follow-up: a randomised controlled trial. Lancet 2006; 368: 2053–2060.
12. Pisano ED, Gatsonis C, Hendrick E, et al. Digital Mammographic Imaging Screening Trial (DMIST) Investigators Group: diagnostic performance of digital versus film mammography for breast-cancer screening. New England Journal of Medicine 2005; 353(17): 1773–1783.
13. Törnberg S, Kemetli L, Ascunce N, Hofvind S, Anttila A et al. A pooled analysis of interval cancer rates in six European countries. European Journal of Cancer Prevention 2010; 19: 87–93.
14. Bennett RL, Sellars SJ, Moss SM. Interval cancers in the NHS breast cancer screening programme in England Wales and Northern Ireland. British Journal of Cancer 2011; 104: 571–577.
15. Zackrisson S, Andersson I, Janzon L, Manjer J, Garne JP. Rate of over-diagnosis of breast cancer 15 years after end of Malmo mammographic screening trial: follow-up study. British Medical Journal 2006; 332: 689–92.
16. Jones JL. Overdiagnosis and overtreatment of breast cancer: progression of ductal carcinoma in situ: the pathological perspective. Breast Cancer Research 2006; 8: 204.
17. Bennett RL, Evans AJ, Kutt E, Record C, Bobrow LG et al. Pathological and mammographic prognostic factors for screen detected cancers in a multi-centre randomised, controlled trial of mammographic screening in women from age 40 to 48 years. Breast 2011; 20(6): 525–528.
18. Tabar L, Tony Chen HH, Amy Yen MF, Tot T, Tung TH et al. Mammographic tumour features can predict long-term outcomes reliably in women with 1–14mm invasive breast carcinoma. Cancer 2004; 101: 1745–1759.
19. Evans AJ, Rakha EA, Pinder SE, Green AR, Paish C et al. Basal phenotype: a powerful prognostic factor in small screen-detected invasive breast cancer with long term follow-up. Journal of Medical Screening 2007; 14: 210–214.

20. Jellema P, van der Windt DA, Bruinvels DJ, Mallen CD, van Weyenberg SJ et al. Value of symptoms and additional diagnostic tests for colorectal cancer in primary care; systematic review and meta-analysis. British Medical Journal 2010; 340: c1269. doi:10.1136/bmj.c1269

21. Hewitson P, Glasziou P, Watson E, Towler B, Irwig L. Cochrane systematic review of colorectal cancer screening using the faecal occult blood test (hemoccult): an update. American Journal of Gastroenterology 2008; 103: 1541–1549.

22. UK Colorectal Cancer Screening Pilot Group. Results of the first round of a demonstration pilot of screening for colorectal cancer in the United Kingdom. British Medical Journal 2004; 329: 133–135.

23. Steele RJC, McClements P L, Libby G, Black R, Morton C et al. Results from the first three rounds of the Scottish demonstration pilot of FOBT screening for colorectal cancer. Gut 2009; 58; 530–535

24. Logan RFA, Patnick J, Nickerson C, Coleman L, Rutter MD et al. Outcomes of the Bowel Cancer Screening Programme (BCSP) in England after the first 1 million tests. Gut 2011; 61(10): 1439–1446.

25. Fraser CG, Digby J, McDonald PJ, Strachan JA, Carey FA et al. Experience with a two-tier reflex gFOBT/FIT strategy in a national bowel screening programme. Journal of Medical Screening 2012; 19: 8–13.

26. Guittet L, Bouvier V, Mariotte N, Vallee JP, Arsène D et al. Comparison of a guaiac based and an immunochemical faecal occult blood test in screening for colorectal cancer in a general average risk population. Gut 2007; 56: 210–214.

27. Van Rossum LG, van Rijn AF, Laheij RJ, van Oijen MG, Fockens P et al. Random comparison of guaiac and immunochemical fecal occult blood tests for colorectal cancer in a screening population. Gastroenterology 2008; 135: 82–90.

28. Segnan N, Armaroli P, Bonelli L, Risio M, Sciallero S, Zappa M et al. Journal of the National Cancer Institute 2011; 193: 1310–1322.

29. Atkin WS, Edwards R, Kralj-Hans I, Wooldrage K, Hart AR et al. Once-only flexible sigmoidoscopy screening in prevention of colorectal cancer: a multicentre randomised controlled trial. Lancet; 2010; 375: 1624–1633.

30. Schoen RE, Pinsky PF, Weissfeld JL, Yokochi LA, Church T et al. Colorectal-cancer incidence and mortality with screening flexible sigmoidoscopy. New England Journal of Medicine 2012; 366(25): 2345–2357.

31. Hoff G, Grotmol T, Skovlund E, Bretthauer M for the Norwegian Colorectal Cancer Prevention Group. Risk of colorectal cancer seven years after flexible sigmoidoscopy screening: randomised controlled trial. British Medical Journal 2009; 338: b1846.

32. Hol L, van Leerdam ME, van Ballegooijen M, van Vuuren AJ, van Dekken H et al. Screening for colorectal cancer: a randomised trial comparing guaiac-based and immunochemical faecal occult blood testing and flexible sigmoidoscopy. Gut 2010; 59: 62–68.

33. Segnan N, Senore C, Andreoni B, Azzoni A, Bisanti L et al. Comparing attendance and detection rate of colonoscopy with sigmoidoscopy and FIT for colorectal cancer screening. Gastroenterology 2007; 132: 230.

34. Zauber AG, Winawer SJ, O'Brien MJ, Landsdorp-Vogelaar I, van Ballegooijen M et al. Colonoscopic polypectomy and long-term prevention of colorectal-cancer deaths. New England Journal of Medicine 2012; 366: 687–696.

35. Baxter NN, Goldwasser MA, Paszat LF, Saskin R, Urbach DR et al. Association of colonoscopy and death from colorectal cancer. Annals of Internal Medicine 2009; 150: 1–8.

36. Stoop EM, de Haan MC, de Wijkersloooth TR, Bossuyt PM, van Ballegooijen M et al. Participation and yield of colonoscopy versus non-cathartic CT colonography in population-based screening for colorectal cancer: a randomised controlled trial. Lancet Oncology 2012; 13: 55–64.

37. Steele RJC, Kostourou I, McClements P, Watling C, Libby G et al. Effect of gender, age and deprivation on key performance indicators in a FOBT based colorectal screening programme. Journal of Medical Screening 2010; 17: 68–74.

38. Steele RJC, Kostourou I, McClements P, Watling C, Libby G et al. Effect of repeated invitations on uptake of colorectal cancer screening using faecal occult blood testing: analysis of prevalence and incidence screening. British Medical Journal 2010: 341:c5531.

39. Young GP, St John DJB, Cole SR, Bielecki BE, Pizzey C, et al. Prescreening evaluation of a brush-based faecal immunochemical test for haemoglobin. Journal of Medical Screening 2003; 10: 123–128.

40. Tinmouth J, Ritvo P, McGregor SE, Claus D, Pasut G et al. A qualitative evaluation of strategies to increase colorectal cancer uptake. Canadian Family Physician 2011; 57:e7–e15

41. Hewitson P, Ward AM, Heneghan C, Halloran SP, Mant D. Primary care endorsement letter and a patient leaflet to improve participation in colorectal cancer screening: results of a factorial randomised trial. British Journal of Cancer: 2011; 105: 475–480.

42. Libby G, Bray J, Champion J, Brownlee LA, Birrell J et al. Pre-notification increases uptake of colorectal cancer screening in all demographic groups: a randomised controlled trial. Journal of Medical Screening 2011: 18: 24–29

43. Steele RJC, McClements P, Watling C, Libby G, Weller D et al. Interval cancers in a FOBT-based colorectal cancer population screening programme: implications for stage, gender and tumour site. Gut 2012; 61: 576–581.

44. MacDonald PJ, Strachan JA, Digby J, Steele RJC, Fraser CG. Faecal haemoglobin concentrations by gender and age: implications for population-based screening for colorectal cancer. Clinical Chemistry and Laboratory Medicine 2012; 50(5): 935–940.

45. Steele RJC, Brewster D. Should we judge cancer screening programmes by their effect on total mortality rather on cancer specific mortality? British Medical Journal 2011; 343: 938–939.

46. Duffy MJ, van Rossum LGM, van Turenhout ST, Malminiemi O, Sturgeon C et al. Use of faecal markers in screening for colorectal neoplasia: a European group on tumor markers position paper. International Journal of Cancer 2011; 128(1): 3–11.

47. Hundt S, Haug U, Brenner H. Blood markers for early detection of colorectal cancer: a systematic review. Cancer Epidemiology, Biomarkers & Prevention 2007; 16: 1935–1953.

48. Grützmann R, Molnar B, Pilarsky C, Habermann JK, Schlag PM et al. Sensitive detection of colorectal cancer in peripheral blood by Septin 9 DNA methylation assay. Plos One 2008; 3: e3759.

49. Sonoda H, Kohnoe S, Yamazato T, Satoh Y, Morizono G et al. Colorectal cancer screening with odour material by canine scent detection. Gut 2011. doi:10.1136/gut2010.218305

50. NHS Cervical Screening Programme (NHSCSP). <http://www.cancer-screening.nhs.uk/cervical/index.html>, accessed on 29 May 2012.

51. Cervical Screening Northern Ireland. Available from: <http://www.cancerscreening.hscni.net/cervical/toc.html>, accessed on 29 May 2012.

52. Cervical Screening Scotland. <http://www.healthscotland.com/topics/health-topics/screening/cervical.aspx>, accessed on 29 May 2012.

53. Cervical Screening Wales. <http://www.screeningservices.org.uk/csw/pub/index.asp>, accessed on 29 May 2012.

54. Cervical Screening Republic of Ireland. <http://www.cervicalcheck.ie/>, accessed on 29 May 2012.

55. Walboomers J, Jacobs M, Manos M, Bosch FX, Kummer JA et al. Human papillomavirus is a necessary cause of invasive cervical cancer worldwide. Journal of Pathology 1999; 189: 12–19.

56. Harper DM, Franco EL, Wheeler C, Ferris DG, Jenkins D et al. Efficacy of a bivalent L1 virus-like particle vaccine in prevention of infection with human papillomavirus types 16 and 18 in young women: a randomised controlled trial. Lancet 2004; 364: 1757–1765.

57. Garland S, Hernandez-Avila M, Wheeler C, Perez G, Harper DM et al. Quadrivalent vaccine against human papillomavirus to prevent anogenital diseases. New England Journal of Medicine 2007; 356: 1928–1943.

58. de Villiers E-M, Fauquet C, Broker TR, Bernard HU, zur Hausen H et al. Classification of papillomaviruses. Virology 2004; 324: 17–27.

59. Bernard H-U, Burk RD, Chen Z, van Doorslaer K, zur Hausen H et al. Classification of papillomaviruses (PVs) based on 189 PV types and proposal of taxonomic amendments. Virology 2010; 401: 70–79.

60. Kmietowicz Z. UK will use Gardasil in its HPV vaccination programme from next September. British Medical Journal. 2011; 343:d7694.

61. Kelly RS, Patnick J, Kitchener HC, Moss SM. HPV testing as a triage for borderline or mild dyskaryosis on cervical cytology: results from the Sentinel Sites study. British Journal of Cancer 2011; 105: 983–988.

62. Kocken M, Uijterwaal MH, de Vries ALM, Berkhof J, Ket JC et al. High-risk human papillomavirus testing versus cytology in predicting post-treatment disease in women treated for high-grade cervical disease: a systematic review and meta-analysis. Gynecologic Oncology 2012; 125: 500–507.

63. Evaluation of Sentinel Sites for HPV triage and test of cure. Available from: <http://www.cancerscreening.nhs.uk/cervical/hpv-sentinel-sites.html> accessed on 29 May 2012.

64. Almonte M, Sasieni P, Cuzick J. Incorporating human papillomavirus testing into cytological screening in the era of prophylactic vaccines. Best Practice & Research Clinical Obstetrics & Gynaecology 2011; 25: 617–629.

65. Ilic D, O'Connor D, Green S, Wilt TJ. Screening for prostate cancer: an updated Cochrane systematic review. BJU International 2011; 107: 882–891.

66. The National Lung Screening Trial Research Team. Reduced lung-cancer mortality with low-dose computed tomographic screening. New England Journal of Medicine 2011; 365: 395–409.

CHAPTER 31

Familial cancer syndromes and genetic counselling

Henry T. Lynch, Carrie L. Snyder, and Jane F. Lynch

Introduction to familial cancer syndromes and genetic counseling

Genetic counselling is truly mandatory for patient education, surveillance, and management of all forms of hereditary cancer. Indeed, it has become the clinical bedrock for these disorders, wherein it has constantly been stimulated by the veritably logarithmic advances in molecular genetics with the identification of an increasing number of cancer-causing germline mutations. Table 31.1 lists known hereditary cancer syndromes, with the caveat that new syndromes and new information on known syndromes are constantly being recognized. This chapter represents more than 50 years of the authors' experience in diagnosing, DNA testing, and counselling thousands of families representing more than 100,000 affected and/or high-risk cancer-prone patients. Using colorectal cancer (CRC) as a model, Table 31.2 points out the magnitude of CRC and its familial and most common hereditary forms, both worldwide and in the US. Figure 31.1 shows the hereditary CRC syndromes that have been identified to date, as an example of the complexity of differential diagnoses.

Family history

The genetic counsellor's responsibility will be the compilation of a comprehensive cancer family history. Ideally, this will involve three or four generations of the proband's family covering both maternal and paternal lineages. It must include cancer of *all* anatomic sites, with verification whenever possible. Clearly, the family history is the linchpin in this effort. Figure 31.2 shows a modified nuclear pedigree which, when completed, will, in most cases, aid significantly in identifying a hereditary cancer syndrome should one be present in the family.

The genetic counsellor's role is exceedingly important, given substantial evidence that among the physician community the family history is often ignored or insufficiently recorded, thereby compromising an opportunity for identifying and targeting those patients who are at high risk for hereditary cancer syndromes and who would benefit from DNA testing, screening, and potential life-saving management. DNA testing will, therefore, enable more certainty for its diagnosis, with furtherance of targeted clinical translation, surveillance, and personalized medical management.

The discipline of evidence-based genetic counselling, particularly as it relates to genomic medicine, which encompasses the roles of medical geneticists with evidence-based genetic counselling, has been more clearly defined in terms of its service obligation for high-risk patients [1–3]. The genetic counselling discipline is clearly a challenging one which harbours an intense thirst among genetic counsellors for its clinical expansion given the incredibly rapid progress in the identification of an increasing number of patients with virtually all forms of hereditary cancer syndromes [4]. When there is germline mutation evidence in a patient/family, there will be a clear need to focus on its genetic counselling implications.

Berliner and Fay [5] have discussed genetic counselling recommendations with a particular bent towards their medical, psychosocial, and ethical implications relevant to the identification of individuals at risk for the hereditary breast-ovarian cancer (HBOC) syndrome and, in turn, embracing genetic susceptibility concerns, as developed by the Practice Issues Subcommittee of the National Society of Genetic Counselors' Familial Cancer Risk Counseling Special Interest Group. This knowledge is based upon an extensive review of the current literature dealing with cancer genetic risk assessment in addition to the professional expertise embodied in the genetic counselling discipline.

Personalized cancer medicine

Disease-related gene identification such as *BRCA1* and *BRCA2* in HBOC syndrome and the mismatch repair (MMR) germline mutations, namely *MLH1*, *MSH2*, *MSH6*, *PMS2*, and deletions in the *EPCAM* gene that silence MSH2 in Lynch syndrome (LS), provide the stimulus for a scientifically-based study design with a highly targeted focus on patients whose lifetime cancer risk, with considerations for differences in their heterogeneity and penetrance, can be more carefully defined than programmes which exist for their so-called sporadic counterparts. The power inherent in the identification of cancer-causing germline mutations harbours further advantage in that it provides benefit which can be effectively derived from individualized therapeutic development, all in concert with this personalized cancer medicine phenomenon. Therefore, with the help of pathologists, medical geneticists, medical oncologists, surgeons, genetic counsellors, and molecular genetic colleagues, we are now merging our cancer control efforts towards the development of newly-derived disease risk classifications in concert with innovative molecular-based cancer treatment. Clearly, this new molecular approach to cancer diagnosis, screening, and therapy means that we are in the midst of a new era for cancer control. Its ultimate success will be seen in the ability to identify family members who fit the particular hereditary cancer

Table 31.1 Hereditary cancer syndromes

Hereditary cancer syndrome	Organs affected	Genes	Frequency
Hereditary breast-ovarian cancer	Breast, ovary, possibly gastric and prostate cancer	BRCA1, BRCA2	exact is unknown; ~4–6% of breast and ovarian cancers
Lynch syndrome	Most commonly the colorectum, followed by the endometrium, ovary, uroepithelial tract, small bowel, stomach, pancreas, hepatobiliary tract, probably breast and prostate; skin in Muir-Torre variant, brain in Turcot variant	mismatch repair genes: MSH2, MLH1, MSH6, PMS2; also silencing of MSH2 by deletion in EPCAM gene	~3% of all colorectal cancer; ~2% of all endometrial cancer; other related cancers less common
Familial CRC type X	Colorectum	unknown	unknown
Familial adenomatous polyposis and attenuated FAP	Colorectum, desmoid tumour, hepatoblastoma, thyroid carcinoma, medulloblastoma	APC	1:6,000–1:13,000
MUTYH-associated polyposis	Colorectum	MUTYH	1.5% of individuals are heterozygous for this recessive trait
Hereditary juvenile polyposis	Colorectum, stomach, small bowel, pancreas	SMAD4, BMPR1A	1:15,000–1:50,000
Peutz–Jeghers syndrome	Breast, colon, pancreas, stomach, ovary (including sex-cord tumours), Sertoli-cell tumours, gall bladder, urinary bladder, genitourinary tract, respiratory tract	STK11	1:29,000–1:120,000
Cowden's syndrome	Breast, follicular thyroid, endometrium	PTEN	1:200,000
Bannayan–Riley–Ruvalcaba syndrome	Thyroid cancer, hamartomatous colon polyps	PTEN	rare
Gorlin syndrome	Basal cell, gastric hamartomas	PTCH	1:40,000–1:57,000
Multiple endocrine neoplasia I	Parathyroid, enteropancreatic endocrine, and pituitary tumours	MEN1	2:100,000
Multiple endocrine neoplasia II B	Medullary thyroid, pheochromocytoma, mucosal neuromas, ganglioneuromas, gastrointestinal hamartomatous polyps	RET	25% of all medullary thyroid carcinoma
Hereditary diffuse gastric cancer	Stomach, lobular breast cancer	CDH1	<3% of gastric cancer
Familial atypical multiple mole melanoma syndrome	Skin, pancreas	CDKN2A	~6%–8% of melanomas; ~5% of pancreatic carcinoma
von Hippel-Lindau	Kidney, liver, pancreas, renal cell carcinoma, pheochromocytoma, retinal and cerebellar hemangioblastoma	VHL	1:36,000
Li–Fraumeni	Sarcoma, breast cancer, brain tumours, leukaemia, lymphoma, laryngeal carcinoma, lung cancer, adrenal cortical carcinoma	P53	unknown
CHEK2 1100delC	Breast, colorectum	CHEK2	unknown
Neurofibromatosis type 1	Neurofibromas, optic nerve gliomas, iris hamartomas, neurofibrosarcoma, pheochromocytoma, duodenal carcinoid, neuroblastoma, ependymoma, rhabdomyosarcoma, and Wilms' tumour; in children: juvenile myelomonocytic leukaemia (juvenile chronic myelogenous leukaemia) and myelodysplasia.	NF1	1:3,000
Neurofibromatosis type 2	central nervous system tumours	NF2	1:35,000
Retinoblastoma	Intraocular	RB	1:13,500–1:25,000
Wilms' tumour	Kidneys, leukaemia, non-cancerous developmental anomalies	WT1, WT2	1:10,000
Ataxia telangiectasia	Breast cancer in heterozygotes; non-Hodgkin lymphoma, leukaemia, gastric cancer, medulloblastoma, glioma	ATM	1.4% of population carry recessive trait; disease incidence 1:30,000–1:100,000
Bloom's syndrome	Leukaemia, lymphoma, carcinomas of larynx, lung, esophagus, colon, breast, cervix, noncancerous anomalies	BLM	Unknown in general population; 1:48,000 among Ashkenazi Jews

(continued)

Table 31.1 Continued

Hereditary cancer syndrome	Organs affected	Genes	Frequency
Fanconi's anaemia	Myelodysplastic syndromes, leukaemia (usually acute myelogenous leukaemia), squamous carcinomas of the upper aerodigestive tract, cervix, vulva, and anus; hepatocellular carcinoma, possibly secondary to anabolic steroid treatment	*FA-A, FA-B, FA-C, FA-D, FA-E*	Estimated 1:300 are heterozygous for this recessive disorder
Werner syndrome	Sarcoma, melanoma, and carcinoma of the thyroid, stomach, liver, breast, and bile duct	*WRN*	1:50,000–1:100,000
Gastrointestinal stromal tumours	Sometimes malignant	KIT/PDGFRA	Hereditary component unknown
Hereditary prostate cancer	Prostate; possible involvement of other sites	Multiple proposed candidate genes	Unknown
Haematologic	Blood-related malignancies	Under investigation	Estimated 5% of the aggregate of haematologic cancers

syndrome's molecular-based diagnosis and thereby can become candidates for full participation in cancer control measures driven by genomic medicine [6, 7].

Demand for genetic counsellors

There is an increasing service demand for genetic counsellors but, unfortunately, the supply of individuals with this expertise is severely limited. Clearly, the need may vary in different geographical regions. A genetic counsellor in a specific geographic location may often be located by clicking on 'find a counselor' in the National Society of Genetic Counselors' website at http://www.nsgc.org.

It is clear that genetic counsellors must assume the role of the 'family teacher and cancer guardian' with responsibility for educating the proband and ideally his/her at-risk relatives. At a minimum, the educational plan must constitute the following:

1. Advice in lay terms about DNA, genetic testing, and its cancer risk significance.

2. Take-home message on screening and management benefits.

3. Legal protection against insurance/employment discrimination as embodied in the Genetic Information Nondiscrimination Act (GINA).

Contact at-risk relatives

Ideally, the counsellor will emphasize the importance of the proband's role to inform close relatives of their cancer risk status with practical input about their need to become committed to

the dicta of this educational process. For most, this will involve the sharing of cancer risk data, DNA testing, and its cancer control implications, so that close relatives can achieve potential lifelong benefit; they must also be made aware of sources of help, for example genetic counselling, medical geneticists, centres of genetic expertise, all in concert with knowledge and participation in this process with their family physicians.

Cancer germline mutations and patient benefit

Mutations may cause cancer in several ways. The main types of gene involved in hereditary carcinogenesis are oncogenes, tumour

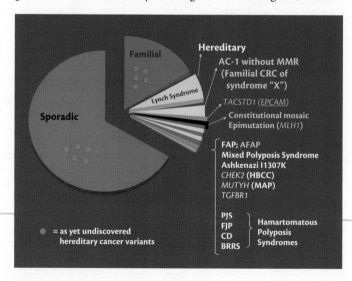

Fig. 31.1 Circle graph depicting the marked genotypic and phenotypic heterogeneity in hereditary colorectal cancer syndromes.

Abbreviations: AC-1, Amsterdam Criteria 1; MMR, mismatch repair; FAP, familial adenomatous polyposis; AFAP, attenuated familial adenomatous polyposis; HBCC, hereditary breast and colorectal cancer; PJS, Peutz–Jeghers syndrome; FJP, familial juvenile polyposis; CD, Cowden's disease; BRRS, Bannayan–Ruvalcaba–Riley syndrome.

Adapted from Lynch et al., Hereditary nonpolyposis colorectal carcinoma (HNPCC) and HNPCC-like families: Problems in diagnosis, surveillance, and management, *Cancer*, Volume 100, Issue 1, pp. 53–64, Copyright © 2003 American Cancer Society, with permission from John Wiley & Sons, Inc. doi: 10.1002/cncr.11912

Table 31.2 Worldwide and US annual CRC syndrome estimates

	Annual CRC incidence	Lynch syndrome (3-5% of all CRC)	FAP (<1% of all CRC)	Familial (20% of all CRC)
Worldwide	1,233,711	37,011–61686	<12,337	246,742
United States	132,700	3,81–6,635	<1,327	26,540

Source: data from The International Agency for Research on Cancer, GLOBOCAN, 2010, available from http://www.iarc.fr/; and Jemal et al., Cancer Statistics, 2010, *CA: A Cancer Journal for Clinicians*, Volume 60, Issue 5, pp. 277–300, Copyright © 2010 American Cancer Society, Inc. doi:10.1002/caac.20073

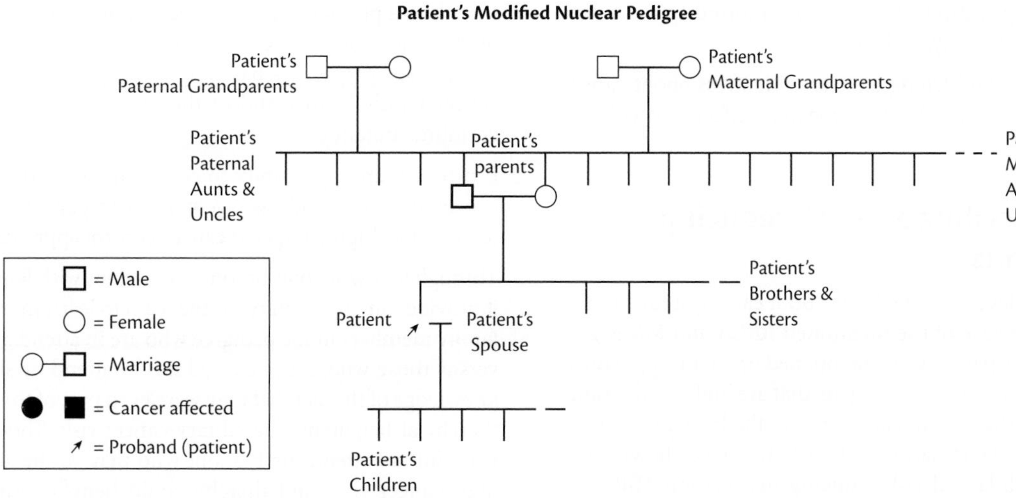

Patient's Modified Nuclear Pedigree

Fig. 31.2 Diagram representing a simple, modified nuclear pedigree for clinical use.
Reproduced from Lynch HT, Schuelke GS, Lynch JF, Hereditary Colorectal Cancer Review: Colonic Polyposis and Nonpolyposis Colonic Cancer (Lynch Syndrome I and II), *Survey of Digestive Diseases*, Volume 2, Number 4, pp. 244–260, Copyright © 1984, with permission from S. Karger AG, doi:10.1159/000171107

suppressor genes, and DNA repair genes. Oncogenes are genes that normally participate in cellular growth pathways, and that become abnormally activated in cancer. Tumour suppressor genes normally suppress cellular growth or cause cells to become differentiated, and are inactivated in cancers. DNA repair genes participate in repair of DNA damage and their inactivation leads to numerous mutations in target genes, including oncogenes and tumour suppressor genes. The 'two-hit' hypothesis of hereditary cancer indicates that when a person inherits an abnormal gene in one allele, an acquired mutation in the other allele will lead to cancer.

Germline mutations which predispose to some of the more common cancers, particularly in the case of the HBOC syndrome and *BRCA* mutations, and CRC with multiple extracolonic cancers in LS, prominently abetted by discovery of the MMR germline mutations, namely *MLH1, MSH2, MSH6,* and *PMS2,* provide excellent models for life-saving benefit from genetic counselling. These well-known and now time-honoured mutation discoveries took place in the mid-1990s [8–10]. Commercial laboratories providing sequencing data for these mutations rapidly emerged throughout the world as patient and physician knowledge expanded and became immersed in a brand new and indeed novel era of patient-centred genetic counselling. This process has rapidly evolved largely due to the cloning of these germline mutations.

Prior to these mutation discoveries, we had to rely solely on an individual's family history and the patient's position in the pedigree to estimate lifetime cancer risk. Thanks to prodigious clinical research on these mutations in patients/families, the cancer spectrum has been broadened in many hereditary cancer-prone syndromes. The vulnerable cancer sites may be extensive as with *BRCA2* mutations, which, in addition to breast and ovarian cancer, may show a pattern of cancer types involving an excess risk of male breast cancer, in addition to cancers of the colon, prostate, pancreas, and malignant melanoma. In the example of LS with MMR germline mutations one may find CRC and extracolonic cancers involving the endometrium, ovary, upper uroepithelial tract, small bowel, breast, prostate, adrenocortical carcinoma, sebaceous carcinomas in the Muir-Torre variant of LS, and glioblastoma in the Turcot's variant. Predictably,

we believe *other* cancers will ultimately be identified as being integral to these hereditary cancer syndromes. These findings, coupled with germline mutations segregating in the families, have allowed us to estimate patients' lifetime risk for these cancers. Importantly, this enables patients to make more informed cancer control decisions, in concert with advice from their physicians and genetic counsellors, about cancer screening, prophylactic (risk-reducing) surgery, or chemoprevention strategies such as tamoxifen as breast cancer chemoprevention in *BRCA* mutation carriers.

The carrier of a cancer-causing mutation may avoid cancer morbidity and mortality through engaging in a variety of preventive options. Non-carriers of a deleterious mutation can avoid the economic and emotional stress of a lifetime of preventive activities and will revert to general population cancer screening guidelines.

Psychosocial factors

Ideally, genetic counsellors must be prepared to work with the patient on the following potential psychosocial and economic issues:

1. Concern about insurance and employment discrimination.

2. The need for the counsellor and physician to keep active communication with the patient current.

3. 'Scapegoating' by family members, such as 'Why did you bring me into the world knowing our family cancer risk was so enormously high?'

4. Fear of manifesting cancer, particularly if found to harbour a cancer-causing mutation, which may be reflected by the query, 'Do I really want to know my molecular genetic test results?' In our experience in the context of our research protocols, at least 20% of our patients who have been tested for a deleterious mutation have declined to receive this information about their gene status, thereby generating an unresolved deep-seated emotional state of anxiety and apprehension about their germline status [11].

5. Emotional stress surrounding the need to tell loved ones about the family history, for example, a fiancé in advance of marriage.

This issue has implications for cancer's morbidity/mortality, long-term risk to progeny, and cost.

6. Finally, there may be lifelong anxiety with stress about cancer risk and the need to know how to cope more effectively with this distress.

Genetic counselling and risk reducing surgical options

Thanks to the high level of knowledge about cancer predictability and certainty in the case of the mentioned BRCA and MMR germline mutations, the past decade has opened up many opportunities for risk-reducing removal of organs that are highly vulnerable to cancer. Thus, in the case of carcinoma of the breast in BRCA1 patients, studies by Hartmann et al. [12, 13] have shown high lifetime benefit of bilateral risk-reducing mastectomy (BRRM). Contralateral risk-reducing mastectomy (CRRM) increased by more than 150% from 1993 to 2003, based upon HBOC's natural history showing an excess of bilateral breast cancer in BRCA mutation carriers. However, Brewster and Parker [14] have shown that while this CRRM reduces the risk for contralateral breast cancer, there is nevertheless conflicting evidence as to why there is not reduced breast cancer mortality. Nevertheless, risk for distant metastatic disease outweighs risk of contralateral breast cancer [14].

Risk-reducing bilateral salpingo-oophorectomy (RRSO) provides an excellent opportunity for prevention of ovarian cancer (OC), which affects approximately 20% of patients with BRCA2 and between 40–68% of those with BRCA1 mutations. Identification and management of at-risk families harbours major public health implications, bridging gynaecologic and clinical genetic practice, given the fact that screening for OC is currently of unproven benefit [15]. An added benefit of RRSO is an approximate 50% reduction in breast cancer in BRCA mutation carriers, particularly when RRSO is performed premenopausaly [16, 17]. We therefore recommend the option of RRSO in women with BRCA mutations who have completed their families and have been provided acceptable genetic counselling and referral to a knowledgeable gynaecologic oncologist [17, 18].

These clinical and molecular genetic considerations mandate the need for genetic counsellors to remain abreast of the multitude of new developments, including newly developed 'next generation' DNA sequencing (NGS) technologies which provide remarkable power for genome study [19, 20].

Family information service (FIS): maximization of personalized medicine

An FIS is a cost-effective, highly efficient way of educating and counselling all available and interested family members from a geographic catchment area in a single setting. It makes the best use of the physician's and genetic counsellor's time and effort, has group therapy potential, and patients welcome it. It has become an extremely valuable application of an expanded genetic counselling model, enabling effective communication with many family members who have gathered together as a group, particularly once a deleterious germline mutation has been identified in the family [21]. This approach to hereditary cancer education, DNA testing, and cancer control has many advantages:

1. It enables a physician, genetic counsellor, or other key members of the cancer genetics team, to explain fully what it means to be at increased cancer risk based upon the presence of a significant cancer family history and/or the presence of a cancer-causing germline mutation.

2. It provides an opportunity to cover highly pertinent aspects of cancer screening and management, with particular focus given to available, highly targeted cancer control approaches.

3. Through follow-up one-on-one discussions with family members, it provides an opportunity for the team to learn more about those family members in the pedigree who are in attendance at the FIS, versus those who either elected not to attend or simply had no knowledge of the fact that they were even part of the pedigree and thereby at heightened hereditary cancer risk. Those individuals who did *not* attend the FIS, but who may yet be at inordinately high cancer risk, and thereby could benefit immensely from appropriate education and individual personalized counselling, should be informed of the team's willingness to assist them. Their more genetically informed close relatives in attendance at the FIS may be in a position to help in this process [22].

4. This entire process allows for collection of consenting patients' DNA for genetic testing following genetic counselling where the pros and cons of germline mutation testing are presented in depth so that the patient can be fully informed about all facets of DNA testing. In this way, the patient will be in the best possible position to follow his/her wishes to provide written informed consent.

5. It supports those high-risk family members who may otherwise be reluctant to express concerns about some of the multifaceted issues involved in their cancer risk status and its assessment through DNA testing. They may be able to discuss more freely any emotionally threatening concerns which may not previously have been broached in a one-on-one genetic counselling session.

6. The FIS may be one of the most cost-effective and emotionally sound approaches known to the hereditary cancer educational process.

Logistics of the FIS

In preparation for the FIS, key family members will often volunteer to help inform their relatives about the objectives of the FIS, encourage their attendance, and identify a meeting place such as their physician's waiting room or their local hospital's outpatient department. These FISs often take place on a weekend when such facilities are less likely to be in use. Indeed, once a convenient time and place are decided, family members can set up individual appointments, should they wish to meet with the physician and/or genetic counsellors for individualized genetic counselling. If DNA had been previously collected and results of testing are available, coupled with informed consent, they can be given their results at the time of an FIS in a private one-on-one result disclosure session.

Importance of proband's close relatives

Rubin et al. [23] investigated whether CRC-affected patients were aware of the increased cancer risk to their close family members and whether sufficient help was delivered to them. Their findings, based upon 253 CRC patients showed that only 120 (47.7%) knew that their first-degree relatives were at increased risk for CRC. A mailed educational brochure, designed to improve their knowledge about their familial cancer risk, did not improve their understanding. These authors [23] therefore concluded that the majority of patients lacked knowledge about their family members' risk and provided a clear indication that more effective educational tools were required. We believe that personal interaction with the family is an optimal way of providing so-called 'hands on' education during meeting with the family information service. Rubin et al. [23] summarize this in the rather terse statement that most CRC-affected patients simply do not know about their family members' risk.

In another study pertaining to cancer risk among probands' relatives, van Dijk et al. [24] investigated the extent to which medical specialists derive information from the family history in concert with the Amsterdam Criteria and Bethesda Guidelines in the case of LS, and subsequently apply recommended cancer control criteria to patients with CRC and a suspicion of LS. Their research involved 244 patients from the Netherlands who satisfied at least one of the Bethesda Guidelines. It was noteworthy that a complete family history was recorded for only 38 of the 244 patients (16%). Those patients with a more complete family history were more likely to be referred to the clinical genetic centre than those with an incomplete or absent family history (53% versus 13% and 4%, respectively; P = 0.0001) and were more likely to be analysed for microsatellite instability (MSI) (34% versus 6% and 1%, respectively; P < 0.001). These authors concluded that the family history is neglected in the majority of patients with CRC. Furthermore, MSI is pursued in only a small proportion of patients who meet the guidelines for this testing.

Tranø et al. [25] studied medical records of CRC patients in Norway and found a striking lack of attention to family history. Sixty-nine percent of patients had no family history recorded on the medical chart. The family history information of the 31.0% who did have it included in their medical record had not been clinically assessed, adding up to 0.0% whose records had been beneficially utilized.

This is not a new observation. Thirty years previous to the Tranø paper, a study was published in *JAMA* [26] that followed a similar design, although the earlier study looked at outpatient cancer clinic records of oncology patients: 'In most cases, the family history of cancer had been either omitted altogether, reported as negative despite substantial evidence to the contrary, or, if noted as positive, not pursued or acted on' [26].

This 1979 study found, as did Tranø's 2009 study, that interviews with the patients whose records had been studied turned up enough positive family histories to be of real concern, as did investigations during the intervening years [27–29].

What the genetic counsellor needs to know about Lynch syndrome

Box 31.1 provides a description of the natural history of LS. Clearly, this reflects the need for the genetic counsellor's knowledge base.

Cancer-prone pedigrees frequently present challenges to the physician/genetic counsellor due to their often diverse genotypic and phenotypic heterogeneity. Often, failure in their interpretation with ultimate problems in diagnosis may result from a lack of extension, reduced penetrance, or failure to search for genealogic and pathologic confirmation of cancer as well as non-cancer phenotypic features such as those so abundant in hereditary disorders such as familial adenomatous polyposis (FAP).

Figure 31.3 depicts a family with the classical phenotype of LS spanning six generations with four generations of affected family members. The proband (IV-3) was diagnosed with three different LS associated cancers: colon cancer at the hepatic flexure at age 53,

---

Box 31.1. Cardinal features of Lynch syndrome

- Autosomal dominant inheritance pattern seen for syndrome cancers in the family pedigree.

- Earlier average age of CRC onset than in the general population. Average age of 45 years in Lynch syndrome versus 63 years in the general population.

- Proximal (right-sided) colonic cancer predilection: 70–85% of Lynch syndrome CRCs are proximal to the splenic flexure.

- Accelerated carcinogenesis: tiny adenomas can develop into carcinomas more quickly, within two to three years in Lynch syndrome versus eight to ten years in the general population.

- High risk of additional CRCs: 25–30% of patients having surgery for a Lynch syndrome-associated CRC will have a second primary CRC within ten years of surgical resection if the surgery was less than a subtotal colectomy

- Increased risk for malignancy at certain extracolonic sites:
  - endometrium (40–60% lifetime risk for female mutation carriers)
  - ovary (12–15% lifetime risk for female mutation carriers)
  - stomach (higher risk in families indigenous to the Orient, reason unknown at this time)
  - small bowel
  - hepatobiliary tract
  - pancreas
  - upper uroepithelial tract (transitional cell carcinoma of the ureter and renal pelvis)
  - prostate cancer
  - breast cancer
  - adrenal cortical carcinomas
  - brain (glioblastomas in the Turcot's syndrome variant of the Lynch syndrome)
  - sebaceous adenomas, sebaceous carcinomas, and multiple keratoacanthomas in the Muir–Torre syndrome variant of Lynch syndrome.

- Pathology of CRCs is more often poorly differentiated, with an excess of mucoid and signet-cell features, a Crohn's-like reaction, and a significant excess of infiltrating lymphocytes within the tumour.

- Increased survival from CRC.

- The sine qua non for diagnosis of LS is the identification of a germline mutation in a mismatch repair gene (most commonly *MLH1*, *MSH2*, or *MSH6*) that segregates in the family, i.e. members who carry the mutation show a much higher rate of syndrome-related cancers than those who do not carry the mutation.

Source: data from The International Agency for Research on Cancer, GLOBOCAN, available from http://www.iarc.fr/ and Jemal et al., Cancer Statistics: A Cancer Journal for Clinicians, Volume 60, Issue 5, pp.277-300, Copyright © 2010 American Cancer Society, Inc. doi:10.1002/caac.20073

ureter cancer at age 56, and then kidney cancer at age 57. Sadly, one of his sons (V-4) developed colon cancer at age 19 and died from this at age 20. Endometrial and ovarian cancers are also expressed in this family in individuals III-1, III-4, III-12, IV-23, IV-24, IV-26, and IV-27. A deleterious *MSH2* mutation was identified within this family in 1995. Genetic testing and counselling of several family members ensued, with education regarding cancer control screening and preventive measures.

Figure 31.4 depicts a contrast to classical LS. Unfortunately, when the proband (V-2) in this family was diagnosed with CRC at the extremely early age of 19 she had no family history to alert her to this possibility. Upon her diagnosis, genetic counselling and testing was done which revealed an *MSH6* mutation. Once the family history was compiled, only a few cases of CRC were discovered on the proband's paternal lineage. Surprisingly, the proband's paternal grandmother (III-22) was found to be positive for the *MSH6* mutation. The grandmother had not been having frequent colonoscopies and yet, fortunately, has not been affected with CRC at the age of 80, giving an example of incomplete penetrance.

Figure 31.5 demonstrates the effectiveness of a multidisciplinary approach to identifying and properly recommending screening based on clinical features. The proband (III-5) was fortunate to have a very astute dermatologist recognize the association between sebaceous adenomas with the risk of CRC due to its association with LS. When the dermatologist diagnosed the proband with a sebaceous adenoma he immediately recommended that the proband have a colonoscopy 'right away'. The proband followed his recommendation and the first two colonoscopies were clear of lesions but the third colonoscopy, done five years after the sebaceous adenoma diagnosis, identified cancer in the ascending colon. If the proband had not been diagnosed with a sebaceous adenoma he would have never been alerted to his risk for developing CRC at such a young age, since the family history is negative.

Figure 31.6 depicts the pedigree of an extremely large family containing more than 700 individuals wherein 50 individuals manifested CRC [30]. The *EPCAM* mutation was identified in this highly extended kindred who was under study by us for more than 35 years [30]. Deletion in the epithelial cell adhesion molecule (*EPCAM*) gene results in hypermethylation and incomplete silencing of *MSH2* [31, 32] *EPCAM* mutation carriers may have phenotypic features that differ from carriers of *MSH2* mutations, namely an almost exclusive expression of site-specific CRC, and so a paucity of extracolonic cancers. However, it should be noted that the larger the deletion and the closer its proximity to the *MSH2* gene, the higher the risk of extracolonic cancers [33]. The breadth and size of the family shown in Figure 31.6 is testament to the potential impact of a single mutation event.

Missed opportunities for DNA testing, screening, and management: genetic counselling implications

Our experience and those discussed in the literature indicate that all too many patients at increased hereditary cancer risk experience confounding factors which contribute unnecessarily to their morbidity and mortality, collectively posing missed cancer prevention opportunities. This problem appears to be one that may be heightened among African Americans (AAs) and other minorities who,

unfortunately, sustain multiple healthcare disparities when compared with European Americans (EAs). One such example is that given by Hall et al. [34] which shows how screening has lowered CRC mortality but, nevertheless, compliance gaps persist among AAs (Table 31.3).

A large LS family studied by Hes [35], with 15 affected family members, provides an excellent example of this problem. This study indicated a deficit of awareness and knowledge about the natural history of LS and its screening and management implications among physicians as well as their high-risk patients. Soberingly, none of the family members underwent pre-symptomatic screening based upon their family history. We must conclude that in spite of the hereditary features indicating LS's natural history of its cancer phenotype, which should have led to referral of high-risk patients for genetic counselling and diagnosis, these were unfortunately totally ignored. Clearly, genetic counselling coupled with family support and encouragement could have diminished consequential high morbidity and mortality [35].

Maximum genetic testing benefit

Should we test all women with breast cancer?

Goodwin et al. [36] ask whether or not all women with breast cancer should be tested for the presence of a *BRCA* mutation, since the finding could be of major clinical significance. For example, information about prognosis can help women make better-informed decisions regarding treatment, risk-reducing surgery inclusive of risk-reducing bilateral mastectomy, and risk-reducing salpingo-oophorectomy. In an editorial on the Goodwin et al. paper, Narod [37] considers this to be an excellent reason to determine one's genetic status. For example, a patient with a *BRCA* mutation can then ask, 'If I develop breast cancer and it's identified by MRI screening, will its prognosis be so good that I'm nearly assured of a cure?' Clearly, if the answer is yes, risk-reducing surgery may be unnecessary. However, Narod suggests that we might test all patients with breast cancer soon after diagnosis, but recognizes fully that the test is expensive. He suggests that the simplest recommendation would be to test women diagnosed with breast cancer younger than 50 years old, as well as those with triple-negative breast cancer and women with a family history of early-onset breast and/or ovarian cancer. Hopefully, in the future the cost of genetic sequencing will decline and so it may be reasonable to test *all* breast cancer patients before a surgical and medical treatment plan is decided.

Should we test all CRC affecteds?

Hampel et al. [38] raise the same DNA-testing question for the identification of LS in all CRC affecteds; they give a resounding 'yes' based upon the evidence they have accumulated. Specifically, they investigated 500 consecutive patients with CRC and identified 18 (3.6%) that had LS. Of these 18, all had high microsatellite instability (MSI-H) while 17 (94%) were correctly predicted by immunohistochemistry (IHC). Their findings disclosed that one in 35 cases of CRC showed LS. These investigators also took the position that all endometrial cancer cases should be molecularly screened for LS [39]. They concluded that IHC is the preferred method to screen for LS.

Mvundura et al. [40] estimated the cost-effectiveness of genetic testing strategies to identify LS among newly- diagnosed CRC

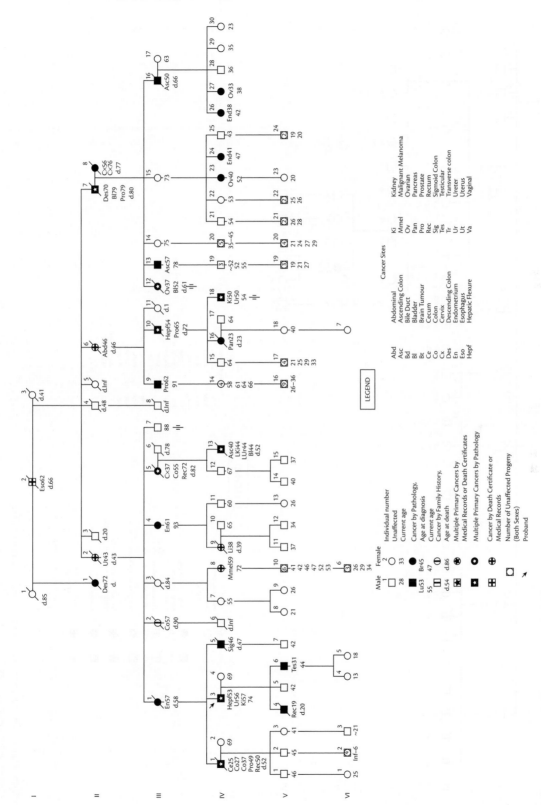

Fig. 31.3 Pedigree showing a classical LS family, with colonic and extracolonic cancers.

Image drawn by Tami Richardson-Nelson, Copyright © Dr Henry T. Lynch 2015.

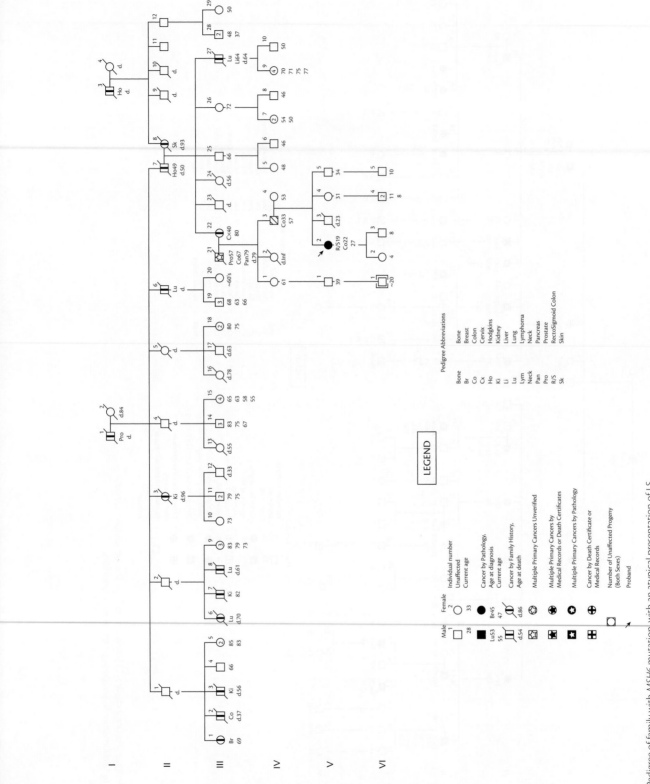

Fig. 31.4 Pedigree of family with *MSH6* mutation, with an atypical presentation of LS.

Image drawn by Tami Richardson-Nelson, Copyright © Dr Henry T. Lynch 2015.

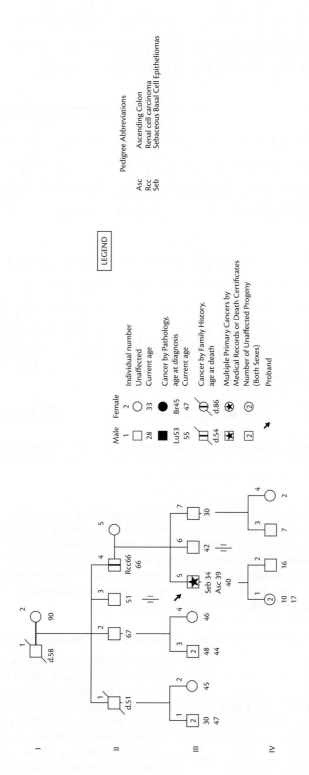

Fig. 31.5 Pedigree of a Muir–Torre syndrome family wherein the proband was diagnosed with a sebaceous carcinoma, leading the dermatologist to recommend regular colonoscopies; a subsequent colonoscopy detected CRC at an early stage.

Image drawn by Tami Richardson-Nelson, Copyright © Dr Henry T. Lynch 2015.

LEGEND

Male	Female	
1	2	Individual number
□ 28	○ 33	Unaffected / Current age
■ Lu53 55	● Br45 47	Cancer by Pathology, age at diagnosis
⌀ d.54	⌀ d.86	Cancer by Family History, Current age / age at death
▣	✦	Multiple Primary Cancers by Medical Records or Death Certificates
2	2	Number of Unaffected Progeny (Both Sexes)
➤		Proband

Pedigree Abbreviations

Asc — Ascending Colon
Rcc — Renal cell carcinoma
Seb — Sebaceous Basal Cell Epitheliomas

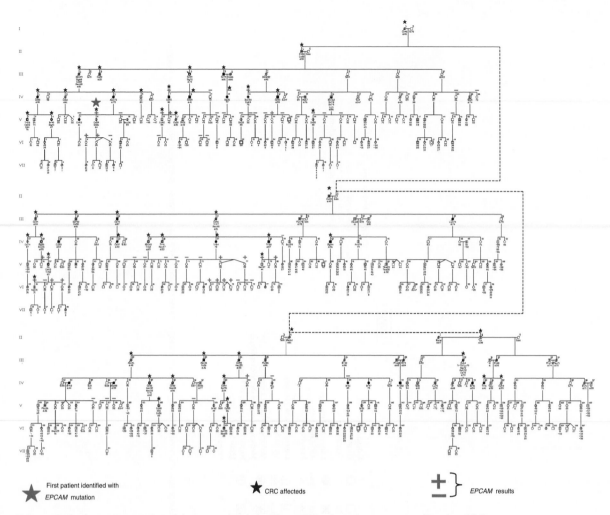

First patient identified with
EPCAM mutation

★ CRC affecteds

+
−
} EPCAM results

Fig. 31.6 Pedigree of a family carrying an *EPCAM* deletion. Numbers below the symbols refer to the age in years of last clinical follow up.
Reproduced with permission from Lynch et al, Lynch Syndrome-Associated Extracolonic Tumors Are Rare in Two Extended Families with the Same *EPCAM* Deletion, *The American Journal of Gastroenterology*, Volume 106, pp. 1829–1839, Copyright © 2011 The American College of Gastroenterology.

patients using MSI and IHC, which appeared to be cost-effective from the perspective of the US healthcare system. Their findings showed that detection involved twice as many cases of LS as would be found by targeting younger patients. Ladabaum et al. [41] also provided further evidence of how widespread CRC testing for LS could yield substantial benefits at acceptable cost. The cost effectiveness depended upon the participation rate among relatives at risk for LS.

These findings, involving more comprehensive testing for HBOC and LS, will immediately define the need for appropriate

genetic counselling among those high-risk individuals who are identified as harbouring the respective HBOC and LS disorders. These data are presented in order to define better the emerging need for genetic counselling in an ever-widening array of hereditary disorders that are highly likely to be identified through rapidly emerging diagnostic genomic and computer-generated technology.

Direct-to-consumer (DTC) genetic testing

The genetic revolution which has impacted the practice of medicine and healthcare has made patients increasingly aware of genetic testing and its benefits. However, unfortunately, many physicians and patients are being misled by DTC test offerings of questionable accuracy and utility [42]. This results in patients' receipt of mundane information based on potentially important results but in the *absence* of appropriate genetic counselling by professionals. This problem has been addressed by the US General Accounting Office which concluded that such DTC tests were 'misleading and of little or no practical use' [43]. Risk profiles provided by such testing companies have been described as having 'no predictive value' and may falsely alarm or reassure consumers [44].

Table 31.3 CRC screening by race [33]

Test	AAs	EAs	P value
Faecal occult blood testing	49.0%	60.7%	0.035
Lower endoscopy	44.1%	58.5%	0.011
Any CRC screening	66.2%	76.3%	0.053

Abbreviations: AAs, African Americans; EAs, European Americans.

Source: data from Hall et al, Rates and predictors of colorectal cancer screening by race among motivated men participating in a prostate cancer risk assessment program, *Cancer*, Volume 118, Issue 2, pp. 478-484, Copyright © 2012, DOI:10.1002/cncr.26315

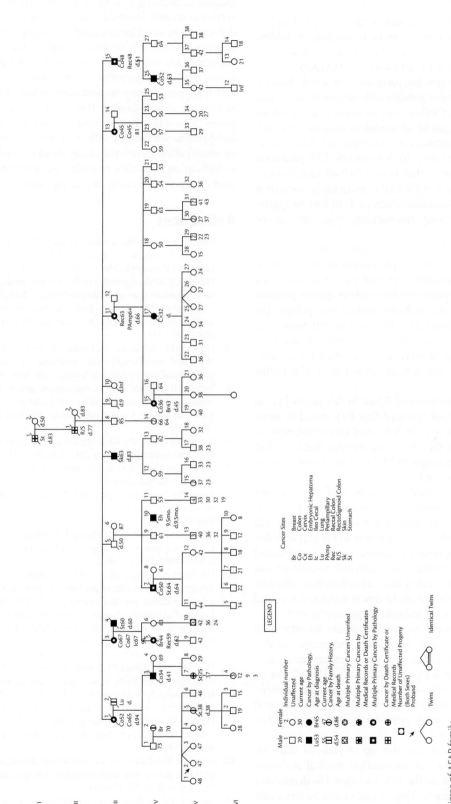

Fig. 31.7 Pedigree of AFAP family.

Reproduced with permission from Lynch HT, FAP, gastric cancer, and genetic cancer featuring children and young adults: a family study and review, *Familial Cancer*, Volume 9, Issue 4, pp. 581–588, Copyright © 2010 Springer Science and Business Media.

Genetic counselling featuring children and young adults

Several forms of hereditary cancer show early clinical and pathology manifestations, and so require genetic counselling of children and youth. The classic example is FAP. Lynch et al. [45] described a variant of this disorder known as attenuated FAP (AFAP).

When evaluating FAP in families, particularly in at-risk children, one must remain cognizant of patients with extremely early onset of colonic adenomas and CRCs as well as upper gastrointestinal fundic gland polyps and gastric adenomas in addition to a variety of other extracolonic tumours. For example, hepatoblastomas, although relatively rare, are more likely to involve FAP patients at an early age. It is noteworthy that among FAP-affected children younger than 10 years, the risk for FAP is more likely to occur at codon 1309 in the *APC* mutation, which leads to a more aggressive phenotype in which early risk-reducing colectomy can be indicated [46].

In one AFAP family, in addition to CRC, gastric cancer occurred, which was heavily influenced by the presence of numerous fundic gland polyps. The study involved more than two decades of investigation in which gastric cancer posed an early diagnostic problem since it was obscured by the multiple fundic gland polyps. The pedigree is depicted in Figure 31.7. Fear and anxiety were rampant among many of these high-cancer-risk patients, based upon the recognizable phenotype of precancerous multiple colonic adenomatous polyps coupled with a highly penetrant *APC* germline mutation.

We provided *APC* results to the children in this family [47] in a group FIS setting, since we reasoned that they would be more likely to express their concerns freely in such an environment. In the educational portion of the FIS, we emphasized that the colon was the major cancer-prone organ in FAP. Cancer control issues in the family were also emphasized.

Special attention was focused on a subset of this pedigree (Figure 31.7), in which progeny, namely individuals VI-6, VI-7, VI-8, VI-9, VI-10, of an *APC* mutation-positive mother (V-12) with a 426delAT *APC* mutation participated in an FIS [21] with disclosure of their *APC* testing results. Informed consent was obtained from non-minors, while among minors parental permission and the minor's assent for genetic testing and counselling were obtained. The importance of early average age of cancer onset and the need for surveillance among affected individuals was emphasized.

The first of V-12's progeny to receive *APC* results during the FIS was individual VI-10, an 8-year-old girl. She understood our discussion but appeared to realize that FAP was rampant throughout her family. After her blood draw, she asked her mother almost on a weekly basis if her test results were ready. Interestingly, however, she did not show any emotion save that for nervous giddiness and laughter when told that she was negative for the *APC* mutation. She did state that she was 'happy'.

The next to receive results was VI-8, an 18-year-old male. He had been born prematurely and had multiple medical problems. He was told he was positive for the *APC* mutation. His demeanour throughout was one of being strikingly negative and he repeatedly said 'I don't care' whenever the issue of *APC* results was discussed. He was informed of the importance of getting a baseline colonoscopy but appeared to be reticent about considering that option.

Conclusion: genetic counselling limitations

Genetic counselling is labour intensive, and remuneration for this service is severely limited by many insurance carriers, resulting in decreased physician involvement. Fortunately, much of this service is being provided by genetic counsellors who are highly experienced and knowledgeable about the natural history of hereditary cancer syndromes, germline mutation testing, as well as screening and management recommendations which are melded into the syndrome's natural history. They often have an educational background in psychology, which may contribute to preparing them for compassionately dealing with the emotional burden experienced by many patients when they learn about the lifelong consequences of harbouring a germline mutation and its potential need for a lifetime of targeted screening and management.

References

1. Baty BJ, Biesecker BB. Seminars in medical genetics: toward evidence-based genetic counseling. American Journal of Medical Genetics (Seminars in Medical Genetics) 2006; 142C: 207–208.
2. Epstein CJ. Medical genetics in the genomic medicine of the 21st century. American Journal of Human Genetics 2006; 79: 434–438.
3. Guttmacher AE, Collins FS. Realizing the promise of genomics in biomedical research. Journal of the American Medical Association 2005; 294: 1399–1402.
4. Lindor NM, McMaster ML, Lindor CJ, Greene MH. Concise handbook of familial cancer susceptibility syndromes: second edition. Journal of the National Cancer Institute Monographs 2008; 2008: 1–93.
5. Berliner JL, Fay AM. Risk assessment and genetic counseling for hereditary breast and ovarian cancer: recommendations of the National Society of Genetic Counselors. Journal of Genetic Counseling 2007; 16: 241–260.
6. Green ED, Guyer MS. Charting a course for genomic medicine from base pairs to bedside. Nature 2011; 470: 204–213.
7. Tajik P, Bossuyt PM. Genomic markers to tailor treatments: waiting or initiating? Human Genetics 2011; 130: 15–18.
8. Narod SA, Feunteun J, Lynch HT, Watson P, Conway T et al. Familial breast-ovarian cancer locus on chromosome 17q12-q23. Lancet 1991; 388: 82–83.
9. Peltomäki P, Aaltonen L, Sistonen P, Pylkkänen L, Mecklin J-P et al. Genetic mapping of a locus predisposing to human colorectal cancer. Science 1993; 260: 810–812.
10. Lindblom A, Tannergard P, Werelius B, Nordenskjold M. Genetic mapping of a second locus predisposing to hereditary nonpolyposis colorectal cancer. Nature Genetics 1993; 5: 279–282.
11. Lerman C, Hughes C, Lemon SJ, Main D, Snyder C et al. What you don't know can hurt you: adverse psychologic effects in members of BRCA1-linked and BRCA2-linked families who decline genetic testing. Journal of Clinical Oncology 1998; 16: 1650–1654.
12. Hartmann LC, Schaid DJ, Woods JE, Crotty TP, Myers JL et al. Efficacy of bilateral prophylactic mastectomy in women with a family history of breast cancer. New England Journal of Medicine 1999; 340: 77–84.
13. Hartmann LC, Sellers TA, Schaid DJ, Frank TS, Soderberg CL et al. Efficacy of bilateral prophylactic mastectomy in BRCA1 and BRCA2 gene mutation carriers. Journal of the National Cancer Institute 2001; 93: 1633–1637.
14. Brewster AM, Parker PA. Current knowledge on contralateral prophylactic mastectomy among women with sporadic breast cancer. Oncologist 2011; 16: 935–941.
15. Rosenthal A, Jacobs I. Familial ovarian cancer screening. Best Practice & Research Clinical Obstetrics & Gynaecology 2006; 20: 321–338.
16. Rebbeck TR, Kauff ND, Domchek SM. Meta-analysis of risk reduction estimates associated with risk-reducing salpingo-oophorectomy in

BRCA1 or BRCA2 mutation carriers. Journal of the National Cancer Institute 2009; 101: 80–87.

17. Kauff ND, Domchek SM, Friebel TM, Robson ME, Lee J et al. Risk-reducing salpingo-oophorectomy for the prevention of BRCA1- and BRCA2-associated breast and gynecologic cancer: a multicenter, prospective study. Journal of Clinical Oncology 2008; 26: 1331–1337.

18. Rebbeck TR, Lynch HT, Neuhausen SL, Narod SA, van't Veer L et al. The prevention and observation of surgical end points study group: prophylactic oophorectomy in carriers of BRCA1 or BRCA2 mutations. New England Journal of Medicine 2002; 346: 1616–1622.

19. Ng SB, Turner EH, Robertson PD, Flygare SD, Bigham AW et al. Targeted capture and massively parallel sequencing of 12 human exomes. Nature 2009; 461: 272–276.

20. Choi M, Scholl UI, Ji W, Tikhonova IR, Zumbo P et al. Genetic diagnosis by whole exome capture and massively parallel DNA sequencing. Proceedings of the National Academy of Sciences USA 2009; 106: 19096–19101.

21. Lynch HT. Family Information Service and hereditary cancer. Cancer 2001; 91: 625–628.

22. Lynch HT, Snyder C, Lynch J, Ghate S, Thome S. Family Information Service (FIS) in a BRCA1 extended family. Journal of Clinical Oncology 2006; 24(18S): 1028.

23. Rubin DT, Gandhi RK, Hetzel JT, Kinnear SH, Aronsohn A et al. Do colorectal cancer patients understand that their family is at risk? Digestive Diseases and Sciences 2009; 54: 2473–2483.

24. van Dijk DA, Oostindiër MJ, Kloosterman-Boele WM, Krijnen P, Vasen HFA et al. Family history is neglected in the work-up of patients with colorectal cancer: a quality assessment using cancer registry data. Familial Cancer 2007; 6: 131–134.

25. Tranø G, Wasmuth HH, Sjursen W, Hofsli E, Vatten LJ. Awareness of heredity in colorectal cancer patients is insufficient among clinicians: a Norwegian population based study. Colorectal Disease 2009; 11: 456–461.

26. Lynch HT, Follett KL, Lynch PM, Albano WA, Mailliard JL et al. Family history in an oncology clinic: implications for cancer genetics. Journal of the American Medical Association 1979; 242: 1268–1272.

27. Tyler CV, Jr, Snyder CW. Cancer risk assessment: examining the family physician's role. Journal of the American Board of Family Medicine 2006; 19: 468–477.

28. Sifri RD, Wender R, Paynter N. Cancer risk assessment from family history: gaps in primary care practice. Journal of Family Practice 2002; 51: 856 (Abstract).

29. Guttmacher AE, Collins FS, Carmona RH. The family history: more important than ever. New England Journal of Medicine 2004; 351: 2333–2336.

30. Lynch H, Riegert-Johnson D, Snyder C, Lynch J, Hagenkord J et al. Lynch syndrome associated extracolonic tumors are rare in two extended families with the same EPCAM deletion. American Journal of Gastroenterology 2011; 106: 1829–1836.

31. Kovacs ME, Papp J, Szentirmay Z, Otto S, Olah E. Deletions removing the last exon of TACSTD1 constitute a distinct class of mutations predisposing to Lynch syndrome. Human Mutation 2009; 30: 197–203.

32. Ligtenberg MJL, Kuiper RP, Chan TL, Goossens M, Hebeda KM et al. Heritable somatic methylation and inactivation of MSH2 in families with Lynch syndrome due to deletion of the 3′ exons of TACSTD1. Nature Genetics 2009; 41: 112–117.

33. Kempers MJE, Kuiper RP, Ockeloen CW, Chappuis PO, Hutter P et al. Risk of colorectal and endometrial cancers in EPCAM deletion-positive Lynch syndrome: a cohort study. Lancet Oncology 2011; 12: 49-55.

34. Hall MJ, Ruth K, Giri VN. Rates and predictors of colorectal cancer screening by race among motivated men participating in a prostate cancer risk assessment program. Cancer 2012; 118: 478–484.

35. Hes FJ. Lynch syndrome: still not a familiar picture. World Journal of Surgical Oncology 2008; 6: 21.

36. Goodwin PJ, Phillips K-A, West DW, Ennis M, Hopper JL et al. Breast cancer prognosis in BRCA1 and BRCA2 mutation carriers: an international prospective breast cancer family registry population-based cohort study. Journal of Clinical Oncology 2012; 30: 19–26.

37. Narod SA. Should all women with breast cancer be tested for BRCA mutations at the time of diagnosis? Journal of Clinical Oncology 2012; 30: 2–3.

38. Hampel H, Frankel WL, Martin E, Arnold M, Khanduja K et al. Feasibility of screening for Lynch syndrome among patients with colorectal cancer. Journal of Clinical Oncology 2008; 26: 5783–5788.

39. Hampel H, Frankel W, Panescu J, Lockman J, Sotamaa K et al. Screening for Lynch syndrome (hereditary nonpolyposis colorectal cancer) among endometrial cancer patients. Cancer Research 2006; 66: 7810–7817.

40. Mvundura M, Grosse SD, Hampel H, Palomaki GE. The cost-effectiveness of genetic testing strategies for Lynch syndrome among newly diagnosed patients with colorectal cancer. Genetics in Medicine 2010; 12: 93–104.

41. Ladabaum U, Wang G, Terdiman J, Blanco A, Kuppermann M et al. Strategies to identify the Lynch syndrome among patients with colorectal cancer: a cost-effectiveness analysis. Annals of Internal Medicine 2011; 155: 69–79.

42. Pirzadeh-Miller S, Bellcross C, Robinson L, Matloff ET. Direct-to-consumer genetic testing: helpful, harmful, or pure entertainment? Community Oncology 2011; 8: 263–268.

43. US Government Accounting Office. GAO report: Direct-to-consumer genetic tests: misleading test results are further complicated by deceptive marketing and other questionable practices. US Government Accounting Office 2010. Available from: <http://www.gao.gov/products/GAO-10-847T>, accessed on 9 June 2015.

44. Udesky L. The ethics of direct-to-consumer genetic testing. Lancet 2010; 376: 1377–1378.

45. Lynch HT, Smyrk T, McGinn T, Lanspa S, Cavalieri J et al. Attenuated familial adenomatous polyposis (AFAP): a phenotypically and genotypically distinctive variant of FAP. Cancer 1995; 76: 2427-2433.

46. Attard TM, Tajouri T, Peterson KD, Tinley S, Thorson AG et al. Familial adenomatous polyposis in children younger than age ten years: a multidisciplinary clinic experience. Diseases of the Colon & Rectum 2008; 51: 207–212.

47. Lynch HT, Snyder C, Davies JM, Lanspa S, Lynch J et al. FAP, gastric cancer, and genetic counseling featuring children and young adults: a family study and review. Familial Cancer 2010; 9: 581–588.

SECTION 5

Support for the cancer patient

32 **Supportive and palliative care** *293*
David Hui and Eduardo Bruera

33 **Quality of life** *302*
Neil K. Aaronson and Peter M. Fayers

34 **Cancer survivorship and rehabilitation** *312*
Rachel L. Yung and Ann H. Partridge

CHAPTER 32

Supportive and palliative care

David Hui and Eduardo Bruera

Introduction to supportive and palliative care

Cancer patients often experience significant symptom burden starting before the time of diagnosis, during cancer treatments and with disease progression [1, 2]. Indeed, patients with advanced cancer report an average of eight to 12 symptoms in cross-sectional surveys [3, 4]. These symptoms may be caused by the tumour itself resulting in obstruction, compression, direct infiltration, or effusions and various complications such as inflammation, thrombosis, infections, and paraneoplastic syndromes. Treatments aimed at reducing the tumour burden can also result in significant side effects. Moreover, patients often experience significant deterioration in their bodily function, sexuality, body image, family dynamics, jobs, financial status and spirituality, resulting in psychological distress. Cancer-related symptoms, treatment side effects, and psychological stressors, coupled with pre-existing comorbidities, significantly decrease patients' quality of life and increase caregiver burden.

In addition to symptom burden, cancer patients often have informational needs regarding their disease, symptoms, prognosis, investigation findings, therapeutic options, and coping strategies. They also require assistance with complex decision-making surrounding treatment choices and advance care planning. As patients approach the end of life (i.e. six months or less of life expectancy), their care needs increase dramatically [2].

Palliative care is an interprofessional discipline that specifically addresses the symptom management, communication, and decision-making aspects of care. It aims at improving 'the quality of life of patients and families who face life-threatening illness by providing pain and symptom relief with spiritual and psychosocial support from diagnosis to the end of life and bereavement' [5]. The terms 'supportive care' and 'Hospice Care' have similar, yet distinct, meanings (Figure 32.1). 'Palliative care' focuses on caring for patients with advanced diseases and includes both hospital-based acute palliative care services and community-based hospice care programmes that are limited to patients with a life expectancy of six months or less. 'Supportive care' encompasses not only palliative and hospice care, but also care for patients with early disease and survivorship [6]. A recent survey of oncologists and mid-level providers suggested that they were more comfortable with the term 'supportive care' than 'palliative care' [7], and referred more patients after our palliative care programme adopted the name 'supportive care' [8]. Given the significant overlap between 'supportive care' and 'palliative care', we will use the term 'supportive and palliative care' for the purpose of this book chapter.

Recognizing the role of supportive and palliative care in optimizing patient care, the Institute of Medicine (IOM) [9], the National Comprehensive Cancer Network (NCCN) [10], the American College of Surgeons Commission on Cancer (CoC) [11], and the American Society of Clinical Oncology (ASCO) [12, 13] all support increased integration of palliative care into oncologic care. Oncologists caring for cancer patients should be familiar with the principles of palliative care and should be equipped with some core skills of symptom management, communication, and decision-making. They should also know when to refer cancer patients to a specialist palliative care team (see Table 32.1). The aim of this chapter is to describe the structure, processes, and outcomes of palliative care, and to discuss contemporary models of integration between oncology and palliative care.

Structure of supportive and palliative care programmes

Palliative care is, by definition, interprofessional. Palliative care programmes typically consist of nurses, physicians, mid-level providers, social workers, psychologists, counsellors, chaplains, physiotherapists, occupational therapists, and a wide number of other disciplinarians including art therapists, music therapists, and volunteers.

Acute palliative care programmes are located within acute care facilities. The four major branches of acute palliative care are (1) inpatient consultation teams, (2) acute palliative care units, (3) outpatient clinics and (4) palliative home care programmes [14]. Each has a unique function and complements the other branches.

Inpatient palliative care consultation teams represent the backbone of palliative care. In a survey of US cancer centres, 92% of National Cancer Institute designated cancer centres reported having a palliative care inpatient consultation team [15]. The consultation team provides advice in symptom management and transition of care for hospitalized patients. Because patients are often acutely ill, the time from referral to death is short (days to weeks) [16, 17].

Patients in severe physical and/or emotional distress seen by the consultation team may be transferred to an acute palliative care unit, which provides intensive symptom management and psychosocial counselling with an interdisciplinary team. Through impeccable communication, education about end-of-life care, family meetings, and goals of care discussions, the palliative care team plays an important role in facilitating transitions of care and discharge planning. In a study of our palliative care unit, approximately one-third of all admissions died in the hospital and the remainder was discharged to the community, mostly with hospice care in place. The median survival from discharge to death was 21 days [18]. In addition to end-of-life care, acute

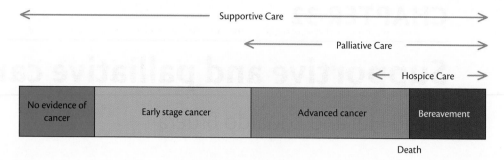

Fig. 32.1 Scope of supportive care, palliative care, and hospice care. Based on a recent systematic review, hospice care provides community-based care for patients at the end of life with a prognosis of six months or less. Palliative care provides care for patients with advanced cancer in the acute care setting through inpatient consultation teams, acute palliative care units, outpatient clinics, and home care services. Supportive care is the most expansive and addresses the need for both early-stage and advanced cancer patients. It includes survivorship care, palliative care, and hospice care programmes.

palliative care units can facilitate simultaneous care by effectively addressing cancer treatment-related adverse effects and complications [19].

Palliative care outpatient clinics aim at providing care to patients earlier in the disease trajectory, with months between referral to death [15, 20]. Outpatient clinics represent the ideal setting for integration between oncology and palliative care. Symptoms may be managed or prevented effectively before crisis occurs, and recommendations can be given to optimize patients' nutritional and functional status during concurrent cancer treatments. Multiple clinic visits also allow the palliative care team to establish a long-term relationship with patients and their families, to establish trust, to provide longitudinal counselling, and to initiate discussions regarding goals of care and advance care planning.

Table 32.1 Palliative care referral

Why should we refer?	To improve the symptom burden, satisfaction, quality of life, and potentially quantity of life of patients with advanced cancer.
Who should be referred?	Studies suggest that patients with advanced cancer should be referred within two months of diagnosis, regardless of their distress level. However, given that few palliative care programmes have the infrastructure to accommodate a large number of patients, selective referral is recommended at this time.
	The National Comprehensive Cancer Network suggested that patients with uncontrolled symptoms, moderate to severe distress, serious comorbidities, life expectancy less than or equal to 12 months, patient/family concerns about the course of disease and decision making, or self-expressed interest should be referred to interdisciplinary palliative care teams for further management [10].
Who should be providing palliative care?	Oncologists (primary palliative care) and palliative care team (secondary palliative care) should work together to deliver comprehensive cancer care.
When should patients be referred?	Earlier is better to facilitate symptom detection and treatment, longitudinal counselling and advance care planning.
How comprehensive should palliative care programmes be?	Studies suggest that interdisciplinary palliative care programmes providing comprehensive services are more effective than when only a few disciplines are involved.

Palliative home care teams deliver healthcare services to patients' homes for those who are not already enrolled onto hospice programmes. In the US, palliative home care is an extension of services from the acute care system, while hospice enrolment means that the patients receive only community-based care. By conducting home visits, the palliative care team can assess symptoms and home safety, delivery medications, address psychosocial issues, while at the same time, minimize patient travel and wait time.

Processes of supportive and palliative care programmes

Principles of symptom management

Symptom management is one of the most important aspects of palliative care. Over the past few decades, multiple principles related to symptom assessment and management have emerged based on an increased understanding of the pathogenesis and natural history of symptom development.

First, symptoms are highly prevalent. In a systematic review of symptom prevalence in patients with advanced cancer, 74% had fatigue, 71% had pain, 53% had appetite loss, and 48% had nervousness [21]. Thus, symptoms should be routinely screened and treated.

Second, symptoms often occur together. Patients with advanced cancer experience on average eight to 12 symptoms at any one time. This may be related to common pathogenesis (e.g., inflammatory cytokines could result in fatigue, anorexia, cachexia and depression) or the fact that symptoms often exacerbate each other (e.g., pain can cause insomnia and anxiety, and anxiety could, in turn, worsen pain). Identification of the cause(s) is an important part of the assessment. Validated symptom batteries are available for clinic use; for instance, the Edmonton Symptom Assessment Scale (ESAS) consists of ten symptoms assessed by numeric rating scale ranging from 0 (no symptom at all) to 10 (worst possible) [22].

Third, symptoms often have multiple etiologies. For instance, cancer-related fatigue may be due to cytokine dysregulation, electrolyte abnormalities, anaemia, deconditioning, and depression in a particular patient [23]. The implication is that multidimensional assessments and interventions are needed. In this example, successful interprofessional intervention may include use of dexamethasone and correction of hypernatremia and anaemia by the palliative care physician, exercise with physiotherapy, and counselling sessions with psychology. Importantly, recommendations should be tailored to the individual's needs.

Fourth, symptom expression can be modulated by multiple factors, such as age, sex, culture, delirium, psychological distress, and secondary gain. Figure 32.2 illustrates how the generation, perception, and expression of various symptoms are related to each other. For instance, pain expression may be 10/10 in a patient with advanced cancer with minimal nociceptive pain but severe psychological distress. Proper management in such patients would include counselling, rather than escalating the opioid dose and nerve blocks.

Fifth, symptom expression fluctuates over time and increases steadily in the last months of life. Seow et al. serially examined the symptom burden in advanced cancer patients in the ambulatory setting. In the last few weeks of life, they found a significant increase in dyspnoea, fatigue, drowsiness, anorexia, and a decrease in well-being [2]. Patients should be educated to anticipate an increased symptom burden and that effective treatment options are available for many symptoms, resulting in more resources needed at the end of life (i.e. last six months).

Sixth, symptom expression is subjective by definition and should be assessed with validated patient reported outcomes tools. No objective measures can replace subjective reporting. Caregivers generally overestimate the symptom burden, while health

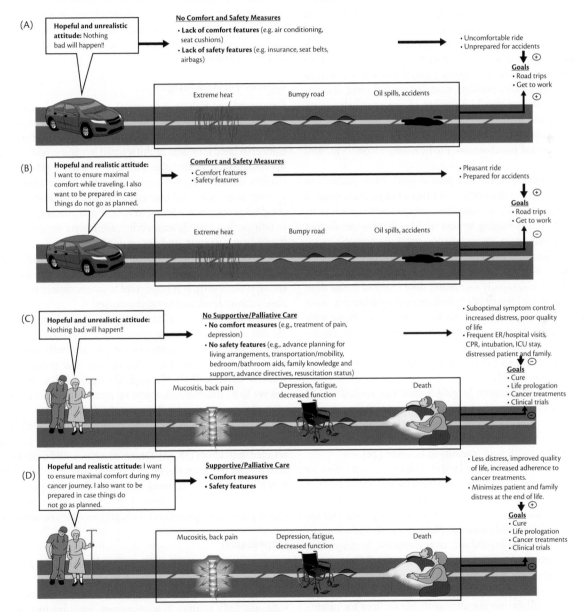

Fig. 32.2 Goals of care discussions [71]. Palliative care referral and advance care planning are analogous to comfort features and safety features in a car. (A) A hopeful and optimistic driver going on a road trip believes that nothing bad will happen along the way, and may not worry about comfort and safety. (B) A hopeful and realistic driver is aware of challenges along the way, and would want to have maximal comfort features, as well as safety measures and car insurance to ensure he can get to his destination comfortably and safely. (C) Similarly, a hopeful and optimistic patient may only want to seek cancer treatments without addressing symptom control and advance-care planning. This lack of preparation may negatively affect the patient's ability to attain his goal. (D) In contrast, a hopeful and realistic patient understands the role of concurrent supportive care. He is more likely to attain his goal of getting more cancer therapies and life prolongation, while maximizing quality of life. He also has peace of mind because of advance care planning.

professionals often underestimate the symptom profile. Studies utilizing patient-reported outcomes found that they provide more information than healthcare professional's assessments and even correlate with survival.

Seventh, more research is needed to examine pathophysiology, assessment and interventions for various symptoms [24, 25].

Cancer pain

Pain is one of the most common symptoms reported by cancer patients, and is associated with decreased function, appetite, sleep, mood, and quality of life. Proper evaluation of pain should include characterization of its location, intensity (0–10 numeric rating scale), nature, duration, and previous therapies. It is also important to conduct a comprehensive assessment of potential causes and to identify modulating factors such as cognitive failure and psychological distress. For patients on opioids, it is also critical to monitor patients for opioid-related side effects, such as nausea, drowsiness, hallucinations, myoclonus, and vivid dreams. Furthermore, clinicians should be aware of aberrant behaviours suggestive of opioid misuse, including unusually high doses, frequent use of breakthrough doses, recurrent loss of prescriptions, as well as concurrent psychotropic medications, alcoholism, and illicit drug use.

Over time, it becomes clear that pain is much more difficult to control in some patients than others. A number of pain assessment tools have been developed to assist clinicians to identify such individuals. The Edmonton Staging System (ESS) includes seven factors (mechanism of pain, pain characteristics, previous narcotic exposure, cognitive function, psychological distress, tolerance, and past history). Patients with any one of neuropathic pain, incidental pain, psychological distress, rapidly increasing dose (>5% of initial dose per day), and positive history of alcoholism or drug addiction were considered to have a poor prognosis for pain control; those with mixed or unknown pain syndrome, >300 mg of morphine equivalent daily dose per day, and altered cognitive function have an intermediate prognosis for pain control; and the remaining patients have a good prognosis [26].

Subsequently, the Edmonton Staging System was revised (rESS) to include five factors only: pain mechanism, incidental pain, psychological distress, addiction, and cognition to facilitate daily practice [27]. This has been found to be predictive of pain control to a certain extent along with pain intensity at baseline [28].

According to the WHO pain ladder, mild pain can often be treated with non-opioids such as non-steroidal anti-inflammatory drugs (NSAIDs) and acetaminophen. Moderate and severe pain may warrant the use of opioids. Common weak opioids include hydrocodone, codeine, and tramadol. Strong opioids include morphine, hydromorphone, oxycodone, oxymorphone, fentanyl, and methadone. Importantly, adjuvant treatments should always be considered to optimize pain management and to minimize the dose of opioids. For example, tricyclic antidepressants, gabapentin, pregabalin, and venlafaxine are all reasonable choices for neuropathic pain. NSAIDs, steroid, bisphosphonates, or radiation may be considered for bone pain. Involvement of services such as palliative care, pain services, and radiation oncology may be helpful.

A working knowledge of opioids is essential for good pain management. With the exception of methadone, all strong opioids are available in extended release and immediate release formulations. Methadone has a long half-life and is fast acting, and is appropriate for both long- and short-acting purposes. All strong opioids have similar efficacy in pain relief at equianalgesic doses. Furthermore, extended-release opioids are similarly as efficacious as immediate-release opioids given around the clock, with the only advantage being fewer doses [29]. When used as a rescue dose, immediate-release opioids should be dosed at 10–20% of the total opioid daily dose, given every one to two hours on an as-needed basis. Because opioids can have serious long- and short-term side effects, it is crucial that patients are educated about their proper use and potential adverse reactions. Importantly, constipation, drowsiness, and nausea can be prevented with laxatives, methylphenidate, and metoclopramide, respectively. Opioid rotation is important for patients who have developed severe opioid toxicity, who have poor pain control despite high doses of opioids, or need to switch opioids for logistic reasons (e.g., cost or change of route of administration).

Cancer-related fatigue

Cancer-related fatigue is the most common concern among cancer patients, particularly among those on cancer treatments and at the end of life [30]. It does not typically improve with rest. Cancer-related fatigue is multifactorial in nature, related to cytokine upregulation, hypothalamic pituitary axis dysregulation, circadian rhythm disturbance, serotonin neurotransmitter alterations, vagal afferent activation, and changes in muscle metabolism [23]. Other conditions commonly found in cancer patients may also contribute to fatigue, and include immobility, electrolyte abnormalities, hypothyroidism, anaemia, and depression.

Routine screening of cancer-related fatigue will improve its detection and treatment. A simple approach is to use a numeric rating scale (0–10). It is important to assess patient function, weakness, activity level, and potential causes.

Treatment of cancer-related fatigue includes both pharmacological and non-pharmacological measures. Specifically, exercise is the most evidence-based treatment for patients both during and after cancer treatment. Aerobic exercises may offer greater benefit than resistive exercise [31]. Although the optimal duration of exercise has yet to be determined, a general recommendation is 30 minutes of moderate exercise per day most days [32].

Medications such as methylphenidate and modafinil have mixed evidence for reducing cancer-related fatigue and may be effective for selected individuals [33, 34]. Dexamethasone could modulate cytokine activity and has been shown to improve fatigue in one randomized, controlled trial [35]. Ginseng may also offer some potential benefits and is being actively investigated [36]. Finally, it is important to correct any reversible causes such as hypothyroidism or severe anaemia.

Depression

Cancer patients experience many psychological stressors throughout their cancer journey. In the first week of cancer diagnosis, the rates of suicide and death from cardiovascular events increase significantly [37]. With each appointment, investigation, or treatment, patients have to face bad news, disappointments, and uncertainties. Furthermore, cancer patients experience significant changes in regard to their body image, sexuality, bodily function, ability to work, ability to engage in their hobbies, family relationships, self-esteem, self-identity, and spirituality. Understandably, psychiatric conditions occur in approximately half of cancer patients and may include adjustment disorder, depression, and anxiety [38, 39].

Psychological distress is associated with increased symptom expression and decreased quality of life [40]. The ESAS consists of two numeric rating scales on depression and anxiety. Other screening questions, including 'Are you depressed?', for anhedonia may also be used [41]. A proper diagnosis of depression is based on the DSM-IV criteria.

Patients with mild to moderate depression would benefit from counselling such as short-term psychotherapy, expressive supportive counselling, and cognitive behavioural therapy [42–44]. Supervised exercise programmes are also useful for depressive symptoms [45]. Patients with severe depressive symptoms would require antidepressants such as selective serotonin reuptake inhibitors (SSRIs) and tricyclic antidepressants. Psychostimulants also have a role in treating depression because of their rapid onset [46]. Referral to psychiatry may be warranted.

Communication and decision-making

Studies have found that most cancer patients are interested in learning more about their disease status, therapeutic options, and prognosis [47]. This information is essential for them to make many personal and financial decisions, as well as various healthcare decisions such as stopping chemotherapy or hospice enrolment. For instance, cancer patients who were aware that they had a poor prognosis were less likely to choose chemotherapy [48]. Surprisingly, a recent study showed that a majority of patients with metastatic lung and colorectal cancer were not aware that their disease is incurable, highlighting a communication gap [49].

Communication is a key determinant of patient satisfaction [50, 51]. Specific techniques such as prompting, non-verbal cues, empathic statements, use of silence and listening may improve the quality of communication [52]. However, studies have found that physicians consistently miss empathic opportunities [53, 54], and that few of them routinely discussed prognosis [55]. This may partly be related to oncologists' concern that prognostic disclosure could negatively affect hope; however, studies have found that patients were able to maintain their level of hope after prognosis discussions [56, 57]. The relative lack of training in communication for oncologists may also contribute to the communication gap [12].

End-of-life discussions address many topics relevant to patient care in the last six months of life, including expected survival, symptom profile, functional changes, goals of care, advanced care planning (i.e. surrogate decision maker(s), advance directives, and out-of-hospital do-not-resuscitate orders). These discussions are important to facilitate end-of-life decision-making and to ensure that patients receive care consistent with their preference. Furthermore, these discussions have been shown to be associated with increased hospice enrolment, higher quality of life, and fewer aggressive measures at the end of life [58, 59]. End-of-life discussions should occur longitudinally, tailored to patients' understanding and readiness. Various communication aids such as recording of the interview, information pamphlets and educational videos may also facilitate the complex decision-making process [60, 61]. The involvement of palliative care teams can facilitate goals of care discussions and advanced care planning [62].

Figure 32.2 illustrates an approach to initiate end-of-life discussions. We use the examples of comfort features and safety features in a car to describe the need to involve palliative care and advanced care planning for cancer patients, respectively. The presence of these would help the patient to better attain the goals of getting more cancer treatments and living longer, while having peace of mind.

Outcomes of supportive and palliative care programmes

Through the provision of comprehensive holistic care, supportive and palliative care programmes have a positive impact on many outcomes, including symptom burden, quality of life, quality of care, satisfaction, and healthcare costs [63]. However, because of heterogeneous study design, inception cohort, palliative care interventions and outcome measures among existing studies, the optimal model of palliative care delivery remains a topic of active investigation.

A meta-analysis found that specialist palliative care was associated with reduced symptom burden [64]. Several randomized controlled trials further demonstrated superiority of palliative care compared to routine oncologic care for depressive symptoms and quality of life among patients with advanced cancer [65, 66].

Through end-of-life discussions, advanced care planning and documentation of care goals [58], palliative care also has a significant impact on improving the quality while reducing the cost of end-of-life care, predominantly by decreasing aggressive interventions in the last days of life, such as emergency room visits, hospital admissions, intensive care unit stays, chemotherapy use, intubations, and resuscitations. The increased use of hospice care also contributes to improved end-of-life care [67, 68].

Systemic reviews on palliative care as an intervention have shown increased patient and caregiver satisfaction [64, 69]. Furthermore, palliative care involvement is associated with improved caregiver bereavement [58].

Integration between oncology and palliative care

With an ageing population, there is an increased number of patients with a cancer diagnosis. Furthermore, patients with advanced cancer are living longer with improved cancer treatment options. Oncologists are faced with an increased demand to coordinate both cancer treatments and support measures. Because of the lack of time, routine screening, interprofessional input, and specific training in supportive and palliative care, many symptoms and patient needs are under-detected, under-diagnosed, and under-treated [70]. To improve the quality of care for cancer patients, we urgently need to integrate palliative care with oncology.

Integration may take place at three levels: primary, secondary and tertiary. At the primary level, oncologists provide front-line supportive care for patients. To ensure a good standard of care, oncologists need to include basic symptom management, communication skills, prognosis-driven patient-centred decision-making, and advance care planning discussions as part of their core training. Furthermore, they need to know when to involve secondary palliative care.

Secondary palliative care is delivered by interprofessional palliative care teams. Patients and family members in severe physical or emotional distress, or those with high care needs, are best managed by an interdisciplinary team with multidimensional interventions. Rather than referral to multiple disciplines for each symptom (e.g., pain service for pain, fatigue clinic for fatigue, physiotherapy

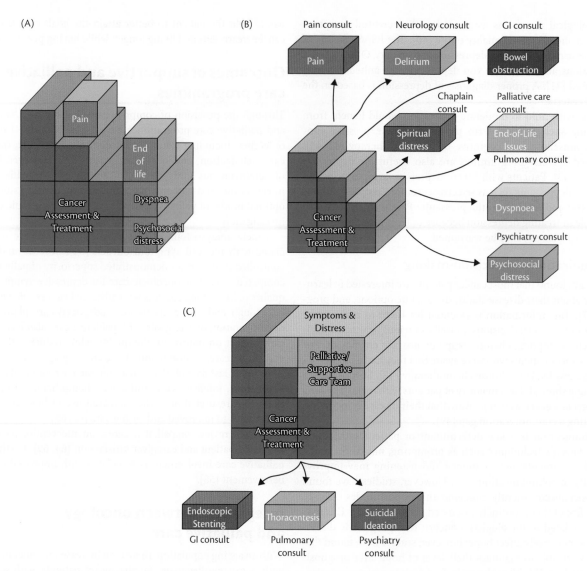

Fig. 32.3 The cancer care package [71]. (A) In the solo practice model, the oncologist is responsible for both cancer treatments and supportive care. The supportive care needs may not be addressed fully because of limited time, expertise, and resources. (B) In the congress model, each supportive care need is contracted out to various specialists. This can be extremely expensive and inefficient. (C) In the integrated care model, the oncologist collaborates with the palliative care team to delivery comprehensive cancer care.

for weakness), the palliative care team can address many of the patients' concerns comprehensively while minimizing overlap.

Tertiary palliative care involves research collaborations between palliative care specialists and oncologists further to advance our knowledge in symptom management, communication, and decision-making. It requires specialized centres with fully developed palliative care and oncology services.

Figure 32.3 illustrates how oncologists can provide supportive care in everyday practice [71]. In the solo approach, the oncologist is the only provider of both oncologic treatments and primary palliative care (Figure 32.3A). The comprehensiveness of cancer care is dependent on the oncologist's time, expertise, attitude, and resources, and may sometimes be limited. To compensate for this, the oncologist may choose to consult various specialists for each supportive care need under the congress approach (Figure 32.3B). Although patients may receive expert care, this approach is expensive and time consuming, and may result in

conflicting recommendations by different teams. The integrated care approach involves palliative care referral early in the disease trajectory (Figure 32.3C). The oncologist focuses on providing cancer management recommendations and may deliver as much primary palliative care as they are able, knowing that the palliative care team will address a majority of patients' supportive care needs. This model allows patients to access timely and expert supportive care through a coherent team while minimizing confusion when many other specialties are involved.

Summary

Patients with advanced cancer often experience significant physical and psychological symptoms. They also have tremendous communication and decision-making needs. Palliative care is an interdisciplinary team with expertise in addressing the care needs for patients with life-limiting illness and their families. Early involvement of palliative care is associated with significant improvement in symptom control, patient and caregiver satisfaction, quality of life and—potentially—quantity of life. Oncologists equipped with basic palliative care skills can deliver effective front-line supportive care. Patients in distress may also benefit from early referral to specialist palliative care teams.

Further reading

Back AL, Anderson WG, Bunch L, Marr LA, Wallace JA et al. Communication about cancer near the end of life. Cancer 2008; 113(7 Suppl.): 1897–1910.

Bruera E, Hui D. Integrating supportive and palliative care in the trajectory of cancer: establishing goals and models of care. Journal of Clinical Oncology 2010; 28(25): 4013–4017.

Hui D, De La Cruz M, Mori M, Parsons HA, Kwon JH et al. Concepts and definitions for 'supportive care,' 'best supportive care,' 'palliative care,' and 'hospice care' in the published literature, dictionaries, and textbooks. Support Care Cancer 2013; 21(3): 659–685.

Hui D, Elsayem A, De la Cruz M, Berger A, Zhukovsky DS et al. Availability and integration of palliative care at US cancer centers. Journal of the American Medical Association 2010; 303(11): 1054–1061.

Levy MH, Adolph MD, Back A, Block S, Codada SN et al. NCCN clinical practice guidelines in oncology. Palliative care. Available from: <http://www.nccn.org/professionals/physician_gls/f_guidelines.asp>, accessed on 20 January 2013.

Seow H, Barbera L, Sutradhar R, Howell D, Dudgeon D et al. Trajectory of performance status and symptom scores for patients with cancer during the last six months of life. Journal of Clinical Oncology 2011; 29(9): 1151–1158.

Smith TJ, Temin S, Alesi ER, Abernethy AP, Balboni TA et al. American Society of Clinical Oncology provisional clinical opinion: the integration of palliative care into standard oncology care. Journal of Clinical Oncology 2012; 30(8): 880–887.

Temel JS, Greer JA, Muzikansky A, Gallagher ER, Admane S et al. Early palliative care for patients with metastatic non-small-cell lung cancer. New England Journal of Medicine 2010; 363(8): 733–742.

Weeks JC, Catalano PJ, Cronin A, Finkelman MD, Mack JW et al. Patients' expectations about effects of chemotherapy for advanced cancer. New England Journal of Medicine 2012; 367(17): 1616–1625.

Wright AA, Zhang B, Ray A, Mack JW, Trice E et al. Associations between end-of-life discussions, patient mental health, medical care near death, and caregiver bereavement adjustment. Journal of the American Medical Association 2008; 300(14): 1665–1673.

References

1. Solano JP, Gomes B, Higginson IJ. A comparison of symptom prevalence in far advanced cancer, AIDS, heart disease, chronic obstructive pulmonary disease and renal disease. Journal of Pain and Symptom Management 2006; 31(1): 58–69.

2. Seow H, Barbera L, Sutradhar R, Howell D, Dudgeon D et al. Trajectory of performance status and symptom scores for patients with cancer during the last six months of life. Journal of Clinical Oncology 2011; 29(9): 1151–1158.

3. Portenoy RK, Thaler HT, Kornblith AB, Lepore JM, Friedlander-Klar H et al. Symptom prevalence, characteristics and distress in a cancer population. Quality of Life Research 1994; 3(3): 183–189.

4. Chang VT, Hwang SS, Feuerman M, Kasimis BS. Symptom and quality of life survey of medical oncology patients at a veterans affairs medical center: a role for symptom assessment. Cancer 2000; 88(5): 1175–1183.

5. WHO Definition of Palliative Care. Available from: http://www.who.int/cancer/palliative/definition/en/, accessed on 21 March 2013.

6. Hui D, De La Cruz M, Mori M, Parsons HA, Kwon JH et al. Concepts and definitions for 'supportive care,' 'best supportive care,' 'palliative

7. Fadul N, Elsayem A, Palmer JL, Del Fabbro E, Swint K et al. Supportive versus palliative care: what's in a name? A survey of medical oncologists and midlevel providers at a comprehensive cancer center. Cancer 2009; 115(9): 2013–2021.

8. Dalal S, Palla S, Hui D, Nguyen L, Chacko R et al. Association between a name change from palliative to supportive care and the timing of patient referrals at a comprehensive cancer center. Oncologist 2011; 16(1): 105–111.

9. Board IOMNCP. Improving Palliative Care for Cancer. Washington, DC: Institute of Medicine, 2001.

10. Levy MH, Adolph MD, Back A, Block S, Codada SN et al. NCCN clinical practice guidelines in oncology. Palliative care. Available from: <http://www.nccn.org/professionals/physician_gls/f_guidelines.asp>, accessed on 20 January 2013.

11. Fashoyin-Aje LA, Martinez KA, Dy SM. New patient-centered care standards from the commission on cancer: opportunities and challenges. Journal of Community and Supportive Oncology 2012; 10(3): 107–111.

12. Ferris FD, Bruera E, Cherny N, Cummings C, Currow D et al. Palliative cancer care a decade later: accomplishments, the need, next steps. Journal of Clinical Oncology 2009; 27(18): 3052–3058.

13. Smith TJ, Temin S, Alesi ER, Abernethy AP, Balboni TA et al. American Society of Clinical Oncology provisional clinical opinion: the integration of palliative care into standard oncology care. Journal of Clinical Oncology 2012; 30(8): 880–887.

14. Bruera E, Hui D. Conceptual models for integrating palliative care at cancer centers. Journal of Palliative Medicine 2012; 15(11): 1261–1269.

15. Hui D, Elsayem A, De la Cruz M, Berger A, Zhukovsky DS et al. Availability and integration of palliative care at US cancer centers. Journal of the American Medical Association 2010; 303(11): 1054–1061.

16. Hui D, Kim SH, Kwon JH, Tanco KC, Zhang T et al. Access to palliative care before death among patients treated at a comprehensive cancer center. Oncologist 2012; 17(12): 1574–1580.

17. Cheng WW, Willey J, Palmer JL, Zhang T, Bruera E. Interval between palliative care referral and death among patients treated at a comprehensive cancer center. Journal of Palliative Medicine 2005; 8(5): 1025–1032.

18. Hui D, Elsayem A, Palla S, De La Cruz M, Li Z et al. Discharge outcomes and survival of patients with advanced cancer admitted to an acute palliative care unit at a comprehensive cancer center. Journal of Palliative Medicine 2010; 13(1): 49–57.

19. Hui D, Elsayem A, Li Z, De La Cruz M, Palmer JL et al. Antineoplastic therapy use in patients with advanced cancer admitted to an acute palliative care unit at a comprehensive cancer center: a simultaneous care model. Cancer 2010; 116(8): 2036–2043.

20. Hui D, Parsons H, Nguyen L, Palla SL, Yennurajalingam S et al. Timing of palliative care referral and symptom burden in phase 1 cancer patients: a retrospective cohort study. Cancer 2010; 116(18): 4402–4409.

21. Teunissen SC, Wesker W, Kruitwagen C, de Haes HC, Voest EE et al. Symptom prevalence in patients with incurable cancer: a systematic review. Journal of Pain and Symptom Management 2007; 34(1): 94–104.

22. Bruera E, Kuehn N, Miller MJ, Selmser P, Macmillan K. The Edmonton Symptom Assessment System (ESAS): a simple method for the assessment of palliative care patients. Journal of Palliative Care 1991; 7(2): 6–9.

23. Ryan JL, Carroll JK, Ryan EP, Mustian KM, Fiscella K et al. Mechanisms of cancer-related fatigue. Oncologist 2007; 12(Suppl. 1): 22–34.

24. Hui D, Arthur J, Dalal S, Bruera E. Quality of the supportive and palliative oncology literature: a focused analysis on randomized controlled trials. Support Care Cancer 2012; 20(8): 1779–1785.

25. Hui D, Parsons HA, Damani S, Fulton S, Liu J et al. Quantity, design, and scope of the palliative oncology literature. Oncologist 2011; 16: 694–703.

26. Bruera E, MacMillan K, Hanson J, MacDonald RN. The Edmonton staging system for cancer pain: preliminary report. Pain 1989; 37(2): 203–209.

27. Fainsinger RL, Nekolaichuk CL. A 'TNM' classification system for cancer pain: the Edmonton Classification System for Cancer Pain (ECS-CP). Support Care Cancer 2008; 16(6): 547–555.

28. Fainsinger RL, Fairchild A, Nekolaichuk C, Lawlor P, Lowe S et al. Is pain intensity a predictor of the complexity of cancer pain management? Journal of Clinical Oncology 2009; 27(4): 585–590.

29. Bruera E, Sloan P, Mount B, Scott J, Suarez-Almazor M. A randomized, double-blind, double-dummy, crossover trial comparing the safety and efficacy of oral sustained-release hydromorphone with immediate-release hydromorphone in patients with cancer pain. Canadian Palliative Care Clinical Trials Group. Journal of Clinical Oncology 1996; 14(5): 1713–1717.

30. Hofman M, Ryan JL, Figueroa-Moseley CD, Jean-Pierre P, Morrow GR. Cancer-related fatigue: the scale of the problem. Oncologist 2007; 12(Suppl. 1): 4–10.

31. Cramp F, Byron-Daniel J. Exercise for the management of cancer-related fatigue in adults. Cochrane Database of Systemic Reviews 2012; 11: CD006145.

32. Berger AM, Abernethy AP, Atkinson A, Barsevick AM, Breitbart WS et al. Cancer-related fatigue. Journal of the National Comprehensive Cancer Network 2010; 8(8): 904–931.

33. Breitbart W, Alici Y. Psychostimulants for cancer-related fatigue. Journal of the National Comprehensive Cancer Network 2010; 8(8): 933–942.

34. Minton O, Richardson A, Sharpe M, Hotopf M, Stone P. Drug therapy for the management of cancer-related fatigue. Cochrane Database of Systemic Reviews 2010; 7: CD006704.

35. Yennurajalingam S, Frisbee-Hume S, Delgado-Guay MO, Bull J, Phan AT et al. Dexamethasone (DM) for cancer related fatigue: a double-blinded, randomized, placebo-controlled trial. 48th American Society of Clinical Oncology Annual Meeting, Chicago, USA: Journal of Clinical Oncology, 2012: Abstract #9002.

36. Barton DL, Soori GS, Bauer BA, Sloan JA, Johnson PA et al. Pilot study of Panax quinquefolius (American ginseng) to improve cancer-related fatigue: a randomized, double-blind, dose-finding evaluation: NCCTG trial N03CA. Support Care Cancer 2010; 18(2): 179–187.

37. Fang F, Fall K, Mittleman MA, Sparen P, Ye W et al. Suicide and cardiovascular death after a cancer diagnosis. New England Journal of Medicine 2012; 366(14): 1310–1318.

38. Derogatis LR, Morrow GR, Fetting J, Penman D, Piasetsky S et al. The prevalence of psychiatric disorders among cancer patients. Journal of the American Medical Association 1983; 249(6): 751–757.

39. Mitchell AJ, Chan M, Bhatti H, Halton M, Grassi L et al. Prevalence of depression, anxiety, and adjustment disorder in oncological, haematological, and palliative-care settings: a meta-analysis of 94 interview-based studies. Lancet Oncology 2011; 12(2): 160–174.

40. Delgado-Guay M, Parsons HA, Li Z, Palmer JL, Bruera E. Symptom distress in advanced cancer patients with anxiety and depression in the palliative care setting. Support Care Cancer 2009; 17(5): 573–579.

41. Chochinov HM, Wilson KG, Enns M, Lander S. 'Are you depressed?' Screening for depression in the terminally ill. American Journal of Psychiatry 1997; 154(5): 674–676.

42. Akechi T, Okuyama T, Onishi J, Morita T, Furukawa TA. Psychotherapy for depression among incurable cancer patients. Cochrane Database of Systemic Reviews 2008; (2)(2): CD005537.

43. Roth AJ, Massie MJ. Anxiety and its management in advanced cancer. Current Opinion in Supportive and Palliative Care 2007; 1(1): 50–56.

44. Greer JA, Traeger L, Bemis H, Solis J, Hendriksen ES et al. A pilot randomized controlled trial of brief cognitive-behavioral therapy for anxiety in patients with terminal cancer. Oncologist 2012; 17(10): 1337–1345.

45. Craft LL, Vaniterson EH, Helenowski IB, Rademaker AW, Courneya KS. Exercise effects on depressive symptoms in cancer survivors: a systematic review and meta-analysis. Cancer Epidemiology, Biomarkers & Prevention 2012; 21(1): 3–19.

46. Rayner L, Price A, Evans A, Valsraj K, Higginson IJ et al. Antidepressants for depression in physically ill people. Cochrane Database of Systemic Reviews 2010(3): CD007503.

47. Hagerty RG, Butow PN, Ellis PA, Lobb EA, Pendlebury S et al. Cancer patient preferences for communication of prognosis in the metastatic setting. Journal of Clinical Oncology 2004; 22(9): 1721–1730.

48. Weeks JC, Cook EF, O'Day SJ, Peterson LM, Wenger N et al. Relationship between cancer patients' predictions of prognosis and their treatment preferences. Journal of the American Medical Association 1998; 279(21): 1709–1714.

49. Weeks JC, Catalano PJ, Cronin A, Finkelman MD, Mack JW et al. Patients' expectations about effects of chemotherapy for advanced cancer. New England Journal of Medicine 2012; 367(17): 1616–1625.

50. Bredart A, Bouleuc C, Dolbeault S. Doctor–patient communication and satisfaction with care in oncology. Current Opinion in Oncology 2005; 17(4): 351–354.

51. Ong LM, Visser MR, Lammes FB, de Haes JC. Doctor–patient communication and cancer patients' quality of life and satisfaction. Patient Education and Counseling 2000; 41(2): 145–156.

52. Back AL, Anderson WG, Bunch L, Marr LA, Wallace JA et al. Communication about cancer near the end of life. Cancer 2008; 113(7 Suppl.): 1897–1910.

53. Pollak KI, Arnold RM, Jeffreys AS, Alexander SC, Olsen MK et al. Oncologist communication about emotion during visits with patients with advanced cancer. Journal of Clinical Oncology 2007; 25(36): 5748–5752.

54. Fine E, Reid MC, Shengelia R, Adelman RD. Directly observed patient-physician discussions in palliative and end-of-life care: a systematic review of the literature. Journal of Palliative Medicine 2010; 13(5): 595–603.

55. Daugherty CK, Hlubocky FJ. What are terminally ill cancer patients told about their expected deaths? A study of cancer physicians' self-reports of prognosis disclosure. Journal of Clinical Oncology 2008; 26(36): 5988–5993.

56. Smith TJ, Dow LA, Virago E, Khatcheressian J, Lyckholm LJ et al. Giving honest information to patients with advanced cancer maintains hope. Oncology (Williston Park) 2010; 24(6): 521–525.

57. Mack JW, Smith TJ. Reasons why physicians do not have discussions about poor prognosis, why it matters, and what can be improved. Journal of Clinical Oncology 2012; 30(22): 2715–2717.

58. Wright AA, Zhang B, Ray A, Mack JW, Trice E et al. Associations between end-of-life discussions, patient mental health, medical care near death, and caregiver bereavement adjustment. Journal of the American Medical Association 2008; 300(14): 1665–1673.

59. Mack JW, Weeks JC, Wright AA, Block SD, Prigerson HG. End-of-life discussions, goal attainment, and distress at the end of life: predictors and outcomes of receipt of care consistent with preferences. Journal of Clinical Oncology 2010; 28(7): 1203–1208.

60. El-Jawahri A, Podgurski LM, Eichler AF, Plotkin SR, Temel JS et al. Use of video to facilitate end-of-life discussions with patients with cancer: a randomized controlled trial. Journal of Clinical Oncology 2010; 28(2): 305–310.

61. Leighl NB, Butow PN, Tattersall MH. Treatment decision aids in advanced cancer: when the goal is not cure and the answer is not clear. Journal of Clinical Oncology 2004; 22(9): 1759–1762.

62. Peppercorn JM, Smith TJ, Helft PR, Debono DJ, Berry SR et al. American society of clinical oncology statement: toward individualized care for patients with advanced cancer. Journal of Clinical Oncology 2011; 29(6): 755–760.

63. Rocque GB, Cleary JF. Palliative care reduces morbidity and mortality in cancer. Nature Reviews Clinical Oncology 2013; 10(2): 80–89.

64. Higginson IJ, Finlay IG, Goodwin DM, Hood K, Edwards AG et al. Is there evidence that palliative care teams alter end-of-life experiences of patients and their caregivers? Journal of Pain and Symptom Management 2003; 25(2): 150–168.

65. Temel JS, Greer JA, Muzikansky A, Gallagher ER, Admane S et al. Early palliative care for patients with metastatic non-small-cell lung cancer. New England Journal of Medicine 2010; 363(8): 733–742.

66. Bakitas M, Lyons KD, Hegel MT, Balan S, Barnett KN et al. The project ENABLE II randomized controlled trial to improve palliative care for rural patients with advanced cancer: baseline findings, methodological challenges, and solutions. Palliat Support Care 2009; 7(1): 75–86.

67. Greer JA, Pirl WF, Jackson VA, Muzikansky A, Lennes IT et al. Effect of early palliative care on chemotherapy use and end-of-life care in patients with metastatic non-small-cell lung cancer. Journal of Clinical Oncology 2012; 30(4): 394–400.

68. Dudgeon DJ, Knott C, Eichholz M, Gerlach JL, Chapman C et al. Palliative Care Integration Project (PCIP) quality improvement strategy evaluation. Journal of Pain and Symptom Management 2008; 35(6): 573–582.

69. Zimmermann C, Riechelmann R, Krzyzanowska M, Rodin G, Tannock I. Effectiveness of specialized palliative care: a systematic review. Journal of the American Medical Association 2008; 299(14): 1698–1709.

70. Fisch MJ, Lee JW, Weiss M, Wagner LI, Chang VT et al. Prospective, observational study of pain and analgesic prescribing in medical oncology outpatients with breast, colorectal, lung, or prostate cancer. Journal of Clinical Oncology 2012; 30(16): 1980–1988.

71. Bruera E, Hui D. Integrating supportive and palliative care in the trajectory of cancer: establishing goals and models of care. Journal of Clinical Oncology 2010; 28(25): 4013–4017.

CHAPTER 33

Quality of life

Neil K. Aaronson and Peter M. Fayers

Introduction to quality of life

In the medical context, the question: 'How are you?' represents more than a simple social ritual. It is usually the first question that is asked by the doctor in the consulting room. It represents an informal invitation to the patient to talk about his or her health. In clinical research we cannot afford to rely on such informal means of collecting information about the patients' health and well-being. In evaluating the effect of a treatment, we need to define what we consider to be the most important outcomes of interest. In clinical oncology, these have traditionally been objective outcomes, including tumour response, disease-free survival, and overall survival. In other words, the question 'How are you?' has usually been posed in purely biologic terms.

There has been a growing recognition that these traditional markers of therapeutic success are often insufficient for evaluating the effect of cancer treatment, and that it may be appropriate—and even essential—to broaden our focus to include formal and systematic assessments of the extent to which cancer and its treatment impact on the quality of life (QoL) of the patient.

What lies behind this shift of focus? In part, it reflects general trends in the distribution of disease in the modern, industrialized world from acute towards chronic health conditions. In contrast to infectious diseases, where cure is often a realistic goal of treatment, chronic diseases typically require a moderation of both patients' and physicians' expectations. While slowing of the disease process may be possible, the patient often must learn to adjust to long-term functional limitations. The primary goals of treatment become symptom relief and minimizing the impact of the disease on the patient's physical and psychosocial functioning.

Although treatment is often directed initially towards cure, it may be important to weigh any gains in survival time against the morbidity caused by the treatment. Many treatments aimed at tumour control are quite aggressive, with a range of side effects. The introduction of formal QoL evaluations in such situations helps us weigh treatment costs and benefits. A substantial percentage of patients will eventually receive treatment with palliative intent. In this context, assessing QoL as part of the evaluation of the effectiveness of palliation is perhaps even more important.

Who should assess the QoL of patients with cancer?

In most clinical studies in oncology, the clinical investigator is asked to assess the patient's performance status, using a rating scale that summarizes the patient's symptom levels and ability to perform normal, everyday activities at home and at work. However, performance status measures such as the Karnofsky, ECOG, and WHO scales assess only a few issues related to physical health and activities of daily living, and ignore psychosocial health. Methodologically, inconsistencies have been noted in performance status ratings provided by different physicians of the same patient, and in ratings of physicians versus patients [1, 2]. Physician-based performance status ratings cannot substitute for more direct measures of patients' QoL. It is today widely accepted that the patient must be the *primary* source of information about his or her QoL.

How do we define QoL?

Although most of us have some intuitive sense of what QoL means, a precise definition remains elusive. QoL is an omnibus term summarizing a broad range of issues. As Alvan Feinstein, one of the early advocates of a patient-centred approach to clinical medicine, once put it: 'the idea has become a kind of umbrella under which are placed many different indexes dealing with whatever the user wants to focus on' [3].

One way of avoiding this problem of definition is to view QoL as a Gestalt that can best be measured at a global level. Some years ago, Ian Gough and his colleagues suggested that one need only ask a single question to evaluate the QoL of patients with cancer: 'How would you rate your QoL today?' [4]. They supported their position by demonstrating a relatively strong correlation between answers to this single question and scores derived from a more extensive battery of questionnaires. H.L. Mencken, the American author and pundit, once said: 'There is an easy solution to every human problem—neat, plausible, and wrong' [5]. What, then, is wrong with this approach?

In choosing an appropriate therapy for an individual patient, or in developing treatment guidelines for a specific diagnostic group, physicians require very specific information on which to base their decisions. For example, it is expected that results of a blood test will be reported in appropriate detail (including calcium, iron, pH, and cholesterol levels), and not as a single value representing a summary of the findings. The same holds true for evaluation of the QoL of patients. How are we to interpret a patient reporting a low overall QoL? Is the patient in pain? Is he so tired that he can no longer carry out his normal daily activities? Is he very anxious or depressed? Or, more likely, is it a combination of such factors? For this reason, QoL assessment should be approached from a multidimensional perspective. Such an approach allows us to disentangle the positive and negative effects of a given treatment.

This still leaves the question of what should be measured. An important limiting factor is that the focus be on 'health-related QoL' or 'health status assessment'. The 1948 constitution of the

World Health Organization defined health as: 'a state of complete physical, mental and social well-being, and not merely the absence of disease and infirmity' [6]. This definition offers a holistic alternative to the classic medical model in which disease and illness are defined in strictly biologic terms.

Also in 1948, Karnofsky and Burchenal [7] identified four sets of criteria necessary to establish the therapeutic value of anti-cancer treatment. The first of these was described as: 'The patient's subjective improvement … in his mood and attitude, his general feelings of well-being, his activity, appetite, and the alleviation of distressing symptoms such as pain, weakness and dyspnoea.'

Taken together, the WHO definition of health and Karnofsky and Burchenal's subjective improvement criteria provided the elements that today, some 50 years later, form the core of QoL measurement in oncology. These include: (1) common disease-related and treatment-related symptoms and (2) the patient's level of functioning, defined in physical, psychological, and social terms [8]. Beyond this core set of domains, there are many additional issues that may be of importance when studying specific groups of patients. Body image may be of particular relevance in studies of patients with breast cancer, head and neck cancer, and other forms of cancer where treatment often involves mutilating surgery. Sexual functioning may be at issue in gynaecological and genitourinary tract cancers. Cognitive functioning may be of particular concern in studies of childhood cancer or of adults with brain tumours. Ultimately, the QoL issues that should be assessed in a given study depend on the patient population, the nature of the applied treatments, and the specific research questions (e.g., whether we are interested in short-term or long-term effects).

How should QoL be measured?

QoL instruments used in clinical oncology can be placed along a continuum reflecting their intended spectrum of application: (1) generic instruments for both the general population and for a wide range of patient populations; (2) disease-specific measures for use with cancer patients in general; and (3) diagnosis-specific measures (e.g., for use with patients with breast cancer, prostate cancer, etc.).

Generic QoL instruments

Generic QoL measures allow comparison of results across studies of different patient populations and facilitate comparison of patient groups with normative data from the general population. This is particularly relevant for issues of health policy and resource allocation. While there are a number of well-known, generic QoL measures, including the Sickness Impact Profile (SIP) [9], the Nottingham Health Profile [10], and the World Health Organization QoL Questionnaire [11], the Medical Outcomes Study Short-Form Health Survey (SF-36) [12] dominates the health outcomes field.

The SF-36 has 36 items forming eight subscales assessing: physical functioning, role limitations due to physical health problems, pain, general health perceptions, vitality, social functioning, role limitations due to emotional problems, and general mental health. Two higher-order summary scores for physical and mental health can also be calculated. Extensive background information on the SF-36, as well as standard scoring algorithms and interpretation guides, are available elsewhere [13].

Cancer-specific QoL instruments

Generic instruments may be limited in their ability to detect small, yet clinically meaningful group differences in QoL, or in detecting changes in QoL over time. Sensitive, cancer-targeted QoL questionnaires include the Functional Living Index—Cancer (FLIC), the Edmonton Symptom Assessment Scale (ESAS), the Rotterdam Symptom Checklist (RSCL), the Cancer Rehabilitation Evaluation System (CARES), the European Organization for Research and Treatment of Cancer Core QoL Questionnaire (EORTC QLQ-C30), the Functional Assessment of Cancer Therapy (FACT-G). Of these, the QLQ-C30, the FACT-G and the ESAS are perhaps the most widely used, and are described in more detail below.

The European Organization for Research and Treatment of Cancer QLQ-C30

The QLQ-C30 [14] was developed by the EORTC QoL Study Group specifically for use in international clinical trials in oncology. Originally published in 1993, the current version (version 3.0; see Figure 33.1) contains 30 items organized into five functional scales (physical, role, emotional, cognitive, and social), three symptom scales (fatigue, nausea and vomiting, and pain), and an overall QoL scale. Additional single items assess other common symptoms of cancer and its treatment (e.g., dyspnoea, loss of appetite, constipation and diarrhoea, etc.). The questionnaire employs a one-week time-frame, and four-point categorical response choices. It has been translated into more than 80 languages and has been tested extensively in multinational research settings. More recently, an abbreviated version of the QLQ-C30, the QLQ-C15-PAL has been generated for use in palliative care settings [15].

The Functional Assessment of Cancer Therapy—General

The FACT-G [16], originally published by Cella and colleagues in 1993, is also designed primarily for use in clinical trials. The current version of the questionnaire (version 4; see Figure 33.2) contains 27 items grouped into four primary domains: physical well-being, social/family well-being, emotional well-being, and functional well-being. A total, summary score can also be generated. The questionnaire employs a one-week time-frame, and five-point categorical response choices. It has been translated into a wide range of languages, which facilitate its use in oncology multinational clinical trials and observational studies in many regions of the world.

The Edmonton Symptom Assessment Scale (ESAS)—palliative care

The ESAS [17] is a standard one-page screening tool of symptoms in palliative care. It contains ten items, each assessed on a numerical rating scale from 0 to 10, and takes about two to five minutes to complete. It is widely used for individual patient management, in which case the scores for each symptom are used, as well as for clinical trials and other research, where the focus may be either on individual symptoms or the total score. Richardson and Jones provide an extensive review of the reliability and validity of the ESAS [18].

Condition-specific and treatment-specific instruments

Both the EORTC and the FACT measurement systems employ a 'modular approach' to QoL assessment whereby supplemental questionnaire modules are developed to assess condition-specific or treatment-specific issues not (sufficiently) addressed by their core instruments. Information on currently available modules and on modules under development can be found via the EORTC and the FACT groups. Both groups provide news of their activities via internet sites [19, 20].

EORTC QLQ-C30 (version 3)

We are interested in some things about you and your health. Please answer all of the questions yourself by circling the number that best applies to you. There are no "right" or "wrong" answers. The information that you provide will remain strictly confidential.

Please fill in your initials: ☐☐☐☐
Your birthdate (Day, Month, Year): ☐☐ ☐☐ ☐☐☐☐
Today's date (Day, Month, Year): 31 ☐☐ ☐☐ ☐☐☐☐

		Not at All	A Little	Quite a Bit	Very Much
1.	Do you have any trouble doing strenuous activities, like carrying a heavy shopping bag or a suitcase?	1	2	3	4
2.	Do you have any trouble taking a <u>long</u> walk?	1	2	3	4
3.	Do you have any trouble taking a <u>short</u> walk outside of the house?	1	2	3	4
4.	Do you need to stay in bed or a chair during the day?	1	2	3	4
5.	Do you need help with eating, dressing, washing yourself or using the toilet?	1	2	3	4

During the past week:		Not at All	A Little	Quite a Bit	Very Much
6.	Were you limited in doing either your work or other daily activities?	1	2	3	4
7.	Were you limited in pursuing your hobbies or other leisure time activities?	1	2	3	4
8.	Were you short of breath?	1	2	3	4
9.	Have you had pain?	1	2	3	4
10.	Did you need to rest?	1	2	3	4
11.	Have you had trouble sleeping?	1	2	3	4
12.	Have you felt weak?	1	2	3	4
13.	Have you lacked appetite?	1	2	3	4
14.	Have you felt nauseated?	1	2	3	4
15.	Have you vomited?	1	2	3	4
16.	Have you been constipated?	1	2	3	4

<u>Please go on to the next page</u>

Fig. 33.1 EORTC QLQ-C30 version 3.0.
Reproduced by permission of the EORTC Study Group on Quality of Life.

During the past week:

	Not at All	A Little	Quite a Bit	Very Much
17. Have you had diarrhea?	1	2	3	4
18. Were you tired?	1	2	3	4
19. Did pain interfere with your daily activities?	1	2	3	4
20. Have you had difficulty in concentrating on things, like reading a newspaper or watching television?	1	2	3	4
21. Did you feel tense?	1	2	3	4
22. Did you worry?	1	2	3	4
23. Did you feel irritable?	1	2	3	4
24. Did you feel depressed?	1	2	3	4
25. Have you had difficulty remembering things?	1	2	3	4
26. Has your physical condition or medical treatment interfered with your <u>family</u> life?	1	2	3	4
27. Has your physical condition or medical treatment interfered with your <u>social</u> activities?	1	2	3	4
28. Has your physical condition or medical treatment caused you financial difficulties?	1	2	3	4

For the following questions please circle the number between 1 and 7 that best applies to you

29. How would you rate your overall <u>health</u> during the past week?

1	2	3	4	5	6	7

Very poor   Excellent

30. How would you rate your overall <u>quality of life</u> during the past week?

1	2	3	4	5	6	7

Very poor   Excellent

Fig. 33.1 EORTC QLQ-C30 version 3.0. (continued)
Reproduced by permission of the EORTC Study Group on Quality of Life

Other groups are also developing condition-specific questionnaires. For example, in the area of prostate cancer, at least four instruments, in addition to those developed by the EORTC and FACT groups, have been published [21–24].

Computer-adaptive testing (CAT)

Self-administered questionnaires have traditionally been paper-based. Apart from groups of items that are skipped over as not applicable, all patients complete the same questionnaire items. Computer-adaptive testing, in contrast, enables questions to be tailored to the individual patient, offering two advantages: questionnaires can be shorter and the scale scores can be estimated more precisely for any given test length. A CAT involves the use of a large item bank of calibrated questions and a computer program that selects the most appropriate and informative items for each patient. The CAT system mimics a clinical interview in that the choice of successive questions depends on the patient's response to previous questions. Despite the apparent simplicity of a CAT, the mathematical algorithms underpinning the process can be quite complex and involve item response theory (IRT) to ensure that the results for all patients are on a common metric that enables comparisons between patients.

CAT versions are being developed for standard instruments such as the EORTC QLQ-C30 [25], while the Patient-Reported Outcome Measurement Information System (PROMIS) is an initiative funded by the US National Institutes of Health to create 'a national resource for precise and efficient measurement of patient-reported symptoms, functioning, and health-related quality of life, appropriate for patients with a wide variety of chronic disease conditions' [26].

Application of QoL assessments in clinical oncology research and practice

The substantial investment of time, energy, and resources in developing reliable, valid, and practical tools for assessing the QoL of cancer patients can only be justified if these measures are put to good use. Have QoL studies advanced our understanding of the burden of disease and the impact of treatment on patients' lives? Have they contributed to evaluating the effectiveness of anti-cancer treatments? Can they be used in the day-to-day care of our patients? How can they contribute to establishing clinical practice guidelines?

Observational QoL studies

Langendijk and colleagues assessed the effect of radiotherapy-induced toxicity on the quality of life of patients with head and neck cancer [28]. Although xerostomia (dry mouth) was the most prevalent side effect of radiotherapy, the QoL of patients was most affected by swallowing problems. These results suggested that future radiotherapy in this patient population should employ a lower radiation dose to minimize the effects on the salivary glands, and should avoid the anatomical structures involved in swallowing.

In observational studies of mid- to long-term cancer survivors, comparisons are often made between the cancer survivors and age- and gender-matched peers from the general population. For example, Rossen et al. [28] conducted a long-term follow-up of 400 Danish testicular cancer survivors as compared to men from

FACT-G (Version 4)

Below is a list of statements that other people with your illness have said are important. **Please circle or mark one number per line to indicate your response as it applies to the <u>past 7 days</u>.**

	PHYSICAL WELL-BEING	Not at all	A little bit	Some-what	Quite a bit	Very much
GP1	I have a lack of energy	0	1	2	3	4
GP2	I have nausea	0	1	2	3	4
GP3	Because of my physical condition, I have trouble meeting the needs of my family	0	1	2	3	4
GP4	I have pain	0	1	2	3	4
GP5	I am bothered by side effects of treatment	0	1	2	3	4
GP6	I feel ill	0	1	2	3	4
GP7	I am forced to spend time in bed	0	1	2	3	4

	SOCIAL/FAMILY WELL-BEING	Not at all	A little bit	Some-what	Quite a bit	Very much
GS1	I feel close to my friends	0	1	2	3	4
GS2	I get emotional support from my family	0	1	2	3	4
GS3	I get support from my friends	0	1	2	3	4
GS4	My family has accepted my illness	0	1	2	3	4
GS5	I am satisfied with family communication about my illness	0	1	2	3	4
GS6	I feel close to my partner (or the person who is my main support)	0	1	2	3	4
Q1	*Regardless of your current level of sexual activity, please answer the following question. If you prefer not to answer it, please mark this box* ☐ *and go to the next section.*					
GS7	I am satisfied with my sex life	0	1	2	3	4

Fig. 33.2 FACT-G (version 4).

Reproduced with permission from FACIT.org.

FACT-G (Version 4)

Please circle or mark one number per line to indicate your response as it applies to the <u>past 7 days</u>.

EMOTIONAL WELL-BEING

		Not at all	A little bit	Some-what	Quite a bit	Very much
GE1	I feel sad	0	1	2	3	4
GE2	I am satisfied with how I am coping with my illness	0	1	2	3	4
GE3	I am losing hope in the fight against my illness	0	1	2	3	4
GE4	I feel nervous	0	1	2	3	4
GE5	I worry about dying	0	1	2	3	4
GE6	I worry that my condition will get worse	0	1	2	3	4

FUNCTIONAL WELL-BEING

		Not at all	A little bit	Some-what	Quite a bit	Very much
GF1	I am able to work (include work at home)	0	1	2	3	4
GF2	My work (include work at home) is fulfilling	0	1	2	3	4
GF3	I am able to enjoy life	0	1	2	3	4
GF4	I have accepted my illness	0	1	2	3	4
GF5	I am sleeping well	0	1	2	3	4
GF6	I am enjoying the things I usually do for fun	0	1	2	3	4
GF7	I am content with the quality of my life right now	0	1	2	3	4

Fig. 33.2 FACT-G (version 4) (continued)
Reproduced with permission from FACIT.org.

the general population, and found their QOL was not significantly different. Although patients treated with chemotherapy reported higher levels of peripheral neuropathy, ototoxicity, and Raynaud-like phenomena, treatment strategies were generally unrelated to QoL.

For many patient groups, however, we still know very little about the short- and long-term effects of the disease and its treatment. Only by carrying out well-designed, descriptive studies can we identify areas where support and rehabilitation services are most needed.

It is important to look beyond average effects: the 'average' patient is a statistical convenience, not someone seen in the doctor's office. Descriptive studies should aim to identify subgroups of patients who are particularly 'at risk' for psychosocial morbidity. Conversely, there may be much to learn from those patients who do well.

Evaluative QoL studies: phase III clinical trials

An important application of QoL measures is in comparing the effects of two or more cancer treatments. QoL measures have sometimes been useful in confirming clinical impressions or expectations

about the psychosocial benefits of one treatment over another. For example, many trials comparing breast-conserving therapy with mastectomy in the treatment of early-stage breast cancer confirm that saving a woman's breast helps her maintain a sense of femininity and preserves a positive body image [29].

The useful half-life of QoL studies would probably be very short if they merely confirmed clinical expectations. That the results of such studies sometimes challenge widely held beliefs explains, in part, the growing enthusiasm for their use. Drawing again on the example of operable breast cancer, it has often been suggested that breast-conserving therapy, while holding certain psychosocial advantages over mastectomy, might increase a woman's fear that the cancer will recur. Yet empirical investigations have not supported this hypothesis [30].

Assessment of QoL is essential in palliative care. In a study of metastatic non-small-cell lung cancer, patients were randomly assigned to receive either early palliative care integrated with standard oncologic care or standard oncologic care alone [31]. The primary outcome was the change in the QoL at 12 weeks. Early palliative care led to significant improvements in both QoL and mood. Compared with patients receiving standard care, patients receiving early palliative care had less aggressive care at the end of life but, interestingly, longer survival.

A final example is a clinical trial that compared medroxyprogesterone acetate (MPA) to a placebo in increasing appetite and promoting weight gain in patients with advanced-stage cancer [32]. MPA had a significant, albeit modest, beneficial effect on both endpoints. However, these gains in appetite and weight did not translate into improvement in QoL. Rather, a decline in the mean QoL scores of *both* the MPA and placebo groups was observed over the 12-week study period. Direct indicators of treatment success do not necessarily translate into improved functioning or sense of well-being.

Interestingly, patients' ratings of their functioning, symptoms and overall well-being obtained *prior* to the start of treatment are significant, independent predictors of survival. Gotay and colleagues [33] reviewed 39 cancer clinical trials that included data relevant to assessing the prognostic value of baseline (i.e. pre-treatment) patient-reported outcomes (primarily QoL measures). QoL was a significant predictor of survival, after adjusting for other known prognostic indicators such as performance status, stage of disease, weight loss, and serum markers. Similarly, Quinten and colleagues reviewed 14 EORTC clinical trials with more than 2200 patients. Patient-reported symptoms added significantly to the prediction of survival in multivariate models that also employed clinicians' ratings of these symptoms [34]. These results should not be over-interpreted; they do not indicate that the emotional state or personality of patients can affect the course of the disease. They do suggest that our current health status is one of the best predictors of future morbidity and mortality, and that patients can be quite accurate in rating their current health [35, 36].

Incorporating QoL assessment in clinical trials

QoL assessment is only relevant to some types of clinical trial. It is rarely necessary in phase I or phase II trials, where the primary aim is to determine tumour response and toxicity. The main role for QoL instruments lies in phase III trials. There are four settings in which QoL assessment is particularly relevant:

1. Palliative studies in which improved QoL may be the principal aim of the intervention and thus QoL assessment may provide the principal endpoint.

2. Equivalence trials, in which little difference is anticipated in terms of improved survival or cure, but where there may be differences in side effects, symptomatology, or morbidity.

3. Trials in which a difference in survival or cure rate might be anticipated, but where the improvement may be small and accompanied by major toxicity or side effects.

4. Studies involving health economic cost-effectiveness.

Various guidance documents have been published on incorporating QoL assessments into clinical trials, including those of the US Food and Drug Administration [37], the European Medicines Agency [38], and the Center for Medical Technology Policy [39]. Additionally, an extension of the CONSORT (Consolidated Standards of Reporting Trials) has recently been published to improve the reporting of QoL results from randomized controlled trials [40].

Interpretation and clinical significance of QoL results

One topic that deserves particular attention is the interpretation and clinical significance of QoL data generated in clinical trials. Typical conclusions from a clinical trial might be that one treatment resulted in 'statistically significant' reduction (or increase) in a QoL scale. But what does such a statement mean? Statistical significance tests only examine whether the differences observed in a clinical trial might be due to chance fluctuations, and tell us nothing about the clinical importance of the results. A large-sized trial will be able to detect trivially small differences in QoL, and results may be (statistically) highly significant even though the differences could be regarded as clinically unimportant. How, therefore, can we decide what is clinically important?

Percentage of 'cases'

Perhaps the simplest method is to report the percentage (or proportion) of patients with particular QoL scores. Many people find it relatively easy to obtain a feeling for percentages (e.g., '30% of patients reported quite a bit of problem with tiredness'), but it is more difficult to use this approach for multi-item scales such as those that summate several items and produce a scale score between, say, 0 and 100.

Reference against normative data from healthy subjects

For many of the more widely used instruments, *normative* data are available, showing the results that may be expected in a random sample of the general population. For example, Ware et al. have provided norm-based interpretations of SF-36 scores based on percentile rankings obtained from large, representative samples from the US general population [13]. Similarly, Hjermstad et al. [41] report normative data for the QLQ-C30 in a randomly selected sample of 3000 people from the Norwegian population. These normative data may serve as a guideline when interpreting QoL in groups of cancer patients.

Contrast with reference data from patient groups

Reference values are often available for groups of patients with different cancer diagnoses. For example, the EORTC Quality of Life Study Group has produced a manual of reference data [42], based upon pooled data from many clinical trials and observational studies. The manual tabulates age- and gender-specific values for the QLQ-C30 and its scales. Investigators can contrast their results with those found in comparable groups of patients.

Measurement of minimal changes that are important to patients

Osoba and colleagues have suggested guidelines for interpreting the 'subjective significance' of change scores on the EORTC QLQ-C30, based on a comparison with direct estimates of change provided by patients retrospectively using so-called 'health transition' or 'global rating of change' questions [43]. In their study, patients were asked to complete the QLQ-C30 on two occasions. At the time of the second administration, they were also asked about *perceived changes* in physical, emotional, and social functioning and in global QL, using a 7-point scale ranging from 'much worse' to 'no change' to 'much better'. Patients who reported 'a little' change for better or worse on a particular SSQ scale had corresponding pre-test/post-test QLQ-C30 changes of about 5 to 10 points, those reporting 'moderate' change on the SSQ had QLQ-C30 changes of about 10 to 20 points, and those reporting 'very much' change on the SSQ had QLQ-C30 changes of greater than 20 points. Other studies, [44, 45] have employed related strategies for defining a palliative response or 'clinical response benefit' based, in part, on patients' self-reported changes in symptom burden.

Anchor-based interpretations

Anchor-based interpretations compare the changes seen in QoL scores ('anchored') against other clinical changes. In a study by King and colleagues [46], 'known groups' of patients who were expected to differ in terms of QoL scores were compared. For example, patients with limited disease were compared to those with advanced disease. For most scales a difference of 5 or less was a 'small' difference, but the definition of a 'large' difference varied for each scale: for example, large differences were 16 for global QoL, 27 for physical functioning, and 7 for emotional functioning. This approach has subsequently been extended for many cancer sites and for both the EORTC QLQ-C30 [47, 48] and the FACT-G [49].

Distribution-based interpretations

Distribution-based interpretations are based on the statistical distributions of results. The most commonly used statistic is the *effect size* (ES), which relates the observed change to the baseline standard deviation [50] or the *standardized response mean* (SRM), which uses the standard deviation of the change. Norman et al. [51] reviewed 38 studies that reported some 62 effect sizes and confirmed that in most cases the thresholds deemed to be clinically significant corresponded to an ES of approximately 0.5 (half a standard-deviation).

Conclusion: future directions

The many years of effort devoted to developing the science of QoL assessment are now bearing fruit. What are the important questions for future research? In the area of measurement, there are a number of methodological challenges. First, efforts should be continued to develop supplemental questionnaires for use with specific groups of patients. More specific instruments are best able to detect treatment effects in clinical studies. Second, we need to develop a much better understanding of the clinical significance of QoL scores. We can accelerate our learning curve by generating normative or reference data for groups of patients with different diagnoses, stages of disease, and treatment experiences. Third, we need to evaluate the performance of questionnaires in diverse cultural settings, including ethnic and cultural minorities within countries. Fourth, research is needed to develop QoL instruments with very high degrees of precision for use at the level of the individual patient in daily clinical

practice. The current efforts of the PROMIS group in the US and the EORTC Quality of Life Group in Europe to develop sophisticated CAT measurement systems are anticipated to usher in a new era of QoL assessment, with measures that are flexible and powerful when used in both clinical research and clinical practice settings.

In the realm of clinical trials, funding agencies and review committees should require that clinical investigators provide an explicit, well-argued rationale for *including* or *not including* QoL outcomes in their trial protocols. When QoL assessment is appropriate, sufficient funding should be made available to facilitate the additional data collection. The most expensive study is that which fails to meet its objectives because of an inadequate research infrastructure. Effective ways are required for communicating the results of QoL studies, both for presenting results so that doctors can interpret and use them in counselling their patients, and so that patients can draw on such information to make more informed choices.

Finally, allocation of healthcare resources is increasingly based on considerations of QoL and survival data, yielding quality-adjusted life years (QALYs). Such an approach arguably oversimplifies a very heterogeneous set of considerations. The process of deciding which medical treatments society is willing to pay for, and which it is not, is rather complex. Those working in the QoL field can perhaps best inform the public debate over healthcare financing by generating high-quality data on the full range of effects that our medical technologies have on patients' functioning and well-being. This will ensure that the patients' perspective is represented in healthcare policy decisions.

References

1. Hutchinson TA, Boyd NF, Feinstein AR, Gonda A, Hollomby D et al. Scientific problems in clinical scales, as demonstrated in the Karnofsky index of performance status. Journal of Chronic Diseases 1979; 32(9-10): 661–666.
2. Taylor AE, Olver IN, Sivanthan T, Chi M, Purnell C. Observer error in grading performance status in cancer patients. Supportive Care in Cancer 1999; 7(5): 332–335.
3. Feinstein AR. Clinimetric perspectives. Journal of Chronic Diseases 1987; 40(6): 635–640.
4. Gough IR, Furnival CM, Schilder L, Grove W. Assessment of the quality of life of patients with advanced cancer. European Journal of Cancer and Clinical Oncology 1983; 19(8): 1161–1165.
5. Mencken, H.L. A Mencken Chrestomathy. New York: Alfred A Knopf, 1949.
6. WHO. Constitution of the World Health Organization. Geneva: Word Health Organization, 1948. Updated text available online at: <http://www.who.int/governance/eb/who_constitution_en.pdf>, accessed on 23 May 2015.
7. Karnofsky D, Abelmann W, Craver L, Burchenal J. The use of the nitrogen mustards in the palliative treatment of carcinoma. With particular reference to bronchogenic carcinoma. Cancer 1948; 1(4): 634–656.
8. Aaronson NK. Quality of life: what is it? How should it be measured? Oncology (Williston Park) 1988; 2(5): 69–76, 64.
9. Bergner M, Bobbitt RA, Carter WB, Gilson BS. The sickness impact profile: development and final revision of a health status measure. Medical Care 1981; 19(8): 787–805.
10. Hunt SM, McEwen J, McKenna SP. Measuring health status: a new tool for clinicians and epidemiologists. Royal College of General Practitioners 1985; 35(273): 185–188.
11. Development of the World Health Organization WHOQOL-BREF Quality of Life Assessment. Psychological Medicine 1998; 28(3): 551–558.

12. McHorney CA, Ware JE, Jr, Raczek AE. The MOS 36-Item Short-Form Health Survey (SF-36): II. Psychometric and clinical tests of validity in measuring physical and mental health constructs. Medical Care 1993; 31(3): 247–263.

13. Ware JE, Snow KK, Kosinski M, Gandek B. SF-36 health survey manual and interpretation guide. Boston, MA: New England Medical Center, The Health Institute, 1993.

14. Aaronson NK, Ahmedzai S, Bergman B, Bullinger M, Cull A et al. The European Organization for Research and Treatment of Cancer QLQ-C30: a quality-of-life instrument for use in international clinical trials in oncology. Journal of the National Cancer Institute 1993; 85(5): 365–376.

15. Groenvold M, Petersen MA, Aaronson NK, Arraras JI, Blazeby JM et al. The development of the EORTC QLQ-C15-PAL: a shortened questionnaire for cancer patients in palliative care. European Journal of Cancer 2006; 42(1): 55–64.

16. Cella DF, Tulsky DS, Gray G, Sarafian B, Linn E et al. The Functional Assessment of Cancer Therapy scale: development and validation of the general measure. Journal of Clinical Oncology 1993; 11(3): 570–579.

17. Bruera E, Kuehn N, Miller MJ, Selmser P, Macmillan K. The Edmonton Symptom Assessment System (ESAS): a simple method for the assessment of palliative care patients. Journal of Palliative Care 1991; 7(2): 6–9.

18. Richardson LA, Jones GW. A review of the reliability and validity of the Edmonton Symptom Assessment System. Current Oncology 2009; 16(1).

19. European Organization for Research and Treatment of Cancer (EORTC), <http://groups.eortc.be/qol>, accessed on 15 May 2015.

20. Functional Assessment of Cancer Therapy (FACT), <http://www.facit.org/FACITOrg/Questionnaires>, accessed on 15 May 2015.

21. Stockler MR, Osoba D, Goodwin P, Corey P, Tannock IF. Responsiveness to change in health-related quality of life in a randomized clinical trial: a comparison of the Prostate Cancer Specific Quality of Life Instrument (PROSQOLI) with analogous scales from the EORTC QLQ-C30 and a trial specific module. European Organization for Research and Treatment of Cancer. Journal of Clinical Epidemiology 1998; 51(2): 137–145.

22. Litwin MS, Hays RD, Fink A, Ganz PA, Leake B et al. The UCLA Prostate Cancer Index: development, reliability, and validity of a health-related quality of life measure. Medical Care 1998; 36(7): 1002–1012.

23. Sommers SD, Ramsey SD. A review of quality-of-life evaluations in prostate cancer. Pharmacoeconomics 1999; 16(2): 127–140.

24. Wei JT DR, Litwin MS, Sandler HM, Sanda MG. Development and validation of the expanded prostate cancer index composite (EPIC) for comprehensive assessment of health-related quality of life in men with prostate cancer (Research support, Non-U.S. Government Research Support). Urology 2000; 56(6): 899–905.

25. Petersen MA, Groenvold M, Aaronson NK, Chie W-C, Conroy T et al. Development of computerised adaptive testing (CAT) for the EORTC QLQ-C30 dimensions—General approach and initial results for physical functioning. European Journal of Cancer 2010; 46(8): 1352–1358.

26. Cella D, Riley W, Stone A, Rothrock N, Reeve B et al. The Patient-Reported Outcomes Measurement Information System (PROMIS) developed and tested its first wave of adult self-reported health outcome item banks: 2005–2008. Journal of Clinical Epidemiology 2010; 63(11): 1179–1194.

27. Langendijk JA, Doornaert P, Verdonck-de Leeuw IM, Leemans CR, Aaronson NK et al. Impact of late treatment-related toxicity on quality of life among patients with head and neck cancer treated with radiotherapy. Journal of Clinical Oncology 2008; 26(22): 3770–3776.

28. Rossen PB, Pedersen AF, Zachariae R, von der Maase H. Health-related quality of life in long-term survivors of testicular cancer. Journal of Clinical Oncology 2009; 27(35): 5993–5999.

29. Irwig L, Bennetts A. Quality of life after breast conservation or mastectomy: a systematic review. Australian and New Zealand Journal of Surgery 1997; 67(11): 750–754.

30. Lasry JC, Margolese RG. Fear of recurrence, breast-conserving surgery, and the trade-off hypothesis. Cancer 1992; 69(8): 2111–2115.

31. Temel JS, Greer JA, Muzikansky A, Gallagher ER, Admane S et al. Early palliative care for patients with metastatic non-small-cell lung cancer. New England Journal of Medicine 2010; 363(8): 733–742.

32. Simons JP, Aaronson NK, Vansteenkiste JF, ten Velde GP, Muller MJ et al. Effects of medroxyprogesterone acetate on appetite, weight, and quality of life in advanced-stage non-hormone-sensitive cancer: a placebo-controlled multicenter study. Journal of Clinical Oncology 1996; 14(4): 1077–1084.

33. Gotay C, Kawamoto C, Bottomley A, Efficace F. The prognostic significance of patient-reported outcomes in cancer clinical trials. Journal of Clinical Oncology 2008; 26(8): 1355–1363.

34. Quinten C, Maringwa J, Gotay CC, Martinelli F, Coens C et al. Patient self-reports of symptoms and clinician ratings as predictors of overall cancer survival. Journal of the National Cancer Institute 2011; 103(24): 1851–1858.

35. Idler EL, Benyamini Y. Self-rated health and mortality: a review of twenty-seven community studies: a reviwe of twenty-seven community studies. Journal of Health and Social Behaviour 2005; 38(1): 21–37.

36. DeSalvo KB, Fan VS, McDonell MB, Fihn SD. Predicting mortality and healthcare utilization with a single question. Health Services Research 2005; 40(4): 1234–1246.

37. US Food and Drug Administration. Guidance for industry: patient-reported outcome measures: use in medical product development to support labeling claims. Silver Spring, MD: FDA, 2009. Available from: <http://www.fda.gov/downloads/Drugs/GuidanceComplianceRegulatoryInformation/Guidances/UCM193282.pdf>, accessed on 15 May 2015.

38. Agency EM. Reflection paper on the regulatory guidance for the use of health-related quality of life (HRQL) measures in the evaluation of medicinal products. London: EMA, 2005. Available from: <www.ema.europa.eu/docs/en_GB/document_library/Scientific_guideline/2009/09/WC500003637.pdf>, accessed on 23 May 2015.

39. Basch E, Abernethy AP, Mullins CD, Reeve BB, Smith ML et al. Recommendations for Incorporating patient-reported outcomes into clinical comparative effectiveness research in adult oncology. Journal of Clinical Oncology 2012; 30(34): 4249–4255.

40. Calvert M, Blazeby J, Altman DG, Revicki DA, Moher D et al. Reporting of patient-reported outcomes in randomized trials: the consort pro extension. Journal of the American Medical Association 2013; 309(8): 814–822.

41. Hjermstad MJ, Fayers PM, Bjordal K, Kaasa S. Health-related quality of life in the general Norwegian population assessed by the European Organization for Research and Treatment of Cancer Core Quality-of-Life Questionnaire: the QLQ=C30 (+ 3). Journal of Clinical Oncology 1998; 16(3): 1188–1196.

42. Fayers PM, Weeden S, Curran D. EORTC QLQ-C30 reference values. Brussels: EORTC; 1998.

43. Osoba D, Rodrigues G, Myles J, Zee B, Pater J. Interpreting the significance of changes in health-related quality-of-life scores. Journal of Clinical Oncology 1998; 16(1): 139–144.

44. Rothenberg ML, Moore MJ, Cripps MC, Andersen JS, Portenoy RK et al. A phase II trial of gemcitabine in patients with 5-FU-refractory pancreas cancer. Annals of Oncology 1996; 7(4): 347–353.

45. Tannock IF, Osoba D, Stockler MR, Ernst DS, Neville AJ et al. Chemotherapy with mitoxantrone plus prednisone or prednisone alone for symptomatic hormone-resistant prostate cancer: a Canadian randomized trial with palliative end points. Journal of Clinical Oncology 1996; 14(6): 1756–1764.

46. King MT. The interpretation of scores from the EORTC quality of life questionnaire QLQ-C30. Quality of Life Research 1996; 5(6): 555–567.

47. Cocks K, King M, Velikova G, Martyn St-James M, Fayers P et al. Evidence-based guidelines for determination of sample size and interpretation of the European Organisation for the Research and Treatment of Cancer Quality of Life Questionnaire Core 30. Journal of Clinical Oncology 2011; 29(1): 89–96.

48. Cocks K, King MT, Velikova G, de Castro G Jr, Martyn St-James M et al. Evidence-based guidelines for interpreting change scores for the European Organisation for the Research and Treatment of Cancer Quality of Life Questionnaire Core 30. European Journal of Cancer 2012; 48(11): 1713–1721.

49. King MT, Stockler MR, Cella DF, Osoba D, Eton DT et al. Meta-analysis provides evidence-based effect sizes for a cancer-specific quality-of-life questionnaire, the FACT-G. Journal of Clinical Epidemiology 2010; 63(3): 270–281.

50. Cohen HJ. Statistical power analysis for the behavioral sciences. Hillsdale NJ: Lawrence Erlbaum, 1988.

51. Norman GR, Sloan JA, Wyrwich KW. Interpretation of changes in health-related quality of life: the remarkable universality of half a standard deviation. Medical Care 2003; 41(5): 582–592.

CHAPTER 34

Cancer survivorship and rehabilitation

Rachel L. Yung and Ann H. Partridge

Introduction to cancer survivorship and rehabilitation

Cancer survivorship is a relatively new area of clinical focus and research. Although practising oncology providers have long contended with the issues that burden their patients with a history of cancer, survivorship has only recently gained recognition as an important and unique component of cancer care and research. In a pivotal editorial on the topic, Mullan described the concept of survivorship in terms of seasons in the cancer trajectory and helped to galvanize efforts to 'map the middle ground of survivorship and minimize medical and social hazards' after cancer [1]. Over the past three decades there has been a slow but steady recognition of the importance of cancer survivorship in the biomedical community, including the launching of the Office of Cancer Survivorship at the National Cancer Institute (NCI) in 1996. Today, survivorship has received international attention in cancer organizations. There are burgeoning survivorship programmes within cancer centres and an increased body of research and quality improvement initiatives focus on issues salient to cancer survivors. Nevertheless, given the heterogeneity of cancer types, treatments, latency periods for issues to arise, and funding constraints, coordinated efforts in this area have been challenging. Much of the research to date has defined the relatively short-term issues that survivors face, with more limited available evidence-based information regarding how to optimally follow cancer survivors or make interventions to improve outcomes.

When is a patient considered a survivor?

The NCI's Office of Cancer Survivorship adopted the National Coalition for Cancer Survivorship's (NCCS) definition of survivorship, defining someone as a cancer survivor from the time of diagnosis and for the balance of life [2]. Survivorship often also refers to the period in the cancer continuum after the completion of active treatment and before end of life. Although family and loved ones have sometimes been included as survivors, the focus for this chapter will be on those with a cancer diagnosis who have completed active treatment.

In the US alone, there are now approximately 12 million adult cancer survivors, a dramatic increase since 1971 when there were fewer than three million [3]. This number is anticipated to grow to 18 million by 2022 [4]. This reflects the increased life expectancy of those with cancer: in 2003, 67% of adult cancer patients lived longer than five years compared to fewer than 50% in the 1970s

[3]. The distribution of cancer survivors reflects both the incidence and survival of different cancer subtypes. Those with breast, colorectal, and prostate cancers make up over half of all survivors (Figure 34.1). Most cancer survivors are over 65 years old (60%), 35% are 40 to 64 years old, 4% are 19 to 39 years old, and 1% are less than 19 years old [3]. Mirroring population demographics, incident cancer cases in people over the age of 65 are projected to double over the next 40 years [5]. This will result in an ageing of the survivorship population. While special attention is clearly needed for younger cancer survivors who have unique concerns, such as employment and fertility, caring for older survivors who are more likely to have comorbidity makes care coordination between their oncologists and primary care doctors paramount. This highlights the need for personalized survivorship care that mirrors the direction of all of cancer care.

Worldwide, the demographics of survivorship are harder to estimate and this in fact is a significant research question. In developed countries with cancer programmes, an interest in survivorship issues has motivated better prevalence estimates. Data from the UK puts their figure at two million survivors [6]. Estimates of survivors in developing countries have been calculated given a country's unique distribution of type of cancer, average survival after treatment, and general life expectancy [7]. Therefore, much of the evidence base has grown out of initial research done in North America; however, recently the research has been global in nature. There is international agreement that survivorship is a key part of cancer treatment.

The essential components of survivorship care include: (1) surveillance, screening, and prevention of recurrence and new cancers, including adherence to clinical guidelines and risk-reducing treatments; (2) identification and management of late and long-term effects; (3) improving modifiable health behaviours; and (4) coordination of care between providers to ensure that individual patients' health needs are met [8]. While great strides have been made in each of these areas, there is much work to be done to improve our understanding of the needs of cancer survivors as well as optimizing cancer survivorship care to improve patient disease and quality of life outcomes.

Surveillance, screening, and prevention

Surveillance for recurrent cancers and screening for new primary cancers are important survivor issues. Cancer-specific recommendations exist (please see the appropriate disease-oriented chapters for cancer-specific details); however, the weight of the evidence

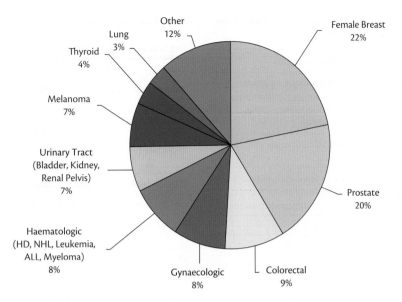

Fig. 34.1 Distribution of primary cancer type of survivors.

Source: data from Howlader N, Noone AM, Krapcho M, Neyman N, Aminou R, Waldron W, Altekruse SF, Kosary CL, Ruhl J, Tatalovich Z, Cho H, Mariotto A, Eisner MP, Lewis DR, Chen HS, Feuer EJ, Cronin KA, Edwards BK (Eds.), *SEER Cancer Statistics Review, 1975–2008*, National Cancer Institute, Bethesda, Maryland, USA, available from <http://seer.cancer.gov/csr/1975_2008/>. Based on November 2010 SEER data submission, posted to the SEER website, 2011.

behind them varies. We do have some data from prospective randomized studies; these results have been incorporated into guideline recommendations and should be followed. For example, surveillance for recurrence with imaging and tumour markers has been shown not to be beneficial in breast cancer [9–12] or ovarian cancer [13] where recurrence is usually incurable and early detection does not improve outcomes. In contrast, intensive surveillance for recurrence is used in colorectal cancer, lymphoma, and testicular cancer where recurrent disease is potentially treatable with curative intent. Surveillance is critical for risk-adapted treatment that limits therapy (and side effects), such as for patients with low-stage seminoma treated with surgery only [14]. Ideal surveillance strategies for many cancer types have yet to be proven in a rigorous manner, but research is ongoing. For example, a Cochrane meta-analysis reported an overall survival benefit for high-intensity versus low-intensity follow-up for colorectal cancer. However, they were unable to comment on the ideal modalities (i.e. imaging, blood tumour markers, and endoscopy) [15]. Currently, there are three large ongoing prospective, randomized controlled trials in Europe evaluating the optimal surveillance for colorectal patients [16–18]. For most diseases, however, there are only limited data to inform follow-up care and future research is necessary.

Screening for new primary malignancies is another priority for survivorship care. Screening in survivors is appropriate where evidence exists to recommend screening for the general population (e.g., breast, colon) and for those patients at higher risk secondary to environmental risks (e.g., smoking and lung cancer), genetic risk factors (e.g., frequent enteroscopy for patients with Lynch syndrome), or at increased risk secondary to previous cancer treatment (e.g., breast cancer screening for women who received mantle irradiation for Hodgkin lymphoma). However, evidence has suggested limited uptake of cancer screening among survivors, bringing to light the gaps in implementation of survivorship care [19–21].

Prevention of recurrence and second primaries is cancer type-specific, but falls into the general categories of optimization of modifiable health behaviours (discussed later in the chapter) and

adherence to chemoprevention, such as adjuvant hormone therapy for breast cancer. There is a large literature demonstrating that, despite the well-known benefit from adjuvant hormone therapy for breast cancer, there are many women who do not initiate or complete a full course of treatment [22–24].

Long-term and late effects of cancer and cancer treatment

There are myriad long-term and late effects that can result from cancer and cancer treatment. Technically, long-term effects are those which appear during treatment and persist, while late effects are those that manifest after cancer treatment has ended [25]. Long-term and late effects can be physical as well as psychosocial. Future survivorship research will also likely reveal additional concerns as well as help develop better management strategies.

Physical late and long-term effects

People with a history of cancer compared to those without a history of cancer have a two-fold higher rate of functional disability, impaired independent activities of daily living [26] and lower ratings for their health status [27]. Tables 34.1, 34.2, and 34.3, list many of the common late and long-term physical effects associated with specific cancer type and treatment. Many patients receive multimodality cancer treatment and late effects can result from combination therapy.

Fatigue

Fatigue is often multifactorial and can be associated with pain, medications, psychosocial distress, anaemia, hypothyroidism, poor nutritional status, or sleep disturbance/insomnia [28]. Although fatigue is a common side effect during active treatment, the prevalence of fatigue after active treatment is more difficult to determine. Fatigue is also common in the general population, making it difficult to determine how much is attributable to cancer and its treatment. However, a comprehensive review reported slightly higher average

Table 34.1 Potential long-term and late effect of systemic anti-cancer therapy (chemotherapy, hormonal, and targeted therapy)

Organ system	Effect	Causative agents
General	Second cancers	Steroids, alkylating agents, nitrosoureas, topoisomerase inhibitors, anthracyclines, tamoxifen
Bone and soft tissue	Osteoporosis, avascular necrosis	Steroids, aromatase inhibitors
Cardiovascular	Inflammation of the heart, congestive heart failure	Anthracyclines, high-dose cyclophosphamide, cisplatin, taxanes, trastuzumab, sunitinib
Endocrine	Diabetes	Steroids
Gastrointestinal	Motility disorders	Vinca alkaloids
Genitourinary	Haemorrhagic cystitis	Cyclophosphamide, ifosfamide, transplant therapy
	Erectile dysfunction	GnRH agonists
Gonadal	Infertility, premature menopause, low testosterone	Cyclophosphamide, nitrosoureas, procarbazine hydrochloride, combination chemotherapy, GnRH agonists
Haematologic	Low blood counts, myelodysplastic syndrome, acute leukaemia	Alkylating agents, anthracyclines, nitrosoureas, topoisomerase inhibitors, purine analogs, any high-dose therapy with autologous transplantation
Hepatic	Abnormal liver function, cirrhosis, liver failure	Methotrexate, carmustine (BCNU)
Immune system	Impaired immune function or immune suppression	Steroids, anti-thymocyte globulin (ATG), methotrexate, rituximab, alemtuzumab, purine analogs, any high-dose therapy with autologous transplantation
Nervous	Cognitive effects	Combination chemotherapy, methotrexate, bortezomib
	Neuropathy	Taxanes, vinca alkaloids, oxaliplatin, cisplatin
	Hearing loss	Cisplatin
Ophthalmologic	Cataracts	Steroids, tamoxifen
Pulmonary	Pulmonary oedema	Imatinib, dasatinib,
	Pulmonary fibrosis	Bleomycin, carmustine, methotrexate
Renal	Renal dysfunction/failure	Cisplatin, methotrexate, nitrosoureas

Adapted with permission from *From Cancer Patient to Cancer Survivor Lost in Transition*, National Academy of Sciences, Washington, DC, USA, Copyright © 2006.

Table 34.2 Potential long-term and late effects of radiation

Organ system	Effect
General	Second cancers
Bone and soft tissue	Atrophy, deformation, fibrosis, and bone death
Cardiovascular	Scarring or inflammation, coronary artery disease
Dental/Oral	Caries, dry mouth
Endocrine	Hypopituitary, hypothyroidism, infertility, premature menopause, testosterone deficiency
Gastrointestinal	Malabsorption, stricture, fistulas
Genitourinary	Bladder scarring, cystitis, fistulas, urinary incontinence
Haematologic	Low blood counts, myelodysplastic syndrome, acute leukaemia
Hepatic	Abnormal liver function, liver failure
Immune system	Impaired immune function, immune suppression
Lymphatic	Lymphoedema
Nervous	Problems with memory, thinking, learning
Ophthalmologic	Cataracts, dry eyes, visual impairment
Pulmonary	Lung scarring, decreased lung function, radiation pneumonitis
Renal	Hypertension, impaired kidney function

Adapted with permission from *From Cancer Patient to Cancer Survivor Lost in Transition*, National Academy of Sciences, Washington, DC, USA, Copyright © 2006.

showed that the rates of fatigue had diminished slightly in the survivor group [34]. Risk factors for chronic fatigue in survivors include depression, pain, multimodality cancer therapy, and other comorbidities [30, 31]. Evaluation and treatment of underlying causes of fatigue, if detected, may improve symptoms. Exercise, behavioural therapy, sleep interventions, and medications such as antidepressants and psychostimulants may help in the management of fatigue. See the National Comprehensive Cancer Network (NCCN) guidelines for additional recommendations for evaluation and treatment of cancer-related fatigue in patients post-treatment [37].

Chronic pain

Acute pain management for patients being actively treated for cancer and with advanced disease is more extensively covered in Chapter 43 on 'Supportive palliative care'. Chronic pain can be characterized as nocioceptic (visceral and somatic) neuropathic, idiopathic, psychogenic, and mixed [38]. It can be secondary to the cancer itself (i.e. compressive neuropathies), cancer treatments (e.g., radiation-induced plexopathies, chemotherapy-induced neuropathy, arthralgias from anti-hormonal agents, or post-surgical pain), or unrelated to the cancer diagnosis (e.g., low back pain). The prevalence of chronic pain in survivors varies by treatment modality. For example, post-surgical series show patients may experience pain at one year up to 50% after breast surgery, 60% after thoracotomy, and 40% after head and neck surgery [39, 40]. In populations that included both cancer and non-cancer patients, predictors of chronic post-surgical pain include chronic preoperative pain, repeat surgeries, passive coping skills, anxiety, depression, worker's compensation claims, risk of nerve damage for a given surgical approach, poorly controlled postoperative

fatigue scores in those with a history of cancer (who had completed active treatment) compared to the non-cancer population, suggesting long-lasting effects of the cancer or treatment [29]. Prevalence estimates of fatigue in the survivor population range from 17% to 56% [30–36]. Fatigue can be persistent. In a population of Hodgkin lymphoma survivors the prevalence was 24–27% at 12 years, compared to 9–12% in controls [35]; however, follow-up at 20 years

Table 34.3 Potential long-term and late effects of surgery

Procedure	Late effect
General	Pain, cosmetic defects, scaring, psychosocial
Neurosurgery	Impairment of any body function
Head and neck	Difficulties with communication, eating, breathing; cosmetic
Endocrine surgery (i.e. pituitary/thyroid)	Endocrinopathies/hypofunction: hypopituitarism, hypothyroidism, hypoparathyroidism
Lymphatic	Lymphoedema, retrograde ejaculation
Abdominal	Risk of obstruction, hernia, fistula
Splenectomy	Impaired immune function, predisposition to sepsis
Pelvic surgery	Sexual dysfunction, infertility, incontinence, hernia, bowel obstruction
Amputation	Functional changes, cosmetic, psychosocial impact, phantom limb pain, arthritis, neuropathic pain
Lung resection	Breathing difficulty, fatigue, general weakness
Prostatectomy	Urinary incontinence, sexual dysfunction
Oophorectomy	Premature menopause and Infertility
Orchiectomy	Infertility, testosterone deficiency
Ostomy	Bowel obstruction or incontinence, sexual dysfunction, poor body image

Adapted with permission from *From Cancer Patient to Cancer Survivor Lost in Transition*, National Academy of Sciences, Washington D.C, USA, Copyright © 2006.

pain, radiation, or chemotherapy [40]. Rates of radiation-induced plexopathies are estimated at 1–5% for breast cancer patients, while 20% of patients with pelvic radiation complain of dysuria at one year [39]. Chronic pain management in the cancer survivor population has been mostly based on data from the non-cancer population and uses a multidisciplinary approach with pharmacological, behavioural and physical interventions. Pharmacologic interventions include traditional opiate and non-opiate analgesics as well as anti-depressants and anti-convulsants for treatment of neuropathic pain [41, 42]. Additionally, cognitive behavioural therapy, physical therapy, and rehabilitation therapy focused on functional outcomes can be effective strategies for patients with chronic pain.

Cognitive effects

Long-term cognitive effects of intrathecal or intraventricular chemotherapy and cranial irradiation for CNS malignancy are widely acknowledged. Cognitive dysfunction after systemic treatment of chemotherapy for non-CNS malignancies, sometimes referred to as 'chemobrain', has been less widely accepted, potentially because of difficulty measuring it. There are some data supporting cognitive dysfunction of patients during or shortly after systemic cytotoxic cancer treatment. Persistent or late cognitive effects of chemotherapy have been more difficult to evaluate. Cognitive dysfunction includes domains such as attention, memory, and processing speed. Early studies lacked standardized tests and cut-offs defining cognitive dysfunction [43] which is reflected in the wide variation in estimated incidence (13–70%) [44]. Therefore, recent task force recommendations call for standard testing and definition criteria

[44]. Incidence of self-reported cognitive impairment tends to be higher than that measured by neuropsychiatric testing. This might reflect recall bias, but it is also plausible that testing has not been sensitive for true changes that might be perceptible to patients. Adding to the difficulty investigating this topic are the potential confounders, including fatigue, insomnia, anxiety, depression, and stress that are common among cancer patients [43]. It is reasonable to acknowledge that this is likely a long-term side effect of cancer therapy and try to improve function with treatment of compounding conditions as well as considering referral to occupational therapy. To date, pharmacological agents have not been shown to be effective.

Cardiotoxicity

Many cancer treatments, including cytotoxic chemotherapies (e.g., anthracycline use), radiation, and newer targeted agents such as trastuzumab and sunitinib are known to cause cardiac side effects, including accelerated atherosclerotic disease as well as cardiomyopathies (Tables 34.1 and 34.2). Risk factors for developing cardiac dysfunction with anthracyclines are cumulative dose, age (both <18 and >65), pre-existing cardiac disease and concomitant administration of other cardiotoxic agents or mediastinal radiation [45, 46]. Treatment is generally similar to that of nonanthracycline-induced cardiomyopathies; however, this has not been extensively evaluated in the survivor population. Survivors who received cisplatin, for instance for testicular cancer, have accelerated atherosclerosis [47, 48]. Despite ongoing investigation, currently there is no standard for monitoring asymptomatic survivors for development of cardiac toxicity caused by these agents [49]. Strategies evaluated include imaging, such as echocardiograms or MUGA, serum testing for B-type naturetic peptide (BNP) or troponin levels, exercise testing, or more invasive testing such as endocardial biopsies or cardiac angiography.

The cardiac dysfunction seen with trastuzumab is usually not fatal and usually reversible with discontinuation and/or treatment with cardiac medications [50]. Early studies demonstrated marked increased rates of cardiac toxicity when it is given concurrently with an anthracycline, which is no longer regularly done. Other risk factors include increasing age and cardiac dysfunction after receiving anthracyclines [51, 52]. Generally, cardiac functioning is monitored with echocardiogram or MUGA during treatment and treatment is held for asymptomatic reduction in left ventricular ejection fraction [53]. Less is known about the late cardiac effects or how patients at risk should be followed. Cardiac toxicity is also seen with other targeted agents, such as the tyrosine kinase inhibitors, that can cause oedema, hypertension, and occasionally heart failure [54].

Radiation can cause damage to all of the anatomical parts of the heart resulting in pericarditis, myocarditis, valvular damage, atherosclerosis, and conduction abnormalities. This is most pronounced in patients who have undergone chest radiation, but has been documented in breast cancer as well as head and neck cancer survivors. More modern radiation techniques such as limited radiation fields, conformational techniques, image-guided therapies, and lower radiation doses have decreased the burden of cardiac side effects; however, follow-up is limited [55]. Few studies have evaluated cardiac screening in this population. The incidence of asymptomatic disease is not known, and it is also not known if treatment of asymptomatic disease would improve outcomes [49].

Pulmonary toxicity

Pulmonary toxicity can be caused by many types of chemotherapy (Table 34.1) or radiation (Table 34.2). The most studied agents include bleomycin and taxanes, which can result in acute pneumonitis. Risk factors for bleomycin-induced pneumonitis include age, smoking, renal dysfunction, mediastinal radiation, and use of oxygen [56, 57]. Additionally, an interstitial pneumonitis has been described with newer targeted therapies such as erlotinib; this occurs generally during or soon after treatment and can be responsive to steroids and discontinuation [58]. Radiation pneumonitis is not uncommon in the treatment of lung cancer, occurring in 5–15% of patients receiving external beam radiation therapy [59] but is much less common in patients with lymphoma (3–11%) [60] or breast cancer who receive radiation (<1% for breast-conserving approach) [61]. Rarely, these patients go on to develop progressive pulmonary fibrosis. Interstitial pneumonitis, due to idiopathic pneumonia syndrome or bronchiolitis obliterans, is common in survivors of bone marrow transplantation, occurring in up to 34% [62].

Endocrine effects

Primary hypothyroidism can be caused by external radiation [63] or tyrosine kinase inhibitors [64] and is well-documented in patients undergoing hematopoietic stem cell transplant [65, 66]. NCCN recommends that survivors of head and neck cancer who have a history of neck irradiation should have screening for hypothyroidism every six to 12 months after completing treatment [67]. Additionally, hypothyroidism is a treatable cause of cancer fatigue and should be evaluated in patients complaining of this symptom [37].

Bone health/osteoporosis

Osteopenia and osteoporosis are common side effects of cancer treatments such as aromatase inhibitors, androgen-deprivation, corticosteroids, radiation, and premature menopause from chemotherapy, radiation, surgery, or ovarian suppression. NCCN, the American Society of Clinical Oncology (ASCO), and the European Society of Medical Oncology (ESMO) guidelines recommend monitoring of bone mineral density (BMD) measurements with dual-energy X-ray absorptiometry (DEXA) for patients on treatment that lowers sex steroids (including premature menopause) at initiation of treatment and with periodic follow up [68–72]. NCCN further recommends the addition of risk calculators, such as FRAX^{TM}, which incorporate other clinical characteristics to help guide management [71]. Treatment for osteopenia/osteoporosis includes vitamin D and calcium supplementation, weight-bearing exercise, smoking cessation, antiresorptive agents (e.g., bisphosphonates, oestrogen, raloxifene) and newer agents such as teriparatide and denosumab. Bisphosphonates are the mainstay of medical treatment. Use of hormones and anabolic agents such as teriparatide should be used cautiously in the cancer population, as they are contraindicated in certain cancer types.

Weight gain/metabolic syndrome

Weight gain is common in cancer survivors and can be secondary to inactivity, ageing, medication side effects (i.e. corticosteroids), low androgen levels (from androgen-depleting medication, radiation, or surgery), or smoking cessation. Additionally, those who have had stem cell transplantation (especially those with a history of chronic graft versus host disease) are at higher risk of developing diabetes than their siblings [66]. Counselling and education interventions have been modestly successful, with those that address multiple components (e.g., diet, exercise, and behavioural modification) having better results than those that focus on only one aspect [73].

Lymphoedema

Lymphoedema is fluid accumulation secondary to disruption of lymphatic vessels, usually in a limb, and is a common side effect of surgery (Table 34.3), radiation (Table 34.2), or a combination of both. It is measured with circumferential or volumetric methods. Although commonly associated with breast cancer, it can occur any time lymphatic drainage is disturbed, such as in nodal evaluation for melanoma, surgery for sarcoma, or any pelvic treatment. It can result in pain, dysfunction, and a propensity to infections. Rates of lymphoedema vary based on the type of surgery, the use of adjuvant radiation, and lymph node evaluation. In breast cancer survivors, the incidence of lymphoedema is decreasing as sentinel lymph node biopsy is used more in place of a full axillary node dissection. Lymphoedema rates for patients having sentinel lymph node biopsy compared to axillary node dissection are <10% versus >10% [74].

Effective treatment includes complete decompressive physiotherapy, compression (bandages/garments/pneumatic devices), manual lymphatic drainage, and exercise. Complete decompressive physiotherapy is a regimen that combines compression and manual lymphatic drainage and is superior to compression alone [75]. Additionally, careful weight-based exercise improves outcomes [76]. Early recognition and treatment are felt to be important.

Bowel and bladder dysfunction

Patients undergoing treatment for prostate, colorectal, bladder, and gynaecological surgeries are at risk for bowel and bladder dysfunction (Table 34.3). Treatment for prostate cancer with surgery can result in urinary incontinence and erectile dysfunction, whereas treatment with radiation can result in both urinary and faecal incontinence. Newer nerve-sparing surgeries reduce the risk of erectile dysfunction for men. Similarly, improvements in the treatment of bladder cancer have been made with research underway in the use of bladder-sparing treatments and continent urinary ostomies.

Patients can have ostomies after many types of pelvic surgeries (rectal, gynaecological, bladder). There is some evidence that ostomies result in more sexual dysfunction, psychological distress, and restrictions on social functioning than sphincter-preserving surgeries [77]. In contrast, a newer Cochrane Review did not find consistent results in the published literature and concluded that quality of life might not be worse for those rectal cancer patients treated with surgery that included creation of a colostomy [78].

Sexuality

Sexuality is multifaceted and influenced by physical, hormonal, psychological, and social factors even without a cancer diagnosis. Cancer can affect each of these aspects. Local treatment such as surgery or radiation for gynaecological, urinary, or gastrointestinal cancers can result in loss or dysfunction of sexual anatomy or in bowel or bladder incontinence. Hormonal therapies can affect erectile function, libido, and vaginal plasticity and dryness. Changes in appearance or emotional state can result in less confidence and comfort in intimate situations. Because of the complexity of issues that often underlie sexual dysfunction, a multidisciplinary team including psychiatric/psychological and medical evaluations and lifestyle and cognitive behavioural therapy techniques is recommended [79–81].

Premature menopause

Premature menopause can result at the time of treatment or years later. It results in infertility (discussed below separately), vasomotor symptoms such as hot flashes and sleep disturbance, hormonal changes resulting in dyspareunia, and other health effects such as accelerated cardiovascular disease and osteoporosis. Management of vasomotor symptoms includes treatment with hormone replacement if appropriate oncologically, antidepressants such as venlafaxine, as well as complementary treatments such as acupuncture. It is important to encourage healthy habits such as sufficient vitamin D and calcium intake combined with weight-bearing exercise for bone health in conjunction with regular interval screening for osteoporosis and appropriate treatment if found. Management of these symptoms is described in Table 34.4. All of these effects should be monitored and managed.

Infertility

Fertility is an important and often inadequately addressed issue for many younger patients facing a new cancer diagnosis. Although many survivorship issues might be best addressed at the time that the effects become evident, fertility is a survivorship issue that is most appropriately addressed prior to cancer treatment if at all possible. Chances of treatment-induced infertility depend on

Table 34.4 Management of premature menopause

Issue	Management
Hot flashes	Antidepressants
	◆ SSRIs (selective serotonin reuptake inhibitors)
	◆ (avoid strong cyp2da inhibitors with concurrent tamoxifen)
	◆ Venlafaxine
	◆ Gabapentin
	Hormone replacement therapy (if oncologically appropriate)
	Complementary treatments (e.g., acupuncture)
Sleep disturbance	Zolpidem
	Exercise
Dyspareunia	Water-based lubricants
	Hormone replacement therapy (if oncologically appropriate)
Bone Health	Sufficient vitamin D and calcium intake
	Weight bearing exercise
	Regular osteoporosis screening
	Tobacco cessation
	Recommendations for alcohol in moderation
Cardiovascular health	Age and risk-based assessment and primary prevention
	Encourage optimal health behaviours (e.g., tobacco cessation)

Table 34.5 Fertility preservation strategies for men and women undergoing cancer treatment

Status	Men	Women
Clinically available	Sperm banking Embryo cryopreservation	Embryo cryopreservation Conservative gynaecological surgery Oophoropexy
Investigational	Testicular tissue cryopreservation	Oocyte cryopreservation Ovarian tissue cryopreservation Gonadal suppression with GnRH antagonists

sex, age, prediagnosis factors, and specific treatment regimens. Standard techniques for fertility preservation include sperm and embryo cryopreservation, but many others are under investigation (Table 34.5). Conservative gynaecological surgery and oophoropexy, which is a procedure to shield the ovaries from radiation, are other methods of preserving fertility in appropriate patients [82]. Given that there are viable options available for patients it is important to be proactive in addressing fertility early in a diagnosis. Published guidelines recommend discussion of fertility as part of informed consent and stress that this should be done as early as possible [82]. Although data are limited, fertility preservation does not appear to increase cancer recurrence, even for hormonally sensitive tumours. Very little is published about adoption after a cancer diagnosis, although it does appear that there can be hurdles for those who chose this option [83]. There are several patient-centred informational websites that provide information and help with decision-making [84, 85].

Improvements in treatment over time

Recognition of these late and long-term effects has resulted in the modification of treatment regimens with the purpose of improving survivorship while maintaining similar efficacy/cure rates. Widely adopted predictive testing of the effectiveness of chemotherapy for individual women with hormone-sensitive breast cancers allows women to forgo chemotherapy in situations in which they are unlikely to benefit [86]. Furthermore, surgical approaches minimizing morbidity, such as limb-sparing [87] and larynx-sparing surgeries [88], are increasingly achieved, as is the omission of radiation for low-risk Hodgkin lymphoma [89].

Psychosocial long-term and late effects

Cancer can have a profound effect on an individual's psychosocial health (Table 34.6). Survivors can experience long-lasting psychological effects including depression, anxiety, body image concerns, and loss of social role functioning, including partnering, parenting, and working. Recently, psychosocial late effects have been better recognized and are actively being researched with increased focus on patient-centred outcomes.

Depression

Depression is not uncommon in the survivor population. Risk factors for distress (depression and/or anxiety) are younger age, more advanced disease, more physical symptoms, and shorter time since

Table 34.6 Potential Psychosocial Late Effects

Potential psychosocial late effects	Population/details	Recommendations/management*
Depression and Anxiety	At higher risk: Younger age More advanced disease Physical symptoms Shorter time since diagnosis Rates of 20–30% at five years	Treatments: Antidepressants Individual and group therapy Psycho-education Relaxation Non-pharmacological treatments appears more effective for patients with anxiety
Fear of recurrence	At higher risk: Younger age White or Hispanic (versus Black) Less education Shorter time since diagnosis Treatment with chemotherapy Depression	Recognition of the problem by physicians Identification of patients at higher risk
Personal Growth	Approximately one-half of patients report personal growth after a diagnosis of cancer. More likely in women and younger patients.	Provide positive reinforcement.
Finances	Younger survivors are at particularly high risk to not be employed. Cancer expenses are high. Many survivors forgo care secondary to expense.	Routine questioning about financial concerns and referral to appropriate resources including social workers, occupational therapists, etc. Educating patients about important survivorship follow up
Disability	Rates are higher than in the general population.	Newer treatment approaches might help prevent disability. Referral to physical and occupational therapy.
Social Role Functioning	Marriage: Interpersonal relationships, such as marriage, are stressed. Parenting: 24% of cancer survivors have children under 18 years of age.	Routine questioning and involvement of social workers and other psychotherapists. Specialized social work care targeted at parents that assists with conversations about disclosure and coping.

* Recommendations are largely based on clinical practice rather than evidence-based because of lack of supporting studies.

diagnosis [90]. Depression rates range from 3% to 17% for survivors, but are higher in those with active cancer [32, 90, 91]. Survivors more than five years out from diagnosis frequently still report symptoms of depression or anxiety (20–30%) [92]. Depression is inversely correlated with quality of life [90]. Furthermore, depression has been associated with poorer cancer outcomes [93]. Cancer survivors have also recently been shown to have increased rates of suicidality [94]. Thus, routine screening for distress in survivors is important as effective treatments are available, such as antidepressants as well as non-pharmacological treatments including individual and group therapy, cognitive behavioural therapy, psychoeducation, and relaxation [95, 96].

Anxiety

The prevalence of anxiety in cancer survivors appears close to that in the general population; however, there is likely a subgroup that experiences considerable anxiety secondary to cancer diagnosis and treatment. Risk factors for anxiety are similar to that of depression. Non-pharmacological interventions appear to be slightly more beneficial in survivors with anxiety rather than depression [96].

Fear of recurrence

Survivors and their families often experience a fear of cancer recurrence that can result in interpretation of somatic stimuli to be symptoms of recurrence, increased general anxiety or limited planning for the future [97, 98]. Most long-term survivors (>5 years from diagnosis) have some concern about recurrence, with a smaller percentage (10–31%) having high levels of fear of recurrence [99]. Factors associated with higher levels of fear of recurrence are younger age, white or Hispanic race (versus black), less education, fewer years since diagnosis, and treatment with chemotherapy. Fear of recurrence is also associated with lower quality of life, fatigue, and depression. Potential strategies to address this fear are education and psychotherapy. The goal is not to eliminate worry, but to reduce maladaptive fear of recurrence and to redirect worry into positive self-care. Patient–provider interactions are likely critical.

Personal growth

In contrast to studies suggesting worse psychological state after cancer, there is also a literature that suggests improvement, which has aptly been named post-traumatic growth [100, 101]. A survey study of survivors reported that their cancer experience had provided new philosophy of life (59% of respondents), greater appreciation of life (47%), and emotional growth of the family (38%) [101]. This effect appears to depend on gender and age: women and younger patients report more personal growth after a cancer diagnosis, whereas men and older patients tend to minimize the impact of cancer on their lives [102].

Social role functioning

Social roles, including partnering, parenting, and working, change considerably over a person's lifetime and a cancer diagnosis can have a profound effect on these roles. Much of the literature looking at partnering and parenting is in survivors of childhood cancer. However, a diagnosis of cancer in young adulthood can also have significant effects on these roles and subsequently on quality of life [103]. Although survivors of childhood cancer have lower marriage rates, there appears no consistent difference in marital status between adult cancer survivors and the general population [104–107]. However, the effect of a cancer diagnosis on quality of life depends on both the gender and coping strategies of the survivor and their spouse in married cancer survivors [108–110]. Better studied is the effect of social support, specifically in marriage, on cancer outcomes; a large meta-analysis demonstrated better social support is associated with lower cancer mortality [111].

Although 24% of cancer survivors have children younger than 18 years of age in the US, accounting for 2.85 million children [112], relatively little has been published about either the children or the survivor parents. Most of the studies are small and qualitative, but do describe important themes of disclosure, communication, and family life [113]. Recently, quantitative scales evaluating parenting-specific distress have been developed [115]. Appropriately, NCI has designated family issues a top research priority [115].

Economics/disability

A diagnosis of cancer can have profound financial effects. Cancer survivors are more likely to be unable to work [26, 27] and to have public rather than private medical insurance [116] compared to those with no cancer history. Out-of-pocket medical expenses for cancer patients are high [117, 118]. Many survivors (up to 21%) forgo medical care secondary to cost [116, 118].

Health behaviours

Survivorship focuses on prevention of recurrent disease, new primary malignancies, and improving functionality. Central to these goals are modifiable health behaviours (Table 34.7). Encounters with the medical profession are 'teachable moments' that can be used to influence patients to choose healthy behaviours, such as tobacco cessation, diet, physical activity, and weight management [8]. Indeed there is a power of suggestion as demonstrated by a randomized controlled trial in which an oncologist's recommendation to exercise after an early diagnosis of breast cancer increased rates of exercise significantly compared to control [120]. Timing also appears critical, with early intervention (within three months of diagnosis for tobacco cessation) being more effective than later recommendations [121].

Smoking cessation

Of modifiable behaviours, tobacco cessation may be the one that physicians are best poised to affect (Table 34.7). A physician's recommendation to quit is an important motivator for many smokers. Tobacco cessation is important in prevention of second primary tumours and primary prevention of heart and lung disease. Smoking at diagnosis is related to worse cancer-specific morbidity and survival [122]. Evidence-based methods to improve abstinence among the general population should be effective in cancer survivors as well [123]. Among smokers diagnosed with cancer, several interventions have been effective including those with nurse-delivered interventions, telephone counselling, peer counselling, education, and nicotine replacement.

Smoking prevalence in cancer survivors varies by age and cancer type. Of considerable concern is the stunningly high rate in adult survivors aged 18–40 compared to the general population who smoke (38–45% compared to 26–30%) [124–126]. In this young adult population our efforts should include a focus on prevention as well as cessation [127]. Although lung cancer patients have higher smoking rates at diagnosis, there is a higher proportion that quit compared to colorectal cancer survivors [128] suggesting specific opportunities to improve care.

Physical activity, diet, and weight management

Physical activity/exercise, diet, and weight management are interconnected and are all emerging as important factors in cancer prevention. Exercise has been fairly well studied in cancer survivors and is associated with better quality of life, physical functioning [129], anthropometric measures, and social functioning, and with less sleep disturbance. Despite the myriad of improvements exercise can provide to survivors, the effect of exercise on cancer recurrence is unknown. More data is emerging showing that weight is independently associated with cancer outcomes. Given its integral part in weight management, along with diet, exercise becomes a target for cancer treatment.

To date, no specific diet has been found definitively to prevent cancer or cancer recurrence [130]. Several diet interventions have been carried out. The largest two are Women's Intervention Nutrition Study (WINS) randomizing 2437 postmenopausal breast cancer survivors to the intervention of a low-fat diet [131] and the Women's Healthy Eating and Living (WHEL) study of high vegetable and fruit intake in 3088 breast cancer survivors [133]. Encouragingly, both studies showed improvement in diet in the intervention arms, but the cancer endpoints were mixed. In the WINS trial, patients on the low-fat diet had lower breast cancer recurrence; however, there was no overall survival benefit. No difference in breast cancer recurrence or overall survival was seen in the WHEL study. Post hoc analyses suggested potential benefit for those who lost weight or those who were more physically active, underscoring the intrinsic relationship between diet, exercise, and weight management and their effects on cancer. Although more research is needed to understand these effects and to determine effective interventions, the American Cancer Society (ACS) has published general recommendations on nutrition and physical activity for survivors (Table 34.7) [130].

A diagnosis of cancer is often a life-changing event; patients can feel a loss of control and often explore ways to regain a sense of well-being. Improving lifestyle behaviours is one possible way of doing this, and this can have significant effects on their physical functioning, quality of life, and even cancer outcomes. Additionally, it is recognized that cancer survivors are also at increased risk of

Table 34.7 Modifiable health behaviours to consider in cancer survivors

	Evidence/situation	Recommendation
Tobacco cessation	Smoking is a carcinogen.	5As: Ask, Advise, Assess willingness to quit, Assist, Arrange follow-up
	Depression and alcohol/substance abuse may require more intense interventions	Both brief and intensive interventions are effective.
		National quit hotline
		Pharmacological treatment which reliably improved abstinence rates:
		◆ Buproprion SR
		◆ Nicotine replacement therapy
		◆ Varenicline
Alcohol use	Alcohol is a primary risk factor for head and neck, oesophageal and hepatocellular cancers.	Screening questions for at risk patients
		Physician recommendations
	It possibly increases risk of primary breast and colorectal.	Referral to counselling
		Pharmacologic deterrents:
	Moderate alcohol intake is likely safe.	◆ Naltrexone
		◆ Disulfiram
		ACS Guideline:
		Limit alcohol consumption to one drink/day for women and two drinks/day for men.
High-risk sexual behaviours and illicit drug abuse	HIV and HPV related cancers	Take a sexual history
		Counsel on risk reduction if appropriate
Diet	Mixed results on benefit of low fat/high fibre	ACS guidelines:
		Consume a healthy diet with emphasis on plant sources:
		◆ maintain healthy weight
		◆ 5+ vegetables and fruits/day
		◆ choose whole grains over processed
		◆ limit consumption of processed and red meats
		Focus on weight management
Physical activity/ exercise	Benefits include weight management, improves distress measures, and functional status.	ACS guidelines:
		Recommend 30+ minutes of vigorous exercise daily 5/week.
		Refer to physical and occupational therapy when appropriate to improve functional outcomes.
Weight management	Obesity is a risk factor for primary breast, colorectal, oesophagus, liver, gallbladder, pancreas, kidney, uterus, and advanced prostate cancer.	ACS guidelines:
		◆ Balance caloric intake with physical exercise
	Evidence suggests that obesity at diagnosis and weight gain may increase the risk of cancer recurrence for some types of cancer (breast, colorectal cancer).	◆ Avoid weight gain over time
		◆ Achieve and maintain a healthy weight if current overweight or obese.

Note: ACS guidelines are for cancer prevention (not specific to survivors).

Source: data from American Cancer Society, *Survivorship: During and After Treatment*, Copyright © 2015 American Cancer Society, Inc. All rights reserved. Available from http://www.cancer.org/Treatment/SurvivorshipDuringandAfterTreatment/index.

other diseases including heart disease, diabetes, and osteoporosis, all of which benefit from improved health behaviours.

Coordination of care

One area of active research is optimal follow-up care for survivors. Some survivors' needs are unique, but not generally out of the purview of primary care providers. Randomized controlled trials of early stage breast cancer patients have demonstrated no difference in cancer outcomes regardless of whether an oncologist or a primary care doctor who is educated about patients' cancer-related

concerns provides follow-up care [133]. Surveys of both Canadian and US primary care physicians consistently show that there is reasonable willingness to care for survivors, even exclusively, but that most want specific guidelines, open communication with the oncologist, and specific survivorship training [134–136]. This model of care-sharing by primary care doctors has been readily adopted for many medical subspecialties including psychiatry, cardiology, neurology, nephrology, and endocrinology. The willingness of primary care doctors, stipulated upon need for guidance, underscores the need for development of comprehensive evidenced-based survivorship guidelines. Taking this a step further, countries with nationalized healthcare that recognize the importance of self-management in the process of recovery from cancer have begun to develop programmes in this area [137].

Survivorship care planning

One proposal to assist in coordination of care has been survivorship care plans [8]. It has been recommended that every cancer survivor receive a care plan which contains a personal treatment summary, as well as possible late/long-term effects, signs of recurrence, guidelines on follow-up care, identification of a patient's providers, lifestyle recommendations, and supportive resources [8, 138–140]. Early studies of survivorship care plans have been mixed; one randomized controlled trial evaluating the effects of care plans showed no difference in patient-reported outcomes [141]. Further, the ideal structures for provider–patient and provider–provider communications in survivorship remain unknown. Regardless, there is clearly a need for improved communications: in practice, it appears that little information is provided to patients who have completed active treatment. A population-based survey found that only 40% received written summary of treatment, and only 74% received follow-up instructions [142], suggesting significant room for improvement. There are resources available to assist providers and patients in care planning from the office of cancer survivorship at NCI [143], through the Lance Armstrong Foundation [144], and through ACS [145]. These resources are being developed internationally and country-specific resources are mounting (e.g., National Cancer Survivorship Institute in the UK [146]) [137].

Clinical practice guidelines

Guidelines for survivorship care are cancer-type specific and can be tailored for the individual's cancer subtype, stage, and treatment received. There are a myriad of different guidelines published by reputable cancer organizations, which were compiled and reviewed by Committee on Cancer Survivorship and published in *Cancer Patient to Cancer Survivor* [8]. Ideally guidelines would address all aspects of survivorship issues, namely: (1) surveillance for recurrent disease; (2) monitoring/prevention of a second primary; (3) management of late sequelae of disease; (4) management of late complications of treatment; (5) management of psychological, social, and spiritual issues; (6) management of genetic issues (reviewed in Chapter 31) and 7) locus of care [8]. However, existing guidelines tend to focus on surveillance and screening with far fewer addressing issues of physical late effects and fewer addressing psychosocial concerns. Furthermore, many recommendations rely on expert consensus/opinion rather than high-quality evidence. Recently, ASCO launched a survivorship committee that plans to develop guidelines focused on survivorship care.

Conclusion: future directions

As cancer incidence and life expectancy after a cancer diagnosis continue to increase, a higher proportion of the population will be cancer survivors. Survivors face unique challenges in terms of disability, chance of recurrence, or second primary malignancy and long-term or late effects of disease or treatment (physical and psychosocial) that are important to recognize and address. Much of the research thus far has been focused on documenting these issues.

Providing optimal survivorship care to all patients with a history of cancer requires evidence-based clinical practice guidelines and systems to implement them. At present, however, there are substantial limitations to the evidence base, available guidelines, and current care delivery systems for cancer survivors. To address these significant gaps, the NCI has delineated several priorities for survivorship research including: (1) chronic and late effects; (2) interventions; (3) healthy lifestyles and behavior; and (4) family issues [115]. Continued efforts to coordinate survivorship care, incorporating new information as it comes along, is also paramount to enhance the lives of the growing population of cancer survivors.

Further reading

Carver JR, Shapiro CL, Ng A, Jacobs L, Schwartz C et al. American Society of Clinical Oncology clinical evidence review on the ongoing care of adult cancer survivors: cardiac and pulmonary late effects. Journal of Clinical Oncology 2007; 25(25): 3991–4008.

de Moor JS, Mariotto AB, Parry C, Alfano CM, Padgett L et al. Cancer survivors in the United States: prevalence across the survivorship trajectory and implications for care. Cancer Epidemiology, Biomarkers & Prevention 2013; 22(4): 561–570.

Foster C, Wright D, Hill H, Hopkinson J, Roffe L. Psychosocial implications of living 5 years or more following a cancer diagnosis: a systematic review of the research evidence. .European Journal of Cancer Care (Engl) 2009; 18(3): 223–247.

From Cancer Patient to Cancer Survivor Lost in Transition. Washington, DC: National Academy of Sciences, 2006.

Hewitt M, Rowland JH, Yancik R. Cancer survivors in the United States: age, health, and disability. Journals of Gerontology Series A: Biological Sciences and Medical Sciences 2003; 58(1): 82–91.

Jones LW, Courneya KS, Fairey AS, Mackey JR. Effects of an oncologist's recommendation to exercise on self-reported exercise behavior in newly diagnosed breast cancer survivors: a single-blind, randomized controlled trial. Annals of Behavioral Medicine 2004; 28(2): 105–113.

Koch L, Jansen L, Brenner H, Arndt V. Fear of recurrence and disease progression in long-term (>/=5 years) cancer survivors-a systematic review of quantitative studies. Psychooncology 2012; 22(1): 1–11.

Lee SJ, Schover LR, Partridge AH, Patrizio P, Wallace WH et al. American Society of Clinical Oncology recommendations on fertility preservation in cancer patients. Journal of Clinical Oncology 2006; 24(18): 2917–2931.

Palli D, Russo A, Saieva C, Ciatto S, Rosselli Del Turco M et al. Intensive vs clinical follow-up after treatment of primary breast cancer: 10-year update of a randomized trial. National Research Council Project on Breast Cancer Follow-up. Journal of the American Medical Association 1999; 281(17): 1586.

Weaver KE, Rowland JH, Alfano CM, McNeel TS. Parental cancer and the family: a population-based estimate of the number of US cancer survivors residing with their minor children. Cancer 2010; 116(18): 4395–4401.

References

1. Mullan F. Seasons of survival: reflections of a physician with cancer. New England Journal of Medicine 1985; 313(4): 270–273.
2. National Coalition for Cancer Survivorship, 2012. Available from: <http://www.canceradvocacy.org/>, accessed on 8 March 2012.
3. Howlader N, Noone AM, Krapcho M, Neyman N, Aminou R et al. eds. SEER Cancer Statistics Review. National Cancer Institute based on November 2010 SEER data submission, posted to the SEER website, 2011. Available from: <http://seer.cancer.gov/csr/1975_2008/>, accessed on March 8, 2012.
4. de Moor JS, Mariotto AB, Parry C, Alfano CM, Padgett L et al. Cancer survivors in the United States: prevalence across

the survivorship trajectory and implications for care. Cancer Epidemiology, Biomarkers & Prevention 2013; 22(4): 561–570.

5. Edwards BK, Howe HL, Ries LA, Thun MJ, Rosenberg HM et al. Annual report to the nation on the status of cancer, 1973–1999, featuring implications of age and aging on US cancer burden. Cancer 2002; 94(10): 2766–2792.

6. Maddams J, Brewster D, Gavin A, Steward J, Elliott J et al. Cancer prevalence in the United Kingdom: estimates for 2008. British Journal of Cancer 2009; 101(3): 541–547.

7. Pisani P, Bray F, Parkin DM. Estimates of the world-wide prevalence of cancer for 25 sites in the adult population. International Journal of Cancer 2002; 97(1): 72–81.

8. From Cancer Patient to Cancer Survivor Lost in Transition. Washington, DC: National Academy of Sciences, 2006.

9. Impact of follow-up testing on survival and health-related quality of life in breast cancer patients. A multicenter randomized controlled trial. The GIVIO Investigators. Journal of the American Medical Association 1994; 271(20): 1587–1592.

10. Palli D, Russo A, Saieva C, Ciatto S, Rosselli Del Turco M et al. Intensive vs clinical follow-up after treatment of primary breast cancer: 10-year update of a randomized trial. National Research Council Project on Breast Cancer Follow-up. Journal of the American Medical Association 1999; 281(17): 1586.

11. Rojas MP, Telaro E, Russo A, Moschetti I, Coe L et al. Follow-up strategies for women treated for early breast cancer. Cochrane Database Systemic Reviews 2005(1): CD001768.

12. Rosselli Del Turco M, Palli D, Cariddi A, Ciatto S, Pacini P et al. Intensive diagnostic follow-up after treatment of primary breast cancer. A randomized trial. National Research Council Project on Breast Cancer follow-up. Journal of the American Medical Association 1994; 271(20): 1593–1597.

13. Rustin GJ, van der Burg ME, Griffin CL, Guthrie D, Lamont A et al. Early versus delayed treatment of relapsed ovarian cancer (MRC OV05/EORTC 55955): a randomised trial. Lancet 2010; 376(9747): 1155–1163.

14. Testicular cancer. NCCN clinical practice guidelines in Oncology 2012; 1.2012. Available from: <http://www.nccn.org/professionals/physician_gls/pdf/testicular.pdf>, accessed on 11 April 2012.

15. Jeffery M, Hickey BE, Hider PN. Follow-up strategies for patients treated for non-metastatic colorectal cancer. Cochrane Database Systemic Reviews 2007(1): CD002200.

16. Follow up after Colorectal Surgery (FACS) Trial. Available from: <http://www.facs.soton.ac.uk/>, accessed on 14 March 2012.

17. Grossmann EM, Johnson FE, Virgo KS, Longo WE, Fossati R. Follow-up of colorectal cancer patients after resection with curative intent-the GILDA trial. Surgical Oncology 2004; 13(2-3): 119–124.

18. Wille-Jorgensen P, Laurberg S, Pahlman L, Carriquiry L, Lundqvist N et al. An interim analysis of recruitment to the COLOFOL trial. Colorectal Disease 2009; 11(7): 756–758.

19. Hodgson DC, Grunfeld E, Gunraj N, Del Giudice L. A population-based study of follow-up care for Hodgkin lymphoma survivors: opportunities to improve surveillance for relapse and late effects. Cancer 2010; 116(14): 3417–3425.

20. Snyder CF, Earle CC, Herbert RJ, Neville BA, Blackford AL et al. Preventive care for colorectal cancer survivors: a 5-year longitudinal study. Journal of Clinical Oncology 2008; 26(7): 1073–1079.

21. Nathan PC, Ness KK, Mahoney MC, Li Z, Hudson MM et al. Screening and surveillance for second malignant neoplasms in adult survivors of childhood cancer: a report from the childhood cancer survivor study. Annals of Internal Medicine 2010; 153(7): 442–451.

22. Partridge AH, LaFountain A, Mayer E, Taylor BS, Winer E et al. Adherence to initial adjuvant anastrozole therapy among women with early-stage breast cancer. Journal of Clinical Oncology 2008; 26(4): 556–562.

23. Partridge AH, Wang PS, Winer EP, Avorn J. Nonadherence to adjuvant tamoxifen therapy in women with primary breast cancer. Journal of Clinical Oncology 2003; 21(4): 602–606.

24. Demissie S, Silliman RA, Lash TL. Adjuvant tamoxifen: predictors of use, side effects, and discontinuation in older women. Journal of Clinical Oncology 2001; 19(2): 322–328.

25. Aziz NM, Rowland JH. Trends and advances in cancer survivorship research: challenge and opportunity. Seminars in Radiation Oncology 2003; 13(3): 248–266.

26. Hewitt M, Rowland JH, Yancik R. Cancer survivors in the United States: age, health, and disability. Journals of Gerontology Series A: Biological Sciences and Medical Sciences 2003; 58(1): 82–91.

27. Yabroff KR, Lawrence WF, Clauser S, Davis WW, Brown ML. Burden of illness in cancer survivors: findings from a population-based national sample. Journal of the National Cancer Institute 2004; 96(17): 1322–1330.

28. Palesh OG, Roscoe JA, Mustian KM, Roth T, Savard J et al. Prevalence, demographics, and psychological associations of sleep disruption in patients with cancer: University of Rochester Cancer Center-Community Clinical Oncology Program. Journal of Clinical Oncology 2010; 28(2): 292–298.

29. Braun IM, Greenberg DB, Pirl WF. Evidenced-based report on the occurrence of fatigue in long-term cancer survivors. Journal of the National Comprehensive Cancer Institute 2008; 6(4): 347–354.

30. Bower JE, Ganz PA, Desmond KA, Bernaards C, Rowland JH et al. Fatigue in long-term breast carcinoma survivors: a longitudinal investigation. Cancer 2006; 106(4): 751–758.

31. Bower JE, Ganz PA, Desmond KA, Rowland JH, Meyerowitz BE et al. Fatigue in breast cancer survivors: occurrence, correlates, and impact on quality of life. Journal of Clinical Oncology 2000; 18(4): 743–753.

32. Carr D, Goudas L, Lawrence D, Pirl W, Lau J et al. Management of Cancer Symptoms: Pain, Depression, and Fatigue. Evidence Report/Technology Assessment No. 61 (Prepared by the New England Medical Center Evidence-based Practice Center under Contract No 290-97-0019). Rockville, MD: Agency for Healthcare Research and Quality, 2002.

33. Cella D, Davis K, Breitbart W, Curt G. Cancer-related fatigue: prevalence of proposed diagnostic criteria in a United States sample of cancer survivors. Journal of Clinical Oncology 2001; 19(14): 3385–3391.

34. Hjermstad MJ, Fossa SD, Oldervoll L, Holte H, Jacobsen AB et al. Fatigue in long-term Hodgkin's Disease survivors: a follow-up study. Journal of Clinical Oncology 2005; 23(27): 6587–6595.

35. Loge JH, Abrahamsen AF, Ekeberg O, Kaasa S. Hodgkin's disease survivors more fatigued than the general population. Journal of Clinical Oncology 1999; 17(1): 253–261.

36. Okuyama T, Akechi T, Kugaya A, Okamura H, Imoto S et al. Factors correlated with fatigue in disease-free breast cancer patients: application of the Cancer Fatigue Scale. Supportive Care in Cancer 2000; 8(3): 215–222.

37. Cancer-Related Fatigue NCCN clinical practice guidelines in Oncology 2012; <http://www.nccn.org/professionals/physician_gls/pdf/fatigue.pdf>, accessed on 14 March 2012.

38. Knudsen AK, Aass N, Fainsinger R, Caraceni A, Klepstad P et al. Classification of pain in cancer patients—a systematic literature review. Palliative Medicine 2009; 23(4): 295–308.

39. Burton AW, Fanciullo GJ, Beasley RD, Fisch MJ. Chronic pain in the cancer survivor: a new frontier. Pain Medicine 2007; 8(2): 189–198.

40. Perkins FM, Kehlet H. Chronic pain as an outcome of surgery: a review of predictive factors. Anesthesiology 2000; 93(4): 1123–1133.

41. WHO's Pain Relief Ladder, 2012. Available from: <http://www.who.int/cancer/palliative/painladder/en/>, accessed on 3 April 2012.

42. Adult Cancer Pain, 2011, version 2.2011. Available from: <http://www.nccn.org/professionals/physician_gls/pdf/pain.pdf>, accessed on 3 April 2012.

43. Vardy J, Tannock I. Cognitive function after chemotherapy in adults with solid tumours. Critical Reviews in Oncology/Hematology 2007; 63(3): 183–202.

44. Wefel JS, Vardy J, Ahles T, Schagen SB. International Cognition and Cancer Task Force recommendations to harmonise studies of cognitive function in patients with cancer. Lancet Oncology 2011; 12(7): 703–708.

45. Hequet O, Le QH, Moullet I, Pauli E, Salles G et al. Subclinical late cardiomyopathy after doxorubicin therapy for lymphoma in adults. Journal of Clinical Oncology 2004; 22(10): 1864–1871.

46. Doyle JJ, Neugut AI, Jacobson JS, Grann VR, Hershman DL. Chemotherapy and cardiotoxicity in older breast cancer patients: a population-based study. Journal of Clinical Oncology 2005; 23(34): 8597–8605.

47. Gietema JA, Sleijfer DT, Willemse PH, Schraffordt Koops H, van Ittersum E et al. Long-term follow-up of cardiovascular risk factors in patients given chemotherapy for disseminated nonseminomatous testicular cancer. Annals of Internal Medicine 1992; 116(9): 709–715.

48. Zagars GK, Ballo MT, Lee AK, Strom SS. Mortality after cure of testicular seminoma. Journal of Clinical Oncology 2004; 22(4): 640–647.

49. Carver JR, Shapiro CL, Ng A, Jacobs L, Schwartz C et al. American Society of Clinical Oncology clinical evidence review on the ongoing care of adult cancer survivors: cardiac and pulmonary late effects. Journal of Clinical Oncology 2007; 25(25): 3991–4008.

50. Ewer MS, Vooletich MT, Durand JB, Woods ML, Davis JR et al. Reversibility of trastuzumab-related cardiotoxicity: new insights based on clinical course and response to medical treatment. Journal of Clinical Oncology 2005; 23(31): 7820–7826.

51. Tan-Chiu E, Yothers G, Romond E, Geyer CE Jr, Ewer M et al. Assessment of cardiac dysfunction in a randomized trial comparing doxorubicin and cyclophosphamide followed by paclitaxel, with or without trastuzumab as adjuvant therapy in node-positive, human epidermal growth factor receptor 2-overexpressing breast cancer: NSABP B-31. Journal of Clinical Oncology 2005; 23(31): 7811–7819.

52. Perez EA, Suman VJ, Davidson NE, Sledge GW, Kaufman PA et al. Cardiac safety analysis of doxorubicin and cyclophosphamide followed by paclitaxel with or without trastuzumab in the North Central Cancer Treatment Group N9831 adjuvant breast cancer trial. Journal of Clinical Oncology 2008; 26(8): 1231–1238.

53. Telli ML, Hunt SA, Carlson RW, Guardino AE. Trastuzumab-related cardiotoxicity: calling into question the concept of reversibility. Journal of Clinical Oncology 2007; 25(23): 3525–3533.

54. Richards CJ, Je Y, Schutz FA, Heng DY, Dallabrida SM et al. Incidence and risk of congestive heart failure in patients with renal and nonrenal cell carcinoma treated with sunitinib. Journal of Clinical Oncology 2011; 29(25): 3450–3456.

55. Demirci S, Nam J, Hubbs JL, Nguyen T, Marks LB. Radiation-induced cardiac toxicity after therapy for breast cancer: interaction between treatment era and follow-up duration. International Journal of Radiation Oncology * Biology * Physics 2009; 73(4): 980–987.

56. Sleijfer S. Bleomycin-induced pneumonitis. Chest 2001; 120(2): 617–624.

57. O'Sullivan JM, Huddart RA, Norman AR, Nicholls J, Dearnaley DP et al. Predicting the risk of bleomycin lung toxicity in patients with germ-cell tumours. Annals of Oncology 2003; 14(1): 91–96.

58. Barber NA, Ganti AK. Pulmonary toxicities from targeted therapies: a review. Targeted Oncology 2011; 6(4): 235–243.

59. McDonald S, Rubin P, Phillips TL, Marks LB. Injury to the lung from cancer therapy: clinical syndromes, measurable endpoints, and potential scoring systems. International Journal of Radiation Oncology * Biology * Physics 1995; 31(5): 1187–1203.

60. Tarbell NJ, Thompson L, Mauch P. Thoracic irradiation in Hodgkin's disease: disease control and long-term complications. International Journal of Radiation Oncology * Biology * Physics 1990; 18(2): 275–281.

61. Harris S. Radiotherapy for early and advanced breast cancer. International Journal of Clinical Practice 2001; 55(9): 609–612.

62. Granena A, Carreras E, Rozman C, Salgado C, Sierra J et al. Interstitial pneumonitis after BMT: 15 years experience in a single institution. Bone Marrow Transplantation 1993; 11(6): 453–458.

63. Hancock SL, Cox RS, McDougall IR. Thyroid diseases after treatment of Hodgkin's disease. New England Journal of Medicine 1991; 325(9): 599–605.

64. Desai J, Yassa L, Marqusee E, George S, Frates MC et al. Hypothyroidism after sunitinib treatment for patients with gastrointestinal stromal tumors. Annals of Internal Medicine 2006; 145(9): 660–664.

65. Littley MD, Shalet SM, Morgenstern GR, Deakin DP. Endocrine and reproductive dysfunction following fractionated total body irradiation in adults. QJ: International Journal of Medicine 1991; 78(287): 265–274.

66. Baker KS, Gurney JG, Ness KK, Bhatia R, Forman SJ et al. Late effects in survivors of chronic myeloid leukemia treated with hematopoietic cell transplantation: results from the Bone Marrow Transplant Survivor Study. Blood 2004; 104(6): 1898–1906.

67. Head and Neck. NCCN clinical practice guidelines in oncology 2012, version 1.2012. Available from: <http://www.nccn.org/professionals/physician_gls/f_guidelines.asp>, accessed on 21 May 2015.

68. Hillner BE, Ingle JN, Chlebowski RT, Gralow J, Yee GC, et al. American Society of Clinical Oncology 2003 update on the role of bisphosphonates and bone health issues in women with breast cancer. Journal of Clinical Oncology2003; 21(21): 4042–4057.

69. Breast Cancer. NCCN clinical practice guidelines in oncology 2012. Available from: <http://www.nccn.org/professionals/physician_gls/pdf/breast.pdf>, accessed on 14 March 2012.

70. Prostate Cancer. NCCN clinical practice guidelines in ncology 2012. Available from: <http://www.nccn.org/professionals/physician_gls/pdf/breast.pdf>, accessed on 14 March 2012.

71. Gralow JR, Biermann JS, Farooki A, et al. NCCN Task Force Report: Bone Health in Cancer Care. Journal of the National Comprehensive Cancer Institute 2009; 7(Suppl. 3): S1–S32; quiz S33–S35.

72. Aebi S, Davidson T, Gruber G, Cardoso F. Primary breast cancer: ESMO Clinical Practice Guidelines for diagnosis, treatment and follow-up. Annals of Oncology 2011; 22(Suppl. 6): vi12–24.

73. Demark-Wahnefried W, Campbell KL, Hayes SC. Weight management and its role in breast cancer rehabilitation. Cancer 2012; 118(8 Suppl.): 2277–2287.

74. Lawenda BD, Mondry TE, Johnstone PA. Lymphedema: a primer on the identification and management of a chronic condition in oncologic treatment. CA: A Cancer Journal for Clinicians 2009; 59(1): 8–24.

75. Didem K, Ufuk YS, Serdar S, Zumre A. The comparison of two different physiotherapy methods in treatment of lymphedema after breast surgery. Breast Cancer Research and Treatment 2005; 93(1): 49–54.

76. Schmitz KH, Ahmed RL, Troxel A, Cheville A, Smith R et al. Weight lifting in women with breast-cancer-related lymphedema. New England Journal of Medicine 2009; 361(7): 664–673.

77. Sprangers MA, Taal BG, Aaronson NK, te Velde A. Quality of life in colorectal cancer. Stoma vs. nonstoma patients. Diseases of the Colon & Rectum 1995; 38(4): 361–369.

78. Pachler J, Wille-Jorgensen P. Quality of life after rectal resection for cancer, with or without permanent colostomy. Cochrane Database Systemic Reviews 2005(2): CD004323.

79. Krychman ML, Pereira L, Carter J, Amsterdam A. Sexual oncology: sexual health issues in women with cancer. Oncology 2006; 71(1–2): 18–25.

80. Park ER, Norris RL, Bober SL. Sexual health communication during cancer care: barriers and recommendations. Cancer Journal 2009; 15(1): 74–77.

81. Ganz PA, Greendale GA, Petersen L, Zibecchi L, Kahn B et al. Managing menopausal symptoms in breast cancer survivors: results of a randomized controlled trial. Journal of the National Cancer Institute 2000; 92(13): 1054–1064.

82. Lee SJ, Schover LR, Partridge AH, Patrizio P, Wallace WH et al. American Society of Clinical Oncology recommendations on fertility preservation in cancer patients. Journal of Clinical Oncology 2006; 24(18): 2917–2931.

83. Gardino SL, Russell AE, Woodruff TK. Adoption after cancer: adoption agency attitudes and perspectives on the potential to parent post-cancer. Cancer Treatment Research 2010; 156: 153–170.

84. Livestrong.com, <http://www.livestrong.com/fertility>.

85. MyOncofertility.org <http://myoncofertility.org/>.

86. Paik S, Tang G, Shak S, Kim C, Baker J et al. Gene expression and benefit of chemotherapy in women with node-negative, estrogen receptor-positive breast cancer. Journal of Clinical Oncology 2006; 24(23): 3726–3734.

87. Bacci G, Forni C, Longhi A, Ferrari S, Mercuri M et al. Local recurrence and local control of non-metastatic osteosarcoma of the extremities: a 27-year experience in a single institution. Journal of Surgical Oncology 2007; 96(2): 118–123.

88. Induction chemotherapy plus radiation compared with surgery plus radiation in patients with advanced laryngeal cancer. The Department of Veterans Affairs Laryngeal Cancer Study Group. New England Journal of Medicine 1991; 324(24): 1685–1690.

89. Cote GM, Canellos GP. Can low-risk, early-stage patients with Hodgkin lymphoma be spared radiotherapy? Current Hematologic Malignancy Reports 2011; 6(3): 180–186.

90. Arden-Close E, Gidron Y, Moss-Morris R. Psychological distress and its correlates in ovarian cancer: a systematic review. Psychooncology 2008; 17(11): 1061–1072.

91. Pirl WF. Evidence report on the occurrence, assessment, and treatment of depression in cancer patients. Journal of the National Cancer Institute Monographs 2004(32): 32–39.

92. Foster C, Wright D, Hill H, Hopkinson J, Roffe L. Psychosocial implications of living 5 years or more following a cancer diagnosis: a systematic review of the research evidence. .European Journal of Cancer Care (Engl) 2009; 18(3): 223–247.

93. Falagas ME, Zarkadoulia EA, Ioannidou EN, Peppas G, Christodoulou C et al. The effect of psychosocial factors on breast cancer outcome: a systematic review. Breast Cancer Research 2007; 9(4): R44.

94. Fang F, Fall K, Mittleman MA, Sparén P, Ye W et al. Suicide and cardiovascular death after a cancer diagnosis. New England Journal of Medicine 2012; 366(14): 1310–1318.

95. Rodin G, Lloyd N, Katz M, Green E, Mackay JA et al. The treatment of depression in cancer patients: a systematic review. Supportive Care in Cancer 2007; 15(2): 123–136.

96. Sheard T, Maguire P. The effect of psychological interventions on anxiety and depression in cancer patients: results of two meta-analyses. British Journal of Cancer 1999; 80(11): 1770–1780.

97. Smith K, Lesko LM. Psychosocial problems in cancer survivors. Oncology (Williston Park) 1988; 2(1): 33–44.

98. Lee-Jones C, Humphris G, Dixon R, Hatcher MB. Fear of cancer recurrence—a literature review and proposed cognitive formulation to explain exacerbation of recurrence fears. Psychooncology 1997; 6(2): 95–105.

99. Koch L, Jansen L, Brenner H, Arndt V. Fear of recurrence and disease progression in long-term (>/=5 years) cancer survivors-a systematic review of quantitative studies. Psychooncology 2012; 22(1): 1–11.

100. Bower JE, Meyerowitz BE, Desmond KA, Bernaards CA, Rowland JH et al. Perceptions of positive meaning and vulnerability following breast cancer: predictors and outcomes among long-term breast cancer survivors. Annals of Behavioral Medicine 2005; 29(3): 236–245.

101. Fromm K, Andrykowski MA, Hunt J. Positive and negative psychosocial sequelae of bone marrow transplantation: implications for quality of life assessment. Journal of Behavioral Medicine 1996; 19(3): 221–240.

102. Foley KL, Farmer DF, Petronis VM, Smith RG, McGraw S et al. A qualitative exploration of the cancer experience among long-term survivors: comparisons by cancer type, ethnicity, gender, and age. Psychooncology 2006; 15(3): 248–258.

103. Eiser C, Penn A, Katz E, Barr R. Psychosocial issues and quality of life. Seminars in Oncology 2009; 36(3): 275–280.

104. Abrahamsen AF, Loge JH, Hannisdal E, Holte H, Kvaloy S. Socio-medical situation for long-term survivors of Hodgkin's disease: a survey of 459 patients treated at one institution. European Journal of Cancer 1998; 34(12): 1865–1870.

105. Gilbert E, Ussher JM, Perz J. Sexuality after breast cancer: a review. Maturitas 2010; 66(4): 397–407.

106. Glantz MJ, Chamberlain MC, Liu Q, Hsieh CC, Edwards KR et al. Gender disparity in the rate of partner abandonment in patients with serious medical illness. Cancer 2009; 115(22): 5237–5242.

107. Koch SV, Kejs AM, Engholm G, Moller H, Johansen C et al. Marriage and divorce among childhood cancer survivors. Journal of Pediatric Hematology/Oncology 2011; 33(7): 500–505.

108. Goldzweig G, Hubert A, Walach N, et al. Gender and psychological distress among middle- and older-aged colorectal cancer patients and their spouses: an unexpected outcome. Critical Reviews in Oncology/Hematology 2009; 70(1): 71–82.

109. Kraemer LM, Stanton AL, Meyerowitz BE, Rowland JH, Ganz PA. A longitudinal examination of couples' coping strategies as predictors of adjustment to breast cancer. Journal of Family Psychology 2011; 25(6): 963–972.

110. Kim Y, Kashy DA, Wellisch DK, Spillers RL, Kaw CK et al. Quality of life of couples dealing with cancer: dyadic and individual adjustment among breast and prostate cancer survivors and their spousal caregivers. Annals of Behavioral Medicine 2008; 35(2): 230–238.

111. Pinquart M, Duberstein PR. Associations of social networks with cancer mortality: a meta-analysis. Critical Reviews in Oncology/Hematology 2010; 75(2): 122–137.

112. Weaver KE, Rowland JH, Alfano CM, McNeel TS. Parental cancer and the family: a population-based estimate of the number of US cancer survivors residing with their minor children. Cancer 2010; 116(18): 4395–4401.

113. Semple CJ, McCance T. Parents' experience of cancer who have young children: a literature review. Cancer Nursing 2010; 33(2): 110–118.

114. Muriel AC, Moore CW, Baer L, Park ER, Kornblith AB et al. Measuring psychosocial distress and parenting concerns among adults with cancer: The Parenting Concerns Questionnaire. Cancer 2012; 118(22): 5671–5678.

115. National Cancer Institute: Cancer Survivorship Research, 2012. Available from: <http://dccps.nci.nih.gov/ocs/>, accessed on 21 May 2015.

116. Sabatino SA, Coates RJ, Uhler RJ, Alley LG, Pollack LA. Health insurance coverage and cost barriers to needed medical care among U.S. adult cancer survivors age<65 years. Cancer 2006; 106(11): 2466–2475.

117. Arozullah AM, Calhoun EA, Wolf M, Finley DK, Fitzner KA et al. The financial burden of cancer: estimates from a study of insured women with breast cancer. Journal of Supportive Oncology 2004; 2(3): 271–278.

118. Langa KM, Fendrick AM, Chernew ME, Kabeto MU, Paisley KL et al. Out-of-pocket health-care expenditures among older Americans with cancer. Value in Health 2004; 7(2): 186–194.

119. Weaver KE, Rowland JH, Bellizzi KM, Aziz NM. Forgoing medical care because of cost: assessing disparities in healthcare access among cancer survivors living in the United States. Cancer 2010; 116(14): 3493–3504.

120. Jones LW, Courneya KS, Fairey AS, Mackey JR. Effects of an oncologist's recommendation to exercise on self-reported exercise behavior in newly diagnosed breast cancer survivors: a single-blind, randomized controlled trial. Annals of Behavioral Medicine 2004; 28(2): 105–113.

121. Garces YI, Schroeder DR, Nirelli LM, Croghan GA, Croghan IT et al. Tobacco use outcomes among patients with head and neck carcinoma treated for nicotine dependence: a matched-pair analysis. Cancer 2004; 101(1): 116–124.

122. Gritz ER, Dresler C, Sarna L. Smoking, the missing drug interaction in clinical trials: ignoring the obvious. Cancer Epidemiology, Biomarkers & Prevention 2005; 14(10): 2287–2293.

123. A clinical practice guideline for treating tobacco use and dependence: 2008 update. A US Public Health Service report. American Journal of Preventive Medicine 2008; 35(2): 158–176.

124. Bellizzi KM, Rowland JH, Jeffery DD, McNeel T. Health behaviors of cancer survivors: examining opportunities for cancer control intervention. Journal of Clinical Oncology 2005; 23(34): 8884–8893.

125. Coups EJ, Ostroff JS. A population-based estimate of the prevalence of behavioral risk factors among adult cancer survivors and noncancer controls. Preventive Medicine 2005; 40(6): 702–711.

126. Tseng TS, Lin HY, Martin MY, Chen T, Partridge EE. Disparities in smoking and cessation status among cancer survivors and non-cancer individuals: a population-based study from National Health and Nutrition Examination Survey. Journal of Cancer Survivorship 2010; 4(4): 313–321.

127. Klosky JL, Tyc VL, Garces-Webb DM, Buscemi J, Klesges RC et al. Emerging issues in smoking among adolescent and adult cancer survivors: a comprehensive review. Cancer 2007; 110(11): 2408–2419.

128. Park ER, Japuntich SJ, Rigotti NA, Traeger L, He Y et al. A snapshot of smokers after lung and colorectal cancer diagnosis. Cancer 2012; 118(12): 3153–3164.

129. Morey MC, Snyder DC, Sloane R, Cohen HJ, Peterson B et al. Effects of home-based diet and exercise on functional outcomes among older, overweight long-term cancer survivors: RENEW: a randomized controlled trial. Journal of the American Medical Association 2009; 301(18): 1883–1891.

130. Doyle C, Kushi LH, Byers T, Courneya KS, Demark-Wahnefried W et al. Nutrition and physical activity during and after cancer treatment: an American Cancer Society guide for informed choices. CA: A Cancer Journal for Clinicians 2006; 56(6): 323–353.

131. Chlebowski RT, Blackburn GL, Thomson CA, Nixon DW, Shapiro A et al. Dietary fat reduction and breast cancer outcome: interim efficacy results from the Women's Intervention Nutrition Study. Journal of the National Cancer Institute 2006; 98(24): 1767–1776.

132. Pierce JP, Natarajan L, Caan BJ, Parker BA, Greenberg ER et al. Influence of a diet very high in vegetables, fruit, and fiber and low in fat on prognosis following treatment for breast cancer: the Women's Healthy Eating and Living (WHEL) randomized trial. Journal of the American Medical Association 2007; 298(3): 289–298.

133. Grunfeld E, Levine MN, Julian JA, Coyle D, Szechtman B et al. Randomized trial of long-term follow-up for early-stage breast cancer: a comparison of family physician versus specialist care. Journal of Clinical Oncology 2006; 24(6): 848–855.

134. Bober SL, Recklitis CJ, Campbell EG, Park ER, Kutner JS et al. Caring for cancer survivors: a survey of primary care physicians. Cancer 2009; 115(18 Suppl.): 4409–4418.

135. Del Giudice ME, Grunfeld E, Harvey BJ, Piliotis E, Verma S. Primary care physicians' views of routine follow-up care of cancer survivors. Journal of Clinical Oncology 2009; 27(20): 3338–3345.

136. Nissen MJ, Beran MS, Lee MW, Mehta SR, Pine DA et al. Views of primary care providers on follow-up care of cancer patients. Family Medicine 2007; 39(7): 477–482.

137. Jefford M, Rowland J, Grunfeld E, Richards M, Maher J, Glaser A. Implementing improved post-treatment care for cancer survivors in England, with reflections from Australia, Canada and the USA. British Journal of Cancer 2013; 108(1): 14–20.

138. Earle CC. Failing to plan is planning to fail: improving the quality of care with survivorship care plans. Journal of Clinical Oncology 2006; 24(32): 5112–5116.

139. Grunfeld E, Earle CC. The interface between primary and oncology specialty care: treatment through survivorship. Journal of the National Cancer Institute Monographs 2010; 2010(40): 25–30.

140. Miller R. Implementing a survivorship care plan for patients with breast cancer. Clinical Journal of Oncology Nursing 2008; 12(3): 479–487.

141. Grunfeld E, Julian JA, Pond G, Maunsell E, Coyle D et al. Evaluating survivorship care plans: results of a randomized, clinical trial of patients with breast cancer. Journal of Clinical Oncology 2011; 29(36): 4755–4762.

142. Underwood JM, Townsend JS, Stewart SL, Buchannan N, Ekwueme DU et al. Surveillance of demographic characteristics and health behaviors among adult cancer survivors—Behavioral Risk Factor Surveillance System, United States, 2009. MMWR Surveillance Summaries 2012; 61(1): 1–23.

143. NCI, Office of Cancer Survivorship, <http://dccps.nci.nih.gov/ocs/>.

144. Lance Armstrong Foundation, <http://www.livestrong.org/>.

145. American Cancer Society, Surviorship: During and After Treatment, <http://www.cancer.org/Treatment/SurvivorshipDuringandAfterTreatment/index>.

146. National Cancer Survivorship Institute, <http://www.ncsi.org.uk/>.

SECTION 6

Disease orientated chapters

35 Head and neck cancer *329*

Christine H. Chung, Andreas Dietz, Vincent Gregoire, Marco Guzzo, Marc Hamoir, C. René Leemans, Jean-Louis Lefebvre, Lisa Licitra, Adel K. El-Naggar, Brian O'Sullivan, I. Bing Tan, Vincent Vandecaveye, Vincent Vander Poorten, Jan B. Vermorken, and Michelle D. Williams

36 Oesophageal cancer *365*

Piet Dirix, Karin Haustermans, Eric Van Cutsem, Xavier Sagaert, Christophe M. Deroose, Philippe Nafteux, Hans Prenen, and Toni Lerut

37 Gastric cancer *388*

Hideaki Bando, Takahiro Kinoshita, Yasutoshi Kuboki, Atsushi Ohtsu, and Kohei Shitara

38 Rectal cancer and systemic therapy of colorectal cancer *408*

Regina Beets-Tan, Bengt Glimelius, and Lars Påhlman

39 Colorectal cancer *444*

Alex Boussioutas, Stephen B. Fox, Iris Nagtegaal, Alexander Heriot, Jonathan Knowles, Michael Michael, Sam Ngan, Kathryn Field, and John Zalcberg

40 Pancreatic cancer *478*

Jürgen Weitz, Markus W. Büchler, Paul D. Sykes, John P. Neoptolemos, Eithne Costello, Christopher M. Halloran, Frank Bergmann, Peter Schirmacher, Ulrich Bork, Stefan Fritz, Jens Werner, Thomas B. Brunner, Elizabeth Smyth, David Cunningham, Brian R. Untch, and Peter J. Allen

41 Hepatobiliary cancers *508*

Graeme J. Poston, Nicholas Stern, Jonathan Evans, Priya Healey, Daniel Palmer, and Mohandas K. Mallath

42 Peritoneal mesothelioma *533*

H. Richard Alexander, Jr., Dario Baratti, Terence C. Chua, Marcello Deraco, Raffit Hassan, Marzia Pennati, Federica Perrone, Paul H. Sugarbaker, Anish Thomas, Keli Turner, Tristan D. Yan, and Nadia Zaffaroni

43 Cancer of the breast *546*

Martine Piccart, Toral Gathani, Dimitrios Zardavas, Hatem A. Azim, Jr., Christos Sotiriou, Giuseppe Viale, Emiel J.T. Rutgers, Mechthild Krause, Monica Arnedos, Suzette Delaloge, Fabrice Andre, and Felipe Ades Moraes

44 Gynaecological cancers *576*

Richard Pötter, Shujuan Liu, Bolin Liu, Sebastien Gouy, Sigurd Lax, Eric Leblanc, Philippe Morice, Fabrice Narducci, Alexander Reinthaller, Maximilian Paul Schmid, Catherine Uzan, and Pauline Wimberger

45 Genitourinary cancers *602*

John Fitzpatrick, Asif Muneer, Jean de la Rosette, and Thomas Powles

46 Lung cancer *628*

Rafał Dziadziuszko, Michael Baumann, Tetsuya Mitsudomi, Keith M. Kerr, Solange Peters, and Stefan Zimmermann

47 Neoplasms of the thymus *655*

Rebecca Bütof, Axel Denz, Gustavo Baretton, Jan Stöhlmacher-Williams, and Michael Baumann

48 Pleural mesothelioma *659*

Andrea S. Wolf, Assunta de Rienzo, Raphael Bueno, Lucian R. Chirieac, Joseph M. Corson, Elizabeth H. Baldini, David Jackman, Ritu Gill, Walter Weder, Isabelle Opitz, Ann S. Adams, and David J. Sugarbaker

49 Skin cancer: melanoma *674*

John F. Thompson, Richard A. Scolyer,
and Richard F. Kefford

50 Skin cancer: non-melanoma *690*

Diona L. Damian, Richard A. Scolyer, Graham Stevens,
Alexander M. Menzies, and John F. Thompson

51 Acute leukaemias *699*

Adele K. Fielding, Charles G. Mullighan, Dieter Hoelzer,
Eytan M. Stein, Ghada Zakout, Martin S. Tallman,
Yishai Ofran, Jacob M. Rowe, and Ross L. Levine

52 Chronic leukaemias *754*

Hemant Malhotra, Lalit Kumar, Pankaj Malhotra,
Devendra Hiwase, and Ravi Bhatia

53 Myeloma *782*

Charlotte Pawlyn, Faith Davies, and Gareth Morgan

54 Malignant lymphomas *808*

Frank Kroschinsky, Friedrich Stölzel, Stefano A. Pileri,
Björn Chapuy, Rainer Ordemann, Christian Gisselbrecht,
Tim Illidge, David C. Hodgson, Mary K. Gospodarowicz,
Christina Schütze, and Gerald G. Wulf

**55 Sarcomas of soft tissues
and bone** *844*

Alessandro Gronchi, Angelo P. Dei Tos,
and Paolo G. Casali

56 Craniospinal malignancies *867*

Puneet Plaha, Allyson Parry, Pieter Pretorius,
Michael Brada, Olaf Ansorge, and Claire Blesing

**57 Tumours of the eye
and orbit** *904*

Daniel G. Ezra, Geoffrey E. Rose, Jacob Pe'er,
Sarah E. Coupland, Stefan Seregard, G.P.M. Luyten,
and Annette C. Moll

58 Endocrine cancers *918*

Andrew Weaver, Anthony P. Weetman,
Oliver Gimm, Ashley Grossman, Petra Sulentic,
Bertram Wiedenmann, Ursula Plöckinger,
Ulrich-Frank Pape, John Wass, Angela Rogers,
and Wouter de Herder

59 Cancer of unknown primary site *965*

Nicholas Pavlidis and George Pentheroudakis

CHAPTER 35

Head and neck cancer

Christine H. Chung, Andreas Dietz,
Vincent Gregoire, Marco Guzzo, Marc Hamoir,
C. René Leemans, Jean-Louis Lefebvre, Lisa Licitra,
Adel K. El-Naggar, Brian O'Sullivan, I. Bing Tan,
Vincent Vandecaveye, Vincent Vander Poorten,
Jan B. Vermorken, and Michelle D. Williams

Epidemiology

Head and neck squamous cell carcinoma (HNSCC) is a heterogeneous disease arising from the mucosal epithelium of the oral cavity, pharynx, and larynx. The most common risk factors for HNSCC development are tobacco and alcohol use, as well as high-risk human papillomavirus (HPV) infection [1, 2]. Concomitant use of tobacco and alcohol also appear to contribute synergistically to HNSCC carcinogenesis. Human papillomavirus-associated squamous cell carcinoma typically occurs in the oropharynx and its incidence is increasing in the Western world [3]. HPV-negative and -positive HNSCC are demographically, biologically and clinically distinct entities with more favourable outcomes associated with HPV-positive tumours of the oropharynx [4–6].

Molecular biology of head and neck cancer

Molecular progression

Human papillomavirus-negative HNSCC develops predominantly in smokers, and a stepwise progression of molecular alterations in the squamous epithelium has been well-established (see Figure 35.1) [7]. It is currently believed that the molecular progression model associated with the phenotypic transformation of normal epithelium to dysplasia and invasive carcinoma constitute stepwise genetic and epigenetic alterations that include gene amplification, deletion, mutation, and methylation [7]. Although the primary events remained unknown, the early alterations associated with increased genomic instability in the squamous mucosal field comprise of frequent loss of heterozygosity, functional loss of tumour suppressors and/or a functional gain of oncogenic activity [7].

In contrast to the HPV-negative HNSCC, the molecular progression of HPV-associated cancer remains largely unknown. HPVs are small, non-enveloped DNA viruses, and their genome encodes various oncoproteins (E5, E6, and E7) and two capsid proteins (L1 and L2) for virion production [8]. The integration of the virus and the human genome entails the disruption of the early exons of the HPV leading to the activities of the E6 and E7, as the critical drivers of carcinogenesis through the degradation of p53 and pRb, respectively (see Figure 35.2) [9, 10]. Loss of p53 and pRb, two potent tumour suppressors, initiates genomic instability and leads to cell cycle deregulation [9]. Although the E6 and E7 are clearly deleterious, the simple expression of these oncoproteins is not sufficient to transform reticular epithelial crypt cells into invasive cancer. Additional genetic aberrations must be acquired. Thus, the genetic alterations required for further malignant transformation after initial HPV infection still need to be elucidated.

Loss of tumour suppressor genes

Based on the current genomic data, it is clear that the majority of HNSCC-related mutations or deletions occur within critical tumour suppressors, resulting in loss of function. Additionally, these alterations are particularly inherent to HPV-negative disease. Among the compromised tumour suppressors, *TP53* and *CDKN2A* (p16) are well established as poor prognostic biomarkers in HNSCC.

Wild type p53 is involved in a wide range of cellular processes including autophagy, DNA damage response, cell cycle regulation, senescence, apoptosis, and ATP generation by oxidative phosphorylation [11]. Mutated p53 accumulates in the nucleus as its altered tertiary structure does not allow for proper folding, ubiquitination, and degradation. Recent data indicate mutations that affect p53 DNA binding (disruptive mutations) are associated with worst clinical outcome compared to non-disruptive mutations. However, the presence of any *TP53* mutation is associated with worse outcome compared to wild-type *TP53* patients treated with surgery for curative intent [12]. Thus, further delineation of TP53 mutant functional complexity is of critical importance for the incorporation of these biomarkers into the development of novel HNSCC therapeutics [11].

Another important tumour suppressor gene in HNSCC is *CDKN2A*, which encodes p16. *CDKN2A* is located at Chr 9p21 and inhibits the kinase activity of CDK4 and CDK6, which induces cell cycle arrest [13]. p16 protein expression is cell cycle dependent and is focally expressed in only 5–10% of normal squamous epithelium. In HNSCC, p16 function is frequently lost by either mutation,

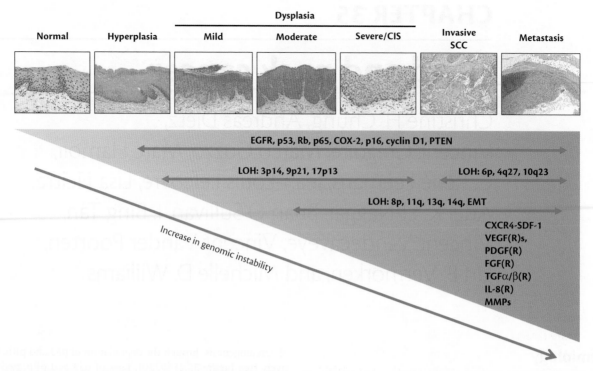

Fig. 35.1 Molecular progression of human papillomavirus-negative head and neck squamous cell carcinoma. Each step is associated with increased genomic instability or aneuploidy involving frequent loss of heterozygosity (i.e. chromosome 3p14, 9p21, 17p13, 8p, 11q, 13q, 14q, 6p, 4q27 and 10q23), functional loss of tumour suppressors (i.e. p53, NOTCH1, p16, PTEN and pRb) and/or functional gain of oncogenes (i.e. cyclin D1, EGFR, RAS and PI3K).

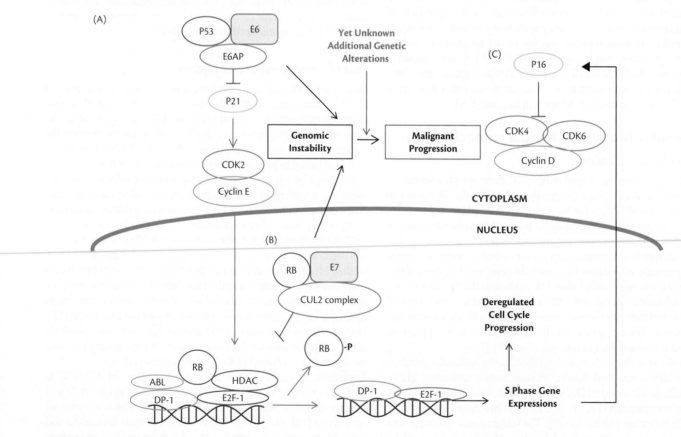

Fig. 35.2 Carcinogenesis induced by human papillomavirus. (A) E6-mediated degradation of p53; (B) E7-mediated degradation of pRb; and (C) upregulation of p16 through feedback loop induced by pRb loss and uncontrolled cell cycle progression.

gene/chromosome deletion, or promoter hyper-methylation of the *CDKN2A* gene [14]. Collectively, deregulation of p16 can occur in up to 90% of HPV-negative HNSCC, while p16 up-regulation is observed in HPV-positive tumours due to E7-related pRb loss (see Figure 35.2) [9, 15]. This results in diffuse over-expression of p16 in tumour cells and is considered a reliable surrogate biomarker for HPV positivity in oropharyngeal HNSCC.

Gain of oncogenic function

HNSCC-specific oncogene characterization is important for targeted therapies. Three common oncogenic alterations are observed in HNSCC: *CCND1* (cyclin D1), *EGFR*, and *PIK3CA*. Although these modifications are shared between HPV-positive and -negative HNSCC, differences in the frequency of their distribution are evident. In HPV-negative tumours, *CCND1*, *EGFR*, and *PIK3CA* mutation/amplification are seen in 32%, 15%, and 34%, respectively [16]. Meanwhile, the same alterations occur in 8%, 3%, and 56% of HPV-positive tumours [16], respectively [15]. Consequently, these data may have therapeutic implications and further clinical research targeting these alterations is required.

Genetic characterization

Recent whole exome sequencing studies of HNSCC have further validated the separation of HPV-negative and -positive HNSCC into molecularly distinct entities [5, 6]. When tumours were stratified by HPV status, HPV-positive tumours had significantly fewer mutations compared to HPV-negative tumours (4.8 versus 20.6 mutations per tumour). Commonly mutated genes included *TP53*, *NOTCH1*, *CDKN2A*, *HRAS*, *PTEN*, and *PIK3CA* [5, 6]. Of these, *TP53* is the most commonly mutated gene, disrupted in 62–78% of HPV-negative tumours while it was not detected in HPV-positive tumours to any appreciable degree [5, 6]. These mutations would functionally disrupt epithelial differentiation and cell cycle regulations and lead to an increase in cellular proliferation. Additional mutations were observed in pathways that regulate nuclear polarity, calcium sensing, and suppression of apoptosis, which would collectively arrest maturation and provide a proliferative advantage [5].

Molecular and growth factor characterization

At the expression level, Chung, et al. described four subtypes of HNSCC based on gene expression with distinct molecular characteristics: Group 1 tumours with high EGFR and ligand (TGFA) expression demonstrating significant EGFR activation; Group 2 tumours demonstrating epithelial-to-mesenchymal transition (EMT) with high expression of vimentin; Group 3 tumours with normal mucosal epithelium-like features; and Group 4 tumours with an up-regulation of xenobiotic metabolism, mostly observed in heavy smokers [17]. Subsequently, these four subtypes were validated by two independent datasets and each group was termed the Basal, Mesenchymal, Atypical, and Classical subtypes, respectively [15, 18]. The Atypical subtype included the majority of the HPV-positive HNSCC. In addition, various aspects of the HPV-negative HNSCC progression model could be associated with the subtypes defined above [18].

In addition, a recent gene expression study enriched with HPV-positive HNSCC (44% compared to 10–19% in other studies) revealed that tumours in the Atypical subtype can be further subdivided into two groups, resulting in five potential molecular subtypes of HNSCC [19]. Current evidence suggests the Atypical subtype

should be reclassified as HPV-Mesenchymal and HPV-Classical subtypes due to the gene expression these tumours share with the Mesenchymal and Classical subtypes. However, these tumours that are aetiologically distinct harbour HPV-specific gene expression. Further delineation of the molecular characteristics associated with HNSCC through functional genomics is expected greatly to advance the development of targeted therapeutics by identifying and characterizing subtype-specific prognostic and predictive biomarkers.

Summary of molecular biology of head and neck cancers

Using the current technological advancements in genomic analysis, we have gained comprehensive knowledge and insight into the molecular biology of HNSCC. In every respect, HNSCC is a heterogeneous disease which has now been molecularly characterized into five subtypes. Predominantly, these alterations are defined by tumour suppressor loss in HPV-negative disease, which is associated with poor prognosis and therapeutic challenges. In contrast, HPV-positive patients have good overall prognosis; however, a subset of these patients associated with worse outcome has been identified. The challenge facing future investigations is efficiently to translate what we have learned with these tools into clinically meaningful advancements in patient treatment. These are challenging goals and will require the concerted effort of HNSCC investigators from a variety of disciplines.

Pathology of head and neck tumours

The histopathologic neoplastic entities of the head and neck region are widely diverse and complex. The most common tumours arise from lining epithelium, salivary glands, and sinonasal sites. This section will focus on the most frequently encountered malignancies at these locations.

Squamous mucosal tumorigenesis

Carcinoma arising from the squamous and metaplastic mucosal lining of the head and neck sites can be broadly classified into conventional and viral-associated squamous carcinoma.

Conventional squamous carcinoma

Squamous tumorigenesis develops from the squamous mucosa of the larynx and sinonasal sites, of the oral cavity, larynx, and squamous metaplasia of respiratory epithelium [20]. These lesions are typically seen in relatively older individuals with history of exposure to and/or abuse of tobacco products and alcohol. Squamous carcinoma at these sites is typically preceded by premalignant lesions [21]. The incidence of progression of these lesions to invasive carcinoma varies considerably from patient to patient and it is currently believed to range from 10–45% [21, 22].

Premalignant squamous lesions

The progression of premalignant lesions to invasive squamous carcinoma is a multistep process resulting from progressive accumulation of genetic and epigenetic alterations [22–24] leading to invasive carcinoma (Figure 35.1).

Squamous carcinoma

Histopathologically, squamous carcinoma are classified into conventional and non-conventional forms. The conventional form is the most dominant, and is graded based on the level of squamous

Table 35.1 Head and neck squamous subtypes

Factor	Verrucous	Papillary	Basaloid	Sarcomatoid
Age	>50	30–50	>50	30–50
Grade	Low	Low	High	High
Sex	>Male	>Male	>Male	>Male
Gross	Exophytic	Exophytic	Endophytic	+/−polyploid
Site	Oral, larynx	Larynx, nasal cavity	Hypo-, oro-pharynx	Larynx, lip, oral cavity
Viral	No	?	Yes in oropharynx	No
Metastasis	No	Low	High	High when endophytic

manifestations and keratin differentiation into well, moderate, and poorly differentiated. The pathologic features associated with aggressive outcome include finger-like invasive pattern, perineural invasion, depth of invasion, and distance of tumour to resection margins.

There are several less frequent phenotypic variants of squamous carcinoma; some are also shared with viral associated carcinoma of the oro- and nasopharyngeal sites (see Table 35.1 and Figure 35.3).

Verrucous carcinoma (VC)

VC is a locally aggressive, well-differentiated squamous carcinoma characterized by a warty-like appearance and broad-base rete ridges with downward growth into the stroma. In its pure form this lesion does not metastasize while hybrid verrucous and conventional squamous carcinoma may retain the potential for metastasis. The differentiation of these lesions is from verrucous hyperplasia and is difficult on small biopsies or partial excisions. The distinction can be made, however, by en bloc excision of the lesion with the adjacent mucosal shoulders. Both lesions should be excised completely.

Papillary squamous carcinoma

This is a rare type of squamous carcinoma that is generally restricted to certain locations including the larynx and the nasal cavity. It is characterized by papillae lined by neoplastic cells and an exophytic appearance with and without invasion. Evidence from an association with high- and low-risk human papilloma virus (HPV) infection has been reported.

Basaloid squamous carcinoma

This is a high-grade variant that typically presents in the pyriform sinus, tonsils/oropharyngeal sites. In non-oropharyngeal sites they are negative for HPV and associated with premalignant non-invasive lesions. The significance of recognizing this variant is important in the differential diagnosis with solid adenoid cystic carcinoma, basal cell carcinoma, small-round-cell tumours, and melanoma on small biopsy materials. A selective panel of immunohistochemical markers can be used to establish the diagnosis.

Sarcomatoid squamous carcinoma

This rare form assumes sarcoma-like morphology and represents a transformation of conventional squamous carcinoma. The most common presentation is in the larynx, which may present as an

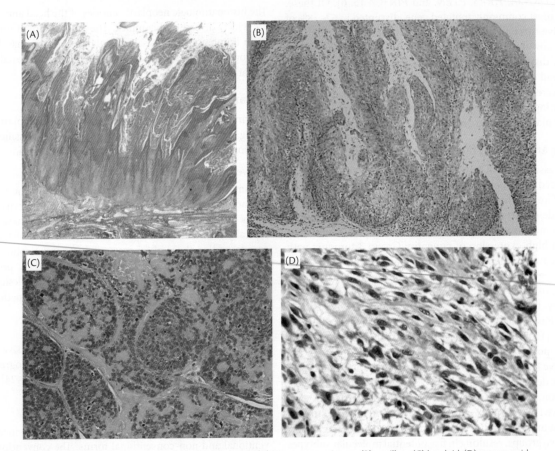

Fig. 35.3 Non-conventional squamous carcinoma subtypes in head and neck. (A) Verrucous carcinoma; (B) papillary; (C) basaloid; (D) sarcomatoid.

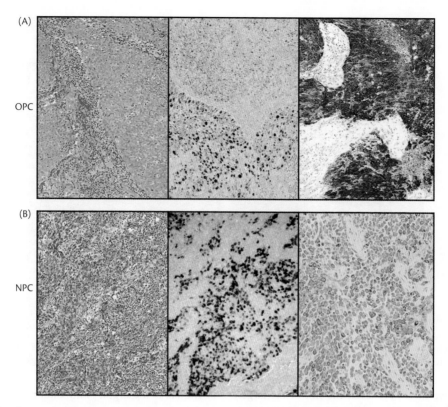

Fig. 35.4 Oropharyngeal (OPC) and nasopharyngeal carcinoma (NPC). (A) Light microscopic, HPV in-situ positivity in tumour cell nuclei, and p16 immunostaining note strong homogeneous (cytoplasmic and nuclear) positivity in tumour; (B) light microscopic and EBV (EBER, Epstein–Barr virus-encoded small RNA) in-situ image of typical undifferentiated squamous carcinoma highlighted also by keratin.

exophytic polypoid mass or with deeply infiltrative endophytic growth. These lesions may cause differential diagnostic challenges with sarcoma, spindle cell melanoma, and pseudosarcomatous lesions. Immunohistochemical positivity for keratin may allow for the exclusion of sarcoma and melanoma. Negative results, however, may occur and close interaction between pathologists and head and neck surgeons are critical to the diagnosis and management of these lesions.

Viral associated head and neck carcinoma

These entities are commonly seen as undifferentiated/basaloid squamous carcinoma morphologies. Both arise in neighbouring structures that are lined by respiratory or squamous epithelium that covers and overlies lymphoid rich stroma. The distinctions between these forms may often be arbitrary if the tumour presents at the boundary of the naso- and oro pharynx.

Nasopharyngeal carcinoma

The nasopharyngeal carcinoma is linked to the Epstein–Barr virus (EBV) especially in endemic locations (see Figure 35.4). Occasionally both EBV and HPV testing may be required for their differentiating. These tumours are histologically classified by WHO into keratinizing (type I) and undifferentiated subtypes (types II and III).

HPV-associated squamous cell carcinoma (oropharyngeal)

In contrast, to conventional squamous carcinoma which accounts for only a subset of tumours in this region, this form occurs in a different demographic population and frequency varies by country. The vast majority of these tumours are non-keratinizing/basaloid squamous carcinoma but keratinizing squamous carcinoma may also occur at these sites. The most common locations are at

the base of the tongue and tonsils. These sites are characterized by invagination of squamous epithelium within the lymphoid stroma. Tumour, therefore, arise in the hidden crypts at these sites especially the tonsils. Conventional premalignant dysplastic lesions, therefore, are rarely identified. Not uncommonly, because of their location, a neck metastasis may precede the identification of the primary and may show cystic features. The majority of these cases are caused by occult primary at the base of the tongue or the tonsils. Tonsillectomy is therefore advised if the primary tumour cannot be identified by imaging. HPV in situ hybridization of high-risk variants of HPV and immunostaining by p16 are sufficient to confirm the diagnosis [25] (see Figure 35.4).

Pathology evaluation

Intraoperative evaluation

Frozen sections are central to the evaluation of depth of invasion and of oral and lingual lesions, and in assessing the status of margins. Margins assessment requires a close cooperation between surgeon and specialized pathologist. Margins can be submitted from the defect by the surgeon or by the pathologist from the specimen. Intraoperative assessment is considered the final evaluation of margins. It is generally acceptable that a distance of 5 mm from the edge of the tumour to closet margin is a safe margin [26]. The final pathologic evaluation of the primary tumour should include positive or negative statements of the following features: size, differentiation, pattern of invasion, depth of invasion, perineural involvement, status of margins, and distance from nearest margin. If lymph node dissection is performed, the report should include the type of dissection, the number

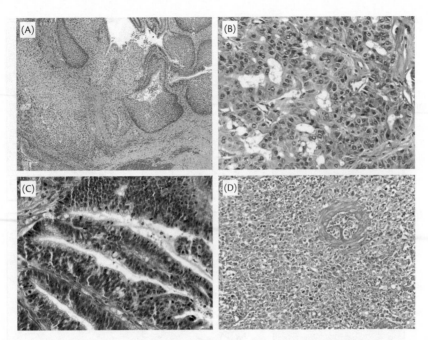

Fig. 35.5 Morphologically diverse sinonasal malignancies. (A) Squamous carcinoma (left) rising in an inverted Schneiderian papilloma (right); (B) non-enteric sinonasal adenocarcinoma, low-grade; (C) High-grade enteric sinonasal adenocarcinoma (intestinal/colonic type); (D) NK/T-cell lymphoma (angiocentric).

of positive and negative nodes per level, the size of the largest positive node, and whether extra-nodal extension is present or absent [27–29]. Other information that can also be included such a degree of immune response and vascular invasion. Since large numbers of squamous carcinoma undergo induction and/or adjuvant therapy prior to resection, the pathologic measurement should be adjusted to reflect the therapeutic effect on the resected tumour [30].

Pathologic reporting
Primary
The pathology report of conventional squamous carcinoma must include certain gross and microscopic features for accurate staging and clinical management. Typically the initial diagnosis is based on a core or biopsy of the index lesion. The biopsy evaluation should include the phenotype, the differentiation status, the presence or lack of submucosal invasion, and, if present, the depth.

The report of surgically excised specimens must include the following information: the histologic type, differentiation status, size of the tumour (three-dimensional), depth of invasion, perineural involvement, pattern of invasion (finger-like/pushing), distance of the closest margin (in mm), and involvement of adjacent structures cartilage/bone, and skeletal muscle.

Lymph node dissection
Close cooperation between the surgeon and the pathologist handling the case is critical to accurate orientation and proper reporting of the node status. Neck lymph nodes should either be submitted intact and then oriented on a template, or submitted as individual levels separately by the surgeon. The latter method is preferred.

Reporting should include the following information:

1. Total number of lymph nodes identified and the number of positive nodes.

2. The location/level of each positive node and the total lymph nodes in that level.

3. The size of the largest positive node.

4. The presence or absence of extracapsular spread (focal or extensive).

Sinonasal and paranasal sinuses
The spectrum of tumours arising in the sinonasal region is diverse arising from specialized Schneiderian respiratory mucosa, seromucous glands, and underlying supporting cells giving rise to some distinctly unique tumour types in this region (Figures 35.5 and 35.6). As sinonasal tumours except squamous carcinoma are rare, careful morphologic evaluation and more importantly immunophenotyping to confirm lineage is usually required [31].

NUT midline carcinoma (a genetic subtype of squamal cell carcinoma (SCC))
This molecularly defined tumour (rearrangement of the NUT gene on Chr 15) is favoured to be a subtype of SCC. Often midline, though not exclusively, this highly aggressive malignancy requires ancillary testing (immunohistochemistry or fluorescence in situ hybridization [FISH]) for definitive classification which is essential for prognostic implications [32].

Adenocarcinoma
Adenocarcinomas of the sinonasal region comprise 10–20% of sinonasal malignancies and are divided into three categories based on differentiation: enteric (intestinal type), non-enteric, and salivary. They are compared in Table 35.2. Prognosis is based on the tumour subtype, grade (if applicable), and stage at presentation.

Sinonasal undifferentiated carcinoma (SNUC)
This rare, aggressive tumour of still debated origin often presents as locally advanced disease morphologically showing high-grade features including frequent mitoses and prominent necrosis (see Figure 35.6C). The differential includes squamous carcinoma (often keratinizing), nasopharyngeal carcinoma (usually EBV+), neuroendocrine carcinoma, high-grade adenocarcinoma, as well as the

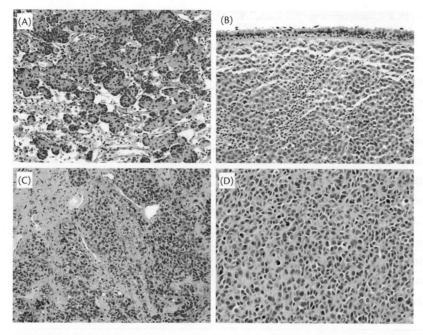

Fig. 35.6 Sinonasal 'small' round cell tumours morphologically overlap particularly on small biopsies. (A) Olfactory neuroblastoma with prominent Homer Wright 'pseudorosettes'; (B) sinonasal mucosal melanoma; (C) sinonasal undifferentiated carcinoma; (D) rhabdomyosarcoma, alveolar subtype.

'small blue cell tumours' [33]. A comparison of the clinicopathologic features of undifferentiated carcinomas is shown in Table 35.3.

Olfactory neuroblastoma (aesthesioneuroblastoma)

The most common neuroendocrine tumour in the sinonasal region is olfactory neuroblastoma (ONB) often a polypoid mass in the region of the cribriform plate [34] (Figure 35.6A). The Hyam's grading system (I–IV) utilizes histologic tumour features of differentiation to define risk (necrosis, mitoses, pleomorphism, architecture, rosettes, gland formation, matrix, and calcification). However, this system is currently undergoing revalidation to exclude the newer pathologic entity of SNUC [35]. As one of the 'small round blue cell' primitive tumours, ONB must be differentiated from rhabdomyosarcoma, Ewing's sarcoma, mucosal

melanoma, and the rare pituitary adenoma extending to this region. Clinicopathologic features of the small-round-cell tumours and the Immunohistochemical evaluation essential to confirm tumour lineage for treatment are highlighted in Table 35.4.

Non-epithelial tumours of the head and neck

Mucosal melanoma

Mucosal melanomas of the upper aerodigestive tract are histologically variable (small cells, rhabdoid, spindled, and pleomorphic), overlapping other tumour types particularly in the sinonasal region [36]. Risk factors, staging, and molecular profile are distinct for mucosal melanomas contrary to skin origin (see Table 35.4 and Figure 35.6B).

Table 35.2 Clinicopathologic features of sinonasal adenocarcinomas

Factor	Salivary	Non-salivary	
		Intestinal	Seromucinous type
Origin	Minor salivary gland	Respiratory mucosa	Minor salivary gland
Age (years)	30 to 70	60 to 70	30 to 70
Gender	Equal	> Males	Equal
Prognosis	Subtype/ stage ~50%	Grade/stage	Grade/stage
Recurrence	High (60%)	High	Yes
Risk factors	?	Wood & leather workers	?
Caveats	Classified as in major salivary glands	Usually high grade	Usually low-grade
		Exclude metastatic colon	

Table 35.3 Clinicopathologic features of undifferentiated carcinomas of the skull base

Feature	SNUC	NEC	NPC
Grade	High	High	High
Incidence	Rare	Rare	<0.5%
M/F	3:1	?	3:1
LN mets	30%	?	Common
Mortality	80%	50–60%	50–60%
Risk factor	?	?	EBV
Site	Nasal cavity & sinuses	Maxillary sinus	Nasopharynx
IHC/marker	Keratin 7	Synaptophysin/ chromogranin, keratin	EBV (EBER in situ)

Abbreviations: EBER, Epstein–Barr virus-encoded small RNA; F, female; IHC, immunohstiochemistry; LN, lymph node; M, male; mets, metastases; NEC, neuroendocrine carcinoma; NPC, nasopharyngeal carcinoma.

Table 35.4 Clinicopathologic and immunohistochemical markers useful in the differential diagnosis of undifferentiated skull-base neoplasms

Feature	ONB	Ewing/PNET	Rhabdo	Lymph-oma	NEC	Melanoma
Age (yrs)	10–20+50	<30	<20	50–60	>40	>50
Site	Cribriform plate	Maxillary	Any	Any	Any	Any
Markers:						
Keratin	-/focal	–	–/rare	–	+	–/rare
Synap	+	–/rare	–/rare	–	+	–/rare
HMB45	–	–	–	–	–	+
CD99	–	+	+/–	–	–	–
Desmin	–	–	+	–	–	–
Myogenin	–	–	+	–	–	–
S–100	Focal	–	–	–	Focal	+
CD45	–	–	–	+	–	–
Molecular	?	t(11;22)	t(2;13)*	EBV+^	?	C-kit 10–15%' BRAF 5%'

'up to 50% of alveolar subtype may expression keratin and neuroendocrine markers; desmin is a sensitive screening marker' [39].

* translocation in the alveolar subset of rhabdomyosarcoma.

^ NK/T-cell lymphoma associated with Epstein–Barr virus (EBV).

' molecular profile of mucosal melanoma differs from cutaneous/sun-exposed melanoma.

Abbreviations: ONB, olfactory neuroblastoma; PNET, peripheral neuroectodermal tumour; rhabdo, rhabdomyosarcoma; synap, synaptophysin.

Sarcoma

Essentially any sarcoma may arise in the head and neck, larynx, sinonasal, and skull base regions including chondrosarcomas, osteosarcomas, rhabdomyosarcoma, Ewing's sarcoma, and chordomas, as well as rare subtypes including mesenchymal chondrosarcoma, which morphologically mimics a small-round-cell tumour in the sinonasal region [37]. Pathologic review by an experienced pathologist, in conjunction with the clinical history and radiographs, aids in a timely optimized diagnosis for treatment of these rare entities.

Rhabdomyosarcoma

Rhabdomyosarcoma, a primitive malignant tumour of skeletal muscle derivation, accounts for 45% of all head and neck sarcomas with the orbit and nasopharynx being most common. There are three subtypes with variability in differential age of onset, site predilection, and prognosis. The embryonal subtype (including spindled and botryoid variants) represents the majority of cases in children. The alveolar subtype is the prevalent morphology seen in the sinonasal region, often shows a molecular translocation, and may express aberrant markers leading to misdiagnosis [38, 39] (see Table 35.4 and Figure 35.6C). Pleomorphic rhabdomyosarcoma is rare in adults and mimics other high-grade tumours including carcinomas, melanomas and other sarcomas.

Lymphoma

The spectrum of lymphomas may involve the head and neck, often presenting in lymphoid-rich areas (tonsil, base of tongue, nasopharynx, neck and parotid lymph nodes). Three prominent subtypes of lymphoma occur in the sinonasal region: B-cell derived, T-cell derived (EBV-), and NK/T-cell (angiocentric) lymphoma, which is an EBV-positive tumour of the sinonasal region often presenting as a midline destructive process [40] (see Figure 35.5D). Lymphomas must be differentiated from other tumours and non-tumorous conditions (Wegener's granulomatosis and cocaine abuse), which may show similarly presenting destructive symptoms.

Salivary gland tumours

Salivary gland tumours represent approximately 10% of all head and neck neoplasms [41, 42]. Histopathologically, they comprise of widely varied subtypes with often overlapping features that may lead to differential diagnostic difficulties. The WHO classification of these neoplasms recognizes numerous benign and malignant subtypes. The primary assessment of salivary neoplasms is generally by fine needle aspiration cytology. This procedure is less sensitive in differentiating benign and malignant tumours. It is very helpful, however, in excluding reactive metastatic, infectious, and lymphoreticular malignancies. Primary benign and malignant salivary neoplasms are primarily managed by surgery. The pathological evaluation of the received mass may require intraoperative evaluation for assessment of malignancy and margins.

Pleomorphic adenoma

The most common benign tumour encountered clinically is pleomorphic adenoma. These tumours may not uncommonly recur or develop carcinoma. Careful histologic examination of the cellularity and malignant transformation is necessary. Of the 24 well-recognized salivary carcinomas, mucoepidermoid, adenoid cystic, and adenocarcinoma are the most common.

Mucoepidermoid carcinoma (MEC)

MEC is the most common salivary malignancy in both adults and children. It is formed of epidermoid, transitional, and mucinous cells and graded into low, intermediate, and high based on the presence of cystic, cellular, and cytological features. The low grade is predominantly cystic and runs a benign course if completely excised. The intermediate and high-grade MEC are more aggressive and may recur and/or develop metastasis. Therefore, grading of these tumours is important for management.

Adenoid cystic carcinoma (ACC)

This is the second most common salivary malignancy and the most biologically relentless subtype [43–46]. Histologically, the tumour is generally composed of dual epithelial and myoepithelial cell formations to form tubular, cribriform, and solid patterns. At least two of these forms exist in a given tumour. The presence of a solid component is considered an ominous feature. ACC tumours are not graded and their dominant pattern typically reflects the clinical course. ACC invariability manifest perineural invasion.

Adenocarcinoma/salivary duct carcinoma

This is generally a high-grade malignancy with poor prognosis. They may present as de novo or as a malignant transformation of pleomorphic adenoma [41, 47, 48]. This entity is characterized by a remarkable morphologic and normal resemblance to mammary duct carcinoma. The following pathologic features are critical to the management of patients with these neoplasms: tumour type, grade if appropriate, size, perineural involvement, and encapsulation and margins status. In general, the tumour type and adverse features including perineural invasion, soft tissue extension, and margins status determine the postoperative therapy.

Imaging techniques for head and neck tumours

Ultrasound

Main applications include salivary and thyroid gland and lymph nodes. For salivary and thyroid gland lesions, ultrasound should aim to differentiate benign from malignant lesions, guide biopsy or the need for further imaging evaluation by computed tomography (CT) or magnetic resonance imaging (MRI), respectively, assessing lesion number and location, texture and/or cystic content, and providing an anatomical background for nuclear imaging [49, 50]. Usually, ultrasound-guided fine needle aspiration cytology (FNAC) or biopsy is mandatory for definitive diagnosis. Ultrasound (US) is the primary modality for nodal staging in thyroid cancer and complementary in HNC. In papillary thyroid cancer, an accuracy of 89% can be obtained in 6 mm lymph nodes (see Figure 35.7) [51]. In HNC, US has variable accuracy compared to

CT and MRI; which can be increased by additional FNAC, reaching specificities of 100% and sensitivities to 73% [52, 53].

Computed tomography–magnetic resonance imaging

CT is performed after injection of an iodinated contrast agent using multidetector technology. MRI is performed with high-resolution T1- and T2-weighted sequences. T1-weighted imaging is repeated after contrast injection with Gadolinium. Recently, functional diffusion-weighted MRI (DWI) is progressively included in the imaging protocol. Technical advances enable MRI to cover the entire head and neck, similarly to CT [54]. CT and MRI balance each other's advantages and disadvantages. CT has a short examination time, and has straightforward execution. MRI shows superior contrast resolution, absent radiation exposure, and allows easy integration of functional imaging.

CT is preferred for evaluation of laryngeal, hypopharyngeal, and oropharyngeal cancer, while MRI is preferred for sinonasal, nasopharyngeal, oral, salivary gland and thyroid cancer, as well as skull base tumours and sarcomas.

Pretreatment imaging

Imaging should provide information about the anatomic subsite of the tumour, deep tumour extent over the (sub)mucosa, muscles, and skeleton, and the neurovascular bundles and nodal stage. CT better depicts subtle cortical skeletal invasion whereas MRI is stronger for detecting bone marrow infiltration [55, 56]. MRI surpasses CT to detect perineural spread for which imaging signs include obliteration of fat in or widening of the bony foramina and enlargement and contrast-enhancement of the affected nerves. Muscle invasion is best evaluated by CT or T1-weighted MRI.

In laryngeal and hypopharyngeal cancer, anatomical parameters predict local control after radiotherapy. Pretreatment tumour volume in supraglottic, glottis, and hypopharyngeal cancers identifies patients with higher likelihood of local control to radiotherapy, with tumour volume showing an inverse correlation to local control [57–60]. CT-determined cartilage abnormalities are not an independent predictor of outcome [60]. In patients with supraglottic and glottic carcinoma examined by MRI, invasion of the pre-epiglottic space, thyroid and cricoid cartilage, and hypopharynx are strong predictors of local outcome post radiotherapy [61, 62].

For detection of nodal metastases, sensitivities between 48% and 97% and specificities between 39% and 96% [63] are reached using the criterion of 10 mm for short axis diameter. Morphological criteria like necrosis and extracapsular spread improve sensitivity but are rare in subcentimetric nodal metastases. Therefore, anatomical imaging criteria lack sufficient accuracy to stage the N0-neck.

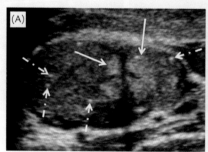
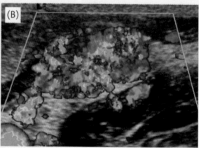

Fig. 35.7 Patient with papillary thyroid cancer. (A) ultrasound shows lymph node with heterogeneous reflective architecture (arrows) and dispersed microcalcifications (dashed arrows); (B) marked hypervascularity of the lymph node can be seen at Colour Doppler ultrasound. Diagnosis is compatible with metastatic lymph node.

Post-treatment imaging

Tumour recurrence appears as a contrast-enhancing soft tissue mass originating at the irradiated primary site or along the resection margin [64]. In contrast, mucosal necrosis is characterized by absent contrast enhancement and sometimes the occurrence of gas bubbles (see Figure 35.8). Laryngeal necrosis shows variable soft tissue swelling, fluid around the necrotic cartilage and/or cartilage fragmentation, collapse, dislocation, lysis or sclerosis [64].

Combining post-treatment baseline and three-months CT or MRI during follow-up improves detection of tumour recurrence in laryngeal and hypopharyngeal cancer. CT can detect tumour recurrence with sensitivity of 83% and specificity of 95% [64]. In contrast, for oropharyngeal cancer, CT scan six weeks post treatment does not have major incremental value to clinical evaluation. MRI six to eight weeks post treatment can predict local control with 48% sensitivity and 85% specificity [51].

For lymphadenopathies, CT eight weeks post treatment may avoid neck dissection. A decrease ratio of more than 50% measured on CT imaging tends to result in a negative hemineck, while high negative predictive value (NPV) up to 95% can be reached based on nodal diameter and absence of focal lucency. However, anatomical imaging criteria suffer from low discriminative value in enlarged lymph nodes [65, 66].

Functional CT and MRI

Functional CT and MRI provide a surrogate marker for perfusion (CT perfusion and perfusion MRI) and cellularity (DWI).

Perfusion imaging is acquired by continuous scanning during contrast injection. Main applications include prediction and early response assessment. Pretreatment CT perfusion may predict response after induction chemotherapy, chemoradiation or surgery [66]. CT perfusion after 40 and 70 Gy of radiation in patients treated with chemoradiation allows treatment monitoring [67]. Pretreatment perfusion MRI parameters are predictive for outcome in stage IV nodal disease and differentiate complete versus partial response to chemoradiation at six months follow-up [68].

DWI probes water mobility changes related to tissue cellularity, quantified by the apparent diffusion coefficient (ADC) being used for nodal staging, post-treatment imaging and response assessment [54]. DWI shows sensitivities between 83% and 98% and specificities between 97% and 87% for detecting nodal metastases [54, 69]. For detecting post-(chemo)radiotherapeutic recurrence, DWI shows sensitivities between 84% and 94% and specificities between 90% and 100% (Figures 35.8 and 35.9) [70, 71]. For response assessment during chemoradiation, absent ADC-changes (ΔADC) relative to baseline, one week, two weeks, and fours weeks during CRT were predictive for tumour recurrence during six months follow-up, respectively. At two years follow-up, significant increase of ADC was a strong predictor of clinical remission [72, 73]. Sensitivities to predict tumour relapse ranged from 86% to 100% and specificities from 83% to 96%. In a study, evaluating the ΔADC, three weeks after completion of chemoradiation, DWI showed a positive predictive value (PPV) of 89% and negative predictive value (NPV) of 100% to predict local control and PPV of 70% and NPV of 96% to predict nodal regional control [74].

^{18}F-FDG PET/CT

^{18}F-FDG is the most commonly used tracer for clinical PET imaging and has gained major advances with hybrid PET/CT, integrating metabolical and morphological information. Typically, PET/CT is initiated 60 to 90 minutes after injection of the radiotracer after scanning the CT portion. High-dose CT with intravenous contrast is recommended. A dedicated CT of the head and neck

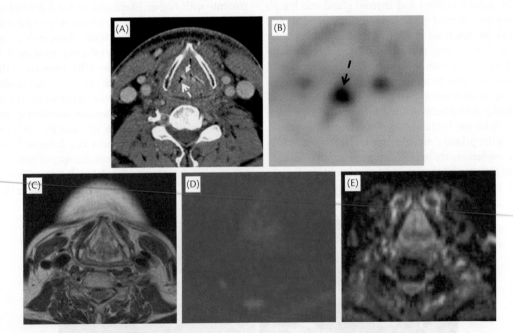

Fig. 35.8 Patient four months after chemoradiotherapy for laryngeal cancer: (A) CT-scan shows diffuse swelling of the soft tissues, dislocation and sclerosis of the right arytenoid (arrow) and small air bubbles adjacent to the arytenoid (dashed arrow). (B) ^{18}F-FDG-PET shows marked hypermetabolism in the larynx not able to distinguish tumour recurrence from inflammation. (C) T2-weighted MRI shows diffuse laryngeal hyperintensity indicating oedema. (D) No focal abnormalities are seen at the b1000 DWI while the (E) calculated ADC-map is bright. Histopathology showed laryngeal necrosis.

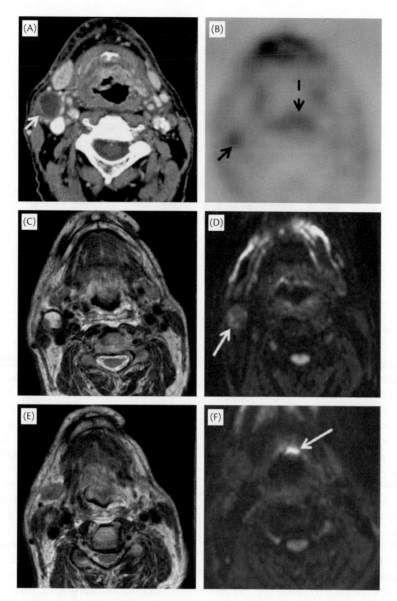

Fig. 35.9 Patient five months after chemoradiotherapy for supraglottic laryngeal cancer shows (A,B) metastatic adenopathy in level 2 of the right neck at PET/CT. Inflammatory changes are seen in the tonsillar area (dashed arrow). (C) T2-weighted and (D) DWI confirm the adenopathy where the viable tumour deposits appear hyperintense at DWI (bright; arrow). In correlation to (E) contrast-enhanced MRI, (F) DWI shows a small hyperintense lesion in the left epiglottis suspect for recurrent primary tumour; confirmed at biopsy after endoscopy.

can be performed prior to whole body imaging, increasing sensitivity for detecting small lesions such as small nodal metastases [75].

Pretreatment imaging

In general, PET or PET/CT improves the detection of primary tumours reaching sensitivities and specificities of 95% and 92% compared to 68% and 69% for CT [76]. PET detects unknown primaries in 10% to 60% of patients with neck lymphadenopathy [77]. In patients with negative physical examination and MRI, PET detects up to 27% of unknown primaries. Baseline FDG-PET characteristics may hold prognostic value. Patients with high FDG uptake have significantly lower control rate (55% versus 86%) and disease-free survival (42% versus 72%) than patients with low uptake [78].

For nodal staging, PET increases sensitivity ranging between 70% to 100% and specificity between 82% and 94% for PET compared to contrast-enhanced CT showing sensitivities between 48%

and 97% and specificities between 39% and 96% [78]. PET complements anatomical imaging by detecting subcentimetre lymphadenopathy. However, the low spatial resolution of PET restricts its use in the N0 neck.

Staging of distant metastases is a core application for PET/CT (Figure 35.10). PET can detect unknown distant metastases in up to 10% of patients during screening [79]. In addition, PET/CT can detect synchronous lung or upper digestive tract tumours. In a study by Schwartz et al., FDG-PET detected distant metastases or second primary in 30% of patients [80]. In a prospective multicentre study by Lonneux et al, FDG-PET detected unknown metastases or second primary tumours in 13 of 233 patients [81].

Post-treatment imaging and response assessment

^{18}F-FDG-PET/CT more accurately detects tumour recurrence than anatomical imaging with sensitivities between 83% and 100% and

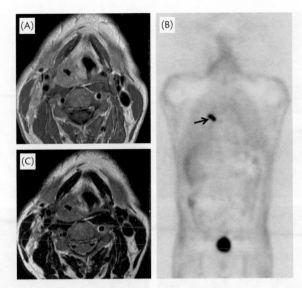

Fig. 35.10 Patient presenting with new diagnosis of (A) and (B) right-sided pyriform sinus cancer with multiple lymphadenopathies in the right neck at T1-weighted contrast enhanced MRI and T2-weighted MRI. (C) Additional ^{18}F-FDG-PET shows hypermetabolic lymph node in the right hilum of the lung (arrow) confirmed as nodal metastasis after endobronchial ultrasound guided biopsy.

specificities between 61% and 94% compared to 38% to 75% sensitivities and 44% to 100% specificities for CT or MRI [77]. It is generally considered that ^{18}F-FDG-PET two to four months post treatment allows better assessment of possible tumour recurrence than scanning at an earlier phase [77]. Four months ^{18}F-FDG-PET is a better predictor of tumour recurrence, while the specificity of ^{18}F-FDG-PET decreases significantly when performed earlier than 12 weeks post chemoradiation (see Figure 35.8) [81, 82]. For imaging surveillance post chemoradiation, ^{18}F-FDG-PET shows sensitivities between 93% and 100%, with specificities between 63% and 94% [83].

Data on ^{18}F-FDG-PET response assessment during non-surgical treatment are relatively scarce. ^{18}F-FDG-PET four weeks after start of radiotherapy shows an NPV of 100% but a low PPV of only 17% to predict local control [84]. In ^{18}F-FDG-PET before and one to three weeks after radical non-surgical treatment, high metabolic ratio post treatment is associated with 62% complete remission rate and 35% five-years' overall survival, while a low metabolic ratio is correlated to a 96% complete remission rate and a 72% overall survival [85].

Summary of imaging for head and neck tumours

Various imaging techniques are available for diagnostic evaluation of head and neck cancer patients, and the choice of imaging technique is usually based on clinical presentation and stage as well as patient tolerance and technique availability. Ultrasound, CT, and MRI remain the primary imaging modalities for HNC, providing lesion characterization, staging, and prognostication. Functional imaging improves the diagnostic yield in HNC.

Tumours of the nasal cavity and paranasal sinuses

Introduction to tumours of the nasal cavity and paranasal sinuses

Tumours of the nasal cavity and paranasal sinuses are rare and include a wide spectrum of malignancies, squamous cell carcinoma being the most frequent in the adult population and sarcoma in children. They account for 0.2–0.8 of all malignant tumours and 3% of those arising in the head and neck. Males are twice as affected as females. The peak incidence ranges between 50 to 70 years of age [86, 87]. Sinonasal tumours originate most frequently in the maxillary sinus (60%) followed by the nasal cavity (20–30%), ethmoid sinus (10–15%), and sphenoid sinus and frontal sinuses (less than 1%). Differences in histology distribution relate to the site of occurrence. Moreover, adenocarcinoma prevails in the ethmoid sinus in all the European series [88, 89], whereas the American series often report a higher prevalence of squamous cell carcinoma [90, 91].

Wood and leather workers have an increased risk of developing an ethmoid adenocarcinoma (5- to 50-fold). Tobacco smokers have a consistent association with sinonasal cancer and particularly with SCC. Exposure to formaldehyde, diisopropyl sulfate, or thorium oxide (Thorotrast), a radioactive thorium-containing contrast material used for radiographic study of the maxillary sinuses represents an additional risk factor [92]. These tumours tend to spread from one sinus to another through the foramina and fissures of the surrounding bone and show vascular, perineural, and lymphatic extension. Finally, they can involve the whole sinus complex and extend to vital structures such as the carotid artery, the cavernous sinus, the orbit skull base, and the brain.

Sinonasal tumours are usually asymptomatic in an early stage. Tumours often masquerade as a chronic inflammatory condition until they are advanced. The extension of the disease at diagnosis and the complexity of the anatomic field make the treatment of these tumours a challenging task.

Complete surgical resection followed by radiotherapy or radio-chemotherapy are widely recognized as the gold standard for these tumours. Despite refinement of surgical techniques and more sophisticated chemoradiation protocols, the prognosis of these tumours continues to be disappointing.

Diagnosis and staging

Sinonasal tumours are often diagnosed at an advanced stage. Initial symptoms are generally non-specific including nasal obstruction, moderate epistaxsis, and hypoanosmia. Once the neoplasm increases in volume, the clinical appearance depends on structures that have been involved by tumour extension. Swelling of the cheek or palate and loose teeth may be associated with oral cavity invasion; diplopia, impaired ocular motion, and proptosis when the orbit is invaded; trismus when tumour extends to the masticatory space and pterygoid; neurologic deficit, headache or cerebrospinal leakage when tumour erodes the skull base and involves dura and brain.

Bone destruction is found in up to 80% of the cases. About 60% of ethmoidal tumours present with intracranial involvement [93] and 66–82% show orbital wall invasion [94]. Orbital invasion occurs in 60–80% of maxillary sinus malignancies and in about 45% of nasal tumours. Cervical lymph node enlargement can also be detected.

Biopsy is mandatory to define the nature of the lesion and to plan the proper clinical approach. The exact definition of the anatomical margins of the tumour has significant implication for staging, treatment selection and prognosis. Consequently computed CT and MRI of the head and neck along with investigations to demonstrate distant metastases are always required. CT scans provide important evaluation of bony cortical erosion and information about the extent of the tumour through the surrounding bone such as orbital floor, lamina papiracea, cribriform plate, hard palate, and skull base. Better distinction of the tumour from the adjacent soft tissue can be achieved with MRI. In particular, MRI gives better indication about tumour invasion of the orbital contents, carotid artery encasement, perineural invasion and perineural tumour spread, dura mater, and brain and cavernous sinus involvement. MRI and CT scan are both useful to asses posterior spread of tumour into the pterygopalatine fossa [95]. Paranasal tumours are staged according to TNM–AJCC classification (TNM, 7thed.). In 2005 Cantù and coworkers validated on a large series of patients a new classification (INT classification) for malignant ethmoid tumours based on the most commonly accepted prognostic factors. This classification does not include N status but in comparison with the TNM staging system seems to provide a better prognostic discrimination among T classification [96].

Treatment

The choice of treatment strictly depends on site and extension of the disease and histology. Surgery associated with radiation or radio-chemotherapy therapy is the gold standard in many cases.

For certain tumours with very poor prognosis such as melanoma, neuroendocrine carcinomas including undifferentiated carcinoma (SNUC) and sarcomas, the role of surgery is questionable. Usually, these malignancies are well treated with radiochemotherapy therapy and surgery is considered for palliation or sometimes for rescue after locoregional recurrences.

Surgery

Limited tumours of the maxillary sinus or nasal vestibule can usually be treated with surgery alone. Advanced tumours of the maxillary sinus are treated according to the extension and location of the neoplasm with an anterior craniofacial resection or tailored maxillectomy. The surgical management of the orbital involvement is still controversial. Any attempt should be made preoperatively to distinguish between erosion of the bony orbital wall, involvement of the periosteum, and deeper penetration involving the orbital soft tissue. The orbital contents can usually be spared when there is no invasion of orbital fat and musculature or involvement of the orbital apex [94].

The invasion of the pterygopalatine fossa and the infratemporal fossa can be dominated by an anterolateral craniofacial approach. Ethmoid tumours growing far from the lamina cribrosa can be treated by transfacial ethmoidectomy. Ketcham in 1963 described the technique of craniofacial resection for a large tumour involving the nasal cavity and the ethmoid sinus approaching or involving the skull base [97]. For many years this combined transcranial-transfacial approach remained the gold standard of anterior skull base tumours [93, 98]. In the late 1990s, these tumours were also treated by an innovative endoscopic technique with or without craniotomy [99, 100]. The comparison between the techniques in terms of outcome and complications is difficult to make. However, recent reports seem to support that endoscopic resection results in a low complication rate and acceptable disease-free survival in selected cases.

The current contraindications to classical craniofacial resection are far less stringent compared to those outlined by Ketcham in his experience. Large brain involvement, encasement/invasion of the internal carotid artery, extensive skull base erosion, and invasion of the cavernous sinus are usually considered a contraindication for surgery.

The contraindications for endoscopic surgery are extensive lacrimal pathway infiltration, involvement of the anterior wall and lateral portion of the frontal sinus, hard palate, nasal bone, and infiltration of the bony walls of the maxillary sinus, with the exception of the medial one.

Neck dissection is indicated only when positive nodes have been clinically detected.

Radiotherapy

Depending on the location and the histopathology of the tumour, treatment using radiation therapy is either in the definitive or adjuvant setting. Because multiple critical normal tissues are located within or near the skull base (e.g., frontal and temporal lobes of the brain, the optic chiasm, the cranial nerves, the orbits, the lacrimal glands, and the brainstem), radiotherapy techniques are focused on treating the tumour while minimizing toxicities and complications. Using conventional radiotherapy techniques, the lacrimal apparatus and the optic pathway structures (retina, optic nerves, chiasm) often received doses equal to the target prescription dose. Conventional radiation therapy for sinonasal cancer resulted in significant ocular toxicity [101, 102]. Local control rates of 90–70% in stages T1–T2 and below 50% in stages T3–T4 were, however, achieved with prescription doses of 56–75 Gy [103].

In this framework, the use of intensity modulated radiation therapy (IMRT) has progressively emerged as the method of choice. IMRT allows selective under-dosage of organs at risk by creating concave dose distributions around the optic pathway structures together with steep cranial, lateral, and caudal gradients outside the planning target volumes to spare the lacrimal apparatus and the central nervous system. In a series of 62 patients with sinonasal tumours (ethmoid sinus, maxillary sinus, and nasal cavity) with adenocarcinoma and squamous cell carcinoma, the four-year actuarial local control after surgery and IMRT was above 80% for patients with T1-T4aN0M0 disease [104]. Eleven patients had T4b tumours with invasion of the dura or brain through the cribriform plate. Fatal relapses occurred within a year after treatment in all of those patients. IMRT implementation was clearly not able to reverse the dismal local control rates that are known to exist in stage T4b with cribriform plate invasion. In this series, severe dry-eye syndrome could be avoided in almost all patients if attempted. Severe optic pathway injury occurred in about 5% of patients. Such complication rates were much lower in comparison to patients previously treated in the same institution prior to the implementation of the IMRT technique.

Chemotherapy

Overall, there are very few reports on the use of chemotherapy in sinonasal carcinomas, and sinonasal squamous cell cancer is not included in the typical head and neck prospective randomized trials on chemotherapy (and/or radiotherapy). Nevertheless, the principles of chemotherapy as outlined in the section on locoregionally advanced larynx and hypopharynx cancer and the section on recurrent/metastatic squamous cell carcinoma of the head and neck are also applicable for sinonasal squamous cell carcinoma. Different schedules have been used in the locoregionally advanced disease setting, but regimens most often applied were platinum based, with a response rate ranging from 36% to 87% [105–107]. Survival figures of different treatments of advanced squamous cell carcinoma of the paranasal sinuses have not changed significantly in the last 20 years. Local recurrence at the primary site and distant metastases are the most common patterns of treatment failure. New approaches should therefore focus on these issues. The incorporation of induction chemotherapy (ICT) in the multimodality treatment of advanced cancer of the paranasal sinuses has shown some promise in this regard [106, 107]. Tumour response to ICT in such patients was suggested to be predictive of treatment outcome and prognosis, giving, moreover, a reasonable chance of organ preservation [106]. Data from the Milan Cancer Institute suggests that sinonasal adenocarcinomas are also chemosensitive, and that patients with such tumours might also be candidates for primary chemotherapy [108]. In the subgroup of patients with ethmoidal intestinal-type adenocarcinomas it was found that those patients who reached a pathologic complete response showed significantly less recurrences in follow-up than those who did not. Moreover, they found that p53 status could be a promising biomarker to predict response to chemotherapy [109, 110].

Sinonasal malignancies with neuroendocrine differentiation (with the exception of esthesioneuroblastomas (ENB) might also benefit from trimodality management, given the higher rates of systemic failure for patients with SNUC, sinonasal neuroendocrine tumours (SNEC) and those with small-cell cancers (smCC) than for those with ENB [111, 112]. In contemporary studies cisplatin is the drug of choice when given concurrently with radiation, and taxane/platinum based regimens for induction, such as TPF (docetaxel, cisplatin, 5-fluorouracil).

A different approach for adenocarcinoma (often found in patients with a woodworker's history) of the ethmoid sinus has been described by the Rotterdam group [113], using a techniques modified from that originally described by Sato et al in 1970 [113, 114]. Surgical debulking performed via an extended anterior maxillary antrostomy is followed by a combination of repeated topical chemotherapy (5-fluorouracil) and necrotomy [113]. Of the 62 patients treated, eight (13%) required additional radiotherapy for local recurrence, while one patient needed surgery for regional lymph node metastases. Results were surprisingly good. Adjusted disease-free survival at five and ten years was 87% and 74%, respectively. Periorbital swelling occurred in 40%, cerebrospinal fluid

leakage in 8%, and meningitis in one patient. A similar observation has been made by another research group [115].

Prognosis

Histology, tumour stage, margin status (where applicable), and site of occurrence affect the prognosis of sinonasal malignancies.

Despite the improvement of surgical techniques and novel radiochemotherapy regimens, the prognosis of these malignancies remains poor with an overall treatment five-years' survival ranging between 30% and 50%. Esthesioneuroblastoma has the best prognosis of all paranasal sinus tumours with a five-year disease-free survival (DFS) of up to 84% to 100%. The prognosis is good for minor salivary gland tumours and low-grade sarcomas with a five-year DFS of about 70%, while patients with adenocarcinoma have a better DFS than those with squamous cell carcinoma (52% versus 43.6%). Sinonasal undifferentiated carcinoma show a five-year DFS less than 20%, while all the patients with mucosal melanoma die of disease within two years after treatment. Intracranial and orbital involvement are also significant predictors. The tumour invasion of the skull base, dura, and brain progressively decreases the five-year DFS from 55.1% to 28.4%. Orbital invasion correlates with poor prognosis with a five-year DFS of 75% in patients with no orbital involvement compared with a DFS when there is periosteum/bone involvement of 40.7%. The importance of a proper surgical approach is well demonstrated by the effect of surgical margins status on disease-specific survival. Complete removal of the tumour with clear margins results in a five-year DFS of 68% compared with less than 30% when surgical margins are positive at histology [98].

Nasopharyngeal carcinoma

Introduction and epidemiology

Nasopharyngeal carcinoma (NPC) differs in many respects from other mucosal head and neck cancers. Its complicated location juxtaposed to the central skull base, and extremely high propensity to develop lymph node metastases in surgically inaccessible sites (e.g., retropharyngeal) means that the role for surgery in initial treatment is limited. The geographic and ethnic distribution is also distinct with the overwhelming majority of patients presenting in Asia, particularly in southern China (including Hong Kong, where the incidence is 25 cases per 100,000 per year, compared to 1–3 per 100,000 in Europe and North America) [116, 117], with high rates also found in Indonesia and neighbouring countries. Unexpected and intermediate rates are also evident among Inuit peoples of North America and certain regions in North Africa and the Mediterranean littoral regions. While all ages and gender are at risk, the peak is in the 40–60-year range in high-risk regions and bimodal peaks at 15–24 and 65–79 years in low-risk regions [118]. The incidence is two-to-threefold higher in men compared to women. A multifactorial aetiology includes inherited genetic predisposition, viral infection, and exposure to dietary/environmental factors in the first decade of life.

Histopathology classification of the nasopharynx includes non-keratinizing, keratinizing, and basaloid types according to the World Health Organization (2005) system. Most patients, especially in high-risk regions, have the non-keratinizing type, which is almost invariably associated with EBV, irrespective of patient ethnicity. It is further subclassified into undifferentiated and differentiated subtypes, although this distinction confers no obvious clinical significance. Human papillomavirus and/or smoking may contribute to cases in lower risk populations [119].

Presentation and primary disease assessment

The most common presenting symptom is a painless enlarging upper neck mass, classically in level 2, but any regional lymph node area is a candidate for involvement. Retropharyngeal nodes are very common and usually require imaging to detect them. Level 1 and parotid lymph nodes may be uncommonly involved. The primary tumour is often asymptomatic or may be associated with blood-stained postnasal secretion and nasal obstruction. Symptoms of tinnitus or impaired hearing are frequent and should prompt specific workup in an Asian patient. More advanced presentations may include aural pain or discharge, headache, facial numbness, diplopia, trismus, dysphagia, and dysarthria.

Initial assessment involves a detailed history and physical examination with special focus on cranial nerves (sixth being most common). Diagnosis is often established by nasopharyngoscopy and biopsy in the ambulatory setting. Preferred initial imaging is MRI, but if unavailable, contrast-enhanced CT is an alternative. Unfortunately, CT is less effective in evaluating perineural intracranial extension without bone erosion, cavernous sinus involvement, and in differentiating retropharyngeal nodal disease from posterolateral extension of primary disease.

Additional staging and supportive approaches

Audiometry and dental assessment are required. Additional workup should include complete blood count, serum biochemistry (including liver and renal function tests) to address disease-related issues but to also prepare for the use of chemotherapy. This should include hepatitis screening in risk patients, since polymerase inhibitors to block hepatitis B replication may be needed to address associated compromise in delivering chemotherapy. For stage III–IV, metastatic workup should include PET with CT; a CT of chest and abdomen and isotope bone scan may be used instead. Pre- and post-treatment plasma/serum load of EBV-DNA measured by copy number can prognosticate in the early phase of management, including attention to the rate of clearance of the viral load [120]. EBV copy number may also augment traditional TNM staging with evidence that it may surpass the prognostic value of some subsets of anatomic stage [121]. This test also facilitates early detection of disease recurrence, especially distant metastasis [122]. Serum EBV serology to assess the IgA response to the viral capsid antigen may be useful for screening and diagnosis, but studies suggest less value for prognostication and post-treatment surveillance [123, 124].

Radiotherapy for NPC

Definitive IMRT, generally with chemotherapy, is the primary treatment for NPC because it is radiosensitive and its anatomic location makes surgery technically difficult. This results from the need to eradicate insidious disease in the base of skull and to address the retropharyngeal nodes. Initially, institutional reports more than a decade ago showed dramatically improved tumour control with IMRT compared to historical expectation. These investigators demonstrated four-year estimates of locoregional and distant progression-free rates of 98% and 66% respectively [125] which has effectively changed the standard of care for this

disease while recognizing that distant disease remained the predominant problem. These observations were coupled with the observation of dramatic reversal of xerostomia rates, due to the salivary sparing capability of IMRT, with only very few suffering from grade 3 xerostomia after two years. The Radiation Therapy Oncology Group (RTOG) confirmed these results in a multicentre single-arm phase II trial showing two-year locoregional, and distant metastasis-free rates of 89.3%, and 84.7%, respectively. Only two patients complained of grade 3 xerostomia at one year [126].

Subsequently, randomized phase II trials were designed to demonstrate the ability of IMRT to ameliorate normal tissue-related sequelae (xerostomia and quality of life) in early disease [127, 128] but were underpowered to address efficacy. Locally advanced disease was presumably not included in these randomized studies due to the challenges in protecting adjacent critical anatomy with non-IMRT techniques. However, these results were recently corroborated in a large phase III trial involving 616 patients that also showed a survival advantage (80% versus 67%, p = 0.001) for IMRT compared to two-dimensional conformal treatment (2D-CRT) [129]. The five-year actuarial local control rate was 90.5%, 91%, and 81.5% for IMRT versus 84.7%, 80%, 62.2% for 2D-CRT for all cases, T3, and T4, respectively, with corresponding improvements in xerostomia and hearing loss favouring IMRT.

General treatment approaches

Early disease

Stage I disease should be treated by radiotherapy alone (preferably IMRT) with an excellent expectation of outcome.

In stage II, concurrent chemoradiotherapy is often recommended without induction or adjuvant chemotherapy. Supporting data are limited but evident from a single randomized trial [130]; however, concerns remain since many low-risk patients can be safely treated by radiotherapy alone.

Locally advanced disease
Concurrent chemotherapy

Stage III IVB disease is universally accepted as requiring combined modality treatment with both IMRT and chemotherapy. In the only individual patient data (IPD) meta-analysis of chemotherapy in NPC (MAC-NPC), an 18% risk reduction in overall survival, representing a five-year absolute reduction in death of 6% from 56% to 62%, was seen [131]. The main contribution was from concurrent chemotherapy (risk reduction of 40% with only modest contributions from induction and adjuvant chemotherapy). Other literature-based meta-analyses and the embodied contributing clinical trials have also supported this. There is therefore no doubt that concurrent cisplatin-based chemotherapy in addition to radiotherapy is absolutely necessary if the best chances of disease control and survival are to be achieved. However, controversies continue regarding the other aspects of treatment sequencing which are the focuses of future clinical trials.

Adjuvant chemotherapy

The need for subsequent adjuvant chemotherapy, a traditional component of management, has recently been challenged by a negative phase III multicentre randomized trial that compared concurrent chemoradiotherapy with or without adjuvant chemotherapy in locoregionally advanced disease [132]. Progress may be realized from the design of future biomarker-guided trials that stratify patients at completion of concurrent chemoradiotherapy according to residual EBV load before randomization to address the need for and intensity of adjuvant chemotherapy in different risk groups. Multicentre trials of this kind will also require attention to collaborative efforts to harmonize such quantitative plasma EBV DNA assays [133].

Induction chemotherapy

Induction chemotherapy is attractive in very advanced disease because its pre-emptive use may eradicate micro-metastasis while also reducing the size of overt gross locoregional disease; this may permit safer delivery of high-dose radiotherapy to ensuing gross disease close to critical structures (e.g., brainstem, optic chiasm), but should not reduce the dose to the elective target regions at risk of harbouring microscopic disease [134]. However, an ongoing concern is whether full-dose induction chemotherapy could compromise the delivery of the essential concurrent phase in terms of total dose of chemotherapy, numbers of cycles, and the delivery of radiotherapy to its intended completion, and whether such compromises are meaningful from a clinical outcomes perspectives. These are the focus of ongoing randomized trials that especially address newer agents, such as taxanes that were not traditionally used for induction approaches in NPC. Promising results are suggested by a small phase II randomized trial that compared neoadjuvant docetaxel and cisplatin versus cisplatin alone [135].

Very advanced disease

Stage IVC requires individualized approaches. Radical treatment should be considered for patients with good performance status and disease confined to oligometastasis [136–138].

Management of treatment failure

Patients should be closely monitored because early detection of recurrence significantly affects the chance of survival. Aggressive salvage should be considered for patients with local/regional recurrence or oligometastasis.

Management of local and/or regional failure

Options for local failure include surgery, external beam re-irradiation (EBRT), brachytherapy, stereotactic radiosurgery, chemotherapy, and photodynamic therapy. The choice of treatment is determined by the extent and location of the tumour, the availability of local resources and expertise.

Surgery is generally considered the treatment of choice if the tumour is resectable. For small and superficial recurrence, resection via the endoscopic approach, or by transoral robotic surgery, is preferred [139]. When the tumour extends across the midline or invades the parapharyngeal space, open surgical approach is indicated; approaches include a lateral infratemporal approach, and inferior transpalatal, transmaxillary, and transcervical approaches [139–141]. For regional failure, neck dissection is indicated. When resection margins are positive or there is extracapsular disease, post-operative re-irradiation is recommended.

If salvage surgery is not feasible, re-irradiation with or without concurrent chemotherapy may be considered. Smaller than usual radiotherapy fraction sizes delivered twice daily may reduce late toxicity.

Brachytherapy has shown good results for small recurrences with a five-year control of 62% [142]. With radioactive gold implants

five-year local control of 70% and overall survival of 64% are achieved [140, 143].

Stereotactic radio surgery can be delivered in one fraction or fractionated. Local control rates do not differ significantly from the results of brachytherapy, but there is a wide range [143]. In addition, severe complications including massive epistaxis, cranial nerve palsies, and temporal lobe necrosis occur. Tumours near the fossa of Rosenmuller and foramen lacerum have the highest risk of haemorrhage due to the location of the carotid artery. Complication rates for fractionated stereotactic surgery are marginally lower than stereotactic surgery, but survival rates do not differ. Long-term results are awaited to evaluate superiority.

A relative new approach is photodynamic therapy (PDT). After intravenous administration of a photosensitive drug, illumination of the tumour will result in cell death with a penetration depth of 0.5–1 cm. Although only small studies are available, preliminary results are promising [144, 145]. Pain is the worst side effect and sometimes 'sunburn' is evident if the patient is exposed to sunlight too soon. A gradual return to sun exposure over two to three weeks is necessary.

Management of distant metastasis

Distant metastasis is the main form of failure. For oligometastasis, surgery, radiation and chemotherapy can be used, and cure is possible in a small subset of patients [138]. For extensive metastasis, palliative chemotherapy with/without radiotherapy to symptomatic sites can be considered. When patients are chemo-naive, cisplatinum-based regimens give the best responses. Otherwise combinations of platinum-based chemotherapy with gemcitabine, capecitabine, or docetaxel could be used [146].

Tumours of the oral cavity

Introduction to tumours of the oral cavity

Therapy of squamous cell carcinoma of the oral cavity (OCSCC), including tumours of the anterior two-thirds of the tongue, hard palate and buccal mucosa, upper and lower alveolar process, and lips is an interdisciplinary task but mainly guided by primary surgical approaches. Radiotherapy and systemic therapies have additional character and are relevant (but not leading) parts in therapy concepts. Therefore, the main task for decision-making in therapy for OCSCC is to answer the question whether the tumour is resectable (with good functional outcome after reconstruction) or not. The following section is related to the German evidence-based clinical Guidelines [147] which are based on the current literature until 2012, analysed for evidence according to the evidence-graduation system of the Scottish Intercollegiate Guidelines Network (SIGN [148]). Furthermore, diagnostics and treatment strategies are based on the criteria of GCP (good clinical practice) which are currently emphasized and recommended in high-evidence-level clinical trials.

Role of surgery

Due to the diagnostic procedure, the role of surgery is to confirm the histological entity of the lesion. Therefore, biopsies have to be taken in the marginal sites of the lesion including panendoscopy in total anaesthesia to exclude metachronous or secondary primary carcinomas of the upper aerodigestive tract. The pathologist should be provided with sufficient information including extension and clear localization of the lesion including clinical TNM (UICC) definition of the staging result. The pathological report must include histological analysis according to the WHO classification: grading, depth of invasion [149], lymphatic, blood vessel, and perineural microinvasion, and other locally infiltrated structures [150]. After completion of the staging procedure, the individual tumour situation should be presented and discussed at the interdisciplinary tumour board (minimum composition of the entire board: medical (or clinical) oncologist, radiation oncologist, radiologist, pathologist, and head and neck surgeon). In case the patient has an acceptable performance status and resectable disease, surgery is recommended as first-choice treatment and first-step procedure in multimodality treatment concepts in OCSCC. Criteria for reasonable resectability are: individual situation of the patient, accessibility of clear resection margins (R0 resection margin according to TNM, UICC), and predictable post-operative quality of life after surgery including functional reconstruction. According to GCP the best available tumour distance to the resection margin should measure not less than 3–5 mm at the formalin fixed resection specimen and there should be a palpable approximately 1 cm tumour border in the patient while in surgery. In the case of R+ or a less than 3 mm resection margin described in the pathology report, localized re-resection is recommended. Continuity of the mandible should be preserved if no infiltration of the bone intra-operatively and in pretherapeutic imaging has been shown. Techniques of reconstruction should be planed related to the individual oncologic situation and as an integrated part of the primary surgical procedure. The extent of reconstruction should be balanced in relation to functional and aesthetic outcomes. For reconstruction of the oral cavity microvascular free flaps have been shown to be feasible and are recommended worldwide for excellent defect closure and functional outcomes. In OCSCC, 20–40% of neck nodes present occult metastases in the neck at level I–III, less often at level IV,V. Consequently, surgical treatment of the neck is recommended according to the worldwide accepted Robbins neck dissection classification guidelines [151]. Additional to invasive definitive OCSCC, squamous intraepithelial neoplasia 3 (SIN 3) lesions also have to be surgically treated since the probability of malignant transformation is nearly 90% [152].

Role of radiation oncology

In OCSCC, the main role of radiotherapy is in the adjuvant setting since response to primary radiotherapy and concurrent chemoradiation is poor compared to the other head and neck sites. Adjuvant radiotherapy is following the degree of the resection margins (R0, R1, R2) or the extent of the primary tumour (>T3) and the N+– neck situation according to the post-surgical staging results. The more recent metanalysis, conducted on all head and neck sites, showed that there is a significant improvement of overall survival and event-free survival by adding systemic therapy to radiation, and this is true both for the curative and the post-operative setting with a five-year overall survival benefit of 6.5%. It was also shown that cisplatin alone, given concomitantly with radiation, is able to achieve the same results as a combination of antineoplastic drugs [153]. In this context, concomitant chemoradiation is considered the state-of-the-art treatment when surgery is not feasible, or post-operatively when high-risk features are present in the pathological report, such as R1 or R0 <5mm (intermediate risk) resection or the presence of nodal disease with extracapsular spread. It should be recognized that this form of treatment may be associated with

severe toxicity, and for this reason its indication should be reviewed on an individual basis by an expert multidisciplinary team.

Potential role of primary systemic therapy

Only a small benefit was shown by induction chemotherapy that included cisplatin and fluorouracil (PF). Based on these encouraging results, induction chemotherapy was further studied by adding a third drug: taxotere to PF (TPF). The triple regimen was superior to PF in terms of overall survival; however, we still lack the evidence that induction chemotherapy is adding to standard locoregional treatment [154]. For this reason this is not considered a standard treatment. Induction chemotherapy has been specifically used in advanced operable oral cavity cancer where patients were treated either with induction chemotherapy followed by surgery and radiation, or surgery followed by radiation. The first randomized study included PF [155] and a more recent one TPF [156]. Both trials were negative with respect to the primary endpoint, which was overall survival, but there was an interesting signal of the potential role of response to induction chemotherapy in terms of sparing mandibulectomies and/or post-operative radiation. In both studies patients achieving a major pathological response with induction chemotherapy had the best prognosis. This observation has been done in other neoplasms treated with induction chemotherapy, such as breast cancer and osteosarcomas. It is clear that a better recognition of chemosensitive patients, for example by exploiting high-throughput techniques together with better drugs, is warranted for future treatment developments.

Tumours of the oropharynx

Introduction and clinical assessment

Oropharyngeal cancer (OPC) originates from the mucosa of the oropharynx, which includes the base of tongue and vallecula anteriorly, the posterior oropharyngeal wall, the tonsillar region and lateral oropharyngeal walls, and the soft palate and uvula superiorly. The incidence is approximately ten per 100,000 inhabitants. They are classified into two disease entities: smoking/alcohol-related and human papillomavirus-related (HPV-positive) OPC squamous cell carcinomas. The former generally have well to moderately differentiated keratinizing morphology, whereas HPV-associated lesions are typically poorly differentiated with a non-keratinizing or basaloid morphology (see also the section 'Pathology of head and neck tumours').

Frequent initial symptoms are a sensation of a foreign body in the throat or pharyngitis, followed by otalgia or odynophagia. Palpable lymph nodes in the neck are very frequent and may be the first and sole symptom. The traditional smoking/alcohol-related case often has a larger primary tumour size, less advanced nodal disease, and a correspondingly less advanced stage group. In contrast the HPV-positive case will generally have a smaller and less infiltrative primary but more extensive nodal disease (and often cystic appearance that may erroneously be considered a 'branchial cleft cyst').

The initial workup requires a comparative evaluation of the local extension with endoscopy, often under general anaesthesia, and imaging. For details on imaging, see 'Imaging techniques for head and neck tumours'.

Epidemiology and disease behaviour

The past decades have witnessed an unprecedented worldwide increase in the emergence of the HPV-positive cases. The traditional form is generally seen in a more debilitated population with less social support and with ongoing comorbidities largely related to lifestyle and the exposure to alcohol and tobacco. The HPV-positive cancers occur in younger patients with a much better performance status, and less intense or even minimal tobacco/alcohol consumption. Males are more commonly affected in both diseases. Aetiology through the sexual transmission of the HPV 16 or 18 viruses is suggested in these lesions.

Irrespective of treatment modality, the HPV-positive variant has a better prognosis, except for distant metastases. Concern has been raised that contemporary treatments developed for the traditional form of the disease may be 'over-treating' the more favourable HPV-associated variant. As a consequence, although treatment does not differ at present, de-intensification clinical trials are in design or ongoing to address treatment options for the different risk groups of HPV-positive and HPV-negative OPC. These include studies addressing the role of radiotherapy alone, transoral surgical techniques (including laser or robotic surgery), and different forms of systemic treatment.

Contemporary standard for locally advanced disease: chemotherapy and radiation

The interaction between chemotherapy and radiation specifically in locoregionally advanced OPC has only been studied to a limited extent. There is a single phase III trial that showed a survival benefit to using induction chemotherapy prior to local treatments [157], and only two trials showed survival improvement with the use of concurrent chemoradiation (CCRT) when compared with conventional radiotherapy alone [158, 159]. Although specific data on OPC are limited, the literature is replete with trials where the oropharynx is the predominant subsite, thereby underpinning the results of the meta-analysis of chemotherapy in head and neck cancer (MACH-NC) reported by Pignon et al. [160, 153]. This meta-analysis showed a significant interaction between the timing of chemotherapy and outcome (CCRT being superior to either induction or adjuvant regimens) and provides the foundation for considering CCRT as the contemporary gold standard for management in the locally advanced (stage III/IV) OPC, irrespective of the HPV status.

An alternative strategy for improving the outcome of 'favourable' locally advanced head and neck cancer is targeting the EGFR based on the improvement in survival from cetuximab delivered concurrently with radiotherapy compared to radiotherapy alone in a randomized trial [161]. Approximately 60% of this trial's population comprised OPC, which was also the subgroup with the most benefit from concurrent cetuximab in this setting, and with a toxicity profile that seemed to be less than that expected from traditional concurrent chemotherapy. While the latter has been disputed, approaches using cetuximab have led initial attempts to reduce toxicity and de-intensify treatments for the HPV-associated cancers by potentially replacing concurrent cisplatin with cetuximab or other anti-EGFR agents in ongoing trials. Another approach is using induction chemotherapy to select patients for a reduced radiotherapy dose (e.g., the completed single-arm ECOG 1308 phase II trial). The induction strategy provides an intriguing possibility for the subset of the HPV-positive population with the greatest risk of distant metastasis, now the leading cause of death for this disease. An induction chemotherapy strategy (e.g., a combination of docetaxel, cisplatin, and 5-fluorouracil (TPF)) with response assessment to minimize or omit concurrent chemotherapy seems a strategy that could be incorporated into future trials when one considers the impact of this approach on distant metastases, as shown in a more recent MACH-NC analysis, 39% of which consisted of OPC (although not HPV-specific) [154].

Risk-stratified management

Considering OPC as a single group of tumours has proved problematic. In the first publication of the RTOG 0129 trial, Ang and colleagues reported that HPV negative status, >10 pack-year tobacco exposure, T4, and N2b-N3 status were adverse predictors for overall and progression-free survival for OPC, and three risk groups could be constructed using these parameters based on risk of death in patients undergoing concurrent chemoradiotherapy [4]. Subsequently O'Sullivan and colleagues performed a similar analysis on an institutional cohort of prospectively compiled HPV-positive stage III/IV patients but addressed distant metastasis risk, rather than survival outcomes alone, in patients treated with either radiotherapy alone or CCRT [162]. Risk of distant metastases was significantly associated with T4 category disease, the degree of nodal involvement, and the same intriguing relationship with smoking history observed in RTOG 0129. Thus, heavy or light smokers with T1–T3, N0–N2a disease seemed relatively immune to the risk of distant metastases whether or not chemotherapy was used, but a smoking history of >10 pack years was important in N2b disease, and N2c and N3 disease were at risk of distant metastases irrespective of smoking history. Recognition of such characteristics has begun to guide contemporary clinical trial designs with several evolved protocols emerging that address different risk groups based on whether the patients belong to a favourable risk group with minimal risk of distant metastases, or require more intense locoregional treatment.

The only phase III randomized trial of an intensive concomitant boost altered fractionation RT alone regimen compared to CCRT with cisplatin in OPC of unknown HPV status was recently reported, and found no difference in DFS or OS [163]. In fact, tolerance was better with altered fractionation and a subset analysis suggested that the efficacy of altered fractionation appeared more pronounced in stage III disease. However, in stage IV, CCRT with cisplatin fared better and was most obvious in more extensive lymph node disease. Garden et al. recently reported a large single institution experience, also of unknown HPV status, indicating that low volume disease (e.g., T1–T2, N1–N2), has extremely favourable outcome with RT alone (exceeding 90%) despite being nominally classified as stage III or IV [164]. Thus, radiotherapy alone may provide very effective control for low-volume 'locally advanced' HPV-positive cases, but as the nodal disease stage increases, especially among heavy smokers, outcome is compromised due predominantly to the risk of distant metastases in the HPV-positive population, though the risk may be mitigated with chemotherapy [162].

Radiotherapy approaches

IMRT is usually used because of its ability to relatively spare normal tissues, most obviously salivary tissues. Pharyngeal constrictor muscles and mandibular regions can often be protected to some degree as well. Eisbruch et al. reported an RTOG multicentre single-arm phase II study of IMRT in OPC which validated one of the major reasons for using IMRT, the reliable and important ability to protect salivary function while achieving high locoregional control [165]. This benefit was confirmed in the PARSPORT trial, a UK multicentre randomized controlled study of IMRT versus conventional radiotherapy in pharyngeal cancer patients (85% OPC), showing reduced incidence of xerostomia with IMRT and significantly better recovery of saliva secretion with improvements in associated quality of life [166].

Contemporary radiotherapy approaches typically employ treatment intensification by the use of chemotherapy as discussed earlier, or hyperfractionation with dose intensification supported by meta-analysis data [167]. In addition, the observed benefit of moderately accelerated radiotherapy was also found to be independent of HPV status in the DAHANCA 6 and 7 trials, suggesting that this strategy should be maintained if the intensity of chemotherapy is reduced [168].

Surgery for oropharyngeal tumours

Although most oropharyngeal tumours are treated by a non-surgical approach, surgery remains important, either for initial treatment or salvage. Careful attention to the goals and needs of each case will provide the rationale, and indication for different surgical approaches for the primary site are summarized below. Elective neck surgery must also be considered if there is doubt about disease eradication, based on clinical and imaging initially or eight to 12 weeks following radiotherapy.

Transoral surgery is an attractive approach for tumours limited to the site of origin. Electrocautery was used initially followed by the laser CO_2 knife in the mid-70s, which became the most common approach. Although providing alternatives to open surgery in selected cases, these techniques remained limited due to the restricted access to the base of the tongue and the glossotonsillar sulcus. More recently, transoral robotic surgery (TORS) has been developed, providing excellent global visualization, with a magnified three-dimensional view, allowing access to difficult areas, and this has expanded the indications for using TORS [169].

There are two main approaches to open surgery: firstly, the mandibular swing approach that provides the same access to the lateral oropharynx as the traditional hemi-mandibulectomy but preserving the mandibular arch via the osteosynthesis performed after tumour resection. Submandibular approaches represent the second group. Thus resection of the posterior wall of the oropharynx may be performed via the opening of the larynx by anterior access between the hyoid bone and the base of tongue. Vallecular tumours may be resected by a supraglottic laryngectomy extended to the base of tongue.

Although limited resections do not ordinarily require reconstruction, reconstruction underpins the ability to undertake much modern head and neck surgery. Improvements in reconstructive surgery have substantially reduced the post-surgical functional and cosmetic sequelae. Local mucosal flaps (such as the FAMM, facial artery musculo-mucosal, flap) may be used in some cases. Pedicled flaps (dorsal flap, trapezius flap, or the most commonly used, the major pectoralis myo-cutaneous flap) have significantly improved volume and surface reconstruction as well as prevention of post-operative complications in the case of salvage surgery in irradiated fields. The introduction of microvascularized free flaps was an important milestone in oropharyngeal surgery. Some flaps are able to reconstruct a mucosal surface (radial forearm free flap) or tongue volume (dorsal free flap, anterolateral thigh free flap) or

the mandible (iliac crest free flap, scapular free flap, or preferably the fibula free flap) [170].

Tumours of the larynx and hypopharynx (including organ preservation)

Introduction and clinical assessment

The large majority of larynx and hypopharynx cancers are SCC. The few other cases comprise glandular carcinomas, sarcomas, melanomas, and lymphomas. The annual world incidence of head and neck cancer is estimated to be nearly 700,000 and globally, with some variations between countries, 20–25% are larynx cancers and 10% are hypopharynx cancers. The incidence of larynx cancer is decreasing in North America and in Western Europe; it is stable or slightly increasing in other countries. The incidence of hypopharynx cancer seems rather stable [171]. The incidence is much higher in males (85–90%) with a peak incidence between 50 and 60 years.

The larynx is divided in three levels: the glottis (true vocal cords), the supraglottic (epiglottis, aryepiglottic folds, false vocal cords, and the ventricles), and the subglottis (between the glottis and the trachea). The hypopharynx is divided into pyriform fossae, the post-cricoid area, and the posterior wall. These cancers are the result of tobacco consumption possibly associated with alcohol abuse for supraglottic and hypopharyngeal cancers.

The presenting symptoms are a sore throat, dysphonia, or a referred otalgia. Dysphagia and dyspnoea occur later. Metastatic lymph nodes are frequent in supraglottic and hypopharyngeal cancers. The initial workup consists of a clinical examination, an endoscopy under general anaesthesia (in 95%; and with biopsy), and imaging. CT is the most useful imaging for detecting in depth extension (cartilages, paraglottic spaces, pre-epiglottic space) and metastatic lymph nodes that are missed by the clinical examination. For details on imaging, see section 'Imaging techniques for head and neck tumours'. Staging should be carried out according to the TNM classification of malignant tumours, with stage groupings I, II, III, IVA, IVB, and IVC.

Management issues

When the initial workup is completed all cases must be discussed during a tumour board meeting (including surgeons, radiation oncologists, medical oncologists, radiologists, pathologists, etc.) in order to select the most appropriate treatment for each patient. Treatment choices depend on patient characteristics (age, occupation, comorbidities) and preferences, tumour characteristics, as well as local expertise and resources.

Early disease

For early disease, the choice is between conservative surgery or radiotherapy, which seem comparable in outcome (although never prospectively compared), while chemotherapy has no role to play.

Locoregionally advanced disease

For advanced disease, the choice is between 'mutilating' surgery (with or without post-operative irradiation) or definitive irradiation with or without chemotherapy or biotherapy (cetuximab), and with surgery in reserve as salvage therapy. There is no randomized study comparing both attitudes that could help in selecting one or the other. Clearly the choice is mainly institution-dependent and must be considered in the light of clinical trials on larynx preservation (see below). For more advanced and unresectable disease, the choice is between irradiation alone with different fractionation schedules and chemo- or bioradiotherapy under different settings. Such approaches are frequently studied in the framework of clinical research.

Recurrent/metastatic disease

For recurrent and/or metastatic disease, for each case one should consider whether a potentially curative option (surgery or re-irradiation) is still feasible. For other options see 'Management of recurrent and/or metastatic squamous cell carcinoma of the head and neck'.

Treatment options

Surgical options

There is a large surgical armamentarium for laryngeal and hypopharyngeal cancers [172]. Transoral CO_2 laser is a widely accepted approach for early diseases pending an excellent endoscopic access and a complete view of the tumour in all directions. This type of surgery is sometimes advocated for larger tumours, particularly in Germany, but is directly linked to the surgeon's expertise. More recently, TORS has been proposed by some teams but should be considered at the moment to be experimental, requiring larger series and cost-effectiveness evaluation.

Open partial surgery ranges from very limited resections (such as cordectomy, epiglottectomy, or lateral pharyngectomy) to large resections (such as supracricoid partial laryngectomy or supracricoid hemi-laryngopharyngectomy) allowing the surgeon to cope with all local extensions.

Total laryngectomy is required for large tumours and may be associated with either partial or circumferential pharyngectomy, requiring either pedicled or free flaps for closure.

A neck dissection is systematically performed (except for tumours confined to true vocal cords).

Radiation therapy options

For early-stage tumours (T1–N0), a standard fractionation regimen delivering a therapeutic dose of 64–66 Gy and a prophylactic neck dose in the order of 50 Gy in daily fractions of 2 Gy, five times a week is recommended. For T1 glottic carcinoma, a dose of 60–64 Gy to the glottic larynx without nodal irradiation is standard. For moderately advanced tumours (T2–N0 or N1), hyperfractionation or accelerated fractionation schedules have shown to be more effective than standard radiotherapy [168]. For these tumour stages, there is no compelling evidence for the use of induction or concomitant systemic treatment (chemotherapy or biotherapy). For locally advanced disease (T3 or T4, more than N1), a therapeutic dose of 70 Gy in daily fractions of 2 Gy, five times a week, and a prophylactic dose of 50 Gy are recommended, in particular when concomitant chemotherapy or biotherapy is used [153]. In case of contraindication to systemic treatment, the use of hyperfractionation, accelerated fractionation, or simultaneous integrated boost radiation therapy is recommended.

Post-operative RT is recommended in the case of inadequate resection margins, T3 or T4 tumour, multiple positive lymph nodes, and in the case of extracapsular spread of disease [173, 174]. Typically, a dose of 60–66 Gy will be delivered with daily fractions of 2 Gy, five times a week. In case of R1 resection and/or presence of extracapsular extension, the use of CCRT has been demonstrated to be superior to radiation alone [175].

Regarding the radiation technique, as demonstrated in randomized trials, the use of IMRT should be standard to decrease the incidence of late morbidity, especially the incidence of xerostomia [167]. For T1 glottic, however, conformal radiation therapy still remains a standard. Consensus guidelines on target volume selection and delineation for a state-of-the-art delivery of IMRT have been provided [176].

However, even in the IMRT era, the use of modified fractionation regimens and the use of CCRT or bioradiotherapy (BRT) is associated with an increased incidence of acute and late toxicity compared to standard radiotherapy alone, with unexplained deaths reported in up to 10% of cases with adequate follow-up after CCRT [177]. Variables that seem to correlate with the development of late severe toxicity are older age, advanced T stage, larynx/hypopharynx site, and neck dissection after CCRT [177]. These alarming data need specific attention and are a further plea to treat head and neck cancer patients in referral centres that meet all the requirement for an optimal care for such patients.

Chemotherapy and biotherapy options

The role of chemotherapy is slowly moving towards a more prominent position within the different treatment paradigms in patients with squamous cell carcinoma of the head and neck. The use of CCRT is generally accepted as a standard therapy post-surgery in high-risk patients (see above), in patients with resectable disease, when the anticipated functional outcome and/or prognosis is so poor that multilating surgery is not justified, and in patients with unresectable disease [178]. The optimal chemotherapy regimen for that approach is cisplatin 100 mg/m^2 days on 1, 22, and 43 during RT. CCRT improves survival and locoregional control over RT alone in patients with locoregionally advanced squamous cell carcinoma of the head and neck [153, 179]. Alternative non-surgical approaches in such patients are BRT with cetuximab (the only approved anti-EGFR monoclonal antibody) and the use of induction chemotherapy (ICT) before local therapies. The addition of cetuximab to RT improved survival and locoregional control over RT alone in one single randomized phase III study [161]. The hazard ratios for survival with RT plus cetuximab versus RT alone were comparable to those reported for CCRT versus RT alone in nearly 10,000 patients included in the MACH-NC meta-analysis [153]. However, there has been no direct comparison between RT plus cetuximab and CCRT in phase III reported. Despite that, there are sufficient data available suggesting that compliance with RT plus cetuximab seems to be better than with CCRT. The MACH-NC meta-analysis indicates that the role of ICT is less than that of platinum-based CCRT. However, the optimal ICT was not part of that analysis. The optimal ICT regimen has been defined by two major phase III trials, TAX 323 and TAX 324, both showing improved survival and progression-free survival with docetaxel, cisplatin and 5-fluorouracil (TPF) compared to PF in patients with resectable and unresectable locoregionally advanced head and neck cancer [180, 181]. In addition, a more recent meta-analysis on TPF versus PF indicated significantly less distant metastases and significantly less locoregional failure with TPF [154]. However, a direct comparison of CCRT versus TPF induction followed by RT has not been performed. So far, randomized trials of sequential therapy, i.e. ICT followed by CCRT versus CCRT alone, have not shown a clear benefit for the sequential approach and this approach should not be considered standard therapy for the moment. It is also unclear whether replacing 5-fluorouracil with cetuximab in the triple regimen might lead to better outcome. Further studies for both approaches are needed. With respect to larynx preservation procedures, platinum-based chemotherapy given during RT (CCRT), preceding RT (ICT→RT), or alternating with RT are all acceptable approaches (see below).

Larynx preservation

At the beginning of the twentieth century two major options were available: surgery (partial or total) and external beam irradiation. Up until the 1980s the surgeons tried to extend the indications of partial surgery with larger procedures and to improve rehabiliation after total laryngectomy with voice prostheses. At the same time radiation oncologists improved the efficacy of irradiation with a better delineation of the irradiated area and with modification of the fractionation. But there was no direct comparison of total laryngectomy and definitive irradiation.

In the 1980, the results of studies with ICT using the PF combination concluded that ICT was able to produce notable tumour regression and that this regression was predicting a high radiosensitivity [182]. This supported the initiation of a period of challenging clinical research on larynx preservation.

The first two adequately powered trials validating the concept of larynx preservation were the Veterans trial in the US for laryngeal cancer and the EORTC 24891 trial in Europe for hypopharyngeal cancer. Both trials compared total laryngectomy with ICT (with PF) followed by RT in good responders or by total laryngectomy in poor responders [183, 184]. Both survival and disease control were found similar in both arms of the respective studies and 56% of patients could retain their larynx in the ICT arm.

The next two trials compared ICT (with PF) to alternating chemoradiotherapy (EORTC 24954 in laryngeal and hypopharyngeal cancer), and ICT (with PF) to cisplatin-based CCRT and to RT alone (RTOG 91-11 in laryngeal cancer) [185, 186]. The first trial failed to find any difference in survival or larynx preservation between both arms. The long-term results of the RTOG 91-11 trial concluded that induction PF followed by RT and CCRT showed similar efficacy for the composite endpoint of laryngectomy-free survival. Locoregional control and larynx preservation were significantly improved with CCRT compared with the ICT arm or the RT alone arm. Overall survival did not differ significantly, although there was a trend towards a worse outcome with CCRT relative to ICT and deaths not attributed to laryngeal cancer were higher with CCRT (30.8% versus 20.8% with ICT and 16.9% with RT alone) [187].

The fifth trial compared two ICT regimens (TPF versus PF) in patients with locally advanced laryngeal and hypopharyngeal cancer as an alternative to total laryngectomy (GORTEC 2000-01). Responding patients received RT with or without additional chemotherapy. Larynx preservation was significantly higher in the TPF arm of the study (70.3% versus 57.5%), without any difference in overall survival [188].

The last trial compared CCRT and biotherapy (RT + cetuximab) in patients responding to ICT with TPF (GORTEC TREMPLIN trial). The overall toxicity was substantial, there was no signal that one arm could be superior to the other, or in favour of RT alone as found in the previous trials [189].

Evidently, the optimal approach for larynx preservation has still not been identified. Several treatment options are available, each with different levels of tolerability but little difference in outcome. CCRT with three courses of cisplatin and TPF induction followed by RT in good responders is the treatment now mostly used. Superiority of one over the other can only be assessed by a randomized trial.

Squamous cell carcinoma of unknown primary site

Introduction to squamous cell carcinoma

Cervical nodal metastasis from clinically undetectable SCC primary sites accounts for approximately 3% of all head and neck malignancies [190], and most frequently manifests in the upper jugular and mid-jugular lymph nodes. Histologically, SCC accounts for the majority of cases, particularly when masses are situated in the upper two-thirds of the neck, and generally indicates an origin from a hidden primary somewhere in the head and neck region. It constitutes a favourable-risk cancer of unknown primary (CUP) group compared to patients with less favourable histologies, such as adenocarcinomas.

Diagnostic workup

Physical examination, including comprehensive nasofibroscopy and endoscopic assessment under general anaesthesia conducted by experienced otolaryngologists or head and neck surgeons, detects primary head and neck SCC in over 50% of patients presenting with cervical lymph node metastases [191]. Locoregional imaging should ideally be performed before endoscopy as it may identify suspicious mucosal areas guiding biopsy sampling. Systematic tonsillectomy has been advocated by some authors as up to 45% of occult primary have been reported [190]. The role of FDG-PET has been extensively studied over the last few years, with detection rate of a primary tumour in up to 30% of patients, and a systematic review has recommended its routine use in patient management [192]. To optimize the yield of guided biopsies, FDG-PET/CT should be performed before the endoscopy. This examination, however, needs to be considered as an adjunct to comprehensive clinical examination, and not as a replacement. Another advantage of FDG-PET examination is that it gives the metastatic workup a higher accuracy than CT or MRI [192].

For pathological confirmation of the disease in the neck, fine needle aspirate is the preferred modality. In case of repetitive negative examination, a surgical procedure removing the entire node, possibly followed by a neck node dissection, is recommended. For pathological examination, in case of poorly differentiated or undifferentiated carcinoma, EBV testing should be routinely performed to exclude the presence of an undifferentiated carcinoma, which has a different prognosis and requires a different treatment approach. HPV testing could also be performed, although no study has so far demonstrated that HPV-positive SCC should be differently managed than HPV-negative SCC. More advanced molecular techniques performed on the lymph node and the random mucosal biopsies have been described, but so far none of these studies has profoundly altered the clinical management of patients with CUP [193].

The staging of CUP follows the staging of the neck for head and neck primaries. It should, however, be emphasized that the 'T'-site should be classified as 'T0' and not as 'Tx', the latter depicting a primary tumour staging that has not been performed, rather than a staging which did not identify any primary tumour.

Therapeutic strategies

In the past, treatment of CUP commonly consisted of lymph node dissection and elective irradiation of the putative mucosal sites and bilateral neck plus supraclavicular nodes. Recently, however, primary concomitant chemoradiotherapy, followed by a selective neck node dissection only in case of residual node disease, has been introduced. In addition, the dogma that radiotherapy for CUP should always include irradiation of both sides of the neck and the oropharyngeal, hypopharyngeal, and laryngeal mucosa has been challenged.

Neck node dissection with or without post-operative radiotherapy

In non-CUP series, for limited disease in the neck (i.e. pN1), neck node dissection procedures (typically selective neck node dissection or modified radical neck node dissection) without post-operative radiotherapy in the absence of extracapsular extension has shown control above the clavicles in the order of 95% plus (see review in [194]). Applied to selected CUP patients, such policy has shown high neck control, but with a significantly higher rate of emergence of primary tumours in the untreated mucosa compared to patients who benefited from post-op or primary radiotherapy [195]. In this series from Denmark, however, there was no difference in disease-specific survival among patient groups. It will always remain impossible to differentiate between the emergence of the putative primary and a subsequent head and neck primary, which typically occurs with a frequency of 1–2% per year.

For patients treated by surgery for a known primary tumour and who presented with multiple nodes and/or capsular rupture, post-operative radiotherapy or chemoradiotherapy (in case of capsular rupture) has been recognized as evidence-based practice [196]. There is thus no reason not to apply such policy to patients with CUP. The question of prophylactic treatment on both sides of the neck and the oropharyngeal, hypopharyngeal, and laryngeal mucosa however still remains unanswered.

Primary radiotherapy

In non-CUP series, it is recognized that radiotherapy alone yields a high rate of regional control above the clavicle around 90–95% for patients with N1 disease (see review in [194]). For patients with advanced neck disease, it has also been reported that altered fractionation radiotherapy or concomitant chemoradiotherapy followed by selective neck node dissection for residual disease yielded neck control rate in the same order of magnitude than after primary neck node dissection. Along this line, there has been a progressive change in the management of patients with CUP towards more use of primary radiotherapy or concomitant chemoradiotherapy. In a large retrospective review of 1726 patients with CUP treated either by surgery and post-operative radiotherapy or chemoradiotherapy (based on extracapsular extension) or by primary chemoradiotherapy, no statistically significant difference in five-year overall survival was observed between the two groups [197]. In this latter series, as reported in non-CUP series, the extent of the nodal disease and the presence of extracapsular extension were strong independent prognostic factors.

Indications for post-radiotherapy neck node dissection

The use of radiotherapy or concomitant chemoradiotherapy as primary treatment modality raises the question of the role of node dissection following radiotherapy for patients with N2–N3 disease at initial diagnosis. Residual neck mass may be present in up to 30–60% of patients after completion of chemoradiotherapy. For those patients, irrespective of the neck stage, there seems to be a consensus in the literature favouring an immediate neck node dissection because of the low probability of achieving a neck control with salvage surgery when recurrence develops [198]. For patients with complete neck response after radiotherapy or chemoradiotherapy, there are currently many arguments supporting the position that systematic planned neck dissection is no longer justified, and many institutions have switched to neck dissection for residual disease in the neck only [199]. Improvement in assessing the neck status with imaging has contributed enormously to this change in paradigm. Very high negative predictive values of CT, MRI, and more recently FDG-PET have indeed been reported for assessing the neck after radiotherapy or concomitant chemoradiotherapy [200, 201]. All the data mentioned above are from series of patients with a known primary tumour; there is however no reason not to extrapolate them to the situation of the CUP patients.

Target volumes in radiotherapy

As already alluded, the choice of the appropriate target volumes for radiotherapy of CUP remains controversial. First, the potential gain with comprehensive radiotherapy in controlling the putative primary carcinoma should be weighed, even in the new IMRT area, against its effect on quality of life resulting from increased acute and persistent morbidity such as xerostomia. Second, as already mentioned, it is possible that a head and neck carcinoma detected later in this patient subset is actually a second primary tumour instead of the putative cancer. Last, the possibility of conservative surgical approaches and the feasibility of re-irradiating the head and neck region (especially in the non-treated areas) are being recognized should a cancer emerge after ipsilateral radiotherapy. In the series from Denmark, although the rate of subsequent mucosal primary was higher in patients who did not receive comprehensive radiotherapy on both side of the neck and on the mucosa, no difference in disease-specific survival could be observed [195]. When all data from small retrospective series are put together totalling up to 1000 patients, no difference in the rate of subsequent head and neck primaries could be detected between patients who got surgery alone, unilateral radiotherapy, or bilateral radiotherapy including the head and neck mucosa (personal data).

Conclusion

The diagnosis of CUP is made after exclusion of the presence of a mucosal primary. There are two mains options for the primary treatment of CUP: either a neck node dissection followed by post-operative radiotherapy or chemoradiotherapy, or a primary radiotherapy or chemoradiotherapy depending on the nodal stage, followed in case of residual neck disease by a selective neck dissection (see Figure 35.11). There is no data to suggest the superiority of one over the other. For radiotherapy, unilateral neck or bilateral neck, including the oropharyngeal, hypopharyngeal, and laryngeal mucosa are possible options. There is no definite data to demonstrate the superiority of one over the other, but owing to the reduced toxicity of unilateral irradiation, and the possibility of salvage treatment in

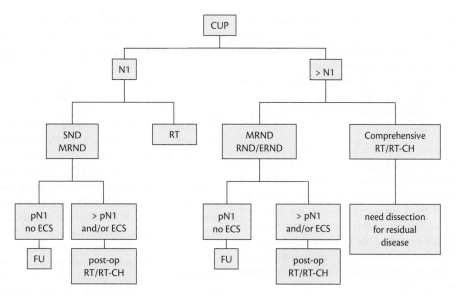

Fig. 35.11 Treatment algorithm of carcinoma of unknown primary (CUP).
Abbreviations: ECS, extracapsular spread; ERND, extended radical neck dissection; FU, follow-up; MRND, modified radical neck dissection; RND, radical neck dissection; RT, radiotherapy; RT-CH, concomitant chemoradiotherapy; SND, selective neck dissection.

case of emergence of a mucosal primary and/or a contralateral neck node development, the former is becoming the preferred option.

Recurrent and/or metastatic squamous cell carcinoma of the head and neck

Extent of the problem

Squamous cell carcinoma of the head and neck (SCCHN) is in great majority a locoregional complex disease, with evidence of dissemination in 10% or less at first presentation. Therefore, achieving adequate locoregional disease control of this primary disease, whether by surgery, radiation (with or without the additional use of systemic treatment), or a combination of these, is of central importance when managing patients with SCCHN. Failing to do so will lead to persistant disease (disease left behind after completion of primary treatment), recurrent disease (to be differentiated from second primary tumours (SPTs) in time and location [202]) and/or distant metastases. Moreover, past and current lifestyle choices in many cases increase the risk for new primary cancers even when the initial tumour has been cured. According to the MACH-NC data from 50 CCRT trials and 30 ICT trials, the rates of local and/or regional recurrences (LRRs) at five years were 50.8% and 47.5% in the experimental arms, respectively, and 60.1% and 46.5% in the control (RT alone) arms of the trials, respectively [203]. The corresponding rates of distant metastases (DM) were below 20%. Factors to be considered when choosing treatment in these circumstances include the extent of the recurrence, the type of initial curative treatment and the time interval between that treatment and the recurrence, the patient's performance status comorbidities and preferences after being well informed. Curative intent strategies in case of local and/or regional recurrences will be possible only in 50% or less [204].

Retreatment strategies

Surgery

Salvage surgery is the treatment of choice for all patients with resectable LRRs or second primary tumours and sufficient good health,

and therefore should be considered first at all times. Goodwin reported that based on a meta-analysis of 32 studies a survival rate of 39% could be expected at five years with salvage surgery [205]. However, the best chances of cure were in those patients with early-stage recurrent tumours and in those with recurrent cancer of the larynx, whereby the treated site seemed to be of less importance than the recurrence stage [205]. Unfortunately, those with limited tumour bulk (after adequate staging with PET or PET/CT) who are also medically fit comprise only 20% or less of the LRRs. Consultation with a radiologist and a careful examination under general anaesthesia is needed. Not only the extent of the recurrence is of importance but also the original extent of the tumour, since it is generally considered mandatory to excise the original extent of the tumour with a generous margin to obtain microscopic radicality. Major salvage surgery nearly always requires flap reconstruction for adequate wound healing and to permit the best post-operative function and quality of life. After (chemo-) radiotherapy, microvascular surgery is often possible and probably still the favoured method, especially for oral and oropharyngeal cancers because pedicled flaps may result in less optimal wound healing and yield inferior functional results. Tonsillar defects can often be reconstructed well with a relatively thin fasciocutaneous flap, whereas base-of-tongue reconstruction often requires an intermediate thickness flap. Laryngectomy defects require a free or pedicled flap as reinforcement of the suture line or as a patch. As to surgery for isolated residual or recurrent disease in the neck, there is a tendency to perform (super)selective neck dissections that remove only the level(s) that contain disease. This does not seem to compromise control of disease, obviates the need for flap surgery, and limits complication rates. Most authors reserve salvage neck surgery for those patients that have evidence of regional recurrence, and refrain from planned neck dissections even for the higher N stages. Salvage laryngectomy for laryngeal cancer recurrence offers survival in the range of 35–66%, albeit with a substantial risk of complications [206–208]. Good function outcome can be expected; the vast majority of patients are able to produce speech using a voice prosthesis, and have a 'normal' or 'soft' diet. Major salvage surgery for other sites yields results that are less favourable (27–40% survival) and likewise carry a fairly high complication rate [205]. Positive surgical margins are the main negative prognostic factor in multivariate analysis, pointing to the great importance of appropriate selection of patients. Regional control after salvage neck dissection can be achieved at five years in the order of 80% [209].

Re-irradiation

Proper selection of patients for re-irradiation is also of major importance. Only those with no or insignificant organ dysfunction and comorbities should be considered candidates for re-irradiation [210]. If possible, the functional status of the patient should be assessed by using standardized measures, such as the Charlson comobidity index or ACE-27 grading [204]. Favourable prognostic factors are the possibility of removing the recurrence beforehand, having a long interval between the recurrence and the initial treatment, and being able to give an adequate radiation dose, while prior CCRT is an unfavourable condition [211].

Patients with resectable recurrences or new primary cancers in a previously irradiated area who undergo salvage surgery should be considered for re-irradiation plus concurrent systemic treatment (whether cytotoxic or non-cytotoxic) when histopathology is showing high-risk features such as positive margins or extracapsular extension. This will lead to a better locoregional control rate, but at the expense of a higher toxicity (grade 3–4 late toxicity in >1/3 of patients and up to 8% treatment-related deaths) and no clear survival advantage compared to no post-operative reirradiation [205, 212, 213]. Expected OS rates at two years are in the order of 40–50% [205].

Patients with unresectable disease, as expected, do less well. Reviews have suggested that one-quarter to one-third of the patients will be free of locoregional disease at two years and two-year OS will be in the order of 10–30%. Grade 3–4 late toxicity in these cases will occur in up to 40%, and nearly 10% of patients will have treatment-related deaths. In general, a radiation dose in the range of ≥60 Gy is recommended, delivered by using conventional fractionation (1.8–2 Gy/fx), hyperfractionation or hypofractionation (in case of stereotactic RT). General advice is to irradiate the gross tumour volume with a sufficient margin (around 5 mm) and no elective treatment of adjacent regions.

Alternative local therapies

Photodynamic therapy involves the use of a light-sensitive drug or photosensitizer (given systemically or topically), in combination with light of a visible wavelength, to destroy the target cells. Patients with early recurrences in the oral cavity, nasopharynx, and larynx might be candidates for such treatment when conventional treatments are not available or not appropriate [214, 215]. In addition electrochemotherapy (ECT) can be seen as an alternative. ECT is the local application of pulses of electric current to tumour tissue to render the cell membranes permeable to otherwise non-permeant or poorly permeant anticancer drugs, thereby facilitating a potential localized cytotoxic effect [216, 217]. However, experience with ECT is still rather limited and the optimal indication is rather uncertain. Both approaches suffer from lack of comparative data versus adequate salvage surgery or re-irradiation.

Systemic treatment

Unfortunately, most patients with recurrent/metastatic (R/M) SCCHN are only eligible for palliative treatment. Treatment options in these patients include supportive care only or supportive care plus single-agent chemotherapy, combination chemotherapy, or targeted therapies, either alone or in combination with cytotoxic agents. Negative prognostic factors for survival are a poor performance status, severe weight loss, tumours originating in the oral cavity or hypopharynx, well/moderately differentiated disease, and prior radiotherapy [218]. Response to cytotoxic chemotherapy also proves to be a favourable characteristic and is of prognostic significance. SCCHN is a chemosensitive disease, as is evident from responses observed with various drugs of different classes of cytotoxic agents [219]. The four most extensively studied single cytotoxic agents are bleomycin (which is hardly used anymore), methotrexate, 5-fluorouracil, and cisplatin. Newer agents from the same or other classes of cytotoxic agents also sometimes showed promising results, but when tested in randomized trials never surpassed the efficacy of methotrexate or cisplatin alone. Taxanes (when combined with platinum compounds) seem more favourable than 5-fluorouracil in the R/Ms disease setting, because they induce less mucositis, a troublesome side effect in particular in patients that have been previously treated with radiation. Table 35.5 summarizes the development of systemic therapy in R/M SCCHN and shows that 30 years after the first use of cisplatin in this disease, survival advantage was observed for the first time when platinum-based cytotoxic chemotherapy was combined with cetuximab, a chimeric IgG1 monoclonal antibody (MoAb) targeting the EGFR [220]. The safety profile of this PFE (platinum/5-FU/ Erbitux®) regimen was quite acceptable, with no negative effect on quality of life and an improved response that coincided with a better symptom control [221].

Recent taxane/platinum/cetuximab combinations suggest that further response and survival improvement might be possible, but a phase III trial is necessary to prove this [222]. Unfortunately, phase III trials with other EGFR targeting agents, whether MoAbs (zalutumumab, panitumumab, nimotuzumab) or reversible selective

Table 35.5 Development of chemotherapy in R/M SCCHN. 1977: cisplatin shows efficacy in first-line SCCHN

Research group	N	Regimen	ORR (%)	Median OS (months)	Significant OS benefit
Grose et al. 1985	100	Methotrexate	16	5.0	No
		Cisplatin	8	4.5	
Forastiere et al. 1992	277	Cisplatin + 5-FU	32*	6.6	No
		Carboplatin + 5-FU	21	5.0	
		Methotrexate	10	5.6	
Clavel et al. 1994	382	CABO	34*	7.3	No
		Cisplatin + 5-FU	31*	7.3	
		Cisplatin	15	7.3	
Gibson et al. 2005	218	Cisplatin + 5-FU	27	8.7	No
		Cisplatin + paclitaxel	26	8.1	
Vermorken et al. 2008	442	Platinum + 5-FU	20	7.4	Yes
		Platinum + 5-FU + Cetuximab	36*	10.1*	

*significant.

CABO, cisplatin, methotrexate, bleomycin, vincristine.

EGFR tyrosine kinase inhibitors (TKIs, such as erlotinib and gefitinib), failed to show significant survival benefit [223]. Therefore, cetuximab is the only targeted agent approved for use in R/M SCCHN in first-line in combination with platinum/5-FU, and in some countries also in platinum-refractory disease in second-line cases. Response rate with cetuximab is rather low, while EGFR expression generally is high. Identification of biomarkers predicting response to cetuximab and other anti-EGFR therapeutics is pressing, as well as unravelling of the underlying mechanisms of resistance [224]. In line with this are studies with a new generation of irreversible small molecule pan-EGFR inhibitors as well as dual targeting MoAbs and a mixture of MoAbs targeting non-overlapping epitopes on the EGFR with the hope of overcoming resistance and to further improve outcome [223]. In addition, other targeted agents, such as c-Met inhibitors, IGF-1R inhibitors, antiangiogenic agents, drugs that block the PI3K/Akt/mTOR pathway, drugs that block the STAT pathway, and drugs that target nuclear and regulatory mechanisms, such as proteasome inhibitors, HDAC inhibitors, and heat shock protein inhibitors are all being studied. It is clear that combinations or sequential targeted therapies needs to be further studied and that identification of predictive markers should get high priority.

Salivary gland cancer and paragangliomas

Salivary gland cancer

Epithelial malignancies of the paired major (parotid, submandibular, and sublingual) and minor salivary glands (MiSG) are most complicated, due to their low incidence. The incidence in the US is ten patients per 10^6 per year. In Europe, Belgium, the Netherlands, the UK, and Finland have approximately six to seven new cases per 10^6 per year. Up to 70% arise in the parotid, 10–25% in the MiSG; the rest are submandibular carcinomas, with sublingual carcinomas being very rare [225].

Clinical presentation—imaging—pretreatment tissue diagnosis

Most parotid tumours present as an asymptomatic peri-auricular lump. Malignancy is suspected by rapid volume increase, pain, enlarged cervical lymph nodes, fixation to deep structures or facial skin, or facial nerve (VIIN) dysfunction. Surgery with or without adjuvant therapy being the treatment of choice, the workup evaluates the likelihood of malignancy and the extent and location of a tumour. Imaging is needed when tumour mobility is impaired, the tumour is >4 cm, and there is any sign of malignancy. MRI outperforms CT for the retromandibular parotid, the stylomastoid foramen area, and for identifying perineural extension. PET with or without CT is performed to exclude distant metastases. The resulting information, summarized in the TNM classification, combined with other clinical, histopathological, patient, and tumour characteristics, determines treatment options [226].

A submandibular gland cancer patient mostly presents with a slow-growing, painless mass under the jaw, occasionally with distortion of the floor of the mouth. Pain (30%) suggests local tissue extension. Cervical lymphadenopathy is present in 25% of patients. Radiological evaluation of submandibular salivary gland cancer (SGC) does not differ from the parotid subsite as mentioned above.

MiSG carcinomas (MiSGCs) are found throughout the entire upper aerodigestive tract and symptoms depend upon the anatomical site involved. Most frequently the oral cavity and oropharynx are affected, with the classical presentation of a painless submucosal swelling, sometimes altering denture positioning. In the nose and pharynx, MiSGC mostly causes obstructive symptoms. Pain is reported in one in four, regional metastasis in one in six patients [227]. To estimate the anatomical involvement, imaging (CT +/− MRI) is mandatory. For MiSGC an incisional biopsy provides the histological information needed to plan further treatment. As for major SGC, the TNM-components and stage grouping are the strongest prognosticators [225].

Before embarking on treatment, for major SGC, FNAC reasonably differentiates between malignant and benign lesions (accuracy 79%). Even if FNAC suggests benign disease, removal of the tumour for further histopathology remains mandatory. In MiSGC, the submucosal tumour is accessible for incisional biopsy, providing a more representative specimen for histopathologic subclassification. The caveat to interpreting these biopsies is that many of the 24 SGC types (Table 35.6) have overlapping histological features. Increasingly, molecular biological studies are performed, on the incisional biopsy material as well [225, 228].

Table 35.6 The WHO 2005 histologic classification of malignant salivary gland tumours

Type WHO	Abbreviation
1. Acinic cell carcinoma	AcCC
2. Mucoepidermoid carcinoma	MEC
3. Adenoid cystic carcinoma	AdCC
4. Polymorphous low grade adenocarcinoma	PLGA
5. Epithelial myoepithelial carcinoma	
6. Clear cell carcinoma, Not Otherwise Specified (NOS)	
7. Basal cell adenocarcinoma	
8. Sebaceous carcinoma	
9. Sebaceous lymphadenocarcinoma	
10. Cystadenocarcinoma	
11. Low grade cribriform cystadenocarcinoma	
12. Mucinous adenocarcinoma	
13. Oncocytic carcinoma	
14. Salivary duct carcinoma	SDC
15. Adenocarcinoma NOS	ACNOS
16. Myoepithelial carcinoma	
17. Carcinoma in pleomorphic adenoma	
18. Carcinosarcoma	
19. Metastasizing pleomorphic adenoma	
21. Small cell carcinoma	
22. Large cell carcinoma	
23. Lymphoepithelial carcinoma	
24. Sialoblastoma	

Adapted with permission from Barnes L, Eveson JW, Reichart P, Sidransky D, World Health Organization Classification of Tumours, *Pathology and Genetics of Head and Neck Tumours*, Volume 9, IARC, Lyon Copyright © 2005.

Treatment: surgery yields post-operative histopathological information

For parotid cancer the best chance of cure follows primary excision, the extent of which depends on the tumour size, the relationship to the VIIN, and extraparotid tissue invasion. For the majority of cancers with a normal functioning VIIN that are located in the superficial parotid lobe (80%), a standard superficial parotidectomy is adequate. Tumours >4 cm, located in the parapharyngeal or deep lobe, or with VIIN involvement should have a total or radical parotidectomy, considering that in high-stage, high-grade parotid cancer, the intraparotid lymph nodes may harbour metastatic disease. Alternatively, one may choose to rely on post-operative radiotherapy to control these possible microscopic deep lobe lymph node deposits [229]. In the same way, it is accepted that microscopical disease left behind on a non-involved spared VIIth branch can be controlled by post-operative radiotherapy. Regional metastasis is seen in one in three patients with parotid cancer, involves mostly levels II, III, and IV, and requires a (modified) radical neck dissection, removing levels I to V; radicality towards the non-lymphatic structures (nerve XI, jugular vein, sternocleidomastoid muscle) depends on proximity of the lymph node metastasis. In pN+ patients, radiotherapy improves locoregional control and survival [230, 231]. In patients with a cN0 neck at presentation, elective treatment (elective neck dissection or radiotherapy) depends on risk factors for occult neck disease (tumour size >4 cm, histology with clinical high-grade behaviour, age >54, perilymphatic and extraparotid extension) [8]. In our practice, we fine-tune the surgical approach to the N0 neck using preoperative USgFNAC and perioperative frozen section of the level II lymph nodes; if the latter reveal macrometastases, a modified neck dissection follows [226]. The MD Anderson approach is elective radiotherapy to the cN0 neck in high-risk patients, relying on definitive histopathology of the resected primary, because the indications for elective neck treatment concur with the indications for post-operative radiotherapy to the primary, and because pre- and perioperative typing of SGC is difficult (accuracy 51–62%) [232].

For submandibular gland cancer, treatment has shifted in the last decades from aggressive surgery, including the submandibular gland in a radical neck dissection, often with en bloc excision of the floor of mouth and lower rim of the mandible as monotherapy [233], to more limited surgery, supplemented by post-operative radiotherapy (level I–II–III dissection comprising the submandibular gland, only to be extended if disease extension dictates so) [234, 235].

For MiSGC, the treatment of choice is resection of the primary with free margins, resection margin status being the most important prognosticator, correlating strongly with anatomical extent and histological type [225]. The neck in MiSGC should be only addressed surgically for cN+ disease, for a cN0 neck when the risk of subclinical disease exceeds 20%, or when the neck is surgically entered as an approach to the primary [227]. Except in high-grade MEC, the occult metastasis rate is too low to justify elective treatment. For patients with pN+ disease, post-operative radiotherapy improves locoregional control and survival [231].

Following resection, the pathologist types the tumour using the 2005 WHO classification (Table 35.6) and identifies grade and negative prognostic factors such as perineural, vascular, and perilymphatic growth, and involved margins. Increasingly, molecular markers including chromosomal translocations with their protein products, improve accurate histological diagnosis. Some tumours express androgen receptors (AR) that could be also therapeutically exploited. There is no clear relationship between histotypes and biological behaviour, as commented by Leivo [236]. In population-based studies, the majority of major SGC are acinic cell carcinoma (AcCC) (15–17%), adenoid cystic carcinoma (AdCC) (16–27%), and MEC (14.5–19.2%). For MiSGC, AdCC (32–71%) and MEC (15–38%) outnumber adenocarcinoma not otherwise specified (ACNOS), AcCC, polymorphous low-grade adenocarcinoma (PLGA), epithelial myoepithelial carcinoma, and carcinoma ex-pleomorphic adenoma [225, 226].

Post-operative radiotherapy for parotid and submandibular carcinomas

Indicated in stage III and IV disease, and in case of adverse histopathological factors (perineural and vascular invasion, close or positive margins, high-grade pathology), IMRT is now the 'standard of care' that minimizes complications. Typically a dose of 60 Gy in 30 fractions of 2 Gy in six weeks will be delivered on the parotid bed and the neck node levels (when pathologically invaded). In case of AdCC infiltrating the facial nerve, a comprehensive coverage of the nerve up to the base of the skull is recommended. The Dutch Head and Neck Oncology Cooperative Group found a 9.7-fold reduction of local recurrence in patients receiving combined surgery and radiotherapy as compared to surgery-only patients. Post-operative radiotherapy can only be omitted for stage I–II lesions in AcCC and low-grade MEC if complete resection does not reveal adverse pathological factors [226]. For high-risk major SGC, two reports recently suggested the benefit of a post-operative platinum-based concomitant chemoradiation scheme [237, 238].

Post-operative radiotherapy for MiSGC

For MiSGC, post-operative radiotherapy to the primary site is recommended for most patients, only to be omitted in 'clear margin' stage I and II disease without lymphovascular or perineural invasion [225, 227, 231].

Radiotherapy and chemotherapy in unresectable disease

For patients who are inoperable, who refuse surgery, or who have an unresectable tumour, primary photon-based radiotherapy (dose of 66 to 70 Gy) results in 17–57% locoregional control at ten years. In a randomized trial conducted 30 years ago, neutron radiotherapy reached up to 75% five-year local control, especially for AdCC, but remains unattractive because of no survival benefit and severe late side effects [239]. More recently, encouraging results have been reported with the use of heavy ion therapy (carbon ion), which combines both the biological advantage of neutrons and an exquisite dose distribution [240].

In SGC chemotherapy remains of palliative use only, resulting in a temporary benefit in about 20% of treated patients. The most active drugs are cisplatin and doxorubicin [241–243]. Taxanes are not active in AdCC. In this latter histotype it is worthwhile suggesting a watchful approach in indolent diseases. Table 35.7 lists the targeted therapies that have been explored clinically. Unfortunately, none has significantly improved results.

AR expressing tumours might be treated with androgen deprivation.

Treatment results according to site

The treatment results for parotid carcinoma in major treatment centres, listed in Table 35.8, have to be appreciated in their specific

Table 35.7 Molecular targets and corresponding therapies studied in salivary gland carcinoma

Molecular target	Salivary gland carcinoma type	Molecular therapy
c-KIT	AdCC	imatinib
ErbB–1	All types	cetuximab gefinitib
ErbB–2	All types	trastuzumab lapatinib
VEGF –family	AcCC	axinitib
NFκB – proteasomes degrading its inhibitor (I-κB)-α	AdCC	bortezomib

context of stage, percentage high-grade, treatment period and corresponding treatment regimens, patient inclusion criteria, and adequacy of follow-up. Many univariate and multivariate statistical analyses have focused on prognostic factors in SGC to fine-tune the individual patient's prognostic estimate [226].

Treatment results for submandibular gland cancer have increased recently as compared to the earlier series where post-operative radiotherapy was not yet customary. The five-year disease-free survival (DSS) of 61% and the ten-year DSS of 51% in Amsterdam [234] are similar to the findings in Toronto with a five-year DSS of 60% and a ten-year DSS of 48% [244].

Table 35.8 Disease-specific survival (DSS) for Parotid Carcinoma (multiple histologies together)

Research group	Publication year	Number of patients	DSS five years	DSS ten years
Spiro	1986	623	55%	47%
Spiro et al.	1989	62	63%	47%
Kane et al.	1991	194	69%	68%
Poulsen et al.	1992	209	71%	65%
Leverstein et al.	1998	65	75%	67%
Therkildsen et al.	1998	251	76%	72%
Renehan et al.	1999	103	78%	65%
Vander Poorten et al.	1999	168	59%	54%
Harbo et al.	2002	152	57%	51%
Godballe et al.	2003	85	52%	
Vander Poorten et al.	2003	231	62%	
Lima et al.	2005	126	72%	69%
Mendenhall et al.	2005	224		57%
Vander Poorten et al.	2009	237	69%	58%

For MiSGC, five-year survival ranges from 66% to 80% and ten-year survival from 56% to 70%, whereas initial tumour control is expected to be 56–62%. MSGCs overall do not imply a poorer prognosis than their submandibular and parotid counterparts, although specific subsites (e.g., the skull base) imply a worse outcome [225].

Summary

Every step in the management of SGC is complicated: the clinical and radiological evaluation, the pathology, the ablative and reconstructive surgery, the radiotherapy and eventual chemotherapy, and the management of complications. The best care can undoubtedly be provided when these patients are centralized in specialized tertiary referral centres.

Cervical paragangliomas

Cervical paragangliomas (PG) are highly vascular soft tissue tumours, originating from the paraganglia receptors in the vascular adventitia. They follow the course of cranial nerve X in the skull base and the parapharyngeal space lower down. With decreasing frequency they arise from the carotid body, jugular, tympanic, and vagal locations. The incidence of these rare head and neck tumours remains unclear, since most are benign tumours, not registered by cancer registries. About 6–19% are reportedly malignant, evidenced only by imaging studies showing local invasion, regional or distant metastasis, since the histological appearance of malignant PG is identical to that of benign tumours [245].

Genetics

About nine in ten PGs are sporadic; in one in ten patients a mutation in the succinate dehydrogenase (SDH) subunits (SDHD, SDHB, SDHC) genes typically causes development of multifocal PG at age <40, and in combination with pheochromocytomas [246].

Clinical presentation—workup

Most patients with carotid PG present with an asymptomatic pulsatile neck mass which patients report to vary in volume. At other sites, symptoms of PG reflect the cranial nerves they interfere with, ranging from vague pain through hearing loss, pulsatile tinnitus (n VIII), velopharyngeal insufficiency (n IX), chronic cough, dysphagia, dysphonia, aspiration (n X) and shoulder weakness (n XI). Up to 3% of PGs secrete catecholamines, detected by urinalysis. CT+/– MRI+/–MR angiography of the head and neck are so typical (salt and pepper appearance, flow voids, splaying of the carotid bifurcation for carotid body tumours, anterior displacement of both internal and external carotid artery in vagal paraganglioma) that they are sufficient for diagnosis, obviating a (hazardous) biopsy. Imaging studies reveal location, extent, relation to the great vessels, and eventual coexistent PG at other sites. For the latter, a somatostatin receptor scanning (octreotide scan) is also useful.

Treatment and outcome

There are three valid options to choose from. The slow growth rate, with half of the tumours not showing volume increase during long-term follow-up, supports an initial wait-and-scan policy for many patients [247, 248]. Alternatively, in volume-increasing lesions, both surgery and radiotherapy (IMRT: moderate-dose RT of 44–50 Gy over 22–25 fractions or in selected very small skull base lesions, stereotactic radiosurgery) are valid options [245, 249]. Given the potential complications, surgery is usually reserved for limited PG where minimal morbidity is expected. Typically, these are the 70% of carotid body tumours that are Shamblin class I (small and easily dissected from the vessels) and class II (glomus tumour partially surrounds the vessels). For all other tumours (class III carotid body tumours and vagal—jugular –tympanic PG), new post-operative cranial deficits are hard to avoid. A recent review looking at 'all surgically treated carotid PG' observed 22% new cranial nerve deficits, 3% stroke, and 1% peroperative deaths [250]. The same authors reviewed the literature on vagal and jugular PG and concluded that on average 1 extra post-operative cranial nerve deficit is observed per patient operated, as opposed to eight post-treatment cranial nerve deficits per 100 patients treated with RT, at a comparable local control rate of 80–90% for both modalities. Ten-year local control rates using RT of 94% and higher are reported [251, 252]. It can be concluded that RT has comparable tumour control and significantly less morbidity than surgery. A choice for surgery should put in the balance the patient's age, tumour size, predicted tumour growth, and cranial nerve function in order maximally to safeguard quality of life.

Further reading

Bauer DE, Mitchell CM, Strait KM, Lathan CS, Stelow EB et al. Clinicopathologic features and long-term outcomes of NUT midline carcinoma. Clinical Cancer Research 2012; 18(20): 5773–5779.

Bisdas S, Rumboldt Z, Surlan-Popovic K, Baghi M, Koh TS et al. Perfusion CT in squamous cell carcinoma of the upper aerodigestive tract: long-term predictive value of baseline perfusion CT measurements. American Journal of Neuroradiology 2010; 31: 576–581.

Cordes B, Williams MD, Tirado Y, Bell D, Rosenthal DI et al. Molecular and phenotypic analysis of poorly differentiated sinonasal neoplasms: an integrated approach for early diagnosis and classification. Human Pathology 2009; 40(3): 283–292.

Dauer EH, Lewis JE, Rohlinger AL, Weaver AL, Olsen KD. Sinonasal melanoma: a clinicopathologic review of 61 cases. Otolaryngology Head and Neck Surgery 2008; 138(3): 347–352.

de Bondt RB, Nelemans PJ, Hofman PA, Casselman JW, Kremer B et al. Detection of lymph node metastases in head and neck cancer: a meta-analysis comparing US, USgFNAC, CT and MR imaging. European Journal of Radiology 2007; 64: 266–272.

Di Martino E, Nowak B, Hassan HA, Hausmann R, Adam G et al. Diagnosis and staging of head and neck cancer: a comparison of modern imaging modalities (positron emission tomography, computed tomography, color-coded duplex sonography) with panendoscopic and histopathologic findings. Archives of Otolaryngology—Head & Neck Surgery 2000; 126: 1457–1461.

Ducic Y, Young L, McIntyre J. Neck dissection: past and present. Minerva Chirurgica 2010; 65(1): 45–58.

Ejaz A, Wenig BM. Sinonasal undifferentiated carcinoma: clinical and pathologic features and a discussion on classification, cellular differentiation, and differential diagnosis. Advances in Anatomic Pathology 2005; 12: 134–143.

El-Naggar AK, Westra WH. p16 expression as a surrogate marker for HPV-related oropharyngeal carcinoma: a guide for interpretative relevance and consistency. Head & Neck 2012; 34(4): 459–461.

Etges A, Pinto DS Jr, Kowalski LP, Soares FA, Araújo VC. Salivary duct carcinoma: immunohistochemical profile of an aggressive salivary gland tumour. Journal of Clinical Pathology 2003; 56(12): 914–918.

Frates MC, Benson CB, Charboneau JW, Cibas ES, Clark OH et al. Management of thyroid nodules detected at US: Society of Radiologists in Ultrasound consensus conference statement. Radiology 2005; 237: 794–800.

Frierson HF Jr, El-Naggar AK, Welsh JB, Sapinoso LM, Su AI et al. Large scale molecular analysis identifies genes with altered expression in salivary adenoid cystic carcinoma. American Journal of Pathology 2002; 161(4): 1315–1323.

Hermans R. Posttreatment imaging in head and neck cancer. European Journal of Radiology 2008; 66: 501–511.

Hermans R, Van den Bogaert W, Rijnders A, Doornaert P, Baert AL. Predicting the local outcome of glottic cancer treated by definitive radiation therapy: value of computed tomography determined tumor parameters. Radiotherapy & Oncology 1999; 50: 39–46.

Howlett DC. High resolution ultrasound assessment of the parotid gland. British Journal of Radiology 2003; 76: 271–277.

Ingeholm P, Theilgaard SA, Buchwald C, Hansen HS, Francis D. Esthesioneuroblastoma: a Danish clinicopathological study of 40 consecutive cases. APMIS 2002; 110(9): 639–645.

Kane SV, Gupta M, Kakade AC, D' Cruz A. Depth of invasion is the most significant histological predictor of subclinical cervical lymph node metastasis in early squamous carcinomas of the oral cavity. European Journal of Surgical Oncology 2006; 32(7): 795–803.

Kim S, Loevner L, Ouon H, Sherman E, Weinstein G et al. Diffusion-weighted magnetic resonance imaging for predicting and detecting early respons to chemoradiation therapy of squamous cell carcinomas of the head and neck. Clinical Cancer Research 2009; 15: 986–994.

King AD. Imaging for staging and management of thyroid cancer. Cancer Imaging 2008; 8: 57–69.

Lango MN, Andrews GA, Ahmad S, Feigenberg S, Tuluc M et al. Postradiotherapy neck dissection for head and neck squamous cell carcinoma: pattern of pathologic residual carcinoma and prognosis. Head & Neck 2009; 31(3): 328–337.

Li S, Feng X, Li T, Zhang S, Zuo Z et al. Extranodal NK/T-cell lymphoma, nasal type: a report of 73 cases at MD Anderson Cancer Center. American Journal of Surgical Pathology 2013; 37(1): 14–23.

Ljumanović R, Langendijk JA, Schenk B, Van Wattingen M, Knol DL et al. Supraglottic carcinoma treated with curative radiation therapy: identification of prognostic groups with MR imaging. Radiology 2004; 232: 440–448.

Lonneux M, Hamoir M, Reychler H, Maingon P, Duvillard C et al. Positron emission tomography with [18F]fluorodeoxyglucose improves staging and patient management in patients with head and neck squamous cell carcinoma: a multicenter prospective study. Journal of Clinical Oncology 2010; 28: 1190–1195.

Lonneux M, Lawson G, Ide C, Bausart R, Remacle M et al. Positron emission tomography with fluorodeoxyglucose for suspected head and neck tumor recurrence in the symptomatic patient. Laryngoscope 2000; 110: 1493–1497.

Myers JN, Greenberg JS, Mo V, Roberts D, Extracapsular spread. A significant predictor of treatment failure in patients with squamous carcinoma of tongue. Cancer 2001 15; 92(12): 3030–3036.

O'Neill JP, Bilsky MH, Kraus D. Head and neck sarcomas: epidemiology, pathology, and management. Neurosurgery Clinics of North America 2013; 24(1): 67–78.

Pameijer FA, Mancuso AA, Mendenhall WM, Parsons JT, Kubilis MS. Can pretreatment computed tomography predict local control in T3 squamous cell carcinoma of the glottis larynx treated with definitive radiotherapy? International Journal of Radiation Oncology Biology Physics 1997; 37: 1011–1021.

Vandecaveye V, De Keyzer F, Nuyts S, Deraedt K, Dirix P, Hamaekers P, Vander Poorten V, Delaere P, Hermans R. Detection of head and neck squamous cell carcinoma with diffusion weighted MRI after (chemo) radiotherapy: correlation between radiologic and histopathologic findings. Int J Radiat Oncol Biol Phys 2007; 67: 960–971.

Kim S, Loevner L, Ouon H et al. Diffusion-weighted magnetic resonance imaging for predicting and detecting early respons to chemoradiation therapy of squamous cell carcinomas of the head and neck. Clin Cancer Res 2009; 15: 986–994.

Quon A, Fischbein NJ, McDougall IR, Le QT, Loo BW Jr et al. Clinical role of 18F-FDG PET/CT in the management of squamous cell carcinoma of the head and neck and thyroid carcinoma. Journal of Nuclear Medicine 2007; 48(Suppl. 1): 58S–67S.

Rao PH, Roberts D, Zhao YJ, Bell D, Harris CP et al. Deletion of 1p32-p36 is the most frequent genetic change and poor prognostic marker in adenoid cystic carcinoma of the salivary glands. Clinical Cancer Research 2008; 14(16): 5181–5187.

Schöder H, Yeung HW. Positron emission imaging of head and neck cancer, including thyroid carcinoma. Seminars in Nuclear Medicine 2004; 34: 180–197.

Schwartz DL, Rajendran J, Yueh B, Coltrera M, Anzai Y et al. Staging of head and neck squamous cell cancer with extended-field FDG-PET. Archives of Otolaryngology—Head & Neck Surgery 2003; 129: 1173–1178.

Shukla-Dave A, Lee NY, Jansen JF, Thaler HT, Stambuk HE et al. Dynamic contrast-enhanced magnetic resonance imaging as a predictor of outcome in head-and-neck squamous cell carcinoma patients with nodal metastases. International Journal of Radiation Oncology Biology Physics 2012; 82: 1837–1844.

Thoeny HC, De Keyzer F, King AD. Diffusion-weighted MR imaging in the head and neck. Radiology 2012; 263: 19–32.

Tshering Vogel DW, Zbaeren P, Geretschlaeger A, Vermathen P, De Keyzer F et al. Diffusion-weighted MR imaging including bi-exponential fitting for the detection of recurrent or residual tumour after (chemo) radiotherapy for laryngeal and hypopharyngeal cancers. European Radiology 2013; 23: 562–569.

van der Waal I. Potentially malignant disorders of the oral and oropharyngeal mucosa; present concepts of management. Oral Oncology 2010; 46(6): 423–425.

Vandecaveye V, De Keyzer F, Dirix P, Lambrecht M, Nuyts S et al. Applications of diffusion-weighted magnetic resonance imaging in head and neck squamous cell carcinoma. Neuroradiology 2010; 52: 773–784.

Vandecaveye V, De Keyzer F, Nuyts S, Deraedt K, Dirix P et al. Detection of head and neck squamous cell carcinoma with diffusion weighted MRI after (chemo)radiotherapy: correlation between radiologic and histopathologic findings. International Journal of Radiation OncologyBiology Physics 2007; 67: 960–971.

Yamamoto Y, Wong TZ, Turkington TG, Hawk TC, Coleman RE. Head and neck cancer: dedicated FDG PET/CT protocol for detection—phantom and initial clinical studies. Radiology 2007; 244: 263–272.

Yeung AR, Liauw SL, Amdur RJ, Mancuso AA, Hinerman RW et al. Lymph node-positive head and neck cancer treated with definitive radiotherapy: can treatment response determine the extent of neck dissection? Cancer 2008; 112: 1076–1082.

References

1. Maier H, Dietz A, Gewelke U, Heller WD, Weidauer H. Tobacco and alcohol and the risk of head and neck cancer. Clnical Investigations 1992; 70(3–4): 320–327.

2. D'Souza G, Kreimer AR, Viscidi R, Pawlita M, Fakhry C et al. Case-control study of human papillomavirus and oropharyngeal cancer. New England Journal of Medicine 2007; 356(19): 1944–1956.

3. Chaturvedi AK, Engels EA, Pfeiffer RM, Hernandez BY, Xiao W et al. Human papillomavirus and rising oropharyngeal cancer incidence in the United States. Journal of Clinical Oncology 2011; 29(32): 4294–4301.

4. Ang KK, Harris J, Wheeler R, Weber R, Rosenthal DI et al. Human papillomavirus and survival of patients with oropharyngeal cancer. New England Journal of Medicine 2010; 363(1): 24–35.

5. Stransky N, Egloff AM, Tward AD, Kostic AD, Cibulskis K et al. The mutational landscape of head and neck squamous cell carcinoma. Science 2011; 333(6046): 1157–1160.

6. Agrawal N, Frederick MJ, Pickering CR, Bettegowda C, Chang K et al. Exome sequencing of head and neck squamous cell carcinoma reveals inactivating mutations in NOTCH1. Science 2011; 333(6046): 1154–1157.

7. Haddad RI, Shin DM. Recent advances in head and neck cancer. New England Journal of Medicine 2008; 359(11): 1143–1154.

8. zur Hausen H. Papillomaviruses and cancer: from basic studies to clinical application. Nature Reviews Cancer 2002; 2(5): 342–350.

9. Chung CH, Gillison ML. Human papillomavirus in head and neck cancer: its role in pathogenesis and clinical implications. Clinical Cancer Researchearch 2009; 15(22): 6758–6762.

10. Howard JD, Chung CH. Biology of human papillomavirus-related oropharyngeal cancer. Seminars in Radiation Oncology 2012; 22(3): 187–193.

11. Maslon MM, Hupp TR. Drug discovery and mutant p53. Trends in Cellular Biology 2010; 20(9): 542–555.

12. Poeta ML, Manola J, Goldwasser MA, Forastiere A, Benoit N et al. TP53 mutations and survival in squamous-cell carcinoma of the head and neck. New England Journal of Medicine 2007; 357(25): 2552–2561.

13. Lukas J, Parry D, Aagaard L, Mann DJ, Bartkova J et al. Retinoblastoma-protein-dependent cell-cycle inhibition by the tumour suppressor p16. Nature 1995; 375(6531): 503–506.

14. Ha PK, Califano JA. Promoter methylation and inactivation of tumour-suppressor genes in oral squamous-cell carcinoma. Lancet Oncology 2006; 7(1): 77–82.

15. Hayes DN, Grandis JR, El-Naggar AK. The Cancer Genome Atlas Network: comprehensive genomic characterization of head and neck squamous cell carcinomas. Nature 2015; 517: 576–582

16. cBioportal for Cancer Genomics, <http://www.cbioportal.org>.

17. Chung CH, Parker JS, Karaca G, Wu J, Funkhouser WK et al. Molecular classification of head and neck squamous cell carcinomas using patterns of gene expression. Cancer Cell 2004; 5(5): 489–500.

18. Walter V, Yin X, Wilkerson MD, Cabanski C, Zhao N et al. Molecular subtypes in head and neck cancer exhibit distinct patterns of chromosomal gain and loss of canonical cancer genes. PLOS One 2013; 8(2):e56823.

19. Keck MK, Zuo Z, Khattri A, Brown CD, Stricker T et al. Integrative analysis of head and neck cancer identifies two biologically distinct HPV and three non-HPV subtypes eerch 2015 Feb 15; 21(4): 870–881

20. Barnes L, Eveson JW, Reichart P et al eds. Head and Neck Tumours. Lym: IARC, 2005.

21. Napier SS, Speight PM. Natural history of potentially malignant oral lesions and conditions: an overview of the literature: an overview of the literature. Journal of Oral Pathology & Medicine 2008; 37(1): 1–10.

22. van der Waal I. Potentially malignant disorders of the oral and oropharyngeal mucosa; present concepts of management. Oral Oncology 2010; 46(6): 423–425.

23. Slaughter DP, Southwick HW, Smejkal W. Field cancerization in oral stratified squamous epithelium; clinical implications of multicentric origin. Cancer 1953; 6(5): 963–968.

24. Lee JJ, Hong WK, Hittelman WN, Mao L, Lotan R et al. Predicting cancer development in oral leukoplakia: ten years of translational research. Clinical Cancer Research 2000 May; 6(5): 1702–1710.

25. El-Naggar AK, Westra WH. p16 expression as a surrogate marker for HPV-related oropharyngeal carcinoma: a guide for interpretative relevance and consistency. Head & Neck 2012; 34(4): 459–461.

26. Kane SV, Gupta M, Kakade AC, D' Cruz A. Depth of invasion is the most significant histological predictor of subclinical cervical lymph node metastasis in early squamous carcinomas of the oral cavity. European Journal of Surgical Oncology 2006; 32(7): 795–803.

27. Myers JN, Greenberg JS, Mo V, Roberts D, Extracapsular spread. A significant predictor of treatment failure in patients with squamous carcinoma of tongue. Cancer 2001 15; 92(12): 3030–3036.

28. Woolgar JA, Scott J. Prediction of cervical lymph node metastasis in squamous cell carcinoma of the tongue/floor of mouth. Head & Neck 1995; 17(6): 463–472.

29. Ducic Y, Young L, McIntyre J. Neck dissection: past and present. Minerva Chirurgica 2010; 65(1): 45–58.

30. Lango MN, Andrews GA, Ahmad S, Feigenberg S, Tuluc M et al. Postradiotherapy neck dissection for head and neck squamous cell carcinoma: pattern of pathologic residual carcinoma and prognosis. Head & Neck 2009; 31(3): 328–337.

31. Cordes B, Williams MD, Tirado Y, Bell D, Rosenthal DI et al. Molecular and phenotypic analysis of poorly differentiated sinonasal neoplasms: an integrated approach for early diagnosis and classification. Human Pathology 2009; 40(3): 283–292.

32. Bauer DE, Mitchell CM, Strait KM, Lathan CS, Stelow EB et al. Clinicopathologic features and long-term outcomes of NUT midline carcinoma. Clinical Cancer Research 2012; 18(20): 5773–5779.

33. Ejaz A, Wenig BM. Sinonasal undifferentiated carcinoma: clinical and pathologic features and a discussion on classification, cellular differentiation, and differential diagnosis. Advances in Anatomic Pathology 2005; 12: 134–143.

34. Ingeholm P, Theilgaard SA, Buchwald C, Hansen HS, Francis D. Esthesioneuroblastoma: a Danish clinicopathological study of 40 consecutive cases. APMIS 2002; 110(9): 639–645.

35. Hyams VJ, Batsakis JG, Michaels L eds. Olfactory neuroblastoma. In Hyams VJ, Baksakis JG, Michaels L eds, Tumors of the Upper Respiratory Tract and Ear. Washington, DC: Armed Forces Institute of Pathology, 1988, 240–248.

36. Dauer EH, Lewis JE, Rohlinger AL, Weaver AL, Olsen KD. Sinonasal melanoma: a clinicopathologic review of 61 cases. Otolaryngology Head and Neck Surgery 2008; 138(3): 347–352.

37. O'Neill JP, Bilsky MH, Kraus D. Head and neck sarcomas: epidemiology, pathology, and management. Neurosurgery Clinics of North America 2013; 24(1): 67–78.

38. Ahmed AA, Tsokos M. Sinonasal rhabdomyosarcoma in children and young adults. International Journal of Surgical Pathology 2007 Apr; 15(2): 160–165.

39. Bahrami A, Gown AM, Baird GS, Hicks MJ, Folpe AL. Aberrant expression of epithelial and neuroendocrine markers in alveolar rhabdomyosarcoma: a potentially serious diagnostic pitfall. Modern Pathology 2008; 21(7): 795–806.

40. Li S, Feng X, Li T, Zhang S, Zuo Z et al. Extranodal NK/T-cell lymphoma, nasal type: a report of 73 cases at MD Anderson Cancer Center. American Journal of Surgical Pathology 2013; 37(1): 14–23.

41. Spiro IJ, Wang CC, Montgomery WW. Carcinoma of the parotid gland: analysis of treatment results and patterns of failure after combined surgery and radiation therapy. Cancer 1993; 71(9): 2699–2705.

42. Spiro RH. Salivary neoplasms: overview of a 35-year experience with 2,807 patients. Head & Neck Surgery 1986; 8(3): 177–184.

43. Mani RS, Chinnaiyan AM. Triggers for genomic rearrangements: insights into genomic, cellular and environmental influences. Nature Reviews Genetics 2010; 11(12): 819–829.

44. Frierson HF Jr, El-Naggar AK, Welsh JB, Sapinoso LM, Su AI et al. Large scale molecular analysis identifies genes with altered expression in salivary adenoid cystic carcinoma. American Journal of Pathology 2002; 161(4): 1315–1323.

45. Rao PH, Roberts D, Zhao YJ, Bell D, Harris CP et al. Deletion of 1p32-p36 is the most frequent genetic change and poor prognostic marker in adenoid cystic carcinoma of the salivary glands. Clinical Cancer Research 2008; 14(16): 5181–5187.

46. Jeng YM, Lin CY, Hsu HC. Expression of the c-kit protein is associated with certain subtypes of salivary gland carcinoma. Cancer Letters 2000; 154(1): 107–111.

47. Murrah VA, Batsakis JG. Salivary duct carcinoma. Annals of Otology, Rhinology & Laryngology 1994; 103(3): 244–247.

48. Etges A, Pinto DS Jr, Kowalski LP, Soares FA, Araújo VC. Salivary duct carcinoma: immunohistochemical profile of an aggressive salivary gland tumour. Journal of Clinical Pathology 2003; 56(12): 914–918.

49. Howlett DC. High resolution ultrasound assessment of the parotid gland. British Journal of Radiology 2003; 76: 271–277.

50. Frates MC, Benson CB, Charboneau JW, Cibas ES, Clark OH et al. Management of thyroid nodules detected at US: Society of Radiologists in Ultrasound consensus conference statement. Radiology 2005; 237: 794–800.

51. Ojiri H, Mendenhall WM, Mancuso AA. CT findings at the primary site of oropharyngeal squamous cell carcinoma within 6–8 weeks after definitive radiotherapy as predictors of primary site control. International Journal of Radiation Oncology Biology Physics 2002; 52: 748–754.

52. King AD. Imaging for staging and management of thyroid cancer. Cancer Imaging 2008; 8: 57–69.

53. de Bondt RB, Nelemans PJ, Hofman PA, Casselman JW, Kremer B et al. Detection of lymph node metastases in head and neck cancer: a meta-analysis comparing US, USgFNAC, CT and MR imaging. European Journal of Radiology 2007; 64: 266–272.

54. Vandecaveye V, De Keyzer F, Dirix P, Lambrecht M, Nuyts S et al. Applications of diffusion-weighted magnetic resonance imaging in head and neck squamous cell carcinoma. Neuroradiology 2010; 52: 773–784.

55. Brockenbrough JM, Petruzzelli GJ, Lomasney L. DentaScan as an accurate method of predicting mandibular invasion in patients with squamous cell carcinoma of the oral cavity. Archives of Otolaryngology—Head & Neck Surgery 2003; 129: 113–117.

56. Imaizumi A, Yoshino N, Yamada I, Nagumo K, Amagasa T et al. A potential pitfall of MR imaging for assessing mandibular invasion of squamous cell carcinoma in the oral cavity. American Journal of Neuroradiology 2006; 27: 114–122.

57. Mancuso AA, Mukherji SK, Schmalfuss I, Mendenhall W, Parsons J et al. Preradiotherapy computed tomography as a predictor of local control in supraglottic carcinoma. Journal of Clinical Oncology 1999; 17: 631–637.

58. Pameijer FA, Mancuso AA, Mendenhall WM, Parsons JT, Kubilis MS. Can pretreatment computed tomography predict local control in T3 squamous cell carcinoma of the glottis larynx treated with definitive radiotherapy? International Journal of Radiation Oncology Biology Physics 1997; 37: 1011–1021.

59. Pameijer FA, Mancuso AA, Mendenhall WM, Parsons JT, Mukherji SK et al. Evaluation of pretreatment computed tomography as a predictor of local control in T1/T2 piriform sinus carcinoma treated with definitive radiotherapy. Head & Neck 1998; 20: 159–68.

60. Hermans R, Van den Bogaert W, Rijnders A, Doornaert P, Baert AL. Predicting the local outcome of glottic cancer treated by definitive radiation therapy: value of computed tomography determined tumor parameters. Radiotherapy & Oncology 1999; 50: 39–46.

61. Ljumanović R, Langendijk JA, Schenk B, Van Wattingen M, Knol DL et al. Supraglottic carcinoma treated with curative radiation therapy: identification of prognostic groups with MR imaging. Radiology 2004; 232: 440–448.

62. Ljumanovic R, Langendijk JA, van Wattingen M, Schenk B, Knol DL et al. MR imaging predictors of local control of glottic squamous cell carcinoma treated with radiation alone. Radiology 2007; 244: 205–212.

63. de Bondt RB, Nelemans PJ, Hofman PA, Casselman JW, Kremer B et al. Detection of lymph node metastases in head and neck cancer: a meta-analysis comparing US, USgFNAC, CT and MR imaging. European Journal of Radiology 2007; 64: 266–272.

64. Hermans R. Posttreatment imaging in head and neck cancer. European Journal of Radiology 2008; 66: 501–511.

65. Yeung AR, Liauw SL, Amdur RJ, Mancuso AA, Hinerman RW et al. Lymph node-positive head and neck cancer treated with definitive radiotherapy: can treatment response determine the extent of neck dissection? Cancer 2008; 112: 1076–1082.

66. Bisdas S, Rumboldt Z, Surlan-Popovic K, Baghi M, Koh TS et al. Perfusion CT in squamous cell carcinoma of the upper aerodigestive tract: long-term predictive value of baseline perfusion CT measurements. American Journal of Neuroradiology 2010; 31: 576–581.

67. Surlan-Popovic K, Bisdas S, Rumboldt Z, Koh TS, Strojan P. Changes in perfusion CT of advanced squamous cell carcinoma of the head and neck treated during the course of concomitant chemoradiotherapy. American Journal of Neuroradiology 2010; 31: 570–575.

68. Shukla-Dave A, Lee NY, Jansen JF, Thaler HT, Stambuk HE et al. Dynamic contrast-enhanced magnetic resonance imaging as a predictor of outcome in head-and-neck squamous cell carcinoma patients with nodal metastases. International Journal of Radiation Oncology Biology Physics 2012; 82: 1837–1844.

69. Thoeny HC, De Keyzer F, King AD. Diffusion-weighted MR imaging in the head and neck. Radiology 2012; 263: 19–32.

70. Vandecaveye V, De Keyzer F, Nuyts S, Deraedt K, Dirix P et al. Detection of head and neck squamous cell carcinoma with diffusion weighted MRI after (chemo)radiotherapy: correlation between radiologic and histopathologic findings. International Journal of Radiation Oncology Biology Physics 2007; 67: 960–971.

71. Tshering Vogel DW, Zbaeren P, Geretschlaeger A, Vermathen P, De Keyzer F et al. Diffusion-weighted MR imaging including bi-exponential fitting for the detection of recurrent or residual tumour after (chemo)radiotherapy for laryngeal and hypopharyngeal cancers. European Radiology 2013; 23: 562–569.

72. Kim S, Loevner L, Ouon H, Sherman E, Weinstein G et al. Diffusion-weighted magnetic resonance imaging for predicting and detecting early respons to chemoradiation therapy of squamous cell carcinomas of the head and neck. Clinical Cancer Research 2009; 15: 986–994.

73. Vandecaveye V, Dirix P, De Keyzer F, de Beeck KO, Vander Poorten V et al. Predictive value of diffusion-weighted magnetic resonance imaging during chemoradiotherapy for head and neck squamous cell carcinoma. European Radiology 2010; 20: 1703–1714.

74. Vandecaveye V, Dirix P, De Keyzer F, Op de Beeck K, Vander Poorten V et al. Diffusion-weighted magnetic resonance imaging early after chemoradiotherapy to monitor treatment response in head-and-neck squamous cell carcinoma. International Journal of Radiation Oncology Biology Physics 2012; 82: 1098–1107.

75. Yamamoto Y, Wong TZ, Turkington TG, Hawk TC, Coleman RE. Head and neck cancer: dedicated FDG PET/CT protocol for detection—phantom and initial clinical studies. Radiology 2007; 244: 263–272.

76. Di Martino E, Nowak B, Hassan HA, Hausmann R, Adam G et al. Diagnosis and staging of head and neck cancer: a comparison of modern imaging modalities (positron emission tomography, computed tomography, color-coded duplex sonography) with panendoscopic and histopathologic findings. Archives of Otolaryngology—Head & Neck Surgery 2000; 126: 1457–1461.

77. Schöder H, Yeung HW. Positron emission imaging of head and neck cancer, including thyroid carcinoma. Seminars in Nuclear Medicine 2004; 34: 180–197.

78. Allal AS, Dulguerov P, Allaoua M, Haenggeli CA, El-Ghazi el A et al. Standardized uptake value of 2-[(18)F] fluoro-2-deoxy-D-glucose in predicting outcome in head and neck carcinomas treated by radiotherapy with or without chemotherapy. Journal of Clinical Oncology 2002; 20: 1398–1404.

79. Quon A, Fischbein NJ, McDougall IR, Le QT, Loo BW Jr et al. Clinical role of 18F-FDG PET/CT in the management of squamous cell carcinoma of the head and neck and thyroid carcinoma. Journal of Nuclear Medicine 2007; 48(Suppl. 1): 58S–67S.

80. Schwartz DL, Rajendran J, Yueh B, Coltrera M, Anzai Y et al. Staging of head and neck squamous cell cancer with extended-field FDG-PET. Archives of Otolaryngology—Head & Neck Surgery 2003; 129: 1173–1178.

81. Lonneux M, Hamoir M, Reychler H, Maingon P, Duvillard C et al. Positron emission tomography with [18F]fluorodeoxyglucose improves staging and patient management in patients with head and neck squamous cell carcinoma: a multicenter prospective study. Journal of Clinical Oncology 2010; 28: 1190–1195.

82. McGuirt WF, Williams DW 3rd, Keyes JW Jr, Greven KM, Watson NE Jr et al. A comparative diagnostic study of head and neck nodal metastases using positron emission tomography. Laryngoscope 1995; 105: 373–375.

83. Lonneux M, Lawson G, Ide C, Bausart R, Remacle M et al. Positron emission tomography with fluorodeoxyglucose for suspected head and neck tumor recurrence in the symptomatic patient. Laryngoscope 2000; 110: 1493–1497.

84. Kishino T, Hoshikawa H, Nishiyama Y, Yamamoto Y, Mori N. Usefulness of 3'-deoxy-3'-18F-fluorothymidine PET for predicting early response to chemoradiotherapy in head and neck cancer. Journal of Nuclear Medicine 2012; 53: 1521–1527.

85. Brun E, Kjellén E, Tennvall J, Ohlsson T, Sandell A et al. FDG PET studies during treatment: prediction of therapy outcome in head and neck squamous cell carcinoma. Head & Neck 2002; 24: 127–135.

86. Sisson GA, Becket SP. Cancer of the nasal cavity and paranasal sinuses In Suen JY, Myers EN ed., Cancer of the Head and Neck. New York: Churchill Livingstone, 1981, 242–279.

87. Carrau R, Myers E, Johnson J. Paranasal sinus carcinoma, diagnosis, treatment andprognosis. Oncology 1992; 6: 43–50.

88. Cheesman A, Lund V, Howard D. Craniofacial resection for tumors of the nasal cavity and paranasal sinuses. Head & Neck Surgery 1986; 8: 429–435.

89. Lund V, Harrison D. Craniofacial resection for tumors of the nasal cavity and paranasal sinuses. American Journal of Surgery 1988; 156: 187–190.

90. Irish J, Gullane P, Gentili F, Freeman J, Boyd JB et al. Tumors of the skull base: outcome and survival analysis of 77 cases. Head & Neck 1994; 16(1): 3–10.

91. Shah J, Kraus D, Arbit E, Galicich J, Strong E. Craniofacial resection for tumor involving the anterior skull. Otolaryngology—Head & Neck Surgery 1992; 106: 387–393.

92. Cantu G, Solero CL, Mariani L, Lo Vullo S, Riccio S et al. Intestinal type adenocarcinoma of the ethmoid sinus in wood and leather workers: a retrospective study of 153 cases. Head & Neck 2011; 33(4): 535–542.

93. Cantu G, Solero CL, Miceli R, Mattana F, Riccio S et al. Anterior craniofacial resection for malignant paranasal tumors: a monoinstitutional experience of 366 cases. Head & Neck 2012; 34(1): 78–87.

94. Suarez C, Ferlito A, Lund VJ, Silver CE, Fagan JJ et al. Management of the orbit in malignant sinonasal tumors. Head & Neck 2008; 30(2): 242–250.

95. Singh N, Eskander A, Huang, Curtin H, Bartlett E et al. Imaging and resectability issues of sinonasal tumors. Expert Review of Anticancer Therapy 2013; 13(3): 297–312.

96. Cantu G, Solero C. L, Miceli R, Bolzoni Villaret A et al. Which classification for ethmoid malignant tumors involving the anterior skull base? Head & Neck 2005; 27(3): 224–231.

97. Ketcham AS, Wilkins RH, Van Buren JM, Mariani L, Mattavelli F et al. A combined intracranial facial approach to the paranasal sinuses. American Journal of Surgery 1963; 106: 698–703.

98. Ganly I, Patel SG, Singh B, Kraus DH, Bridger PG et al. Craniofacial resection for malignant paranasal sinus tumors: report of an international collaborative study. Head & Neck 2005; 27(7): 575–584.

99. Nicolai P, Battaglia P, Bignami M, Bolzoni Villaret A, Delù G et al. Endoscopic surgery for malignant tumors of the sinonasal tract and adjacent skull base: a 10-year experience. American Journal of Rhinology 2008; 22(3): 308–316.

100. Batra PS, Luong A, Kanowitz SJ, Sade B, Lee J et al. Outcomes of minimally invasive endoscopic resection of anterior skull base neoplasms. Laryngoscope 2010; 120(1): 9–16.

101. Parsons JT, Bova FJ, Fitzgerald, Mendenhall WM, Million RR. Severe dry-eye syndrome following external beam irradiation. International Journal of Radiation Oncology Biology Physics 1994; 30; 775–780.

102. Parsons JT, Bova FJ, Mendenhall WM, Million RR, Fitzgerald CR. Response of the normal eye to high dose radiotherapy. Oncology (Huntington) 1996; 10; 837–847.

103. Dulguerov P, Jacobsen MS, Allal, Lehmann W, Calcaterra T et al. Nasal and paranasal sinus carcinoma: are we making progress? A series of 220 patients and a systematic review. Cancer 2001; 92; 3012–3029.

104. Duthoy W, Boterberg T, Claus, Ost P, Vakaet L et al. Postoperative intensity-modulated radiotherapy in sinonasal carcinoma: clinical results in 39 patients. Cancer 2005; 104; 71–82.

105. Licitra L, Locati LD, Bossi P, Cantù G. Head and neck tumors other than squamous cell carcinoma. Current Opinions in Oncology 2004; 16: 236–241.

106. Hanna EY, Cardenas AD, DeMonte F, Roberts D, Kupferman M et al. Induction chemotherapy for advanced squamous cell caricnoma of the paranasal sinuses. Archives of Otolaryngology—Head & Neck Surgery 2011; 137(1): 78–81.

107. Lee MM, Vokes EE, Rosen A, Witt ME, Weichselbaum RR et al. Multimodality therapy in advanced paranasal sinus caricnoma: superior long-term results. Cancer Journal from Scientific American 1999; 5(4): 219–223.

108. Licitra L, Locati LD, Cavina R, Garassino I, Mattavelli F et al. Primary chemotherapy followed by anterior craniofacial resection and radiotherapy for paranasal cancer. Annals of Oncology 2003; 14: 367–372.

109. Licitra L, Suardi S, Bossi P, Locati LD, Mariani L et al. Prediction of TP53 status for primary cisplatin, fluorouracil, and leucovorin chemotherapy in ethmoid sinus intestinal-type adenocarcinoma. Journal of Clinical Oncology 2004; 22: 4901–4906.

110. Bossi P, Perrone F, Miceli R, Cantù G, Mariani L et al. TP53 status as guide for the management of ethmoid sinus intestinal-type adenocarcinoma. Oral Oncology 2013; 49: 413–419.

111. Rosenthal DI, Barker JL, El-Naggar AK, Aggarwal JP, Kane SV et al. Sinonasal malignancies with neuroendocrine differentiation. Patterns of failure according to histologic phenotype. Cancer 2004; 101: 2567–2573.

112. Mourad WF, Hauerstock D, Shourbaji RA, Hu KS, Culliney B et al. Trimodality management of sinonasal undifferentiated carcinoma and review of the literature. American Journal of Clinical Oncology 2013; 36: 584–588.

113. Knegt PP, Ah-See KW, vd Velden LA, Kerrebijn J. Adenocarcinoma of the ethmoidal sinus complex: surgical debulking and topical fluorouracil may be the optimal treatment. Archives of Otolaryngology—Head & Neck Surgery 2001; 127: 141–146.

114. Sato Y, Morita M, Takahashi H, Watanabe N, Kirikae I. Combined surgery, radiotherapy, and regional chemotherapy of the paranasal sinuses. Cancer 1970; 25; 571–579.

115. Almeyda R, Capper J. Is surgical debridement and topical 5-fluorouracil the optimum treatment for woodworkers' adenocarcinoma of the ethmoid sinuses? A case-controlled study of a 20 years experience. Clinical Otolaryngology 2008; 33(5): 435–441.

116. Van Dijk BA, Gatta G, Capocaccia R, Pierannunzio D, Strojan P et al. Rare cancers of the head and neck area in Europe. European Journal of Cancer 2012; 48: 783–796.

117. Chang ET, Adami HO. The enigmatic epidemiology of nasopharyngeal carcinoma. Cancer Epidemiology, Biomarkers & Prevention 2006; 15: 1765–1777.

118. Bray F, Haugen M, Moger TA, Tretli S, Aalen OO et al. Age-incidence curves of nasopharyngeal carcinoma worldwide: bimodality in low-risk populations and aetiologic implications. Cancer Epidemiology, Biomarkers & Prevention 2008; 17: 2356–2365.

119. Robinson M, Suh YE, Paleri V, Devlin D, Ayaz B et al. Oncogenic human papillomavirus-associated nasopharyngeal carcinoma: an observational study of correlation with ethnicity, histological subtype and outcome in a UK population. Infectious Agents and Cancer 2013; 8: 30.

120. Hsu CL, Chang KP, Lin CY, Chang HK, Wang CH et al. Plasma Epstein–Barr virus DNA concentration and clearance rate as novel prognostic factors for metastatic nasopharyngeal carcinoma. Head & Neck 2012; 34: 1064–1070.

121. Leung SF, Zee B, Ma BB, Hui EP, Mo F et al. Plasma Epstein-Barr viral deoxyribonucleic acid quantitation complements tumor-node-metastasis staging prognostication in nasopharyngeal carcinoma. Journal of Clinical Oncology 2006; 24: 5414–5418.

122. Hsu CL, Chan SC, Chang KP, Lin TL, Lin CY et al. Clinical scenario of EBV DNA follow-up in patients of treated localized nasopharyngeal carcinoma. Oral Oncology 2013; 49: 620–625.

123. Twu CW, Wang WY, Liang WM, Jan JS, Jiang RS et al. Comparison of the prognostic impact of serum anti-EBV antibody and plasma EBV DNA assays in nasopharyngeal carcinoma. International Journal of Radiation Oncology Biology Physics 2007; 67: 130–137.

124. Feng M, Wang W, Fan Z, Fu B, Li J et al. Tumor volume is an independent prognostic indicator of local control in nasopharyngeal carcinoma patients treated with intensity-modulated radiotherapy. Radiation Oncology 2013; 8: 208.

125. Lee N, Xia P, Quivey JM, Chau RM, Suen JJ et al. Intensity-modulated radiotherapy in the treatment of nasopharyngeal carcinoma: an update of the UCSF experience. International Journal of Radiation Oncology Biology Physics 2002; 53: 12–22.

126. Lee N, Harris J, Garden AS, Straube W, Glisson B et al. Intensity-modulated radiation therapy with or without chemotherapy for nasopharyngeal carcinoma: radiation therapy oncology group phase II trial 0225. Journal of Clinical Oncology 2009; 27: 3684–3690.

127. Kam MK, Leung SF, Zee B, Chau RM, Suen JJ et al. Prospective randomized study of intensity-modulated radiotherapy on salivary gland function in early-stage nasopharyngeal carcinoma patients. Journal of Clinical Oncology 2007; 25: 4873–4879.

128. Pow EH, Kwong DL, McMillan AS, Wong MC, Sham JS et al. Xerostomia and quality of life after intensity-modulated radiotherapy vs. conventional radiotherapy for early-stage nasopharyngeal carcinoma: initial report on a randomized controlled clinical trial. International Journal of Radiation Oncology Biology Physics 2006; 66: 981–991.

129. Peng G, Wang T, Yang KY, Zhang S, Zhang T et al. A prospective, randomized study comparing outcomes and toxicities of intensity-modulated radiotherapy vs. conventional two-dimensional radiotherapy for the treatment of nasopharyngeal carcinoma. Radiotherapy & Oncology 2012; 104: 286–293.

130. Chen QY, Wen YF, Guo L, Liui H, Huang P-Y et al. Concurrent chemoradiotherapy vs radiotherapy alone in stage II nasopharyngeal carcinoma: phase III randomized trial. Journal of the National Cancer Institute 2011; 103: 1761–1770.

131. Baujat B, Audry H, Bourhis J, et al. Chemotherapy in locally advanced nasopharyngeal carcinoma: an individual patient data meta-analysis of eight randomized trials and 1753 patients. International Journal of Radiation Oncology Biology Physics 2006; 64: 47–56.

132. Chen L, Hu CS, Chen XZ, Chan AT, Onat H et al. Concurrent chemoradiotherapy plus adjuvant chemotherapy versus concurrent chemoradiotherapy alone in patients with locoregionally advanced nasopharyngeal carcinoma: a phase 3 multicentre randomised controlled trial. Lancet Oncology 2012; 13: 163–171.

133. Le QT, Zhang Q, Cao H, Cheng AJ, Pinsky BA et al. An international collaboration to harmonize the quantitative plasma Epstein-Barr virus DNA assay for future biomarker-guided trials in nasopharyngeal carcinoma. Clinical Cancer Research 2013; 19: 2208–2215.

134. Lee WM, Ng WT, Chan OS, et al. If concurrent-adjuvant chemoradiotherapy is beneficial for locoregionally advanced nasopharyngeal carcinoma, would changing the sequence to induction-concurrent achieve better outcome? Journal of Radiation Oncology 2012; 1: 107–115.

135. Hui EP, Ma BB, Leung SF, King AD, Mo F et al. Randomized phase II trial of concurrent cisplatin-radiotherapy with or without neoadjuvant docetaxel and cisplatin in advanced nasopharyngeal carcinoma. Journal of Clinical Oncology 2009; 27: 242–249.

136. Lin H, Lin H, Cai X, Jin T, Guo LB et al. Chemotherapy plus radiotherapy makes curability a possibility in nasopharyngeal carcinoma patients with distant metastasis at diagnosis. Head & Neck Oncology 2013; 5: 1.

137. Ma J, Wen ZS, Lin P, Wang X, Xie FY. The results and prognosis of different treatment modalities for solitary metastatic lung tumor from nasopharyngeal carcinoma: a retrospective study of 105 cases. Chinese Journal of Cancer 2010; 29: 787–795.

138. Fandi A, Bachouchi M, Azli N, Taamma A, Boussen H et al. Long-term disease-free survivors in metastatic undifferentiated carcinoma of nasopharyngeal type. Journal of Clinical Oncology 2000; 18: 1324–1330.

139. Hao SP, Tsang NM. Surgical management of recurrent nasopharyngeal carcinoma. Chang Gung Medical Journal 2010; 33: 361–369, 2010.

140. Wei WI, Kwong DL. Current management strategy of nasopharyngeal carcinoma. Clinical & Experimental Otorhinolaryngology 2010; 3: 1–12.

141. Wei WI, Sham JS. Nasopharyngeal carcinoma. Lancet 365: 2041–2054, 2005.

142. Suarez C, Rodrigo JP, Rinaldo A, Langendijk JA, Shaha AR et al. Current treatment options for recurrent nasopharyngeal cancer. European Archives of Otorhinolaryngology 2010; 267: 1811–1824.

143. Chua DT, Wei WI, Sham JS, Hung KN, Au GK. Stereotactic radiosurgery versus gold grain implantation in salvaging local failures of nasopharyngeal carcinoma. International Journal of Radiation Oncology Biology Physics 2007; 69: 469–474.

144. Indrasari SR, Timmermans AJ, Wildeman MA, Karakullukcu MB, Herdini C et al. Remarkable response to photodynamic therapy in residual T4N0M0 nasopharyngeal carcinoma: a case report. Photodiagnosis and Photodynamic Therapy 2012; 9: 319–320.

145. Wildeman MA, Nyst HJ, Karakullukcu B, Tan BI. Photodynamic therapy in the therapy for recurrent/persistent nasopharyngeal cancer. Head & Neck Oncology 2009; 1: 40.

146. Bensouda Y, Kaikani W, Ahbeddou N, Rahhali R, Jabri M et al. Treatment for metastatic nasopharyngeal carcinoma. European Annals of Otorhinolaryngology–Head & Neck Diseases 2011; 128: 79–85.

147. Wolff K-D, Bootz F, Beck J, Bikowski K, Böhme P et al. Carcinoma of the oral cavity [Mundhöhlenkarzinom, Diagnostik und Therapie des Mundhöhlenkarzinoms] AWMF-Register-Number 007-100OL, Version 2.0 11.2012.

148. Scottish Intercollegiate Guidelines Network (SIGN), <http://www. sign.ac.uk>.

149. O'Brien CJ, Lauer CS, Fredricks S, Clifford AR, McNeil EB et al. Tumor thickness influences prognosis of T1 and T2 oral cavity cancer—but what thickness? Head & Neck 2003; 25(11): 937–945.

150. Royal College of Pathologists. Standards and Datasets for Reporting Cancers: Datasets for Histopathology Reports on Head and Neck Carcinomas and Salivary Neoplasms, 2nd ed. London: Royal College of Pathologists, 2005. Available from url: http://www.rcpath.org/ Resources/RCPath/Migrated%20Resources/Documents/G/G112_ NeckDissectionDataset_Nov13.pdf, accessed on 21 May 2015.

151. Robbins KT, Clayman G, Levine PA, Medina J, Sessions R et al. Neck dissection classification update: revisions proposed by the American Head and Neck Society and the American Academy of Otolaryngology—Head and Neck Surgery. Archives of Otolaryngology—Head & Neck Surgery 2002; 128(12117328): 751–758.

152. Küffer R, Lombardi T. Premalignant lesions of the oral mucosa: a discussion about the place of oral intraepithelial neoplasia (OIN). Oral Oncologyog 2002; 38(2): 125–130.

153. Pignon JP, le Maitre A, Maillard E, Bourhis J on behalf of the MACH-NC Collaborative Group. Meta-analysis of chemotherapy in head and neck cancer (MACH_NC): an update on 93 randomised trials and 17,346 patients. Radiotherapy and Oncology 2009; 92: 4–14.

154. Blanchard P, Bourhis J, Lacas B, Posner MR, Vermorken JB et al. Taxane-cisplatin-fluorouracil as induction chemotherapy in locally advanced head and neck cancers: an individual patient data meta-analysis of the meta-analysis of chemotherapy in head and neck cancer group. Journal of Clinical Oncology 2013; 31(23): 2854–2860.

155. Licitra L, Grandi C, Guzzo M, Mariani L, Lo Vullo S et al. Primary chemotherapy in resectable oral cavity squamous cell cancer: a randomized controlled trial. Journal of Clinical Oncology 2003; 21(2): 327–333.

156. Zhong LP, Zhang CP, Ren GX, Guo W, William WN Jr et al. Randomized phase III trial of induction chemotherapy with docetaxel, cisplatin, and fluorouracil followed by surgery versus up-front surgery in locally advanced resectable oral squamous cell carcinoma. Journal of Clinical Oncology 2013; 31(6): 744–751.

157. Domenge C, Hill C, Lefebvre JL, De Raucourt D, Rhein B et al. Randomized trial of neoadjuvant chemotherapy in oropharynx carcinoma. French Groupe d'Etude des Tumeurs de la Tête et du Cou (GETTEC). British Journal of Cancer 2000; 83: 1594–1598.

158. Denis F, Garaud P, Bardet E, Alfonsi M, Sire C et al. Final results of the 94-01 French Head and Neck Oncology and Radiotherapy Group randomized trial comparing radiotherapy alone with concomitant radiochemotherapy in advanced-stage oropharynx carcinoma. Journal of Clinical Oncology 2004; 22: 69–76.

159. Fallai C, Bolner A, Signor M, Gava A, Franchin G et al. Long-term results of conventional radiotherapy versus accelerated hyperfractionated radiotherapy versus concomitant radiotherapy and chemotherapy in locoregionally advanced carcinoma of the oropharynx. Tumori 2006; 92: 41–54.

160. Pignon JP, Bourhis J, Domenge C, De Raucourt D, Rhein B et al. Chemotherapy added to locoregional treatment for head and neck squamous-cell carcinoma: three meta-analyses of updated individual data. MACH-NC Collaborative Group. Meta-Analysis of Chemotherapy on Head and Neck Cancer. Lancet 2000; 355: 949–955.

161. Bonner JA, Harari PM, Giralt J, Azarnia N, Shin DM et al. Radiotherapy plus cetuximab for squamous-cell carcinoma of the head and neck. New England Journal of Medicine 2006; 354: 567–578.

162. O'Sullivan B, Huang SH, Siu LL, Waldron J, Zhao H et al. Deintensification candidate subgroups in human papillomavirus-related oropharyngeal cancer according to minimal risk of distant metastasis. Journal of Clinical Oncology 2013; 31: 543–550.

163. Rishi A, Ghoshal S, Verma R, Oinam AS, Patil VM et al. Comparison of concomitant boost radiotherapy against concurrent chemoradiation in locally advanced oropharyngeal cancers: a phase III randomised trial. Radiotherapy & Oncology 2013; 107: 317–324.

164. Garden AS, Kies MS, Morrison WH, Weber RS, Frank SJ et al. Outcomes and patterns of care of patients with locally advanced oropharyngeal carcinoma treated in the early 21st century. Radiation Oncology 2013; 8: 21.

165. Eisbruch A, Harris J, Garden AS, Chao CK, Straube W et al. Multi-institutional trial of accelerated hypofractionated intensity-modulated radiation therapy for early-stage oropharyngeal cancer (RTOG 00-22). International Journal of Radiation Oncology Biology Physics 2010; 76: 1333–1338.

166. Nutting CM, Morden JP, Harrington KJ, Urbano TG, Bhide SA et al. Parotid-sparing intensity modulated versus conventional radiotherapy in head and neck cancer (PARSPORT): a phase 3 multicentre randomised controlled trial. Lancet Oncology 2011; 12: 127–136.

167. Bourhis J, Overgaard J, Audry H, Ang KK, Saunders M et al. Hyperfractionated or accelerated radiotherapy in head and neck cancer: a meta-analysis. Lancet 2006; 368: 843–854.

168. Lassen P, Eriksen JG, Krogdahl A, Therkildsen MH, Ulhøi BP et al. The influence of HPV-associated p16-expression on accelerated fractionated radiotherapy in head and neck cancer: evaluation of the randomised DAHANCA 6&7 trial. Radiotherapy & Oncology 2011; 100: 49–55.

169. Adelstein DJ, Ridge JA, Brizel DM, et al. Transoral resection of pharyngeal cancer: summary of a National Cancer Institute Head and Neck Cancer Steering Committee Clinical Trials Planning Meeting, November 6–7, 2011, Arlington, Virginia. Head & Neck 2012; 34: 1681–1703.

170. Bozec A, Poissonet G, Chamorey E, Casanova C, Laout C et al. Quality of life after oral and oropharyngeal reconstruction with a radial forearm free flap: propsective study. Journal of Otolaryngology—Head & Neck Surgery 2009; 38: 401–408.

171. Curado MP, Edwards B, Storm H, Ferlay J, Heanue M et al eds. Cancer Incidence in Five Continents, vol. IX. IARC Scientific Publications No. 160. Lyon, France: International Agency for Research on Cancer, 2007.

172. Chevalier D, Lefebvre JL. Laryngeal cancer. In Anniko M, Bernal-Sprekelsen M, Bonkowsky V, Bradley PJ eds. Otorhinolaryngology, Head and Neck Surgery, European Manuel of Medicine. Berlin-Heidelberg: Springer-Verlag, 2010, 499–502.

173. Bernier J, Domenge C, Ozsahin M, Matuszewska K, Lefèbvre JL et al. European Organization for Research and Treatment of Cancer Trial 22931. Postoperative irradiation with or without concomitant

chemotherapy for locally advanced head and neck cancer. New England Journal of Medicine 2004; 350: 1945–1952.

174. Cooper JS, Pajak TF, Forastiere AA, Jacobs J, Campbell BH et al. Radiation Therapy Oncology Group 9501/Intergroup. Postoperative concurrent radiotherapy and chemotherapy for high-risk squamous-cell carcinoma of the head and neck. New England Journal of Medicine 2004; 350: 1937–1944.

175. Bernier J, Cooper JS, Pajak TF, van Glabbeke M, Bourhis J et al. Defining risk levels in locally advanced head and neck cancers: a comparative analysis of concurrent postoperative radiation plus chemotherapy trials of the EORTC (#22931) and RTOG (# 9501). Head & Neck 2005; 27: 843–850.

176. Grégoire V, Ang K, Budach W, Grau C, Hamoir M et al. Delineation of the neck node levels for head and neck tumors: A 2013 update. DAHANCA, EORTC, HKNPCSG, NCIC CTG, NCRI, RTOG, TROG consensus guidelines. Radiotherapy & Oncology 2013; 110(1): 172–181.

177. Machtay M, Moughan J, Trotti A, Garden AS, Weber RS et al. Factors associated with severe late toxicity after concurrent chemoradiation for locally advanced head and neck cancer: an RTOG analysis. Journal of Clinical Oncology 2008; 26: 3582–3589.

178. Gregoire V, Lefebvre JL, Licitra L, Felip E. Squamous cell carcinoma of the head and neck. EHNS-ESMO-ESTRO Clinical Practice Guidelines for diagnosis, treatment and follow-up. Annals of Oncology 2010; 21(Suppl. 5): v184–v186.

179. Blanchard P, Baujat B, Holostenco V, Baey C, Bauhis J et al. Meta-analysis of chemotherapy in head and neck (MACH-NC): a comprehensive analysis by tumour site. Radiotherapy & Oncology 2011; 100: 33–40.

180. Vermorken JB, Remenar E, van Herpen C. Cisplatin, fluorouracil, and docetaxel in unresectable head and neck cancer. New England Journal of Medicine 2007; 357; 1695–1704.

181. Posner MR, Hershock DM, Blajman CR, Mickiewicz E, Winquist E et al. Cisplatin and fluorouracil alone or with docetxe l in head and neck cancer. New England Journal of Medicine 2007; 357: 1705–1715.

182. Ensley JF, Jacobs JR, Weaver A, Kinzie J, Crissman J et al. Correlation between response to cisplatinum-combination chemotherapy and subsequent radiotherapy in previously untreated patients with advanced squamous cell cancers of the head and neck. Cancer 1984; 54(5): 811–814.

183. The Department of Veterans Affairs Laryngeal Cancer Study Group. Induction chemotherapy plus radiation compared with surgery plus radiation in patients with advanced laryngeal cancer. New England Journal of Medicine 1991; 324: 1685–1690.

184. Lefebvre JL, Chevalier D, Luboinski B, Kirkpatrick A, Collette L et al. Larynx preservation in pyriform sinus cancer: Preliminary results of a European Organization for Research and Treatment of Cancer phase III trial. EORTC Head and Neck Cancer Cooperative Group. Journal of the National Cancer Institute 1996; 88: 890–899.

185. Lefebvre JL, Horiot J, Rolland F, Tesselaar M, Leemans CR et al. Phase III study on larynx preservation comparing sequential versus alternating chemoradiotherapy in hypopharynx and larynx cancer. Journal of the National Cancer Institute 2009; 101: 142–152.

186. 21. Forastiere AA, Goepfert H, Maor M, Pajak TF, Weber R et al. Concurrent chemotherapy and radiotherapy for organ preservation in advanced laryngeal cancer. New England Journal of Medicine 2003; 349: 2091–2098.

187. Forastiere AA, Zhang G, Weber RS, Maor MH, Goepfert H et al. Long-term results of RTOG 91-11: a comparison of three non-surgical treatment strategies to preserve the larynx in patients with locally advanced larynx cancer. Journal of Clinical Oncology 2013; 31: 845–852.

188. Pointreau Y, Garaud P, Chapet S, Sire C, Tuchais C et al. Randomized trial of induction chemotherapy with cisplatin and5-fluorouracil with or without docetaxel for larynx preservation. Journal of the National Cancer Institute 2009; 101: 498–506.

189. Lefebvre JL, Pointreau Y, Rolland F, Alfonsi M, Baudoux A et al. Induction chemotherapy followed by either cemoradiotherapy or bioradiotherapy for larynx preservation: the TREMPLIN randomized phase II study. Journal of Clinical Oncology 2013; 31: 853–859. Erratum in Journal of Clinical Oncology 2013; 31: 1702.

190. Strojan P, Ferlito A, Medina JE, Woolgar JA, Rinaldo A et al. Contemporary management of lymph node metastases from an unknown primary to the neck: I. A review of diagnostic approaches. Head & Neck 2013; 35(1): 123–132.

191. Cianchetti M, Mancuso AA, Amdur RJ, Werning JW, Kirwan J et al. Diagnostic evaluation of squamous cell carcinoma metastatic to cervical lymph nodes from an unknown head and neck primary site. Laryngoscope 2009; 119: 2348–2354.

192. Yoo J, Henderson S, Walker-Dilks C. Evidence-based guideline recommendations on the use of positron emission tomography imaging in head and neck cancer. Clinical Oncology (Royal College of Radiologists) 2013; 25(4): e33–e66.

193. Hasina R, Lingen MW. Head and neck cancer: the pursuit of molecular diagnostic markers. Semin Oncol 2004 Dec; 31(6): 718–725.

194. Grégoire V, Duprez Th, Lengelé B, Hamoir M. Management of the neck. In: Gunderson LL, Tepper JE eds, Clinical Radiation Oncology. Philadelphia: Churchill Livingstone, 2007, 827–852.

195. Grau C, Johansen LV, Jakobsen J, Geertsen P, Andersen E et al. Cervical lymph node metastases from unknown primary tumours. Results from a national survey by the Danish Society for Head and Neck Oncology. Radiotherapy & Oncology 2000 May; 55(2): 121–129.

196. Bernier J, Pfister DG, Cooper JS. Adjuvant chemo- and radiotherapy for poor prognosis head and neck squamous cell carcinomas. Critical Reviews Oncology Hematology 2005; 56(3): 353–364.

197. Balaker AE, Abemayor E, Elashoff D, St John MA. Cancer of unknown primary: does treatment modality make a difference? Laryngoscope 2012; 122(6): 1279–1282.

198. Narayan K, Crane CH, Kleid S, Hughes PG, Peters LJ. Planned neck dissection as an adjunct to the management of patients with advanced neck disease treated with definitive radiotherapy: for some or for all? Head Neck 1999; 21: 606–613.

199. Hamoir M, Ferlito A, Schmitz S, Hanin FX, Thariat J et al. The role of neck dissection in the setting of chemoradiation therapy for head and neck squamous cell carcinoma with advanced neck disease. Oral Oncology 2012; 48: 203–210.

200. Bar-Ad V, Mishra M, Ohri N, Intenzo C. Positron emission tomography for neck evaluation following definitive treatment with chemoradiotherapy for locoregionally advanced head and neck squamous cell carcinoma. Reviews on Recent Clinical Trials 2012; 7(1): 36–41.

201. Clavel S, Charron MP, Bélair M, Delouya G, Fortin B et al. The role of computed tomography in the management of the neck after chemoradiotherapy in patients with head-and-neck cancer. International Journal of Radiation Oncology Biology Physics 2012; 82: 567–573.

202. Warren S, Gates O. Multiple primary malignant tumors: a survey of the literature and a statistical study. American Journal of Cancer 1932; 16: 1358–1414.

203. Blanchard P, Baujat B, Holostenco V, et al. Meta-analysis of chemotherapy in head and neck cancer (MACH-NC): a comprehensive analysis by tumour site. Radiation Oncology 2011; 100: 33–40

204. Strojan P, Corry J, Eisbruch A, Vermorken JB, Mendenhall WM et al. Recurrent and second primary squamous cell carcinoma of the head and neck: when and how to re-irradiate. Head & Neck 2013; 37(1):134–150.

205. Goodwin WJ JR. Salvage surgery for patients with recurrent squamous cell carcinoma of the upper aerodigestive tract: when do the ends justify the means? Laryngoscope 2000; 110(3 Pt 2 Suppl. 93): 1–18.

206. Stoeckli SJ, Pawlik AB, Lipp M, Huber A, Schmid S. Salvage surgery after failure of nonsurgical therapy for carcinoma of the larynx and

hypopharynx. Archives of Otolaryngology—Head & Neck Surgery 2000; 126: 1473–1477.

207. Parsons JT, Mendenhall WM, Stringer SP, Cassisi NJ, Million RR. Salvage surgery following radiation failure in squamous cell carcinoma of the supraglottic larynx. International Journal of Radiation Oncology Biology Physics 1995; 32: 605–609.

208. Van der Putten L, de Bree R, Kuik DJ, Rietveld DH, Buter J et al. Salvage laryngectomy: oncological and functional outcome. Oral Oncology 2011; 47: 296–301.

209. Van der Putten L, van den Broek GB, de Bree R, van den Brekel MW, Balm AJ et al. Effectiveness of selective and radical neck dissection for regional pathological lymphadenopathy after chemoradiation. Head & Neck 2009; 31: 593–603.

210. Tanvetyanon T, Padhya T, McCaffrey J, Zhu W, Boulware D et al. Prognostic factors for survival after salvage reirradiation of head and neck cancer. Journal of Clinical Oncology 2009; 27: 1983–1991

211. Choe KS, Haraf DJ, Solanski A, Cohen EE, Seiwert TY et al. Prior chemoradiotherapy adversely impacts outcomes of recurrent and second primary head and neck cancer treated with concurrent chemotherapy and reirradiation. Cancer 2011; 117(20): 4671–4678.

212. Paleri V, Kelly CG. Re-irradiation with concurrent chemotherapy in re current head and neck cancer: a decision analysis model based on a systemic review. Clin Otolaryngol 2008; 33: 331–337

213. Sher DJ, Haddad RI, Norris CM Jr, Posner MR, Wirth LJ et al. Efficacy and toxicity of re-irradiation using intensity-modulated radiotherapy for recurrent or second primary head and neck cancer. Cancer 2010; 116: 4761–4768.

214. Nyst HJ, Tan IB, Stewart FA, Balm AJ. Is photodynamic therapy a good alternative to surgery and radiotherapy in the treatment of head and neck cancer? Photodiagnostic Photodynamic Therapy 2009; 6(1): 3–11.

215. Stoker SD, van Diessen JN, de Boer JP, Karakullukcu B, Leemans CR et al. Current treatment options for local residual nasopharyngeal caricnoma. Current Treatment Options in Oncology 2013; 14(4): 475–791.

216. Tijink BM, De Bree R, Van Dongen GA, Leemans CR. How we do it: Chdemo-eletroporation in the head and neck for otherwise untreatable patients. Clinical Otolaryngology 2006; 31(5): 447–451.

217. Mevio N, Bertino G, Occhini A, Scelsi D, Tagliabue M et al. Electrochemotherapy for the treatment of recurrent head and neck cancers: preliminary results. Tumori 2012; 98(3): 308–313

218. Argiris A, Li Y, Forastiere A. Prognostic factors and long-term survivorship in patients with recurrent or metastatic carcinoma of the head and neck. Cancer 2004; 101 (10): 2222–2229

219. Vermorken JB, Specenier P. Optimal treatment for recurrent/metastatic head and neck cancer. Annals of Oncology 2010; 21 (Suppl. 7): vii252–vii261

220. Vermorken JB, Mesia R, Rivera F, Remenar E, Kawecki A et al. Platinum-based chemotherapy plus cetuximab in head and neck cancer. New England Journal of Medicine 2008; 359 (11): 1116–1127.

221. Mesia R, Rivera F, Kawecki A, Rottey S, Hitt R et al. Quality of life of patients receiving plastinum-based chemotherapy plus cetuximab first line for recurrent and/or metastatic squamous cell carcinoma of the head and neck. Annals of Oncology 2010; 21 (10): 1967–1973.

222. Guigay J, Fayette J, Dillies A-F, Sire C, Kerger JN et al. Cetuximab, docetaxel, and cisplatin (TPEx) as first-line treatment in patients with recurrent or metastatic (R/M) squamous cell carcinoma of the head and neck (SCCHN): final results of phase II trial GORTEC 2008-03. Journal of Clinical Oncology 2012; 30 (15S): 357s (abstract#5505).

223. Schmitz S, Ang KK, Vermorken J, Haddad R, Suarez C et al. Targeted therapies for squamous cell carcinoma of the head and neck: current knowledge and future directions. Cancer Treat Rev 2013; 40(3): 390–404.

224. Boeckx C, Baay M, Wouters, Specenier P, Vermorken JB et al. Anti-epidermal growth factor receptor therapy in head and neck squamous cell carcinoma: focus on potential molecular mechanisms of drug resistance. Oncologist 2013; 18(7): 850–864,

225. Vander Poorten V, Hunt J, Bradley PJ et al. Recent trends in the management of minor salivary gland carcinoma. Head Neck 2013.

226. Vander Poorten V, Bradley PJ, Takes RP, Rinaldo A, Woolgar JA, et al. Diagnosis and management of parotid carcinoma with a special focus on recent advances in molecular biology. Head Neck 2012; 34: 429–440.

227. Vander Poorten VLM, Balm AJM, Hilgers FJM, Tan IB, Keus RB et al. Stage as major long term outcome predictor in minor salivary gland carcinoma. Cancer 2000; 89: 1195–1204.

228. Barnes L, Eveson JW, Reichart P, Sidranski P. Pathology and genetics of head and neck tumours. World Health Classification of Tumours. In IARC, ed. Lyon: IARC press; 2005;210.

229. Kirkbride P, Liu FF, O'Sullivan B et al. Outcome of curative management of malignant tumours of the parotid gland. Journal of Otolaryngology 2001; 30: 271–279.

230. Armstrong JG, Harrison LB, Spiro RH, Fass DE, Strong EW et al. Malignant tumors of major salivary gland origin: a matched-pair analysis of the role of combined surgery and postoperative radiotherapy. Archives of Otolaryngology – Head and Neck Surgery 1990; 116: 290–293.

231. Terhaard CH, Lubsen H, Rasch CR, Levendag PC, Kaanders HH et al. The role of radiotherapy in the treatment of malignant salivary gland tumors. International Journal of Radiation Oncology Biology Physics 2005; 61: 103–111.

232. Frankenthaler RA, Byers RM, Luna MA, Callender DL, Wolf P et al. Predicting occult lymph node metastasis in parotid cancer. Archives of Otolaryngology – Head and Neck Surgery 1993; 119: 517–520.

233. Conley J, Myers E, Cole R. Analysis of 115 patients with tumors of the submandibular gland. Annals of Otology, Rhinology & Laryngology 1972; 81: 323–330.

234. Vander Poorten VLM, Balm AJM, Hilgers FJM, Tan IB, Loftus-Coll BM et al. Prognostic factors for long term results of the treatment of patients with malignant submandibular gland tumors. Cancer 1999; 85: 2255–2264.

235. Weber RS, Byers RM, Petit B, Wolf P, Ang K et al. Submandibular gland tumors. Adverse histologic factors and therapeutic implications. Archives of Otolaryngology – Head and Neck Surgery 1990; 116: 1055–1060.

236. Leivo I. Insights into a complex group of neoplastic disease: advances in histopathologic classification and molecular pathology of salivary gland cancer. Acta Oncologica 2006; 45: 662–668.

237. Tanvetyanon T, Qin D, Padhya T, McCaffrey J, Zhu W et al. Outcomes of postoperative concurrent chemoradiotherapy for locally advanced major salivary gland carcinoma. Archives of Otolaryngology – Head and Neck Surgery 2009; 135: 687–692.

238. Pederson AW, Salama JK, Haraf DJ, Witt ME, Stenson KM et al. Adjuvant chemoradiotherapy for locoregionally advanced and high-risk salivary gland malignancies. Head and Neck Oncology 2011; 3: 31.

239. Laramore GE, Krall JM, Griffin TW, Duncan W, Richter MP et al. Neutron versus photon irradiation for unresectable salivary gland tumors: final report of an RTOG-MRC randomized clinical trial. Radiation Therapy Oncology Group. Medical Research Council. International Journal of Radiation Oncology Biology Physics 1993;27:235–240.

240. Jensen AD, Nikoghosyan AV, Lossner K, Herfarth KK, Debus J et al. IMRT and carbon ion boost for malignant salivary gland tumors: interim analysis of the COSMIC trial. BMC Cancer 2012; 12: 163.

241. Licitra L, Cavina R, Grandi C et al. Cisplatin, doxorubicin and cyclophosphamide in advanced salivary gland carcinoma: a phase II trial of 22 patients. Annals of Oncology 1996; 7: 640–642.

242. Laurie SA, Ho AL, Fury MG, Sherman E, Pfister DG. Systemic therapy in the management of metastatic or locally recurrent adenoid cystic carcinoma of the salivary glands: a systematic review. Lancet Oncology 2011; 12: 815–824.

243. Laurie SA, Licitra L. Systemic therapy in the palliative management of advanced salivary gland cancers. Journal of Clinical Oncology 2006;24:2673–2678.

244. Bissett RJ, Fitzpatrick PJ. Malignant submandibular gland tumors. A review of 91 patients [published erratum appears in American Journal of Clinical Oncology 1988; 11(4): 514]. American Journal of Clinical Oncology 1988; 11: 46–51.

245. Mendenhall WM, Amdur RJ, Vaysberg M, Mendenhall CM, Werning JW. Head and neck paragangliomas. Head & Neck 2011; 33: 1530–1534.

246. Martin TP, Irving RM, Maher ER. The genetics of paragangliomas: a review. Clinical Otolaryngology 2007; 32: 7–11.

247. van der Mey AG, Frijns JH, Cornelisse CJ, Brons EN, van Dulken H et al. Does intervention improve the natural course of glomus tumors? A series of 108 patients seen in a 32-year period. Annals of Otology, Rhinology & Laryngology 1992; 101: 635–642.

248. Langerman A, Athavale SM, Rangarajan SV, Sinard RJ, Netterville JL. Natural history of cervical paragangliomas: outcomes of observation

249. Foote RL, Pollock BE, Gorman DA, Schomberg PJ, Stafford SL et al. Glomus jugulare tumor: tumor control and complications after stereotactic radiosurgery. Head & Neck 2002; 24: 332–338.

250. Suarez C, Rodrigo JP, Mendenhall WM, Hamoir M, Silver CE et al. Carotid body paragangliomas: a systematic study on management with surgery and radiotherapy. European Archives of Oto-Rhino-Laryngology 2013.

251. Verniers DA, Keus RB, Schouwenburg PF, Bartelink H. Radiation therapy, an important mode of treatment for head and neck chemodectomas. European Journal of Cancer 1992; 28A: 1028–1033.

252. Suarez C, Rodrigo JP, Bodeker CC, Llorente JL, Silver CE et al. Jugular and vagal paragangliomas: systematic study of management with surgery and radiotherapy. Head & Neck 2013; 35(8): 1195–1204.

of 43 patients. Archives of Otolaryngology – Head and Neck Surgery 2012; 138: 341–345.

CHAPTER 36

Oesophageal cancer

Piet Dirix, Karin Haustermans, Eric Van Cutsem,
Xavier Sagaert, Christophe M. Deroose,
Philippe Nafteux, Hans Prenen, and Toni Lerut

Epidemiology

Worldwide, oesophageal cancer, including cancer of the gastro-oesophageal junction (GEJ), is the sixth leading cause of death from cancer [1]. The vast majority of oesophageal cancers occur as either squamous cell carcinoma (SCC) in the middle or upper third of the oesophagus or as adenocarcinoma in the distal third or at the gastro-oesophageal junction, with other tumour types occurring only very rarely. Epidemiologic data show that the incidence of oesophageal cancer varies considerably from one country to another and often within a single country. The geographic diversity of oesophageal cancer worldwide, of which over 70% are SCC, underscores the multifactorial aetiology of this group of diseases. The highest rates are found in southern and eastern Africa and eastern Asia. An 'oesophageal cancer belt' extends from northeast China to the Middle East, where more than 90% of cases are SCC [2]. In Western industrialized countries, however, there has been a slight decline in SCC over the past three decades, while a dramatic rise in adenocarcinoma has been observed. Overall incidence of oesophageal adenocarcinoma is highest in white men over the age of 60. Mortality rates are very similar to incidence rates due to the relatively late stage of diagnosis and the poor efficacy of treatment with a survival rate at five years below 10%.

The pathogenesis of oesophageal cancer remains unclear. Data from animal studies suggest that damage from factors such as smoking or gastro-oesophageal reflux, which cause inflammation, oesophagitis, and increased cell turnover, may initiate the carcinogenic process. SCC most commonly develops in patients with a long-standing history of alcohol and/or tobacco consumption, whereas adenocarcinoma virtually always arises against a background of Barrett mucosa in the oesophagus (Table 36.1). Familial aggregation of both squamous cell as well as adenocarcinoma has been described, but the extent to which hereditary factors are involved in the development of oesophageal cancer is unclear [1, 2].

Squamous cell carcinoma: molecular biology and pathology

Definition

SCC of the oesophagus is a malignant epithelial tumour with squamous cell differentiation, which is defined as the penetration of neoplastic squamous epithelium through the epithelial basement membrane and extension into the lamina propria or deeper tissue layers. Oesophageal SCC is located predominantly in the middle and the upper third of the oesophagus and develops in flat cells that line the oesophagus.

Pathogenesis

Any factor that causes chronic irritation and inflammation of the oesophageal mucosa appears to increase the incidence of SCC. The two major risk factors for SCC are tobacco and alcohol (Table 36.1). Recurrent thermal injury to the oesophageal mucosa caused by the consumption of large amounts of hot beverages has also been consistently speculated to be a risk factor for SCC. Other causes of chronic oesophageal irritation include achalasia and oesophageal diverticuli, in which food is retained and decomposed by bacteria, releasing various chemical irritants. Genetic predisposition is found in non-epidermolytic palmoplantar keratoderma, or tylosis, a rare autosomal dominant disorder defined by a genetic abnormality at chromosome 17q25. Tylosis is characterized by hyperkeratosis of the palms and soles, as well as by thickening of the oral mucosa. In affected families, it confers up to a 95% risk of SCC of the oesophagus by the age of 70. Low socio-economic status is also linked to a higher risk of SCC of the oesophagus. Finally, several dietary factors have been associated with SCC, such as foods containing N-nitroso compounds and red meat [3, 4].

Histology

Oesophageal SCC is thought to develop through a multistep process, which involves basal cell hyperplasia, intraepithelial neoplasia (dysplasia and carcinoma in situ), and finally invasive carcinoma (see Figure 36.1). These tumours frequently present as fungating, ulcerating, or infiltrating lesions in the oesophageal epithelium. The fungating pattern is characterized by a predominantly exophytic growth, whereas in the ulcerative and infiltrating pattern the tumour growth is predominantly intramural, with a central ulceration and elevated ulcer edges. An infiltrating pattern of the cancer will only cause a small mucosal defect.

Basal cell hyperplasia

The basal layer is the deepest layer of the epidermis, containing basal cells. Basal cells divide continuously, forming new keratinocytes, replacing the old ones that are shed from the surface. Basal cell hyperplasia is diagnosed when the basal zone thickness is

Table 36.1 Risk factors for oesophageal cancer

Risk Factor	Squamous cell carcinoma	Adenocarcinoma
Tobacco use	++++	++
Alcohol use	++++	/
Barrett's Esophagus	/	++++
Weekly reflux symptoms	/	+++
Obesity	/	++
Poverty	++	/
Achalasia	+++	/
Caustic injury to the oesophagus	++++	/
Nonepidermolytic palmoplantar keratoderma (tylosis)	++++	/
Plummer-Vinson syndrome	++++	/
History of head and neck cancer	++++	/
History of breast cancer treated with radiotherapy	+++	+++
Frequent consumption of extremely hot beverages	+	/
Prior use of beta-blockers, anticholinergics, aminophyllines	/	±

greater than 15% of the total epithelial thickness, without elongation of lamina propria papillae.

Intraepithelial neoplasia

Intraepithelial neoplasia includes both architectural and cytological abnormalities. The architectural abnormality is characterized by a disorganization of the epithelium and loss of normal cell polarity. Cytologically, the cells exhibit irregular and hyperchromatic nuclei, an increase in nuclear/cytoplasmic ratio, and increased mitotic activity. Dysplasia is usually graded as low- or high-grade dysplasia. In carcinoma in situ, the atypical cells are present throughout the full thickness of the epithelium without invasion.

Invasive SCC

Neoplastic squamous cells are present and invade through the basement membrane. A mix of undifferentiated or primitive basal cells, large flat squamous cells, and keratinized foci is often observed. Tumour clusters may be found distant from the main mass due to lymphatic spread through the submucosa. The tumour cells often exhibit keratinization and have intercellular bridges. Cytologically, the cells have enlarged nuclei, multiple and enlarged nucleoli, and loss of nuclear polarity in cell clusters. Variants of SCC are basaloid SCC, verrucous carcinoma, and spindle cell carcinoma [4]. Immunohistochemical markers that are often used in the diagnosis of SCC are p63 and cytokeratin 5/6.

Molecular biology

Genetic changes associated with the development of oesophageal SCC include activation of oncogenes (e.g., cyclin D1, epidermal growth factor receptor (EGFR)) and inactivation of several tumour suppressor genes (e.g., p53, p16, retinoblastoma (Rb)). Loss of heterozygosity (LOH) on chromosome 17q25 has been linked with tylosis.

Proto-oncogenes

Cyclin D1

Gene amplification and the subsequent over-expression of cyclin D1 were commonly demonstrated in cell lines from oesophageal SCC. The product of cyclin D1 gene forms a complex with cyclin-dependent protein kinase (CDK) that governs a key in the cell cycle G1/S transition. Amplification of the gene has potential for growth advantage and enhances tumourigenesis.

EGFR

The ErbB family comprises four structurally related receptor tyrosine kinases, which are HER1 (EGFR, ErbB1), HER2 (Neu, ErbB2), HER3 (ErbB3), and HER4 (ErbB4). EGFR is expressed in many SCC cell lines and tumours [5]. Signal transduction by the EGFR induces tumour cell proliferation, migration, inhibition of apoptosis and angiogenesis (see Figure 36.2). EGFR has also been described as a prognostic marker in several tumours, including oesophageal cancer [6].

Tumour suppressor genes

p53

The p53 mutation is the most common genetic alteration in human cancers and the most frequently studied genetic alteration in oesophageal SCC. The p53 tumour suppressor gene, located on the short arm of chromosome 17, appears to have an important effect on cellular growth control. The p53 gene product is known to regulate cell growth and proliferation. The wild-type p53 protein suppresses cell growth by controlling the G1 checkpoint. The wild-type p53 protein also has several additional physiologic functions, including control of the G2 cell cycle checkpoint and mediation of apoptosis.

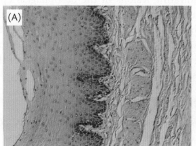
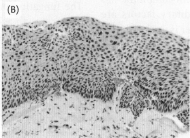
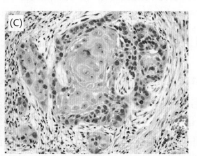

Fig. 36.1 The development of oesophageal SCC: (A) basal cell hyperplasia, (B) intraepithelial neoplasia, (C) invasive oesophageal SCC.
Images reproduced courtesy of Prof. Dr. Xavier Sagaert, Department of Pathology, University Hospital Leuven, Belgium.

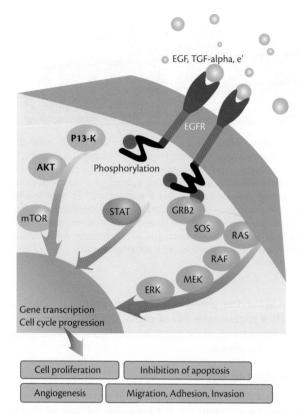

Fig. 36.2 EGFR signalling pathway. EGF and TGFα binding to EGFR typically promote cell survival, growth, and differentiation via the activation of several integrated signalling pathways.

p16

Methylation of the p16 gene is common in oesophageal SCC, and tends to increase in prevalence in mucosal foci as the histological severity of the disease increases. Gene methylation means the addition of methyl groups to cytosines in CpG islands. Methylation of these CpG islands has been reported to be a critical mechanism for the inactivation and silencing of several genes including transcription factors and genes involved in apoptosis, which promotes the development of cancers, including oesophageal squamous cell carcinogenesis. p16, acting as a cyclin-dependent kinase inhibitor, binds to and inhibits the activity of CDK4 and CDK6 and arrests the cell cycle in the G1/S phase in a p53-dependent pathway.

Rb

The LOH at the Rb locus is frequently detected in oesophageal SCC. LOH at the Rb locus causes a reduced expression of Rb protein (pRb). The retinoblastoma gene product controls cell proliferation through regulation of the cell cycle at the G1/S-phase transition. The pRb is bound to transcription factor E2F during the G1 phase. However, when pRb is phosphorylated by the cyclin-dependent kinase complexes, E2F is released, and the cell can initiate DNA synthesis.

Adenocarcinoma

Definition

Adenocarcinoma is a malignant epithelial tumour of the oesophagus with glandular differentiation arising predominantly from Barrett mucosa in the lower third of the oesophagus. Infrequently, adenocarcinoma originates from heterotopic gastric mucosa in the upper oesophagus, or from mucosal and submucosal glands.

Pathogenesis

Most adenocarcinomas arise from a region of Barrett metaplasia (Table 36.1). Barrett oesophagus, which is most commonly attributable to gastro-oesophageal reflux disease, occurs as an adaptive response to injury from refluxed acid and bile, as intestinal columnar epithelium is protected by mucus secretion (see Figure 36.3). The adenocarcinoma incidence increase may also be related to the Western obesity epidemic, either through direct physical effects increasing reflux or indirectly through a metabolic syndrome. Recently, a genome-wide association study in patients with Barrett oesophagus found evidence that SNP alleles predisposing to obesity also increased risk for Barrett oesophagus [7]. Adenocarcinoma is more frequently seen in males. The reasons for a male preponderance are unclear but an increased incidence in postmenopausal women raises questions about hormones and iron status.

Histology

Adenocarcinoma arises through a Barrett metaplasia/dysplasia sequence. Barrett metaplasia refers to a condition in which the normal stratified squamous mucosa is replaced by columnar-lined epithelium that extends upward from the GEJ. The condition is an acquired process that develops in response to an oesophageal mucosal injury that heals in the setting of the inflammatory stimulus of continued gastro-oesophageal reflux (Figure 36.4A). Barrett oesophagus may progress to dysplasia (Figure 36.4B and 36.4C) and adenocarcinoma (Figure 36.4D). The degree of dysplasia is determined by evaluating the architecture (relationship of glands and lamina propria), the cytology (nuclear and cytoplasmic features), and degree of surface maturation (comparison of nuclear size within crypts to nuclear size at the mucosal surface), and interpreting these findings in conjunction with the amount of background inflammation. A revised Vienna classification system is frequently used to score the degree of dysplasia (Table 36.2): (1) negative for neoplasia/dysplasia; (2) indefinite for neoplasia/dysplasia; (3) low-grade dysplasia; and (4) high-grade dysplasia.

Negative for neoplasia/dysplasia

This includes metaplastic epithelium showing reactive/regenerative changes. The nuclei may be slightly enlarged, hyperchromatic, with

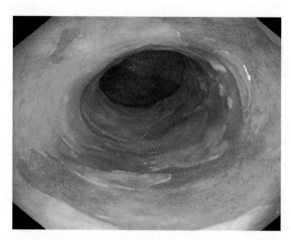

Fig. 36.3 Barrett oesophagus.

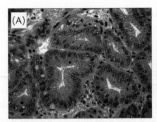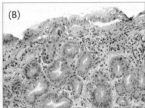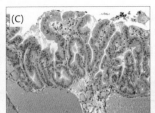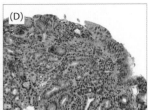

Fig. 36.4 Histopathology of the oesophagus. (A) Barrett metaplasia. (B) Low-grade dysplasia—this type of dysplasia more commonly shows an 'adenomatous' cytological appearance, resembling low-grade tubular adenomata of the large bowel, where nuclei are elongated, slightly enlarged and hyperchromatic with inconspicuous nucleoli. There may be mild pleomorphism, mucin depletion, mild loss of polarity, nuclear crowding, and stratification of nuclei up to three-quarters of the height of the cell, but not touching the luminal surface. (C) High grade dysplasia—the cytologic changes are severe with markedly enlarged nuclei at the surface, pronounced pleomorphism, and at least focal loss of nuclear polarity. Surface maturation is lost. Mild to marked architectural distortion is a frequent finding, with crowded glands, loss of lamina propria, focal budding, and/or cribriform glands. (D) Adenocarcinoma—invasive adenocarcinoma is usually well to moderately differentiated cancer, with the malignant cells producing mucin and sometimes with foci of squamous or endocrine differentiation. Adjacent Barrett mucosa with high-grade dysplasia may be present and rarely signet-ring cells or papillary structures are observed. Variants of adenocarcinoma are (1) adenoacanthoma, (2) mucoepidermoid carcinoma, and (3) adenoid cystic carcinoma [4]. Immunohistochemical markers used for adenocarcinoma are periodic acid staining (PAS) and cytokeratin 7 and 20. PAS staining is based on the presence of neutral mucins in adenocarcinomas.
Images reproduced courtesy of Prof. Dr. Xavier Sagaert, Department of Pathology, University Hospital Leuven, Belgium.

smooth nuclear membranes, prominent nucleoli, and eosinophilic cytoplasm. There may be some stratification of the nuclei at the base. Neutrophils may also be present. Regenerative changes can be more pronounced at the squamo-columnar junction; therefore, the threshold for making a diagnosis of low grade dysplasia should be raised at this site.

Indefinite for neoplasia/dysplasia

This category is applied to biopsies where changes cannot be definitively described as reactive or neoplastic. It is most often used in the presence of pronounced inflammation or the loss of surface epithelium. Cytologic atypia characterized by hyperchromasia, overlapping nuclei, irregular nuclear borders, and nuclear stratification can

be seen in the deep glands or the sides of villiform structures while the surface epithelium is free of atypia. The architecture should be largely normal with, at the most, minimal gland crowding. Surface maturation is present.

Molecular Biology

Although a clearly defined sequence of genetic alterations leading to adenocarcinoma has not been defined, several changes in gene structure, gene expression, and protein structure are associated with the progression of Barrett oesophagus to adenocarcinoma. An accumulation of abnormalities has been identified in a wide range of genes that regulate proliferation, apoptosis, invasion, metastasis, angiogenesis, and growth and cell cycle regulation. Alterations in tumour suppressor genes, including p53, are early events in the metaplasia–dysplasia–adenocarcinoma sequence, followed by loss of cell cycle checkpoints. The activation of proto-oncogenes and inactivation of tumour suppressor genes as the result of genetic instability lead to cumulative genetic errors and thereby the generation of multiple clones of transformed cells, which form the key genetic foci contributing to tumour development.

Proto-oncogenes

EGFR

Expression of the EGFR increases as Barrett oesophagus progresses to adenocarcinoma. The over-expression of erbB-2 is usually noted in adenocarcinoma but only rarely in SCC. ErbB-2 is located at chromosome 7p12-13, a frequently amplified region in oesophageal SCC and adenocarcinomas. TGFα binds to EGFR and stimulates cell division. Amplification of the TGFα gene at chromosome 2p13 has been found in the progression of oesophageal adenocarcinoma. In Barrett tissue, TGFα has been found to activate vascular endothelial growth factor (VEGF), which plays a role in the vascularization of adenocarcinomas. Expression of VEGF is indeed increased in Barrett adenocarcinomas.

bFGF

bFGF expression levels are significantly increased in Barrett adenocarcinomas and dysplastic tissues as compared to normal oesophageal mucosa and metaplasia. The fibroblast growth factors are

Table 36.2 Vienna classification system of gastrointestinal epithelial neoplasia

Category		Histology
Negative for dysplasia	A	Normal with well-spaced glands
	C	Regular nuclei, smooth membranes
	M	Complete
Indefinite for dysplasia	A	Normal to mild distortion, often inflamed
	C	Hyperchromasia, overlapping nuclei, irregular nuclei borders
	M	Complete when intact surface epithelium present
Low-grade dysplasia	A	Normal to mild distortion, gland crowding
	C	Minimal pleomorphism, maintained polarity, increased mitotic activity
	M	Minimal to none
High-grade dysplasia	A	Mild to marked distortion, crowded and budding glands
	C	Loss of polarity, markedly enlarged nuclei, prominent pleomorphism
	M	None

Abbreviations: A, architecture; C, cytology; M, maturation.

Reproduced with permission from Schlemper RJ et al., The Vienna classification of gastrointestinal epithelial neoplasia, *Gut*, Volume 47, Issue 2, pp. 251–255, Copyright © 2000 BMJ Publishing Group Ltd.

important pro-angiogenic factors with the capability to regulate growth and differentiation of various cell types.

Tumour suppressor genes

p53

p53 is mutated in more than 50% of oesophageal adenocarcinomas [7]. p53 protein over-expression is reported early in the transformation of Barrett oesophagus to adenocarcinoma and increases with histologic progression. Therefore, p53 immunostaining is often used in the pathology lab to detect dysplasia in Barrett oesophagus.

Surgical management

Clinical presentation

Signs and Symptoms

Both adenocarcinoma and SCC have similar clinical presentations except that adenocarcinoma arises much more commonly in the distal oesophagus or at the GEJ. Early-stage oesophageal cancer has no typical symptoms. Difficult transit through the oesophageal tube of harder ingredients (e.g., French fries or bread crusts), which can be overcome by the patient with careful chewing or frequent drinking, may precede outright dysphagia. Patients may also notice retrosternal discomfort or a burning sensation. Among patients with locally advanced cancer, obstruction of the oesophagus by the tumour causes progressive solid food dysphagia often accompanied by weight loss. Dysphagia indicates that the oesophageal lumen has been reduced by at least 50–75% of its normal diameter and that about two-thirds of the circumference of the oesophageal wall is involved. Regurgitation of food uncontaminated by gastric secretions can also occur in patients with advanced disease. Hoarseness may arise if the recurrent laryngeal nerve is invaded or due to chronic aspiration. Ultimately, oesophageal obstruction becomes complete for both solid food and fluids.

Chronic gastrointestinal blood loss from oesophageal cancer is common and may result in iron deficiency anaemia. However, patients seldom notice melena, haematemesis or blood in regurgitated food. Similarly, acute upper gastrointestinal bleeding is rare and is a result of tumour erosion into the aorta or pulmonary or bronchial arteries. Tracheo-bronchial fistulas are a late complication of oesophageal cancer. The fistulas are caused by direct invasion through the oesophageal wall and into the main stem bronchus. Such patients often present with intractable coughing or frequent pneumonias.

Clinical examination

Clinical examination is usually normal in localized disease, although supraclavicular or neck lymph nodes can be present in more advanced disease. Obviously, thorough clinical examination should be performed to exclude metastatic disease (e.g., malignant pleural effusion or ascites) or concurrent liver disease, since many patients have a history of alcohol abuse.

Diagnosis and staging

Diagnosis

Timely diagnosis of oesophageal cancer is hampered by the usually late occurrence of tumour-related symptoms. Most early oesophageal cancers are detected serendipitously or during screening for or surveillance of Barrett oesophagus. Patients with more advanced disease are often symptomatic for two to four months before seeking professional help. The diagnostic algorithm for oesophageal cancer includes establishing the definite diagnosis as well as evaluation of oncological and functional operability.

Initially, existence of a clinically suspected carcinoma should be either confirmed or ruled out. Previously, contrast medium swallow studies were most commonly applied for this purpose, but this has been largely replaced with endoscopy. A 2009 survey among surgeons regularly performing oesophagectomy showed that endoscopy and barium oesophagography are routinely used by 98% and 51% of surgeons, respectively [8].

Nowadays, patients with suggestive symptoms should preferably undergo endoscopy with biopsies. In addition to achieving a biopsy, the endoscopist should document tumour location relative to both the teeth and the GEJ, tumour length, extent of circumferential involvement, degree of obstruction, and any evidence of Barrett oesophagus to assist with treatment planning.

Gastro-oesophageal junction adenocarcinoma

A specific problem is the diagnosis, and especially the definition, of gastro-oesophageal junction tumours (usually adenocarcinoma). Because tumours originating at the GEJ are often differently defined and classified by surgeons, endoscopists, and pathologists alike, significant debate on the optimal multimodality treatment of these tumours persists.

According to the seventh-edition TNM staging system of the American Joint Committee on Cancer/International Union Against Cancer (AJCC/UICC) for oesophageal and gastric cancer, tumours whose midpoint is in the lower thoracic oesophagus, gastro-oesophageal junction, or within the proximal 5 cm of the stomach that extends into the gastro-oesophageal junction or oesophagus are classified as adenocarcinoma of the oesophagus for the purposes of staging [9]. These tumours are staged (and consequently treated) as oesophageal rather than as gastric adenocarcinomas. All other tumours, i.e. with a midpoint in the stomach lying more than 5 cm from the gastro-oesophageal junction or within 5 cm of the gastro-oesophageal junction but without extension into the oesophagus, are staged (and probably treated) as gastric cancers. This approach remains a subject of debate.

Siewert classified adenocarcinoma of the gastro-oesophageal junction in 1987 into three distinct types, based purely on the anatomic location of the epicentre of the tumour or the location of the tumour mass [10]. According to this classification, GEJ adenocarcinomas encompass all tumours with an epicentre within 5 cm proximal or distal to the anatomical Z-line, the 'squamo-columnar junction' visible as the transition between the reddish columnar epithelium lining the gastric cardia and the pale squamous epithelium lining the oesophagus.

Siewert Type I adenocarcinoma

If the epicentre of the tumour or more than 66% of the tumour mass is located more than 1 cm above the anatomic GEJ, then the tumour is classified as an adenocarcinoma of the distal oesophagus, type I. According to Siewert, these should be considered as typical adenocarcinomas of the distal oesophagus that infiltrate the gastro-oesophageal junction from above. Siewert type I tumours also have epidemiologic and histological characteristics that are similar to distal thoracic oesophageal adenocarcinomas, including a strong male predominance, association with a history of reflux symptoms, and a predominance of intestinal-type histology, having arisen from Barrett metaplasia secondary to gastro-oesophageal reflux. In general, type I cancers more frequently involve lymph nodes in the upper mediastinum (tracheal bifurcation and above).

Siewert Type II adenocarcinoma

If the epicentre of the tumour or tumour mass is located within 1 cm proximal and 2 cm distal to the anatomic GEJ, it is classified as type II. These could be considered as 'true' gastro-oesophageal junction adenocarcinomas, arising from the cardiac epithelium or short segments with intestinal metaplasia at the gastro-oesophageal junction. There is increasing evidence to suggest that Siewert type II tumours have two distinct aetiologies, some being oesophageal adenocarcinomas probably arising from Barrett oesophagus, and others gastric adenocarcinomas caused by Helicobacter pylori infection and atrophic gastritis (as with type III tumours).

Siewert Type III adenocarcinoma

If the epicentre of the tumour or more than 66% of the tumour mass is located more than 2 cm below the anatomic gastro-oesophageal junction, the tumour is classified as type III. Type III tumours resemble distal (subcardiac) gastric cancers, with a similar proportion of diffuse and intestinal histologic types and no association with reflux, which infiltrate the gastro-oesophageal junction from below. They arise from the gastric mucosa, and their origin might be associated with Helicobacter pylori and atrophic gastritis.

Staging

After diagnosis is confirmed, pretreatment staging should be initiated (see Figure 36.5). The questions to be addressed are the potential resectability of the primary tumour with its locoregional lymphatic drainage as well as the presence of distant metastases.

Endoscopic ultrasonography (EUS), computed tomography (CT), and positron emission tomography (PET) are currently the procedures of choice.

A sophisticated diagnostic workup and staging must be performed in order to allow for an accurate treatment choice. Oesophageal cancer patients are grouped in different stages depending on tumour location, grade and histological type in combination with the tumoural extension according to the TNM principle. The staging system can be accessed at the website of the American Cancer Society [11].

While the TNM classification is essentially the same for adenocarcinoma and SCC, one of the major changes between the 2002 (6th) and the 2010 (7th) editions was the development of separate stage groupings according to histology [11]. This change was based upon an analysis of worldwide data on 4627 patients with cancer of the oesophagus or gastro-oesophageal junction who underwent surgery alone; this showed that among patients with lymph-node-negative tumours, prognosis was dependent on T-classification as well as histology, grade, and tumour location [12]. While the new AJCC/UICC staging system provides a better separation of prognostic groups for both histologies as determined by the TNM categories at the time of initial diagnosis, it was based on pTNM data from patients who were treated by oesophagectomy alone, without induction chemotherapy and/or radiotherapy. As a result, its prognostic utility in patients who receive multimodality therapy is unclear [12].

Stage is the most important factor in prognosis and choice of treatment and thus reliable non-invasive methods for accurate staging are very important. Staging usually begins with a CT scan of the thorax and abdomen to evaluate for the presence of metastatic

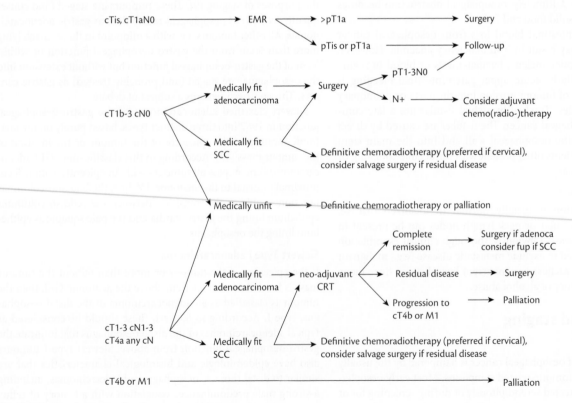

Fig. 36.5 Proposed treatment flow for oesophageal cancer.

disease. Patients without evidence of metastatic disease undergo EUS, which uses a high-frequency ultrasound transducer to provide detailed images of oesophageal masses and their relationship with the five-layered structure of the oesophageal wall. EUS allows assessment of both perigastric and mediastinal lymph nodes, which can potentially be sampled during the evaluation with a fine needle aspiration biopsy if the result would impact treatment decisions. PET and integrated PET-CT scans are useful to detect metastatic disease in patients who are otherwise believed to be surgical candidates after routine staging with conventional contrast-enhanced CT. The role of staging laparoscopy is controversial, and there is no consensus on this issue from expert groups.

Modalities

Oesophagography

Barium studies are well established in the diagnosis of oesophageal disorders, including carcinoma of the oesophagus and the GEJ. In general, a double-contrast examination is preferred to a single-contrast study. Barium swallow is considered safe, easy to perform, readily available, and inexpensive. Barium studies have a low sensitivity for early tumoral lesions and have a moderate positive predictive value but can be useful in the determination of the relationship between the tumour and the proximal sphincter (cricoid muscle).

Endoscopy

The role of endoscopy, consisting of upper endoscopy and endoscopic ultrasound, in diagnosis and staging of oesophageal cancer is crucial. Obviously, standard endoscopy with biopsies provides histological confirmation of the diagnosis. EUS for T and N staging has been well studied and is indicated to assess local disease extent in the absence of metastasis. Conventional EUS with a 7.5–12 MHz probe is able to visualize five oesophageal layers but does not discriminate between T1a and T1b disease. In general, the accuracy of EUS for T staging is reported to be 89% and this increases with increasing disease stage, thereby outperforming CT scan [13, 14].

In the era of neoadjuvant therapy, N staging often determines preoperative management. EUS characteristics suggestive of nodal disease include a diameter of more than 10 mm, a hypoechoic, homogeneous appearance, a round shape, and sharp demarcation. If all these features are present, the lymph node is very likely to be malignant [15]. However, all four features are only simultaneously present in 25% of malignant lymph nodes. In general, the accuracy of EUS for lymph node metastasis ranges between 64% and 90% [15]. It should be noted that specificity can affect patient management considerably: in a study including 214 patients, EUS was correct in only 64.5% of patients to predict final N staging, with a very good sensitivity (93.8%) but a poor specificity of 20%. Based on the N stage, 32% of the patients who underwent primary surgery should have received neoadjuvant chemoradiotherapy and 36% of the patient staged as N1 would have been wrongly assigned to neoadjuvant chemoradiotherapy [16]. Fine needle aspiration significantly helps to improve lymph node staging and increases specificity to more than 90% and should be considered mandatory if technically possible [17].

CT imaging

The penetration depth of EUS is limited to approximately 5 cm. Therefore, CT is generally added to the pretreatment workup in an effort to improve detection of metastases in distant lymph nodes and other organs. According to a recent meta-analysis, CT scans of the chest show a reduced sensitivity for detecting regional lymph-node metastases (0.50, 95% CI 0.41–0.60) compared with EUS [15]. However, the specificity of CT (0.83, 95% CI 0.77–0.89) is superior. Regarding malignant abdominal lymph nodes, the sensitivity is 0.42 (95% CI 0.29–0.54) with a specificity of 0.93 [95% CI 0.86–1.00]. As in many other organs, sensitivity of CT is hampered by its inevitable reliance on nodal size and shape as a diagnostic criterion. Obviously, metastases can be found in subcentimetric lymph nodes. Even if enlarged lymph nodes are visible, CT images do not always enable a distinction between enlargement due to metastatic spread or due to inflammation.

PET and PET-CT imaging

PET allows accurate non-invasive molecular characterisation of tissues, thereby adding a complement to the structural information on conventional imaging. Making use of the increased glucose metabolism now recognized as a key feature of a great range of malignancies, PET imaging with the glucose analogue 2-^{18}F-fluoro-2-deoxy-D-glucose (FDG) allows a better distinction between malignant and benign tissues [18]. SCC are typically strongly FDG-avid; in adenocarcinomas this is usually lower with ~25% of tumours that are not FDG-avid, mainly tumours with poor differentiation, diffuse growth pattern, or high mucus content [19].

Modern PET cameras in use for oncological imaging are typically hybrid devices that combine a PET camera with a CT resulting in a fusion dataset. FGD-PET/CT is widely accepted for TNM determination in oesophageal cancer. For the primary tumour, FGD-PET/CT can help to determine the longitudinal extent of the tumour, which can be useful for radiation treatment planning. For detection of regional lymph node involvement, a recent meta-analysis showed that EUS has a better sensitivity (80%) than CT or FDG-PET (50% and 57%, respectively), but the specificity of FDG-PET and CT is higher (83% and 85%, respectively) than that of EUS (70%) [15]. The main advantages of FDG-PET are the detection of normal-size lymph nodes with tumoural involvement and the fact that PET can detect malignant lymph nodes in areas that are not assessed with EUS. In a recent meta-analysis, for the detection of distant metastases FDG-PET showed a higher sensitivity than CT (71% versus 52%) with a comparable specificity (93% versus 91%), leading to detection of unsuspected M1 stage in up to 20% of patients [20].

The use of FDG-PET/CT leads to changes in stage in up to 40% of patients, and results in clinical management changes in up to one-third of patients [21]. Incorporating FDG-PET/CT leads to a better selection of patients with poor long-term prognosis as measured by five-year overall survival. In 5–10% of patients synchronous primary tumours can be detected [22].

Evolving role of surgery

Resection is generally considered integral to achieving cure in patients with oesophageal cancer. In very early stages, i.e. in cancers limited to the mucosal layer, endoscopic resection is an accepted alternative to surgery [23, 24]. In intermediate stages (T1b and T2 categories), primary surgical resection undoubtedly remains the treatment of choice. In locally advanced categories (T3 and T4a), surgery alone has shown rather disappointing survival rates.

Consequently, surgery is usually performed as part of a multimodal treatment strategy and commonly follows neoadjuvant chemoradiotherapy (CRT). The landmark paper by Herskovic was the first to demonstrate that definite CRT could result in survival rates comparable to what is achieved with surgery [25]. Consequently, some institutions prefer this approach, especially in SCC, to avoid the high morbidity and mortality associated with surgery in such patients. However, in a study from the linked Surveillance, Epidemiology and End Results (SEER)–Medicare database, five-year survival rates for patients with stages I–III oesophageal cancer treated with and without surgery were 28% and 10%, respectively [26]. Obviously, these data must be interpreted cautiously. The longer survival in the surgically treated patients could represent selection bias in that younger and healthier patients may have been selected to undergo more aggressive, multimodality treatment with surgery. Evidently, in patients with potentially operable cancer who are unfit for major surgery owing to an impaired functional status, definitive CRT is the procedure of choice. In cases of advanced disease or distant metastases palliative measures are indicated.

Endoluminal therapy

The first choice treatment for early neoplastic oesophageal lesions has shifted from surgery to endoluminal therapy over the last decade. In well-selected patients with well to moderately differentiated mucosal cancer without signs of lymphovascular invasion on histology, endoscopic resection (ER) has an excellent long-term outcome and survival, comparable to surgery [23, 24]. The rationale for this approach originates from the inherent morbidity and mortality of surgery on the one hand, and the low risk of nodal involvement in T1a cancers. The prevalence of nodal disease in mucosal cancer is estimated to be 0.7% and 1.4% in adenocarcinoma and SCC, respectively [27]. Unfortunately, conventional EUS is not suited for differentiating between T1a and T1b disease. High-frequency EUS probes (12–30 MHz) permit viewing a more detailed architecture, although several studies have shown that the accuracy for T staging in early cancer is insufficient in comparison to staging ER, with a sensitivity and specificity for diagnosing T1a disease of 62–100% and 65–94%, respectively [27]. In addition, a recent study showed that if a lesion looks endoscopically amenable for endoscopic resection, a staging ER can be performed, providing a final pathological staging. A study on high-resolution endoscopy compared the endoscopic appearance of early lesions to high-frequency EUS in 100 patients with early oesophageal neoplasia for predicting submucosal invasion. The accuracy was not different for high-resolution endoscopy or high-frequency EUS (83.4% and 79.6%, respectively) [28].

Endoscopic resection is the basis of proper risk stratification and patient selection as it allows the assessment of the histopathological prerequisites for a curative treatment. Only lesions limited to the mucosa that are well- to moderately-differentiated and without signs of lymphovascular infiltration can be considered as cured after ER, with a good oncological outcome, comparable to surgery [24, 27, 29]. However, in particular in Barrett disease, metachronous disease can occur in up to 30% of patients. Therefore, the preferred strategy in patients with a long enough life expectancy is to provide additional ablation with radiofrequency ablation (RFA) [30]. This is a recently introduced new ablative therapy for Barrett oesophagus during which radiofrequency energy is delivered through a balloon-based system for circumferential ablation or with a cap-electrode attached to the tip of an endoscope for focal ablation. The generated heat will destroy remaining dysplastic and non-dysplastic epithelium with a high success rate [31]. It has to be emphasized that RFA is only indicated to ablate flat dysplasia and not for ablation of mucosal cancer [30, 32]. Pre-ER biopsies insufficiently predict final staging after ER, with upgrading of 20% of lesions with only high- or low-grade dysplasia on biopsy to a carcinoma after ER [33]. In the era of RFA it is therefore crucial to resect any small visible lesion for proper histological assessment and patient selection.

Principles of surgical treatment

The first direct transthoracic oesophagectomy for cancer was performed by Franz Thorek in 1913 in New York [34]. He carried out a left thoracic subtotal resection of the oesophagus for a SCC of the middle third in a 67-year-old patient. The patient subsequently survived for 13 years and was fed orally via an external rubber tube connecting the cervical oesophagus with the stomach.

It took another two decades to finally accomplish a successful oesophagectomy with an intrathoracic oesophagogastrostomy; Osawa has been given the credit for this pioneering success [35]. With the further improvements of thoracic anaesthesia and surgery, oesophagectomy became the mainstay of therapy for operable cancer of the oesophagus and remains so today.

The surgical treatment strategy of oesophageal carcinoma is complex and the long-term outcome of surgical therapy is often disappointing. A malignancy arising from the oesophagus may easily invade the adjacent organs, which makes the tumour surgically unresectable. Additionally, lymphatic dissemination is an early event and has a negative influence on survival. Lymph node metastases are found in less than 5% of intramucosal tumours, but in as many as 30–40% of submucosal tumours [36]. Furthermore, the oesophageal wall is characterized by an extensive submucosal lymphatic plexus, which supplies a drainage route for early dissemination and gives rise to jump-metastases (i.e. lymph nodes adjacent to the primary tumour are not affected, but more distantly located lymph nodes contain metastases) [37]. As a result, transmural tumours show lymph node involvement in over 80% and the number of involved nodes increases with the volume of the tumour.

Further adding to the complexity are the tumours of the GEJ which are classified by some as gastric cancer by others as oesophageal cancer. This explains in part the continuing controversy as to which strategy to follow when it comes to surgical approach and surgical techniques.

It is generally accepted that surgical resection should only be performed with curative intent. Resection is ill advised when macroscopically incomplete, because invasion of adjacent structures and/or non-resectable metastases are to be expected. Absolute contraindications for oesophagectomy include local tumour invasion of non-resectable neighbouring structures (T4b), carcinomatosis peritonei, haematogenous parenchymatous metastases, and non-resectable metastatic lymph nodes.

The pattern of lymphatic dissemination is difficult to predict, but carcinomas of the proximal and middle thirds of the oesophagus preferably metastasize to the cervical region, whereas more distal-lying tumours and tumours of the gastro-oesophageal junction more commonly metastasize to the lymph nodes around the celiac trunk. Resectable metastatic lymph nodes in the region of the primary tumour, including the celiac trunk and its trifurcation for distal third tumours and cervical nodes for middle and proximal tumours, are not necessarily a contraindication for surgery. The presence of such lymph node metastases, however, has a negative influence on survival, even following extensive lymphadenectomy.

Macroscopic as well as microscopic completeness (R0) is the ultimate goal of oesophagectomy for cancer. Consequently, optimal preoperative staging is of paramount importance as well as individual case presentation and discussion at a multidisciplinary tumour board.

Before embarking on such major surgery, careful evaluation of medical operability is equally important. Indeed, many patients present with a history of alcohol and tobacco abuses requiring careful evaluation of cardiovascular, pulmonary, and liver function. An even more careful assessment of the operability of the older patient is essential when an operation of such magnitude is considered. An advanced age, in and of itself, is however not a contraindication for extensive surgical procedures for oesophageal carcinoma [38, 39].

The early-stage lymphatic dissemination as well as completeness of tumoural resection pose challenges for radical surgical treatment and are still a matter of debate. The concept of extensive en bloc resections was initially reported in 1963, but its associated mortality of more than 20% in that original report discouraged general acceptance [40]. Skinner and Akiyama reintroduced the concept of en bloc resection combined with extensive lymphadenectomy [41, 42]. Ultimately, they were able to reduce operative mortality to 5%, with five-year survival rates of 18 and 42%, respectively.

The radical en bloc resection, as opposed to the standard resection, aims at performing a wide as possible peritumoural with an en bloc lymph-node resection of the middle and distal thirds of the posterior mediastinum.

The two-field lymph node dissection incorporates, besides a wide local excision of the primary tumour, a lymphadenectomy of the entire posterior mediastinum, including the subcarinal nodes and up to the nodes along the left recurrent nerve and the brachiocephalic trunk. In the abdomen it includes the lymph nodes along the celiac trunk, common hepatic and splenic arteries, as well as the lymph nodes along the lesser gastric curvature and in the lesser omentum (the so-called DII lymphadenectomy).

The three-field lymph node dissection. The pattern of lymphatic dissemination is not restricted to the thorax and abdomen. About 20% of the patients with a distal tumour present with metastasis in the cervical region [36, 37]. In this operation, besides the already mentioned removal of thoracic and abdominal nodes, the cervical field includes the para-oesophageal nodes and the nodes lateral to the carotid vessel as well as the supraclavicular nodes.

These considerations on radicality of resection and extent of lymphadenectomy are the rationale to justify a transthoracic approach as opposed to the transhiatal approach for which the rationale is merely based on an effort to decrease perioperative morbidity and possibly postoperative mortality.

Techniques

Transhiatal oesophagectomy

The transhiatal oesophagectomy without thoracotomy has a number of practical advantages, i.e. a short operative duration, probably lower incidence of pulmonary complications and the avoidance of post-thoracotomy pain [43]. The method is particularly applicable to tumours of the distal oesophagus and GEJ where, via a surgically widened hiatus, the lower mediastinum can be approached. The organ for reconstruction is preferably the stomach, which is anastomosed to the remaining cervical oesophagus via the oesophageal bed (the so-called pre-vertebral route) or via the retrosternal route.

Transthoracic oesophagectomy

Oesophageal tumours situated in the proximal and middle thirds of the intrathoracic oesophagus are probably best approached via the right thoracic cavity. In contrast, distal tumours and tumours of the gastro-oesophageal junction may be better approached from the left side. The most commonly used transthoracic approaches are the Ivor Lewis (two-hole) and Mc Keown (three-hole) right thoracic approach and the left-sided approach through a left thoracophrenotomy [44–47].

Minimally invasive oesophagectomy (MIE)

In an effort to limit the physiologic stress of oesophagectomy while preserving the principle of en bloc resection, a minimally invasive approach to oesophageal resection allowing the same type of resection compared to the transthoracic approach has been developed [48]. The best indications for MIE are Barrett high-grade dysplasia or small tumours (T1a or T1b without suspicious nodes) although it is also increasingly used for more advanced cancers [49, 50].

Surgical Results

Over the years, controversy remained as to the radicality of resection and extent of lymphadenectomy. Those who believe that lymph node involvement equals systemic disease will advocate a simple resection and reconstruction typically through a transhiatal approach. Others believe that the natural course of the disease may be influenced by radical oesophagectomy and extensive (two- or three-field) lymphadenectomy. Although several publications both from Japan and from the West seem to indicate a benefit in favour of the more radical approach, definitive proof is lacking. More radical resections seem to result in overall survival rates between 35% and 50%, as shown in Table 36.3, whereas standard resection has five-year survival rates between 15% and 20%, as shown in Table 36.4, but these non-randomized data might have been influenced by selection bias [51–60].

But perhaps an even more important finding is the influence of hospital volume indicating a potential beneficial effect of centralization of oesophagectomy as suggested by an increasing number

Table 36.3 Survival after radical surgery

Author	N pat.	Three-year survival	Five-year survival
Ando et al. [51]	419	52%	40%
Akiyama et al. [42]	913	52.6%	42.4%
Isono et al. [52]	1740	42%	34.3%
Lerut, Nafteux et al. [53]	174	55%	42%
Collard et al. [54]	235 R0	65%	49%
	324 R0-2	50%	35%
Hagen et al. [55]	100	60%	52%
Altorki N et al. [56]	111	52%	40%
Hulscher et al. [57]	114	42%	40%

Table 36.4 Survival after radical surgery stage III (T3-4 N+)

Author	N pat.	Five-year survival
Ando et al. [51]	201	37.6%
Akiyama et al. [42]	175	27% (2F) / 56% (3F)
Baba et al. [58]	22	30%
Lerut, Coosemans et al. [60]	162	26%
Collard et al. [54]	98	30%
Hagen et al. [55]	32	26%
Altorki NK et al. [59]	33	34.5% (4-year)

of publications [61, 62]. From these data, it must be clear that the results as obtained today in centres of experience with primary surgery are to be seen as the gold standard to which all other therapeutic options, and in particular the multimodality therapies, should be compared. In all trials, no standard quality criteria for the surgical arm have been determined. Not surprisingly, the mean Jadad quality score in different prospective randomized trials is rather low (2.1 on the scale of 5 points) [63, 64].

Surgical Complications

As for any other major surgical intervention, postoperative complications occur frequently after oesophagectomy. Postoperative morbidity, often major morbidity, is seen in up to 30% to 50% [65]. These complications can be divided in medical complications (e.g., cardiac arrhythmias, pulmonary infections, renal insufficiency, CVA, etc.) and surgical complications (e.g., anastomotic leak, chyle leak, and wound infection). A correlation between complications and early recurrence and its timing has been reported [65]. Achieving oesophagectomy without postoperative complications, therefore, is of utmost importance for oncologic reasons, underscoring the need to have this type of surgery performed in centres of experience.

Anastomostic Complications

Anastomotic complications are considered to be the Achilles heel of oesophageal surgery, in particular anastomotic leaks. The incidence of anastomotic leaks reported in literature is between 0% and 50%. However, recent studies have demonstrated that the incidence of leakage after cervical anastomosis can be kept well below 5% [66]. Orringer et al. and Collard et al. introduced the concept of a semi-mechanical side-to-side anastomosis. The authors claim that with this technique there is a significant reduction both in early anastomotic leaks and late strictures [67, 68].

Anastomotic strictures occur in approximately 15% to 30% of the patients. Early postoperative endoscopy in order to monitor healing, followed when necessary by early dilatations may reduce the incidence of benign strictures [69, 70].

Pulmonary complications

Pulmonary infections are the most important cause of early postoperative mortality [71]. Because of the high incidence in pulmonary complications after an oesophagectomy, transhiatal oesophagectomy was reintroduced in the 1970s [72]. A large randomized trial confirmed the short-term advantage of the transhiatal technique [57]. Similar results have been obtained in a randomized trial comparing MIE versus open oesophagectomy with 34% versus 12% pulmonary infections, respectively [73].

Chylothorax

The incidence of chylothorax following oesophagectomy is 1–4% and the management is still controversial. There is a place for short conservative treatment, which consists of drainage of the pleural cavity. Suspending enteral feeding and starting total parenteral nutrition can dramatically reduce the production of chyle. Failure of reduction within three to five days in the chyle output to less than 1 litre per 24 hours is an indication for surgery [74]. Postoperative identification of the site of leakage is facilitated by administering enteral lipids. Thoracoscopic ligation is technically feasible and in skilled hands is preferred over thoracotomy [75]. Percutaneous CT-guided embolization is another way to stop chyle leaks [76].

Vocal cord paralysis

Vocal cord paralysis is a well-known complication, causing hoarseness, dysphagia, weight loss, aspiration, dyspnoea, and pneumonia [77]. Dissection alongside both recurrent nerves may cause damage followed by a temporary or definitive vocal cord paralysis. Besides aspiration during eating and drinking, patients with vocal cord paralysis may also be at risk of reflux-induced aspiration and subsequent pneumonia. Because of these potentially life-threatening consequences, a number of authors advocate the early and aggressive treatment of vocal cord paralysis that does not recover within a few weeks of surgery. Teflon injection of the vocal cord is an easy and safe procedure resulting in substantial improvement of phonation and swallowing in the majority of patients [78]. Another technique reported to be successful is the use of silicone elastomere [79].

Reflux oesophagitis

Despite a significant reduction of acid output related to truncal vagotomy, persistent acid secretion has been reported, originating from an autonomous acid secretion in the gastric antrum cells [80]. Consequently, a substantial number of patients will suffer from reflux symptoms. There is a significantly higher incidence of reflux oesophagitis in patients with an intrathoracic anastomosis than in patients with a cervical anastomosis [81]. Gutschow et al reported that 38% of patients had reflux in the remnant oesophagus at three years or more after oesophagectomy [82]. In more recent years, the introduction of potent anti-acid medication (i.e. proton pump inhibitors) has probably resulted in a major decrease of reflux-related problems, although objective data are not available in the literature.

Gastric-emptying-related problems

Vagal denervation can result in chronic dysmotility of the gastric remnant and an outlet dysfunction of the pylorus, which may cause delayed emptying. This may induce a wide spectrum of symptoms: early satiety, postprandial fullness, heartburn, high dysphagia, aspiration, and pneumonia. The addition of a gastric drainage procedure has been advocated. However, the need for such drainage procedure has been criticized as being harmful because of pyloroplasty-related technical complications (leaks), dumping, and biliary reflux. The largest randomized study has been performed by Fok et al, with a meticulous analysis of eating abilities and gastric emptying function [83]. In this study, the whole stomach had been used for reconstruction in all patients. From this study, gastric drainage procedures are recommended when using the whole stomach.

Gastric outlet obstruction

Irrespective of whether or not a pyloric drainage procedure has been performed, a number of patients may suffer from gastric outlet obstruction. Balloon dilatation of the pylorus can be an effective procedure to solve this problem. Bemelman et al. reported a successful outcome with balloon dilatation in six out of 18 patients [84]. An alternative is to administer erythromycin. Erythromycin is a motilin agonist and has been demonstrated to improve gastric emptying in normal subjects and in patients with diabetic gastroparesis or post-vagotomy gastroparesis [85]. More recently, botox injection into the pylorus has been successfully used [86].

Intestinal metaplasia in the oesophageal remnant

The ablation of the lower oesophageal sphincter mechanism and the vagotomy-induced pyloric dysfunction with possible enterogastric biliary reflux are of increasing concern in relation to the risk of development of Barrett metaplasia, especially in long-term survivors. In a series of 39 patients, Oberg et al. noticed a 47% prevalence of metaplastic columnar mucosa within the cervical oesophagus [87]. It is currently unknown whether these patients have the same risk of developing adenocarcinoma as is seen in the classic reflux-induced Barrett population [88].

Dumping, diarrhoea

After oesophagectomy followed by gastroplasty, many patients complain of dumping symptoms, with a reported incidence of between 10% and 50% [89, 90]. Diarrhoea, abdominal cramps, nausea, dizziness, postprandial sweating, and hypotension are the main complaints [91]. An effective relief of dumping symptoms can be achieved with dietary modifications to minimize the ingestion of simple carbohydrates and to exclude fluid intake during the ingestion of the solid portion of a meal. More severely affected patients may respond to agents such as pectin and guar, which increase the viscosity of the intraluminal contents, or to drugs such as the glucosidase inhibitor acarbose, which decreases the rapid absorption of glucose, or native somatostatin or the somatostatin analogue octreotide, which alter gut transit and inhibit the release of vasoactive mediators into the bloodstream [92].

Quality of life after operation

The nature of the operation, transhiatal versus transthoracic, or the position of the proximal anastomosis, high thoracic versus cervical, has only a limited effect on quality of life. Gastro-oesophageal reflux and dumping syndrome are encountered in more than half of the patients. 20–25% of patients also encounter stenosis of the proximal anastomosis. An anastomosis at the cervical level has a significantly lower chance of symptomatic reflux than one lying within the thorax, but has a higher chance of suture-line leakage and benign stricturing [93]. Global quality scores reveal a significant decrease in physical and role functional scales and an increase in fatigue, nausea, pain, dyspnoea, deglutition, and gastrointestinal symptoms in the initial postoperative phase. However, a gradual improvement is noticed over time, and one year after resection, patients not suffering from tumour recurrence consider their quality of life comparable to that of their predisease state. Ten years after

surgery, two-thirds of surviving patients appear to maintain satisfactory ability for solid-food ingestion [93].

Radiotherapy (RT)

When radiation is used with curative intent in the treatment for oesophageal cancer, either alone or in combination with surgery and/or chemotherapy, the radiation volume should encompass the detectable tumour and the anatomic areas at risk for metastatic spread. In oesophageal cancer it is hard to determine these areas for the individual tumour. Moreover, the areas at risk are very large and this implies that if all areas at risk need to be covered, large radiation volumes are necessary.

Guidelines for selection of target volumes

According to the International Commission on Radiation Units and Measurements (ICRU) 50 guidelines, radiation oncologists use three different target volumes for radiotherapy planning: (1) gross tumour volume (GTV): gross extent of the malignancy as determined by all available means; (2) clinical target volume (CTV): GTV together with areas of possible subclinical microscopic disease; (3) planning target volume (PTV): CTV plus a margin to ensure that the CTV receives the prescribed dose [94].

When delineating the target volumes for oesophageal cancer, the radiation oncologist should make sure that the clinical target volume adequately encompasses all gross disease (whether primary tumour or macroscopically invaded lymph nodes) as well as lymph node areas at risk. Due to the anatomy of the oesophagus this will inevitably lead to large radiation volumes. Many of these more distant nodes are only microscopically invaded and the total dose given to these regions at risk does not need to be as high as the dose needed to treat macroscopic disease. The use of shrinking volumes is a logical approach to eliminate distant microscopically invaded lymphatics and nodes from the irradiated volume while limiting toxicity.

Delineation of the GTV

The GTV is delineated on planning CT, taking all clinical, endoscopic, and radiological information into account. FDG-PET/CT can play an important role in the planning of RT. The high-dose volume should be extended to include lymph nodes that are PET-positive without suspicion on CT or EUS [95]. The FDG uptake in the primary tumour can also be useful in the delineation of the primary tumour, with good correlation between PET-based length and pathological specimens [95]. Use of FDG-PET has been shown to reduce inter-observer variability with reduction of geographical miss of gross tumour. The dose distribution in normal tissue will change in a large majority of cases compared to CT-only planning, with a reduction of dose to the heart and lungs [96].

CTV margins around the primary tumour

Oesophageal cancer is notorious for its ability to spread intramurally distant from the main lesion. Oesophageal cancer can spread longitudinally and radially. Longitudinal spread occurs in both distal and proximal directions along the intramural lymphatic network and perineural spaces, with intramural localizations up to 5–6 cm from the primary tumour. In a study of 393 patients with SCC in the thoracic oesophagus, 60 were found by histological examination to have intramural metastasis [97].

The CTV should probably include 4–5 cm margins beyond the macroscopic tumour extent in the anterio-caudal direction and less (1.5–2.0 cm) horizontally around the GTV [98]. For adenocarcinoma of the lower third of the oesophagus and GEJ, the caudal extension of the CTV includes a 3–4 cm margin of gastric cardia below the lower border of GTV [99].

Elective nodal CTV

The oesophagus has a dual longitudinal interconnecting system of lymphatics in the lamina propria and the other in the muscularis mucosae. As a result of this system, lymph fluid can travel over the entire length of the oesophagus before draining into the lymph nodes [100]. Although upper oesophageal tumours spread mainly to the cervical and supraclavicular regions, involvement of the celiac nodes can occur in 10–30% of these tumours. The opposite is also true: involvement of the supraclavicular nodes can occur in 10–30% of patients with lower oesophageal tumours [100].

It is generally accepted that lymph node regions with a probability of 15–20% or more to be microscopically invaded should be included in the CTV. This would mean that the celiac trunk nodes do not need to be included in the CTV for all tumours of the upper and middle oesophagus. However, most cases referred for radiation have an advanced stage at diagnosis and are referred for preoperative, i.e. neoadjuvant, treatment. So the estimated percentage of involved nodes deduced from surgical series is probably lower than the probability among those patients referred for radiotherapy.

A recent meta-analysis pooled results from 45 observational studies with a total of 18,415 oesophageal carcinoma patients, > 90% with SCC [101]. The pooled estimates of lymph node metastasis rate in upper, middle, and lower thoracic oesophageal cancer were 30.7%, 16.8%, and 11.0% cervical; 42.0%, 21.1%, and 10.5% upper mediastinal; 12.9%, 28.1%, and 19.6% middle mediastinal; 2.6%, 7.8%, and 23.0% lower mediastinal; and 9%, 21.4%, and 39.9% abdominal, respectively. Lymph node metastases were most frequent in the paratracheal (31.7%) and perigastric (30.0%) lymph node areas, suggesting that these should always be included in the CTV [101].

For upper oesophageal cancer, cervical and upper mediastinal nodes should probably be included in the CTV, especially the supraclavicular, upper thoracic paraoesophageal, and thoracic paratracheal lymph nodes. Tumours located in the mid-oesophagus can skip not only up to the cervical lymph nodes, but also down to the abdomen. Thus, the CTV should include cervical, upper, middle mediastinal and abdominal portions, especially thoracic paratracheal, subcarinal, middle thoracic paraoesophageal, and lymph node stations around the cardia and the left gastric artery. As to the lower oesophagus, the CTV should cover the middle, lower mediastinal, and abdominal regions, especially including the lower thoracic paraoesophageal lymph nodes and the stations around the cardia, greater and lesser curvature, and the left gastric artery [101].

Regarding gastro-oesophageal junction adenocarcinoma, the European Organization for Research and Treatment of Cancer (EORTC) developed expert guidelines for target volume delineation in 2009. They advocate including the para-oesophageal lymph nodes in the lower thorax, the supra-diaphragmatic lymph nodes, the lymph nodes in the oesophageal hiatus of the diaphragm, the infra-diaphragmatic lymph nodes, those along the left gastric artery and around the celiac artery, as well as the right and left paracardial lymph nodes in all cases. For Siewert type I tumours, i.e. distal oesophageal tumours, the posterior mediastinal lymph nodes should also be included. In Siewert type II tumours, the lymph nodes along the lesser curvature, the short gastric vessels and the proximal splenic artery should be incorporated into the CTV. Siewert type III tumours should be delineated as gastric tumours and the CTV should at the very least include the lymph nodes along the lesser curvature, the short gastric vessels and the proximal as well as distal splenic artery, and the lymph nodes at the splenic hilum [99].

Techniques

The thoracic and upper abdominal region is a complex site for radiotherapy, because normal (e.g., lungs, heart, and spinal cord) and tumoural structures generally lie in close proximity to each other. The introduction of conformal radiotherapy with three-dimensional treatment planning (3D-RT) on CT scans signified a first major improvement over conventional two-dimensional radiotherapy (2D-RT), where the treatment portals are based on a radiographic simulation film. Forward treatment planning is employed for both 2D-RT and 3D-RT, which essentially consists of the radiation oncologist designing the RT fields and the radiation physicist generating an optimized dose distribution. In contrast, inverse treatment planning is employed with intensity-modulated radiotherapy (IMRT) and consists of identifying the target volumes and organs at risk on the planning CT. The dose to the tumour is specified, as well as the maximum acceptable doses to adjacent normal structures, and the physicist uses that information to produce the optimal plan, i.e. one that ensures target coverage by the prescribed radiation dose while reducing doses to the organs at risk. It may be expected that treatment with IMRT will result in fewer side effects [102].

Close patient monitoring and aggressive supportive care are essential during radiation treatment. Management of acute toxicities is necessary to avoid treatment interruptions or dose reductions. Anti-emetics should be given on a prophylactic basis when appropriate. Antacid and antidiarrhoeal medications may be prescribed when needed. If the caloric intake is inadequate, oral and/or enteral nutrition should be considered. Feeding jejunostomies or nasogastric feeding tubes may be placed if clinically indicated. Adequate enteral and/or intravenous hydration is necessary throughout CRT and early recovery.

Dose and fractionation schedules

Total radiation dose and daily fraction size are obviously important determinants for locoregional tumour control as well as acute and late toxicity. Definitive radiation therapy (i.e. without further surgery) requires a total dose of at least 59.4 to 66.6 Gy in daily fractions of 1.8 to 2.0 Gy. Smaller daily fractions (i.e. 1.8 instead of 2.0 Gy) potentially reduce the likelihood of late toxicity [98, 103].

The optimal radiation dose and fractionation schedule for pre- or postoperative radiotherapy has never been prospectively defined, although a total dose of at least 45.0 to 50.4 Gy is usually administered in 25 to 28 daily fractions of 1.8 Gy, five days per week, with adequate locoregional control and acceptable toxicity [98, 103].

Dose constraints for organs at risk

The complete volumes of the lungs, the liver, the kidneys, and the heart have to be delineated. Spinal cord must be outlined along the whole volume interested by the beams plus 2 cm above or below this volume.

Every effort should be made to keep the lung volume and doses to a minimum. Normal lung (>2 cm outside the target volume) should never receive more than 40 Gy. To reduce the incidence of postoperative pulmonary complications, a possible guideline is to limit the proportion of total lung receiving 20 Gy or more to 20% (V20 <20%) and 10 Gy or more to 40% (V10 <40%). Furthermore, the combined lung volume receiving less than 5 Gy should be higher than 2300 cc [98].

Further attention should be devoted to reduce unnecessary dose to other normal structures [98]. The maximal spinal cord dose must not exceed a total dose of 45 Gy. In case of combined modality treatment with concomitant chemotherapy this dose should probably be lowered. The whole heart must not have more than 30% exposed to a total dose of 40–50 Gy and not more than 50% exposed to a total dose of 25 Gy. Special effort should be made to keep the left ventricle doses to a minimum. At least 70% of one physiologically functioning kidney should receive a total dose of less than 20 Gy (V20 <60–70%). For the contralateral kidney, the volume exposed to more than 20 Gy has to be less than 30% (V20 <30%). Overall, not more than 50% of the combined functional renal volume should receive more than 20 Gy. Caution is required if the treatment is combined with chemotherapy, as there are no reports of the effect of concomitant treatment on renal function. The liver must not have more than 30% of its volume exposed to more than 30 Gy (V30 <30%). However, it is recognized that these guidelines may be exceeded as needed to achieve other important planning goals [98].

Brachytherapy

Brachytherapy permits treatment of a localized area of the oesophagus to high radiation doses with relative sparing of surrounding structures. This technique may be used alone or in combination with external beam radiotherapy with or without chemotherapy.

Brachytherapy involves intraluminal placement of a radioactive source into the oesophagus with a nasogastric applicator. With the introduction of small sources like Iridium-192 into afterloading brachytherapy, treatment of advanced obstructive tumours became possible using applicators with a small diameter (down to 1.7 mm).

For patient comfort, high dose rate (HDR) brachytherapy is common practice, although there is also some experience with low dose rate (LDR) brachytherapy. Modern HDR equipment delivers radiation much faster than 0.2 Gy/minute, permitting the delivery of a planned dose within minutes. Since HDR delivers a high dose of radiotherapy in a short period of time, fractionation is necessary; typically two to four fractions are administered for treatment of oesophageal cancer.

Total dose, fractionation, and overall treatment time of radiotherapy depend on the intent of treatment. For treatment with curative intent, a dose of 50–60 Gy (2 Gy per fraction) by external beam radiotherapy is followed by one or two brachytherapy applications with 5 to 6 Gy (HDR). The total dose for brachytherapy alone in a palliative setting is 15–25 Gy given in three to four HDR brachytherapy applications (4-6 Gy per fraction).

Brachytherapy alone is a palliative modality and results in a local control rate of 25–35% and a median survival of approximately five months. In the randomized trial from Sur et al., no significant difference was seen in local control or survival with high-dose brachytherapy compared with external beam [104].

Regarding combined modality treatment, no randomized data are available and results from retrospective analyses are mixed. The Radiation Therapy Oncology Group (RTOG) 92-07 trial prospectively combined CRT (5-FU and cisplatin with 50 Gy of external beam radiotherapy) with an intraluminal brachytherapy boost (20 Gy LDR or 15 Gy HDR) in 75 patients [105]. The HDR boost dose was reduced to 10 Gy after an interim analysis suggested high levels of treatment-related toxicity. Local failure was 27%, and acute toxicity included 58% of patients with grade 3 toxicity, 26% with grade 4, and 8% with grade 5. The cumulative incidence of fistula was 18% per year, and the crude incidence was 14%. Therefore, the benefit of adding intraluminal brachytherapy to curative radiotherapy, although theoretically interesting, remains unclear.

Medical management

Chemotherapy

Although there is a clear role for chemotherapy in oesophageal cancer, many studies have shortcomings. The strategy can be grouped into different potential indications: (1) peri-operative chemotherapy in resectable gastro-oesophageal junction adenocarcinoma, based on studies in gastric cancer, including gastro-oesophageal adenocarcinoma; (2) post-operative chemotherapy in gastro-oesophageal junction adenocarcinoma, also based on studies in gastric cancer, including gastro-oesophageal adenocarcinoma; (3) combined strategy with radiotherapy in the neoadjuvant treatment; (4) combined strategy with radiotherapy in the post-operative treatment of gastro-oesophageal junction adenocarcinoma based on studies in gastric cancer, including gastro-oesophageal adenocarcinoma; (5) metastatic squamous cell adenocarcinoma; and (6) metastatic adenocarcinoma. There is no evidence-based role as single modality for chemotherapy in the preoperative or post-operative treatment setting of SCC [106–108].

Amongst the shortcomings of published trials are the simultaneous inclusion of SCC and adenocarcinoma in many combined modality trials of locally advanced disease and in some trials in metastatic disease, the inclusion of locally advanced and metastatic disease, the heterogeneity of the chemotherapy and CRT regimens, and the relatively small sample size of many trials, with resulting weak statistical hypotheses.

Although there is no single standard regimen in combination regimens with radiotherapy, most modern studies and recommendations include combinations of two classic cytotoxic agents [109]. In combination with radiotherapy, the most frequently recommended regimens include a fluoropyrimidine/platinum based combination (often 5-FU and cisplatin). Recently, however, the combination of carboplatin and paclitaxel seems to be an excellent alternative with limited toxicity in combination with radiotherapy as demonstrated by Dutch investigators in the CROSS trial [110]. Potential valid alternatives to these cytotoxics include oxaliplatin, irinotecan, docetaxel, and capecitabine in different combinations, although these combinations have been evaluated less extensively in adequate phase III studies.

In patients with metastatic SCC, the number of high-quality randomized phase III studies remains limited. Often a combination of a fluoropyrimidine (5-FU or capecitabine) and a platinum (cisplatin or oxaliplatin) is proposed. There are, however, also limited data suggesting some activity of the taxanes (docetaxel and paclitaxel) and irinotecan.

Metastatic GEJ adenocarcinoma has been studied more extensively, since most of these patients are treated similar to patients with metastatic adenocarcinoma of the stomach in a large number of well performed phase II trials (see Chapter on Gastric cancer). The evidence is, however, growing that there may be clear molecular differences between gastro-oesophageal junction adenocarcinoma and gastric adenocarcinoma (e.g., higher HER2 positivity rate in GEJ cancer and potentially different benefit from bevacizumab in Western patients) [111]. Although oesophageal adenocarcinoma is often treated in the same way as GEJ adenocarcinoma, it has never been demonstrated that these patients derive a similar benefit from chemotherapy. The regimens in metastatic adenocarcinoma often include a doublet and sometimes a triplet: the doublet often consists of a fluoropyrimidine (5-FU, capecitabine or S1) and a platinum (cisplatin or oxaliplatin). The triplets include these drugs added with docetaxel or epirubicin. The data on epirubicin are controversial and there is wide geographic difference in the addition of epirubicin to a fluoropyrimidine/platinum backbone. The taxanes docetaxel and paclitaxel and irinotecan are alternatives in first-line combinations or are options in second-line chemotherapy for patients with metastatic disease [112].

Targeted agents

There is ongoing activity on the unravelling of the molecular targets and pathways playing a role in SCC and adenocarcinoma and on the evaluation of novel targeted agents, especially in adenocarcinoma: trastuzumab has been approved for HER2 positive metastatic GEJ and gastric adenocarcinoma [111]. Trastuzumab is now also under investigation in peri-operative chemotherapy studies and in preoperative CRT regimens. Amongst the other agents under investigation, mainly in metastatic adenocarcinoma (in part because adenocarcinomas are more frequent in developed countries that have the ability to perform clinical trials), the new HER2 blockers TDM-1 and pertuzumab, the EGFR and HER2 tyrosine kinase inhibitor lapatinib, the angiogenesis inhibitors bevacizumab and ramucirimab, the cMET inhibitors (antibodies and tyrosine kinase inhibitors), mTOR inhibitors, and fibroblast growth factor receptor inhibitors are of research interest. Disappointing results were reported recently on the anti-EGFR antibodies cetuximab and panitumumab in metastatic adenocarcinoma of the stomach and GEJ [113, 114]. However, further evaluation is ongoing in SCC of the oesophagus in combination with chemotherapy, analogous to SCC of the head and neck region.

Multidisciplinary management

Surgery remains the standard treatment for early stage oesophageal cancer, with good overall survival rates (Table 36.3). Still, its utility as a monotherapy has been rightly challenged, especially in more advanced disease [115]. Data from contemporary surgical series in those patients are relatively disappointing (Table 36.4), even in high-volume centres. In an analysis of 4627 patients with oesophageal cancer who were treated with surgery alone without adjuvant or neoadjuvant therapy, five-year survival rates were <50% for all disease stages except stage I, and they were 15% for any patient with node-positive disease [116]. Consequently, neoadjuvant (pre-operative), adjuvant (post-operative), and non-operative strategies aimed at improving survival in patients with apparently localized disease have been developed.

(Chemo-)radiotherapy alone

Definitive radiotherapy

Before the seminal paper by Herskovic et al., radiotherapy alone was sometimes performed in patients without distant metastases who were medically or surgically inoperable. Results were generally disappointing: in a meta-analysis of 49 historical series involving more than 8400 patients treated with radiotherapy alone, survival rates at one, two, and five years were only 18%, 8%, and 6%, respectively [117]. However, it should be noted that with modern radiotherapy and staging techniques, better results can be achieved. In a more recent retrospective analysis of 101 patients (only 11 adenocarcinomas) treated between 1985 to 1994, definitive radiotherapy was associated with a five-year survival rate up to 21% [118]. In that analysis, survival was better for adenocarcinoma than for SCC, though not statistically significantly. The only significant prognostic factor was the use of diagnostic CT scanning (42% versus 13% five-year survival with or without CT scanning, respectively, p = 0.01), which was associated with an increase in field size. This suggests that older, more unsatisfactory outcomes with definitive radiotherapy could be related to inadequate staging and patient selection, as well as outdated radiation techniques.

The potential of modern radiation techniques can be illustrated by a Chinese randomized trial in which surgery was compared to radiotherapy alone in 269 patients with oesophageal SCC [119]. Obviously, the quality of the surgery cannot be assessed, but lymph node dissection appears to have been limited. In the radiotherapy group, patients received a rather high total dose of 68.4 to 71.0 Gy without concomitant chemotherapy. The five-year overall survival rate was 36.9% in the surgery group versus 34.7% in the radiotherapy group, without statistical difference between the two groups. Obviously, such results cannot be extrapolated to patients with adenocarcinoma.

Still, the role for definitive radiotherapy alone appears limited, and concomitant chemotherapy should be prescribed whenever possible.

Definitive CRT

Theoretically, concurrent CRT should permit maximal tumour control through (1) higher locoregional control because of the additive, so-called radiosensitizing, effect of the chemotherapy on radiotherapy; (2) higher systemic control since the chemotherapy potentially reduces (micro-) metastatic disease.

As mentioned before, the seminal Herskovic paper was the landmark RTOG 85-01 trial, comparing radiotherapy alone (64 Gy in 32 fractions over 6.5 weeks) versus radiotherapy (50 Gy in 25 fractions over five weeks) with concurrent CRT (two cycles of 5-FU plus cisplatin) in patients with thoracic oesophageal cancer [25]. The CRT group received two additional chemotherapy courses, three weeks apart, after RT. Surgery was not part of the treatment schedule. It should be noted that the overall majority of patients (>90%) had SCC. The trial was stopped after the accumulated results in 121 patients demonstrated a significant advantage for survival in the patients who received CRT. In the radiotherapy group, two-year survival rate was 10%; the concomitant CRT group had a two-year survival rate of 38% (p <0.001]. The patients who received combined treatment had significantly fewer local and distant recurrences. Severe toxicity was higher in the combined treatment arm (44% versus 25%). The trial was updated in 1999, confirming the important survival advantage of concomitant chemotherapy: five-year survival with CRT was 26% versus 0% with RT alone [120]. Persistence of disease was the most common mode of treatment failure; however, it was less common in the groups receiving combined therapy (26%) than in the group treated with radiotherapy only (37%). There were no significant differences in severe late toxic effects between the groups.

In order to assess the optimal radiation dose in definitive CRT, the RTOG 94–05 trial compared a total dose of 50.4 versus 64.5 Gy (in daily 1.8 Gy fractions), both given in combination with cisplatin and 5-FU [121]. The higher radiation dose failed to show superiority compared to the lower dose with regards to local tumour control, overall survival, and relapse-free survival. On the other hand, acute adverse effects and treatment-associated deaths were significantly more common with the higher dose. Therefore, the regimen from RTOG 85–01 is still regarded as a reference regimen [25]. In many experienced centres, variations of this protocol have been developed and higher radiation doses are applied as a boost to smaller target volumes.

Combined approaches

Preoperative CRT

The often disappointing results with surgery alone and the apparent success and feasibility of definitive CRT have provided the motivation for the evaluation of combining CRT with surgery in an effort to further improve survival. Consequently, neoadjuvant CRT has been the most commonly investigated approach in the treatment of resectable oesophageal cancer in recent years.

At least nine trials compared surgery alone to some sort of preoperative CRT schedule for patients with potentially resectable oesophageal cancer [110, 122–129]. The most recent and largest meta-analysis included 1932 patients from 13 randomized trials [109]. The hazard ratio (HR) for the reduction of the overall mortality was 0.78 in favour of CRT (p = 0.002), resulting in an absolute two-year survival benefit of 8.7%. The benefit for patients with oesophageal SCC and patients with oesophageal adenocarcinoma was comparable.

Preoperative CRT increases the post-operative morbidity and mortality, according to some, but not all, studies. Three meta-analyses report on significantly increased post-operative morbidity and mortality following preoperative CRT [130–132]. However, the post-operative mortality was not increased when studies with dose per fraction above 2 Gy were not included [130].

The potential deleterious effects of preoperative CRT are only partly understood. Radiation in higher doses causes a disruption of the alveolar diffusion capacity and thereby deteriorates the pulmonary gas exchange. As a consequence, post-operative respiratory insufficiency occurs more often in irradiated patients [133]. Therefore, as emphasized above, current concepts of preoperative radiation treatment confine the target volumes to a necessary extent, limiting especially the exposure of the lungs. In this context, currently available techniques of intensity-modulated radiation treatment planning may have additional benefit.

The recently published CROSS trial is a prospective randomized controlled trial comparing surgery alone with neoadjuvant CRT followed by surgery [110]. It is the largest study investigating preoperative CRT in oesophageal cancer. Dutch investigators randomly assigned 363 patients with potentially resectable cancer (24% SCC, 76% adenocarcinoma) of the oesophagus or the gastro-oesophageal junction (in 11% of cases) to preoperative radiotherapy of 41.4 Gy

over five weeks with weekly paclitaxel plus carboplatin or surgery alone. Preoperative CRT was well tolerated, with grade 3 or worse hematologic toxicity in 7%, and grade 3 or higher non-hematologic toxicity in <13%; there were also no differences in post-operative morbidity or mortality between the two groups. The complete (R0) resection rate was higher with CRT (92% versus 69%, p < 0.001), and 29% of those treated with CRT had a pathological complete remission (pCR). At a median follow-up of 32 months, median overall survival was significantly better with preoperative CRT (three-year survival rate 58% versus 44%, p = 0.003). Therefore, CROSS certainly defines the new standard of care for advanced (T3-4 or N+) disease.

In less advanced disease, upfront surgery will remain the standard of care, and preoperative CRT appears to add little. A French randomized trial by the Fédération Francophone de Cancérologie Digestive (FFCD) tried to assess whether preoperative CRT improves outcomes for patients with localized (stages I or II) oesophageal cancer [129]. In the FFCD 9901 trial, 195 patients were randomized from 2000 to 2009: 98 were assigned to surgery alone and 97 to neoadjuvant CRT, consisting of a dose to 45 Gy in 25 daily fractions of 1.8 Gy with 2 courses of concomitant chemotherapy (5-FU and cisplatin). After a median follow-up of 5.7 years, median overall survival was 43.8 months in the surgery group versus 31.8 months (p = 0.66) in the combined modality arm. Post-operative mortality rates were 1.1% in the surgery group versus 7.3% in the CRT group (p = 0.054), respectively. These data strongly suggest that neoadjuvant CRT does not improve overall survival but enhances post-operative mortality rate with this regimen for patients with early oesophageal cancer compared with surgery alone.

A consistent finding in many studies is that response to preoperative CRT, particularly the absence of residual disease in the surgical specimen, is an indication of better disease-free and overall survival. In a comprehensive literature review of 22 studies in which patients with oesophageal or gastro-oesophageal junction cancer underwent oesophagectomy after neoadjuvant CRT, patients with a pCR were two- to three-fold more likely to survive as were those with residual disease in the oesophagectomy specimen [134]. Overall survival for patients with pCR was 93.1%, 75.0%, and 50.0% at 2, 3, and 5 years, respectively, whereas it was 36.8%, 29.0%, and 22.6% for patients with residual tumour (p < 0.025).

These results provide the rationale for intensification of preoperative treatment. Apparently, escalation of the radiation dose will not be the answer [121]. Perhaps intensification of the chemotherapy schedule could further improve results. Several groups have reported their experience with sequential induction chemotherapy followed by CRT. Encouraging as some of these results might be, it should be noted that no randomized trial to date has compared sequential induction chemotherapy followed by CRT to standard CRT. Moreover, it remains to be seen whether the added toxicity of any of these approaches is balanced by substantial survival gains.

Preoperative chemotherapy

Multiple randomized trials have evaluated the benefit of chemotherapy administered prior to surgery. A survival benefit for neoadjuvant chemotherapy relative to surgery alone was shown in the recent meta-analysis on neoadjuvant treatments, including nine randomized comparisons (n = 1981) of neoadjuvant chemotherapy versus surgery alone for oesophageal or gastro-oesophageal junction cancer [109]. The HR for all-cause mortality for neoadjuvant chemotherapy was 0.87 (95% CI 0.70–0.88), and this translated into an absolute survival benefit at two years of 5.1% and a number needed to treat to prevent one death of 19. The potential benefit of neoadjuvant chemotherapy was not offset by a higher post-operative mortality. The HR for SCC was 0.92 (0.81–1.04; p = 0.18) and for adenocarcinoma it was 0.83 (0.71–0.95; p = 0.01).

Preoperative chemotherapy or chemoradiotherapy?

Only one published trial, the German POET trial, directly compared preoperative CRT to neoadjuvant chemotherapy alone followed by surgery [135]. A total of 119 patients with locally advanced adenocarcinoma of the lower oesophagus or gastric cardia were randomly allocated to one of two treatment groups: induction chemotherapy (15 weeks of cisplatin plus 5-FU) followed by surgery; or chemotherapy (12 weeks of identical chemotherapy) followed by low-dose radiotherapy (30.0 Gy in 15 daily fractions of 2.0 Gy) concurrent with cisplatin and etoposide, followed by surgery. The study was prematurely closed due to low accrual. Although consequently underpowered, patients in the radiotherapy arm had a significantly higher probability of showing pCR (15.6% versus 2.0%) at resection. Preoperative radiotherapy improved three-year survival rate from 27.7% to 47.4% (p = 0.07]. Post-operative mortality was non-significantly increased in the CRT group (10.2% versus 3.8%; p = 0.26). Considering the importance of achieving pCR, these results demonstrate that radiotherapy is an indispensable component of the neoadjuvant treatment schedule for adenocarcinoma of the lower oesophagus and gastro-oesophageal junction. Whether these results can be extrapolated to SCC of the thoracic oesophagus is uncertain, but results from the CROSS trial strongly suggest that the benefit in those patients might be even larger [110].

The Sjoquist meta-analysis showed HR for all-cause mortality was 0.77 in favour of CRT compared to chemotherapy alone, but this was not statistically significant [109].

A randomized trial, the TOPGEAR trial, has been initiated to directly compare preoperative chemotherapy alone (consisting of epirubicin, cisplatin, and 5-FU [ECF]) versus CRT (two cycles of ECF followed by concurrent fluoropyrimidine-based CRT) in patients with resectable adenocarcinoma of the stomach and gastro-oesophageal junction. Both groups will receive three further cycles of ECF post-operatively.

Response assessment after neoadjuvant therapy

The early evaluation of response to neoadjuvant therapy (chemotherapy alone or CRT) has been extensively studied for oesophageal carcinoma. The therapy-induced reduction in FDG uptake is more pronounced than the morphological changes and precedes them by several weeks [136]. Patients with more pronounced reduction in uptake ('metabolic responders') have a better outcome than patients without or with a less pronounced reduction in FDG uptake ('metabolic non-responders'). For example, in one study the three-year survival rate was 70% versus 35%, respectively [137, 138]. In one prospective study (the Municon trial), after two weeks of initial cisplatin-based induction therapy metabolic non-responders were treated with immediate surgery whereas metabolic responders received a full course of neoadjuvant chemotherapy before surgery [139]. Compared to metabolic non-responders, the metabolic responders had a better median event-free survival (29.7 months versus not reached) and overall survival (14.1 and

25.8 months). In a follow-up study, the Municon II trial, metabolic non-responders after 14 days of chemotherapy were treated with salvage CRT whereas metabolic responders were treated with only chemotherapy, with surgery at the end of treatment in both groups [140]. The outcome in the metabolic non-responder group was significantly worse than in the metabolic responders, despite the more intense treatment. In other studies, early response prediction with FDG-PET was less accurate, with sensitivity and specificity of 70% in a recent meta-analysis, so that routine clinical adoption of PET-based treatment decisions is not warranted, and should only be done within the scope of prospective clinical trials [141]. In the US, a trial of PET-directed neoadjuvant therapy (NCT01333033) is being performed, in which metabolic non-responders will have their induction chemotherapy changed to a different regimen during radiation.

Is surgery still necessary?

Clearly, neoadjuvant treatment with chemotherapy and especially CRT improves survival in advanced, but not early-stage, oesophageal cancer. Particularly striking is the large percentage of patients with pCR in modern series (e.g., up to 30% in the recent CROSS trial [110]). Similarly remarkable is the observation that with modern definitive CRT series long-term overall survival rates can be achieved that are quite high, up to 30–40% [121, 142]. This raises the interesting question as to whether surgery is still always necessary and if concomitant CRT might not one day become the standard of care in selected patients [143].

Historical, non-randomized results from the 1992–1994 Patterns of Care study and the 1988–2006 SEER regional database suggest a survival benefit for post-CRT oesophagectomy [144, 145]. In addition, locoregional disease persistence is not uncommon in older series on CRT without surgery [25].

At least two randomized trials directly comparing CRT alone to CRT followed by surgery have failed to demonstrate better survival, although both show better locoregional control and a lesser need for palliative procedures when surgery is a component of multimodality treatment. It should be noted that the patient populations in both were either exclusively or predominantly SCC.

Stahl et al. randomly allocated 172 patients with locally advanced SCC of the oesophagus to either induction chemotherapy (3 cycles of 5-FU, leucovorin, etoposide, and cisplatin) followed by CRT (total dose to 40.0 Gy with cisplatin plus etoposide) followed by surgery or the same induction chemotherapy followed by CRT (at least 65.0 Gy with cisplatin plus etoposide) without surgery [146]. Treatment-related mortality was higher in the trimodality arm (12.8% versus 3.5%). After a median follow-up time of six years, the surgically treated patients had significantly better local control (two-year local progression-free survival 64% versus 41%; p = 0.003), but this did not translate into significantly better overall survival at three (31% versus 24%) or five (28% versus 17%) years. In comparison to other trials using concomitant CRT alone or followed by surgery, radiotherapy doses and the intensity of chemotherapy were low. This may in part explain the lower survival rate in the non-surgically treated patients when compared to the results of RTOG 85-01 [25].

In the French FFCD 9102 trial, 444 patients with potentially resectable (cT3N0-1) thoracic oesophageal SCC (89%) or adenocarcinoma (11%) received two cycles of 5-FU and cisplatin and either conventional (46 Gy in 4.5 weeks) or split-course (15 Gy, days 1 to 5 and 22 to 26) concomitant radiotherapy [147]. Patients with response and no contraindication to either treatment were randomly assigned to surgery or continuation of CRT (three more cycles of 5-FU/cisplatin and either conventional (20 Gy) or split-course (15 Gy) radiotherapy). Two-year survival rate was 34% in the surgery group versus 40% in the CRT group (p = 0.44). Two-year local control rate was 66.4% in the surgical arm compared with 57.0% in the CRT arm, and stents were less required in the surgical arm (5% versus 32%, p <0.001). Again, the initial (three-months) mortality rate was 9.3% in the surgical arm compared with 0.8% in the CRT arm (p = 0.002).

In conclusion, although no significant survival advantage of surgical treatment was proven in these studies, there is a significant advantage for locoregional control in favour of surgical treatment. Therefore, surgical resection should be recommended in patients without contraindications and willing to take the risk of post-operative morbidity and mortality, particularly in adenocarcinoma patients since there are few data on non-surgical management and the rate of pCR is relatively low for adenocarcinoma as compared to SCC. Until now, there are scarce data on the efficacy of definitive CRT in oesophageal adenocarcinoma. Therefore, CRT alone is not a proven and established alternative to surgery. For patients with SCC who have an endoscopic complete response, non-operative management is an option balancing the risks of surgical mortality versus improved locoregional control.

Adjuvant therapies

Clearly, patients with cT3-4a and/or clinically node-positive oesophageal or gastro-oesophageal junction cancer should ideally be offered induction therapy with chemotherapy or CRT before surgical resection. Still, some patients will go immediately to surgery, usually because the extent of the disease was underestimated on preoperative EUS or imaging. For patients who are found to have advanced disease after surgery alone, the addition of post-operative, additional therapy (chemotherapy with or without radiotherapy) should be considered in an effort to improve outcome.

Adjuvant chemotherapy

Since trials of post-operative chemotherapy in oesophageal cancer did not show any benefit and suffered from many shortcomings, post-operative chemotherapy in SCC cannot be recommended routinely. The data in GEJ adenocarcinoma are, however, more difficult to interpret, since the trials of post-operative chemotherapy usually include both gastric as well as GEJ adenocarcinoma. Most individual trials in Western patients did not show benefit, while the trials in Asia with adjuvant chemotherapy (predominantly S1) in mainly gastric adenocarcinoma showed benefit. A few relatively small combined analyses showed conflicting results. A large meta-analysis on adjuvant chemotherapy in adenocarcinoma based on individual patient data, however, showed a statistically significant and relevant benefit in favour of post-operative chemotherapy compared to surgery alone [148]. In that analysis from 17 trials (3838 patients) with a median follow-up exceeding seven years, adjuvant chemotherapy was associated with a statistically significant benefit in terms of overall survival (HR 0.82; p <0.001) and disease-free survival (HR 0.82; p < 0.001). Five-year overall survival increased from 49.6% to 55.3% with chemotherapy. The authors concluded that, post-operative adjuvant chemotherapy based on fluorouracil

regimens was associated with reduced risk of death compared with surgery alone [148]. Since this is a meta-analysis, and since numerically the benefit remains smaller than that of perioperative chemotherapy and of post-operative chemoradiotherapy in GEJ and gastric adenocarcinoma, the level of recommendation of post-operative CRT remains lower and this option is only recommended in patients with high-risk tumours who were not offered a preoperative treatment and who are not good candidates for post-operative CRT.

Adjuvant chemoradiotherapy

For patients with node-positive adenocarcinoma of the GEJ, post-operative CRT is a well-established approach. The large Intergroup trial (INT-0116) by Macdonald et al. is undoubtedly the most important study in that respect [149]. A total of 556 patients with pT1-4 pN0-1 resected adenocarcinoma of the stomach (80%) or gastro-oesophageal junction (20%) were randomly assigned to active surveillance or post-operative CRT (one cycle of 5-FU with leucovorin (LV), followed by 45 Gy in 25 fractions of 1.8 Gy with 5-FU and LV during the first and last week, followed by two more cycles of 5-FU/LV) or surgery alone. The median overall survival in the surgery-only group was 27 months, as compared with 36 months in the CRT group (p = 0.005), although only 64% of patients could finish the combined modality arm as planned. Patients with gastro-oesophageal junction adenocarcinoma appeared to derive the same benefit as those with non-cardia gastric cancer.

Fuchs et al. tried to improve on the INT-0116 trial by prescribing ECF (epirubicin, cisplatin, and 5-FU) instead of 5-FU/LV before and after radiotherapy to 45 Gy with concomitant 5-FU [150]. They included 546 patients with resected gastric or gastro-oesophageal junction adenocarcinoma, but median disease-free survival was nearly identical (30 months in the 5-FU/LV group versus 28 months in the ECF group) in both arms.

In the current Dutch CRITICS trial, all patients will receive induction chemotherapy followed by surgery and randomization to post-operative chemotherapy versus CRT.

For other patients, particularly those with an oesophageal SCC, the optimal approach is uncertain. Some uncontrolled trials and retrospective comparisons of patients treated with and without CRT suggest potential benefit for post-operative CRT. However, others do not, and there are no randomized trials proving benefit as compared to surgery alone, or indeed post-operative chemotherapy [151].

Palliative treatment

Palliative systemic therapy

The prognosis of patients with metastatic oesophageal cancer remains very poor. It has been shown that patients in good condition and with good organ function treated with chemotherapy may derive a survival benefit from chemotherapy combinations, which remains, however, modest: the median survival of patients treated with best supportive care (BSC) is usually around three to four months, while with BSC plus chemotherapy it is around nine to 12 months. The development of regimens for therapy in oesophageal cancer is impeded, in part, by two histologies (squamous cell and adenocarcinoma) as well as the relatively small number of patients fit for clinical trials in developed countries.

Adenocarcinoma patients with advanced oesophageal adenocarcinoma or gastro-oesophageal adenocarcinoma are typically included in gastric cancer trials. For that reason, more extensive discussion of treatment options can be found in the text and tables dedicated to that disease (see Chapter on 'Gastric cancer'). For squamous cell cancers, regimens are typically selected that are used in squamous cell cancer of the lung or head and neck cancer, such as platinum compounds and taxanes, or regimens from trials which included both oesophageal histologies. An exhaustive search of clinical trial registries in late 2013 revealed no large trials of systemic therapies alone for oesophageal squamous cell cancers. In general, doublet therapy is preferred in first-line treatment, with second-line treatments comprising those drugs/classes not previously used. For example, a patient treated initially with capecitabine/oxaliplatin (± epirubicin) should subsequently receive a single-agent taxane, such as docetaxel.

The ECF (epirubicin, cisplatin, infusional 5-FU) and DCF (docetaxel, cisplatin, infusional 5-FU) combinations are considered standard regimens for first-line treatment in Western countries [152, 153]. In Japan, there is a significant benefit for the oral fluoropyrimidine S1 plus cisplatin over S1 alone in terms of response survival [154]. Therefore, S-1 plus cisplatin is the Japanese standard chemotherapy.

In the UK in particular, the REAL-2 phase III study in advanced gastric cancer were assigned to three weekly cycles of epirubicin plus cisplatin and either capecitabine or infusional 5-FU, or epirubicin plus oxaliplatin and either capecitabine or infusional 5-FU [155]. Based on the data from this study, and on clinical experience, oxaliplatin and capecitabine are frequently substituted in place of cisplatin and parenteral 5-FU in metastatic oesophageal cancer.

For HER2 positive metastatic gastro-oesophageal cancers, the benefits from trastuzumab apply from the ToGA trial, in which HER2 positivity more often found in gastro-oesophageal cancers than body of stomach (33.2 versus 20.9%) [156]. With trastuzumab combined with cisplatin plus either capecitabine or 5-FU, the median overall survival was 13.8 months (95% CI 12-16) in those assigned to trastuzumab plus chemotherapy compared with 11.1 months [10, 12, 13] in those assigned to chemotherapy alone (hazard ratio 0.74; 95% CI 0.60–0.91; p = 0.0046).

Explorations of the VEGF agent (bevacizumab) and the EGFR agents (panitumumab and cetuximab) combined with chemotherapy in gastrointestinal cancer have failed to show benefit (bevacizumab in combination with chemotherapy as first-line therapy in advanced gastric cancer; a randomized double-blind placebo-controlled phase III study [157 - 159].

For refractory or second-line therapies, active single agents are frequently used if not already given in first-line treatment. Ramucirumab, a monoclonal antibody VEGFR-2 antagonist, has been compared to BSC alone in this setting for gastro-oesophageal cancers (ramucirumab monotherapy for previously treated advanced gastric or gastro-oesophageal junction adenocarcinoma (REGARD: an international, randomized, multicentre, placebo-controlled, phase III trial) [160]. Median overall survival was 5.2 months in patients in the ramucirumab group and 3.8 months in those in the placebo group (hazard ratio 0.776, 95% CI 0.603–0.998; p = 0.047). This drug is likely to be approved in many countries, as a non-chemotherapy approach for this patient population.

Palliative local therapy

Dysphagia is undoubtedly the most important symptom in patients with advanced oesophageal cancer. Palliative resection is nowadays only seldom considered, and should probably be avoided. Endoscopic interventions include dilatation, laser therapy, endoscopic mucosal resection, and placement of self-expanding metal or plastic stents.

In a pivotal randomized trial by Homs et al., 209 patients with dysphagia from inoperable oesophageal carcinoma were assigned to metal stent placement or single-dose (12 Gy) HDR brachytherapy [161]. Dysphagia improved more rapidly after stent placement than after brachytherapy, but long-term relief of dysphagia was better after brachytherapy. Stent placement also had more complications than brachytherapy (33% versus 21%, p = 0.02), which was mainly due to an increased incidence of late haemorrhage. Quality-of-life scores were also in favour of brachytherapy. However, both groups did not significantly differ for persistent or recurrent dysphagia, or for median survival.

For patients with complete oesophageal obstruction, surgical or radiologic placement of jejunostomy or gastrostomy tubes may be necessary to provide adequate hydration and nutrition.

Further reading

Ding X, Zhang J, Li B, Wang Z, Huang W et al. A meta-analysis of lymph node metastasis rate for patients with thoracic oesophageal cancer and its implication in delineation of clinical target volume for radiation therapy. British Journal of Radiology 2012; 85: 1110–1119.

Herskovic A, Martz K, al-Sarraf M. Combined chemotherapy and radiotherapy compared with radiotherapy alone in patients with cancer of the esophagus. New England Journal of Medicine 1992; 326: 1593–1598.

Homs MYV, Steyerberg EW, Eijkenboom WMH, Tilanus HW, Stalpers LJ et al. Single-dose brachytherapy versus metal stent placement for the palliation of dysphagia from oesophageal cancer: multicentre randomised trial. Lancet 2004; 364: 1497–1504.

Nafteux P, Moons J, Coosemans W, Decaluwé H, Decker G et al. Minimally invasive oesophagectomy: a valuable alternative to open oesophagectomy for the treatment of early oesophageal and gastro-oesophageal junction carcinoma. European Journal of Cardio-Thoracic Surgery 2011; 40(6): 1455–1463.

Prasad GA, Wu TT, Wigle DA, Buttar NS, Wongkeesong LM et al. Endoscopic and surgical treatment of mucosal (T1a) esophageal adenocarcinoma in Barrett's esophagus. Gastroenterology 2009; 137(3): 815–823.

Rice TW, Rusch VW, Ishwaran H, Blackstone EH, Worldwide Esophageal Cancer Collaboration. Cancer of the esophagus and esophagogastric junction: data-driven staging for the seventh edition of the American Joint Committee on Cancer/International Union Against Cancer Cancer Staging Manuals. Cancer 2010; 116: 3763.

Sjoquist KM, Burmeister BH, Smithers BM, Zalcberg JR, Simes RJ et al. Australasian Gastro-Intestinal Trials Group. Survival after neoadjuvant chemotherapy or chemoradiotherapy for resectable oesophageal carcinoma: an updated meta-analysis. Lancet Oncology 2011; 12(7): 681.

Skinner DB. En bloc resection for neoplasms of the esophagus and cardia. Journal of Thoracic and Cardiovascular Surgery 1983; 85(1): 59–71.

van Vliet EP, Heijenbrok-Kal MH, Hunink MG, Kuipers ET, Siersma PD. Staging investigations for oesophageal cancer: a meta-analysis. British Journal of Cancer 2008; 98(3): 547–57.

van Hagen P, Hulshof MC, van Lanschot JJ, Steyerberg EW, van Berge Henegouwen MI et al. Preoperative chemoradiotherapy for esophageal or junctional cancer. New England Journal of Medicine 2012; 366(22): 2074–2084.

References

1. Chak A, Lee T, Kinnard MF, Brock W, Faulx A et al. Familial aggregation of Barrett's oesophagus, oesophageal adenocarcinoma, and oesophagogastric junctional adenocarcinoma in Caucasian adults. Gut 2002; 51(3): 323–328.

2. Chang-Claude J, Becher H, Blettner M, Qiu S, Yang G et al. Familial aggregation of oesophageal cancer in a high incidence area in China. International Journal of Epidemiology 1997; 26(6): 1159–1165.

3. Islami F, Malekshah AF, Kimiagar M, Pourshams A, Wakefield J et al. Patterns of food and nutrient consumption in northern Iran, a high-risk area for esophageal cancer. Nutrition and Cancer 2009; 61(4): 475–483.

4. Keszei AP, Schouten LJ, Goldbohm RA, van den Brandt PA. Red and processed meat consumption and the risk of esophageal and gastric cancer subtypes in The Netherlands Cohort Study. Annals of Oncology 2012; 23(9): 2319–2326.

5. Yang YL, Xu KL, Zhou Y, Gao X, Chen LR. Correlation of epidermal growth factor receptor overexpression with increased epidermal growth factor receptor gene copy number in esophageal squamous cell carcinomas. Chinese Medical Journal 2012; 125(3): 450–454.

6. Nicholson RI, Gee JM, Harper ME. EGFR and cancer prognosis. European Journal of Cancer 2001; 37(Suppl. 4): S9–S15.

7. Su Z, Gay LJ, Strange A, Palles C, Band G, et al. Common variants at the MHC locus and at chromosome 16q24.1 predispose to Barrett's esophagus. Nature Genetics 2012; 44(10): 1131–1136.

8. Boone J, Livestro DP, Elias SG, Borel Rinkes IH, van Hillegersberg R et al. International survey on esophageal cancer: part II staging and neoadjuvant therapy. Diseases of the Esophagus 2009; 22: 203–210.

9. Edge SB, Byrd DR, Compton CC, Fritz AG, Greene FL, et al. AJCC Cancer Staging Manual, 7th ed. New York: Springer; 2010.

10. Siewert JR, Holscher AH, Becker K, Gossner W. Cardia cancer: attempt at a therapeutically relevant classification. Der Chirurg 1987: 25–32.

11. American Cancer Society, 2014. Esophagus cancer. <http://www.cancer.org/cancer/esophaguscancer/detailedguide/esophagus-cancer-staging>.

12. Rice TW, Rusch VW, Ishwaran H, Blackstone EH, Worldwide Esophageal Cancer Collaboration. Cancer of the esophagus and esophagogastric junction: data-driven staging for the seventh edition of the American Joint Committee on Cancer/International Union Against Cancer Cancer Staging Manuals. Cancer 2010; 116: 3763.

13. Rösch T. Endosonographic staging of esophageal cancer: a review of literature results. Gastrointestinal Endoscopy Clinics of North America 1995; 5(3): 537–547.

14. Lightdale CJ, Kulkarni KG. Role of endoscopic ultrasonography in the staging and follow-up of esophageal cancer. Journal of Clinical Oncology 2005; 23(20): 4483–4489.

15. van Vliet EP, Heijenbrok-Kal MH, Hunink MG, Kuipers ET, Siersma PD. Staging investigations for oesophageal cancer: a meta-analysis. British Journal of Cancer 2008; 98(3): 547–57.

16. Kutup A, Link BC, Schurr PG, Strate T, Kaifi JT et al. Quality control of endoscopic ultrasound in preoperative staging of esophageal cancer. Endoscopy 2007; 39(8): 715–719.

17. Vazquez-Sequeiros E, Levy MJ, Clain JE, Schwartz DA, Harewood GC et al. Routine vs. selective EUS-guided FNA approach for preoperative nodal staging of esophageal carcinoma. Gastrointestinal Endoscopy 2006; 63(2): 204–211.

18. Vander Heiden MG, Cantley LC, Thompson CB. Understanding the Warburg effect: the metabolic requirements of cell proliferation. Science 2009; 324(5930): 1029–1033.

19. Ott K, Weber WA, Fink U, Helmberger H, Becker K et al. Fluorodeoxyglucose-positron emission tomography in adenocarcinomas of the distal esophagus and cardia. World Journal of Surgery 2003; 27(9): 1035–1039.

20. Bar-Shalom R, Guralnik L, Tsalic M, Fu Z, Yin Y et al. The additional value of PET/CT over PET in FDG imaging of oesophageal cancer. European Journal of Nuclear Medicine and Molecular Imaging 2005; 32(8): 918–924.

21. Barber TW, Duong CP, Leong T, Bressel M, Drummond EG et al. 18F-FDG PET/CT has a high impact on patient management and provides powerful prognostic stratification in the primary staging of esophageal cancer: a prospective study with mature survival data. Journal of Nuclear Medicine 2012; 53(6): 864–871.

22. Malik V, Johnston C, Donohoe C, Claxton Z, Lucey J et al. (18) F-FDG PET-detected synchronous primary neoplasms in the staging of esophageal cancer: incidence, cost, and impact on management. Clinical Nuclear Medicine 2012; 37(12): 1152–1158.

23. Pech O, Bollschweiler E, Manner H, Leers J, Ell C et al. Comparison between endoscopic and surgical resection of mucosal esophageal adenocarcinoma in Barrett's esophagus at two high-volume centers. Annals of Surgery 2011; 254(1): 67–72.

24. Prasad GA, Wu TT, Wigle DA, Buttar NS, Wongkeesong LM et al. Endoscopic and surgical treatment of mucosal (T1a) esophageal adenocarcinoma in Barrett's esophagus. Gastroenterology 2009; 137(3): 815–823.

25. Herskovic A, Martz K, al-Sarraf M. Combined chemotherapy and radiotherapy compared with radiotherapy alone in patients with cancer of the esophagus. New England Journal of Medicine 1992; 326: 1593–1598.

26. Paulson E, Ra J, Armstrong K, Wirtalla C, Spitz F et al. Underuse of esophagectomy as treatment for resectable esophageal cancer. Archives of Surgery 2008; 143: 1198.

27. Pech O, Günter E, Ell C. Endosonography of high-grade intra-epithelial neoplasia/early cancer. Best Practice & Research Clinical Gastroenterology 2009; 23(5): 639–647.

28. May A, Günter E, Roth F, Gossner L, Stolte M et al. Accuracy of staging in early oesophageal cancer using high resolution endoscopy and high resolution endosonography: a comparative, prospective, and blinded trial. Gut 2004; 53(5): 634–640.

29. Pech O, Behrens A, May A, Nachbar L, Gossner L et al. Long-term results and risk factor analysis for recurrence after curative endoscopic therapy in 349 patients with high-grade intraepithelial neoplasia and mucosal adenocarcinoma in Barrett's oesophagus. Gut 2008; 57(9): 1200–1206.

30. Bennett C, Vakil N, Bergman J. Consensus statements for management of Barrett's dysplasia and early-stage esophageal adenocarcinoma, based on a Delphi process. Gastroenterology 2012; 143(2): 336–346.

31. Shaheen NJ, Sharma P, Overholt BF. Radiofrequency ablation in Barrett's esophagus with dysplasia. New England Journal of Medicine 2009; 360(22): 2277–2288.

32. Pouw RE, Wirths K, Eisendrath P, Sondermeijer CM, Ten Kate FJ et al. Efficacy of radiofrequency ablation combined with endoscopic resection for Barrett's esophagus with early neoplasia. Clinical Gastroenterology and Hepatology 2010; 8(1): 23–29.

33. Moss A, Bourke MJ, Hourigan LF, Gupta S, Williams SJ et al. Endoscopic resection for Barrett's high-grade dysplasia and early esophageal adenocarcinoma: an essential staging procedure with long-term therapeutic benefit. American Journal of Gastroenterology 2010; 105(6): 1276–1283.

34. Thorek F. The first successful case of resection of the thoracic portion of the oesophagus for carcinoma. Surgery, Gynecology & Obstetrics 1913; 16: 614–617.

35. Kakegawa T., Fujita H. A history of esophageal surgery in the twentieth century. General Thoracic and Cardiovascular Surgery 2009; 57(2): 55–63.

36. Clark GW, Peters JH, Ireland AP, Ehsan A, Hagen JA et al. Nodal metastasis and sites of recurrence after en bloc esophagectomy for adenocarcinoma. Annals of Thoracic Surgery 1994; 58(3): 646–653.

37. Akiyama H, Tsurumaru M, Kawamura T, Ono Y. Principles of surgical treatment for carcinoma of the esophagus: analysis of lymph node involvement. Annals of Surgery 1981; 194(4): 438–446.

38. Thomas P, Doddoli C, Neville P, Pons J, Lienne P et al. Esophageal cancer resection in the elderly. European Journal of Cardio-Thoracic Surgery 1996; 10(11): 941–946.

39. Poon RT, Law SY, Chu KM, Branicki FJ, Wong J. Esophagectomy for carcinoma of the esophagus in the elderly: results of current surgical management. Annals of Surgery 1998; 227(3): 357–364.

40. Logan A. The surgical treatment of carcinoma of the esophagus and cardia. Journal of Thoracic and Cardiovascular Surgery 1963 Aug; 46: 150–161.

41. Skinner DB. En bloc resection for neoplasms of the esophagus and cardia. Journal of Thoracic and Cardiovascular Surgery 1983; 85(1): 59–71.

42. Akiyama H, Tsurumaru M, Udagawa H, Kajiyama Y. Radical lymph node dissection for cancer of the thoracic esophagus. Annals of Surgery 1994; 220(3): 364–372.

43. Orringer MB. Transhiatal esophagectomy without thoracotomy for carcinoma of the thoracic esophagus. Annals of Surgery 1984; 200(3): 282–288.

44. Lewis I. The surgical treatment of carcinoma of the oesophagus; with special reference to a new operation for growths of the middle third. British Journal of Surgery 1946; 34: 18–31.

45. McKeown KC. Total three-stage oesophagectomy for cancer of the oesophagus. British Journal of Surgery 1976; 63(4): 259–262.

46. Sweet RH. Carcinoma of the esophagus and cardiac end of the stomach: immediate and late results of treatment by resection of primary esophagogastric anastomosis. Journal of the American Medical Association 1947; 135: 485.

47. Belsey RH. Surgical exposure of the esophagus. In: Skinner DBJ, Belsey RH eds, Management of Esophageal Disorders. Philadelphia: WB Saunders, 1988. p. 192–201, 757.

48. Luketich JD, Alvelo-Rivera M, Buenaventura PO, Christie NA, McCaughan JS et al. Minimally invasive esophagectomy: outcomes in 222 patients. Annals of Surgery 2003; 238(4): 486–494.

49. Nafteux P, Moons J, Coosemans W, Decaluwé H, Decker G et al. Minimally invasive oesophagectomy: a valuable alternative to open oesophagectomy for the treatment of early oesophageal and gastro-oesophageal junction carcinoma. European Journal of Cardio-Thoracic Surgery 2011; 40(6): 1455–1463.

50. Luketich JD, Pennathur A, Awais O, Levy RM, Keeley S et al. Outcomes after minimally invasive esophagectomy: review of over 1000 patients. Annals of Surgery 2012; 256(1): 95–103.

51. Ando N, Ozawa S, Kitagawa Y, Shinozawa Y, Kitajima M. Improvement in the results of surgical treatment of advanced squamous esophageal carcinoma during 15 consecutive years. Annals of Surgery 2000; 232(2): 225–232.

52. Isono K, Sato H, Nakayama K. Results of a nationwide study on the three-field lymph node dissection of esophageal cancer. Oncology 1991; 48(5): 411–420.

53. Lerut T, Nafteux P, Moons J, Coosemans W, Decker G et al. Three-field lymphadenectomy for carcinoma of the esophagus and gastroesophageal junction in 174 R0 resections: impact on staging, disease-free survival, and outcome: a plea for adaptation of TNM classification in upper-half esophageal carcinoma. Annals of Surgery 2004; 240(6): 962–972.

54. Collard JM, Otte JB, Fiasse R, Laterre PF, De Kock M et al. Skeletonizing en bloc esophagectomy for cancer. Annals of Surgery 2001; 234(1): 25–32.

55. Hagen JA, DeMeester SR, Peters JH, Chandrasoma P, DeMeester TR. Curative resection for esophageal adenocarcinoma: analysis of 100 en bloc esophagectomies. Annals of Surgery 2001; 234(4): 520–530.

56. Altorki N, Skinner D. Should en bloc esophagectomy be the standard of care for esophageal carcinoma? Annals of Surgery 2001; 234(5): 581–587.

57. Hulscher JB, van Sandick JW, de Boer AG, Wijnhoven BP, Tijssen JG et al. Extended transthoracic resection compared with limited transhiatal resection for adenocarcinoma of the esophagus. New England Journal of Medicine 2002; 347(21): 1662–1669.

58. Baba M, Aikou T, Yoshinaka H, Natsugoe S, Fukumoto T et al. Long-term results of subtotal esophagectomy with three-field lymphadenectomy for carcinoma of the thoracic esophagus. Annals of Surgery 1994; 219(3): 310–316.

59. Altorki NK, Girardi L, Skinner DB. En bloc esophagectomy improves survival for stage III esophageal cancer. Journal of Thoracic and Cardiovascular Surgery 1997; 114(6): 948–955.

60. Lerut T, Coosemans W, Decker G, De Leyn P, Ectors N et al. Extracapsular lymph node involvement is a negative prognostic factor in T3 adenocarcinoma of the distal esophagus and gastroesophageal junction. Journal of Thoracic and Cardiovascular Surgery 2003; 126(4): 1121–1128.

61. Birkmeyer JD, Siewers AE, Finlayson EV, Stukel TA, Lucas FL et al. Hospital volume and surgical mortality in the United States. New England Journal of Medicine 2002; 346(15): 1128–1237.

62. van Lanschot JJ, Hulscher JB, Buskens CJ, Tilanus HW, Ten Kate FJ et al. Hospital volume and hospital mortality for esophagectomy. Cancer 2001; 91(8): 1574–1578.

63. Lerut T, Decker G, Coosemans W, De Leyn P, Decaluwé H et al. Quality indicators of surgery for adenocarcinoma of the esophagus and gastroesophageal junction. Recent Results in Cancer Research 2010; 182: 127–142.

64. Jadad AR, Moore RA, Carroll D, Jenkinson C, Reynolds DJ et al. Assessing the quality of reports of randomized clinical trials: is blinding necessary? Controlled Clinical Trials 1996; 17(1): 1–12.

65. Lerut T, Moons J, Coosemans W, Van Raemdonck D, De Leyn P et al. Postoperative complications after transthoracic esophagectomy for cancer of the esophagus and gastroesophageal junction are correlated with early cancer recurrence: role of systematic grading of complications using the modified Clavien classification. Annals of Surgery 2009; 250(5): 798–807.

66. Bardini R, Bonavina L, Asolati M, Ruol A, Castoro C et al. Single-layered cervical esophageal anastomoses: a prospective study of two suturing techniques. Annals of Thoracic Surgery 1994; 58(4): 1087–1089.

67. Orringer MB, Marshall B, Iannettoni MD. Eliminating the cervical esophagogastric anastomotic leak with a side-to-side stapled anastomosis. Journal of Thoracic and Cardiovascular Surgery 2000; 119(2): 277–288.

68. Collard JM, Romagnoli R, Goncette L, Otte JB, Kestens PJ. Terminalized semimechanical side-to-side suture technique for cervical esophagogastrostomy. Annals of Thoracic Surgery 1998; 65(3): 814–817.

69. Pierie JP, de Graaf PW, Poen H, van der Tweel I, Obertop H. Incidence and management of benign anastomotic stricture after cervical oesophagogastrostomy. British Journal of Surgery 1993; 80(4): 471–474.

70. Trentino P, Pompeo E, Nofroni I, Francioni F, Rapacchietta S et al. Predictive value of early postoperative esophagoscopy for occurrence of benign stenosis after cervical esophagogastrostomy. Endoscopy 1997; 29(9): 840–844.

71. Gillinov AM, Heitmiller RF. Strategies to reduce pulmonary complications after transhiatal esophagectomy. Diseases of the Esophagus 1998; 11(1): 43–47.

72. Hulscher JB, Tijssen JG, Obertop H, van Lanschot JJ. Transthoracic versus transhiatal resection for carcinoma of the esophagus: a meta-analysis. Annals of Thoracic Surgery 2001; 72(1): 306–313.

73. Biere SS, van Berge Henegouwen MI, Maas KW, Bonavina L, Rosman C et al. Minimally invasive versus open oesophagectomy for patients with oesophageal cancer: a multicentre, open-label, randomised controlled trial. Lancet 2012; 379(9829): 1887–1892.

74. Paul S, Altorki NK, Port JL, Stiles BM, Lee PC. Surgical management of chylothorax. The Thoracic and Cardiovascular Surgeon 2009; 57(4): 226–228.

75. Graham DD, McGahren ED, Tribble CG, Daniel TM, Rodgers BM. Use of video-assisted thoracic surgery in the treatment of chylothorax. Annals of Thoracic Surgery 1994; 57(6): 1507–1511.

76. Marcon F, Irani K, Aquino T, Saunders JK, Gouge TH et al. Percutaneous treatment of thoracic duct injuries. Surgical Endoscopy 2011; 25(9): 2844–2848.

77. Hulscher JB, van Sandick JW, Devriese PP, van Lanschot JJ, Obertop H. Vocal cord paralysis after subtotal oesophagectomy. British Journal of Surgery 1999; 86(12): 1583–1587.

78. Isshiki N, Morita H, Okamura H, Hiramoto M. Thyroplasty as a new phonosurgical technique. Acta Oto-Laryngologica 1974 Nov; 78(5–6): 451–457.

79. Kraus DH, Ali MK, Ginsberg RJ, Hughes CJ, Orlikoff RF et al. Vocal cord medialization for unilateral paralysis associated with intrathoracic malignancies. Journal of Thoracic and Cardiovascular Surgery 1996; 111(2): 334–339.

80. Shibuya S, Fukudo S, Shineha R, Miyazaki S, Miyata G et al. High incidence of reflux esophagitis observed by routine endoscopic examination after gastric pull-up esophagectomy. World Journal of Surgery 2003; 27(5): 580–583.

81. De Leyn P, Coosemans W, Lerut T. Early and late functional results in patients with intrathoracic gastric replacement after oesophagectomy for carcinoma. European Journal of Cardio-Thoracic Surgery 1992; 6(2): 79–84.

82. Gutschow C, Collard JM, Romagnoli R, Salizzoni M, Holscher A. Denervated stomach as an esophageal substitute recovers intraluminal acidity with time. Annals of Surgery 2001; 233(4): 509–514.

83. Fok M, Cheng SW, Wong J. Pyloroplasty versus no drainage in gastric replacement of the esophagus. American Journal of Surgery 1991; 162(5): 447–452.

84. Bemelman WA, Taat CW, Slors JF, van Lanschot JJ, Obertop H. Delayed postoperative emptying after esophageal resection is dependent on the size of the gastric substitute. Journal of the American College of Surgeons 1995; 180(4): 461–464.

85. Burt M, Scott A, Williard WC, Pommier R, Yeh S et al. Erythromycin stimulates gastric emptying after esophagectomy with gastric replacement: a randomized clinical trial. Journal of Thoracic and Cardiovascular Surgery 1996; 111(3): 649–654.

86. Nguyen NT, Dholakia C, Nguyen XM, Reavis K. Outcomes of minimally invasive esophagectomy without pyloroplasty: analysis of 109 cases. American Journal of Surgery 2010; 76(10): 1135–1138.

87. Oberg S, Johansson J, Wenner J, Walther B. Metaplastic columnar mucosa in the cervical esophagus after esophagectomy. Annals of Surgery 2002; 235(3): 338–345.

88. Franchimont D, Covas A, Brasseur C, Laethem JL, El-Nakadi I et al. Newly developed Barrett's esophagus after subtotal esophagectomy. Endoscopy 2003; 35(10): 850–853.

89. McLarty AJ, Deschamps C, Trastek VF, Allen MS, Pairolero PC et al. Esophageal resection for cancer of the esophagus: long-term function and quality of life. Annals of Thoracic Surgery 1997; 63(6): 1568–1572.

90. Humphrey CS, Johnston D, Walker BE, Pulvertaft CN, Goligher JC. Incidence of dumping after truncal and selective vagotomy with pyloroplasty and highly selective vagotomy without drainage procedure. British Medical Journal 1972; 3(5830): 785–788.

91. Sinha S, Padhy AK, Chattopadhyay TK. Dumping syndrome in the intra-thoracic stomach. Tropical Gastroenterology 1997; 18(3): 131–133.

92. Hasler WL. Dumping syndrome. Current Treatment Options in Gastroenterology 2002; 5(2): 139–145.

93. Scarpa M, Valente S, Alfieri R, Cagol M, Diamantis G et al. Systematic review of health-related quality of life after esophagectomy for esophageal cancer. World Journal of Gastroenterology 2011; 17(42): 4660–4674.

94. ICRU Report 50. Dose specification for reporting external beam therapy with photons and electrons. International Commission on Radiation Units and Measurements, Washington, DC: ICRU, 1978 (ICRU Report issued September 1993).

95. Muijs CT, Beukema JC, Pruim J, Mul VE, Groen H et al. A systematic review on the role of FDG-PET/CT in tumour delineation and radiotherapy planning in patients with esophageal cancer. Radiotherapy & Oncology 2010; 97(2): 165–171.

96. Leong T, Everitt C, Yuen K, Condron S, Hui A et al. A prospective study to evaluate the impact of FDG-PET on CT-based radiotherapy treatment planning for oesophageal cancer. Radiotherapy & Oncology 2006; 78(3): 254–261.

97. Kato H, Tachimori Y, Watanabe H, Itabashi M, Hirota T et al. Intramural metastasis of thoracic esophageal carcinoma. International Journal of Cancer 1992; 50(1): 49–52.

98. Czito BG, Denittis AS, Willett CG. Esophagus. In: Halperin EC, Perez CA, Brady LW, Wazer DE. Perez and Brady's Principles and Practice of Radiation Oncology, 5th ed. Philadelphia: Lippincott Williams & Wilkins, 2007: 1131–1153.

99. Matzinger O, Gerber E, Bernstein Z, Maingon P, Haustermans K et al. EORTC-ROG expert opinion: radiotherapy volume and treatment guidelines for neoadjuvant radiation of adenocarcinomas of the gastroesophageal junction and the stomach. Radiotherapy & Oncology 2009; 92: 164–175.

100. Hosch SB, Stoecklein NH, Pichlmeier U, Rehders A, Scheunemann P et al. Esophageal cancer: the mode of lymphatic tumor cell spread and its prognostic significance. Journal of Clinical Oncology 2001; 19(7): 1970–1975.

101. Ding X, Zhang J, Li B, Wang Z, Huang W et al. A meta-analysis of lymph node metastasis rate for patients with thoracic oesophageal cancer and its implication in delineation of clinical target volume for radiation therapy. British Journal of Radiology 2012; 85: 1110–1119.

102. Tu L, Sun L, Xu Y. Paclitaxel and cisplatin combined with intensity-modulated radiotherapy for upper esophageal carcinoma. Radiation Oncology 2013; 27: 75.

103. Haustermans K, Withers HR. The biological basis of fractionation. Rays 2004; 29(3): 231–236.

104. Sur RK, Donde B, Levin VC, Mannell A. Fractionated high dose rate intraluminal brachytherapy in palliation of advanced esophageal cancer. International Journal of Radiation Oncology Biology Physics 1998; 40: 447–453.

105. Gaspar LE, Qian C, Kocha WI, Coia LR, Herskovic A et al. A phase I/II study of extrenal beam radiation, brachytherapy and concurrent chemotherapy in localized cancer of the esophagus (RTOG 92-07): preliminary toxicity report. International Journal of Radiation Oncology Biology Physics 1997; 37: 593–599.

106. Pennathur A, Gibson M.K, Jobe B.A, Luketich J.D. Oesophageal carcinoma. Lancet 2013; 381: 400–412.

107. Schweigert M, Dubecz A, Stein HJ Oesophageal cancer—an overview. Nature Reviews Gastroenterology & Hepatology 2013; 10: 230–244.

108. Lutz MP, Zalcberg JR, Ducreux M, Ajani JA, Allum W et al. Highlights of the EORTC St. Gallen International Expert Consensus on the primary therapy of gastric, gastroesophageal and oesophageal cancer—differential treatment strategies for subtypes of early gastroesophageal cancer. European Journal of Cancer 2012; 48: 2941–2953.

109. Sjoquist KM, Burmeister BH, Smithers BM, Zalcberg JR, Simes RJ et al. Australasian Gastro-Intestinal Trials Group. Survival after neoadjuvant chemotherapy or chemoradiotherapy for resectable oesophageal carcinoma: an updated meta-analysis. Lancet Oncology 2011; 12(7): 681.

110. van Hagen P, Hulshof MC, van Lanschot JJ, Steyerberg EW, van Berge Henegouwen MI et al. Preoperative chemoradiotherapy for esophageal or junctional cancer. New England Journal of Medicine 2012; 366(22): 2074–2084.

111. Bang YJ, Van Cutsem E, Feyereislova A, Chung HC, Shen L et al. Trastuzumab in combination with chemotherapy versus chemotherapy alone for treatment of HER2-positive advanced gastric or gastro-oesophageal junction cancer (ToGA): a phase 3, open-label, randomised controlled trial. Lancet 2010; 376: 687–697.

112. Van Cutsem E, Dicato M, Geva R, Arber N, Bang Y et al. The diagnosis and management of gastric cancer: expert discussion and recommendations from the 12th ESMO/World Congress on Gastrointestinal Cancer, Barcelona, 2010. Annals of Oncology 2011; 22: 1–9.

113. Waddell T, Chau I, Cunningham D, Gonzalez D, Okines AF et al. Epirubicin, oxaliplatin, and capecitabine with or without panitumumab for patients with previously untreated advanced oesophagogastric cancer (REAL3): a randomised, open-label phase 3 trial. Lancet Oncology 2013; 14: 481–489.

114. Lordick F, Kang YK, Chung HC, Salman P, Oh SC et al. Capecitabine and cisplatin with or without cetuximab for patients with previously untreated advanced gastric cancer (EXPAND): a randomised, open-label phase 3 trial. Lancet Oncology 2013; 14: 490–499.

115. O'Reilly S, Forastiere AA. Is surgery necessary with multimodality treatment of oesophageal cancer. Annals of Oncology 1995; 6(6): 519.

116. D'Amico TA. Outcomes after surgery for esophageal cancer. Gastrointestinal Cancer Research 2007; 1(5): 188–196.

117. Earlam R, Cunha-Melo JR. Oesophageal squamous cell carcinoma: II. A critical review of radiotherapy. British Journal of Surgery 1980; 67(7): 457.

118. Sykes AJ, Burt PA, Slevin NJ, Stout R, Marss JE. Radical radiotherapy for carcinoma of the oesophagus: an effective alternative to surgery. Radiotherapy & Oncology 1998; 48(1): 15.

119. Sun XD, Yu JM, Fan XL, Ren RM, Li MH et al. Randomized clinical study of surgery versus radiotherapy alone in the treatment of resectable esophageal cancer in the chest. Zhonghua Zhong Liu Za Zhi 2006; 28(10): 784–787.

120. Cooper JS, Guo MD, Herskovic A. Chemoradiotherapy of locally advanced esophageal cancer: long-term follow-up of a prospective randomized trial (RTOG 85-01). Journal of the American Medical Association 1999; 281(17): 1623.

121. Minsky BD, Pajak TF, Ginsberg RJ, Pisansky TM, Martenson J et al. INT 0123 (Radiation Therapy Oncology Group 94-05) phase III trial of combined-modality therapy for esophageal cancer: high-dose versus standard-dose radiation therapy. Journal of Clinical Oncology 2002; 20: 1167–1174.

122. Nygaard K, Hagen S, Hansen HS, Hatlevoll R, Hultborn R et al. Pre-operative radiotherapy prolongs survival in operable esophageal carcinoma: a randomized, multicenter study of pre-operative radiotherapy and chemotherapy. The second Scandinavian trial in esophageal cancer. World Journal of Surgery 1992; 16(6): 1104.

123. Le Prise E, Etienne PL, Meunier B, Maddern G, Ben Hassel M et al. A randomized study of chemotherapy, radiation therapy, and surgery versus surgery for localized squamous cell carcinoma of the esophagus. Cancer 1994; 73(7): 1779.

124. Walsh TN, Noonan N, Hollywood D, Kelly A, Keeling NP et al. A comparison of multimodal therapy and surgery for esophageal adenocarcinoma. New England Journal of Medicine 1996; 335(7): 462.

125. Bosset JF, Gignoux M, Triboulet JP, Tiret E, Mantion G et al. Chemoradiotherapy followed by surgery compared with surgery alone in squamous-cell cancer of the esophagus. New England Journal of Medicine 1997; 337(3): 161.

126. Urba SG, Orringer MB, Turrisi A, Iannettoni M, Forastiere A et al. Randomized tial of pre-operative chemoradiation versus surgery alone in patients with locoregional esophageal carcinoma. Journal of Clinical Oncology 2001; 19(2): 305.

127. Burmeister BH, Smithers BM, Gebski V, Fitzgerald L, Simes RJ et al. Surgery alone versus chemoradiotherapy followed by surgery for resectable cancer of the oesophagus: a randomised controlled phase III trial. Lancet Oncology 2005; 6(9): 659.

128. Tepper J, Krasna MJ, Niedzwiecki D, Hollis D, Reed CE et al. Phase III trial of trimodality therapy with cisplatin, fluorouracil, radiotherapy, and surgery compared with surgery alone for esophageal cancer: CALGB 9781. Journal of Clinical Oncology 2008; 26(7): 1086.

129. Mariette C, Seitz JF, Maillard E, Mornex F, Thomas PA et al. Surgery alone versus chemoradiotherapy followed by surgery for localized esophageal cancer: analysis of a randomized controlled phase III trial FFCD 9901. Journal of Clinical Oncology 2010; 28(15 Suppl.): 4005.

130. Fiorica F, Di BD, Schepis F, Licata A, Shahied L et al. Preoperative chemoradiotherapy for oesophageal cancer: a systematic review and meta-analysis. Gut 2004; 53(7): 925–930.

131. Greer SE, Goodney PP, Sutton JE, Birkmeyer JD. Neoadjuvant chemoradiotherapy for esophageal carcinoma: a meta-analysis. Surgery 2005; 137(2): 172–177.

132. Urschel JD, Vasan H. A meta-analysis of randomized controlled trials that compared neoadjuvant chemoradiation and surgery to surgery alone for resectable esophageal cancer. American Journal of Surgery 2003; 185(6): 538–543.

133. Abou-Jawde RM, Mekhail T, Adelstein DJ, Rybicki LA, Mazzone PJ et al. Impact of induction concurrent chemoradiotherapy on pulmonary function and postoperative acute respiratory complications in esophageal cancer. Chest 2005; 128(1): 250–255.

134. Scheer RV, Fakiris AJ, Johnstone PA. Quantifying the benefit of a pathologic complete response after neoadjuvant chemoradiotherapy in the treatment of esophageal cancer. International Journal of Radiation Oncology Biology Physics 2011; 80(4): 996.

135. Stahl M, Walz MK, Stuschke M. Phase III comparison of preoperative chemotherapy compared with chemoradiotherapy in patients with locally advanced adenocarcinoma of the esophagogastric junction. Journal of Clinical Oncology 2009; 27(6): 851.

136. Wieder HA, Beer AJ, Lordick F, Ott K, Fischer M et al. Comparison of changes in tumor metabolic activity and tumor size during chemotherapy of adenocarcinomas of the esophagogastric junction. Journal of Nuclear Medicine 2005; 46(12): 2029–2034.

137. Flamen P, Van Cutsem E, Lerut A, Cambier JP, Haustermans K et al. Positron emission tomography for assessment of the response to induction radiochemotherapy in locally advanced oesophageal cancer. Annals of Oncology 2002; 13(3): 361–368.

138. Ott K, Weber WA, Lordick F, Becker K, Busch R et al. Metabolic imaging predicts response, survival, and recurrence in adenocarcinomas of the esophagogastric junction. Journal of Clinical Oncology 2006; 24(29): 4692–4698.

139. Lordick F, Ott K, Krause BJ, Weber WA, Becker K et al. PET to assess early metabolic response and to guide treatment of adenocarcinoma of the oesophagogastric junction: the MUNICON phase II trial. Lancet Oncology 2007; 8(9): 797–805.

140. zum Buschenfelde CM, Herrmann K, Schuster T, Geinitz H, Langer R et al. (18)F-FDG PET-guided salvage neoadjuvant radiochemotherapy of adenocarcinoma of the esophagogastric junction: the MUNICON II trial. Journal of Nuclear Medicine 2011; 52(8): 1189–1196.

141. Chen YM, Pan XF, Tong LJ, Shi YP, Chen T. Can (1)(8) F-fluorodeoxyglucose positron emission tomography predict responses to neoadjuvant therapy in oesophageal cancer patients? A meta-analysis. Nuclear Medicine Communications 2011; 32(11): 1005–1010.

142. al-Sarraf M, Martz K, Herskovic A, Leichman L, Brindle JS et al. Progress report of combined chemoradiotherapy versus radiotherapy alone in patients with esophageal cancer: an intergroup study. Journal of Clinical Oncology 1997; 15(1): 277.

143. Lordick F, Ebert M, Stein HJ. Current treatment approach to locally advanced esophageal cancer: is resection mandatory? Future Oncology 2006 Dec; 2(6): 717–721.

144. Coia LR, Minsky BD, Berkey BA, John MJ, Haller D et al. Outcome of patients receiving radiation for cancer of the esophagus: results of the 1992–1994 Patterns of Care Study. Journal of Clinical Oncology 2000; 18(3): 455.

145. McKenzie S, Mailey B, Artinyan A, Metchikian M, Shibata S et al. Improved outcomes in the management of esophageal cancer with the addition of surgical resection to chemoradiation therapy. Annals of Surgical Oncology 2011; 18(2): 551.

146. Stahl M, Stuschke M, Lehmann N, Meyer HJ, Walz MK et al. Chemoradiation with and without surgery in patients with locally advanced squamous cell carcinoma of the esophagus. Journal of Clinical Oncology 2005; 23(10): 2310.

147. Bonnetain F, Bouché O, Michel P, Mariette C, Conroy T et al. A comparative longitudinal quality of life study using the Spitzer quality of life index in a randomized multicenter phase III trial (FFCD 9102): chemoradiation followed by surgery compared with chemoradiation alone in locally advanced squamous resectable thoracic esophageal cancer. Annals of Oncology 2006; 17(5): 827.

148. GASTRIC (Global Advanced/Adjuvant Stomach Tumor Research International Collaboration) Group, Paoletti X, Oba K, Burzykowski T, Michiels S et al. Benefit of adjuvant chemotherapy for resectable

gastric cancer: a meta-analysis. Journal of the American Medical Association 2010; 303: 1729–1737.

149. Macdonald JS, Smalley SR, Benedetti J, Hundahl SA, Estes NC et al. Chemoradiotherapy after surgery compared with surgery alone for adenocarcinoma of the stomach or gastroesophageal junction. New England Journal of Medicine 2001; 345: 725.

150. Fuchs CS, Tepper JE, Niedzwiecki D, Hollis D, Mamon HJ et al. Postoperative adjuvant chemoradiation for gastric or gastroesophageal junction (GEJ) adenocarcinoma using epirubicin, cisplatin, and infusional (CI) 5-FU (ECF) before and after CI 5-FU and radiotherapy (CRT) compared with bolus 5-FU/LV before and after CRT: Intergroup trial CALGB 80101. Journal of Clinical Oncology 2011; 29; 4003.

151. Tachibana M, Yoshimura H, Kinugasa S, Shibakita M, Dhar DK et al. Postoperative chemotherapy vs. chemoradiotherapy for thoracic esophageal cancer: a prospective randomized clinical trial. European Journal of Surgical Oncology 2003; 29: 580.

152. Waters JS, Norman A, Cunningham D, Scarffe JH, Webb A et al. Long-term survival after epirubicin, cisplatin and fluorouracil for gastric cancer: results of a randomized trial. British Journal of Cancer 1999; 80(1–2): 269–272.

153. Ajani JA, Moiseyenko VM, Tjulandin S, Majlis A, Constenla M et al. Clinical benefit with docetaxel plus fluorouracil and cisplatin compared with cisplatin and fluorouracil in a phase III trial of advanced gastric or gastroesophageal cancer adenocarcinoma: the V-325 Study Group. Journal of Clinical Oncology 2007; 25(22): 3205–3209.

154. Koizumi W, Narahara H, Hara T, Takagane A, Akiya T et al. S-1 plus cisplatin versus S-1 alone for first-line treatment of advanced gastric cancer (SPIRITS trial): a phase III trial. Lancet Oncology 2008; 9(3): 215–221.

155. Cunningham D, Starling N, Rao S, Iveson T, Nicolson M et al. Upper Gastrointestinal Clinical Studies Group of the National Cancer Research Institute of the United Kingdom. New England Journal of Medicine 2008; 358(1): 36–46

156. Bang YJ, Van Cutsem E, Feyereislova A, Chung HC, Shen L et al. Trastuzumab in combination with chemotherapy versus chemotherapy alone for treatment of HER2-positive advanced gastric or gastro-oesophageal junction cancer (ToGA): a phase 3, open-label, randomised controlled trial. Lancet 2010; 376(9742): 687–697

157. Ohtsu A, Shah MA, Van Cutsem A, Rha SY, Sawaki A et al. Bevacizumab in combination with chemotherapy as first-line therapy in advanced gastric cancer: a randomized, double-blind, placebo-controlled phase III study. Journal of Clinical Oncology 2011; 29: 3968–3976

158. Waddell T, Chau I, Cunningham D, Gonzalez D, Okines AF et al. Epirubicin, oxaliplatin, and capecitabine with or without panitumumab for patients with previously untreated advanced oesophagogastric cancer (REAL3): a randomised, open-label phase 3 trial. Lancet Oncology 2013; 14(6): 481–499.

159. Lordick F, Kang YK, Chung HC, Salman P, Oh SC et al. Capecitabine and cisplatin with or without cetuximab for patients with previously untreated advanced gastric cancer (EXPAND): a randomised, open-label phase 3 trial. Lancet Oncology 2013; 14(6): 490–499.

160. Fuchs CS., Tomasek J, Yong CJ., et al. Ramucirumab monotherapy for previously treated advanced gastric or gastro-oesophageal junction adenocarcinoma (REGARD): an international, randomised, multicentre, placebo-controlled, phase 3 trial. Lancet 2013; e-pub ahead of print.

161. Homs MYV, Steyerberg EW, Eijkenboom WMH, et al. Single-dose brachytherapy versus metal stent placement for the palliation of dysphagia from oesophageal cancer: multicentre randomised trial. Lancet 2004; 364: 1497-504.

CHAPTER 37

Gastric cancer

Hideaki Bando, Takahiro Kinoshita, Yasutoshi Kuboki, Atsushi Ohtsu, and Kohei Shitara

Epidemiology

Gastric cancer is a malignant epithelial neoplasia which remains a common cause of cancer death worldwide, despite the recent steady decline in both the incidence and mortality of the disease. Several risk factors for gastric cancer have been reported. It has been suggested that *Helicobactor pylori* infection and diets containing N-nitroso compounds and salty foods may play important roles in the pathogenesis of this cancer. Several precancerous conditions (chronic gastritis and intestinal metaplasia) and precancerous lesions (adenoma and dysplasia) have been described in the stomach. Gastric adenocarcinoma has been morphologically classified into two types by Lauren (intestinal type and diffuse type) and by Nakamura (differentiated type and undifferentiated type). It has been shown that while the intestinal type adenocarcinoma predominates in high-risk areas, the diffuse type of gastric cancer is less likely to be related to environmental influences. According to the WHO classification, gastric adenocarcinoma can be subclassified into five subtypes: (1) tubular, (2) papillary, (3) poorly differentiated, (4) mucinous, and (5) mixed. Some morphological features are associated with genetic alterations with characteristic pattern of tumour spread and clinicopathological features. Hereditary diffuse gastric cancer, which is an autosomal-dominant cancer susceptibility syndrome having germline E-cadherin gene mutations, is characterized by the presence of multiple signet-ring cell carcinomas in the stomach.

Stomach cancer has been reported to be among the most frequently diagnosed malignancies in the world and remains the leading cause of cancer death worldwide. The incidence is high in eastern Asian countries such as Japan, China, and Korea, as well as Eastern Europe and Central and Latin America. North America, northern Europe and most countries in Africa and Southeast Asia represent areas of low incidence. There has been a steady decline in both the incidence and mortality of gastric carcinoma in the last three decades. The male–female ratio is 2:1, and the incidence of gastric cancer increases with age.

The major factors considered to be involved in the pathogenesis of gastric cancer have been classified into the following three categories: (1) environmental factors, (2) host factors, and (3) genetic factors. Environmental and host factors are thought to be the most important for intestinal-type gastric cancer, since families migrating from high-risk to low-risk areas acquire the level of risk that prevails in the new area [1]. Among the environmental factors, diet including smoked and salted foods and pickled vegetables appears to be the most significant [2]. The presence of N-nitroso compounds and benzopyrene in the diet may play an important role in gastric carcinogenesis [3]. In addition to the diet, *H. pylori* infection, which commonly takes place in early childhood and persists throughout adult life causing chronic atrophic gastritis, is important as a host factor [4, 5]. Inflammation induced by *H. pylori* causes chronic atrophic gastritis followed by intestinal metaplasia which is one of the precursor conditions prior to the development of gastric cancer.

Molecular biology of gastric cancer

There are two distinct types of gastric adenocarcinoma—intestinal (well-differentiated) and diffuse (undifferentiated)—which have distinct morphologic appearance, epidemiology, pathogenesis, and genetic profiles [6].

Intestinal-type cancers are causally related to *H. pylori*. While the infection usually starts in infancy or early childhood, there is a long latency period and cancers are typically clinically diagnosed four or more decades later [7]. During this period, a prolonged precancerous process takes place, represented by a cascade of events with the following well-characterized, sequential histopathologic stages: chronic active non-atrophic gastritis, multifocal atrophic gastritis, intestinal metaplasia, dysplasia (adenoma), and invasive carcinoma [8]. The manner in which environmental risk factors contribute to or influence the progression of *H. pylori*-induced gastric carcinogenesis is unclear.

Diffuse-type gastric cancers can also be induced by *H. pylori* infection, much as intestinal-type cancers. However, there are also prominent differences between these two variants. *H. pylori*-associated invasive intestinal-type cancers are characterized by a defined series of preneoplastic stages which are not seen in diffuse-type cancers. From an epidemiologic standpoint, both diffuse- and intestinal-type cancers have been decreasing in incidence in most countries, although the decline is more marked for intestinal-type cancers. Intestinal-type cancers are also more frequent in men and they are associated with a slightly better prognosis. Diffuse-type cancers are highly metastatic and characterized by rapid disease progression and a poorer prognosis than intestinal cancers. They also have a greater tendency to invade the gastric wall, sometimes extending to the lower oesophagus or to the duodenum. Occasionally, a broad region of the gastric wall or even the entire stomach is extensively infiltrated, resulting in a rigid thickened stomach, termed 'linitis plastica'. The main carcinogenic event in diffuse carcinomas is loss of expression of E-cadherin, a key cell surface protein for establishing intercellular connections and maintaining the organization of epithelial tissues [9].

Association between *Helicobacter pylori* infection and gastric cancer

The International Agency for Research on Cancer (IARC) has declared *H. pylori* to be a group I human carcinogen for gastric adenocarcinoma [10]. *H. pylori* can cause chronic active gastritis and atrophic gastritis, early steps in the carcinogenesis sequence. Furthermore, a number of studies in humans have demonstrated a clear association between *H. pylori* infection and gastric adenocarcinoma. The link has been demonstrated in both the intestinal and diffuse subtypes of gastric cancer. Two meta-analyses of cohort and case-control studies examining the relationship between *H. pylori* seropositivity and gastric cancer found that *H. pylori* infection was associated with a twofold increased risk for developing gastric adenocarcinoma [11, 12]. One of the largest prospective studies addressing *H. pylori* and cancer risk included 1526 Japanese patients, of whom 1246 had *H. pylori* infection [13]. Patients underwent endoscopy with biopsy at enrolment and then at one and three years. During a mean follow-up of 7.8 years, 36 patients developed gastric cancer (2.9%), all of whom were *H. pylori* infected. No uninfected patient developed cancer. Despite the clear association between *H. pylori* and gastric adenocarcinomas, only a minority of infected individuals will develop gastric cancer. Several hypotheses have been proposed to explain the role of *H. pylori* in carcinogenesis, although the exact mechanism is incompletely understood [14]. Initiation of the carcinogenesis process has been linked to oxidative stress brought about by inducible nitric oxide synthase (iNOS) which is produced by inflammatory cells responding to *H. pylori* infection. Nitric oxides are mutagenic and may induce abnormalities in the DNA of epithelial cells [3, 15]. Furthermore, two processes important in carcinogenesis are apoptosis (programmed cell death) and hyperproliferation. Following severe DNA damage, apoptosis occurs as a protective mechanism to prevent replication of mutated DNA. The mechanism by which *H. pylori* induces apoptosis is unclear. Proliferating cells may be resistant to apoptosis. This would upset the balance between cell growth and death, leading to hyperproliferation and the promotion of neoplasia. There is evidence of an increased amount of the anti-apoptosis protein, Bcl-2, in the setting of gastric dysplasia. Other reports have found that apoptosis may be due to plasminogen activator inhibitor (PAI)-2, the expression of which is increased by *H. pylori* and is increased in gastric cancer. An uncoupling of epithelial proliferation and apoptosis may be a strain-dependent phenomenon [16, 17].

In addition, certain polymorphisms in IL-1 beta and other cytokines may confer an increased susceptibility to non-cardia gastric adenocarcinoma caused by *H. pylori* by inducing a hypochlorhydric and atrophic response to *H. pylori* infection. An illustrative study compared IL-1 beta polymorphisms in 393 patients with gastric cancer compared with 430 controls. Two specific polymorphisms (IL-1B-31T and IL-1RN*2) were associated with low acid secretion and gastric atrophy. The authors concluded that 38% of *H. pylori*-related gastric cancer could be attributed to the presence of these alleles. IL-1 beta, a potent inhibitor of gastric acid secretion, is upregulated by the presence of *H. pylori* [18]. In addition, pro-inflammatory genotypes of tumour necrosis factor alpha (TNFα) and IL-10 were associated with more than a doubling of the risk of non-cardia gastric cancer. Carriage of multiple pro-inflammatory polymorphisms of IL-1 beta, IL-1 receptor antagonist, TNFα, and IL-10 conferred even greater risk. By contrast, these polymorphisms were not associated with an increased risk of oesophageal or gastric cardia cancers. These data suggest that gene polymorphisms influence cytokine expression, gastric inflammation, and risk for development of precancerous lesions in those infected with *H. pylori* [19].

Molecular biology of intestinal type cancer

Abnormalities in oncogenes, tumour suppressor genes, growth factors/receptors, cell cycle regulators, and epigenetic alterations have been identified. Some of these have been linked to *H. pylori* infection, while the relationship of many to *H. pylori* infection remains unresolved. Canonical oncogenic pathways such as E2F, RAS, p53, and Wnt/β-catenin signalling are also known to be deregulated with varying frequencies, suggesting a high degree of molecular heterogeneity.

Oncogenes, growth factors/receptors

Several oncogenes are over-expressed in various stages of gastric carcinogenesis, although none has consistently been shown to be present in any one particular stage.

KRAS/BRAF

The Ras–Raf–MEK–ERK–MAP kinase pathway plays a critical role in cell proliferation, and is frequently activated in cancer cells. Early involvement of KRAS mutations is suggested by their being found in invasive cancers, dysplasia, and intestinal metaplasia [20]. On the other hand, several studies have reported a low incidence of Ras gene mutation (codons 12, 13, and 61) in gastric carcinoma (roughly 0–10%). BRAF mutation is less common than Ras gene mutation. There seems to be no difference between Asian and Western gastric cancer [21].

EGFR

The epidermal growth factor receptor (EGFR) gene is located at chromosomal region 7p12 and encodes a 170-kDa transmembrane tyrosine kinase receptor. EGFR is activated by binding to its ligands such as epidermal growth factor or TGFα, resulting in homodimerization or heterodimerization with another member of the EGFR family. This receptor activation is followed by phosphorylation of specific tyrosine residues within the cytoplasmic tail, stimulating the downstream signalling pathway that regulates cell proliferation, migration, adhesion, differentiation, and survival. Gene amplification and/or protein over-expression of EGFR have been observed in a variety of solid tumours. The frequency of EGFR over-expression and/or amplification in gastric cancers has been variously reported to be 0–38% [22]. EGFR over-expression is associated with advanced gastric cancer, the presence of lymph node metastasis, a higher stage, and lymphatic invasion. The EGFR/MAPK pathway has also been shown to be activated in gastric carcinomas with microsatellite instability.

HER2

The proto-oncogene ERBB2 (also known as HER2) is a member of the ERBB/HER RTK family, additionally comprised of EGFR, HER3/ERBB3, and HER4/ERBB4 [23]. Upon extracellular ligand binding, these four receptors mediate normal cell proliferation and cell survival via two major signalling pathways: Ras-Raf-MAPK and PI3K/Akt/mTOR. Whereas EGFR and ERBB4 have known extracellular ligands and possess active tyrosine kinase domains, no direct high-affinity ligand has been identified for HER2 [24, 25].

Furthermore, ERBB3 binds several different ligands, but has little or no tyrosine kinase activity, and is possibly able only to weakly autophosphorylate [26]. HER2 is amplified or over-expressed in as many as 25% of gastric cancer cases. HER2 amplification or over-expression is most prevalent in intestinal gastric cancer (~30% HER2 positivity rate) and least prevalent in diffuse-type gastric cancer (~5% HER2 positivity rate). Assessment of HER2 positivity rates, therefore, depends entirely on the constituent population studied, and will be higher in areas where proximal gastric cancers prevail and less frequent where diffuse gastric cancers are common. HER2 mutations have been reported in breast cancer, lung cancer, and colorectal cancer. However, few reports are available on HER2 mutations in gastric cancer.

c-MET

c-MET is one of the tyrosine kinase receptors family, encoding a receptor for hepatocyte growth factor (HGF). Activation of c-MET by HGF and its signalling pathways is pivotal for cellular morphogenesis, regeneration, proliferation, migration, angiogenesis, and invasion. c-MET is expressed in a variety of normal epithelial and endothelial cells and mediates the biological activities of HGF [27, 28]. In vitro, highly virulent strains of *H. pylori* that make the effector protein CagA appear to modulate c-MET receptor signal transduction pathways, and this might influence cancer initiation and/or tumour progression [29]. c-MET over-expression and amplification have been reported in 18–82% of gastric carcinoma studied by immunofluorescence, immunohistochemistry (IHC), reverse transcription polymerase chain reaction (RT-PCR), Northern blot analysis and Southern blot analysis. However, MET mutation is quite low in gastric cancer.

Tumour suppressor genes

Approximately 50% of intestinal-type gastric cancers have alterations in genes that are thought to function as tumour suppressor genes, including TP53, TP73, APC (adenomatous polyposis coli), etc. [30].

TP53

The p53 gene (TP53) is an important regulator of the cell cycle, in particular at the point at which damaged cells must progress through cell cycle arrest and repair versus apoptosis [31]. Loss of TP53 expression by LOH or mutational inactivation is the most frequent genetic alteration in gastric cancer, occurring in over 60% of invasive tumours [32]. Abnormalities are also found in *H. pylori*-associated chronic gastritis, intestinal metaplasia, and dysplasia. p53 appears to be a key regulatory molecule in the response to microenvironmental chronic inflammatory stress. Furthermore, at least some data suggest that inactivation of p53 in gastric epithelial cells may reduce their ability to undergo apoptosis in response to injury caused by *H. pylori* [33].

TP73

LOH in TP73, a transcription factor related to TP53 that also functions as a tumour suppressor gene, can be detected in gastric carcinomas, and loss of expression has also been reported via epigenetic mechanisms (promoter methylation) in EBV-associated gastric cancers [34]. Over-expression of p73 and the oncogenic isoform DeltaNp73 suppresses p73 transcriptional and apoptotic activity in gastroepithelial cancer cells, and increases intracellular beta-catenin levels, an effect that is inhibited in the presence of wild-type but not mutant p53 [35].

APC

Mutations in the APC gene are identified in significantly more intestinal-type than diffuse-type gastric cancers. These mutations are also found in *H. pylori*-associated dysplasia and intestinal metaplasia. APC mutations modulate the Wnt/catenin signalling pathway [36, 37].

Cyclin E/CDKN1B

Cyclin E and cyclin-dependent kinase inhibitor 1B (CDKN1B) part in the G1/S transition. Cyclin E over-expression is a frequent event in gastric carcinomas, and it might be an indicator for malignant transformation of dysplasia, and/or tumour aggressiveness once an invasive cancer develops [38]. Decreased expression of cyclin-dependent kinase inhibitor 1B also correlates with an adverse prognosis in invasive gastric cancer. Furthermore, loss of CDKN1B expression increases susceptibility to gastric carcinogenesis in *H. pylori*-infected CDKN1B-knockout mice. The E2F family of transcription factors also plays a key role in the control of cell cycle progression, and over-expression of E2F-1 protein was confirmed in many of the gastric cancers [39].

Beta-catenin/Wnt signalling

Beta-catenin mutation is a frequent cause of Wnt pathway activation in gastric cancer [40]. Beta-catenin is important in mediating the E-cadherin-related cell adhesion and also in participating in Wnt signalling pathways. The Wnt signalling pathway regulates several processes during development, such as determination of cell fate, morphology, polarity, adhesion, and growth. Wnt signalling can be divided into canonical and non-canonical pathways. In the canonical pathway, Wnt signals (extracellular ligands, such as Wnt-1) stabilize beta-catenin, therefore activating gene transcription by interaction of beta-catenin with transcriptional factors. In gastric cancer tissues, in the expression of Wnt-1, beta-catenin has been found to be increased when compared to normal gastric tissue, and related to tumour size, tumour invasive depth, lymph node metastasis, pTNM stage, differentiation, and prognosis [41].

Epigenetic events

Epigenetic alterations such as DNA methylation of gene promoters can silence the expression of certain genes. At least some data suggest that aberrant promoter methylation may be closely associated with *H. pylori* infection and that higher methylation levels correlate with higher risk for invasive cancers [42]. Tumour suppressor genes such as CDKN2A, CDH1, MLH1, and RUNX3 are inactivated more frequently by aberrant DNA methylation than by mutations, indicating that gastric cancer is an epigenetic disease [43, 44]. In addition to methylation silencing of driver tumour suppressor genes, recent genome-wide analyses have revealed that hundreds of passenger genes are also methylated in gastric cancers. The fact that *H. pylori* infection induces epigenetic alterations provides the missing link between the causal role of *H. pylori* infection in gastric carcinogenesis and the deep involvement of epigenetic alterations in gastric cancers. It is currently speculated that infection by *H. pylori* induces H3K27me3 and removes RNA polymerase II at its target genes, and that these genes then become methylated [45]. Gastric cancer is a typical example of a disease in which infection, chronic inflammation, and epigenetic alterations are interconnected.

Genetic instability causes an accumulation of genetic alterations and participates in the early stage of gastric cancers. Cases in which two or more of five microsatellite loci show replication error are considered to be showing high-frequency microsatellite instability (MSI-H), and those with only one locus showing replication error are considered to show low-frequency MSI (MSI-L). MSI-H is observed in only 4% of gastric carcinomas, in particular in the well-differentiated type in elderly patients [46]. The frequency of MSI-L is about 30% in primary gastric cancers, including early cancers. Some intestinal metaplasias and adenomas also show MSI-L, and these should be considered 'true precancerous lesions'. MSI-H is used as an indicator of HNPCC, which is caused by the germline mutation of mismatch repair genes, including hMLH1 and hMSH2. In sporadic gastric cancers with MSI-H, CpG island hypermethylation of hMLH1 is associated with loss of hMLH1 protein [47–49].

Diffuse-type cancer

Like intestinal-type cancers, diffuse-type gastric cancers can be induced by *H. pylori* infection. However, there are also prominent differences between these two variants. In most cases, this results from loss of expression of the cell adhesion protein E-cadherin. It has been reported that some of other signalling pathways or epigenetic events are important in diffuse-type gastric cancers.

E-cadherin

The main carcinogenic event in diffuse carcinomas is loss of expression of E-cadherin, a key cell surface protein for establishing intercellular connections and maintaining the organization of epithelial tissues. Biallelic inactivation of the gene encoding E-cadherin, CDH1, can occur through germline or somatic mutation, allelic imbalance events (e.g., loss of heterozygosity), or epigenetic silencing of gene transcription through aberrant methylation of the CDH1 promoter. Germline truncating mutations of the CDH1 gene, located on chromosome 16q22.1, were originally described in three Maori families from New Zealand that were predisposed to diffuse gastric cancer [50]. Subsequently germline mutations have been identified in many other kindreds worldwide. These mutations are not concentrated in a single hotspot, but rather evenly distributed along the gene in several different exons. The trigger and molecular mechanism by which the second allele of E-cadherin is inactivated appears to be diverse, and includes promoter hypermethylation, mutation, and loss of heterozygosity [51]. Abnormalities in CDH1 have also been linked to sporadic diffuse (and intestinal) carcinomas. Somatic mutations in the CDH1 gene are identified in 40–83% of sporadic diffuse-type gastric cancers, and promoter hypermethylation is also reported. Thus, the CDH1 gene appears to function as a tumour suppressor gene and its inactivation follows the classical 'two-hit' model [52, 53].

FGFR2

Fibroblast growth factors (FGFs) and their receptors are considered to be associated with multiple biological activities, including fundamental developmental pathways, cellular proliferation, differentiation, motility, and transforming activities. FGF signalling is also involved in many physiological roles in the adult organism, such as the regulation of angiogenesis and wound repair. FGF receptors (FGFRs) are expressed on many different cell types and regulate key cell behaviours of cancer cells. Emerging evidence has demonstrated that the deregulation of FGF signalling is frequently observed in various solid cancers and haematological malignancies. The K-sam gene was first identified and characterized as an amplified gene in the human gastric cancer cell line KATO-III [54], and its product was later found to be identical to the bacteria-expressed kinase, or keratinocyte growth factor receptor, and FGF receptor 2 (FGFR2). FGFR2 mutations are reportedly rare in gastric cancers. On the other hand, FGFR2 amplification has been found in diffuse-type gastric cancer-derived cell lines and amplification was preferentially detected in diffuse-type gastric cancer. FGFR2 protein expression was positively correlated with scirrhous cancer, diffuse type, invasion depth, infiltration type, and poor prognosis [55].

c-MET

Frequent amplification of the c-Met gene in carcinogenesis and progression of scirrhous-type gastric cancers has been reported. With regard to the complex interaction between tumour cells and stromal cells, human HGF, whose receptor is a c-Met protein, may play an important role in progression and morphogenesis of gastric carcinoma. HGF is expressed by stromal fibroblasts and stimulates proliferation of gastric carcinoma cells which express c-Met protein [20].

IL-1a

IL-la, which is mainly produced by activated macrophages, mediates many of the local and systemic responses to infection and inflammation. IL-la activates T cells, B cells, and endothelial cells, increases number of neutrophilic cells, and affects the expression of various adhesion molecules. On fibroblasts, IL-la stimulates proliferation, prostaglandin production, and collagenase secretion.

IL-la may be involved in the multi-autocrine loops of the growth factor/cytokine system in gastric carcinoma. Therefore, there is a high possibility that IL-la produced by gastric carcinoma cells may act as a paracrine factor and cause stromal fibrosis and activation of the cytokine network. In fact, scirrhous gastric carcinomas characterized by productive fibrosis expressed IL-la mRNA at high levels. On the other hand, IL-la is well known to be produced by stromal cells, such as activated macrophages, fibroblasts, and vascular endothelial cells. IL-la secreted by the stromal cells could exert a great influence on cell proliferation, differentiation, and necrosis of gastric carcinoma in a paracrine manner [56].

Epigenetic events

In addition to CDH1, RAR-beta promoter hypermethylation was observed more frequently in diffuse-type gastric carcinoma than in other types. Moreover, hypermethylation of the CDH1 and RAR-beta promoters occurred concordantly. It was reported that retinoic acid induces expression of nm23- H1, which is known to reduce cell motility. Silencing of RAR-beta by promoter followed by hypermethylation-reduced nm23-H1 may occur frequently in carcinomas of the diffuse type [57].

Other oncogenic signalling pathway
Hedgehog pathway

Hedgehog (Hh) signalling plays an important role during embryonic development and differentiation, proliferation, and maintenance of adult tissues through the maintenance of stem cell population. Alterations in Hh signalling pathway activation are related to gastric cancers [58]. The expression of Hh ligands, Ptch1, Smo, and the three Gli transcription factors (Gli1, Gli2, and Gli3) has been related with more than two-thirds of primary gastric cancers and correlated with poorly differentiated and more aggressive tumours [59].

Notch pathway

The Notch signalling pathway is evolutionarily conserved and plays a role in many important and fundamental processes in cell and tissues such as proliferation, differentiation, apoptosis, cell fate determination, and maintenance of stem cells. Recently, an association between Notch signalling and progression of gastric cancer has been described. Three Notch receptors (Notch1–Notch3) and Notch ligand Jagged1 are expressed in human gastric cancer and the Notch signalling pathway is activated after infection with *H. pylori* in gastric cancer. Gastric cancer patients with Jagged1 expression in tumour tissues have more aggressive tumours and poor survival, suggesting an important role of this pathway in gastric cancer progression [60].

Transforming growth (TGF) factor-β pathway

Transforming growth factor (TGF) is a multifunctional cytokine that controls differentiation, apoptosis, cell growth, and immune reactions. TGF-β1, -β2, and -β3 are three isoforms of TGF-β that are present in mammals. In most types of cells, TGF-β is a potent growth inhibitor, so alterations on TGF-β signalling lead to tumour progression by the induction of angiogenesis, extracellular matrix accumulation, and immunosuppression.

Several studies have demonstrated that the over-expression of TGF-β in gastric cancer is correlated with lymph node metastasis and poor prognosis, as well as promotion of invasion and metastasis [60]. TGF-β induces RUNX3. RUNX3 interacts with FoxO3a/FKHRL1 to activate Bim and induce apoptosis. RUNX3 is expressed in glandular stomach epithelial cells; however, the loss of expression of this gene is associated with the progression, differentiation, metastasis, and poor prognosis of gastric cancer. *H. pylori* causes methylation of the RUNX3 gene and its loss of expression in gastric epithelial cells. Moreover, RUNX3 Smad4 inactivation has been documented in gastric cancer [62].

Cancer stem cells (CSCs)

Stem cells are functional units of growth that regenerate tissues and organs and play a role in tissue homoeostasis and repair after damage or loss. Stem cells have the unlimited ability to self-renew and the capacity to differentiate into several specialized cell types. Tumours may originate from a small subpopulation of CSCs that are able to maintain long-term tumour growth, tumour recurrence, and apoptosis and chemotherapy resistance. The results from some studies suggest that CD44, CD54, CD90, CD71, aldehyde dehydrogenase 1 (ALDH1), ATP-binding cassette subfamily B member 1 (ABCB1), ATP-binding cassette subfamily G member 2 (ABCG2), and CD133 etc. are potential biomarkers for gastric CSCs. Recent study has shown that expression of CD44, in particular that of a variant isoform (CD44v), contributes to reactive oxygen species (ROS) defence by promoting the synthesis of reduced glutathione (GSH), a primary intracellular antioxidant, namely that CD44v plays a role in the protection of CSCs from high levels of ROS in the tumour microenvironment [63]. In addition, some studies suggest that several signalling pathways, including Hedgehog and Wnt/beta-catenin, are essential for maintaining gastric CSCs [64, 65]. CSCs, which have already received great attention in the field of cancer research, are potential novel therapeutic targets in the treatment of gastric cancer.

Summary of the molecular biology of gastric cancers

In summary, gastric cancers that have epidemiologic and histologic distinction can also be distinguished by genomic and molecular analysis. As we improve our understanding of gastric cancer heterogeneity and its clinical consequences, our hope is to improve patient outcomes with improved prevention, screening and treatment options, using distinct biologic subtypes.

Pathology of gastric cancer: anatomy and histology of the stomach

The gastric wall consists of the mucosa, submucosa, muscularis propria, and serosa. The gastric mucosa lining the five regions of the stomach (cardia, fundus, corpus or body, antrum, and pylorus) measures 0.5–1.5 mm in thickness, and is composed of mucosal epithelium and a delicate stroma of connective tissue (lamina propria) occupying the space between the glands and the muscularis mucosae. Histologically, each mucosa is composed of surface foveolar epithelium and mucous secreting glands corresponding to the upper half and the lower half of the mucosa, respectively. The cardiac glands contain mucus-secreting cells. The fundic mucosa is characterized by the foveola representing one-fourth of the thickness mucosa, and straight fundic gland cells including chief cells, parietal cells, mucous neck cells, and endocrine cells. The chief cells produce pepsinogen I, and parietal cells produce acid and intrinsic factor, the latter of which binds to and facilitates the absorption of vitamin B12. Mucous neck cells are found at the junction of the gastric glands with the foveolar epithelial cells and produce a PAS-positive, diastase-resistant mucus. The antral mucosa and pyloric mucosa contain pyloric glands which are simple or branched tubules.

Most of the surface glandular cells express and secrete mucin that protects gastric epithelial cells from acid and proteinase secreted from chief and parietal cells. The mucin secreted by the foveolar epithelial cells is mainly PAS-positive neutral mucin, MUC1 and MUC5AC, and the glands secrete MUC6.

H. pylori infection and chronic gastritis

H. pylori infection

H. pylori infection is the most important predisposing factor for distal gastric carcinoma [4]. Patients with persistent *H. pylori* infection for prolonged periods of time exhibit typical phenotypic changes as chronic atrophic gastritis, focal intestinal metaplasia, and diffuse intestinal metaplasia and adenoma, which may be followed by the development of intestinal-type adenocarcinoma of the stomach. In *H.pylori*-positive subjects tested at least ten years prior to cancer diagnosis, the odds ratio was 5.9 (95% confidence interval 3.4–10.3) as compared to the non-infected population [5]. The cancer-preventive role of antibiotic therapy has been reported in patients free of atrophy or metaplasia. A randomized controlled trial study of 544 *H. pylori*-positive patients with early gastric cancer revealed a significant reduction in the recurrence rate of cancer in the group administrated eradication therapy after endoscopic resection [66].

Chronic atrophic gastritis

Chronic gastritis is pathologically divided into (1) chronic superficial gastritis and (2) chronic atrophic gastritis, based on the degree of inflammatory cell infiltration and presence of atrophy of the glandular epithelium. In chronic superficial gastritis, the inflammatory cell infiltration is limited to the foveolar epithelium, with no evidence of glandular atrophy. When the inflammatory cell infiltration is associated with glandular atrophy, this condition is referred to as chronic atrophic gastritis. Persistent chronic atrophic gastritis causes atrophy of gastric mucosa showing cystic dilatation of the gastric glands and intestinal metaplasia where few inflammatory cells infiltrate.

Precancerous conditions and precancerous lesions

The precursors of gastric cancer have been divided into two categories: (1) precancerous conditions and (2) precancerous lesions [67]. Precancerous conditions are clinical entities associated with an increased risk of gastric cancer development, such as chronic atrophic gastritis, intestinal metaplasia, and chronic gastric ulcer, whereas precancerous lesions are pathological lesions that may show malignant transformation, such as dysplasia, adenoma, Menetrier's disease, hyperplastic polyp, and gastric stump. A list of precancerous conditions and lesions is given in Table 37.1.

Intestinal metaplasia

'Metaplasia' refers to the replacement of one type of adult tissue by another. Intestinal metaplasia of the stomach is morphologically and enzymatically defined as replacement of the antral or fundic gastric mucosa by glands resembling those of the intestine. Intestinal metaplasia has been classified into the complete type (small intestine) and incomplete (large intestine) type based on morphological, histochemical, and immunohistochemical studies. Complete metaplastic glands contain Paneth cells and exhibit sucrose trehalase, leucine aminopeptidase, and alkaline phosphatase activity, while incomplete metaplastic glands exhibit no histochemical evidence of trehalase or alkaline phosphatase activity. Incomplete-type intestinal metaplasia has drawn attention as a precursor for intestinal-type gastric cancer. P53 gene alterations and degree of DNA methylation have also been reported in the metaplastic glands [68, 69].

Adenoma, intraepithelial neoplasia/dysplasia

The term 'adenoma' is used to refer to a protruding neoplastic proliferative lesion by Western pathologists, whereas Japanese pathologists use the term to refer to all gross lesions that may be elevated, flat, or depressed. According to the WHO 2010 definition of dysplasia, dysplasia is an unequivocal lesion for neoplasia [70]. However, it is sometimes difficult to distinguish dysplasia from reactive or regenerative mucosal epithelium associated with active inflammation, especially in small biopsy samples. At least one of these three categories should be considered for the diagnosis of dysplasia/adenoma in gastric mucosal specimen. (1) Negative for intraepithelial

neoplasia/dysplasia—this category may include benign mucosal processes corresponding regenerative or metaplastic changes. (2) Indefinite for intraepithelial neoplasia/dysplasia—this is not a final diagnosis of the samples. (3) Intraepithelial neoplasia/dysplasia unequivocally comprising epithelial neoplasia characterized by cellular and structural abnormalities but no evidence of invasion.

Intraepithelial neoplasia/dysplasia has been classified low- or high-grade: (1) low-grade intraepithelial neoplasia/dysplasia is characterized by minimal structural abnormalities and mild to moderate cytologic atypia, including elongated but polarized nuclei and low to moderate mitoses. (2) High-grade intraepithelial neoplasia/dysplasia is characterized by both cytological abnormalities including a high nuclear/cytoplasm ratio with hyperchromatic nuclei and amphophilic nucleoli, and more prominent architectural disarray characterized by a high nuclear–cytoplasmic ratio, loss of nuclear polarity, and numerous mitoses. Lesions such as high-grade dysplasia/intraepiethelial neoplasia require medical management such as endoscopic mucosal resection (EMR) or rebiopsy to confirm the morphological grading.

Fundic gland polyps

Fundic gland polyps are neoplastic polypoid lesions of the stomach and may occur sporadically in patients with familial adenomatous polyposis (FAP) and in patients under long-term treatment with proton-pump inhibitors. Patients with FAP may develop dysplasia in the fundic gland polys; however, carcinoma is rare. Genetic alterations of the CTNNB1 (beta-catenin) and APC genes affecting the Wnt signalling pathway are observed. The detection of mutations of CTNNB1 and APC observed in the sporadic fundic gland polyps strongly support the contention that fundic-gland polyps are neoplastic.

Adenocarcinoma

Among the most common malignant tumours of the stomach is a gastric carcinoma, followed in frequency by lymphomas (4%), carcinoids (3%), and malignant stromal cell tumour (GIST) (2%). Gastric carcinomas are malignant epithelial neoplasms of the stomach including adenocarcinoma, adenosquamous carcinoma, carcinoma with lymphoid stroma (medullary carcinoma), hepatoid adenocarcinoma, squamous cell carcinoma, and undifferentiated carcinoma. The most frequent site of gastric adenocarcinoma is the lesser curvature of the antropyloric region. However, the incidence of upper gastric cancer has been reported as increasing in recent years.

Since gastric cancer has heterogeneous morphology and biology, there have been several classifications of gastric cancer. Gastric carcinoma is clinicopathologically classified on the basis of (1) macroscopic type, (2) depth of invasion, and 3) histologic subtype.

Macroscopic type

The macroscopic types of advanced gastric cancer are based on Borrmann's classification (see Figure 37.1) There are four types; type 1 (protruding type); type 2 (circumscribed excavating type); type 3 (ulcerated with infiltrating spread type); and type 4 (diffuse infiltrating without ulceration type). Each macroscopic type depends on the location of the tumours and the histological type. Type 1 and type 2 frequently occur in the antrum and correspond to the intestinal type. Type 4 is a scirrhous-type cancer that occurs in the antrum or fundus; type 4 has been termed 'linitis plastic'

Table 37.1 Precancerous conditions and lesions

Precancerous conditions	Chronic atrophic gastritis Intestinal metaplasia
Precancerous lesions	Dysplasia/adenoma
	Gastric polyps
	Hyperplastic polyp
	Fundic gland polyp
	Chronic gastric ulcer
	Ménétrier's disease
	Post-resection gastric stump

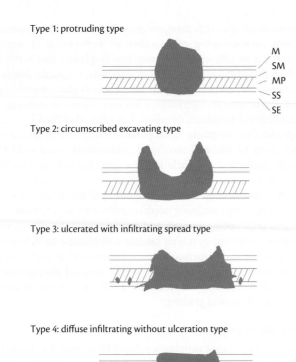

Type 1: protruding type

Type 2: circumscribed excavating type

Type 3: ulcerated with infiltrating spread type

Type 4: diffuse infiltrating without ulceration type

Fig. 37.1 Macroscopic type of gastric adenocarcinoma.
Source: data from Borrmann R, *Geschweulste des Magens und Duodenums*, Volume 4, pp. 812–1054, Copyright © 1926 Springer-Verlag Berlin Heidelberg.

> **Box 37.1** Classification of depth of invasion in gastric cancer
>
> Tis: Carcinoma in situ (intraepiethelial tumour without invasion of the lamina propria, high-grade dysplasia)
>   T1: Tumour invades lamina propria, muscularis mucosae or submucosa.
>   T1a: Tumour invades lamina propria or muscularis mucosae.
>   T1b: Tumour invades submucosa.
>   T2: Tumour invades the muscularis propria.
>   T3: Tumour invades the subserosa.
>   T4: Tumour perforates serosa or invades adjacent structures.
>   T4a: Tumour perforates the serosa.
>   T4b: Tumour invades adjacent structures.
>
> Reproduced with permission from Sobin L. et al. (Eds.), *TNM Classification of Malignant Tumours*, 7th ed., John Wiley & Sons Ltd, UK, Copyright © 2010 by Blackwell Publishing Ltd.

characterized by diffuse thickening and hardening of almost the entire gastric wall. This scirrhous-type cancer is often encountered in the younger age group and the male–female ratio is almost the same. The features of type 3 are intermediate between type 2 and type 4.

Depth of invasion

The tumour staging for the gastric carcinoma was based on the depth of invasion based on the classification proposed by the UICC (International Union Against Cancer); see Box 37.1. The T categorization is now identical to that for other gastrointestinal carcinomas such as those of oesophagus, duodenum, and colon.

Histological classification of gastric adenocarcinoma

Since the histological features of gastric carcinoma are markedly heterogeneous, there are several histological classifications for gastric adenocarcinomas. Figures 37.2 and 37.3 that show the representative histological subtypes of gastric adenocarcinoma based on the WHO classification, Lauren's classification, and Nakamura's classification.

WHO classification

The WHO histological classification is strictly descriptive for the morphology [70]. The five main types of gastric adenocarcinoma are identified in the WHO classification according to the morphological patterns: (1) tubular, (2) papillary, (3) mucinous, (4) poorly differentiated, including signet-ring-cell carcinoma, and (5) mixed carcinomas (Figures 37.2 and 37.3).

1. Tubular adenocarcinoma is composed of dilated or branching tubules of disarrayed glandular structures. It can be classified into well-differentiated and moderately differentiated subtypes. Acinar and solid structures are also present in various amounts. Individual neoplastic cells are columnar, cuboidal, or flattened and show high nuclear/cytoplasmic ratio with various atypical nucleus.

2. Papillary adenocarcinoma is characterized by the presence of papillary or villous structures mainly composed of cuboidal to cylindrical tumour cells. This type is often associated with tubular structures (papillotubular adenocarcinoma). The degree of cellular atypia and mitotic index vary.

3. Poorly differentiated adenocarcinoma, including signet-ring-cell carcinoma, is composed of poorly cohesive carcinoma cells occurring as isolated cells or arranged in small clusters with few distinct glandular structures. Signet-ring cells are characterized by a central clear globoid droplet of cytoplasmic mucin with an eccentrically placed nucleus. This type of cancer cell is often observed in 'linitis plastica'-type tumours.

4. Mucinous adenocarcinoma is composed of cancer cells that are composed of either differentiated or poorly differentiated adenocarcinoma cells with large amounts of extracellular mucinous pools. The tumour shows more than 50% extracellular mucin area.

5. Mixed carcinoma displays a mixture of the differentiated glandular and poorly cohesive cancers in a single tumour.

6. Rare histological variants represent about 5% of all gastric cancers and include adenosquamous carcinoma, squamous cell carcinoma, hepatoid adenocarcinoma, carcinoma with lymphoid stroma (medullary carcinoma), choriocarcinoma, carcinosarcoma, and undifferentiated carcinoma.

Lauren classification and other classification

Lauren was the first to classify gastric cancer into two distinct morphological types, the intestinal type and diffuse type [6]. Tumours containing approximately equal amounts of intestinal and diffuse components are termed mixed.

Carcinoma of the intestinal type may arise from the metaplastic epithelium and show various degrees of differentiation from well-differentiated glandular structures to poorly differentiated solid cell nests. Carcinoma of this type preferentially metastasizes

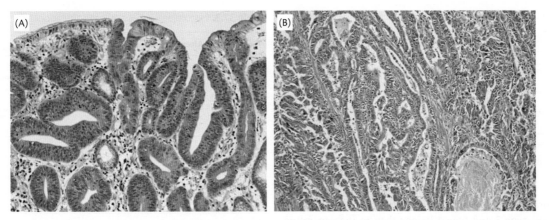

Fig. 37.2 Histological classification of gastric adenocarcinoma. Intestinal type (Lauren [6])/differentiated type (Nakamura [71]). (A) Tubular adenocarcinoma; (B) papillary adenocarcinoma.

hematogenously to the liver. However, diffuse-type gastric cancer frequently occurs in the antropyloric region and body of the stomach and is composed of poorly cohesive cells with little or no gland formation, and preferentially metastasizes to the peritoneal cavity. The representative gastric cancer of diffuse-type cancer is known as 'linitis plastica', which is characterized by occurring predominantly in young females. Penetration of the serosa by carcinoma frequently results in peritoneal seeding. Bilateral massive involvement of the ovaries (Krukenberg tumour) can result from transperitoneal or hematogenous spread.

Nakamura categorized all gastric carcinomas into the differentiated or undifferentiated types, which vaguely correspond to the intestinal type and diffuse types classified by Lauren [71]. As Nakamura's classification is based on the different morphological structure of the tumour, the differentiated type is composed of well differentiated and moderately differentiated tubular adenocarcinoma and papillary adenocarcinoma, and the undifferentiated type represents poorly differentiated, signet-ring-cell, and mucinous carcinoma. However, some cases of poorly differentiated adenocarcinoma with solid growth could be differently classified as the intestinal type by Lauren's classification but as the undifferentiated type according to Nakamura's classification.

The TNM classification of malignant tumours by the UICC proposed the histopathological grading as G categories, which apply to all digestive system tumours except those of the liver (see Table 37.2).

Early gastric cancer

Based on the clinicopathological behaviour, 'early gastric cancer' is defined as an invasive carcinoma that is limited to the mucosa or the mucosa and submucosa regardless of the nodal status. Most cases of early gastric cancer show a low incidence of lymph node and distant metastasis; however, if left untreated, they progress over a few months to several years.

Early gastric cancers are classified endoscopically into the three following categories according to their macroscopic appearance, protruded (type 0-I), superficial (type 0-II) and excavated (type 0-III). The most predominant of these type, 0-II, is further subdivided elevated (0-IIa), flat (0-IIb), and depressed (0-IIc) lesions. The risk of deep and multifocal penetration of the submucosa or lymphatic invasion varies from case to case, so the surgical and endoscopic submucosal resection specimens must be pathologically examined in detail in order to select the most suitable treatment.

Tumour spread

Gastric cancer arises from the mucosa and spreads by direct extension to adjacent organs, metastasizes to lymph nodes or distant organs, or shows peritoneal dissemination. The presence of serosal

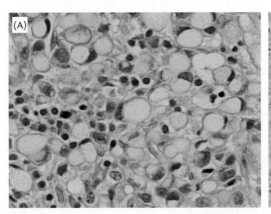
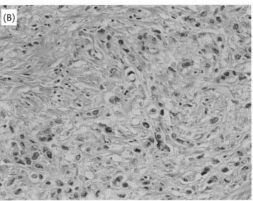

Fig. 37.3 Histological classification of gastric adenocarcinoma. Diffuse type (Lauren [6])/undifferentiated type (Nakamura [71]). (A) Signet-ring-cell carcinoma; (B) poorly differentiated adenocarcinoma.

Table 37.2 Histopathological grading of gastric cancers

GX	Grade of differentiation cannot be assessed
G1	Well differentiated
G2	Moderately differentiated
G3	Poorly differentiated
G4	Undifferentiated

Reproduced with permission from Sobin L. et al. (Eds.), *TNM Classification of Malignant Tumours, Seventh Edition*, John Wiley & Sons Ltd, UK, Copyright © 2010 by Blackwell Publishing Ltd.

Table 37.3 Histological types and gene alterations

Gene	Alteration	Frequency
APC	LOH, Mutation	intestinal (30-40%) > diffuse (<2%)
DCC	LOH	intestinal (60%) > diffuse (<1%)
P53	LOH, Mutation	intestinal (25–40%) > diffuse (0-21%)
RB1	Reduced expression	diffuse (30%)
CDKN1B	Reduced expression	40–50%
CDH1	LOH, Mutation Reduced expression	diffuse (>50%)
CTNNB1	Mutation	17–27%
BLC2	Over-expression	diffuse (10–30%)
c-MYC	Over-expression	40–45%
Cyclin E	Over-expression	15–20%
KRAS	Mutation	intestinal (1-28%) > diffuse (<1%)
EGFR	Amplification Over-expression	30%
ERBB2	Amplification Over-expression	intestinal (15–25%) > diffuse (0–5%)
FGFR2	Amplification Over-expression	30%
MET	Amplification Over-expression	intestinal (7%) > diffuse (7%)

Abbreviation: LOH, loss of heterozygosity.

spread is more common in tumours with infiltrative growth such as macroscopic type 3 and type 4 lesions than in the expanding growth type tumours, such as type 1 and type 2. The presence of mucosal (submucosal) lymph vessel infiltration is statistically associated with lymph node metastasis. Vascular invasion is also strongly associated with a high frequency of distant metastasis. The most frequent sites of metastasis from gastric carcinoma are the liver, peritoneum, and lung, followed by adrenal gland, ovary, and bone marrow.

Close association has been observed between the histological type and the sites of metastasis: intestinal-type carcinomas preferentially metastasize hematogenously to the liver, whereas diffuse-type carcinomas tend to be associated with peritoneal dissemination.

Molecular targets in gastric cancer

Recent advances in molecular biological techniques have clarified the presence of some molecular genetic alterations of gastric cancer. Table 37.3 shows a list of gene alterations in gastric cancer. Some of them are closely associated with the histological subtypes. While APC gene mutations and LOH, p53 gene mutation, KRAS gene mutations, and ErbB 2 gene amplification have been reported to occur more frequently in intestinal-type gastric cancer, RB1 loss of expression, FGFR2, K-SAM gene amplification are more frequently observed in diffuse-type gastric cancer. Cell adhesion molecule abnormalities have been reported in the poorly-cohesive-type gastric cancer. CDH-1 (E-cadherin) and CTNNB1 (βeta-catenin) gene alterations have been reported in both gastric cancer cell lines and human gastric cancer [72]. These findings are good examples of gene-morphological consistency, wherein disruption of cell adhesion by gene mutations is frequently detected in poorly cohesive adenocarcinoma including signet-ring cell carcinoma.

Anti-c-erbB2 (HER2) antibody is now used as a molecular target therapy for c-erbB2-positive gastric cancer. HER2 testing is now recommended to all advanced and recurrent gastric cancer patients. Compared to the HER2 testing in breast cancer, more heterogenous HER2 expression has been reported in gastric cancer (Figure 37.4) [73]. In addition to ERBB2, some receptor type tyrosine-kinases, such as EGFR, FGFR2, c-MET, and VEGFR are drawing attention as new targets for therapy.

Whole exon analysis has been introduced recently as an advanced molecular technique and revealed new genetic profiles of many cancers including gastric cancer [74, 75]. However, so-called driver gene mutations have not been identified yet in gastric cancer.

Hereditary diffuse gastric cancer

Hereditary diffuse gastric cancer is an autosomal-dominant cancer-susceptibility syndrome that is characterized by signet-ring-cell gastric cancer and lobular carcinoma of the breast. The genetic basis for this syndrome was discovered in 1998, and consisted of germline mutations of the E-cadherin (CDH-1) gene. The International Gastric Cancer Linkage Consortium (IGCLC) defined criteria for genetic analysis of the CHD-1 gene mutation to detect the hereditary diffuse gastric cancer syndrome. The age at onset of clinically significant diffuse gastric cancer varies even within families. The cancer is characterized morphologically by the presence of multifocal invasive lesions of signet-ring-cell carcinoma, with no mass lesion. Histological examination of the entire gastric mucosa is necessary before the absence of neoplasia can be claimed. Early invasive carcinoma is not restricted to any topographic region of the stomach. The signet-ring-cell carcinomas observed in asymptomatic CDH-1 mutation show absent or reduced E-cadherin staining.

Surgical management of gastric cancer

The current role of surgical therapy in the treatment of gastric cancer includes staging, resection with curative intent, and palliation or tumour reduction in patients with stage IV disease. Surgical treatment remains the best treatment modality for a potential cure. The primary goal of surgery is to accomplish complete removal with negative margins (R0 resection). The extent of prophylactic or curative lymph node dissection remains controversial, and the surgical strategy of lymph node dissection differs between the East (countries with a higher incidence, such as Japan or South Korea) and the West (countries with a lower incidence, such as the

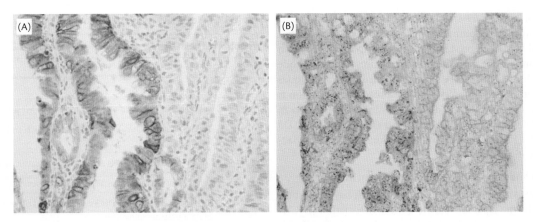

Fig. 37.4 Heterogeneous expression of HER2 protein and gene amplification. (A) HER2 IHC; (B) HER2 ISH.

US). During the past decade, laparoscopic surgery has played an increasingly important role—not only in staging, but also in radical gastrectomy with lymph node dissection, especially in East Asian countries.

Extent of gastric resection in curative surgery: surgical margin

In surgery with curative intent, a sufficient resection margin should be ensured to determine the resection line. The length of the proximal margin recommended by the Japanese guideline according to cancer type is indicated below [76].

Advanced-stage cancer

In tumours with an expansive growth pattern, at least 3 cm is recommended for the proximal margin. In tumours with an infiltrative growth pattern, 5 cm is recommended. However, for tumours invading the oesophagus, a 5 cm proximal margin is not necessary. To ensure safe surgical margins, intraoperative frozen section examination is desirable.

Early-stage cancer

For T1 tumours, 2 cm is the recommended safety margin. When the border is unclear in superficial tumours, preoperative marking clips placed by gastroendoscopy may be helpful to confirm the resection line during the operation.

Type of gastric resection

The various types of gastric resection currently performed include: total gastrectomy, distal gastrectomy (subtotal gastrectomy), proximal gastrectomy, pylorus-preserving gastrectomy, and segmental gastrectomy or local gastrectomy.

If the tumour is located within the distal two-thirds of the stomach and an adequate proximal margin can be obtained, distal gastrectomy is preferred in Japan. If the tumour involves the upper third of the stomach, total gastrectomy is chosen. Although the same opinion is held outside Japan [77], total gastrectomy is generally accepted rather than subtotal gastrectomy in European countries for better local control [78]. There is controversy regarding whether splenectomy is mandatory in combination with total gastrectomy for the purpose of complete clearance of lymph nodes at the splenic hilum (at least 10 lymph nodes). A randomized controlled trial is currently ongoing in the Japan Clinical Oncology Group (JCOG) to estimate the impact of splenectomy on long-term survival [79]. In

general, pancreas-preserving total gastrectomy with splenectomy is considered for tumours located along the greater curvature of the upper stomach in Japan.

Function-preserving gastric resection has also become an important consideration in the treatment of early-stage gastric cancer. Some articles have reported that preservation of the pylorus, vagal nerve, and gastric reservoir significantly improves patients' gastrointestinal function and quality of life. Pylorus-preserving gastrectomy is performed for tumours located in the middle stomach, ensuring a margin of at least 4 cm from the pylorus. Proximal gastrectomy is performed for tumours located in the proximal third of the stomach, ensuring that more than half of the stomach can be preserved. At present, these procedures are only recommended for cT1N0 cancer. Local excision gastrectomy plays little role currently because of the progression of peroral endoscopic interventions. However, it is possible that the utility of local gastrectomy will be re-evaluated if innovative diagnostic technologies such as sentinel node diagnosis are developed.

Lymph node dissection

History in Japan

In the 1960s, Japanese surgeons established D2 lymphadenectomy, which includes systematic dissection of the perigastric nodes (first tier) and the nodes around the celiac artery and its branches (second tier). Early studies demonstrated that the five-year survival rate of patients with positive lymph node metastasis including the second-tier nodes ranged from 30% to 40% after D2 dissection [80]. No randomized clinical trials have compared D1 and D2 dissections in Japan, but since the aforementioned early studies were performed, D2 dissection has been recognized as standard surgery in Japan. Since the 1980s, more radical extended lymphadenectomy, namely extended para-aortic node dissection (D3 or PAND), has been performed in many high-volume centres for patients with positive nodes. However, a multi-institutional randomized trial conducted by the JCOG showed no survival benefits of D3 compared with D2, at least in patients with curable gastric cancer (JCOG 9501) [81]. In JCOG 9501, a total of 523 patients were randomized to either D2 lymphadenectomy or D3 (D2 + PAND) lymphadenectomy. The results demonstrated higher morbidity with D2 + PAND (28.1% versus 20.9%, P = 0.07); however, there was no difference in mortality (0.8% in both groups). There was also no difference in survival between the two groups, with five-year survival rates of 70% and 69%, respectively (P = 0.85). Thus, to date, the Japanese guideline recommends that potentially curable gastric cancers should be treated by standard gastrectomy with D2 lymph node dissection, but for early-stage cancer, minimal lymph node dissection such as D1 or D1+ is recommended. The techniques of D2 dissection in open surgery are widespread. D2 dissection is performed not only in community hospitals in Japan, but also in Eastern countries such as South Korea and China. However, D3 dissection (D2 + PAND) is not routinely performed for prophylactic lymph node dissection in Japan.

Nodal station and lymphadenectomy definition in Japan

The lymph node stations surrounding the stomach have been precisely defined by the Japanese Gastric Cancer Association (JGCA) [82]. The JGCA previously divided these stations into four levels (first through fourth tier) based on analysis of the lymphatic flow from the stomach, and these designations were defined on the location of the primary tumour (i.e., upper third, middle third, and lower third) [83]. The anatomic definitions and numbering of the lymph node stations have remained constant during further revisions of the JGCA classification system. There have been several revisions, and in 2010 the JGCA abandoned the designation of nodal stations to more closely adopt and avoid confusion with the staging of the UICC/American Joint Committee on Cancer (AJCC). Lymph node stations 1 to 12 and 14v are defined as regional gastric lymph nodes (Table 37.4); metastasis to any other nodes is classified as M1. Nodal stations for D1 and D2 are now defined by the type of operation performed rather than the tumour location (Table 37.4).

D1 versus D2 studies in Western Countries

In contrast, in Western countries, most surgeons avoid extensive lymph node dissection as performed in Eastern countries; instead, D1 lymph node dissection (perigastric nodes only) is performed in the majority of institutions. This difference between Eastern and Western countries may exist for several reasons. First, the incidence of gastric cancer is much higher in Eastern countries; therefore, surgeons are more familiar with gastric cancer surgery and the surgical anatomy surrounding the stomach. It is unquestionable that the controversy regarding the extent of lymph node dissection stems from differences in the global epidemiology of gastric cancer. Second, Western general populations have higher body mass indices and more visceral adipose tissue, which may increase post-operative complications after intensive lymph node dissection around the pancreas. Third, proximal tumours, which tend to behave more aggressively, are less common in Japan than in the West.

In an attempt to clarify the effectiveness of D2 dissection established in Japan, two large European randomized controlled trials comparing D1 and D2 dissection were carried out in the 1990s (Table 37.5). In the UK, a multicentre randomized controlled trial (Medical Research Council (MRC) trial) which enrolled 400 patients was performed to compare D1 and D2 lymphadenectomy [84, 85]. The study showed significantly higher morbidity (46% versus 28%, P <0.001) and mortality (13% versus 6.5%, P = 0.04) in the D2 group. No difference in overall survival or disease-specific survival was observed between D1 and D2 lymph node dissection. This study was highly criticized because of the quality of lymph node dissection: the median number of retrieved lymph nodes was 13 in the D1 group and 17 in the D2 group. In addition, many Eastern surgeons pointed out that the mortality rate was unacceptably high, which

Table 37.4 Regional lymph node stations of the stomach

Number and definitions	
1	Right paracardial LNs
2	Left paracardial LNs
3a	Lessor curvature LNs along the branches of left gastric artery
3b	Lessor curvature LNs along the second branch and distal part of right gastric artery
4sa	Left greater curvature LNs along the short gastric arteries
4sb	Left greater curvature LNs along the left gastroepiploic artery
4d	Right greater curvature LNs long the second branch and distal part of right gastroepiploic artery
5	Suprapyloric LNs along the first branch and proximal part of right gastric artery
6	Infrapyloric LNs along the first branch and proximal part of right gastroepiploic artery down to the confluence of the right gastroepiploic vein
7	LNs along the trunk of the left gastric artery
8a	Anterosuperior LNs along the common hepatic artery
8p	Posterior LNs along the common hepatic artery
9	Celiac artery LNs
10	Splenic hilar LNs
11b	Proximal splenic artery LNs
11d	Distal splenic artery LNs
12a	Hepatoduodenal ligament LNs along the proper hepatic artery
12b	Hepatoduodenal ligament LNs along the bile duct
12p	Hepatoduodenal ligament LNs along the portal vein
14v	LNs along the superior mesenteric vein

Abbreviation: LN, lymph node.

Reproduced from Springer, *Gastric Cancer*, Volume 1, Issue 1, pp. 10–24, Japanese Classification of Gastric Carcinoma, Second English Edition, Japanese Gastric Cancer Association, Table 2, Copyright © 1998 by International and Japanese Gastric Cancer Associations. With kind permission from Springer Science and Business Media.

was mainly caused by inappropriate distal pancreaticosplenectomy in D2 total gastrectomy. The second major European study was the Dutch Gastric Cancer trial (Dutch trial), in which 711 patients were randomized to either D2 or D1 lymph node dissection [86–88]. All surgeons were instructed by an expert from Japan, and all D2 lymph node dissections were supervised by a specialized surgeon. In spite of this setting, non-compliance was encountered in 36% of D1 and 51% of D2 dissections. Likewise, as in the MRC trial, the D2 arm showed higher morbidity (43% versus 25%, P <0.001) and mortality (10% versus 4%, P = 0.004). The survival data were reported for three separate time intervals. In the first two publications, there was no difference overall or disease-specific survival, with a reported 11-year overall survival rate of 35% in the D2 arm versus 30% in the D1 arm (P = 0.53). At that time, management of gastric cancer in the West was greatly influenced by these disappointing outcomes, and surgeons in the West became even more reluctant to perform D2 dissection. Many Japanese surgeons considered the results of these two trials to have an unacceptably high operative mortality

Table 37.5 Extent of lymph node dissection in main gastric resection

Total gastrectomy	
D0	less than D1
D1	Nos 1–7
D1+	D1 + Nos 8a, 9, 11p
D2	D1 + Nos. 8a, 9, 10, 11p, 11d, 12a
Distal gastrectomy	
D0	less than D1
D1	Nos 1, 3, 4sb, 4d, 5, 6, 7
D1+	D1 + Nos 8a, 9
D2	D1 + Nos 8a, 9, 11p, 12a

Reproduced from Springer, *Gastric Cancer*, Volume 1, Issue 1, pp. 10–24, Japanese Classification of Gastric Carcinoma, Second English Edition, Japanese Gastric Cancer Association, Table 3, Copyright © 1998 by International and Japanese Gastric Cancer Associations. With kind permission from Springer Science and Business Media.

rate, which had likely masked any potential survival advantage. Perioperative mortality in the JCOG 9501 trial was 0.8%, and the five-year survival rate was 70%; in the European trials, however, the mortality rate was 4–6% and the five-year survival rate was 33–35%. However, the five-year results of the Dutch trial were published in 2010, indicating that there remains no significant difference in overall survival [89]. Interestingly, there was improved locoregional control in the D2 arm and improved gastric cancer mortality in the D2 arm (37% versus 48%, respectively; P = 0.01). Thus, in the West, the NCCN guidelines recommend that gastric cancer surgery should be performed by experienced surgeons in high-volume centres and should include removal of perigastric lymph nodes (D1) and those along the named vessels of the celiac axis (D2), with a goal of examining 15 or more lymph nodes. To avoid perioperative morbidity and mortality, the NCCN guideline also recommends modified D2 lymphadenectomy (without distal pancreatectomy or splenectomy), which is standard in the West [90]. The Italian Gastric Cancer Study Group recently published their randomized clinical trial comparing D1 and D2 gastrectomy in 267 patients treated at specialized hospitals and revealed that specialized centres may have lower rates of morbidity and mortality (12% versus 17.9% and 3% versus 2.2%, respectively) with D2 dissection, even in Western countries [91].

Study of D1 versus D3 in Asia

In the East, another randomized trial was performed in Taiwan comparing D1 and D3 lymphadenectomy in 211 patients, although it was a single-institution study involving three highly trained surgeons [92]. This study showed that the morbidity rate was higher in the D3 group (17.1% versus 7.3%, P = 0.012); however, no operative mortality was reported in either group. More lymph nodes were retrieved in the D3 group than in the D1 group (37.2 versus 19.4, respectively). The study demonstrated improved survival with D3 lymphadenectomy, although the difference was small (59.5% versus 53.6%, P = 0.041). This study suggests that in the hands of highly experienced surgeons, D3 lymphadenectomy is superior to D1 with low operative mortality.

Laparoscopic gastrectomy with lymph node dissection

Laparoscopic gastrectomy is now widely accepted in many communities, mainly in Japan and South Korea. When compared with open surgery, advantages regarding short-term outcomes, such as faster recovery, decreased blood loss, and less pain with minimal wounds, have been reported. Laparoscopic surgery for gastric cancer was launched in the early 1990s [93]. Its techniques, including meticulous lymph node dissection under a magnified endoscopic view and intracorporeal intestinal reconstruction, were subsequently developed in Eastern countries, especially in Japan. Laparoscopic surgery is currently regarded as the treatment of choice for early gastric cancer. The feasibility and safety of laparoscopic distal gastrectomy in the treatment of stage I gastric cancer have been proven by several prospective studies that investigated post-operative complications (JCOG 0703 and Korean Laparoscopic Gastrointestinal Surgery Study 01 trials [KLASS 01]) [94, 95]. However, laparoscopic distal gastrectomy is recognized as investigational treatment, not as a standard procedure, in the Japanese guideline because the oncological outcomes have not been clearly demonstrated in any prospective studies. At present, the long-term outcomes of laparoscopic distal gastrectomy in early-stage gastric cancer have been assessed in randomized clinical trials in Japan and South Korea (JCOG 0912 and KLASS 01 trials).

The majority of these studies have been performed in Japan and South Korea, where more patients present with early gastric cancer; applicability to Western countries, where patients present at more advanced stages, remains to be seen. The safety and oncologic validity of laparoscopic gastrectomy with D2 dissection for advanced gastric cancer are still being debated because of the technical difficulties of this procedure. Only one meta-analysis has reported on the comparison of laparoscopic gastrectomy with D2 dissection [96]. Although this report was based mostly on case-controlled studies, laparoscopic gastrectomy with D2 dissection resulted in a longer duration of operation by approximately one hour, reduced blood loss, fewer total post-operative complications, less pain, faster bowel function recovery, and shorter hospital stay, with similar numbers of harvested lymph nodes and a similar overall survival rate compared with open gastrectomy with D2 dissection.

Laparoscopic total gastrectomy was first reported in 1999 [97], but it is still considered to be a technically demanding procedure. Long-term follow-up data for validation of oncological outcomes are still lacking. Robotic gastrectomy is also currently performed by Japanese and Korean experts in laparoscopic surgery, but, again, conclusive data are lacking.

Non-curative surgery

Palliative surgery

Palliative gastric resection is performed to improve symptoms such as stenosis or haemorrhage due to tumour-related haemorrhage in patients with stage IV non-resectable gastric cancer. When the tumour is expected to be relatively easy to remove without risks, palliative resection is selected. When palliative resection seems difficult or the operation is risky, bypass surgery such as gastrojejunostomy may be elected to improve the patient's quality of life.

Reduction surgery

Gastrectomy as reduction surgery is performed in an attempt to decrease the tumour volume in patients with other non-curative factors, such as liver metastasis or peritoneal dissemination. The purpose of this surgery is to prolong survival time by reducing tumour volume; however, there is insufficient scientific evidence to support the effectiveness of this kind of surgery in patients with gastric cancer. A randomized clinical trial is currently ongoing to compare reduction surgery and systemic chemotherapy with the cooperation of both Japan and South Korea (JCOG 0705/REGATTA).

Staging laparoscopy

Even current CT scan devices of the highest quality have limitations in the detection of metastases on peritoneal surfaces. Numerous studies have demonstrated the effectiveness of staging laparoscopy in the management of patients with gastric cancer. Laparoscopic inspection should include full inspection of peritoneal surfaces and the liver to detect metastases. Suspicious peritoneal lesions should undergo biopsy. In addition, peritoneal cytology using normal saline should be performed. Positive biopsy or peritoneal cytology results are considered indicative of the presence of metastatic disease.

Medical management of gastric cancer

In Japan or Korea, where screening is performed widely, early detection of gastric cancer is often possible. In other countries, most cases are diagnosed in advanced stage. Overall, gastric cancer is a fatal malignancy with the one of the worst five-year survival rates. According to data from the US National Cancer Institute Surveillance, Epidemiology and End Results (SEER) programme, the five-year survival for patients with gastric cancer was 22% [98]. Based on population-based cancer registries, the survival rate is higher in Japan than in other countries (approximately 50–60% versus 20–25%) [99, 100].

Treatment strategies for localized but advanced gastric cancer vary in different geographic regions. Primary gastrectomy with lymph node dissection followed by adjuvant chemotherapy is standard in Asian countries. Neoadjuvant chemotherapy and chemoradiotherapy is standard in Western countries. For patients with metastatic disease, cytotoxic chemotherapy is the most effective treatment modality to prolong survival and alleviate symptoms. The addition of targeted agents has also been recently investigated.

Adjuvant chemoradiotherapy

Between 1991 and 1998, the US Intergroup INT-0116 randomly assigned 556 patients with curatively resected gastric or EGJ adenocarcinoma (Stage IB–IV, M0) to surgery only and surgery plus post-operative chemoradiotherapy. Adjuvant treatment consisted of 45 Gy radiotherapy, with bolus fluorouracil (FU) plus leucovorin. One cycle of bolus FU plus leucovorin before chemoradiation and two cycles after chemoradiation were also given [101]. Median overall survival (OS) was significantly longer (36 versus 27 months) in the chemoradiotherapy group (P = 0.005). Benefits were maintained with ten-year median follow-up (the hazard ratio (HR) for OS 1.32; P = 0.0046) and no increases in late toxic effects were noted [102]. Current consensus guidelines in the US recommend post-operative chemoradiotherapy as a treatment option. However, this study has been criticized, mainly for the limited extent of the surgical procedure. Although D2 lymph node dissection was recommended, it was performed in only 10% of patients and 54% of patients underwent a limited lymph node dissection (D0), which could have undermined survival.

In Korea, additional data for chemoradiotherapy has been provided by the ARTIST trial. 458 patients with curatively resected gastric cancer by D2 lymph node dissection (Stage IB–IV, M0) were randomly assigned to six courses of post-operative capecitabine plus cisplatin (XP) or two courses of post-operative XP followed by chemoradiotherapy (45 Gy RT with concurrent daily capecitabine) and two additional courses of XP [103]. Compared to chemotherapy alone, the addition of RT to XP chemotherapy did not significantly improve the three-year disease-free survival (DFS) rate (78.2% versus 74.2%; p = 0.0862). For the patients with completely resected gastric cancer and a D2 lymph node dissection, the role of adjuvant radiotherapy is still unclear.

Key clinical trials of Adjuvant and Neoadjuvant therapy are briefly discussed in Table 37.6.

Neoadjuvant/perioperative chemotherapy

In contrast to the US, perioperative (preoperative plus post-operative) chemotherapy has become the main approach in European countries.

The British Medical Research Council (MRC) conducted the first well-powered phase III trial (MAGIC trial) that evaluated perioperative chemotherapy for patients with resectable gastroesophageal cancer. In this trial, 503 patients with potentially resectable gastric (74%), distal oesophageal (11%), or EGJ adenocarcinomas (15%) were randomly assigned to surgery alone or surgery plus perioperative chemotherapy. Chemotherapy consisted of three preoperative and three post-operative cycles of epirubicin, cisplatin, and infusional 5-fluorouracil (ECF) [104]. Although chemotherapy was well tolerated and fewer than 12% of all patients developed grade 3 or 4 toxic effects, only 104 (42%) completed all protocol treatment. The extent of lymph node dissection was determined by the surgeon's discretion, and the reported rates of D2 dissection were 41% in the perioperative-chemotherapy group and 40% in the surgery group. As compared with the surgery group, the perioperative-chemotherapy group showed a significantly better OS (HR 0.75; P = 0.009; five-year rate, 36.3% versus 23.0%) and progression-free survival (PFS) (HR 0.66; P<0.001).

In a more recent FNCLCC/FFCD trial, the benefit of perioperative chemotherapy (infusional FU plus cisplatin, every four weeks) was also shown in patients with potentially resectable adenocarcinoma of the stomach, EGJ, or the lower third of the oesophagus [105]. Patients undergoing perioperative chemotherapy showed a significantly better OS (HR 0.69; P = 0.02; five-year rate, 38% versus 24%) and a better DFS (HR 0.65; P = 0.003; five-year rate 34% versus 19%).

Based on these results, perioperative chemotherapy, particularly with ECF, in addition to D1 surgery has become the standard treatment in European countries.

Adjuvant chemotherapy

Although more than 30 randomized trials have compared adjuvant chemotherapy to surgery alone in curatively resected gastric cancer up to the present time, most studies were negative for OS. The reasons for these negative results were considered to be due to poor statistical power, inferior surgical techniques, and ineffective regimens. An individual patient-level meta-analysis of randomized control trials was performed by the GASTRIC (Global Advanced/Adjuvant Stomach Tumour Research International Collaboration) Group to quantify the potential benefit of chemotherapy after complete resection over surgery alone [106]. From 17 randomized controlled trials, 3838 patients were included in their analyses; they

Table 37.6 Results of pivotal Randomized Trials of Adjuvant and Neoadjuvant therapy for resected Gastric Cancer

Study	Stage	Treatment	No. of Patients	Three-year RFS (%)	Three-year survival (%)
Adjuvant chemoradiotherapy					
INT-0016	Stage IB-IV, M0	FU/Leucovorin +RT	281	48	50
		Surgery alone (D0 >D1)	275	31 P<0.001	41 P = 0.005
ARTIST	Stage IB-IV, M0	2 of XP, Capecitabine+RT, 2 of XP	230	78.2	Not reported
		6 of XP	228	74.2 P = 0.0862	
Perioperative chemotherapy					
MAGIC	Stage II or higher, M0	Perioperative ECF	250	Not reported	36.3[†]
		Surgery alone	253	P <0.001	23.0 P = 0.009
FNCLCC/FFCD	Judged resectable	Perioperative FU/Cisplatin	113	34[†]	38[†]
		Surgery alone	111	19 P = 0.003	24 P = 0.02
Post-operative chemotherapy					
ACTS-GC	Stage II–III	S-1	529	65.4[†]	71.7[†]
		Surgery alone (D2)	530	53.1 HR:0.653	61.1 HR:0.669
CLASSIC	Stage II–IIIB	Capecitabine/Oxaliplatin	520	74	83
		Surgery alone (D2)	515	59 p <0.0001	78 p = 0.0493

[†]At 5 years.

RT, radiotherapy; XP, capecitabine plus cisplatin; ECF, epirubicin, cisplatin and infusional 5-fluorouracil; RFS, relapse-free survival.

concluded that adjuvant chemotherapy was associated with a statistically significant benefit in terms of OS (HR 0.82; P < 0.001) and DFS (HR 0.82; <0.001).

In Japan, the ACTS-GC trial evaluated the benefit of adjuvant treatment with S-1 monotherapy in patients with stage II or III gastric cancer who had undergone curative surgery with D2 lymphadenectomy. In this study, 1059 patients were randomly assigned to one year of S1 versus surgery alone [107]. Five-year OS and relapse-free survival (RFS) were significantly better with S-1 (five-year OS 71.7% versus 61.1%; HR 0.669 and five-year RFS 65.4% versus 53.1%; HR 0.653) [108]. In comparing the results among the ACTS-GC, INT-0116, and MAGIC trials, there are remarkable differences in survival rates: even the surgery alone group in the ACTS-GC trial resulted in remarkably higher rates than the treatment groups in other studies (INT-0116 (three-year); 50% versus 41%, and MAGIC trial (five-year); 36.3% versus 23.0% for the treatment and control groups, respectively) [109, 101].

The CLASSIC trial investigated the benefit of adjuvant therapy with capecitabine plus oxaliplatin. In this trial, 1035 patients with stage II–IIIB gastric cancer were randomly assigned to eight cycles of capecitabine plus oxaliplatin for six months or surgery alone after D2 gastrectomy [110]. The study was conducted in South Korea, China, and Taiwan. At a median follow-up of 34.2 months, chemotherapy was associated with a significant improvement in three-year DFS, which met its primary endpoint (74% versus 59%, HR 0.56, P<0.0001). In a subgroup analysis, three-year DFS benefits of capecitabine plus oxaliplatin were consistently shown for all disease stages (stage II, IIIa, and IIIb). Although a robust estimate of median OS is not yet available, the improvement of three-year OS was a borderline statistically significant (83% versus 78%, HR 0.72, P = 0.0493). Further follow-up is needed to confirm the impact in

OS and whether two-drug combinations in this study were better than monotherapy in future comparison with the results of ACTS-GC.

The results of these two studies strongly support that the use of post-operative chemotherapy after curative surgery with D2 lymph node dissection is standard treatment in Asia. The role of intensive perioperative chemotherapy or chemoradiation in patients who undergo D2 surgery remains undetermined.

Summary of medical management of gastric cancer

Gastrectomy with D2 lymph node dissection is the standard treatment for resectable gastric cancer in the East Asia. On the contrary, in Western countries, D2 lymph node dissection is considered a recommended standard procedure, but not uniformly performed. These facts might affect the geographical variations of the standard treatment and the survival rate.

In the US, D0 or D1 surgery plus fluorouracil-based post-operative chemoradiotherapy is a standard of care. In Europe, perioperative chemotherapy is established as a standard option for patients with resectable gastric cancer who have undergone curative surgery with limited lymph node dissection (D1). In eastern Asia, the results of two large trials support the use of post-operative chemotherapy after curative surgery with D2 lymph node dissection in patients with resectable gastric cancer.

Medical management for unresectable and metastatic gastric cancer

Chemotherapy for unresectable gastric cancer

The goals of chemotherapy in patients with advanced gastric cancer are to palliate symptoms and prolong survival. Even with combination chemotherapy it is difficult to cure patients with met-astatic gastric cancer. A number of small randomized trials and a meta-analysis provide evidence for the benefit of systemic chemo-therapy as compared to supportive care alone for patients with advanced gastric cancer. In a meta-analysis of three trials compar-ing chemotherapy versus best supportive care, there was a signifi-cant benefit of chemotherapy in terms of overall survival (OS, HR 0.37), which translated into an improvement in median OS from 4.3 to 11 months. Effective cytotoxic agents for advanced gastric cancer include 5-fluorouracil (5-FU), oral fluoropyrimidines (S-1, capecit-abine), platinum agents (cisplatin, oxaliplatin), taxanes (docetaxel, paclitaxel), irinotecan, and anthracyclines, with reported response rate as single agents ranging between 10% and 40%.

First-line chemotherapy for gastric cancer

Systemic chemotherapy is indicated to patients with good general status, sufficient organ function, and without significant comorbid-ity. Since efficacy of chemotherapy is still limited and the purpose of chemotherapy is to prolong the OS, the indication of chemother-apy for patients with poor performance status, organ dysfunction, and comorbidity should be discussed cautiously.

Combination chemotherapy regimens are the treatment of choice in clinical practice based on meta-analysis of several ran-domized trials which showed a modest but statistically significant survival benefit of combination chemotherapy when compared to single-agent therapy, where the HR for death was 0.82. First-line regimens have resulted in median PFS of four to six months and median OS of around ten to 13 months. Doublet chemotherapy is currently the standard in many Asian countries, with preferred

regimens containing of a platinum compound, typically cisplatin, in combination with either infusion 5-FU or an oral fluoropyri-midines (S-1, capecitabine). In contrast, the ECF (epirubicin, cis-platin, infusional 5-FU) and DCF (or TCF, docetaxel, cisplatin, infusional 5-FU) combinations have regarded as standard regimens for first-line treatment in Western countries, primarily in Europe [111]. Oxaliplatin, a newer platinum agent is used in place of cis-platin in approved countries since at least comparable efficacy of oxaliplatin is reported in randomized studies.

Treatment regimens should be cautiously selected based on a patient's status. For example, cisplatin is contradicted to patients with severe renal dysfunction. The use of oral agents requires both patient sufficient compliance and gastrointestinal tract function. Patients with poor performance status might be a candidate for single-agent systemic chemotherapy or supportive care alone. The duration of chemotherapy for patients with advanced gastric cancer has not yet been specifically studied. In general, chemotherapies are given until the patient has progressive disease or unacceptable toxicities, although individualization is important based on each patient's tolerance and response to the treatment regimen, as well as the patient's preferences.

After the establishment of HER2 protein (human epidermal growth factor receptor type-2) as a new target of treatment for gastric cancer, HER2 positive gastric cancer has been treated with HER2 targeting therapy (i.e. trastuzumab). Patients with advanced gastric cancer should be screened for HER2 status. Detail of HER2 targeting treatment will be described later ('Targeting HER2').

Key clinical trials of cytotoxic chemotherapy are briefly discussed in Table 37.7.

Table 37.7 Results of pivotal phase III studies of first-line chemotherapy for unresectable gastric cancer (UGC)

Study	Main study area	N	Chemotherapy	OS (months)	PFS or TTP (months)	ORR (%)
V325	Europe, USA	445	5-FU+cisplatin	8.6	3.7	25
			5-FU+Cisplatin+docetaxel	9.2	5.6	37
JCOG9912	Japan	703	5-FU	10.8	2.2	9
			S-1	11.4	3.8	28
			Irinotecan+Cisplatin	12.3	4.8	38
SPIRITS	Japan	298	S1	11	4	31
			S1+cisplatin	13	6	54
FLAGS	Europe, USA	1053	5-FU+cisplatin	7.9	4.8	31.9
			S1+cisplatin	8.6	5.5	29.1
REAL-2	Europe	1002	epirubicin+5-FU+cisplatin	9.9	6.2	41
			epirubicin+capecitabine+cisplatin	9.9	6.7	46
			epirubicin+5-FU+oxaliplatin	9.3	6.5	42
			epirubicin+capecitabine+oxaliplatin	11.2	7	48
ML17032	Korea	316	5-FU+cisplatin	9.3	5	32
			capecitabine+cisplatin	10.5	5.6	46
ToGA	Global	584	capecitabine+cisplatin	11	5.5	34.5
			capecitabine+cisplatin+trastuzumab	13.8	6.7	47.3

OS, overall survival; PFS, progression-free survival: TTP, time-to progression: ORR, overall response rate.

In the V325 study, docetaxel plus cisplatin and 5-FU showed superior response rates, time to tumour progression, and survival in comparison with 5-FU and cisplatin [112]. Although DCF is approved by the US Food Drug Administration (FDA), a high incidence of febrile neutropenia is problematic. Various modifications of DCF have been evaluated in clinical trials.

The efficacy of the oral fluoropyrimidine derivative S-1 was shown in the Japanese phase III (JCOG 9912 trial) which evaluated non-inferiority of S-1 alone and superiority of irinotecan plus cisplatin over infusional 5-FU [113]. The response rate was higher with S1 than with 5-FU and median OS was 11.4 versus 12.3 months. The SPIRITS trial in Japan showed a significant benefit for combined S1 plus cisplatin over S1 alone in terms of both response rate and median survival [114]. Therefore, S-1 plus cisplatin is the Japanese standard chemotherapy. The FLAGS (First-Line Advanced Gastric Cancer Study) trial as a global phase III study did not show the superiority of S-1 plus cisplatin compared to infusional 5-FU plus cisplatin, although it showed a more favourable toxicity profile with S-1 plus cisplatin [115].

Capecitabine is another oral fluoropyrimidine. REAL-2 is a randomized phase III study in which 1002 patients with advanced gastric cancer were assigned, using a 2 x 2 factorial design, to three-weekly cycles of epirubicin plus cisplatin and either capecitabine or infusional 5-FU, or epirubicin plus oxaliplatin and either capecitabine or infusional 5-FU [109]. This study clearly showed non-inferiority of capecitabine to 5-FU and oxaliplatin to cisplatin. Oxaliplatin is associated with less neutropenia, anaemia, alopecia, and thromboembolic events than cisplatin. Sensory neuropathy and diarrhoea is more common with oxaliplatin. Similar results of non-inferiority of capecitabine to 5-FU were reported in another randomized trial (ML17032) which compared cisplatin plus either capecitabine or infusional 5-FU [116]. Based on these data, in clinical practice, many physicians select doublet combinations with either infusional 5-FU, capecitabine or S-1 combined with oxaliplatin (i.e. FOLFOX, XELOX, or S-1+oxaliplatin).

Second-line chemotherapy

For patients with an adequate performance status, utilization of other active agents not used in the first-line regimen is a reasonable option, either in combination or as serial single agents. At this time, there is no single standard approach for second-line therapy. Commonly used second-line agents after first-line 5-FU/fluoropyrimidines and platinum agents include irinotecan and taxanes. The survival benefit of second-line therapy was recently confirmed in randomized trials. In a Korean trial, patients with advanced gastric cancer and prior exposure to fluoropyrimidines and a platinum agent with good performance status were randomly assigned to best supportive care with or without chemotherapy (docetaxel or irinotecan). Second-line chemotherapy was associated with a significant improvement in median overall survival (5.3 versus 3.8 months) and patients were also significantly more likely to receive further salvage chemotherapy [117]. Similar survival befits with docetaxel compared with BSC was observed in another phase III trials in EU (COUGAR-02 [118]). Japanese trials (WJOG4407G) showed similar efficacy with weekly paclitaxel and irinotecan [119].

Recently, ramucirumab, an anti-vascular endothelial growth factor (VEGF) receptor antibody is reported to improve the prognosis of previously treated advanced gastric cancer. Detail of ramcirumab will be discussed below ('Targeting VEGF').

Biologic agents for gastric cancer
Targeting HER2

HER2 protein, also known as HER2/neu or ErbB2, is a transmembrane receptor with a molecular weight of 185 kDa, and its positivity is important for gastric cancer since HER2 positive patients are candidates for HER2 targeting agents. The HER family, after the activation of its receptor, enables transmission of the growth factor activation signal through the downstream signalling pathways, inducing cellular responses including cell proliferation, differentiation, and migration. Approximately 10–30% of gastric cancers over-express HER2, a similar percentage to that seen in breast cancer, although the definition of HER2 positivity is slightly different from that of breast cancer. HER2 status in gastric cancers is assessed in terms of HER2 protein expression by IHC and HER2 gene amplification by fluorescence in situ hybridization (FISH). HER2 expression is categorized into one of four levels (0, 1+, 2+, 3+) based upon a composite score that incorporates the intensity of staining and the percentage of cancer cells demonstrating that intensity. Patients with IHC +3 are considered to be HER2 positive. Patients with equivocal results (+2) should undergo FISH testing to confirm gene amplification. For interpretation of FISH, a HER2–CEP17 ratio of 2 or greater is considered to be HER2 amplified (FISH positive). HER2 positivity is more common in oesophagogastric cancer than distal gastric cancer. In addition, HER2 positivity is more common with intestinal-type than with diffuse-type gastric cancers.

Trastuzumab is an IgG1 monoclonal antibody against HER2 protein. Trastuzumab can specifically recognize the extracellular domain of HER2 and inhibit signalling. An antitumour activity of trastuzumab has also been reported and is due to antibody-depended cellular cytotoxicity.

The ToGA multiregional randomized trial was conducted to verify the clinical benefits of combination therapy with trastuzumab and standard chemotherapy (cisplatin and fluoropyrimidine (5-FU or capecitabine), FC) for patients with HER2-positive gastric cancers [120]. Among the samples screened, 22.1% were HER2 positive. The intestinal type exhibited a higher rate of HER2 positive than did the diffuse type (34% versus 6%); in addition, HER2 positivity was higher for adenocarcinoma of the oesophagogastric junction compared to gastric cancer (33.2% versus 20.9%). In the ToGA study, the median OS was significantly longer in the combination arm: 11.0 months for the FC arm versus 13.8 months for the FC + trastuzumab arm (HR 0.71, P = 0.0046). Both PFS and response rate were also significantly improved in the combination arm: 6.7 versus 5.5 months (HR 0.71, P = 0.0002) and 47.3% versus 34.5% (P = 0.0017), respectively. In the subset analysis of HER2 status, the effect of trastuzumab was more prominent for IHC2+/FISH+ or IHC3+ patients. The toxicities in the two arms were comparable, except that a higher number of trastuzumab-treated patients had grade 3 or 4 diarrhoea (9% versus 4%) and an asymptomatic decrease in left ventricular ejection fraction (5% versus 1%). From these results, for HER2-positive cases, trastuzumab showed a clear survival benefit, and the use of trastuzumab was approved in many countries. Additionally, results of retrospective subset analysis suggest that it is applicable for the group that is IHC2+/ IHC3+ and FISH positive. Controversy exists on whether to recommend trastuzumab in IHC 0-1+ cases that are FISH-positive. Randomized studies of several new agents (lapatinib, trastuzumab/emtansine and pertuzumab) are currently ongoing.

Targeting VEGF

The VEGF pathway is reported to play a role in tumour growth and is associated with poor prognosis in patients with several types of malignancies. The anti-VEGF monoclonal antibody has proven efficacy in several types of malignancies such as colon cancer, lung cancer, renal cancer, and ovarian cancer.

Ramucirumab is a fully humanized monoclonal antibody of VEGF receptor 2 (VEGFR-2). The REGARD trial was conducted in 30 countries to compare ramucirumab and best supportive care (BSC) with placebo as second-line treatment (following disease progression on first-line platinum or fluoropyrimidine-containing combination therapy) in a total of 355 patients [121]. The ramucirumab arm was associated with longer OS (5.2 versus 3.8 months; HR = 0.776; P = 0.04) and prolonged PFS.

Palliative care

The majority of patients with advanced gastric cancer will require palliative treatment at some point in the course of their disease. To alleviate tumour-related symptoms is an important aspect of treatment for advanced gastric cancer. For patients with poor performance status or patients who cannot tolerate intensive chemotherapy, supportive care alone is an appropriate treatment. Assessment of severity of the disease-related symptoms is essential to initiate appropriate palliative interventions that will prevent and relieve symptoms. Treatment options used for palliation of symptoms in patients with advanced gastric cancer include: gastrojejunostomy, endoscopic placement of a self-expandable metallic stent for gastric stenosis or obstruction; and pain control with pain medications and radiotherapy (especially for bone metastasis).

References

1. Fuchs CS, Mayer RJ. Gastric carcinoma. New England Journal of Medicine 1995; 333: 32–41.
2. Sugimura T. Studies on environmental chemical carcinogenesis in Japan. Science 1986; 233: 312–318.
3. Mannick E, Bravo L, Zarama G, Realpe JL, Zhang XJ et al. Inducible nitric oxide systhase, nitrotyrosine, and apoptosis in Helicobactor pylori gastritis: effect of antibiotics and antioxidants. Cancer Research 1996; 56: 3238–3243.
4. Correa P. Human gastric carcinogenesis: A mustistep and multifactorial process. First American Cancer Society Award Lecture on Cancer Epidemiology and Prevention. Cancer Research 1992; 52: 6735–6740.
5. Correa P, Houghton J. Carcinogenesis of Helicobactor pylori. Gastroenterology 2007; 133: 659–672.
6. Lauren PA. The two type histological main types of gastric carcinoma: diffuse and so-called intestinal type carcinoma. Acta pathologica, microbiologica, et immunologica Scandinavica 1965; 64: 31–49.
7. Solcia E, Fiocca R, Luinetti O, Villani L, Padovan L et al. Intestinal and diffuse gastric cancers arise in a different background of Helicobacter pylori gastritis through different gene involvement. American Journal of Surgical Pathology 1996; 20(Suppl. 1): S8.
8. Correa P, Haenszel W, Cuello C, Tannenbaum S, Archer M. A model for gastric cancer epidemiology. Lancet 1975; 2: 58.
9. Machado JC, Soares P, Carneiro F, Rocha A, Beck S et al. E-cadherin gene mutations provide a genetic basis for the phenotypic divergence of mixed gastric carcinomas. Laboratory Investigation 1999; 79: 459.
10. IARC Monographs on the Evaluation of Carcinogenic Risks to Humans. Schistosomes, Liver Flukes and Helicobacter pylori. Volume 61. Lyon: IARC, 1994, 177.
11. Huang JQ, Sridhar S, Chen Y, Hunt RH. Meta-analysis of the relationship between Helicobacter pylori seropositivity and gastric cancer. Gastroenterology 1998; 114: 1169.
12. Eslick GD, Lim LL, Byles JE, Xia HH, Talley NJ. Association of Helicobacter pylori infection with gastric carcinoma: a meta-analysis. American Journal of Gastroenterology 1999; 94: 2373.
13. Uemura N, Okamoto S, Yamamoto S, Matsumura N, Yamaguchi S et al. Helicobacter pylori infection and the development of gastric cancer. New England Journal of Medicine 2001; 345: 784.
14. Crowe SE. Helicobacter infection, chronic inflammation, and the development of malignancy. Current Opinion in Gastroenterology 2005; 21: 32.
15. Pignatelli B, Bancel B, Estève J, et al. Inducible nitric oxide synthase, anti-oxidant enzymes and Helicobacter pylori infection in gastritis and gastric precancerous lesions in humans. European Journal of Cancer Prevention 1998; 7: 439.
16. Lauwers GY, Scott GV, Hendricks J. Immunohistochemical evidence of aberrant bcl-2 protein expression in gastric epithelial dysplasia. Cancer 1994; 73: 2900.
17. Varro A, Noble PJ, Pritchard DM, Kennedy S, Hart CA et al. Helicobacter pylori induces plasminogen activator inhibitor 2 in gastric epithelial cells through nuclear factor-kappaB and RhoA: implications for invasion and apoptosis. Cancer Research 2004; 64: 1695.
18. El-Omar EM, Carrington M, Chow WH, McColl KE, Bream JH et al. Interleukin-1 polymorphisms associated with increased risk of gastric cancer. Nature 2000; 404: 398.
19. El-Omar EM, Rabkin CS, Gammon MD, Vaughan TL, Risch HA et al. Increased risk of noncardia gastric cancer associated with proinflammatory cytokine gene polymorphisms. Gastroenterology 2003; 124: 1193.
20. Yasui W, Oue N, Kuniyasu H, Ito R, Tahara E et al. Molecular diagnosis of gastric cancer: present and future. Gastric Cancer 2001; 4: 113.
21. van Grjeken NC, Aoyma T, Chambers PA, Bottomley D, Ward LC et al. KRAS and BRAF mutations are rare and related to DNA mismatch repair deficiency in gastric cancer from the East and the West: results from a large international multicentre study. British Journal of Cancer 2013; 108: 1495–1501.
22. Kim MA, Lee HS, Kim WH, Jeon YK, Yang HK et al. EGFR in gastric carcinomas: prognostic significance of protein overexpression and high gene copy number. Histopathology 2008; 52(6): 738–746.
23. Hynes NE, Lane HA. ERBB receptors and cancer: the complexity of targeted inhibitors. Nature Reviews Cancer 2005; 5, 341–354.
24. Carraway KL III, Sliwkowski MX, Nuijens A, Platko JV, Guy PM et al. The erbB3 gene product is a receptor for heregulin. Journal of Biological Chemistry 1994; 269: 14303–14306.
25. Burgess AW, Cho HS, Eigenbrot C, Ferguson KM, Garrett TP et al. An open-and-shut case? Recent insights into the acti- vation of EGF/ErbB receptors. Molecular Cell 2003; 12: 541–552.
26. Shi F, Telesco SE, Liu Y, Lemmon MA, Radhakrishnan R, Lemmon MA. ErbB3/HER3 intracellular domain is competent to bind ATP and catalyze autophosphorylation. Proceedings of the National Academy of Sciences USA 2010; 107: 7692–7697.
27. Birchmeier C, Birchmeier W, Gherardi E, Vande Woude GF. Met, metastasis, motility and more. Nature Reviews Molecular Cell Biology 2003; 4: 915–925.
28. Prat M, Narsimhan RP, Comoglio PM, Malaveille C, Calmels S et al. The receptor encoded by the human c-MET oncogene is expressed in hepatocytes, epithelial cells and solid tumors. International Journal of Cancer 1991; 49: 323–328.
29. Churin Y, Al-Ghoul L, Kepp O, Meyer TF, Birchmeier W et al. (2003). Helicobacter pylori CagA protein targets the c-Met receptor and enhances the motogenic response. Journal of Cell Biology 2003; 161: 249.
30. Yasui W, Sentani K, Motoshita J, Nakayama H. Molecular pathobiology of gastric cancer. Scandinavian Journal of Surgery 2006; 95: 225.
31. Morgan C, Jenkins GJ, Ashton T, Griffiths AP, Baxter JN et al. Detection of p53 mutations in precancerous gastric tissue. British Journal of Cancer 2003; 89: 1314.
32. Mingchao, Devereux TR, Stockton P, Sun K, Sills RC. Loss of E-cadherin expression in gastric intestinal metaplasia and later stage

p53 altered expression in gastric carcinogenesis. Experimental and Toxicologic Pathology 2001; 53: 237.

33. Ashktorab H, Ahmed A, Littleton G, Wang XW, Allen CR et al. p53 and p14 increase sensitivity of gastric cells to H. pylori-induced apoptosis. Digestive Diseases and Sciences 2003; 48: 1284.

34. Ushiku T, Chong JM, Uozaki H, Hino R, Chang MS et al. p73 gene promoter methylation in Epstein-Barr virus-associated gastric carcinoma. International Journal of Cancer 2007; 120: 60.

35. Tomkova K, Belkhiri A, El-Rifai W, Zaika AI. p73 isoforms can induce T-cell factor-dependent transcription in gastrointestinal cells. Cancer Research 2004; 64: 6390.

36. Fang DC, Luo YH, Yang SM, Li XA, Ling XL et al. Mutation analysis of APC gene in gastric cancer with microsatellite instability. World Journal of Gastoenterology 2002; 8: 787.

37. Staib F, Robles AI, Varticovski L, Wang XW, Zeeberg BR et al. The p53 tumor suppressor network is a key responder to microenvironmental components of chronic inflammatory stress. Cancer Research 2005; 65: 10255.

38. Akama Y, Yasui W, Yokozaki H, Kuniyasu H, Kitahara K et al. Frequent amplification of the cyclin E gene in human gastric carcinomas. Japanese Journal of Cancer Research 1995; 86: 617.

39. Takano Y, Kato Y, van Diest PJ, Masuda M, Mitomi H et al. (2000). Cyclin D2 overexpression and lack of p27 correlate positively and cyclin E inversely with a poor prognosis in gastric cancer cases. American Journal of Pathology 2000; 156: 585.

40. Clements WM, Wang J, Sarnaik A, Kim OJ, MacDonald J et al. beta-Catenin mutation is a frequent cause of Wnt pathway activation in gastric cancer. Cancer Research 2002; 62: 3503.

41. Kurayoshi M, Oue N, Kikuchi A, Kishida M, Inoue A et al. Expression of Wnt-5a is correlated with aggressiveness of gastric cancer by stimulating cell migration and invasion. Cancer Research 2006; 66: 10439–10448.

42. Tahara T, Arisawa T, Shibata T, Wang FY, Nakamura M et al. Risk prediction of gastric cancer by analysis of aberrant DNA methylation in non-neoplastic gastric epithelium. Digestion 2007; 75: 54.

43. Ushijima T, Sasako M. Focus on gastric cancer. Cancer Cell 2004; 5: 121–125.

44. Yamashita S, Tsujino Y, Ushijima T, Tatematsu M, Ushijima T et al. Chemical genomic screening for methylation-silenced genes in gastric cancer cell lines using 5-aza-2¢-deoxycytidine treatment and oligonucleotide microarray. Cancer Science 2006; 97: 64–71.

45. Takeshima H, Yamashita S, Ushijima T, Niwa T, Ushijima T et al. The presence of RNA polymerase II, active or stalled, predicts epigenetic fate of promoter CpG islands. Genome Research 2009; 19: 1974–1982.

46. Yokozaki H, Yasui W, Tahara E. Genetic and epigenetic changes in stomach cancer. International Review of Cytology 2001; 204: 49–95.

47. Hamamoto T, Yokozaki H, Miyazaki K, Yasui W, Yunotani S et al. Altered microsatellites in incomplete-type intestinal metaplasia adjacent to primary gastric cancers. Journal of Clinical Pathology 1997; 50: 841–846.

48. Toyota M, Ahuja N, Imai K, Itoh F, Ohe-Toyota M et al. Aberrant methylation in gastric cancer associated with the CpG island methylator phenotype. Cancer Research 1999; 59: 5438–5442.

49. Fleisher AS, Esteller M, Wang S, Tamura G, Suzuki H et al. Hypermethylation of the hMLH1 gene promoter in human gastric cancers with microsatellite instability. Cancer Research 1999; 59: 1090–1095.

50. Guilford, P, Hopkins, J, Harraway J, McLeod, M, McLeod N et al. E-cadherin germline mutations in familial gastric cancer. Nature 1998; 392: 402–405.

51. Barber M, Murrell A, Ito Y, Maia AT, Hyland S et al. Mechanisms and sequelae of E-cadherin silencing in hereditary diffuse gastric cancer. Journal of Pathology 2008; 216: 295.

52. Humar B, Graziano F, Cascinu S, Catalano V, Ruzzo AM et al. Association of CDH1 haplotypes with susceptibility to sporadic diffuse gastric cancer. Oncogene 2002; 21: 8192.

53. Tamura G, Yin J, Wang S, Fleisher AS, Zou T et al. E-Cadherin gene promoter hypermethylation in primary human gastric carcinomas. Journal of the National Cancer Institute 2000; 92: 569.

54. Hattori Y, Odagiri H, Terada M, Miyagawa K, Naito K et al. K-sam, an amplified gene in stomach cancer, is a member of the heparin-binding growth factor receptor genes. Proceedings of the National Academy of Sciences USA 1990; 87: 5983–5987.

55. Toyokawa T, Yashiro M, Hirakawa K. Co-expression of keratinocyte growth factor and K-sam is an independent prognostic factor in gastric carcinoma. Oncology Reports 2009; 21(4): 875–880.

56. Ito R, Kitadai Y, Kyo E, Yokozaki H, Yasui W et al. Interleukin 1 alpha acts as an autocrine growth stimulator for human gastric carcinoma cells. Cancer Research 1993; 53(17): 4102–4106.

57. Oue N, Motoshita J, Yasui W, Hayashi K, Tahara E et al. Distinct promoter hypermethylation of p16INK4a, CDH1, and RAR-beta in intestinal, diffuse-adherent, and diffuse-scattered type gastric carcinomas. Journal of Pathology 2002; 198(1): 55–59.

58. Yang L, Xie G, Fan Q, Xie J. Activation of the hedgehog-signaling pathway in human cancer and the clinical implications. Oncogene 2010; 29: 469–481.

59. Fukaya, M, Sasaki, H, Aoyagi K, Ochiya T et al. Hedgehog signal activation in gastric pit cell and in diffuse-type gastric cancer. Gastroenterology 2006; 131, 14–29.

60. Yeh TS, Wu CW, Chi CW, Liao WJ, Yang MC et al. The activated Notch1 signal pathway is associated with gastric cancer progression through cyclooxygenase-2. Cancer Research 2009; 69: 5039–5048.

61. Maehara Y, Kakeji Y, Sugimachi K, Rocha A, Beck S et al. Role of transforming growth factor-beta 1 in invasion and metastasis in gastric carcinoma. Journal of Clinical Oncology 1999; 17(2): 607–614.

62. Wu WK, Cho CH, Lee CW, Fan D, Wu K et al. Dysregulation of cellular signaling in gastric cancer. Cancer Letters 2010; 295(2): 144–153.

63. Ishimoto T, Nagano O, Saya H, Tamada M, Motohara T et al. CD44 variant regulates redox status in cancer cells by stabilizing the xCT subunit of system xc(-) and thereby promotes tumor growth. Cancer Cell 2011; 19(3): 387–400.

64. Cai C, Zhu X. The Wnt/b-catenin pathway regulates self-renewal of cancer stem-like cells in human gastric cancer. Molecular Medicine Report 2012; 5: 1191–1196.

65. Ishimoto T, Saya H, Nagano O, Kai K, Torii R et al. CD44+ slow-cycling tumor cell expansion is triggered by cooperative actions of Wnt and prostaglandin E2 in gastric tumorigenesis. Cancer Science 2010; 101(3): 673–678.

66. Fukase K, Kato M, Kikuchi S, Inoue K, Uemura N et al. Effect of eradication of Helicobacter pylori on incidence of metachronous gastric carcinoma after endoscopic resection of early gastric cancer: an openlabel, randomized controlled trial. Lancet 2008; 372: 392–397.

67. Morson BC, Sobin LH, Grundmann, E, Johansen A, Nagayo T et al. Precancerous conditions and epithelial dysplasia in the stomach. Journal of Clinical Pathology 1980; 33: 711–721.

68. Ochiai A, Yamauchi U, and Hirohashi S. p53 mutations in the non-neoplastic mucosa of the human stomach showing intestinal metaplasia. International Journal of Cancer 1996, 69: 28–33.

69. Ushijima T, Hattori N. Molecular pathways: involvement of Helicobacter pylori-triggered inflammation in the formation of an epigenetic field defect, and its usefulness as cancer risk and exposure markers. Clinical Cancer Research 2012; 18: 923–929.

70. Bosman, BT, Carneiro, F, Hruban, RH, Theise ND. WHO Classification of Tumors of the Digestive System. Lyon: International Agency for Research on Cancer, 2010.

71. Nakamura K, Sugano H Takagi, K, Kumakura K. Histogenesis of carcinoma of the stomach with special reference to 50 primary microcarcinomas. Light- and electron-microscopic and statistical studies. Japanese Journal of Clinical Oncology 1967; 15: 627–647.

72. Hirohashi S. Inactivation of the E-cadherin-mediated cell adhesion system in human cancers. American Journal of Pathology 1998, 153: 333–339.

73. Aizawa M, Nagatsuma AK, Kitada K, Kuwata T, Fujii S, et al. Evaluation of HER2-based biology in 1,006 cases of gastric cancer in a Japanese population. Gastric Cancer 2014; 17(1): 34–42.

74. Zang ZJ, Cutcutache I, Poon SL, Zang SL, McPherson JR et al. Exome sequencing of gastric adenocarcinoma identifies recurrent somatic mutations in cell adhesion and chromatin remodeling genes. Nature Genetics 2012; 44(5): 570–574.

75. Nagarajan N, Bertrand D, Hillmer AM, Zang ZJ, Yao F et al. Whole-genome reconstruction and mutational signatures in gastric cancer. Genome Biology 2012; 13(12): R115.

76. Japanese Gastric Cancer Association. Japanese gastric cancer treatment guidelines 2010 (ver. 3). Gastric Cancer 2011; 14: 113–123.

77. Bozzetti F, Marubini E, Bonfanti G, Miceli R, Piano C et al. Subtotal versus total gastrectomy for gastric cancer: five-year survival rates in a multicenter randomized Italian trial. Italian Gastrointestinal Tumor Study Group. Annals of Surgery 1999; 230: 170–178.

78. Ott K, Lordick F, Blank S, Buechler M. Gastric cancer: surgery in 2011. Langenbeck's Archives of Surgery 2011; 396: 743–758.

79. Sano T, Yamamoto S, Sasako M. Randomized controlled trial to evaluate splenectomy in total gastrectomy for proximal gastric carcinoma: Japan clinical oncology group study JCOG 0110-MF. Japanese Journal of Clinical Oncology 2002; 32: 363–364.

80. Sano T, Sasako M, Yamamoto S, Nashimoto A, Kurita A. Gastric cancer surgery: morbidity and mortality results from a prospective randomized controlled trial comparing D2 and extended para-aortic lymphadenectomy—Japan Clinical Oncology Group study 9501. Journal of Clinical Oncology 2004; 22: 2767–2773.

81. Sasako M, Sano T, Yamamoto S, Kurokawa Y, Nashimoto A et al. D2 lymphadenectomy alone or with para-aortic nodal dissection for gastric cancer. New England Journal of Medicine 2008; 359: 453–462.

82. Japanese Gastric Cancer Association. Japanese classification of gastric carcinoma, 3rd English ed. Gastric Cancer 2011; 14: 101–112.

83. Nishi M, Omori Y, Miwa K. Japanese Classification of Gastric Carcinoma. Tokyo: Kanehara & Co, 1995.

84. Cuschieri A, Fayers P, Fielding J, Craven J, Bancewicz J et al. Postoperative morbidity and mortality after D1 and D2 resections for gastric cancer: preliminary results of the MRC randomised controlled surgical trial. The Surgical Cooperative Group. Lancet 1996; 347: 995–999.

85. Cuschieri A, Weeden S, Fielding J, Bancewicz J, Craven J et al. Patient survival after D1and D2 resections for gastric cancer: long-term results of the MRC randomized surgical trial. Surgical Co-operative Group. British Journal of Cancer 1999; 79: 1522–1530.

86. Bonenkamp JJ, Songun I, Hermans J, Sasako M, Welvaart K et al. Randomised comparison of morbidity after D1 and D2 dissection for gastric cancer in 996 Dutch patients. Lancet 1995; 345: 745–748.

87. Bonenkamp JJ, Hermans J, Sasako M, van de Velde CJ, Welvaart K et al. Extended lymph-node dissection for gastric cancer. New England Journal of Medicine 1999; 340: 908–914.

88. Hartgrink HH, van de Velde CJ, Putter H, Bonenkamp JJ, Klein Kranenbarg E et al. Extended lymph node dissection for gastric cancer: who may benefit? Final results of the randomized Dutch gastric cancer group trial. Journal of Clinical Oncology 2004; 22: 2069–2077.

89. Songun I, Putter H, Kranenbarg EM, Sasako M, van de Velde CJ. Surgical treatment of gastric cancer: 15-year follow-up results of the randomised nationwide Dutch D1D2 trial. Lancet Oncology 2010; 11: 439–449.

90. NCCN Guidelines Version 2. Gastric Cancer. NCCN, 2011, <http://www.nccn.org/professionals/physician_gls/f_guidelines.asp>.

91. Degiuli M, Sasako M, Ponti A. Morbidity and mortality in the Italian Gastric Cancer Study Group randomized clinical trial of D1 versus D2 resection for gastric cancer. British Journal of Surgery 2010; 97: 643–649.

92. Wu CW, Hsiung CA, Lo SS, Hsieh MC, Chen JH et al. Nodal dissection for patients with gastric cancer: a randomised controlled trial. Lancet Oncology 2006; 7: 309–315.

93. Kitano S, Iso Y, Moriyama M, Sugimachi K. Laparoscopy-assisted Billroth I gastrectomy. Surgical Laparoscopy Endoscopy & Percutaneous Techniques 1994; 4: 146–148.

94. Katai H, Sasako M, Fukuda H, Nakamura K, Hiki N et al. Safety and feasibility of laparoscopy-assisted distal gastrectomy with suprapancreatic nodal dissection for clinical stage I gastric cancer: a multicenter phase II trial (JCOG 0703). Gastric Cancer 2010; 13: 238–244.

95. Kim HH, Hyung WJ, Cho GS, Kim MC, Han SU et al. Morbidity and mortality of laparoscopic gastrectomy versus open gastrectomy for gastric cancer: an interim report—a phase III multicenter, prospective, randomized Trial (KLASS Trial). Annals of Surgery 2010; 251(3): 417–420.

96. Wei HB, Wei B, Qi CL, Chen TF, Huang Y et al. Laparoscopic versus open gastrectomy with D2 lymph node dissection for gastric cancer: a meta-analysis. Surgical Laparoscopy Endoscopy & Percutaneous Techniques 2011; 21: 383–390.

97. Uyama I, Sugioka A, Fujita J, Komori Y, Matsui H et al. Laparoscopic total gastrectomy with distal pancreatosplenectomy and D2 lymphadenectomy for advanced gastric cancer. Gastric Cancer 1999; 2: 230–234.

98. SEER Cancer Statistics, <http://www.seer.cancer.gov/statistics/>, accessed on 24 May 2012.

99. Matsuda T, Ajiki W, Marugame T, Ioka A, Tsukuma H et al. Population-based survival of cancer patients diagnosed between 1993 and 1999 in Japan: a chronological and international comparative study. Japanese Journal of Clinical Oncology 2011; 41(1): 40–51.

100. Parkin DM. Global cancer statistics in the year 2000. Lancet Oncology 2001; 2(9): 533–543.

101. Macdonald JS, Smalley SR, Benedetti J, Hundahl SA, Estes NC et al. Chemoradiotherapy after surgery compared with surgery alone for adenocarcinoma of the stomach or gastroesophageal junction. New England Journal of Medicine 2001; 345(10): 725–730.

102. Smalley SR, Benedetti JK, Haller DG, Hundahl SA, Estes NC. Updated analysis of SWOG-Directed Intergroup Study 0116: a phase III trial of adjuvant radiochemotherapy versus observation after curative gastric cancer resection. Journal of Clinical Oncology 2012; 30(19): 2327–2333.

103. Lee J, Lim DH, Kim S, Park SH, Park JO et al. Phase III trial comparing capecitabine plus cisplatin versus capecitabine plus cisplatin with concurrent capecitabine radiotherapy in completely resected gastric cancer with d2 lymph node dissection: the ARTIST trial. Journal of Clinical Oncology 2011; 30(3): 268–273.

104. Cunningham D, Allum WH, Stenning SP, Thompson JN, Van de Velde CJ et al. Perioperative chemotherapy versus surgery alone for resectable gastroesophageal cancer. New England Journal of Medicine 2006; 355(1): 11–20.

105. Ychou M, Boige V, Pignon JP, Conroy T, Bouche O et al. Perioperative chemotherapy compared with surgery alone for resectable gastroesophageal adenocarcinoma: an FNCLCC and FFCD multicenter phase III trial. Journal of Clinical Oncology 2011; 29(13): 1715–1721.

106. Paoletti X, Oba K, Burzykowski T, Michiels S, Ohashi Y et al. Benefit of adjuvant chemotherapy for resectable gastric cancer: a meta-analysis. Journal of the American Medical Association 2010; 303(17): 1729–1737.

107. Sakuramoto S, Sasako M, Yamaguchi T, Kinoshita T, Fujii M et al. Adjuvant chemotherapy for gastric cancer with S-1, an oral fluoropyrimidine. New England Journal of Medicine 2007; 357(18): 1810–1820.

108. Sasako M, Sakuramoto S, Katai H, Kinoshita T, Furukawa H et al. Five-year outcomes of a randomized phase III trial comparing adjuvant chemotherapy with s-1 versus surgery alone in stage II or III gastric cancer. Journal of Clinical Oncology 2011; 29(33): 4387–4393.

109. Cunningham D, Starling N, Rao S, Iveson T, Nicolson M et al. Capecitabine and oxaliplatin for advanced esophagogastric cancer. New England Journal of Medicine 2008; 358: 36–46.

110. Bang YJ, Kim YW, Yang HK, Chung HC, Park YK et al. Adjuvant capecitabine and oxaliplatin for gastric cancer after D2 gastrectomy (CLASSIC): a phase 3 open-label, randomised controlled trial. Lancet 2012; 379(9813): 315–321.

111. National Comprehensive Cancer Network. NCCN Guidelines for Gastric Cancer 2013 ver. 3. Fort Washington, PA: NCCN, 2013.

112. Van Cutsem E, Moiseyenko VM, Tjulandin S, Majlis A, Constenia M et al. Phase III study of docetaxel and cisplatin plus fluorouracil compared with cisplatin and fluorouracil as first-line therapy for advanced gastric cancer: a report of the V325 Study Group. Journal of Clinical Oncology 2006; 24: 4991–4997.

113. Boku N, Yamamoto S, Fukuda H, Shirao K, Doi T et al. Fluorouracil versus combination of irinotecan plus cisplatin versus S-1 in metastatic gastric cancer: a randomised phase 3 study. Lancet Oncology 2009; 10: 1063–1069.

114. Koizumi W, Narahara H, Hara T, Takagane A, Akiya T et al. S-1 plus cisplatin versus S-1 alone for first-line treatment of advanced gastric cancer (SPIRITS trial): a phase III trial. Lancet Oncology 2008; 9: 215–221.

115. Ajani JA, Rodriguez W, Bodoky G, Moiseyenko V, Lichinitser M et al. Multicenter phase III comparison of cisplatin/S-1 with cisplatin/infusional fluorouracil in advanced gastric or gastroesophageal adenocarcinoma study: the FLAGS trial. Journal of Clinical Oncology 2010; 28: 1547–1553.

116. Kang YK, Kang WK, Shin DB, Chen J, Xiong J et al. Capecitabine/cisplatin versus 5-fluorouracil/cisplatin as first-line therapy in patients with advanced gastric cancer: a randomised phase III noninferiority trial. Annals of Oncology 2009; 20: 666–673.

117. Kang JH, Lee SI, Lim DH, Park KW, Oh SY et al. Salvage chemotherapy for pretreated gastric cancer: a randomized phase III trial comparing chemotherapy plus best supportive care with best supportive care alone. Journal of Clinical Oncology 2012; 30, 1513–1518.

118. Ford H, Marshall A, Wadsley J, Coxon FY, Mansoor W. A randomized phase III study of docetaxel versus active symptom control in advanced esophagogastric adenocarcinoma. Journal of Clinical Oncology 2013; 30(Suppl. 34): abs. LBA4.

119. Ueda S, Hironaka S, Yasui H, Nishina T, Tsuda M et al. Randomized phase III study of irinotecan (CPT-11) versus weekly paclitaxel (wPTX) for advanced gastric cancer (AGC) refractory to combination chemotherapy (CT) of fluoropyrimidine plus platinum (FP): WJOG4007 trial. Journal of Clinical Oncology 2012; 30(suppl.): abs. 4002.

120. Bang YJ, Van Cutsem E, Feyereislova A, Chung HC, Shen L et al. Trastuzumab in combination with chemotherapy versus chemotherapy alone for treatment of HER2-positive advanced gastric or gastro-oesophageal junction cancer (ToGA): a phase 3, open-label, randomised controlled trial. Lancet 2010; 376: 687–697.

121. Fuchs CS, Tomasek J, Cho JY, Dumitru F, Passalacqua R et al. REGARD: A phase III, randomized, double-blind trial of ramucirumab and best supportive care (BSC) versus placebo and BSC in the treatment of metastatic gastric or gastroesophageal junction (GEJ) adenocarcinoma following disease progression on first-line platinum- and/or fluoropyrimidine-containing combination therapy. Journal of Clinical Oncology 2013; 30(Suppl. 34): abs. LBA5.

CHAPTER 38

Rectal cancer and systemic therapy of colorectal cancer

Regina Beets-Tan, Bengt Glimelius, and Lars Påhlman

Introduction to rectal cancer

Approximately every third colorectal cancer (CRC) starts in the rectum. There is no clear demarcation border between rectum and colon although the likely most used definition is that cancers starting up to 15 cm above the anal verge are referred to as rectal cancers. The great majority of CRC are adenocarcinoma and there are great similarities in many aspects between the two anatomical regions. Therefore, in order to avoid overlap, the epidemiology, risk factors, molecular genetics, inherited syndromes, pathology and screening are described in the chapter on colon cancer, whereas staging, follow-up, and treatment of metastatic disease are dealt with in this chapter on rectal cancer.

Surgical removal of all known disease is basically the only therapy that can cure a patient with CRC. The exception is small rectal cancers that can either be treated with endoluminal contact radiotherapy/brachytherapy or that are sufficiently sensitive to chemoradiotherapy.

The cured fraction can be slightly elevated by additional pre- or post-operative radiotherapy and/or post-operative chemotherapy. Surgery is not always possible, either because the disease cannot be resected (inextirpable primary or multiple secondaries), or for general reasons (very high age or severe concomitant diseases). Today, approximately 40% of the patients with rectal cancer are left with palliative treatments, either primarily or because of a recurrence later during the course of the disease. The treatment armamentarium has markedly expanded during the past decade, partly because of significant increased knowledge about the genetic pathways of CRC development. This has resulted in improved overall survival, although the survival gains have been rather modest.

For an explanation of the epidemiology, molecular biology, and pathology of rectal cancer, please refer to Chapter 39.

Surgical management of rectal cancer

Diagnosis and staging of colorectal cancer

CRC is presently staged according to TNM7 from 2010 [1]. A new version of TNM is presented every five to ten years based on new knowledge. There are presently controversies as to the best version, and some countries use TNM5, mainly because of concerns about stage migration caused by different criteria for lymph node metastases [2]. The major criteria for staging colorectal cancer can be found on the website of the American Cancer Society [3].

Most patients with rectal cancer have some type of symptoms like bleeding, without or with anaemia, mucous discharge, or changes in bowel habits. Pain may be a sign of a large tumour growing outside the bowel wall into the pelvic sidewall, and weight loss a sign of distant metastases. Some villous adenomas have a profound mucous production leading to symptoms of diarrhoea and problems with major discharge with decreased serum potassium and sodium.

Once there is a suspicion of a rectal adenoma or malignancy, endoscopy should be performed. The whole rectum can, without any problem, be examined with a flexible sigmoidoscope and is preferable. However, when measuring the distance from the anal verge to the tumour it is more accurate to use a rigid rectoscope. Biopsies taken with a flexible sigmoidoscope are often too small and for this reason it is also preferable to change to a rigid rectoscope to take larger biopsies for diagnosis. Small polyps, less than 1 cm, are rarely malignant but the larger the polyp the higher the risk of malignancy. Adenomas larger than 2.5 cm have malignant transformation in about 25% [4]. Sometimes it is difficult to distinguish whether or not large villous adenomas are malignant.

A digital examination is of outmost importance to evaluate whether or not the tumour is fixed to the wall, tethered to the surrounding fat, or is an early tumour confined to the bowel wall [5]. The relation to the pelvic floor and the puborectal sling gives important information as to whether a sphincter-preserving procedure can be carried out or if the patient requires an abdominoperineal resection [5]. Based on the digital examination, endorectal ultrasonography (ERUS) for an early lesion will disclose whether the tumour is growing into or through muscularis propria [6]. If the tumour is more advanced, the mesorectal fascia (MRF) is of greatest interest and a magnetic resonance imaging (MRI) investigation is essential [7, 8].

Preoperatively, a 'clean colon' examination has to be done to rule out whether synchronous lesions are present. Preferably this is done with colonoscopy, but computed tomography (CT) colonography is also used [9]. Moreover, the liver and lungs have to be examined to disclose distant metastatic disease. This is done with CT of thorax and abdomen; in cases of equivocal CT findings PET/CT may give more information.

See Chapter 30 'Population cancer screening' for a discussion of screening in colorectal cancer.

Imaging of rectal cancer

Introduction to imaging of rectal cancer

The treatment of rectal cancer had been plagued by high local recurrence rates until the role of a good surgical technique and additional (chemo)radiotherapy ((C)RT) was fully appreciated. (C)RT is more effective when given before, rather than after the resection [10–12]. Previously, decisions on post-operative treatment were based on the risk assessment for recurrence through histological evaluation of the surgical specimen. Decisions on preoperative treatment must be based on risk assessment through clinical evaluation and imaging. Although modern CT techniques can provide information for locoregional and distant staging, ERUS and MRI are the two best imaging methods for rectal cancer local staging and recommended as part of standard workup. The radiologist's role in the multidisciplinary management has become crucial. In addition to a reliable prediction of certain risk factors for local recurrence, the imaging findings will have clinical consequences and dictate both treatment strategy and treatment details such as surgical approach and radiotherapy volumes.

Risk factors for local recurrence

Histopathological risk factors for local and distant recurrence are T stage, N stage, distance of the tumour to the circumferential resection margin (CRM), perineural invasion, lymph and blood vessel invasion, and grade [13–15]. It is unrealistic to expect 100% accuracy from any imaging technology in predicting the histological classification; imaging is, however, helpful in predicting risks for recurrence with volume and relation to anatomical structures as main prognostic variables.

Tumour stage

Since the mid-1980s ERUS has been used to assess tumour growth into the bowel [16, 17]. It is superior to all other imaging techniques in visualizing all layers of the rectal wall, with three hyperechoic and two hypoechoic bands, corresponding to the anatomic layers and the interfaces between them. It is generally considered that ERUS is good in imaging smaller tumours. For large lesions, ERUS can identify ingrowth in surrounding structures that are within the field of view such as vagina, prostate, and seminal vesicles. Difficulties of ERUS arise with tumours located high in the rectum and stenosing tumours that are beyond the reach of the endosonography probe. The overall limited field of view provides insufficient anatomical information on the posterior extent of the tumour into the mesorectal fascia and pelvic wall.

The distinction between a T2 and a T3 tumour is usually straightforward histologically. This does not always easily transfer to staging through imaging. Although imaging may provide accurate information on the size of the tumour, both MRI and ERUS will have difficulties in predicting the exact microscopic relationship to a histological interface. Reports have shown MRI accuracies for T staging varying between 65% and 86%. MRI is accurate for identifying large T3 and T4 tumours with sensitivities for prediction of T3 varying between 80% and 86% and specificities between 71% and 76%. MRI is the technique of preference to map the tumour and, in contrast to ERUS, anatomical information from MRI is less subject to interobserver variations [18]. Most staging failures with MRI occur in the differentiation of tumours at the interface of rectal wall layers, i.e. the distinction between T1 and T2 lesions and between T2 and borderline T3 lesions. A T1 tumour cannot be reliably distinguished from T2 because the submucosal layer is generally not visualized on MRI. MRI has difficulties in determining lesions on the border of T2 and T3 if the tumour shows spiculations corresponding with desmoplastic reaction. In a large

European study (MERCURY), MRI was accurate in predicting the extramural depth of tumour ingrowth in the mesorectum, a prognostic factor that is not part of the TNM staging system.

Mesorectal fascia (MRF)

The importance of the involvement of the MRF as a prognostic factor has been recognized and confirmed in the past 20 years [14]. The ideal plane of resection in a total mesorectal excision (TME) is just outside MRF, and a positive CRM can be the result of inadequate TME surgery. An involved MRF is defined as a closest distance of ≤ 1 mm between tumour and the MRF, as this represents an important prognostic cut-off point.

While a positive CRM is a problem of surgical technique, an involved MRF is a matter of preoperative identification of the advanced tumours for an adequate preoperative treatment. These patients should be identified with MRI. Furthermore, regardless of the preoperative treatment, it is important for the surgeon to know the exact anatomical relation of the tumour to the MRF and surrounding structures in order to obtain a complete resection.

Many single-centre studies have shown that MRI is highly accurate for the prediction of an involved MRF [18–20]. Because of the accurate depiction of the tumour mass in relation to the MRF it is often said that with MRI 'what you see is what you get' (Figure 38.1).

A systematic review confirms the high performance of MRI, showing sensitivities between 60% and 88% and specificities between 73% and 100% [7]. The MERCURY study [8] showed a sensitivity of 59% and specificity of 92%. Centres can report a decrease in the number of positive margins after the incorporation of MRI and discussion of all rectal cancer patients in multidisciplinary meetings [21, 22].

Nodal stage

Identifying nodal disease with imaging remains difficult because using size criteria alone results in only moderate accuracy. Lymph nodes with a diameter of ≥10 mm are invariably malignant, but the majority of involved nodes are smaller than 5 mm [23]. In addition to size, with 5 mm as the cut-off, ERUS also uses roundness, border irregularity, and hypoechoic nature as criteria for malignancy. For MRI the same criteria of roundness and border irregularity are used, and heterogeneous signals provide additional accuracy over size alone [24, 25]. This can be of help in evaluating nodes that are larger than 5 mm, but characterization of smaller nodes is not reliable. The difficulties in nodal staging with the standard imaging methods are illustrated by a multicentre report in which cT3N0 tumours, staged with ERUS or MRI were node positive at histology in 22%, despite preoperative CRT [26].

MRI techniques are continuously improving, and with modern machines, new sequences, and lymph-node-specific MR contrast agents the accuracy will improve. An example is ultrasmall superparamagnetic particles of iron oxide (USPIO) that showed higher accuracy for lymph node characterization in prostate and rectal cancer [27]. USPIO is not available for regular use because it is not FDA approved.

How does one work in practice with a suboptimal accuracy of preoperative lymph node imaging? One approach is to rely on imaging information on nodal status only when the tumour is associated with round large nodes (>5 mm) that are irregular in border and/or heterogeneous in signal or echogenicity. Whenever these criteria for node positivity are absent on ERUS or MRI, information on nodal

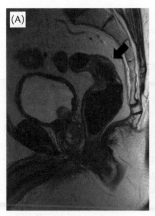
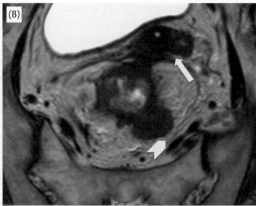

Fig. 38.1 (A) A sagittal MR image of a male patient with a high rectal tumour (black arrow) confined to the bowel wall. MRI visualizes a resectable tumour at distance from the TME resection plane. (B) An axial MR image of a female patient with a T4 rectal tumour, invading the cervix anteriorly (white arrow). Laterodorsal on the left side the tumour threatens but does not invade the mesorectal fascia (white arrow head).

status is not reliable. Another approach is to disregard the imaging data on nodal status and give preoperative treatment in most patients according to T (sub)stage, accepting over-treatment rather than under-treatment. A third approach is to take into account the prevalence of nodal metastases according to T (sub)stage and give neoadjuvant therapy for T3NX lesions, regardless of nodal imaging results, but not for T2 (or T3a/b) N0 lesions [26]. It can be argued that the small volume nodal disease that is easily missed by imaging is prognostically less important for local recurrence and may be controlled by good TME surgery [28]. Although there are no real data to support or refute any of the above approaches, the most practical strategy seems to be to use the information on lymph node staging in the preoperative decision making, keeping in mind the suboptimal accuracy. Erring on the safe side, large tumours or tumours extending deep into the subserosa or close to MRF can be treated preoperatively irrespective of the nodal status.

Restaging after chemoradiotherapy

For rectal tumours that respond well to preoperative CRT, restaging by MRI is useful but only if the surgeon will act upon the imaging findings. If the latter is the case, the surgeon needs to know whether the tumour has regressed from an anticipated involved resection plane, so a less extensive resection can be considered. Accurate restaging is becoming more relevant nowadays with discussions on organ-saving treatment.

Tumour regression from the MRF

Literature shows consistent results on the performance of MRI for assessment of tumour regression from the MRF. The overall accuracy for prediction of MRF involvement after (C)RT is around 80% with NPVs up to 90% [29, 30]. The high NPV is at the expense of 50% positive predictive value (PPV), mainly due to the difficulties in interpretation of fibrosis. A fibrotic thickening of the MRF is in 50% associated with viable small clusters of tumour in the fibrosis. To be on the safe side and prevent under-treatment a high false positivity is more acceptable than a high false negativity.

Tumour and nodal downstaging

The same difficulties in interpreting fibrosis also occur with a fibrotic tumour bed after irradiation. If morphological MRI only is used, it leads to inaccurate assessment of tumour downstaging

and over-estimation of tumour remnant. If morphologic MR features and MR volumetric changes of the tumour are combined, the assessment of an ypT0-2 tumour can increase the accuracy from 78% to 87% [31, 32]. PPV in these studies increases to 94%. One should bear in mind, however, that a learning curve exists. A general radiologist who has no previous training in pelvic MRI reaches the level of an expert reader after 60 to 80 MRIs.

Crucial in the selection of organ-saving treatment is the identification of node negativity. Up to 45% of visible nodes disappear and another 40% decrease in size (unpublished data). Sterilization of nodes is reported in a significant proportion after (C)RT. Restaging the nodes with MRI is more accurate than with ERUS [26]. MRI studies from recent years have reported accuracies of 67–90% and negative predictive values (NPVs) of 83–93% for MR nodal staging after (C)RT. Accepting some false positives, patients with sterilized nodes can be reliably identified on standard MRI.

Future perspectives and conclusions

The most promising development is the non-invasive assessment of imaging biomarkers by metabolic and functional imaging. FDG-PET/CT is promising for assessment of response during and after CRT. MRI is evolving as a competitive alternative because of its versatility and higher cost-efficiency. In addition to detailed information on morphology, MRI provides information on tumour heterogeneity by evaluating local tumour perfusion (dynamic contrast enhanced MRI) and diffusional capacity (diffusion weighted MRI) [33]. The introduction of new hybrid MR/PET machines in clinics will speed up the availability of a fast and accurate whole body staging process. Image reconstruction technology also evolves rapidly by automatically reconstructing and calculating complex quantification data.

In the multidisciplinary treatment of rectal cancer there is an increased demand for accurate selection of patients for individual tailoring of treatment, both at primary staging and at restaging after preoperative treatment. MRI has a prominent role in this decision-making strategy. While ERUS remains the most cost-efficient method in the workup of small superficial tumours, MRI is the preferred modality to assess the extent of large tumours. Nodal staging is at present not sufficiently reliable, although slightly more accurate in the restaging setting. Restaging MRI after (C)RT is useful, if alteration of treatment plan is considered. MRI can evaluate tumour downsizing and downstaging and can predict tumour regression from the planned surgical resection plane.

Principles of surgery

Management of rectal polyps

It is essential to evaluate the histopathological features of polyps in the rectum. Hyperplastic polyps can most often be ignored whereas adenomas have to be followed up. If there are several hyperplastic polyps (more than five) in the rectum, many claim that the whole colon has to be investigated, to secure that no malignancy further proximally is present [34]. There is no good study that shows that proximal neoplasms are found more often if several hyperplastic polyps are seen during sigmoidoscopy than if no pathology is detected. If adenomas are found, the whole colon must be examined to detect proximal tumours. If there are numerous adenomas, familiar adenomatous polyposis (FAP) must be suspected and the family history should be explored. Patients with FAP should be screened for mutations in the APC gene and based upon that mutation it is possible to screen the whole family with a simple blood test.

The majority of the polyps and adenomas can be handled by endoscopic removal. Sessile adenomas with a broad base (more than 1 cm) should preferably be removed with a TEM (transanal endoscopic microsurgery) technique [35]. Very experienced endoscopists can remove such an adenoma with the EMR (endoscopic mucosa resection) technique [36]. With TEM, a full thickness biopsy into the fat can be done. It is then possible to evaluate how deep a cancer has grown.

Management of rectal cancers

The gold standard treatment for rectal cancer is resection of the diseased bowel segment. The technique in the upper and middle rectum is exactly the same whether or not a sphincter-preserving procedure or an abdominoperineal excision is carried out. However, in small tumours confined to the mucosa or bowel wall, a local excision preferably with the TEM technique can be considered.

Preoperative preparation

The distance from the anal verge to the tumour and the relation to the pelvic floor and the puborectal sling are the landmarks for the decision as to whether or not a sphincter-preserving procedure can be carried out. With this information together with the preoperative MRI it is possible to evaluate if the tumour can be radically (R0) resected without a stoma. This is especially important in low-lying tumours if an intersphincteric procedure is planned. Preoperative bowel preparation is important, particularly if a sphincter-preserving procedure is to be carried out, since the majority of these patients today will have a functioning ileostomy and the bowel should be empty during the healing period of the anastomosis [37, 38]. If an abdominoperineal excision is planned, an enema to empty the left colon is sufficient. The day before surgery it is important to mark the stoma site. The patient should have prophylactic antibiotic cover before surgery [39] and prophylaxis for venous thromboembolism. The thrombosis prophylaxis should be longer than the hospital stay, preferably until one month after surgery, since longer prophylaxis than eight to ten days reduces the thrombosis risk even further without causing more adverse effects [40].

Surgical technique

There should be no difference in the procedure whether the operation is carried out as open surgery or laparoscopically, but both approaches must follow the TME technique (Figure 38.2) [41]. In the open technique, it is most often easier to start to mobilize the sigmoid from the left side and identify the ureter and also the hypogastric nerves and enter the correct plane under the sigmoid colon. Having carried out the same procedure on the right side, the vessels to the rectum can be divided. If working laparoscopically, most surgeons prefer to start on the right side, but the mobilization

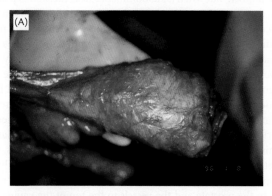

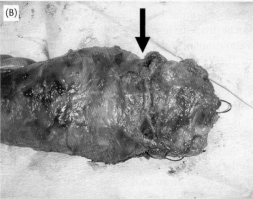

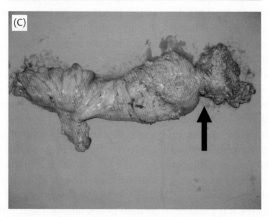

Fig. 38.2 (A) Surgical specimen after a low anterior resection for a rectal cancer using the TME-technique with dissection outside the mesorectal fascia (shining on the picture). (B) Surgical specimen after an abdominal excision where the abdominal dissection was stopped appropriately prior to the perineal dissection to avoid coning. (C) Coning into the puborectal muscle creating a waist was done, increasing the risk of a non-radical resection.

in the abdomen, control of the nerves, and vessel ligation are identical. Some prefer a 'high tie' division of the vessels, which means that the inferior mesenteric artery is divided flush to the aorta. 'Low tie' indicates that the first branch of the inferior mesenteric artery, arteria rectalis superior, is divided. It has been debated whether a 'low tie' will change the cancer outcome. However, cancer positive lymph nodes in that short distance, from the aorta to the first division of the inferior mesenteric artery (1–2 cm), indicate disseminated disease beyond any chance of surgical cure and therefore most surgeons divide the vessel dependent upon what is needed for the surgery [42]. If a low anterior resection is planned, it is often convenient to do a 'high tie' in order to have sufficient bowel length to reach down, but when an abdominoperineal excision is planned, where the sigmoid colon is taken out as a stoma, a 'low tie' is enough.

Once the vessels have been divided and the hypogastric nerves identified, the non-vascular plane dorsally around the MRF is identified and followed down into the pelvis. Most often it is easy to do this posteriorly first and then go laterally on both sides. Anteriorly, in men, part of the bladder peritoneum should be included in the resection. The vesicles are identified and it is often easy to find the correct plane anterior to the Denonvilliers' fascia. In women, the posterior fornix of the vagina should be identified in a similar way but this is often more difficult with some bleeding from veins. Once the anterior or posterior plane is released, the lateral part of the dissection will continue. Care has to be taken not to destroy the nerves going to the prostate and the vessels to the top of the vagina. This area has been called the 'lateral ligaments' but they are nerves and should not be divided. However, in approximately 10% a mid-rectal artery is also running in this structure, which can be easily handled with care. There should not be any sexual disturbances after a rectal cancer dissection provided that the nerves are moved aside [43]. If the tumour grows into the nerves, they of course must be sacrificed.

If an anterior resection is planned, the dissection will continue down to the top of the pelvic floor. The rectum is then divided below the tumour with a straight stapler. Before this, an enema to wash out the rectal stump is advisable since data support that this decreases the risk of local recurrence [44]. The question is whether it is necessary to go down to the pelvic floor in all rectal cancer patients when a sphincter-preserving procedure is planned. Often it is easier to do a TME. But in cancers in the upper rectum, particularly in females, one can stop the dissection below the tumour if the division is done at least 5 cm distally of the tumour. The 5 cm rule is essential in high rectal cancers in order to remove all potential tumour deposits in the mesorectum [45], but in low rectal cancers one can accept a lesser margin provided that a TME is done [46]. In the bowel wall, a 1 cm margin is enough if a sphincter-preserving procedure is carried out [47].

If an abdominoperineal excision is planned, the abdominal dissection should be stopped at the level of the top of the vagina or the seminal vesicles. Otherwise there is a risk of coning into the puborectal muscle and creating a wrist on the specimen with a high risk of positive CRM (Figure 38.2). By stopping the abdominal phase in this area it is possible to go from below outside the sphincters, follow the levator muscles, and come to the abdominal resection plane without coning. The risk of CRM positivity and consequently a local recurrence will then be less. The perineal part of the procedure can be done in patients in lithotomy or prone position [48]. Most surgeons advocate the prone position mainly because it is then easier to teach others how to do it.

Open or laparoscopic surgery

There is still a debate as to whether rectal cancer surgery should be carried out laparoscopically or not. Data from a randomized trial indicates that both the short-term and long-term results are the same [49–52]. A new trend is to do these operations with robotics [53]. One randomized trial is finished, the ROLARR-trial, and preliminary data are awaited in the Fall 2015 [54]. A completely new way to perform the mesorectal excision is to do it from below. Several reports have found this feasible, but new complications have been seen, like the risk of ureteral damage if the dissection goes too lateral [55, 56].

Results of surgery for rectal cancers

Important endpoints after rectal cancer surgery are the immediate complication rate, i.e. post-operative mortality and morbidity, local recurrence rate, and cancer-specific survival. CRM positivity is a good surrogate endpoint for both local recurrence and cancer-specific survival [14].

Overall post-operative mortality in the Western world should not be more than 1–2% since rectal cancer surgery is elective [57]. The mortality will increase in an elderly population with more comorbidity but should on average be below 2%. The post-operative morbidity is more complex. If all types of complications are counted, approximately 35% of the patients will have a complication [57]. These could be anything from serious wound infections, perineal wound infections, deep vein thrombosis, and pulmonary embolism to more superficial problems such as urinary infection and pneumonia. A dreadful complication is an anastomotic leakage, which has been described in 10% to 25% [58]. A randomized trial showed that a diverting ileostomy decreases the frequency and the consequences of a leakage after an anterior resection; despite a covering ileostomy, approximately 10% will have a leakage [58].

The local recurrence rate has historically been high with reported figures of 30–50% [59]. With the TME technique this has been diminished and with selective use of appropriate radiotherapy the local recurrence rate in the population who undergo radical surgery should not be higher than 5–10% [60, 61].

Survival has also improved and, in many Western countries, a relative survival above 60% is possible to reach [57, 62]. The most likely reasons for this improvement are the efforts to decrease rectal cancer local recurrence rates by better staging, improved surgery, and incorporation of (C)RT.

Role of radiotherapy

Introduction to the role of radiotherapy

Improved surgery is likely responsible for about half of the reduction in local recurrence rates in population-based materials from 30% to 50% a few decades ago down to about 5% to 10%, and the addition of RT is likely responsible for the other half. The different surgical approaches have not been subject to randomized studies, whereas additional RT has. The studies collectively show that pre-operative RT is more efficient than post-operative RT, even when given with concomitant chemotherapy (CRT), and reduces the risk of local recurrence by slightly more than half (see Table 38.1) [63, 64]. The relative effect of RT is higher the lower the absolute risk of local recurrence after surgery alone, i.e. RT is relatively more effective with better surgery. This may be because improved surgery

Table 38.1 Major randomized radiotherapy trials in primary rectal cancer[1]

Study	Inclusion time	No of patients	Treatments — Surgery alone	Treatments — Preop (C)RT	Treatments — Postop (C)RT	Patient group[3]	Radiation technique[4]	Increased death	Local recurrence (%) — Surgery alone	Local recurrence (%) — Preop RT + surgery	Local recurrence (%) — Postop RT	Increased survival	Comments
pre-TME era													
Uppsala [11]	1980–1985	471	-	5,1 x 5[2]	2 x 30	Intermediate	3D-CRT	No	-	13*[5]	22	No	Preop 5 Gy x 5 is better than post-op RT (60 Gy). Increased risk of late complications after post-op RT
Stockholm I [282]	1980–1987	849	Yes	5 x 5	-	Intermediate	AP-PA	Yes	28	14**	-	No	Increased post-op death (8% versus 2%), large target, suboptimal technique, decreased local recurrence risk. Increased risk late complications.
SRCT [67, 70]	1987–1990	1110	Yes	5 x 5	-	Intermediate	3D-CRT	No	27	12***	-	Yes	Decreased local recurrence risk, no increased acute toxicity, some late toxicity after 10–15 years.
Stockholm II [283]	1987–1993	557	Yes	5 x 5	-	Intermediate	3D-RT	Yes?	25	12***	-	(Yes)	Overlaps to a large part SRCT, simplified radiation technique, tendency to increased post-op mortality (4% versus 1%). Lower local recurrence risk, increased survival as in SRCT. Increased risk late complications.
Post-TME era													
TME [68, 72]	1996–1999	1861	Yes	5 x 5		Intermediate	3D-CRT	No	11	5***		No	No increased post-op mortality. Decreased local recurrence risk even with TME, no improved survival, some risk for increased late complications after five to ten years.
MRC-CR07 [69]	1998–2005	1350	-	5 x 5	CRT if CRM+	Intermediate	3D-CRT	No		5**	11	Yes	Preop 5 Gy x 5 better than post-op CRT if CRM+, marginally increased survival. No increase in late complications (3–5 years).
Polish [74]	1999–2002	312	-	5 x 5 / CRT		Intermediate (low)	3D-CRT	No		11 / 16		No	First study that shows less risk of acute toxicity from 5 x 5 compared with preop CRT, no difference local recurrence and survival or late complications (three to five years).
TROG [284]		326	-	5 x 5 / CRT		Intermediate	3D-CRT	No		7 / 4		No	Same design as the Polish study, same results.
EORTC 22921 [78]	1993–2003	1011	-	RT / CRT	RT / CRT	Intermediate	3D-CRT	No		15 / 8		No	2 x 2 design, chemotherapy in addition to RT (CRT) gives fewer local recurrences than RT alone, increased toxicity, no increased survival

(continued)

Table 38.1 Continued

Study	Years	N									Comments
FFCD 9203 [77]	1993–2003	742	-	RT CRT	Intermediate	3D-CRT	No	17 / 10		No	Preop CRT results in fewer local recurrences than preop RT, increased toxicity, no survival difference
LARCS [79]	1998–2003	207	-	RT CRT	Locally advanced (ugly)	3D-CRT	No	33 / 18*		Yes	The only study in ugly rectal cancers, preop CRT gives better local control and better disease and cancer specific survival, tendency better survival (66% versus 53% after five years). Increased acute and possibly late toxicity from CRT.
AIO-94 [10, 285]	1995–2002	823	-	CRT CRT	Intermediate	3D-CRT	No	6** / 13		No	Preop CRT is less toxic and gives fewer local recurrences than post-op CRT, no difference in survival

[1] Only large studies of relevance for present treatment recommendations are included.

[2] 5 x 5 means 5 Gy daily for five days during one week. CRT means chemoradiotherapy with 1.8–2 Gy daily to 45–50.4 Gy. RT means the same radiotherapy as in the CRT arm without chemotherapy.

[3] Inclusion criteria in the studies. In the early studies patients who had a resectable tumour, excluding the polyp cancers, were included. In later studies, intermediate (bad) tumours were included except in LARCS that included 'non-resectable' (ugly) tumours.

[4] 3D-CRT means 3D-conformed radiotherapy, three or four beams with blocking of normal tissues that did not contain tumour cells. 3D-RT (in the Stockholm II study) means four beams but no blocking. AP-PA means anterior posterior beams with no blocking, meaning high radiation doses to large normal tissue volumes.

5* P <0.05, ** P <0.01, *** P <0.001. Only statistically significant values have been presented.

results in leaving fewer and smaller tumour deposits behind, which can then be more easily eradicated by the RT covering a larger tissue volume than has been surgically removed. The relation between the risk of local recurrence after surgery alone versus after preoperative RT and surgery is illustrated in Figure 38.3. There is a gain from preoperative RT even in early tumours operated on by the best surgeons, but the number of patients needed to treat to prevent one local recurrence becomes too high considering the adverse effects from the RT.

The importance of local control in rectal cancer

Radical removal of the primary rectal cancer and no local recurrence are prerequisites for cure, although secondary surgery and/or CRT can salvage occasional local recurrences. Avoidance of persistent or recurrent tumour in the pelvis is important, even if cure cannot be achieved, since uncontrolled pelvic growth is usually associated with severe, disabling symptoms.

Thus, an important aim is to treat so that the risk of residual disease in the pelvis is very low or preferably less than about 5% in the population in which locally curative treatment is intended. This should be possible in all but the few (≤5%) who present with a fixed tumour growing into a non-readily resectable organ (less than half of those with clinical stage T4 (cT4)). At the same time,

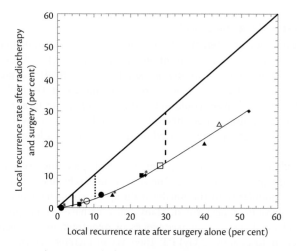

Fig. 38.3 Local recurrence risk after preoperative RT and surgery in relation to surgery alone (solid line from origin at a 45-degree angle) for primary rectal cancer. The symbols around the downwards convex line are from randomized studies where preoperative RT with surgery was compared with surgery alone. The results from studies after 2001 also fit along this line. The vertical bars illustrate the difference in local recurrence-risk between non-irradiated and irradiated groups. The solid line to the left illustrates an early (good) tumour where the local recurrence-risk is decreased from about 4% to about 1%. The dotted line in the middle illustrates a tumour belonging to the intermediate (bad) group where the local recurrence-risk is decreased from approximately 10% to 3%. The hatched line to the right illustrates the decrease in locally advanced (ugly) tumours where the decrease can be from some 30% down to 15%. The relative difference is about 70% in early tumours and about 50% in locally advanced tumours. The absolute difference should be put in relation to the problems that local recurrences give raise to in terms of morbidity and mortality and the late adverse effects RT can cause.

Reprinted with permission from *Radiotherapy and Oncology*, Volume 61, Issues 1, Glimelius B, Pre- or post-operative radiotherapy in rectal cancer—more to learn?, pp. 1–5, Copyright © 2001 Published by Elsevier Ireland Ltd, with permission from Elsevier, http://www.sciencedirect.com/science/journal/01678140

as little acute and late morbidity as possible should be aimed at. Surgery, particularly if extensive, may give substantial morbidity, and additional treatments like RT or CRT, whether given pre- or post-operatively, increase morbidity. Thus, the additional treatments should be given selectively, i.e. when they benefit sufficiently many.

Tumours with distal extension to 15 cm or less (as measured by rigid sigmoidoscopy) from the anal margin are classified as rectal. Whether this 15 cm limit is the best for choosing a 'rectal cancer strategy' or a 'colon cancer strategy' is open to discussion. Others prefer to separate colon and rectal cancers at the peritoneal reflection, or about 9–12 cm from the anal verge. The localization of the tumour in relation to adjacent organs and structures and, thus, the distance from the anal verge are important for outcome and treatment. Cancers between 10 cm and 15 cm are best discussed as rectal cancers since RT is an important component of therapy to decrease the risk of local failure, even if less often than for lower rectal cancers (0–10 cm) [57].

From a practical point of view, rectal cancers can be divided into three groups, early (cT1–2, some cT3, where c indicates clinical), intermediate (most cT3–, some cT4) and locally advanced (some cT3, most cT4). Other factors than cT-stage, such as tumour height, closeness to the MRF (potentially the CRM; preoperatively, the term MRF is better than CRM, since the CRM cannot be defined until after surgery [65]), nodal (cN) stage, and extramural vascular invasion are also relevant. It is at present not possible to provide a precise description of which T and N substages belong to these groups. The terms 'favourable or early or good', 'intermediate or bad', and 'locally advanced or ugly' are used for categorizing the rectal cancers into these clinical subgroups (Figure 38.4). In clinical practice and in many recent studies, the term 'locally advanced' has been commonly used for the 'intermediate/bad' group, but is best reserved for the truly 'locally advanced/ugly' tumours [63].

Differences in treatment strategy in the world

There is a difference in how lateral lymph node metastases outside the mesorectum, frequently seen in intermediate/locally advanced tumours below the peritoneal reflection, are managed. Surgical removal of these nodes has been the preferred option in Asia, whereas the rest of the world has explored the value of radiation in addition to surgery for the primary, to kill the tumour deposits. Both extensive surgery (i.e. more than TME) and additional RT increase morbidity. There are no randomized studies that compare the two strategies. Comparisons between trials reveal that the results are equally good at specialized centres, although patient selection precludes firm conclusions. In clinical practice, it is more efficient to 'remove' subclinical cancer deposits using radiation rather than surgery unless it is dissected in a surgical plane. This is not possible outside the MRF. The resultant morbidity is very different although the impact of this on patient well-being differs between cultures.

In the Western world, preoperative RT has been mainly explored in Europe, whereas post-operative RT has been explored in the US. A few small studies have indicated that post-operative CRT was better than post-operative RT in preventing local recurrence and that treatment was more effective than no additional treatment. Based upon this, a National Cancer Institute (NCI) report in 1991 stated that post-operative CRT should be standard treatment in rectal cancer stages II and III [66].

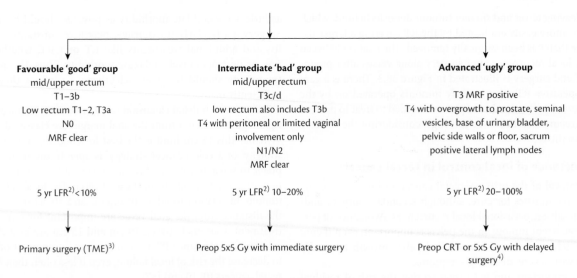

Fig. 38.4 Subgrouping of localized rectal cancer assessed by MRI and recommended primary treatment.

[1]The algorithm does not primarily address the risk of systemic disease, although this risk also increases with the presence of many of the risk factors, however, not necessarily parallel to the local failure rate (LFR). The algorithm is also 'too simplified' in that other factors like size of the mesorectum, anterior or posterior location, extramural vascular invasion (EMVI+) are relevant. Note that the distinction between subgroups is not between T2 and T3 and between T3 and T4 but rather within T3.

[2]Calculated in the group of patients planned for surgery, i.e. irrespective of the surgical outcome. The figures are valid if the surgeon is an experienced rectal cancer surgeon and no pre-treatment is given.

[3]A local procedure is possible in a few patients (chiefly pT1, sm1(2), N0). This group is in the text referred to as 'very favourable'.

[4]CRT means chemoradiotherapy to 45–50.4 Gy in 1.8–2 Gy fractions with 5-fluorouracil (capecitabine). 5 x 5 Gy in one week with delayed surgery is used in patients not fit for CRT.

In Europe, in contrast, large randomized trials compared surgery alone versus preoperative RT and surgery. These studies showed that, particularly if short-course RT was used, i.e. the Swedish 5 x 5 Gy schedule in one week with immediate surgery, there was a relative reduction in local failure rates of 50–60% [67–69]. Long-term follow-up of the trials have shown that the recurrences are prevented, not just delayed [70–72]. Based upon these results, preoperative RT was recommended early on as routine therapy in many countries, but not until quite recently in most countries.

Pre- or post-operative RT—short- or long-course RT—RT with or without chemotherapy—sphincter preservation?

For about two decades, several research questions have dominated the arena: (1) should the RT be given before or after surgery; (2) should it be long-course or short-course; and (3) should the long-course RT be given alone or with chemotherapy? In Europe researchers were not convinced of the advantages of concomitant chemotherapy, as stated in the US documents. In addition, (4) sphincter-preserving surgery was considered important, and whether this could be increased after preoperative (C)RT was debated extensively, and subject to trials.

Pre- or post-operative RT?

Multiple randomized trials have shown that preoperative RT is more effective than post-operative RT, whether the RT is given alone or with chemotherapy [10–12]. It is also less toxic. Most of the world has now accepted that additional (C)RT in rectal cancer should be given before rather than after surgery. An analysis of data from all randomized studies also indicated that preoperative RT is more dose-efficient than post-operative RT [73], i.e. a lower radiation dose is needed to give the same effect.

Short- or long-course RT?

The question of whether a short-course (5 x 5 Gy) schedule in one week or a long-course conventionally fractionated RT (1.8–2.0 Gy x 25–28 in five to six weeks) in the intermediate (bad) risk group is not yet settled. Two randomized trials including 316 and 326 patients, respectively, could not find any difference in local recurrence rates, disease-free survival (DFS) and overall survival (OS) between the groups randomized to short-course RT or long-course CRT (Table 38.1) [74, 75].

Differences between and potential advantages of the two schedules are given in Table 38.2. The short-course schedule has gained much popularity in the northern European countries where the trials have been performed. Many concerns have been expressed about the long-term consequences of hypofractionated (giving fraction doses above 2 Gy) RT. There is considerable evidence that the short-course schedule results in long-term morbidity, and the scale of that morbidity is well known [76]. The long-term morbidity of CRT whether given pre- or post-operatively has not been studied systematically, with the result that the extent of late morbidity is not known. Both options, short-course 5 x 5 Gy and long-course CRT, are considered valid in the intermediate group of rectal cancers [63], although the short-course schedule is much less resource demanding and has less acute toxicity.

RT without or with chemotherapy?

If long-course RT is combined with 5-FU-based chemotherapy, local control is improved (9% versus 17% in the intermediate group and 18% versus 33% in the locally advanced group) based upon the results of three randomized studies [77–79]. A significant survival gain was only seen in the trial including locally advanced cancers [79, 80]. Whenever a patient with a locally advanced rectal cancer receives preoperative treatment, CRT should be used unless the patient cannot tolerate this treatment. It should, however, be

Table 38.2 Main differences between and potential advantages of short-course and long-course preoperative radiotherapy in intermediate (bad) rectal cancers[1]

	Short course	Long course
Total (physical) radiation dose	25 Gy	45–50.4 Gy
Fraction size/number of fractions	5 Gy/5	1.8–2 Gy/23–28
Radiation duration	1 week	4.5–5.5 weeks
BED[2], acute effects	37.5 Gy	37.5–44.4 Gy
BED[2], late effects	66.7	72–84 Gy
Overall treatment time	About 10 days	10–14 weeks
Demands of radiation resources	Planning + 5 fractions	Planning + 23–28 fractions
Concomitant chemotherapy[3]	No	Yes
Acute toxicity	Minimal	More
Late toxicity	Present, limited in the "bad" group	Present, but not extensively studies. Anticipated higher than after short course
Down-sizing/ Down-staging	No[4]	Yes[5]

[1]In locally advanced (ugly) tumours, long-course CRT is the evidence-based and preferred option although short-course RT with a delay to surgery is an option if CRT is not tolerated because of high age or co-morbidity.

[2]Biologically effective dose according to the time-corrected linear quadratic model. Major uncertainties exist in the relative biological efficacy of the fractionation schedules concerning particularly the acute (antitumour) effects. The parameters selected for the acute effects were those used in the meta-analyses from 2001 [12], even if they can be criticized and probably are incorrect. For late effects, an α/β of 3 Gy with no time correction is used. The important message is that the anticipated antitumour effects do not differ substantially and that late toxicity is at least not higher using short-course RT.

[3]Improves local control with long-course CRT, increases acute toxicity and probably also late toxicity. Should not be given with short-course RT.

[4]Seen after short-course RT with delayed surgery.

[5]Not relevant in these intermediate tumours (unless organ-preservation is aimed at), however, relevant in locally advanced (ugly) tumours.

recognized that the gains from the chemotherapy addition are limited and come at a rather high price in terms of more acute toxicity (grade 3–4 gastrointestinal toxicity of about 15%) and potentially also more late toxicity.

Sphincter preservation, organ preservation

Trials, again chiefly run in Europe, have explored whether long-course CRT with a delay of four to eight weeks before surgery could increase sphincter preservation rates, whereas others took it for granted that this was the case. The trials have shown that this effect did not occur to any meaningful extent [81, 82]. It is possible that better restaging of the tumour using MRI after long-course CRT could have influenced the possibilities of performing sphincter-preserving surgery. Hopes about improved chances of sphincter preservation influenced routines in many countries, particularly in southern Europe, Germany, and the US. At present, hopes about organ preservation influence treatment decisions.

Risk-adapted treatment

Very favourable rectal cancer

In the earliest, most favourable cases, chiefly the malignant polyps (Haggitt 1–3, T1 sm1(-2)N0), a local procedure (e.g., using the TEM technique) is appropriate [83]. The resection should be radical (R0) without signs of vessel invasion or poor differentiation. If this is not the case or if the tumour infiltrates deeper into the submucosa (Haggit 4, T1 sm(2-)3) or is a T2 tumour, the risk of recurrence is too high (≥10%) and the patient should have post-operative CRT or, more safely, be recommended major (TME) surgery. If the cancer is biopsy verified, presurgery CRT is preferred if the intent is to perform a local procedure. As an alternative to local surgery, alone or with (preoperative) CRT, local RT (brachytherapy or contact X-ray therapy [Papillon technique]) can be used. Experience of these treatments is limited outside specialized centres [84] and more prospective studies are required before they can become part of clinical routines.

Early 'good' rectal cancers

In the early favourable cases (cT1-2, some early cT3a(-b)N0(1) and clear MRF (MRF−) according to MRI, 'good' group) above the levator muscle plane, surgery alone, using the TME technique is appropriate, since the risk of local failure is low [63]. Although the randomized trials using short-course RT have shown that this treatment even further reduces local recurrence rates (from 5–10% to 2–5%) [61–63], surgery alone is recommended since the addition of preoperative RT results in over-treatment of too many individuals [63]. The balance between the reduction in local recurrence rates and long-term morbidity is intricate (Figure 38.4).

Intermediate 'bad' rectal cancers

In the intermediate 'bad' group (most cT3 (cT3(b)c+, MRF− according to MRI), some cT4 (e.g., limited vaginal or peritoneal involvement only), preoperative RT is recommended, since this reduces local recurrence rates. Even in the absence of signs of extramural growth on ERUS or MRI (cT2) in very low tumours (0–5 cm), preoperative RT may be indicated because the distance to the MRF is very small. Twenty-five Gy delivered during one week followed by immediate surgery (<10 days from the first radiation fraction) is convenient and of low toxicity [67–69]. Trials have shown that the risk of local failure in the randomized population has been reduced by 50–70% versus surgery alone (Table 38.1). A more demanding, but not proven to be more effective, alternative is 46–50.4 Gy, 1.8–2 Gy/fraction with 5-FU (bolus, continuous infusion or oral) [63]. Two European trials [77, 78] showed that the addition of 5-FUFA improves local control with reduced local failure rates after five years. These were 16–17% in the preoperative RT arms alone and 8–10% in the CRT arms. In the EORTC trial, the same reduction was seen irrespective of whether the chemotherapy was administered concomitantly or post-operatively. Two trials (Polish, TROG 01.04) have compared preoperative 5 x 5 Gy and preoperative CRT (5-FUFA + 50.4 Gy) without detecting any difference in local recurrence rates, DFS and OS [74, 75]. In the MRC-CR07 trial, preoperative 5 x 5 Gy was compared with post-operative CRT if CRM was positive. Local recurrence rates (5% versus 17%, P<0.001) and DFS (hazard ratio (HR) 0.76, P = 0.01) favoured the preoperative arm whereas OS did not differ significantly (HR 0.91, P = 0.04) [69].

Locally advanced 'ugly' rectal cancers

In the locally advanced, sometimes non-resectable cases (cT3 MRF+, cT4 with overgrowth to other organs), preoperative CRT, 50.4 Gy, 1.8 Gy/fraction with concomitant 5-FU-based therapy should be used [63, 79] followed by radical surgery six to eight weeks later. In the Nordic randomized trial (cT4NXM0), local control was significantly better after five years in the CRT arm (50 Gy + bolus 5-FUFA) than in the RT-only arm (50 Gy) (82% versus 67%, P = 0.03). In addition, DFS and cancer-specific survival were better in the combined modality arm, whereas OS did not significantly differ (66% versus 53% at five years, P = 0.09) [79].

In very old patients (≥80–85 years) and in patients not fit for CRT, 5 x 5Gy with a delay of approximately eight weeks before surgery is an alternative option, after favourable reports from several centres [85–87].

What chemoradiation schedule? Targeted drugs?

Standard preoperative CRT means a dose of 46–50.4 Gy together with 5-FU given either as bolus injections together with leucovorin six to ten times during the radiation (as in the trials proving that CRT provides better local control than RT alone) [77–80], prolonged continuous infusion (likely better than bolus) or oral capecitabine [88]. Combinations of 5-FU or other antifolates with other cytotoxics like oxaliplatin or irinotecan or targeted biological drugs have been extensively explored in phase I–II trials, which have claimed more favourable results (more downsizing, higher pathological complete remission (pCR) rates), but also more acute toxicity. Several comparative randomized trials using oxaliplatin have been performed. Mature data are reported from one of the studies, the German AIO-04 trial [89]. The trial included 1265 patients belonging to what here is named intermediate rectal cancers (in the article locally advanced). At three years, DFS in the investigational arm receiving preoperative CRT with infused 5-FU and oxaliplatin and postoperatively likewise infused 5-FUFA with oxaliplatin was 76% compared with 71% (HR 0.79, P = 0.03) in the control arm receiving 5-FU only. The 5-FU-schedules, however, varied between the two arms. Local and distant recurrences did not significantly differ between arms, although a slight advantage for the experimental arm may be present. It is too early to consider the addition of oxaliplatin as a new reference treatment, at least for the cancer stages included in the trial (chiefly cT3). The initial results of the other studies are not favourable, although pCR rates may be slightly increased [90, 91], and these combinations are thus still experimental. Nor are the initial results of adding targeted drugs like cetuximab, panitumumab, or bevacizumab favourable. When cetuximab was added to neoadjuvant oxaliplatin–capecitabine and preoperative CRT in the randomized phase II EXPERT-C trial, more radiological responses were seen in the cetuximab arm (89% versus 72%, P = 0.003) in the KRAS wild-type population (N = 90) [92]. OS was also improved (96% versus 81% at three years, P = 0.04, which was, however, not significantly at five years (84% and 72%), P = 0.20 [93]).

Post-operative chemoradiotherapy

Post-operative CRT (about 50.4–54 Gy, 1.8–2.0Gy/fraction) with concomitant 5-FU-based chemotherapy is no longer recommended, but could be used in patients with positive CRM, perforation in the tumour area, or in other cases with high risk of local recurrence if preoperative RT was not given. The strategy of giving post-operative CRT to CRM+ tumours was, however, inferior to giving preoperative 5 x 5 Gy to all [68].

Organ preservation

Apart from the earliest tumours that can be treated with local surgery or local RT, as previously described, it has become increasingly popular to first deliver CRT, restage the tumour and, if it has disappeared completely at palpation, endoscopy, and MRI (complete clinical remission, cCR) to postpone surgery (organ preservation) [94, 95]. If there are questions as to whether the tumour has completely disappeared, an excision biopsy of the previous tumour area can be carried out [92, 94]. If no viable tumour cells are found, no further therapy is delivered and the patient is monitored closely for at least five years. It is then assumed that potential lymph node metastases have been eradicated parallel with the excellent response of the primary tumour. Although this may undoubtedly occur in some patients, this strategy has not been subject to properly controlled prospective studies. It is likely that this excellent response will not be frequently seen in the intermediate and locally advanced cases [95], except if the tumour is small and located at the sphincter or levator plane, but rather only in the early cases. The advantages, no major surgery and no rectal excision if the tumour is very low, are apparent for certain individuals who run a high risk from surgery or who cannot accept a stoma. However, the disadvantages for many others are seldom discussed. In most patients with an early 'good' rectal cancer, a low anterior resection alone is the preferred therapeutic option. Cure rates are high and morbidity is only a result of the surgery, although this may be problematic with long-term bowel dysfunction for some patients (low anterior resection syndrome, LARS [99]). If these patients are instead treated with the aim of organ preservation, all will receive CRT with its acute morbidity. Those responding well clinically (cCR) could then be cared for with a watch-and-wait policy. These are the patients who have a potential benefit from this approach, although they would all suffer from the long-term toxicity that can be seen after CRT. If the tumour is located in the lower rectum, at least part of the sphincters must be included in the irradiated volume, and poor anal function can be a result. For those not responding well or those recurring during follow-up, major surgery is required. These patients will thus suffer the morbidity inherent in both CRT and surgery. No study has so far had a prospective design so it is not possible to estimate the proportion of patients who do not require major surgery [97].

Evaluation of response after preoperative (chemo) radiotherapy

Since the response to preoperative CRT influences prognosis [98] and thus subsequent therapy, attempts clinically and pathologically to restage the tumours have been made. The increasing experience in evaluating tumour response by repeat MRI is described in the previous section. Using FDG-PET, decrease in uptake can also be seen [100, 101]. At present, knowledge about the relevance of these changes is too uncertain to modify the extent of surgery.

Several systems for pathological tumour regression grading have been used. The best approach as regards reproducibility, prognostic information, etc. is not yet known. The tumours should at least be graded into three groups, complete response (pCR), some (potentially in the future good, moderate, and poor) response and no response. The proportion of pCRs is influenced by the intensity of dissection. Standardization of the dissection is required before pCR rates can be used as a valid endpoint.

Radiation therapy volumes and doses

Whenever RT is indicated to lower the risk of local failure in the 'intermediate/bad' group or to cause downsizing to allow radical surgery in 'locally advanced/ugly' tumours, the primary tumour with mesorectum and lymph nodes outside the mesorectum at risk of containing tumour cells more than exceptionally should be irradiated. In the 'early/good' group before or after a local procedure, only mesorectal nodes are at sufficient risk to be involved. The appropriate dose to subclinical disease is not precisely known, but with 5-FU chemotherapy should be at least 45 Gy in 1.8–2 Gy fractions. The relative reduction in local failure rates is then in the order of 50–60%, and subsequently there is room for improvement. A boost of about 4–6 Gy in 2–4 fractions to the primary tumour can be given.

The entire mesorectum is at risk of having tumour deposits, often in the mesorectal lymph nodes, in all tumours except the very earliest (T1 sm1–2) and should be included in the clinical target volume (CTV). An exception is high tumours where it is sufficient to include the 4–5 cm distal to the tumour. Besides the mesorectal nodes, the presacral nodes along aa rectales superiores up to the level of S1–2 (if presacral nodes are radiologically involved, the upper border should be even higher). Local recurrences above S1–2 are seldom seen [102, 103]. The lateral nodes along aa rectales inferiores and aa obturatorii and the internal iliac nodes up to the bifurcation from aa iliac communes should be included in tumours below the peritoneal reflection, i.e. up to about 9–12 cm from the anal verge [104]. The risk of lateral node involvement in the Western world is not properly known, but studies from Asia show that these lymph nodes are rarely involved in low-mid-rectal pT1-2 tumours and in high tumours irrespective of T stage [105]. External iliac nodes should only be included if an anterior organ like the urinary bladder, prostate, or female sexual organs is involved. The medial inguinal nodes need only to be prophylactically irradiated when the tumour grows below the dentate line [106]. When lymph nodes are metastatic so that this can be seen on imaging, there is a risk of aberrant spread, and CTV can be enlarged to include other nodal stations than those described.

Fossae ischiorectales should only be included when the levator muscles and the internal and external sphincters are involved, since the fascia inside the levators is a strong barrier to tumour cell penetration [107].

Late toxicity from rectal cancer radiotherapy

The prevention of local failures, with the severe morbidity they may have, must be weighed against the morbidity from (C)RT that all treated patients can develop. Studies have tried to estimate what minimal absolute gain should be present for patients to prefer RT alone. These studies are difficult to interpret, although many patients accept an absolute 3% difference for the known morbidity risks of RT [108].

From the randomized trials, we have good evidence of morbidity after 5 x 5 Gy [76]. Increased risks of poor anal and sexual function, small bowel toxicity with obstruction, and secondary malignancies have been reported. These are increased roughly between 50–100%. For example, if the risk of any anal incontinence is 40% after surgery alone, it is about 60% after RT + surgery. If more severe

incontinence problems are seen after 8%, it is increased to about 12%. Late bowel obstruction was seen in 6% after surgery alone and in 8–10% after combined therapy. Finally, the risk of second malignancy after a follow-up between 14 to 20 years was 9% versus 4% (relative risk 1.85 (95% confidence interval (CI) 1.23–2.78) in two Swedish studies [109]. No increased risk of secondary malignancies was seen in the Dutch TME-study [110]. With these figures in mind for those who survive at least eight to ten years, an absolute reduction in the risk of a local failure of approximately 5% motivates the recommendation to irradiate (Figure 38.3). Importantly, the RT given today will mean less late toxicity than that seen in the follow-up studies of the RT delivered during the 1980s and 1990s.

An important question as yet unresolved is the late toxicity from 5 x 5 Gy compared with the toxicity seen after 46–50 Gy in 25–28 fractions, usually administered with 5-FU. We know the long-term morbidity from 5 x 5 Gy up to at least ten years follow-up (with yesterday's techniques) from studies including thousands of patients. We do not have this knowledge from CRT. The Polish [74] and MRC-CR07 trials [69] have reported late toxicity after four years of follow-up, without being able to detect any differences between 5 x 5 Gy and CRT to 46–50 Gy. The short-course schedule uses a high fraction size of 5 Gy, compared with 1.8–2.0 Gy, whereas the total dose is less (25 Gy compared to 46–50 Gy). Both the fraction size and the total dose are relevant. The relationship between total dose, fraction size, and late toxicity is, however, complex (Table 38.2).

Another yet unresolved question is whether the addition of 5-FU, or in the future other drugs, increases late toxicity [111]. In one of the two randomized trials in the intermediate risk group [77, 78], the addition of 5-FU affected global QoL, social functioning and diarrhoea negatively. Almost 60% of the patients suffered faecal incontinence, impairing their social life [112]. In the trial in locally advanced/ugly cancers, more patients had stoma or poor anal function in the CRT group than in the RT group (89% versus 70%, P = 0.046) [113], but no differences in QoL were seen after four to eight years [114]. Whether this means that the chemotherapy addition results in more late toxicity or if this difference reflects survival of patients with more advanced tumours in the CRT group cannot be deduced.

Medical management

Adjuvant chemotherapy

In colon cancer there is high scientific evidence for significant gains in both DFS and OS from adjuvant biochemically modulated 5-FU or capecitabine. The addition of oxaliplatin further improves DFS and possibly OS [115]. The relative reduction in recurrences by fluoropyrimidines in stage III is in the order of 30–35% and a further 15–20% by the addition of oxaliplatin, resulting in an overall relative reduction of 40–45%. Based on these results, adjuvant systemic chemotherapy is standard treatment in colon cancer stage III and in stage II if the risk of recurrence is high.

In rectal cancer, the scientific evidence for convincing gains in DFS and OS from adjuvant chemotherapy is much less. The large adjuvant trials have included comparatively few patients with rectal cancer or have focused on colon cancer alone. The trials evaluating the value of oxaliplatin have so far only included colon cancer patients. Most patients with rectal cancer have also received locoregional treatment with pre- or post-operative RT or CRT, whereas this is not done in colon cancer. This more complex treatment scenario and the evolvement over time of the local treatment strategies (better surgery and more often RT or CRT) have made the effects of adjuvant chemotherapy in rectal cancer more difficult to evaluate. The low level of scientific evidence for benefit from adjuvant chemotherapy in rectal cancer is acknowledged in authoritative treatment guidelines and by expert groups that still often conclude that such treatment should be considered based on the principles used for colon cancer [63, 116].

A Cochrane report [117], based on 21 clinical trials including 9221 patients treated over several decades, during which locoregional treatment has undergone considerable changes, concluded that statistically significant gains are present in both DFS and OS (Table 38.3). Based on this report, it is possible to conclude that adjuvant treatment for rectal cancer could be given as it is for colon cancer. A systematic review, however, concluded that adjuvant chemotherapy after surgery for rectal cancer following RT or CRT is not 'evidence-based' [118]. The trial data were then divided based on whether surgery was the only locoregional treatment or was accompanied by pre- or post-operative RT or CRT. Based upon the report of a few randomized studies in 2014 and 2015, two additional meta-analyses, one of which was based on individual patient data, have been published in 2015 [119, 120]. They both reach the conclusion that there is no evidence of benefit from adjuvant chemotherapy in patients who preoperatively received RT/CRT. The trial results are summarized in Table 38.3.

Adjuvant chemotherapy following surgery alone

This treatment setting, in most cases not relevant today in the Western world, except for the early stages, has mostly been studied in Japan. The trials, in total including more than 2000 rectal cancer patients, showed statistically significant benefit in DFS and/or OS with risk reductions in the 15–30% range from adjuvant oral UFT (uracil/tegafur) or carmofur, sometimes together with mitomycin C [121–125]. Similar observations were also observed in two Western world trials, including the QUASAR trial, which explored the value of adjuvant 5-FUFA in patients with colon or rectal cancer where the benefit of adjuvant chemotherapy was considered uncertain [125].

Of 3239 patients in the QUASAR trial, 984 had rectal cancer. In this group, OS at five years was 78% in the group randomized to 5-FUFA compared with 74% in the control group (HR 0.77, P = 0.05). Subgroup analyses with patients divided into those with surgery alone (N = 549) or pre- (N = 198) or post-operative RT (N = 201) did not show significant heterogeneity between the groups. The groups were too small to show statistically significant differences but all showed point estimates indicating benefit from adjuvant chemotherapy.

Adjuvant chemotherapy following surgery and post-operative RT or CRT

Four moderately sized trials showed no benefit in DFS or OS from adjuvant 5-FU for six to 12 months [126–129]. This treatment setting was also part of the QUASAR trial [125].

Adjuvant chemotherapy following preoperative RT or CRT and surgery

This was investigated in the 2 x 2 factorially designed EORTC 22921 trial. In total, 1011 patients were randomized to preoperative RT or CRT and to post-operative adjuvant 5-FUFA for three months or observation [78]. Adjuvant chemotherapy tended to

provide benefit in DFS and OS following preoperative RT or CRT, but the differences were not statistically significant. However, in patients given adjuvant chemotherapy, the local recurrence rate was reduced from 17% to 9% (P = 0.002). In an update of the trial after 10 years [130], there was still a gain from adjuvant chemotherapy in the risk of local recurrences (22% versus 12–15%) but no difference in DFS and OS. In the QUASAR trial, an obvious trend to benefit from adjuvant chemotherapy was seen among the 198 patients who had preoperative RT [125].

The Dutch/Swedish PROCTOR/SCRIPT trial randomized patients following short-course RT and immediate surgery or long-course CRT to six months of 5-FU/leucovorin (PROCTOR) or capecitabine (SCRIPT) or observation only, and the UK Chronicle trial randomized patients after preoperative CRT to observation or adjuvant capecitabine and oxaliplatin [131, 132]. Both trials closed patient inclusion prematurely due to poor recruitment. None of the studies reveal any significant gains in OS or DFS however, the trials lack statistical power to exclude meaningful gains. In an Italian trial [133], 635 patients were randomized to 4.5 months of adjuvant 5-FUFA or observation alone after preoperative CRT. No differences in OS, DFS, distant metastasis rates or local recurrence rates were detected.

Adding 5-FU-based adjuvant chemotherapy after surgery alone thus seems to provide meaningful benefit in terms of OS and DFS, and perhaps also local recurrence rate. This is in correspondence with colon cancer. From a clinical practice point of view, however, this has limited relevance since probably very few patients today with more advanced rectal cancer up to the level of about 10 cm have surgery without preoperative (C)RT. This knowledge is of use when a patient has been operated on without prior (C)RT based on favourable clinical and radiology findings at staging, but with high-risk features in the histopathology report. It is then reasonable to consider adjuvant chemotherapy as an alternative to post-operative CRT, since it may provide both improved local and systemic control. It is acknowledged, however, that these data are not strong, particularly not for the use of an oxaliplatin–fluoropyrimidine combination where no mature trial data exist. If the local recurrence risk is high (e.g., non-radical surgery (R1+R2 or CRM+), CRT are more relevant than if the risk criteria indicate higher risk of systemic relapse (e.g., N2 or EMVI+). However, a beneficial effect from adjuvant chemotherapy on local recurrences is also supported by pooled analyses of several trials [134, 135], but pooling of data from different trials may easily introduce bias.

The overall picture gets complicated when preoperative CRT has been used. For such therapy given post-operatively, most data show that adjuvant chemotherapy provides no major benefit [136, 137]. Most data indicate that when preoperative (C)RT has been given, the benefit from adding adjuvant chemotherapy is likely also very small or absent, with the QUASAR trial as an exception [119, 120]. By adding preoperative (C)RT, which has an obvious effect on small tumour deposits locoregionally, as indicated by reduced local recurrence rates, the effect from adjuvant chemotherapy is in some way reduced. The chemotherapy added to RT could theoretically have an adjuvant systemic effect although this is unlikely considering the lack of benefit in OS and DFS from preoperative CRT compared with RT alone [74–78] and the low total systemic exposure to chemotherapy compared with conventional adjuvant chemotherapy.

Table 38.3 Major randomized clinical trials and summary of recent meta-analyses on the role of systemic adjuvant chemotherapy after locoregional treatment of rectal cancer for cure

Locoregional treatment	Study/reference	No of pts	Stages, treatments	Results	Comments
Surgery alone	Sakamoto/Japanese meta-analysis [123]	2310 from 3 old trials	Stages I–III, 5-FU, UFT or carmofur 6 m, mitoC 6 m added in two trials	HR for OS 0.86 (P = 0.049), for DFS 0.77 (P = 0.0003)	No gain in colon cancer (n = 2380)
	JSCCR/Japanese meta-analysis [124]	2385 from 3 trials	Stages I–III, UFT or carmofur 12 m, mitoC 6 m	HR for OS 0.92 (P = 0.04), for DFS 0.83 (NS)	2 trials probably included in [111]
	Sakamoto/Japanese meta-analysis [121]	2091 from 5 trials	Stages I–III, UFT or carmofur 12–24 m, mitoC 6 m added in three trials	HR for OS 0.82 (P = 0.02), for DFS 0.73 (P < 0.0001) and for LRFS 0.68 (P = 0.003)	Some trials overlapping with [111] and [112]
	NSAS-CC [122]	274	Stage III, UFT 12 m	HR for OS 0.60 (P = 0.034), for DFS 0.66 (P = 0.033)	Included in [112] updated results. No gain in colon cancer (n = 334), HR 0.82, P = 0.4).
	Nordic trials [286]	691	Stages II–III, 5-FU (various) 4–12 m	OS at 5 y 73% versus 81% for AC in stage II (P = 0.09) and 51% versus 48% for AC in stage III (P = 0.91)	A gain was seen in colon cancer stage III (n = 708, OS at 5 y 48 versus 55%, P = 0.15)
	NSABP-R01 [287]	371	Stage II–III, 5-FU, semustine and vincristine	OS and DFS improved (43% versus 53% for AC at 5 y, P = 0.05 and 30% versus 42% for AC, 0.006, respectively	Postop RT alone had no effect on OS or DFS
	QUASAR uncertain [125]	549	Stage II, III, 5-FU 6 m	HR for OS approx 0.85 (NS), for DFS approx 0.75 (NS)	Subgroup analysis. In all 948 RC patients included HR for OS was 0.77 (95% CI 0.54–1.00), for DFS 0.68 (0.4–0.96). 86% of all pts included had stage II
Surgery and post-op RT/CRT	Hellenic Group [126]	220	Stage II, III, post-op CRT w/wo 5-FUFA four cycles	AC NS improved DFS at 5 y from 68 to 70% and OS from 73 to 77%	
	Cafiero et al [129]	218	Stage II, III, post-op RT w/wo 5-FU/Leva 6 m	HR for OS 1.04 (P = 0.9), for DFS 1.12 (P = 0.6)	Low compliance with adjuvant chemotherapy, NS improvement in compliant pts
	Dutch group [128]	299	Stage II, III, post-op RT w/wo 5-FU/Leva 12 m	HR for OS approx 0.95, for DFS approx 0.90 (NS)	Approx 75% of pts had at least 6 m treatment. Significant effect seen in colon cancer in the same trial
	ECOG Est 4276 [126]	237	Stages II–III, post-op RT, CT or CRT	5-yr OS RT 46%, CT 47%, CRT, 50% (NS)	Abstract only
	QUASAR uncertain [125]	201	Stage II, III, post-op RT w/wo 5-FU 6 m	HR for OS approx 0.80 (NS), for DFS approx 0.65 (NS)	See comment on QUASAR above
Preop RT and surgery	EORTC 22921 [78]	505	cT3, T4, preop RT w/wo 5-FU 3 m	HR for OS for AC versus no AC 0.85 (0.68–1.04) and for DFS 0.87 (0.72–1.04). LR at 5 y was 17 and 10% in the RT and RT/AC groups, respectively	Represents 2 of the 4 arms in this trial. Results not separated for preop RT and CRT (see below) groups. 27% of pts scheduled for AC never started. Difference in LR between preop RT only and the other 3 groups, P = 0.002
	QUASAR uncertain [125]	198	Stage II, III, 5-FU 6 m	HR for OS and DSF approx 0.55 (NS)	See comment on QUASAR above
	PROCTOR/SCRIPT [131]	470	Stage II, III, preop RT (5x5) or CRT 5-FU (PROCTOR), Cap (SCRIPT) 6 m	OS at 5 y 79% versus 80% for AC (HR 0.93 (0.60–1.39), DFS HR 0.80 (0.60–1.07), P = 0.13). No diff in LR	61 patients had preop CRT, 376 preop RT, prematurely broken

(continued)

Table 38.3 Continued

Preop CRT and surgery	EORTC 22921 [78, 130] l	506	cT3, T4, 5-FU 3 m post-op	See above. LR was 9% and 8% in the CRT and CRT/AC groups, resp	See above. Long-term follow-up after 10 years did not alter the results
	Italian Group [133]	655	Fixed/tethered RC. 5-FU 4.5 m post-op	OS 69% for CRT only and 68% when AC added (NS). No difference in DFS or LR	28% never started AC
	Chronicle [132]	113	Preop CRT, Xelox 4.5 m	OS 3 y, 89% versus 88%. (HR 1.18), DFS 78% versus 71%, HR 0.80 (0.38–1.69)	Prematurely closed, 93% started AC, 48% completed 6 cycles
	Individual meta-analysis [119]	1196 from 4 trials	Preop RT or CRT	OS HR 0.97 (0.81–1.17), distant rec, HR 0.94 (0.78–1.14)	Overall no gain. In tumors 10–15 cm, DFS HR 0.59 (0.40-0.85, P = 0.005)
	Systematic Overview [120]	2431 in 5 trials	Preop CRT/RT versus observation	OS HR 0.94 (0.81–1.09), DFS 0.93 (0.81–1.06)	
		2710 in 4 trials	Preop CRT with or without oxaliplatin, AC±oxaliplatin	DFS HR 0.84 (0.66–1.06, P = 0.15)	3 trials short follow-up, 1 trial published [89] sign gain in DFS and OS. Not the same 5-FU in controls and experimental group
All	Cochrane analysis [108]	9221 from 21 trials	All stages, all treatments, all settings	HR for OS 0.88 (0.76–0.91), for DFS 0.75 (0.68–0.83)	Great heterogeneity between trials running during several decades

Abbreviations: preop, preoperative; Postop, post-operative; AC, systemic adjuvant chemotherapy; RT, radiotherapy; CRT, chemoradiotherapy; pts, patients; UFT, uracil-tegafur; carmofur, 1-hexylcarmobyl-5-fluorouracil; m, months; HR, hazard ratio; OS, overall survival; DFS, disease free survival; LRFS, local relapse-free survival; JSCCR, Japanese Society for Cancer of the Colon and Rectum; HCFU, 1-hexylcarbomoyl-5-fluorouracil; NS, not statistically significant; 5-FU, 5-fluorouracil (modulated with folinic acid in most trials); mitoC, mitomycin C; y, year; w/wo, with or without; Leva, levamisole; approx., approximately; CI, confidence interval; resp, respectively.

Source: data from Hoirup Petersen S et al., Post-operative adjuvant chemotherapy in rectal cancer operated for cure, *Cochrane Database of Systematic Reviews*, Issue 3, Art. No.: CD004078, Copyright © 2012 The Cochrane Collaboration. Published by John Wiley & Sons, Ltd.

One possibility is a lower sensitivity of rectal cancer compared with colon cancer in the adjuvant setting based on differences in tumour biology. Similar activity of chemotherapy in terms of tumour response rates and benefit in PFS and OS in metastatic CRC argue against this possibility. However, colon cancer differs from rectal cancer in several aspects relevant to tumour biology, and although such differences may not materialize when metastatic, they may be important in putative tumour 'stem cells', responsible for establishment and growth of metastasis in different organs.

Yet another explanation to the small or absent effect from adjuvant chemotherapy in rectal cancer treated with preoperative CRT would be the timing of adjuvant chemotherapy, i.e. that adjuvant chemotherapy starts later than in colon cancer due to the time spent on CRT and waiting for surgery and/or post-operative complications. In colon cancer the efficacy of adjuvant chemotherapy is attenuated by time of start after surgery [138].

Starting with the systemic rather than the locoregional treatment in rectal cancer could approach the relevance of the timing effect. Apparently favourable findings in the EXPERT(-C) trials, where four cycles of XELOX were given prior to CRT, indicate that this approach may be beneficial [92, 139]. This approach seems feasible and well tolerated [139, 140], and is being investigated in the RAPIDO trial in which patients with poor-prognosis rectal cancer are randomized to conventional CRT followed by surgery and optional adjuvant chemotherapy or short-course RT followed immediately by neoadjuvant chemotherapy (six cycles of XELOX) and surgery [141].

Subgroup analyses of the EORTC 22921 trial have indicated that patients with tumour downstaging from cT_{3-4} to pT_{0-2} compared with those with tumours remaining as pT_{3-4} following (C)RT had

better prognosis but also showed benefit from adjuvant chemotherapy [142]. However, this effect seemed restricted to preoperative RT and not to CRT, and was not related to nodal status after treatment. Additional methodological problems with the subgroup analysis are present [118]. Thus, although response to neoadjuvant CRT provides prognostic information in rectal cancer, it cannot, based on current knowledge, be used to predict the efficacy of adjuvant chemotherapy.

Follow-up

The rationale for follow-up of patients after rectal cancer surgery is to find metachronous tumours for quality control and audit.

Metachronous metastases and new primary colorectal tumours

The most common places for a recurrence are the liver or the lungs. Therefore follow-up programmes include scanning of these organs, potentially allowing radical metastasectomy if recurrence occurs. Preoperatively, the liver and the lungs are scanned, preferably with CT. Post-operatively the patient should be investigated with the same type of scan so that it is possible to compare the findings. There is a debate as to how often patients should be scanned. In many centres worldwide patients are seen every sixth month or sometimes even more often during the first years, but the literature is very scarce and there is no data to support intense follow-up. The COLOFOL trial randomized 2500 patients with stages II and III CRC to intensive follow-up (every sixth month the first two years and then a three-year follow-up) or a 'standard' follow-up (one and three years after surgery). In both groups, scanning of the liver and lungs and a CEA value were done. Follow-up is ongoing. The primary endpoint is survival [143].

Between 3–4% of patients who have had CRC will later have another colorectal tumour [144]. Therefore, a follow-up programme with colonoscopies has been recommended. Again, no consensus about the frequency exists. Based upon a Danish trial, where 600 patients were randomized to colonoscopy every year or every fifth year it is sufficient to investigate most patients every fifth year [145].

Quality control

Since rectal cancer surgery is a major procedure with many complications, it behooves patients to be seen post-operatively. In many countries nurse practitioners perform this in cooperation with the surgeon [146]. An enterostomal therapy nurse is essential for all patients with a stoma. The patient has to be checked by the operating surgeon some weeks after discharge to disclose problems which can hopefully then be corrected. Based upon that follow-up visit it might be necessary to see the patient several times, if post-operative complications persist. Once the post-operative period is over a follow-up programme for metachronous metastases should be followed, as outlined previously.

Audit

Another important aim is to use follow-up as an audit for the department. It is important that all departments handling rectal cancer patients are aware of their results concerning both early and late complications and oncology outcome, and can break down the data on the individual surgeons. A good audit system allows changing procedures and improving the results [147].

Treatment of metastatic disease

In colon and rectum cancer, about 20% of the patients in Western populations have synchronous metastases, and another 20% will later develop metastases. The most common site is the liver, but lung metastases are also frequent, particularly if the primary is in the rectum. If the disease is metastatic, the primary tumour site is less important since it has not been possible to detect any clinically relevant differences in tumour behaviour or response to medical therapy. The primary tumour site is of relevance in synchronous disease if surgery of the primary, for cure or for palliation, is planned.

During the past 20–25 years scientific activities in metastatic CRC (mCRC) have markedly increased. Definite improvements have also been seen. Although one may question whether the gains achieved have been sufficient in proportion to the efforts, the gains have markedly influenced clinical routines. In spite of the apparently marked progress in medical treatments of mCRC, surgical removal of all known disease is in practice the only therapy that can cure a patient with mCRC. Alternatives to surgical removal of metastases, if technically possible and the tumour is biologically sound, are radiofrequency ablation (RFA), other invasive ablative procedures, and stereotactic body radiotherapy (SBRT). Progress in medical oncology has, however, contributed to potential cure for some patients with mCRC.

Advances in systemic treatment of patients with metastatic colorectal cancer

In the absence of tumour-controlling treatments, the prognosis for patients with mCRC is poor with, on a population level, a median survival of less than six months and a very low probability of surviving beyond one or two years. Median survival in most recent trials is at least three times longer than it was two decades ago. The impression is also that these patients mostly do well during those extra months. This impression has been substantiated in trials where quality of life (QoL) estimations have been performed. A number of small steps have been taken, together resulting in median survival of patients included in trials being prolonged from about six to eight months to about 24 months or even slightly longer if molecular selection is done (Table 38.4).

Survival in population-based materials of patients with newly diagnosed stage IV CRC is presently about one year [148]. The discrepancy between survival of about one year in the entire population and above two years in the most recent trials clearly indicates that patients included in trials are selected [149]. It is important to focus on reasons for this selection and develop treatments that not only benefit the fittest patients.

Balancing gains and costs

The effects of chemotherapy on objective response rates (RRs), progression-free survival (PFS), OS and QoL are well documented in mCRC. Most gains with high statistical significance have been shown in individual trials or in meta-analyses of the trials [150, 151]. More toxicity and higher economic costs have accompanied each improvement in treatment results. The cost increase is particularly true for the development that has taken place in the past decade. The overall gains in terms of longer PFS and OS, and

Table 38.4 Chemotherapy in advanced colorectal cancer, development with time

Decade	Median survival	Action taken
1970	4–5 months	Supportive care, unselected patients
1980	6–7 months	Supportive care, trial patients
	10–12 months	5-FU/folinic acid (FA), trial patients
1990	12–14 months	5-FUFA, good performance trial patients
	14–15 months	5-FUFA + new drug[1], good performance trial patients
2000	15–17 months	5-FUFA + new drug, first- and second-line treatment
	18–20 months	5-FUFA + new drug, sequential treatments, local methods (chiefly surgery)
	20–22 months	5-FUFA + new drug, sequential treatments, local methods + targeted drugs[2], good performance trials patients
2010	22–26+ months	5-FUFA + new drug, sequential treatments, local methods + targeted drugs used in subgroups potentially benefiting from therapy, very good performance trials patients that could potentially be resected
2015	26–30+	Everything above, triplet+beva or doublet +EGFR in RAS wild-type tumours

Patient selection and better treatments are most important for this prolongation in median survival.

Follow-up routines are also of importance. About 2–4 months may be explained by earlier diagnosis of metastases in recent compared with older patient series.

[1] irinotecan or oxaliplatin

[2] bevacizumab, cetuximab, or panitumumab

QoL improvements of palliative chemotherapy in mCRC are sufficiently large to merit such changes being made to routine therapy [152]. What may need further discussion is whether all incremental gains are sufficiently large in relation to toxicity, other inconveniences, and costs to qualify as routine therapy. Since trial methodology has improved, including recognition to perform large trials, there is danger that 'too small' gains are proven to have statistical significance.

Most clinicians agree that statistical significance does not necessarily indicate clinical relevance. Still, this conclusion is controversial. There is no consensus on whether a minimum size of any gain, in relation to toxicity, inconvenience, and other costs, in fact exists. Further, there is no consensus as to the most relevant parameter for treatment efficacy. Most importance is given to OS, although PFS has replaced OS as primary endpoint in most clinical trials, at least in the first-line situation [153]. Of great relevance is also the individual patient's judgement of whether a particular gain is sufficient to accept therapy in the light of anticipated treatment burden. However, research and clinical experience have shown that patients generally also want to be treated for small gains [154], and sometimes for gains too small for doctors or healthcare providers to accept. Many patients facing the outcome of progressive cancer accept very short survival prolongation or limited probabilities of symptom relief, even at the cost of considerable toxicity.

Costs have increased substantially on anticancer drug budgets, and mCRC is no exception [155]. The number of studies of costs in patients with mCRC is limited [152, 156], and, although there may be claims that one treatment is cost-effective in comparison with other treatments, it is difficult to draw firm conclusions. Some of the recent development seen in mCRC is very close to or above the limit of what may be acceptable, at least in healthcare systems that have the ambition to offer equality to all individuals. This is also reflected in, for example, the guidelines published by the National Institute for Health and Clinical Excellence (NICE) [152, 157].

Necessity of continuous good supportive care

Even if the death of many patients with mCRC has been postponed by several months or years, the ultimate fate is clear from the very beginning for the majority of them. This knowledge and the fear of problematic symptoms later in the course of the disease may be a burden to the patients, their relatives, and close friends. Even if the palliative treatments appear to function well, with tumour regressions and limited toxicity, there is need for continuous support. This need increases when fewer treatments with sufficient probability to work remain. The requirements of palliative care when death is approaching are likely the same whether they occur a few months or a few years after the diagnosis of incurable disease.

Chemotherapy can prolong life and improve the well-being of patients with metastatic colorectal cancer

Until the late 1980s there was no evidence that treatment had any meaningful influence on the well-being of many patients. Single patients had short-lived benefit from being treated, but the impression was that it did not prolong survival [158]. In 1989, two randomized trials comparing 5-FU alone, the mainstay of treatment for decades, with biochemically modulated 5-FU, reported prolonged survival (median about three months) and improved QoL by the

combined regimen [159, 160]. A meta-analysis [150] and a systematic overview [161] of 11 trials, including overall 796 patients, reported that 5-FU-based treatment (systemic or regional administration) prolonged median survival by four to six months compared with a control group (no or delayed chemotherapy). Supportive evidence for survival gains also comes from trials in the second- and third-line situation after failure on previous regimens [162].

Trials randomizing between chemotherapy and no/delayed chemotherapy or comparing different schedules have shown that the QoL of individual patients can be improved by treatment, or at least remain stable even if the treatment may cause disabling toxicity [162, 163]. Using fluoropyrimidines alone, an objective response (complete and partial remission, CR + PR) and stationary disease (SD) with a duration exceeding four months to 5-FU-based therapy is usually associated with a favourable QoL outcome (Table 38.5). This is the same using combinations of drugs, which more frequently result in objective responses, although increased toxicity to the treatments may temporarily counterbalance this [164, 165]. A response to treatment is also an independent predictor of survival [166, 167], although this relation is not always strong, since survival prolongation is also seen in those with SD. The arbitrarily set criteria for an objective response (30% in the sum of the longest diameters using RECIST) [168] are not optimal for survival prediction [169]. Further, subsequent lines of therapy also influence OS.

The elderly and comorbid patients represent a therapeutic challenge. Even if age per se is not a prognostic factor in most of the trials [170, 171], the great majority of the elderly population is never evaluated for trial participation. Thus, selection among the elderly is extensive [162]. Many patients above an age of 75–80 years do not tolerate present treatments particularly well, even if they are in a very good shape at diagnosis of mCRC. However, there are exceptions and a reasonably high chronological age should not be an absolute contraindication to initiating therapy.

5-fluorouracil (5-FU), biochemically modulated 5-FU, oral fluoropyrimidines

Among the drugs tested for antineoplastic activity in mCRC, 5-FU is still the individually most active agent. During the 1990s, chemotherapy for mCRC using fluoropyrimidines evolved along several paths; potentiation of 5-FU bolus activity by biochemical modulators, particularly methotrexate and folinic acid (FA, leucovorin), protracted venous infusion of low daily doses, infusions during one or a few days of comparatively high 5-FU doses alone or modified by FA, and combinations of the alternatives. 5-FU likely acts differently depending upon schedule [172]. Biochemically modulated 5-FU results in more tumour regressions than 5-FU alone, at least when given as bolus injections. This has not been translated into considerable survival prolongation. Since toxicity is not substantially increased, biomodulated 5-FU is considered to be a better palliative treatment than 5-FU alone unless prolonged infusions (three days or longer) are given. There is at present no firm evidence showing that any of the modulated 5-FU regimens (Table 38.6) is superior to the others, although the 'infused' regimen is considered superior to bolus regimen, since it gives more tumour regressions, longer PFS, and less toxicity [173–175]. The comparator in those trials was the Mayo Clinic regimen. This regimen is, however, associated with a high degree of toxicity, and generally considered

Table 38.5 Relations between an objective response and quality of life changes (patient defined/independently categorized) to 5-FU-based chemotherapy alone (above) or in combination with irinotecan in advanced colorectal cancer (below)

Quality of life	Objective response		
	CR + PR + SD4	SD2+PD	All
Improved	38	4	42
Unchanged	8	4	12
Worse	4	60	64
All	50	68	118

Quality of life	Objective response		
	CR + PR + SD4	SD2+PD	All
Improved	61	8	69
Unchanged	54	7	61
Worse	26	12	38
All	141	27	168

Data are pooled from three Nordic trials run during the 1980s and 1990s where symptomatic patients were treated with 5-FU alone or biochemically modulated 5-FU, or from the Nordic 7 study where patients were treated with FUFA + irinotecan [152] (not all centres participated in the QoL substudies).

Abbreviations: CR, complete remission, PR, partial remission, SD4, stationary disease for at least 4 months, SD2, stationary disease between 2 and 4 months, PD, progressive disease. Using the comparably low-toxic single agent 5-FU, a response was in most patients associated with improved well-being, whereas this was not always the case with a more toxic treatment where particularly diarrhoea, fatigue, and hair loss at least temporarily resulted in poorer global quality of life. The lack of response was usually not associated with improved well-being.

Reproduced with permission from Glimelius B, Quality of life and methodology in colorectal cancer studies, in H Bleiberg et al. (Eds.), *Colorectal Cancer: A Clinical Guide to Therapy*, Copyright © 2002 Martin Dunitz.

Table 38.6 Palliative chemotherapy regimen in colorectal cancer: selection of 'evidence-based' treatment options

First and second line	
Fluoropyrimidines alone	
Bolus 5-FU+folinic acid (FA)	Mayo Clinic, Roswell-Park, Machover, Nordic FLv
Infused± FA	German AIO, Spanish TTD, Lokich
Hybrid bolus/infused+FA	deGramont (Lv5-FU2, several simplified variants)
Oral	Capecitabine, UFT+FA, S1
Raltitrexed	
Combinations of a fluoropyrimidine and another cytotoxic drug	
	5-FUFA + oxaliplatin (like FOLFOX 4-7, FLOX)
	5-FUFA + irinotecan (like Lv5-FU2-Iri, FOLFIRI, FLIRI)
	5-FUFA + oxaliplatin + irinotecan (FOLFOXIRI)
	Capecitabine + oxaliplatin (XELOX)
	Capecitabine + irinotecan (XELIRI)
	Lokich + Mitomycin C (seldom used any more)
Other combinations	Irinotecan and oxaliplatin (IROX) (inferior to fluoropyrimidine-combinations)
Combinations with targeted drugs	
	5-FUFA + bevacizumab
	Capecitabine + bevacizumab
	5-FUFA + irinotecan or oxaliplatin + bevacizumab
	Capecitabine + irinotecan or oxaliplatin + bevacizumab
	5-FUFA + irinotecan or oxaliplatin + cetuximab or panitumumab
	5-FUFA + irinotecan + aflibercept
	5-FUFA+irinotecan+oxaliplatin+bevacizumab
Third and fourth line	
EGFR-inhibitor	Cetuximab
	Panitumumab
	Irinotecan + cetuximab (or panitumumab)
Multikinase inhibitor	Regorafenib
Fluoropyrimidine	TAS102

Abbreviations: FA, folinic acid (leucovorin); 5-FU, 5-fluorouracil.

unacceptable as palliative treatment [176]. Other bolus schedules are better tolerated [177].

Several oral alternatives were also developed. Capecitabine is converted to 5-FU, preferentially in tumour tissue, by thymidine phosphorylase. Studies have shown that results are similar to intravenous 5-FUFA in metastatic disease [178]. UFT is composed of tegafur, a fluorouracil prodrug, and uracil that competes with 5-FU as a substrate for dihydropyrimidine dehydrogenase (DPD), responsible for 5-FU catabolism. Again the efficacy and safety profile of UFT + leucovorin is similar to 5-FUFA in mCRC. S1, a combination of tegafur, oteracil, and dihydroxypyrimidine, also has activity in mCRC [179]. Oral 5-FU prodrugs (best explored using capecitabine) can replace 5-FUFA in all lines of therapy since they are more convenient and have the same efficacy [180]. The level of toxicity is about the same, although the toxicity profiles are not identical.

New drugs and drug combinations

During the late 1990s, two other drugs were introduced in the treatment of mCRC. Oxaliplatin is a third-generation platinum that has low activity as single agent. However, when combined with 5-FUFA (or capecitabine) [181], it is superior to 5-FUFA alone. The lack of a clear OS benefit in the trials is likely obscured by crossover for salvage therapy. Although primarily tested with the

bi-monthly de Gramont schedule [181], it has been combined with other infused regimen [182], bolus 5-FUFA [183], oral fluoropyrimidines [184], raltitrexed, and irinotecan. Oxaliplatin with capecitabine (XELOX) results in similar PFS and OS to infused 5-FUFA/oxaliplatin-combinations [184].

Irinotecan, CPT-11, is a topoisomerase I inhibitor which showed activity in patients who had failed 5-FUFA treatment. Irinotecan was superior to best supportive care (BSC) (OS median three months, P <0.001) and best estimated chemotherapy regimen

(Lv5FU2) (OS median two months, P = 0.04) in two randomized studies [162, 185]. The addition of irinotecan to infused 5-FUFA (48-hour bimonthly and weekly 24-hour) in first line gave more responses than 5-FUFA alone (about 40% versus 20%; P < 0.001), longer PFS and OS, median about two months [186, 187].

Combinations of either oxaliplatin or irinotecan with 5-FUFA have higher antitumour activity than 5-FUFA alone with more objective responses, longer PFS, and slightly prolonged OS. It also appears that the superiority is independent of the chosen 5-FUFA regimen, although one irinotecan/bolus 5-FUFA combination (IFL) was too toxic [187, 188]. IFL, at a reduced initial dose (rIFL), was inferior to bolus/infused 5-FUFA/oxaliplatin (FOLFOX-4) [189].

We have lived without knowledge of the best 5-FUFA schedule for the past decades. Presently, the best combination schedule is not known, although many consider either oxaliplatin or irinotecan with the de Gramont schedule (including several simplified variants) to be reference schedules (FOLFOX and FOLFIRI). Head-to-head comparisons between the many 5-FUFA/irinotecan or 5-FUFA/oxaliplatin combinations have hardly been done. The bolus FLIRI regimen resulted in the same PFS and OS and had the same toxicity as bolus/infused Lv5-FU2-Iri (FOLFIRI is a variant), but slightly lower RR (35% versus 49%, P <0.001) [190]. In a pooled analysis of six randomized studies of 3 494 patients comparing oxaliplatin with 5-FUFA (any FLOX/FOLFOX variant) or capecitabine, similar OS and PFS were found, whereas RRs were slightly lower using XELOX (odds ratio 0.85 (95% CI 0.74–0.97, P = 0.02)) [184]. The toxicity profiles differ between XELOX and 5-FUFA/oxaliplatin, but overall toxicity is similar [191]. As palliative treatments, a more convenient XELOX regimen can be used [184, 192, 193], whereas it has been argued that a 5-FUFA/oxaliplatin combination (like FOLFOX) should be used when tumour cell kill is to be maximized, as in the neo-adjuvant/adjuvant and conversion situations. The same can probably also be said about combinations of capecitabine and irinotecan (XELIRI) [194]. Initially, XELIRI gave rather too much unpredictable toxicity and shorter PFS, but more recent studies indicate that it is effective and tolerable [194–197]. The differences between the more convenient oral alternatives and the entirely intravenous schedules are small, and the alternatives can likely be used interchangeably for palliation according to patient and doctor preferences.

Both irinotecan and oxaliplatin add toxicity and cost to the 5-FUFA treatment. The toxicity profiles of irinotecan (preferentially diarrhoea, some alopecia) and oxaliplatin (preferentially paraesthesias) are entirely different, and it is not possible to state that one of the drug combinations can be favoured over the other. Several randomized phase II studies have compared the combinations (5-FUFA/IRI and 5-FUFA/OX, alone or with targeted drugs) without detecting any significant difference in efficacy [196, 198–200]. The regimen to choose must individually be evaluated and discussed with the patient.

Second-line treatment

After failure on one 5-FU-containing regimen, patients could respond to another 5-FU-based regimen. If the first regimen was bolus 5-FU, infused 5-FU was frequently used based upon the assumption that the antitumour activity was different [172]. It was not until irinotecan, with a different mode of action, appeared

that conclusive trials were performed. Irinotecan significantly prolonged survival in patients refractory to 5-FU when compared with either BSC [162] or bolus-infused 5-FU (Lv5FU2) [172]. These two randomized trials greatly influenced the use of several lines of chemotherapy in patients still in good shape in spite of failing one regimen. Slightly later, oxaliplatin with 5-FUFA (FOLFOX-4) showed superior activity to either drug alone following bolus IFL [201]. About 35–40% of the patients had symptom relief, compared with 10–15% in the control groups, and median PFS was prolonged from two to four months. Objective responses were seen in about 10% of the patients treated with FOLFOX-4 compared with 0–2% in those treated with Lv5-FU2 or oxaliplatin alone.

In a large MRC-FOCUS study, irinotecan alone after failure on 5-FUFA was slightly inferior to a combination of 5-FUFA with either irinotecan or oxaliplatin in second-line (RR 11% versus 16–23%, disease-control at 12 weeks (CR + PR + SD) 40% versus 57–60%, P < 0.005) [202]. In 491 patients failing on 5-FUFA, FOLFOX-4 resulted in more responses (28% versus 16%, P = 0.009) and longer PFS (6.2 versus 4.4 months, P = 0.009) than irinotecan alone, but OS was the same (median about 14 months) [203]. About half of the patients received the mandated third-line therapy. The trials show that it appears important to keep 5-FUFA in the second-line situation and that there is no major difference if an irinotecan or an oxaliplatin combination is used upfront.

Sequential treatment

Once it was established that a cytotoxic drug with another mode of action had activity after failure on a previous regimen and that combination chemotherapy was more efficient than 5-FUFA, sequential administration was explored. Trials have shown that OS is similar whether the first-line regimen is a 5-FUFA (capecitabine) combination with irinotecan or with oxaliplatin [196, 198, 200, 202]. The non-chosen combination is given in second line. OS has, in trials including patients in good performance and with no laboratory abnormalities precluding therapy, been up to 20–22 months using either of the two sequences. Objective responses can be expected in about 50% to the first-line combination and in 10–15% to the second-line combination. Median PFS in first line is eight to nine months and three to four months in second line. The toxicity profiles of the combinations are entirely different and it is up to the individual patient to prefer either sequence. Since oxaliplatin frequently causes disabling and persistent peripheral neurotoxicity, there is some rationale starting with an irinotecan combination since time to progression, and thus treatment duration, is much longer in first than in second line. The time to death, during which the patient potentially has to live with neuropathy, is then longer. Irinotecan combinations, however, result in alopecia more often than oxaliplatin combinations (about 60% versus 5%).

Single-agent fluoropyrimidine as initial treatment

Combinations of two cytotoxic drugs result in more toxicity than modulated 5-FU alone. Therefore, in order to postpone the occurrence of severe toxicity, several trials have started with 5-FUFA in first line and given combination chemotherapy in second and third lines as opposed to starting with one combination in first line and giving the other combination in second line. The largest of these trials (MRC FOCUS [202]) randomized 2135 patients to three strategies: A—single 5-FUFA, then single irinotecan; B—single 5-FUFA, then combination with FUFA/IRI or FUFA/OXA; C—combination upfront, either FUFA/OXA or FUFA/IRI. Median OS was 14 months using strategy A, i.e. providing only single-agent therapy. It was between 15 and 17 months in strategies B and C whether the choice of first-line combination included irinotecan or oxaliplatin. There was no overall difference between strategies B and C, i.e. it is non-inferior to start with single-agent 5-FUFA provided the patients do not have an initially aggressive clinical course, prompting upfront combination therapy. Patients, who could be surgically resected, if sufficient tumour regression is obtained, should not initially receive fluoropyrimidine alone. Similar results were seen in a subsequent study in elderly and frail patients (FOCUS-2) [204], another UK study [205], the Dutch CAIRO-1 study (N = 820) [195], and the FFCD 2000-05 study (N = 410) [206]. A staged approach of initial single-agent treatment upgraded to combination after failure is thus not worse than upfront combination therapy in properly selected patients, but only initially less toxic, postponing more severe toxicity.

Triple combination as initial treatment

In situations where initially it may be important to induce responses as frequently as possible (e.g., in the liver conversion situation) all three active drugs (5-FU, irinotecan, and oxaliplatin) have been combined. In a randomized study including 244 patients, patients who received the triple combination FOLFOXIRI compared to the reference regimen FOLFIRI responded more frequently (66% versus 41%, P = 0.002), and had longer PFS (median 9.6 versus 6.9 months, P = 0.006) and OS (median 23 versus 17 months, P = 0.03) [207]. Toxicity was substantially increased (e.g., grade 3 to 4 neutropenia 50% versus 28%, P = 0.001). After long-term follow-up [208], an absolute benefit in OS of 7% (15% versus 8%) at five years was seen. In a follow-up study including 508 patients comparing the same regimen with the addition of the targeted drug bevacizumab, the triplet again was significantly superior (e.g. PFS median 12 versus 10 months, P = 0.003) [209]. A Greek study including 283 patients compared a slightly dose-reduced FOLFOXIRI with FOLFIRI and found similar results, albeit not statistically significant [210]. Chemotherapy triplets are not yet routine therapy in palliative treatment of patients with mCRC due to the much higher toxicity, but could be used if it important to induce tumour regressions as efficiently as possible, e.g. in the conversion situation and in a clearly symptomatic patient. In the conversion situation, a small randomized phase II study (OLIVIA, n=80) the triplet FOLFOXIRI + bevacizumab was superior to the doublet mFOLFOX-6 with bevacizumab [211].

Targeted drugs

Prior to around 2000, clinical development was concentrated on 'conventional' cytotoxic drugs, the fluoropyrimidines, irinotecan, and oxaliplatin. Different combinations of these drugs, including a triplet combination have been further explored since 2000. Further improvements in patient outcomes have been noted although most of the improvements were already being seen around 2000. During the past decade, most clinical research efforts have concentrated on the exploration of drugs targeting specific molecules associated with CRC cells. Knowledge about molecular events initiating or promoting cancer cell growth in general and CRC in particular had grown substantially during the previous decades.

The development in mCRC has concentrated on targeting vascular endothelial growth factor (VEGF) and the epidermal growth factor receptor (EGFR, HER-1). Clinical progress has been seen, and four monoclonal antibodies are approved for mCRC. Other molecular entities, also aiming at other targets, have been tested, so far without any major success. The improvements seen with the approved drugs bevacizumab and aflibercept, targeting VEGF, and cetuximab and panitumumab, targeting EGFR, as well as those that may be approved in the coming year, have been at best modest when explored in populations with tumours non-screened for certain molecular changes. The inability to identify subpopulations enriched for response has so far prevented substantial improvement. Exclusion of patients with tumours containing RAS mutations for treatment with EGFR inhibitors is an important exception.

Antiangiogenic drugs

Bevacizumab

Bevacizumab (Avastin®) is a recombinant, humanized monoclonal antibody against VEGF. In the pivotal trial, 813 patients received the bolus IFL regimen with placebo or bevacizumab (5 mg/kg) [212] (Table 38.7). Initially, a third arm with 5-FUFA + bevacizumab was included. Median OS and PFS increased and RRs were improved. The increased efficacy came at limited toxicity. Hypertension was seen in 22% of IFL+bevacizumab-treated patients compared to 8% with IFL+placebo. Bowel perforation was more common in bevacizumab-treated patients (1.5% versus 0.0%).

Supportive findings were reported from randomized phase II studies. A pooled analysis of patients (N = 490) from three studies showed statistically significant gains in RR and OS when bevacizumab was added to 5-FUFA [213]. Tolerability was the same in these studies preferably including patients older than 65 years. The efficacy of bevacizumab to either 5-FUFA or IFL in elderly patients (≥65 years) was separately shown in another analysis of the studies (OS 19.3 versus 14.3 months, HR = 0.70 (95% CI 0.55–.90, P = 0.006)). RRs did not differ (34% versus 29%, ns [214]). Patients randomized to capecitabine with bevacizumab had longer PFS, but not longer OS, than patients treated with capecitabine in another study [215] (Table 38.7). Mitomycin-C did not further improve the results.

The good tolerability of bevacizumab was subsequently confirmed in observational studies [216–219]. The risks of arterial events and bowel perforation are about 2% in patients fulfilling inclusion criteria for clinical trials.

In a subsequent first-line study, 1401 patients were randomly assigned to FOLFOX-4 or XELOX and bevacizumab/placebo in a 2 x 2 factorial design [220]. The primary endpoint, PFS, favoured bevacizumab (9.4 versus 8.0 months; HR 0.83, 95% CI 0.72–0.95, P = 0.002), but the effect was much smaller than in the IFL study [212]. RRs were identical (38%) and OS differed, although not significantly. The reasons for the much less impressive data have been speculated upon. FOLFOX-4 is more effective than IFL [189]. Oxaliplatin has cumulative toxicity that sooner or later requires discontinuation of the drug. Bevacizumab was then frequently also withdrawn, particularly in the placebo arm (71% versus 53%). Retrospective analyses of observational studies [216, 217] have indicated that prolonged exposure to bevacizumab may be beneficial, but such comparisons can be biased. Continuous treatment with bevacizumab after chemotherapy withdrawal either pre-planned or because of toxicity has been explored in a randomized TML trial in patients with metastatic colorectal cancer progressing up to three months after discontinuing first-line

Table 38.7 Benefit of bevacizumab or aflibercept targeting angiogenesis to chemotherapy in metastatic colorectal cancer, major studies only

	Number of patients	RR (%)		PFS (months)		OS (months)	
First line			**+ beva**		**+ beva**		**+ beva**
5-FUFA [288]	104[a]	17	32	5.2	7.4	13.8	18.0
5-FUFA [289]	209	15	26	5.5	9.2***	12.9	16.6
Capecitabine [215]	313	30	38	5.7	8.5***	18.9	16.5
IFL [212]	813	35	45**	6.2	10.6***	15.6	20.3***
Xelox/FOLFOX [221]	1401	38	38	8.0	9.4**	19.9	21.3
FOLFIRI [224]	222	37	35	NR	NR	22.0	25.0
mIFL [290]	214	17	35*	4.2	8.3***	13.4	18.7*
FOLFIRI/FOLFOX [291]	376	51	50	8.4	9.6		
2nd line							
FOLFOX [222]	829	9	23***	4.7	7.3***	10.8	12.9**
Any combination[b] [223]	820	4	5	4.1	5.7***	9.8	11.2**
			+afliber		**+afliber**		**+afliber**
FOLFIRI [229]	1226	11	20***	4.7	6.9***	12.1	13.5
FOLFIRI [292]	1072		**+ramu**		**+ramu**		**+ramu**
						11.7	13.3*

[a] Two doses of bevacizumab were given, 5 mg/kg versus 10 mg/kg with no statistically significant difference; however, the 5 mg/kg dose was numerically better.

[b] Patients received bevacizumab in first line.

** = P < 0.01; *** = P < 0.001; beva = bevacizumab; afliber = aflibercept; ramu=ramucirumab.

bevacizumab plus chemotherapy who were randomly assigned to second-line chemotherapy with or without bevacizumab 2.5 mg/kg per week equivalent (either 5 mg/kg every two weeks or 7.5 mg/kg every three weeks, intravenously). The choice between oxaliplatin-based or irinotecan-based second-line chemotherapy depended on the first-line regimen (switch of chemotherapy) [221]. The primary endpoint, OS, was improved from 9.8 months for placebo to 11.2 months for bevacizumab, which has led to approval by agencies for so-called 'bevacizumab beyond progression' (see 'Aflibercept', below).

After failure on an irinotecan–5-FUFA combination, 829 patients were randomized to FOLFOX-4 with or without bevacizumab (10 mg/kg) [222]. The addition of bevacizumab resulted in improved RRs (23% versus 8%, P < 0.001), PFS (7.3 versus 4.7 months, P < 0.001) and OS (12.9 versus 10.8 months, P = 0.001). Bevacizumab thus improved outcomes together with an oxaliplatin combination in the second-line situation in a better way than it did in the first-line situation (Table 38.7). Bevacizumab alone had no activity (RR 3%, median PFS 2.7 months). When bevacizumab was added to combination chemotherapy in the second-line situation after failure on the other combination with bevacizumab, a small gain in PFS (5.7 versus 4.1 months, P < 0.001), and OS (11.2 versus 9.8 months, P < 0.01) was seen [223].

The effect of bevacizumab appears relatively better in combination with 'less effective chemotherapy' (fluoropyrimidine, IFL), but this statement is only based upon intertrial comparisons. No improved outcome was seen in a small Greek study (N = 222)

comparing 5-FUFAIri±bevacizumab given every third week (OS 22 versus 25 months, P = 0.13, similar RRs) [224]. No differences in outcomes were seen in a subgroup analysis of a German study where patients with KRAS-mutant tumours (N = 100) were randomized between FOLFIRI + cetuximab (EGFR-inhibitors are not active in these tumours, see 'EGFR inhibitors') and FOLFIRI + bevacizumab [225].

No predictive factors for efficacy have been identified. Hypertension during treatment has been suggested as relevant for long PFS and OS [226], but this is controversial [227]. There is an urgent need to understand the mechanism of action for bevacizumab and to identify predictive markers. Current data do not, for example, support efficacy in all regimens [228].

Aflibercept

After failure on an oxaliplatin combination in first-line, aflibercept (VEGF-trap, Zaltrap®), a recombinant human fusion protein that acts as a decay receptor preventing VEGF-A, VEGF-B, and PlGF from interacting with their receptors with FOLFIRI was superior to FOLFIRI alone [229]. Of the 1226 patients, 30% had received prior bevacizumab. Median OS was 13.5 months for FOLFIRI + aflibercept versus 12.1 months for FOLFIRI + placebo (HR 0.82 (0.71–0.97, P = 0.003). In addition, PFS (6.9 versus 4.7 months, HR 0.76, P < 0.001) and RR (20 versus 11%, P < 0.001) favoured aflibercept. Diarrhoea, fatigue, stomatitis, infection, hypertension, and neutropenia were among the toxicities seen more frequently in the aflibercept-treated group. As with bevacizumab, aflibercept has also been approved for patients progressing on first-line antiangiogenic therapy.

EGFR inhibitors

Cetuximab

Cetuximab (Erbitux®) is a human-murine chimeric monoclonal antibody inhibiting EGFR. It was first explored in patients with chemotherapy refractory disease. Initially, the tumours should express EGFR immunohistochemically in at least some cells, but this was later found not to be necessary for a therapeutic effect. In the pivotal randomized phase II BOND-1 study [230], patients (N = 329) had failed treatment with irinotecan. The trial showed that this resistance could be overcome by adding cetuximab. RRs to the combination was 23% compared to 12% (P = 0.007) with cetuximab only. PFS was also significantly longer (median 4.1 versus 1.5 months, P <0.001), but not OS.

A randomized phase III study in 572 chemotherapy-refractory patients showed that cetuximab alone compared to BSC prolonged PFS (median 2.0 months, HR 0.68, P < 0.001) and OS (6.1 versus 4.6 months, HR 0.77, P = 0.005) [231]. Similar effects have been shown using the other EGFR-inhibiting antibody panitumumab (see 'Panitumumab') [232]. The predominant toxicity of EGFR inhibition is skin toxicity. Patients who get an acne-like rash of grade 2 or more have better RRs and longer survival. Further analyses have shown that the antitumour effects are restricted to patients with tumours with wild-type KRAS [233, 234]. In these studies, mutations were investigated in codon 12 and 13. The evidence is most solid for mutations in exon 2, codon 12, being by far most common (almost 80% of the approximately 40% who have a mutated KRAS). Mutations in codon 13 (almost 20%) do not necessarily indicate total resistance to EGFR inhibition [235]. More recent knowledge using both cetuximab and panitumumab has revealed that rarer KRAS mutations in exon 3 and 4 and NRAS mutations in exons 2–4 also confer resistance to EGFR inhibition [236, 237]. Altogether, between 55% and 60% of metastatic CRC carry a mutation in the RAS gene, and these patients should not be treated with an EGFR inhibitor.

Cetuximab has also been tested with combination chemotherapy in first-line treatment (Table 38.8). The CRYSTAL study [238–240] compared FOLFIRI with FOLFIRI + cetuximab in 1198 patients with EGFR-positive tumours. Retrospectively, the analyses were performed according to first KRAS mutation status and subsequently RAS mutation status, and all benefit from cetuximab was seen in the RAS wild-type group, constituting about half of the analysed population. In the wild-type group, OS (median 28.4 versus 20.2 months, HR 0.69, P = 0.002), PFS and RR (66% versus 39%, OR 3.1, P < 0.001) favoured cetuximab-treated patients. RAS mutation was not prognostic, whereas the presence of a BRAF V600E mutation was similar to other studies [241]. It was not established whether BRAF mutations were predictive for response to EGFR inhibition [240].

A beneficial effect from the addition of cetuximab was also seen in the randomized phase II study OPUS [242], but not in two more recently reported phase-III studies [243, 244] (Table 38.8). In the MRC-COIN study, 1630 patients received FOLFOX or XELOX with no overall benefit of the cetuximab addition in the KRAS wild-type population. A tendency to better results in cetuximab-treated patients was seen with FOLFOX but not with XELOX [243]. No beneficial effect was seen in the Nordic 7 study where the bolus Nordic FLOX regimen was used [244]. The reasons for the lack of efficacy from cetuximab in these two large studies are not known, although it has been speculated that oxaliplatin, bolus 5-FUFA, or capecitabine are not optimal partners for EGFR-inhibition, whereas irinotecan and infused 5-FUFA are. In a meta-analysis of 14 randomized trials (cetuximab and panitumumab), it was seen that the heterogeneity between first- and second-line trials was best explained by the fluoropyrimidine used [245].

Two large trials, FIRE-3 and C80405, comparing first-line cetuximab versus bevacizumab with combination chemotherapy have been reported in various stages of maturity and with some differing conclusions [246, 246]. The trials cannot be directly compared for many reasons, including the types and quantities of therapy beyond first progression, and planned surgery for resections of liver metastases in C80405, among others. In FIRE-3, there was no difference in RR (65% versus 59%, P = 0.18, PFS (10 months both groups), whereas a significant improvement in overall survival was seen (median 33 versus 25 months, HR 0.70, P = 0.006) in the RAS wild-type group. The survival gain was not shown in C80405. Importantly, in these trials, when only the patients with all RAS wild-type tumours were evaluated, overall survival in excess of 30 months was seen.

Panitumumab

Panitumumab (Vectibix®) is a human monoclonal antibody inhibiting EGFR. Compared to cetuximab, which is a chimeric antibody, it gives rise to fewer infusion-related allergic reactions. When the two antibodies were compared in a randomized study in third line (the ASPECCT study, N = 999), OS (median about ten months), PFS (median four months), and response rates (20–22%) were similar [248]. Toxicity was also similar, with the exception of infusion reactions, which were more common with cetuximab (1.8% versus 0.2%).

The results seen using panitumumab in first line together with FOLFOX [249] or in third line against BSC [235] appear similar to the results seen in the corresponding trials using cetuximab (Table 38.8). Panitumumab has also been explored in second line with FOLFIRI after failing FOLFOX (± bevacizumab) [250]. A statistically significant gain was seen in the primary endpoint PFS (median 5.9 versus 3.9 months, HR 0.73 (P = 0.004), RR (35% versus 10%, P <0.001)) but not in OS (14.5 versus 12.5 months, HR 0.85, P = 0.1) in patients with KRAS wild-type tumours.

Taken all evidence reported from clinical trials together, it is likely that cetuximab, being studied more extensively, and panitumumab have similar anti-tumour activity and that none of them has any efficacy in RAS-mutant tumours. It is also likely that BRAF-mutation indicates resistance to these inhibitors [251], meaning that only about one-third of the mCRC population is eligible for therapy. The effects from the drugs seen in the trials including patients with molecularly unselected tumours are then restricted to the wild-type population, meaning that the gains are potentially larger than reported from the old trials.

Antiangiogenic and anti-EGFR treatment in combination

Since both bevacizumab and cetuximab have efficacy with chemotherapy or, in the case of cetuximab, alone, it was a natural step to combine the two biological agents. This was explored in two first-line studies, the CAIRO-2 study [252] and the PACCE trial [253]. Both trials showed that the addition of an EGFR-inhibitor to chemotherapy with bevacizumab resulted in worse outcomes. The mechanism behind this negative interaction is not known.

Table 38.8 Benefit of EGFR-inhibitors to chemotherapy in metastatic colorectal cancer in the major studies

	Number of patients	KRAS	RR (%)		PFS (months)		OS (months)	
First line				+ cetuximab		+ cetuxi		+ cetuxi
FOLFIRI (CRYSTAL) [238, 239]	1198	all	39	47	8.0	8.9	18.6	19.9*
	666	wt	40	57***	8.4	9.9**	20.0	23.5**
	397	mt	36	31	7.7	7.4	16.7	16.2
FOLFOX/XELOX[1] (COIN) [243]	1630	all	45	49	8.1	7.5	15.8	15.3
	729	wt	50	59	8.6	8.6	17.9	17.0
	565	mt	41	40	6.9	6.5	14.8	13.6
FOLFOX (OPUS) [242]	337	all	36	46	7.2	7.2		
	134	wt	37	61*	7.2	7.7*		
	99	mt	49	33	8.6*	5.5		
FLOX (Nordic 7) [244]	566	all	41	49	7.9	8.3	20.4	19.7
	303	wt	47	46	8.7	7.9	22.0	20.1
	195	mt	40	49	7.8	9.2	20.4	21.1
Third line								
[231, 233]	572	all	0	8***	2.0	2.0***	4.6	6.1**
	230	wt	0	13***	1.9	3.6***	4.8	9.5***
	164	mt	0	1	1.8	1.8	4.6	4.5
	Number of patients	KRAS	RR (%)		PFS (months)		OS (months)	
First line				+ panitumumab		+ panitumumab		+ panitumumab
FOLFOX (PRIME) [249]	1183	all						
	656	wt	48	55	8.0	9.6*	19.7	23.9
	440	mt	40	40	8.8*	7.3	19.3	15.5
Second line								
FOLFIRI [250]	1186	all						
	597	wt	10	36***	4.9	6.7*	12.5	14.5
	486	mt	14	13	4.9	5.0	11.1	11.8
Third line								
[232, 234]	463	all	0	10	1.7	1.9		
	243	wt	0	17***	1.7	2.8***	7.6	8.1
	184	mt	0	0	1.7	1.7	4.4	4.9

[1] Numerically, a benefit from cetuximab was seen using FOLFOX but not using XELOX.

** = P <0.01; *** = P <0.001.

When bevacizumab was added to irinotecan + cetuximab or to cetuximab alone in the randomized phase-II BOND-2 trial in chemotherapy refractory patients [254], apparently better results were seen than in the preceding BOND-1 trial [230]. The study included only 83 patients and the comparison was with a historical control, which is why the results are only hypothesis-generating.

Two small retrospective studies have reported that the addition of bevacizumab to irinotecan and cetuximab in patients resistant to other treatments, i.e. basically in fourth-line situations, results in apparently favourable results with several responses: PFS of about eight months and OS of 12 months [255, 256]. Although these results speak against the results of the two randomized first-line studies, they are intriguing, indicating that tumours previously exposed to chemotherapy may act differently than previously non-exposed tumours. They prompt further mechanistic studies of the activity of bevacizumab and EGFR inhibitors.

Regorafenib

Regorafenib is a small-molecule multikinase inhibitor that prolonged OS by median 1.4 months (from 5.0 to 6.4 months, HR 0.77 (95% CI 0.64–0.94), P = 0.005) in a trial including 760 patients who had failed all available standard therapy (fluoropyrimidine, oxaliplatin, irinotecan, bevacizumab, and an EGFR-inhibitor in KRAS wild-type tumours) [257]. Hand-foot skin reactions, fatigue, diarrhoea, hypertension, and rash or desquamation were common adverse events in relation to regorafenib.

TAS-102

TAS-102 is a novel nucleoside antitumor agent consisting of trifluridine and tipiracil hydrochloride. Trifluridine is the active component of TAS-102 and is directly incorporated into DNA. However, when trifluridine is taken orally it is largely degraded to an inactive form. Tiperacil hydrochloride prevents the degradation of trifluridine. In a large phase-III RECOURSE trial tested in a refractory population similar to the regorafenib study, TAS-102 prolonged overall survival compared to placebo (HR = 0.68); median overall survival was 7.1 months for TAS-102 and 5.3 months for placebo. TAS-102 also improved PFS compared to placebo (HR = 0.48), results comparable to regorafenib [258]. Neutropenia was the most common adverse event. This drug has been designated for fast-track approval in the US.

Ramucirumab

Ramucirumab is a human IgG1 monoclonal antibody that targets the extracellular domain of VEGFR-2, classifying it as an antiangiogenic agent. This drug has shown to be of benefit in second-line therapy in gastric and lung cancers, alone and with chemotherapy. Recently, data from the RAISE trial were presented in patients progressing on fluoropyrimidine, oxaliplatin, and bevacizumab who were randomize to FOLFIRI with or without ramucirumab [259]. The results were quite similar in the same setting as bevacizumab and aflibercept. In 1072 eligible patients who were randomized, the OS HR was 0.84 (95% CI: 0.73, 0.98; log-rank P = 0.0219). Median OS was 13.3 months for RAM versus 11.7 months for PBO. The PFS HR was 0.79 (95% CI: 0.70, 0.90; log-rank P = 0.0005). Median PFS with RAM was 5.7 months and 4.5 months for PBO. ORR was 13.4% RAM; 12.5% PBO (P = 0.6336). Significant toxicities included neutropenia, fatigue, hypertension, and diarrhoea.

Treatment intention

When deciding what treatment an individual patient with mCRC should receive of the many evidence-based options (Table 38.6), the treatment intention is of greatest relevance. At present, it is important to discuss this in the following terms: (1) neoadjuvant, (2) conversion, (3) immediate palliation, and (5) palliation.

Neoadjuvant

In this situation, the patient has one or a few metastases, possibly with a primary tumour that are technically all resectable. The primary aim of chemotherapy is to eradicate microscopic tumour cells to decrease the risk of recurrence after resection. The traditional way is to resect and give adjuvant chemotherapy. This has been explored in two small French trials (N = 278) that found a slight OS gain (HR 1.32 (95% CI 0.95–1.82, P = 0.1) using 5-FUFA [260]. The concept of early systemic treatment to kill subclinical disease, operate, and then give the rest of the chemotherapy afterwards was explored in the EPOC trial (N = 364) where six cycles of FOLFOX

were given preoperatively and six cycles post-operatively [261]. The primary endpoint DFS was improved (35.4% versus 28.1% at three years) in the randomized population; however, it was not statistically significant (HR = 0.79, P = 0.058). In the resected population, the gain was 9.2% units, P = 0.025. OS at five years was insignificantly improved (from 48% to 51% in all randomized patients, P = 0.3). Preoperative chemotherapy increased post-operative morbidity, but did not increase post-operative mortality in the study.

The presently best documented and likely most efficient treatment in this neoadjuvant situation is FOLFOX. As adjuvant treatment, an irinotecan combination is not sufficiently superior to 5-FUFA alone [262]. The addition of bevacizumab or cetuximab to FOLFOX does not improve outcome in colon cancer stage III and has presently no role as neoadjuvant therapy. When cetuximab was added to FOLFOX in the randomized New-EPOC trial including patients with resectable liver metastases (KRAS exon 2 wild-type tumours), shorter PFS was seen in the group treated with cetuximab [263]. The interpretation of the results has been much discussed.

Conversion

In this situation, the metastatic disease burden is limited, usually confined to the liver, but not (readily) resectable. It is then important both to cause tumour regression to allow surgery and to kill micrometastases, i.e. to maximize the chances for the patients to remain disease-free after potential resection. Macroscopic liver metastases generally contain 10^9–10^{10} tumour cells and subclinical foci may contain up to this number. Since CR to medical therapy in mCRC is rare and PR only means about one log of cell kill, the present therapy is far from being curative, even if subclinical foci are more likely to be eradicated than macroscopic disease. The regression of visible liver metastases has sometimes been impressive, and has indicated that liver surgery or an ablative procedure, removing remaining metastatic lesions, may potentially cure some. It is attractive to combine the best of local and systemic treatment, but the weakest component of this is the systemic treatment.

In retrospective analyses of multiple trials, correlation between response rates to chemotherapy and the proportion of patients who could be resected has been seen [264]. The most effective treatment (highest RR, longest PFS) in metastatic disease should thus be given. Since the many alternatives have frequently not been compared to each other, it is impossible to identify that regimen. In RAS wild-type tumours, one choice is FOLFIRI + cetuximab based upon the CRYSTAL study [239]. In the study, the differences in RR (57% versus 40%) and PFS (9.9 versus 8.4 months) between the chemotherapy doublet or the doublet with an antibody were among the largest seen in a phase III trial. This does not automatically mean that this treatment is the most effective in inducing responses, although it is presently a preferred option [116]. In RAS-mutant tumours, where an EGFR inhibitor has no role, FOLFOXIRI is likely the most active option [207], potentially in combination with bevacizuma [209, 211]. In both RAS wild-type and mutated tumours, a doublet without or with bevacizumab is likely not substantially inferior and all combinations are valid options.

Most experience with 'conversion' of liver metastases came initially from a French group at Hôpital Paul Brousse, Villejuif [265, 266], but was later reported from numerous sites and from large collaborative trials. In unselected groups of patients with mCRC, up to about 10% can presently have radical surgery. In groups of patients with potentially resectable liver metastases only, as many as 20–50% have had secondary liver surgery [199, 267]. Patient selection, rather than more efficient treatment is responsible for these figures.

The distinction between resectable and non-resectable liver metastases is far from clear and probably interpreted differently at different hospitals. A common definition of non-resectable metastases is large size, poor location, multinodularity, and/or extrahepatic disease. A sufficiently large volume of the liver must remain after resection. None of these factors necessarily implies that surgery could not remove all tumour lesions without any pretreatment but they all indicate poor prognosis [267], and most teams likely hesitate to operate upfront even if some of those patients could have been long-term survivors after primary surgery. Patients operated upon for cure after conversion chemotherapy have a prognosis that is almost in line with those with less advanced disease having surgery alone, suggesting that their survival has been improved. However, the magnitude of the survival gain is not precisely known. Even if the magnitude of gain in the EPOC trial [261] was limited, disappointing to many, the study tells that combinations of local and systemic treatments are here to stay.

Preoperative chemotherapy increases toxicity at liver surgery and there is a wish to restrict the number of cycles before resection [267]. However, even if this is valid, the inability of present systemic treatments to eradicate all subclinical disease is what ultimately kills most patients. The balance between the number of cycles before resection, toxicity at surgery, and the possibility of curing as many as possible is not properly known. Since preoperative treatment is likely the most relevant part for OS, the number of cycles given should not be too few even if 'resectability' is rapidly achieved. Six to eight cycles of a fortnightly regimen before and four to six after is probably better than three to four before, although this statement is not universally agreed upon.

Immediate palliation

In these patients with progressive, usually symptomatic, disease, there is a need rapidly to induce antitumour activity, and tumour regression, without necessarily fulfilling criteria for an objective response. At the same time, treatment is palliative since the disease burden is too extensive to allow future surgery, even if good regression is seen, and excessive toxicity should be avoided. A prolonged time to progression and as long and as good a life as possible are the ultimate aims. A chemotherapy doublet (see Table 38.6 for examples), alone or with bevacizumab, is the currently preferred choice. In the light of the results of the FIRE-3 trial described above showing prolonged survival with the addition of cetuximab if the tumour was RAS wild-type, some would argue that an EGFR-inhibitor should be the preferred first-line treatment. In analogy, if the tumour is RAS-mutated, a triplet, alone or with bevacizumab, is an option since this treatment also prolongs PFS and OS. If starting with a doublet, it does not matter whether oxaliplatin or an irinotecan doublet is used for survival. Toxicity is important, and one has to choose between the risk of getting disturbing peripheral neuropathy, possibly for the rest of the patient's life, from the point of diagnosis or at a later time, and initial hair loss, which is seen more frequently after irinotecan. In the second-line situation, the other combination is used. If bevacizumab were not part of first-line treatment, it could then be added. In the third-line situation, an EGFR inhibitor can be used, alone or preferably with irinotecan, in KRAS wild-type tumours.

Palliation

In many patients with recently detected disseminated disease, no or only mild tumour-related symptoms are present. If, in addition, there are no signs of rapidly progressive disease, such as leucocytosis, thrombocytosis, or increased alkaline phosphatase, and the extent of disease and/or comorbidity precludes secondary surgery, an initial period of wait-and-see or fluoropyrimidines alone is a valid option. If no initial treatment is chosen, close monitoring is recommended. Clinical evaluation with simple laboratory tests every month and imaging every other month may be appropriate. A strategy to wait until symptoms or other signs of progression appear, with clinical evaluation every other month, may compromise OS, as was seen in a randomized trial [163]. In the trial, OS was almost median five months longer (14 versus nine months, P <0.02, N = 183) in the primary chemotherapy group. During this initial wait-and-see period, the patient could be eligible for 'window-of-opportunity' trials exploring new molecular compounds [268]. Otherwise, a fluoropyrimidine (5-FUFA or capecitabine) alone or with bevacizumab is indicated since this strategy postpones severe toxicity and does not compromise survival [195, 202]. When this treatment no longer controls disease, one of the doublets is given followed by the other after progression. In RAS wild-type tumours, an EGFR-inhibitor could be used in the fourth line and possibly regorafenib or TAS102 in the fifth and so far last evidence-based line.

Treatment interruptions, maintenance therapy

Breaks in the treatment should be utilized frequently whenever tumour growth is retarded. Several trials have shown that (toxic) chemotherapy holidays in one or another way in properly selected patients do not compromise OS [243, 244, 269–273]. A systematic review of 11 studies including 4854 patients concluded that 'intermittent strategies of delivering systemic treatment of mCRC do not result in a clinically significant reduction in OS compared with a continuous strategy of delivery, and should be part of an informed discussion of treatment options with patients with mCRC' [274]. Several details, such as the proper duration of the (intensive) chemotherapy phase, the duration of the interruption, and whether or not maintenance is of value, are still missing. The French GERCOR group randomized 620 patients to FOLFOX-4 continuously or FOLFOX-7 with oxaliplatin in a stop-and-go fashion [269]. OS was similar in the two groups (19 versus 21 months, ns). In a subsequent trial (OPTIMOX-2, N = 202), 5-FUFA was not used in the oxaliplatin-free periods [275]. Since OS tended to be worse in the stop-and-go group (median 19 versus 26 months, P = 0.055), it has been suggested that maintenance with 5-FUFA is better than a chemotherapy-free period. Whether targeted drugs have a role during the maintenance has been explored in trials. The Cairo3 trial [276] randomized 558 patients to either a maintenance group receiving capecitabine and bevacizumab or an observation group who had reached at least stable disease after six cycles of 3-weekly capecitabin, oxaliplatin and bevacizumab (CAPOX-B). Time to the primary endpoint, secondary progression (PFS2), was 11.7 months in the maintenance group and 8.5 months in the observation group (HR 0.67, P = 0.0001). Global quality of life did not deteriorate during maintenance treatment. A German study (AIO KRK 0207) has preliminarily reached similar results [277]. In the trial, bevacizumab alone was not inferior to a fluoropyrimidine with bevacizumab as maintenance treatment. OS was not improved.

Two trials have evaluated erlotinib, a small molecule against EGFR as maintenance treatment. In the GERCOR-DREAM study [278] including 452 patients PFS (4.9 months with bevacizumab alone and 5.9 months with bevacizumab/erlotinib (HR 0.77, P = 0.01). OS was also prolonged (median 22.1 months versus 24.9 months (HR 0.79, P = 0.04). In the other trial (Nordic ACT) [279] enrolling 249 patients median PFS was 4.2 months in the group of patients who received bevacizumab alone and 5.7 months in those receiving bevacizumab and erlotinib (HR 0.79, P = 0.2). Collectively, the trials show that interruptions in the administration of intensive chemotherapy should be used and indicate that if the breaks are filled with less intensive treatment, at least time to progression will be prolonged. The best maintenance treatment is not established.

Concluding remarks and remaining issues

The results of chemotherapy have improved substantially during the past several years. From being a treatment of unproven value, benefiting very few, during the 1980s, it is now a well-documented treatment prolonging survival, relieving, or postponing symptoms in many, and potentially curing a few if combined with local methods, particularly surgery. Median survival has been prolonged from about six months to above 22–24 months in some patient series (Table 38.4). Earlier detection of metastatic disease, generally because of routinely performed imaging with methods like spiral CT and MRI, detecting smaller lesions than possible before, is responsible for some of the longer survival seen. Selection of patients with more limited disease spread, for example only or predominantly liver metastases, is another important reason for the apparently much better results. Medical oncology is not solely responsible for the progress.

The extra months, or years, gained are generally good months in spite of the toxicity seen. Future improvements are probable using a multidisciplinary approach, together with the hope that new treatments, based upon recent tumour-biological knowledge, will eventually yield clinically meaningful effects. The exploration of new and better response predictors has highest priority. So far, only RAS mutation status is relevant for routine use prior to EGFR inhibition [280]. Besides likely predicting resistance to EGFR-inhibition, the presence of a BRAF-mutation also indicates poor survival, and it is possible that this should influence the choice of initial therapy, e.g. not to start with a fluoropyrimidine alone but rather with a doublet or rather give a triplet instead of a doublet. There are no trial data to guide in this decision. The lack of predictors is particularly critical for antiangiogenesis treatments. The gains seen so far with the 'biologics' have, however, been modest, sometimes minute. Trial designs other than performing large randomized studies to, hopefully, find those incremental gains must be explored. Target-driven small randomized phase-II studies and window trials are some examples [268, 281].

Multidisciplinary management of complex cases

For a general discussion of multidisciplinary management, see Chapter 39.

Patients presenting with an intermediate or locally advanced rectal cancer and synchronous metastases are particularly challenging cases, both if they are potentially curable should all disease ultimately be resected radically and if this is not possible, i.e. the intent is palliative from diagnosis. Two case presentations will illustrate the therapeutic dilemmas.

Case 1

A 69-year-old previously healthy man has noted blood in his stool for a few months. Minor problems with defecation. No weight loss. A 5 cm large rectal tumour 5 cm from the anal verge is discovered. Biopsies show infiltrating mucinous adenocarcinoma. Pelvic MRI reveals a cT3dN2 tumour, EMVI+, MRF+, i.e. locally advanced (ugly) requiring preoperative (C)RT to be resected with high probability of local control. CT of the thorax and abdomen shows three three to five large liver metastases, all in the right lobe. The liver metastases require a right-sided hepatectomy to be radically resected, even if they are diminished in size. The patient is potentially curable.

The greatest threat to this patient's life is the liver metastases. For this reason, initial combination therapy can be advocated. The primary tumour may also respond to systemic therapy, but radiation has a higher probability for response. Conventional CRT over five to sex weeks is an option, but the systemic chemotherapy component is then weak during those weeks and during the recovery period, i.e. up to ten weeks overall. Higher dose intensity of the systemic treatment can be achieved if 5 x 5 Gy is given, allowing full-dose chemotherapy from ten to 12 days later. The patient requires all modalities, and an attractive sequence is 5 x 5 Gy, combination chemotherapy, surgery of the liver metastases and the primary, and possibly more chemotherapy up to about six months in all if regression was seen during the induction phase.

Case 2

The same case as above. An MRI of the liver reveals eight additional small metastases involving all segments. There is thus no potential for cure and the situation is palliative. The liver metastases are still the greatest threat to the length of life, which is why upfront chemotherapy is the preferred option. The primary tumour does not require immediate intervention, and surgery without prior radiation and a delay is suboptimal. If the patient responds, the chemotherapy may continue. If the primary tumour does not become symptomatic, chemotherapy through the second and third lines may continue. If symptoms cannot be controlled by chemotherapy, local RT may be given, often controlling symptoms for six to eight months. Surgery for the primary may often not be needed, but should always be considered if it is expected to cause local problems not controlled by the non-surgical therapies. With the extent of liver metastases at diagnosis, liver surgery is not relevant even if a good response is seen.

Further reading

Birgisson H, Påhlman L, Gunnarsson U, Glimelius B. Late adverse effects of radiation therapy for rectal cancer—a systematic overview. Acta Oncologica 2007; 46: 504–516.

Bujko K, Glynne-Jones R, Bujko M. Does adjuvant fluoropyrimidine-based chemotherapy provide a benefit for patients with resected rectal cancer who have already received neoadjuvant radio(chemo)therapy? A systematic review of randomized trials. Annals of Oncology 2010; 21: 1743–1750.

Burton S, Brown G, Daniels IR, Norman AR, Mason B et al. MRI directed multidisciplinary team preoperative treatment strategy: the way to eliminate positive circumferential margins? British Journal of Cancer 2006; 94: 351–357.

Colorectal Cancer Collaborative Group. Adjuvant therapy for rectal cancer: a systematic overview of 8507 patients from 22 randomised trials. Lancet 2001; 358: 1291–1304.

Folkesson J, Birgisson H, Påhlman L, Cedermark B, Glimelius B et al. Swedish Rectal Cancer Trial: Long lasting benefits from radiotherapy on survival and local recurrence rate. Journal of Clinical Oncology 2005; 23: 5644–5650.

Glimelius B. Multidisciplinary treatment of patients with rectal cancer: Development during the past decades and plans for the future. Upsala Journal of Medical Sciences 2012; 117: 225–236.

Glynne-Jones R, Hughes R. Critical appraisal of the 'wait and see' approach in rectal cancer for clinical complete responders after chemoradiation. British Journal of Surgery 2012; 99: 897–909.

Habr-Gama A, Perez RO, Nadalin W, Sabbaga J, Ribeiro U Jr et al. Operative versus nonoperative treatment for stage 0 distal rectal cancer following chemoradiation therapy: long-term results. Annals of Surgery 2004; 240: 711–717.

Heald RJ, Husband EM, Ryall RD. The mesorectum in rectal cancer surgery—the clue to pelvic recurrence? British Journal of Surgery 1982; 69: 613–616.

Hoirup Petersen S, Harling H, Kirkeby LT, Wille-Jorgensen P, Mocellin S. Postoperative adjuvant chemotherapy in rectal cancer operated for cure. Cochrane Database of Systematic Reviews 2012: CD004078.pub2.

Köhne C-H, Cunningham D, Di Costanzo F, Glimelius B, Blijham G et al. Clinical determinants of survival in patients with 5-fluorouracil-based treatment for metastatic colorectal cancer: results of a multivariate analysis of 3825 patients. Annals of Oncology 2002; 13: 308–317.

Lahaye MJ, Engelen SM, Nelemans PJ, Beets GL, van de Velde CJ et al. Imaging for predicting the risk factors—the circumferential resection margin and nodal disease—of local recurrence in rectal cancer: a meta-analysis. Seminars in Ultrasound, CT and MRI 2005; 26: 259–268.

Macedo LT, da Costa Lima AB, Sasse AD. Addition of bevacizumab to first-line chemotherapy in advanced colorectal cancer: a systematic review and meta-analysis, with emphasis on chemotherapy subgroups. BMC Cancer 2012; 12: 89.

Matthiessen P, Hallbook O, Rutegard J, Simert G, Sjodahl R. Defunctioning stoma reduces symptomatic anastomotic leakage after low anterior resection of the rectum for cancer: a randomized multicenter trial. Annals of Surgery 2007; 246: 207–214.

National Institute for Health and Clinical Excellence. Bevacizumab and cetuximab for the treatment of metastatic colorectal cancer 2009; 118. Available from: <https://www.nice.org.uk/guidance/ta118>, accessed on 24 May 2015.

Påhlman L, Bohe M, Cedermark B, Dahlberg M, Lindmark G et al. The Swedish rectal cancer registry. British Journal of Surgery 2007; 94: 1285–1292.

Schmoll HJ, Van Cutsem E, Stein A, Valentini V, Glimelius B et al. ESMO Consensus Guidelines for management of patients with colon and rectal cancer. a personalized approach to clinical decision making. Annals of Oncology 2012; 23: 2479–2516.

Sebag-Montefiore D, Stephens RJ, Steele R, Monson J, Grieve R et al. Preoperative radiotherapy versus selective post-operative chemoradiotherapy in patients with rectal cancer (MRC CR07 and NCIC-CTG C016): a multicentre, randomised trial. Lancet 2009; 373: 811–820.

Sobin LH, Gospodarowics MK, Wittekind C. TNM classification of malignant tumours. New York: Wiley-Blackwell, 2009.

Valentini V, Aristei C, Glimelius B, Minsky BD, Beets-Tan R et al. Multidisciplinary rectal cancer management. Radiotherapy & Oncology 2009; 92: 148–163.

van Gijn W, Marijnen CA, Nagtegaal ID, Kranenbarg EM, Putter H et al. Preoperative radiotherapy combined with total mesorectal excision for resectable rectal cancer: 12-year follow-up of the multicentre, randomised controlled TME trial. Lancet Oncology 2011; 12: 575–582.

Vale CL, Tierney JF, Fisher D, Adams RA, Kaplan R et al. Does anti-EGFR therapy improve outcome in advanced colorectal cancer? A systematic review and meta-analysis. Cancer Treatment Reviews 2012; 38: 618–625.

References

1. Sobin LH, Gospodarowics MK, Wittekind Ch. TNM classification of malignant tumours. New York: Wiley-Blackwell, 2009.

2. Quirke P, Cuvelier C, Ensari A, Glimelius B, Laurberg S, Ortiz H, et al. Evidence-based medicine: the time has come to set standards for staging. Journal of Pathology 2010; 221: 357–360.

3. How is colorectal cancer staged? http://www.cancer.org/cancer/colonandrectumcancer/detailedguide/colorectal-cancer-staged. American Cancer Society, 2014.

4. Jass JR. Colorectal polyposes: from phenotype to diagnosis. Pathology, Research and Practice 2008; 204: 431–447.

5. Nicholls RJ, Mason AY, Morson BC, Dixon AK, I Kelsey Fry. The clinical staging of rectal cancer. British Journal of Surgery 1982; 69: 404–409.

6. Bipat S, Glas AS, Slors FJ, Zwinderman AH, Bossuyt PM et al. Rectal cancer: local staging and assessment of lymph node involvement with endoluminal US, CT, and MR imaging—a meta-analysis. Radiology 2004; 232: 773–783.

7. Lahaye MJ, Engelen SM, Nelemans PJ, Beets GL, van de Velde CJ et al. Imaging for predicting the risk factors—the circumferential resection margin and nodal disease—of local recurrence in rectal cancer: a meta-analysis. Seminars in Ultrasound, CT and MRI 2005; 26: 259–268.

8. Extramural depth of tumor invasion at thin-section MR in patients with rectal cancer: results of the MERCURY study. Radiology 2007; 243: 132–139.

9. Copel L, Sosna J, Kruskal JB, Raptopoulos V, Farrell RJ et al. CT colonography in 546 patients with incomplete colonoscopy. Radiology 2007; 244: 471–478.

10. Sauer R, Becker H, Hohenberger W, Rodel C, Wittekind C et al. Preoperative versus postoperative chemoradiotherapy for rectal cancer. New England Journal of Medicine 2004; 351: 1731–1740.

11. Frykholm G, Glimelius B, Påhlman L. Pre- or postoperative irradiation in adenocarcinoma of the rectum: Final treatment results of a randomized trial and an evaluation of late secondary effects. Diseases of the Colon & Rectum 1993; 36: 564–572.

12. Colorectal Cancer Collaborative Group. Adjuvant therapy for rectal cancer: a systematic overview of 8507 patients from 22 randomised trials. Lancet 2001; 358: 1291–1304.

13. Gunderson LL, Sargent DJ, Tepper JE, O'Connell MJ, Allmer C et al. Impact of T and N substage on survival and disease relapse in adjuvant rectal cancer: a pooled analysis. International Journal of Radiation Oncology Biology Physics 2002; 54: 386–396.

14. Nagtegaal ID, Quirke P. What is the role for the circumferential margin in the modern treatment of rectal cancer? Journal of Clinical Oncology 2008; 26: 303–312.

15. Marijnen CA, Nagtegaal ID, Kapiteijn E, Kranenbarg EK, Noordijk EM et al. Radiotherapy does not compensate for positive resection margins in rectal cancer patients: report of a multicenter randomized trial. International Journal of Radiation Oncology Biology Physics 2003; 55: 1311–1320.

16. Hildebrandt U, Feifel G, Schwarz HP, Scherr O. Endorectal ultrasound: instrumentation and clinical aspects. International Journal of Colorectal Diseasesease 1986; 1: 203–207.

17. Beynon J, Foy DM, Roe AM, Temple LN, Mortensen NJ. Endoluminal ultrasound in the assessment of local invasion in rectal cancer. British Journal of Surgery 1986; 73: 474–477.

18. Beets-Tan R, Beets G, Vliegen R, Kesels A, Van Boven H et al. Accuracy of magnetic resonance imaging in prediction of tumour-free resection margin in rectal cancer surgery. Lancet 2001; 357: 497–504.

19. Blomqvist L, Machado M, Rubio C, Gabrielsson N, Granqvist S et al. Rectal tumour staging: MR imaging using pelvic phased-array and endorectal coils vs endoscopic ultrasonography. European Radiology 2000; 10: 653–660.

20. Peschaud F, Cuenod CA, Benoist S, Julie C, Beauchet A et al. Accuracy of magnetic resonance imaging in rectal cancer depends on location of the tumor. Diseases of the Colon & Rectum 2005; 48: 1603–1609.

21. Beets-Tan RG, Lettinga T, Beets GL. Pre-operative imaging of rectal cancer and its impact on surgical performance and treatment outcome. European Journal of Surgical Oncology 2005; 31: 681–688.

22. Burton S, Brown G, Daniels IR, Norman AR, Mason B et al. MRI directed multidisciplinary team preoperative treatment strategy: the way to eliminate positive circumferential margins? British Journal of Cancer 2006; 94: 351–357.

23. Wang C, Zhou Z, Wang Z, Zheng Y, Zhao G et al. Patterns of neoplastic foci and lymph node micrometastasis within the mesorectum. Langenbeck's Archives of Surgery 2005; 390: 312–318.

24. Brown G, Richards CJ, Bourne MW, Newcombe RG, Radcliffe AG et al. Morphologic predictors of lymph node status in rectal cancer with use of high-spatial-resolution MR imaging with histopathologic comparison. Radiology 2003; 227: 371–377.

25. Kim JH, Beets GL, Kim MJ, Kessels AG, Beets-Tan RG. High-resolution MR imaging for nodal staging in rectal cancer: are there any criteria in addition to the size? European Journal of Radiology 2004; 52: 78–83.

26. Guillem JG, Diaz-Gonzalez JA, Minsky BD, Valentini V, Jeong SY et al. cT3N0 rectal cancer: potential overtreatment with preoperative chemoradiotherapy is warranted. Journal of Clinical Oncology 2008; 26: 368–373.

27. Lahaye MJ, Engelen SM, Kessels AG, de Bruine AP, von Meyenfeldt MF et al. USPIO-enhanced MR imaging for nodal staging in patients with primary rectal cancer: predictive criteria. Radiology 2008; 246: 804–811.

28. Cecil TD, Sexton R, Moran BJ, Heald RJ. Total mesorectal excision results in low local recurrence rates in lymph node-positive rectal cancer. Diseases of the Colon & Rectum 2004; 47: 1145–1149; discussion 9–50.

29. Vliegen RF, Beets GL, Lammering G, Dresen RC, Rutten HJ et al. Mesorectal fascia invasion after neoadjuvant chemotherapy and radiation therapy for locally advanced rectal cancer: accuracy of MR imaging for prediction. Radiology 2008; 246: 454–462.

30. Kulkarni T, Gollins S, Maw A, Hobson P, Byrne R et al. Magnetic resonance imaging in rectal cancer downstaged using neoadjuvant chemoradiation: accuracy of prediction of tumour stage and circumferential resection margin status. Colorectal Diseases 2008; 10: 479–489.

31. Dresen RC, Beets GL, Rutten HJ, Engelen SM, Lahaye MJ et al. Locally advanced rectal cancer: MR imaging for restaging after neoadjuvant radiation therapy with concomitant chemotherapy. Part I. Are we able to predict tumor confined to the rectal wall? Radiology 2009; 252: 71–80.

32. Barbaro B, Fiorucci C, Tebala C, Valentini V, Gambacorta MA et al. Locally advanced rectal cancer: MR imaging in prediction of response after preoperative chemotherapy and radiation therapy. Radiology 2009; 250: 730–739.

33. Curvo-Semedo L, Lambregts DM, Maas M, Thywissen T, Mehsen RT et al. Rectal cancer: assessment of complete response to preoperative combined radiation therapy with chemotherapy—conventional MR volumetry versus diffusion-weighted MR imaging. Radiology 2011; 260: 734–743.

34. Cafferty FH, Wong JM, Yen AM, Duffy SW, Atkin WS et al. Findings at follow-up endoscopies in subjects with suspected colorectal abnormalities: effects of baseline findings and time to follow-up. Cancer Journal 2007; 13: 263–270.

35. Qi Y, Stoddard D, Monson JR. Indications and techniques of transanal endoscopic microsurgery (TEMS). Journal of Gastrointestinal Surgery 2011; 15: 1306–1308.

36. Barendse RM, van den Broek FJ, Dekker E, Bemelman WA, de Graaf EJ et al. Systematic review of endoscopic mucosal resection versus transanal endoscopic microsurgery for large rectal adenomas. Endoscopy 2011; 43: 941–949.

37. Guenaga KK, Matos D, Wille-Jorgensen P. Mechanical bowel preparation for elective colorectal surgery. Cochrane Database of Systemic Reviews 2009: CD001544.

38. Slim K, Vicaut E, Launay-Savary MV, Contant C, Chipponi J. Updated systematic review and meta-analysis of randomized clinical trials on the role of mechanical bowel preparation before colorectal surgery. Annals of Surgery 2009; 249: 203–209.

39. Nelson RL, Glenny AM, Song F. Antimicrobial prophylaxis for colorectal surgery. Cochrane Database of Systemic Reviews 2009:CD001181.

40. Rasmussen MS, Jorgensen LN, Wille-Jorgensen P, Nielsen JD, Horn A et al. Prolonged prophylaxis with dalteparin to prevent late thromboembolic complications in patients undergoing major abdominal surgery: a multicenter randomized open-label study. Journal of Thrombosis and Haemostasis 2006; 4: 2384–2390.

41. Heald RJ, Husband EM, Ryall RD. The mesorectum in rectal cancer surgery—the clue to pelvic recurrence? British Journal of Surgery 1982; 69: 613–616.

42. Pezim ME, Nicholls RJ. Survival after high or low ligation of the inferior mesenteric artery during curative surgery for rectal cancer. Annals of Surgery 1984; 200: 729–733.

43. Lange MM, Marijnen CA, Maas CP, Putter H, Rutten HJ et al. Risk factors for sexual dysfunction after rectal cancer treatment. European Journal of Cancer 2009; 45: 1578–1588.

44. Kodeda K, Holmberg E, Jorgren F, Nordgren S, Lindmark G. Rectal washout and local recurrence of cancer after anterior resection. British Journal of Surgery 2010; 97: 1589–1597.

45. Williams NS, Dixon MF, Johnston D. Reappraisal of the 5 centimetre rule of distal excision for carcinoma of the rectum: a study of distal intramural spread and of patients' survival. British Journal of Surgery 1983; 70: 150–154.

46. Rullier E, Laurent C, Bretagnol F, Rullier A, Vendrely V et al. Sphincter-saving resection for all rectal carcinomas: the end of the 2-cm distal rule. Annals of Surgery 2005; 241: 465–469.

47. Karanjia ND, Schache DJ, North WR, Heald RJ. 'Close shave' in anterior resection. British Journal of Surgery 1990; 77: 510–512.

48. Holm T, Ljung A, Haggmark T, Jurell G, Lagergren J. Extended abdominoperineal resection with gluteus maximus flap reconstruction of the pelvic floor for rectal cancer. British Journal of Surgery 2007; 94: 232–238.

49. Laurent C, Leblanc F, Wutrich P, Scheffler M, Rullier E. Laparoscopic versus open surgery for rectal cancer: long-term oncologic results. Annals of Surgery 2009; 250: 54–61.

50. Jayne DG, Guillou PJ, Thorpe H, Quirke P, Copeland J et al. UK MRC CLASICC Trial Group. Randomized trial of laparoscopic-assisted resection of colorectal carcinoma: 3-year results of the UK MRC CLASICC Trial Group. Journal of Clinical Oncology 2007; 25: 3061–3068.

51. Choi DJ, Kim SH, Lee PJ, Kim J, Woo SU. Single-stage totally robotic dissection for rectal cancer surgery: technique and short-term outcome in 50 consecutive patients. Diseases of the Colon & Rectum 2009; 52: 1824–1830.

52. Green BL, Marshall HC, Collinson F, Quirke P, Guillou P et al. Long-term follow-up of the Medical Research Council CLASICC trial of conventional versus laparoscopically assisted resection in colorectal cancer. British Journal of Surgery 2013; 100: 75–82.

53. van der Pas MH, Haglind E, Cuesta MA, Fürst A, Lacy AM et al. COlorectal cancer Laparoscopic or Open Resection II (COLOR II) Study Group. Laparoscopic versus open surgery for rectal cancer (COLOR II): short-term outcomes of a randomised, phase 3 trial. Lancet Oncology 2013; 14: 210–218.

54. Collinson FJ1, Jayne DG, Pigazzi A, Tsang C, Barrie JM et al. An international, multicentre, prospective, randomised, controlled, unblinded, parallel-group trial of robotic-assisted versus standard laparoscopic surgery for the curative treatment of rectal cancer. International Journal of Colorectal Disease 2012; 27(2): 233–241.

55. Rouanet P, Mourregot A, Azar CC, Carrere S, Gutowski M et al. Transanal endoscopic proctectomy: an innovative procedure for difficult resection of rectal tumors in men with narrow pelvis. Diseases of the Colon Rectum. 2013; 56: 408-15.

56. Velthuis S, van den Boezem PB, van der Peet DL, Cuesta MA, Sietses C. Feasibility study of transanal total mesorectal excision. Br J Surg. 2013; 100: 828-31.

57. Påhlman L, Bohe M, Cedermark B, Dahlberg M, Lindmark G et al. The Swedish rectal cancer registry. British Journal of Surgery 2007; 94: 1285–1292.

58. Matthiessen P, Hallbook O, Rutegard J, Simert G, Sjodahl R. Defunctioning stoma reduces symptomatic anastomotic leakage after low anterior resection of the rectum for cancer: a randomized multi-center trial. Annals of Surgery 2007; 246: 207–214.

59. Påhlman L, Glimelius B. Local recurrences after surgical treatment for rectal carcinoma. Acta Chirurgica Scandinavica 1984; 150: 331–335.

60. MacFarlane JK, Ryall RDH, Heald RJ. Mesorectal excision for rectal cancer. Lancet 1993; 341: 457–460.

61. Martling AL, Holm T, Rutqvist LE, Moran BJ, Heald RJ et al. Effect of a surgical training programme on outcome of rectal cancer in the County of Stockholm. Lancet 2000; 356: 93–96.

62. Birgisson H, Talback M, Gunnarsson U, Påhlman L, Glimelius B. Improved survival in cancer of the colon and rectum in Sweden. European Journal of Surgical Oncology 2005; 31: 845–853.

63. Valentini V, Aristei C, Glimelius B, Minsky BD, Beets-Tan R et al. Multidisciplinary rectal cancer management. Radiotherapy & Oncology 2009; 92: 148–163.

64. Glimelius B. Multidisciplinary treatment of patients with rectal cancer: Development during the past decades and plans for the future. Upsala Journal of Medical Sciences 2012; 117: 225–236.

65. Glimelius B, Beets-Tan R, Blomqvist L, Brown G, Nagtegaal I et al. Mesorectal fascia instead of circumferential resection margin in pre-operative staging of rectal cancer. Journal of Clinical Oncology 2011; 29: 2142–2143.

66. NCI. Clinical Announcement. Adjuvant therapy of rectal cancer, 14 March. National Cancer Institute, Bethesda, Maryland, US, 1991.

67. Swedish Rectal Cancer Trial. Improved survival with preoperative radiotherapy in resectable rectal cancer. New England Journal of Medicine 1997; 336: 980–987.

68. Kapiteijn E, Marijnen CAM, Nagtegaal ID, Putter H, Steup WH et al. Preoperative radiotherapy in combination with total mesorectal exci-sion improves local control in resectable rectal cancer. Report from a multicenter randomized trial. New England Journal of Medicine 2001; 345: 638–646.

69. Sebag-Montefiore D, Stephens RJ, Steele R, Monson J, Grieve R et al. Preoperative radiotherapy versus selective postoperative chemoradiotherapy in patients with rectal cancer (MRC CR07 and NCIC-CTG C016): a multicentre, randomised trial. Lancet 2009; 373: 811–820.

70. Folkesson J, Birgisson H, Påhlman L, Cedermark B, Glimelius B et al. Swedish Rectal Cancer Trial: Long lasting benefits from radiotherapy on survival and local recurrence rate. Journal of Clinical Oncology 2005; 23: 5644–5650.

71. Peeters KCMJ, Marijnen CAM, Nagtegaal ID, Kranenberg EK, Putter H et al. For the Dutch Colorectal Cancer Group. The TME trial after a median follow-up of 5 years: increased local control but no survival benefit in irradiated patients with resectable rectal carcinoma. Annals of Surgery 2007; 246: 693–701.

72. van Gijn W, Marijnen CA, Nagtegaal ID, Kranenbarg EM, Putter H et al. Preoperative radiotherapy combined with total mesorectal excision for resectable rectal cancer: 12-year follow-up of the mul-ticentre, randomised controlled TME trial. Lancet Oncology 2011; 12: 575–582.

73. Glimelius B, Isacsson U, Jung B, Påhlman L. Radiotherapy in addition to radical surgery in rectal cancer: evidence for a dose-response effect favouring preoperative treatment. International Journal of Radiation Oncology Biology Physics 1997; 37: 281–287.

74. Bujko K, Nowacki MP, Nasierowska-Guttmejer A, Michalski W, Bebenek M et al. Long-term results of a randomised trial comparing preoperative short-course radiotherapy vs preoperative convention-ally fractionated chemoradiation for rectal cancer. British Journal of Surgery 2006; 93: 1215–1223.

75. Ngan SY, Burmeister B, Fisher RJ, Solomon M, Goldstein D et al. Randomized trial of short-course radiotherapy versus long-course chemoradiation comparing rates of local recurrence in patients with t3 rectal cancer: trans-tasman radiation oncology group trial 01.04. Journal of Clinical Oncology 2012; 30: 3827–3833.

76. Birgisson H, Påhlman L, Gunnarsson U, Glimelius B. Late adverse effects of radiation therapy for rectal cancer—a systematic overview. Acta Oncologica 2007; 46: 504–516.

77. Gerard JP, Conroy T, Bonnetain F, Bouche O, Chapet O et al. Preoperative radiotherapy with or without concurrent fluorouracil and leucovorin in T3-4 rectal cancers: results of FFCD 9203. Journal of Clinical Oncology 2006; 24: 4620–4625.

78. Bosset JF, Collette L, Calais G, Mineur L, Maingon P et al. Chemotherapy with preoperative radiotherapy in rectal cancer. New England Journal of Medicine 2006; 355: 1114–1123.

79. Braendengen M, Tveit KM, Berglund Å, Birkemeyer E, Frykholm G et al. A randomized phase III study (LARCS) comparing preoperative radiotherapy alone versus chemoradiotherapy in non-resectable rectal cancer. Journal of Clinical Oncology 2008; 26: 3687–3694.

80. Glimelius B, Holm T, Blomqvist L. Chemotherapy in addition to preop-erative radiotherapy in locally advanced rectal cancer—a systematic overview. Reviews on Recent Clinical Trials 2008; 3: 204–211.

81. Bujko K, Kepka L, Michalski W, Nowacki MP. Does rectal cancer shrinkage induced by preoperative radio(chemo)therapy increase the likelihood of anterior resection? A systematic review of randomised trials. Radiotherapy & Oncology 2006; 80: 4–12.

82. Gerard JP, Rostom Y, Gal J, Benchimol D, Ortholan C et al. Can we increase the chance of sphincter saving surgery in rectal cancer with neoadjuvant treatments: lessons from a systematic review of recent randomized trials. Critical Reviews in Oncology/Hematology 2012; 81: 21–28.

83. Baatrup G, Endreseth BH, Isaksen V, Kjellmo A, Tveit KM et al. Preoperative staging and treatment options in T1 rectal adenocarci-noma. Acta Oncologica 2009; 48: 328–342.

84. Gerard JP, Ortholan C, Benezery K, Ginot A, Hannoun-Levi JM et al. Contact X-ray therapy for rectal cancer: experience in Centre Antoine-Lacassagne, Nice, 2002-2006. International Journal of Radiation Oncology Biology Physics 2008; 72: 665–670.

85. Radu C, Berglund Å, Påhlman L, Glimelius B. Short course preopera-tive radiotherapy with delayed surgery in rectal cancer—a retrospective study. Radiotherapy & Oncology 2008; 87: 343–349.

86. Hatfield P, Hingorani M, Radhakrishna G, Cooper R, Melcher A et al. Short-course radiotherapy, with elective delay prior to surgery, in patients with unresectable rectal cancer who have poor performance status or significant co-morbidity. Radiotherapy & Oncology 2009; 92: 210–214.

87. Pettersson D, Holm T, Iversen H, Blomqvist L, Glimelius B et al. Preoperative short-course radiotherapy with delayed surgery in pri-mary rectal cancer. British Journal of Surgery 2012; 99: 577–583.

88. Hofheinz RD, Wenz F, Post S, Matzdorff A, Laechelt S et al. Chemoradiotherapy with capecitabine versus fluorouracil for locally advanced rectal cancer: a randomised, multicentre, non-inferiority, phase 3 trial. Lancet Oncology 2012; 13: 579–588.

89. Rödel C, Graeven U, Fietkau R, et al. Oxaliplatin added to fluorouracil-based preoperative chemoradiotherapy and postoperative chemotherapy of locally advanced rectal cancer: the German CAO/ARO/AIO-04 randomised phase 3 trial. Lancet Oncology 2015; in press.

90. Gerard JP, Azria D, Gourgou-Bourgade S, Martel-Laffay I, Hennequin C et al. Comparison of two neoadjuvant chemoradiotherapy regi-mens for locally advanced rectal cancer: results of the phase III trial ACCORD 12/0405-Prodige 2. Journal of Clinical Oncology 2010; 28: 1638–1644.

91. Aschele C, Cionini L, Lonardi S, Pinto C, Cordio S et al. Primary tumor response to preoperative chemoradiation with or without oxaliplatin in locally advanced rectal cancer: pathologic results of the STAR-01 randomized phase III trial. Journal of Clinical Oncology 2011; 29: 2773–2780.

92. Dewdney A, Cunningham D, Tabernero J, Capdevila J, Glimelius B et al. Multicenter randomized phase II clinical trial comparing

neoadjuvant oxaliplatin, capecitabine, and preoperative radiotherapy with or without cetuximab followed by total mesorectal excision in patients with high-risk rectal cancer (EXPERT-C). Journal of Clinical Oncology 2012; 30: 1620–1627.

93. Sclafani F, Gonzalez D, Cunningham D, Hulkki Wilson S, Peckitt C et al. TP53 mutational status and cetuximab benefit in rectal cancer: 5-year results of the EXPERT-C trial. Journal of the National Cancer Institute 2014; 106(7).

94. Habr-Gama A, Perez RO, Nadalin W, Sabbaga J, Ribeiro U Jr et al. Operative versus nonoperative treatment for stage 0 distal rectal cancer following chemoradiation therapy: long-term results. Annals of Surgery 2004; 240: 711–717.

95. Maas M, Beets-Tan RG, Lambregts DM, Lammering G, Nelemans PJ et al. Wait-and-see policy for clinical complete responders after chemoradiation for rectal cancer. Journal of Clinical Oncology 2011; 29: 4633–4640.

96. Hughes R, Harrison M, Glynne-Jones R. Could a wait and see policy be justified in T3/4 rectal cancers after chemo-radiotherapy? Acta Oncologica 2010; 49: 378–381.

97. Glynne-Jones R, Hughes R. Critical appraisal of the 'wait and see' approach in rectal cancer for clinical complete responders after chemoradiation. British Journal of Surgery 2012; 99: 897–909.

98. Bujko K, Kolodziejczyk M, Nasierowska-Guttmejer A, Michalski W, Kepka L et al. Tumour regression grading in patients with residual rectal cancer after preoperative chemoradiation. Radiotherapy & Oncology 2010; 95: 298–302.

99. Chen TY, Emmertsen KJ, Laurberg S. What are the best questionnaires to capture anorectal function after surgery in rectal cancer? Current Colorectal Cancer Reports 2015; 11: 37–43.

100. Martoni AA, Di Fabio F, Pinto C, Castellucci P, Pini S et al. Prospective study on the FDG-PET/CT predictive and prognostic values in patients treated with neoadjuvant chemoradiation therapy and radical surgery for locally advanced rectal cancer. Annals of Oncology 2011; 22: 650–656.

101. Yoon MS, Ahn SJ, Nah BS, Chung WK, Song JY et al. The metabolic response using 18F-fluorodeoxyglucose-positron emission tomography/computed tomography and the change in the carcinoembryonic antigen level for predicting response to pre-operative chemoradiotherapy in patients with rectal cancer. Radiotherapy & Oncology 2011; 98: 134–138.

102. Syk E, Torkzad MR, Blomqvist L, Nilsson PJ, Glimelius B. Local recurrence in rectal cancer: Anatomic localization and effect on radiation target. International Journal of Radiation Oncology Biology Physics 2008; 72: 658–664.

103. Nijkamp J, Kusters M, Beets-Tan RG, Martijn H, Beets GL et al. Three-dimensional analysis of recurrence patterns in rectal cancer: the cranial border in hypofractionated preoperative radiotherapy can be lowered. International Journal of Radiation Oncology Biology Physics 2011; 80: 103–110.

104. Kusters M, Wallner C, Lange MM, Deruiter MC, van de Velde CJ et al. Origin of presacral local recurrence after rectal cancer treatment. British Journal of Surgery 2010; 97: 1582–1587.

105. Yano H, Moran BJ. The incidence of lateral pelvic side-wall nodal involvement in low rectal cancer may be similar in Japan and the West. British Journal of Surgery 2008; 95: 33–49.

106. Taylor N, Crane C, Skibber J, Feig B, Ellis L et al. Elective groin irradiation is not indicated for patients with adenocarcinoma of the rectum extending to the anal canal. International Journal of Radiation Oncology Biology Physics 2001; 51: 741–747.

107. West NP, Finan PJ, Anderin C, Lindholm J, Holm T et al. Evidence of the oncologic superiority of cylindrical abdominoperineal excision for low rectal cancer. Journal of Clinical Oncology 2008; 26: 3517–3522.

108. Bakx R, Emous M, Legemate DA, Zoetmulder FA, van Tienhoven G et al. Harm and benefits of short-term pre-operative radiotherapy in patients with resectable rectal carcinomas. European Journal of Surgical Oncology 2006; 32: 520–526.

109. Birgisson H, Påhlman L, Gunnarsson U, Glimelius B. Occurrence of second cancers in patients treated with radiotherapy for rectal cancer. Journal of Clinical Oncology 2005; 23: 6126–6131.

110. Wiltink LM, Nout RA, Fiocco M, Meershoek-Klein Kranenbarg E, Jurgenliemk-Schulz IM et al. No increased risk of second cancer after radiotherapy in patients treated for rectal or endometrial cancer in the randomized TME, PORTEC-1, and PORTEC-2 trials. Journal of Clinical Oncology 2015; 33: 1640–1646.

111. Kripp M, Wieneke J, Kienle P, Welzel G, Brade J et al. Intensified neoadjuvant chemoradiotherapy in locally advanced rectal cancer—impact on long-term quality of life. European Journal of Surgical Oncology 2012; 38: 472–477.

112. Bosset JF, Puyraveau M, Mineur L, Calais G, Bardet E et al. EORTC 22921 Rectal Cancer Trial: Quality of life (QoL) and functional outcome 5 years after treatment. ECCO 16 2011: abs. 6018.

113. Braendengen M, Tveit KM, Bruheim K, Cvancarova M, Berglund Å et al. Late patient-reported toxicity after preoperative radiotherapy or chemoradiotherapy in nonresectable rectal cancer: Results from a randomized phase III study. International Journal of Radiation Oncology Biology Physics 2011; 81: 1017–1024.

114. Braendengen M, Tveit KM, Hjermstad MJ, Johansson H, Berglund K et al. Health-related quality of life (HRQoL) after multimodal treatment for primarily non-resectable rectal cancer. Long-term results from a phase III study. European Journal of Cancer 2012; 48: 813–819.

115. Jonker DJ, Spithoff K, Maroun J. Adjuvant systemic chemotherapy for Stage II and III colon cancer after complete resection: an updated practice guideline. Clinical Oncology (Royal College of Radiologists) 2011; 23: 314–322.

116. Schmoll HJ, Van Cutsem E, Stein A, Valentini V, Glimelius B et al. ESMO Consensus Guidelines for management of patients with colon and rectal cancer. a personalized approach to clinical decision making. Annals of Oncology 2012; 23: 2479–2516.

117. Hoirup Petersen S, Harling H, Kirkeby LT, Wille-Jorgensen P, Mocellin S. Postoperative adjuvant chemotherapy in rectal cancer operated for cure. Cochrane Database of Systematic Reviews 2012: CD004078.pub2.

118. Breugom AJ, Swets M, Bosset JF, Collette L, Sainato A et al. Adjuvant chemotherapy after preoperative (chemo)radiotherapy and surgery for patients with rectal cancer: a systematic review and meta-analysis of individual patient data. Lancet Oncology 2015;16: 200–207.

119. Bujko K, Glimelius B, Valentini V, Michalski W, Spalek M. Postoperative chemotherapy in patients with rectal cancer receiving preoperative radio(chemo)therapy: A meta-analysis of randomized trials comparing surgery +/– a fluoropyrimidine and surgery + a fluoropyrimidine +/– oxaliplatin. European Journal of Surgical Oncology 2015; 41: 713–723.

120. Bujko K, Glynne-Jones R, Bujko M. Does adjuvant fluoropyrimidine-based chemotherapy provide a benefit for patients with resected rectal cancer who have already received neoadjuvant radio(chemo)therapy? A systematic review of randomized trials. Annals of Oncology 2010; 21: 1743–1750.

121. Sakamoto J, Hamada C, Yoshida S, Kodaira S, Yasutomi M, Kato T, et al. An individual patient data meta-analysis of adjuvant therapy with uracil-tegafur (UFT) in patients with curatively resected rectal cancer. British Journal of Cancer 2007; 96: 1170–1177.

122. Hamaguchi T, Shirao K, Moriya Y, Yoshida S, Kodaira S et al. Final results of randomized trials by the National Surgical Adjuvant Study of Colorectal Cancer (NSAS-CC). Cancer Chemotherapy and Pharmacology 2011; 67: 587–596.

123. Sakamoto J, Hamada C, Kodaira S, Nakazato H, Ohashi Y. Adjuvant therapy with oral fluoropyrimidines as main chemotherapeutic agents after curative resection for colorectal cancer: individual patient data meta-analysis of randomized trials. Japanese Journal of Clinical Oncology 1999; 29: 78–86.

124. Meta-Analysis Group of the Japanese Society for cancer of the colon and rectum and the Meta-Analysis Group in cancer. Efficacy of oral adjuvant

therapy after resection of colorectal cancer: 5-year results from three randomized trials. Journal of Clinical Oncology 2004; 22: 484–492.

125. Quasar Collaborative Group, Gray R, Barnwell J, McConkey C, Hills RK et al. Adjuvant chemotherapy versus observation in patients with colorectal cancer: a randomised study. Lancet 2007; 370: 2020–2029.

126. Fountzilas G, Zisiadis A, Dafni U, Konstantaras C, Hatzitheoharis G et al. Postoperative radiation and concomitant bolus fluorouracil with or without additional chemotherapy with fluorouracil and high-dose leucovorin in patients with high-risk rectal cancer: a randomized phase III study conducted by the Hellenic Cooperative Oncology Group. Annals of Oncology 1999; 10: 671–676.

127. Mansour EG, Lefkopoulou M, Johnson R, Douglass H. A comparison of postoperative adjuvant chemotherapy, radiotherapy or combination therapy in potentially curable resectable rectal carcinoma. An ECOG study Est 4276. Proceedings of the American Society of Clinical Oncology 1991; 10: 154 abs.

128. Taal BG, Van Tinteren H, Zoetmulder FA. Adjuvant 5FU plus levamisole in colonic or rectal cancer: improved survival in stage II and III. British Journal of Cancer 2001; 85: 1437–1443.

129. Cafiero F, Gipponi M, Peressini A, Bertoglio S, Lionetto R. Preliminary analysis of a randomized clinical trial of adjuvant postoperative RT vs. postoperative RT plus 5-FU and levamisole in patients with TNM stage II-III resectable rectal cancer. Journal of Surgical Oncology 2000; 75: 80–88.

130. Bosset JF, Calais G, Mineur L, Maingon P, Stojanovic-Rundic S et al. Fluorouracil-based adjuvant chemotherapy after preoperative chemoradiotherapy in rectal cancer: long-term results of the EORTC 22921 randomised study. Lancet Oncology 2014; 15: 184–190.

131. Breugom AJ, van Gijn W, Muller EW, Berglund A, van den Broek CB et al. Adjuvant chemotherapy for rectal cancer patients treated with preoperative (chemo)radiotherapy and total mesorectal excision: a Dutch Colorectal Cancer Group (DCCG) randomized phase III trial. Annals of Oncology 2015; 26: 696–701.

132. Glynne-Jones R, Counsell N, Quirke P, Mortensen N, Maraveyas A et al. Chronicle: results of a randomised phase III trial in locally advanced rectal cancer after neoadjuvant chemoradiation randomising postoperative adjuvant capecitabine plus oxaliplatin (XELOX) versus control. Annals of Oncology 2014; 25: 1356–1362.

133. Sainato A, Cernusco Luna Nunzia V, Valentini V, De Paoli A, Maurizi ER et al. No benefit of adjuvant Fluorouracil Leucovorin chemotherapy after neoadjuvant chemoradiotherapy in locally advanced cancer of the rectum (LARC): long term results of a randomized trial (I-CNR-RT). Radiotherapy and Oncology 2014; 113: 223–229.

134. Kusters M, Valentini V, Calvo FA, Krempien R, Nieuwenhuijzen GA et al. Results of European pooled analysis of IORT-containing multimodality treatment for locally advanced rectal cancer: adjuvant chemotherapy prevents local recurrence rather than distant metastases. Annals of Oncology 2010; 21: 1279–1284.

135. Valentini V, van Stiphout RG, Lammering G, Gambacorta MA, Barba MC et al. Nomograms for predicting local recurrence, distant metastases, and overall survival for patients with locally advanced rectal cancer on the basis of European randomized clinical trials. Journal of Clinical Oncology 2011; 29: 3163–3172.

136. National Comprehensive Cancer Network. Rectal Cancer. NCCN Clinical Practice Guidelines in Oncology 2011, ver. 3. NCCN, 2011.

137. Valentini V, Glimelius B. Rectal cancer radiotherapy: towards European consensus. Acta Oncologica 2010; 49: 1206–1216.

138. Biagi JJ, Raphael MJ, Mackillop WJ, Kong W, King WD et al. Association between time to initiation of adjuvant chemotherapy and survival in colorectal cancer: a systematic review and meta-analysis. Journal of the American Medical Association 2011; 305: 2335–2342.

139. Chua YJ, Barbachano Y, Cunningham D, Oates JR, Brown G et al. Neoadjuvant capecitabine and oxaliplatin before chemoradiotherapy and total mesorectal excision in MRI-defined poor-risk rectal cancer: a phase 2 trial. Lancet Oncology 2010; 11: 241–248.

140. Fernandez-Martos C, Pericay C, Aparicio J, Salud A, Safont M et al. Phase II, randomized study of concomitant chemoradiotherapy followed by surgery and adjuvant capecitabine plus oxaliplatin (CAPOX) compared with induction CAPOX followed by concomitant chemoradiotherapy and surgery in magnetic resonance imaging-defined, locally advanced rectal cancer: Grupo cancer de recto 3 study. Journal of Clinical Oncology 2010; 28: 859–865.

141. Nilsson PJ, van Etten B, Hospers GAP, Påhlman L, van de Velde CJH et al. Short-course radiotherapy followed by neo-adjuvant chemotherapy in locally advanced rectal cancer—the RAPIDO trial. BMC Cancer 2013; 13: 279.

142. Collette L, Bosset JF, den Dulk M, Nguyen F, Mineur L et al. Patients with curative resection of cT3-4 rectal cancer after preoperative radiotherapy or radiochemotherapy: does anybody benefit from adjuvant fluorouracil-based chemotherapy? Journal of Clinical Oncology 2007; 25: 4379–386.

143. Wille-Jorgensen P, Laurberg S, Pahlman L, Carriquiry L, Lundqvist N et al. An interim analysis of recruitment to the COLOFOL trial. Colorectal Diseases 2009; 11: 756–758.

144. Jorgensen OD, Kronborg O, Fenger C, Rasmussen M. Influence of long-term colonoscopic surveillance on incidence of colorectal cancer and death from the disease in patients with precursors (adenomas). Acta Oncologica 2007; 46: 355–360.

145. Kjeldsen BJ, Kronborg O, Fenger C, Jörgensen OD. A prospective randomized study of follow-up after radical surgery for colorectal cancer. British Journal of Surgery 1997; 84: 666–669.

146. Strand E, Nygren I, Bergkvist L, Smedh K. Nurse or surgeon follow-up after rectal cancer: a randomized trial. Colorectal Diseases 2011; 13: 999–1003.

147. van Gijn W, van de Velde CJ. Improving quality of cancer care through surgical audit. European Journal of Surgical Oncology 2010; 36(Suppl. 1): S23–S26.

148. Lemmens VE, de Haan N, Rutten HJ, Martijn H, Loosveld OJ et al. Improvements in population-based survival of patients presenting with metastatic rectal cancer in the south of the Netherlands, 1992–2008. Clinical & Experimental Metastasis 2011; 28: 283–290.

149. Sorbye H, Pfeiffer P, Cavalli-Bjorkman N, Qvortrup C, Holsen MH et al. Clinical trial enrollment, patient characteristics, and survival differences in prospectively registered metastatic colorectal cancer patients. Cancer 2009; 115: 4679–4687.

150. Colorectal Cancer Collaborative Group. Palliative chemotherapy for advanced colorectal cancer: systematic review and meta-analysis. British Medical Journal 2000; 321: 531–535.

151. Golfinopoulos V, Salanti G, Pavlidis N, Ioannidis JP. Survival and disease-progression benefits with treatment regimens for advanced colorectal cancer: a meta-analysis. Lancet Oncology 2007; 8: 898–911.

152. Hind D, Tappenden P, Tumur I, Eggington S, Sutcliffe P et al. The use of irinotecan, oxaliplatin and raltitrexed for the treatment of advanced colorectal cancer: systematic review and economic evaluation. Health Technology Assessment 2008; 12: iii–ix, xi–162.

153. Allegra C, Blanke C, Buyse M, Goldberg R, Grothey A et al. End points in advanced colon cancer clinical trials: a review and proposal. Journal of Clinical Oncology 2007; 25: 3572–3575.

154. Slevin ML, Stubbs L, Plant HJ, Wilson P, Gregory WM et al. Attitudes to chemotherapy: comparing views of patients with cancer with those of doctors, nurses, and general public [see comments]. British Medical Journal 1990; 300: 1458–1460.

155. McCabe C, Bergmann L, Bosanquet N, Ellis M, Enzmann H, von Euler M, et al. Market and patient access to new oncology products in Europe: a current, multidisciplinary perspective. Annals of Oncology 2009; 20: 403–412.

156. Krol M, Koopman M, Uyl-de Groot C, Punt CJ. A systematic review of economic analyses of pharmaceutical therapies for advanced colorectal cancer. Expert Opinion on Pharmacotherapy 2007; 8: 1313–1328.

157. National Institute for Health and Clinical Excellence. Bevacizumab and cetuximab for the treatment of metastatic colorectal cancer 2009; 118. Available from: <https://www.nice.org.uk/guidance/ta118>, accessed on 24 May 2015.

158. Moertel CG. Chemotherapy for colorectal cancer. New England Journal of Medicine 1994; 16: 1136–1142.

159. Nordic Gastrointestinal Tumour Adjuvant Therapy Group. Sequential methotrexate/5-fluorouracil/leucovorin (MFL) is superior to 5-fluorouracil alone in advanced symptomatic colorectal carcinoma. A randomized trial. Journal of Clinical Oncology 1989; 7: 1437–1446.

160. Poon MA, O'Connell MJ, Moertel CG, Wieand HS, Cullinan SA et al. Biochemical modulation of fluorouracil: Evidence of significant improvement of survival and quality of life in patients with advanced colorectal carcinoma. Journal of Clinical Oncology 1989; 7: 1407–1418.

161. Ragnhammar P, Hafström Lo, Nygren P, Glimelius B. A systematic overview of chemotherapy effects in colorectal cancer. Acta Oncologica 2001; 40: 282–308.

162. Cunningham D, Pyrhönen S, James RD, Pant CJA, Hickish TF et al. Randomised trial of irinotecan plus supportive care versus supportive care alone after fluorouracil failure for patients with metastatic colorectal cancer. Lancet 1998; 352: 1413–1418.

163. Nordic Gastrointestinal Tumour Adjuvant Therapy Group. Expectancy or primary chemotherapy in patients with advanced asymptomatic colorectal cancer: a randomized trial. Journal of Clinical Oncology 1992; 10: 904–911.

164. Funaioli C, Longobardi C, Martoni AA. The impact of chemotherapy on overall survival and quality of life of patients with metastatic colorectal cancer: a review of phase III trials. Journal of Chemotherapy 2008; 20: 14–27.

165. Byström P, Johansson B, Bergström I, Berglund Å, Sorbye H et al. Health-related quality of life as therapeutic guidance in patients with advanced colorectal cancer receiving palliative combination chemotherapy. Acta Oncologica 2013; 3(2): 57–71.

166. Graf W, Glimelius B, Påhlman L, Bergström R. The relationship between an objective response to chemotherapy and survival in advanced colorectal cancer. British Journal of Cancer 1994; 70: 559–563.

167. Buyse M, Thirion P, Carlson RW, Burzykowski T, Molenberghs G et al. Relation between tumour response to first-line chemotherapy and survival in advanced colorectal cancer: a meta-analysis. Meta-Analysis Group in Cancer. Lancet 2000; 356: 373–378.

168. Therasse P, Eisenhauer EA, Verweij J. RECIST revisited: a review of validation studies on tumour assessment. European Journal of Cancer 2006; 42: 1031–1039.

169. Suzuki C, Blomqvist L, Sundin A, Jacobsson H, Bystrom P et al. The initial change in tumor size predicts response and survival in patients with metastatic colorectal cancer treated with combination chemotherapy. Annals of Oncology 2012; 23: 948–954.

170. Blanke CD, Bot BM, Thomas DM, Bleyer A, Kohne CH et al. Impact of young age on treatment efficacy and safety in advanced colorectal cancer: a pooled analysis of patients from nine first-line phase III chemotherapy trials. Journal of Clinical Oncology 2011; 29: 2781–2786.

171. Köhne C-H, Cunningham D, Di Costanzo F, Glimelius B, Blijham G et al. Clinical determinants of survival in patients with 5-fluorouracil-based treatment for metastatic colorectal cancer: results of a multivariate analysis of 3825 patients. Annals of Oncology 2002; 13: 308–317.

172. Sobrero AF, Aschele C, Bertino JR. Fluorouracil in colorectal cancer—a tale of two drugs: implications for biochemical modulation. Journal of Clinical Oncology 1997; 15: 368–381.

173. de Gramont A, Bosset JF, Milan C, Rougier P, Bouche O et al. Randomized trial comparing monthly low-dose leucovorin and fluorouracil bolus with bimonthly high-dose leucovorin and fluorouracil bolus plus continuous infusion for advanced colorectal cancer: a French intergroup study. Journal of Clinical Oncology 1997; 15: 808–815.

174. Aranda E, Diaz-Rubio E, Cervantes A, Antón-Torres A, Carrato A et al. Randomized trial comparing monthly low-dose leucovorin and fluorouracil bolus with weekly high-dose 48-hour continuous-infusion fluorouracil for advanced colorectal cancer: A Spanish Cooperative Group for Gastrointestinal Tumor Therapy (TTD) study. Annals of Oncology 1998; 9: 727–731.

175. Weh HJ, Zschaber R, Braumann D, Hoelzer P, Hoffmann R et al. A randomized phase III study comparing weekly folinic acid (FA) and high-dose 5-fluorouracil (5-FU) with monthly 5-FU/FA (days 1-5) in untreated patients with metastatic colorectal carcinoma. Onkologie 1998; 21: 403–407.

176. Vincent M, Ho C, Tomiak A, Winquist E, Whiston F et al. Toxicity analysis of the 5-day bolus 5-fluorouracil/folinic acid regimen for the treatment of colorectal carcinoma from 2 randomized controlled trials: a concern about dose. Clinical Colorectal Cancer 2002; 2: 111–118.

177. Nordic Gastrointestinal Tumor Adjuvant Therapy Group. Biochemical modulation of 5-fluorouracil: A randomized comparison of sequential methotrexate, 5-fluorouracil and leucovorin versus sequential 5-fluorouracil and leucovorin in patients with advanced symptomatic colorectal cancer. Annals of Oncology 1993; 4: 235–241.

178. Van Cutsem E, Twelves C, Cassidy J, Allman D, Bajetta E et al. Oral capecitabine compared with intravenous fluorouracil plus leucovorin in patients with metastatic colorectal cancer: results of a large phase III study. Journal of Clinical Oncology 2001; 19: 4097–4106.

179. Satoh T, Sakata Y. S-1 for the treatment of gastrointestinal cancer. Expert Opinion on Pharmacotherapy 2012; 13: 1943–1959.

180. Kurtz JE, Andres E, Natarajan-Ame S, Noel E, Dufour P. Oral chemotherapy in colorectal cancer treatment: review of the literature. European Journal of Internal Medicine 2003; 14: 18–25.

181. de Gramont A, Figer A, Seymour M, Homerin M, Hmissi A et al. Leucovorin and fluorouracil with or without oxaliplatin as first-line treatment in advanced colorectal cancer. Journal of Clinical Oncology 2000; 18: 2938–2947.

182. Martoni A, Mini E, Pinto C, Nobili S, Gentile AL et al. Oxaliplatin and protracted continuous 5-fluorouracil infusion in patients with pretreated advanced colorectal carcinoma. Annals of Oncology 2001; 12: 519–524.

183. Sørbye H, Glimelius B, Berglund Å, Fokstuen T, Tveit KM et al. Multicentre phase II study of Nordic 5-fluorouracil/Leucovorin bolus schedule combined with oxaliplatin (FLOX) as first-line treatment of metastatic colorectal cancer. Journal of Clinical Oncology 2004; 22: 31–38.

184. Arkenau HT, Arnold D, Cassidy J, Diaz-Rubio E, Douillard JY et al. Efficacy of oxaliplatin plus capecitabine or infusional fluorouracil/leucovorin in patients with metastatic colorectal cancer: a pooled analysis of randomized trials. Journal of Clinical Oncology 2008; 26: 5910–5917.

185. Rougier P, Van Cutsem E, Bajetta E, Niederle N, Possinger K et al. Randomised trial of irinotecan versus fluorouracil by continuous infusion after fluorouracil failure in patients with metastatic colorectal cancer. Lancet 1998; 352: 1407–1412.

186. Douillard JY, Cunningham D, Roth AD, Navarro M, James RD et al. Irinotecan combined with fluorouracil compared with fluorouracil alone as first-line treatment for metastatic colorectal cancer: a multicentre randomised trial. Lancet 2000; 355: 1041–1047.

187. Saltz LB, Cox JV, Blanke C, Rosen LS, Fehrenbacher L et al. Irinotecan plus fluorouracil and leucovorin for metastatic colorectal cancer. Irinotecan Study Group. New England Journal of Medicine 2000; 343: 905–914.

188. Rothenberg ML, Meropol NJ, Poplin EA, Van Cutsem E, Wadler S. Mortality associated with irinotecan plus bolus fluorouracil/leucovorin: summary findings of an independent panel. Journal of Clinical Oncology 2001; 19: 3801–3807.

189. Goldberg RM, Sargent DJ, Morton RF, Fuchs CS, Ramanathan RK et al. Randomized controlled trial of reduced-dose bolus fluorouracil plus leucovorin and irinotecan or infused fluorouracil plus leucovorin and oxaliplatin in patients with previously untreated metastatic colorectal cancer: a North American Intergroup Trial. Journal of Clinical Oncology 2006; 24: 3347–3353.

190. Glimelius B, Sorbye H, Balteskard L, Bystrom P, Pfeiffer P et al. A randomized phase III multicenter trial comparing irinotecan in combination with the Nordic bolus 5-FU and folinic acid schedule or the bolus/infused de Gramont schedule (LV5FU2) in patients with metastatic colorectal cancer. Annals of Oncology 2008; 19: 909–914.

191. Ducreux M, Bennouna J, Hebbar M, Ychou M, Lledo G et al. Capecitabine plus oxaliplatin (XELOX) versus 5-fluorouracil/leucovorin plus oxaliplatin (FOLFOX-6) as first-line treatment for metastatic colorectal cancer. International Journal of Cancer 2011; 128: 682–690.

192. Cassidy J, Clarke S, Diaz-Rubio E, Scheithauer W, Figer A et al. XELOX vs FOLFOX-4 as first-line therapy for metastatic colorectal cancer: NO16966 updated results. British Journal of Cancer 2011; 105: 58–64.

193. Rothenberg ML, Cox JV, Butts C, Navarro M, Bang YJ et al. Capecitabine plus oxaliplatin (XELOX) versus 5-fluorouracil/folinic acid plus oxaliplatin (FOLFOX-4) as second-line therapy in metastatic colorectal cancer: a randomized phase III noninferiority study. Annals of Oncology 2008; 19: 1720–1726.

194. Kohne CH, De Greve J, Hartmann JT, Lang I, Vergauwe P et al. Irinotecan combined with infusional 5-fluorouracil/folinic acid or capecitabine plus celecoxib or placebo in the first-line treatment of patients with metastatic colorectal cancer. EORTC study 40015. Annals of Oncology 2008; 19: 920–926.

195. Koopman M, Antonini NF, Douma J, Wals J, Honkoop AH et al. Sequential versus combination chemotherapy with capecitabine, irinotecan, and oxaliplatin in advanced colorectal cancer (CAIRO): a phase III randomised controlled trial. Lancet 2007; 370: 135–142.

196. Moosmann N, von Weikersthal LF, Vehling-Kaiser U, Stauch M, Hass HG et al. Cetuximab plus capecitabine and irinotecan compared with cetuximab plus capecitabine and oxaliplatin as first-line treatment for patients with metastatic colorectal cancer: AIO KRK-0104—a randomized trial of the German AIO CRC study group. Journal of Clinical Oncology 2011; 29: 1050–1058.

197. Ducreux M, Adenis A, Pignon JP, Francois E, Chauffert B et al. Efficacy and safety of bevacizumab-based combination regimens in patients with previously untreated metastatic colorectal cancer: final results from a randomised phase ii study of bevacizumab plus 5-fluorouracil, leucovorin plus irinotecan versus bevacizumab plus capecitabine plus irinotecan (FNCLCC ACCORD 13/0503 study). European Journal of Cancer 2013; 49: 1236–1245.

198. Tournigand C, Andre T, Achille E, Lledo G, Flesh M et al. FOLFIRI followed by FOLFOX6 or the reverse sequence in advanced colorectal cancer: a randomized GERCOR study. Journal of Clinical Oncology 2004; 22: 229–237.

199. Folprecht G, Gruenberger T, Bechstein WO, Raab HR, Lordick F et al. Tumour response and secondary resectability of colorectal liver metastases following neoadjuvant chemotherapy with cetuximab: the CELIM randomised phase 2 trial. Lancet Oncology 2010; 11: 38–47.

200. Ocvirk J, Brodowicz T, Wrba F, Ciuleanu TE, Kurteva G et al. Cetuximab plus FOLFOX6 or FOLFIRI in metastatic colorectal cancer: CECOG trial. World Journal of Gastroenterology 2010; 16: 3133–3143.

201. Rothenberg ML, Oza AM, Bigelow RH, Berlin JD, Marshall JL et al. Superiority of oxaliplatin and fluorouracil-leucovorin compared with either therapy alone in patients with progressive colorectal cancer after irinotecan and fluorouracil-leucovorin: interim results of a phase III trial. Journal of Clinical Oncology 2003; 21: 2059–2069.

202. Seymour MT, Maughan TS, Ledermann JA, Topham C, James R et al. Different strategies of sequential and combination chemotherapy for patients with poor prognosis advanced colorectal cancer (MRC FOCUS): a randomised controlled trial. Lancet 2007; 370: 143–152.

203. Kim GP, Sargent DJ, Mahoney MR, Rowland KM, Jr, Philip PA et al. Phase III noninferiority trial comparing irinotecan with oxaliplatin, fluorouracil, and leucovorin in patients with advanced colorectal carcinoma previously treated with fluorouracil: N9841. Journal of Clinical Oncology 2009; 27: 2848–2854.

204. Seymour MT, Thompson LC, Wasan HS, Middleton G, Brewster AE et al. Chemotherapy options in elderly and frail patients with metastatic colorectal cancer (MRC FOCUS2): an open-label, randomised factorial trial. Lancet 2011; 377: 1749–1759.

205. Cunningham D, Sirohi B, Pluzanska A, Utracka-Hutka B, Zaluski J et al. Two different first-line 5-fluorouracil regimens with or without oxaliplatin in patients with metastatic colorectal cancer. Annals of Oncology 2009; 20: 244–250.

206. Ducreux M, Malka D, Mendiboure J, Etienne PL, Texereau P et al. Sequential versus combination chemotherapy for the treatment of advanced colorectal cancer (FFCD 2000-05): an open-label, randomised, phase 3 trial. Lancet Oncology 2011; 12: 1032–1044.

207. Falcone A, Ricci S, Brunetti I, Pfanner E, Allegrini G et al. Phase III trial of infusional fluorouracil, leucovorin, oxaliplatin, and irinotecan (FOLFOXIRI) compared with infusional fluorouracil, leucovorin, and irinotecan (FOLFIRI) as first-line treatment for metastatic colorectal cancer: the Gruppo Oncologico Nord Ovest. Journal of Clinical Oncology 2007; 25: 1670–1676.

208. Masi G, Vasile E, Loupakis F, Cupini S, Fornaro L et al. Randomized trial of two induction chemotherapy regimens in metastatic colorectal cancer: an updated analysis. Journal of the National Cancer Institute 2011; 103: 21–30.

209. Loupakis F, Cremolini C, Masi G, Lonardi S, Zagonel V, Salvatore L, et al. Initial therapy with FOLFOXIRI and bevacizumab for metastatic colorectal cancer. New England Journal of Medicine 2014; 371: 1609–1618.

210. Souglakos J, Androulakis N, Syrigos K, Polyzos A, Ziras N et al. FOLFOXIRI (folinic acid, 5-fluorouracil, oxaliplatin and irinotecan) vs FOLFIRI (folinic acid, 5-fluorouracil and irinotecan) as first-line treatment in metastatic colorectal cancer (MCC): a multicentre randomised phase III trial from the Hellenic Oncology Research Group (HORG). British Journal of Cancer 2006; 94: 798–805.

211. Gruenberger T, Bridgewater J, Chau I, Garcia Alfonso P, Rivoire M et al. Bevacizumab plus mFOLFOX-6 or FOLFOXIRI in patients with initially unresectable liver metastases from colorectal cancer: the OLIVIA multinational randomised phase II trial. Annals of Oncology 2015; 26: 702–708.

212. Hurwitz H, Fehrenbacher L, Novotny W, Cartwright T, Hainsworth J et al. Bevacizumab plus Irinotecan, Fluorouracil, and Leucovorin for Metastatic Colorectal Cancer. New England Journal of Medicine 2004; 350: 2335–2342.

213. Kabbinavar FF, Hambleton J, Mass RD, Hurwitz HI, Bergsland E et al. Combined analysis of efficacy: the addition of bevacizumab to fluorouracil/leucovorin improves survival for patients with metastatic colorectal cancer. Journal of Clinical Oncology 2005; 23: 3706–3712.

214. Kabbinavar FF, Hurwitz HI, Yi J, Sarkar S, Rosen O. Addition of bevacizumab to fluorouracil-based first-line treatment of metastatic colorectal cancer: pooled analysis of cohorts of older patients from two randomized clinical trials. Journal of Clinical Oncology 2009; 27: 199–205.

215. Tebbutt NC, Wilson K, Gebski VJ, Cummins MM, Zannino D et al. Capecitabine, bevacizumab, and mitomycin in first-line treatment of metastatic colorectal cancer: results of the Australasian Gastrointestinal Trials Group Randomized Phase III MAX Study. Journal of Clinical Oncology 2010; 28: 3191–3198.

216. Kozloff M, Yood MU, Berlin J, Flynn PJ, Kabbinavar FF et al. Clinical outcomes associated with bevacizumab-containing treatment of metastatic colorectal cancer: the BRiTE observational cohort study. Oncologist 2009; 14: 862–870.

217. Van Cutsem E, Rivera F, Berry S, Kretzschmar A, Michael M et al. Safety and efficacy of first-line bevacizumab with FOLFOX, XELOX, FOLFIRI and fluoropyrimidines in metastatic colorectal cancer: the BEAT study. Annals of Oncology 2009; 20: 1842–1847.

218. Hammerman A, Greenberg-Dotan S, Battat E, Feldhamer I, Bitterman H et al. The 'real-life' impact of adding bevacizumab to first-line therapy in metastatic colorectal cancer patients: a large Israeli retrospective cohort study. Acta Oncologica 2015; 54: 164–170.

219. Stein A, Petersen V, Schulze M, Seraphin J, Hoeffkes HG et al. Bevacizumab plus chemotherapy as first-line treatment for patients with metastatic colorectal cancer: results from a large German community-based observational cohort study. Acta Oncologica 2015; 54: 171–178.

220. Saltz LB, Clarke S, Diaz-Rubio E, Scheithauer W, Figer A et al. Bevacizumab in combination with oxaliplatin-based chemotherapy as first-line therapy in metastatic colorectal cancer: a randomized phase III study. Journal of Clinical Oncology 2008; 26: 2013–2019.

221. Bennouna J, Sastre J, Arnold D, Österlund P, Greil R et al. Continuation of bevacizumab after first progression in metastatic colorectal cancer (ML18147): a randomised phase 3 trial. Lancet Oncology 2013; 14(1): 29–37.

222. Giantonio BJ, Catalano PJ, Meropol NJ, O'Dwyer PJ, Mitchell EP et al. Bevacizumab in combination with oxaliplatin, fluorouracil, and leucovorin (FOLFOX4) for previously treated metastatic colorectal cancer: results from the Eastern Cooperative Oncology Group Study E3200. Journal of Clinical Oncology 2007; 25: 1539–1544.

223. Bennouna J, Sastre J, Arnold D, Osterlund P, Greil R et al. Continuation of bevacizumab after first progression in metastatic colorectal cancer (ML18147): a randomised phase 3 trial. Lancet Oncology 2013; 14: 29–37.

224. Stathopoulos GP, Batziou C, Trafalis D, Koutantos J, Batzios S et al. Treatment of colorectal cancer with and without bevacizumab: a phase III study. Oncology 2010; 78: 376–381.

225. Stintzing S, Fischer von Weikersthal L, Decker T, Vehling-Kaiser U, Jager E et al. FOLFIRI plus cetuximab versus FOLFIRI plus bevacizumab as first-line treatment for patients with metastatic colorectal cancer-subgroup analysis of patients with KRAS: mutated tumours in the randomised German AIO study KRK-0306. Annals of Oncology 2012; 23: 1693–1699.

226. Osterlund P, Soveri LM, Isoniemi H, Poussa T, Alanko T et al. Hypertension and overall survival in metastatic colorectal cancer patients treated with bevacizumab-containing chemotherapy. British Journal of Cancer 2011; 104: 599–604.

227. Hurwitz HI, Douglas PS, Middleton JP, Sledge GW, Johnson DH et al. Analysis of early hypertension and clinical outcome with bevacizumab: results from seven phase III studies. Oncologist 2013; 18: 273–280.

228. Macedo LT, da Costa Lima AB, Sasse AD. Addition of bevacizumab to first-line chemotherapy in advanced colorectal cancer: a systematic review and meta-analysis, with emphasis on chemotherapy subgroups. BMC Cancer 2012; 12: 89.

229. Van Cutsem E, Tabernero J, Lakomy R, Prenen H, Prausova J et al. Addition of aflibercept to fluorouracil, leucovorin, and irinotecan improves survival in a phase III randomized trial in patients with metastatic colorectal cancer previously treated with an oxaliplatin-based regimen. Journal of Clinical Oncology 2012; 30: 3499–506.

230. Cunningham D, Humblet Y, Siena S, Khayat D, Bleiberg H et al. Cetuximab monotherapy and cetuximab plus irinotecan in irinotecan-refractory metastatic colorectal cancer. New England Journal of Medicine 2004; 351: 337–345.

231. Jonker DJ, O'Callaghan CJ, Karapetis CS, Zalcberg JR, Tu D et al. Cetuximab for the treatment of colorectal cancer. New England Journal of Medicine 2007; 357: 2040–2048.

232. Van Cutsem E, Peeters M, Siena S, Humblet Y, Hendlisz A et al. Open-label phase III trial of panitumumab plus best supportive care compared with best supportive care alone in patients with chemotherapy-refractory metastatic colorectal cancer. Journal of Clinical Oncology 2007; 25: 1658–1664.

233. Karapetis CS, Khambata-Ford S, Jonker DJ, O'Callaghan CJ, Tu D et al. K-ras mutations and benefit from cetuximab in advanced colorectal cancer. New England Journal of Medicine 2008; 359: 1757–1765.

234. Amado RG, Wolf M, Peeters M, Van Cutsem E, Siena S et al. Wild-type KRAS is required for panitumumab efficacy in patients with metastatic colorectal cancer. Journal of Clinical Oncology 2008; 26: 1626–1634.

235. Modest DP, Jung A, Moosmann N, Laubender RP, Giessen C et al. The influence of KRAS and BRAF mutations on the efficacy of cetuximab-based first-line therapy of metastatic colorectal cancer: an analysis of the AIO KRK-0104-trial. International Journal of Cancer 2012; 131: 980–986.

236. Douillard JY, Oliner KS, Siena S, Tabernero J, Burkes R et al. Panitumumab-FOLFOX4 treatment and RAS mutations in colorectal cancer. New England Journal of Medicine 2013; 369: 1023–1034.

237. Stintzing S, Jung A, Rossius L, Modest DP, Fischer von Weikersthal L et al. Analysis of KRAS/NRAS and BRAF mutations in FIRE-3: A randomized phase III study of FOLFIRI plus cetuximab or bevacizumab as first-line treatment for wild-type (WT) KRAS (exon 2) metastatic colorectal cancer (mCRC) patients. European Journal of Cancer 2013; 49(Suppl 3): abs. LBA17.

238. Van Cutsem E, Kohne CH, Hitre E, Zaluski J, Chang Chien CR et al. Cetuximab and chemotherapy as initial treatment for metastatic colorectal cancer. New England Journal of Medicine 2009; 360: 1408–1417.

239. Van Cutsem E, Kohne CH, Lang I, Folprecht G, Nowacki MP et al. Cetuximab Plus Irinotecan, Fluorouracil, and Leucovorin As First-Line Treatment for Metastatic Colorectal Cancer: Updated Analysis of Overall Survival According to Tumor KRAS and BRAF Mutation Status. Journal of Clinical Oncology 2011; 29: 2011–2019.

240. Van Cutsem E, Lenz HJ, Kohne CH, Heinemann V, Tejpar S et al. Fluorouracil, leucovorin, and irinotecan plus cetuximab treatment and RAS mutations in colorectal cancer. Journal of Clinical Oncology 2015; 33: 692–700.

241. Richman SD, Seymour MT, Chambers P, Elliott F, Daly CL et al. KRAS and BRAF mutations in advanced colorectal cancer are associated with poor prognosis but do not preclude benefit from oxaliplatin or irinotecan: results from the MRC FOCUS trial. Journal of Clinical Oncology 2009; 27: 5931–5937.

242. Bokemeyer C, Cutsem EV, Rougier P, Ciardiello F, Heeger S et al. Addition of cetuximab to chemotherapy as first-line treatment for KRAS wild-type metastatic colorectal cancer: pooled analysis of the CRYSTAL and OPUS randomised clinical trials. European Journal of Cancer 2012; 48: 1466–1475.

243. Maughan TS, Adams RA, Smith CG, Meade AM, Seymour MT et al. Addition of cetuximab to oxaliplatin-based first-line combination chemotherapy for treatment of advanced colorectal cancer: results of the randomised phase 3 MRC COIN trial. Lancet 2011; 377: 2103–2114.

244. Tveit KM, Guren T, Glimelius B, Pfeiffer P, Sorbye H et al. Phase III trial of cetuximab with continuous or intermittent fluorouracil, leucovorin, and oxaliplatin (Nordic FLOX) census FLOX alone in first-line treatment of metastatic colorectal cancer: the NORDIC-VII Study. Journal of Clinical Oncology 2012; 30: 1755–1762.

245. Vale CL, Tierney JF, Fisher D, Adams RA, Kaplan R et al. Does anti-EGFR therapy improve outcome in advanced colorectal cancer? A systematic review and meta-analysis. Cancer Treatment Reviews 2012; 38: 618–625.

246. Heinemann V, von Weikersthal LF, Decker T, Kiani A, Vehling-Kaiser U et al. FOLFIRI plus cetuximab versus FOLFIRI plus bevacizumab as first-line treatment for patients with metastatic colorectal cancer (FIRE-3): a randomised, open-label, phase 3 trial. Lancet Oncology 2014; 15(10): 1065–1075.

247. Venook AP, Niedzwiecki D, Lenz H-J, Innocenti F, Mahoney MR. CALGB/SWOG 80405: Phase III trial of irinotecan/5-FU/leucovorin (FOLFIRI) or oxaliplatin/5-FU/leucovorin (mFOLFOX6) with bevacizumab (BV) or cetuximab (CET) for patients (pts) with KRAS wild-type (wt) untreated metastatic adenocarcinoma of the colon or rectum (MCRC). Journal of Clinical Oncology 2014; 25(Suppl. 4): abs. LBA3. doi:10.1093/annonc/mdu438.13

248. Price T, Peeters M, Kim TW, Li J, Cascinu S et al. ASPECCT: A randomized, multicenter, open-label, phase 3 study of panitumumab (pmab) vs cetuximab (cmab) for perviously treated wild-type (WT) KRAS metastatic colorectal cancer (mCRC). European Journal of Cancer 2013; 49:(Suppl 3): abs. LBA18.

249. Douillard JY, Siena S, Cassidy J, Tabernero J, Burkes R et al. Randomized, phase III trial of panitumumab with infusional fluorouracil, leucovorin, and oxaliplatin (FOLFOX4) versus FOLFOX4 alone as first-line treatment in patients with previously untreated metastatic colorectal cancer: the PRIME study. Journal of Clinical Oncology 2010; 28: 4697–4705.

250. Peeters M, Price TJ, Cervantes A, Sobrero AF, Ducreux M et al. Randomized phase III study of panitumumab with fluorouracil, leucovorin, and irinotecan (FOLFIRI) compared with FOLFIRI alone as second-line treatment in patients with metastatic colorectal cancer. Journal of Clinical Oncology 2010; 28: 4706–4713.

251. Therkildsen C, Bergmann TK, Henrichsen-Schnack T, Ladelund S, Nilbert M. The predictive value of KRAS, NRAS, BRAF, PIK3CA and PTEN for anti-EGFR treatment in metastatic colorectal cancer: a systematic review and meta-analysis. Acta Oncologica 2014; 53: 852–864.

252. Tol J, Koopman M, Cats A, Rodenburg CJ, Creemers GJ et al. Chemotherapy, bevacizumab, and cetuximab in metastatic colorectal cancer. New England Journal of Medicine 2009; 360: 563–572.

253. Hecht JR, Mitchell E, Chidiac T, Scroggin C, Hagenstad C et al. A randomized phase IIIB trial of chemotherapy, bevacizumab, and panitumumab compared with chemotherapy and bevacizumab alone for metastatic colorectal cancer. Journal of Clinical Oncology 2009; 27: 672–680.

254. Saltz LB, Lenz HJ, Kindler HL, Hochster HS, Wadler S et al. Randomized phase II trial of cetuximab, bevacizumab, and irinotecan compared with cetuximab and bevacizumab alone in irinotecan-refractory colorectal cancer: the BOND-2 study. Journal of Clinical Oncology 2007; 25: 4557–4561.

255. Feliu Batlle J, Cuadrado E, Castro J, Caldes T, Belda C et al. Irinotecan-cetuximab-bevacizumab as a salvage treatment in heavily pretreated metastatic colorectal cancer patients: a retrospective observational study. Chemotherapy 2011; 57: 138–144.

256. Larsen FO, Pfeiffer P, Nielsen D, Skougaard K, Qvortrup C et al. Bevacizumab in combination with cetuximab and irinotecan after failure of cetuximab and irinotecan in patients with metastatic colorectal cancer. Acta Oncologica 2011; 50: 574–577.

257. Grothey A, Van Cutsem E, Sobrero A, Siena S, Falcone A et al. Regorafenib monotherapy for previously treated metastatic colorectal cancer (CORRECT): an international, multicentre, randomised, placebo-controlled, phase 3 trial. Lancet 2013; 381: 303–312.

258. Mayer RJ, Van Cutsem E, Falcone A, Yoshino T, Garcia-Carbonero R et al. Randomized trial of TAS-102 for refractory metastatic colorectal cancer. New England Journal of Medicine 2015; 372: 1909–1919.

259. Tabernero J, Cohn AL, Obermannova R, Bodoky G, Garcia-Carbonero R et al. RAISE: A randomized, double-blind, multicenter phase III study of irinotecan, folinic acid, and 5-fluorouracil (FOLFIRI) plus ramucirumab (RAM) or placebo (PBO) in patients (pts) with metastatic colorectal carcinoma (CRC) progressive during or following first-line combination therapy with bevacizumab (bev), oxaliplatin (ox), and a fluoropyrimidine (fp). Journal of Clinical Oncology 2015; 33 (Suppl. 3): abs. 512.

260. Mitry E, Fields AL, Bleiberg H, Labianca R, Portier G et al. Adjuvant chemotherapy after potentially curative resection of metastases from colorectal cancer: a pooled analysis of two randomized trials. Journal of Clinical Oncology 2008; 26: 4906–4911.

261. Nordlinger B, Sorbye H, Glimelius B, Poston GJ, Schlag PM et al. Perioperative chemotherapy with FOLFOX4 and surgery versus surgery alone for resectable liver metastases from colorectal cancer (EORTC Intergroup trial 40983): a randomised controlled trial. Lancet 2008; 371: 1007–1016.

262. Papadimitriou CA, Papakostas P, Karina M, Malettou L, Dimopoulos MA et al. A randomized phase III trial of adjuvant chemotherapy with irinotecan, leucovorin and fluorouracil versus leucovorin and fluorouracil for stage II and III colon cancer: a Hellenic Cooperative Oncology Group study. BMC Medicine 2011; 9: 10.

263. Primrose J, Falk S, Finch-Jones M, Valle J, O'Reilly D et al. Systemic chemotherapy with or without cetuximab in patients with resectable colorectal liver metastasis: the New EPOC randomised controlled trial. Lancet Oncology 2014; 15: 601–611.

264. Folprecht G, Cunningham D, Ross P, Glimelius B, Di Costanzo F et al. Efficacy of 5-fluorouracil-based chemotherapy in elderly patients with metastatic colorectal cancer: a pooled analysis of clinical trials. Annals of Oncology 2004; 15: 1330–1338.

265. Giacchetti S, Itzhaki M, Gruia G, Adam R, Zidani R et al. Long-term survival of patients with unresectable colorectal cancer liver metastases following infusional chemotherapy with 5-fluorouracil, leucovorin, oxaliplatin and surgery. Annals of Oncology 1999; 10: 663–669.

266. Adam R, Delvart V, Pascal G, Valeanu A, Castaing D et al. Rescue surgery for unresectable colorectal liver metastases downstaged by chemotherapy: a model to predict long-term survival. Annals of Surgery 2004; 240: 644–657; discussion 57–58.

267. Nordlinger B, Van Cutsem E, Gruenberger T, Glimelius B, Poston G et al. Combination of surgery and chemotherapy and the role of targeted agents in the treatment of patients with colorectal liver metastases: recommendations from an expert panel. Annals of Oncology 2009; 20: 985–992.

268. Glimelius B, Lahn M, Gawande S, Cleverly A, Darstein C et al. A window of opportunity phase II study of enzastaurin in chemonaive patients with asymptomatic metastatic colorectal cancer. Annals of Oncology 2010; 21: 1020–1026.

269. Tournigand C, Cervantes A, Figer A, Lledo G, Flesch M et al. OPTIMOX1: a randomized study of FOLFOX4 or FOLFOX7 with oxaliplatin in a stop-and-go fashion in advanced colorectal cancer—a GERCOR study. Journal of Clinical Oncology 2006; 24: 394–400.

270. Maughan TS, James RD, Kerr DJ, Ledermann JA, Seymour MT et al. Comparison of intermittent and continuous palliative chemotherapy for advanced colorectal cancer: a multicentre randomised trial. Lancet 2003; 361: 457–464.

271. Lal R, Dickson J, Cunningham D, Chau I, Norman AR et al. A randomized trial comparing defined-duration with continuous irinotecan until disease progression in fluoropyrimidine and thymidylate synthase inhibitor-resistant advanced colorectal cancer. Journal of Clinical Oncology 2004; 22: 3023–3031.

272. Labianca R, Sobrero A, Isa L, Cortesi E, Barni S et al. Intermittent versus continuous chemotherapy in advanced colorectal cancer: a randomised 'GISCAD' trial. Annals of Oncology 2011; 22: 1236–1242.

273. Adams RA, Meade AM, Seymour MT, Wilson RH, Madi A et al. Intermittent versus continuous oxaliplatin and fluoropyrimidine combination chemotherapy for first-line treatment of advanced colorectal cancer: results of the randomised phase 3 MRC COIN trial. Lancet Oncology 2011; 12: 642–653.

274. Berry SR, Cosby R, Asmis T, Chan K, Hammad N et al. Continuous versus intermittent chemotherapy strategies in metastatic colorectal cancer: a systematic review and meta-analysis. Annals of Oncology 2015; 26: 477–485.

275. Chibaudel B, Maindrault-Goebel F, Lledo G, Mineur L, Andre T et al. Can chemotherapy be discontinued in unresectable metastatic colorectal cancer? The GERCOR OPTIMOX2 Study. Journal of Clinical Oncology 2009; 27: 5727–5733.

276. Simkens LH, van Tinteren H, May A, ten Tije AJ, Creemers GJ et al. Maintenance treatment with capecitabine and bevacizumab in metastatic colorectal cancer (CAIRO3): a phase 3 randomised controlled trial of the Dutch Colorectal Cancer Group. Lancet 2015; 385: 1843–1852.

277. Arnold D, Graeven U, Lerchenmuller C, Killing B, Depenbusch R et al. Maintenance strategy with fluoropyrimidines (FP) plus Bevacizumab (Bev), Bev alone, or no treatment, following a standard

combination of FP, oxaliplatin (Ox), and Bev as first-line treatment for patients with metastatic colorectal cancer (mCRC): a phase III non-inferiority trial (AIO KRK 0207). Journal of Clinical Oncology 2014; 32: 5s (suppl; abstr 3503).

278. Chibaudel B, Tournigand C, Samson B, Scheithauer W, Mesange P et al. Bevacizumab-erlotinib as maintenance therapy in metastatic colorectal cancer. Final results of the GERCOR DREAM study. ESMO 2014; abstr 4970.

279. Johnsson A, Hagman H, Frodin JE, Berglund A, Keldsen N et al. A randomized phase III trial on maintenance treatment with bevacizumab alone or in combination with erlotinib after chemotherapy and bevacizumab in metastatic colorectal cancer: the Nordic ACT Trial. Annals of Oncology 2013; 24: 2335–2341.

280. Asghar U, Hawkes E, Cunningham D. Predictive and prognostic biomarkers for targeted therapy in metastatic colorectal cancer. Clinical Colorectal Cancer 2010; 9: 274–281.

281. Freidlin B, McShane LM, Polley MY, Korn EL. Randomized phase II trial designs with biomarkers. Journal of Clinical Oncology 2012; 30: 3304–3309.

282. Stockholm Rectal Cancer Study Group. Preoperative short-term radiation therapy in operable rectal carcinoma. A prospective randomized trial. Cancer 1990; 66: 49–55.

283. Martling A, Holm T, Johansson H, Rutqvist LE, Cedermark B. The Stockholm II trial on preoperative radiotherapy in rectal carcinoma: long-term follow-up of a population-based study. Cancer 2001; 92: 896–902.

284. Ngan SY, Burmeister B, Fisher RJ, Solomon M, Goldstein D et al. Randomized trial of short-course radiotherapy versus long-course chemoradiation comparing rates of local recurrence in patients with T3 rectal cancer: Trans-Tasman Radiation Oncology Group Trial 01.04. Journal of Clinical Oncology 2012; 30(31): 3827–3833.

285. Sauer R, Liersch T, Merkel S, Fietkau R, Hohenberger W et al. Preoperative versus postoperative chemoradiotherapy for locally advanced rectal cancer: results of the German CAO/ARO/AIO-94 randomized phase III trial after a median follow-up of 11 years. Journal of Clinical Oncology 2012; 30: 1926–1933.

286. Glimelius B, Dahl O, Cedermark B, Jakobsen A, Bentzen SM et al. Adjuvant chemotherapy in colorectal cancer: a joint analysis of randomised trials by the Nordic Gastrointestinal Tumour Adjuvant Therapy Group. Acta Oncologica 2005; 44: 904–912.

287. Fisher B, Wolmark N, Rockette H, Redmond C, Deutsch M et al. Postoperative adjuvant chemotherapy or radiation therapy for rectal cancer: results from NSABP Protocol R-01. Journal of the National Cancer Institute 1988; 80: 21–29.

288. Kabbinavar F, Hurwitz HI, Fehrenbacher L, Meropol NJ, Novotny WF et al. Phase II, randomized trial comparing bevacizumab plus fluorouracil (FU)/leucovorin (LV) with FU/LV alone in patients with metastatic colorectal cancer. Journal of Clinical Oncology 2003; 21: 60–65.

289. Kabbinavar FF, Schulz J, McCleod M, Patel T, Hamm JT et al. Addition of bevacizumab to bolus fluorouracil and leucovorin in first-line metastatic colorectal cancer: results of a randomized phase II trial. Journal of Clinical Oncology 2005; 23: 3697–3705.

290. Guan ZZ, Xu JM, Luo RC, Feng FY, Wang LW et al. Efficacy and safety of bevacizumab plus chemotherapy in Chinese patients with metastatic colorectal cancer: a randomized phase III ARTIST trial. Chinese Journal of Cancer 2011; 30: 682–689.

291. Passardi A, Nanni O, Tassinari D, Turci D, Cavanna L et al. Effectiveness of bevacizumab added to standard chemotherapy in metastatic colorectal cancer: final results for first-line treatment from the ITACa randomized clinical trial. Annals of Oncology 2015; 26: 1201–1207.

292. Tabernero J, Yoshino T, Cohn AL, Obermannova R, Bodoky G et al. Ramucirumab versus placebo in combination with second-line FOLFIRI in patients with metastatic colorectal carcinoma that progressed during or after first-line therapy with bevacizumab, oxaliplatin, and a fluoropyrimidine (RAISE): a randomised, double-blind, multicentre, phase 3 study. Lancet Oncology 2015; 16: 499–508.

CHAPTER 39

Colorectal cancer

Alex Boussioutas, Stephen B. Fox, Iris Nagtegaal, Alexander Heriot, Jonathan Knowles, Michael Michael, Sam Ngan, Kathryn Field, and John Zalcberg

Epidemiology of colorectal cancer

Colorectal cancer (CRC), which includes primary cancers of the colon and rectum, is the third most common cancer in men and second for women in the world, based on GLOBOCAN statistics current at 2012 [1]. This accounts for 1.36 million new cases of CRC per year and 694,000 deaths attributed to this disease.

When comparing developed regions and developing regions according to United Nations criteria, the age standardized rates (ASR) per 100,000 for incidence of CRC was 36.3 in males from developed regions and 13.6 from less developed regions. Female patterns were similar with 23.6 in developed regions and 9.8 in less developed regions. Particularly high incidence was found in Australia and New Zealand, Southern and Western Europe and North America. The incidence is higher in men than women (based on sex ratio of ASR of 1.4:1) [1].

The risk for developing CRC increases with age and there are suggestions that the distribution of incident cancers in the colorectum is becoming more proximal [2–4]. Age has been suggested as being a contributing factor to this observation [5] as well as female gender [6] and possible use of screening that may detect more lesions of the left colon. Recent observations of the prevalence of colon cancer from Surveillance, Epidemiology and End Results (SEER) Medicare data in the US show 67% were right-sided lesions [7] consistent with older studies. However, there has been a decline in incidence of CRC since the mid-1980s in the US; it has been suggested this may, in part, be the result of screening for CRC, particularly the emergence of endoscopic screening [8]. It is notable, however, that the decline in incidence commenced before the widespread implementation of endoscopic screening in the US, attesting to alternative explanations.

There has been a related reduction in mortality attributed to CRC in US over a similar time frame [9]. The survival at one year and five years after therapy for CRC is 83.2% and 64.3%, respectively [10]. This raises the issue of survivorship, which will be dealt with later in this chapter. Estimates of the prevalence of CRC survivors in the US in 2012 make this the second commonest cancer diagnosis among survivors, at 9% for males and 8% females [10].

Risk factors for CRC

Chronic inflammation/inflammatory bowel disease

Chronic inflammation plays a critical role in initiating, sustaining, and advancing tumour growth. Chronic inflammation alters the microenvironment by soluble mediators (cytokine networks) through recruitment of cells that stimulate tumour growth. The production of reactive oxygen and nitrogen species by inflammatory cells can cause DNA damage in epithelial cells, which may lead to activation of oncogenes and inactivation of tumour suppressor genes. Indeed, these oxygen forms reduce expression and activity of mismatch repair proteins including MLH1, MSH2, and MSH6 by direct enzyme damage, transcription factor displacement, or up-regulation of DNA methyltransferase. Structural DNA damage, such as strand breaks and cross-links can lead to chromosomal instability. In addition, increased methylation and aberrant microRNA expression are present in chronic inflammatory conditions. Inflammation can also supply bioactive molecules to the tumour microenvironment. In addition to local effects, increasing evidence suggests that the presence of chronic inflammation can cause genotoxicity affecting mainly leucocytes that might decrease antitumour responses. Several genetic and epigenetic changes in epithelial cells have been described in ulcerative colitis that might be responsible for colon carcinogenesis. Early events in colitis-associated cancer often involve microsatellite instability (MSI) and p53 mutations, which are already present in non-dysplastic, chronically inflamed tissue. Accelerated colon aging has been suggested as one of the main contributions to the increased cancer risk in patients with ulcerative colitis, based on premature telomere shortening and increased age-related CpG island methylation.

Thus, both ulcerative colitis and Crohn's disease are a significant risk factor for the development of CRC, after inherited syndromes like Familial Adenomatous Polyposis (FAP) and Lynch syndrome with a relative risk of 19x and 18x, respectively. For ulcerative colitis there are cumulative probabilities of 8% at 20 years, and 18% at 30 years (without surveillance or chemoprophylaxis) and for Crohn's disease there is a cumulative risk for CRC of ~7% at 20 years and these tend to be related to the degree of colonic involvement. Although rare, after continued inflammation, pouch-related carcinomas occur in patients with inflammatory bowel disease. The tumours that develop are more likely to be well-differentiated adenocarcinomas of mucinous or signet-ring-cell type compared with sporadic CRC and may demonstrate differences in molecular characteristics.

Radiation

Radiation-induced neoplasia is a well-recognized effect of either sunlight, ionizing or particulate radiation. Different tissues react differently to these types of radiation and despite the severe acute effects of radiation, the gastrointestinal tract is fairly resistant to radiation-induced neoplasia as shown by the rare secondary tumours that develop after treatment of prostate, cervix and bladder.

Diet and lifestyle

There is a burgeoning literature on the association of diet and dietary components with risk of developing CRC. The role of diet as a contributory factor to the development of CRC has been estimated to be as high as 50% of sporadic CRC [11, 13].

Burkitt reported the association with fibre intake in 1971, attributing the observation of lower incidence in Africans to their high-fibre diet [12]. Since that time, there have been multiple studies that have investigated the effect of dietary fibre on incidence of CRC. Case control studies have suggested a mild protective effect [13, 14] but the results from cohort studies have been mixed [15–17] with reports of confounding due to lifestyle and non-fibre food groups [18] that were not incorporated in the earlier study designs. It has been suggested that the protective effect of dietary fibre may be due to specific subtypes of fibre such as cereal fibre [19] and may explain some of the mixed results in other studies that grouped all types of fibre.

Red meat or processed meat consumption and the fat content of diets have been associated with the risk of developing CRC [20–23]. Willet et al. reported that a diet high in animal fat was particularly associated with increased risk of CRC [23]. The initial positive associations between these diets and CRC risk have been brought into question and the magnitude of the risk is also questionable based on other prospective studies and large meta-analyses [24–26].

There are several hypotheses linking a diet high in animal fat and risk of CRC. One mechanistic link involves increased exposure of the colon to bile acids, which acts as a mutagen or carcinogen [27–29]. There are reports of increased levels of excreted bile acids in populations that are at increased risk of CRC [30, 31]. One of the prevailing theories is that bacterial flora may produce carcinogens from animal fat or bile acids in the colon [32]. There have also been suggestions of bacterial or viral effects that may contribute to the risk of CRC through multiple mechanisms but involving inflammation of the epithelium [33].

Lifestyle often confounds analysis of studies investigating diet and CRC risk. There have been attempts to clarify the role of lifestyle in the risk for CRC. A recent large prospective cohort trial in Denmark addressed this issue and suggested adherence to recommendations for physical activity, waist circumference, smoking, alcohol intake, and diet may reduce the risk of CRC by up to 23% [34]. This is compelling data that a significant proportion of CRC risk can be modified by lifestyle measures.

On the balance of evidence it would appear that lifestyle and certain dietary modification may be beneficial in reducing the risk of CRC, but the degree of benefit remains to be determined. Given the negligible health risks of such positive lifestyle changes, it makes practical sense for health professionals to advocate these changes for those deemed to be at risk of CRC. The data on specific diets remains inconclusive, particularly with respect to red meat and dietary fibre. However, a number of studies and at least one large meta-analysis have suggested Vitamin D intake and blood 25(OH)D levels were inversely associated with the risk of CRC [35]. The VITamin D and OmegA-3 TriaL (VITAL) is an ongoing randomized clinical trial in 25,875 US men and women investigating whether taking daily dietary supplements of vitamin D3 (2000 IU) or omega-3 fatty acids (Omacor® fish oil, 1 g) reduces the risk of developing cancer, heart disease, and stroke in people who do not have a prior history of these illnesses (NLM Identifier NCT01169259).

Post-cholecystectomy

Another link to the role of bile acids and CRC comes from observational data suggesting an association of cholecystectomy and risk of developing CRC [36]. Two meta-analyses of predominantly case-control studies suggested an increased risk of CRC in the proximal colon [37, 38] and both raised concerns about the quality of the data.

A relatively recent study from Sweden suggested a higher-than-expected incidence of proximal CRC and proximal carcinoids [39]. A concern with these data was raised in earlier studies suggesting that there was more enriched risk after 15 years post-cholecystectomy [37]. The Swedish study measured potential latency and found the majority of cases of CRC occurred earlier than 15 years, which is contrary to earlier studies. They concluded that the risk of CRC post-cholecystectomy is low.

Diabetes, obesity, and insulin resistance

There is consistent evidence of an association of obesity [40, 41] and type II diabetes mellitus and risk of CRC [42–44]. Early studies were small and difficult to interpret the risk of type II diabetes mellitus in the context of confounders such as BMI and physical inactivity [45, 46].

Prospective studies showed an independent association between type II diabetes mellitus and onset of CRC in men and women [44, 47]. Other studies have found the same trend in increased risk in both males and females, but the result did not reach statistical significance in women [48]. In an analysis of the Nurses Health Study, adult onset type II diabetes mellitus was also found to be a risk factor for the development of CRC [49] with a multivariate adjusted relative risk of 1.30 (95% CI 1.20–1.40). This relative risk is consistent with the risk for men. A Japanese prospective cohort study of more than 90,000 individuals also made an association of diabetes mellitus and colon cancer with an adjusted relative risk of 1.36 (95% CI 1.00–1.85). However, when they excluded diagnoses of colon cancer within five years, which may have antedated the diagnosis of diabetes mellitus, the risk for CRC was not significant 1.14 (95% CI 0.74–1.75) [50].

There are a number of hypotheses posed for the mechanism of type II diabetes mellitus accounting for an increased risk of CRC. There is data suggesting a causal role of hyperinsulinaemia and insulin-like growth factors (IGF) in colorectal carcinogenesis. Colorectal cancer cells are found to express insulin and IGF-1 receptors [51, 52] and there is animal data implicating insulin as a promoter of growth of aberrant crypt foci which are thought to be the earliest precursor lesion of CRC [53]. Indeed, high endogenous insulin has been suggested as a risk factor for CRC when levels of C-peptide are measured in high-risk populations [54, 55].

There is a suggestion that exogenous insulin therapy may also lead to higher risk of CRC [56] although data are conflicting, with the association of type II diabetes probably accounting for the excess risk rather than insulin therapy [48].

As yet, screening guidelines have not specifically targeted individuals with diabetes mellitus for more intensive screening interventions, but this may be a consideration in populations with endemic obesity and increasing prevalence of type II diabetes mellitus.

Cigarette smoking

A meta-analysis of observational data [57] has found those individuals that have ever smoked have a relative risk of 1.18 (95% CI 1.11–1.25) of developing CRC over those individuals who have never smoked. This study found an equally significant increase in mortality from CRC in smokers. Previous studies also made the association between cigarette smoking and CRC incidence [58].

Alcohol

The association between alcohol consumption and CRC risk has been made in a number of studies. A recent meta-analysis summarizes the potential risk for moderate to heavy consumers up to a relative risk (RR) of 1.52; 95% CI 1.27–1.81 for persons consuming more than four standard drinks per day [59]. In support of no association with low alcohol intake, a study investigating consumption of up to 30 g alcohol per day (one standard drink) in the UK Dietary Cohort Consortium found no association with CRC [60]. There are ongoing studies investigating the potential beneficial role of specific types of alcoholic beverages and the risk of CRC. Red wine has been postulated to lower the risk of CRC due to its content of polyphenols but this work needs further study.

Ureterocolic anastomosis

The practice of ureterosigmoidostomy has been reported to increase the risk of CRC at the anastomosis. This is an uncommon complication of an uncommon procedure and has a long latency [61–63].

Genetic risk factors

There are a number of dominant and recessively inherited predispositions for CRC. These will be covered in the section 'Molecular biology'.

Screening for CRC

There are now well-established guidelines that address screening issues for patients deemed at average or population-level risk and those at high risk due to high penetrance genetic syndromes through many gastroenterological associations (the American Gastroenterological Association, the British Society of Gastroenterologists, and Australian National Health and Medical Research Council are some examples).

As mentioned earlier, the incidence of CRC in the US has been declining over the last three decades [9, 64]. Screening has been determined as a factor accounting for up to 50% of the decreasing incidence using microsimulation modelling methods, particularly with the removal of adenomatous polyps [64]. Screening may also have contributed to the reduction in mortality due to earlier diagnosis and management of CRC.

Risk factors that are considered in the allocation of appropriate screening recommendations include: (1) genetic risk such as Lynch syndrome or FAP mutation carriers; (2) personal history of colorectal carcinoma or adenomatous polyps of the colon; (3) inflammatory bowel disease with colonic involvement for over eight years;

(4) family history of CRC but not meeting criteria for a diagnosis of a known genetic syndrome; and (5) demographic and clinical risk factors that are known to attribute higher risk for CRC. These have included race/ethnicity in the US, where black persons have highest incidence and mortality from CRC [65].

While recommendations vary slightly according to country, average risk persons are advised to consider a number of options for screening strategies as outlined in greater detail in Chapter 30, 'Population cancer screening':

1. Faecal immunochemical test (FIT) which has largely replaced the guaiac-based faecal occult blood test (gFOBT) annually or biennially.

2. Faecal DNA testing.

3. Flexible sigmoidoscopy.

4. Colonoscopy.

5. CT colonography (although this is not widely adopted yet).

Chemoprevention of CRC

Aspirin and NSAIDs

Epidemiological associations of a negative correlation with CRC incidence and regular use of aspirin [66, 67] stimulated significant research into its use as a potential chemoprevention agent.

These initial studies led to intervention studies into aspirin as a chemoprevention for CRC. A systematic review of the literature prepared for the US Preventive Services Taskforce [68] suggested regular aspirin use reduces the incidence of CRC with a pooled relative risk reduction of 22%, especially with longer duration of therapy and at relatively high dosage. The study did acknowledge the potential harms of aspirin when given at dosage above 200 mg/day with an approximate gastrointestinal bleed rate of 2.69% per year. This study acknowledged a discrepancy in data from randomized controlled studies that did not show as significant an effect as observational studies.

Another meta-analysis of radiochemotherapy (RCT) data suggested the effect of aspirin was seen in the first 12 months after the intervention [69]. There have also been mixed effects on the incidence of colonic adenoma with studies suggesting a reduction in incidence of new adenomas in patients with a prior CRC or adenoma that was treated with regular aspirin [70, 71].

Follow-up data from British-led intervention trials of aspirin have been analysed suggesting a reduction in the incidence of CRC of approximately 24% in patients taking aspirin [72]. This also led to improved prognosis.

A randomized control trial of daily aspirin in Lynch syndrome patients has shown a reduction in incidence of CRC after a treatment period of at least two years' duration [73]. The initial analysis of this data did not show a significant difference at one year [74]. A peculiarity of this data was that there was no difference in the incidence of adenomas between the control group and treatment group during the follow-up period.

Studies have also shown that NSAID drugs reduce the burden of colorectal adenomas in familial adenomatous polyposis (FAP) patients, with sulindac being the best studied, showing up to 40% reduction in polyp burden [75–77]. Although there is benefit from COX2 selective inhibitors, their potential cardiovascular toxicity at high dose has caused concern. Generally, NSAID drugs are advocated to delay definitive colectomy in FAP patients but do not replace prophylactic surgery [78].

Molecular biology and pathology of CRC

Molecular biology

Genomic integrity in normal cells is maintained by a comprehensive array of DNA repair machinery. However, mutations in genes coding for elements in the different repair pathways leads to genomic instability, the 'mutator' phenotype, which facilitates the development of cancers. There are three main molecular pathways [79–80] leading to genomic instability in CRC development. First, the conventional adenoma-carcinoma sequence characterized by chromosomal instability (CIN), as reported by Vogelstein et al. [81] which accounts for ~60% of colorectal carcinoma. Second, defects in DNA repair that accounts for ~5% and lead to the microsatellite instability pathway (as seen in the prototypical HNPCC/Lynch syndrome) and third, aberrant DNA methylation that leads to the so-called CpG island methylated phenotype (CIMP+), which accounts for the remaining ~35% [82–84]. Since there is no consensus on the precise criteria of these pathways they are not mutually exclusive.

Chromosomal instability (CIN)

This is characterized by large and frequent changes in chromosomal copy number and structure that result in inactivation of tumour suppressor genes (the so-called suppressor pathway) [85]. The tumour karyotype is complex with numerous chromosomal gains and losses that differ between tumour cells. The definition of CIN has not been standardized, with many different methodologies and criteria being used such as karyotyping, FISH, LOH, array CGH, and more recently next-generation sequencing. Indeed, some authors have suggested that there are sub-categories within CIN with low and high subtypes that may be prognostic [86, 87].

There are many proposed mechanisms that could be responsible for the CIN phenotype [85]. See Figure 39.1. The aneuploidy could result from chromosomal segregation disorders from perturbations in the spindle assembly that control the mitotic checkpoint or centrosomes and anchor the microtubules [88–91]. Other potential causes of CIN include telomere dysfunction through shortening, resulting in repetitive breakage–fusion–bridge cycles, amplification of DNA sequences genomic alteration [92] and abnormalities in the DNA damage response [93]. All these processes, therefore, lead to unbalanced structural rearrangements leading to the numerous mutations in CRC demonstrating CIN; however, only a small proportion will be driver mutations, with the majority being passenger mutations [94].

DNA-repair abnormalities

Cells have developed a vast array of different mechanisms of DNA repair to ensure genomic integrity [90, 95]. Indeed, ~30% of the genes in the human genome encode for proteins that regulate DNA fidelity [96]. One such DNA repair apparatus is the mismatch repair pathway, which removes replication errors in a strand-specific manner, to remove mismatched nucleotides from the newly replicated strand of DNA. The major proteins involved in this process are MLH1, MSH2, MSH6, PMS2, which form functional heterodimers [97, 98]. Mutations in these genes lead to loss of function leading to strand slippage or looping in repetitive regions present in introns, untranslated terminal regions, and the coding exons throughout the genome [98]. This results in increases in sequence length in daughter cells during DNA synthesis or shortening if there is slippage during DNA replication. This can be assessed in the pathology laboratory using MSI testing (see Figure 39.2) [99, 100]. The degree of MSI can be categorized as high MSI (MSI-H) when two or more panel markers are involved, low MSI (MSI-L) if only one marker is involved, and microsatellite stable (MSS) if none [101, 102]. The value of a MSI-L category remains questionable [84] since the clinical presentation of MSI-L tumours has yet to be fully determined.

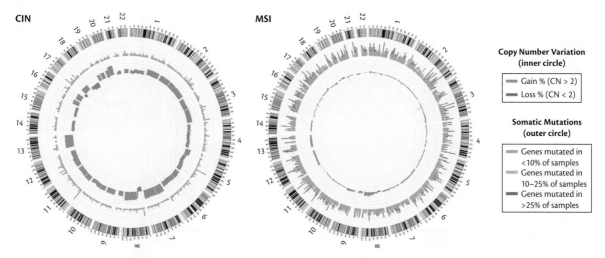

Fig. 39.1 CIRCOS plot demonstrating inherent difference between the two broad molecular subtypes of CRC: MSI-H and CIN. While CIN tumours are characterized by genome-wide copy number aberrations, MSI-H tumours remain largely chromosomally stable (inner circles represent the proportion of tumours with copy number gain/loss at a given chromosomal location). Conversely, MSI-H tumours exhibit elevated number of non-synonymous mutations (both single nucleotide polymorphisms and indels, especially around simple sequence repeats), when compared to CIN tumours (outer circle represents proportion of samples with a non-synonymous mutation at a given gene).

Figure kindly provided with the permission of Dr D Mouradov and Dr Seiber.

Since there are repetitive sequences in a number of oncogenes including growth factor receptors (EGFR, TGFβ type II), cell cycle and apoptosis (BAX, caspase-5), and DNA repair (CHK1, MLH3, MSH3) subsequent alterations in these genes lead to further accumulation of genetic changes [96].

The preferred test for MMR deficiency is the combination of MSI testing with immunohistochemistry to MMR proteins (see Figure 39.3), since this can identify the likely candidate gene for subsequent germline testing which testing for MSI cannot. MLH1 methylation can be responsible for aberrant MLH1 staining and

MSI (~15% of all MSI tumours and >80% of sporadic MSI CRCs) with similar morphology as the other MSI tumours and a good prognosis [102, 103].

A further DNA repair pathway mechanism of CRC development results from mutation in the Mut Y homolog (MUTYH) gene (see section on MUTYH below).

Aberrant DNA methylation

DNA methylation is more frequent in tumorigenesis than DNA mutation [104]. Although aberrant methylation occurs throughout

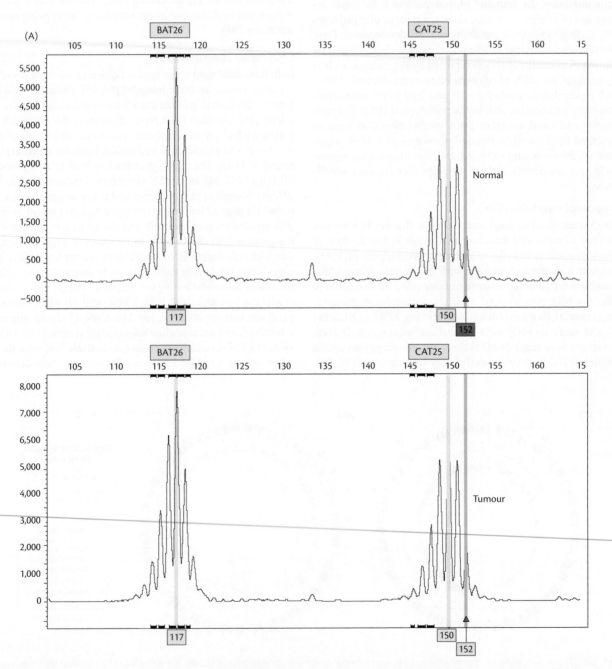

Fig. 39.2 Microsatellite electropherograms following multiplex PCR amplification of fluoresceinated microsatellite markers from a microsatellite stable (A) and unstable (B) CRC. Normal and tumour DNA product from the same individual are amplified for each microsatellite marker and the product lengths are compared to determine MSI status. Amplification normally gives rise to a central peak plus a Gaussian distribution of stuttering peaks from slippage of the polymerase during the amplification reaction. The appearance of additional shorter peaks from shortening of the repeats occurs in the tumour cells. Residual normal peaks are often present in the tumour electropherogram due to contamination of non-neoplastic cells within the tumour sample.

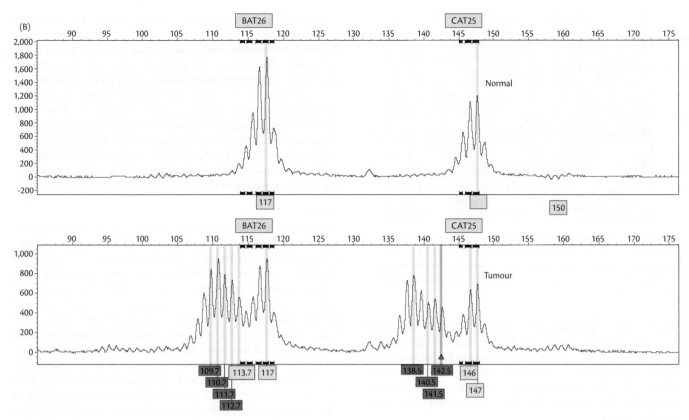

Fig. 39.2 Continued

the genome, methylation that leads to transcriptional silencing occurs preferentially at CpG islands present in up to 60% of the 5' promoter region. There is a group of ~35% CRCs that become aberrantly and extensively methylated that have been termed CpG island methylator phenotype (CIMP) [84, 105]. Methylation appears to occur early in CRC development as it is identified in adenomas [106–110]. The precise definition of this group is unclear with different classification schemes using different markers for CIMP [105]. It is also unclear whether such CRC are a true molecular subtype or represent the end of a spectrum of methylation.

Nevertheless, there are data to suggest that there are qualitative as well as quantitative differences within CIMP that are determined by the molecular pathway of tumourigenesis, either the traditional adenoma-carcinoma or serrated adenoma-carcinoma [84, 111–113]. Thus, CIMP1 is predominantly associated with methylation of multiple genes including MLH1 through the increased susceptibility to methylation from a BRAF mutation, which results in MSI. CIMP2, another category, is characterized by KRAS and is associated with methylation of a restricted number of genes including the DNA repair gene, O-6-methylguanine DNA methyltransferase (MGMT) that results in base excision and repair defects leading to the observed chromosomal instability and LOH; these are MSI-low. The third CIMP negative category is rarely methylated but demonstrates p53 mutation [114]. The CIMP1 and CIMP2 categories are proposed to arise from an alternative serrated adenoma pathway. The BRAF serrated pathway is better defined than the KRAS mediated pathway.

Key genes involved in CRC

In CRC, the presence of repeating molecular aberrations in copy number, expression profile, methylation patterns, and mutations support a common underlying biology. Several pathways are central to CRC carcinogenesis, the Wnt signalling pathways being the most important [115]. The tumour suppressor gene APC is frequently mutated, in a minority of cases beta catenin is mutated, and in rare cases, functional analogues of APC like AXIN 1 and 2, and NKD1 are the first step towards CRC. Consecutive steps towards tumour development are the inactivation of additional tumour suppression genes in the p53 and TGFβ pathways. Activation of oncogenes such as KRAS, BRAF, and PI3CKA are necessary for the development of the tumour. When DNA repair defects are the initial step for carcinogenesis, the sequence of events can be modified and frequencies of affected genes are different. Recent data from massive parallel sequencing demonstrate that by including these commonly affected genes and pathways a total number of 24 genes are repeatedly mutated in CRC [116] but the frequency may differ between primary and metastases [117].

Inherited aspects of colorectal carcinoma

Approximately 25% of all colorectal carcinoma is estimated to have an hereditary element (see Figure 39.4). The major CRC genetic syndromes that account for ~5% of the hereditary effect and include FAP, attenuated FAP (AFAP), MUTYH-associated polyposis (MAP), and Lynch syndrome (hereditary nonpolyposis CRC, HNPCC) [118]. Rarer syndromes include hamartomatous polyposis conditions (Peutz–Jeghers syndrome (PJS), juvenile polyposis syndrome (JPS), and others) [119–121] and hyperplastic polyposis [122]; they contribute a further small proportion of cases together with a number of genetic syndromes including Li–Fraumeni (p53) [123] and Bloom's (BLM) [124] that are associated with multiple tumour types and sites, including the colon. Additionally, familial CRCs that do not meet the clinical criteria for a diagnosis of known

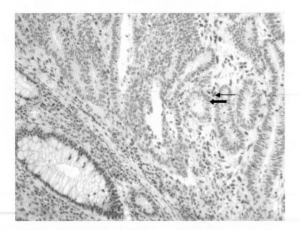

Fig. 39.3 Mismatch repair immunohistochemistry. Immunohistochemistry for MSH6. One of the mismatch repair proteins, showing the loss of staining for protein in the tumour cells (large arrow) with retention of expression in the non-neoplastic elements including normal intestinal crypts, stromal cells (thin arrow) and lymphocytes.

hereditary CRC syndromes have up to a sixfold increased risk that is dependent on the age and number of affected family members. A component of this increased risk is likely to be due to a number of low-penetrance risk genes that account for ~10% of the familial association have been identified using genome wide association studies [125, 126] which might also act as modifiers of other more penetrant genes.

Major hereditary syndromes
Familial adenomatous polyposis (FAP)

FAP is an autosomal dominantly transmitted disease caused by a mutation of the APC gene located on 5q21, which is a negative regulator of the Wnt pathway [127–129]. Most mutations are nonsense type, leading to the formation of a truncated protein. FAP is characterized by up to thousands of adenomatous polyps in the large intestine that develop in childhood and inevitably transform to CRC by 40 years of age [130]. However, there are FAP variants

that depend on the region and the type of mutation (i.e. frameshift mutation versus missense mutation) in the APC gene. These include (1) attenuated FAP, a variant that has a later presentation with polyps that are fewer in number compared with conventional FAP (up to 100 polyps), and a lower (~70%) lifetime risk of CRC [131]; (2) Gardner's syndrome, in which individuals also develop extracolonic tumours including upper GI polyps, small intestinal tumours, desmoid tumours, osteomas, and cysts; and (3) one form of Turcot's syndrome in which patients develop CRC and medulloblastoma [132–134]. Thus, for example, a mutation between codons 1250–1464 is associated with usual-type FAP whereas mutations at the 3' end are associated with desmoid tumours [130, 133].

MUTYH

MUTYH is located on chromosome 1p, and encodes a protein of the DNA base excision repair (BER) pathway, mutations of which predispose to the development of CRC [135]. The BER system is responsible for repairing one of the most stable deleterious products of oxidative DNA damage, that of 8-oxo-7,8-dihydro-2-deoxyguanosine. Formation of such damaged DNA predisposes to point mutations particularly increased G:C to T:A transversions [135], but even though the genomic instability effects individual base pairs the tumours demonstrate CIN [136]. MUTYH polyposis is autosomal recessive and is associated with variable adenomatous polyposis from only a few to several hundred that can mimic FAP; it has a significant increase in susceptibility to CRC that approaches 100% by the age of 60 years [137–139]. Two common variants have been reported—Tyr165Cys and Gly382Asp, which account for ~80% of cases. Affected individuals also have an increased incidence of developing other tumour types [135].

Lynch syndrome

Lynch syndrome is an autosomally dominant disease characterized by colorectal, endometrial, ureteric, gastric, ovarian, biliary, urinary tract, small bowel, brain, and pancreatic carcinomas that result from germline inactivation of DNA mismatch repair genes (see Chapter 31, 'Familial cancer syndromes and genetic counselling'). Lynch syndrome is largely (~80%) due to mutations in

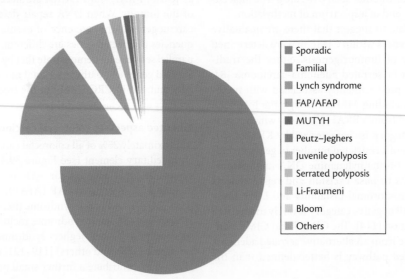

■ Sporadic
■ Familial
■ Lynch syndrome
▨ FAP/AFAP
■ MUTYH
■ Peutz–Jeghers
▨ Juvenile polyposis
▨ Serrated polyposis
▨ Li-Fraumeni
▨ Bloom
■ Others

Fig. 39.4 Frequencies of hereditary CRC. The majority of CRC have a sporadic origin (75%), 15% of cases have an increased risk of CRC (familial CRC), but no defined underlying gene mutation. The remaining 10% of cases originate from patients with a known hereditary cancer syndrome, of which Lynch syndrome is the most frequent (5%).

MLH1 and MSH2 with alterations in MSH6 (10%), PMS2, and MLH3 accounting for the remainder. A rare germline deletion in TACSTD1, resulting in TACSTD1/MSH2 fusion transcripts generation with epigenetic inactivation of the corresponding MSH2 allele, also causes Lynch syndrome. The overall lifetime risk of CRC is 80%, but risks vary depending on the gene affected (e.g., PMS2 has only a 15–20% risk for CRC). Although mutations can be identified spanning these genes, founder mutations have been identified, accounting for up to 10% of all Lynch syndrome patients. Variants of Lynch syndrome include (1) Turcot syndrome, the result of mutation in the mismatch repair genes hMLH1 or hPMS2 characterized by CRC and glioblastoma and (2) Muir–Torre syndrome, which results from mutations in MLH1 and MSH2 and is characterized by the presence of sebaceous gland neoplasms and visceral malignancies, usually CRC. Screening for Lynch syndrome includes using immunohistochemistry for MMR proteins on CRC or endometrial carcinomas (other Lynch-associated tumours have low specificity and sensitivity) for absence of staining and MSI [100]. Since absent staining of MLH1 protein might be due to methylation, BRAF mutation status by mutational analysis or use of mutation-specific antibodies may be required. If negative, directed germline mutation analysis can be performed; in the future, clinical massive parallel sequencing may alter this testing algorithm.

Hamartomatous polyposis syndromes
Peutz–Jeghers syndrome
Peutz-Jeghers syndrome is an autosomal dominant disorder that presents in childhood, characterized by mucocutaneous pigmented lesions around and within the mouth, and hamartomatous polyps in the gastrointestinal tract, particularly the small bowel [121]. Most patients have a germline truncation or missense mutation in the tumour suppressor STK11 gene, located at 19p13.3 that encodes a serine threonine kinase (STK) protein [140], although other genes may be implicated (e.g., MYH11 [141]). Mutation results in tumour suppressor activity as LKB1-AMPK signalling negatively regulates the mTOR pathway [142]. Activation of mTOR signalling leads to hamartoma formation, which predisposes to a number of malignancies in the gastrointestinal tract and other organs including pancreatic, lung, breast, uterine, ovarian, and testicular tumours [143, 144].

Juvenile polyposis
Juvenile polyposis is rare and has three main subtypes comprising juvenile polyposis of infancy, juvenile polyposis of the colon, and generalized juvenile polyposis, all of which have different modes of presentation [119, 120]. Patients with juvenile polyposis of infancy have no family history and present with diffuse gastrointestinal polyposis that is associated with macrocephaly, digital clubbing, and hypotonia. Individuals usually die from non-neoplastic complications of the condition such as haemorrhage, malnutrition, or and intussusception before the age of 2 years.

Juvenile polyposis of the colon and generalized juvenile polyposis usually present by the age of 10 with acute or chronic gastrointestinal haemorrhage, anaemia, and polyps that can number in the hundreds. Patients have a cumulative life-time risk for CRC of 39–68% and an increased risk of other intestinal tumours, dependent on the location of the polyps. They are associated in 50–60% with an inherited or new mutation (usually point mutations or small deletions but also large deletions in 5–15%) in SMAD4 and BMPR1A. Mutations of PTEN, the gene responsible for Cowden syndrome, have also been reported, and some individuals with

SMAD4 germline mutations have hereditary haemorrhagic telangiectasia [145]. All these genes encode proteins in the TGFβ signalling pathway and thus might represent be a spectrum of phenotypes.

Mixed polyposis syndrome
Mixed polyposis syndrome is a relatively recent recognized entity, without any clear definition, caused by a mutation in BMPR1A and thus, might be part of the spectrum of TGFβ-pathway-associated polyposes. This mutation shows an autosomal dominant inheritance and carriers have an increased risk of CRC [146, 147] on a background of adenomas and hyperplastic and juvenile polyps.

Others
Polyps closely resembling juvenile polyps are found in other conditions such as Cowden disease, an autosomal dominant condition of the phosphatase and tensin homolog (PTEN) gene or rarely SDHB. However, although polyps are identified in the gastrointestinal tract in ~80% there is no apparent cancer risk [121]. Bannayan–Riley–Ruvalcaba syndrome, characterized by juvenile polyps, mental retardation, macrocephaly, lipomatosis, haemangiomas, and genital pigmentation was originally thought to be a distinct entity but also harbour a PTEN mutation in 60% of individuals. Thus, an aggregate term of PTEN hamartoma syndrome has been suggested [148], the phenotypic differences being due to ascertainment bias. Cronkhite–Canada syndrome is a further gastrointestinal polyposis of unknown aetiology but is non-hereditary [149].

Hyperplastic polyposis syndrome
Hereditary non-polyposis colon cancer/hyperplastic polyposis is a rare condition defined by arbitrary criteria that are likely to represent a spectrum of conditions. They are characterized by the WHO as having (1) at least five histologically diagnosed hyperplastic polyps proximal to the sigmoid colon of which two are greater than 10 mm in diameter; (2) any number of hyperplastic polyps occurring proximal to the sigmoid colon in an individual who has a first-degree relative with hyperplastic polyposis; or (3) more than 30 hyperplastic polyps of any size, but distributed throughout the colon [150–152]. Individuals develop CRC (baseline 25–37% of patients [150, 153]) on a background of hyperplastic polyps, other serrated adenomas, and even traditional adenomas. The molecular genetics of this condition(s) is unknown.

Pathology of colorectal carcinoma
Precursor lesions of CRC

Aberrant crypt foci (ACF)
ACF are microscopic mucosal abnormalities [154], some of which may be precursors to CRC [155]. ACF are most frequent in the rectum, descending and sigmoid colon and microscopically have the morphology of dysplastic microadenomas (single crypt adenomas) or hyperplastic crypts with or without a serrated luminal pattern. Although reported in FAP and sporadic CRC they are also identified in ~40% of patients with benign colonic diseases such as diverticular disease, rectal prolapse, and volvulus [155]. The number of ACF increases with age and correlate with the presence of adenomas. The adenomas that form from ACF in the context of FAP have APC mutations, whereas those in the sporadic setting harbour KRAS mutations (and lack of methylation). The non-dysplastic ACF might be precursors of CRC through the alternate serrated

adenoma pathway associated with BRAF and occasionally KRAS mutations [156, 157].

Adenomas

These are largely polypoid neoplasms characterized by dysplastic large intestinal-type epithelium, although some show a flat or sessile configuration. They can show a tubular, villous, or mixed architecture and most are <10mm. Villous adenomas >10mm with severe dysplasia are associated with synchronous or metachronous carcinoma associated with the CIN pathway. The pathology is similar whether the patient has FAP or its variants, with MUTYH-associated polyposis or sporadic. KRAS rather than BRAF mutations are associated with adenomas.

Serrated polyps

Serrated polyps [84, 113] are a heterogeneous collection of lesions characterized by serrated epithelium and account for a ~40% of colorectal polyps. There are many forms, some forms of which, through genetic and epigenetic changes akin to the traditional adenoma-carcinoma sequence, progress along a 'serrated pathway' as an alternate mechanism of CRC development.

Hamartomatous polyps

These are malformations of the mucosa, lamina propria, and sometimes muscularis propria that form a polyp. They have varied morphologies depending on the underlying pathogenesis but include polyps with a central smooth muscle core that arborizes and is covered by mucosa with a villous pattern, as in Peutz–Jegher, to simple tags and mixtures of connective tissue with oedematous stroma, cystic gland formation, variable inflammation, lobulation, and branching.

Colorectal carcinoma

The histological biopsy forms the basis for therapeutic decisions for the patient and, for rectal cancer, is a requirement for the commencement of neoadjuvant therapy. After surgery, pathological evaluation [158] of the characteristics of the primary tumour, the presence of lymph node metastases, and the evaluation of treatment (surgery and neoadjuvant therapy) form the basis for subsequent adjuvant therapy. Primary tumour characteristics that are suggestive of hereditary cancer syndromes might necessitate additional testing, such as MSI testing and MMR immunohistochemistry. In case of advanced or metastatic disease, additional molecular testing can be performed in order to test suitability for targeted therapies (e.g., RAS testing) [159].

The macroscopic appearances of CRC are varied with tumours having an appearance that is endophytic, exophytic, or annular with or without ulceration or a combination; a rare form of diffuse infiltration has also been described. The presence of carcinoma is defined as invasion through the muscularis mucosa to the submucosa. Histological classification follows the World Health Organization. There are also other non-epithelial tumour types, which might be encountered in the colon and rectum: lymphomas, sarcomas, and melanomas [160].

Particular histological tumour types are associated with particular molecular characteristics. For example MSI-H tumours, whether Lynch or sporadic, tend to be well circumscribed, proximally located, and demonstrate two patterns: (1) well-differentiated mucinous and (2) poorly-differentiated with tumour-infiltrating lymphocytes, a Crohn's-like reaction (also classified as medullary carcinoma), which despite their poor differentiation have a good prognosis.

Location

The majority of CRCs are located in the distal colon and rectum, although the frequencies at different sites depend on the underlying molecular genetics. Thus, tumours demonstrating MSI or CIMP are generally right-sided (caecum, ascending and transverse colon) whereas CIMP-positive and MSS cancers occur on right and left; MSS without CIMP are located mainly in the left colon. Although location has been used to aid classification of the underlying pathogenesis of CRC, recent data suggests that non-MSI tumours are similar irrespective of their origin, whereas a continuum model may apply for MSI tumours as frequencies of CIMP, MSI, and BRAF mutation increase in a linear manner distal to proximal [161].

Pathologic prognostic markers

Stage

The staging system of choice is the TNM or AJCC classification [162, 163]. The three pillars of this system are depth of **T**umour penetration (TNM I and II), presence of lymph **N**ode metastases (TNM III) and distant **M**etastases (TNM IV). This system can adequately predict local recurrence, distant metastases, and survival rates, although stage II patients do show a large variation in prognosis. A special high-risk stage II group has been defined, characterized by the presence of perforation, T4, obstruction, less than ten examined lymph nodes, extramural vascular invasion, or poor differentiation [164].

Lymph node burden

One of the most important factors in patients' prognosis is the presence of nodal metastases. Approximately ~70% of the patients with no lymph node metastases are alive five years after surgery, while those with metastases have a five-year survival rate of 40%. Standard guidelines are provided for the number and location of the examined lymph nodes, but ideally 12 lymph nodes should be examined before a patient can be classified as N0. Nevertheless, in daily practice, even 12 lymph nodes can be challenging to acquire, as the number of nodes is influenced by preoperative radiotherapy and in the type of resection performed, as well as variation between patients [165]. Differences in the quality of pathological examination using a combination of visual inspection, palpation, and dissection is another important factor determining the yield of lymph nodes isolated from the perirectal fat.

Early CRC cancer

With the widespread introduction of population screening for CRC, the number of early CRCs is expected to increase from the ~25% that currently present with early disease (stage I). Local excision is an attractive option for early disease in both colon and rectal cancer, since it is associated with considerably less surgery-related morbidity and almost no post-operative mortality compared with colectomy and total mesorectal excision (TME) (mortality rates of 1.9–6.5% (rectum) and 3.2–9.8% (colon) have been reported). Patient selection through careful histological analysis of local excision specimens can be very useful to avoid over- and under-treatment. Several pathologic features of the primary tumour have been associated with presence of LNM, such as poor differentiation, tumour budding, presence of lymphatic or vascular invasion, and submucosal invasion depth.

Histological prognostic factors

Mucinous carcinomas have a slightly poorer prognosis than adenocarcinomas, mainly from presentation at advanced stage. Signet-ring-cell carcinomas, as well as mucinous carcinomas with signet ring cells, are associated with poor prognosis. In contrast, medullary carcinomas have a very good prognosis. Histological grading of cancer though the assessment of tumour differentiation is used as a surrogate for tumour aggressiveness. There are a variety of systems [166] but the majority of studies use a two-tiered stratification. Growth pattern is another feature that has prognostic value in CRC. The circumscript/pushing configuration is associated with a good prognosis, while diffuse infiltration is associated with a poor prognosis [167]. A closely-associated feature is the presence of tumour budding [168], where tumour cells at the invasive front of CRC detach into single cells or clusters of up to five cells. The presence of budding is associated with lymph node metastases and metastatic disease. Other histological features that have prognostic relevance are (1) lymphatic invasion (tumour cells in the submucosal lymphatic vessels), which is mainly related to the risk of lymph node metastases; (2) extramural vascular invasion (tumour cells in the subserosal blood vessels), which is associated with the development of blood-borne distant metastases; and (3) perineural invasion (tumour cells in and around nerves), which is associated with local as well as distant recurrence [169].

Tumour regression grading after neoadjuvant therapy

Various methods have been developed to grade tumour regression to assess neoadjuvant treatment, and although using differing criteria, each generally show increased regression is associated with a prolonged survival. However, the lack of standardization of grading together with inter- and intra-observer variation make regression grading a less reliable indication of tumour response such that other factors, such as circumferential radial margin involvement, are more important [170]. Nevertheless, although response grading is of some utility, the main purpose of neoadjuvant therapy is downstaging of the tumour, facilitating surgical excision.

Other prognostic markers

Despite the numerous publications about prognostic markers in CRC, few are used in practice such as an inflammatory infiltrate in and around the tumour [171]. Recent developments have standardized this analysis in the Immunoscore® [172], which is currently under investigation in a multicentre study. There is consistent evidence for the favourable prognosis of MSI tumours [80] whereas BRAF mutation is associated with a poor prognosis [173].

Predictive markers

The presence of MSI has previously been considered a contraindication for 5-FU-based therapy, although again conflicting studies have been published. In a meta-analysis [174] no clear conclusion could be drawn about the effects of MSI on 5-FU response, due to significant inter-study heterogeneity. However, with the relative good prognosis of these tumours, the potential for beneficial effects is small. For targeted therapy, the predictive marker is KRAS mutation. In the presence of an activating KRAS mutation, inhibition of the EGF receptor does not have the desired effect on tumour cells and thus there is no indication for this therapy. It is expected that the increased use of targeted drugs will lead to the identification of additional predictive markers.

Surgical management

Surgery is the mainstay of treatment for colon cancer. If a patient is fit enough to undergo surgery, resection of the primary tumour with excision of the draining lymph nodes provides the only option for cure, with around two-thirds of the patients disease-free at five years [175], and recurrence after this time is rare. The introduction of laparoscopic colorectal surgery over the last decade has reduced the traumatic impact of surgical resection, improving patient recovery. Advanced colonoscopic techniques such as endoscopic mucosal resection have facilitated removal of adenomas that would previously have required surgical resection. These are being identified more frequently with the advent of national bowel cancer screening programs.

Survival rates following surgery remained static for some time, but the introduction of adjuvant chemotherapy has resulted in an improvement in survival and a reduction in the development of metastatic disease. The surgical approach to metastatic disease, either metachronous or synchronous, has evolved to become increasingly proactive. Resection of liver, lung, and peritoneal metastases can be curative and improve survival outcomes. The increased survival of patients with stage IV disease through improvements in chemotherapy has also led to an increased role for surgery to control palliative symptoms.

Diagnosis

Colonoscopy is the gold standard diagnostic test for colon cancer, with a sensitivity of 95% [176]. Cancers can be visually assessed and biopsied to provide tissue for histological diagnosis. Histology may be inconclusive due to sampling of tumour slough and inflammation or if a malignant core is surrounded by adenoma. If further biopsies are inconclusive or the lesion is not reachable endoscopically, it should be considered to be malignant. CT pneumocolonography provides a diagnostic alternative to endoscopy. The sensitivity for cancers is equal to that of colonoscopy [176]; however, identified abnormalities need endoscopic evaluation.

With the increase in minimally invasive surgery, lesions should be marked at their distal border with Indian or carbon particle suspension 'ink'. Lesions impassable with an endoscope are at risk of obstruction and early surgery or colonic stenting should be considered. If there is an impassable lesion, the remainder of the colon should be examined for synchronous lesions by CT pneumocolonography.

Preoperative staging

This aims to identify metastatic spread and local invasion. The mainstay of staging in colonic cancer is high-resolution CT scanning. This should include the chest, abdomen, and pelvis. The two commonest sites of haematogenous spread are to the liver and the lungs. Incidental liver lesions may cause diagnostic uncertainty and further imaging with ultrasound or MRI may be required. FDG-PET scanning is being used more frequently, as it has a higher sensitivity for recurrent and metastatic disease than CT [177]. It can also help differentiate between benign and malignant lesions seen on standard CT. In patients with metastatic disease being considered for curative resection, it may identify otherwise occult metastases.

Identification of locally advanced disease allows planning of en-bloc resection of the invaded organ along with the primary tumour, if the patient is fit enough. In colon cancer, the proximity of the small bowel and the mobility of the colon make the use of neoadjuvant chemoradiotherapy mostly impractical.

Preoperative assessment

Prior to elective cancer resection there is a window to investigate the patient's general health. The stress of abdominal surgery places the patient at risk of ischaemic vascular events, thromboembolism, and hypostatic and invasive-line-related infections. Preoperative assessment aims to find unidentified or undertreated medical conditions and assess the likelihood of surviving the procedure. This is usually started with a pre-anaesthetic assessment and may then be aided by a number of objective measures of patient 'fitness'.

Ischaemic and valvular heart disease, respiratory conditions, hypertension, and diabetes mellitus should be optimally medically managed prior to surgery. Medical conditions such as cardiac ischaemia, which would normally require intervention, should be treated and surgery delayed to allow this [178].

An objective measure of risk can be gained with scores such as the acute physiology and chronic health evaluation score or physiological testing such as cardio-pulmonary exercise testing. These can help to identify patients who require more aggressive and invasive perioperative care [179]. They can also identify patients in whom surgery has a high risk of complications or death. If patients are found to have poor performance with physiological testing, then preoperative optimization of haematinics, nutrition, and exercise programmes may improve their outcome [180].

The multidisciplinary team

Once diagnostic, staging, and preoperative assessment have taken place, cases should be presented to a CRC multidisciplinary team. These groups review the radiology and histology, ensuring quality control and allowing a consensus opinion on the appropriate management of individual cases.

Perioperative care

Colonic cancer surgery has led the way in the healthcare trend towards early mobilization and reduced inpatient stay. The work by Kehlet [181] in open intestinal surgery has become the cornerstone of enhanced recovery programmes. These are often combined with the reduced surgical stress of minimally invasive techniques to facilitate early discharge.

Perioperative care should start prior to admission. Consent is best gained away from the stress of the surgical environment. Patients can meet stoma therapists, nurse specialists, and enhanced recovery coordinators prior to their stay. Education on thromboembolic prevention, physiotherapy, and pain control can be provided. Bowel preparation and preoperative nutritional supplements can all be taken at home prior to admission. In most cases, it is safe for patients to be admitted on the morning of surgery [182].

Enhanced recovery tries to facilitate the normal return of gut and motor function. This combines early feeding and mobilization with reduced opiates and nauseating anaesthetic agents. Pain control with local or regional anaesthetic blocks and non-steroidal anti-inflammatories are combined to reduce opiates. Tubes which reduce mobility such as abdominal drains, nasogastric and urinary catheters are avoided or used for short periods. Intravenous fluid replacement is 'targeted' [183] intraoperatively and in the post-operative period replaced at maintenance volumes only, until full oral nutrition has returned. Enteral nutrition is encouraged from day one in the post-operative period.

Thromboprophylaxis is particularly important in patients with a cancer diagnosis and undergoing abdominal surgery. Anti-thromboembolism stockings, pneumatic compression devices, and early low-molecular-weight heparin should all be utilized if possible, aided by early return to mobility.

Surgical techniques

Colonic resection

The underlying principle of surgery for colon cancer is resection of the bowel where the tumour has originated along with the lymph nodes draining that area. The two ends of bowel are then joined together with an anastomosis to restore bowel 'continuity'. Lymph node involvement is usually unknown until the resected specimen is reviewed by the pathologist. Hence, the extent of resection is determined by the lymphatic anatomy of the colon. Lymphatic colonic drainage channels follow the arterial blood supply. By ligating and dividing the relevant artery close to its origin, 'high ligation', removal of the draining lymph nodes is ensured. Turnbull proposed a 'no-touch technique' [184], where ligation of the feeding vessels is undertaken prior to mobilization of the tumour, reducing tumour spread. In fact, this was a surrogate for 'proper' high arterial ligation and adequate resection of the lymph node containing colonic mesentery. See Figure 39.5.

Division of the artery will define an area of colon which will become ischaemic. This should contain the tumour and margins of 'normal' colon of at least 5 cm proximally and distally. The two ends of intestine should have adequate blood supply from the adjacent arterial vessels via the marginal artery to allow healing. The marginal artery runs around the length of the colon and is supplied by branches of both the superior mesenteric and inferior mesenteric arteries. The blood flow in this artery is determined by the distance from the feeding vessel and the quality of those vessels. This is affected by factors such as atherosclerosis, hypotension, vasoconstriction, and cardiac output. The quality of blood flow in the marginal artery can be demonstrated by pulsatile flow on division of the vessel [185]. If the blood supply is poor, further resection of colon may be required. Other factors influencing anastomotic healing include tension across the anastomosis, radiotherapy, or bowel disease. Healing is also influenced by global patient factors such as poor nutrition, immunosuppression, and concurrent illness. Despite this, most colonic surgery can be anastomosed safely. In obstructed or severely malnourished patients a de-functioning or temporary-end ileostomy can be life-saving. In most cases, the risk of anastomotic leaks is not enough to warrant their formation.

When performing a right hemicolectomy, the ileocolic artery is high ligated, along with the right colic artery which is present in 10% of patients. This resection will allow removal of caecal, ascending colon, and hepatic flexure tumours. For tumours of the descending and sigmoid colon high ligation of the inferior mesenteric artery is performed as part of a left hemicolectomy or high anterior resection. Tumours of the transverse colon are predominantly supplied by the middle colic artery but may include supply from the ileocolic vessels. These tumours are removed with an

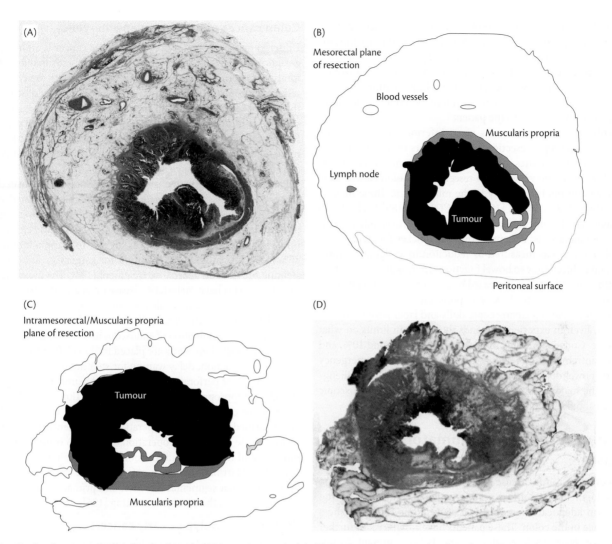

Fig. 39.5 Quality of surgery and relation to the circumferential resection margin. (A)–(B) Good quality of surgery, the plane of resection is on the mesorectal fascia, the CRM is free. (C)–(D) The plane of surgery is on the muscularis propria, the CRM is threatened.

extended right hemicolectomy, where ligation of the middle colic is added to that of the ileocolic artery. Transverse colon resections are rarely performed as they may compromise the oncological resection and have been associated with a higher anastomotic leak rate [186].

The steps required to undertake a colonic resection remain fairly constant. The right and left colon are retroperitoneal with their vessel containing mesentery draped over the retroperitoneal structures, whilst the transverse and sigmoid colon are freely mobile on their respective mesenteries. The right and left colon are mobilized by division of their peritoneal attachments. Once mobilized, the supplying vascular pedicle is divided high and the mesentery divided up to the points on the bowel appropriate for the resection. After resection, the bowel is usually reanastomosed using one of a number of configurations. These include end-to-end, end-to-side, and side-to-side anastomoses, all of which can be performed using hand-sewn or stapled techniques.

Treatment of splenic flexure tumours

The surgical management of tumours near the splenic flexure remains difficult. This area is a watershed between the middle colic and left colic artery and branches of both will supply most of these tumours. If the inferior mesenteric artery is taken high then the whole of the left colon needs to be resected unless one relies on marginal artery supply to maintain the remaining left colon. The alternative is to perform an extended right hemicolectomy and anastomose the ileum to the left colon. This doesn't take as much of the left-sided lymphatic drainage but replaces poorly vascularized left colon with ileum to form an anastomosis. There remains no good evidence to favour one approach, and surgeons commonly make the decision based on the position of the tumour intraoperatively.

Laparoscopic colonic resection

The advent of laparoscopic or minimally invasive approaches has been the major change in surgery for CRC over the last ten years. There remains a spectrum of uptake for these techniques. The fundamental steps and principles of colonic resection are the same as for open surgery but are performed via small incisions in the abdominal wall through which 5 mm or 10 mm 'ports' are inserted. The laparoscopic instruments are then inserted through these ports. Division of the mesentery can be undertaken intra- or extra-corporally. The bowel division and subsequent anastomosis may also be undertaken intra- or extra-corporally, the mobilized specimen being delivered through a small incision using a wound protector to minimize wound or port site implantation. The end result is the same operation as an open resection but with a reduction in iatrogenic trauma to the patient.

Initially, there were concerns of an inferior oncological outcome for laparoscopic resection as well as fears of implantation of tumour cells at port sites. A number of multicentre randomized trials of laparoscopic versus open resection for colon cancer were completed and published early in the millennium. These include the CLASSIC [187], COST [188], and COLOR [189] trials. These have demonstrated oncological equivalence and no significant risk of port site metastasis. Patient recovery is quicker following laparoscopic resection as measured by reduction in analgesic requirements and reduced time to bowel function. There is also a reduction in length of inpatient stay, increased by combining minimally invasive surgery with enhanced recovery programmes. There is a learning curve for attaining laparoscopic skills and laparoscopic colonic resection. Even in experienced hands there remain limits on what is possible. Conversion rates to open surgery are around 10%, and relative contraindications such as previous laparotomy, emergency cases, or bowel obstruction make laparoscopic surgery challenging. For the majority of elective colonic resections a laparoscopic approach should be considered the approach of choice.

Colonic cancer and inflammatory bowel disease

Colitis due to Crohn's disease and ulcerative colitis predisposes to the development of colonic cancer. In patients with pancolitis who develop an adenocarcinoma or area of dysplasia there may be a field change in the colon. These patients have a high risk of further tumours or dysplasia developing or already being present. In this situation it is safest to remove the whole colon and rectum [190]. In ulcerative colitis the patient can be left with either an end ileostomy or a restorative ileoanal pouch.

If the patient has segmental colitis then a balance needs to be struck between segmental resection and colectomy. In patients with mild, burnt-out, or very limited disease it may be possible to perform a standard segmental resection. Prior to this, careful evaluation of patients' symptoms and endoscopic evaluation of the mucosa is essential. Patients with limited disease but troublesome urgency and frequency will have a poor functional result with a segmental resection. For these patients an end stoma or pouch may well give a better quality of life.

Colonic cancer and polyposis or HNPCC

Patients with familial adenomatous polyposis coli should be managed in specialist centres. Following a period of endoscopic surveillance started in their late teens, they should have a colectomy and pouch or ileoanal anastomosis formed in their twenties prophylactically.

Patients with hereditary non-polyposis coli are best treated with a subtotal colectomy and ileorectal or ileosigmoid anastomosis [191]. The remainder of the colon should then be regularly examined with flexible sigmoidoscopy to prevent metachronous disease developing.

Colon cancer presenting as an emergency

Undergoing emergency surgery for colonic cancer is an independent poor prognostic factor [192]. In patients with malignant perforation the aim should be to treat the emergency expediently to reduce peritoneal contamination time. The aim should be to allow the patient to receive adjuvant chemotherapy, if required, soon after surgery to improve its efficacy. It may be more sensible to perform a Hartmann's, removing the attendant risks of anastomotic leak and reducing operative time. This can be reversed once the patient has completed chemotherapy.

Patients presenting with obstructing tumours may be treated with surgery or stenting. Right-sided tumours should be treated with a right hemicolectomy. Although this is considered a low-morbidity procedure, the complications rates are higher than the elective setting, with anastomotic leak rates as high as 10% and a mortality of 17% [193]. In patients who are unfit for surgery or are palliative, stenting provides an alternative treatment [194]. The use of stenting in patients who have metastatic disease or as a bridge to surgery in obstruction is still being evaluated with prospective trials, but has been shown to be safe in retrospective studies [195]. Stents should be placed using a combination of endoscopy and radiological guidance. Results are best when stents are placed in short left-sided strictures. In acute obstruction, delay waiting for stenting must be avoided as there is a risk of perforation and caecal ischaemia. If stenting is not available or appropriate then emergency resection should be undertaken. If the caecum is not viable then a subtotal colectomy should be performed. This is a safe operation but an ileorectal anastomosis as a single or two-stage operation can lead to troublesome loose motions and nocturnal call to stool. If the remainder of the colon is viable, a Hartmann's or segmental resection can be used. Studies have shown that segmental resection and primary anastomosis is a safe operation in the emergency setting [196].

Treatment of polyp or early cancers

Improvements in endoscopic polypectomy techniques have allowed bigger polyps to be excised. Early cancers or 'polyp' cancers (stage 1 or T1/T2) are being found more commonly in these resected polyps. Early cancers that have not already been excised at colonoscopy should be treated with standard resection techniques.

Colonic adenomas are polyps with areas of cellular dysplasia. They have a risk of malignancy broadly related to size, with polyps smaller than 1 cm having less than a 1% chance of containing a malignant focus [197]. All polyps larger than 1 cm and those with suspicious features should be tattooed prior to polypectomy or tattooed and biopsied if not excisable. Polypectomy can be performed using endoscopic mucosal resection, where the polyp is lifted away from the submucosa with saline/gelatine or hyaluronate solution. The polyp is then excised with a diathermy snare. Endoscopic submucosal dissection is a modification using an endoscopic diathermy knife to resect the lesion en bloc, which can reduce recurrence [198, 199].

Resected polyp cancers cannot be fully staged. To determine if further resection is required, features that increase the risk of lymph node spread or local recurrence are identified. If the polyp cancer is incompletely excised or within 1–2 mm of the diathermy margin, further excision should be undertaken. The risk of spread or invasion is also related to the levels of invasion towards the base of the polyp: see Haggitt [200] for stalked and Kikuchi [201] for flat polyps. If the patient is unfit for surgery, then endoscopic surveillance

Table 39.1 Risk factors for lymph node positivity in early CRCs [200]: high-grade, lymphovascular invasion, budding, cribriform cellular pattern

Risk factors	Lymph node metastasis	Micromets in 'negative' node
0	0.7%	6.8%
1	27%	14.3%
>2	36%	16.7%

Source: data from Ueno H et al., Risk factors for an adverse outcome in early invasive colorectal carcinoma, *Gastroenterology*, Volume 127, Issue 2, pp. 385–394, Copyright © 2004.

can be used. Features which suggest more aggressive cancer types with a greater likelihood of metastasis are high grade, lymphovascular invasion, budding, and cribriform cellular pattern, which are shown in Table 39.1.

Liver and lung metastasis

There has been a change in the philosophy of metastatic colon cancer management over the last 20 years. The two most common sites of metastasis, liver and lungs, can now be treated curatively with resection. Improvements in imaging have allowed metastases to be identified earlier and improvements in surgical technique and haemostatic technology have reduced the physiological insult of the surgery. Liver resection has now become the standard of care for hepatic metastasis, with five-year disease free survival of 26–34% [202]. Whilst hepatic resection was initially limited to one to three metastatic deposits, the indications for resection are now much broader. Hepatic resection can be considered if the metastatic disease can be resected with clear margins, leaving enough functional liver—around 30%—for survival. Factors such as the volume of metastatic disease and time of recurrence are predictive of long-term outcome [203].

Patients who present with liver metastasis and a primary colon tumour may undergo synchronous resection or have their liver metastasis resected in a separate operation. Synchronous resection is usually reserved for patients having a simple colonic resection and a simple liver resection. The morbidity with simultaneous resection can be significantly increased, with higher rates of anastomotic leaks making complex resections unsafe [204].

Strategies have also developed to address initially unresectable hepatic disease. Chemotherapy may downstage unresectable disease to resectable disease. A recent European Organisation for Research and Treatment of Cancer (EORTC) randomized trial has demonstrated the benefit in progression-free survival of preoperative chemotherapy in the majority of resectable cases [205]. Lack of adequate functional liver post resection can be addressed by staged liver resection. This can be combined with portal vein embolization to generate hypertrophy of one side of the liver, increasing residual liver volume. Even unresectable liver deposits can be controlled by radiofrequency or microwave ablation.

Pulmonary resection of colorectal metastatic disease is a more recent development but has also demonstrated survival benefits. This has been facilitated by the advent of improved imaging and surveillance leading to higher detection rates and the use of minimally invasive thoracoscopic techniques, reducing the morbidity of pulmonary resection [206].

Peritoneal disease

Up to 10% of colon cancer cases have peritoneal spread at the time of presentation, and its treatment remains one of the challenges in colon cancer management. Cytoreductive surgery and perioperative intraperitoneal hyperthermic chemotherapy (HIPEC) has provided a treatment option for these patients [207]. The principle is to surgically resect the macroscopic peritoneal disease leaving microscopic or minimal visible disease only. Heated intraperitoneal chemotherapy, either oxaliplatin or mitomycin C, is then added to the abdominal cavity to control any remaining malignant cells. Patient selection is important as the surgery can be extensive, involving resection of a number of organs and stripping of large areas of peritoneum. It is usually reserved for patients with good performance status and low volumes of disease. A single randomized trial demonstrated a survival advantage, with a median survival of 22 months [208]. This data is being increasingly supported by large cohort studies [209].

Results of surgery and treatment for colon cancer

Elective colon cancer surgery is considered to have a low mortality and morbidity, with good postoperative quality of life. Results from large prospective multicentre trials show mortality figures of 1–4%, and morbidity of 1–20% [210, 211]. The surgery still has significant risks of adverse events. This is in part because even very elderly patients and those with multiple comorbidities will be offered surgical treatment. The quality of life following surgery is excellent, even in older populations, often with scores as good as or better than before surgery [212].

The results of colon cancer treatment have been improving steadily over the last 30 years, with 22% five-year survival for colon cancer in 1971–1975 compared with 51% in 2001–2006 [213]. Outcomes in the UK are not as good as for those with equivalent disease in the rest of Western Europe. The reasons for this remain poorly understood [214, 215]. The main determinant of survival is still cancer stage (Table 39.2); other independent poor prognostic features include presentation as an emergency and poor socioeconomic groups [216], and cancer features associated with more aggressive phenotypes such as lymphovascular and perineural invasion, tumour budding, mucinous, and poorly differentiated cell types.

Table 39.2 Percentage of cases and five-year relative survival (%) by stage at diagnosis, CRC patients diagnosed 1996–2002, England [213]

AJCC/Dukes' stage	Percentage of cases	Five-year survival
Stage 1/A	8.7%	93.2%
Stage 2/B	24.2%	77%
Stage 3/C	23.6%	47.7%
Stage 4/D	9.2%	6.6%

Source: data from Cancer Research UK, *CancerStats*, Copyright © Cancer Research UK 2013. All rights reserved, available from http://www.cancerresearchuk.org/cancer-info/cancerstats/

Medical management of early-stage disease

See Chapter 38 for the management of stage IV disease. Approximately 70–80% of newly diagnosed cases of CRC undergo curative resection; however, 40% of these develop incurable recurrent disease due to undetected micrometastases [217, 218]. Patients with stage III (A (T1, 2N1M0), B (T3, 4N1M0), C (T x N2M0) or Dukes' C) disease have a five-year survival rate from 83% to 44%, respectively, with three-year disease-free survival (DFS) ranging from 45% to 52%. Those with stage II (A (T3N0M0) or B (T4N0M0)) colon cancer after surgical resection have a five-year survival rate of 45–60% and 64–75%, respectively [217, 219]. The inability to cure all such patients is a direct consequence of residual occult disease.

Adjuvant chemotherapy is offered to such high-risk patients with the aim of decreasing relapse and improving overall survival (OS) by attempting to eliminate microscopic residual disease. It is offered where the benefits outweigh the risks from chemotherapy-related toxicities. Adjuvant therapy has been offered to patients with stage III disease as standard therapy for over two decades [220], a practice strongly reinforced by two recent meta-analyses [221, 222].

In the case of patients with stage II disease, the role of adjuvant therapy is controversial given the difficulty in identifying patients at the highest of risk who would benefit the most from adjuvant therapy [223]. The recognized clinical/pathological poor prognostic markers for patients with stage II disease include (1) poorly differentiated histology [224], obstruction or perforation at presentation [225], lymphovascular invasion [226]; (2) fewer than 12 lymph nodes retrieved during primary resection [225, 227, 228]; and (3) tumoural stage, including T4 disease (with invasion into adjacent organs) [224, 229]. From the SEER database, it was observed that the five-year OS rates between T3N0 and T4N0 patients was 87.5%±0.4% versus 71.5%±0.8% and between T4a (penetration through visceral peritoneum) and T4b (penetration of other organs or structures) 79.6%±1% versus 58.4%±1.3%, respectively [229]. These high-risk factors have not been evaluated in prospective trials in which such patients were randomized to treatment versus no treatment [230].

Adjuvant chemotherapy for stage III disease (T1–4, N1–2M0)

Adjuvant chemotherapy has been the standard of care for stage III disease for the last two decades. Initial efforts concentrated on the evaluation of 5-fluorouracil (5-FU)-based regimens and 5FU biochemical modulation. With the advances in the treatment of metastatic disease including oral 5-FU prodrugs, oxaliplatin, irinotecan, and the biologicals (including EGFR and anti-vascular endothelial growth factor (VEGF) monoclonal antibodies), these agents have also been evaluated and—in some cases—are now standard of care in patients with stage III disease. These new agents either provided a more favourable administration or toxicity profile (as in the case of the oral 5-FU prodrugs) or increase in DFS or OS (in the case of oxaliplatin).

During this time, three-year DFS rate has been validated as an appropriate endpoint for adjuvant trials given its strong correlation with five-year OS (correlation coefficient 0.86, HR = 0.91) [231]. On a subsequent analysis of six additional phase III trials, the two- or three-year DFS HRs were highly predictive of five- and six-year OS

HRs in stage III, but not stage II patients. In all patients, the DFS/OS association is stronger for six-year OS; thus at least six years' follow-up was recommended to assess OS benefit [232]. However, extended survival after recurrence reduces the association between treatment effects on thee-year DFS and five-year OS, particularly in stage II patients [233]. In modern adjuvant trials, six or seven years may now be required to demonstrate OS improvements [233].

5-FU-based therapy

The major advances in adjuvant chemotherapy for resected CRC were made in the early 1990s, with the biochemical modulation of 5-FU with either levamisole (Lev) or LV. Two recent meta-analyses have shown that the reduction in mortality by modulation of 5-FU by LV or Lev (29%, P < 0.007; 22%, P < 0.01, respectively) was significantly larger than that for unmodulated 5-FU (6%, P < 0.11) [221, 222].

The NCCTG study demonstrated the benefit of 5-FU-Lev relative to observation or Lev alone in reducing tumour recurrence and improving OS in patients with Dukes' C disease [234]. The IMPACT, NSABP-C03, and NCCTG trials have all demonstrated the advantage of 5-FU-LV relative to their respective control arms [235–237]. Since then, several large multicentre randomized trials have been performed to define the optimal 5-FU-based regimen: that is, the combination with high- or low-dose LV (HDLV, LDLV, respectively) and/or Lev in patients with stage III colon cancer. One of the largest was the Intergroup-0089 trial, a four-arm trial involving 3760 patients with high-risk stage II/III disease [238]. The other large trial, the QUASAR study, evaluated the role of Lev (versus placebo) and LV dose (175 mg versus 25 mg) in stage I–III CRC [239–240]. These large studies demonstrated the following: (1) 5-FU/HDLV is equivalent to 5-FU/LDLV at least as administered in the daily by 5, four-weekly regimen; (2) the weekly regimen of 5-FU-LV is equivalent but less toxic compared with a four-weekly regimen; (3) the addition of Lev provided no additional survival benefit [237–241]; and (4) the efficacy of adjuvant chemotherapy for 12 months provided no further benefit compared with six months.

The efficacy of 5-FU-LV or -Lev in the adjuvant setting has been evaluated specifically in terms of the elderly with stage III disease [242–244]. The lack of significant interaction between age and treatment efficacy has been demonstrated by the results of a meta-analysis (seven trials involving 3351 patients) [242], a population analysis using NCI SEER and the US Medicare database [243], and a prospective analysis of 85,934 patients from 1990 to 2002 [244].

Oral 5-FU prodrugs

The most widely available is capecitabine, a prodrug that undergoes final conversion to 5-FU through tumoural thymidine phosphorylase. In terms of adjuvant therapy, capecitabine (24 weeks, 1250 mg/m^2 twice daily, day 1–14, one week rest) was compared to the six-months' bolus 5-FU-LV as adjuvant therapy for stage III colon cancer in the randomized phase III X-ACT trial [245]. The DFS (primary study endpoint) in the capecitabine arm was at least equivalent to that in the 5-FU-LV arm (HR = 086, P = 0.04); the upper limit of the HR was significantly (P < 0.001) below the predefined margins for non-inferiority. Capecitabine was also associated with significantly fewer 5-FU-related grade 3/4 adverse events (AEs; P < 0.001) and fewer adverse-event (AE)-related hospital admissions. Pharmacoeconomic analyses performed in several countries showed that the savings in direct costs (drug administration and AE-related costs) associated with capecitabine versus

5-FU-LV offset the drug acquisition costs [245]. A follow-up report with a median follow-up of 6.9 years again confirmed these earlier results with regards to DFS [246].

Oxaliplatin and 5-FU or capecitabine

The efficacy of oxaliplatin plus 5-FU in the adjuvant setting was demonstrated by two pivotal trials: the MOSAIC [247] and the NSABP C07 trials. In the MOSAIC trial, 2246 patients who had stage II or III colon cancer were randomized to receive a combined bolus and infusional 5-FU regimen (LV5-FU2) alone or with oxaliplatin (FOLFOX4) for six months. The primary endpoint was 3-year DFS [247]. A total of 1123 patients were randomly assigned to each group. The rate of DFS at three years was 78.2% in the group given FOLFOX4 versus 72.9% in the LV5-FU2 group (P = 0.002). In the group given FOLFOX4, the incidence of grade 3 sensory neuropathy was 12.4% during treatment, decreasing to 1.1% at one year of follow-up [247].

With longer follow-up, the final results of the study, including six-year OS and five-year updated DFS were reported [248]. The five-year DFS rates were 73.3% and 67.4% in the FOLFOX4 and LV5-FU2 groups, respectively (HR = 0.80; P = 0.003). Six-year OS rates were 78.5% and 76.0% in the FOLFOX4 versus LV5-FU2 groups, respectively (HR = 0.84; P = 0.046). The corresponding six-year OS rates for patients with stage III disease were 72.9% and 68.7%, respectively (HR = 0.80; P = 0.023). Of note was that no difference in OS was seen in the stage II population [248].

In the NSABP C07 trial, 2492 patients with stage II and III colon cancer were randomly assigned to either 5-FU 500 mg/m^2 bolus weekly for six weeks plus LV 500 mg/m^2 IV weekly for six weeks during each eight-week cycle (Roswell Park regimen) for three cycles (5-FU-LV), or the same 5-FU-LV regimen with oxaliplatin 85 mg/m^2 IV administered on weeks 1, 3, and 5 of each eight-week cycle for three cycles (FLOX) [249]. The DFS hazard ratio (FLOX versus 5-FU-LV) was 0.80 (P <0.004). The four-year DFS rates were 67.0% for 5-FU-LV and 73.2% for FLOX, respectively. In terms of stage II and III patients: for stage II the four-year DFS was 81% versus 84.2%, and stage III 61.1% versus 68.9% for 5-FU-LV and FLOX, respectively [249].

A subsequent trial compared capecitabine plus oxaliplatin (XELOX; oxaliplatin 130 mg/m^2 on day 1 plus capecitabine 1000 mg/m^2 twice daily on days 1 to 14, every three weeks for 24 weeks) with bolus 5-FU-LV (Mayo Clinic for 24 weeks or Roswell Park for 32 weeks) as adjuvant therapy for patients with stage III colon cancer [250]. The primary study endpoint was DFS. After 57 months of follow-up, the three-year DFS rate was 70.9% with XELOX and 66.5% with 5-FU-LV (HR = 0.80, P = 0.0045). The HR for OS for XELOX compared to 5-FU-LV was 0.87 (P = 0.1486). The five-year OS for XELOX and 5-FU-LV were 77.6% and 74.2%, respectively. It was thus concluded that the addition of oxaliplatin to capecitabine improves DFS in patients with stage III colon cancer. XELOX is thus considered an additional adjuvant treatment option for these patients [250].

The efficacy of adjuvant oxaliplatin therapy has also been confirmed, albeit inconsistently, in the elderly. Subgroup analyses of DFS of the NO1968 trial comparing XELOX to 5-FU-LV, demonstrated reduced risk of recurrence in all subgroups receiving oxaliplatin including patients <65 years of age and those ≥65 years of age; however, in the latter group the trend was not significant [250]. A post hoc analysis of the effect of oxaliplatin in the NSABP

CO7 trials did vary by age for OS (younger than age 70 versus 70+, interaction P = 0.039), with a similar trend for DFS (interaction P = 0.073). Oxaliplatin significantly improved OS in patients younger than age 70 (HR, 0.80; P = 0.013), but no positive effect was evident in older patients [251].

An analysis of the ACCENT database, derived from six phase III adjuvant trials comparing IV 5-FU to combinations with irinotecan, oxaliplatin, or oral FU in stage II/III colon cancer, evaluated data from 10,499 patients younger than 70 and 2170 patients ≥70 years. OS, DFS, and TTR were not significantly improved for those patients older than 70 years of age in the experimental versus control arms. The interaction between age and treatment was statistically significant for all endpoints (P = 0.01 for OS, DFS, and TTR) [252]. A further analysis evaluated the benefit of the oxaliplatin combination in patients above and below 70 years of age (overall, 3742 patients; 614 ≥ 70 years of age) from four clinical trials in the adjuvant and metastatic setting [253]. OS and DFS rates did not differ by age, though data from patients older than 80 was sparse [253].

Irinotecan and 5-FU

Despite the activity of irinotecan in the treatment of advanced CRC, randomized phase III trials in the adjuvant setting (including CALBG 89803, PETACC3, ACCORD 2 trials) have failed to demonstrate an added benefit relative to 5-FU-LV alone [254–256]. Further trials evaluating this agent in this setting have not progressed.

Biological agents and combination chemotherapy

In the metastatic setting the antiangiogenic agent, bevacizumab, a monoclonal antibody to VEGF, and the anti-EGFR monoclonal antibodies cetuximab and panitumumab have shown added benefit when added to conventional chemotherapy backbones, whether oxaliplatin- or irinotecan-based or 5-FU-LV [257]. However, recent phase III trials in the adjuvant setting have demonstrated that these biological agents provide no additional benefit and may actually be detrimental when added to a chemotherapy backbone, usually oxaliplatin-5-FU.

In the case of bevacizumab, the NSABP C08 [258] and the AVANT trials [259] have shown no additional benefit. In the former trial, 2672 patients with stage II/III disease were randomized to mFOLFOX6 for six months versus the same regimen with 12 months of bevacizumab. The primary endpoint of three-year DFS was 75.5% versus 77.4% for the control and experimental arms, respectively (HR = 0.89, P = 0.15). There was a transient effect of bevacizumab during treatment whereby the impact on DFS was significant before versus after a 15-month landmark: HR = 0.61 (P < 0.001) and HR = 1.22 (P = 0.076), respectively [258]. The reason for this transient benefit of bevacizumab is unclear [258, 260].

The lack of benefit with bevacizumab was, however, confirmed by the AVANT trial, in which high-risk stage II/III patients were randomized to FOLFOX4 for six months ± bevacizumab for 48 weeks or XELOX for six months ± bevacizumab for 48 weeks [259]. The addition of bevacizumab did not prolong DFS or OS in stage III patients, with efficacy favouring the chemotherapy-alone arm [259]. Two other large relevant trials are yet to be reported. These include the QUASAR 2 study, randomizing patients to capecitabine ± bevacizumab, and ECOG E5202 [260].

In terms of cetuximab, the NCCTG-N0147 trial randomized patients with stage III KRAS wild-type disease to six month of mFOLFOX6 ± cetuximab [261]. Three-year DFS for mFOLFOX6 alone was 74.6% versus 71.5% with the addition of cetuximab (HR = 1.21; P = 0.08), with no significant benefit in any subgroups assessed [260]. The PETTAC8 trial was of similar design: a pre-specified interim analysis did not support a benefit in DFS for patients given cetuximab plus FOLFOX-4 compared with patients treated with FOLFOX-4 alone. The FoxTROT trial evaluating FOLFOX or XELOX ± panitumumab is yet to be reported [262].

The mechanisms for this lack of synergy with chemotherapy and the biological agents in this setting as compared to advanced disease are not clear but may be explained by the induction of compensatory/alternate mechanisms and pro-survival pathway activation by VEGF or EGFR inhibition, which have been discussed elsewhere [263].

Adjuvant therapy of patients with resected stage II colon cancer

The case for and against

In the case of patients with stage II disease the role of adjuvant therapy is controversial given the difficulty in identifying patients at the highest risk who would benefit the most from adjuvant therapy whilst avoiding potential toxicity in patients who would not benefit [223].

The efficacy of systemic adjuvant chemotherapy for patients with stage II cancer has still not been confirmed. A pooled analysis of 1016 patients with B2 colon cancer from the IMPACT trial, in which patients were randomized to 5-FU-LV versus observation, found chemotherapy did not provide a significant advantage in terms of event-free survival (EFS) (82% versus 80%, respectively) or OS (76% versus 73%, respectively) after a median follow-up of 5.75 years [264]. However, in contrast, when the results from the NSABP C01–4 trials were pooled to compare the efficacy of chemotherapy in 1565 patients with Dukes' B relative to Dukes' C disease, regardless of stage, there was a reduction in mortality, DFS, and recurrence after chemotherapy. The reduction for Dukes' B was of a similar magnitude to that seen for Dukes' C disease [265].

The large phase III QUASAR trial randomized 6668 patients with resected stage II and III colon cancer to 5-FU (370 mg/m^2) with HD (175 mg) or LD (25 mg), LV and either Lev or placebo. The primary outcome was all-cause mortality [239–240]. Overall, 28% of the patients entered had stage B (or stage II) disease, selected for high risk features, such as T4, obstruction, and perforation. The relative risk of recurrence for colon cancer was reduced with an HR of 0.78 (P = 0.004), and the relative risk for cancer-related death was also reduced, HR = 0.84 (P = 0.06). Treatment efficacy did not differ significantly by tumour site, stage, sex, age, or chemotherapy schedule [239–240].

In terms of modern combination therapy there is relevant data from the MOSAIC and the NSABP C07 trials in patients with stage II disease. In terms of the MOSAIC trial, 899 patients with stage II disease were randomized between LV5U2 versus oxaliplatin-LV5U2. With a median follow-up of 6.8 years: five-year DFS was 79.9% versus 83.7% (HR = 0.84, P = 0.258) and the six-year OS 86.8% versus 86.9% (P = 0.986), respectively [248]. For the NSABP CO7 trial, 29% overall had resected stage II disease; the four-year DFS was 81% versus 84.2% in favour of FLOX [249].

A recent Cochrane analysis considered all randomized trials or meta-analyses containing data on stage II colon cancer patients undergoing adjuvant therapy versus surgery alone; overall 8642 patients were considered [262]. In terms of the effect of adjuvant therapy on stage II colon cancer, the pooled relative risk ratio for OS was 0.96 (95% CI 0.88–1.05), and for DFS 0.83 (95% CI 0.75–0.92). Hence the benefit was in terms of DFS only. The authors concluded that it was reasonable to discuss the benefits of adjuvant systemic chemotherapy with those stage II patients who have high-risk features. The comorbidities and likelihood of tolerating adjuvant systemic chemotherapy should be considered as well [266].

Identifying high-risk stage II patients

Given the modest benefit for adjuvant therapy in patients with resected stage II disease, there is thus an urgent need to better characterize high-risk patients who would gain the greatest benefit. At present, the identifiers of high risk relate to the tumour as well as clinical factors, albeit inconsistently [223]. Considerable effort has been directed to identify molecular prognostic and predictive factors; however, as expected, there is considerable heterogeneity in terms of the cohorts evaluated, prospective versus retrospective analyses, and analytical methodology.

The markers evaluated thus far include aneuploidy/tetraploidy DNA, 18q allelic loss, as well as microsatellite status (MS), p53, KRAS, BRAF, and thymidylate synthase [230, 277–270]. A detailed review of these molecular factors with regard to stage II disease has been published recently [271]. These factors, however, may not be mutually exclusive: for example, the molecular analysis of the PETACC-3 study found that in stage II–III colon cancer, KRAS mutation status did not have major prognostic value, but BRAF was prognostic for OS in MS-L/MSS tumours [268].

Microsatellite instability (MSI)

The assessment of MSI, which serves as a marker for DNA mismatch repair (MMR) system function, has emerged as a useful tool for risk stratification of patients with stage II colon cancer. It seems clear, from retrospective studies and meta-analyses, that patients with stage II and III tumours classified as MSI-H (or defective MMR (dMMR)) have a better prognosis, independent of adjuvant therapy, relative to MSS tumours [272–274].

Whilst the prognostic importance of MSI has been confirmed, however, its importance in predicting response to adjuvant chemotherapy is unclear [267]. It appears that patients with dMMR do not benefit from adjuvant 5-FU therapy [275, 276]. The largest study involved 457 patients who were previously randomized to 5-FU-based therapy adjuvant therapy (n = 229) versus no post-surgical treatment (n = 228) [276]. Overall, 70 (15%) of 457 patients exhibited dMMR. Adjuvant therapy significantly improved DFS (HR = 0.67; P = 0.02) in patients with preserved MMR tumours. Patients with dMMR tumours receiving 5-FU had no improvement in DFS (HR = 1.10; P = 0.85) compared to surgery alone. A parallel analysis of a pooled data set of 1027 patients confirmed these findings [276].

The data thus far support MMR status assessment for patients being considered for 5-FU therapy alone. Based on the body of current data, with the caveat that MSI status is still to be validated prospectively as a predictive biomarker, the current NCCN guidelines recommend that where adjuvant therapy is being considered in patients with stage II disease, MSI status must be assessed; those with MSI-H tumours should not be offered 5-FU-based therapy [225, 260].

It is unclear whether this also applies to oxaliplatin-5-FU adjuvant regimens. A recent study investigated the clinical implication of MSI-H/dMMR and p53 expression in resected colon cancer patients who received post-operative FOLFOX therapy [277]. Overall, in 135 patients there were 13 (9.6%) patients with stage II disease and 108 (80%) patients with stage III. MMR status was not significantly associated with DFS or OS in patients receiving adjuvant FOLFOX. It was concluded, albeit in this small heterogeneous study, that adding oxaliplatin to adjuvant chemotherapy may overcome the negative impact of 5-FU on colon cancers with MSI-H/dMMR [277].

18q allelic imbalance (18qAI)

The chromosome 18q contains the tumour suppressor genes deleted in colon cancer (DCC) and the SMAD4 gene, which are lost in the oncogenic development of CRC [278]. The allelic loss of 18q is manifested as a loss of heterozygosity (LOH). The 18qLOH or 18 allelic imbalance (18qAI) have been correlated with a poorer prognosis in patients with stage II and III disease, albeit inconsistently [279, 280].

In a landmark study, LOH from chromosomes 18q, 17p, and 8p, cellular levels of p53 and p21 (WAF1/CIP1) proteins, TGF-beta1 type II receptor gene mutation, and MSI status were analysed in 460 patients with stage III and high-risk stage II colon cancer who had been treated with 5-FU-based therapy [280]. Among patients with MSS stage III cancer, five-year OS after 5-FU-based chemotherapy was 74% in those whose cancer retained 18q alleles and 50% in those with 18q LOH (RR for death with 18q LOH was 2.75; P = 0.006). The five-year OS among patients whose cancer had MSI-H was 74% in the presence of a mutated gene for the TGF-beta1 type II receptor and 46% if the tumour did not have this mutation (RR of death, 2.90; P = 0.03). It was concluded in this retrospective study that retention of 18q alleles in MSS cancers and TGF-beta1 type II receptor gene mutation in cancers with high levels of MSI-H point to a favourable outcome with 5-FU-based regimens for stage III colon cancer [280].

The recently closed ECOG E5202 study is also relevant in this regard. It assigned stage II patients, stratified by MSI status and 18q allele imbalance, to observation for low-risk patients (MSS or MSI-L with retention of 18q or MSI-H) and high-risk patients (MSS/18qLOH or MSI-L/18qLOH) to FOLFOX4 +/ bevacizumab. It was closed early following the reports of the AVANT and NSABP C08 trials that demonstrated the lack of benefit of bevacizumab in the adjuvant setting [260].

Gene expression approaches

Quantitative gene expression assays have been evaluated to assess recurrence risk, though with less utility for the benefits from chemotherapy in patients with stage II disease. There are at present two commercially available gene expression classifiers (ColoPrint® and Oncotype DX®) that have been developed and are being subsequently validated prognostically to classify patients with early-stage colon cancer at high risk of relapse, rather than to determine their predictive ability in terms of outcomes from adjuvant chemotherapy [281, 282]. Others have also been reported and are being validated [283, 284].

ColoPrint® is an 18-gene prognostic classifier that was developed to predict disease relapse in patients with early-stage CRC. It was derived from fresh frozen tumour tissue from 188 patients with stage I to IV CRC undergoing surgery, whereby the majority (83.6%) did not receive adjuvant chemotherapy, and were analysed using Agilent 44K oligonucleotide arrays [281]. The classifier components were identified for their association with five-year distant metastasis-free survival. The classifier was validated on an independent set of 206 samples from patients with stages I–III CRC, whereby the signature classified 60% of patients as low risk and 40% as high risk. Five-year relapse-free survival (RFS) rates were 87.6% and 67.2% for low- and high-risk patients, respectively, with a HR of 2.5 (P = 0.005). In a multivariate analysis, including pathological stage and MSI status, the signature remained one of the most significant prognostic factors, with a HR of 2.69 (P = 0.003). In patients with stage II CRC, the signature had an HR of 3.34 (P = 0.017). Thus, ColoPrint® significantly improved the prognostic accuracy of pathologic factors and MSI in patients with stage II and III CRC and may identify patients with stage II disease who may be managed without chemotherapy [281].

ColoPrint® has subsequently been validated in an independent dataset, comprising of 320 stage II patients, 227 of which were T3/MSS [285]. In the analysis of all stage II patients, ColoPrint® classified two-thirds of stage II patients as being at lower risk. The three-year RFS was 91% for low risk and 74% for patients at higher risk, HR of 2.9 (P = 0.001). Standard poor prognostic clinicopathological parameters did not predict a differential outcome for high-risk patients (P <0.20). In the subgroup of patients with T3 and MSS phenotype, ColoPrint® classified 61% of patients at lower risk with a three-year RFS of 91% and 39% of patients at higher risk with a three-year RFS of 73% (P = 0.002) [285].

The second type of commercial assay is the Oncotype DX®. It was developed to quantify the risk of recurrence, as well as the likelihood of differential treatment benefit, of 5-FU/LV adjuvant chemotherapy for patients with resected stage II and III disease [282]. Fixed, paraffin-embedded tumour blocks were analysed from 1086 patients with stage II or III colon cancer treated as part of the NSABP C-01, -02, -04, and -06 trials. In its final development, the assay comprised of an 18-gene panel that included seven genes for RFS prognosis in colon cancer to yield a prognostic recurrence score (RS), six genes to predict response to 5-FU/LV chemotherapy to yield a predictive treatment score (TS), and five reference genes. Subsequent algorithms were developed to identify groups of patients with low, intermediate, and high likelihood of recurrence and benefit from 5-FU/LV [282].

Oncotype DX® has been subsequently validated in the stage II CRC dataset from the QUASAR study [273]. RNA was extracted from fixed paraffin-embedded primary colon tumour blocks from 1436 patients. Both RS and TS were calculated from gene expression levels of the 13 cancer-related genes described previously. The risk of recurrence was significantly associated with RS: recurrence risks at 3 years were 12%, 18%, and 22% for predefined low-, intermediate-, and high-recurrence risk groups, respectively. T stage (HR 1.94; P <0.001) and MMR status (HR 0.31; P <0.001) were the strongest histopathologic prognostic factors. There was no trend for increased benefit from chemotherapy at higher RS (P = 0.95). It was concluded that this continuous 12-gene RS provided prognostic value that complements T stage and MMR. The TS was not predictive of chemotherapy benefit [273]. The Oncotype DX® assay has also been validated in the dataset derived from the PETACC-3 trial [284].

In conclusion, adjuvant therapy is recommended for patients with resected stage III colon cancer. Patients, based on fitness and preference, with completely resected stage III cancer should be offered six months of adjuvant chemotherapy, which optimally should start within eight weeks of surgery. The optimal regimen is oxaliplatin in combination with 5-FU-LV or capecitabine, based on relevant consideration of the therapeutic ratio, especially in regard to neurotoxicity. Patients not considered suitable for oxaliplatin should be offered 5-FU-LV (weekly bolus, or Roswell Park regimen, or LV5-FU2 bolus-infusional regimen) or capecitabine [230]. Patient compliance in terms of cumulative toxicity and the differing toxicity profile for capecitabine must be carefully considered. Current trials are now investigating the optimal length of therapy, i.e. three versus six months (IDEA trial, multinational intergroup trial) and the SCOT (Short Course Oncology Therapy), a study of adjuvant chemotherapy in colorectal cancer by the CACTUS and QUASAR 3 Groups, and the additional benefit of the EGFR monoclonal antibody panitumumab (the FOxTROT trial), which is also testing the role of neoadjuvant therapy [263].

In terms of patients with resected stage II disease, adjuvant chemotherapy may be discussed with patients at high risk of disease relapse, based upon clinicopathological factors discussed above and whilst considering the patients' comorbidities, age, as well as the risk of therapy-related adverse events. MSI status must be assessed for those patients being considered for adjuvant therapy, and those with an MSI-H tumour should not be offered 5-FU-based therapy alone [225, 260]. The utility of oxaliplatin-based therapy in this setting is controversial, given the marginal benefit and greater risk of toxicity. Where available, commercial gene expression classifiers may also be considered to further classify patients based on risk of relapse. However, at his stage they cannot predict which patients are likely to respond to therapy.

Radiotherapy for colon cancer

In contrast to rectal cancer, the role of adjuvant radiotherapy is not well established in the management of colon cancer. The colon is a much longer structure than the rectum. It begins with the caecum in the right iliac fossa, and continues as the ascending colon in the retroperitoneal region on the right side of abdomen. It then becomes the transverse colon with its mesentery attached to the posterior abdominal wall, running from the right side to the left side of the abdomen. It runs further as the descending colon in the retroperitoneal position on the left side of the abdomen, and then as the sigmoid colon with its mesentery in the lower abdomen.

Colon cancer may recur locally in several different ways: anastomotic recurrence, tumour bed recurrence, and nodal recurrence [286]. The risk of local recurrence is, however, lower compared with rectal cancer. Anastomotic recurrence is not common, possibly because, at surgery, wide proximal and distal resection margins are achievable in most situations. The extent of proximal and distal resection margins is determined not only by the tumour extent, but also by the amount of vascular supply of the colon that is resected during clearance of the lymphatic drainage.

The risk of tumour bed recurrence varies for different parts of the colon. The high-risk portion is the immobile part of the colon in the retroperitoneal position—the ascending colon and the descending colon. The risk is particularly high when the tumour involves the posterolateral wall of the colon where the serosa is lacking. The low-risk portion is the mobile part of the colon with complete peritoneal covering attached to the posterior abdominal wall with its mesentery, the transverse colon, and the sigmoid colon. Wide circumferential margins are achievable in these areas. The risk of local recurrence also depends on whether the adjacent organs, when invaded by the tumour, can be sacrificed for an extended resection.

Adjuvant radiotherapy was found to decrease local recurrence for locally advanced tumours [287]. It was found to be beneficial for patients with T4 lesions, tumours associated with abscess or fistula formation, and residual local disease after subtotal resection [288]. It was also found in a retrospective study that post-operative radiotherapy decreased the risk of local recurrence in patients with T3–4 tumours of the caecum, ascending colon, or descending colon [289].

In view of the high risk of local recurrence in the autopsy and reoperation series, a randomized controlled study was performed to evaluate the benefit of adjuvant radiation in addition to adjuvant chemotherapy after complete resection of the colon cancer [290]. Patients suitable for the Intergroup Protocol 0130 were those with resected colon cancer where there was tumour adherence or invasion to the surrounding structures and with T3N1 or T3N2 tumours of the ascending or descending colon. The experimental arm included treatment with radiation to a total dose of 45 to 50.4 Gy in 1.8 Gy per fraction, in addition to adjuvant chemotherapy consisting of 5-FU and levamisole. This study was terminated because of slow accrual after the enrolment of 222 patients, which was less than a third of the accrual target. Data from assessable patients (n = 187) showed that patients who received chemotherapy or chemoradiation had similar overall survival and disease-free survival rates. Toxicity was higher among chemoradiation patients. These results, however, must be interpreted with caution because of the high number of ineligible patients and the limited power of the study to detect potentially meaningful differences.

Several deficiencies in the study methodology were subsequently identified. Radio-opaque surgical clips for guiding the radiation field were used only in a minor proportion of patients. Preoperative imaging was not available for most patients. The completeness of the resection could not be confirmed because of the lack of information about the radial margins. It highlights the importance of close cooperation among surgeons, radiation and medical oncologists, pathologists, and radiologists in selection of patients for adjuvant radiotherapy.

In order to evaluate the area at risk for adjuvant radiotherapy planning, availability of a preoperative CT scan, operation notes, and pathology report are essential. In addition, surgeons can assist in localization of the tumour bed by inserting radio-opaque surgical clips at the time of surgery. Accurate localization of the tumour bed improves tumour control by reducing the risk of marginal miss. It also limits unnecessary radiation exposure to the nearby critical structures at low risk for involvement.

The organs that limit radiation dose vary according to the location of the colon cancer. These organs include small intestine, liver, kidneys, spinal cord, urinary bladder, and gynaecological structures. Improvement of radiotherapy technique allows treatment to be delivered safely. Radiation side effects have been significantly reduced with conformal radiotherapy and intensity-modulated radiation therapy (IMRT).

Adjuvant chemoradiation is to be considered for selected patients with T4 disease penetrating to a fixed structure or for patients with recurrent disease. Preoperative chemoradiation is also a consideration for patients with clinical T4 or recurrent disease to increase the chance of complete resection. In addition, highly selected cases of T3 cancers on the posterolateral wall of the ascending and descending colon, where wide resection margins cannot be achieved, are to be considered. The common dose regimen for adjuvant chemoradiation is 45–50.4 Gy in 1.8 Gy per fraction over 5–5.5 weeks with concurrent infusion chemotherapy 5-FU. The radiotherapy target volume includes the primary tumour bed with a margin. There is no evidence that enlarging the radiotherapy target volume to include the regional lymph nodes improves outcomes [287]. Radiation can also be delivered intraoperatively in specialized centres after resection of the colon cancer [291]. Intraoperative radiation therapy (IORT) is a highly conformal form of radiotherapy. Special equipment and dedicated operation theatres are necessary for this procedure. Two forms of IORT are available. One form of delivery is with electrons from a dedicated linear accelerator located in a shielded theatre. IORT can also be delivered by brachytherapy with the flap technique. Brachytherapy is a form of radiotherapy where a radiation source is placed inside or next to the area requiring treatment. The radiation target volume is tailored according to the area at risk at the time of surgery. Side effects are kept to a minimum by displacing normal organs away from the radiation field during treatment. In addition, lead shields are used to protect tissue close to the radiation target. The effective depth of radiation is approximately 1 cm. It is reserved for situations where a wide circumferential resection margin is not achievable. In order to select suitable cases for IORT, thorough preoperative workup is necessary.

Whole abdominal radiation therapy (WART) has also been attempted to reduce the risk of intra-abdominal recurrence. A pilot clinical study of WART was performed in patients with locally advanced colon cancer, in view of the high incidence of peritoneal metastasis in this group of patients [292]. The inclusion criteria of the Southwest Oncology Group study were patients with completely resected T3N1–2M0 colon cancer. Infusion chemotherapy 5-FU was administered with concomitant 30 Gy of WART in 1 Gy per fraction. An additional 16 Gy boost to the tumour bed was administered in 1.6 Gy per fraction. There were no treatment-related fatalities but 17% of patients had severe toxicity and 7% had life-threatening toxicity of any kind. Its efficacy has not been confirmed in randomized studies.

Radiation therapy for liver metastasis

In a selected group of patients, resection of liver metastasis provides long-term tumour control and improved survival [293]. Recently, high-dose radiotherapy has been used to eradicate liver metastasis; this is a treatment option available in specialized centres. Technological improvements in radiation delivery have allowed liver irradiation to be delivered safely up to doses of 90 Gy in 1.5 Gy per fractions [294].

Stereotactic body radiotherapy (SBRT) is an emerging technique employed in the treatment of liver metastasis. It delivers high doses of radiation to the liver metastasis with multiple fields, resulting in highly conformal dose gradients that can spare normal structures from high risk of toxicity. High accuracy and precision of treatment is ensured by use of image-guided radiotherapy at every treatment course (usually one to six treatments). Insertion of radio-opaque markers in the liver can facilitate localization of the metastasis at every treatment. 4-dimensional CT imaging is used in planning the position of the metastasis during different phases of the respiratory cycle. Accordingly, internal motion of the lesion can be accounted for in the radiotherapy plan. Various methods to control respiratory motion are used. Abdominal compression is used to reduce abdominal movement during the respiratory cycle. Active or voluntary breathholding during simulation and treatment

allows treatment to be delivered at either an inhale or exhale phase of breathing. Gated radiotherapy can be performed by obtaining a respiratory signal or position of the tumour by use of either an internal or external fiducial marker. These methods allow smaller margins to be used in radiotherapy delivery and hence reduce rates of normal tissue toxicity while obtaining ablative doses of radiotherapy to the tumour.

In a multi-institutional phase I/II study, patients with one to three hepatic lesions and maximum individual tumour diameters less than 6 cm were included. Radiation dose was escalated from 36 Gy to 60 Gy, in three fractions, in increments of 6 Gy, during phase I study. The phase II dose was 60 Gy in three fractions. Thirteen patients were treated to a dose less than 60 Gy, and 36 patients received 60 Gy. Forty-seven patients with 63 lesions were treated. Grade 3 or higher toxicity was 2%. Actuarial in-field local control rates at one and two years after SBRT were 95% and 92%, respectively. Among lesions with maximal diameter of 3 cm or less, two-year local control was 100%. Median survival was 20.5 months [295].

A different approach is individualizing total radiation dose according to the normal tissue tolerance of the liver. In a phase I study, 68 patients with inoperable liver metastases were treated with individualized SBRT. Median radiation dose was 41.8 Gy (range 27.7 to 60 Gy) in six fractions over two weeks. Median tumour volume was 75.2 ml (range 1.19 to 3,090 ml). Two grade 3 liver toxicity enzyme changes occurred, but no radiation-induced liver disease or other grade 3 or higher liver toxicity. The one-year local control rate was 71% (95 CI, 58% to 85%) [296].

New treatment strategies are being explored. A dose-escalating phase I study is being performed to investigate the maximum tolerated dose of single-fraction SBRT (NCT01162278). A phase I/II trial combines liver SBRT with sorafenib (NCT00892424). Proton beam SBRT is being investigated in treating liver metastasis (NCT01239381). Proton beam radiation uses tiny particles to deliver radiation to tumours. A phase II with individualized SBRT for liver tumours is being conducted with patients who have had previous liver treatment (NCT01522937). The development of SBRT for liver metastasis has been promising. Conformal external beam radiotherapy can be considered in highly selected cases or in the setting of a clinical trial but it should not be used indiscriminately in patients who are potentially surgically resectable.

Multidisciplinary care of early stage colon cancer

Introduction to multidisciplinary care

As management strategies for colon cancer become increasingly refined and personalized medicine becomes the rule rather than the exception, complexity arises when optimizing the treatment for individuals. The treatment of colon cancer has evolved over the last several decades from what was originally primarily a surgical disease, to one where it is expected that doctors and allied health professionals from several disciplines will be involved in patient management from the outset. A multidisciplinary approach is essential from the point of diagnosis, through treatment, and beyond. While the role of multidisciplinary involvement is most obvious in challenging and complex scenarios, every patient in fact requires expertise from several medical and allied health disciplines—a biopsychosocial approach for optimal outcomes after the diagnosis of colon cancer. Many (over 60%) are cured from their colon cancer, and thus surveillance and survivorship issues are particularly pertinent in the setting of colon cancer.

This section will outline the multidisciplinary nature of early-stage colon cancer care. As several aspects of such care are addressed in other chapters within this textbook, a general overview will be presented in these circumstances.

Role of multidisciplinary meetings and team management—consensus and controversies

Multidisciplinary team meetings and strategies have been implemented in many cancer centres throughout the world. Multiple doctors are involved in an individual's care; a prior UK study of 50 cancer patients found that within the first year of diagnosis, patients saw an average of 28 doctors [297]. Clearly, communication between these doctors is of critical importance. A multidisciplinary approach can help to streamline a patient's personal navigation through the system of colonoscopies, blood work, radiological investigation, surgery with or without perioperative chemotherapy or radiotherapy, stomal care, and timely post-operative oncological review, and appropriate follow-up. Aside from the 'physical' aspects of multidisciplinary care, the involvement of a multidisciplinary team can also identify potential psychosocial or comorbidity-related issues which may need to be considered and addressed during the patient's care. Finally and most importantly, discussion in a multidisciplinary context may help to identify patients who are suitable for clinical trials [298].

A more formalized approach to multidisciplinary care, including multidisciplinary team meetings, documentation, and care planning, is a concept increasingly embraced worldwide. The UK National Institute for Health and Clinical Excellence (NICE) guidelines recommend that patients with CRC should be treated by a multidisciplinary team [299]. Effective, coordinated, universal multidisciplinary care, although desirable, is not as prevalent in some centres as others [300].

The literature regarding the effectiveness of a formalized multidisciplinary approach is largely supportive [301], but while this is certainly felt to improve timeliness of referral, communication between specialists, and quality of patient care, it has been more difficult to demonstrate objective evidence that the multidisciplinary team improves patient outcome, especially in the context of changing and improving proposed therapies. An international literature review in 2010 of 21 studies investigating the impact of multidisciplinary care on patient survival could not demonstrate a positive relationship between the two, largely due to significant heterogeneity in the definition of multidisciplinary care, but noted that 12 of the studies did report a statistically significant association between multidisciplinary care and patient survival [302]. Specifically for CRC, a single-centre study from China comparing outcomes before and after the introduction of an MDT concluded that MDT discussion was an independent variable associated with improved overall survival [303]. Similarly, a single-surgeon audit from the UK of cases before and after the implementation of an MDT meeting reported a significant association between MDT status and survival, as well as a prognostic indicator of chemotherapy prescription [304].

Where possible, all patients with newly diagnosed CRC should be discussed and managed in a formalized multidisciplinary setting, while nevertheless recognizing that hospitals and centres may have differing capacities for multidisciplinary care depending on location and resources. A good outline of the 'ideal' MDT system is provided in the NICE guidelines.

Multidisciplinary management of colon cancer in special groups

Elderly patients

The current consensus is that the management of older cancer patients needs to be multidisciplinary—and ideally involves a geriatrician, where possible, as well as the patient's community doctor. A formalized comprehensive geriatric assessment is ideal, but may be resource intensive [305, 306]. Even without the resources to implement a comprehensive geriatric assessment, the role of social work, physiotherapy, and occupational therapy practitioners is clearly of value when assessing the ability of an older person to live well in the community. A decision about adjuvant chemotherapy must be made with this in mind, being aware that the balance between recurrence risk and quality of life is perhaps a more delicate one in the very old.

Young patients

Two to three percent of CRC is diagnosed in individuals less than 40 years of age. A diagnosis of any malignancy in a young person is associated with specific issues—in particular fertility and the possibility of a genetic cause or familial cancer. Concurrent illness such as inflammatory bowel disease, known to be associated with increased risk of CRC, may be present and need treatment, usually by a gastroenterologist. Concomitant immunosuppressive drugs used to treat inflammatory bowel disease may increase the risk of chemotherapy-associated myelosuppression. Additionally, many young people are working rather than retired at the time of diagnosis—thus the need for social work involvement with respect to the economic consequences of being away from the workplace during treatment. Disability-adjusted life years are rarely accounted for when considering the cost of CRC to the community, but are pertinent in this patient group.

There is ongoing dissent in the literature regarding whether young age at diagnosis is a poor prognostic factor itself in CRC. One American study utilizing a prospective clinical database concluded that patients under 40 did not have inferior DFS, but were more likely to have higher surgical lymph node yield and receive adjuvant chemotherapy; the authors postulated that more aggressive management may result in similar survival outcomes [307]. A UK retrospective review of young patients found that although no differences in survival overall was seen, younger patients had a higher rate of T4 disease and vascular invasion, both of which led to inferior outcomes [308]. A study from Scotland reported on ten-year survival outcomes for over 2000 patients, concluding that young age did not have an adverse impact on cancer-specific survival [309]. A Canadian retrospective study over 20 years, however, concluded that young patients with early-stage CRC had survival outcomes inferior to expectation [310]. Similarly, a Taiwanese study found inferior survival outcomes in young patients with CRC [311]. It may be stage at diagnosis rather than age itself that may contribute to what may appear to be worse overall outcomes in young patients with CRC.

Fertility may be affected by surgery, radiotherapy, and chemotherapy. While radiotherapy is generally not a consideration for early-stage colon cancer, chemotherapy in many cases will be considered in particular in a young person where much is at stake. The implications of fluoropyrimidines on gonadal function are thought to be minimal; however, oxaliplatin may be moderately gonadotoxic [312, 313]. Pregnancy should be avoided during chemotherapy and for several months afterwards. In male patients who are considering having children, the option of sperm collection and storage prior to chemotherapy must be discussed. In female patients, there are several options to consider for oocyte or ovarian preservation [312–314]. Expedited referral to a fertility expert is essential if fertility preservation is desired in young women diagnosed with CRC. The timing of fertility preservation techniques must be balanced with the need to commence adjuvant chemotherapy ideally within six to eight weeks of surgery.

Role of allied health teams and lifestyle factors in multidisciplinary management

Nurse practitioner

With the advent of screening faecal occult blood tests, and the universal recognition that CRC screening reduces mortality from the disease, comes the ever-increasing need for endoscopists to perform diagnostic lower gastrointestinal endoscopy. To this end, nurse practitioners have been involved in some centres for several years [315, 316]. A more recent randomized controlled trial comparing screening colonoscopy performed by nurse practitioners (n = 50) or gastroenterologists (n = 100) found that the nurse practitioner group were as safe and accurate as the gastroenterologist group [317]. The use of nurse practitioners for this purpose has been advocated by many as a way of safely, efficiently, and effectively addressing the need for endoscopic services [318]. Nurse practitioners are also involved in follow-up clinics after CRC diagnosis in some centres, again addressing the demand for timely and appropriate follow-up methods given the high prevalence of survivors [319]. Since the advent of capecitabine, an oral 5-FU analogue, for the management of both early-stage and metastatic CRC, nurse-led hospital and home-based care has been shown to be effective in monitoring and delivering oral chemotherapy safely [320, 321].

Stomal therapist

Depending on the type of bowel surgery required, a temporary or permanent stoma may be necessary for individuals undergoing resection of colon or rectal cancer. A stoma may have significant adverse effects on patient quality of life and body image [322, 323], although an earlier Cochrane review did not conclude firmly that quality of life with a stoma was significantly inferior [324]. Where possible, preoperative assessment and education by a stomal therapist is ideal. A study across 12 colorectal surgical units in Spain showed that patients who did see a therapist preoperatively had significantly less stoma complications and anxiety than those who did not [325]. Ongoing physical and psychological support from a stomal therapist while a stoma is present is appropriate.

Dietetics

Weight loss is significantly associated with decreased survival in colon cancer. Conversely, obesity places a person at increased risk of not only developing CRC but also having inferior outcomes [326–332]. The role of a dietician in the management of early-stage colon cancer is important at three steps: the acute phase of perioperative care and surgical recovery, the medium-term phase during adjuvant chemotherapy treatment, and the longer-term phase of healthy eating to maintain a healthy weight range. In the metastatic setting, managing cancer-related cachexia also requires the expertise of a dietician.

To demonstrate a positive association between particular dietary constituents and cancer incidence requires large cohort studies over long periods of time, and definitive evidence may remain elusive. Meat consumption, in particular processed meats, has been associated with increased risk of colon cancer in one meta-analysis [331]. A high-fibre diet was shown to be protective in the EPIC prospective cohort study, involving over 510,000 people [332]. A prospective observational study of over 1000 patients enrolled in an adjuvant stage III colon cancer trial found that a Western-pattern diet was associated with higher recurrence and mortality compared with a prudent dietary pattern, as has low levels of vitamin D [333]. It is important to be aware of these and other similar studies, in order comprehensively to advise patients on strategies to reduce their risk of CRC development and recurrence.

Exercise

Exercise is protective against the development of colon cancer [334]. Greater levels of exercise both pre- and post-diagnosis of CRC have been positively associated with improved survival in several observational studies. The Melbourne Collaborative Cohort Study, involving over 41,000 Australians, found that of the 528 people diagnosed with CRC over the follow-up period, those who exercised regularly had significantly improved disease-specific survival, in particular for stage II–III cancers, where the HR for DFS was 0.49 (P = 0.01) [335]. This finding, if related to a new anti-cancer agent, would be practice-changing if confirmed in a prospective study, which is understandably difficult to achieve in an intervention such as exercise, although intervention trials are underway. Nevertheless, exercising more and maintaining a healthy body weight are most likely the two most influential lifestyle modifications an individual can address in order to reduce their lifetime risk of CRC; and at least in the case of exercise, to reduce the risk of recurrence and death from their disease.

An oncologist, surgeon, or family practitioner alone can only partly influence an individual's decision to address issues such as weight loss and exercise, Similarly to the anti-smoking message and campaign, a multidisciplinary approach will surely be required to help effect the increasing body of evidence regarding the adverse effects of obesity and lack of exercise in the risk of CRC and other malignancies. A team effort, including government and non-government as well as doctors, dieticians, physiotherapists, and exercise physiologists will be required. Importantly, strategies are needed for the purposes of prevention as well as post-diagnosis health and, as such, addressing these risk factors is a large-scale effort and extends well beyond the individual and into the realms of public health and health policy.

Surveillance and follow-up—a multidisciplinary pathway

The aim of surveillance after curative-intent treatment of early-stage colon cancer is to improve survival by detecting early (curable) recurrence or small-volume asymptomatic metastatic disease that may be amenable to curative-intent resection. Additionally, colonoscopic surveillance for precancerous adenomas and polyps can reduce the risk of a second primary malignancy developing. As the majority of recurrences will recur within three to five years, this is when surveillance is most beneficial.

Several systematic reviews or meta-analyses, including a Cochrane review, have demonstrated significantly improved overall survival for patients who have more intensive post-surgical follow up for early-stage CRC, although, notably, not all randomized trials comparing 'intensive' with 'minimal' surveillance have shown a survival advantage for the 'intensive' arm [336–339]. Interestingly, the optimal methods or timings of surveillance investigations are not definitively established. A more recent systematic review of 15 studies comparing different surveillance programmes was inconclusive, largely due to the heterogeneity of surveillance programmes among studies, and recommended future randomized trials with larger sample sizes to help establish the best surveillance practices [340]. In fact, 'intensive' surveillance in one study may be akin to 'minimal' surveillance in another; hence, the difficulty when attempting to ascertain which practice is optimal. Several such trials are currently underway at the time of writing including the GILDA, FACS, and COLOFOL randomized studies.

As such, to date, clinical practice guidelines for optimal surveillance vary somewhat between countries. Surveillance generally includes clinical examination, colonoscopic surveillance, imaging (most commonly CT), and testing of serum carcino-embryonic antigen (CEA) [313]. FDG-PET imaging is currently not used as a surveillance tool, but rather when investigating suspected recurrence, for example in the setting of an increased CEA without CT changes. A randomized trial of 130 patients from France comparing PET with conventional surveillance found that recurrences were found after a shorter time in the PET group, and these were more frequently cured by surgery [341]. Another single-arm European surveillance study in 132 patients found that CT/PET had the highest sensitivity and specificity for detection of recurrence [342]. However, from a practical and financial perspective, PET is unlikely to be part of routine surveillance in most centres and is not currently recommended as part of evidence-based guidelines [343].

By nature of the methods of regular surveillance recommended, multidisciplinary involvement already exists in that surgeons and radiologists are involved; not uncommonly, a medical oncologist will also continue to follow the patient, especially if adjuvant chemotherapy has been administered. In some models of care, a family physician, general practitioner, or nurse specialist may assume a dominant role in overseeing patient follow-up [319, 344]; in others, this rests with the patient's primary specialist centre.

A number of guidelines are now available, each based on a literature review and expert opinion. It should be noted that these guidelines are for standard-risk patients; higher-risk patients such as those with a familial cancer syndrome or inflammatory bowel disease should have more frequent colonoscopic surveillance, again available using the various guidelines [345, 346–349].

Beyond the physical: the multidisciplinary approach to psychosocial sequelae and survivorship

The majority of patients diagnosed with early-stage colon cancer will survive the disease. Stage I and II disease have a 90% five-year survival rate and stage III up to 70% [350]. Even in metastatic disease, a small percentage of patients are alive years later due to the aggressive surgical management of oligometastatic disease and improved drug strategies. Overall, close to 65% of patients with CRC are considered 'cured' after five to ten years [351]. As such, there are tens of thousands of colon cancer survivors in the community, and this number is sure to increase given, firstly, advances in CRC screening and, secondly, improved survival outcomes for those diagnosed with the disease. However, the term 'management' should not extend only to the duration of adjuvant chemotherapy or the completion of recommended surveillance tests. Colonoscopies, serum CEA tests, and CT scans are only one (physical) component of the ongoing patient management after a diagnosis of colon cancer. To be diagnosed with any malignancy is understandably challenging for an individual and their family, and both symptom management and psychological support both during and after the diagnosis should be, in ideal circumstances, readily available. A systematic review of ten studies detailing long-term quality of life in CRC survivors (more than five years) concluded that overall quality of life was good, although depression scores were worse than the general population and ongoing bowel symptoms and cancer-related distress remained prominent [352]. A five-year prospective study of quality of life in CRC survivors found that although quality of life measures improved with increasing time from diagnosis, psychological distress measures remained static [353]. Ongoing healthcare provision for CRC survivors should continue to be addressed [354]. Aside from standard surveillance strategies, a more holistic approach to CRC survivorship should ideally address the role of diet, exercise, and maintaining a healthy body weight, as, in particular for exercise and body mass index, evidence indicates maintaining a healthy weight range and exercising regularly may reduce the risk of cancer recurrence or even second primary cancers [355, 356].

Conclusion

The management of early-stage colon cancer continues to evolve as science and medicine grow a deeper appreciation of not only the molecular, cellular, and genetic aspects of this disease, but also its effect on the individual, the family, the medical system, and society as a whole. Colorectal cancer will continue to be one of the most common malignancies in the developed world and increasingly in the developing world, and due to significant advances in screening, diagnosis, and management over the last several decades, there are increasing numbers of people surviving or living with the disease, rather than dying from it. These promising advances necessitate a multidisciplinary approach to CRC across the spectrum from prevention, through diagnosis and treatment, to palliative care. We need to encompass appreciation of the genetic makeup of a single cell from an individual's tumour, but also understand the impact of CRC from a global public health perspective, and everything in between these two extremes. Multidisciplinary management is the way forward in the optimal management of CRC.

Further reading

Andre T, Boni C, Mounedji-Boudiaf L, Navarro M, Tabernero J et al. Oxaliplatin, fluorouracil, and leucovorin as adjuvant treatment for colon cancer. New England Journal of Medicine 2004; 350(23): 2343–2351.

Atkin WS, Edwards R, Kralj-Hans I, et al. Once-only flexible sigmoidoscopy screening in prevention of colorectal cancer: a multicentre randomised controlled trial. Lancet 2010; 375: 1624–1633.

Benson AB, III, Schrag D, Somerfield MR, Cohen AM, Figueredo AT et al. American Society of Clinical Oncology recommendations on adjuvant chemotherapy for stage II colon cancer. Journal of Clinical Oncology: Official Journal of the American Society of Clinical Oncology 2004; 22(16): 3408–3419.

Bingham SA, Day NE, Luben R, Ferrari P, Slimani N et al. Dietary fibre in food and protection against colorectal cancer in the European Prospective Investigation into Cancer and Nutrition (EPIC): an observational study. Lancet 2003; 361: 1496–1501.

Chua TC, Morris DL, Saxena A, Esquivel J, Liauw W et al. Influence of modern systemic therapies as adjunct to cytoreduction and perioperative intraperitoneal chemotherapy for patients with colorectal peritoneal carcinomatosis: a multicenter study. Annals of Surgical Oncology 2011; 18(6): 1560–1567.

de Gramont A, Hubbard J, Shi Q, O'Connell MJ, Buyse M et al. Association between disease-free survival and overall survival when survival is prolonged after recurrence in patients receiving cytotoxic adjuvant therapy for colon cancer: simulations based on the 20,800 patient ACCENT data set. Journal of Clinical Oncology 2010; 28(3): 460–465.

Edwards BK, Ward E, Kohler BA, et al. Annual report to the nation on the status of cancer, 1975-2006, featuring colorectal cancer trends and impact of interventions (risk factors, screening, and treatment) to reduce future rates. Cancer 2010; 116: 544–573.

Elias D, Gilly F, Boutitie F, Quenet F, Bereder JM et al. Peritoneal colorectal carcinomatosis treated with surgery and perioperative intraperitoneal chemotherapy: retrospective analysis of 523 patients from a multicentric French study 3. Journal of Clinical Oncology 2010; 28(1): 63–68.

Figueredo A, Coombes ME, Mukherjee S. Adjuvant therapy for completely resected stage II colon cancer. Cochrane Database Systemic Reviews 2008(3): CD005390.

Franko J, Shi Q, Goldman CD, Pockaj BA, Nelson GD et al. Treatment of colorectal peritoneal carcinomatosis with systemic chemotherapy: a pooled analysis of north central cancer treatment group phase III trials N9741 and N9841. Journal of Clinical Oncology 2012; 30(3): 263–267.

Gill S, Loprinzi CL, Sargent DJ, Thomé SD, Alberts SR et al. Pooled analysis of fluorouracil-based adjuvant therapy for stage II and III colon cancer: who benefits and by how much? Journal of Clinical Oncology 2004; 22(10): 1797–1806.

Glehen O, Kwiatkowski F, Sugarbaker PH, Elias D, Levine EA et al. Cytoreductive surgery combined with perioperative intraperitoneal chemotherapy for the management of peritoneal carcinomatosis from colorectal cancer: a multi-institutional study. Journal of Clinical Oncology 2004; 22(16): 3284–3292.

Gunderson LL, Sosin H, Levitt S. Extrapelvic colon—areas of failure in a reoperation series: implications for adjuvant therapy. International Journal of Radiation Oncology Biology Physics 1985; 11(4): 731–741.

Hardcastle JD, Chamberlain JO, Robinson MH, et al. Randomised controlled trial of faecal-occult-blood screening for colorectal cancer. Lancet 1996; 348: 1472–1477.

Hong N, Wright F, Gagliardi F, Paszat LF. Examining the potential relationship between multidiscipinary cancer care and patient survival: an international literature review. Journal of Surgical Oncology 2010; 102(2): 125–132.

Ihemelandu CU, Shen P, Stewart JH, Votanopoulos K, Levine EA. Management of peritoneal carcinomatosis from colorectal cancer. Seminars in Oncology 2011; 38(4): 568–575.

Jansen L, Koch L, Brenner H, Arndt V et al. Quality of life among long-term (>/=5 years) colorectal cancer survivors—systematic review. European Journal of Cancer 2010; 46: 2879–2888.

Jayne DG, Guillou PJ, Thorpe H, Quirke P, Copeland J et al. Randomized trial of laparoscopic-assisted resection of colorectal carcinoma: 3-year results of the UK MRC CLASICC Trial Group 2. Journal of Clinical Oncology 2007; 25(21): 3061–3068.

Jeffery M, Hickey BE, Hider PN. Follow-up strategies for patients treated for non-metastatic colorectal cancer. Cochrane Database Systemic Reviews 2007: CD002200.

Klaver YL, Leenders BJ, Creemers GJ, Rutten HJ, Verwaal VJ et al. Addition of biological therapies to palliative chemotherapy prolongs survival in patients with peritoneal carcinomatosis of colorectal origin. American Journal of Clinical Oncology 2012; 36(2): 157–161.

Kronborg O, Fenger C, Olsen J, Jorgensen OD, Sondergaard O. Randomised study of screening for colorectal cancer with faecal-occult-blood test. Lancet 1996; 348: 1467–1471.

Laparoscopically assisted colectomy is as safe and effective as open colectomy in people with colon cancer. Abstracted from: Nelson H, Sargent D, Wieand HS, et al; for the Clinical Outcomes of Surgical Therapy Study Group. A comparison of laparoscopically assisted and open colectomy for colon cancer. New England Journal of Medicine 2004; 350: 2050–2059.

Lee MT, Kim JJ, Dinniwell R, Brierley J, Lockwood G et al. Phase I study of individualized stereotactic body radiotherapy of liver metastases. Journal of Clinical Oncology 2009; 27(10): 1585–1591.

Markowitz SD, Bertagnolli MM. Molecular origins of cancer: Molecular basis of colorectal cancer. New England Journal of Medicine 2009; 361(25): 2449–2460.

Martenson JA Jr, Willett CG, Sargent DJ, Maillard JA, Donohue JH et al. Phase III study of adjuvant chemotherapy and radiation therapy compared with chemotherapy alone in the surgical adjuvant treatment of colon cancer: results of intergroup protocol 0130. Journal of Clinical Oncology 2004; 22(16): 3277–3283.

Meyerhardt J. Energy balance and other modifiable host factors on colorectal cancer prognosis. Energy Balance and Cancer 2012; 4: 141–156.

Nagtegaal ID, Quirke P. What is the role for the circumferential margin in the modern treatment of rectal cancer? Journal of Clinical Oncology: Official Journal of the American Society of Clinical Oncology 2008; 26(2): 303–312.

Nagtegaal ID, van de Velde CJ, Marijnen CA, van Krieken JH, Quirke P et al. Low rectal cancer: a call for a change of approach in abdominoperineal resection. Journal of Clinical Oncology: Official Journal of the American Society of Clinical Oncology 2005; 23(36): 9257–9264.

Nordlinger B, Sorbye H, Glimelius B, Poston GJ, Schlag PM et al. Perioperative chemotherapy with FOLFOX4 and surgery versus surgery alone for resectable liver metastases from colorectal cancer (EORTC Intergroup trial 40983): a randomised controlled trial 1. Lancet 2008; 371(9617): 1007–1016.

O'Connell MJ, Lavery I, Yothers G, Paik S, Clark-Langone KM et al. Relationship between tumor gene expression and recurrence in four independent studies of patients with stage II/III colon cancer treated with surgery alone or surgery plus adjuvant fluorouracil plus leucovorin. Journal of Clinical Oncology 2010; 28(25): 3937–3944.

Rothwell PM, Wilson M, Elwin CE, Norrving B, Algra A et al. Long-term effect of aspirin on colorectal cancer incidence and mortality: 20-year follow-up of five randomised trials. Lancet 2010; 376: 1741–1750.

Rusthoven KE, Kavanagh BD, Cardenes H, Stieber VW, Burri SH et al. Multi-institutional phase I/II trial of stereotactic body radiation therapy for liver metastases. Journal of Clinical Oncology 2009; 27(10): 1572–1578.

Salazar R, Roepman P, Capella G, Moreno V, Simon I et al. Gene expression signature to improve prognosis prediction of stage II and III colorectal cancer. Journal of Clinical Oncology 2011; 29(1): 17–24.

Sargent DJ, Marsoni S, Monges G, Thibodeau SN, Labianca R et al. Defective mismatch repair as a predictive marker for lack of efficacy of fluorouracil-based adjuvant therapy in colon cancer. Journal of Clinical Oncology 2010; 28(20): 3219–3226.

Screening for colorectal cancer: U.S. Preventive Services Task Force recommendation statement. Annals of Internal Medicine 2008; 149: 627–637.

Sinicrope FA, Sargent DJ. Molecular pathways: microsatellite instability in colorectal cancer: prognostic, predictive, and therapeutic implications. Clinical Cancer Research 2012; 18(6): 1506–1512.

Snover DC. Update on the serrated pathway to colorectal carcinoma. Human Pathology 2011; 42(1): 1–10.

Sugarbaker PH. Peritoneal carcinomatosis: natural history and rational therapeutic interventions using intraperitoneal chemotherapy. Cancer Treatment Research 1996; 81: 149–168.

Sugarbaker PH. Peritonectomy procedures. Cancer Treat Research 2007; 134: 247–264.

Verwaal VJ, Bruin S, Boot H, van Slooten G, van Tinteren H. 8-year follow-up of randomized trial: cytoreduction and hyperthermic intraperitoneal chemotherapy versus systemic chemotherapy in patients with peritoneal carcinomatosis of colorectal cancer. Annals of Surgical Oncology 2008; 15(9): 2426–2432.

Verwaal VJ, van RS, de BE, van Sloothen GW, van TH et al. Randomized trial of cytoreduction and hyperthermic intraperitoneal chemotherapy versus systemic chemotherapy and palliative surgery in patients with peritoneal carcinomatosis of colorectal cancer 1. Journal of Clinical Oncology 2003; 21(20): 3737–3743.

Yan TD, Black D, Savady R, Sugarbaker PH. Systematic review on the efficacy of cytoreductive surgery combined with perioperative intraperitoneal chemotherapy for peritoneal carcinomatosis from colorectal carcinoma. Journal of Clinical Oncology 2006; 24(24): 4011–4019.

Young JP, Parry S. Risk factors: hyperplastic polyposis syndrome and risk of colorectal cancer. Nature Reviews Gastroenterology & Hepatology 2010; 7(11): 594–595.

Chronic inflammation/inflammatory bowel disease

Baxter NN, Tepper JE, Durham SB, Rothenberger DA, Virnig BA. Increased risk of rectal cancer after prostate radiation: a population-based study. Gastroenterology 2005; 128(4): 819–824.

Choi PM, Zelig MP. Similarity of colorectal cancer in Crohn's disease and ulcerative colitis: implications for carcinogenesis and prevention. Gut 1994; 35(7): 950–954.

Colotta F, Allavena P, Sica A, Garlanda C, Mantovani A. Cancer-related inflammation, the seventh hallmark of cancer: links to genetic instability. Carcinogenesis 2009; 30(7): 1073–1081.

Eaden JA, Abrams KR, Mayberry JF. The risk of colorectal cancer in ulcerative colitis: a meta-analysis. Gut 2001; 48(4): 526–535.

Friedman S. Cancer in Crohn's disease. Gastroenterology Clinics of North America 2006; 35(3): 621–639.

Gillen CD, Walmsley RS, Prior P, Andrews HA, Allan RN. Ulcerative colitis and Crohn's disease: a comparison of the colorectal cancer risk in extensive colitis. Gut 1994; 35(11): 1590–1592.

Harpaz N, Polydorides AD. Colorectal dysplasia in chronic inflammatory bowel disease: pathology, clinical implications, and pathogenesis. Archives of Pathology & Laboratory Medicine 2010; 134(6): 876–895.

Hartnett L, Egan LJ. Inflammation, DNA methylation and colitis-associated cancer. Carcinogenesis 2012; 33(4): 723–731.

Kulaylat MN, Dayton MT. Ulcerative colitis and cancer. Journal of Surgical Oncology 2010; 101(8): 706–712.

M'Koma AE, Moses HL, Adunyah SE. Inflammatory bowel disease-associated colorectal cancer: proctocolectomy and mucosectomy do not necessarily eliminate pouch-related cancer incidences. International Journal of Colorectal Disease 2011; 26(5): 533–552.

Munkholm P. Review article: the incidence and prevalence of colorectal cancer in inflammatory bowel disease. Alimentary Pharmacology & Therapeutics 2003; 18 Suppl 2: 1–5.

Sountoulides P, Koletsas N, Kikidakis D, Paschalidis K, Sofikitis N. Secondary malignancies following radiotherapy for prostate cancer. Therapeutic Advances in Urology 2010; 2(3): 119–125.

Trinchieri G. Innate inflammation and cancer: Is it time for cancer prevention? F1000 Medicine Reports 2011; 3: 11.

Weber DC, Wang H, Bouchardy C, Rosset A, Rapiti E, Schmidlin F, et al. Estimated dose to the rectum and colon in prostate cancer patients treated with exclusive radiation therapy presenting a secondary colorectal malignancy. Clinical Oncology (The Royal College of Radiologists) 2009; 21(9): 687–694.

Weedon DD, Shorter RG, Ilstrup DM, Huizenga KA, Taylor WF. Crohn's disease and cancer. The New England Journal of Medicine 1973; 289(21): 1099–1103.

Alcohol

Cai H, Scott E, Kholghi A, Andreadi C, Rufini A, Karmokar A, Britton RG, Horner-Glister E, Greaves P, Jawad D, James M, Howells L, Ognibene T, Malfatti M, Goldring C, Kitteringham N, Walsh J, Viskaduraki M, West K, Miller A, Hemingway D, Steward WP, Gescher AJ, Brown K. Cancer chemoprevention: Evidence of a nonlinear dose response for the protective effects of resveratrol in humans and mice. Science Translational Medicine 2015; 7(298): 298ra117.

Kontou N, Psaltopoulou T, Soupos N, Polychronopoulos E, Xinopoulos D, Linos A, Panagiotakos D. Alcohol consumption and colorectal cancer in a Mediterranean population: a case-control study. Diseases of the Colon & Rectum 2012; 55(6): 703–710.

Patel KR, Brown VA, Jones DJ, Britton RG, Hemingway D, Miller AS, West KP, Booth TD, Perloff M, Crowell JA, Brenner DE, Steward WP, Gescher AJ, Brown K. Clinical pharmacology of resveratrol and its metabolites in colorectal cancer patients. Cancer Research 2010; 70(19): 7392–7399.

Wolter F, Ulrich S, Stein J. Molecular mechanisms of the chemopreventive effects of resveratrol and its analogs in colorectal cancer: key role of polyamines? Journal of Nutrition 2004; 134(12): 3219–3222.

References

1. Ferlay J, Soerjomataram I, Dikshit R, Eser S, Mathers C. Cancer incidence and mortality worldwide: sources, methods and major patterns in GLOBOCAN 2012. International Journal of Cancer 2015;136(5): E359–386. doi: 10.1002/ijc.29210. [Epub 2014 Oct 9.]

2. Jessup JM, McGinnis LS, Steele GD Jr, Menck HR et al. The National Cancer Data Base. Report on colon cancer. Cancer 1996; 78: 918–926.

3. Thorn M, Bergstrom R, Kressner U, Sparen P, Zack M et al. Trends in colorectal cancer incidence in Sweden 1959-93 by gender, localization, time period, and birth cohort. Cancer Causes Control 1998; 9: 145–152.

4. Troisi RJ, Freedman AN, Devesa SS. Incidence of colorectal carcinoma in the U.S.: an update of trends by gender, race, age, subsite, and stage, 1975-1994. Cancer 1999; 85: 1670–1676.

5. Schub R, Steinheber FU. Rightward shift of colon cancer. A feature of the aging gut. Journal of Clinical Gastroenterology 1986; 8: 630–634.

6. Stewart RJ, Stewart AW, Turnbull PR, Isbister WH. Sex differences in subsite incidence of large-bowel cancer. Diseases of the Colon & Rectum 1983; 26: 658–660.

7. Weiss JM, Pfau PR, O'Connor ES, King J, LoConte N et al. Mortality by stage for right- versus left-sided colon cancer: analysis of surveillance, epidemiology, and end results—Medicare data. Journal of Clinical Oncology 2011; 29: 4401–4409.

8. Siegel RL, Ward EM, Jemal A. Trends in colorectal cancer incidence rates in the United States by tumor location and stage, 1992–2008. Cancer Epidemiology, Biomarkers & Prevention 2012; 21: 411–416.

9. Howlader N, Noone A, Krapcho M, et al. SEER Cancer Statistics Review, 1975–2009 (Vintage 2009 Populations). Available from: <http://seer.cancer.gov/archive/csr/1975_2009_pops09/>, accessed on 25 May 2015. National Cancer Institute, 2012.

10. Siegel R, Desantis C, Virgo K, Stein K, Mariotto A et al. Cancer treatment and survivorship statistics, 2012. CA: A Cancer Journal for Clinicians 2012; 62: 220–241.

11. Kune GA, Bannerman S, Watson LF. Attributable risk for diet, alcohol, and family history in the Melbourne Colorectal Cancer Study. Nutrition and Cancer 1992; 18: 231–235.

12. Burkitt DP. Epidemiology of cancer of the colon and rectum. Cancer 1971; 28: 3–13.

13. Howe GR, Benito E, Castelleto R, Cornée J, Estève J et al. Dietary intake of fiber and decreased risk of cancers of the colon and rectum: evidence from the combined analysis of 13 case-control studies. Journal of the National Cancer Institute 1992; 84: 1887–1896.

14. Trock B, Lanza E, Greenwald P. Dietary fiber, vegetables, and colon cancer: critical review and meta-analyses of the epidemiologic evidence. Journal of the National Cancer Institute 1990; 82: 650–661.

15. Bingham SA, Day NE, Luben R, Ferrari P, Slimani N et al. Dietary fibre in food and protection against colorectal cancer in the European Prospective Investigation into Cancer and Nutrition (EPIC): an observational study. Lancet 2003; 361: 1496–1501.

16. Kato I, Akhmedkhanov A, Koenig K, Toniolo PG, Shore RE et al. Prospective study of diet and female colorectal cancer: the New York University Women's Health Study. Nutrition and Cancer 1997; 28: 276–281.

17. Park Y, Hunter DJ, Spiegelman D, et al. Dietary fiber intake and risk of colorectal cancer: a pooled analysis of prospective cohort studies. Journal of the American Medical Association 2005; 294: 2849–2857.

18. Michels KB, Fuchs CS, Giovannucci E, Colditz GA, Hunter DJ et al. Fiber intake and incidence of colorectal cancer among 76,947 women and 47,279 men. Cancer Epidemiology, Biomarkers & Prevention 2005; 14: 842–849.

19. Aune D, Chan DS, Lau R, Vieira R, Greenwood DC et al. Dietary fibre, whole grains, and risk of colorectal cancer: systematic review and dose-response meta-analysis of prospective studies. British Medical Journal 2011; 343:d6617.

20. Chan DS, Lau R, Aune D, Vieira R, Greenwood DC et al. Red and processed meat and colorectal cancer incidence: meta-analysis of prospective studies. PLoS One 2011; 6: e20456.

21. Chao A, Thun MJ, Connell CJ, McCullough ML, Jacobs EJ et al. Meat consumption and risk of colorectal cancer. Journal of the American Medical Association 2005; 293: 172–182.

22. Norat T, Bingham S, Ferrari P, Slimani N, Jenab M et al. Meat, fish, and colorectal cancer risk: the European Prospective Investigation into cancer and nutrition. Journal of the National Cancer Institute 2005; 97: 906–916.

23. Willett WC, Stampfer MJ, Colditz GA, Rosner BA et al. Relation of meat, fat, and fiber intake to the risk of colon cancer in a prospective study among women. New England Journal of Medicine 1990; 323: 1664–1672.

24. Alexander DD, Weed DL, Cushing CA, Lowe KA. Meta-analysis of prospective studies of red meat consumption and colorectal cancer. European Journal of Cancer Prevention 2011; 20: 293–307.

25. Jarvinen R, Knekt P, Hakulinen T, Rissanen H, Heliovaara M. Dietary fat, cholesterol and colorectal cancer in a prospective study. British Journal of Cancer 2001; 85: 357–361.

26. Truswell AS. Meat consumption and cancer of the large bowel. European Journal of Clinical Nutrition 2002; 56 Suppl 1:S19–S24.

27. Cheah PY, Bernstein H. Colon cancer and dietary fiber: cellulose inhibits the DNA-damaging ability of bile acids. Nutrition and Cancer 1990; 13: 51–57.

28. Watabe J, Bernstein H. The mutagenicity of bile acids using a fluctuation test. Mutation Research 1985; 158: 45–51.

29. Wilpart M, Mainguet P, Maskens A, Roberfroid M. Mutagenicity of 1,2-dimethylhydrazine towards Salmonella typhimurium, co-mutagenic effect of secondary biliary acids. Carcinogenesis 1983; 4: 45–48.

30. Imray CH, Radley S, Davis A, Barker G, Hendrickse CW et al. Faecal unconjugated bile acids in patients with colorectal cancer or polyps. Gut 1992; 33: 1239–1245.

31. Reddy BS, Wynder EL. Large-bowel carcinogenesis: fecal constituents of populations with diverse incidence rates of colon cancer. Journal of the National Cancer Institute 1973; 50: 1437–1442.

32. Hill MJ, Drasar BS, Hawksworth G, Aries V, Crowther JS et al. Bacteria and aetiology of cancer of large bowel. Lancet 1971; 1: 95–100.

33. Collins D, Hogan AM, Winter DC. Microbial and viral pathogens in colorectal cancer. Lancet Oncology 2011; 12: 504–512.

34. Kirkegaard H, Johnsen NF, Christensen J, Frederiksen K, Overvad K et al. Association of adherence to lifestyle recommendations and risk of colorectal cancer: a prospective Danish cohort study. British Medical Journal 2010; 341: c5504.

35. Ma Y, Zhang P, Wang F, Liu Z, Qin H. Association between vitamin D and risk of colorectal cancer: a systematic review of prospective studies. Journal of Clinical Oncology 2011; 29(28): 3775–3782.

36. Linos D, Beard CM, O'Fallon WM, Dockerty MB, Beart RW Jr et al. Cholecystectomy and carcinoma of the colon. Lancet 1981; 2: 379–381.

37. Giovannucci E, Colditz GA, Stampfer MJ. A meta-analysis of cholecystectomy and risk of colorectal cancer. Gastroenterology 1993; 105: 130–141.

38. Reid FD, Mercer PM, Harrison M, Bates T. Cholecystectomy as a risk factor for colorectal cancer: a meta-analysis. Scandinavian Journal of Gastroenterology 1996; 31: 160–169.

39. Lagergren J, Ye W, Ekbom A. Intestinal cancer after cholecystectomy: is bile involved in carcinogenesis? Gastroenterology 2001; 121: 542–547.

40. Giovannucci E, Ascherio A, Rimm EB, Colditz GA, Stampfer MJ et al. Physical activity, obesity, and risk for colon cancer and adenoma in men. Annals of Internal Medicine 1995; 122: 327–334.

41. Martinez ME, Giovannucci E, Spiegelman D, Hunter DJ, Willett WC et al. Leisure-time physical activity, body size, and colon cancer in women. Nurses' Health Study Research Group. Journal of the National Cancer Institute 1997; 89: 948–955.

42. Deng L, Gui Z, Zhao L, Wang J, Shen L. Diabetes mellitus and the incidence of colorectal cancer: an updated systematic review and meta-analysis. Digestive Diseases and Sciences 2012; 57: 1576–1585.

43. Giovannucci E, Michaud D. The role of obesity and related metabolic disturbances in cancers of the colon, prostate, and pancreas. Gastroenterology 2007; 132: 2208–2225.

44. Larsson SC, Orsini N, Wolk A. Diabetes mellitus and risk of colorectal cancer: a meta-analysis. Journal of the National Cancer Institute 2005; 97: 1679–1687.

45. O'Mara BA, Byers T, Schoenfeld E. Diabetes mellitus and cancer risk: a multisite case-control study. Journal of Chronic Diseases 1985; 38: 435–441.

46. Williams JC, Walsh DA, Jackson JF. Colon carcinoma and diabetes mellitus. Cancer 1984; 54: 3070–3071.

47. Will JC, Galuska DA, Vinicor F, Calle EE. Colorectal cancer: another complication of diabetes mellitus? American Journal of Epidemiology 1998; 147: 816–825.

48. Campbell PT, Deka A, Jacobs EJ, Newton CC, Hildebrand JS et al. Prospective study reveals associations between colorectal cancer and type 2 diabetes mellitus or insulin use in men. Gastroenterology 2010; 139: 1138–1146.

49. Hu FB, Manson JE, Liu S, Hunter D, Colditz GA et al. Prospective study of adult onset diabetes mellitus (type 2) and risk of colorectal cancer in women. Journal of the National Cancer Institute 1999; 91: 542–547.

50. Inoue M, Iwasaki M, Otani T, Sasazuki S, Noda M et al. Diabetes mellitus and the risk of cancer: results from a large-scale population-based cohort study in Japan. Archives of Internal Medicine 2006; 166: 1871–1877.

51. Guo YS, Narayan S, Yallampalli C, Singh P. Characterization of insulin-like growth factor I receptors in human colon cancer. Gastroenterology 1992; 102: 1101–1108.

52. Watkins LF, Lewis LR, Levine AE. Characterization of the synergistic effect of insulin and transferrin and the regulation of their receptors on a human colon carcinoma cell line. International Journal of Cancer 1990; 45: 372–375.

53. Corpet DE, Jacquinet C, Peiffer G, Tache S. Insulin injections promote the growth of aberrant crypt foci in the colon of rats. Nutrition and Cancer 1997; 27: 316–320.

54. Ma J, Giovannucci E, Pollak M, Leavitt A, Tao Y et al. A prospective study of plasma C-peptide and colorectal cancer risk in men. Journal of the National Cancer Institute 2004; 96: 546–553.

55. Schoen RE, Tangen CM, Kuller LH, Burke GL, Cushman M et al. Increased blood glucose and insulin, body size, and incident colorectal cancer. Journal of the National Cancer Institute 1999; 91: 1147–1154.

56. Yang YX, Hennessy S, Lewis JD. Insulin therapy and colorectal cancer risk among type 2 diabetes mellitus patients. Gastroenterology 2004; 127: 1044–1050.

57. Botteri E, Iodice S, Bagnardi V, Raimondi S, Lowenfels AB et al. Smoking and colorectal cancer: a meta-analysis. Journal of the American Medical Association 2008; 300: 2765–2778.

58. Giovannucci E, Colditz GA, Stampfer MJ, Hunter D, Rosner BA et al. A prospective study of cigarette smoking and risk of colorectal adenoma and colorectal cancer in U.S. women. Journal of the National Cancer Institute 1994; 86: 192–199.

59. Fedirko V, Tramacere I, Bagnardi V, et al. Alcohol drinking and colorectal cancer risk: an overall and dose-response meta-analysis of published studies. Annals of Oncology 2011; 22: 1958–1972.

60. Park JY, Dahm CC, Keogh RH, Mitrou PN, Cairns BJ et al. Alcohol intake and risk of colorectal cancer: results from the UK Dietary Cohort Consortium. British Journal of Cancer 2010; 103: 747–756.

61. Harford FJ, Fazio VW, Epstein LM, Hewitt CB. Rectosigmoid carcinoma occurring after ureterosigmoidostomy. Diseases of the Colon & Rectum 1984; 27: 321–324.

62. Stewart M, Macrae FA, Williams CB. Neoplasia and ureterosigmoidostomy: a colonoscopy survey. British Journal of Surgery 1982; 69: 414–416.

63. Urdaneta LF, Duffell D, Creevy CD, Aust JB. Late development of primary carcinoma of the colon following ureterosigmoidostomy: report of three cases and literature review. Annals of Surgery 1966; 164: 503–513.

64. Ekbom A, Helmick C, Zack M, Adami HO. Ulcerative colitis and colorectal cancer. A population-based study. New England Journal of Medicine 1990; 323: 1228–1233.

65. Ward E, Jemal A, Cokkinides V, Singh GK, Cardinez C et al. Cancer disparities by race/ethnicity and socioeconomic status. CA: A Cancer Journal for Clinicians 2004; 54: 78–93.

66. Kune GA, Kune S, Watson LF. Colorectal cancer risk, chronic illnesses, operations, and medications: case control results from the Melbourne Colorectal Cancer Study. Cancer Research 1988; 48: 4399–4404.

67. Thun MJ, Namboodiri MM, Heath CW Jr. Aspirin use and reduced risk of fatal colon cancer. New England Journal of Medicine 1991; 325: 1593–1596.

68. Dubé C, Rostom A, Lewin G, Tsertsvadze A, Barrowman N et al. The use of aspirin for primary prevention of colorectal cancer: a systematic review prepared for the U.S. Preventive Services Task Force. Annals of Internal Medicine 2007; 146: 365–375.

69. Cole BF, Logan RF, Halabi S, et al. Aspirin for the chemoprevention of colorectal adenomas: meta-analysis of the randomized trials. Journal of the National Cancer Institute 2009; 101: 256–266.

70. Baron JA, Cole BF, Sandler RS, Benamouzig R, Sandler RS et al. A randomized trial of aspirin to prevent colorectal adenomas. New England Journal of Medicine 2003; 348: 891–899.

71. Sandler RS, Halabi S, Baron JA, Budinger S, Paskett E et al. A randomized trial of aspirin to prevent colorectal adenomas in patients with previous colorectal cancer. New England Journal of Medicine 2003; 348: 883–890.

72. Rothwell PM, Wilson M, Elwin CE, Norrving B, Algra A et al. Long-term effect of aspirin on colorectal cancer incidence and mortality: 20-year follow-up of five randomised trials. Lancet 2010; 376: 1741–1750.

73. Burn J, Gerdes AM, Macrae F, Mecklin J-P, Moeslein G et al. Long-term effect of aspirin on cancer risk in carriers of hereditary colorectal cancer: an analysis from the CAPP2 randomised controlled trial. Lancet 2011; 378: 2081–2087.

74. Burn J, Bishop DT, Mecklin JP, Macrae F, Möslein G et al. Effect of aspirin or resistant starch on colorectal neoplasia in the Lynch syndrome. New England Journal of Medicine 2008; 359: 2567–2578.

75. Cruz-Correa M, Hylind LM, Romans KE, Booker SV, Giardiello FM. Long-term treatment with sulindac in familial adenomatous polyposis: a prospective cohort study. Gastroenterology 2002; 122: 641–645.

76. Giardiello FM, Hamilton SR, Krush AJ, Piantadosi S, Hylind LM et al. Treatment of colonic and rectal adenomas with sulindac in familial adenomatous polyposis. New England Journal of Medicine 1993; 328: 1313–1316.

77. Labayle D, Fischer D, Vielh P, Drouhin F, Pariente A et al. Sulindac causes regression of rectal polyps in familial adenomatous polyposis. Gastroenterology 1991; 101: 635–639.

78. Vasen HF, Moslein G, Alonso A, Aretz S, Bernstein I et al. Guidelines for the clinical management of familial adenomatous polyposis (FAP). Gut 2008; 57: 704–713.

79. Migliore L, Migheli F, Spisni R, Coppede F. Genetics, cytogenetics, and epigenetics of colorectal cancer. Journal of Biomedicine and Biotechnology 2011: 792362.

80. Sinicrope FA, Sargent DJ. Molecular pathways: microsatellite instability in colorectal cancer: prognostic, predictive, and therapeutic implications. Clinical Cancer Research 2012; 18(6): 1506–1512.

81. Vogelstein B, Fearon ER, Hamilton SR, Kern SE, Preisinger AC et al. Genetic alterations during colorectal-tumor development. New England Journal of Medicine 1988; 319(9): 525–532.

82. Cunningham D, Atkin W, Lenz HJ, Lynch HT, Minsky B et al. Colorectal cancer. Lancet 2010; 375(9719): 1030–1047.

83. Fearon ER. Molecular genetics of colorectal cancer. Annual Review of Pathology 2011; 6: 479–507.

84. Jass JR. Classification of colorectal cancer based on correlation of clinical, morphological and molecular features. Histopathology 2007; 50(1): 113–130.

85. Pino MS, Chung DC. The chromosomal instability pathway in colon cancer. Gastroenterology 2010; 138(6): 2059–2072.

86. Watanabe T, Kobunai T, Yamamoto Y, Matsuda K, Ishihara S et al. Chromosomal instability (CIN) phenotype, CIN high or CIN low, predicts survival for colorectal cancer. Journal of Clinical Oncology: Official Journal of the American Society of Clinical Oncology 2012; 30(18): 2256–2264.

87. Walther A, Houlston R, Tomlinson I. Association between chromosomal instability and prognosis in colorectal cancer: a meta-analysis. Gut 2008; 57(7): 941–950.

88. Janssen A, van der Burg M, Szuhai K, Kops GJ, Medema RH. Chromosome segregation errors as a cause of DNA damage and structural chromosome aberrations. Science 2011; 333(6051): 1895–1898.

89. Rao CV, Yamada HY, Yao Y, Dai W. Enhanced genomic instabilities caused by deregulated microtubule dynamics and chromosome segregation: a perspective from genetic studies in mice. Carcinogenesis 2009; 30(9): 1469–1474.

90. Xu H, Tomaszewski JM, McKay MJ. Can corruption of chromosome cohesion create a conduit to cancer? Nature Reviews Cancer 2011; 11(3): 199–210.

91. Barber TD, McManus K, Yuen KW, Reis M, Parmigiani G et al. Chromatid cohesion defects may underlie chromosome instability in human colorectal cancers. Proceedings of the National Academy of Sciences USA 2008; 105(9): 3443–3448.

92. Murnane JP. Telomere dysfunction and chromosome instability. Mutation Research 2012; 730(1–2): 28–36.

93. Lukas J, Lukas C, Bartek J. More than just a focus: The chromatin response to DNA damage and its role in genome integrity maintenance. Nature Cell Biology 2011; 13(10): 1161–1169.

94. Wood LD, Parsons DW, Jones S, Lin J, Sjoblom T et al. The genomic landscapes of human breast and colorectal cancers. Science 2007; 318(5853): 1108–1113.

95. Negrini S, Gorgoulis VG, Halazonetis TD. Genomic instability—an evolving hallmark of cancer. Nature Reviews Molecular Cell Biology 2010; 11(3): 220–228.

96. Grady WM, Carethers JM. Genomic and epigenetic instability in colorectal cancer pathogenesis. Gastroenterology 2008; 135(4): 1079–1099.

97. Poulogiannis G, Frayling IM, Arends MJ. DNA mismatch repair deficiency in sporadic colorectal cancer and Lynch syndrome. Histopathology 2010; 56(2): 167–179.

98. Hewish M, Lord CJ, Martin SA, Cunningham D, Ashworth A. Mismatch repair deficient colorectal cancer in the era of personalized treatment. Nature Reviews Clinical Oncology 2010; 7(4): 197–208.

99. Boland CR, Goel A. Microsatellite instability in colorectal cancer. Gastroenterology 2010; 138(6): 2073–2087 e3.

100. Bedeir A, Krasinskas AM. Molecular diagnostics of colorectal cancer. Archives of Pathology & Laboratory Medicine 2011; 135(5): 578–587.

101. Kanthan R, Senger J, Kanthan S. Molecular events in primary and metastatic colorectal carcinoma: a review. Pathology Research International 2012; 2012 (Article ID 597497).

102. Baudhuin LM, Burgart LJ, Leontovich O, Thibodeau SN. Use of microsatellite instability and immunohistochemistry testing for the identification of individuals at risk for Lynch syndrome. Familial Cancer 2005; 4(3): 255–265.

103. Hong SP, Min BS, Kim TI, Cheon JH, Kim NK et al. The differential impact of microsatellite instability as a marker of prognosis and tumour response between colon cancer and rectal cancer. European Journal of Cancer 2012; 48(8): 1235–1243.

104. Jones PA. Functions of DNA methylation: islands, start sites, gene bodies and beyond. Nature Reviews Genetics 2012; 13(7): 484–492.

105. Hughes LA, Khalid-de Bakker CA, Smits KM, van den Brandt PA, Jonkers D et al. The CpG island methylator phenotype in colorectal cancer: progress and problems. Biochimica et Biophysica Acta 2012; 1825(1): 77–85.

106. Bahar A, Bicknell JE, Simpson DJ, Clayton RN, Farrell WE. Loss of expression of the growth inhibitory gene GADD45gamma, in human pituitary adenomas, is associated with CpG island methylation. Oncogene 2004; 23(4): 936–944.

107. Kakar S, Deng G, Cun L, Sahai V, Kim YS. CpG island methylation is frequently present in tubulovillous and villous adenomas and correlates with size, site, and villous component. Human Pathology 2008; 39(1): 30–36.

108. Park SJ, Rashid A, Lee JH, Kim SG, Hamilton SR et al. Frequent CpG island methylation in serrated adenomas of the colorectum. American Journal of Pathology 2003; 162(3): 815–822.

109. Psofaki V, Kalogera C, Tzambouras N, Stephanou D, Tsianos E et al. Promoter methylation status of hMLH1, MGMT, and CDKN2A/p16 in colorectal adenomas. World Journal of Gastroenterology 2010; 16(28): 3553–3560.

110. Wynter CV, Kambara T, Walsh MD, Leggett BA, Young J et al. DNA methylation patterns in adenomas from FAP, multiple adenoma and sporadic colorectal carcinoma patients. International Journal of Cancer 2006; 118(4): 907–915.

111. Shen L, Toyota M, Kondo Y, Lin E, Zhang L et al. Integrated genetic and epigenetic analysis identifies three different subclasses of colon cancer. Proceedings of the National Academy of Sciences USA 2007; 104(47): 18654–18659.

112. Snover DC. Update on the serrated pathway to colorectal carcinoma. Human Pathology 2011; 42(1): 1–10.

113. Leggett B, Whitehall V. Role of the serrated pathway in colorectal cancer pathogenesis. Gastroenterology 2010; 138(6): 2088–2100.

114. Issa JP. Colon cancer: it's CIN or CIMP. Clinical Cancer Research 2008 October 1; 14(19): 5939–5940.

115. Segditsas S, Tomlinson I. Colorectal cancer and genetic alterations in the Wnt pathway. Oncogene 2006; 25(57): 7531–7537.

116. Comprehensive molecular characterization of human colon and rectal cancer. Nature 2012; 487(7407): 330–337.

117. Vakiani E, Janakiraman M, Shen R, Sinha R, Zeng Z et al. Comparative genomic analysis of primary versus metastatic colorectal carcinomas. Journal of clinical oncology: official journal of the American Society of Clinical Oncology 2012; 30(24): 2956–2962.

118. Buchanan DD, Roberts A, Walsh MD, Parry S, Young JP. Lessons from Lynch syndrome: a tumor biology-based approach to familial colorectal cancer. Future Oncology 2010; 6(4): 539–549.

119. Chow E, Macrae F. A review of juvenile polyposis syndrome. Journal of gastroenterology and hepatology 2005; 20(11): 1634–1640.

120. Brosens LA, Langeveld D, van Hattem WA, Giardiello FM, Offerhaus GJ. Juvenile polyposis syndrome. World Journal of Gastroenterology 2011; 17(44): 4839–4844.

121. Schreibman IR, Baker M, Amos C, McGarrity TJ. The hamartomatous polyposis syndromes: a clinical and molecular review. American Journal of Gastroenterology 2005; 100(2): 476–490.

122. Kalady MF, Jarrar A, Leach B, LaGuardia L, O'Malley M et al. Defining phenotypes and cancer risk in hyperplastic polyposis syndrome. Diseases of the Colon and Rectum 2011; 54(2): 164–170.

123. Wong P, Verselis SJ, Garber JE, Schneider K, DiGianni L et al. Prevalence of early onset colorectal cancer in 397 patients with classic Li-Fraumeni syndrome. Gastroenterology 2006; 130(1): 73–79.

124. Lowy AM, Kordich JJ, Gismondi V, Varesco L, Blough RI, et al. Numerous colonic adenomas in an individual with Bloom's syndrome. Gastroenterology 2001; 121(2): 435–439.

125. Houlston RS, Cheadle J, Dobbins SE, Tenesa A, Jones AM et al. Meta-analysis of three genome-wide association studies identifies susceptibility loci for colorectal cancer at 1q41, 3q26.2, 12q13.13 and 20q13.33. Nature Genetics 2010; 42(11): 973–977.

126. Peters U, Hutter CM, Hsu L, Schumacher FR, Conti DV et al. Meta-analysis of new genome-wide association studies of colorectal cancer risk. Human genetics 2012; 131(2): 217–234.

127. Fodde R. The APC gene in colorectal cancer. European Journal of Cancer 2002; 38(7): 867–871.

128. Aoki K, Taketo MM. Adenomatous polyposis coli (APC): a multi-functional tumor suppressor gene. Journal of Cell Science 2007; 120(Pt 19): 3327–3335.

129. Schneikert J, Behrens J. The canonical Wnt signalling pathway and its APC partner in colon cancer development. Gut 2007; 56(3): 417–425.

130. Half E, Bercovich D, Rozen P. Familial adenomatous polyposis. Orphanet Journal of Rare Diseases 2009; 4: 22.

131. Knudsen AL, Bisgaard ML, Bulow S. Attenuated familial adenomatous polyposis (AFAP). A review of the literature. Familial Cancer 2003; 2(1): 43–55.

132. Hamilton SR, Liu B, Parsons RE, Papadopoulos N, Jen J et al. The molecular basis of Turcot's syndrome. The New England Journal of Medicine 1995; 332(13): 839–847.

133. Foulkes WD. A tale of four syndromes: familial adenomatous polyposis, Gardner syndrome, attenuated APC and Turcot syndrome. QJM: Monthly Journal of the Association of Physicians 1995; 88(12): 853–863.

134. Bulow S, Berk T, Neale K. The history of familial adenomatous polyposis. Familial Cancer 2006; 5(3): 213–820.

135. Nielsen M, Morreau H, Vasen HF, Hes FJ. MUTYH-associated polyposis (MAP). Critical Reviews in Oncology/Hematology 2011; 79(1): 1–16.

136. Cardoso J, Molenaar L, de Menezes RX, van Leerdam M, Rosenberg C et al. Chromosomal instability in MYH- and APC-mutant adenomatous polyps. Cancer Research 2006; 66(5): 2514–2519.

137. Al-Tassan N, Chmiel NH, Maynard J, Fleming N, Livingston AL et al. Inherited variants of MYH associated with somatic G:C—>T:A mutations in colorectal tumors. Nature Genetics 2002; 30(2): 227–232.

138. Jones S, Emmerson P, Maynard J, Best JM, Jordan S et al. Biallelic germline mutations in MYH predispose to multiple colorectal adenoma and somatic G:C—>T:A mutations. Human Molecular Genetics 2002; 11(23): 2961–2967.

139. Nielsen M, Joerink-van de Beld MC, Jones N, Vogt S, Tops CM et al. Analysis of MUTYH genotypes and colorectal phenotypes in patients With MUTYH-associated polyposis. Gastroenterology 2009; 136(2): 471–476.

140. Launonen V. Mutations in the human LKB1/STK11 gene. Human Mutation 2005; 26(4): 291–297.

141. Alhopuro P, Phichith D, Tuupanen S, Sammalkorpi H, Nybondas M et al. Unregulated smooth-muscle myosin in human intestinal neoplasia. Proceedings of the National Academy of Sciences of the USA 2008; 105(14): 5513–5518.

142. Shaw RJ, Bardeesy N, Manning BD, Lopez L, Kosmatka M et al. The LKB1 tumor suppressor negatively regulates mTOR signaling. Cancer Cell 2004; 6(1): 91–99.

143. Giardiello FM, Brensinger JD, Tersmette AC, Goodman SN, Petersen GM et al. Very high risk of cancer in familial Peutz-Jeghers syndrome. Gastroenterology 2000; 119(6): 1447–1453.

144. Lim W, Olschwang S, Keller JJ, Westerman AM, Menko FH et al. Relative frequency and morphology of cancers in STK11 mutation carriers. Gastroenterology 2004; 126(7): 1788–1794.

145. Gallione CJ, Repetto GM, Legius E, Rustgi AK, Schelley SL et al. A combined syndrome of juvenile polyposis and hereditary haemorrhagic telangiectasia associated with mutations in MADH4 (SMAD4). Lancet 2004; 363(9412): 852–859.

146. Cao X, Eu KW, Kumarasinghe MP, Li HH, Loi C, Cheah PY. Mapping of hereditary mixed polyposis syndrome (HMPS) to chromosome 10q23 by genomewide high-density single nucleotide polymorphism (SNP) scan and identification of BMPR1A loss of function. Journal of Medical Genetics 2006; 43(3): e13.

147. O'Riordan JM, O'Donoghue D, Green A, Keegan D, Hawkes LA et al. Hereditary mixed polyposis syndrome due to a BMPR1A mutation. Colorectal Disease 2010; 12(6): 570–573.

148. Marsh DJ, Kum JB, Lunetta KL, Bennett MJ, Gorlin RJ et al. PTEN mutation spectrum and genotype-phenotype correlations in Bannayan–Riley–Ruvalcaba syndrome suggest a single entity with Cowden syndrome. Human Molecular Genetics 1999; 8(8): 1461–1472.

149. Burke AP, Sobin LH. The pathology of Cronkhite-Canada polyps. A comparison to juvenile polyposis. The American Journal of Surgical Pathology 1989; 13(11): 940–946.

150. Young JP, Parry S. Risk factors: hyperplastic polyposis syndrome and risk of colorectal cancer. Nature Reviews Gastroenterology & Hepatology 2010; 7(11): 594–595.

151. Lynch PM. Hyperplastic polyposis: semantics, biology, and endoscopy. Gut 2010; 59(8): 1019–1021.

152. Guarinos C, Sanchez-Fortun C, Rodriguez-Soler M, Alenda C, Paya A et al. Serrated polyposis syndrome: molecular, pathological and clinical aspects. World Journal of Gastroenterology 2012; 18(20): 2452–2461.

153. Boparai KS, Mathus-Vliegen EM, Koornstra JJ, Nagengast FM, van Leerdam M et al. Increased colorectal cancer risk during follow-up in patients with hyperplastic polyposis syndrome: a multicentre cohort study. Gut 2010; 59(8): 1094–1100.

154. Fenoglio-Preiser CM, Noffsinger A. Aberrant crypt foci: A review. Toxicologic Pathology 1999; 27(6): 632–642.

155. Stevens RG, Swede H, Rosenberg DW. Epidemiology of colonic aberrant crypt foci: review and analysis of existing studies. Cancer Letters 2007; 252(2): 171–183.

156. Suehiro Y, Hinoda Y. Genetic and epigenetic changes in aberrant crypt foci and serrated polyps. Cancer Science 2008; 99(6): 1071–1076.

157. Rosenberg DW, Yang S, Pleau DC, Greenspan EJ, Stevens RG et al. Mutations in BRAF and KRAS differentially distinguish serrated versus non-serrated hyperplastic aberrant crypt foci in humans. Cancer Research 2007; 67(8): 3551–3554.

158. Lanza G, Messerini L, Gafa R, Risio M. Colorectal tumors: the histology report. Digestive and Liver Disease 2011; 43(Suppl. 4): S344–S355.

159. De Hertogh G, Geboes KP. Practical and molecular evaluation of colorectal cancer: new roles for the pathologist in the era of targeted therapy. Archives of Pathology & Laboratory Medicine 2010; 134(6): 853–863.

160. DiSario JA, Burt RW, Kendrick ML, McWhorter WP. Colorectal cancers of rare histologic types compared with adenocarcinomas [published erratum appears in Diseases of the Colon and Rectum 1995; 38(11): 1227]. Diseases of the Colon and Rectum 1994; 37(12): 1277–1280.

161. Yamauchi M, Lochhead P, Morikawa T, Huttenhower C, Chan AT et al. Colorectal cancer: a tale of two sides or a continuum? Gut 2012; 61(6): 794–797.

162. TNM classification of malignant tumours. New York: Wiley-Blackwell, 2009.

163. AJCC Cancer Staging Manual. New York: Springer-Verlag, 2010.

164. Benson AB, III, Schrag D, Somerfield MR, Cohen AM, Figueredo AT et al. American Society of Clinical Oncology recommendations on adjuvant chemotherapy for stage II colon cancer. Journal of Clinical Oncology: Official Journal of the American Society of Clinical Oncology 2004; 22(16): 3408–3419.

165. Nagtegaal ID, van Krieken JHJM. Role of pathologists in quality control of diagnosis and treatment of rectal cancer. Eur J Cancer Mekenkamp LJ, Van Krieken JH, Marijnen CA, van dV, Nagtegaal ID. Lymph node retrieval in rectal cancer is dependent on many factors-the role of the tumor, the patient, the surgeon, the radiotherapist, and the pathologist. American Journal of Surgical Pathology 2009; 33(10): 1547–1553.

166. Thomas GDH, Dixon MF, Smeeton NC, Williams NS. Observer variation in the histological grading of rectal carcinoma. Journal of Clinical Pathology 1983; 36: 385–391.

167. Jass JR, Ajioka Y, Allen JP, Chan YF, Cohen RJ et al. Assessment of invasive growth pattern and lymphocytic infiltration in colorectal cancer. Histopathology 1996; 28(6): 543–548.

168. Ueno H, Murphy J, Jass JR, Mochizuki H, Talbot IC. Tumour 'budding' as an index to estimate the potential of aggressiveness in rectal cancer. Histopathology 2002; 40(2): 127–132.

169. Ueno H, Hase K, Mochizuki H. Criteria for extramural perineural invasion as a prognostic factor in rectal cancer. British Journal of Surgery 2001; 88: 994–1000.

170. Nagtegaal ID, Marijnen CAM. The future of TNM in rectal cancer—the era of neoadjuvant therapy. Current Colorectal Cancer Reports 2008; 4(3): 147–154.

171. Jass JR. Lymphocytic infiltration and survival in rectal cancer. Journal of Clinical Pathology 1986; 39: 585–589.

172. Galon J, Costes A, Sanchez-Cabo F, Kirilovsky A, Mlecnik B et al. Type, density, and location of immune cells within human colorectal tumors predict clinical outcome. Science 2006; 313(5795): 1960–1964.

173. Tol J, Nagtegaal ID, Punt CJ. BRAF mutation in metastatic colorectal cancer. New England Journal of Medicine 2009; 361(1): 98–99.

174. Guastadisegni C, Colafranceschi M, Ottini L, Dogliotti E. Microsatellite instability as a marker of prognosis and response to therapy: a meta-analysis of colorectal cancer survival data. European Journal of Cancer 2010; 46(15): 2788–2798.

175. Gordon NL, Dawson AA, Bennett B, Innes G, Eremin O et al. Outcome in colorectal adenocarcinoma: two seven-year studies of a population. British Medical Journal 1993; 307(6906): 707–710.

176. Pickhardt PJ, Hassan C, Halligan S, Marmo R. Colorectal cancer: CT colonography and colonoscopy for detection—systematic review and meta-analysis Radiology 2011; 259(2): 393–405.

177. Whiteford MH, Whiteford HM, Yee LF, Ogunbiyi OA, Dehdashti F et al. Usefulness of FDG-PET scan in the assessment of suspected metastatic or recurrent adenocarcinoma of the colon and rectum 2. Diseases of the Colon & Rectum 2000; 43(6): 759–767.

178. Fleisher LA, Beckman JA, Brown KA, Calkins H, Chaikof EL et al. ACC/AHA 2007 guidelines on perioperative cardiovascular evaluation and care for noncardiac surgery: a report of the American College of Cardiology/American Heart Association Task Force on Practice Guidelines (Writing Committee to Revise the 2002 Guidelines on Perioperative Cardiovascular Evaluation for Noncardiac Surgery) developed in collaboration with the American Society of Echocardiography, American Society of Nuclear Cardiology, Heart Rhythm Society, Society of Cardiovascular Anesthesiologists, Society for Cardiovascular Angiography and Interventions, Society for Vascular Medicine and Biology, and Society for Vascular Surgery. Journal of the American College of Cardiology 2007 Oct 23; 50(17):e159-e241.

179. Older P, Hall A, Hader R. Cardiopulmonary exercise testing as a screening test for perioperative management of major surgery in the elderly. Chest 1999; 116(2): 355–362.

180. Valkenet K, van de Port IG, Dronkers JJ, de Vries WR, Lindeman E et al. The effects of preoperative exercise therapy on postoperative outcome: a systematic review 1. Clinical Rehabilitation 2011; 25(2): 99–111.

181. Bardram L, Funch-Jensen P, Jensen P, Crawford ME, Kehlet H. Recovery after laparoscopic colonic surgery with epidural analgesia, and early oral nutrition and mobilisation. Lancet 1995; 345(8952): 763–764.

182. Rothwell LA, Bokey EL, Keshava A, Chapuis PH, Dent OF. Outcomes after admission on the day of elective resection for colorectal cancer 1. ANZ Journal of Surgery 2006; 76(1–2): 14–19.

183. Noblett SE, Snowden CP, Shenton BK, Horgan AF. Randomized clinical trial assessing the effect of Doppler-optimized fluid management on outcome after elective colorectal resection 1. British Journal of Surgery 2006 Sep; 93(9): 1069–1076.

184. Turnbull RB Jr, Kyle K, Watson FR, Spratt J. Cancer of the colon: the influence of the no-touch isolation technic on survival rates 6. Annals of Surgery 1967; 166(3): 420–427.

185. Novell JR, Lewis AA. Peroperative observation of marginal artery bleeding: a predictor of anastomotic leakage 3. British Journal of Surgery 1990; 77(2): 137–138.

186. Bouwman DL, Weaver DW. Colon cancer: surgical therapy 1. Gastroenterology Clinics of North America 1988; 17(4): 859–872.

187. Jayne DG, Guillou PJ, Thorpe H, Quirke P, Copeland J et al. Randomized trial of laparoscopic-assisted resection of colorectal carcinoma: 3-year results of the UK MRC CLASICC Trial Group 2. Journal of Clinical Oncology 2007; 25(21): 3061–3068.

188. Laparoscopically assisted colectomy is as safe and effective as open colectomy in people with colon cancer Abstracted from: Nelson H, Sargent D, Wieand HS, et al; for the Clinical Outcomes of Surgical Therapy Study Group. A comparison of laparoscopically assisted and open colectomy for colon cancer. New England Journal of Medicine 2004; 350: 2050–2059.

189. Hazebroek EJ. COLOR: a randomized clinical trial comparing laparoscopic and open resection for colon cancer. Surgery Endoscopy 2002; 16(6): 949–953.

190. Bernstein CN, Shanahan F, Weinstein WM. Are we telling patients the truth about surveillance colonoscopy in ulcerative colitis? 8. Lancet 1994; 343(8889): 71–74.

191. de Vos tot Nederveen Cappel WH, Buskens E, van DP, Cats A, Menko FH, et al. Decision analysis in the surgical treatment of colorectal cancer due to a mismatch repair gene defect. Gut 2003 Dec; 52(12): 1752–1755.

192. Wrigley H, Roderick P, George S, Smith J, Mullee M et al. Inequalities in survival from colorectal cancer: a comparison of the impact of deprivation, treatment, and host factors on observed and cause specific survival 1. Journal of Epidemiology & Community Health 2003; 57(4): 301–309.

193. Zorcolo L, Covotta L, Carlomagno N, Bartolo DC. Safety of primary anastomosis in emergency colo-rectal surgery. Colorectal Disease 2003; 5(3): 262–269.

194. Meyer F, Marusch F, Koch A, Meyer L, Fuhrer S, Kockerling F, et al. Emergency operation in carcinomas of the left colon: value of Hartmann's procedure 1. Techniques in Coloproctology 2004; 8(Suppl. 1): s226–s229.

195. Saida Y, Sumiyama Y, Nagao J, Uramatsu M. Long-term prognosis of preoperative 'bridge to surgery' expandable metallic stent insertion for obstructive colorectal cancer: comparison with emergency operation. Diseases of the Colon & Rectum 2003; 46(10 Suppl.): S44–S49.

196. de Aguilar-Nascimento JE, Caporossi C, Nascimento M. Comparison between resection and primary anastomosis and staged resection in obstructing adenocarcinoma of the left colon 1. Arquivos de Gastroenterologia 2002; 39(4): 240–245.

197. Yamaji Y, Mitsushima T, Yoshida H, Watabe H, Okamoto M et al. The malignant potential of freshly developed colorectal polyps according to age 1. Cancer Epidemiology, Biomarkers & Prevention 2006; 15(12): 2418–2421.

198. Puli SR, Kakugawa Y, Saito Y, Antillon D, Gotoda T et al. Successful complete cure en-bloc resection of large nonpedunculated colonic polyps by endoscopic submucosal dissection: a meta-analysis and systematic review. Annals of Surgical Oncology 2009; 16(8): 2147–2151.

199. Saito Y, Sakamoto T, Fukunaga S, Nakajima T, Kiriyama S et al. Endoscopic submucosal dissection (ESD) for colorectal tumors. Digestive Endoscopy 2009; 21(Suppl. 1): S7–S12.

200. Ueno H, Mochizuki H, Hashiguchi Y, Shimazaki H, Aida S et al. Risk factors for an adverse outcome in early invasive colorectal carcinoma. Gastroenterology 2004; 127(2): 385–394.

201. Kikuchi R, Takano M, Takagi K, Fujimoto N, Nozaki R et al. Management of early invasive colorectal cancer. Risk of recurrence and clinical guidelines 1. Diseases of the Colon & Rectum 1995; 38(12): 1286–1295.

202. Abbas S, Lam V, Hollands M. Ten-year survival after liver resection for colorectal metastases: systematic review and meta-analysis 2. ISRN Oncology 2011; 2011: 763245.

203. Rees M, Tekkis PP, Welsh FK, O'Rourke T, John TG. Evaluation of long-term survival after hepatic resection for metastatic colorectal cancer: a multifactorial model of 929 patients 4. Annals of Surgery 2008; 247(1): 125–135.

204. Nakajima K, Takahashi S, Saito N, Kotaka M, Konishi M et al. Predictive factors for anastomotic leakage after simultaneous resection of synchronous colorectal liver metastasis 9. Journal of Gastrointestinal Surgery 2012; 16(4): 821–827.

205. Nordlinger B, Sorbye H, Glimelius B, Poston GJ, Schlag PM et al. Perioperative chemotherapy with FOLFOX4 and surgery versus surgery alone for resectable liver metastases from colorectal cancer (EORTC Intergroup trial 40983): a randomised controlled trial 1. Lancet 2008; 371(9617): 1007–1016.

206. Villeneuve PJ, Sundaresan RS. Surgical management of colorectal lung metastasis 2. Clinics in Colon and Rectal Surgery 2009; 22(4): 233–241.

207. Koppe MJ, Boerman OC, Oyen WJ, Bleichrodt RP. Peritoneal carcinomatosis of colorectal origin: incidence and current treatment strategies 2. Annals of Surgery 2006; 243(2): 212–222.

208. Verwaal VJ, van RS, de BE, van Sloothen GW, van TH et al. Randomized trial of cytoreduction and hyperthermic intraperitoneal chemotherapy versus systemic chemotherapy and palliative surgery in patients with peritoneal carcinomatosis of colorectal cancer 1. Journal of Clinical Oncology 2003; 21(20): 3737–3743.

209. Elias D, Gilly F, Boutitie F, Quenet F, Bereder JM et al. Peritoneal colorectal carcinomatosis treated with surgery and perioperative intraperitoneal chemotherapy: retrospective analysis of 523 patients from a multicentric French study 3. Journal of Clinical Oncology 2010; 28(1): 63–68.

210. Guillou PJ, Quirke P, Thorpe H, Walker J, Jayne DG et al. Short-term endpoints of conventional versus laparoscopic-assisted surgery in patients with colorectal cancer (MRC CLASICC trial): multicentre, randomised controlled trial 1. Lancet 2005; 365(9472): 1718–1726.

211. Neudecker J, Klein F, Bittner R, Carus T, Stroux A et al. Short-term outcomes from a prospective randomized trial comparing laparoscopic and open surgery for colorectal cancer 1. British Journal of Surgery 2009; 96(12): 1458–1467.

212. Amemiya T, Oda K, Ando M, Kawamura T, Kitagawa Y et al. Activities of daily living and quality of life of elderly patients after elective surgery for gastric and colorectal cancers. Annals of Surgery 2007; 246(2): 222–228.

213. Cancer Research UK. CancerStats. Cancer Research UK, n.d. Available from: <http://www.cancerresearchuk.org/cancer-info/cancerstats/>, accessed on 26 May 2015.

214. Gatta G, Faivre J, Capocaccia R, Ponz de LM. Survival of colorectal cancer patients in Europe during the period 1978–1989. EUROCARE Working Group. European Journal of Cancer 1998; 34(14 Spec. No.): 2176–2183.

215. Gatta G, Zigon G, Aareleid T, Ardanaz E, Bielska-Lasota M et al. Patterns of care for European colorectal cancer patients diagnosed 1996–1998: a EUROCARE high resolution study 1. Acta Oncologica 2010; 49(6): 776–783.

216. Coleman MP, Rachet B, Woods LM, Mitry E, Riga M et al. Trends and socioeconomic inequalities in cancer survival in England and Wales up to 2001. British Journal of Cancer 2004; 90(7): 1367–1373.

217. Lombardi L, Gebbia V, Silvestris N, Testa A, Colucci G et al. Adjuvant therapy in colon cancer. Oncology 2009; 77(Suppl. 1): 50–56.

218. Chou JF, Row D, Gonen M, Liu YH, Schrag D et al. Clinical and pathologic factors that predict lymph node yield from surgical specimens in colorectal cancer: a population-based study. Cancer 2010; 116(11): 2560–2570.

219. O'Connell JB, Maggard MA, Ko CY. Colon cancer survival rates with the new American Joint Committee on Cancer sixth edition staging. Journal of the National Cancer Institute 2004; 96(19): 1420–1425.

220. NIH consensus conference. Adjuvant therapy for patients with colon and rectal cancer. Journal of the American Medical Association 1990; 264(11): 1444–1450.

221. Dube S, Heyen F, Jenicek M. Adjuvant chemotherapy in colorectal carcinoma: results of a meta-analysis. Diseases of the Colon & Rectum 1997; 40(1): 35–41.

222. Gray R. 5'fluorouracil (FU) and folinic acid (FA) in either the weekly 'Roswell Park' or the 4-weekly 'Mayo' regimen should be standard chemotherapy for colon cancer. European Journal of Cancer 2003; 39(14): 2110.

223. Dotan E, Cohen SJ. Challenges in the management of stage II colon cancer. Seminars in Oncology 2011; 38(4): 511–520.

224. Gill S, Loprinzi CL, Sargent DJ, Thomé SD, Alberts SR et al. Pooled analysis of fluorouracil-based adjuvant therapy for stage II and III colon cancer: who benefits and by how much? Journal of Clinical Oncology 2004; 22(10): 1797–1806.

225. Engstrom PF, Arnoletti JP, Benson AB, 3rd, et al. NCCN Clinical Practice Guidelines in Oncology: colon cancer. Journal of the National Comprehensive Cancer Network 2009; 7(8): 778–831.

226. Ouchi K, Sugawara T, Ono H, Fujiya T, Kamiyama Y et al. Histologic features and clinical significance of venous invasion in colorectal carcinoma with hepatic metastasis. Cancer 1996; 78(11): 2313–2317.

227. Berger AC, Sigurdson ER, LeVoyer T, Hanlon A, Mayer RJ et al. Colon cancer survival is associated with decreasing ratio of metastatic to examined lymph nodes. Journal of Clinical Oncology 2005; 23(34): 8706–8712.

228. Le Voyer TE, Sigurdson ER, Hanlon AL, Mayer RJ, Macdonald JS et al. Colon cancer survival is associated with increasing number of lymph nodes analyzed: a secondary survey of intergroup trial INT-0089. Journal of Clinical Oncology 2003; 21(15): 2912–2919.

229. Gunderson L, Jessup J, Sargent D, Greene F, Stewart A. Revised TN categorization for colon cancer based on national survival outcomes data. Journal of Clinical Oncology 2010; 28: 264–271.

230. Jonker DJ, Spithoff K, Maroun J. Adjuvant systemic chemotherapy for Stage II and III colon cancer after complete resection: an updated practice guideline. Journal of Clinical Oncology (Royal College of Radiologists) 2011; 23(5): 314–322.

231. Sargent D, Shi Q, Yothers G, Van Cutsem E, Cassidy J et al. Two or three year disease-free survival (DFS) as a primary end-point in stage III adjuvant colon cancer trials with fluoropyrimidines with or without oxaliplatin or irinotecan: data from 12,676 patients from MOSAIC, X-ACT, PETACC-3, C-06, C-07 and C89803. European Journal of Cancer; 47(7): 990–996.

232. Franko J, Shi Q, Goldman CD, Pockaj BA, Nelson GD et al. Treatment of colorectal peritoneal carcinomatosis with systemic chemotherapy: a pooled analysis of north central cancer treatment group phase III trials N9741 and N9841. Journal of Clinical Oncology 2012; 30(3): 263–267.

233. de Gramont A, Hubbard J, Shi Q, O'Connell MJ, Buyse M et al. Association between disease-free survival and overall survival when survival is prolonged after recurrence in patients receiving cytotoxic adjuvant therapy for colon cancer: simulations based on the 20,800 patient ACCENT data set. Journal of Clinical Oncology 2010; 28(3): 460–465.

234. Moertel CG, Fleming TR, Macdonald JS, Haller DG, Laurie JA et al. Intergroup study of fluorouracil plus levamisole as adjuvant therapy for stage II/Dukes' B2 colon cancer. Journal of Clinical Oncology 1995; 13(12): 2936–2943.

235. Efficacy of adjuvant fluorouracil and folinic acid in colon cancer. International Multicentre Pooled Analysis of Colon Cancer Trials (IMPACT) investigators. Lancet 1995; 345(8955): 939–944.

236. Wolmark N, Rockette H, Fisher B, Wickerham DL, Redmond C et al. The benefit of leucovorin-modulated fluorouracil as postoperative adjuvant therapy for primary colon cancer: results from National Surgical Adjuvant Breast and Bowel Project protocol C-03. Journal of Clinical Oncology 1993; 11(10): 1879–1887.

237. O'Connell MJ, Laurie JA, Kahn M, Fitzgibbons RJ Jr, Erlichman C et al. Prospectively randomized trial of postoperative adjuvant chemotherapy in patients with high-risk colon cancer. Journal of Clinical Oncology 1998; 16(1): 295–300.

238. Haller DG, Catalano PJ, Macdonald JS, O'Rourke MA, Frontiera MS et al. Phase III study of fluorouracil, leucovorin, and levamisole in high-risk stage II and III colon cancer: final report of Intergroup 0089. Journal of Clinical Oncology 2005; 23(34): 8671–8678.

239. Comparison of flourouracil with additional levamisole, higher-dose folinic acid, or both, as adjuvant chemotherapy for colorectal cancer: a randomised trial. QUASAR Collaborative Group. Lancet 2000; 355(9215): 1588–1596.

240. Kerr DJ, Gray R, McConkey C, Barnwell J. Adjuvant chemotherapy with 5-fluorouracil, L-folinic acid and levamisole for patients with colorectal cancer: non-randomised comparison of weekly versus four-weekly schedules—less pain, same gain. QUASAR Colorectal Cancer Study Group. Annals of Oncology 2000; 11(8): 947–955.

241. Wolmark N, Rockette H, Mamounas E, Jones J, Wieand S et al. Clinical trial to assess the relative efficacy of fluorouracil and leucovorin, fluorouracil and levamisole, and fluorouracil, leucovorin, and levamisole in patients with Dukes' B and C carcinoma of the colon: results from National Surgical Adjuvant Breast and Bowel Project C-04. Journal of Clinical Oncology 1999; 17(11): 3553–3559.

242. Sargent DJ, Goldberg RM, Jacobson SD, Macdonald JS, Labianca R et al. A pooled analysis of adjuvant chemotherapy for resected colon cancer in elderly patients. New England Journal of Medicine 2001; 345(15): 1091–1097.

243. Sundararajan V, Mitra N, Jacobson JS, Grann VR, Heitjan DF et al. Survival associated with 5-fluorouracil-based adjuvant chemotherapy among elderly patients with node-positive colon cancer. Annals of Internal Medicine 2002; 136(5): 349–357.

244. Jessup JM, Stewart A, Greene FL, Minsky BD. Adjuvant chemotherapy for stage III colon cancer: implications of race/ethnicity, age, and differentiation. Journal of the American Medical Association 2005; 294(21): 2703–2711.

245. Twelves CJ. Xeloda in Adjuvant Colon Cancer Therapy (X-ACT) trial: overview of efficacy, safety, and cost-effectiveness. Clinical Colorectal Cancer 2006; 6(4): 278–287.

246. Twelves C, Scheithauer W, McKendrick J, Seitz JF, Van Hazel G et al. Capecitabine versus 5-fluorouracil/folinic acid as adjuvant therapy for stage III colon cancer: final results from the X-ACT trial with analysis by age and preliminary evidence of a pharmacodynamic marker of efficacy. Annals of Oncology 2012; 23(5): 1190–1197.

247. Andre T, Boni C, Mounedji-Boudiaf L, Navarro M, Tabernero J et al. Oxaliplatin, fluorouracil, and leucovorin as adjuvant treatment for colon cancer. New England Journal of Medicine 2004; 350(23): 2343–2351.

248. Andre T, Boni C, Navarro M, Tabernero J, Hickish T et al. Improved overall survival with oxaliplatin, fluorouracil, and leucovorin as adjuvant treatment in stage II or III colon cancer in the MOSAIC trial. Journal of Clinical Oncology. Jul 1 2009; 27(19): 3109–3116.

249. Kuebler JP, Wieand HS, O'Connell MJ, Smith RE, Colangelo LH et al. Oxaliplatin combined with weekly bolus fluorouracil and leucovorin as surgical adjuvant chemotherapy for stage II and III colon

cancer: results from NSABP C-07. Journal of Clinical Oncology 2007; 25(16): 2198–2204.

250. Haller DG, Tabernero J, Maroun J, de Braud F, Price T et al. Capecitabine plus oxaliplatin compared with fluorouracil and folinic acid as adjuvant therapy for stage III colon cancer. Journal of Clinical Oncology 2011; 29(11): 1465–1471.

251. Yothers G, O'Connell MJ, Allegra CJ, Kuebler JP, Colangelo LH et al. Oxaliplatin as adjuvant therapy for colon cancer: updated results of NSABP C-07 trial, including survival and subset analyses. Journal of Clinical Oncology 2011; 29(28): 3768–3774.

252. Jackson McCleary N, Meyerhardt J, Green E, Yothers A, de Gramont A et al. Impact of older age on the efficacy of newer adjuvant therapies in >12,500 patients (pts) with stage II/III colon cancer: findings from the ACCENT Database. Journal Clinical Oncology 2009; 27(15s Suppl); abs. 4010.

253. Goldberg RM, Tabah-Fisch I, Bleiberg H, de Gramont A, Tournigand C et al. Pooled analysis of safety and efficacy of oxaliplatin plus fluorouracil/leucovorin administered bimonthly in elderly patients with colorectal cancer. Journal of Clinical Oncology 2006; 24(25): 4085–4091.

254. Saltz LB, Niedzwiecki D, Hollis D, Goldberg RM, Hantel A et al. Irinotecan fluorouracil plus leucovorin is not superior to fluorouracil plus leucovorin alone as adjuvant treatment for stage III colon cancer: results of CALGB 89803. Journal of Clinical Oncology 2007; 25(23): 3456–3461.

255. Van Cutsem E, Labianca R, Bodoky G, Barone C, Aranda E et al. Randomized phase III trial comparing biweekly infusional fluorouracil/leucovorin alone or with irinotecan in the adjuvant treatment of stage III colon cancer: PETACC-3. Journal of Clinical Oncology 2009; 27(19): 3117–3125.

256. Ychou M, Hohenberger W, Thezenas S, Navarro M, Maurel J et al. A randomized phase III study comparing adjuvant 5-fluorouracil/folinic acid with FOLFIRI in patients following complete resection of liver metastases from colorectal cancer. Annals of Oncology 2009; 20(12): 1964–1970.

257. Kabbinavar FF, Schulz J, McCleod M, Patel T, Hamm JT et al. Addition of bevacizumab to bolus fluorouracil and leucovorin in first-line metastatic colorectal cancer: results of a randomized phase II trial. Journal of Clinical Oncology 2005; 23(16): 3697–3705.

258. Allegra CJ, Yothers G, O'Connell MJ, Sharif S, Petrelli NJ et al. Phase III trial assessing bevacizumab in stages II and III carcinoma of the colon: results of NSABP protocol C-08. Journal of Clinical Oncology 2011; 29(1): 11–16.

259. De Gramont A, Van Cutsem E, Tabernero J, Moore MJ, Cunningham D et al. AVANT: Results from a randomized, three-arm multinational phase III study to investigate bevacizumab with either XELOX or FOLFOX4 versus FOLFOX4 alone as adjuvant treatment for colon cancer. Journal of Clinical Oncology 2011; 29(Suppl. 4): abstr 362.

260. Van Loon K, Venook AP. Adjuvant treatment of colon cancer: what is next? Current Opinion in Oncology 2011; 23(4): 403–409.

261. Alberts SR, Sargent DJ, Nair S, Mahoney MR, Mooney M et al. Effect of oxaliplatin, fluorouracil, and leucovorin with or without cetuximab on survival among patients with resected stage III colon cancer: a randomized trial. Journal of the American Medical Association 2012; 307(13): 1383–1393.

262. Graham JS, Cassidy J. Adjuvant therapy in colon cancer. Expert Review of Anticancer Therapy 2012; 12(1): 99–109.

263. de Gramont A, de Gramont A Chibaudel B, Bachet JB, Larsen AK et al. From chemotherapy to targeted therapy in adjuvant treatment for stage III colon cancer. Seminars in Oncology 2011; 38(4): 521–532.

264. Efficacy of adjuvant fluorouracil and folinic acid in B2 colon cancer. International Multicentre Pooled Analysis of B2 Colon Cancer Trials (IMPACT B2) Investigators. Journal of Clinical Oncology 1999; 17(5): 1356–1363.

265. Mamounas E, Wieand S, Wolmark N, Bear HD, Atkins JN et al. Comparative efficacy of adjuvant chemotherapy in patients with Dukes' B versus Dukes' C colon cancer: results from four National Surgical Adjuvant Breast and Bowel Project adjuvant studies (C-01, C-02, C-03, and C-04). Journal of Clinical Oncology. May 1999; 17(5): 1349–1355.

266. Figueredo A, Coombes ME, Mukherjee S. Adjuvant therapy for completely resected stage II colon cancer. Cochrane Database Systemic Reviews 2008(3): CD005390.

267. Tejpar S, De Roock W, Jonker D. KRAS genotypes and outcome in patients with chemotherapy-refractory metastatic colorectal cancer treated with cetuximab-reply. Journal of the American Medical Association 2011; 305(6): 564–566.

268. Donada M, Bonin S, Nardon E, De Pellegrin A, Decorti G et al. Thymidilate synthase expression predicts longer survival in patients with stage II colon cancer treated with 5-flurouracil independently of microsatellite instability. Journal of Cancer Research and Clinical Oncology 2011; 137(2): 201–210.

269. Roth AD, Tejpar S, Delorenzi M, Yan P, Fiocca R et al. Prognostic role of KRAS and BRAF in stage II and III resected colon cancer: results of the translational study on the PETACC-3, EORTC 40993, SAKK 60-00 trial. Journal of Clinical Oncology 2010; 28(3): 466–474.

270. Farina-Sarasqueta A, van Lijnschoten G, Moerland E, Creemers GJ, Lemmens VE et al. The BRAF V600E mutation is an independent prognostic factor for survival in stage II and stage III colon cancer patients. Annals of Oncology 2010; 21(12): 2396–2402.

271. Tejpar S, Bertagnolli M, Bosman F, Lenz HJ, Garraway L et al. Prognostic and predictive biomarkers in resected colon cancer: current status and future perspectives for integrating genomics into biomarker discovery. Oncologist 2010; 15(4): 390–404.

272. Gryfe R, Kim H, Hsieh ET, Aronson MD, Holowaty EJ et al. Tumor microsatellite instability and clinical outcome in young patients with colorectal cancer. New England Journal of Medicine 2000; 342(2): 69–77.

273. Gray RG, Quirke P, Handley K, Lopatin M, Magill L et al. Validation study of a quantitative multigene reverse transcriptase-polymerase chain reaction assay for assessment of recurrence risk in patients with stage II colon cancer. Journal of Clinical Oncology 2011; 29(35): 4611–4619.

274. Popat S, Hubner R, Houlston RS. Systematic review of microsatellite instability and colorectal cancer prognosis. Journal of Clinical Oncology 2005; 23(3): 609–618.

275. Ribic CM, Sargent DJ, Moore MJ, Thibodeau SN, French AJ et al. Tumor microsatellite-instability status as a predictor of benefit from fluorouracil-based adjuvant chemotherapy for colon cancer. New England Journal of Medicine 2003; 349(3): 247–257.

276. Sargent DJ, Marsoni S, Monges G, Thibodeau SN, Labianca R et al. Defective mismatch repair as a predictive marker for lack of efficacy of fluorouracil-based adjuvant therapy in colon cancer. Journal of Clinical Oncology 2010; 28(20): 3219–3226.

277. Kim ST, Lee J, Park SH, Park JO, Lim HY et al. Clinical impact of microsatellite instability in colon cancer following adjuvant FOLFOX therapy. Cancer Chemotherapy and Pharmacology 2010; 66(4): 659–667.

278. Fearon ER, Cho KR, Nigro JM, Kern SE, Simons JW et al. Identification of a chromosome 18q gene that is altered in colorectal cancers. Science 1990; 247(4938): 49–56.

279. Jen J, Kim H, Piantadosi S, Liu ZF, Levitt RC et al. Allelic loss of chromosome 18q and prognosis in colorectal cancer. New England Journal of Medicine 1994; 331(4): 213–221.

280. Watanabe T, Wu TT, Catalano PJ, Ueki T, Satriano R et al. Molecular predictors of survival after adjuvant chemotherapy for colon cancer. New England Journal of Medicine 2001; 344(16): 1196–1206.

281. Salazar R, Roepman P, Capella G, Moreno V, Simon I et al. Gene expression signature to improve prognosis prediction of stage II and III colorectal cancer. Journal of Clinical Oncology 2011; 29(1): 17–24.

282. O'Connell MJ, Lavery I, Yothers G, Paik S, Clark-Langone KM et al. Relationship between tumor gene expression and recurrence in four independent studies of patients with stage II/III colon cancer treated

with surgery alone or surgery plus adjuvant fluorouracil plus leucovorin. Journal of Clinical Oncology 2010; 28(25): 3937–3944.

283. Van Laar RK. An online gene expression assay for determining adjuvant therapy eligibility in patients with stage 2 or 3 colon cancer. British Journal of Cancer 2010; 103(12): 1852–1857.

284. Roth A, Di Narzo AF, Tejpar S, Bosman F, Popoviciet VC et al. Validation of two gene-expression risk scores in a large colon cancer cohort and contribution to an improved prognostic method. Journal of Clinical Oncology 2012; 30 (Suppl.): abs. 3509.

285. Salazar R, Tabernero J, Moreno V, Nitsche U, Bachleitner-Hofmannet T al. Validation of a genomic classifier (ColoPrint) for predicting outcome in the T3-MSS subgroup of stage II colon cancer patients. Journal of Clinical Oncology 2012; 30 (suppl.); abs. 3510.

286. Gunderson LL, Sosin H, Levitt S. Extrapelvic colon—areas of failure in a reoperation series: implications for adjuvant therapy. International Journal of Radiation Oncology Biology Physics 1985; 11(4): 731–741.

287. Mendenhall WM, Amos EH, Rout WR, Zlotecki RA, Hochwald SN et al. Adjuvant postoperative radiotherapy for colon carcinoma. Cancer 2004; 101(6): 1338–1344. 5

288. Willett CG, Fung CY, Kaufman DS, Efird J, Shellito PC. Postoperative radiation therapy for high-risk colon carcinoma. Journal of Clinical Oncology 1993; 11(6): 1112–1127.

289. Kopelson G. Adjuvant postoperative radiation therapy for colorectal carcinoma above the peritoneal reflection. II. Antimesenteric wall ascending and descending colon and cecum. Cancer 1983; 52(4): 633–636.

290. Martenson JA Jr, Willett CG, Sargent DJ, Mailliard JA, Donohue JH et al. Phase III study of adjuvant chemotherapy and radiation therapy compared with chemotherapy alone in the surgical adjuvant treatment of colon cancer: results of intergroup protocol 0130. Journal of Clinical Oncology 2004; 22(16): 3277–3283.

291. Willett CG, Czito BG, Tyler DS. Intraoperative radiation therapy. Journal of Clinical Oncology 2007; 25(8): 971–977.

292. Fabian C, Giri S, Estes N, Tangen CM, Poplin E et al. Adjuvant continuous infusion 5-FU, whole-abdominal radiation, and tumor bed boost in high-risk stage III colon carcinoma: a Southwest Oncology Group Pilot study. International Journal of Radiation Oncology Biology Physics 1995 May 15; 32(2): 457–464.

293. Ben-Josef E, Normolle D, Ensminger WD, Walker S, Tatro D et al. Phase II trial of high-dose conformal radiation therapy with concurrent hepatic artery floxuridine for unresectable intrahepatic malignancies. Journal of Clinical Oncology 2005; 23(34): 8739–8747.

294. Abdalla EK, Vauthey JN, Ellis LM, Ellis V, Pollock R et al. Recurrence and outcomes following hepatic resection, radiofrequency ablation, and combined resection/ablation for colorectal liver metastases. Annals of Surgery 2004; 239(6): 818–825; discussion 825–827.

295. Rusthoven KE, Kavanagh BD, Cardenes H, Stieber VW, Burri SH et al. Multi-institutional phase I/II trial of stereotactic body radiation therapy for liver metastases. Journal of Clinical Oncology 2009; 27(10): 1572–1578.

296. Lee MT, Kim JJ, Dinniwell R, Brierley J, Lockwood G et al. Phase I study of individualized stereotactic body radiotherapy of liver metastases. Journal of Clinical Oncology 2009; 27(10): 1585–1591.

297. Smith SD, Nicol KM, Devereux J, Cornbleet MA. Encounters with doctors: quantity and quality. Palliative Medicine 1999; 13: 217–223.

298. McNair AG, Choh CT, Metcalfe C, Littlejohns D, Barham CP et al. Maximising recruitment into randomised controlled trials: the role of multidisciplinary cancer teams. European Journal of Cancer 2008; 44: 2623–2626.

299. Improving outcomes in colorectal cancer. National Institute for Health and Clinical Excellence (NICE). Available from: <http://guidance.nice.org.uk/CSGCC>, accessed 26 May 2015.

300. Walsh J, Harrison JD, Young JM, Butow PN, Solomon MJ et al. What are the current barriers to effective cancer care coordination? A qualitative study. BMC Health Services Research 2010; 10: 132.

301. Fleissig A, Jenkins V, Catt S, Fallowfield L. Multidisciplinary teams in cancer care: are they effective in the UK? Lancet Oncology 2006; 7: 935–943.

302. Hong N, Wright F, Gagliardi F, Paszat LF. Examining the potential relationship between multidiscipinary cancer care and patient survival: an international literature review. Journal of Surgical Oncology 2010; 102(2): 125–132.

303. Ye YJ, Shen ZL, Sun XT, Wang ZF, Shen DH et al. Impact of multidisciplinary team working on the management of colorectal cancer. Chinese Medical Journal (Engl) 2012; 125: 172–177.

304. MacDermid E, Hooton G, MacDonald M, McKay G, Grose D et al. Improving patient survival with the colorectal cancer multi-disciplinary team. Colorectal Disease 2009; 11: 291–295.

305. Hurria A, Lichtman SM, Gardes J, et al. Identifying vulnerable older adults with cancer: integrating geriatric assessment into oncology practice. Journal of the American Geriatrics Society 2007; 55: 1604–1608.

306. Pal SK, Katheria V, Hurria A. Evaluating the older patient with cancer: understanding frailty and the geriatric assessment. CA: A Cancer Journal for Clinicians 2010; 60: 120–132.

307. Quah HM, Joseph R, Schrag D, Shia J, Guillem JG et al. Young age influences treatment but not outcome of colon cancer. Annals of Surgical Oncology 2007; 14: 2759–2765.

308. Ganapathi S, Kumar D, Katsoulas N, Melville D, Hodgson S et al. Colorectal cancer in the young: trends, characteristics and outcome. International Journal of Colorectal Diseaseease 2011; 26: 927–934.

309. McMillan DC, McArdle CS. The impact of young age on cancer-specific and non-cancer-related survival after surgery for colorectal cancer: 10-year follow-up. British Journal of Cancer 2009; 101: 557–560.

310. Al-Barrak J, Gill S. Presentation and outcomes of patients aged 30 years and younger with colorectal cancer: a 20-year retrospective review. Medical Oncology 2011; 28: 1058–1061.

311. Chou CL, Chang SC, Lin TC, Chen WS, Jiang JK et al. Differences in clinicopathological characteristics of colorectal cancer between younger and elderly patients: an analysis of 322 patients from a single institution. American Journal of Surgery 2011; 202: 574–582.

312. Spanos CP, Mamopoulos A, Tsapas A, Syrakos T, Kiskinis D et al. Female fertility and colorectal cancer. International Journal of Colorectal Disease 2008; 23: 735–743, 2008

313. O'Neill MT, Ni Dhonnchu T, Brannigan AE. Topic update: effects of colorectal cancer treatments on female fertility and potential methods for fertility preservation. Diseases of the Colon & Rectum 2011; 54: 363–569.

314. Redig AJ, Brannigan R, Stryker SJ, Woodruff TK, Jeruss JS et al. Incorporating fertility preservation into the care of young oncology patients. Cancer 2011; 117: 4–10.

315. Rosevelt J, Frankl H. Colorectal cancer screening by nurse practitioner using 60-cm flexible fiberoptic sigmoidoscope. Digestive Diseases and Sciences 1984; 29: 161–163.

316. Maule WF. Screening for colorectal cancer by nurse endoscopists. New England Journal of Medicine 1994; 330: 183–187.

317. Limoges-Gonzalez M, Mann NS, Al-Juburi A, Tseng D, Inadomi J et al. Comparisons of screening colonoscopy performed by a nurse practitioner and gastroenterologists: a single-center randomized controlled trial. Gastroenterology Nursing 2011; 34: 210–216.

318. Limoges-Gonzalez M. Opening doors for nonphysician colonoscopists. Nurse Practitioner 2012; 37: 35–40.

319. McFarlane K, Dixon L, Wakeman CJ, Robertson GM, Eglinton TW et al. The process and outcomes of a nurse-led colorectal cancer follow-up clinic. Colorectal Disease 2012; 14:e245–e249.

320. MacLeod A, Branch A, Cassidy J, McDonald A, Mohammed N et al. A nurse-/pharmacy-led capecitabine clinic for colorectal cancer: results of a prospective audit and retrospective survey of patient experiences. European Journal of Oncology Nursing 2007; 11: 247–254.

321. Molassiotis A, Brearley S, Saunders M, Craven O, Wardley A et al. Effectiveness of a home care nursing program in the symptom

management of patients with colorectal and breast cancer receiving oral chemotherapy: a randomized, controlled trial. Journal of Clinical Oncology 2009; 27: 6191–6198.

322. Sharpe L, Patel D, Clarke S. The relationship between body image disturbance and distress in colorectal cancer patients with and without stomas. Journal of Psychosomatic Research 2011; 70: 395–402.

323. Ross L, Abild-Nielsen AG, Thomsen BL, Karlsen RV, Boesen EH et al. Quality of life of Danish colorectal cancer patients with and without a stoma. Support Care Cancer 2007; 15: 505–513.

324. Pachler J, Wille-Jorgensen P. Quality of life after rectal resection for cancer, with or without permanent colostomy. Cochrane Database Systemic Reviews 2004: CD004323.

325. Millan M, Tegido M, Biondo S, García-Granero E, García-Granero E. Preoperative stoma siting and education by stomatherapists of colorectal cancer patients: a descriptive study in twelve Spanish colorectal surgical units. Colorectal Disease 2010; 12: e88–e92.

326. Moghaddam AA, Woodward M, Huxley R. Obesity and risk of colorectal cancer: a meta-analysis of 31 studies with 70,000 events. Cancer Epidemiology, Biomarkers & Prevention 2007; 16: 2533–2547.

327. Renehan AG, Tyson M, Egger M, Heller RF, Zwahlen M. Body-mass index and incidence of cancer: a systematic review and meta-analysis of prospective observational studies. Lancet 2008; 371: 569–578.

328. Sinicrope FA, Foster NR, Sargent DJ, O'Connell MJ, Rankin C. Obesity is an independent prognostic variable in colon cancer survivors. Clinical Cancer Research 2010; 16: 1884–1893.

329. Larsson SC, Wolk A. Obesity and colon and rectal cancer risk: a meta-analysis of prospective studies. American Journal of Clinical Nutrition 2007; 86: 556–565.

330. Dignam JJ, Polite BN, Yothers G, Raich P, Colangelo L et al. Body mass index and outcomes in patients who receive adjuvant chemotherapy for colon cancer. Journal of the National Cancer Institute 2006; 98: 1647–1654.

331. Sandhu MS, White IR, McPherson K. Systematic review of the prospective cohort studies on meat consumption and colorectal cancer risk: a meta-analytical approach. Cancer Epidemiology, Biomarkers & Prevention 2001; 10: 439–446.

332. Bingham SA, Day NE, Luben R, Ferrari P, Slimani N et al. Dietary fibre in food and protection against colorectal cancer in the European Prospective Investigation into Cancer and Nutrition (EPIC): an observational study. Lancet 2003; 361: 1496–1501.

333. Meyerhardt JA, Niedzwiecki D, Hollis D, Saltz LB, Hu FB et al. Association of dietary patterns with cancer recurrence and survival in patients with stage III colon cancer. Journal of the American Medical Association 2007; 298: 754–764.

334. Meyerhardt J. Energy Balance and other modifiable host factors on colorectal cancer prognosis. Energy Balance and Cancer 2012; 4: 141–156.

335. Haydon AM, Macinnis RJ, English DR, Giles GG. Effect of physical activity and body size on survival after diagnosis with colorectal cancer. Gut 2006; 55: 62–67.

336. Renehan AG, Egger M, Saunders MP, O'Dwyer ST. Impact on survival of intensive follow up after curative resection for colorectal cancer: systematic review and meta-analysis of randomised trials. British Medical Journal 2002; 324: 813.

337. Figueredo A, Rumble RB, Maroun J, Earle CC, Cummings B et al. Follow-up of patients with curatively resected colorectal cancer: a practice guideline. BMC Cancer 2003; 3: 26.

338. Tjandra JJ, Chan MK. Follow-up after curative resection of colorectal cancer: a meta-analysis. Diseases of the Colon & Rectum 2007; 50: 1783–1799.

339. Jeffery M, Hickey BE, Hider PN. Follow-up strategies for patients treated for non-metastatic colorectal cancer. Cochrane Database Systemic Reviews 2007: CD002200.

340. Baca B, Beart RW Jr, Etzioni DA. Surveillance after colorectal Cancer Researchection: a systematic review. Diseases of the Colon & Rectum 2011; 54: 1036–1048.

341. Sobhani I, Tiret E, Lebtahi R, Aparicio T, Itti E et al. Early detection of recurrence by 18FDG-PET in the follow-up of patients with colorectal cancer. British Journal of Cancer 2008; 98: 875–880.

342. Sorensen NF, Jensen AB, Wille-Jorgensen P, Friberg L, Rørdam L et al. Strict follow-up programme including CT and (1)(8)F-FDG-PET after curative surgery for colorectal cancer. Colorectal Disease 2010; 12: e224–e228

343. Chan K, Welch S, Walker-Dilks C, Raifu A, Ontario provincial Gastrointestinal Disease Site Group. Evidence-based guideline recommendations on the use of positron emission tomography imaging in colorectal cancer. Clinical Oncology (Royal College of Radiologists) 2012; 24: 232–249.

344. Knowles G, Sherwood L, Dunlop MG, Dean G, Jodrell D et al. Developing and piloting a nurse-led model of follow-up in the multidisciplinary management of colorectal cancer. European Journal of Oncology Nursing 2007; 11: 212–223; discussion 224–227.

345. Colorectal cancer: National Institute for Health and Clinical Education (NICE) guidelines, November 2011. Available from: http://www.nice.org.uk/guidance/CG131/NICEGuidance Accessed May 2012.

346. Cairns SR, Scholefield JH, Steele RJ, Dunlop MG, Thomas HJW et al. Guidelines for colorectal cancer screening and surveillance in moderate and high risk groups (update from 2002). Gut 2010; 59: 666–689.

347. Desch CE, Benson AB III Somerfield MR, Flynn PJ, Krause C et al. Colorectal cancer surveillance: 2005 update of an American Society of Clinical Oncology practice guideline. Journal of Clinical Oncology 2005; 23: 8512–8519.

348. National Comprehensive Cancer Network (NCCN) Guidelines Version 3.2012 Colon Cancer. Available from: <http://www.nccn.org>, accessed in May 2012.

349. LaBianca R, Nordlinger B, Beretta D, Brouquet A, Cervantes A. Primary colon cancer: ESMO Clinical Practice Guidelines for diagnosis, adjuvant treatment and follow-up. Annals of Oncology 2010; 21(Suppl. 5): v70–v77.

350. Surveillance Epidemiology and End Results (SEER) Stat Fact Sheets: Colon and Rectum. Available from: <http://seer.cancer.gov/statfacts/html/colorect.html>, accessed in May 2012.

351. Francisci S, Capocaccia R, Grande E, Santaquilani M, Simonetti A et al. The cure of cancer: a European perspective. European Journal of Cancer 2009; 45: 1067–1079.

352. Jansen L, Koch L, Brenner H, Arndt V et al. Quality of life among long-term (>/=5 years) colorectal cancer survivors—systematic review. European Journal of Cancer 2010; 46: 2879–2888.

353. Chambers SK, Meng X, Youl P, Aitken J, Dunn J et al. A five-year prospective study of quality of life after colorectal cancer. Quality of Life Research 2011; 21(9): 1551–1564.

354. Denlinger CS, Barsevick AM. The challenges of colorectal cancer survivorship. Journal of the National Comprehensive Cancer Network 2009; 7: 883–893; quiz 894.

355. Davies NJ, Batehup L, Thomas R. The role of diet and physical activity in breast, colorectal, and prostate cancer survivorship: a review of the literature. British Journal of Cancer 2011; 105(Suppl. 1): S52–S73.

356. Rock CL, Doyle C, Demark-Wahnefried W, Meyerhardt J, Courneya KS et al. Nutrition and physical activity guidelines for cancer survivors. CA: A Cancer Journal for Clinicians 2012; 62(4): 242–274.

CHAPTER 40

Pancreatic cancer

Jürgen Weitz, Markus W. Büchler, Paul D. Sykes, John P. Neoptolemos, Eithne Costello, Christopher M. Halloran, Frank Bergmann, Peter Schirmacher, Ulrich Bork, Stefan Fritz, Jens Werner, Thomas B. Brunner, Elizabeth Smyth, David Cunningham, Brian R. Untch, and Peter J. Allen

Introduction to pancreatic cancer

Pancreatic cancer comprises several different exocrine and endocrine malignant diseases. The most common form is pancreatic adenocarcinoma, the tenth most common solid cancer in most of the Western countries [1], which is discussed in this chapter. The lifetime risk of developing such a disease is 1.5% with a mean age of diagnosis in the seventh decade [2]. Unfortunately, no specific symptoms of this disease exist. Typically patients present with unspecific abdominal discomfort, weight loss, and early satiety. More specific symptoms are painless jaundice and signs of endocrine or exocrine pancreatic insufficiency. Management of pancreatic cancer is complex and should best be performed by a multidisciplinary team. The individual components of such an approach are described in this chapter.

Epidemiology and risk factors

Pancreatic cancer is estimated to result in about 269,000 deaths per year worldwide (153,500 in developed countries) [3]. Incidence rates only slightly exceed the mortality rates of the disease (48,960 estimated new cases versus 40,560 deaths in the USA in 2015) which reflects the poor prognosis of pancreatic cancer, resulting in an overall five-year survival rate of 4-6% [4]. In the USA, pancreatic cancer represents the fourth leading cause of cancer-related death for women and men, affecting the latter slightly more often [4]. Since the 1970s, in the US population there have been no significant trend changes in the death rate of pancreatic cancer [4]. Pancreatic cancer typically affects patients in their later adult life, most frequently occurring in their seventh and eight decades [5]. Unlike other pancreatic neoplasms, it is exceptionally rare before the age of 40 years [5, 6]. Globally increased lifespan, especially in Asian countries, are likely to result in higher absolute numbers of pancreatic cancer [7].

Pancreatic cancer usually arises sporadically. Nevertheless, a hereditary etiology of pancreatic cancer has been estimated for about 10% of patients [8]. Autosomal dominant hereditary syndromes associated with pancreatic cancer include, among others, hereditary pancreatitis (PRSS1, SPINK1 genes; cumulative risk of 25–70%), familial atypical multiple mole melanoma syndrome (CDKN2A; risk 13–17%), hereditary breast and ovarian cancer syndrome (BRCA2, PALB2, BRCA1; risk 1.2–6.9%), Peutz–Jeghers syndrome (STK11/ LKB1; risk 5–36%), and hereditary non-polyposis colorectal cancer syndrome (MLH1, MLH2, MSH6 etc; risk 3.7%) [8]. Furthermore, a familial pancreatic cancer syndrome has been described, whose underlying genetic alterations are yet to be defined [9].

Beyond hereditary syndromes and family history, smoking has been identified as a dominant risk factor for pancreatic cancer. Cigarette smoking has been reported to double the risk and account for 20% to 25% of pancreatic cancers [7, 10]. Although the smoking–carcinoma linkage seems to be less pronounced than in lung cancer, pancreatic cancers from smokers were shown to harbour more mutations than those from non-smokers [10]. Further risk factors for pancreatic cancer include chronic pancreatitis for more than five years, long-term diabetes mellitus type 2, obesity, and high caloric intake, and a non-0-bloodgroup [7].

Molecular biology

Knowledge of the molecular changes and pathways involved in tumorigenesis is essential for exploration of new methods of detection, diagnosis, and treatment of cancer in pancreatic ductal adenocarcinoma, which has one of the poorest survival rates of all carcinomas.

While there are fundamental similarities in the series of molecular events required for the development of cancer, some cancer types have specific profiles [11]. This section will discuss the series of events that led to the development of pancreatic ductal adenocarcinoma, the pathways that are involved in proliferation and the complex interaction between the tumour cells and the surrounding stroma (desmoplastic reaction) that characterizes this killer disease (see Figure 40.1).

Profile of genetic disruption

Whole genomic analysis of pancreatic cancer tissue has revealed the genetic alteration of 12 core pathways in the majority of cases,

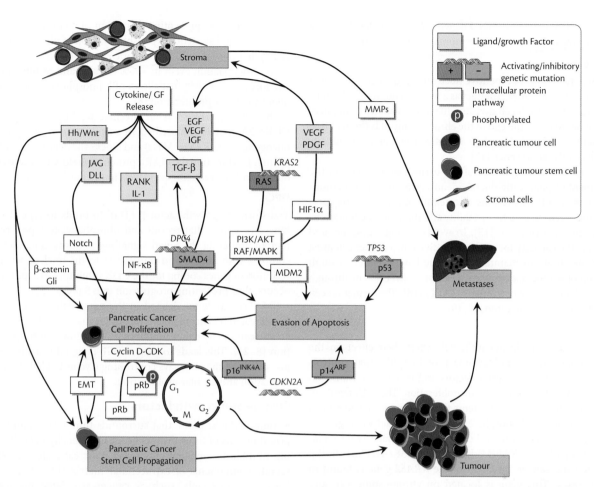

Fig. 40.1 A summary of the key pathways involved in the development of pancreatic adenocarcinoma and their interaction with surrounding stroma. Signature lesions, such as KRAS2, TP53, CDKN2A, and DPC4 mutations result in uncontrolled cellular proliferation and upregulation of cytokines. The cytokines stimulate stroma and lead to the activation of other paracrine signalling pathways (Hh, Notch, Wnt, and NF-κB) that further propagate cellular proliferation, epithelial-to-mesenchymal transition (EMT) and tumour cells capable of metastatic dissemination.

although the specific genes involved vary widely [6]. Order can be brought to this complex disease process by focusing on the following key signature pathways that are almost universally disrupted [12], rather than the many individual mutations that alter their normal signal transduction:

- Regulation of G1/S phase transition (KRAS and p16^{INK4A}).
- Apoptosis and DNA damage control (p53 and p14^{ARF}).
- TGF-β signalling (SMAD proteins).
- Cellular organization pathways (Hedgehog, Notch, Wnt and NF-κB).

Next-generation sequencing of metastatic disease has revealed the genomic instability present during pancreatic cancer development persists following dissemination, resulting in metastatic colonies that are genetically distinct from the original tumour [13]. Detailed analysis of primary and metastatic tumours from the same patient has demonstrated that the majority of mutations are present in all metastases, suggesting they are early events that occurred before the tumour spread [14]. Mutations found only in metastases may indicate the events required tumour cells to become capable of dissemination and seeding a distant site [12, 13].

Precursor lesions

There is evidence that pancreatic intraepithelial neoplasia (PanIN), intraductal papillary mucinous neoplasms (IPMNs) and mucinous cystic neoplasm (MCNs) can lead to the development of pancreatic ductal adenocarcinoma. PanINs are the most common lesions believed to precede development of pancreatic adenocarcinoma [10]. They are classified under histological examination by the extent and type of hyperplasia present as: PanIN-1(A/B), PanIN-2, and finally PanIN-3, which represents carcinoma in situ [15]. Quantification of the genetic mutations present in these lesions has indicated a series of events that lead to the development of pancreatic cancer. Activating *KRAS* mutations are found in all forms of PanIN lesion and even some benign pancreatic cells, suggesting that this defect alone is not sufficient for tumorigenesis. Further mutations and progressive shortening of telomeres occur with increasing PanIN grade: inactivation of *CDKN2A* is observed from PanIN-2 onwards and alterations in the *TP53* gene in PanIN-3 lesions. Finally, mutations of the *DPC4* gene resulting in inactivation of the SMAD4 protein are associated with invasive carcinoma and correlate with poor prognosis.

Similarly to PanINs, KRAS activation is an early event in IPMN and MCN and is associated with dysplasia; inactivation of CDKN2A is also important early in IPMN. Likewise, *TP53* and *DPC4* are seen later in IPMN and in invasive carcinoma from MCN [16].

Telomere shortening

Telomeres are regions of repetitive nucleotide sequences, present at the ends of chromosomes. They act as a mitotic counter by shortening naturally with each cell division due to an inability of duplication enzymes to reach the end of the chromosome. It is thought that this progressive shortening plays an anticancer role by eventually inducing cellular senescence [17].

Telomeric shortening is one of the earliest events seen in the development of pancreatic ductal adenocarcinoma and is demonstrated in 90% of PanIN lesions. Shortening of telomeres may predispose these cells to genetic instability and therefore the mutations necessary for tumorigenesis [15]. To avoid entering senescence and to promote the capacity for continuous division, a cancer cell must develop the ability to maintain telomeric length, either through expression of telomerase reverse transcriptase (hTERT) or through alternative lengthening of telomeres (ALT) [18]. The former is seen in 85–90% of pancreatic tumours [19].

KRAS

Growth signalling pathways ultimately exert their effect on the tumour suppressor, retinoblastoma protein (pRb) that controls the release of E2F transcription factors and thereby the transition from G1 into S phase and cellular proliferation. The RAS family of proteins are early upstream proteins that exist in an inactive form bound to guanosine diphosphate (GDP) and an activated guanosine triphosphate (GTP)-bound complex that initiates two cellular proliferation pathways: RAF/MEK/ERK and PI3K/AKT/mTOR [6].

In pancreatic cancer, mutation of the *KRAS2* gene is found in >90% of cases. This gene is located on chromosome 12p and encodes for Kirsten rat sarcoma protein (KRAS). The mutations are most commonly point mutations of codons 12, 13, or 61 and inhibit the hydrolyzing effect of GTPase, resulting in a persistently activated KRAS protein and cellular proliferation [8]. Initiation of the RAF/MEK/ERK pathway results in G1 to S-phase transition by phosphorylation of pRb. Activation of the PI3K/AKT/mTOR pathway inhibits GSK-3, which stabilizes Cyclin D assembly with CDK 4/6 and allows cellular proliferation. Evasion of apoptosis is the result of p53 inhibition via activation of the murine double minute protein (Mdm2).

TP53

The TP53 gene located on chromosome 17 codes for the tumour suppressor protein p53, which acts as a molecular check for DNA damage and, if detected, forces the cell into senescence or apoptosis. Under normal conditions, p53 levels are kept low by Mdm2, which acts in two ways: the first is to transport p53 from the nucleus into the cytosol and the second is the ubiquitination of p53, thus marking it for proteasome degradation [20]. Mdm2 is inhibited under conditions of cellular stress, such as DNA damage or oncogenic activation, and p53 levels increase, resulting in cell cycle arrest and initiation of apoptosis or cellular senescence. *TP53* is found to be mutated in 50–75% of tumours resulting in cells that are susceptible to further genomic instability as DNA damage-control checks are bypassed and apoptosis evaded [8].

CDKN2A

The CDKN2A gene is located on chromosome 9p and codes for two protein products: p16^{INK4A} and p14^{ARF}. Normally, p16^{INK4A} inhibits CDK4/6, preventing formation of a complex with Cyclin D complex and subsequent phosphorylation of pRb, thus impeding cell cycle progression. In pancreatic cancer, *CDKN2A* is subject to a hypermethylation event in >95% of cases and results in an inactive form of p16^{INK4A} that allows pRb phosphorylation and consequently cellular proliferation [8].

The protein, p14^{ARF}, is an alternate reading frame product of CDKN2A that is transcribed in response to overexpression of oncogenes (e.g., *RAS* or *MYC*) and blocks the degradation of p53 by Mdm2. Dysfunctional p14ARF protein therefore promotes evasion of apoptosis by reducing p53 levels in the nucleus [21].

DPC4

Transforming growth factor-β (TGF-β) binds to type II tyrosine kinase receptors that recruit and phosphorylate type I receptors thereby initiating the Smad signalling pathway. Smad2/3 form a complex with Smad4 and translocate to the nucleus where transcription of genes coding for the CDK inhibitors p15, p21, and p27 occurs, thus preventing progression into S phase [22].

SMAD4 stands for deleted in the pancreatic cancer 4 (*DPC4*) gene located on chromosome 18q and is inactivated in 55% of pancreatic cancers by either homozygous deletion or intragenic mutation [8, 23]. This leads to loss of TGF-β signal transduction, and loss of one of the pathways controlling Cyclin D-CDK4/6 complex formation and cellular proliferation.

Stroma and growth factors

Stroma is the 'scaffold' that surrounds tumour cells and is comprised of cells of three distinct groups: mesenchymal cells, including fibroblasts, myofibroblasts and pancreatic stellate cells that secrete components of extracellular matrix (ECM) such as collagen; immune cells, such as cancer-associated macrophages, lymphocytes, mast cells, and neutrophils that respond to inflammatory cytokines such is IL1/6; and finally, endothelial cells that form the vasculature and lymphatics and respond to growth factors expressed by tumour cells. Stromal cells interact with tumour cells through growth factors and developmental signalling pathways that form a complex paracrine loop that stimulates tumour proliferation and invasion [3].

Growth factors are often over-expressed in cancers as they play an important role in cellular proliferation and evasion of apoptosis. Increased sensitivity to growth factors can be as a result of up-regulation by tumour cells of the factors themselves or their receptors. More recently, it been demonstrated that the surrounding stroma plays an important role through complex paracrine interaction with the tumour mediated in part by growth factors [24].

Epidermal growth factor receptor (EGFR or HER1) is a member of the ErbB family of tyrosine kinase receptors of which EGFR, ErbB2, and ErbB3 are over-expressed in pancreatic cancer [25]. Up-regulation of *EGFR* is seen in 70% of pancreatic cancer cases with two principal binding ligands that are similarly over-expressed: epidermal growth factor (EGF) and transforming growth factor-α (TGF-α) [20]. On binding of EGF or TGF-α to the extracellular domain, phosphorylation of the receptor occurs providing a binding site for an SOS/GRB2/SHC protein complex that triggers exchange of GDP for GTP on RAS proteins and subsequent activation of RAF/MAPK and PI3K/AKT pathways [26].

Vascular endothelial growth factor (VEGF) is an angiogenesis-inducing agent that is expressed in response to hypoxic stimuli or oncogenic signalling [9]. As the tissue environment of pancreatic cancer is typically hypovascular, up-regulation of VEGF is found in 90% of pancreatic cancers [7]. In addition, VEGF binds to VEGF receptors (VEGFR1–3) on the surface of the tumour cell, promoting cell growth and survival through induction of RAF/MEK and PI3K/AKT pathways [26]. Hypoxia-inducible factor 1α (HIF-1α) expression is induced by both the PI3K/AKT and RAF/MEK pathways, which in turn stimulates further VEGF expression [27].

Insulin-like growth factor receptor 1 (IGF1R) is a further tyrosine kinase receptor that acts via insulin receptor substrate (IRS) proteins to recruit PI3K to the cellular membrane, resulting in the phosphorylation of PIP2 and initiation of the PI3K/AKT pathway [4]. IGF1R is overexpressed in up to 60% of pancreatic cancers [28]. These receptors are activated by the insulin-like growth factor protein (IGF), which is likewise elevated in pancreatic cancer [29].

Platelet-derived growth factor (PDGF) has been implicated in many pathways that signal for tumour growth, angiogenesis, invasion, and metastasis. Although this is not completely understood, upstream regulators of PDGF secretion include urokinase plasminogen activator (uPA), interleukin-1β (IL1β), and reactive oxygen species (ROS) such as hydrogen peroxide [30]. Up-regulation of PDGF acts to drive tumour cell proliferation via pathways including RAS (PI3K/AKT and RAF/ERK), NFκB and Notch. More importantly, associations have been made with matric metalloproteinases (MMPs), enzymes that are capable of degrading basement membranes and ECM, a process thought to be crucial in the development of metastatic spread [31].

EMT, stem cells, and signalling pathways

Epithelial-to-mesenchymal transition (EMT) describes the process whereby tumour cells lose their epithelial characteristics and acquire invasive stem cell-like features that expand their ability for local invasion and metastases. These changes have even been described in PanIN-2 and -3 lesions in mice, challenging the classical model that metastases occur late in development of cancer. Genetic mutation that enables cells to invade and seed distant sites was previously considered a late event [32, 33].

Pancreatic stem cells (PSCs) account for 0.2–0.8% of pancreatic tumour cell population and exhibit up to a 100-fold increase in tumorigenic potential [34]. Additionally, they possess properties such as self-renewal, ability to produce differentiated progeny, and up-regulation of the embryonic signalling molecule sonic hedgehog, which that are usually associated with typical stem cells [35]. They could, however, offer new treatment opportunities as depleting the PSCs in a tumour can almost entirely deplete the metastatic potential of a tumour in a mouse xenograft model [36].

Notch

Notch is an important cell-to-cell developmental signalling pathway that is inappropriately activated in pancreatic cancer and leads to tumour initiation and progression [37]. In the normal adult pancreas, Notch signalling is largely inactive, although reactivation has been observed following pancreatic injury, such as in pancreatitis, and is thought to be involved in cellular regeneration [38]. Notch signalling occurs through binding of five known ligands (delta-like—DLL1/3/4 or jagged—JAG1/2) to Notch receptors (NOTCH1-4) and results in a series of proteolytic steps that release the Notch receptor intracellular domain (NICD). Following translocation to the nucleus, the NICD initiates a transcriptional cascade that includes the oncogenes *CCND1* (Cyclin D), *MYC*, and *BCL-2* [39].

Inappropriate activation of the Notch pathway in pancreatic cancer is thought to occur via growth factor signalling, such as TGF-α, and therefore stromal cells are likely to play in important role [40]. It has been shown that Notch signalling is involved in both acinar-to-ductal metaplasia, thought to occur early in development of pancreatic adenocarcinoma, and epithelial-to-mesenchymal transition, leading to cells with the ability invade surrounding tissue and metastasize [40, 41].

Hedgehog

Hedgehog (Hh) is an embryonic signalling pathway that is employed in the gastrointestinal tract for normal organ development. Three subgroups of Hh ligands (sonic, Indian, and desert) combine with two transmembrane receptors, patched (PTCH) and smoothened (SMO), to direct cellular development via the glioma-associated oncogene homologue (GLI) family of proteins [35]. In the majority of adult tissues the pathway is inactivated by the absence of ligand, allowing inhibition of SMO through the binding of PTCH, although it remains important in the proliferation of adult stem cells, such as the haematopoetic system [42].

Although inactivating mutations of the PTCH receptor occur, it is ligand over-expression that is thought to be the major contributor to the abnormal Hh signalling that is implicated in initiation and growth of the pancreatic tumours [35]. Abnormal Hh ligand expression is seen in approximately 75% of pancreatic cancers and is thought to be an early event as it has been detected in PanIN lesions [43]. The contribution of stromal cells that secrete growth factors in response to increased Hh ligand, initiating RAS-mediated tumour cell proliferation also appears important [44]. Finally, aberrant Hh signalling is thought to be essential for the proliferation of pancreatic cancer stem cells, as blockade of the Hh pathway eliminates these cells and prolongs survival in mice [45].

Wnt-β-catenin

Wnt-β-catenin signalling is another developmental pathway involved in the proliferation and differentiation of several organs. Wnt ligands bind to Frizzled receptors and trigger the release of intracellular Dishevelled (Dvl) protein that blocks the degradation of β-catenin by a complex comprised of adenomatous polyposis coli (APC), Axin, and GSK-3β proteins [35]. B-catenin accumulates in the nucleus as a result and activates target genes through the transcription factors of the TCF/LEF family, thus driving proliferation.

The role of Wnt-β-catenin remains contentious in pancreatic cancer as, although accumulation of β-catenin has been demonstrated, genetic lesions affecting the proteins involved in β-catenin signalling are rare [35]. Although the exact mechanism of β-catenin accumulation is currently unknown, increasing levels of β-catenin correlate with PanIN grade, and inhibition of β-catenin moderates proliferation and prompts apoptosis in pancreatic cancer cells [46, 47].

NF-κB

The nuclear factor of κ-light-chain-enhancer of activated B cells (NF-κB) protein complex controls transcription factors that are rapidly activated in by harmful cellular stimuli and play an important role in the cellular response to inflammation. The principal components are the receptor activator of nuclear factor κB (RANK), a type of tumour necrosis factor receptor (TNFR), and the interleukin 1 receptor (IL1R). Upon binding of their respective ligands (RANKL/IL1), receptor activation is mediated via TNF receptor associated factor (TRAF) proteins that activate IκB kinase (IKK) enzymes and release NFκB from inhibitor of κB proteins (IκB). Nuclear gene transcription then occurs, resulting in cellular proliferation, and protects the cell from apoptosis.

In 95% of pancreatic cancer, this pathway is activated in either of two ways. The first is in an autocrine loop instigated by KRAS, causing direct activation of IKK via the PI3K/AKT pathway and production of the transcription factor activator protein 1 (AP-1), which is responsible for transcription of several cytokines, including IL1 [8, 48]. The second is paracrine activation of RANK and IL1R by cytokines, such as TNF-α, which is synthesized by stromal cells, such as macrophages and emphasizes the importance of the desmoplasia that characterizes pancreatic cancer [49].

Pathology

Gross findings

The term 'pancreatic cancer' comprises a number of various malignant epithelial pancreatic neoplasms. Most commonly, however, it refers to pancreatic ductal adenocarcinoma, which will be the focus of this chapter. Pancreatic cancer most frequently arises in the pancreatic head (60–70% of cases), where it is typically located in the superior part between the bile duct and the main pancreatic duct. Of tumours 5–15% arise in the body, 10–15% in the tail, and 5–15% affect the entire gland [50]. In rare instances, pancreatic cancer has been reported to arise from ectopic pancreas [51]. On the cut surface, pancreatic cancer characteristically imposes as firm, solid, white-yellow mass with ill-defined borders. The lobulated architecture of the pancreas is lost within most tumours. Necrosis is not typical but may occur, as well as areas of small cystic transformation, the latter frequently displaying obstructed, dilated non-neoplastic pancreatic ducts. In resected specimens, tumours show a median size of approximately 3 cm (1.5–5 cm), and the vast majority display infiltration of the peripancreatic fatty tissue [51, 52]. When located in the pancreatic head, tumours frequently infiltrate the duodenal wall and the intrapancreatic bile duct. Furthermore, infiltration of the portal vein and the stomach are common, the latter especially when tumours arise from the pancreatic body or tail. Small tumours that are restricted to the pancreas are rare and typically represent incidental findings in specimens of chronic pancreatitis, or areas of invasive cancer within larger cystic pancreatic neoplasms such as intraductal papillary mucinous neoplasms or mucinous cystic neoplasms [52].

Microscopic findings

See Figure 40.2. The majority of pancreatic cancers are well to moderately differentiated and consist of glandular and duct-like epithelial formations that are embedded in a usually abundant desmoplastic stroma [51]. As summarized in Table 40.1, grading is based on histological and cytological criteria, such as the mucin production and nuclear features, and the mitotic activity. Well-differentiated carcinomas display glandular and duct-like formations of neoplastic epithelia that are typically well formed and of angular or irregular shape. They consist of cuboidal to columnar mucinous cells with little polymorphism. The cytoplasm is eosinophilic but may also be pale or with a clear cell appearance. Mitoses are rare [51]. Moderately differentiated carcinomas resemble well-differentiated tumours; however, the growth pattern and the cytology are more variable. Thus, moderately differentiated carcinomas consist of medium-sized duct-like structures and small tubular glands of variable size and shape, including incompletely formed glands and cribriform patterns. The tumour cells show a moderate polymorphism; nucleoli may be prominent. The mitotic rate is increased. The cytoplasm is usually eosinophilic, but a clear cell aspect may occur [51]. In poorly differentiated pancreatic cancer, the tumours display densely packed, small irregular glands, solid sheets and nests, and isolated tumour cells [51]. There is a marked nuclear pleomorphism and high mitotic activity [51]. In contrast to well and moderately differentiated ductal adenocarcinomas, poorly differentiated tumours frequently show only little or no desmoplastic stroma, which may cause difficulties in the gross detection of the masses. In case of intratumoural heterogeneity, the highest tumour grade must be reported, even if only present in a minor fraction of the neoplasm [51].

Distinction of pancreatic cancer from non-neoplastic ducts may be difficult in the setting of chronic pancreatitis. As a rule, neoplastic glands display an irregular, haphazard architecture while a lobular architecture is maintained in chronic pancreatitis. On the cellular level, even well-differentiated adenocarcinomas display some loss of polarity, the nuclei of neoplastic cells are greater than in non-neoplastic ducts, and there is some variation in size. Close proximity of ductal structures to muscular vessels suggests the diagnosis of pancreatic cancer [50].

Immunhistochemical and molecular markers

Pancreatic cancer shows immunoreactivity for keratins 7, 8, 18, 19, and less frequently keratin 20 [52, 53]. CEA, B72.3, CA125, CA19-9, MUC1, MUC3, MUC4, and MUC5AC usually stain positive, in contrast to MUC2 [51]. Pancreatic cancer may contain scattered synaptophysin and chromogranin A-positive neuroendocrine cells [51]. Their immunohistochemical profile discriminates pancreatic ductal adenocarcinoma from other exocrine and neuroendocrine pancreatic neoplasms. However, distinction from non-neoplastic ducts or bile duct cancer is not possible based on immunohistochemistry alone.

Several other molecular markers, such as Smad4 or p53 may be assessed immunohistochemically, as discussed in detail in the chapter on 'Molecular Biology'.

Tumour spread

Pancreatic cancer is a highly aggressive neoplasm that typically shows extensive local spread at the time of the clinical diagnosis. Depending on the tumour location within the pancreas, this may include, among others, infiltration of the peripancreatic fatty tissue, the duodenal wall, mesenteric vessels, the stomach, the spleen, the mesentery and peritoneum, as well as the large bowel. Besides direct infiltrative growth of the tumour cells, the infiltration of nerves may significantly contribute to the local spread, showing intense tumour-nerve interactions [55]. Further common findings are infiltration of blood vessels and lymphatics, and about 75% of resected pancreatic cancers reveal lymph node metastases [52]. Distant metastases most frequently affect the liver, as well as the peritoneum, lung, bones, and adrenals [51, 56].

The staging of pancreatic cancer considers size and extent of the tumours for the local stage [57, 58]. A full explanation of the TNM staging for pancreatic cancer can be accessed at the website of the American Cancer Society [59]

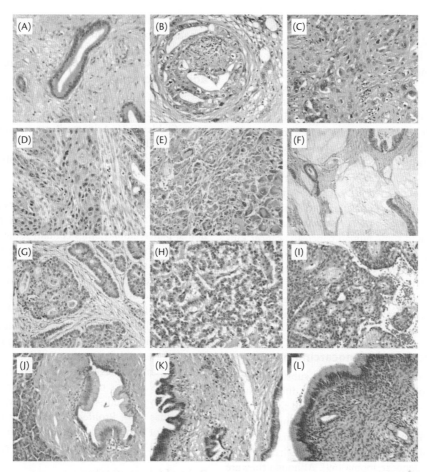

Fig. 40.2 Microscopic findings of: (A) well-differentiated pancreatic ductal adenocarcinoma; (B) moderately differentiated pancreatic ductal adenocarcinoma with perineural invasion; (C) poorly differentiated pancreatic ductal adenocarcinoma; (D) adenosquamous carcinoma showing ductal and solid, squamous differentiation; (E) anaplastic carcinoma with osteoclast-like giant cells (right bottom); (F) noncystic mucinous adenocarcinoma; (G) acinar cell carcinoma; (H) neuroendocrine tumor; (I) solid-pseudopapillary neoplasm with regressive changes; (J) pancreatic intraepithelial neoplasia grade 1; (K) intraductal-papillary mucinous neoplasm with heterogeneous grade of dysplasia; (L) mucinous cystic neoplasm with ovarian-type stoma and low-grade dysplasia.

Table 40.1 Grading of pancreatic ductal adenocarcinoma

Grade	Glandular differentiation	Mucin production	Mitoses (per 10 HPF)	Nuclear features
G1	Well-differentiated	intensive	5	Little pleomorphism, polar arrangement
G2	Moderately differentiated duct-like and tubular structures	irregular	6–10	Moderate polymorphism
G3	Poorly differentiated glands, abortive mucoepidermoid and pleomorphic structures	abortive	<10	Marked polymorphism, increased size

Abbreviation: HPF, high power fileld.

Reproduced with permission from Lüttges J. et al., The grade of pancreatic ductal carcinoma is an independent prognostic factor and is superior to the immuno-histochemical assessment of proliferation, *Journal of Pathology*, Volume 191, Issue 2, pp. 154–161, Copyright © 2000 John Wiley and Sons Ltd.

Remarkably, the T4 stage is defined by infiltration of the celiac axis or the superior mesentery artery, which usually implements inoperability of the patients. The regional lymph node status should be determined on examination of at least ten lymph nodes [57].

Prognosis and predictive factors

Inoperable tumours, which make up about 90% of cases, result in median survival times of three to five months [51]. In resected pancreatic cancer the median survival is ten to 20 months, with five-year-survival of 15–25% [51]. Prognostic factors, identified in larger series of resected pancreatic cancer, include the TNM system, resection status, grade, age, preoperative insulin-dependant diabetes mellitus, CA19-9 levels, and a stratification of risk factors leads to an improved survival prognostication [52, 60]. Concerning R status, a revised R0-classification, defined by tumour-free distance of 1 mm to the margins, has been shown significantly to improve the prognostic value [52]. Therefore, resected specimens should be examined systematically, considering the transection margins of the pancreas, bile duct, duodenum/stomach, resected large vessels, and the peripancreatic margins, inked for topographic orientation [61, 62].

Precursor lesions

PanIN are morphologically well-characterized precursor lesions of pancreatic cancer [63]. It has been suggested that PanIN originate from the centroacinar compartment [64, 65]. Paralleling an increase of dysplasia grade (PanIN 1A/B, 2, 3) they accumulate mutations, epigenetic changes, and microRNA phenoytypes that are typical for pancreatic cancer [63, 66]. The evolution from PanIN lesions to invasive pancreatic cancer could also be reproduced in genetically engineered mice [63]. The frequency of PanIN lesions increases with age and in chronic pancreatitis [63]. As especially low-grade PanIN lesions are by far more frequently detected than pancreatic cancer and may already be seen in children, a 1% probability of a single PanIN lesion progressing to invasive cancer has been estimated [67]. More recently, flat atypical lesions have been reported as precursor lesions in animal models and some human pancreatic cancer kindreds with a strong family history [68]. Furthermore, lobulocentric atrophy with associated PanIN was reported to accumulate in pancreatic cancer patients with familial predisposition [51].

Cystic neoplasms, intraductal papillary mucinous neoplasm and mucinous cystic neoplasms, may progress to pancreatic cancer (Table 40.2).

Variants of pancreatic ductal adenocarcinoma

Pancreatic ductal adenocarcinoma may contain substantial areas of mixed squamous, neuroendocrine and/or acinar differentiation. Non-cystic mucinous carcinomas are characterized by extensive mucin production. Rarely, tumours contain signet ring cells [50]. Anaplastic carcinomas which may lose their epithelial and gain mesenchymal characteristics were shown to evolve from PanIN and conventional ductal adenocarcinoma [69]. Although they are highly aggressive neoplasms, long-term survivors were observed in cases containing osteoclast-like giant cells [70]. Medullary and hepatoid carcinomas are exceedingly rare.

Pancreatic cancer other than pancreatic ductal adenocarcinoma

Besides pancreatic ductal adenocarcinoma and its variants, various neuroendocrine and exocrine malignancies arise from the pancreas (Table 40.3). Acinar cell carcinomas typically show acinar, solid, or trabecular growth patterns, express acinar markers (e.g., trypsin) and lack a marked desmoplastic stroma [50, 41]. They metastasize early to lymph nodes and/or liver. The overall five-year survival rate is poor (6%), but it has been suggested that patients with limited metastatic disease may benefit from surgery [71]. In addition to an epithelial component resembling acinar cell carcinoma, pancreatoblastomas contain squamoid bodies and eventually neuroendocrine or primitive-appearing small cell areas [51]. The overall survival is 50%, with a highly unfavourable outcome in non-resectable patients [51]. Solid pseudopapillary neoplasms display solid-appearing cell-rich areas containing thick-walled capillaries. Degenerative changes result in cystic changes with pseudopapillary aspect. These low-grade malignant neoplasms predominantly affect young females and have a good prognosis even in cases with liver metastasis [50, 51]. A centroacinar origin of these tumours has been suggested. Neuroendocrine tumours/carcinomas express neuroendocrine markers (Chromogranin A, Synaptophysin) and show similar growth patterns to acinar cell carcinomas [50]. Proliferation activity (mitotic count, Ki67) is essential for tumour classification [51]. In serous cystic neoplasms, malignancy, as defined by metastases, is exceedingly rare [51].

Role of frozen section

Frozen section is primarily useful to examine the pancreatic transection margin. While there is general agreement that this should be free of invasive cancer, the significance of PanIN in the transection

Table 40.2 Intraductal papillary mucinous neoplasms and mucinous cystic neoplasms

Macroscopy	Histology/immunohistochemistry	Comment
Intraductal papillary mucinous neoplasm		
Cystic tumours involving main duct and/or branch ducts, filled with mucin	Mucinous epithelium with low-, intermediate- or high-grade dysplasia or invasive cancer (ductal or colloid phenotype) Gastric (MUC5AC), intestinal (MUC2, MUC5AC), pancreatobiliary (MUC1, MUC5AC, MUC6), and oncocytic (MUC1, MUC6) types	Marked heterogeneity within tumours may require complete sampling
Mucinous cystic neoplasm		
Uni-or multilocular cystic tumours without duct association (>95% tail)	Mucinous epithelium with low, intermediate, or high-grade dysplasia or invasive cancer (ductal or anaplastic phenotype). Ovarian-type stroma. Cytokeratins 7, 8, 18, 19, MUC5AC	Strong preponderance for women

Source: data from Bosman FT et al. (Eds.), *WHO Classification of Tumours of the Digestive System*, 4th ed., IARC press, Lyon, Copyright © 2010; and Hruban RH et al. (Eds.), *Tumours of the Pancreas*, AFIP Atlas of Tumour Pathology Series 4, Fascicle 6, Armed Forces Institute of Pathology, Washington DC, Copyright © 2007.

Table 40.3 Independent prognostic factors for overall survival in patients undergoing resection for pancreatic cancer

Risk factor	Category	Risk assessment
Age	≥70 versus <70 years	+
IDDM	yes versus no	+
CA19-9	≥400 versus <400 U/mL	+
T status	Tis/T1/T2 versus T3	−
	T4 versus T3	+
Lymph node ratio	>0.2 versus 0/≤0.2	+
Distant metastasis	M1 versus M0	+
R status	R0 revised versus R0 old/R1/R2	−
Grading	G1 versus G2	−
	G3/4 versus G2	+

Abbreviations: IDDM, insulin dependent diabetes mellitus; +, adverse prognostic factor; −, good prognostic factor.

Reproduced with permission from Hartwig W et al., Pancreatic cancer surgery in the new millennium: better prediction of outcome, *Annals of Surgery*, Volume 254, Issue 2, pp. 311–319, Copyright © 2011 Wolters Kluwer Health.

margin is debated, and it has been suggested that even the presence of PanIN 3 in the transection margin does not influence the survival of pancreatic cancer patients [72]. Secondly, preoperatively unclear masses and cystic lesions can be diagnosed by frozen sections, helping to plan the extent of operations.

Surgical management of pancreatic adenocarcinoma

In resectable pancreatic adenocarcinoma, surgery remains the cornerstone of therapy; advances in applied surgical technique have led to a decrease of perioperative mortality from more than 30% decades ago to less than 5% in high-volume centres today [73–75]. Unfortunately, about 80% of patients present with an advanced often metastasized disease with surgery not being the primary treatment option [75, 76].

Treatment algorithm

Once a pancreatic malignancy is suspected, patients should be thoroughly examined following standardized algorithms and categorized into one of the three treatment groups described below (see also 'Definitions of resectability') [74, 77, 78]. As a volume–outcome relationship has been confirmed in studies, patients should be offered referral to high-volume centres for further management [79, 80]. The main question that needs to be answered is whether the primary tumour is resectable. It is well known that experienced surgeons will judge cancers as resectable, even with advanced disease and vessel infiltration, which would otherwise be denied the possibility of surgery [81–83].

Pancreatic cancers can be categorized into localized and systemically metastasized disease. The group of patients presenting with systemic disease is treated with systemic chemotherapy, palliative surgery, endoscopic intervention, and best supportive care [77].

Patients in the localized pancreatic cancer group should be divided into resectable, borderline-resectable, and unresectable cases. Treatment will follow a standardized algorithm; patients with resectable tumours will undergo exploration laparotomy and resection of the tumour with the goal of R0 status with curative intent. In case of a borderline-resectable cancer, neoadjuvant therapy should be contemplated. However, some surgeons still opt for a primary surgical approach, as preoperative assessment of resectability is still not optimal and the term 'borderline-resectable' is defined differently among surgeons, despite efforts to standardize these definitions (see 'Definitions of resectability'). Patients primarily categorized as locally unresectable should undergo neoadjuvant (radio)chemotherapy for local downsizing followed by laparotomy with the goal of curative R0 resection [77, 78].

If the intraoperative judgement is that an R0 resection is not possible and/or systemic disease exists (distant metastases, peritoneal seeding), palliation surgery may be performed in the same session, for example by a double bypass (gastro-enterostomy and bilodigestive anastomosis).

Preoperative workup

The standardized preoperative workup always involves an interdisciplinary team approach of a team familiar with routine treatment of this disease. Members of this expert team include surgical oncologists and/or pancreatic surgeons, radiologists, medical oncologists, radiation oncologists, and endoscopy experts [77, 78, 84].

A standardized workup consists of abdominal ultrasound and CT scan according to special pancreas protocols. Pancreas protocol MRI might evolve as an alternative for selected patients. Endoscopic ultrasound (EUS) is optional. The role of PET/CT remains uncertain outside of clinical trials. Histological confirmation of pancreatic adenocarcinoma is contraindicated in patients with resectable and borderline resectable disease if primary surgical resection is planned, due to prolonged waiting time for surgery and risk of tumour cell dissemination and the missing of a therapeutic consequence [77]. However, histological confirmation of pancreatic adenocarcinoma, preferably via EUS-guided fine needle aspiration (FNA), is mandatory before induction of neoadjuvant or palliative treatment options.

Definitions of resectability

The group of patients with locally confined disease can be further divided into resectable, borderline-resectable, and non-resectable cases (see also 'Multidisciplinary management of complex cases'). According to current consensus on definitions, these are defined as follows [77, 85].

Resectable

* Tumours recognized as being locally resectable will present without any signs of distant metastases (including para-aortic lymph node metastases).

* Resectable tumours have no signs of superior mesenteric vein (SMV) or portal vein infiltration, no tumour thrombus, and no venous encasement.

* Resectable tumours have no signs of arterial involvement (clear planes around the superior mesenteric artery (SMA), the celiac trunk and the hepatic artery.

Borderline resectable

* Borderline resectable tumours present without any signs of distant metastases (including para-aortic lymph node metastases).

* Borderline resectable tumours may present with portal vein/ SMV involvement, including impingement, narrowing of the lumen, encasement, occlusion, tumour thrombus, infiltration. Venous involvement has to be with sufficient clear venous vessel allowing for safe venous resection and reconstruction.

* Borderline resectable tumours may present with gastroduodenal artery encasement up to the hepatic artery (including short segment encasement of the hepatic artery), but without any involvement of the celiac trunk.

* Borderline resectable tumours may have tumour abutment of the SMA not exceeding involvement of 180 degree of the vessel wall.

Unresectable

* Any pancreatic adenocarcinoma presenting in the stage of systemic disease (distant metastases).

* Aortic invasion or encasement.

* Involvement of more than 180 degree of the circumference of the SMA.

* Any celiac trunk involvement.

* Unreconstructible SMV and/or portal vein infiltration

Operative technique

Surgery should be performed in specialized high-volume pancreatic cancer centres [79, 80]. The goal of every potentially curative pancreatic resection should be a R0 resection with complete removal of the tumour and a standardized lymphatic dissection with a safe reconstruction technique.

Standard resection techniques are the pylorus-preserving Kausch–Whipple resection (pylorus preserving pancreaticoduodenectomy; PPPD), the pancreatic left (tail) resection and the total pancreatectomy, depending on the location and extent of the tumour.

History of pancreatic surgery

The first documented pancreatic resection has been attributed to Friedrich Trendelenburg, who performed a distal pancreatectomy and splenectomy in a patient with a sarcoma originating from the tail of the pancreas in 1882, more than a century ago [86]. The first modern pancreaticoduodenectomy has been credited to Walther Carl Eduard Kausch, who described a two-staged pancreaticoduodenectomy, which he performed in Berlin, Germany in 1909 [87]. A one-stage pancreaticoduodenectomy had been performed in 1912 by Georg Hirschel of Heidelberg, Germany [88]. In 1935 a landmark article was published by Allen Oldfather Whipple describing his surgical experience in three cases of pancreatic ampullary carcinoma, linking his name to the procedure of pancreaticoduodenectomy [89]. Recent advances have been extended vascular resections, neoadjuvant therapies for primarily unresectable disease, the introduction of laparoscopic techniques as well as stapling devices into the field of pancreatic cancer surgery [83, 90–93].

Standard and pylorus-preserving Kausch–Whipple operation

Nowadays, the pylorus-preserving pancreaticoduodenectomy (PPPD or pp-Whipple surgery) is the option of choice for most adenocarcinomas located in the pancreatic head (see Figure 40.3). The pylorus-preserving modification of the classical Kausch–Whipple operation was described by Traverso and Longmire in 1978 [94, 95]. Current studies have shown the superiority of this modification with respect to operation time and intraoperative blood loss, while maintaining equal morbidity and short- and long-term mortality rates [96]. The classical Kausch–Whipple procedure should still be performed in tumours close to/or infiltrating the proximal duodenum and/or the stomach.

Both the classical Kausch–Whipple surgery and the pylorus-preserving modification start with a meticulous exploration of the abdomen to rule out peritoneal carcinomatosis and/or distant metastases. Any suspicious areas will be biopsied and analysed by a pathologist via frozen sections to exclude systemic disease. The next step is the mobilization of the right colonic flexure, the duodenum, and pancreatic head by a Kocher manoeuvre. After dissection of the gastrocolic ligament or the greater omentum from the transverse colon, access to the lesser sac is obtained. Next the SMV is identified and tumour size, tumour relation to the portal vein, and retroperitoneal infiltration are investigated at this point. Careful preparation of the hepatoduodenal ligament will provide details about potential arterial involvement and any potential accessory hepatic arteries.

The operation continues with the resection phase, which consists of a cholecystectomy, standard lymphadenectomy, and transection of the hepatic duct, gastroduodenal artery, and the duodenum (preserving a short postpyloric segment).

The standard lymphadenectomy includes the lymph nodes within the hepatoduodenal ligament, around the common hepatic artery, portal vein, SMV, right-sided from the celiac trunk and the SMA root. Extended lymphadenectomy has not provided better outcome results with regard to survival, while producing a higher morbidity rate, and should therefore not be performed [97–99].

The pancreas will then be cut above the portal vein via sharp dissection, and pancreas and bile duct resection margins will be sent to immediate histopathological analysis via frozen section to confirm clear resection margins. After complete mobilization of the pancreatic head and uncinate process from the SMA, the horizontal part of the duodenum is cut with a linear stapler and the resection phase ends (Figure 40.3A). The medial resection margin (i.e. the SMA margin) is well known to be the most critical for a margin-positive resection (R1) [100]. It is currently under examination whether alternative surgical strategies (e.g., artery first approach) may lower the high positive margin rate [101].

The most important part of the reconstruction phase is the pancreatic anastomosis. This can be either performed via a pancreaticojejunostomy or pancreaticogastrostomy. Both techniques can be regarded as equal, as long as a tension-free anastomosis in well-perfused tissue without obstruction is performed [102]. The biliodigestive anastomosis is performed as an end-to-end anastomosis approximately 15 cm arborally from the pancreatic anastomosis. The duodenum is anastomosed antecolically with the jejunum 50 cm distally from the hepaticojejunostomy (Figure 40.3B). Antecolic reconstruction has been shown to reduce the incidence of delayed gastric emptying [103]. Drainage placement has not been shown to improve surgical outcome; however, many surgeons still use drains for two to three days post-operatively to measure enzyme activity [104].

The classical Whipple procedure is similar to the modified version with the difference that the distal 1/3 of the stomach is resected and gastrointestinal continuity is reestablished via an antecolic gastrojejunostomy.

Left resection (pancreatic tail resection)

Resection of the pancreatic tail will be performed in tumours of the left side and pancreatic corpus. The lower resection rate in this type of surgery results from the usually more advanced disease in left-sided pancreatic cancer, as symptoms usually only appear in a very late (unresectable) stage of disease. In most cases a splenectomy with resection of the splenic vessels will be performed simultaneously to achieve R0 status.

After transection of the gastrosplenic ligament and mobilization of the left colon the pancreas is undermined above the SMV. After transection of the splenic artery and vein the pancreatic tail can then be removed together with the spleen; care should be taken to obtain a negative retroperitoneal resection margin.

The critical part of this operation is the closure of the remaining pancreas with an incidence of pancreatic fistulas in the literature ranging from 0–70%. A recent trial has compared closure with a stapling device compare to hand suture and found no significant difference with regard to the fistula rate [92].

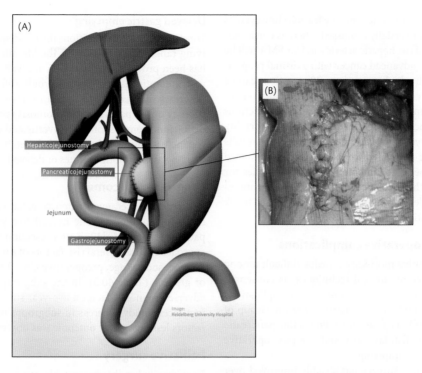

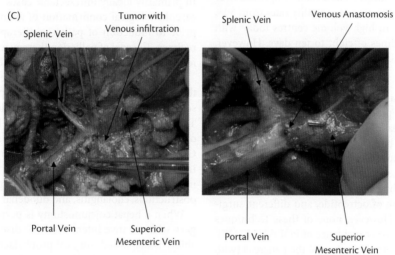

Fig. 40.3 (A) Status after pancreatic head resection with standardized lymph adenectomy; (B) standard reconstruction after a pylorus preserving pancreaticoduodenectomy (inlay: pancreaticojejunostomy); (C) portal vein resection for advanced pancreatic cancer.
Image 40.3(A) reproduced courtesy of Heidelberg University Hospital.

Total pancreatectomy

If a clear resection margin cannot be achieved with a Whipple procedure or for multifocal tumours in the pancreas, a total pancreatectomy might be indicated if R0 resection status can then be achieved. Due to the possibly higher long-term sequelae after total pancreatectomy, indications should be reviewed carefully and PPPD should be preferred whenever possible.

Laparoscopic pancreatic surgery

In recent years laparoscopic pancreatic surgery has evolved in some high-volume centres. Indications should be reviewed critically and laparoscopic surgery for pancreatic malignancies should be performed within clinical trials in high-volume centres only. In

experienced hands good results, even including extended resections with vascular reconstructions, can be achieved [91, 93, 105].

Vascular resection

Venous infiltration is common for pancreatic cancer and results in vascular resections involving the SMV and/or portal vein in 20–25% of the cases. En bloc venous resections can be performed with equal perioperative mortality and morbidity rates as standard resections. Median survival after venous resection is superior to palliative chemotherapy, and long-term survival is a possibility. Therefore venous resection should be performed if necessary and R0 situations can otherwise not be achieved [83] (Figure 40.3C).

Resection of arterial structures is technically feasible; however, its potential benefits are controversially discussed. There is consensus that arterial involvement of the hepatic arteries and/or SMA will be a sign of aggressive and/or advanced cancer with a dismal prognosis. However, there are individual cases where R0 resections can be achieved via hepatic artery resection or SMA resection and reconstruction. A recent meta-analysis has shown that arterial resections are associated with an increased risk of perioperative mortality and poor one- and three-year survival rates. However, the results were still more favourable compared to no resection in advanced cases [106]. There have been documentations of small series for advanced disease within the corpus/cauda with extended pancreatic left resections plus splenectomy, gastrectomy, and celiac trunk resections (Appleby operation) [107].

Management of post-operative complications

Comparison of post-operative morbidity remains difficult among centres and between different surgical techniques, as consensus regarding the definition of typical post-operative complications has only been made recently by the International Study Group of Pancreatic Surgery (ISGPS). Typical morbidities after pancreatic surgery include pancreatic fistulas, early and late post-operative bleeding, and delayed gastric emptying.

Safety of pancreatic cancer surgery has steadily improved over the recent years, shown by a reduction of mortality rates from 30% in the 1970s to less than 5% in high-volume centres today with average hospital admission times of eight to ten days. However, perioperative morbidity remains high at 30–40% [108, 109].

Pancreatic fistula

Pancreatic leakage due to post-operative pancreatic fistula (POPF) represents the major cause for procedure-related perioperative morbidity and mortality in pancreatic surgery [110]. A standard definition of POPF has only recently been agreed upon by the International Study Group on Pancreatic Fistula Definition (ISGPF) [111, 112].

Various techniques have been described in the literature aiming for a lower fistula rate including fibrin glue techniques, drainage, various types of stent, the use of octreotide, and different surgical anastomosis techniques. However, none of these techniques have provided evidence for a lower incidence of POPF [113–117]. Known risk factors for POPF are the texture of the pancreas (with a higher incidence of POPF for soft pancreas), smaller pancreatic ducts, which make anastomosis technically more challenging, and obstructions located distally from the anastomosis [90].

Post-operative haemorrhage

Post-operative haemorrhage after pancreatic surgery has been reported at a rate of 2–15% and is one of the major causes of perioperative mortality [118]. A definition of postpancreatectomy haemorrhage (PPH) has been created by the ISGPS [119]. Bleeding can be divided into early bleeding (<24 hours post-operatively), usually from an anastomotic site or insufficient haemostasis or late bleeding (>24 hours), which is usually due to erosion of vessels by leakage from the pancreatic anastomosis and/or resulting pseudoaneurysms. Late haemorrhage is usually severe and should be thoroughly examined; initial radiological intervention should be performed whenever possibly and necessary. Surgical revision is necessary if radiological intervention cannot be performed or fails [120, 121]. Mortality rates of up to 40% have been described for late post-operative bleeding [122].

Delayed gastric emptying

Due to inconsistent definitions the incidence of delayed gastric emptying ranges from 14–70% in the literature. A standard definition has been provided by the ISGPS and validated [123, 124]. Delayed gastric empting is a common morbidity after pancreatic surgery and describes the inability to return to normal diet after surgery. The patency of the pancreatic anastomosis (gastrojejunostomy or duodenojejunostomy) should be investigated endoscopically and a retropancreatic abscess should be excluded by abdominal cross-section imaging after prolonged times of delayed gastric emptying.

Long-term outcome

Pancreatic cancer, even when resected completely, is known for its dismal prognosis. The overall five-year survival rate for all patients is about 6% [125]; after resection the five-year survival rate approaches 20%. Several risk factors of a worse prognosis have been defined, such as age, preoperative CA 19-9 levels, T status, R status or grading (Table 40.3). In the subgroup of patients without any adverse prognostic factor a five-year survival of 55% was observed in a recent study, whereas in subgroups of patients with more risk factors less favourable outcome was observed [126].

Palliative surgery

In primarily locally unresectable cases or cases with systemic disease, histological confirmation of adenocarcinoma is mandatory prior to induction of palliative therapy or neoadjuvant therapy regimes. The goal of palliation therapy will be to ameliorate the suffering of the patient while ensuring the best possible quality of life.

Most patients undergoing palliative chemo- or chemoradiotherapy after diagnosis of non-curable pancreatic cancer will need some kind of interventional therapy due to disease progression. Typical indications are jaundice caused by biliary obstruction and/or duodenal stenosis due to local tumour infiltration/encasement. Generally, the surgical approach compared to the endoscopic/interventional approach is associated with a higher short-term morbidity but might provide better long-term results, due to stent obstructions, cholangitis, and duodenal stenosis [127–129].

When a hepaticojejunostomy is performed, or if during a surgery with curative intent systemic disease and/or local unresectability is diagnosed, surgical prophylactic double bypass might be indicated—even in the absence of duodenal stenosis. The prophylactic gastrojejunostomy and hepaticojejunostomy can usually be carried out with low morbidity and mortality [127–129].

A primary R2 resection of pancreatic tumours (tumour debulking) is of no survival benefit for the patients, while having a higher risk of post-operative complications, and thus should be avoided.

Surgical management of premalignant lesions

The classic premalignant lesions of ductal adenocarcinoma of the pancreas are PanINs. In addition, premalignant lesions of the pancreas are present in a high percentage of cystic tumours of the pancreas (e.g., IPMNs and MCNs). The knowledge regarding the risk of malignant transformation as well as the diagnosis and treatment of such lesions has developed rapidly over the last decade. The present section summarizes the evidence available on this topic.

With the use of modern multidetector computed tomography (MDCT) and MRI, an increasing number of cystic pancreatic lesions are detected incidentally. Recent studies have shown that in approximately 2% of the general population unsuspected pancreatic cysts are found [130, 131]. Although these lesions are often benign and harmless, about 10% of cystic pancreatic tumours are IPMNs and MCNs. Both lesions are known to have the potential to progress to invasive pancreatic cancer. It is estimated that there is a time lag of at least five years between the first presence of a cystic pancreatic neoplasm and the occurrence of associated invasive carcinoma [132]. It has been reported that pancreatic cancers in general tend to metastasize fairly late in their genetic evolution [133]. Thus, there remains a time window for detection and therapeutic intervention for premalignant lesions at a potentially curable stage.

Although cystic pancreatic lesions are generally detectable with modern abdominal imaging, it remains challenging to predict accurately which cyst can be safely followed conservatively, and which lesion is likely to progress to invasive cancer and therefore should be surgically resected before neoplastic changes occur. A five-year survival of >90% has been reported for patients with non-invasive IPMNs compared to a survival of only 40–50% if the IPMN is associated with invasive carcinoma. Overall, it is estimated that one-third of IPMNs are associated with invasive cancer at the time of surgical resection [134].

The risk of harbouring malignancy of cystic pancreatic neoplasms depends on their morphology and anatomical location. Today, it is well established that IPMNs arising in the main pancreatic duct (main-duct type) display a markedly higher risk of harbouring malignancy (60–70%) compared to IPMNs of the branch-duct type (25–35%) [135]. The prevalence of invasive cancer reported in MCN varied widely between 6% and 36%. In contrast to IPMNs, MCNs are generally solitary and do not recur after complete surgical resection. In 2006, a consortium of the International Association of Pancreatology met in Sendai, Japan and established evidence-based treatment guidelines for IPMNs and MCNs [136]. According to these 'Sendai criteria', surgical resection is recommended for all IPMNs located in the main pancreatic duct (main-duct IPMN and mixed-type IPMN). In patients with suspected branch-duct type IPMN, only those with a cyst diameter of more than 3 cm, with symptoms, with mural nodules or positive cytology should undergo resection. MCNs, unless there are contraindications for surgery, for example due to relevant comorbidity, should always be considered for surgical resection. The reason for this approach is that most MCN patients are relatively young at the time of diagnosis. Considering life expectancy and the ongoing risk for progression to invasive cancer, surgical resection is recommended in most cases. In experienced centres, surgical resection for MCNs can be performed with minimal morbidity and mortality. Since the majority of MCNs are located in the body or tail of the pancreas, resection can often be accomplished by laparoscopic means.

From preoperative imaging and even during intraoperative exploration, it is not always possible to ascertain with reliability the invasiveness of cystic pancreatic lesions. Thus, whenever any doubt exists, a formal oncological resection with lymph node dissection is warranted. Only small lesions without any preoperative signs of malignancy can be treated with limited pancreatic resection, which includes segmental pancreatic resection, middle-segment pancreatectomy, or local enucleation. However, this approach is only recommended when the intraoperative histopathological assessment is negative for malignancy and as long as negative resection margins can be obtained. Whenever intraoperative margins are positive for malignancy (high-grade dysplasia or invasive carcinoma), patients should undergo further resection, and even total pancreatectomy, if necessary. The treatment of patients with resection margins positive for benign IPMN remains debatable. Most pancreatic surgeons refrain from further resection in case IPMN with only low-grade dysplasia is found in the resection margin after pancreatectomy.

Beside from mucinous cystic neoplasms (IPMNs or MCNs), infiltrating carcinomas of the pancreas can arise from histologically defined precursor lesions in the small ducts and ductules of the pancreas [137]. These lesions are PanINs and display precursors for the common ductal adenocarcinoma of the pancreas. In contrast to cystic mucinous neoplasms of the pancreas, PanINs can only be detected by histopathologic examination. Thus, these lesions are found either incidentally in specimens resected for benign pancreatic diseases (e.g., chronic pancreatitis) or in intraoperative frozen sections of resection margins after pancreatectomies. According to the grade of dysplasia, PanINs are divided into three categories. In case PanIN 2 or 3 lesions are found incidentally on histological examination, resection should be tailored to the individual situation.

With regard to the poor prognosis of pancreatic cancer and the lack of an effective chemotherapy, early detection of premalignant lesions is crucial. Even with the use of modern abdominal imaging and fine needle aspiration, it remains difficult reliably to predict malignancy in cystic pancreatic lesions. In future, molecular biomarkers will eventually allow screening for pancreatic cystic lesions in order to enable appropriate treatment stratification.

Radiotherapy in pancreatic cancer

Pancreatic cancer is localized in a region of the body that has been particularly difficult for radiation oncologists to treat. This is due to the organs at risk surrounding the pancreas, namely stomach, duodenum, jejunum, liver, kidneys and spinal cord. However, radiotherapy has recently undergone a dramatic technical revolution in terms of high precision and protection of organs at risk which now allows the safe application of effective doses. Some of the keywords of this progress are intensity-modulated radiotherapy (IMRT) and image-guided radiotherapy (IGRT). Chemoradiotherapy which is standard for most of the situations in which radiotherapy is used in pancreatic cancer has also been refined alongside the technical improvements of radiotherapy. At the time of the publication of this book most of the clinical trials that are available were still using the technical standards prior to the above-described revolution in radiation oncology, which makes it difficult adequately to estimate the value of radiotherapy for the current situation. This is why one of the key messages of this section is that every patient with pancreatic cancer should ideally be treated within a clinical trial. In parallel to technical developments, molecular targeted approaches have also started to contribute to the progress of radiotherapy [138, 139].

Before focusing on the respective stages of pancreatic cancer, it is important briefly to address the overarching understanding of the disease with specific relevance to radiotherapy: again and again it has been shown that surgery is the only potentially curative therapeutic option underscoring the relevance of locoregional treatment. On the other hand, metastatic disease is very frequent in pancreatic cancer which only can be dealt with by systemic treatment. A post-mortem study of pancreatic cancers of all stages from patients who have succumbed to the disease has shown that uncontrolled local growth is the cause of death in 30% of patients with pancreatic cancer and DPC4 immunolabelling status was highly correlated with widespread metastases versus locally destructive tumours [140]. Therefore, finding the right balance between locoregional and systemic treatment is of the highest importance when the radiotherapy is integrated into the treatment of pancreatic cancer (Figure 40.4).

Locally advanced (unresectable) disease and palliation

Locally advanced pancreatic cancer (LAPC) is encountered in about one-third of the patients at initial presentation. LAPC is defined as unresectable disease without any detectable metastases. In the past, LAPC has often not been separated from metastatic disease especially in trials testing chemotherapy and also not from borderline resectable pancreatic cancer (BRPC). BRPC will be discussed below but it is important to remember that practically all trials reported so far have not distinguished between LAPC and BRPC.

Whenever radiotherapy is prescribed for LAPC it should be performed with chemotherapy based on a number of reports. A small prospective randomized trial comparing chemoradiotherapy versus best supportive care detected a median overall survival (mOS) of 13.2 versus 6.4 months. Additionally, quality of life was significantly better and distant metastases were significantly fewer in the chemoradiotherapy group [141]. Following a previous study [142], chemoradiotherapy was compared with radiotherapy only in a three-armed trial of the Gastrointestinal Tumour Study Group (GITSG) comparing split-course radiotherapy (60 Gy) with two arms of chemoradiation (40 Gy, 60 Gy) [143]. Median overall survival time was 8.3 and 11.3 months with chemoradiotherapy compared to 5.5 months with radiotherapy only (P < 0.01). An important detail of this trial was the requirement for laparotomy proof of LAPC and the continuation of 5-FU chemotherapy until further progression. This may explain the conflicting results of another randomized trial accruing between 1983 and 1989 [144]. This ECOG trial compared radiotherapy only to a total dose of 59.4 Gy with additional chemotherapy (5-FU: 1 g/ m2/day by continuous infusion, days 2 to 5 and 28 to 31; mitomycin-C: 10 mg/

m2 day 2) with no additive chemotherapy where median OS was 7.1 versus 8.4 months (P = n.s.). The comparison of the effects of chemoradiotherapy with chemotherapy only in LAPC is currently being intensively investigated. Based on two trials in the 1980s chemoradiotherapy was commonly accepted to be superior to chemotherapy only because these two trials demonstrated improved local control and overall survival [145, 146]. However, a recent randomized phase III trial reported inferiority of chemoradiotherapy versus gemcitabine only [146]. After chemotherapy, mOS was 13 versus 8.6 months after chemoradiotherapy. This result can be explained at least partly by the specific details of the chemoradiotherapy used: of particular importance is an excessively large radiotherapy planning treatment volume (PTV) to an unusual high total and single-dose (60 Gy in 30 fractions). This was combined with an unusual chemotherapy regimen (cisplatin and 5-FU) and resulted not only in a high rate of grade 3/4 toxicities but also of incomplete treatment in the chemoradiation arm (58% versus 27% received less than 75% of chemoradiotherapy versus chemotherapy; six versus ten cycles of maintenance chemotherapy after chemoradiotherapy). This contrasts with the results of the ECOG 4201 phase III trial which employed a much smaller PTV to a lower dose in combination with gemcitabine versus gemcitabine chemotherapy only [148]. Chemoradiotherapy followed by chemotherapy resulted in a higher rate of stable disease compared to chemotherapy only (68% versus 35%) as a result of a reduced rate of progressive disease. This resulted in prolonged overall survival at 12, 18, and 24 months (mOS 11 versus 9.2 months, P = 0.032) at the cost of an elevated rate of mainly haematological grade 4 toxicity but also fatigue and nausea/vomiting. The concomitant dose of gemcitabine at 600 mg/m2/week for six weeks is high compared to a number of other trials using gemcitabine-based chemoradiotherapy, explaining the toxicity. Classically, fluoropyrimidine-based chemoradiotherapy is regarded to be standard in pancreatic cancer [141, 149]. After the publication of a meta-analysis comparing 5-FU with gemcitabine-based chemoradiotherapy [150], gemcitabine can also be recommended for concurrent chemoradiotherapy provided that the specific rules (gemcitabine dose and PTV) for this combination, as described in more detail in the section 'Irradiation techniques', are respected. The meta-analysis comprised 229 patients. Gemcitabine-based compared to 5-FU-based chemoradiation resulted in superior 12-month-overall survival with a relative risk of 1.54 (95% CI: 1.05–2.26). However, the meta-analysis also noted the higher toxicity of gemcitabine-based chemoradiotherapy. The studies included into the meta-analysis were conducted from the late 1990s through to 2005 and no IMRT, high-conformality or systematic gastric mucosa protection were utilized to limit toxicity (see 'Irradiation techniques').

Induction chemotherapy before chemoradiotherapy started to be investigated during the last decade [138, 151–153]. Whilst the results of the first randomized controlled trials are still awaited [153], the collective evidence of early-phase and retrospective studies suggests that induction chemotherapy is suitable to select patients without early distant metastatic progression for chemoradiotherapy. In these trials duration of induction chemotherapy ranged from one to six months. The comparison between two analyses from the GERCOR group points to a minimum of three months of induction chemotherapy required for adequate selection because of the high rate of distant metastases after the completion of the chemoradiation element when only two months of gemcitabine-oxaliplatin

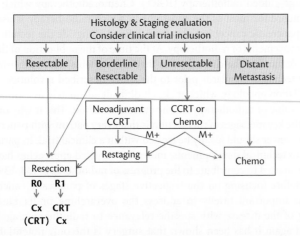

Fig. 40.4 Treatment algorithm for the multidisciplinary treatment of pancreatic cancer; tissue diagnosis should be obtained in primary non-surgical approaches of pancreatic cancer.

Abbreviations: CCRT, induction chemotherapy followed by chemoradiotherapy; Cx, chemotherapy; M+, distant metastasis; R0, R0-resection, i.e. clear margins; R1, R1-resection, i.e. microscopically positive margins.

induction chemotherapy were given [151, 152]. After three months of induction chemotherapy with various gemcitabine-based combinations, almost 30% of 181 patients had developed distant metastases. In the remaining patients mOS was 15 months after chemoradiotherapy (72 patients) versus 11.7 months after continued chemotherapy (56 patients; P = 0.0009). A retrospective report compared 247 patients with primary chemoradiotherapy with 76 patients who had 2.5 months' induction chemotherapy followed by chemoradiotherapy resulting in 11.9 versus 8.5 months mOS (P <0.001). Two months of induction chemotherapy in 69 patients with combined gemcitabine-oxaliplatin-cetuximab followed by capecitabine-cetuximab-based chemoradiotherapy produced a remarkable mOS of 19.2 months and was very well tolerated. Recently, the results of a randomized trial comparing gemcitabine- versus capecitabine-based chemoradiotherapy in patients with locally advanced pancreatic cancer being stable or responding to 12 weeks of induction chemotherapy (gemcitabine and capecitabine) were reported [155]. Even though the primary endpoint (nine-month progression free survival) was not different between the two groups (62.9% versus 51.4%), patients in the capecitabine group had a longer median overall survival (15.2 versus 13.4 months, P = 0.012) and experienced less treatment-associated toxicity.

An important and often missed opportunity after chemoradiotherapy in LAPC is secondary tumour resection. This was analysed in a systematic review and meta-analysis in 2010 [156]. For the patients with initially non-resectable tumours the trial reported a resectability rate of 33%, resulting in a median overall survival rate of 20.5 months, thus giving a similar prognosis compared to patients with initially resectable tumours. Whereas the survival rates of this meta-analysis are relatively robust, the rate of secondary resectability is probably an overestimation because resectability criteria were not clearly defined in more than half of the studies included in the analysis. Resectability criteria are based on the amount of vascular involvement, which is discussed in the section 'Borderline resectable pancreatic cancer' [157–159]. We recommend reevaluating patients six to eight weeks after completion of chemoradiotherapy for potential resection, but tumour response may also appear several months after completion of chemoradiation. CT restaging may underestimate tumour response, as it fails to discriminate adequately residual tumour from fibrosis. It has been suggested that the addition of PET/CT restaging might provide additional information [139, 160, 161]. However, future prospective studies will have to confirm these observations.

Adjuvant treatment

The concept of adjuvant chemoradiotherapy aims to reduce locoregional relapse, which has been identified as an important site of failure of 50–80% in several reports analysing the patterns of failure after surgical resection [162–165]. Most adjuvant studies additionally used systemic chemotherapy to reduce distant relapse. Since positive resection margins are found in 20–75% of the patients [166], chemoradiotherapy also specifically aims to control R1 disease after surgery. However, to date, the use of adjuvant chemoradiotherapy is a matter of great controversy and reflects the fact that all published phase III trials testing chemoradiotherapy have either been subject to serious criticism [167–170] or inadequate to testing the role of adjuvant chemoradiotherapy [171]. Much hope that this issue may be resolved surrounds the RTOG 08-48 trial,

currently recruiting, which randomizes between chemotherapy and chemoradiotherapy for patients without progressive disease after five cycles of adjuvant chemotherapy. Up to now the most convincing level I data are from adjuvant chemotherapy where the CONKO-001 trial validated gemcitabine after surgery compared to best supportive care [172], whereas the ESPAC-3 trial could not find a significant difference between gemcitabine and the Mayo Clinic 5-FU regimen [173]. In summary, the above-mentioned criticisms of the randomized trials were (1) poor recruitment of only 49 patients in eight years into the well-designed, randomized GITSG trial [168] comparing surgery only versus chemoradiotherapy (mOS 21 versus 10.9 months, P = 0.005) followed by chemotherapy which could not be invalidated by registering an additional 30 patients in a non-randomized way despite the confirmation of improved survival [170]. (2) Similarly, a trial conducted by the EORTC was underpowered and additionally confounded by including patients with periampullary cancer (mOS for pancreatic cancer 17.1 versus 12.6 months, P = 0.099) [167]. In this trial, 20% of the patients in the experimental arm never received chemoradiotherapy and no additional chemotherapy after chemoradiotherapy was given. (3) Finally, the ESPAC-1 trial was performed using a complex 2 x 2 factorial design, allowing 'background' therapy in addition to protocol therapy [169]. There were no quality assurance guidelines for radiotherapy. This might explain the poor overall survival rates in this trial of 13.9 months after adjuvant chemoradiotherapy compared with 16.9 months after surgery alone. (4) The RTOG 97-04 trial had chemoradiotherapy in both arms and compared only gemcitabine versus 5-FU in the sandwich chemotherapy, and is therefore inadequate to demonstrate the effect of chemoradiotherapy in adjuvant treatment. Two meta-analyses addressing adjuvant chemoradiotherapy mainly include data from the above-discussed trials and therefore cannot provide a solution to the above-described concerns [174, 175]. However, the meta-analysis from Stocken et al. pointed to an additional aspect of adjuvant therapy: after R1-resections adjuvant chemoradiotherapy showed a reduction of the hazard ratio by 28% whereas chemotherapy showed no significant effect on survival [174]. A retrospective analysis of 30 patients after R1-resections showed a mOS of 22.8 months after adjuvant chemoradiotherapy and consolidation chemotherapy, and appears to confirm this effect on a lower level of evidence [176]. In the absence of appropriate data from appropriately conducted phase III trials the conflicting results of large numbers of non-randomized studies should be highlighted in a recently published collaborative analysis of the Johns Hopkins Hospital and the Mayo Clinic in 1092 patients [177]. Adjuvant treatment was 5-FU-based chemoradiotherapy in 583 patients from the two centres and mOS was 21.1 versus 15.5 months (P <0.001) after adjuvant treatment or surgery only. In order to account for biases associated with non-random allocation of patients to adjuvant therapy or surgery alone, propensity score and matched-pair analyses were performed and the latter resulted in mOS of 21.9 versus 14.3 months (P < 0.001). In summary, adjuvant chemotherapy is currently standard after R0-resections and adjuvant chemoradiotherapy is reserved for clinical trials at this time at least until completion of the RTOG 08-48 trial. Chemoradiotherapy is an option in the R1-situation but requires further investigation. There are also studies of gemcitabine + nab-paclitaxel to gemcitabine alone, as well as the triple regimen FOLFIRINOX compared to gemcitabine alone.

Neoadjuvant treatment

The theoretical advantages of neoadjuvant treatment include possibly increased efficacy due to a more effective chemotherapy delivery with intact blood supply compared to reduced blood flow and increased hypoxia in the post-operative situation. Analogous to the observations made in rectal cancer it is hypothesized to achieve a higher rate of R0 –resections [178, 179], of nodal negative tumour stage (ypN0) [180], and of locoregional control, all of which have prognostic importance. Radiotherapy target volumes are difficult to define after surgery and therefore larger. This has important consequences for the acute toxicity of the treatment and limits the total dose because the gastrointestinal reconstruction receives the full dose of radiotherapy. In addition, post-operative treatment is impeded by delayed recovery after Whipple's resections in 25% of the patients [181, 182]. Moreover, neoadjuvant chemoradiotherapy is being tested in clinical trials with the hope of reducing the rate of patients who are found to be unresectable intraoperatively due to undetected metastatic disease or underestimated tumour contact to peripancreatic vessels [183]. Patients with rapid development of metastatic disease during neoadjuvant treatment can be spared a major surgical procedure. Potential disadvantages of neoadjuvant treatment are that in the absence of laparoscopic staging, patients with metastatic disease will unnecessarily receive radiotherapy. This is a realistic concern as up to 30% of the patients without evidence of metastatic disease at imaging were shown to have distant metastases during staging laparoscopy [184–186]. Concerns that neoadjuvant chemoradiotherapy increases the rate of post-operative complications have not been substantiated [185, 187]. It is also important to stress that a group of patients included in neoadjuvant trials cannot be directly compared with a group of patients treated in adjuvant trials because the intention to resect always relies on imaging which had a negative predictive value of 0.74 only with modern MDCT [186]. Where it is not possible to obtain a tissue diagnosis patients are not eligible for neoadjuvant treatment and this is typically the case in smaller tumours.

Neoadjuvant therapy for resectable disease

Patients with resectable tumours at diagnosis should not be treated with neoadjuvant chemoradiotherapy outside of clinical trials because only one randomized controlled trial has been reported so far as an abstract [185]. This multicentre trial tested primary surgery versus neoadjuvant chemoradiotherapy followed by surgery. The trial aimed to recruit 254 patients but was stopped for pure accrual after 73 patients. Of the 68 patients eligible for analysis 33 had primary tumour resection and 30 the experimental treatment. Four patients refused the allocated chemoradiotherapy and another four had tumour progression thereafter. At explorative laparotomy four versus two tumours were locally not resectable and distant metastases prevented resection in five versus eight patients respectively (primary versus neoadjuvant). Tumour resection was performed in 24 versus 20 patients by intention-to-treat analysis and the R0-resection rate was 67% versus 90% with a pN0 status of 38% versus 70%. Post-operative complications were comparable in both groups with one post-operative fatality in the arm of primary resection due to perioperative myocardial infarction. Intention-to-treat mOS was 14.4 months versus 17.4 months and analysis per protocol showed a mOS of 18 versus 25 months. An important lesson from this trial is that from randomization through to surgery, four versus eight patients were found to have distant metastases in the arm with primary resection versus pretreatment followed by surgery. This is expected with a mainly locoregional therapy where chemotherapeutic agents are administered at reduced doses. The literature for the group of patients with resectable disease is practically devoid of trials testing induction chemotherapy followed by chemoradiotherapy and resection, whereas this sequence has been described to be very active in more advanced disease and this should be a focus of future investigations [138, 151]. A recently published systematic review and meta-analysis identified 35 trials with resectable tumours and 57 trials with tumours non-resectable before treatment, and almost all studies (104/111) contained radiotherapy [156]. The grade 3/4 toxicity for the group with resectable tumours was 26.3%. Response rates after neoadjuvant treatment were comparable between resectable and non-resectable tumours: in all patients, 3.9% had complete response, 29.1% partial response, 43.9% stable disease, and 20.8% progressive disease. In the group of patients deemed resectable prior to treatment 88.1% were explored. There was an estimated rate of 73.6% for resections and 82.1% of these were R0-resections. The estimated median survival was 23.3 months with resection and 8.4 months without resection in this cohort. This is very similar compared to the results after adjuvant chemotherapy (21.7 and 22.1 months after R0 and R1 resection) [188].

Similar rates of distant metastases were reported in a large single-arm neoadjuvant phase II trial including 86 patients: 9.3% had distant disease at restaging and another 10.5% intraoperatively. In total, 74% of the patients underwent resection and achieved a mOS of 36 months [178]. Very recently, Duke University reported a large retrospective comparison of immediately operated patients (92 patients) with patients having preoperative chemoradiotherapy for resectable disease (144 patients) [188]. Resection was not performed because of distant metastases in 19% of the neoadjuvant group and in 17% of the surgery-only group. In patients with tumour resection mOS was 27 months versus 17 months in the other groups (P = 0.04).

Neoadjuvant therapy for unresectable and borderline resectable disease

Classically, neoadjuvant treatment was discriminated for resectable versus non-resectable tumours. Recently, a new category of BRPC has been introduced, which better defines the cohort of patients who might benefit from neoadjuvant therapy [158, 159, 190]. One of the problems of the currently available literature is that there are large undefined discrepancies between the definitions of resectability, and therefore it is highly recommended to use definition of BRPC consistently. On the expert consensus statement published by Callery see 'Definitions of resectability' [190]. Most of the patients reported to have had successful resection after neoadjuvant therapy for non-resectable disease are believed to be part of the group with BRPC but resection rates from such trials are influenced by patients with clearly non-resectable tumours in the literature. The system review and meta-analysis published by Gillen reported on 57 neoadjuvant studies for unresectable disease [156]. In this group 47% of the patients were explored, with an estimated rate of 33.2% resections (79.2% of these were R0 resections). The estimated mOS was 20.5 months with resection and 10.2 months without resection. Therefore, the prognosis of patients with BRPC after resection is equally good compared to those with primary resectable tumours.

Consequently, trials testing adjuvant therapy specifically in BRPC have been activated.

Of particular interest in this context is a prospective comparative study where patients with non-resectable tumours (68 patients; T3, N0-1, M0; third AJCC classification) were treated with split-course chemoradiotherapy (5-FU, streptozocin, and cisplatin) with the plan of subsequent resection compared with patients undergoing immediate resection in less advanced tumour stages (91 patients). In the neoadjuvant group, 20 patients (29.4%) were resectable and had a mOS of 32.3 months compared to 14 months for all patients with initial tumour resection (P = 0.006) and 16 months for the 69% with adjuvant chemo(radiotherapy) therapy. A different retrospective comparison of the same nature reported a mOS of 21 months after immediate resection (58 patients) versus 54 months after neoadjuvant treatment (21 patients) [191].

In summary, neoadjuvant chemoradiotherapy remains experimental. However, especially in the situation of BRPC, resectability should be reevaluated after chemoradiotherapy/chemotherapy as this is the population where the current evidence points to a particularly high impact on survival. For resectable disease, future trials should include induction chemotherapy prior to chemoradiotherapy because of the higher rates of distant metastases described in the literature.

Irradiation techniques

The previous sections have made clear that the technique of radiotherapy is of the highest importance for adequate effectiveness and tolerance, and this has recently been highlighted in a radiation therapy quality analysis of the RTOG 97-04 trial in 416 evaluable patients with adjuvant chemoradiotherapy [192]. The survival of the 52% of the patients treated according to protocol was significantly longer compared to those treated below the standard (20.9 versus 17.5 months mOS, P = 0.019), demonstrating that insufficient quality of radiotherapy can lead to false negative outcomes in the radiotherapy arm of clinical trials. Consequently, consensus panel guidelines for the delineation of the clinical target volume (CTV) in post-operative treatment, including an atlas, have been introduced [193]. Similar guidelines have been developed for the definition of treatment volumes in LAPC and for neoadjuvant therapy derived from the distribution of lymph node metastases in surgical series [194]. In the latter setting, especially, groups using full-dose gemcitabine exclude elective nodal irradiation altogether.

Chemoradiotherapy is standard for definitive, adjuvant, and neoadjuvant therapy, except for rare cases of palliative treatment. Radiotherapy should be conventionally fractionated (1.8–2.0 Gy) and standard total doses range between 50 Gy and 55 Gy. Higher doses up to 60 Gy were reported to be safe with IMRT or highly conformal treatment. Commonly accepted standard concomitant chemotherapy is either continuous infusional 5-FU or capecitabine, and gemcitabine chemoradiotherapy is an emerging alternative standard [150]. Gemcitabine appears to be more effective than fluoropyrimidines but can also be more toxic if the PTV is not carefully restricted [150, 195]. Contouring should be performed on contrast-enhanced CT scans for adequate visualization of the GTV, vessels, and small bowel. 4D treatment planning is useful to limit the expansion margins of the GTV but the recommendation is to use IGRT in parallel to avoid geographical misses [195]. Whenever possible, the classic four-field approach should no longer be used. 3D-conformal or preferably IMRT planning is recommended, as

this was recently shown to have a better toxicity profile [197, 198]. Dose constraints for organs at risk (OAR) are particularly important for the liver, kidneys, and spinal cord, as well as the stomach, duodenum, and small bowel. Gastrointestinal toxicity (acute toxicity and bleeding) is of high importance and critically depends on dosimetric values to these organs [199]. Active supportive therapy is an integral component of radiotherapy and consists of proton-pump inhibitor therapy, anti-emetic therapy, analgesia, and dietary support.

Medical management of pancreatic cancer

Given the high rates of mortality associated with resected pancreatic cancer, significant efforts have been made to improve these outcomes with the addition of chemotherapy and/or chemoradiation to patients who have undergone potentially curative surgical resection. The initial GITSG evaluated the efficacy of the addition of chemoradiation (40 Gy with weekly bolus of 5-FU for two years) versus surgery alone [200]. Median overall and two-year survival were both significantly increased in the chemoradiation group (20 months versus 11 months and 42% versus 15%, respectively). Despite the small number of patients enrolled (43), chemoradiation became a standard of care for resected pancreatic cancer, particularly in the US (Table 40.4). A second, larger EORTC study comparing the addition of infused 5-FU (5-FU dose of 25 mg/kg per

Table 40.4 Malignant epithelial pancreatic tumours

Ductal adenocarcinoma
Adenosquamous carcinoma
Colloid carcinoma (mucinous noncystic carcinoma)
Hepatoid carcinoma
Medullary carcinoma
Signet-ring-cell carcinoma
Undifferentiated carcinoma
Undifferentiated carcinoma with osteoclast-like giant cells
Acinar cell carcinoma
Acinar cell cystadenocarcinoma
Intraductal papillary mucinous neoplasm with an associated invasive carcinoma
Mixed acinar-ductal carcinoma
Mixed acinar-neuroendocrine carcinoma
Mixed acinar-neuroendocrine-ductal carcinoma
Mixed ductal-neuroendocrine carcinoma
Mucinous cystic neoplasm with an associated invasive carcinoma
Pancreatoblastoma
Serous cystadenocarcinoma
Solid-pseudopapillary neoplasm
Neuroendocrine tumour/ neuroendocrine carcinoma

Reproduced with permission from Bosman FT, Carneiro F, Hruban RH, Theise ND (Eds.), *WHO classification of tumours of the digestive system, Fourth edition,* Copyright © 2010 IARC Press.

24 hours) concurrently with 40 Gy radiation was negative [201]. However, as a trend was seen towards a benefit for chemoradiation it has been argued that this trial was underpowered. Finally, the RTOG 9704 study randomized 451 patients with resected pancreas cancer to either pre- and post-chemoradiation infused 5-FU or gemcitabine. Survival was not significantly different between the arms (16.7 months for gemcitabine and 18.8 months for 5-FU, P = 0.34) [202]. Although used to support the principle of chemoradiation, survival in this study is comparable and possibly inferior to that seen in subsequent trials utilizing chemotherapy alone. It is also noteworthy that the majority of patients in each arm received the other chemotherapy as salvage treatment on recurrence, thus potentially confounding these results.

The only study comparing all four potential adjuvant treatment approaches for resected pancreatic cancer is the randomized ESPAC1 (European Study Group for Pancreatic Cancer) study, which was initially conceived as a 2 x 2 factorial analysis of the benefits of chemotherapy ('Mayo-Clinic'-style bolus 5-FU/leucovorin; split course 5-FU-based chemoradiation; both chemotherapy and chemoradiation; or post-operative observation [203]). Analysis of the 289 patients restricted to the original factorial design demonstrated a survival benefit for chemotherapy but not for the addition of radiation. Five-year survival was 29% for patients receiving chemotherapy only, and 13.2% for patients receiving chemoradiation followed by chemotherapy. However, this was superior to those treated with chemoradiation alone (7.3%), which was comparable to the observation arm (10.7%) [204]. However, changes to the study design during the course of recruitment, and concerns regarding radiation quality control and treatment compliance have led to questions regarding the validity of this trial's results [205, 206]. Following this the CONKO-001 study compared the gemcitabine chemotherapy to surgery alone in resected patients (R0 or R1 surgical resection and a preoperative CA 19-9 level <2.5 times the upper limit of normal). The primary endpoint of an improvement in disease-free survival was achieved; this was increased from 6.9 months in the surgery-alone arm to 13.4 months for gemcitabine-treated patients (P <0.001) [207]. A survival update on this study presented in abstract form demonstrated a statistically significant overall survival benefit for the interventional arm (22.8 months versus 20.2 months, P = 0.005, five-year survival 21% versus 9%), confirming the utility of adjuvant chemotherapy in this setting [208]. Building on the perceived success of adjuvant chemotherapy in the ESPAC1 study, the ESPAC3 trial was a large (1088-patient) two-arm randomized trial comparing the benefits of six months of bolus fluorouracil and leucovorin with six months of gemcitabine [209]. Although no significant difference was seen in the two arms with respect to overall survival (23 months for fluorouracil and 23.6 months for gemcitabine, HR 0.94: 95% CI0.81–1.08), toxicity profiles favoured the gemcitabine-containing arm with lower levels of diarrhoea and stomatitis, although this did not appear significantly to impact on quality of life. Thus, both gemcitabine and 5-FU may be considered reasonable options for the adjuvant treatment of resected pancreatic cancer, although, based on tolerability, gemcitabine is more commonly selected. Additions to the gemcitabine backbone design include the current ESPAC4 trial will assess the benefit of a capecitabine/gemcitabine combination versus gemcitabine alone, and the CONK0-005 trial, which examines the addition of erlotinib to standard gemcitabine therapy.

Finally, given the number of patients in whom complete surgical resection is not possible, a neoadjuvant chemotherapy and/or chemoradiation approach is attractive. Potential benefits of this treatment strategy include assessment of chemosensitivity in vivo, reduction in tumour volume presurgery with increased respectability for 'borderline tumours', and selection of those with less aggressive disease biology who do not progress on neoadjuvant therapy to undergo a surgical procedure associated with significant morbidity. However, despite promising single-institution studies and uncontrolled trials, randomized data in this setting is lacking and it remains an experimental treatment approach [210].

Gemcitabine

For patients with advanced pancreatic cancer, meta-analysis demonstrates that chemotherapy is associated with superior survival when compared to best supportive care alone (HR 0.64 months 95%, CI 0.42–0.98) [211]. Gemcitabine (2',2'-difluorodeoxycytidine; Gemzar®, Eli-Lilly), a nucleoside analogue with structures in common with cytarabine, has until recently been the backbone of most cytotoxic chemotherapy regimens for this disease. Early studies in patients with untreated advanced pancreas cancer (800 mg/m2 IV q weekly three of four weeks) demonstrated modest response rates of 6.3–11% [212, 213]. However, given the difficulty associated with radiological assessment of response for patients with pancreatic cancer and the frequent presence of disease-related symptoms in these patients, a separate endpoint of 'clinical benefit rate' has frequently been used to assess the efficacy of chemotherapy regimens in this disease. This endpoint, a composite of changes in pain score, Karnofsky performance status (KPS), and weight was first used in conjunction with traditional measures of radiological response in a study by Rothenberg et al. of gemcitabine (1000 mg/m2 weekly x 7 followed by one week of rest, then weekly x 3 every four weeks thereafter) in 5-fluoropyramidine refractory advanced pancreas cancer patients [214]. Clinical benefit was defined as ≥50% reduction in pain intensity, ≥50% reduction in daily analgesic consumption, or ≥20 point improvement in KPS that was sustained for ≥4 consecutive weeks. Although radiological response rate in this second-line setting was comparable to other studies at 10.3%, 27% of patients derived a clinical benefit, the median duration of which was 14 weeks. Following this, the clinical benefit rate of gemcitabine in the first-line setting was demonstrated in a randomized study comparing both this and traditional measures of response and survival for patients with treatment-naive pancreatic cancer [215]. Gemcitabine was superior to 5-fluorouracil in terms of radiological response (5.3% versus 0%), progression-free survival, and overall survival (nine weeks versus one week and 5.65 months versus 4.41 months, respectively, P = 0.0025). One-year survival was nine times more likely for patients in the gemcitabine-containing cohort (18% versus 2%). Finally, the clinical benefit rate was 23.8% for gemcitabine-treated patients compared to 4.8% for those treated with 5-FU (P = 0.0022). It is of note, however, that assessors of clinical response rate in this study were not blinded to the treatment assignment leading to a potential source of bias. The results of this study led to licensing of gemcitabine for the first-line treatment of advanced pancreatic cancer.

Fixed-dose-rate infusion gemcitabine

In theory, administration of gemcitabine over a longer period may have pharmacokinetic advantages. Deoxycytidine kinase which metabolizes gemcitabine to the active gemcitabine triphosphate becomes saturated at infusion rates of >10 mg/m2/min [216, 217]. That a longer 'fixed-dose rate' infusion could impact on efficacy was suggested by a randomized phase II study of 92 patients with advanced pancreatic cancer, where those treated with gemcitabine (1500 mg/m2 over 150 minutes) compared to those treated with gemcitabine (2200 mg/m2 over 30 minutes, 'dose intense regimen') demonstrated not only elevated levels of gemcitabine triphosphate in peripheral white cells, but also superior survival to those treated with a conventional schedule (eight months versus five months, respectively) [218]. This benefit was not replicated in a larger phase III randomized study of 832 patients in which patients received standard-dose gemcitabine (1000 mg/m2 weekly x 7 followed by one week of rest, then weekly x 3 every four weeks thereafter), fixed-dose rate gemcitabine (1500 mg/m2 over 150 minutes weekly for three weeks of four), or a fixed-dose rate gemcitabine-oxaliplatin combination [219]. Median overall survival were 4.9 months and 6.5 months in the standard and fixed-dose arms, respectively, which did not meet the prespecified criteria for superiority. Thus, administration of gemcitabine outside of standard methodology is not recommended at this time.

Gemcitabine combination chemotherapy regimens

In an effort to improve the modest response rates associated with gemcitabine and to improve survival, multiple gemcitabine-based combination chemotherapy regimens have been investigated. These include the addition of cisplatin [220–223], oxaliplatin [219, 224], taxanes [225–229], fluoroyrimidines [230, 231], and irinotecan [228, 229, 232]. Although most gemcitabine-containing doublets were associated with increased response rate, none of these combinations have been demonstrated to result in a statistically significant improvement in overall survival. A possible exception to this is the combination of gemcitabine and the oral fluoropyrimidine capecitabine; the largest phase III randomized trial conducted by Cunningham et al. examining this regimen demonstrated not only an increase in response rate and progression free survival for the doublet, but when the three studies examining this combination were combined in meta-analysis, the increased number of patients involved moved the difference in overall survival into statistical significance (HR 0.84, 95%, CI 0.75–0.98, P = 0.02) [233]. However, the margin of benefit achieved remains debatable, as the improvement in overall survival seen for patients treated with the gemcitabine–capecitabine combination in these studies ranged from only less than one month to 1.3 months maximally [230, 231, 233].

Two further meta-analyses have examined the utility of adding a second agent to gemcitabine. Heinemann et al. compared gemcitabine + X in a combination of 15 controlled trials and a total of 4465 patients [234]. They found a significant survival benefit for doublet chemotherapy with a pooled hazard ratio (HR) of 0.91 (95% CI 0.85– 0.97, P = 0.004). This benefit was seen for both platinum- and fluoropyrimidine-containing combinations, but not in the group of trials containing gemcitabine with other agents. However, the clinical relevance of this result is again brought into question by a further meta-analysis by Vacarro et al. which compared the results of seven trials containing gemcitabine in combination with only cisplatin, oxaliplatin, and capecitabine [235s]. The conclusions of the authors were that although the addition of a second agent was associated with a statistically significant survival benefit

for all classes of drug examined, the absolute benefit was clinically insignificant, with power calculations outruling a >5% benefit in survival at one year.

5-FU-containing regimens

Prior to the adoption of gemcitabine as the chemotherapy of choice for advanced disease, fluoropyrimidine regimens were in common use. However, in both phase II and randomized controlled trials, both bolus and infusion leucovorin modulated 5-FU-containing regimens are associated with low response rates and survival inferior to that seen with gemcitabine [215, 236–238]. Single-agent capecitabine (1250 mg/m2 BD orally for 14 of 21 days) was associated with a clinical benefit rate of 24% in a phase II study of 42 patients with advanced pancreatic cancer, despite a low radiological response rate of 7%. Capecitabine in combination with oxaliplatin (CapeOx) was examined in a German AIO study in comparison with both GemCap and GemOx regimens [239]. No statistically significant differences between the arms were seen with respect to overall response rate (ORR), progression-free survival (PFS), or OR, implying that the Cape-Ox combination could be considered in gemcitabine-intolerant patients. Irinotecan in combination with 5-FU (modified FOLFIRI) has been investigated in a small phase II study, and was associated with an encouraging ORR response rate of 37.5% and a survival of >12 months [240]. However, these findings have not been confirmed in a controlled setting, and contrast with the failure of irinotecan to improve survival for patients with advanced pancreatic cancer when added to gemcitabine chemotherapy [232, 241].

FOLFIRINOX—a new standard for metastatic pancreatic cancer

A significant advance in the treatment of metastatic pancreatic cancer was demonstrated on the presentation of the recently reported FOLFIRINOX study by Conroy et al. [218]. An initial phase II non-randomized trial of 46 patients treated with oxaliplatin 85 mg/m2 and irinotecan 180 mg/m2 plus leucovorin 400 mg/m2 followed by bolus FU 400 mg/m2 on day 1, then FU 2400 mg/m2 as a 46-hour continuous infusion yielded a response rate of 26%, a time to progression of 8.2 months, a median overall survival of 10.2 months and an impressive one-year survival (for all patients) of 43% [242]. In sharp contrast to the repeated failure of gemcitabine-containing combination regimens FOLFIRINOX demonstrated clear superiority with respect to ORR, PFS, and OS when compared to single-agent gemcitabine (1000 mg/m2 weekly for seven of eight weeks and then weekly for three of four weeks) [243]. Objective response rates were 31.6% in the FOLFIRINOX arm versus 9.4% in the gemcitabine arm (P <0.001), PFS was improved from 3.3 months to 6.4 months, and overall survival from 6.8 months to 11.1 months, respectively (HR 0.57; 95% CI 0.45 to 0.73; P <0.001). This enhanced efficacy did occur at the cost of increased toxicity; ≥grade 3 neutropenia and febrile neutropenia were both increased in the FOLFIRINOX arm (45.7% versus 21%, P <0.001 and 5.4% versus 1.2%, P = 0.03, respectively). However, the rate of toxic death was low, with two occurrences overall, one in each arm. This may be attributed to the high use of granulocyte colony stimulating factor in the FOLFIRINOX arm (42.5%), although this was not a prerequisite at the time of treatment initiation. Importantly, quality of life measurements were not detrimentally affected by the triplet combination regimen, and time to definitive decline in global health status was significantly longer in the FOLFIRINOX arm (31% at six months versus 66% for gemcitabine, HR 0.47; 95% CI 0.30 to 0.70; P <0.001). As this mirrors the benefits seen in PFS this may also reflect that the toxicity associated with an effective treatment in advanced pancreas cancer may be balanced by control of cancer-related symptoms with effective treatment.

FOLFIRINOX selection criteria

It is pertinent to note that the eligibility criteria for this study were particularly stringent. No elevations of bilirubin beyond 1.5x the upper limit of normal were permitted, which led to both low rates of patients with pancreatic head tumours compared to other studies, and to low rates of biliary stents (14%). Furthermore, patients with an ECOG performance status of ≥2 were excluded, as were those over the age of 75 years. This may in part explain the relatively low rates of febrile neutropenia and cholangitis, which have been more common in other studies of combination regimens. As such, the generalizability to the general populace of advanced pancreas cancer patients has been questioned. Although there is no doubt that this combination is superior to gemcitabine (and gemcitabine-containing regimens investigated to date), the potential difficulties associated with the addition of other targeted agents to a polychemotherapy backbone leaves the desirability of this as a basis for future developments in question.

Second-line therapy for pancreatic cancer

Multiple non-randomized studies utilizing fluoropyrimidines, taxanes, platinums, and camptothecins demonstrate overall survivals of between 3.9 months to 7.6 months for single-agent chemotherapy in the second line setting [225]. Until recently, there was a lack of randomized data in this treatment setting; however, a recently reported randomized phase III trial comparing the use of oxaliplatin/5-FU and folinic acid to best supportive care for patients with gemcitabine refractory pancreatic cancer demonstrated a statistically significant benefit with respect to overall survival for the treatment arm of 2.3 months versus 4.8 months (0.45 (95% CI: 0.24–0.83), P = 0.008), despite early closure of the study due to poor recruitment [244]. For good performance-status patients with gemcitabine refractory pancreatic cancer, this regimen could now be considered a standard of care. For patients not suitable for doublet chemotherapy, monotherapy with fluoropyrimidines remains a treatment option. Following treatment with FOLFIRINOX, Conroy et al. reported that 82.5% of patients were treated in the second-line setting with gemcitabine, with a smaller proportion (12.5%) treated with gemcitabine combinations [218]. Interestingly, survival following institution of second-line therapy was comparable at 4.4 months for patients treated initially with either gemcitabine or FOLFIRINOX, implying that first-line therapy did not have appear to have an impact on the efficacy of treatment in the second-line setting.

A novel encapsulation of irinotecan in a long-circulating nanoliposome (MM-398, Merrimack) has been shown to extend OS as well as PFS, when it was added on to 5FU and leucovorin as a second-line therapy [245]. These results come from a 417-patient phase III trial known as NAPOLI-1.The combination of MM-398 with 5-FU and leucovorin improved overall survival to 6.1 months compared with 4.2 months with the control group of 5-FU and leucovorin (P = 0.012; HR 0.67). The addition of MM-398 also improved PFS to 3.1 months compared with 1.5 months in the control group (P = .0001; HR 0.56). This drug has not yet been commercially approved.

Targeted therapy for pancreatic cancer

Several treatment approaches using a gemcitabine backbone plus a novel targeted agent have been pursued; however, to date none have surpassed the OS seen with the FOLFIRINOX regimen. The most promising of these approaches was seen using the oral tyrosine kinase inhibitor erlotinib. In a randomized phase III trial of 569 patients with locally advanced or metastatic pancreatic cancer treated with gemcitabine (1000 mg/m2/week) plus or minus erlotinib (100 mg/day) a statistically significant benefit was seen with respect to overall survival (HR 0.81, P = 0.038) [246]. However, it is arguable whether the absolute benefit seen in survival (an increase from 5.9m in the control arm to 6.2 m in the experimental arm) is of clinical relevance. Of note, ≥ grade 2 rash developing with erlotinib therapy appeared to predict for improved survival with combination therapy (5.3 months versus 10.3 months). Alternate mechanisms of targeting the EGFR pathway in pancreatic cancer using the monoclonal antibody cetuximab have not been successful; one large randomized trial (n = 702) comparing gemcitabine alone to a gemcitabine–cetuximab combination did not demonstrate any benefit with respect to response rate, PFS, or OS, and EGFR expression had no impact on these outcomes [247]. Another phase II study of the addition of cetuximab to gemcitabine and cisplatin produced similar results [248].

Targeting the tumour vasculature using antiangiogenic agents has not proved fruitful to date in pancreatic cancer. This may be due to the relative hypovascularity of this disease. In one large (n = 707) placebo-controlled randomized trial examining the efficacy of the addition of bevacizumab to a gemcitabine–erlotinib doublet, a statistically significant one-month benefit in PFS was seen (3.6 months versus 4.6 months); however, no statistically significant improvement was seen in OS [249]. The orally available multitargeted antiangiogenic axitinib demonstrated no better success in a 632-patient phase III randomized trial in combination with gemcitabine, with identical PFS and OR in both control and experimental arms of the study [250]. A combined approach using gemcitabine, capecitabine, erlotinib, and bevacizumab yielded encouraging results in an initial phase I dose-finding study with an impressive median overall survival of over 12 months [251]. These findings were replicated in a larger phase II study presented in abstract form; however, at this time no controlled data exist to support the use of this regimen outside the experimental setting [252].

Nab-paclitaxel—a novel chemotherapy agent for pancreatic cancer

A more promising approach using a novel chemotherapeutic agent for pancreatic cancer was recently initially demonstrated in a phase I/II study by von Hoff et al. using nab-paclitaxel, an albumin-bound form of the taxane drug [253]. This drug formulation attaches in vivo to SPARC (secreted protein acidic and rich in cysteine) which is over-expressed in pancreatic tissues, in particular in peritumoral fibroblasts which produce the hypovascular desmoplastic stroma in pancreatic cancer, which in turn may be responsible for the decreased rates of intratumoral drug delivery characteristic of this disease [227, 254]. In combination with gemcitabine (1000 mg/m2/

week three out of four weeks), nabpaclitaxel 125 mg/m2/week on the same schedule was associated with a response rate of 48%, a PFS of 7.9 months, and an OS of 12.2 months [253]. A confirmatory phase III study in 861 patients randomised to gemcitabine alone or a gemcitabine-nabpaclitaxel doublet demonstrated a significant improvement in response rate and an overall survival benefit for the combination; median overall survival was 8.5 months in the nab-paclitaxel–gemcitabine group and 6.7 months in the gemcitabine group (HR 0.72; 95% CI, 0.62 to 0.83; P<0.001) [255].

Assessment of response in metastatic disease

Assessment of the primary tumour in pancreatic cancer may be difficult due to tumour hypovascularity and a frequent desmoplastic response in the surrounding tissue. As a result, endpoints other than objective response have been considered useful in many pancreatic cancer trials. These include both CA19-9 levels and 'clinical benefit rate'. Clinical benefit rate may be defined as those who have an improvement in symptoms such as pain, weight loss, and analgesic use whilst demonstrating minimal or no objective radiological response. Data on CA19-9 as a surrogate for tumour response are conflicting; in two series of patients with metastatic pancreatic cancer, decreases in CA19-9 of 20–25% were associated with significantly increased overall survival [256, 257]. In the first of these series, an elevation of CA19-9 above the median was also a poor prognostic marker [255]. However, these findings were not replicated in a larger case series of 175 patients treated with gemcitabine ± capecitabine [257]. The final series may have been influenced, however, by the necessity of demonstrating a 50% reduction in CA19-9 levels over a relatively short period of time (eight weeks), whilst the half-life of the tumour marker is 15 to 33 days [239]. It is also notable that people who do not express Lewis a or b blood antigens are classified as CA19-9 non-secretors; surveillance using this marker in these cases is not useful [243]. For these reasons the use of CA19-9 as a solitary marker of response in pancreatic cancer is not currently recommended [259]. Guidelines suggest that CA19-9 levels should be measured at treatment initiation and then every one to three months during treatment. If progressive disease is suggested by an increase in CA19-9, this should be confirmed radiologically.

Symptomatic care and management of comorbidities

Patients with pancreatic cancer are frequently affected by issues of pain, nutrition, and medical comorbidity such as diabetes and thromboembolism in addition to the devastating psychological effects of a poor-prognosis cancer diagnosis. For this reason, symptomatic and supportive care are an essential component of therapy.

Pain is a frequent occurrence in patients with advanced disease, and may often require opiate-based therapy. The use of celiac nerve blockade with local injection of alcohol to ablate the afferent nerve fibres of the celiac plexus has become more common. This may be achieved intraoperatively, percutaneously, or at endoscopy. This procedure may be more effective for the relief of pain than oral opiates, without the systemic toxicity associated with this form of medication [246]. Palliative radiation therapy may also be considered; however, this has a longer time to onset of action than either oral analgesia or celiac blockade.

Obstructive jaundice may often be the presenting complaint for patients with pancreatic cancer, and ensuring adequate biliary drainage is often a prerequisite to commencing effective therapy.

Placement of expandable metal stents is often sufficient to ensure this, with surgery reserved for those in whom stent placement is not possible [260]. The endoscopic and percutaneous approaches may have equal efficacy, although morbidity is increased with percutaneous placement, which additionally is less convenient for the patient due to the external position of the drain [261–263]. Although stent placement is associated with lower morbidity than surgery, complications such as reocclusion with recurrent jaundice or infection with cholangitis may occur. Plastic stents are more easily placed and removed than metal stents, but are also more prone to recurrent occlusion [260, 264]. Covered metal stents are equivalent to uncovered stents in terms of efficacy; however, may also be more easily removed and are therefore the preferred option [225]. Endoscopically placed expandable stents are also useful in the presence of duodenal obstruction, which occurs in up to 20% of patients with advanced pancreatic cancer. In this setting, stents are associated with shorter hospital stays than surgical bypass procedures and successful outcomes in up to 81% of cases [265].

Patients with pancreatic cancer have an increased (20–30%) risk of thromboembolic complications which are associated with a poor prognosis [221]. However, although the use of prophylactic anticoagulation is associated with a decreased risk of symptomatic thromboembolism, this did not in a randomized clinical trial lead to an improvement in OS, and is not recommended in routine practice [233].

Pancreatic cancer is often associated with significant cachexia and weight loss with subsequent need for intensive nutritional support. This may be complicated in many patients by a concurrent diagnosis of diabetes. Exocrine pancreatic insufficiency is treated with pancreatic enzyme replacement therapy which is associated with a decrease in protein or fat malabsorption and an increase in weight gain [266, 267].

As a result of the complexity of management of these multiple issues in those with pancreatic cancer, early involvement of palliative care services for both medical and psychological support is mandated for these patients.

Medical management of pancreatic cancer summary

Although for most patients, a diagnosis of pancreatic cancer remains associated with a poor prognosis, for selected populations significant improvements in overall survival have been demonstrated with novel chemotherapy combinations such as FOLFIRINOX. Targeted therapy has not yet yielded the benefits seen in other tumour types; however, targeting the tumour stroma may be a promising treatment option for patients with advanced pancreatic cancer. Other future directions of interest include inhibition of Hedgehog and insulin growth factor receptor pathways and anti-mucin-based therapies. Finally, supportive therapies such as pain control and nutritional interventions will also continue to remain paramount for this disease.

Multidisciplinary management of complex cases

Introduction to multidisciplinary management of complex cases

Metastatic disease will be present at the time of diagnosis in approximately 60% of patients with pancreatic adenocarcinoma. In the remaining patients, 25% will present with borderline resectable or locally unresectable tumours, and 15% will have radiographically resectable lesions. The following section will focus on the multidisciplinary approach to patients who present with borderline or locally unresectable tumours. Effective treatment for this patient population requires interaction between experienced diagnostic and interventional radiologists, pancreatic surgeons, gastroenterologists, radiation oncologists, and medical oncologists. This multidisciplinary approach is necessary to optimize patient selection for both operative and multimodal treatment approaches [268, 269]. A combination of definitive chemotherapy, radiation, and/or resection for patients who present with borderline or locally unresectable pancreatic cancer has been suggested as a cause of the reported improvement in overall survival in recent years as compared to historical series.

The multidisciplinary team

The experience and expertise of the members of a multidisciplinary team is one of the most important factors in delivering high-quality care for patients with locally unresectable or borderline resectable pancreatic cancer. A high-volume pancreatic surgeon should first determine if the tumour is locally resectable. This is essential as the subsequent treatment recommendations will vary depending on the determination of local resectability. Unresectable disease typically manifests as circumferential encasement of foregut arterial structures (superior mesenteric artery and hepatic artery) and/or thrombosis of the portal vein and/or superior mesenteric vein for a length of several centimetres that cannot be reconstructed [270]. A hepatobiliary radiologist is extremely important in establishing the designation of 'resectable' with the surgeon. Both the quality of the imaging and the quality of the interpretation is vital, as one without the other may result in misinterpretation of either distant or local sites of disease. A previous study from MSKCC found that the addition of triphasic imaging and interpretation by a hepatobiliary radiologist increased the yield for identification of distant metastatic disease by an additional 10% [271].

Within the group of patients deemed radiographically resectable, the primary management issues include the management of preoperative jaundice and the role of neoadjuvant systemic therapy or chemoradiation. Due to a lack of randomized controlled data, there is substantial variability from surgeon to surgeon and from centre to centre regarding neoadjuvant therapy [272, 273]. Neoadjuvant treatment offers several theoretical advantages over an initial resection and adjuvant treatment paradigm, including the early delivery of systemic therapy for all patients, and thus early intervention on micrometastatic disease, a higher negative margin resection rate (when radiation is included), and enhanced patient selection for surgery, collectively leading to potentially improved survival [274, 275]. This approach, however, has not been subjected to randomized trial design and thus many favour an initial operative approach, with cited concern being the theoretic risk of disease progression during therapy because of unfavourable tumour biology and/or ineffective treatment. The management of preoperative jaundice has been evaluated in prospective and randomized trials, including a recent multi-institutional study evaluating preoperative internal biliary drainage [276]. In general, these trials have demonstrated an increased infectious risk to preoperative biliary drainage in patients with moderate elevation in the bilirubin, and because of this our preference is to avoid biliary stenting when possible. In patients who require prolonged preoperative evaluation, or when resection cannot be done in a timely manner, internal biliary drainage should be considered.

The current treatment recommendation for patients with locally unresectable pancreatic adenocarcinoma is for initial systemic therapy or chemoradiation. Conversion of a locally unresectable patient to resectable status is an uncommon event. However, this appears to be occurring more commonly with systemic regimens such as FOLFIRINOX. In general, locally unresectable patients are treated similarly to patients with metastatic disease, with an initial focus on systemic therapy and radiation reserved for patients who have stable or responsive disease. When response to resectability is observed, resection is generally recommended, as long-term survival has been reported following resection in patients with initially unresectable disease [269]. A similar approach is generally recommended in patients who present with borderline resectable lesions. The National Comprehensive Cancer Network (NCCN) guidelines currently recommend either initial exploration or initial systemic therapy; however, an initial systemic approach appears to be gaining favour.

The MSKCC approach to borderline resectable and locally unresectable tumours

We recommend all patients who present to our institution with a pancreatic mass and suspicion for pancreatic adenocarcinoma to have assessment with high-quality pancreatic protocol CT imaging (non-contrasted then arterial, parenchymal, and portal venous phase contrasted). Patients that have borderline resectable or locally unresectable tumours are presented at a multidisciplinary conference to determine the most appropriate treatment course. At our institution, a dedicated team of hepatobiliary specialists are present at this conference and this includes radiologists, surgeons, medical oncologists, gastroenterologists, and radiation oncologists. Typically, multiple members of each specialty are present to provide opinions. One member of the team leads the conference and the physician who performed the initial evaluation presents the patient. In general, borderline resectable patients with venous involvement undergo surgical exploration with reconstruction of venous structures as needed. Borderline patients with evidence of possible arterial involvement are generally treated initially with systemic therapy, and in selected cases chemoradiation is given. After completion of treatment, repeat CT imaging is performed and the patient is once again assessed for resectability. For patients that demonstrate stable disease, chemoradiation is typically implemented in an attempt to obtain local response. Interval imaging is performed and patients are considered for exploration if and when they are judged to be resectable. For patients who eventually undergo resection, gemcitabine-based adjuvant chemotherapy is generally recommended. Post-operative radiation treatment is typically reserved for those patients with R1 or R2 resections.

Case presentation

In order to demonstrate the complex care of these patients, the following case is presented. A 62-year-old male presented to his local hospital with symptoms of gastric outlet obstruction. CT imaging suggested a mass in the head of the pancreas and the patient underwent upper endoscopy. Visualization was poor and the procedure was aborted. The patient was subsequently transferred to our medical centre for further evaluation. A pancreatic protocol CT scan

Prior to Chemotherapy and Chemoradiation

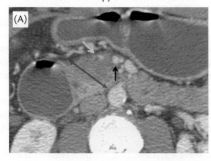

After Treatment

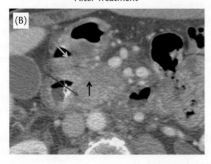

Fig. 40.5 CT scan before and after neoadjuvant chemotherapy followed by gemcitabine-based chemoradiation. Red arrow indicates tumour, yellow arrow indicates SMV, black arrow indicates SMA.

demonstrated a hypoattenuated pancreatic head mass measuring 4.6 x 2.9 cm with compression of the duodenum and encasement of the SMV and ill-defined infiltration around the SMA (Figure 40.5). The patient underwent EGD and was found to have a duodenal obstruction. A duodenal stent was successfully deployed and during the same procedure the patient had an EUS fine needle aspiration biopsy performed of the mass. The EUS also confirmed mesenteric vascular involvement. The gastric outlet symptoms resolved and the patient was discharged home. Fine needle aspiration cytology demonstrated adenocarcinoma. The patient was deemed locally unresectable by the admitting surgeon and subsequently the patient was started on gemcitabine and cisplatin for four cycles. Imaging following this treatment revealed very little change in the mass. Gemcitabine-based chemoradiation was then initiated. A CT scan eight months after initial diagnosis demonstrated a reduction in the size of the mass (from 4.6 x 2.9 cm to 4.2 x 2.0 cm) with regression from the SMV but persistent abutment of the SMA (Figure 40.5). Given the mild but definable radiographic response, the lack of encasement of the SMA, and the lack of systemic disease, the patient was taken to the operating room for attempted pancreaticoduodenectomy. The tumour was dissected free of the mesenteric vessels without difficulty and no vein resection was required. The final pathology was T3N0, with negative surgical margins. The patient suffered a wound infection requiring gauze packing but had no other complications.

This case highlights the importance of a multidisciplinary approach to patients with pancreatic adenocarcinoma. A successful outcome in this patient (i.e. R0 resection) required a team approach across multiple specialties. Unfortunately, the patient developed peritoneal recurrence 1.5 years following resection. However, he was maintained on systemic therapy for another 1.5 years until his death from disease almost four years after initial diagnosis.

Conclusion

In order to obtain optimal patient outcomes in patients with pancreatic adenocarcinoma, an experienced team of physicians is paramount. Borderline resectable and locally unresectable patients represent a unique subset of pancreatic cancer patients that are best served with multidisciplinary care to address their specific challenges. Because of a lack of randomized clinical trials to help guide management decisions, the multidisciplinary team should employ strategies that are most likely to yield successes in their practice setting.

Further reading

Conroy T, Desseigne F, Ychou M, Bouché O, Guimbaud R et al. FOLFIRINOX versus gemcitabine for metastatic pancreatic cancer. New England Journal of Medicine 2011; 364(19): 1817–1825.

Gillen S, Schuster T, Meyer zum Buschenfelde C, Friess H, Kleeff J. Preoperative/neoadjuvant therapy in pancreatic cancer: a systematic review and meta-analysis of response and resection percentages. PLoS Medicine 2010; 7: e1000267.

Hartwig W, Hackert T, Hinz U, Gluth A, Bergmann F et al. Pancreatic cancer surgery in the new millennium: better prediction of outcome. Annals of Surgery 2011; 254(2): 311–319.

Huguet F, Andre T, Hammel P, Artru P, Balosso J et al. Impact of chemoradiotherapy after disease control with chemotherapy in locally advanced pancreatic adenocarcinoma in GERCOR phase II and III studies. Journal of Clinical Oncology 2007; 25: 326–331.

Jones S, Zhang X, Parsons DW, Lin JC, Leary RJ et al. Core signaling pathways in human pancreatic cancers revealed by global genomic analyses. Science 2008; 321(5897): 1801–1806.

Neoptolemos JP, Stocken DD, Friess H, Bassi C, Dunn JA et al. A randomized trial of chemoradiotherapy and chemotherapy after resection of pancreatic cancer. New England Journal of Medicine 2004; 350: 1200–1210.

Oettle H, Post S, Neuhaus P, Gellert K, Langrehr J et al. Adjuvant chemotherapy with gemcitabine vs observation in patients undergoing curative-intent resection of pancreatic cancer: a randomized controlled trial. Journal of the American Medical Association 2007; 297: 267–277.

Siegel R, Naishadham D, Jemal A. Cancer statistics: 2012. CA: A Cancer Journal of Clinicians 2012; 62: 10–29.

Tanaka M, Chari S, Adsay V, Fernandez-del Castillo C, Falconi M et al. International consensus guidelines for management of intraductal papillary mucinous neoplasms and mucinous cystic neoplasms of the pancreas. Pancreatology 2006; 6(1–2): 17–32.

Tempero M, Arnoletti J, Behrman S, Ben-Josef E, Benson AB et al. NCCN clinical practice guidelines in oncology. Pancreatic adenocarcinoma. Journal of the National Comprehensive Cancer Network 2010; 8(9): 972–1017.

Weitz J, Koch M, Friess H, Büchler MW. Impact of volume and specialization for cancer surgery. Digestive Surgery 2004; 21: 253–261.

References

1. Siegel R, Naishadham D, Jemal A. Cancer statistics: 2012. CA: A Cancer Journal of Clinicians 2012; 62: 10–29.
2. Robert Koch Institute, <http://www.rki.de/DE/Home/homepage_node.html>.
3. Neesse A, Michl P, Frese KK, Feig C, Cook N et al. Stromal biology and therapy in pancreatic cancer. Gut 2011; 60(6): 861–868.
4. Tao Y, Pinzi V, Bourhis J, Deutsch E. Mechanisms of disease: signaling of the insulin-like growth factor 1 receptor pathway—therapeutic perspectives in cancer. Nature Cinical Practice Oncology 2007; 4(10): 591–602.
5. SEER, <www.seer.cancer.gov>.

6. Jones S, Zhang X, Parsons DW, Lin JC, Leary RJ et al. Core signaling pathways in human pancreatic cancers revealed by global genomic analyses. Science 2008; 321(5897): 1801–1806.

7. Seo Y, Baba H, Fukuda T, Takashima M. High expression of vascular endothelial growth factor is associated with liver metastasis and a poor prognosis for patients with ductal pancreatic adenocarcinoma. Cancer 2000; 88(10): 2239–2245.

8. Hruban RH, Maitra A, Schulick R, Laheru D, Herman J et al. Emerging molecular biology of pancreatic cancer. Gastrointestinal Cancer Research 2008; 2(Suppl. 4): S10–S15.

9. Ferrara N. Vascular endothelial growth factor. Arteriosclerosis, Thrombosis, and Vascular Biology 2009; 29(6): 789–791.

10. Pérez-Mancera PA, Guerra C, Barbacid M, Tuveson DA. What we have learned about pancreatic cancer from mouse models. Gastroenterology 2012; 142(5): 1079–1092.

11. Hanahan D, Weinberg RA. Hallmarks of cancer: the next generation. Cell 2011; 144(5): 646–674.

12. Tuveson DA, Neoptolemos JP. Understanding metastasis in pancreatic cancer: a call for new clinical approaches. Cell 2012; 148(1–2): 21–23.

13. Campbell PJ, Yachida S, Mudie LJ, Stephens RJ et al. The patterns and dynamics of genomic instability in metastatic pancreatic cancer. Nature 2010; 467(7319): 1109–1113.

14. Yachida S, Jones S, Bozic I, Antal T, Leary R et al. Distant metastasis occurs late during the genetic evolution of pancreatic cancer. Nature 2010; 467(7319): 1114–1117.

15. Hruban RH, Maitra A, Goggins M. Update on pancreatic intraepithelial neoplasia. International Journal of Clinical and Experimental Pathology 2008; 1(4): 306–316.

16. Yonezawa S, Higashi M, Yamada N, Goto M. Precursor lesions of pancreatic cancer. Gut and Liver 2008; 2(3): 137.

17. Hornsby PJ. Cellular aging and cancer. Critical Reviews in Oncology/Hematology 2011; 79(2): 189–195.

18. Sun B, Chen M, Hawks C. Immortal ALT + human cells do not require telomerase reverse transcriptase for malignant transformation. Cancer Research 2005; 65(15): 6512–6515.

19. Middleton G, Ghaneh P, Costello E, Greenhalf W, Neoptolemos JP. New treatment options for advanced pancreatic cancer. Expert Review of Gastroenterology and Hepatology 2008; 2(5): 673–696.

20. Bode AM, Dong Z. Post-translational modification of p53 in tumorigenesis. Nature Reviews Cancer 2004; 4(10): 793–805.

21. Clark PA, Llanos S, Peters G. Multiple interacting domains contribute to p14ARF mediated inhibition of MDM2. Oncogene 2002; 21(29): 4498–4507.

22. Iacobuzio-Donahue CA. Genetic evolution of pancreatic cancer: lessons learnt from the pancreatic cancer genome sequencing project. Gut 2011; 61(7): 1085–1094.

23. Hahn SA, Schutte M, Hoque AT, Moskaluk CA, da Costa LT et al. DPC4, a candidate tumor suppressor gene at human chromosome 18q21.1. Science 1996; 271(5247): 350–353.

24. Mahadevan D, Hoff Von DD. Tumor-stroma interactions in pancreatic ductal adenocarcinoma. Molecular Cancer Therapeutics 2007; 6(4): 1186–1197.

25. Liles JS, Arnoletti JP, Tzeng C-WD, Howard JH, Kossenkov AV et al. ErbB3 expression promotes tumorigenesis in pancreatic adenocarcinoma. Cancer Biology & Therapy 2010; 10(6): 555–563.

26. Yuan TL, Cantley LC. PI3K pathway alterations in cancer: variations on a theme. Oncogene 2008; 27(41): 5497–5510.

27. Wang Y, Li Y, Wang D, Li Y, Chang A, Chan WK. Suppression of the hypoxia inducible factor-1 function by redistributing the aryl hydrocarbon receptor nuclear translocator from nucleus to cytoplasm. Cancer Letters 2012; 320(1): 111–121.

28. Ouban A, Muraca P, Yeatman T, Coppola D. Expression and distribution of insulin-like growth factor-1 receptor in human carcinomas. Human Pathology 2003; 34(8): 803–808.

29. Bergmann U, Funatomi H, Yokoyama M, Beger HG, Korc M. Insulin-like growth factor I overexpression in human pancreatic cancer: evidence for autocrine and paracrine roles. Cancer Research 1995; 55(10): 2007–2011.

30. Wang Z, Ahmad A, Li Y, Kong D, Azmi AS et al. Emerging roles of PDGF-D signaling pathway in tumor development and progression. Biochimica et Biophysica Acta 2010; 1806(1): 122–130.

31. Roy R, Yang J, Moses MA. Matrix metalloproteinases as novel biomarkers and potential therapeutic targets in human cancer. Journal of Clinical Oncology 2009; 27(31): 5287–5297.

32. Haeno H, Gonen M, Davis MB, Herman JM, Iacobuzio-Donahue CA et al. Computational modeling of pancreatic cancer reveals kinetics of metastasis suggesting optimum treatment strategies. Cell 2012; 148(1–2): 362–375.

33. Rhim AD, Mirek ET, Aiello NM, Maitra A, Bailey JM et al. EMT and dissemination precede pancreatic tumor formation. Cell 2012; 148(1–2): 349–361.

34. Li C, Heidt DG, Dalerba P, Burant CF, Zhang L et al. Identification of pancreatic cancer stem cells. Cancer Research 2007; 67(3): 1030–1037.

35. Morris JP, Wang SC, Hebrok M. KRAS, Hedgehog, Wnt and the twisted developmental biology of pancreatic ductal adenocarcinoma. Nature Reviews Cancer 2010; 10(10): 683–695.

36. Hermann PC, Huber SL, Herrler T, Aicher A, Ellwart JW et al. Distinct populations of cancer stem cells determine tumor growth and metastatic activity in human pancreatic cancer. Cell Stem Cell 2007; 1(3): 313–323.

37. Ranganathan P, Weaver KL, Capobianco AJ. Notch signalling in solid tumours: a little bit of everything but not all the time. Nature Reviews Cancer 2011; 11(5): 338–351.

38. Mysliwiec P, Boucher MJ. Targeting Notch signaling in pancreatic cancer patients—rationale for new therapy. Advances in Medical Sciences 2009; 54(2): 136–142.

39. Fortini M. Notch signaling: the core pathway and its posttranslational regulation. Developmental Cell 2009; 16(5): 633–647.

40. Ristorcelli E, Lombardo D. Targeting Notch signaling in pancreatic cancer. Expert Opinion on Therapeutic Targets 2010; 14(5): 541–552.

41. Miyamoto Y, Maitra A, Ghosh B, Zechner U, Argani P et al. Notch mediates TGF alpha-induced changes in epithelial differentiation during pancreatic tumorigenesis. Cancer Cell 2003; 3(6): 565–576.

42. Merchant JL. Hedgehog signalling in gut development, physiology and cancer. Journal of Physiology (London) 2012; 590(Pt 3): 421–432.

43. Thayer SP, di Magliano MP, Heiser PW, Nielsen CM, Roberts DJ et al. Hedgehog is an early and late mediator of pancreatic cancer tumorigenesis. Nature 2003; 425(6960): 851–856.

44. Hidalgo M, Maitra A. The hedgehog pathway and pancreatic cancer. New England Journal of Medicine 2009; 361(21): 2094–2096.

45. Feldmann G, Habbe N, Dhara S, Bisht S, Alvarez H et al. Hedgehog inhibition prolongs survival in a genetically engineered mouse model of pancreatic cancer. Gut 2008; 57(10): 1420–1430.

46. Wang L, Heidt DG, Lee CJ, Yang H, Logsdon CD et al. Oncogenic function of ATDC in pancreatic cancer through Wnt pathway activation and beta-catenin stabilization. Cancer Cell 2009; 15(3): 207–219.

47. Pasca di Magliano M, Biankin AV, Heiser PW, Cano DA, Gutierrez PJ et al. Common activation of canonical Wnt signaling in pancreatic adenocarcinoma. PLoS ONE 2007; 2(11): e1155.

48. Ling J, Kang Y, Zhao R, et al. KrasG12D-induced IKK2/β/NF-κB Activation by IL-1α and p62 feedforward loops is required for development of pancreatic ductal adenocarcinoma. Cancer Cell 2012; 21(1): 105–120.

49. Chu GC, Kimmelman AC, Hezel AF, DePinho RA. Stromal biology of pancreatic cancer. Journal of Cellular Biochemistry 2007; 101(4): 887–907.

50. Hruban RH, Bishop Pitman M, Klimstra DS eds. Tumors of the pancreas. AFIP Atlas of Tumor Pathology Series 4: 6th fascicle. Washington, DC: AFIP, 2007.

51. Bosman FT, Carneiro F, Hruban RH, Theise ND eds. WHO classification of tumours of the digestive system, 4th ed. Lyon: IARC Press, 2010.

52. Hartwig W, Hackert T, Hinz U, Gluth A, Bergmann F et al. Pancreatic cancer surgery in the new millennium: better prediction of outcome. Annals of Surgery 2011; 254(2): 311–319.

53. Moll R, Löwe A, Laufer J, Franke WW. Cytokeratin 20 in human carcinomas. A new histodiagnostic marker detected by monoclonal antibodies. American Journal of Pathology 1992; 140(2): 427–447.

54. Schüssler MH, Skoudy A, Ramaekers F, Real FX. Intermediate filaments as differentiation markers of normal pancreas and pancreas cancer. American Journal of Pathologyy 1992; 140(3): 559–568.

55. Ceyhan GO, Bergmann F, Kadihasanoglu M, Altintas B, Demir IE et al. Pancreatic neuropathy and neuropathic pain—a comprehensive pathomorphological study of 546 cases. Gastroenterology 2009; 136(1): 177–186.

56. Matsuno S, Kato S, Kobari M, Sato T. Clinicopathological study on hematogenous metastasis of pancreatic cancer. Japanese Journal of Surgery 1986; 16(6): 406–411.

57. Edge SB, Byrd SE, Compton CC, Fritz AG, Greene FL et al. eds. AJCC Cancer Staging Manual, 7th ed. New York: Springer, 2010.

58. Sobin LH, Gospodarowicz MK, Wittekind C eds. TNM classification of malignant tumours. Oxford: Wiley-Blackwell, Oxford, 2001.

59. American Cancer Society. How is pancreatic cancer stage?, American Cancer Society, 2014, <http://www.cancer.org/cancer/pancreaticcancer/detailedguide/pancreatic-cancer-staging>.

60. Wasif N, Ko CY, Farrell J, Wainberg Z, Hines OJ et al. Impact of tumor grade on prognosis in pancreatic cancer: should we include grade in AJCC staging? Annals of Surgical Oncology 2010; 17(9): 2312–2320.

61. Esposito I, Kleeff J, Bergmann F, Reiser C, Herpel E et al. Most pancreatic Cancer Researchections are R1 resections. Annals of Surgical Oncology 2008; 15(6): 1651–1660.

62. Verbeke CS, Leitch D, Menon KV, McMahon MJ, Guillou PJ et al. Redefining the R1 resection in pancreatic cancer. British Journal of Surgery 2006; 93(10): 1232–1237.

63. Hruban RH, Maitra A, Goggins M. Update on pancreatic intraepithelial neoplasia. International Journal of Clinical and Experimental Pathology 2008; 1(4): 306–316.

64. Esposito I, Seiler C, Bergmann F, Kleeff J, Friess H et al. Hypothetical progression model of pancreatic cancer with origin in the centroacinar-acinar compartment. Pancreas 2007; 35(3): 212–217.

65. Guerra C, Schuhmacher AJ, Cañamero M, Grippo PJ, Verdaguer L et al. Chronic pancreatitis is essential for induction of pancreatic ductal adenocarcinoma by K-Ras oncogenes in adult mice. Cancer Cell 2007; 11(3): 291–302.

66. Yu J, Li A, Hong SM, Hruban RH, Goggins M. MicroRNA alterations of pancreatic intraepithelial neoplasias. Clinical Cancer Research 2012; 18(4): 981–992.

67. Terhune PG, Phifer DM, Tosteson TD, Longnecker DS. K-ras mutation in focal proliferative lesions of human pancreas. Cancer Epidemiology, Biomarkers & Prevention 1998; 7(6): 515–521.

68. Aichler M, Seiler C, Tost M, Siveke J, Mazur PK et al. Origin of pancreatic ductal adenocarcinoma from atypical flat lesions: a comparative study in transgenic mice and human tissues. Journal of Pathology 2012; 226(5): 723–734.

69. Bergmann F, Esposito I, Michalski CW, Herpel E, Friess H et al. Early undifferentiated pancreatic carcinoma with osteoclastlike giant cells: direct evidence for ductal evolution. American Journal of Surgical Pathology 2007; 31(12): 1919–1925.

70. Strobel O, Hartwig W, Bergmann F, Hinz U, Hackert T et al. Anaplastic pancreatic cancer: Presentation, surgical management, and outcome. Surgery 2011; 149(2): 200–208.

71. Hartwig W, Denneberg M, Bergmann F, Hackert T, Hinz U et al. Acinar cell carcinoma of the pancreas: is resection justified even in limited metastatic disease? American Journal of Surgery 2011; 202(1): 23–27.

72. Matthaei H, Hong SM, Mayo SC, dal Molin M, Olino K et al. Presence of pancreatic intraepithelial neoplasia in the pancreatic transection margin does not influence outcome in patients with R0 resected pancreatic cancer. Annals of Surgical Oncology 2011; 18(12): 3493–3499.

73. van Heek NT, Kuhlmann KFD, Scholten RJ, de Castro SMM, Busch ORC et al. Hospital volume and mortality after pancreatic resection: a systematic review and an evaluation of intervention in the Netherlands. Annals of Surgery 2005; 242: 781–788, discussion 788–790.

74. Adler G, Seufferlein T, Bischoff SC, Brambs H-J, Feuerbach S et al. [S3-Guidelines 'Exocrine pancreatic cancer' 2007]. Zeitung für Gastroenterologie 2007; 45: 487–523.

75. Bilimoria KY, Bentrem DJ, Ko CY, Tomlinson JS, Stewart AK et al. Multimodality therapy for pancreatic cancer in the US: utilization, outcomes, and the effect of hospital volume. Cancer 2007; 110: 1227–1234.

76. Vincent A, Herman J, Schulick R, Hruban RH, Goggins M. Pancreatic cancer. Lancet 2004; 363: 1049–1057.

77. National Comprehensive Cancer Network (NCCN). NCCN Clinical Practice Guidelines in Oncology (NCCN Guidelines) Pancreatic Adenocarcinoma Version 2.2012, 2012.

78. Tempero MA, Arnoletti JP, Behrman SW, Ben-Josef E, Benson AB 3rd et al. Pancreatic Adenocarcinoma, Version 2.2012: Featured Updates to the NCCN Guidelines. Journal of the National Comprehensive Cancer Network: JNCCN 2012; 10: 703–713.

79. Birkmeyer JD, Siewers AE, Finlayson EVA, Stukel TA, Lucas FL et al. Hospital volume and surgical mortality in the United States. New England Journal of Medicine 2002; 346: 1128–1137.

80. Weitz J, Koch M, Friess H, Büchler MW. Impact of volume and specialization for cancer surgery. Digestive Surgery 2004; 21: 253–261.

81. Sohn TA, Lillemoe KD, Cameron JL, Pitt HA, Huang JJ et al. Reexploration for periampullary carcinoma: resectability, perioperative results, pathology, and long-term outcome. Annals of Surgery 1999; 229: 393–400.

82. Andersson R, Vagianos CE, Williamson RCN. Preoperative staging and evaluation of resectability in pancreatic ductal adenocarcinoma. HPB (Oxford) 2004; 6: 5–12.

83. Weitz J, Kienle P, Schmidt J, Friess H, Büchler MW. Portal vein resection for advanced pancreatic head cancer. Journal of the American College of Surgeons 2007: 204: 712–716.

84. Tempero MA, Arnoletti JP, Behrman S, Ben-Josef E, Benson AB et al. Pancreatic adenocarcinoma. Journal of the National Comprehensive Cancer Network 2010: 8: 972–1017.

85. Callery MP, Chang KJ, Fishman EK, Talamonti MS, William Traverso L et al. Pretreatment assessment of resectable and borderline resectable pancreatic cancer: expert consensus statement. Annals of Surgery and Oncology 2009; 16: 1727–1733.

86. Witzel O. Aus der Klinik des Herrn Prof. Trendelenburg. Beitrage zur Chirurgie der Bauchorgane. Deutsche Zeitschrift für Chirurgie 1886; 24: 326–354.

87. Kausch W. Das Carcinom der Papilla duodeni und seine radikale Entfernung. Beitrage zur klinischen Chirurgie 1912; 78: 439–486.

88. Hirschel G. Die Resektion des Duodenums mit der Papille wegen Karzinoms. Münchener Medizinische Wochenschrift 1914; 61: 1728–1729.

89. Whipple AO, Parsons WB, Mullins CR. Treatment of carcinoma of the ampulla of vater. Annals of Surgery 1935: 102: 763–779.

90. Loos M, Kleeff J, Friess H, Büchler MW. Surgical treatment of pancreatic cancer. Annals of the New York Academy of Sciences 2008; 1138: 169–180.

91. Kendrick ML, Cusati D. Total laparoscopic pancreaticoduodenectomy: feasibility and outcome in an early experience. Archives of Surgery 2010; 145: 19–23.

92. Diener MK, Seiler CM, Rossion I, Kleeff J, Glanemann M et al. Efficacy of stapler versus hand-sewn closure after distal pancreatectomy (DISPACT): a randomised, controlled multicentre trial. Lancet 2011; 377: 1514–1522.

93. Kendrick ML, Sclabas GM. Major venous resection during total laparoscopic pancreaticoduodenectomy. HPB (Oxford) 2011; 13: 454–458.

94. Traverso LW, Longmire WP Jr. Preservation of the pylorus in pancreaticoduodenectomy. Surgery, Gynecology & Obstetrics 1978: 146: 959–962.

95. Traverso LW, Longmire WP Jr. Preservation of the pylorus in pancreaticoduodenectomy a follow-up evaluation. Annals of Surgery 1980; 192: 306–310.

96. Diener MK, Heukaufer C, Schwarzer G, Seiler CM, Antes G et al. Pancreaticoduodenectomy (classic Whipple) versus pylorus-preserving pancreaticoduodenectomy (pp Whipple) for surgical treatment of periampullary and pancreatic carcinoma. Cochrane Database of Systemic Reviews 2008: CD006053.

97. Riall TS, Cameron JL, Lillemoe KD, Campbell KA, Sauter PK et al. Pancreaticoduodenectomy with or without distal gastrectomy and extended retroperitoneal lymphadenectomy for periampullary adenocarcinoma—part 3: update on 5-year survival. Journal of Gastrointestinal Surgery 2005; 9: 1191–1204; discussion 1204–1206.

98. Nakao A, Takeda S, Inoue S, Nomoto S, Kanazumi N et al. Indications and techniques of extended resection for pancreatic cancer. World Journal of Surgery 2006; 30: 976–982; discussion 983–984.

99. Michalski CW, Kleeff J, Wente MN, Diener MK, Büchler MW et al. Systematic review and meta-analysis of standard and extended lymphadenectomy in pancreaticoduodenectomy for pancreatic cancer. British Journal of Surgery 2007; 94: 265–273.

100. Esposito I, Kleeff J, Bergmann F, Reiser C, Herpel E et al. Most pancreatic cancer resections are R1 resections. Annals of Surgery and Oncology 2008; 15: 1651–1660.

101. Weitz J, Rahbari N, Koch M, Büchler MW. The 'artery first' approach for resection of pancreatic head cancer. Journal of the American College of Surgeons 2010; 210: e1–e4.

102. Wente MN, Shrikhande SV, Müller MW, Diener MK, Seiler CM et al. Pancreaticojejunostomy versus pancreaticogastrostomy: systematic review and meta-analysis. American Journal of Surgery 2007; 193: 171–183.

103. Tani M, Terasawa H, Kawai M, Ina S, Hirono S et al. Improvement of delayed gastric emptying in pylorus-preserving pancreaticoduodenectomy: results of a prospective, randomized, controlled trial. Annals of Surgery 2006; 243: 316–320.

104. Diener MK, Tadjalli-Mehr K, Mehr K-T, Wente MN, Kieser M et al. Risk-benefit assessment of closed intra-abdominal drains after pancreatic surgery: a systematic review and meta-analysis assessing the current state of evidence. Langenbecks Archives of Surgery 2011; 396: 41–52.

105. Song KB, Kim SC, Park JB, Kim YH, Jung YS et al. Single-center experience of laparoscopic left pancreatic resection in 359 consecutive patients: changing the surgical paradigm of left pancreatic resection. Surgical Endoscopy 2011; 25: 3364–3372.

106. Mollberg N, Rahbari NN, Koch M, Hartwig W, Hoeger Y et al. Arterial resection during pancreatectomy for pancreatic cancer: a systematic review and meta-analysis. Annals of Surgery 2011; 254: 882–893.

107. Gagandeep S, Artinyan A, Jabbour N, Mateo R, Matsuoka L et al. Extended pancreatectomy with resection of the celiac axis: the modified Appleby operation. American Journal of Surgery 2006; 192: 330–335.

108. Venkat R, Puhan MA, Schulick RD, Cameron JL, Eckhauser FE et al. Predicting the risk of perioperative mortality in patients undergoing pancreaticoduodenectomy: a novel scoring system. Archives of Surgery 2011; 146: 1277–1284.

109. Hsu CC, Wolfgang CL, Laheru DA, Pawlik TM, Swartz MJ et al. Early mortality risk score: identification of poor outcomes following upfront surgery for resectable pancreatic cancer. Journal of Gastrointestinal Surgery 2012; 16: 753–761.

110. Berberat PO, Friess H, Kleeff J, Uhl W, Büchler MW. Prevention and treatment of complications in pancreatic cancer surgery. Digestive Surgery 1999; 16: 327–336.

111. Bassi C, Dervenis C, Butturini G, Fingerhut A, Yeo C. Postoperative pancreatic fistula: an international study group (ISGPF) definition. Surgery 2005; 138: 8–13.

112. Dong X, Zhang B, Kang MX, Chen Y, Guo QQ et al. Analysis of pancreatic fistula according to the International Study Group on Pancreatic Fistula classification scheme for 294 patients who underwent pancreaticoduodenectomy in a single center. Pancreas 2011; 40: 222–228.

113. Sahin M, Foulis AA, Poon FW, Imrie CW. Late focal pancreatic metastasis of renal cell carcinoma. Digestive Surgery 1998; 15: 72–74.

114. Ohwada S, Tanahashi Y, Ogawa T, Kawate S, Hamada K et al. In situ vs ex situ pancreatic duct stents of duct-to-mucosa pancreaticojejunostomy after pancreaticoduodenectomy with billroth I-type reconstruction. Archives of Surgery 2002; 137: 1289–1293.

115. Kurosaki I, Hatakeyama K. Omental wrapping of skeletonized major vessels after pancreaticoduodenectomy. International Surgery 2004; 89: 90–94.

116. Lillemoe KD, Cameron JL, Kim MP, Campbell KA, Sauter PK et al. Does fibrin glue sealant decrease the rate of pancreatic fistula after pancreaticoduodenectomy? Results of a prospective randomized trial. Journal of Gastrointestinal Surgery 2004; 8: 766–772; discussion 772–774.

117. Poon RTP, Fan ST, Lo CM, Ng KK, Yuen WK et al. External drainage of pancreatic duct with a stent to reduce leakage rate of pancreaticojejunostomy after pancreaticoduodenectomy: a prospective randomized trial. Annals of Surgery 2007; 246: 425–433; discussion 433–435.

118. Halloran CM, Ghaneh P, Bosonnet L, Hartley MN, Sutton R et al. Complications of pancreatic Cancer Researchection. Digestive Surgery 2002; 19: 138–146.

119. Wente MN, Veit JA, Bassi C, Dervenis C, Fingerhut A et al. Postpancreatectomy hemorrhage (PPH)–An International Study Group of Pancreatic Surgery (ISGPS) definition. Surgery 2007; 142: 20–25.

120. Cullen JJ, Sarr MG, Ilstrup DM. Pancreatic anastomotic leak after pancreaticoduodenectomy: incidence, significance, and management. American Journal of Surgery 1994; 168: 295–298.

121. Stampfl U, Hackert T, Sommer C-M, Klauss M, Bellemann N et al. Superselective embolization for the management of postpancreatectomy hemorrhage: a single-center experience in 25 patients. Journal of Vascular and Interventional Radiology 2012; 23: 504–510.

122. Trede M, Schwall G. The complications of pancreatectomy. Annals of Surgery 1988; 207: 39–47.

123. Wente MN, Bassi C, Dervenis C, Fingerhut A, Gouma DJ et al. Delayed gastric emptying (DGE) after pancreatic surgery: a suggested definition by the International Study Group of Pancreatic Surgery (ISGPS). Surgery 2007; 142: 761–768.

124. Park JS, Hwang HK, Kim JK, Cho SI, Yoon D-S, et al. Clinical validation and risk factors for delayed gastric emptying based on the International Study Group of Pancreatic Surgery (ISGPS) Classification. Surgery 2009; 146: 882–887.

125. Siegel R, Naishadham D, Jemal A: Cancer statistics: 2012. CA: A Cancer Journal for Clinicians 2012; 62: 10–29.

126. Hartwig W, Hackert T, Hinz U, Gluth A, Bergmann F et al. Pancreatic cancer surgery in the new millennium: better prediction of outcome. Annals of Surgery 2011; 254: 311–319.

127. Lillemoe KD, Cameron JL, Hardacre JM, Sohn TA, Sauter PK et al. Is prophylactic gastrojejunostomy indicated for unresectable periampullary cancer? A prospective randomized trial. Annals of Surgery 1999; 230: 322–328; discussion 328–330.

128. Gouma DJ. Stent versus surgery. HPB (Oxford) 2007; 9: 408–413.

129. Moss AC, Morris E, Leyden J, MacMathuna P. Malignant distal biliary obstruction: a systematic review and meta-analysis of endoscopic and surgical bypass results. Cancer Treatment Reviews 2007; 33: 213–221.

130. de Jong K, Nio CY, Hermans JJ, Dijkgraaf MG, Gouma DJ et al. High prevalence of pancreatic cysts detected by screening magnetic resonance imaging examinations. Clinical Gastroenterology and Hepatology 2010; 8(9): 806–811.

131. Laffan TA, Horton KM, Klein AP, Berlanstein B, Siegelman SS. Prevalence of unsuspected pancreatic cysts on MDCT. American Journal of Roentgenology 2008; 191(3): 802–807.

132. Sohn TA, Yeo CJ, Cameron JL, Hruban RH, Fukushima N et al. Intraductal papillary mucinous neoplasms of the pancreas: an

updated experience. Annals of Surgery 2004; 239(6): 788–797; discussion 797–789.

133. Yachida S, Jones S, Bozic I, Antal T, Leary R et al. Distant metastasis occurs late during the genetic evolution of pancreatic cancer. Nature 2010; 467(7319): 1114–1117.

134. Basturk O, Coban I, Adsay NV. Pancreatic cysts: pathologic classification, differential diagnosis, and clinical implications. Archives of Pathology & Laboratory Medicine 2009; 133(3): 423–438.

135. Fernandez-del Castillo C, Adsay NV. Intraductal papillary mucinous neoplasms of the pancreas. Gastroenterology 2010; 139(3): 708–713; 713, e701–702.

136. Tanaka M, Chari S, Adsay V, Fernandez-del Castillo C, Falconi M et al. International consensus guidelines for management of intraductal papillary mucinous neoplasms and mucinous cystic neoplasms of the pancreas. Pancreatology 2006; 6(1–2): 17–32.

137. Hruban RH, Goggins M, Parsons J, Kern SE. Progression model for pancreatic cancer. Clinical Cancer Research 2000; 6(8): 2969–2972.

138. Crane CH, Varadhachary GR, Yordy JS, Staerkel GA, Javle MM et al. Phase II trial of cetuximab, gemcitabine, and oxaliplatin followed by chemoradiation with cetuximab for locally advanced (T4) pancreatic adenocarcinoma: correlation of Smad4(Dpc4) immunostaining with pattern of disease progression. Journal of Clinical Oncology 2011; 29: 3037–3043.

139. Brunner TB, Geiger M, Grabenbauer GG, Lang-Welzenbach M, Mantoni TS et al. Phase I trial of the human immunodeficiency virus protease inhibitor nelfinavir and chemoradiation for locally advanced pancreatic cancer. Journal of Clinical Oncology 2008; 26: 2699–2706.

140. Iacobuzio-Donahue CA, Fu B, Yachida S, Luo M, Abe H et al. DPC4 gene status of the primary carcinoma correlates with patterns of failure in patients with pancreatic cancer. Journal of Clinical Oncology 2009; 27: 1806–1813.

141. Shinchi H, Takao S, Noma H, et al. Length and quality of survival after external-beam radiotherapy with concurrent continuous 5-fluorouracil infusion for locally unresectable pancreatic cancer. International Journal of Radiation Oncology Biology Physics 2002; 53: 146–150.

142. Moertel CG, Childs DS Jr, Reitemeier RJ, Colby MY Jr, Holbrook MA et al. Combined 5-fluorouracil and supervoltage radiation therapy of locally unresectable gastrointestinal cancer. Lancet 2 1969; 865–867.

143. Moertel CG, Frytak S, Hahn RG, O'Connell MJ, Reitemeier RJ et al. Therapy of locally unresectable pancreatic carcinoma: a randomized comparison of high dose (6000 rads) radiation alone, moderate dose radiation (4000 rads + 5-fluorouracil), and high dose radiation + 5-fluorouracil: the Gastrointestinal Tumor Study Group. Cancer 1981; 48: 1705–1710.

144. Cohen SJ, Dobelbower R Jr, Lipsitz S, Catalano PJ, Sischy B et al. A randomized phase III study of radiotherapy alone or with 5-fluorouracil and mitomycin-C in patients with locally advanced adenocarcinoma of the pancreas: Eastern Cooperative Oncology Group study E8282. International Journal of Radiation Oncology Biology Physics 2005; 62: 1345–1350.

145. GITSG. Treatment of locally unresectable carcinoma of the pancreas: comparison of combined-modality therapy (chemotherapy plus radiotherapy) to chemotherapy alone. Gastrointestinal Tumor Study Group. Journal of the National Cancer Institute 1988; 80: 751–755.

146. Klaassen DJ, MacIntyre JM, Catton GE, Engstrom PF, Moertel CG et al. Treatment of locally unresectable cancer of the stomach and pancreas: a randomized comparison of 5-fluorouracil alone with radiation plus concurrent and maintenance 5-fluorouracil—an Eastern Cooperative Oncology Group study. Journal of Clinical Oncology 1985; 3: 373–378.

147. Chauffert B, Mornex F, Bonnetain F, Rougier P, Mariette C et al. Phase III trial comparing intensive induction chemoradiotherapy (60 Gy, infusional 5-FU and intermittent cisplatin) followed by maintenance gemcitabine with gemcitabine alone for locally advanced unresectable pancreatic cancer. Definitive results of the 2000–2001 FFCD/SFRO study. Annals of Oncology 2008; 19(9): 1592–1599.

148. Loehrer PJ, Feng Y, Cardenes HR, Wagner L, Brell JM et al. Gemcitabine alone versus gemcitabine plus radiotherapy in patients with locally advanced pancreatic cancer: an Eastern Cooperative Oncology Group Trial. Journal of Clinical Oncology 2011; 29(31): 4105–4112.

149. McGinn CJ, Zalupski MM, Shureiqi I, Robertson JM, Eckhauser FE et al. Phase I trial of radiation dose escalation with concurrent weekly full-dose gemcitabine in patients with advanced pancreatic cancer. Journal of Clinical Oncology 2001; 19: 4202–4208.

150. Zhu CP, Shi J, Chen YX, Xie WF, Lin Y. Gemcitabine in the chemoradiotherapy for locally advanced pancreatic cancer: a meta-analysis. Radiotherapy & Oncology 2011; 99: 108–1013.

151. Huguet F, Andre T, Hammel P, Artru P, Balosso J et al. Impact of chemoradiotherapy after disease control with chemotherapy in locally advanced pancreatic adenocarcinoma in GERCOR phase II and III studies. Journal of Clinical Oncology 2007; 25: 326–331.

152. Moureau-Zabotto L, Phelip JM, Afchain P, Mineur L, André T et al. Concomitant administration of weekly oxaliplatin, fluorouracil continuous infusion, and radiotherapy after 2 months of gemcitabine and oxaliplatin induction in patients with locally advanced pancreatic cancer: a Groupe Coordinateur Multidisciplinaire en Oncologie phase II study. Journal of Clinical Oncology 2008; 26: 1080–1085.

153. Krishnan S, Rana V, Janjan NA, Varadhachary GR, Abbruzzese JL et al. Induction chemotherapy selects patients with locally advanced, unresectable pancreatic cancer for optimal benefit from consolidative chemoradiation therapy. Cancer 2007; 110: 47–55.

154. Hammel P, Huguet F, Van Laethem JL, Goldstein D, Glimelius B et al. Randomized multicenter phase III study in patients with locally advanced adenocarcinoma of the pancreas: gemcitabine with or without chemoradiotherapy and with or without erlotinib—LAP 07 study. Journal of Clinical Oncology 2011; 29: e14619.

155. Mukherjee S, Hurt CN, Bridgewater J, Falk S, Cummins S et al. Gemcitabine-based or capecitabine-based chemoradiotherapy for locally advanced pancreatic cancer (SCALOP): a multicenter, randomized, phase 2 trial. Lancet Oncology 2013; 14: 317–326.

156. Gillen S, Schuster T, Meyer zum Buschenfelde C, Friess H, Kleeff J. Preoperative/neoadjuvant therapy in pancreatic cancer: a systematic review and meta-analysis of response and resection percentages. PLoS Medicine 2010; 7: e1000267.

157. Lu DS, Reber HA, Krasny RM, Kadell BM, Sayre J. Local staging of pancreatic cancer: criteria for unresectability of major vessels as revealed by pancreatic-phase, thin-section helical CT. American Journal of Roentgenology 1997; 168: 1439–1443.

158. Abrams RA, Lowy AM, O'Reilly EM, Wolff RA, Picozzi VJ et al. Combined modality treatment of resectable and borderline resectable pancreas cancer: expert consensus statement. Annals of Surgical Oncology 2009; 16: 1751–1756.

159. Tempero M, Arnoletti J, Behrman S, Ben-Josef E, Benson AB et al. NCCN clinical practice guidelines in oncology. Pancreatic adenocarcinoma. Journal of the National Comprehensive Cancer Network 2010; 8(9): 972–1017.

160. Topkan E, Parlak C, Kotek A, Yapar AF, Pehlivan B et al. Predictive value of metabolic 18FDG-PET response on outcomes in patients with locally advanced pancreatic carcinoma treated with definitive concurrent chemoradiotherapy. BMC Gastroenterology 2011; 11: 123.

161. Patel M, Hoffe S, Malafa M, Hodul P, Klapman J et al. Neoadjuvant GTX chemotherapy and IMRT-based chemoradiation for borderline resectable pancreatic cancer. Journal of Surgical Oncology 2011; 104: 155–161.

162. Tepper J, Nardi G, Sutt H. Carcinoma of the pancreas: review of MGH experience from 1963 to 1973: analysis of surgical failure and implications for radiation therapy. Cancer 1976; 37: 1519–1524.

163. Griffin JF, Smalley SR, Jewell W, Paradelo JC, Reymond RD et al. Patterns of failure after curative resection of pancreatic carcinoma. Cancer 1990; 66: 56–61.

164. Foo ML, Gunderson LL, Nagorney DM, McLlrath DC, van Heerden JA et al. Patterns of failure in grossly resected pancreatic ductal

adenocarcinoma treated with adjuvant irradiation +/− 5 fluorouracil. International Journal of Radiation Oncology Biology Physics 1993; 26: 483–489.

165. Kayahara M, Nagakawa T, Ueno K, Ohta T, Takeda T et al. An evaluation of radical resection for pancreatic cancer based on the mode of recurrence as determined by autopsy and diagnostic imaging. Cancer 1993; 72: 2118–2123.

166. Verbeke CS, Menon KV. Redefining resection margin status in pancreatic cancer. HPB (Oxford) 2009; 11: 282–289.

167. Klinkenbijl JH, Jeekel J, Sahmoud T, van Pel R, Couvreur ML et al. Adjuvant radiotherapy and 5-fluorouracil after curative resection of cancer of the pancreas and periampullary region: phase III trial of the EORTC gastrointestinal tract cancer cooperative group. Annals of Surgery 1999; 230: 776–782.

168. Kalser MH, Ellenberg SS. Pancreatic cancer. Adjuvant combined radiation and chemotherapy following curative resection [published erratum appears in Archives of Surgery 1986; 121(9): 1045]. Archives of Surgery 1985; 120: 899–903.

169. Neoptolemos JP, Stocken DD, Friess H, Bassi C, Dunn JA et al. A randomized trial of chemoradiotherapy and chemotherapy after resection of pancreatic cancer. New England Journal of Medicine 2004; 350: 1200–1210.

170. GITSG. Further evidence of effective adjuvant combined radiation and chemotherapy following curative resection of pancreatic cancer. Gastrointestinal Tumor Study Group. Cancer 1987; 59: 2006–2010.

171. Regine WF, Winter KA, Abrams RA, Safran H, Hoffman JP et al. Fluorouracil vs gemcitabine chemotherapy before and after fluorouracil-based chemoradiation following resection of pancreatic adenocarcinoma: a randomized controlled trial. Journal of the American Medical Association 2008; 299: 1019–1026.

172. Oettle H, Post S, Neuhaus P, Gellert K, Langrehr J et al. Adjuvant chemotherapy with gemcitabine vs observation in patients undergoing curative-intent resection of pancreatic cancer: a randomized controlled trial. Journal of the American Medical Association 2007; 297: 267–277.

173. Neoptolemos JP, Stocken DD, Bassi C, Ghaneh P, Cunningham D et al. Adjuvant chemotherapy with fluorouracil plus folinic acid vs gemcitabine following pancreatic cancer resection: a randomized controlled trial. Journal of the American Medical Association 2010; 304: 1073–1081.

174. Stocken DD, Buchler MW, Dervenis C, Bassi C, Jeekel H et al. Meta-analysis of randomised adjuvant therapy trials for pancreatic cancer. British Journal of Cancer 2005; 92: 1372–1381.

175. Khanna A, Walker GR, Livingstone AS, Arheart K L, Rocha-Lima C et al. Is adjuvant 5-FU-based chemoradiotherapy for resectable pancreatic adenocarcinoma beneficial? A meta-analysis of an unanswered question. Journal of Gastrointestinal Surgery 2006; 10: 689–697.

176. Wilkowski R, Thoma M, Duhmke E, Rau HG, Heinemann V. Concurrent chemoradiotherapy with gemcitabine and cisplatin after incomplete (R1) resection of locally advanced pancreatic carcinoma. International Journal of Radiation Oncology Biology Physics 2004; 58: 768–772.

177. Hsu CC, Herman JM, Corsini MM, Miller RC. Adjuvant chemoradiation for pancreatic adenocarcinoma: the Johns Hopkins Hospital-Mayo Clinic collaborative study. Annals of Surgical Oncology 2010; 17: 981–990.

178. Evans DB, Varadhachary GR, Crane CH, Sun CC, Lee JE et al. Preoperative gemcitabine-based chemoradiation for patients with resectable adenocarcinoma of the pancreatic head. Journal of Clinical Oncology 2008; 26: 3496–3502.

179. Pingpank JF, Hoffman JP, Ross EA, Cooper HS, Meropol NJ et al. Effect of preoperative chemoradiotherapy on surgical margin status of resected adenocarcinoma of the head of the pancreas. Journal of Gastrointestinal Surgery 2001; 5: 121–130.

180. Tinkl D, Grabenbauer GG, Golcher H, Meyer T, Papadopoulos T et al. Downstaging of pancreatic carcinoma after neoadjuvant chemoradiation. Strahlentherapie und Onkologie 2009; 185: 557–566.

181. Spitz FR, Abbruzzese JL, Lee JE, Pisters PW, Lowy AM et al. Preoperative and postoperative chemoradiation strategies in patients treated with pancreaticoduodenectomy for adenocarcinoma of the pancreas [see comments]. Journal of Clinical Oncology 1997; 15: 928–937.

182. Sohn TA, Yeo CJ, Cameron JL, Koniaris L, Kaushal S et al. Resected adenocarcinoma of the pancreas-616 patients: results, outcomes, and prognostic indicators. Journal of Gastrointestinal Surgery 2000; 4: 567–579.

183. Wayne JD, Wolff RA, Pisters PW, Evans DB. Multimodality management of localized pancreatic cancer. Cancer Journal 2001; 7(Suppl. 1): S35–S46.

184. Rumstadt B, Schwab M, Schuster K, Hagmüller E, Trede M. The role of laparoscopy in the preoperative staging of pancreatic carcinoma. Journal of Gastrointestinal Surgery 1997; 1: 245–250.

185. Brunner TB, Golcher H, Witzigmann H, Marti L, Bechstein W et al. Neoadjuvant chemoradiotherapy versus surgery for pancreatic cancer: a multi-centre randomised phase II trial. Radiotherapy & Oncology 2012; 101: S186–S187.

186. Tamm EP, Loyer EM, Faria S, Raut CP, Evans DB et al. Staging of pancreatic cancer with multidetector CT in the setting of preoperative chemoradiation therapy. Abdominal Imaging 2006; 31: 568–574.

187. Cheng TY, Sheth K, White RR, Ueno T, Hung CF et al. Effect of neoadjuvant chemoradiation on operative mortality and morbidity for pancreaticoduodenectomy. Annals of Surgical Oncology 2006; 13: 66–74.

188. Boeck S, Ankerst DP, Heinemann V. The role of adjuvant chemotherapy for patients with resected pancreatic cancer: systematic review of randomized controlled trials and meta-analysis. Oncology 2007; 72: 314–321.

189. Papalezova KT, Tyler DS, Blazer DG 3rd, et al. Does preoperative therapy optimize outcomes in patients with resectable pancreatic cancer? Journal of Surgical Oncology 2012; 106: 111–118.

190. Callery MP, Chang KJ, Fishman EK, Talamonti MS, William Traverso L et al. Pretreatment assessment of resectable and borderline resectable pancreatic cancer: expert consensus statement. Annals of Surgical Oncology 2009; 16: 1727–1733.

191. Golcher H, Brunner T, Grabenbauer G, Poen JC, Vierra MA et al. Preoperative chemoradiation in adenocarcinoma of the pancreas: a single centre experience advocating a new treatment strategy. European Journal of Surgical Oncology 2008; 34: 756–764.

192. Abrams RA, Winter KA, Regine WF, Safran H, Hoffman JP et al. Failure to adhere to protocol specified radiation therapy guidelines was associated with decreased survival in RTOG 9704—a phase III trial of adjuvant chemotherapy and chemoradiotherapy for patients with resected adenocarcinoma of the pancreas. International Journal of Radiation Oncology Biology Physics 2012; 82: 809–816.

193. Goodman KA, Regine WF, Dawson LA, Ben-Josef E, Haustermans K et al. Radiation therapy oncology group consensus panel guidelines for the delineation of the clinical target volume in the postoperative treatment of pancreatic head cancer. International Journal of Radiation Oncology Biology Physics 2012; 83: 901–908.

194. Brunner TB, Merkel S, Grabenbauer GG, Meyer T, Baum U et al. Definition of elective lymphatic target volume in ductal carcinoma of the pancreatic head based upon histopathologic analysis. International Journal of Radiation Oncology Biology Physics 2005; 62: 1021–1029.

195. Crane CH, Wolff RA, Abbruzzese JL, Evans DB, Milas L et al. Combining gemcitabine with radiation in pancreatic cancer: understanding important variables influencing the therapeutic index. Seminars in Oncology 2001; 28: 25–33.

196. van der Geld YG, van Triest B, Verbakel WF, van Sörnsen de Koste JR, Senan S et al. Evaluation of four-dimensional computed tomography-based intensity-modulated and respiratory-gated radiotherapy techniques for pancreatic carcinoma. International Journal of Radiation Oncology Biology Physics 2008; 72: 1215–1220.

197. Yovino S, Poppe M, Jabbour S, David V, Garofalo M et al. Intensity-modulated radiation therapy significantly improves acute gastrointestinal toxicity in pancreatic and ampullary cancers. International Journal of Radiation Oncology Biology Physics 2011; 79: 158–162.

198. Ben-Josef E, Shields AF, Vaishampayan U, Vaitkevicius V, El-Rayes BF et al. Intensity-modulated radiotherapy (IMRT) and concurrent capecitabine for pancreatic cancer. International Journal of Radiation Oncology Biology Physics 2004; 59: 454–459.

199. Nakamura A, Shibuya K, Matsuo Y, Nakamura M, Shiinoki T et al. Analysis of dosimetric parameters associated with acute gastrointestinal toxicity and upper gastrointestinal bleeding in locally advanced pancreatic cancer patients treated with gemcitabine-based concurrent chemoradiotherapy. International Journal of Radiation Oncology Biology Physics 2012; 84(2): 369–375.

200. Kalser MH, SS Ellenberg. Pancreatic cancer: adjuvant combined radiation and chemotherapy following curative resection. Archives of Surgery 1985; 120(8): 899–903.

201. Klinkenbijl JH, Jeekel J, Sahmoud T, van Pel R, Couvreur ML et al. Adjuvant radiotherapy and 5-fluorouracil after curative resection of cancer of the pancreas and periampullary region: phase III trial of the EORTC gastrointestinal tract cancer cooperative group. Annals of Surgery 1999; 230(6): 776–782; discussion 782–784.

202. Regine WF, Winter KA, Abrams RA, Safran H, Hoffman JP et al. Fluorouracil vs gemcitabine chemotherapy before and after fluorouracil-based chemoradiation following resection of pancreatic adenocarcinoma. Journal of the American Medical Association 2008; 299(9): 1019–1026.

203. Neoptolemos JP, Dunn JA, Stocken DD, Almond J, Link K et al. Adjuvant chemoradiotherapy and chemotherapy in resectable pancreatic cancer: a randomised controlled trial. Lancet 2001; 358(9293): 1576–1585.

204. Neoptolemos JP, Stocken DD, Friess H, Bassi C, Dunn JA et al. A randomized trial of chemoradiotherapy and chemotherapy after resection of pancreatic cancer. New England Journal of Medicine 2004; 350(12): 1200–1210.

205. Abrams RA, Lillemoe KD, Piantadosi S. Continuing controversy over adjuvant therapy of pancreatic cancer. Lancet 2001; 358(9293): 1565–1566.

206. Choti MA. Adjuvant therapy for pancreatic cancer—the debate continues. New England Journal of Medicine 2004; 350(12): 1249–1251.

207. Oettle H, Post S, Neuhaus P, Gellert K, Langrehr J et al. Adjuvant chemotherapy with gemcitabine vs observation in patients undergoing curative-intent resection of pancreatic cancer. Journal of the American Medical Association 2007; 297(3): 267–277.

208. Neuhaus Riess H, Post S. Final results of the randomized, prospective, multicenter phase III trial of adjuvant chemotherapy with gemcitabine vs. observation in patients with resected pancreatic cancer (abstract). Journal of Clinical Oncology 2008; 26: 1009s.

209. Neoptolemos JP, Stocken DD, Bassi C, Ghaneh P, Cunningham D et al. Adjuvant chemotherapy with fluorouracil plus folinic acid vs gemcitabine following pancreatic cancer resection. Journal of the American Medical Association 2010; 304(10): 1073–1081.

210. Lim K-H, Cao D, Linehan D, Smith CT, Cunningham D, Starling N, Neoptolemos JP et al. Neoadjuvant therapy of pancreatic cancer: the emerging paradigm? Oncologist 2012; 17(2): 192–200.

211. Sultana A, Smith CT, Cunningham D, Starling N, Neoptolemos JP et al. Meta-analyses of chemotherapy for locally advanced and metastatic pancreatic cancer. Journal of Clinical Oncology 2007; 25(18): 2607–2615.

212. Carmichael J, Fink U, Russell RC, Spittle MF, Harris AL et al. Phase II study of gemcitabine in patients with advanced pancreatic cancer. British Journal of Cancer 1996; 73(1): 101–105.

213. Casper ES, Green MR, Kelsen DP, Heelan RT, Brown TD et al. Phase II trial of gemcitabine (2,2'-difluorodeoxycytidine) in patients with adenocarcinoma of the pancreas. Investigational New Drugs 1994; 12(1): 29–34.

214. Rothenberg ML, Moore MJ, Cripps MC, Andersen JS, Portenoy RK et al. A phase II trial of gemcitabine in patients with 5-FU-refractory pancreas cancer. Annals of Oncology 1996; 7(4): 347–353.

215. Burris HA, Moore MJ, Andersen J, Green MR, Rothenberg ML et al. Improvements in survival and clinical benefit with gemcitabine as first-line therapy for patients with advanced pancreas cancer: a randomized trial. Journal of Clinical Oncology 1997; 15(6): 2403–2413.

216. Grunewald R, Abbruzzese JL, Tarassoff P, Plunkett W et al. Saturation of 2',2'-difluorodeoxycytidine 5'-triphosphate accumulation by mononuclear cells during a phase I trial of gemcitabine. Cancer Chemotherapy and Pharmacology 1991; 27(4): 258–262.

217. Grunewald R, Kantarjian H, Keating MJ, Abbruzzese J, Tarassoff P et al. Pharmacologically directed design of the dose rate and schedule of 2',2'-difluorodeoxycytidine (gemcitabine) administration in leukemia. Cancer Research 1990; 50(21): 6823–6826.

218. Conroy T, Desseigne F, Ychou M, Bouché O, Guimbaud R et al. FOLFIRINOX versus gemcitabine for metastatic pancreatic cancer. New England Journal of Medicine 2011; 364(19): 1817–1825.

219. Poplin E, Feng Y, Berlin J, Rothenberg ML, Hochster H et al. Phase III, randomized study of gemcitabine and oxaliplatin versus gemcitabine (fixed-dose rate infusion) compared with gemcitabine (30-minute infusion) in patients with pancreatic carcinoma E6201: a trial of the Eastern Cooperative Oncology Group. Journal of Clinical Oncology 2009; 27(23): 3778–3785.

220. Colucci G, Giuliani F, Gebbia V, Biglietto M, Rabitti P et al. Gemcitabine alone or with cisplatin for the treatment of patients with locally advanced and/or metastatic pancreatic carcinoma. Cancer 2002; 94(4): 902–910.

221. Shah MM, Saif MW. Pancreatic cancer and thrombosis. Highlights from the '2010 ASCO Annual Meeting'. Chicago, IL, USA. June 4–8 2010. Journal of Oncology Practice 2010; 11(4): 331–333.

222. Wang X, Ni Q, Jin M, Li Z, Wu Y et al. Gemcitabine or gemcitabine plus cisplatin for in 42 patients with locally advanced or metastatic pancreatic cancer. Zhonghua Zhong Liu Za Zhi 2002; 24(4): 404–407.

223. Reni M. et al. Gemcitabine versus cisplatin, epirubicin, fluorouracil, and gemcitabine in advanced pancreatic cancer: a randomised controlled multicentre phase III trial. Lancet Oncology 2005; 6(6): 369–376.

224. Kahaleh M, Cordio S, Milandri C, Passoni P, Bonetto E et al. Covered self-expandable metal stents in pancreatic malignancy regardless of resectability: a new concept validated by a decision analysis. Endoscopy 2007; 39(4): 319–324.

225. Custodio A, Puente J, Sastre J, Díaz-Rubio E et al. Second-line therapy for advanced pancreatic cancer: a review of the literature and future directions. Cancer Treatment Reviews 2009; 35(8): 676–684.

226. Ryan DP, Bayraktar S, Blaya M, Lopes G, Merchan J et al. A phase II study of gemcitabine and docetaxel in patients with metastatic pancreatic carcinoma. Cancer 2002; 94(1): 97–103.

227. Cengel KA, Edmonds C. Tumor: stroma interactions in pancreatic pancer: Will this sparc prove a raging fire? Cancer Biology & Therapy 2008; 7(11): 1816–1817.

228. Stathopoulos GP, Mavroudis D, Tsavaris N, Kouroussis C, Aravantinos G et al. Treatment of pancreatic cancer with a combination of docetaxel, gemcitabine and granulocyte colony-stimulating factor: a phase II study of the Greek Cooperative Group for Pancreatic Cancer. Annals of Oncology 2001; 12(1): 101–103.

229. Kulke MH, Tempero MA, Niedzwiecki D, Hollis DR, Kindler HL et al. Randomized phase ii study of gemcitabine administered at a fixed dose rate or in combination with cisplatin, docetaxel, or irinotecan in patients with metastatic pancreatic cancer: CALGB 89904. Journal of Clinical Oncology 2009; 27(33): 5506–5512.

230. Herrmann R, Bodovsky, G, Ruhstaller T, Glimelius B, Bajetta E et al. Gemcitabine plus capecitabine compared with gemcitabine alone in advanced pancreatic cancer: a randomized, multicenter, phase III trial of the Swiss Group for Clinical Cancer Research and the Central European Cooperative Oncology Group. Journal of Clinical Oncology 2007; 25(16): 2212–2217.

231. Scheithauer W, Schüll B, Ulrich-Pur H, Schmid K, Raderer M et al. Biweekly high-dose gemcitabine alone or in combination with capecitabine in patients with metastatic pancreatic adenocarcinoma: a randomized phase II trial. Annals of Oncology 2003; 14(1): 97–104.

232. Riess H, Pelzer U, Hilbig A, Stieler J, Opitz B et al. Rationale and design of PROSPECT-CONKO 004: a prospective, randomized trial of simultaneous pancreatic cancer treatment with enoxaparin and chemotherapy. BMC Cancer 2008; 8: 361.

233. Cunningham D, Chau I, Stocken DD, Valle JW, Smith D et al. Phase III randomized comparison of gemcitabine versus gemcitabine plus capecitabine in patients with advanced pancreatic cancer. Journal of Clinical Oncology 2009; 27(33): 5513–5518.

234. Heinemann V, Stefan Boeck, Hinke A, Labianca R, Louvet C. Meta-analysis of randomized trials: evaluation of benefit from gemcitabine-based combination chemotherapy applied in advanced pancreatic cancer. BMC Cancer 2008; 8: 82.

235. Vaccaro V, Sperduti I, Milella M. FOLFIRINOX versus gemcitabine for metastatic pancreatic cancer. New England Journal of Medicine 2011; 365(8): 768–769.

236. Crown J, Casper ES, Botet J, Murray P, Kelsen DP et al. Lack of efficacy of high-dose leucovorin and fluorouracil in patients with advanced pancreatic adenocarcinoma. Journal of Clinical Oncology 1991; 9(9): 1682–1686.

237. DeCaprio JA, Mayer RJ, Gonin R, Arbuck SG et al. Fluorouracil and high-dose leucovorin in previously untreated patients with advanced adenocarcinoma of the pancreas: results of a phase II trial. Journal of Clinical Oncology 1991; 9(12): 2128–2133.

238. Van Rijswijk RE, Jeziorski K, Wagener DJ, Van Laethem JL, Reuse S et al. Weekly high-dose 5-fluorouracil and folinic acid in metastatic pancreatic carcinoma: a phase II study of the EORTC GastroIntestinal Tract Cancer Cooperative Group. European Journal of Cancer 2004; 40(14): 2077–2081.

239. Heinemann V, Schermuly MM, Stieber P, Schulz L, Jüngst D et al. CA19-9: a pedictor of response in pancreatic cancer treated with gemcitabine and cisplatin. AntiCancer Research 1999; 19(4A): 2433–2435.

240. Taïeb J, Lecomte T, Aparicio T, Asnacios A, Mansourbakht T, et al. FOLFIRI.3, a new regimen combining 5-fluorouracil, folinic acid and irinotecan, for advanced pancreatic cancer: results of an Association des Gastro-Entérologues Oncologues (Gastroenterologist Oncologist Association) multicenter phase II study. Annals of Oncology 2007; 18(3): 498–503.

241. Stathopoulos GP, Syrigos K, Aravantinos G, Polyzos A, Papakotoulas P et al. A multicenter phase III trial comparing irinotecan-gemcitabine (IG) with gemcitabine (G) monotherapy as first-line treatment in patients with locally advanced or metastatic pancreatic cancer. British Journal of Cancer 2006; 95(5): 587–592.

242. Conroy T, Paillot B, François E, Bugat R, Jacob JH et al. Irinotecan plus oxaliplatin and leucovorin-modulated fluorouracil in advanced pancreatic cancer—a Groupe Tumeurs Digestives of the Fédération Nationale des Centres de Lutte Contre le Cancer Study. Journal of Clinical Oncology: 2005 23(6): 1228–1236.

243. Tempero MA, Uchida E, Takasaki H, Burnett DA, Steplewski Z et al. Relationship of carbohydrate antigen 19-9 and Lewis antigens in pancreatic cancer. Cancer Research 1987; 47(20): 5501–5503.

244. Pelzer U, Schwaner I, Stieler J, Adler M, Seraphin J et al. Best supportive care (BSC) versus oxaliplatin, folinic acid and 5-fluorouracil (OFF) plus BSC in patients for second-line advanced pancreatic cancer: a phase III-study from the German CONKO-study group. European Journal of Cancer 2011; 47(11): 1676–1681.

245. Von Hoff D, Li CP, Wang-Gillam A, Bodovsky G, Dean A et al. NAPOLI-1: Randomized phase 3 study of MM-398 (nal-iri), with or without 5-fluorouracil and leucovorin, versus 5-fluorouracil and leucovorin, in metastatic pancreatic cancer progressed on or following gemcitabine-based therapy. Annals of Oncology 2014: 25(Suppl. 2): ii105–ii106.

246. Arcidiacono PG, Calori G, Carrara S, McNicol ED, Testoni PA et al. Celiac plexus block for pancreatic cancer pain in adults. Cochrane Database of Systemic Reviews: 2011(3): CD007519.

247. Philip PA, Benedetti J, Corless CL, Wong R, O'Reilly EM et al. Phase III study comparing gemcitabine plus cetuximab versus gemcitabine in patients with advanced pancreatic adenocarcinoma: Southwest Oncology Group–Directed Intergroup Trial S0205. Journal of Clinical Oncology 2010; 28(22): 3605–3610.

248. Cascinu S, Berardi R, Labianca R, Siena S, Falcone A et al. Cetuximab plus gemcitabine and cisplatin compared with gemcitabine and cisplatin alone in patients with advanced pancreatic cancer: a randomised, multicentre, phase II trial. Lancet Oncologyogy 2008; 9(1): 39–44.

249. Van Cutsem E. et al. Phase III Trial of Bevacizumab in Combination With Gemcitabine and Erlotinib in Patients With Metastatic Pancreatic Cancer. Journal of Clinical Oncology 2009; 27(13): 2231–2237.

250. Kindler H, Ioka T, Richel DJ, Bennouna J, Létourneau R et al. Axitinib plus gemcitabine versus placebo plus gemcitabine in patients with advanced pancreatic adenocarcinoma: a double-blind randomised phase 3 study. Lancet Oncology: 2011 12(3): 256–262.

251. Starling N, Watkins D, Cunningham D, Thomas J, Webb J et al. Dose finding and early efficacy study of gemcitabine plus capecitabine in combination with bevacizumab plus erlotinib in advanced pancreatic cancer. Journal of Clinical Oncology 2009; 27(33): 5499–5505.

252. Watkins D, Starling N, Cunninham D, Thomas J, Webb J et al. The combination of a chemotherapy doublet (gemcitabine plus capecitabine) with a biologic doublet (bevacizumab plus erlotinib) in patients with advanced pancreatic adenocarcinoma: the TARGET study. Journal of Clinical Oncology 2010 28: 15s: abs. 4036.

253. Von Hoff DD, Ramanathan RK, Borad MJ, Laheru DA, Smith LS et al. Gemcitabine plus nab-paclitaxel is an active regimen in patients with advanced pancreatic cancer: a phase I/II trial. Journal of Clinical Oncology 2011; 29(34): 4548–4554.

254. Infante JR, Matsubayashi H, Sato N, Tonascia J, Klein AP et al. Peritumoral fibroblast SPARC expression and patient outcome with resectable pancreatic adenocarcinoma. Journal of Clinical Oncology 2007; 25(3): 319–325.

255. Von Hoff DD, Ervin T, Arena FP, Chiorean EG, Infante J et al. Increased survival in pancreatic cancer with nab-paclitaxel plus gemcitabine. New England Journal of Medicine 2013; 369(18): 1691–1703.

256. Maisey NR, Norman AR, Hill A, Massey A, Oates J et al. CA19-9 as a prognostic factor in inoperable pancreatic cancer: the implication for clinical trials. British Journal of Cancer 2005; 93(7): 740–743.

257. Ko AH, Hwang J, Venook AP, Abbruzzese JL, Bergsland EK et al. Serum CA19-9 response as a surrogate for clinical outcome in patients receiving fixed-dose rate gemcitabine for advanced pancreatic cancer. British Journal of Cancer 2005; 93(2): 195–199.

258. Hess V, Glimelius B, Grawe P, Dietrich D, Bodoky G et al. CA 19-9 tumour-marker response to chemotherapy in patients with advanced pancreatic cancer enrolled in a randomised controlled trial. Lancet Oncology 2008; 9(2): 132–138.

259. Locker GY, Hamilton S, Harris J, Jessup JM, Kemeny N et al. ASCO 2006 update of recommendations for the use of tumor markers in gastrointestinal cancer. Journal of Clinical Oncology 2006; 24(33): 5313–5327.

260. Moss AC, Morris E, Mac Mathuna P. Palliative biliary stents for obstructing pancreatic carcinoma. Cochrane Database of Systemic Reviews: 2006(2): CD004200.

261. Speer AG, Cotton PB, Russell RC, Mason RR, Hatfield AR et al. Randomised trial of endoscopic versus percutaneous stent insertion in malignant obstructive jaundice. Lancet 1987; 2(8550): 57–62.

262. Saluja SS, Gulati M, Garg PK, Pal H, Pal S et al. Endoscopic or percutaneous biliary drainage for gallbladder cancer: a randomized trial and quality of life assessment. Clinical Gastroenterology and Hepatology 2008; 6(8): 944–950.

263. Piñol V, Castells A, Bordas JM, Real MI, Llach J et al. Percutaneous self-expanding metal stents versus endoscopic polyethylene

endoprostheses for treating malignant biliary obstruction: randomized clinical Trial. Radiology 2002; 225(1): 27–34.

264. Levy MJ, Baron TH, Gostout CJ, Petersen BT, Farnell MB. Palliation of malignant extrahepatic biliary obstruction with plastic versus expandable metal stents: an evidence-based approach. Clinical Gastroenterology and Hepatology: 2004 2(4): 273–285.

265. Yim HB, Jacobson BC, Saltzman JR, Johannes RS, Bounds BC et al. Clinical outcome of the use of enteral stents for palliation of patients with malignant upper GI obstruction. Gastrointestinal Endoscopy 2001; 53(3): 329–332.

266. Perez MM, Newcomer AD, Moertel CG, Go VL, Dimagno EP et al. Assessment of weight loss, food intake, fat metabolism, malabsorption, and treatment of pancreatic insufficiency in pancreatic cancer. Cancer 1983; 52(2): 346–352.

267. Bruno MJ, Haverkort EB, Tijssen GP, Tytgat GN, van Leeuwen DJ et al. Placebo controlled trial of enteric coated pancreatin microsphere treatment in patients with unresectable cancer of the pancreatic head region. Gut 1998; 42(1): 92–96.

268. Katz MH, Wang H, Fleming JB, Sun CC, Hwang RF et al. Long-term survival after multidisciplinary management of resected pancreatic adenocarcinoma. Annals of Surgical Oncol 2009; 16(4): 836–847.

269. Bickenbach KA, Gonen M, Tang LH, O'Reilly E, Goodman K et al. Downstaging in pancreatic cancer: a matched analysis of patients resected following systemic treatment of initially locally unresectable disease. Annals of Surgical Oncology 2012; 19(5): 1663–1669.

270. Abrams RA, Lowy AM, O'Reilly EM, Wolff RA, Picozzi VJ et al. Combined modality treatment of resectable and borderline resectable pancreas cancer: expert consensus statement. Annals of Surgical Oncology 2009; 16(7): 1751–1756.

271. White R, Winston C, Gonen M, D'Angelica M, Jarnagin W et al. Current utility of staging laparoscopy for pancreatic and peripancreatic neoplasms. Journal of the American College of Surgeons 2008; 206(3): 445–450.

272. Evans DB, Varadhachary GR, Crane CH, Sun CC, Lee JE et al. Preoperative gemcitabine-based chemoradiation for patients with resectable adenocarcinoma of the pancreatic head. Journal of Clinical Oncology 2008; 26(21): 3496–3502.

273. Varadhachary GR, Wolff RA, Crane CH, Sun CC, Lee JE et al. Preoperative gemcitabine and cisplatin followed by gemcitabine-based chemoradiation for resectable adenocarcinoma of the pancreatic head. Journal of Clinical Oncology 2008; 26(21): 3487–3495.

274. Lowy AM. Neoadjuvant therapy for pancreatic cancer. Journal of Gastrointestinal Surgery 2008; 12(9): 1600–1608.

275. Snady H, Bruckner H, Cooperman A, Paradiso J, Kiefer L. Survival advantage of combined chemoradiotherapy compared with resection as the initial treatment of patients with regional pancreatic carcinoma: an outcomes trial. Cancer 2000; 89(2): 314–327

276. van der Gaag NA, Rauws EA, van Eijck CH, Bruno MJ, van der Harst E et al. Preoperative biliary drainage for cancer of the head of the pancreas. New England Journal of Medicine 2010; 362(2): 129–137.

CHAPTER 41

Hepatobiliary cancers

Graeme J. Poston, Nicholas Stern, Jonathan Evans,
Priya Healey, Daniel Palmer, and Mohandas K. Mallath

Introduction to hepatobiliary cancers

The liver, and with it the gall bladder and bile ducts, are some of the most frequent sites of primary and metastatic cancers. Unfortunately, the cancers frequently remain asymptomatic until at an advanced stage and most are therefore detected late, beyond any hope of potentially curative intervention. However, significant advances have been made in detection (particularly radiology), interventional radiological and endoscopic management, surgery, and most significantly in systemic therapies, which means that the prognosis is now brighter than that endured barely a decade ago. This chapter will explore recent advances in radiology and endoscopy before covering the contemporary management of the common primary cancers that affect the liver, gall bladder, and bile ducts.

Epidemiology of hepatocellular carcinoma

The majority of hepatocellular carcinomas (HCCs) occur in patients with underlying parenchymal liver disease, particularly cirrhosis (see Figure 41.1). While chronic liver disease has many aetiologies, cirrhosis per se should be considered the major risk factor for the development of HCC. There are, however, some particular risk factors that have been shown to carry a significantly increased risk for the development of HCC. These include infection with hepatitis B [1, 2] and C [3, 4] viruses, as well as alcoholic liver disease [5, 6]. One of the largest increases in cause of liver disease in the West is non-alcoholic steatohepatitis (NASH)-related cirrhosis. As the liver end-organ disease related to the metabolic

syndrome, NASH-related cirrhosis is associated with diabetes mellitus, dyslipidaemia, hypertension, and the other end-organ diseases of coronary artery disease and cerebrovascular disease. Most cases previously described as cryptogenic cirrhosis are likely to be NASH-related cirrhosis, and this appears to have led to a significant risk for the development of HCC [7]. Common causes of chronic liver disease are shown in Box 41.1.

Epidemiology of biliary cancer

Gall bladder cancer

The incidence rates of gall bladder cancer (GBC) vary widely around the world [8]. Highest rates of GBC are reported from Chile, Bolivia, and Peru. High incidence is also reported from Northern and Eastern India, Pakistan, and Bangladesh, as well as several East Asian countries like Korea and Japan [8, 9]. The incidence of GBC is generally on the lower side in North America and western and northern Europe. However, GBC is more common among Native Americans and Mexican Americans [9]. Some of the lowest incidence rates for GBC are found in African countries as well as among African Americans [8, 10]. Within each ethnic group, the incidence of GBC is several-fold higher in women and steadily increases with age [8–10]. On the whole, the incidence rates for GBC is declining in most parts of the world and much of this is attributed to widespread application of laparoscopic cholecystectomy [11], see also Table 41.1.

Chronic inflammation of the gall bladder mucosa triggered by cholelithiasis is the most common mechanism for the development of GBC [12]. In a small subset of patients having anomalous pancreatic biliary duct (APBD) junction, the carcinogenesis is triggered by the reflux of pancreatic juice into the biliary tree resulting

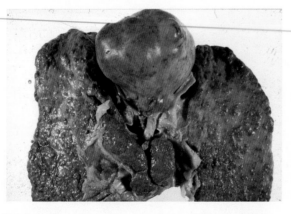

Fig. 41.1 Post-mortem liver specimen showing large HCC arising against background cirrhosis.

Box 41.1 Aetiology of chronic liver disease
Hepatitis B virus
Hepatitis C virus
Alcohol-related liver disease
Non-alcoholic steatohepatitis (NASH)
Hereditary (HFE Gene related) haemochromatosis
Primary biliary cirrhosis
Auto-immune hepatitis
Alpha-one antitrypsin deficiency
Drugs

Table 41.1 Incidence rates of GBC among women worldwide

Incidence rates in women*	Countries
Very low 0.1–1.0	Nigeria, Mongolia, Philippines, Iceland, Uganda, Sri Lanka, United Kingdom, Kenya, Iraq, Egypt
Low 1.1–2.0	Malaysia, Greece, South Africa, Iran, Russian Federation, Norway, Canada, Cuba, USA, Sweden Indonesia, Denmark, The Netherlands, Australia, New Zealand, China, Israel, Spain, Finland, United Arab Emirates, Austria, Switzerland
High 2.1–4.0	Democratic Republic of Korea, Thailand, Germany, Brazil, India, Pakistan, Saudi Arabia, Ireland, Singapore, Argentina, Italy, Qatar, Poland, Colombia, Uruguay
Very high 4.1–13.4	Japan, Czech Republic, Mexico, Republic of Korea, Bangladesh, Peru, Nepal, Bolivia, Chile

* The rates are per 100,000 and adjusted for age.

Source: data from Ferlay J. et al., GLOBOCAN 2008 v2.0, *Cancer Incidence and Mortality Worldwide: IARC CancerBase No. 10*, International Agency for Research on Cancer, Lyon, France, Copyright © 2010, available from <http://globocan.iarc.fr>.

in biliary epithelial damage and chronic inflammation [12]. The molecular alterations found in GBC tissues in patients with an APBD junction are different from those in the setting of gallstone disease. Most GBCs are strongly associated with genetic and environmental factors facilitating the development of gallstones. There is a strong association between gallstones and GBC in numerous studies [12–14]. Gallstones are found in 70 to 90% of patients with GBC. However, the overall incidence of GBC in patients with cholelithiasis is only 0.2 to 3%. Less than 1% of gall bladders removed for symptomatic stone disease show evidence of incidental GBC. The risk of GBC is higher with larger gallstones and of long-standing duration. The risk of GBC in porcelain gall bladder is lower than what was initially reported [15].

There are several other risk factors for GBC including gall bladder polyps, chronic infections, congenital anomalies, exposure to toxins, obesity, diabetes, etc. The proportions of GBC attributable to these risk factors vary widely in different geographic regions. Gall bladder polyps are mucosal protuberances detected incidentally on ultrasonography or after cholecystectomy. The gall bladder polyps mostly occur in the absence of cholelithiasis, and chronic inflammation is usually absent [12]. The benign polyps are sub-classified as non-neoplastic (e.g., cholesterol and inflammatory polyps, adenomyomas) or neoplastic (e.g., adenomas, leiomyomas) depending on the histopathologic features. The malignant potential of an adenoma is variable, and the frequency of progression from adenoma to carcinoma is unclear.

Several reports have associated biliary cysts and APBD junction and GBC. Biliary cysts are congenital or acquired dilatation of the biliary tree, often associated with other anatomic abnormalities of the biliary tract [16]. The APBD and biliary cysts are more common in East Asians. There is a strong association between GBC and chronic infection of the gall bladder and biliary tract by *Salmonella* and *Helicobacter* in endemic regions. Socio-economic factors that facilitate chronic infections of the gall bladder and biliary tract by pathogenic bacteria like *Salmonella* and *Helicobacter* are also

important. The chronic carrier state occurs most often in individuals with cholelithiasis, and gallstones appear to be the primary cause of the ongoing infection and inflammation. While typhoid carrier state is an established strong risk factor for GBC, the causal role of *Helicobacter* infection needs more studies [17]. Cigarette smoking, obesity, and diabetes have been associated with GBC in several large studies [18–20]. A small proportion of GBCs are associated with drugs like methyldopa, isoniazid, and oral contraceptives; exposure to industrial toxins among occupations handling oil, paper, chemicals, shoe, textiles, and cellulose acetate fibres; and manufacturing industries and miners exposed to radon.

Cholangiocarcinoma

The term cholangiocarcinoma is used to include intrahepatic, perihilar, and extrahepatic bile duct cancers. These tumours accounts for about 3% of all digestive cancers. The proportions of intrahepatic cholangiocarcinoma (IHCC) are variable and make up about 15% of all primary liver cancers and the prevalences of extrahepatocellular carcinoma (EHCC) vary in different parts of the world and constitute about one-third of all cancers grouped as gall bladder cancers. The recent time trends for cholangiocarcinoma are noteworthy [21, 22]. The incidence of IHCC has been rising in most parts of Europe, North America, Asia, Japan, and Australia like the HCC trends. The incidence rates of EHCC have been declining like GBC trends. This is partly attributed to changes in the International Classification of Disease classification, and better diagnostic methods [23]. However, part of this trend is related to increase in risk factors such as chronic liver disease. The decreasing incidence of EHCC is largely unexplained, and is attributed to reducing risk factors such as uncontrolled inflammatory bowel disease, smoking, and biliary infestations and infections. In contrast to GBC, the incidence of cholangiocarcinoma is several-fold higher in men [8]. The incidence of cholangiocarcinoma steadily increases with age, but those associated with primary sclerosing cholangitis (PSC) and choledochal cysts occur few decades earlier [24].

The risk factors for cholangiocarcinoma vary widely in different geographical regions [22]. Chronic inflammation is the trigger for the development of cholangiocarcinoma like GBC [25]. IHCC is strongly associated with chronic liver diseases and EHCC is associated with inflammatory conditions of the biliary tract [22–27]. In Western countries, PSC and choledochal cysts are the major risk factors for cholangiocarcinoma [24]. In Asian regions, chronic intrahepatic stone disease, recurrent pyogenic cholangitis, and parasitic infestations are the common causes of EHCC [28].

Chronic inflammation of the biliary tree due to PSC causes fibrosis and stricturing of the intrahepatic and/or extrahepatic bile ducts. Symptomatic or asymptomatic ulcerative colitis is very frequently found in PSC and about 30% of patients with EHCC have ulcerative colitis. The lifetime risk of cholangiocarcinoma in patients with ulcerative colitis has been is estimated to be 10 to 15% but autopsy studies reveal higher risk. Tobacco and alcohol abuse and genetic predispositions also contribute to the risk of cholangiocarcinoma in patients with PSC. Patients with choledochal cysts of various subtypes are at increased risk of developing cholangiocarcinoma at a younger age. The postulated mechanism involves chronic inflammation triggered by biliary stasis, reflux of pancreatic juice, or deconjugation of carcinogens.

Parasitic infection with liver flukes of the genera *Clonorchis* and *Opisthorchis* are associated with IHCC [28]. The highest parasite-related cholangiocarcinomas are reported from Thailand. The fluke larvae present in fish enters the human body by eating undercooked fish and reach maturity in the biliary tract. Adult flukes lay eggs in the biliary tract and initiate a chronic inflammation. Secondary bacterial infection, smoking, and alcohol are found to be cofactors. Increased risk (lower than for GBC) between gallstone disease and cholangiocarcinoma has been reported [14]. Chronic intrahepatic stone disease, also called recurrent pyogenic cholangitis or hepatolithiasis, is associated with cholangiocarcinoma. This disease is endemic in many parts of East Asia and is rare in Western countries. The exact cause of hepatolithiasis is unknown, and is probably related to congenital ductal abnormalities or chronic infection by bacterial or parasitic infestations. The intrahepatic stones are composed of calcium bilirubinate (brown pigment stones), suggesting that bacterial deconjugation of stagnant bile is responsible.

The finding of IHCC in explanted cirrhotic livers indicates that chronic hepatic inflammation is an important mechanism for the development of IHCC. A cohort study from Denmark reported a ten-fold higher risk for IHCC in patients with chronic liver disease compared to the general population. Several studies have reported an increased risk for IHCC (lower than for HCC) in patients with hepatitis C virus (HCV)-related chronic liver disease. An increased risk of IHHC in patients with chronic hepatitis B virus infection has been reported. Chronic liver disease from non-viral etiology is also associated with IHCC. Populations of HIV infected individuals are at increased risk of IHCC, and some of this association is due to coexisting chronic liver disease.

Exposure to Thorotrast (a radiologic contrast now banned) has been associated with the development of cholangiocarcinoma. Other associations include exposure to occupational toxins among those working in the automotive, rubber, chemical, and wood-finishing industries. Hereditary non-polyposis colorectal cancer, biliary papillomatosis, and hemochromatosis are some genetic disorders with increased risk of cholangiocarcinoma. Cigarette smoking, obesity, and diabetes have also been associated with GBC in several large studies.

Microbiology and pathology of hepatobiliary cancer

The majority of hepatobiliary (HB) cancers are caused by chronic inflammation of the liver parenchyma or the epithelium of the bile ducts. Over 80% of the global burden of hepatocellular cancer (HCC) is attributed to chronic hepatitis caused by hepatitis B virus (HBV) or hepatitis C virus (HCV) [29, 30]. A small proportion of HCCs are caused by mixed HBV and HCV infections or co-infection of HBV carriers with hepatitis delta virus (HDV) [30, 31]. Chronic HBV and HCV infections also cause IHCC [32]. Most of the IHCCs in high-incidence regions are caused by chronic infestation of intrahepatic bile ducts with liver flukes [33]. A strong association between gall bladder cancer and carrier state of *Salmonella typhi* and *S. paratyphi* has been reported in many studies. This may be a secondary phenomenon as the majority of these patients harbour gallstones. There are increasing reports associating various Helicobacter species (*H. bilis, H. hepaticus,* and *H. pylori*) with gall bladder cancer. More studies are needed to confirm if this association is causal. The wide variations in the incidence rates of HB cancers are explainable by regional variations in the prevalence of chronic infection with HBV, HCV, other parasites, and other environmental toxins.

Hepatitis B

There is a strong causal association between chronic HBV infection and HCC and the geographical incidence of HCC closely follows the regional HBV carrier rates classified as high, intermediate, and low-prevalence regions. Most of the HBV infection has been acquired vertically by perinatal transmission in high-prevalence regions, while horizontal transmission is more often the mechanism in low-incidence regions. Decades of HBV vaccination has reduced the incidence of HBV-related HCC [34]. Although patients with chronic HBV can develop HCC in the absence of cirrhosis, over 70 to 90% of patients with HBV-associated HCC have cirrhosis. Several HBV-related factors modify the risk of developing HCC. This includes the viral load of HBV, the presence of hepatitis B e antigen (HBeAg), the presence of hepatitis B surface antigen (HBsAg), the genotype of HBV, the presence or absence of cirrhosis, and the use of antiviral therapies [35–40]. The risk of HCC is proportional to the viral load of HBV DNA and the risk is lower in those who have low levels. The HBV DNA load is an independent risk factor for HCC after adjusting for other known risk factors including male sex, older age, smoking, alcohol consumption, HBeAg status, serum alanine transaminase (ALT) level, and the presence of cirrhosis. The HBV DNA load tends to fluctuate and a single measurement can be misleading. Presence of high HBV DNA loads and active inflammation (elevated ALT) are indicators of high risk of developing HCC and such patients are advised to undergo regular surveillance for HCC. Active viral replication suggested by HBeAg positivity is also an independent predictive marker for the progression to HCC after adjustment for other risk factors. Patients with inactive carrier state (HBsAg positive but HBeAg negative) and those having serologically resolved infections (HBsAg negative, HBsAg positive) are also at an increased risk of developing HCC compared to the general population. Suppression of the viral replication with antiviral therapies helps in reducing the incidence of HBV-related HCC. Systematic review of multiple studies indicates that the relative risk for developing HCC is reduced substantially with effective anti-HBV therapies. The development of antibiotic resistance increases the risk for HCC. Dual infection with HCV and co-infection with HDV are associated with a higher risk of developing HCC. Several other risk factors such as older age, family history of HCC, habitual alcohol consumption, cigarette smoking, exposure to aflatoxin, the presence of core and precore mutations, and higher hepatic iron reserves increase the risk of developing HCC in patients with chronic HBV infection.

Hepatitis C

There is a strong causal association between chronic HCV infection and HCC [41]. Chronic HCV is an increasing cause of HCC in developed countries and is responsible for the rising incidence rates of HCC in North America, Europe, and Japan. The cumulative lifetime risk for developing HCC with chronic HCV infection is higher in men. Like HBV-related HCC, patients with higher HCV viral loads have increased risk of developing HCC. It is generally agreed that HCC arises as a result of chronic inflammation caused by the hepatitis C virus and HCV-induced HCC correlates well with the degree of inflammation and necrosis. Advanced stages of hepatic fibrosis or cirrhosis are found in nearly 90% of patients with HCV-associated HCC. HBV-related HCC, on the other hand, does not correlate very well with hepatic inflammation, as oncogene activation by replicating HBV is an important mechanism for the development of HCC. The HCV genotype can modify the risk of developing HCC, and antiviral therapy that reduces the viral load and achieves sustained virologic response (i.e., viral clearance) reduces the risk of developing HCC in these patients [42]. Other cofactors that increase the risk of HCC in patients with chronic HCV include heavy alcohol use, diabetes mellitus, increased hepatic iron, and non-alcoholic fatty liver disease [43]. Reductions of HCV infections are now achievable with interferon, ribavirin, and protease and polymerase inhibitors; although achievable with some toxicity and cost, these treatments could reduce the development of HCC in some populations.

Liver flukes

Several liver flukes (trematodes) infest humans as opportunistic hosts and are an important cause of cholangiocarcinoma [44–45]. They include: *Clonorchis sinensis, Opisthorchis* species, *Metorchis conjunctus*, and *Fasciola hepatica. Clonorchis sinensis* (Chinese liver fluke) is endemic in many regions of the Far East in Japan, China, Korea, Taiwan, Vietnam, and parts of eastern Russia [33, 44–47]. Clonorchis is a fish parasite and infests fish-eating mammals like dogs and cats, which serve as the common reservoirs. It is estimated that there are over 600 million people at risk and more than 35 million people have been infected worldwide. Opisthorchiasis is generally caused by accidental infestation of humans by *O. felineus* or *O. viverrini*, a fish parasite which infests fish-eating mammals that also serve as the common reservoirs. *O. felineus* is seen in South-east Asia and in central and eastern Europe (Siberia and other parts of the former Soviet Union). It has been estimated that over 16 million people have been infested and the prevalence rates are very high up to 40 to 95% in some regions. *O. viverrini* is an endemic liver fluke in Thailand, Cambodia, Laos, and Vietnam. It is estimated that over 23 million people are infected worldwide, with prevalence rates of 24 to 90% in some regions of Thailand and 40 to 80% in Laos. *Metorchis conjunctus* is a liver fluke endemic to North America and Russia. It is in the same Opisthorchiidae family as *C. sinensis, O. viverrini*, and *O. felineus* and share same life cycle. This fluke is common among native Canadians. It is unknown whether prolonged infection and biliary complications can occur with *M. conjunctus*.

The adult flukes take about a month to mature and may range in size from a few millimetres to several centimetres depending on the species. The adult liver flukes can remain in the bile ducts for two or more decades. Repeat infections are frequent as protective immunity is ineffective, and cumulative worm burden can be high in endemic regions. Symptomatic infection is delayed for many years and commonly manifests in older adults. Travellers and immigrants from endemic areas harbouring the flukes may take it to non-endemic areas as demonstrated in surveys of South-east Asian immigrants. Frozen, dried, and pickled fish may contain surviving larvae and infect individuals who have never travelled to endemic areas. Biliary stones may be formed over dead parasites or ova. Obstructive jaundice, pancreatitis, recurrent cholangitis, and pyogenic liver abscesses, cholangiohepatitis, are some of the common clinical manifestations. Chronic irritation of the epithelial cells eventually leads to hyperplasia, dysplasia, and fibrosis. This may result in pigment stone formation, biliary strictures, dilation of intrahepatic bile ducts, with fibrosis of hepatic cells and IHCC as delayed complications. There are community-based programs running in Thailand and other East Asian regions to control liver fluke infestation by various interventions to reduce the incidence of cholangiocarcinoma [45].

Pathology

The World Health Organization (WHO) classification is used for pathological subtyping of HB cancers [48]. Histopathology subtypes of liver cancers include hepatocellular carcinoma (HCC), intrahepatic cholangiocarcinoma (IHCC), combined hepatocellular and cholangiocarcinoma (CHCC), bile duct cyst adenocarcinoma, hepatoblastoma, and undifferentiated carcinoma. The subtypes of extrahepatic bile ducts and gall bladder cancer include: adenocarcinoma, papillary adenocarcinoma, adenocarcinoma, intestinal type adenocarcinoma, gastric foveolar type, mucinous adenocarcinoma, clear cell adenocarcinoma, signet-ring cell carcinoma, adenosquamous carcinoma, squamous cell carcinoma, small cell (oat cell) carcinoma, large cell neuroendocrine carcinoma, undifferentiated carcinoma, and biliary cystadenoma. There is no pathognomonic immunohistochemical stain to confirm the cell type of origin of HB cancers. Immunohistochemical staining for cytokeratin-7 (CK-7) and hepatocyte paraffin 1 monoclonal antibody (Hep Par 1) is used to support the pathological diagnosis of cholangiocarcinoma and HCC.

When patients are on a screening program, most of the HCCs are diagnosed non-invasively using defined radiological criteria. An image-guided biopsy (core biopsy is preferred) is needed in patients with atypical features, when the diagnosis is uncertain and before using chemotherapy or targeted therapy in non-resectable cancers. The HCCs are often multicentric in nature. The microscopic appearance vary from well-differentiated (malignant hepatocytes appearing nearly identical to normal hepatocytes) to poorly-differentiated lesions (large multinucleate anaplastic tumour giant cells). Central necrosis is common in larger cancers. The surrounding liver has features of the primary cause of the chronic liver disease and dysplasia in a cirrhotic liver is the only finding. The cholangiocarcinomas are classified by their location in the biliary tree: IHCC, hilar cholangiocarcinoma, and EHCC. Simultaneous involvement of multiple sites is infrequent. Adenocarcinomas comprise nearly 90% of all cholangiocarcinomas with varying desmoplastic reaction. The gross appearance may be papillary, sclerosing, nodular, and combined type. The cholangiocarcinoma tends to grow slowly, invade locally, produce mucin, invade perineural sheaths, and distant metastases are uncommon. Preoperative diagnosis by biopsy or cytology is difficult due to the desmoplastic fibrosis. Cholangiocarcinoma caused by chronic biliary disease (e.g., hepatolithiasis) may harbour precancerous lesions like dysplasia and carcinoma in situ. Adenocarcinomas comprise nearly 90% of all primary gall bladder cancers. The gross appearance may be papillary, infiltrative, nodular, and combined type. GBC with papillary subtypes have the best prognosis. Gall bladder cancers invade the wall and beyond to the liver and other adjoining organs easily because of the lack of a well-defined muscularis layer.

Imaging of hepatobiliary cancers

Ultrasound is conventionally the first-line modality in imaging the liver and biliary tract for detection of focal liver lesions (FLL) and assessment of biliary tract dilatation. Good quality ultrasound can characterize a definite benign lesion (e.g., cyst), from a definite malignant lesion (e.g., metastasis). However, due to considerable overlap in appearance of benign and malignant lesions, accurate characterization is often not possible using unenhanced ultrasound alone.

Obese patients and those with altered anatomy can be particularly difficult to evaluate with ultrasound. Fatty liver attenuates ultrasound resulting in poor liver penetration, reducing confidence in accurate evaluation of the entire liver; it should not be used when there is a high clinical suspicion of malignancy. Although ultrasound is frequently used to assess biliary dilatation, it is less useful in determining the aetiology. Dilatation of the ducts can suggest the presence of malignancy in a high-risk patient, but due to frequent overlying gastric and duodenal gas, the ducts are rarely seen throughout their entire course.

The advent of ultrasound contrast bubbles (CEUS) has significantly increased the sensitivity and specificity of FLL [49]. CEUS assesses real-time lesion vascularity with a temporal resolution superior to that of other imaging modalities [50]. CEUS enhancement pattern of FLL is similar to that of contrast enhanced computed tomography (CT) and magnetic resonance (MR). Portal venous invasion and tumour thrombus being well depicted [51], CEUS is particularly useful in patients with renal failure, where CT and MR contrast agents are contraindicated due to the risk of increasing renal failure and nephrogenic systemic fibrosis.

CT is widely used to assess HB cancers. The spatial resolution and ability to perform multiphase and multiplanar images result in a high sensitivity and specificity in detecting, characterizing, and staging cancers. It is also the first-line imaging modality used for patients with liver metastases from an unknown primary.

Triphasic scans are conventionally used to assess HB tumours (Figure 41.2). The phase depends on the type of tumour being assessed. An unenhanced, arterial, and portal venous phase scan is used to assess cirrhotic livers. Hyperdense nodules corresponding to iron-rich regenerative nodules appear denser than the surrounding liver, giving false positive readings of arterial enhancement. An unenhanced scan of the liver is performed to assess nodule density before contrast is administered. This phase provides a more accurate assessment of arterial enhancement and washout when assessing small HCCs. Due to the angiogenesis of HCC in cirrhotic livers [52], it can be difficult to differentiate a regenerative nodule from well-differentiated HCC. In these patients, short-term follow-up is often necessary to assess for change in the enhancement characteristics of nodules. Due to the heavy radiation burden of CT, MR or CEUS is considered more appropriate for these patients.

Cholangiocarcinomas are hypovascular, and due to the desmoplastic reaction typically seen within these lesions, and there is progressive enhancement of the lesion with time. Therefore, an arterial, portal, and delayed five-minute scan is performed to assess the full extent of the tumour. Vascular contact and invasion is accurately depicted on CT.

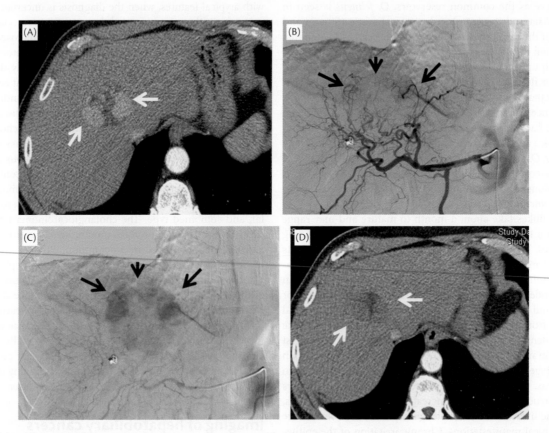

Fig. 41.2 HCC. Arterial phase CT (A) showing lobulated tumour enhancement and fat within the tumour. Arteriography at the time of TACE showing tumour arterialization in the early phase (B) followed by contrast staining a few seconds later. (C) Arterial CT (D) after three TACE procedures over six months showing reduced size and disappearance of arterial enhancement.

Whole body CT is performed to assess for distant metastases. Multiplanar reformats aid the surgeon in assessing the vascular supply to the liver and variants in the vascular and biliary structures. CT is conventionally used in the follow-up of patients post-treatment due to the uniformity and reproducibility of the images for the purposes of RECIST criteria.

MR of the liver can be superior to CT in characterizing liver lesions and detecting small liver metastases [53, 54]. The advent of liver specific contrast agents have significantly improved lesion characterization and detection [55, 56] particularly in differentiating small HCC from regenerative nodules [57]. These contrast agents are taken up by normally functioning hepatocytes. A lesion not containing hepatocytes will not take up contrast, and will appear dark against an enhancing liver. These contrast agents are now being used more frequently due to the ability to detect more lesions on the liver specific phase together with the conventional sequences, than on conventional contrast enhanced CT alone. This is particularly important for colorectal liver metastases prior to consideration of liver resection [58].

Although the biliary tract is seen well on CT, MR is superior in assessment of the biliary tree. Contrast MR and magnetic resonance cholangio-pancreatography (MRCP) is the imaging modality of choice in the assessment of the liver and biliary tree particularly in hilar (mostly infiltrating) and intraductal cholangiocarcinoma for the purposes of resectability [59]. The 3D maximum intensity projection (MIP) image of the biliary tree depicts the extent of duct dilatation, stricturing, and invasion of the intra- and extrahepatic ducts necessary for tumour staging. Contrast enhanced MR depicts the extent of the lesion and vascular contact, and the presence of satellite lesions. Liver-specific MR contrast agents are excreted in bile, providing further assessment of the biliary tract with an enhanced MRCP image. Diffusion weighted imaging of the liver has been shown to be useful in the characterization of FLL. This sequence has found to be particularly useful for the detection of small liver metastases [60] and has proved useful in the identification of an HCC amongst regenerative nodules in the cirrhotic liver [61]. Its role in the assessment of tumour responsiveness to chemotherapy and follow-up is being evaluated [62].

Positron emission tomography (PET) utilizes the increase in glycolysis in cells to depict metabolically active lesions. This is not only seen in tumour cells, but also in normal and inflamed tissue. Therefore PET can be sensitive, but not always specific. The uptake of tracer is variable in HCC, with low sensitivity compared to CT. Regenerative nodules can show increased tracer uptake compared to HCC. Disease staging using PET is only useful if the primary tumour is metabolically avid [63]. Peripheral cholangiocarcinomas are hypermetabolic but hilar and intraductal cholangiocarcinomas demonstrate low uptake of tracer. PET CT may be used in staging and characterizing peripheral tumours but its use is otherwise limited. PET MR is an emerging technique for assessment of colorectal liver metastases and has been shown to be superior to PET CT in their detection [64]. There is limited literature to date about the usefulness of PET MR in primary liver and ductal carcinomas.

Interventional biliary endoscopy

With improved cross-sectional and diagnostic imaging modalities, interventional biliary endoscopy is now rarely required for diagnosis. MRI now provides high quality cholangiography and cross-sectional imaging (65–67). Endoscopic ultrasound (EUS) [68, 69] provides views from the gut lumen which are particularly useful for diagnostic imaging of the extrahepatic biliary tree and pancreas. The improved quality of CT [70–72] provides accurate diagnosis and staging of HB malignancies, thereby avoiding the risks of endoscopic retrograde cholangio-pancreatography (ERCP).

Endoscopic ultrasound

EUS evaluates the extrahepatic biliary tree, including indeterminate lymphadenopathy at the porta hepatis and para-aortic regions. EUS provides detailed views of the bile ducts, ampulla, pancreas, and liver hilum. EUS does not carry the associated risks of ERCP. Radial EUS provides a 360° image, whereas linear EUS provides a view in the plane of the scope and allows for the sampling of tissue via biopsy or fine needle aspiration (FNA) [73, 74]. EUS is also the most sensitive tool for diagnosing small bile duct calculi.

Endoscopic retrograde cholangio-pancreatography

ERCP provides access to the biliary tree and is complimentary to percutaneous transhepatic cholangiography (PTC) in both the investigation and management of biliary tract tumours. Initially a diagnostic tool, ERCP is now largely a therapeutic modality in view of the associated complication rate. At ERCP, a side viewing duodenoscope is passed to the second part of the duodenum, sitting opposite the Ampulla of Vater to enable cannulation. The duct of choice (normally the common bile duct), is then accessed, normally using a wire guided cannulation technique. A 0.035" diameter wire is passed into the duct of choice and a cholangiogram obtained with fluoroscopic screening to provide diagnostic imaging. Tissue acquisition can be performed at the time for suspected malignant disease using brush cytology sampling, which carries a relatively low diagnostic yield [75, 76], or by the passage of small biopsy forceps into the duct to enable formal biopsy, with increasing diagnostic yield.

In biliary malignancy, therapeutic ERCP is often used to investigate obstructive jaundice [77]. The type of intervention depends on the site and stage of tumour, and the planned treatment course. ERCP and biliary drainage must only be performed following high quality cross-sectional diagnostic imaging and discussions regarding operability for patients with proximal cholangiocarcinoma. As the surgical options for hilar cholangiocarcinomas involve major liver resections, communication between the liver surgeon and endoscopist is essential to allow accurate planning of any preoperative ERCP with appropriate drainage of the planned future liver remnant (FLR). There is increasing use of self-expanding metallic stents (SEMS) to decompress obstructed bile ducts prior to such planned liver surgery [78]. Given the complex and multidisciplinary nature of these decisions, drainage procedures for proximal biliary malignancies should only be performed in specialist hepatobiliary units.

The majority of patients undergoing endoscopic stenting for proximal biliary malignancies will not be operable, and in these cases adequate biliary drainage is paramount for good palliation of jaundice, but the decision about whether to drain proximal biliary obstruction endoscopically or percutaneously may be unclear. However, in potentially operable cases, the goal is to enable adequate internal biliary drainage of the appropriate segment(s) of the FLR. It is not uncommon that combined endoscopic and percutaneous interventions will be necessary. The choice about whether these interventions should be primarily endoscopic or percutaneous depends on available local expertise: however, both modalities should be available to maximize the chances of successful biliary drainage for all cases.

When performing ERCP on patients with hilar tumours it is essential to ensure drainage of all opacified segments, as failure to do so increases biliary sepsis and mortality [79, 80]. Adequate biliary drainage can be achieved to palliate jaundice by draining just 30% of the liver, which involves unilateral drainage of the FLR [81, 82]. With more aggressive biliary drainage and reduction of sepsis complicating biliary obstruction, patients will be palliated for longer; therefore, draining just 30% of the liver is unlikely to be adequate long-term, especially given the risks of sepsis associated with systemic chemotherapy. Therefore, drainage of at least 50% of the liver volume should be done, which will often involve bilateral stents. One should avoid drainage of atrophic liver segments, which increases the risks of sepsis, while not providing drainage to the FLR.

Direct endoscopic cholangioscopy

Cholangioscopy enables direct visualization of the bile ducts, either operatively or endoscopically. Originally, mother and baby ERCP cholangioscopy only visualized the biliary mucosa of the common duct, and required two endoscopists to operate. This has changed with the development of the new SpyGlass™ (Boston Scientific) cholangioscope. SpyGlass™ cholangioscopy enables a single operator to visualise the biliary mucosa to at least second and third order ducts, with the benefit of a working channel to allow directly visualised biopsies and therapy applied. Directly targeted biopsies improve the diagnostic yield to >80% in patients with indeterminate biliary strictures [83, 84]. While the use of diagnostic ERCPs has decreased significantly, the benefit of direct ERCP cholangioscopy is clear. In our practice, such cholangioscopy is only performed following a specialized multidisciplinary review of all non-invasive and cross-sectional imaging.

Multidisciplinary management of HCC

Diagnosis and staging: surveillance for HCC in high-risk groups

There is little strong evidence for the surveillance of patients with cirrhosis, or other high-risk groups for HCC. Only one randomized controlled trial has been performed in a Chinese population with predominantly chronic Hepatitis B infection [85]. While this study did show detection of earlier stage disease and better outcomes in the surveillance group, this was only adhered to in about 60% of patients. The authors concluded that the benefit may be greater if surveillance protocols were more rigidly followed. Other uncontrolled (mostly retrospective) studies have shown detection of earlier stage disease and better survival in surveillance groups [86–88]. There are no randomized controlled trials examining HCC surveillance in Western populations.

Despite the lack of grade one evidence, most authorities on liver disease advocate the surveillance of identified high-risk groups (cirrhosis, non-cirrhotic chronic Hepatitis B and C infection) [89–92]. Given the wide use and recommendation of surveillance strategies in managing these patients, it is unlikely that a randomized controlled trial of surveillance for HCC will take place in a Western country. Currently, surveillance is recommended in the form of six-monthly liver ultrasound scans and serum alpha-feto

Table 41.2 Child-Pugh score

	1	2	3
Albumin	>34	28–34	<28
Bilirubin	<34	34–51	>51
INR	<1.7	1.7–2.3	>2.3
Ascites	None	Mild	Moderate to severe
Encephalopathy	None	Grade I–II	Grade III–IV

Child A: ≤6; Child B: 7-9; Child C ≥10.

Reproduced from Pugh RNH et al., Transection of the oesophagus for bleeding oesophageal varices, *British Journal of Surgery*, Volume 60, Issue 8, pp. 646–649, Copyright © 1973 British Journal of Surgery Society Ltd, with permission from John Wiley & Sons Ltd.

protein (AFP) measurement. It is hoped that this regimen will diagnose more tumours in their earlier stages where active treatments are available for either potential cure or disease control. The goal of surveillance is cost-effective monitoring of high-risk groups to diagnose disease at an early and treatable stage. Given current methods, AFP is not raised in a large proportion of HCCs, particularly in those small enough for potentially cure, so while cheap, AFP may not be particularly effective as a sole surveillance marker [93, 94]. Ultrasound, whilst more expensive to perform, has a better sensitivity and specificity for the identification of liver lesions that can then be characterized further using more detailed imaging methods [95]. While surveillance of at risk groups is useful, a significant proportion of patients present with HCC without a known prior history of chronic liver disease and, increasingly, HCC is seen as the presenting problem in patients with NASH cirrhosis.

Assessment of severity of cirrhosis

Assessment of the liver function is necessary to determine the appropriate treatment of patients with HCC with cirrhosis. For patients to be treated with either loco-regional therapies or occasionally surgical resection requires preserved hepatic synthetic function. The severity of liver disease and degree of liver failure can be measured using various clinical and laboratory parameters. The standard bedside assessment, and that used as a part of the Barcelona Clinic for Liver Cancer (BCLC) staging algorithm [96] involves the use of the Child-Pugh score [97]. The Child-Pugh score is detailed in Table 41.2, where a Child-Pugh score ≤6 relates to well-compensated cirrhosis or good liver function with a good prognosis (Child-Pugh A). A Child-Pugh score ≥10 equates to decompensated liver disease or liver failure with a bad prognosis (Child-Pugh C); while Child-Pugh score 7–9 (Child-Pugh B) relates to a prognosis between A and C. When assessing patients for liver transplantation for parenchymal liver failure, transplant centres tend to stratify severity using the model of end-stage liver disease (MELD) [98], or in the UK a variant on this which includes the prognostic value of a serum sodium level, the United Kingdom end-stage liver disease score (UKELD) [99] (Table 41.3).

Decision making in hepatocellular carcinoma

While the decision making algorithm for most cancer patients depends on both staging of the disease and patient fitness (performance status), the severity and stage of liver disease is a third aspect that needs to be taken into consideration in patients with cirrhosis and HCC. The diagnosis of HCC is frequently made

Table 41.3 MELD and UKELD Scores

MELD Score	MELD = 9.57 × log$_e$(creatinine, mg/dl) + 3.78 × log$_e$(total bilirubin, mg/dl) + 11.2 × log$_e$(INR) + 6.43
UKELD Score	5 × [1.5 × log$_e$(INR) + 0.3 × log$_e$(creatinine, μmol/l) + 0.6 × log$_e$(bilirubin, μmol/l) − 13 × log$_e$(serum sodium, mmol/l) + 70]

against a background history of chronic liver disease, an elevated or rising serum AFP and radiology of the liver (see above). Biopsy should only be a last resort, and then only performed at the tertiary liver centre because of the real risk of tumour seeding (see Figure 41.3). For the majority of treatment modalities, synthetic liver function has to be preserved (Child-Pugh A or B). Treatments for HCC are decided largely according to the BCLC criteria (Figure 41.4) [96]. The BCLC staging system encompasses tumour characteristics as well as performance status and liver function. BCLC as a tool to stage and direct treatment has been adopted as the preferential system for both the European (EASL-EORTC) and American (AASLD) guidelines for the treatment of HCC [89, 90, 92].

In those with good performance status and well-compensated liver disease, the options for treatment are based on tumour factors, particularly the number of and size of the HCCs. The other significant tumour factor relates to the presence of extrahepatic disease and vascular involvement which contraindicate resection, transplantation, or loco-regional therapies. Potentially curative options include surgery: resection, transplantation or ablation of the HCC. Many patients are not amenable for curative treatment and benefit from palliative approaches with loco-regional or systemic therapies.

Surgery

Resection

Resection should be considered in all non-cirrhotic patients with HCC. In those fit to undergo liver resection, the site of the tumour

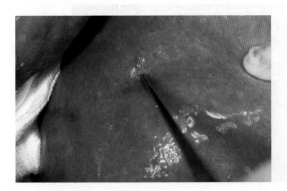

Fig. 41.3 Operative photograph of macroscopically visible liver capsule deposit of HCC at site of previous diagnostic biopsy.

and relationship to vessels will determine operability. In those patients with cirrhosis, the decision to resect is more complex, with an increased risk of parenchymal liver failure (jaundice, ascites, coagulopathy) following resection. This risk of liver failure is greatest in those with portal hypertension complicating their cirrhosis. A small minority of patients, with well compensated (Child-Pugh A) cirrhosis and no portal hypertension may be amenable to undergo liver resection for HCC. With HCC resection, particularly in cirrhosis, as with ablative therapies, the underlying liver disease is not altered and the risk of recurrent disease continues, so ongoing surveillance is necessary [100]. One of the technical challenges in such surgery is the propensity of the tumour to grow down blood vessels and bile ducts (Figure 41.5).

Liver transplantation

Liver transplantation treats both HCC and the underlying liver disease. It should always be considered and is often the treatment of choice. While there is always a risk of recurrent disease in immunosuppressed post-transplant patients, the development of stringent criteria to select patients for transplantation reduces that risk. The widely used Milan criteria have been shown to give good outcomes, with five-year survival in excess of 70% post-transplant [101]. Milan criteria constitute a cirrhotic liver with a single lesion ≤5 cm or three lesions all ≤3 cm with no involvement of the portal vein and no extrahepatic disease [101]. While outcomes from liver transplantation for HCC within Milan criteria are good (and in keeping with those transplanted for non-tumour parenchymal liver failure), it has been felt to be restrictive, since patients with larger volumes of disease are still likely to benefit from transplantation. Extended criteria have been developed that appear to have similar outcomes when considering long-term survival.

The University of California at San Francisco (UCSF) produced and validated an extended criterion, comprising a single lesion ≤6.5 cm in diameter or three nodules, the largest ≤4.5 cm and total diameter ≤8 cm [102, 103]. While this study did not compare those within Milan criteria to those outside of it, the overall survival was comparable [102, 103]. A further, 'up to 7' criteria, based on a large volume review of factors present in those with positive outcomes from transplantation outside of Milan criteria has also been shown to have good post-transplant outcomes with comparable five-year survival rates [104]. The 'up to 7' criteria consist of the sum of size (in cm) and number of tumours for any given patient. This would allow one 6 cm tumour, two 5 cm tumours, three 4 cm tumours, etc. [104].

The major limitation for transplantation, and a significant factor in not extending the transplantation criteria for patients with HCC, is the shortage of available donor organs. It is accepted in both a recent review relating to this subject [105] and a recent published international consensus [106] that liver transplantation should be reserved for HCC patients who have a predicted five-year survival comparable to non-HCC patients, and that the Milan criteria be used as a benchmark for selection of HCC patients for liver transplantation, and as the basis for comparison with other suggested criteria. A caution to increasing the criteria beyond Milan has also been raised regarding the availability of organs for non-malignant indications. Markov modelling has shown that extending the criteria for transplantation for HCC would lead to an increase in deaths amongst those on the transplant waiting list for other indications [107].

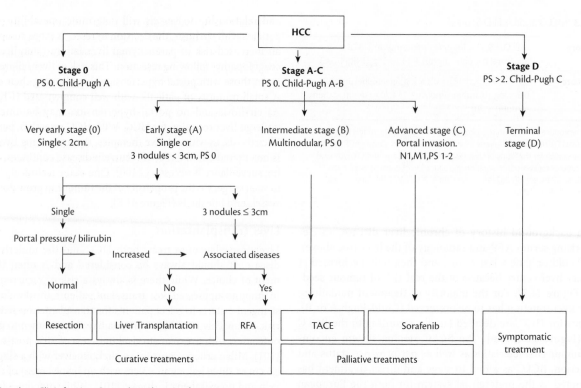

Fig. 41.4 Barcelona Clinic for Liver Cancer (BCLC) staging for HCC.

Reprinted from *The Lancet*, Volume 362, Issue 9399, Llovet J. et al., Hepatocellular carcinoma, pp. 1907–1917, Copyright © 2003 with permission from Elsevier, <http://www.sciencedirect.com/science/journal/01406736>

Loco-regional treatments for hepatocellular carcinomas

Interventional techniques for hepatobiliary malignancy

Interventional radiology plays an ever increasing role in managing HB cancers. Minimally invasive treatment of HB malignancy is delivered either percutaneously using tissue ablative techniques or trans-arterially. Endoscopic therapies are covered elsewhere in this chapter. The liver has distinct attributes that allow targeted treatment, and there is considerable interest in the synergistic effect of systemic chemotherapy and targeted liver treatments for liver dominant disease. Even with significant extrahepatic disease burden, it is disease progression in the liver that determines survival.

HCC often arises against background chronic liver disease where liver resection carries high morbidity and recurrent tumours are common in the residual liver. Targeted treatment such as ablation or trans-arterial chemoembolization (TACE) preserve liver function to a great extent, and can frequently be repeated. HCC surveillance programs are detecting tumours much earlier, allowing more effective ablative techniques. Tumours up to 3 cm in maximal diameter are ablated with very low rates of residual disease leading to tumour recurrence [108]. A combination of ablation and TACE, or TACE alone, is used when the tumour exceeds 3.5 cm.

Thermal ablative technologies such as radiofrequency ablation, laser, microwave, and cryoablation have all become established in routine practice. High intensity focused ultrasound (HIFU) is still under development, but offers the opportunity to thermally ablate tumour without puncturing the skin [109]. Irreversible electroporation (IRE) is a non-thermal technique which may allow

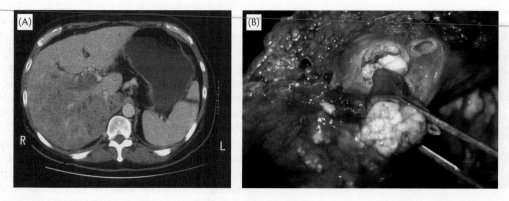

Fig. 41.5 (A) CT scan showing HCC tumour thrombus occluding the portal vein, so causing cavernous transformation and portal venous collaterals. This patient is inoperable. (B) Operative photograph of HCC tumour thrombus retrieved from the common hepatic duct.

treatment of tumours deemed inaccessible for thermal ablative techniques [110].

Image guidance

All targeted treatments require high quality image guidance for maximum treatment efficacy and safety, CT and ultrasound being the most commonly used modalities. CEUS improves tumour visualization and assesses devascularization at the time of treatment [111]. Modern interventional suite fluoroscopy can create CT-like images while intra-arterial contrast is being injected. The exact artery supplying the tumour can be identified and TACE administered accordingly [112].

Catheter delivered treatment

The portal vein provides in excess of 80% of the blood supply to the normal liver, while the hepatic artery is the main supply to both primary and secondary liver tumours. This situation can be exploited when targeting tumours with trans-arterial drug-delivery systems. The venous outflow via the hepatic veins into the inferior vena cava can be occluded. The liver vascular dynamics are therefore relatively easy to manipulate [113].

Technique

Arterial access is usually via the common femoral artery, after which the coeliac and superior mesenteric arteries are imaged using a 4-5F catheter. A microcatheter (2-3F) is advanced within the 4F catheter to allow selection of the appropriate intrahepatic artery. If a solitary tumour is being treated then the catheter should be within the appropriate segmental artery, whereas if there is diffuse lobar disease the catheter is placed in the lobar artery. Total liver treatment with TACE is inadvisable due to the side effects, and most operators would treat individual lobes on separate occasions [114]. Conventional TACE for HCC involves injecting a slurry of particulate matter combining lipiodol (an oil-based contrast agent with a partial embolic effect) with chemotherapy, thereby slowing the passage of the chemotherapeutic agent through the tumour. It is highly visible on fluoroscopy and persists in the malignant microvasculature, due to the lack of Kupffer cells. This also aids targeting treatment at subsequent sessions [115] (see Figure 41.6).

Drug-eluting beads

Drug-eluting beads (DEB) overcome the problems of conventional TACE, where a significant amount of the cytotoxic component passes straight through the tumour capillary bed. The cytotoxic agent is bound to 30 um beads which do not to completely embolize the vessel supplying the tumour, but transport the cytotoxic agent to the tumour. The drug is then released into the surrounding tumour at a steady rate to ensure prolonged exposure and minimal systemic side effects [116, 117]. The bead size is selected to allow deep penetration into the tumour, without the risk of shunting into the systemic circulation. Doxorubicin is the drug of choice when used with DEB TACE for HCC while irinotecan is preferred when using DEB TACE to treat colorectal liver metastases [116, 117].

Selective internal radiation treatment

For many years, external beam radiation has not been used for liver tumours due to the unacceptably high risk of radiation hepatitis and damage to the adjacent soft tissue. However, many primary and secondary tumours are very susceptible to radiation and with improved technology in micro-catheter construction and carrier particles it is now possible to deliver radiation treatment internally.

Either a resin or glass bead is used to carry yttrium 90, a β-emitter, to the tumour capillary bed where it becomes trapped. β photons can penetrate up to 11 mm in soft tissue and so treatment remains localized to the liver. The half-life of yttrium 90 is 64 hours which, combined with the short range of penetration, means that the patient poses little or no radiation risk to others in close proximity. Up to 50% of liver replacement by tumour is considered safe so long as the background liver function is satisfactory, and the portal vein patent [118, 119].

Treatment is usually performed in two stages. An initial arteriogram demonstrates the anatomy, especially vessels that may supply extrahepatic structures. It is very important to identify all such vessels as a single mal-deployed particle will cause tissue necrosis. It is common practice to embolize the gastroduodenal artery (GDA) and the right gastric artery, both of which usually arise close to the origin of the right and left hepatic arteries. Reflux of particles into these vessels is likely to lead to gastroduodenal ulceration or pancreatitis. During the initial angiogram, and after embolization, a bolus of technetium bound to macro-aggregated albumin (MAA) is injected at the same site as the proposed SIRT injection. MAA is roughly the same diameter as SIRT particles and is a good surrogate to predict SIRT distribution. The patient undergoes radionuclide imaging immediately after injection of the technetium-MAA to look for sites of extrahepatic migration, and evidence of significant arterio-venous shunting into the pulmonary capillary bed. If there is significant shunting (>10%) then dose reduction should be considered. The patient returns to the interventional suite within two to three weeks for SIRT treatment. Unlike TACE, the embolic effect of SIRT is low which allows single session whole liver treatment with an acceptable side effect profile.

Chemosaturation

The liver can be excluded from the systemic circulation by placing a double occlusion balloon catheter in the inferior vena cava (IVC); one balloon in the supra-hepatic IVC and the other in the supra-renal IVC. High dose chemotherapy is then delivered to the whole liver via the hepatic artery. As for SIRT, any branches of the coeliac axis that may allow the chemotherapy to enter extrahepatic sites must first be occluded with embolization coils. The liver is remains saturated with chemotherapy for 30 minutes, before being removed from the isolated segment of IVC through a lumen in the balloon catheter. More than 90% of the chemotherapy is removed from the blood using a filtration and pump system, before being returned to the patient via an internal jugular vein sheath. The technique has shown promise in a phase II trial for ocular melanoma and sarcoma liver metastases [120].

Ablative techniques

Thermal ablation causes irreversible cell death by either heating or freezing tissue. Radiofrequency ablation (RFA), laser therapy, and microwave ablation are needle based systems that cause cell death by heating tumour cells to a temperature that produces coagulative necrosis or lesser degrees of irreversible cell death. Prolonged heating of cells at 50–55°C or short exposure to temperatures above 60°C produces irreversible cell death. RFA uses an alternating current to vibrate molecules creating frictional heat [121]. The ablation volume is gradually increased to avoid tissue desiccation which would be detrimental to current flow. A 4 cm diameter ablation can take 20 minutes to achieve with RFA, whereas microwave ablation takes approximately 2–4 minutes to achieve the same tissue

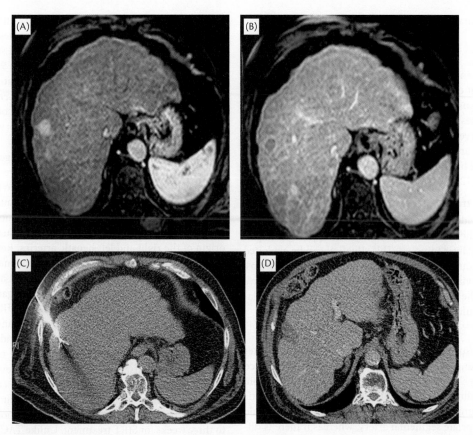

Fig. 41.6 Small HCC segment 7/8. (A) Arterial phase CT showing marked enhancement and (B) venous phase showing rapid washout of contrast. (C) Treated with CT guided RFA and follow-up scan at four weeks and (D) showing low attenuation ablation site.

destruction. As with other types of thermal ablation, the ablation zone size and shape is variable. Proximity of adjacent vessels has a significant adverse effect due to the cooling effect of the flowing blood, preventing adjacent tumour from reaching 60°C (heat sink effect) [122].

Irreversible electroporation

Irreversible electroporation (IRE) is a non-thermal tissue destruction technique which uses short blasts of electric current, passing between two or more parallel needles, to create irreparable holes in the cell membrane. This leads to uncontrollable ion transfer and apoptosis. Unlike thermal ablation, cell death does not depend on temperature-related coagulative necrosis and so the heat sink effect does not apply. There is also very little or no scarring following treatment. IRE destroys only cells, sparing collagen-based structures such as blood vessels, bowel wall, and bile ducts. These inherent qualities mean that it could be used at sites where thermal ablation is too dangerous, or where the heat sink effect is significant. IRE should avoid bile duct and arterial injury, allowing safe treatment of central liver tumours [123]. This is still a very novel technique requiring further evaluation.

Medical management of hepatocellular carcinomas

Surgical therapy, including transplantation, or local ablation may offer the prospect of cure for patients with hepatocellular carcinoma but are applicable to only a minority of patients. For other

patients with preserved liver function and a patent portal venous system, chemoembolization may afford a modest survival benefit. However, as tumour size increases, the frequency of vascular invasion (micro and macroscopic) and the incidence of intrahepatic and extrahepatic spread increases thereby limiting the impact of local control. This forms the basis for guidelines, based on tumour size and number, above which local treatments are inappropriate. For patients beyond these criteria systemic therapy may be appropriate. Traditionally, this has taken the form of cytotoxic chemotherapy or endocrine manipulation although more recently molecular targeted therapies have been employed with some success.

Cytotoxic chemotherapy for advanced hepatocellular carcinoma

A large number of mostly uncontrolled studies have been performed using the major classes of chemotherapeutic drugs alone or in combination. Response rates for single-agent chemotherapy are low and durable remission is rare. The anthracycline, doxorubicin, has been the most studied agent. The overall response rate for more than 700 patients treated in a number of studies was 18%. The small, non-randomized design and patient heterogeneity in these trials make it difficult to assess any effect of doxorubicin on overall survival. One small randomized trial has compared doxorubicin with best supportive care. This reported a statistically significant survival advantage in favour of doxorubicin. However, with median survival of 10.6 weeks versus 7.5, the absolute difference in survival was modest with very short survival in both arms, suggesting inclusion of patients with very advanced disease and/or poor liver function [124].

In five trials involving 118 patients treated with mitoxantrone, an anthracenedione, the response rate was 16%, with less toxicity; this became the first systemic agent to be licensed for use in HCC [125] although it has never been widely adopted as a standard of care.

A randomized trial has compared the oral fluoropyrimidine, UFT, with supportive care. UFT comprises tegafur, an orally active 5-FU prodrug metabolized by the liver to 5-FU, and uracil, a biochemical modulator of 5-FU via inhibition of dihydropyrimidine dehydrogenase (DPD, the rate limiting enzyme of 5-FU metabolism). HCC is reported to have high levels of DPD, which may explain resistance to 5-FU and, therefore, DPD inhibition may enhance 5-FU activity. Although objective responses to UFT were uncommon, there was a significant prolongation of survival (median 51 vs 27 weeks; p <0.01). This was a small study with only 28 patients per arm and larger studies are required, but it does suggest that radiological response may not correlate with survival [126]. In two recent large-scale trials drugs that had shown promising activity in early phase trials, Ti67, a novel tubulin-binding drug [127] and nolatrexed, a thymidylate synthase inhibitor [128], were tested against doxorubicin as the control arm. In the former, there was no survival improvement; in the latter, the patients in the doxorubicin arm survived significantly longer (6.9 compared to 4.7 months, hazard ratio 0.753) suggesting a possible impact of doxorubicin on survival and highlighting the uncertainty in predicting phase III trial outcome based on apparently promising phase II data.

Combination chemotherapy for advanced hepatocellular carcinoma

On the basis of its modest activity as a single agent, doxorubicin has been investigated in combination with a variety of other drugs. A phase II study of cisplatin, interferon alpha-2b, doxorubicin and 5-fluorouracil (PIAF) was encouraging; although the response rate was modest (26%), 9 of 13 partial responders had their disease rendered resectable and, in some of these, there was a complete pathological response [129]. Despite this encouraging activity, a prospective randomized study comparing PIAF to doxorubicin failed to demonstrate any improvement in survival with the combination [130].

Recently, a randomized phase III trial compared FOLFOX with doxorubicin in 371 Chinese patients with predominantly HBV-associated HCC. Although there was a trend to prolonged survival with FOLFOX (6.4 vs 4.9 months; HR 0.797), this difference was not statistically significant (p = 0.085) [131]. Despite some encouraging data, there remains no convincing evidence of survival benefit for systemic chemotherapy for HCC and chemotherapy in this setting may be poorly tolerated due to coexisting chronic liver disease resulting in unpredictable drug metabolism. Thus, many non-cytotoxic systemic therapies have been investigated.

Endocrine therapy for advanced hepatocellular carcinoma

Up to one-third of HCC express oestrogen receptors (ER) and animal models of liver carcinogenesis, as well as epidemiological studies, suggest a role for sex steroids in its pathogenesis. Initial studies suggested promising activity for tamoxifen. For example, a small trial randomizing 38 patients to tamoxifen or supportive care reported one-year survival of 22% and 5% respectively [132]. However, several larger studies have reported no benefit or, in the case of high-dose tamoxifen, a detrimental effect over placebo. For example, the Italian CLIP study including almost 500 patients randomized to tamoxifen or placebo reported median survival of 15 and 16 months, respectively (p = 0.54) [133]. In the setting of breast cancer, it is clear that ER-negative tumours derive no benefit from endocrine therapy. However, these HCC studies did not select patients on the basis of ER status. A randomized trial of tamoxifen compared with placebo has attempted to address this question. Of 119 patients, the ER status was determined in 66 but there was no difference in survival between patients with ER-positive or ER-negative tumours [134].

Targeting angiogenesis

HCC is a highly vascular tumour and, indeed, this forms the therapeutic basis of TACE. More recently, the molecular mechanisms mediating tumour angiogenesis have been elucidated and these have provided potential pharmacological targets. In particular, the fundamental role of angiogenic growth factor receptor signalling, most notably the importance of vascular endothelial growth factor (VEGF) signalling has been recognized. This process can be perturbed in a number of ways. Bevacizumab is a humanized monoclonal antibody against VEGF ligand and phase II trials have indicated activity against HCC, although there are concerns regarding the risk of GI bleeding and recent studies has mandated prophylactic treatment of varices prior to treatment [135]. VEGF receptor signalling can also be inhibited by small molecules targeting receptor tyrosine kinase activity.

Sorafenib for advanced hepatocellular carcinoma

Sorafenib is a small molecule inhibitor of tumour-cell proliferation and angiogenesis and induces apoptosis in a range of tumour models including HCC. It acts by inhibiting the serine–threonine kinases Raf-1 and B-Raf and the receptor tyrosine kinase activity of vascular endothelial growth factor receptors (VEGFRs) 1, 2, and 3 and platelet-derived growth factor receptor β (PDGFR-β). Results of a phase II study involving 137 patients with advanced hepatocellular carcinoma and Child-Pugh class A or B status indicated that sorafenib had encouraging activity [136]. On this basis, it was tested in a large phase III, double-blind, placebo-controlled trial. Median survival was 10.7 months in the sorafenib group and 7.9 months in the placebo group (hazard ratio 0.69; p <0.001) [137]. Diarrhoea, weight loss, hand-foot skin reaction, and hypophosphatemia were more frequent in the sorafenib group. A smaller confirmatory randomized phase III study, with the same eligibility criteria, was conducted in patients from the Asia-Pacific region (with predominantly HBV-driven cancers). Sorafenib again significantly prolonged survival (median 6.5 months vs 4.2 months, hazard ratio 0.68, p = 0.014) compared to placebo [138]. In the Asia-Pacific trial, more patients had extrahepatic disease, a greater number of hepatic lesions, and a poorer performance status which may, in part, explain the lower absolute overall survival and time to progression figures in this trial, although the aetiology of the predisposing liver disease may also be significant.

Sorafenib is thus the first systemic therapy to unequivocally demonstrate a survival advantage in selected patients with advanced HCC, good performance status and well compensated liver disease, with the relative magnitude of benefit being similar to that achieved by targeted therapies in other cancer types, and has been approved by the United States Food and Drug Administration and by the European Medicines Agency for the treatment of advanced HCC.

Notably, there was no statistically significant difference in the median time to symptomatic progression between the two arms in either study. This may be explained by the validity of the assessment tool used, the counterbalance between improving tumour-related symptoms and treatment-related side effects and the additional complexity of cirrhosis-related symptoms, which may not improve despite effective anti-cancer therapy.

Use of sorafenib in patients with compromised liver function

These phase III trials were deliberately restricted to patients with well-preserved liver function in order to capture the potential survival benefit of sorafenib without confounding from deaths related to advanced liver disease and there remain limited data on the safety and efficacy of sorafenib in patients with Child-Pugh class B or C cirrhosis. In the phase II trial, 38 of the 137 patients enrolled had Child-Pugh B cirrhosis and the pharmacokinetic and toxicity profiles were similar to those with Child-Pugh A cirrhosis. However, patients with Child-Pugh class B status had a worse median overall survival (14 weeks vs 41 weeks) and an increased rate of encephalopathy and worsening ascites. For patients with Child-Pugh B cirrhosis, the available data suggest that sorafenib should be used with caution, and further prospective evaluation in this group is required.

Other targeted agents for advanced hepatocellular carcinomas

A growing number of molecules are now in clinical trials in patients with HCC and several large trials have been completed. The first of these investigated sunitinib, a potent inhibitor of VEGF and PDGF receptors as well as c-kit and flt-3, in a 1200 patient study [139]. However, again despite encouraging phase II data, sunitinib was significantly inferior to sorafenib (median survival 7.9 vs 10.2 months, HR 1.3; p = 0.001). There was greater toxicity and, consequently reduced dose intensity, in the sunitinib arm which may have contributed to its inferior efficacy. However, this study may also indicate the importance of *raf* inhibition in mediating the efficacy of sorafenib. Similarly disappointing results were reported from a large phase III trial of the potent VEGFR inhibitor, linifanib, which was terminated early due to toxicity, again reflecting the challenges of investigating systemic therapies in patients with HCC and underlying cirrhosis [140].

Since fibroblast growth factor (FGF) is an important alternative pathway of angiogenesis, it may contribute to resistance to VEGF-targeted drugs and thus brivanib, a VEGF and FGF receptor tyrosine kinase inhibitor, may have the potential to delay the emergence of such resistance. However, a recent large phase III trial of this drug also failed to improve outcomes compared with sorafenib [141].

A number of randomized trials have also been undertaken in the second-line setting and, whilst first-line trials have shown that agents with broadly similar mechanisms of action to sorafenib do not result in clinically significant increments in survival, there may be scope for sequential therapy when resistance emerges to first line treatment. This is exemplified by a small study using bevacizumab following sorafenib failure reported a median survival of 9.5 months despite patients largely having poor performance status and often a Child-Pugh score of 7 [142]. Similar data has been observed using axitinib as a second-line agent in the setting of renal cancer. However, a phase III trial of brivanib following sorafenib failure has failed to demonstrate improved survival compared with best supportive care [143].

A better understanding of the mechanisms of resistance to VEGF-targeted therapies may help improve therapeutic strategies. For example, there is evidence that hepatocyte growth factor (HGF) signalling through its receptor, c-met, may play a role in mediating such resistance and, indeed, may contribute to the emergence of a more aggressive phenotype during anti-VEGF therapy. This suggests a potential role for c-met inhibition as a second line strategy, or in combination with anti-angiogenic therapy. The c-met inhibitor ARQ197 has been investigated in a randomized phase II trial for patients with HCC and significantly prolonged time to progression, the primary endpoint of the study, compared with best supportive care (HR 0.64). An exploratory analysis of survival according to c-met expression assessed by immunohistochemistry on tumour biopsies suggested that c-met was an adverse prognostic factor and that patients with high c-met may derive greatest benefit from ARQ197, although this requires further prospective evaluation [144].

Processes other than angiogenesis also contribute to the pathogenesis of HCC. Specific inhibitors of epidermal growth factor receptors (EGFRs) are growth inhibitory in HCC models in vitro and in vivo and early phase trials of anti-EGFR monoclonal antibody (cetuximab) and of small molecule EGFR tyrosine kinase inhibitor (erlotinib) suggest clinical activity [145, 146]. Downstream pathways of growth factor receptor signalling include the Map Kinase (*ras/raf/mek/erk*) and PI3Kinase/akt/mTOR cascades. Indeed, sorafenib works, in part, through *raf* inhibition. The PI3K pathway is commonly upregulated in HCC leading to activation of mTOR, a key regulator of cell growth and proliferation. Inhibition of mTOR has shown promise in preclinical models and clinical trials using mTOR inhibitors are underway with promising data emerging [147].

There are a number of other pathways that are commonly perturbed in HCC, including wnt/β-catenin and hedgehog signalling cascades but, as yet, these have not lent themselves to pharmacological manipulation.

Combination therapy

Combination of signal transduction inhibitors acting at different points in the same pathway offers the potential to maximise pathway inhibition to produce additive clinical benefit and to reduce potential development of resistance. Thus, EGFR activation results in secretion of angiogenic cytokines, including VEGF, such that EGFR inhibition may also mediate anti-angiogenic effects. Indeed, preclinical models suggest that EGFR signalling is a prerequisite for angiogenesis in HCC via upregulation of VEGF. This process appears to be mediated through phosphorylation of AKT rather than ERK/MAPK and thus may be specifically susceptible to EGFR or mTOR inhibitors [148]. A phase II trial has investigated the combination of bevacizumab with erlotinib, with an objective response rate of 25% (including one complete response), median progression free survival of nine months and median survival 15.6 months [149]. This combination is being further investigated in a phase III trial against sorafenib. Combination of mTOR inhibitors with VEGFR antagonists has synergistic effects in preclinical models and a phase II trial of everolimus with bevacizumab has demonstrated safety of this combination [150]. However, in a phase I trial exploring the combination of everolimus with sorafenib, it was not possible to safely escalate the dose of everolimus to target therapeutic levels [151]. There is also cross-talk between IGF and VEGF receptor signalling suggesting that combining drugs to target both may be beneficial. However, one such study combining an anti-IGF-1 receptor antibody with sorafenib was closed early due to problems with toxicity of the combination [152]. These latter studies emphasize that tolerability, even with so-called targeted agents, can be an issue in the setting of HCC and may limit the use of some regimens despite a strong scientific rationale for their combination.

Targeted therapies in combination with conventional chemotherapy

HCC is generally regarded as resistant to conventional chemotherapeutic drugs. However, pathways that are inhibited by novel targeted therapies, including *raf/mek/erk* may contribute to this resistance and so combination of these agents with chemotherapy may overcome chemoresistance. There is preclinical evidence of synergy between doxorubicin and *raf* inhibition. In a vascular endothelial model, resistance to doxorubicin is, at least in part, mediated via FGF-mediated *raf*-dependent survival signals, and can be overcome by inhibition of *raf*, providing rationale for combining doxorubicin with sorafenib or inhibitors of FGFR such as brivanib [153]. Furthermore, there is clinical evidence of benefit from the combination of anti-angiogenic agents with conventional chemotherapy in other tumour types. A randomized phase II study has investigated the combination of sorafenib and doxorubicin compared to doxorubicin alone [154]. The overall survival in the combination arm was more than double the control arm (13.7 months compared to 6.5 months, HR 0.45) To determine whether this benefit is attributable to synergy between the two agents or to sorafenib alone requires a further randomized trial of the combination using sorafenib as the control arm.

Improving efficacy of systemic therapies through application in earlier stage disease

Although effective local control can be achieved by loco-regional therapies, as tumour size increases, so does the frequency of vascular invasion and with it the risk of metastases thereby limiting the impact of local control. Systemic therapy might be applied in two settings to ameliorate this problem. Firstly, in the neoadjuvant setting it might downstage a non-resectable tumour to resectability and this has occasionally been reported with doxorubicin and doxorubicin based combinations [129]. However, this is less likely to be achieved with drugs such as sorafenib where significant tumour shrinkage is rarely seen. Secondly, use in the adjuvant setting may eradicate micrometastases. The Sorafenib as Adjuvant Treatment in the Prevention of Recurrence of Hepatocellular Carcinoma (STORM) trial is a randomised, double-blind, placebo-controlled phase III study to evaluate the safety and efficacy of sorafenib versus placebo in patients with HCC after potentially curative treatment with surgical resection or local ablation, taken continuously for up to four years. This study has recruited 1100 patients, with

final survival results awaited. The toxicity profile will be of particular interest, as these patients would otherwise be expected to be well and asymptomatic. Unlike other cancers, as well as the risk of disease recurrence through micrometastases (which may conceivably be eradicated by an active systemic therapy) there is also a risk of de novo tumour formation in the remaining diseased liver. It is for this reason that a four-year duration of therapy was selected in this trial, although to date there is no evidence that sorafenib may prevent the progression of premalignant lesions to invasive cancer and, undoubtedly, such prolonged therapy will have significant health economic implications.

The addition of a systemic agent such as sorafenib to chemoembolization may also be beneficial since TACE induces profound tumour hypoxia, activating hypoxia-inducible signalling pathways and angiogenic factors such as VEGF, b-FGF, and IGF-2, which may mediate the revascularization that is characteristic of TACE failure, or stimulate the growth and vascularization of micrometastases. A randomized phase III trial of sorafenib vs placebo after TACE, in Japanese and Korean patients with unresectable HCC, has recently been completed with 458 patients enrolled [155]. No significant prolongation of TTP was observed for patients treated with sorafenib. Notably, over half of patients commenced sorafenib more than nine weeks after chemoembolization, and three-quarters of the sorafenib-treated patients required dose reductions. Since pro-angiogenic mediators are upregulated immediately following TACE, the timing of sorafenib in relation to the TACE procedure may be critically important and may explain the failure of this study. Inhibiting the action of VEGF by administering sorafenib simultaneously with TACE may result in better efficacy and this is being tested in ongoing clinical trials. The sorafenib or placebo in combination with TACE for intermediate stage hepatocellular carcinoma (SPACE) trial is a multinational, randomized, double-blind, placebo-controlled phase II study being conducted that has completed its accrual of 300 patients and has met its primary endpoint of prolonging TTP with the addition of sorafenib given simultaneously with TACE [156]. However, it was not sufficiently powered to determine an overall survival benefit and there remains a need for further phase III trials.

Whether sorafenib, or other systemic therapy, could have a significant impact on recurrence as an adjuvant to liver transplant seems unlikely since with currently employed criteria recurrence is already very rare and any impact would likely be marginal. This may be different if transplant criteria were broadened but at present this is primarily limited by availability of donor organs.

Hepatitis B virus reactivation and chemotherapy

Hepatitis B virus (HBV) carriers are at risk of virus reactivation when receiving cytotoxic chemotherapy. A prospective study of 102 HBsAg-positive patients with HCC receiving doxorubicin-based chemotherapy showed that 32 patients developed hepatitis attributable to HBV reactivation of whom 30% died as a consequence [157]. Reactivation can be reduced by antiviral therapy such as lamivudine. A non-randomized comparison of HBV-positive patients receiving chemotherapy reported reactivation rates of 4% compared to 24% in patients receiving lamivudine or not, respectively. Since lamivudine prophylaxis was not routinely used prior to this, it is quite possible that HBV reactivation contributed to apparent toxicity in earlier chemotherapy studies, especially those conducted in HBV-endemic regions.

Cases of HBV reactivation have also been observed in patients treated with mTOR inhibitors, such that HBV carriers receiving this class of drug may also benefit from prophylaxis [158].

Multidisciplinary management of biliary tract cancer

Surgical management of gall bladder cancer

Population data in the US from 1988 to 2003 suggested more than 95% of surgically resectable gall bladder cancer has been treated with only simple cholecystectomy [159]. Although recent advances in surgical technique and perioperative management have allowed an increased role for radical surgery in appropriately selected cases, the outcomes of majority of patients with advanced gall bladder cancer remains poor.

Patients with gall bladder cancer usually present in one of three ways:

(1) advanced unresectable cancer;

(2) detection of suspicious lesion preoperatively and resectable after staging work-up;

(3) incidental finding of cancer during or after cholecystectomy for benign disease. Advanced is defined as tumour penetrating through gall bladder wall (T3 or greater), metastasizing to regional lymph node (N1) or distant organ (M1). In the AJCC staging system, this is staged as II or higher on 6th edition [160] and as III, IVa, or IVb on the 5th edition system [161].

Clinical presentation and work-up

Most patients with gall bladder cancer present when the disease is at an advanced stage, and majority of patients are diagnosed when the disease is beyond the borders of resection [162–166]. The most common symptoms at presentation are abdominal pain or biliary colic [162, 165, 166]. Patients with advanced disease may also present with jaundice from tumour invasion of the biliary tree or with systemic signs such as malaise and weight loss. Jaundice is well recognized as predictor of worse outcomes. In the series from Memorial Sloan-Kettering from 1995 through to 2005, one-third of patients presented with jaundice and only 7% had resectable disease [163].

The diagnosis is often suspected on an ultrasound done to evaluate right upper quadrant abdominal pain. Echogenic or discontinuous gall bladder mucosa, submucosal echolucency, or a mass should lead one to suspect gall bladder cancer. The presence of gallstones trapped within the tumour during its growth is a useful sign of possible gall bladder cancer [167, 168]. Although the detection of early lesions is challenging, ultrasound has a sensitivity of 85% and accuracy of 80% to diagnose advanced gall bladder cancer [167, 169]. Doppler ultrasound is helpful not only to identify the presence of hepatic arterial or portal venous invasion, but also to improve specificity of US by differentiating malignant tumour from benign lesions by measuring blood flow into the suspected lesions [170].

ERCP or PTC is useful to identify the spread of gall bladder cancer into biliary tree. A mid-bile duct stricture is a classic sign of gall bladder cancer involving bile duct. For patients with jaundice, cholangiography is useful for localizing the obstruction and also facilitating stent placement and establishing a diagnosis of cancer via brush cytology [171].

If gall bladder cancer is suspected, abdominal cross-sectional imaging (CT or MRI) is mandatory to evaluate for nodal or metastatic disease as well as to further define the local extent of disease (see Figure 41.7). Lymph nodes involved by cancer are usually >1 cm diameter and ring-shaped heterogeneous enhancement with IV contrast. Ohtani et al. reported the positive predictive value of conventional CT scan for detecting involvement in various lymph node stations as 75–100% despite of lower sensitivity as 17–78% [172]. These same authors reported the sensitivity of CT scan to detect of tumour invasion into liver, bile duct, or other adjacent organs such as pancreas and transverse colon as 50–65% and the positive predictive value as 77–100% [173]. The use of spiral CT provides a better diagnostic accuracy in both nodal spread as well as in-depth invasion than conventional CT scan [174, 175]. In a report by Yoshimitsu et al., the sensitivity of detecting tumour invasion into liver or other adjacent organ was 80–100%. MRI is less frequently used for staging of gall bladder cancer, but sometimes the use of MRCP or magnetic resonance angiography (MRA) provides more information than ultrasound or CT. Schwartz et al. demonstrated in retrospective analysis of 34 patients with gall bladder cancer that combination of conventional MRI and MRCP achieved a sensitivity of 100% for liver invasion and 92% for lymph node involvement [176].

PET using fluorine-18-labelled fluoro-deoxyglucose (FDG) is an emerging imaging modality that may prove to be of clinical value in the preoperative work-up of patients with gall bladder cancer. Multiple studies have shown that PET scans reliably detect primary and metastatic gall bladder cancer [177, 178] as well as residual tumour after cholecystectomy [179]. Corvera and his colleagues demonstrated that PET added information and altered management in 23% of selected patients with gall bladder who were preoperatively staged using US/CT/MRI [180]. Since PET is not routinely available, and the data for real contribution to preoperative staging is relatively limited, the role of PET in the multimodality work-up of patients with suspected gall bladder cancer is still being defined and its use should be individualized.

Principles of surgery

Although many studies have suggested improved survival in patients with early gall bladder cancer with radical surgery including en bloc resection of gall bladder fossa and regional lymphadenectomy, its role for those with advanced gall bladder cancer remains controversial. First, patients with more advanced disease often require more extensive resections than early stage tumours, and operative morbidity and mortality rates are higher [181]. Secondly, the long-term outcomes after resection, in general, tend to be poorer; long-term survival after radical surgery has been reported only for patients with limited local and lymph node spread. Therefore, the indication of radical surgery should be limited to well-selected patients based on thorough preoperative and intraoperative staging, and the extent of surgery should be determined based on the area of tumour involvement.

Surgical resection is warranted only for those who with loco-regional disease without distant spread. Because of the limited sensitivity of current imaging modalities to detect metastatic lesions of gall bladder cancer, staging laparoscopy prior to proceeding to laparotomy is very useful to assess the abdomen for evidence of discontinuous liver disease or peritoneal metastasis and to avoid unnecessary laparotomy. Weber et al. reported that 48% of patients with potentially resectable gall bladder cancer on preoperative

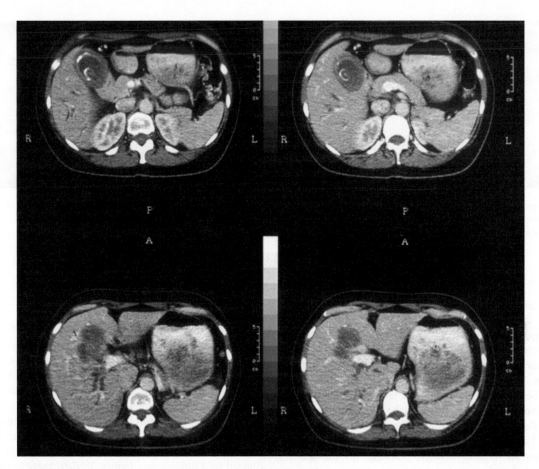

Fig. 41.7 CT scan appearance of T3 gall bladder cancer with invasion into the gall bladder fossa.

imaging work-up were spared laparotomy by discovering unresectable disease by laparoscopy [182]. Laparoscopic cholecystectomy should be avoided when a preoperative cancer is suspected because of the risk of violation of the plane between tumour and liver and the risk of port site seeding.

The goal of resection should always be complete extirpation with microscopic negative margins. Tumours beyond T2 are not cured by simple cholecystectomy and as with most of early gall bladder cancer, hepatic resection is always required. The extent of liver resection required depends upon whether involvement of major hepatic vessels, varies from segmental resection of segment IVb and V, at minimum to formal right hemihepatectomy or even right trisectionectomy. Invasion of the right portal pedicle structures is not considered a contraindication to potentially curative resection, but invasion of the common portal vascular structures is considered a contraindication to surgery by many surgeons (see Figure 41.8). The right portal pedicle is at particular risk for advanced tumour located at the neck of gall bladder, and when such involvement is suspected, right hepatectomy is required. Bile duct resection and reconstruction is also required if tumour involved in bile duct. However, bile duct resection is associated with increased perioperative morbidity [183] and it should be performed only if it is necessary to clear tumour; bile duct resection does not necessarily increase the lymph node yield.

Because of its propensity to spread to regional lymph nodes at early stage, resection of the liver involved and regional lymph node should be included for definitive treatment. In fact, frequency of metastasis to regional lymph nodes (hilar, celiac, peripancreatic, periduodenal) is fairly high for advanced tumours: pT3/4 60–81% vs pT1/2 0–62% [184–187]. The most common lymph nodes involved are pericholedochal (42%) and retropancreatic (37%). Other nodal stations including celiac, SMA, para-aortic are involved in 20–25% of patients [188]. However, optimal extent of lymphadenectomy is ill-defined. It is the authors' practice to include extirpation of lymph nodes within the hepatoduodenal ligament but not retropancreatic or celiac nodes as patients with involvement in these nodal basin are unlikely to benefit from resection. Nodal metastasis beyond the hepatoduodenal ligament on exploration is associated extremely poor outcomes [181] and we generally do not proceed with operation if gross metastasis is discovered on exploration.

In the other hand, direct involvement of colon, pancreas, or duodenum is not an absolute contraindication of surgery. Several authors have reported that en bloc resection of adjacent organs [183, 189–191], such as duodenum or pancreas, can be associated with prolonged survival. In a recent study, resection of adjacent organ was performed in 21 patients for presumable malignant involvement; the resected adjacent organ was histologically involved only in half of the cases and only 16 of 21 cases were node negative, emphasizing that the finding of adherent organs does not necessarily imply advanced disease. Most importantly, adjacent organ resection was not associated with changes in long-term survival of patients [183].

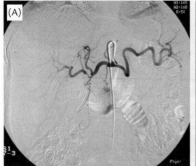
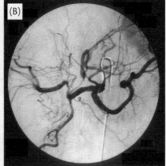
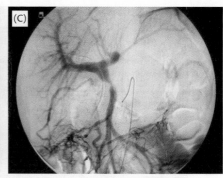

Fig. 41.8 (A) Hepatic arterial angiogram in patient with gall bladder cancer showing involvement of right hepatic artery. This patient is resectable. (B) Hepatic arterial angiogram in patient with gall bladder cancer showing involvement of common hepatic artery. This patient would rarely be considered resectable with curative intent. (C) Indirect portal vein angiogram in patient with gall bladder cancer showing involvement of common portal vein. This patient would rarely be considered resectable with curative intent.

Outcomes

Although advances in surgical technique and improvement in perioperative care allows us to perform radical resection for patients with gall bladder cancer safely, the outcomes for those with advanced cancer remain disappointing. The five-year survival rates for patients having radical surgery ranged from 0% to 51%; most of them fall in 20–30% (Table 41.4). Nodal status and histological margin have been reported as predictive factors of survival after radical resection for this group of patients throughout the literature. For example, Behari and his colleague reported that positive node was associated with incomplete resection and none of the patients with N1 disease survived beyond five years [187]. Endo and his colleague reported in their analysis of 55 patients who underwent complete resection, a 77% five-year survival for patients without nodal involvement, 33% for those with single lymph node involvement and 0% for those with two or more lymph nodes involvement [192]. These findings suggest that radical resection should not be performed for patients with gross lymph nodes involvement or extensive tumour infiltration to adjacent structure on perioperative

Table 41.4 Outcomes of radical surgery for advanced gall bladder cancer

Authors	Year	Number	Stage	5-year survival rate	Note
Fong et al. [156]	2000	58	III/IVa*	28/25%	
Kondo et al. [207]	2002	38	III/IVa**	33/17%	
Behari et al. [181]	2003	24	III/IVa*	28/0%	
Shih et al. [191]	2007	39	II***	34%	
Kayahara et al. [208]	2008	631	III/IVa*	39–51/ 22–24%	Multi-institutional study
D'Angelica et al. [177]	2009	72	II***	22%	

*AJCC 5th ed., **UICC 5th ed., ***AJCC 6th ed.

evaluation, both of which make complete resection with histological negative margin unlikely.

Medical management of gall bladder cancer

Because of its propensity to spread to regional lymph nodes at early stage and high rate of loco-regional recurrence, adjuvant chemotherapy, and/or chemoradiation therapy seems a rational therapeutic option for gall bladder cancer. Traditionally, 5-FU based chemotherapeutic regimen has been used with or without combination of chemoradiation. However, there are few data to support its efficacy. The rarity of gall bladder cancer and further limitation of patients who can undergo complete resection make the randomized trial difficult to conduct. To date, there is only one randomized trial examining the efficacy of adjuvant chemotherapy for gall bladder cancer. This study reported significant improvement in five-year overall survival rate (26% vs 14.4%) with postoperative mitomycin C and 5-FU following surgery compared with surgery alone as well as improvement in five-year disease free survival rate (20.3% vs 11.6%) [193]. However, definitive conclusion from this trial is limited by the small numbers of patients and the inclusion of patients undergoing incomplete (i.e., R1) resections. Indeed, subgroup analysis of patients who underwent a complete resection showed no survival benefit with adjuvant treatment. Most other data for the use of adjuvant or neo-adjuvant therapy in patients with gall bladder cancer is derived from phase II trials, in which treated patients were compared with historical controls [194, 195]. Kreral and his colleagues reported a 64% five-year survival rate of patients who received 5-FU and external beam radiation following surgical resection compared to 33% of those their historical control [195]. In contrast, Houry and his colleagues reported no survival benefit from adjuvant chemoradiation therapy on patients who underwent curative resection [196]. Unfortunately, no study has provided conclusive evidence for benefit of adjuvant chemo or chemoradiation treatment for gall bladder cancer.

Most patients with gall bladder cancer present with advanced, incurable disease and many are not candidates for surgical resection. The median survival of patients with advanced gall bladder cancer who are deemed inoperable ranges between 2 and 4 months [163, 166, 197] and palliation of symptoms should be the primary goal. Symptoms and conditions associated with incurable gall bladder cancer include jaundice, cholangitis, pain, and gastrointestinal obstruction. For obstructive jaundice or gastrointestinal obstruction, palliative intervention may be required. The common procedure for biliary obstruction due to gall bladder cancer is a segment III bypass [198]. In their series of 41 consecutive segment III bypass for patients with advanced gall bladder cancer, Kapoor and his colleagues reported 87% success rate with 12% mortality and 51% morbidity rate [199]. Because of poor survival, biliary stent is a preferred option for most of the patients. It can be placed either via percutaneous transhepatic route or endoscopic approach with minimal morbidity. Intestinal bypass should be performed only in patients who have symptomatic obstruction.

Systemic chemotherapy and radiation therapy have, in general, little impact on unresectable gall bladder cancer. Multiple regimens have been tested including combinations of 5-FU, leucovorin, mitomycin C, doxorubicin, and methotrexate. However, the effects have been mostly disappointing with poor response rates of 10–20% [200]. Recent phase II trials using combination of gemcitabine and oxaliplatin showed an improved response rate ranging 40–50% [211, 212, 215], and large-scale randomized trial is warranted.

Surgical management of cholangiocarcinoma

Cholangiocarcinoma usually arises in the major bile ducts near the porta hepatis and so usually presents as painless obstructive jaundice of insidious onset. Despite recent major advances in surgical and anaesthetic techniques, due to vascular involvement or distant spread the majority remain unresectable at time of presentation. The imaging characteristics of cholangiocarcinoma are discussed earlier, as are the interventional strategies (endoscopic and radiologic) to palliate obstructive jaundice. However, the usual presentation is one of painless obstructive jaundice, and the diagnostic imaging demonstrating a hilar stricture, with associated hepatic parenchymal atrophy of the lobe from which the tumour originally emanated (Figure 41.9). If surgery is not possible, then palliative biliary stenting should employ long-lasting coated metal stents, rather than temporary plastic stents, which have a propensity to silt up, lasting on average only three months (Figure 41.10).

Principles of surgery

Surgery is the only therapeutic modality which offers any chance of cure. Historically, median survival of patients with unresected cholangiocarcinoma remained less than one year. However, good multidisciplinary management, including aggressive and repeated biliary/percutaneous stenting can now achieve median survivals that approach or even surpass two years. No consensus has been achieved with regard to the criteria for surgery because of the small number of patients in each reported series. While, in general, the operative principles are very similar to those required to deal with Stage 3 gall bladder cancer, some authors consider that positive peri-portal lymph nodes detected at frozen section during exploratory laparotomy are a contraindication to resection [201], while others disagree and report long-term survival following resection in such patients [202, 203]. Furthermore, there is no consensus with regard to the optimal surgical procedure, although it is clear that a positive surgical resection margin is associated with a poorer prognosis [201, 204, 205] as is tumour invasion along Glisson's capsule or along neurovascular bundles (see Figure 41.11) [206, 207]. If resection is technically possible then five-year survival rates of over 30% can be achieved [208].

An alternative, but controversial, strategy currently being explored at a number of centres is orthotopic liver transplantation after neoadjuvant chemoradiotherapy. However, the numbers of patients studied remains small, none are randomized, and the treatment only offered to patients with early stage disease, so reported outcomes could be susceptible to selection bias [209].

Medical management of cholangiocarcinoma

Adjuvant strategies

There have been no reported randomized controlled trials to demonstrate any benefit from postoperative adjuvant therapy following apparently curative resection for cholangiocarcinoma, although the CRUK BILCAP study of surgery versus surgery plus adjuvant gemcitabine continues to recruit in the UK.

Systemic therapies

Evidence supporting a role for chemotherapy in advanced biliary cancer (ABC) was until recently limited to small, single arm, phase II trials [210–212]. This was partly due to the relatively low incidence of biliary cancer combined with the challenges of ensuring adequate biliary drainage and managing biliary sepsis. In addition, trials were often hampered by the inability to obtain a histological diagnosis and the lack of radiologically measurable disease. Most of these trials utilised traditional single arm phase II endpoints, and did not allow comparisons between treatment regimens. However,

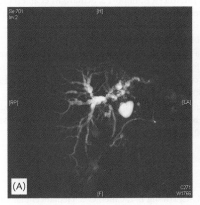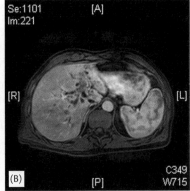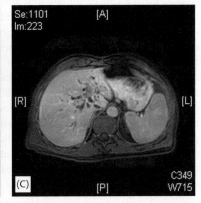

Fig. 41.9 Klatskin cholangiocarcinoma. (A) MRCP demonstrates a tight stricture at the bifurcation of the intrahepatic ducts with a normal calibre common duct. (B) Arterial phase and (C) portal venous phase scans demonstrate a hypovascular lesion in the left lobe of the liver infiltrating the intrahepatic ducts with dilatation of the right and left ducts.

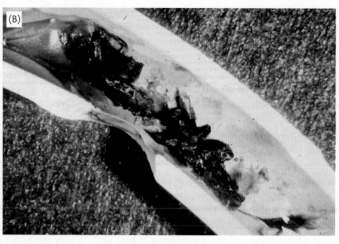

Fig. 41.10 (A) Good long-term biliary drainage achieved with a coated metal wall stent in hilar cholangiocarcinoma presenting with obstructive jaundice. (B) Rapid silting with biliary debris in temporary plastic biliary stent.

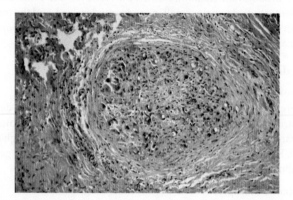

Fig. 41.11 Histological slide of resection margin following surgical resection of hilar cholangiocarcinoma showing neurovascular invasion, predictive of a poorer outcome.

more recently, a small number of randomised phase II and III trials have been successfully performed, due in the main to multi-centre collaborations and technical advances in securing biliary drainage and obtaining tissue diagnosis [213, 214].

The results of the UK ABC-02 trial in 2010 [215] provided a standard of care in the systemic management of locally advanced and metastatic biliary cancer for the first time. This phase III trial demonstrated a significant survival advantage for the combination of gemcitabine and cisplatin over gemcitabine alone. A total of 410 patients were recruited to the trial, making it the largest trial to date in advanced biliary cancer. Progression-free survival and overall survival were both significantly improved in the gemcitabine/cisplatin arm. The median OS was 11.7 months in the combination arm and 8.1 months following single-agent gemcitabine (hazard ratio, 0.64; 95% confidence interval, 0.52 to 0.80; p < 0.001). Importantly, the combination of gemcitabine and cisplatin was not associated with significantly increased toxicity. While the combination increased neutropaenia, this did not translate into an increased infection rate. The good tolerability of this regimen now provides a suitable chemotherapy backbone upon which to investigate the addition of novel therapeutics. However, a better understanding of the molecular pathogenesis of biliary cancers is required in order to select appropriate targeted therapies for clinical trials.

Further reading

Andre T, Tournigand C, Rosmorduc O et al. Gemcitabine combined with oxaliplatin (GEMOX) in advanced biliary tract adenocarcinoma: a GERCOR study. Annals of Oncology 2004; 15(9): 1339–1343.

Cheng AL, Kang YK, Chen Z, Tsao CJ, Qin S et al. Efficacy and safety of sorafenib in patients in the Asia-Pacific region with advanced hepatocellular carcinoma: a phase III randomised, double-blind, placebo-controlled trial. Lancet Oncology 2009; 10(1): 25–34.

DeOliveira ML, Cunningham SC, Cameron JL et al. Cholangiocarcinoma: 31 year experience with 564 patients at a single institution. Annals of Surgery 2007; 245: 755–762.

European Association for the Study of the L, European Organization for R, Treatment of C. EASL–EORTC Clinical Practice Guidelines: Management of hepatocellular carcinoma. Journal of Hepatology 2012; 56(4): 908–943.

Fong Y, Jarnagin W, Blumgart LH. Gallbladder cancer: comparison of patients presenting initially for definitive operation with those presenting after prior noncurative intervention. Annals of Surgery 2000; 232(4): 557–569.

Llovet JM, Brú C, Bruix J. Prognosis of hepatocellular carcinoma: the BCLC staging classification. Seminars in Liver Disease 1999; 19(03): 329–338.

Llovet JM, Ricci S, Mazzaferro V, Hilgard P, Gane E et al. SHARP Investigators Study Group. Sorafenib in advanced hepatocellular carcinoma. New England Journal of Medicine 2008; 359(4): 378–390.

Mazzaferro V, Llovet JM, Miceli R, Bhoori S, Schiavo M et al. Predicting survival after liver transplantation in patients with hepatocellular carcinoma beyond the Milan criteria: a retrospective, exploratory analysis. The Lancet Oncology 2009; 10(1): 35–43.

Mazzaferro V, Regalia E, Doci R, Andreola S, Pulvirenti A et al. Liver transplantation for the treatment of small hepatocellular carcinomas in patients with cirrhosis. New England Journal of Medicine 1996; 334(11): 693–700.

Valle J, Wasan H, Palmer DH et al. Cisplatin plus gemcitabine versus gemcitabine for biliary tract cancer. New England Journal of Medicine 2010; 362(14): 1273–1281.

References

1. Beasley RP, Lin C-C, Hwang L-Y, Chien C-S. Hepatocellular carcinoma and hepatitis B virus: a prospective study of 22 707 men in Taiwan. The Lancet 1981; 318(8256): 1129–1133.

2. Beasley RP. Hepatitis B virus. The major etiology of hepatocellular carcinoma. Cancer 1988; 61(10): 1942–1956.

3. Niederau C, Lange S, Heintges T, Erhardt A, Buschkamp M et al. Prognosis of chronic hepatitis C: results of a large, prospective cohort study. Hepatology 1998; 28(6): 1687–1695.

4. Degos F, Christidis C, Ganne-Carrie N, Farmachidi J-P, Degott C et al. Hepatitis C virus related cirrhosis: time to occurrence of hepatocellular carcinoma and death. Gut 2000; 47(1): 131–136.

5. Hassan MM, Hwang L-Y, Hatten CJ, Swaim M, Li D et al. Risk factors for hepatocellular carcinoma: synergism of alcohol with viral hepatitis and diabetes mellitus. Hepatology 2002; 36(5): 1206–1213.

6. Schöniger-Hekele M, Müller C, Kutilek M, Oesterreicher C, Ferenci P et al. Hepatocellular carcinoma in Austria: aetiological and clinical characteristics at presentation. European Journal of Gastroenterology & Hepatology. 2000; 12(8): 941–948.

7. Baffy G, Brunt EM, Caldwell SH. Hepatocellular carcinoma in non-alcoholic fatty liver disease: an emerging menace. Journal of Hepatology 2012; 56: 1384–1391.

8. Ferlay J, Shin HR, Bray F, Forman D, Mathers C et al. GLOBOCAN 2008 v2.0, Cancer Incidence and Mortality Worldwide: IARC CancerBase No. 10 [Online]. Lyon, France: International Agency for Research on Cancer; 2010. Available from: <http://globocan.iarc.fr>, accessed on 22 September 2013.

9. Ali R, Barnes I, Cairns BJ, Finlayson AE, Bhala N et al. Incidence of gastrointestinal cancers by ethnic group in England, 2001–2007. Gut 2012 [Epub ahead of print]. PubMed PMID: 23092766.

10. Castro FA, Koshiol J, Hsing AW et al. Biliary tract cancer incidence in the United States—demographic and temporal variations by anatomic site. International Journal of Cancer 2013; 133: 1664–1671.

11. Randi G, Franceschi S, La Vecchia C. Gallbladder cancer worldwide: geographical distribution and risk factors. International Journal of Cancer 2006; 118: 1591–1602.

12. Wistuba II, Gazdar AF. Gallbladder cancer: lessons from a rare tumour. Nature Reviews Cancer 2004; 4: 695.

13. Castro FA, Koshiol J, Hsing AW, Devessa SS. Inflammatory gene variants and the risk of biliary tract cancers and stones: a population-based study in China. BMC Cancer 2012; 12: 468. doi:10.1186/1471-2407-12-468

14. Nordenstedt H, Mattsson F, El-Serag H, Lagergren J. Gallstones and cholecystectomy in relation to risk of intra and extrahepatic cholangiocarcinoma. British Journal of Cancer 2012; 106: 1011–1015.

15. Khan ZS, Livingston EH, Huerta S. Reassessing the need for prophylactic surgery in patients with porcelain gallbladder: case series and systematic review of the literature. Archives of Surgery 2011; 146: 1143–1147.

16. Lee SE, Jang JY, Lee YJ, Park T, Lee SY et al. Korean Pancreas Surgery Club choledochal cyst and associated malignant tumors in adults: a multicenter survey in South Korea. Archives of Surgery 2011; 146: 1178–1184.

17. Alvi AR, Siddiqui NA, Zafar H. Risk factors of gallbladder cancer in Karachi-a case-control study. World Journal of Surgical Oncology 2011; 9: 164. doi:10.1186/1477-7819-9-164

18. Pandey M, Mishra RR, Dixit R, Jayswal R, Shukla M et al. Helicobacter bilis in human gallbladder cancer: results of a case-control study and a meta-analysis. Asian Pacific Journal of Cancer Prevention 2010; 11: 343–347.

19. Schlesinger S, Aleksandrova K, Pischon T, Fedirko V, Jenab M et al. Abdominal obesity, weight gain during adulthood and risk of liver and biliary tract cancer in a European cohort. International Journal of Cancer 2013; 132: 645–657.

20. Schlesinger S, Aleksandrova K, Pischon T, Jenab M, Fedirko V et al. Diabetes mellitus, insulin treatment, diabetes duration, and risk of biliary tract cancer and hepatocellular carcinoma in a European cohort. Annals of Oncology 2013; 24: 2449–2455.

21. Yang JD, Kim B, Sanderson SO, Sauver JS, Yawn BP et al. Biliary tract cancers in Olmsted County, Minnesota, 1976–2008. American Journal of Gastroenterology 2012; 107: 1256–1262.

22. Rustagi T, Dasanu CA. Risk factors for gallbladder cancer and cholangiocarcinoma: similarities, differences and updates. Journal of Gastrointestinal Cancer 2012; 43: 137–147.

23. Khan SA, Emadossadaty S, Ladep NG, Thomas HC, Elliott P et al. Rising trends in cholangiocarcinoma: is the ICD classification system misleading us? Journal of Hepatology 2012; 56: 848–854.

24. Suarez-Munoz MA, Fernandez-Aguilar JL, Sanchez-Perez B, Perez-Daga JA, Garcia-Albiach B et al. Risk factors and classification of hilar cholangiocarcinoma. World Journal of Gastrointestinal Oncology 2013; 5: 132–138.

25. Palmer WC, Patel T. Are common factors involved in the pathogenesis of primary liver cancers? A meta-analysis of risk factors for intrahepatic cholangiocarcinoma. Journal of Hepatology 2012; 57: 69–76.

26. Zhou Y, Zhao Y, Li B, Huang J, Wu L et al. Hepatitis viruses infection and risk of intrahepatic cholangiocarcinoma: evidence from a meta-analysis. BMC Cancer 2012; 12: 289. doi:10.1186/1471-2407-12-289. PubMed PMID: 22799744.

27. Fürst T, Keiser J, Utzinger J. Global burden of human food-borne trematodiasis: a systematic review and meta-analysis. The Lancet Infectious Diseases 2012; 12: 210–221.

28. Sripa B. Infectious diseases and tropical disease pathology: SY16-3 opisthorchiasis: from pathogenesis to control. Pathology 2014 (October); 46 (suppl 2): S28. doi: 10.1097/01.PAT.0000454145.24899.b4

29. Perz JF, Armstrong GL, Farrington LA, Hutin YJ, Bell BP. The contributions of hepatitis B virus and hepatitis C virus infections to cirrhosis and primary liver cancer worldwide. Journal of Hepatology 2006; 45: 529.

30. Huang YT, Jen CL, Yang HI, Lee MH, Su J et al. Lifetime risk and sex difference of hepatocellular carcinoma among patients with chronic hepatitis B and C. Journal of Clinical Oncology 2011; 29: 3643.

31. Ji J, Sundquist K, Sundquist J. A population-based study of hepatitis D virus as potential risk factor for hepatocellular carcinoma. Journal of the National Cancer Institute 2012; 104: 790.

32. Chang JS, Tsai CR, Chen LT. Medical risk factors associated with cholangiocarcinoma in Taiwan: a population-based case-control study. PLoS One. 2013; 8: e69981. doi:10.1371/journal.pone.0069981

33. Fürst T, Keiser J, Utzinger J. Global burden of human food-borne trematodiasis: a systematic review and meta-analysis. The Lancet Infectious Diseases 2012; 12: 210–221.

34. Plymoth A, Viviani S, Hainaut P. Control of hepatocellular carcinoma through hepatitis B vaccination in areas of high endemicity: perspectives for global liver cancer prevention. Cancer Letters 2009; 286: 15–21.

35. Chen CF, Lee WC, Yang HI, Chang HC, Jen CL et al. Changes in serum levels of HBV DNA and alanine amino transferase determine risk for hepatocellular carcinoma. Gastroenterology 2011; 141: 1240.

36. Tseng TC, Liu CJ, Yang HC, Su TH, Wang CC et al. High levels of hepatitis B surface antigen increase risk of hepatocellular carcinoma in patients with low HBV load. Gastroenterology 2012; 142: 1140.

37. Chen JD, Yang HI, Iloeje UH, You SL, Lu SN et al. Carriers of inactive hepatitis B virus are still at risk for hepatocellular carcinoma and liver-related death. Gastroenterology 2010; 138: 1747.

38. Simonetti J, Bulkow L, McMahon BJ, Homan C, Snowball M et al. Clearance of hepatitis B surface antigen and risk of hepatocellular carcinoma in a cohort chronically infected with hepatitis B virus. Hepatology 2010; 51: 1531.

39. Liu S, Zhang H, Gu C, Yin J, He Y et al. Associations between hepatitis B virus mutations and the risk of hepatocellular carcinoma: a meta-analysis. Journal of the National Cancer Institute 2009; 101: 1066.

40. Singal AK, Salameh H, Kuo YF, Fontana RJ. Meta-analysis: the impact of oral anti-viral agents on the incidence of hepatocellular carcinoma in chronic hepatitis B. Alimentary Pharmacology & Therapeutics 2013; 38: 98.

41. Lok AS, Seeff LB, Morgan TR, di Bisceglie AM, Sterling RK et al. Incidence of hepatocellular carcinoma and associated risk factors in hepatitis C-related advanced liver disease. Gastroenterology 2009; 136: 138.

42. Morgan RL, Baack B, Smith BD, Yartel A, Pitasi M et al. Eradication of hepatitis C virus infection and the development of hepatocellular carcinoma: a meta-analysis of observational studies. Annals of Internal Medicine 2013; 158: 329.

43. Furutani T, Hino K, Okuda M, Gondo T, Nishina S et al. Hepatic iron overload induces hepatocellular carcinoma in transgenic mice expressing the hepatitis C virus polyprotein. Gastroenterology 2006; 130: 2087.

44. Cai WK, Sima H, Chen BD, Yang GS. Risk factors for hilar cholangiocarcinoma: a case-control study in China. World Journal of Gastroenterology 2011; 17: 249–253.

45. Sripa B, Kaewkes S, Sithithaworn P, Mairiang E, Laha T et al. Liver fluke induces cholangiocarcinoma. PLOS Medicine 2007; 4: 1148–1155.

46. Andrews RH, Sithithaworn P, Petney TN. Opisthorchis viverrini: an underestimated parasite in world health. Trends in Parasitology 2008; 24: 497.

47. Mordvinov VA, Yurlova NI, Ogorodova LM, Katokhin AV. Opisthorchis felineus and Metorchis bilis are the main agents of liver fluke infection of humans in Russia. Parasitology International 2012; 61: 25.

48. Hamilton SR, Aaltonen LA eds. World Health Organization classification of tumours. Pathology and genetics of tumours of the digestive system. Lyon: IARC Press, 2000.

49. Strobel D, Seitz K, Blank W, Schuler A, Dietrich C et al. Contrast-enhanced ultrasound for the characterisation of focal liver lesions—diagnostic accuracy in clinical practice (DEGUM multicentre trial). European Journal of Ultrasound 2008; 29: 499–505.

50. Claudon M, Cosgrove D, Albrecht T, Bolondi L, Bosio M et al. Guidelines and good clinical practice recommendations for contrast enhanced ultrasound (CEUS)—update 2008. European Journal of Ultrasound 2008; 29: 28–44.

51. Salvatore V, Borghi A, Piscaglia F. Contrast-enhanced ultrasound for liver imaging: recent advances. Current Pharmaceutical Design 2012; 18(15): 2236–2252.

52. Chen JA, Shi M, Li JQ, Qian CN. Angiogenesis: multiple masks in hepatocellular carcinoma and liver regeneration. Hepatology International 2010; 4(3): 537–547.

53. Akai H, Kiryu S, Matsuda I, Satou J, Takao H et al. Detection of hepatocellular carcinoma by Gd-EOB-DTPA enhanced liver MRI—comparison with triple phase 64 detector row helical CT. European Journal of Radiology 2011; 80(2): 310–315.

54. Schima W, Kulinna C, Langenberger H, Ba-Ssalamah A. Liver Metastases of colorectal cancer: US, CT or MRI. Cancer Imaging 2005; 5: S149–155.

55. Bluemke DA, Sahani D, Amendola M, Balzer T, Breuer J et al. Efficacy and safety of MR imaging with liver-specific contrast agents: U.S. Multicenter phase III study. Radiology 2005; 237: 89–98.

56. Murakami T Imai Y, Okada M, Hyodo T, Lee WJ et al. Ultrasonography, computed tomography and magnetic resonance imaging of hepatocellular carcinoma: toward improved treatment decisions. Oncology 2011; 81: S1-86–99.

57. Ichikawa SK. Imaging study of early hepatocellular carcinoma: usefulness of gadoxetic acid-enhanced MR imaging. Radiology 2011; 261(3): 834–844.

58. Muhi A, Ichikawa T, Motosugi U, Sou H, Nakajima H et al. Diagnosis of colorectal hepatic metastases: a comparison of contrast-enhanced CT, contrast enhanced US, superparamagneticiron-oxide MRI, and gadoxetic acid-enhanced MRI. Journal of Magnetic Resonance Imaging 2011; 34(2): 326–335.

59. Morana G, Dorigo A. Imaging in cholangiocarcinoma. Cancer Imaging 2011; 11: S72–3.

60. Lowenthal D, Zeile M, Lim WY, Wybranski C, Fischbach F et al. Detection and characterisation of focal liver lesions in colorectal carcinoma patients: comparison of diffusion-weighted and Gd-EOB-DTPA enhanced MR imaging. European Radiology 2011; 21(4): 832–840.

61. Le Moigne F, Durieux M, Bancel B, Boublay N, Boussel L et al. Impact of diffusion-weighted MR imaging on the characterisation of small hepatocellular carcinoma in the cirrhotic liver. Magnetic Resonance Imaging 2012; 30: 656–665.

62. Kele PG, Van der Jagt EJ. Diffusion weighted imaging in the liver. World Journal of Gastroenterology 2010; 16(13): 1567–1576.

63. Blodgett TM, Casagranda B, Townsend DW, Meltzer CC. Issues, controversies, and clinical utility of combined PET/CT imaging: what is the interpreting physician facing? American Journal of Roentgenology 2005 May; 184(5 Suppl): S138–45.

64. Yong TW, Yuan ZZ, Jun Z, Lin Z, He WZ et al. Sensitivity of PET/MR images on liver metastases from colorectal carcinoma. Hellenic Journal of Nuclear Medicine 2011; 14(3): 264–268.

65. Ishizaki Y, Wakayama T, Okada Y, Kobayashi T. Magnetic resonance cholangiography for evaluation of obstructive jaundice. Americal Journal of Gastroenterology 1993; 88(12): 2072–2077.

66. Pavone P, Laghi A, Passariello R. MR cholangiopancreatography in malinant biliary obstruction. Seminars in Ultrasound, CT and MRI 1999; 20(5): 317–323.

67. Vaishali MD, Agarwal AK, Upadhyaya DN, Chauhan VS, Sharma OP et al. Magnetic resonance cholangiopancreatography in obstructive jaundice. Journal of Clinical Gastroenterology 2004; 38(10): 887–890.

68. Rösch T, Lorenz R, Braig C, Feuerbach S, Rudiger Siewert J, et al. Endoscopic ultrasound in pancreatic tumor diagnosis. Gastrointestinal Endoscopy 1991; 37(3): 347–352.

69. Saftoiu A, Vilmann P. Role of endoscopic ultrasound in the diagnosis and staging of pancreatic cancer. Journal of Clinical Ultrasound 2009; 37(1): 1–17.

70. Zandrino F, Benzi L, Ferretti M et al. Multislice CT cholangiography without biliary contrast agent: technique and initial clinical results in the assessment of patients with biliary obstruction. European Radiology 2002; 12(5): 1155–1161.

71. Ochotorena IJL, Kiyosue H, Hori Y, Yokoyama S, Yoshida T et al. The local spread of lower bile duct cancer: evaluation by thin-section helical CT. European Radiology 2000; 10(7): 1106–1113.

72. Zech CJ, Schoenberg SO, Reiser M, Helmberger T. Cross-sectional imaging of biliary tumors: current clinical status and future developments. European Radiology 2004; 14(7): 1174–1187.

73. Vilmann P, Jacobsen GK, Henriksen FW, Hancke S. Endoscopic ultrasonography with guided fine needle aspiration biopsy in pancreatic disease. Gastrointestinal Endoscopy 1992; 38(2): 172–173.

74. Agarwal B, Abu-Hamda E, Molke KL, Correa AM, Ho L. Endoscopic ultrasound-guided fine needle aspiration and multidetector spiral CT in the diagnosis of pancreatic cancer. American Journal of Gastroenterology 2004; 99(5): 844–850.

75. Angelo Paulo F, David RL, Adam S, Catherine C, David LC-L. Brush cytology during ERCP for the diagnosis of biliary and pancreatic malignancies. Gastrointestinal Endoscopy 1994; 40(2): 140–145.

76. Mahmoudi N, Enns R, Amar J, AlAli J, Lam E, Telford J. Biliary brush cytology: factors associated with positive yields on biliary brush cytology. World Journal of Gastroenterology [Original Article] 2008;14(4): 569–573.

77. Walta DC, Fausel CS, Brant B. Endoscopic biliary stents and obstructive jaundice. The American Journal of Surgery 1987; 153(5): 444–447.

78. Lammer J, Hausegger KA, Fluckiger F, Winkelbauer FW, Wilding R et al. Common bile duct obstruction due to malignancy: treatment with plastic versus metal stents. Radiology [Paper] 1996; 201: 167–172.

79. Hochwald S, Burke E, Jarnagin W, Fong Y, Blumgart L. Association of preoperative biliary stenting with increased postoperative infectious complications in proximal cholangiocarcinoma. Archives of Surgery 1999; 134(3): 261–266.

80. Chang W-H, Kortan P, Haber GB. Outcome in patients with bifurcation tumors who undergo unilateral versus bilateral hepatic duct drainage. Gastrointestinal Endoscopy 1998; 47(5): 354–362.

81. DePalma G, Pezzullo A, Rega M, Persico M, Patrone F et al. Unilateral placement of metallic stents for malignany hilar obstruction: a prospective study. Gastrointestinal Endoscopy 2003; 58(1): 50–53.

82. Inal M, Akgul E, Aksungur E, Seydaoglu G. Percutaneous placement of biliary metallic stents in patients with malignant hilar obstruction: unilobar versus bilobar drainage. Journal of Vascular Interventional Radiology 2003; 14: 1409–1416.

83. Draganov PV, Chauhan S, Wagh MS, Gupte AR, Lin T et al. Diagnostic accuracy of conventional and cholangioscopy-guided sampling of indeterminate biliary lesions at the time of ERCP: a prospective, long-term follow-up study. Gastrointestinal Endoscopy 2012; 75(2): 347–353.

84. Kalaitzakis E, Webster G, Oppong K, Kallis Y, Vlavianos N et al. Diagnostic and therapeutic utility of single-operator peroral cholangioscopy for indeterminate biliary lesions and bile duct stones. European Journal of Gastroenterology & Hepatology 2012; 24: 656–664.

85. Zhang B-H, Yang B-H, Tang Z-Y. Randomized controlled trial of screening for hepatocellular carcinoma. Journal of Cancer Research and Clinical Oncology 2004; 130(7): 417–422.

86. McMahon BJ, Bulkow L, Harpster A, Snowball M, Lanier A et al. Screening for hepatocellular carcinoma in Alaska natives infected with chronic hepatitis B: a 16-year population-based study. Hepatology 2000; 32(4): 842–846.

87. Wong LL, Limm WM, Severino R, Wong LM. Improved survival with screening for hepatocellular carcinoma. Liver Transplantation 2000; 6(3): 320–325.

88. Oka H, Kurioka N, Kim K, Kanno T, Kuroki T et al. Prospective study of early detection of hepatocellular carcinoma in patients with cirrhosis. Hepatology 1990; 12(4): 680–687.

89. Bruix J, Sherman M. Management of hepatocellular carcinoma. Hepatology 2005; 42(5): 1208–1236.

90. European Association for the Study of the L, European Organisation for R, Treatment of C. EASL–EORTC Clinical Practice Guidelines: management of hepatocellular carcinoma. Journal of Hepatology 2012; 56(4): 908–943.

91. Ryder S. Guidelines for the diagnosis and treatment of heptocellular carcinoma (HCC) in adults. Gut 2003; 52(Suppl III): iii1–iii8.

92. Bruix J, Sherman M. Management of hepatocellular carcinoma: an update. Hepatology 2011; 53(3): 1020–1022.

93. Marrero JA, Fontana RJ, Barrat A, Askari F, Conjeevaram HS et al. Prognosis of hepatocellular carcinoma: comparison of 7 staging systems in an American cohort. Hepatology 2005; 41(4): 707–715.

94. Trevisani F, D'Intino PE, Morselli-Labate AM, Mazzella G, Accogli E et al. Serum α-fetoprotein for diagnosis of hepatocellular carcinoma in patients with chronic liver disease: influence of HBsAg and anti-HCV status. Journal of Hepatology 2001; 34(4): 570–575.

95. Singal A, Volk ML, Waljee A, Salgia R, Higgins P et al. Meta-analysis: surveillance with ultrasound for early-stage hepatocellular carcinoma in patients with cirrhosis. Alimentary Pharmacology & Therapeutics 2009; 30(1): 37–47.

96. Llovet JM, Brú C, Bruix J. Prognosis of hepatocellular carcinoma: the BCLC staging classification. Seminars in Liver Disease 1999; 19(03): 329–338.

97. Pugh RNH, Murray-Lyon IM, Dawson JL, Pietroni MC, Williams R. Transection of the oesophagus for bleeding oesophageal varices. British Journal of Surgery 1973; 60(8): 646–649.

98. Brown Jr RS, Kumar KS, Russo MW, Kinkhabwala M, Rudow DL et al. Model for end-stage liver disease and Child-Turcotte-Pugh score as predictors of pretransplantation disease severity, posttransplantation outcome, and resource utilization in United Network for Organ Sharing status 2A patients. Liver Transplantation 2002; 8(3): 278–284.

99. Barber K, Madden S, Allen J, Collett D, Neuberger J, Gimson A. Elective liver transplant mortality: development of a United Kingdom end-stage liver disease score. Transplantation 2011; 92(4): 469–476.

100. Ochiai T, Ogino S, Ishimoto T, Toma A, Yamamoto Y et al. Prognostic impact of hepatectomy for patients with non-hepatitis B, non-hepatitis C hepatocellular carcinoma. Anticancer Research 2014 Aug; 34(8): 4399–4410.

101. Mazzaferro V, Regalia E, Doci R, Andreola S, Pulvirenti A et al. Liver transplantation for the treatment of small hepatocellular carcinomas in patients with cirrhosis. New England Journal of Medicine 1996; 334(11): 693–700.

102. Yao FY, Ferrell L, Bass NM, Watson JJ, Bacchetti P et al. Liver transplantation for hepatocellular carcinoma: expansion of the tumor size limits does not adversely impact survival. Hepatology 2001; 33(6): 1394–1403.

103. Yao FY, Xiao L, Bass NM, Kerlan R, Ascher NL et al. Liver transplantation for hepatocellular carcinoma: validation of the UCSF-expanded criteria based on preoperative imaging. American Journal of Transplantation 2007; 7(11): 2587–2596.

104. Mazzaferro V, Llovet JM, Miceli R, Bhoori S, Schiavo M et al. Predicting survival after liver transplantation in patients with hepatocellular carcinoma beyond the Milan criteria: a retrospective, exploratory analysis. The Lancet Oncology 2009; 10(1): 35–43.

105. Silva MF, Sherman M. Criteria for liver transplantation for HCC: what should the limits be? Journal of Hepatology 2011; 55(5): 1137–1147.

106. Clavien P-A, Lesurtel M, Bossuyt PMM, Gores GJ, Langer B et al. Recommendations for liver transplantation for hepatocellular carcinoma: an international consensus conference report. The Lancet Oncology 2012; 13: e11–e22.

107. Volk ML, Vijan S, Marrero JA. A novel model measuring the harm of transplanting hepatocellular carcinoma exceeding Milan criteria. American Journal of Transplantation 2008; 8(4): 839–846.

108. Peng ZW, Chen MS. Transcatheter arterial chemoembolization combined with radiofrequency ablation for the treatment of hepatocellular carcinoma. Oncology 2013; 84 Suppl 1: 40–43.

109. Chan AC, Cheung TT, Fan ST, Chok KS, Chan SC, Poon RT et al. Survival analysis of high-intensity focused ultrasound therapy versus radiofrequency ablation in the treatment of recurrent hepatocellular carcinoma. Annals of Surgery 2013; 257: 686–692.

110. Guo Y, Zhang Y, Klein R, Nijm GM, Sahakian AV et al. Irreversible electroporation therapy in the liver: longitudinal efficacy studies in a rat model of hepatocellular carcinoma. Cancer Research 2010; 70: 1555–1563.

111. Friedrich-Rust M, Klopffleisch T, Nierhoff J, Herrmann E, Vermehren J et al. Contrast-enhanced ultrasound for the differentiation of benign and malignant focal liver lesions: a meta-analysis. Liver International 2013 [Epub ahead of print]. doi:10.1111/liv.12115

112. Takayasu K. Transcatheter arterial chemoembolization for unresectable hepatocellular carcinoma: recent progression and perspective. Oncology 2013; 84 (Suppl 1): 28–33.

113. Minouchehr S, Radtke A, Sotiropoulos GC, Molmenti EP, Braun F et al. Drainage patterns of right and accessory hepatic veins: anatomical-functional classification derived from 3-dimensional CT reconstructions. Hepatogastroenterology 2011; 58: 1664–1669.

114. Kaibori M, Tanigawa N, Kariya S, Ikeda H, Nakahashi Y et al. A prospective randomized controlled trial of preoperative whole-liver chemolipiodolization for hepatocellular carcinoma. Digestive Diseases and Sciences 2012; 57: 1404–1412.

115. Meyer T, Kirkwood A, Roughton M, Beare S, Tsochatzis E et al. A randomised phase II/III trial of 3-weekly cisplatin-based sequential transarterial chemoembolisation vs embolisation alone for hepatocellular carcinoma. British Journal of Cancer 2013 [Epub ahead of print]. doi:10.1038/bjc.2013.85

116. Burrel M, Reig M, Forner A, Barrufet M, de Lope CR et al. Survival of patients with hepatocellular carcinoma treated by transarterial chemoembolisation (TACE) using Drug Eluting Beads. Implications for clinical practice and trial design. Journal of Hepatololgy 2012; 56: 1330–1335.

117. Fiorentini G, Aliberti C, Benea G, Montagnani F, Mambrini A et al. TACE of liver metastases from colorectal cancer adopting irinotecan-eluting beads: beneficial effect of palliative intra-arterial lidocaine and post-procedure supportive therapy on the control of side effects. Hepatogastroenterology 2008; 55: 2077–2082.

118. Prompers L, Bucerius J, Brans B, Temur Y, Berger L et al. Selective internal radiation therapy (SIRT) in primary or secondary liver cancer. Methods 2011; 55: 253–257.

119. Lau WY, Kennedy AS, Kim YH, Lai HK, Lee RC et al. Patient selection and activity planning guide for selective internal radiotherapy with yttrium-90 resin microspheres. International Journal of Radiation Oncology Biology Physics. 2012; 82: 401–407.

120. Deneve JL, Choi J, Gonzalez RJ, Conley AP, Stewart S et al. Chemosaturation with percutaneous hepatic perfusion for unresectable isolated hepatic metastases from sarcoma. Cardiovascular Interventional Radiology 2012; 35: 1480–1487.

121. Takaki H, Yamakado K, Nakatsuka A, Yamada T, Shiraki K, Takei Y et al. Frequency of and Risk Factors for Complications After Liver Radiofrequency Ablation Under CT Fluoroscopic Guidance in 1500 Sessions: single-Center Experience. American Journal of Roentgenology 2013; 200: 658–664.

122. Swan RZ, Sindram D, Martinie JB, Iannitti DA. Operative microwave ablation for hepatocellular carcinoma: complications, recurrence, and long-term outcomes. Journal of Gastrointestinal Surgery 2013; 17: 719–729.

123. Kingham TP, Karkar AM, D'Angelica MI, Allen PJ, Dematteo RP et al. Ablation of perivascular hepatic malignant tumors with irreversible electroporation. Journal of the American College of Surgeons 2012; 215: 379–387.

124. Lai CL, Wu PC, Chan GC, Lok AS, Lin HJ. Doxorubicin versus no antitumor therapy in inoperable hepatocellular carcinoma. A prospective randomized trial. Cancer 1988; 62(3): 479–483.

125. Lai KH, Tsai YT, Lee SD, Ng WW, Teng HC et al. Phase II study of mitoxantrone in unresectable primary hepatocellular carcinoma following hepatitis B infection. Cancer, Chemotherapy and Pharmacology 1989; 23(1): 54–56.

126. Ishikawa T, Ichida T, Sugitani S, Tsuboi Y, Genda T et al. Improved survival with oral administration of enteric-coated tegafur/uracil for advanced stage IV-A hepatocellular carcinoma. Journal of Gastroenterology and Hepatology 2001; 16(4): 452–459.

127. Posey J, Johnson P, Mok T, Hirmand M, Dahlberg S et al. Results of a phase 2/3 open-label, randomized trial of T138067 versus doxorubicin (DOX) in chemotherapy-naïve, unresectable hepatocellular carcinoma (HCC). Journal of Clinical Oncology 2005, ASCO Annual Meeting Proceedings Vol. 23, No. 16S, Part I of II (June 1 Supplement): 4035.

128. Gish RG, Porta C, Lazar L, Ruff P, Feld R et al. Phase III randomized controlled trial comparing the survival of patients with unresectable hepatocellular carcinoma treated with nolatrexed or doxorubicin. Journal of Clinical Oncology 2007; 25(21): 3069–3075.

129. Leung TW, Patt YZ, Lau WY, Ho SK, Yu SC et al. Complete pathological remission is possible with systemic combination chemotherapy for inoperable hepatocellular carcinoma. Clinical Cancer Research 1999; 5(7): 1676–1681.

130. Yeo W, Mok TS, Zee B, Leung TW, Lai PB et al. A randomized phase III study of doxorubicin versus cisplatin/interferon alpha-2b/doxorubicin/fluorouracil (PIAF) combination chemotherapy for unresectable hepatocellular carcinoma. Journal of the National Cancer Institute 2005; 97(20): 1532–1538.

131. Qin S, Bai Y, Ye S, Fan J, Lim H et al. Phase III study of oxaliplatin plus 5-fluorouracil/leucovorin (FOLFOX4) versus doxorubicin as palliative systemic chemotherapy in advanced HCC in Asian patients. Journal of Clinical Oncology 2010; 28: 15s, (suppl; abstr 4008).

132. Farinati F, Salvagnini M, de Maria N, Fornasiero A, Chiaramonte M et al. Unresectable hepatocellular carcinoma: a prospective controlled trial with tamoxifen. Journal of Hepatology 1990; 11(3): 297–301.

133. CLIP investigators. Tamoxifen in treatment of hepatocellular carcinoma: a randomised controlled trial. CLIP Group (Cancer of the Liver Italian Programme). The Lancet 1998; 352(9121): 17–20.

134. Liu CL, Fan ST, Ng IO, Lo CM, Poon RT et al. Treatment of advanced hepatocellular carcinoma with tamoxifen and the correlation with expression of hormone receptors: a prospective randomized study. American Journal of Gastroenterology 2000; 95(1): 218–222.

135. Siegel AB, Cohen EI, Ocean A, Lehrer D, Goldenberg A et al. Phase II trial evaluating the clinical and biologic effects of bevacizumab in unresectable hepatocellular carcinoma. Journal of Clinical Oncology 2008; 26(18): 2992–2998.

136. Abou-Alfa GK, Schwartz L, Ricci S, Amadori D, Santoro A et al. Phase II study of sorafenib in patients with advanced hepatocellular carcinoma. Journal of Clinical Oncology 2006; 24: 4293–4300.

137. Llovet JM, Ricci S, Mazzaferro V, Hilgard P, Gane E et al. SHARP Investigators Study Group. Sorafenib in advanced hepatocellular carcinoma. New England Journal of Medicine 2008; 359(4): 378–390.

138. Cheng AL, Kang YK, Chen Z, Tsao CJ, Qin S et al. Efficacy and safety of sorafenib in patients in the Asia-Pacific region with advanced hepatocellular carcinoma: a phase III randomised, double-blind, placebo-controlled trial. The Lancet Oncology 2009; 10(1): 25–34.

139. Cheng A, Kang Y, Lin D, Park J, Kudo M et al. Phase III trial of sunitinib (Su) versus sorafenib (So) in advanced hepatocellular carcinoma (HCC). Journal of Clinical Oncology 2013; 31: 4067–4075.

140. Johnson PJ, Qin S, Park JW, Poon RT, Raoul JL et al. A phase II study of brivanib vs sorafenib in patients with advanced hepatocellular carcinoma. Journal of Clinical Oncology 2013; 31: 3517–3524.

141. Pazo Cid RA, Esquerdo G, Puertolas T, Calderero V, Gil I et al. Bevacizumab (BVZ) as second-line treatment after sorafenib (SFB) progression in patients (pts) with advanced hepatocellular carcinoma (HCC). Journal of Clinical Oncology 2010; 28 (suppl; abstr e14619).

142. Rimassa L, Santoro A, Daniele B, Germano D, Gasbarrini A et al. Tivantinib, a new option for second-line treatment of advanced hepatocellular carcinoma? The experience of Italian centers. Tumori 2015; 101:139–143.

143. Zhu AX, Stuart K, Blaszkowsky LS, Muzikansky A, Reitberg DP et al. Phase 2 study of cetuximab in patients with advanced hepatocellular carcinoma. Cancer 2007; 110(3): 581–589.

144. Thomas MB, Chadha R, Glover K, Wang X, Morris J et al. Phase 2 study of erlotinib in patients with unresectable hepatocellular carcinoma. Cancer 2007; 110(5): 1059–10567.

145. Zhu AX, Abrams TA, Miksad R, Blaszkowsky LS, Meyerhardt JA et al. Phase 1/2 study of everolimus in advanced hepatocellular carcinoma. Cancer 2011; 117: 5094–5102.

146. Ueda S, Basaki Y, Yoshie M, Ogawa K, Sakisaka S et al. PTEN/Akt signaling through epidermal growth factor receptor is prerequisite for angiogenesis by hepatocellular carcinoma cells that is susceptible to inhibition by gefitinib. Cancer Research 2006; 66(10): 5346–5353.

147. Thomas MB, Morris JS, Chadha R, Iwasaki M, Kaur H et al. Phase II trial of the combination of bevacizumab and erlotinib in patients who have advanced hepatocellular carcinoma. Journal of Clinical Oncology 2009; 27(6): 843–850.

148. Treiber G. Treatment of advanced or metastatic hepatocellular cancer (HCC): interim analysis of a single-arm phase II study of bevacizumab and RAD001. Journal of Clinical Oncology 2010; 28: 15s (suppl; abstr 4102).

149. Finn RS, Poon RT, Yau T, Klümpen HJ, Chen LT et al. Phase I study investigating everolimus combined with sorafenib in patients with advanced hepatocellular carcinoma. Journal of Hepatology 2013; 59: 1271–1277.

150. O'Donnell R, El-Khoueiry AB, Lenz H, Gandara DR. A phase I trial of escalating doses of the anti-IGF-1R monoclonal antibody (mAb) cixutumumab (IMC-A12) and sorafenib for treatment of advanced hepatocellular carcinoma (HCC). Journal of Clinical Oncology 2010; 28: 15s (suppl; abstr TPS212).

151. Alavi A, Hood JD, Frausto R, Stupack DG, Cheresh DA. Role of Raf in vascular protection from distinct apoptotic stimuli. Science 2003; 301(5629): 94–96.

152. Abou-Alfa GK, Johnson P, Knox JJ, Capanu M, Davidenko I et al. Doxorubicin plus sorafenib vs doxorubicin alone in patients with advanced hepatocellular carcinoma: a randomized trial. Journal of the American Medical Association 2010; 304(19): 2154–2160.

153. Okita K, Imanaka N, Chida WY, Tak K, Nakachi, T et al. Phase III study of sorafenib in patients in Japan and Korea with advanced hepatocellular carcinoma (HCC) treated after transarterial chemoembolization (TACE). ASCO 2010 Gastrointestinal Cancers Symposium. LBA 128.

154. Lencioni R, de Baere T, Burrel M, Caridi JG, Lammer J et al. Transcatheter treatment of hepatocellular carcinoma with Doxorubicin-loaded DC Bead (DEBDOX): technical recommendations. Cardiovascular and Interventional Radiology 2012; 35: 980–985.

155. Yeo W, Lam KC, Zee B, Chan PS, Mo FK et al. Hepatitis B reactivation in patients with hepatocellular carcinoma undergoing systemic chemotherapy. Annals of Oncology 2004; 15(11): 1661–1666.

156. Yeo W, Chan PK, Ho WM, Zee B, Lam KC et al. Lamivudine for the prevention of hepatitis B virus reactivation in hepatitis B s-antigen seropositive cancer patients undergoing cytotoxic chemotherapy. Journal of Clinical Oncology 2004; 22(5): 927–934.

157. Sezgin Göksu S, Bilal S, Coşkun HŞ. Hepatitis B reactivation related to everolimus. World Journal of Hepatology 2013; 5(1): 43–45.

158. Teng CF, Wu HC, Tsai HW, Shiah HS, Huang W, Su IJ. Novel feedback inhibition of surface antigen synthesis by mammalian target of rapamycin (mTOR) signal and its implication for hepatitis B virus tumorigenesis and therapy. Hepatology 2011 (October); 54(4): 1199–1207.

159. Coburn NG, Cleary SP, Tan JC, Law CH. Surgery for gallbladder cancer: a population-based analysis. Journal of the American College of Surgeons 2008; 207(3): 371–382.

160. Greene F, Page D, Fleming I, Fritz CM, Balch DG et al. AJCC Cancer Staging Manual, 6th edn. New York: Springer-Verlag, 2002.

161. Fleming I, Cooper J, Henson D, Fritz CM, Balch DG et al. AJCC Cancer Staging Manual, 5th edn. Philadelphia: Lippincott-Raven, 1998.

162. Fong Y, Jarnagin W, Blumgart LH. Gallbladder cancer: comparison of patients presenting initially for definitive operation with those presenting after prior noncurative intervention. Annals of Surgery 2000; 232(4): 557–569.

163. Hawkins WG, DeMatteo RP, Jarnagin WR et al. Jaundice predicts advanced disease and early mortality in patients with gallbladder cancer. Annals of Surgical Oncology 2004; 11(3): 310–315.

164. Chan SY, Poon RT, Lo CM et al. Management of carcinoma of the gallbladder: a single-institution experience in 16 years. Journal of Surgical Oncology 2008; 97(2): 156–164.

165. Dixon E, Vollmer CM Jr, Sahajpal A, Cattral M, Grant D et al. An aggressive surgical approach leads to improved survival in patients with gallbladder cancer: a 12-year study at a North American Center. Annals of Surgery 2005; 241(3): 385–394.

166. Ito H, Matros E, Brooks DC, Osteen RT, Zinner MJ et al. Treatment outcomes associated with surgery for gallbladder cancer: a 20-year experience. Journal of Gastrointestinal Surgery 2004; 8(2): 183–190.

167. Gandolfi L, Torresan F, Solmi L, Puccetti A. The role of ultrasound in biliary and pancreatic diseases. European Journal of Ultrasound 2003; 16(3): 141–159.

168. Levy AD, Murakata LA, Rohrmann CA, Jr. Gallbladder carcinoma: radiologic-pathologic correlation. Radiographics 2001; 21(2): 295–314; questionnaire, 549–555.

169. Onoyama H, Yamamoto M, Takada M, Urakawa T, Ajiki T et al. Diagnostic imaging of early gallbladder cancer: retrospective study of 53 cases. World Journal of Surgery 1999; 23(7): 708–712.

170. Komatsuda T, Ishida H, Konno K, Hamashima Y, Naganuma H et al. Gallbladder carcinoma: color Doppler sonography. Abdominal Imaging 2000; 25(2): 194–197.

171. Gourgiotis S, Kocher HM, Solaini L, Yarollahi A, Tsiambas E et al. Gallbladder cancer. American Journal of Surgery 2008; 196(2): 252–264.

172. Ohtani T, Shirai Y, Tsukada K, Hatakeyama K, Muto T. Carcinoma of the gallbladder: CT evaluation of lymphatic spread. Radiology 1993; 189(3): 875–880.

173. Ohtani T, Shirai Y, Tsukada K, Muto T, Hatakeyama K. Spread of gallbladder carcinoma: CT evaluation with pathologic correlation. Abdominal Imaging 1996; 21(3): 195–201.

174. Kumaran V, Gulati S, Paul B, Pande K, Sahni P et al. The role of dual-phase helical CT in assessing resectability of carcinoma of the gallbladder. European Radiology 2002; 12(8): 1993–1999.

175. Yoshimitsu K, Honda H, Shinozaki K, Aibe H, Kuroiwa T et al. Helical CT of the local spread of carcinoma of the gallbladder: evaluation according to the TNM system in patients who underwent surgical resection. American Journal of Roentgenology 2002; 179(2): 423–428.

176. Schwartz LH, Black J, Fong Y, Jarnagin W, Blumgart L et al. Gallbladder carcinoma: findings at MR imaging with MR cholangiopancreatography. Journal of Computer Assisted Tomography 2002; 26(3): 405–410.

177. Petrowsky H, Wildbrett P, Husarik DB, Hany TF, Tam S et al. Impact of integrated positron emission tomography and computed tomography on staging and management of gallbladder cancer and cholangiocarcinoma. Journal of Hepatology 2006; 45(1): 43–50.

178. Rodriguez-Fernandez A, Gomez-Rio M, Llamas-Elvira JM, Ortega-Lozano S, Ferrón-Orihuela JA et al. Positron-emission tomography with fluorine-18-fluoro-2-deoxy-D-glucose for gallbladder cancer diagnosis. American Journal of Surgery 2004; 188(2): 171–175.

179. Anderson CD, Rice MH, Pinson CW, Chapman WC, Chari RS et al. Fluorodeoxyglucose PET imaging in the evaluation of gallbladder carcinoma and cholangiocarcinoma. Journal of Gastrointestinal Surgery 2004; 8(1): 90–97.

180. Corvera CU, Blumgart LH, Akhurst T, DeMatteo RP, D'Angelica M et al. 18F-fluorodeoxyglucose positron emission tomography influences management decisions in patients with biliary cancer. Journal of the American College of Surgeons 2008; 206(1): 57–65.

181. Kondo S, Nimura Y, Hayakawa N, Kamiya J, Nagino M et al. Regional and para-aortic lymphadenectomy in radical surgery for advanced gallbladder carcinoma. British Journal of Surgery 2000; 87(4): 418–422.

182. Weber SM, DeMatteo RP, Fong Y, Blumgart LH, Jarnagin WR. Staging laparoscopy in patients with extrahepatic biliary carcinoma. Analysis of 100 patients. Annals of Surgery 2002; 235(3): 392–399.

183. D'Angelica M, Dalal KM, Dematteo RP, Fong Y, Blumgart LH et al. Analysis of the extent of resection for adenocarcinoma of the gallbladder. Annals of Surgical Oncology 2008.

184. Matsumoto Y, Fujii H, Aoyama H, Yamamoto M, Sugahara K et al. Surgical treatment of primary carcinoma of the gallbladder based on the histologic analysis of 48 surgical specimens. American Journal of Surgery 1992; 163(2): 239–245.

185. Pawlik TM, Gleisner AL, Vigano L, Kooby DA, Bauer TW et al. Incidence of finding residual disease for incidental gallbladder carcinoma: implications for re-resection. Journal of Gastrointestinal Surgery 2007; 11(11): 1478–1486; discussion, 1486–1487.

186. You DD, Lee HG, Paik KY, Heo JS, Choi SH et al. What is an adequate extent of resection for T1 gallbladder cancers? Annals of Surgery 2008; 247(5): 835–838.

187. Behari A, Sikora SS, Wagholikar GD, Kumar A, Saxena R et al. Longterm survival after extended resections in patients with gallbladder cancer. Journal of the American College of Surgeons 2003; 196(1): 82–88.

188. Shimada H, Endo I, Togo S, Nakano A, Izumi T et al. The role of lymph node dissection in the treatment of gallbladder carcinoma. Cancer 1997; 79(5): 892–899.

189. Doty JR, Cameron JL, Yeo CJ, Campbell K, Coleman J et al. Cholecystectomy, liver resection, and pylorus-preserving pancreaticoduodenectomy for gallbladder cancer: report of five cases. Journal of Gastrointestinal Surgery 2002; 6(5): 776–780.

190. Miyazaki M, Itoh H, Ambiru S, Shimizu H, Togawa A et al. Radical surgery for advanced gallbladder carcinoma. British Journal of Surgery 1996; 83(4): 478–481.

191. Shirai Y, Ohtani T, Tsukada K, Hatakeyama K. Combined pancreaticoduodenectomy and hepatectomy for patients with locally advanced gallbladder carcinoma: long term results. Cancer 1997; 80(10): 1904–1909.

192. Endo I, Shimada H, Tanabe M, Fujii Y, Takeda K et al. Prognostic significance of the number of positive lymph nodes in gallbladder cancer. Journal of Gastrointestinal Surgery 2006; 10(7): 999–1007.

193. Takada T, Amano H, Yasuda H, Nimura Y, Matsushiro T et al. Is postoperative adjuvant chemotherapy useful for gallbladder carcinoma? A phase III multicenter prospective randomized controlled trial in patients with resected pancreaticobiliary carcinoma. Cancer 2002; 95(8): 1685–1695.

194. Czito BG, Hurwitz HI, Clough RW, Tyler DS, Morse MA et al. Adjuvant external-beam radiotherapy with concurrent chemotherapy after resection of primary gallbladder carcinoma: a 23-year

experience. International Journal of Radiation Oncology Biology Physics 2005; 62(4): 1030–1034.

195. Kresl JJ, Schild SE, Henning GT, Gunderson LL, Donohue J et al. Adjuvant external beam radiation therapy with concurrent chemotherapy in the management of gallbladder carcinoma. International Journal of Radiation Oncology Biology Physics 2002; 52(1): 167–175.

196. Houry S, Schlienger M, Huguier M, Lacaine F, Penne F et al. Gallbladder carcinoma: role of radiation therapy. British Journal of Surgery 1989; 76(5): 448–450.

197. Shih SP, Schulick RD, Cameron JL, Lillemoe KD, Pitt HA et al. Gallbladder cancer: the role of laparoscopy and radical resection. Annals of Surgery 2007; 245(6): 893–901.

198. Jarnagin WR, Burke E, Powers C, Fong Y, Blumgart LH. Intrahepatic biliary enteric bypass provides effective palliation in selected patients with malignant obstruction at the hepatic duct confluence. American Journal of Surgery 1998; 175(6): 453–460.

199. Kapoor VK, Pradeep R, Haribhakti SP, Singh V, Sikora SS et al. Intrahepatic segment III cholangiojejunostomy in advanced carcinoma of the gallbladder. British Journal of Surgery 1996; 83(12): 1709–1711.

200. Hejna M, Pruckmayer M, Raderer M. The role of chemotherapy and radiation in the management of biliary cancer: a review of the literature. European Journal of Cancer 1998; 34(7): 977–986.

201. Inoue K, Makuuchi M, Takayama T, Torzilli G, Yamamoto J et al. Long-term survival and prognostic factors in the surgical treatment of mass-forming type cholangiocarcinoma. Surgery 2000; 127: 498–505.

202. Uenishi T, Kubo S, Yamazaki O, Yamada T, Sasaki Y et al. Indications for surgical treatment of intrahepatic cholangiocarcinoma with lymph node metastases. Journal of Hepatobiliary and Pancreatic Surgery 2008; 15: 417–422.

203. Nakagawa T, Kamayama T, Kurauchi N, Matsushita M, Nakanishi K et al. Number of lymph node metastases is a prognostic factor in intrahepatic cholangiocarcinoma. World Journal of Surgery 2005; 29: 728–733.

204. De Oliveira ML, Cunningham SC, Cameron JL, Kamangar F, Winter JM et al. Cholangiocarcinoma: 31 year experience with 564 patients at a single institution. Annals of Surgery 2007; 245: 755–762.

205. Paik KY, Jung JC, Heo JS, Choi SH, Choi DW et al. What prognostic factors are important for resected intrahepatic cholangiocarcinoma? Journal of Gastroenterology and Hepatology 2008: 23; 766–770.

206. Sasaki A, Aramaki M, Kawano K, Morii Y, Nakashima K et al. Intrahepatic peripheral cholangiocarcinoma: mode of spread and choice of surgical treatment. British Journal of Surgery 1998; 85: 1206–1209.

207. Shirabe K, Shimada M, Harimoto N, Sugimachi K, Yamashita Y et al. intrahepatic cholangiocarcinoma: its mode of spreading and therapeutic modalities. Surgery 2002; 131: S159–164.

208. Liver Cancer Study Group of Japan. National Surveillance of Primary Liver Cancer in Japan, 17th Report. Kyoto: Media Planning, 2006.

209. Gores GJ, Nagorney DM, Rosen CB. Cholangiocarcinoma: is transplantation an option? For whom? Journal of Hepatology 2007; 47: 454–475.

210. Harder J, Riecken B, Kummer O, Lohrmann C, Otto F et al. Outpatient chemotherapy with gemcitabine and oxaliplatin in patients with biliary tract cancer. British Journal of Cancer 2006; 95(7): 848–852.

211. Andre T, Tournigand C, Rosmorduc O, Provent S, Maindrault-Goebel F et al. Gemcitabine combined with oxaliplatin (GEMOX) in advanced biliary tract adenocarcinoma: a GERCOR study. Annals of Oncology 2004; 15(9): 1339–1343.

212. Verderame F, Russo A, Di Leo R, Badalamenti G, Santangelo D et al. Gemcitabine and oxaliplatin combination chemotherapy in advanced biliary tract cancers. Annals of Oncology 2006; 17 Suppl 7: vii68–72.

213. Kondo S, Nimura Y, Hayakawa N, Kamiya J, Nagino M et al. Extensive surgery for carcinoma of the gallbladder. British Journal of Surgery 2002; 89(2): 179–184.

214. Kayahara M, Nagakawa T, Nakagawara H, Kitagawa H, Ohta T. Prognostic factors for gallbladder cancer in Japan. Annals of Surgery 2008; 248(5): 807–814.

215. Valle J, Wasan H, Palmer DH, Cunningham D, Anthoney A et al. Cisplatin plus gemcitabine versus gemcitabine for biliary tract cancer. New England Journal of Medicine 2010; 362 (14): 1273–1281.

CHAPTER 42

Peritoneal mesothelioma

H. Richard Alexander, Jr., Dario Baratti, Terence C. Chua, Marcello Deraco, Raffit Hassan, Marzia Pennati, Federica Perrone, Paul H. Sugarbaker, Anish Thomas, Keli Turner, Tristan D. Yan, and Nadia Zaffaroni

Introduction to peritoneal mesothelioma

Mesothelioma is a neoplasm originating from the mesothelial cells lining the human body cavities (Figure 42.1). Mesothelioma may involve the pleura, less frequently the peritoneum, and rarely, the pericardium and tunica vaginalis testes. In the past, peritoneal mesothelioma was a rapidly fatal peritoneal surface malignancy with a median survival of less than one year [1, 2]. It represents about one-fifth to one-third of all forms of mesothelioma; there are approximately 400 new cases in the United States each year [3].

The most common age range at presentation is between 40–60 years [4]. Asbestos exposure appears to be causative in some cases of peritoneal mesothelioma, but a search for other carcinogens continues [5–7]. The initial clinical presentation of patients is usually non-specific with symptoms of abdominal pain and increasing abdominal girth being the most common [8]. The predominance of abdominal symptoms as a clinical feature of malignant peritoneal mesothelioma (MPM) is a reflection of the natural history of the disease, as MPM typically remains confined to the abdominal cavity; morbidity and mortality is a consequence of intra-abdominal disease progression and is characterized by small bowel obstruction and cachexia [9]. Computed tomography (CT) is the most commonly used imaging modality in the diagnostic workup, but tissue biopsy with immunohistochemical staining is obligatory for definitive diagnosis. The use of cytoreductive surgery (CRS) and hyperthermic perioperative chemotherapy (HIPEC) has become the accepted initial management for suitable patients with MPM. MPM treatment centres have shown that CRS and HIPEC is associated with a durable improvement in survival from a historical median survival of six months [10] for patients with untreated disease to 34–92 months for selected patients [11–16]. This chapter describes the most recent experience with MPM and analyzes symptoms, clinicopathologic features, survival after aggressive local-regional treatment, and examines future prospects for improved management.

Epidemiology

In the Washington Cancer Institute data of 51 MPM patients, the mean age was 53 years, with a range of 16 to 78 years. A majority of patients were Caucasian; there was one African American and one Asian American. Sixteen patients had no history of exposure to asbestos, 20 had a positive history, and no data are available on 15 patients. Nineteen patients had a family history of cancer in a parent or sibling and five had more than one first-degree relative with a malignancy; no data are available on nine patients [17]. MPM is strongly linked with prior asbestos exposure with latency period of decades before its formal diagnosis. This disease is mostly observed in countries with a higher socio-economic status due to the historical use of asbestos in the construction industry and the availability of current medical technology that allows its diagnosis [18]. In 2009, there were 2558 patients diagnosed with mesothelioma and this incidence has demonstrated an increasing trend since the 1970s with an exponential increase noted since year 2000 from 0.5 to 3 persons per 100 000 [19]. Peritoneal mesothelioma accounts for one-third of all mesotheliomas [20].

The exact pathogenesis of MPM is unknown; however, several hypotheses have been proposed. It is thought that inhaled asbestos may form expectorate that may subsequently be swallowed. Upon entry into the gastrointestinal tract, it penetrates the luminal surfaces of the intestinal mucosa to enter the lymphatic and splanchnic circulation [21]. This triggers a foreign body reaction resulting in a series of inflammatory responses. Together, the chronicity of this

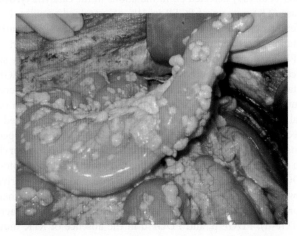

Fig. 42.1 Malignant peritoneal mesothelioma with whitish tumour nodules present on parietal and visceral peritoneal surfaces of the abdomen and pelvis.

inflammatory reaction leads to disruption and alterations of the genetic make-up of mesothelial cells [22]. Evidence from clinical studies to support this association have shown that patients with malignant mesothelioma have higher levels of interleukin (IL)-10, a cytokine that drives further production of transforming growth factor (TGF)-ß. Both IL-10 and TGF-ß are postulated to play a role asbestos-related carcinogenesis [23].

Molecular biology and pathology of peritoneal mesothelioma

Molecular features as prognostic biomarkers

Thus far, the presence and prognostic relevance of a handful of biomarkers, mainly related to cell cycle control, receptor tyrosine kinase (RTK)-mediated signalling and telomere maintenance, have been investigated. These molecular features have been studied as 'prognostic biomarkers'.

Cell cycle-related markers

A reduced expression or loss of p16 protein, a cyclin-dependent kinase (CDK) inhibitor which prevents progression through the G1-S restriction point of the cell cycle by blocking the activity of CDK4/6, has been frequently observed in MPM [24, 25], although the prognostic significance of such an alteration is still controversial. In fact, while Borczuk et al. [24] found that p16 loss was associated with increased risk of death at multivariate analysis, such a finding was not confirmed by Nonaka et al. [25]. Homozygous deletion of the 9p21 locus harbouring the p16 coding gene CDKN2A, which represents one of the most common genetic alterations in pleural mesothelioma, has been also recorded in small but significant percentages of MPMs (25–35%) [26, 27]. In addition, patients with CDKN2A deletions were found to have worse overall and disease-specific survival [27]. Studies aimed to evaluate the prognostic relevance of another cell kinetic parameter, mitotic count (MC), showed that high MC was an indicator of an unfavourable prognosis on univariate [28] and multivariate [29] analyses.

Cell signalling pathway-related markers

Epidermal growth factor receptor (EGFR) was consistently shown to be over-expressed in more than 90% of MPMs examined in different studies [30–32], but its prognostic value is still unclear [25]. Foster et al. [31] detected point mutations in the catalytic tyrosine kinase (TK) domain of EGFR in 31% of examined samples. Nine different mutations were identified: the known L858R activating mutation described in non-small cell lung cancer and eight novel EGFR TK domain point mutations. Although no statistically significant difference in survival was reached, all patients with EGFR mutations were alive with a mean survival of 24 months, whereas 5 out of 18 of the wild-type group died of disease with a mean survival of seven months. However, two subsequent studies failed to detect mutations in the EGFR TK domain of MPM surgical specimens [32, 33]. Specifically, we found the expression/phosphorylation of EGFR as well as of platelet-derived growth factor receptor β (PDGFR-β) in most of the samples analyzed, and platelet-derived growth factor receptor α (PDGFR-α) activation in half of them. Expression of the cognate ligands transforming growth factor α (TGF-α), PDGF β, and PDGF α in the absence of RTK mutation and amplification suggested the presence of an autocrine/paracrine loop. In addition, RTK downstream signalling analysis

demonstrated the activation/expression of AKR mouse thymoma kinase (AKT) and mammalian target of rapamycin (mTOR) in almost all the MPMs [32]. More recently, Varghese et al. [34] reported that the activation of phosphoinositide-3-kinase (PI3K) and mTOR signalling pathways were associated with shortened survival in MPM patients.

Telomere maintenance-associated markers

In a study aimed to investigate the prevalence of the two currently known telomere maintenance mechanisms, telomerase activity (TA) and alternative lengthening of telomeres (ALT), and to assess their prognostic relevance in MPM, we found that 86.4% of the samples expressed at least one mechanism. Specifically, ALT or TA alone was found in 18.2% or 63.6% of lesions, respectively, whereas 4.6% of the cases expressed both mechanisms. In addition, at a median follow-up of 38 months, TA expression correlated at multivariate analysis with both reduced disease-free and cancer-related survival, whereas ALT failed to significantly affect clinical outcome [35].

Based on currently available information, a consensus on which biological factors are specific biomarkers for MPM has not yet been achieved owing to large inconsistencies in the data collected. Discrepancies could depend on diverse experimental variables, including selection of the case series and the experimental assays used. Studies encompassing larger and more homogeneous MPM case series are warranted to properly validate new biomarkers in view of their possible translation into medical practice.

Pathology

The correct pathological diagnosis of MPM is necessary in that a variety of other abdominal and pelvic malignancies will present with peritoneal seeding. Approximately 10% of patients with primary colon cancer will have peritoneal carcinomatosis. Up to 30% of patients with gastric cancer and pancreatic cancer have peritoneal seeding at the time of exploration for resection of the primary malignancy. A majority of patients with papillary serous ovarian cancer have peritoneal seeding. Unless the pathologist carries a high index of suspicion, diffuse peritoneal involvement by cancer can be falsely identified as carcinomatosis; in reality, the proper immunostains would show MPM (Table 42.1).

Also, the simultaneous occurrence of one of these common cancers coincidentally with a primary peritoneal mesothelioma can occur [17]. Interestingly, one patient in our series who was diagnosed with peritoneal carcinomatosis of colorectal origin presented two years later with peritoneal mesothelioma. In a review of the pathology the peritoneal implants were MPM and not colorectal peritoneal metastases [36].

Tumours arising from the mesothelial cells lining the abdominal cavity cover a wide spectrum of biological aggressiveness [37]. Adenomatoid tumour and solitary fibrous tumour are truly benign lesions that very unlikely recur after simple excision. Multicystic peritoneal mesothelioma (MCPM) and well-differentiated papillary peritoneal mesothelioma (WDPPM) are exceedingly rare lesions with uncertain malignant potential and enigmatic natural history. At the other extreme, MPM is a rapidly lethal malignancy, with an overall survival of approximately one year using standard treatments.

Classification of peritoneal mesothelioma according to clinical presentation, biological behaviour, and histopathological features

Table 42.1 Immunostains of adenocarcinoma and malignant peritoneal mesothelioma. The data summarize the percentage of positive staining to be expected

	Gastrointestinal adenocarcinoma	Mesothelioma
VIMENTIN	0–6	40
CEA	90–100	0–10
EMA	83	80–100
PAN-Cytokeratin	100	100
B72.3	81	0–5
BER-EP4	90–100	0–11
CD15 (LEU-MI)	58–100	0–10
PLAP	50	0
Calretinin	6–9	42–100
S-100	31	0–11
CA125	90	14–94
P53	43–53	45

is shown in Table 42.2. Adenomatoid tumour is a solitary asymptomatic lesion which most often involves the peritoneum of the genital region in women of reproductive age. Solitary fibrous tumour affects primarily men in their sixth decade. Recent immunohistochemical and ultrastructural studies have suggested that this lesion arises from sub-mesothelial mesenchymal tissue [38]. The subsequent sections of this chapter centres on borderline and malignant peritoneal mesotheliomas, which attract more interest on the part of the medical community and pose substantial problems in clinical practice.

Malignant peritoneal mesothelioma

MPM is characterized by multiple variably sized grey-white nodules throughout the abdominal cavity. As the disease progresses, the nodules become confluent to form plaques, masses, bowel encasement, or uniformly cover peritoneal surfaces. Abundant effusion is often present.

Similar to the more frequent pleural counterpart, MPM histological features may be classified into three types as described by Battifora and McCaughey: epithelial, sarcomatoid, and biphasic (mixed) [39]. However, the incidence of biphasic tumours is lower than in pleural disease, and pure sarcomatoid MPM is rare. Epithelial MPM is composed of polygonal, oval, or cuboidal cells exhibiting cytonuclear features and architectural formations ranging from well-differentiated to anaplastic/pleomorphic. Sarcomatoid tumours and the sarcomatoid component of biphasic MPM consist of spindle cells arranged in fascicle or storiform pattern [40, 41].

Epithelial MPM can be further categorized by the patterns observed for the malignant epithelial component. The tubulo-papillary pattern is one of the most common patterns. It consists of a mixture of small tubules and papillary structures with fibrovascular cores lined by bland flat, cuboidal, or polygonal cells. The solid pattern consists of nests, cords, or sheets of round, oval, or polygonal cells with abundant eosinophilic cytoplasm and

Table 42.2 Classification of malignant peritoneal mesothelioma by clinical behaviour, biological behaviour, and histopathologic features

Clinical presentation	Biological behaviour	Histological subtype	Histological pattern	Prevalence (%)
Localized	Benign	Adenomatoid tumour		Uncommon
		Solitary fibrous tumour		Uncommon
Diffuse	Borderline	Multicystic		Uncommon
		Papillary well-differentiated		Uncommon
	Malignant	Epithelial	Tubulo-papillary	75–80%
			Solid	
			Small cells	
			Adenomatoid	
			Acinar	
			Clear-cells	
			Signet-ring cells	
			Deciduoid	
			Rhabdoid	
	Biphasic (mixed)		Mixed epithelioid and desmoplastic	10–15%
	Sarcomatoid		Desmoplastic	4–6%
			Linpho-istiocytoid	
			Anaplastic	
			Giant-cell	

round, vesicular nuclei with prominent nucleoli. The adenomatoid (micro-glandular), acinar, clear-cell, decidioid, signet-ring cell, small-cell, and rhabdoid patterns are less common [38–41].

Sarcomatoid MPM may demonstrate anaplastic, giant-cell, and desmoplastic features, or osteosarcomatous/chondrosarcomatous areas. On occasion, atypical histiocytoid-appearing cells within an intense lymphoplasmacytic infiltrate can be seen (lymphohistiocytic pattern).

Lymph node metastases within and outside the abdominal cavity can occur even as the initial manifestation of MPM. Node involvement has been reported in 7–14% of patients undergoing extensive cytoreductive surgery. By contrast, metastatic disease outside the abdominal cavity is uncommon, except for direct invasion of pleural spaces through the hemidiaphragms [42].

Multicystic and well-differentiated papillary peritoneal mesothelioma

Both these rare disease entities generally affect women of reproductive age with no history of asbestos exposure and show indolent clinical behaviors. MCPM is often associated with previous abdominal surgery, inflammation, or endometriosis. However, early recurrences requiring multiple surgical interventions, transformation into truly malignant disease, lymph node involvement, and even death have been described. This, along with the reported clear evidence of diffuse disease distribution throughout the peritoneum and invasion into peritoneal surfaces, suggest that MCPM and WDPPM should be considered as borderline or low-malignant potential conditions, rather than benign tumours [43, 44].

At macroscopic examination, MCPM forms multiple variably sized thin-walled cysts involving primarily the pelvis, but often spreading throughout the abdominal cavity. Microscopically, cysts are separated by fibrous/adipose septa, and lined by single layers of flattened to cuboidal cells with no or little atypia. WDPPM is characterized by multiple small nodules and, at microscopic level, by well-developed papillary structures with fibrovascular core. The papillae are covered by bland cuboidal cells. Mitoses and atypia are rarely present. Because the natural history of WDPPM is distinct from MPM, the differential diagnosis with similar histology but more aggressive clinical behaviour of tubulo-papillary epithelial MPM is important [41].

According to the consensus opinion of expert pathologists from the International Mesothelioma Interest Group (Chicago, October 2006), the diagnosis of MPM must always be based on an adequate biopsy in the context of appropriate clinical, radiologic, and surgical findings [38]. A history of asbestos exposure should not be taken into consideration when diagnosing MPM. There is still limited role of cytology in the primary diagnosis, despite the increased accuracy of immunohistochemical and ultrastructural techniques.

MPM can exhibit highly variable morphological features and grows in a wide range of histological patterns. Accordingly, the disease can be confused with a variety of neoplastic and non-neoplastic conditions. The objectives of an accurate pathological workup are:

◆ Separating benign from malignant mesothelial proliferations.

◆ Differentiating MPM from other metastatic or primary peritoneal malignancies.

◆ Defining the histological subvariant and other relevant prognostic determinants.

The first step for the diagnosis of mesothelioma is haematoxylin-eosin stain. Immunohistochemical studies are adjuncts to diagnosis. Demonstration of stromal invasion into visceral or parietal peritoneum (or beyond) is the key feature in the differential diagnosis with reactive mesothelial proliferations, and can be highlighted with pancytokeratin or calretinin immunostaining. However, invasion must be carefully differentiated from entrapment, and the distinction between the rare desmoplastic MPM and reactive fibrosis may be difficult [45, 46].

Peritoneal (versus pleural) location, sex of the patient, and basic histological type affect the differential diagnosis. Any carcinoma of gastrointestinal origin and, in women, ovarian, primary peritoneal, and, more rarely, lobular breast carcinoma, should be considered for epithelial MPM. The differential diagnosis for sarcomatoid MPM includes sarcoma and other spindle cells neoplasms, such as sarcomatoid renal carcinoma and, particularly for biphasic MPM, synovial sarcoma [38]. Since no immunohistochemical marker is entirely specific and sensitive for mesothelioma, the standard is to use panels of positive and negative markers. Mesothelioma is characterized by positive staining for EMA, calretinin, Wilms Tumour-1 antigen, cytokeratin 5/6, HBME-1, podoplanin, and mesothelin. Depending on the tumour being considered in the differential diagnosis, CEA, Leu-M1, Ber-Ep4, claudine, B72.3, Bg8, and MOC-31 can be used as negative marker. Electron microscopy may help in difficult cases [38–41, 47].

To date peritoneal mesothelioma lacks a grading system. However, histomorphologic parameters can be used to help select treatment options and estimate survival. Biphasic/sarcomatoid histology and MCPM/WDPPM have, respectively, poorer and better prognosis than epithelial MPM. However, the low incidence of biphasic/sarcomatoid and borderline mesotheliomas restricts the clinical utility of this variable. For the same reason, rare secondary histological patterns that seem to have lower survival are of limited utility [42].

An exhaustive clinicopathological analysis of 62 patients undergoing comprehensive treatment at the Washington Cancer Institute revealed that nuclear and nucleolar size (rated by a four-tiered score) correlated with survival [48]. Clinical data from the Milan Peritoneal Malignancy Program demonstrated that both pathologically involved lymph nodes and inadequate nodal sampling correlate with poor prognosis. Accordingly, careful examination of lymph nodes that drain the visceral and parietal peritoneum is recommended, including bilateral iliac, right gastroepiploic, and ileocolic nodes [42]. Proliferative activity has been reported to be useful for prognostic stratification. It may be quantified either by means of mitotic count or immunohistochemical staining with Ki-67 antigen, an excellent marker of cellular proliferation. Proliferative activity is generally low in MPM, but higher rates correlates with poor outcome [49–51].

Surgical management of peritoneal mesothelioma

Diagnosis and staging

The initial symptom that led to a diagnosis of MPM was prospectively recorded in 51 patients. In the past, it was assumed that the initial symptom in virtually all patients was an expanding abdomen from malignant ascites. However, as shown in Table 42.3,

Table 42.3 Symptoms and signs of peritoneal mesothelioma in 51 patients treated at Washington Cancer Institute

Symptom	Total	Men	Women
Increased abdominal girth	16 (31%)	12 (35%)	4 (24%)
Pain	17 (33%)	11 (32%)	6 (35%)
Increased abdominal girth and pain	5 (10%)	3 (9%)	2 (12%)
New onset hernia	6 (12%)	5 (15%)	1 (6%)
Incidental finding	4 (8%)	0	4 (24%)
Other	3 (6%)	3 (9%)	0
Total	51	34	17

Source: data from Acherman YIZ et al., Clinical presentation of peritoneal mesothelioma, *Tumori*, Volume 89, Issue 3, pp. 269–273, Copyright © 2003.

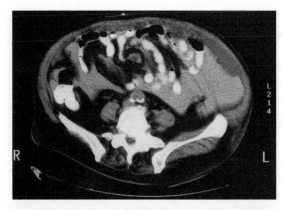

Fig. 42.2 CT of wet type of malignant peritoneal mesothelioma. Fluid conforms to the shape of the small bowel and its mesentery. A small volume of solid tumour is layered out on the parietal peritoneum.

these patients can present with a variety of symptoms. We categorized the patients into three groups based on presenting symptoms: approximately one-third present with abdominal distention, one-third with abdominal pain, usually localized, and the remaining third present with combined symptoms of distention, pain, and other findings. We have designated these three types as a 'wet type' of peritoneal mesothelioma presenting with symptoms of malignant ascites causing increased abdominal girth, a 'dry-painful type' presenting with a focal mass seen on computed tomography (CT) scan causing pain, and a 'combined type' characterized by both pain and ascites. We correlated histologic findings with patient symptoms at presentation but no significant relationships were apparent [52].

Patients may present with an acute abdomen with peritoneal mesothelioma. Four patients had the sudden onset of severe pain requiring evaluation at an emergency treatment facility; three had acute appendicitis, and one of these three had a perforated appendix. A single patient presented with an incarcerated umbilical hernia. In addition to pain, increased abdominal girth and new-onset hernia, signs and symptoms included weight loss, infertility, shortness of breath, fever, and night sweats.

In patients with advanced disease, the increase in peritoneal tumour burden may result in an increase in abdominal compartment pressure leading to the development of a new onset hernia. The masses that develop on the peritoneum may lead to malignant adhesions and fluid production that develop amongst intestinal loops to result in a partial bowel obstruction and ascites [53]. The diagnostic pathway is often tedious and is arrived upon following exclusion of other more common gastrointestinal malignancies.

Computed tomography diagnosis

Park et al. used the terminology of 'dry' and 'wet' as descriptors of the CT features of peritoneal mesothelioma with the dry appearance consisting of peritoneal-based lesions and the wet appearance consisting of ascites, irregular or nodular thickening of the peritoneum, and an omental mass that may scallop or directly invade adjacent abdominal viscera [54]. The two clinical types of peritoneal mesothelioma, wet or dry-painful type, correspond well to these different appearances by CT examination. In the wet type, there is little or no evidence of solid tumour. Occasionally, small nodules lining the parietal peritoneal surfaces are evident,

especially beneath the right hemidiaphragm (Figure 42.2). The CT/radiologic presentation of the dry-painful type of peritoneal mesothelioma may disclose several mass lesions, but often there is a dominant mass isolated to one part of the abdomen. Likewise, the tumour mass is commonly associated with the greater omentum. Usually, the symptomatic mass lesion seen on CT is mistaken for intra-abdominal abscess or a large primary adenocarcinoma. Only at laparotomy is the definitive diagnosis evident in these patients presenting which solid tumour in the absence of ascites (Figure 42.3).

CT imaging of the abdomen and pelvis detect peritoneal tumours as well-defined masses with features that demonstrate omental thickening and nodularity of the mesentery. This predominant central abdominal and pelvic disease burden observed may be a characteristics pattern of presentation [55].

The CT appearance of multicystic peritoneal mesothelioma (MCPM) can be contrasted to CT of MPM. Despite an immense distortion of the abdominal and pelvic space by fluid-filled cysts and ascites, there is no disruption of intestinal function or segmental bowel obstruction. Compartmentalization of small bowel is seen on CT (Figure 42.4).

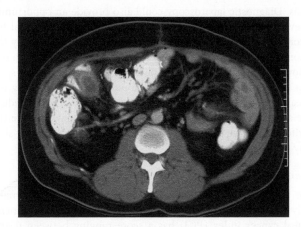

Fig. 42.3 CT of dry painful type of malignant peritoneal mesothelioma. Discrete masses are present at multiple sites around the abdomen. These masses are painful to deep palpation.

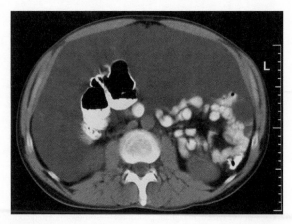

Fig. 42.4 CT of multicystic peritoneal mesothelioma. Thin walled cysts filled with clear fluid fill the abdominal and pelvic spaces. The small bowel is pushed to the side (compartmentalized). This separation of viscera from tumour is associated with a good prognosis with cytoreductive surgery plus intraperitoneal chemotherapy.

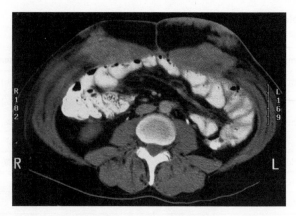

Fig. 42.5 CT of abdomen in a patient who had lateral trochar sites in a laparoscopy to diagnose malignant peritoneal mesothelioma.

Tumour markers for diagnosis

Standard haematological and serological panels including tumour markers (CEA, CA 19-9, CA-125 and mesothelin) are required. CA-125 and mesothelin are observed to be elevated in MPM but are not considered specific for diagnosis as they may be elevated in other malignancies including ovarian cancer and in infective processes such as tuberculosis [56, 57]. These tumour markers are, however, more suited for disease monitoring following treatment rather than for diagnosis. A markedly elevated CA-125 indicates poor prognosis.

Endoscopic procedures

Clinically, the vague nature of the symptoms and signs and the young age of presentation often lead to a delay in diagnosis. Diagnostic procedures include oesophago-gastroduodenoscopy and colonoscopy to exclude a gastrointestinal malignancy following which tumour biopsies may be performed through a diagnostic laparoscopy. Laparoscopy was the most common diagnostic test required for definitively diagnosing mesothelioma (64%). Cytology of fluid removed by paracentesis rarely resulted in a definitive diagnosis. Diagnostic laparoscopy could also provide an opportunity to evaluate the peritoneal disease burden to assess potential for cytoreductive surgery. An important caveat must accompany the recommendation for laparoscopy in the diagnosis of MPM. In our follow-up, port site recurrence is observed at nearly all trochar sites. Our recommendation is to limit the puncture sites to along the linea alba. As seen in the CT scan shown in Figure 42.5, cytoreductive surgery plus intraperitoneal chemotherapy may stabilize the peritoneal surface disease while disease within lateral trochar sites may progress rapidly.

Preoperative workup

The peritoneal disease burden of MPM is assessed systematically using the Sugarbaker's peritoneal cancer index. The peritoneal cancer index (PCI) has a score ranging between 0 and 39. Lesion size is determined as 0 to 3 within 13 abdominopelvic regions (Figure 42.6) [58]. The Peritoneal Surface Oncology Group International (PSOGI) has collaborated to combine their experiences of managing patients with peritoneal mesothelioma. They enrolled patients collectively into a multi-institutional registry database to formulate a clinicopathologic staging system through prognostic parameters identified from patients treated uniformly with CRS and HIPEC at eight international institutions. The staging system adopts the common nomenclature of the tumour-node-metastasis (TNM) system comprising of elements the tumour burden (T) assessed by the PCI subgrouped into four categories: T1 being PCI 1–10, T2 being PCI 11–20, T3 being PCI 21–30, and T4 being PCI 30–39. Abdominal nodal disease commonly affected by peritoneal mesothelioma includes the iliac chain, para-aortic, coeliac axis, mesenteric, and the porto-caval lymph nodes; any involvement of nodes would be classified as N1. The M element refers to the presence or absence of extra-abdominal metastases. Formal stage-wise classification was done in a reverse fashion following analysis of the prognostic impact of the PCI, lymph node, and metastasis status prior to arriving at four clinical stages (Table 42.4). Patients with T1N0M0 were designated as stage I, T2-3N0M0 as stage II and stage III comprised of patients with T4, N1, or M1 disease. From the complete clinicopathologic data of the 294 patients that formed the cohort used to derive this staging system, stratification of stage-based survival was achieved with five-year survival associated with stage I, II, and III disease being 87%, 53%, and 29%, respectively. This proposed TNM staging system is being evaluated in prospective studies and hopefully will be formally endorsed by the American Joint Committee on Cancer in future [59].

Medical management of malignant peritoneal mesothelioma

Systemic therapies

Malignant peritoneal mesothelioma patients with surgically unresectable disease or whose medical co-morbidities preclude surgery are considered for palliative systemic therapy. Due to its relatively low incidence and inherent difficulties of radiologic assessment, few studies of systemic therapy have been conducted. Treatment recommendations are often extrapolated from pleural mesothelioma. A variety of chemotherapeutic drugs have been reported to be effective and used in MPM with the most commonly used agents being cisplatin, gemcitabine, doxorubicin, and pemetrexed.

Peritoneal Cancer Index

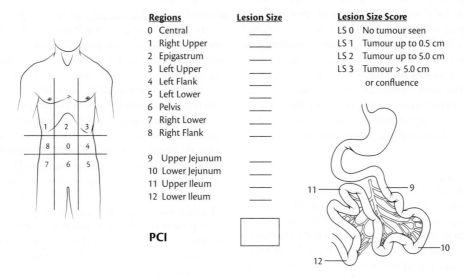

Regions	Lesion Size	Lesion Size Score
0 Central	_____	LS 0 No tumour seen
1 Right Upper	_____	LS 1 Tumour up to 0.5 cm
2 Epigastrum	_____	LS 2 Tumour up to 5.0 cm
3 Left Upper	_____	LS 3 Tumour > 5.0 cm
4 Left Flank	_____	or confluence
5 Left Lower	_____	
6 Pelvis	_____	
7 Right Lower	_____	
8 Right Flank	_____	
9 Upper Jejunum	_____	
10 Lower Jejunum	_____	
11 Upper Ileum	_____	
12 Lower Ileum	_____	

PCI

Fig. 42.6 Sugarbaker's scoring of the peritoneal disease burden using the Peritoneal Cancer Index (PCI).
From Harmon R, Sugarbaker P, Prognostic indicators in peritoneal carcinomatosis from gastrointestinal cancer, *International Seminars in Surgical Oncology*, Volume 2, Issue 3, Copyright © 2005 Harmon and Sugarbaker; licensee BioMed Central Ltd. Reproduced under the Creative Commons Attribution License 2.0, <http://creativecommons.org/licenses/by/2.0/>.

Historical data from the Dana-Farber Cancer Institute and Brigham and Women's Hospital's experience of 180 mesothelioma patients of which 37 patients had MPM reported a median survival of 15 months following a variety of palliative chemotherapy treatments [60]. A randomized trial was performed by the Cancer and Leukemia Group B (CALGB) comparing cisplatin and mitomycin versus cisplatin and doxorubicin in 79 patients with pleural mesothelioma or MPM. This trial reported an overall response rate of 26% and 14%, median time to treatment failure of 3.6 months and 4.8 months, and median overall survival of 7.7 months and 8.8 months in the cisplatin-mitomycin and cisplatin-doxorubicin groups respectively [61]. This study had only 4 of 79 patients with MPM.

Pemetrexed-based therapies

Pemetrexed, a multi-targeted antifolate that inhibits thymidylate synthase (TS), dihydrofolate reductase (DHFR), and glycinamide ribonucleotide formyltransferase (GARFT) was approved

Table 42.4 Proposed TNM staging for malignant peritoneal mesothelioma with corresponding survival rates

Stage	Tumour	Node	Metastasis	Five-year survival rates (%)
I	T1	N0	M0	87
II	T2-3	N0	M0	53
III	T4	N0-1	M0-1	29
	T1-4	N1	M0-1	
	T1-4	N0-1	M1	

T1 (PCI 1–10), T2 (PCI 11–20), T3 (PCI 21–30), T4 (PCI 30–39).

N0—nil lymph node, N1—positive lymph node involvement.

M0—nil metastasis, M1—metastatic disease.

Reproduced from Yan TD et al., A novel tumour-node-metastasis (TNM) staging system of diffuse malignant peritoneal mesothelioma using outcome analysis of a multi-institutional database, *Cancer*, Volume 117, Issue 9, pp. 1855–1863, Copyright © 2011 John Wiley and Sons Ltd.

for use in pleural mesothelioma based on results of a phase III trial which demonstrated improved response rates and overall survival with cisplatin and pemetrexed over cisplatin alone in chemotherapy-naive patients who were not eligible for curative surgery [62]. Activity of pemetrexed in peritoneal mesothelioma was observed in two Expanded Access Programs (EAP) which allowed access to pemetrexed for eligible patients prior to its regulatory approval in pleural mesothelioma [63, 64]. Notwithstanding the many biases of such analyses, for example lack of randomization, absence of uniform response criteria and high censoring rate, data from EAPs suggest a role for pemetrexed-based combination chemotherapy in MPM.

In the international EAP, 109 patients with chemo-naive or previously treated surgically unresectable MPM received pemetrexed (500 mg/m^2) alone or with cisplatin (75 mg/m^2) or carboplatin [area under curve (AUC) 5] every 21 days until disease progression [63]. The response rate and one-year survival rate in the overall population were 18.7% and 47.4%, respectively. Combination chemotherapy was well tolerated. Although response rates were higher with combination treatment (20.0–24.1%) compared with pemetrexed alone (12.5%), patients in the latter group were older and had more prior treatments.

In the United States EAP, 73 patients with chemo-naive or previously treated surgically unresectable MPM received pemetrexed (500 mg/m^2) alone or with cisplatin (75 mg/m^2) every 21 days for six cycles or until disease progression [64]. Response rates were 26%, 19.2%, and 29.8% in the overall population, pemetrexed alone and pemetrexed/cisplatin groups, respectively. Response rates were similar in chemo-naïve and previously treated patients (25% and 23.3%, respectively). Median survival was 13.1 months for patients who received pemetrexed with cisplatin and 8.7 months for pemetrexed alone.

In chemo-naive patients, combination of pemetrexed (500 mg/m^2 on day 8) with gemcitabine (1250 mg/m^2 on days one and eight) administered every 21 days for six cycles or until progressive disease was evaluated in a phase II study [65]. Of the 20 patients with MPM who enrolled, the combination yielded response rates of 15%, median time to disease progression of 10.4 months, median overall survival of 26.8 months and one-year survival rate of 67.5%, but resulted in significant toxicities including one treatment-related death. Grade 3 to 4 neutropenia and febrile neutropenia were observed in 60% and 10% of patients respectively. Myelosuppression is the most significant toxicity associated with the administration of pemetrexed, gemcitabine, or platinum. For pemetrexed, prophylactic supplementation with vitamin B12 and folic acid can abrogate haematologic toxicity without adversely affecting survival [62].

Other systemic therapies

In a retrospective single-institution report of 17 patients, combination of cisplatin and irinotecan yielded a response rate of 24% [66]. Other chemotherapy agents that are used alone or in combination for MPM based on data suggesting efficacy in pleural mesothelioma include vinorelbine [67], doxorubicin, mitomycin, and trimetrexate [68]. There are isolated reports of the role of whole-abdominal radiation; however, this treatment has not been adequately studied naturally owing to the potentially high morbidity. Nonetheless a study on surgery and intraperitoneal chemotherapy with whole abdominal radiation was reported to achieve improved disease-free survival [69].

Limited data are available to guide the sequencing of chemotherapy in relation to surgery, i.e., adjuvant versus neoadjuvant. Since CRS and HIPEC achieve complete cytoreduction in less than 50% of the patients [70] and recurrence is common even among patients who undergo a complete cytoreduction [71], adjuvant systemic chemotherapy is being explored in combination with intraperitoneal chemotherapy [72].

In summary, based on extrapolation from the pleural mesothelioma data and from analyses of EAP data, systemic therapy with pemetrexed and cisplatin should be considered in patients with surgically unresectable MPM [62–64]. Carboplatin may be a reasonable alternative to cisplatin in the elderly and patients with poor performance status considering its better safety profile [63]. In patients who cannot tolerate platinum, combination of pemetrexed and gemcitabine may be considered, although it is associated with significant toxicities [65].

Cytoreductive surgery and intraperitoneal chemotherapy

As MPM is confined within the peritoneal surfaces of the abdominal cavity before metastasizing to lymph nodes and extra-abdominal regions later in the disease history, a proof of concept to treat this disease with intraperitoneal chemotherapy to allow direct targeting of disease by Markman and Kelsen was conducted. They treated 19 patients with intraperitoneal cisplatin and mitomycin [73]. In this study, the treatment was well tolerated with control of ascites achieved in 47% of patients. Amongst the 19 patients, the median survival was nine months; however, four patients with minimal volume peritoneal disease were reported to survive more than three years. This suggested that if peritoneal tumour cytoreduction could be achieved and intraperitoneal chemotherapy may serve as an adjunct to achieve peritoneal disease control and prolong the disease-free survival.

Cytoreductive surgery for peritoneal tumours was introduced by Sugarbaker who described six peritonectomy procedures that allowed removal of all peritoneal lining of the abdominopelvic cavity [74]. Some groups advocate complete peritonectomy be performed even for peritoneal surfaces that are uninvolved by tumour [75]. In a case-control study by Baratti et al. comparing complete peritonectomy versus selective peritonectomy, five-year survival was 63.9% and 40%, respectively, without any difference in morbidity and reoperation rates [76]. The importance of nodal sampling and its impact on outcome has been shown to be important. In a multivariate analysis controlled for other prognostic variables, negative lymph nodes were an independent predictor of improved survival [77]. In their study, negative nodes as compared to positive or non-assessed nodes were associated with increased survival and hence the need for careful nodal sampling when performing cytoreduction. Although node positivity ultimately bears a poorer outcome and survival is unlikely to be modified through extended lymphadenectomy, an approach to standardized lymph node sampling would assist in disease staging [59].

HIPEC has been commonly used as an intraoperative adjunct to cytoreduction. It may be administered using either an open or closed abdomen technique. For MPM, the drugs commonly used include cisplatin alone or cisplatin with doxorubicin with the abdominal cavity being perfused with the chemotherapy solution at a temperature of 40 to 43°C. From the PSOGI registry of 405 patients treated uniformly with CRS and HIPEC, an overall median survival of 53 months, three- and five-year survival rates of 60% and 47%, respectively, were achieved. Epithelioid tumour subtype, absence of lymph node metastasis, optimal cytoreduction, and HIPEC were independently associated with improved outcome [70]. MCPM was also studied as a subgroup analysis from the PSOGI registry. There were 26 patients (6.4%) with MCPM with a large preponderance of females (20 women and 6 men). Following cytoreduction and a median follow up of 54 (range 5 to 129) months, all patients treated are alive and free of disease. Clearly, this represents a distinct subtype with a favourable disease biology where long-term survival may be achieved through complete eradication of the cystic peritoneal lesions [78]. Another interesting finding that emerged from this registry study that was the impact of gender difference [79]. From clinical observation, females tended to have lower PCI and hence lower stage of disease. Post- cytoreduction survival rate was 68% compared to 39% at five years in females compared to males. When the survival was stratified according to the staging criteria and gender, females continued to show superior survival over males for each TNM stage. The five-year survival for females was 97% (Stage I), 70% (Stage II), and 40% (Stage III); and for males was 70%, 40%, and 30%, respectively.

The apparent survival benefits of CRS and HIPEC are obvious over palliative chemotherapy. However, this treatment is highly specialized and has evolved from years of experience and learning to perform the extensive peritonectomy procedures required for CRS and the delivery of HIPEC [80]. Today this treatment is considered to have an acceptable morbidity for the survival benefits it derives. The risk of mortality ranges from 1 to 5% and major morbidity ranges from 12% to 52% which is comparable with other major gastrointestinal oncologic surgery [81].

Adjuvant bidirectional chemotherapy with intraperitoneal pemetrexed combined with intravenous cisplatin

CRS with HIPEC has been used in a number of centres worldwide showing median survivals of 36–92 months and has become the preferred therapy for eligible patients [70]. Yet, a significant proportion of patients with mesothelioma treated with this modality are not able to achieve complete CRS and therefore need further treatment with chemotherapy. Even in patients who have a complete CRS and HIPEC, recurrent disease is common and it usually occurs in the abdomen [71]. Pemetrexed is a multitargeted antifolate agent that was shown in Phase III studies to significantly improve response rates in patients with advanced pleural mesothelioma and MPM. At the Washington Cancer Institute the adjuvant treatment with intraperitoneal pemetrexed combined with intravenous cisplatin in patients with MPM who underwent CRS and HIPEC has become standard of practice.

Peritoneal port placement and maintenance

Peritoneal ports are placed at the time of CRS and HIPEC in all patients. Immediately prior to abdominal closure, the port is placed using the following technique: a 5 cm transverse incision is made lateral to the umbilicus on the left side overlying the lateral border of the rectus sheath. The tissues are dissected to the abdominal fascia and a small opening made in the fascia to accommodate the catheter that is placed in the abdomen with the tip directed at the pelvis. Blunt dissection is used to create a subcutaneous channel and pocket 10 cm cephalad to the skin incision where the port is positioned. A right angle non-coring needle (Gripper Plus, Smith Medical ASD Inc, St Paul, MN) is then used to access the port, secured in position with sutures and left in place for 10 days during post-operative recovery to prevent port twisting [82].

Adjuvant bidirectional chemotherapy

The treatment consists of pemetrexed 500 mg/m^2 given intraperitoneally and cisplatin 50 mg/m^2 given intravenously simultaneously on day one of every 21-day cycle for six cycles. Pemetrexed is mixed in one litre of peritoneal dialysis solution and administered through an implantable peritoneal port (Port-a-Cath, Smith Medical ASD Inc, St Paul, MN) placed at the time of cytoreductive surgery.

All patients receive folic acid 1000 μg orally daily and vitamin B12 1000 μg intramuscularly every nine weeks beginning two weeks before starting therapy and continued through the end of the last cycle of therapy. The patients also receive dexamethasone orally on the day before, the day of and the day after pemetrexed.

Using this regimen, nine of ten patients were able to complete all six cycles of therapy without treatment delays or dosing modifications. One patient developed a catheter infection after cycle three and required catheter removal. He was switched to intravenous pemetrexed and cisplatin for one cycle, then had a new peritoneal catheter placed and subsequently completed cycles five and six according to protocol. The most common toxicities were fatigue, nausea, and abdominal pain but were generally mild. The only grade three toxicity was the above mentioned catheter infection. There were no deaths related to treatment and no hospitalizations due to treatment side effects [72].

Pharmacokinetics of intraperitoneal pemetrexed

In four patients the pharmacokinetics of intraperitoneal pemetrexed was studied on the first cycle of adjuvant treatment (Figure 42.7). The area under the curve (AUC) of peritoneal fluid concentration times time was 84 150 μgmL^{-1}. The AUC of plasma pemetrexed concentrations times time was 1250 μgmL^{-1}. The increased exposure of peritoneal surfaces to chemotherapy as compared to plasma (AUC ratio) was 70. The peak plasma concentration was 6.5±3 μg/ml at 180 minutes. In summary, this study showed that an adjuvant

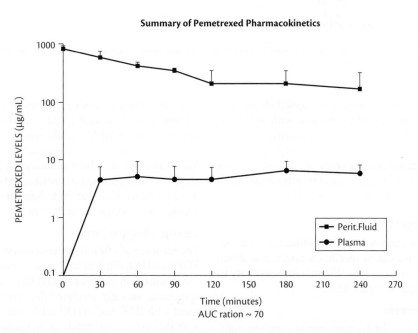

Summary of Pemetrexed Pharmacokinetics

Fig. 42.7 Concentration times time graph of pemetrexed in peritoneal fluid and plasma from four different pharmacologic studies. The AUC ratio of peritoneal fluid to plasma was 70. Peak plasma concentration was 0.05 (+0.02) μg/mL at 30 minutes.

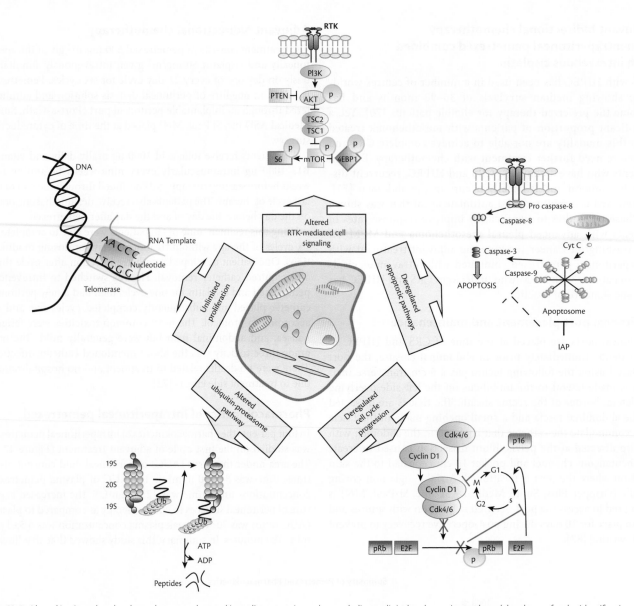

Fig. 42.8 Altered/activated molecular pathways, as detected in malignant peritoneal mesothelioma clinical and experimental models, relevant for the identification of novel prognostic biomarkers and therapeutic targets.

protocol of combined intravenous and intraperitoneal chemotherapy can be successfully implemented for patients with MPM following CRS and HIPEC with low morbidity. Our practice of placing the intraperitoneal port at the end cytoreductive surgery was successful and only one significant catheter problem was observed. We recommend this regimen to be tested as a multi-institutional adjuvant protocol for patients with this rare cancer [83].

Novel therapeutic targets

A few published studies have focused on the identification of deregulated pathways in MPM that can be specifically targeted to obtain a direct therapeutic effect or to increase the tumour sensitivity to conventional anticancer agents (Figure 42.8).

Inhibitors of apoptosis proteins

We initially demonstrated that the dysregulation of apoptotic pathways may play a role in the relative chemoresistance of MPM and

that surviving and other members of the inhibitors of apoptosis protein family (i.e., IAP-1, IAP-2, and X-IAP), which are overexpressed in most MPMs, could represent new therapeutic targets. Indeed, we found that RNAi-mediated survivin knockdown in MPM cells enhanced both spontaneous and drug-induced apoptosis [84], thus supporting the notion that survivin antagonists (such as YM-155, which is currently being tested in clinical trials) may provide new approaches to the treatment of MPMs.

Cell signalling pathways

The existence of a ligand-dependent activation and co-activation of EGFR and PDGFRB, as well as of a connection between them and the downstream pathway of mTOR we observed in clinical MPM specimens, strongly suggested the opportunity of combined treatment with RTK and mTOR inhibitors in the disease. Consistent with this hypothesis, cytotoxicity studies carried out on a human MPM cell line showed a supra-additive antiproliferative effect after sequential treatment with sorafenib and RAD001 [32]. In this context, Varghese et al. [34] recently demonstrated the potential of the combined targeting of PI3K and mTOR signalling pathways for the treatment of MPM. Specifically, using the dual-class PI3K and mTOR inhibitor BEZ235, they observed a significant inhibition of cell proliferation and downstream cell signalling in two human MPM cell lines.

The ubiquitin-proteasome pathway

Searching for differentially expressed functional gene categories in MPM histologic subtypes through a microarray analysis, Borczuk et al. [85] identified the ubiquitin-proteasome pathway as up-regulated in biphasic tumours, suggesting its potential relevance as a therapeutic target in this category of poor prognosis tumours. Indeed, cytotoxicity experiments carried out in 211H cells derived from a human (pleural) biphasic mesothelioma demonstrated a synergistic antitumour effect of sequential treatment regimens containing the proteasome inhibitor bortezomib and oxaliplatin, as a consequence of an increased apoptotic response.

Although experimental evidence of deregulated expression/function suggests a possible role for selective gene pathways in the development of the disease, no definite conclusions can be drawn on their relevance as therapeutic targets. In this context, a major issue to be addressed is related to the development of in vivo MPM experimental models able to properly recapitulate the features of clinical tumours in order to clarify the antitumour potential of novel therapeutic approaches rationally designed on a biological basis in view of possible translation of experimental research advances into the clinical setting.

Further reading

Acherman YIZ, Welch LS, Bromley CM, Sugarbaker PH. Clinical presentation of peritoneal mesothelioma. Tumori 2003; 89: 269–273.

Deraco M, Nonaka D, Baratti D, Casali P, Rosai J et al. Prognostic analysis of clinicopathologic factors in 49 patients with diffuse malignant peritoneal mesothelioma treated with cytoreductive surgery and intraperitoneal hyperthermic perfusion. Annals of Surgical Oncology 2006; 13(2): 229–237.

Husain AN, Colby T, Ordonez N, Krausz T, Attanoos R et al. Guidelines for pathologic diagnosis of malignant mesothelioma: 2012 update of the consensus statement from the International Mesothelioma Interest Group. Archives of Pathology and Laboratory Medicine August 28, 2012. [Epub ahead of print].

Manzini Vde P, Recchia L, Cafferata M, Porta C, Siena S et al. Malignant peritoneal mesothelioma: a multicenter study on 81 cases. Annals of Oncology 2010; 21(2): 348–353.

Park JY, Kim KW, Kwon HJ, Park MS, Kwon GY et al. Peritoneal mesotheliomas: clinicopathologic features, CT findings, and differential diagnosis. American Journal of Roentgenology 2008; 191(3): 814–825.

Van der Speeten K, Govaerts K, Stuart OA, Sugarbaker PH: pharmacokinetics of the perioperative use of cancer chemotherapy in peritoneal surface malignancy patients. Gastroenterology Research and Practice 2012: Article ID 827534.

Yan TD, Brun EA, Cerruto CA, Haveric N, Chang D et al. Prognostic indicators for patients undergoing cytoreductive surgery and perioperative intraperitoneal chemotherapy for diffuse malignant peritoneal mesothelioma. Annals of Surgical Oncology 2007; 14(1): 41–49.

Yan TD, Deraco M, Baratti D, Kusamura S, Elias D et al. Cytoreductive surgery and hyperthermic intraperitoneal chemotherapy for malignant peritoneal mesothelioma: multi-institutional experience. Journal of Clinical Oncology 2010; 27: 6237–6242.

Yan TD, Deraco M, Elias D, Glehen O, Levine EA et al. A novel tumor-node-metastasis (TNM) staging system of diffuse malignant peritoneal mesothelioma using outcome analysis of a multi-institutional database. Cancer 2011; 117(9): 1855–1863.

Zaffaroni N, Costa A, Pennati M, De Marco C, Affini E et al. Survivin is highly expressed and promotes cell survival in malignant peritoneal mesothelioma. Cell Oncology 2007; 29(6): 453–466.

References

1. Battifora H, McCaughey W. Tumors of the Serosal Membranes. Washington, DC: Armed Forces Institute of Pathology, 1994.
2. Robinson BWS, Lake RA. Advances in malignant mesothelioma. New England Journal of Medicine 2005; 353: 1591–1603.
3. Moolgavkar SH, Meza R, Turim J. Pleural and peritoneal mesotheliomas in SEER: age effects and temporal trends, 1973–2005. Cancer Causes Control 2009; 20(6): 935–944.
4. Averbach AM, Sugarbaker PH. Peritoneal mesothelioma: treatment approach based on natural history. Cancer Treatment and Research 1996; 81: 193–211.
5. Welch LS, Acherman YIZ, Haile Haile E, Sokas RK, Sugarbaker PH. Asbestos and peritoneal mesothelioma among college-educated men. International Journal of Occupational and Environmental Health 2005; 11: 254–258.
6. Bocchetta M, Di Resta I, Powers A, Fresco R, Tosolini A et al. Human mesothelial cells are unusually susceptible to simian virus 40-mediated transformation and asbestos carcinogenicity. Proceedings of the National Academy of Sciences USA 2000; 17: 260–271.
7. Sugarbaker PH, Yan TD, Stuart OA, Yoo D. Comprehensive management of diffuse malignant peritoneal mesothelioma. European Journal of Surgical Oncology 2006; 32(6): 686–691.
8. Acherman YI, Welch LS, Bromley CM, Sugarbaker PH. Clinical presentation of peritoneal mesothelioma. Tumori 2003; 89(3): 269–273.
9. Antman KH, Pomfret EA, Aisner J, MacINtyre J, Osteen RT et al. Peritoneal mesothelioma: natural history and response to chemotherapy. Journal of Clinical Oncology 1983; 1(6): 386–391.
10. Eltabbakh GH, Piver MS, Hempling RE, Recio FO, Intengen ME. Clinical picture, response to therapy, and survival of women with diffuse malignant peritoneal mesothelioma. Journal of Surgical Oncology 1999; 70(6): 6–12.
11. Feldman AL, Libutti SK, Pingpank JF, Bartlett DL, Beresnev TH et al. Analysis of factors associated with outcome in patients with malignant peritoneal mesothelioma undergoing surgical debulking and intraperitoneal chemotherapy. Journal of Clinical Oncology 2003; 21(24): 4560–4567.
12. Sugarbaker PH, Yan TD, Stuart OA, Yoo. Comprehensive management of diffuse malignant peritoneal mesothelioma. European Journal of Surgical Oncology 2006; 32(6): 686–691.
13. Loggie BW, Fleming RA, McQuellon RP, Russell GB, Geisinger KR et al. Prospective trial for the treatment of malignant peritoneal mesothelioma. The American Journal of Surgery 2001; 67(10): 999–1003.
14. Brigand C, Monneuse O, Mohamed F, Sayag-Beaujard AC, Isaac S et al. Peritoneal mesothelioma treated by cytoreductive surgery and intraperitoneal hyperthermic chemotherapy: results of a prospective study. Annals of Surgical Oncology 2006; 13(3): 405–412.
15. Yan TD, Brun EA, Cerruto CA, Haveric N, Chang D et al. Prognostic indicators for patients undergoing cytoreductive surgery and perioperative intraperitoneal chemotherapy for diffuse malignant peritoneal mesothelioma. Annals of Surgical Oncology 2007; 14(1): 41–49.
16. Deraco M, Nonaka D, Baratti D, Casali P, Rosai J et al. Prognostic analysis of clinicopathologic factors in 49 patients with diffuse malignant peritoneal mesothelioma treated with cytoreductive surgery and intraperitoneal hyperthermic perfusion. Annals of Surgical Oncology 2006; 13(2): 229–237.
17. Sugarbaker PH, Welch L, Mohamed F, Glehen O. A review of peritoneal mesothelioma at the Washington Cancer Institute. Surgical Oncology Clinics of North America 2003; 12(3): 605–621.

18. Delgermaa V, Takahashi K, Park E-K, Le GV, Hara T et al. Global mesothelioma deaths reported to the World Health Organization between 1994 and 2008. Bulletin of the World Health Organization 2011; 89(10): 716–724C.

19. Hodgson JT, McElvenny MD, Darnton AJ, Price MJ, Peto J. The expected burden of mesothelioma mortality in Great Britain from 2002 to 2050. British Journal of Cancer 2005; 92(3): 587–593.

20. Robinson BW, Musk AW, Lake RA. Malignant mesothelioma. The Lancet 2005; 366(9483): 397–408.

21. Jeong YJ, Kim S, Kwak SW, Lee NK, Lee JW et al. Neoplastic and non-neoplastic conditions of serosal membrane origin: CT findings. Radiographics 2008; 28(3): 801–818.

22. Matsuzaki H, Maeda M, Lee S, Nishimura Y, Kumagai-Takei N et al. Asbestos-induced cellular and molecular alteration of immunocompetent cells and their relationship with chronic inflammation and carcinogenesis. Journal of Biomedicine and Biotechnology 2012:492608. doi:10.1155/2012/492608

23. Maeda M, Nishimura Y, Kumagai N, Hayashi H, Hatayama T et al. Dysregulation of the immune system caused by silica and asbestos. Journal of Immunotoxicology 2010; 7(4): 268–278.

24. Borczuk AC, Taub RN, Hesdorffer M, Hibshoosh H, Chabot JA et al. P16 loss and mitotic activity predict poor survival in patients with peritoneal malignant mesothelioma. Clinical Cancer Research 2005; 11: 3303–3308.

25. Nonaka D, Kusamura S, Baratti D, Casali P, Cabras AD et al. Diffuse malignant mesothelioma of the peritoneum: a clinicopathological study of 35 patients treated locoregionally at a single institution. Cancer 2005; 104: 2181–2188.

26. Chiosea S, Krasinskas A, Cagle PT, Mitchell KA, Zander DS et al. Diagnostic importance of 9p21 homozygous deletion in malignant mesotheliomas. Modern Pathology 2008; 21: 742–747.

27. Krasinskas AM, Bartlett DL, Cieply K, Dacic S. CDKN2A and MTAP deletions in peritoneal mesotheliomas are correlated with loss of p16 protein expression and poor survival. Modern Pathology 2010; 23: 531–538.

28. Yan TD, Brun EA, Cerruto CA, Haveric N, Chang D et al. Prognostic indicators for patients undergoing cytoreductive surgery and perioperative intraperitoneal chemotherapy for diffuse malignant peritoneal mesothelioma. Annals of Surgical Oncology 2007; 14: 41–49.

29. Scattone A, Serio G, Marzullo A, Nazzaro P, Corsi F et al. High Wilms' tumour gene (WT1) expression and low mitotic count are independent predictors of survival in diffuse peritoneal mesothelioma. Histopathology 2012; 60: 472–481.

30. Trupiano JK, Geisinger KR, Willingham MC, Manders P, Zbieranski N et al. Diffuse malignant mesothelioma of the peritoneum and pleura, analysis of markers. Modern Pathology 2004; 17: 476–481.

31. Foster JM, Gatalica Z, Lilleberg S, Haynatzki G, Loggie BW. Novel and existing mutations in the tyrosine kinase domain of the epidermal growth factor receptor are predictors of optimal resectability in malignant peritoneal mesothelioma. Annals of Surgical Oncology 2009; 16: 152–158.

32. Perrone F, Jocollè G, Pennati M, Deraco M, Baratti D et al. Receptor tyrosine kinase and downstream signalling analysis in diffuse malignant peritoneal mesothelioma. European Journal of Cancer 2010; 46: 2837–2848.

33. Kalra N, Ashai A, Xi L, Zhang J, Avital I et al. Patients with peritoneal mesothelioma lack epidermal growth factor receptor tyrosine kinase mutations that would make them sensitive to tyrosine kinase inhibitors. Oncology Reports 2012; 27: 1794–1800.

34. Varghese S, Chen Z, Bartlett DL, Pingpank JF, Libutti SK et al. Activation of the phosphoinositide-3-kinase and mammalian target of rapamycin signaling pathways are associated with shortened survival in patients with malignant peritoneal mesothelioma. Cancer 2011; 117: 361–371.

35. Villa R, Daidone MG, Motta R, Venturini L, De Marco C et al. Multiple mechanisms of telomere maintenance exist and differentially affect clinical outcome in diffuse malignant peritoneal mesothelioma. Clinical Cancer Research 2008; 14: 4134–4140.

36. Alcorn KW, Yan H, Shmookler BM, Sugarbaker PH. Differential diagnosis of the simultaneous occurrence of colon carcinoma and peritoneal mesothelioma by immunohistochemistry. Surgical Rounds 2000; 23(7): 411–417.

37. Churg A, Roggli VL, Galateau-Salle F, Cagle PT, Gibbs AR et al. Tumours of the pleura: mesothelial tumours. In Travis WD, Brambilla E, Harris CC, Muller-Hermelink HK eds, Pathology and Genetics of Tumours of the Lung, Pleura, Thymus and Heart. Lyon, France: IARC Press; 2004; 128–136.

38. Husain AN, Colby T, Ordonez N, Krausz T, Attanoos R et al. Guidelines for Pathologic Diagnosis of Malignant Mesothelioma: 2012 Update of the Consensus Statement from the International Mesothelioma Interest Group. Archives of Pathology and Laboratory Medicine August 28, 2012 [Epub ahead of print].

39. Battifora H, McCaughey WTE. Tumours and pseudotumours of the serosal membranes. In Atlas of Tumour Pathology third series, fascicle 15. Washington DC: Armed Forces Institute of Pathology, 1995: 15–88.

40. Roggli VL, Cagle PT. Pleura, pericardium and peritoneum. In Silverberg SG, DeLellis RA, Frable WJ, LiVolsi VA, Wick MR eds. Silverberg's Principles and Practice of Surgical Pathology fourth edn. New York, NY: Churchill-Livingstone/Elsevier, 2006, 1005–1039.

41. Attanoos RL, Gibbs AR. Pathology of malignant mesothelioma. Histopathology 1997; 30: 403–418.

42. Baratti D, Kusamura S, Cabras AD, Laterza B, Balestra MR et al. Lymph node metastases in diffuse malignant peritoneal mesothelioma. Annals of Surgical Oncology 2010; 17: 45–53.

43. Butnor KJ, Sporn TA, Hammar SP, Roggli VL. Well-differentiated papillary mesothelioma. American Journal of Surgical Pathology 2001; 25: 1304–1309.

44. Baratti D, Kusamura S, Nonaka D, Oliva GD, Laterza B et al. Multicystic and well-differentiated papillary peritoneal mesothelioma treated by surgical cytoreduction and hyperthermic intra-peritoneal chemotherapy (HIPEC). Annals of Surgical Oncology 2007; 14: 2790–2797.

45. Churg A, Colby TV, Cagle P. The separation of benign and malignant mesothelial proliferations. American Journal of Surgical Pathology 2000; 24: 1183–1200.

46. Attanoos RL, Griffin A, Gibbs AR. The use of immunohistochemistry in distinguishing reactive from neoplastic mesothelium: a novel use for desmin and comparative evaluation with epithelial membrane antigen, p53, platelet-derived growth factor-receptor, P-glycoprotein and Bcl-2. Histopathology 2003; 43: 231–238.

47. Ordonez NG. Immunohistochemical diagnosis of epithelioid mesothelioma: an update. Archives of Pathology and Laboratory Medicine 2005; 129: 1407–1414.

48. Cerruto CA, Brun EA, Chang D, Sugarbaker PH. Prognostic significance of histomorphologic parameters in diffuse malignant peritoneal mesothelioma. Archives of Pathology and Laboratory Medicine 2006; 130: 1654–1661.

49. Borczuk AC, Taub RN, Hesdorffer M, Hibshoosh H, Chabot JA et al. P16 loss and mitotic activity predict poor survival in patients with peritoneal malignant mesothelioma. Clinical Cancer Research 2005; 11: 3303–3308.

50. Zaffaroni N, Costa A, Pennati M, De Marco C, Affini E et al. Survivin is highly expressed and promotes cell survival in malignant peritoneal mesothelioma. Cell Oncology 2007; 29: 453–466.

51. Nonaka D, Kusamura S, Baratti D, Casali P, Cabras AD et al. Diffuse malignant mesothelioma of the peritoneum: a clinicopathological study of 35 patients treated locoregionally at a single institution. Cancer 2005; 104: 2181–2188.

52. Acherman YIZ, Welch LS, Bromley CM, Sugarbaker PH. Clinical presentation of peritoneal mesothelioma. Tumori 2003; 89: 269–273.

53. Manzini Vde P, Recchia L, Cafferata M, Porta C, Siena S et al. Malignant peritoneal mesothelioma: a multicenter study on 81 cases. Annals of Oncology 2010; 21(2): 348–353.

54. Park JY, Kim KW, Kwon HJ, Park MS, Kwon GY et al. Peritoneal mesotheliomas: clinicopathologic features, CT findings, and

differential diagnosis. American Journal of Roentgenology 2008; 191(3): 814–825.

55. Whitley N, Brenner D, Antman K, Grant D, Aisner J. CT of peritoneal mesothelioma: analysis of eight cases. American Journal of Roentgenology 1982; 138(3): 531–535.

56. Baratti D, Kusamura S, Martinetti A, Seregni E, Oliva D et al. Circulating CA125 in patients with peritoneal mesothelioma treated with cytoreductive surgery and intraperitoneal hyperthermic perfusion. Annals of Surgical Oncology 2007; 14(2): 500–508.

57. Creaney J, Olsen NJ, Brims F, Dick IM, Musk AW et al. Serum mesothelin for early detection of asbestos-induced cancer malignant mesothelioma. Cancer Epidemiology Biomarkers and Prevention 2010; 19(9): 2238–2246.

58. Jacquet P, Sugarbaker PH. Current methodologies for clinical assessment of patients with peritoneal carcinomatosis. Journal of Experimental and Clinical Cancer Research 1996; 15: 49–58.

59. Yan TD, Deraco M, Elias D, Glehen O, Levine EA et al. A novel tumor-node-metastasis (TNM) staging system of diffuse malignant peritoneal mesothelioma using outcome analysis of a multi-institutional database. Cancer 2011; 117(9): 1855–1863.

60. Antman K, Shemin R, Ryan L, Klegar K, Osteen R et al. Malignant mesothelioma: prognostic variables in a registry of 180 patients, the Dana-Farber Cancer Institute and Brigham and Women's Hospital experience over two decades, 1965–1985. Journal of Clinical Oncology 1988; 6(1): 147–153.

61. Chahinian AP, Antman K, Goutsou M, Corson JM, Suzuki Y et al. Randomized phase II trial of cisplatin with mitomycin or doxorubicin for malignant mesothelioma by the Cancer and Leukemia Group B. Journal of Clinical Oncology 1993; 11(8): 1559–1565.

62. Vogelzang NJ, Rusthoven JJ, Symanowski J, Denham C, Kaukel E et al. Phase III study of pemetrexed in combination with cisplatin versus cisplatin alone in patients with malignant pleural mesothelioma. Journal of Clinical Oncology 2003; 21: 2636–2644.

63. Carteni G, Manegold C, Garcia GM, Siena S, Zielinski CC et al. Malignant peritoneal mesothelioma—results from the International Expanded Access Program using pemetrexed alone or in combination with a platinum agent. Lung Cancer 2009; 64(2): 211–218.

64. Jänne PA, Wozniak AJ, Belani CP, Keohan ML, Ross HJ et al. Open-label study of pemetrexed alone or in combination with cisplatin for the treatment of patients with peritoneal mesothelioma: outcomes of an expanded access program. Clinical Lung Cancer 2005; 7: 40–46.

65. Simon GR, Verschraegen CF, Jänne PA, Langer CJ, Dowlati A et al. Pemetrexed plus gemcitabine as first-line chemotherapy for patients with peritoneal mesothelioma: final report of a phase II trial. Journal of Clinical Oncology 2008; 26: 3567–3572.

66. Le DT, Deavers M, Hunt K, Malpica A, Verschraegen CF. Cisplatin and irinotecan (CPT-11) for peritoneal mesothelioma. Cancer Investigation 2003; 21: 682–689.

67. Steele JP, Shamash J, Evans MT, Gower NH, Tischkowitz MD et al. Phase II study of vinorelbine in patients with malignant pleural mesothelioma. Journal of Clinical Oncology 2000; 18: 3912–3917.

68. Vogelzang NJ, Weissman LB, Herndon JE 2nd, Antman KH, Cooper MR et al. Trimetrexate in malignant mesothelioma: a Cancer and Leukemia Group B Phase II study. Journal of Clinical Oncology 1994; 12: 1436–1442.

69. Hesdorffer ME, Chabot JA, Keohan ML, Fountain K, Talbot S et al. Combined resection, intraperitoneal chemotherapy, and whole abdominal radiation for the treatment of malignant peritoneal mesothelioma. American Journal of Clinical Oncology 2008; 31(1): 49–54.

70. Yan TD, Deraco M, Baratti D, Kusamura S, Elias D et al. Cytoreductive surgery and hyperthermic intraperitoneal chemotherapy for malignant peritoneal mesothelioma: multi-institutional experience. Journal of Clinical Oncology 2010; 27: 6237–6242.

71. Baratti D, Kusamura S, Cabras AD, Dileo P, Laterza B et al. Diffuse malignant peritoneal mesothelioma: failure analysis following cytoreduction and hyperthermic intraperitoneal chemotherapy (HIPEC). Annals of Surgical Oncology 2009; 16: 463–472.

72. Bijelic L, Stuart OA, Sugarbaker PH. Adjuvant bidirectional chemotherapy with intraperitoneal pemetrexed combined with intravenous cisplatin for diffuse malignant peritoneal mesothelioma. Gastroenterology Research and Practice 2012; 2012: Article ID 890450.

73. Markman M, Kelsen D. Efficacy of cisplatin-based intraperitoneal chemotherapy as treatment of malignant peritoneal mesothelioma. Journal of Cancer Research and Clinical Oncology 1992; 118(7): 547–550.

74. Sugarbaker PH. Peritonectomy procedures. Annals of Surgery 1995; 221(1): 29–42.

75. Kusamura S, O'Dwyer ST, Baratti D, Younan R, Deraco M. Technical aspects of cytoreductive surgery. Journal of Surgical Oncology 2008; 98(4): 232–236.

76. Baratti D, Kusamura S, Cabras A, Deraco M. cytoreductive surgery with selective versus complete parietal peritonectomy followed by hyperthermic intraperitoneal chemotherapy in patients with diffuse malignant peritoneal mesothelioma: a controlled study. Annals of Surgical Oncology 2012; 19(5): 1416–1424.

77. Baratti D, Kusamura S, Cabras AD, Laterza B, Balestra MR et al. Lymph node metastases in diffuse malignant peritoneal mesothelioma. Annals of Surgical Oncology 2010; 17(1): 45–53.

78. Chua TC, Yan TD, Deraco M, Glehen O, Moran BJ et al. Multi-institutional experience of diffuse intra-abdominal multicystic peritoneal mesothelioma. British Journal of Surgery 2011; 98(1): 60–64.

79. Cao C, Yan TD, Deraco M, Elias D, Glehen O et al. Importance of gender in diffuse malignant peritoneal mesothelioma. Annals of Oncology 2012; 23(6): 1494–1498.

80. Chua TC, Liauw W, Saxena A, Al-Mohaimeed K, Fransi S et al. Evolution of locoregional treatment for peritoneal carcinomatosis: single-center experience of 308 procedures of cytoreductive surgery and perioperative intraperitoneal chemotherapy. American Journal of Surgery 2011; 201(2): 149–156.

81. Chua TC, Yan TD, Saxena A, Morris DL. Should the treatment of peritoneal carcinomatosis by cytoreductive surgery and hyperthermic intraperitoneal chemotherapy still be regarded as a highly morbid procedure?: a systematic review of morbidity and mortality. Annals of Surgery 2009; 249(6): 900–907.

82. Sugarbaker PH, Bijelic L. Adjuvant bidirectional chemotherapy using an intraperitoneal port. Gastroenterology Research and Practice 2012: Article ID 752643.

83. Van der Speeten K, Govaerts K, Stuart OA, Sugarbaker PH. Pharmacokinetics of the perioperative use of cancer chemotherapy in peritoneal surface malignancy patients. Gastroenterology Research and Practice 2012: Article ID 827534.

84. Zaffaroni N, Costa A, Pennati M, De Marco C, Affini E et al. Survivin is highly expressed and promotes cell survival in malignant peritoneal mesothelioma. Cell Oncology 2007; 29: 453–466.

85. Borczuk AC, Cappellini GC, Kim HK, Hesdorffer M, Taub RN et al. Molecular profiling of malignant peritoneal mesothelioma identifies the ubiquitin-proteasome pathway as a therapeutic target in poor prognosis tumors. Oncogene 2007; 26: 610–617.

CHAPTER 43

Cancer of the breast

Martine Piccart, Toral Gathani, Dimitrios Zardavas, Hatem A. Azim, Jr., Christos Sotiriou, Giuseppe Viale, Emiel J.T. Rutgers, Mechthild Krause, Monica Arnedos, Suzette Delaloge, Fabrice Andre, and Felipe Ades Moraes

Epidemiology of breast cancer

Breast cancer is the most frequent cancer among women with an estimated 1.7 million new cancer cases diagnosed in 2012. Incidence rates vary almost fivefold between more and less developed regions of the world. The disease is now the most common cancer both in developed and developing regions with around 690 000 new cases estimated in each region. Incidence rates for the disease are increasing in less developed regions of the world, and are largely thought to be due to changing lifestyles and reproductive patterns of women in these parts of the world [1].

Reproductive risk factors

There is a large body of evidence from both experimental and epidemiological studies which points to a major influence of ovarian hormones, oestrogen in particular, on breast cancer risk.

An increased risk of breast cancer is associated with early menarche and late menopause. The effects of menarche and menopause are not equivalent, in that the excess risk associated with lengthening a woman's reproductive years by one year at menarche is greater that than the excess associated with one year's lengthening at menopause [2].

Childbearing and breastfeeding are of considerable importance when considering subsequent breast cancer risk. Childbearing reduces the risk of breast cancer; the higher the number of full-term pregnancies, the greater the protection. The risk of breast cancer reduces by 7% with each full-term pregnancy and overall, women who have had children have a 30% lower risk than nulliparous women. Women who breastfeed reduce their risk of developing breast cancer compared with women who do not breastfeed. The longer a woman breastfeeds, the greater the protection: risk is reduced by 4% for every 12 months of breastfeeding [3]. Abortion, either spontaneous or induced, has not been shown to have any effect on subsequent breast cancer risk [4].

The use exogenous hormones such as the oral contraceptive pill in reproductive life and by hormone replacement therapy in non-reproductive life is widespread and both have an influence on breast cancer risk, but the effects are largely reversible. Current users of the combined oral contraceptive pill are at a 25% increased risk of breast cancer but this excess risk falls after cessation of use, such that after ten or more years after use stops no significant increase in risk is seen [5]. Current users of hormone therapy are also at an increased risk of developing breast cancer and the risk is greater for users of oestrogen-progesterone combined hormone therapy than for users of oestrogen-only hormone therapy. Overall, the evidence suggests that the risk is increased whilst the women are taking hormone therapy and that the effect wears off quickly once use has ceased [6].

Non-reproductive factors

The incidence of breast cancer increases with age, with 80% of all breast cancer occurring in women over the age of 50 in the UK [7].

The anthropometric factors of body mass index and height are determinants of breast cancer risk. The incidence of breast cancer in obese postmenopausal women is twice that of the non-obese and is related to increased levels of circulating oestrogens due to the peripheral aromatization of oestrogen in adipose tissue [8] whereas obese pre-menopausal women have a 20% reduction in cancer risk. Taller women are at an increased risk of breast cancer compared to shorter women [9].

The role of diet in the aetiology of breast cancer remains controversial. Interest in the role of diet in the aetiology of breast cancer is stimulated by the observation of the lower incidence of breast cancer in Asian populations where intake of animal products is lower than that of Western populations [10]. Studies to date exploring the relationship of diet and breast cancer incidence and mortality have not demonstrated any difference between vegetarians compared to non-vegetarians [11]. Alcohol consumption does have an effect on breast cancer risk; the relative risk of breast cancer is increased in women who report drinking alcohol compared to women who report no alcohol intake for an intake of 35–44 g per day alcohol [12].

Up to 5% of breast cancer in Western countries may be a result of a genetic predisposition to the disease. High-risk allele mutations probably account for most of the families with four or more cases of breast cancer and for around 20–25% of the familial breast cancer risk overall, but for only 5% of all breast cancers [13, 14]. Women who have a positive history of breast cancer are at a two-fold increased relative risk of breast cancer. However, most of these women will never develop breast cancer and most who do will do so after the age of 50. Furthermore, eight out of nine women who develop breast cancer do not have an affected mother, sister, or daughter [15].

Molecular biology of breast cancer

Personalized cancer medicine, envisioned more than 30 years ago [16], has been exemplified by the discovery of the oestrogen receptor (ER) and its consequent therapeutic targeting, as well as by the therapeutic targeting of HER2 oncogene. Recently, large-scale gene expression profiling studies have shed light onto the complex molecular background of breast cancer (BC), holding the potential for more accurate prognostication and personalized treatment decision-making. This chapter highlights the most important advances made recently in the molecular biology of BC, emphasizing their clinical relevance.

Molecular classification of breast cancer

The advent of DNA microarray platforms enabled BC gene expression profiling, representing a major step towards unravelling its molecular complexity [17, 18]. Initially, four intrinsic molecular subtypes were identified: luminal A (ER-positive, histologically low-grade and slowly proliferative tumours); luminal B (high-grade ER-positive tumours); HER2-positive (tumours driven by amplification of HER2 gene and other genes in the same amplicon); and, finally, basal-like (tumours characterized, although not invariably, by negative expression for ER, progesterone receptor [PR] and HER2, also referred to as the triple negative phenotype).

Despite the recognized importance of this molecular classification, there are important impediments to implementing it clinically. One problem is how to discriminate between the luminal A and B subtypes, with these tumours being defined on the basis of proliferation-related genes, which constitute a continuum of expression levels, rather than a binary set of characteristics. An immunohistochemical (IHC) score based on Ki-67 expression levels has been proposed as a potential tool to distinguish the luminal A and B tumours [19]; however, false-positive and false-negative rates reach up to 25%. Another problem concerns HER2-positive tumours. Defined by microarray assays, they show IHC overexpression of the corresponding protein in 70% of the cases; conversely, however, not all cases of HER2 IHC overexpression are classified as HER2-positive by microarray analysis [20].

Basal-like tumours are associated with several additional challenges. Although they have been approximated by the triple negative phenotype in the clinic, the lack of absolute concordance between basal-like and triple negative BC is well known [21]. Within basal-like tumours, additional molecular subtypes have been reported: (i) the claudin-low subtype [22] displaying a gene expression profile of mesenchymal features, immune response genes, and high enrichment for epithelial-to-mesenchymal transition markers; and (ii) the molecular apocrine class [23], characterized by positivity for the androgen receptor and downstream signalling. The heterogeneity of triple negative BC was recently even further elaborated with the identification of six subtypes overall [24].

Additionally, methodological problems have been identified. The gene expression-based BC classifiers use large sets of intrinsic genes, with questionable stability and quality assessment remaining difficult [25]. An alternative approach to large gene sets has been presented [26], namely a subtype classification model called SCMGENE assessing the expression levels of three key genes: oestrogen regulated gene (ESR1), HER2, and AURKA. This simplified classification model was concordant with its more complex multi-gene counterparts, providing comparable prognostication and representing a readily available alternative approach.

Despite incremental refinements in our ability to classify BC, its molecular complexity leaves much to be explored. This has been recently demonstrated by landmark work investigating the genomic and transcriptomic architecture of almost 2000 breast tumours [27], which identified ten novel molecular groups (intclust 1–10), hence splitting the intrinsic subtypes recognized to date.

Oncogenic signalling pathways in breast cancer

The aforementioned gene expression profiling studies and the advent of high-throughput molecular screening tools has led to the identification of multiple oncogenic molecular alterations in BC. One common characteristic emerging from those studies is the genomic heterogeneity of the disease, both between and within individual tumours. In the following sections we present an overview of the major deregulated oncogenic signalling pathways across the distinct molecular BC subtypes.

Luminal breast cancer

Evidence of activated insulin growth factor (IGF) signalling has been found in up to 90% of BC cases [28], with several lines of evidence supporting its implication in luminal subtypes. IGF activates its target receptor IGF-1R, leading to a cascade of signal transduction via the Ras and phosphatidylinositol 3-kinase (PI3K) pathways. Direct cross-talk between ER and IGF-1R has been demonstrated and found to mediate tamoxifen resistance [28]. Furthermore, an IGF-1R signature was manifest mainly in ER-negative BC and a small subset (around 25%) of ER-positive tumours, suggesting that IGF activation may confer hormone resistance [29].

Fibroblast growth factor (FGF) receptors and their corresponding ligands represent another important molecular network in luminal BC [30]. FGFR1 represents one of the most commonly amplified genes in BC (approximately 10%) particularly in the luminal B subtype (16% to 27%) [31]. FGFR1-amplified BC cells are resistant to endocrine therapy, a feature that is reversible upon FGFR1 knock-down [31].

The PI3K signalling pathway represents a molecular 'highway', transducing oncogenic signals from a plethora of upstream receptors. Increased PI3K activity [32] is conferred by multiple molecular aberrations affecting its key molecular components such as PIK3CA, Akt and/or phosphatase and tensin homolog (PTEN). PIK3CA mutations are common in luminal-A and luminal-B BC, and increased expression of PI3K pathway genes was recently found in luminal-B cases [33], with evidence supporting that hormonal resistance is mediated by PI3K signalling activation. However, the prognostic impact of PI3K pathway activation remains to be defined. In the largest molecular study of PI3K in BC conducted to date [34], genomic and proteomic analyses from a cohort of patients with early luminal BC-associated PIK3CA mutations and a corresponding gene expression signature with better clinical outcome.

HER2-positive breast cancer

The HER2-positive BC subtype is driven by the amplification of the HER2 oncogene. HER2 acts through the formation of homo- or hetero-dimers with other members of the HER family. The HER2/HER3 heterodimer is the most potent activator of the PI3K/Akt signalling pathway, thus making HER3 an attractive therapeutic target [35].

Further molecular aberrations involved in activating signalling pathways such as FGF, IGF, and PI3K/Akt have also been described. These are likely clinically important because they have been shown to mediate resistance to HER2-targeted therapies [36]. Importantly, an unbiased, genome-wide RNA interference screen showed that PIK3CA mutations and PTEN loss were important mediators of resistance to trastuzumab treatment [37]. Furthermore, truncation of the HER2 receptor itself [38] was also suggested to confer resistance to trastuzumab with these findings requiring further clinical validation.

Approximately half of HER2-positive BC cases are also ER-positive, and there is solid data proving bidirectional cross-talk between HER2 and ER-positive signalling pathways [39]. Specifically, activation of the HER2 signalling pathway appears to mediate a decrease in the sensitivity to hormonal manipulations [40]. It has been shown that ER status does not determine the overall genetic profile of HER2-positive BC [41], indicating that HER2 remains the main driver of oncogenesis in ER/HER2 over-expressing tumours.

Basal-like breast cancer

The DNA repair BRCA pathway is responsible for homologous recombination, and it has been found to be commonly deregulated in basal-like BC. Its deregulation may be mediated either through germ-line inactivating mutations or alternatively through BRCA1 gene promoter methylation, BRCA1 transcriptional inactivation, and/or overexpression of BRCA1 negative regulators like ID4 (inhibitor of DNA binding 4). This deregulation offers the potential to exploit therapeutically the concept of synthetic lethality (i.e., the situation whereby two different gene defects lead to cell death, whereas each of them separately does not) through the use of PARP inhibition. PARP-1 is a nuclear enzyme essential for the base-excision repair pathway, an alternative DNA repair pathway. BRCA1-deregulation sensitises breast cancer cells to PARP-inhibition, which causes cell-cycle arrest and apoptotic death [42].

High expression of epidermal growth factor receptor (EGFR) [43]—the first member of the HER family of cytoplasmic receptors, mediating multiple oncogenic effects—has been reported in a subpopulation of basal-like BC. Importantly, PTEN loss is observed with high frequency across this molecular subtype [44], conferring PI3K pathway activation, which can mediate resistance to anti-EGFR treatment.

Several other features are also salient in basal-like BC. The expression of KIT, a cytoplasmic cytokine receptor, has been found in higher frequency across these tumours than in other molecular subtypes [45], and was recently found to be highly expressed in breast tumours from individuals with BRCA1 germline mutations [46]. Basal-like BC also shows a higher incidence of nuclear accumulation of p53 or TP53 gene mutations [47]. Besides these molecular defects, a higher frequency of copy number alterations has been reported in basal-like BC than in the other subtypes [48], indicating genomic instability.

Next generation sequencing in breast cancer

Next generation sequencing (NGS) has numerous advantages over older technologies and has already led to important new insights about BC, ranging from the nature and diversity of gene mutations to early diagnosis and monitoring of disease progression. It allows millions of individual templates to be sequenced in parallel [49]. Moreover, NGS can determine the prevalence of any given DNA sequence within a cell population, thus enhancing scientists' ability to determine the mutational heterogeneity of individual tumours. NGS is also informative with respect to structural alterations in DNA molecules, i.e. point mutations, deletions, insertions, copy numbers, translocations, and gene fusion events.

Studies in BC employing NGS have already led to important conceptual advances. Initial results suggest that a larger than previously anticipated repertoire of cancer gene mutations [50] need to be functionally elucidated. In particular, 'drivers', i.e., mutational events driving oncogenic progression, need to be distinguished from 'passengers', i.e. mutations lacking functional importance. Moreover, the mutational burden has been found to be lower in early-stage lobular BC [51], where a significant mutational evolution parallels disease progression. Importantly, it has been shown that extended somatic mutational heterogeneity was present before the emergence of any selective pressure induced by exposure to anticancer agents. A large-scale, paired-end sequencing strategy recently identified three different patterns of somatic rearrangements in BC genomes and their potential contribution to malignant progression [52].

Other NGS studies have revealed that mutations in BC are non-recurring, with individual tumours exhibiting unique mutational blueprints. For example, a recently reported study of 50 luminal BC cases [53] showed that from among more than 1700 different mutations identified, only three genes were mutated at frequencies approaching or exceeding a threshold of 10%. This inter-tumour heterogeneity was further exemplified in another study exploring the metastatic progression of a basal-like BC [54]; it revealed that, despite the significant overlap of mutational events between the primary tumour and a corresponding brain metastasis, significant changes in the allelic frequencies of those mutations had occurred during the metastatic dissemination.

NGS techniques can contribute with regard to monitoring disease progression and early diagnosis. In one study, circulating nucleic acids were identified in the serum of BC patients [55], with a diagnostic specificity level of 95% and a sensitivity of 90% when compared with healthy and non-malignant controls. This discovery in turn led to the development of a serum-based routine laboratory test for BC screening and monitoring. Similar efforts have been undertaken by other researchers. Using massively parallel sequencing techniques, they identified translocations in BC patients serving as personalized biomarkers [56].

Prognostic gene expression signatures in breast cancer

Gene expression profiling has contributed to the development of genomic tests improving prognostication beyond what is provided by classical clinicopathological parameters, with two different tests having been adopted. The first assessed the epithelial cellular compartment of BC, being mainly proliferation-driven. This approach led to the development of several gene signatures [17], some of which are currently clinically available (MammaPrint®, Oncotype Dx®, MapQuantDx®, Theros®, and EndoPredict®). The second approach took into account not only the epithelial cancer cells, but also the stroma and immune-related compartments.

The proliferation-driven 'first-generation' signatures have led to the identification of a low-risk group of patients, but only within the ER-positive BC population [17]. These signatures assign nearly all patients with HER2 amplification or the triple negative phenotype to high-risk categories [57, 58]. This is not surprising, because most of the assessable genes in the signatures are cell-cycle and proliferation-related, and the ER-negative subtypes are highly proliferative [59]. Despite this limitation, these signatures have been shown to add significant prognostic information to clinical variables like tumour size and nodal size [59]. Because they capture similar biological phenomena, they have similar prognostic ability, and using more than one signature does not improve the ability to predict prognosis [59, 60]. It should be noted that these signatures accurately predict mainly recurrences occurring during the first five years following diagnosis [60]. To date, there is no clear consensus about the clinical utility of the prognostic signatures, with two large phase III randomized trials addressing this issue: the Microarray in Node Negative and 0 to 3 Positive Lymph Node Disease May Avoid Chemotherapy Trial (MINDACT) in Europe (testing MammaPrint®) [61], and the Trial Assigning Individualized Options for Treatment (TAILORx) study in the United States (testing Oncotype DX®) (Figure 43.1) [62].

Several 'second generation signatures' were then developed as the result of efforts to overcome the conceptual drawbacks of their first generation counterparts, with the latter disregarding that ER and HER2 expression status define fundamentally different molecular profiles of BC and that its biological behaviour is influenced by tumour-associated stroma and immune activation status. These concepts were corroborated by a meta-analysis [57] showing that stroma and immune-related gene modules are key determinants of clinical outcome in patients with HER2-positive BC, while immune-gene modules define clinical outcome in basal-like tumours.

Well-conducted studies of separately micro-dissected breast stroma and cancer cells have identified extensive changes in the gene expression profile of BC stroma during tumour progression [63]. Stromal collagen deposition was found to facilitate malignant progression in BC cells, through a β1-integrin-dependent mechanism [64] and through collaboration with COX-2 [65]. Moreover, the presence of tumour-associated-macrophages is associated with aggressive biological behaviour [66], since the macrophages induce increased angiogenic activity through the production of angiogenic factors (e.g., VEGF and IL-8) and matrix metalloproteinases (MMPs). Tumour angiogenesis [67] is an important feature, providing tumours with the nutrients necessary to facilitate metastatic dissemination. In BC, a tumour microenvironment of metastasis was recently identified [68], referring to perivascular macrophages guiding BC cells and facilitating their local invasion in newly formed blood vessels, thus promoting haematogenous metastatic dissemination.

Recently, tumour immune microenvironment was shown to regulate the response to chemotherapy through the recruitment of macrophages [69]. These findings offer hope for new therapeutic avenues, with blockade of macrophage recruitment combined with chemotherapy, significantly decreasing primary tumour formation and reducing metastatic dissemination [69].

Further data supporting the role of the immune system in mediating the response to chemotherapy were recently presented in a study of almost 1000 BC patients treated with neoadjuvant chemotherapy [70]. Gene expression modules describing important biologic processes correlated with response to neoadjuvant chemotherapy, and, independently of other clinical variables, the immune module was found to be predictive for pCR, especially in the HER2-positive subtype.

Finally, cancer-associated fibroblasts are also important mediators of BC malignant progression [71]. This is mainly due to their ability to secrete stroma-derived-factor 1 (SDF-1/CXCL12), a chemokine serving a dual function and facilitating: (1) the recruitment of endothelial precursor cells, thus promoting angiogenesis; and (2) tumour cell invasion in the stroma.

A comparison of tumour stroma and matched normal stroma from BC samples generated a 26-gene signature, called the stroma-derived prognostic predictor (SDPP) [72], being highly prognostic independently of ER, HER2, and clinical prognostic factors. In addition, it provided accurate prognostication in the HER2-positive subtype, out-performing MammaPrint®. In ER-negative BC, an immune-response-related 7-gene module [73] was found to accurately predict prognosis as well. Similar results were obtained by another group using a 14-gene signature [74]. The pivotal role of stromal and tumour cell interaction was further elucidated through the generation of a 12-gene CD10+ stromal signature [75], being prognostic in patients with the HER2-positive subtype and predictive of nonresponse to chemotherapy for those patients.

Additional levels of complexity with respect to the BC genetic heterogeneity have arisen through the identification of microRNAs (miRNAs) [76], which are conserved, noncoding short RNA molecules regulating gene expression. Microarray-based studies using deep sequencing recently led to a 9-miRNA-signature [77], able to identify women with poor prognosis BC.

Apart from the abundance of genomic changes, epigenetic differences (i.e., DNA methylation and histone modifications) have also been observed across different molecular subtypes of BC [78]. Specific DNA methylation patterns were found to identify luminal BC patients with different risks of relapse independently of other clinical variables [79], proving that the profiling of perturbed epigenetic phenomena holds promise for improved prognostication.

Role of gene expression signatures in predicting response to primary systemic therapy

More limited information is available about whether proliferation-related gene expression signatures can predict benefit from chemotherapy. Since conventional cytotoxic agents target highly-proliferating cancer cells, it should come as no surprise that 'first generation signatures' predict chemo-sensitivity [80], particularly in ER-positive BC. Importantly, those gene signatures 'capturing' the generic chemosensitivity of highly-proliferating tumour cells challenge the currently applied clinicopathologic criteria to predict benefit from adjuvant chemotherapy. The 21-gene recurrence score assay (Oncotype DX®) was recently proven to predict benefit from anthracycline-based chemotherapy, irrespectively of the tumour stage [81]. Patients with infiltrated lymph nodes and a low recurrence score did not seem to benefit, whereas patients with a higher recurrence score showed a major benefit, independently of the number of positive nodes. The randomized, prospective RxPONDER trial ('Rx for Positive Node, Endocrine Responsive Breast Cancer') will reveal whether chemotherapy benefits patients

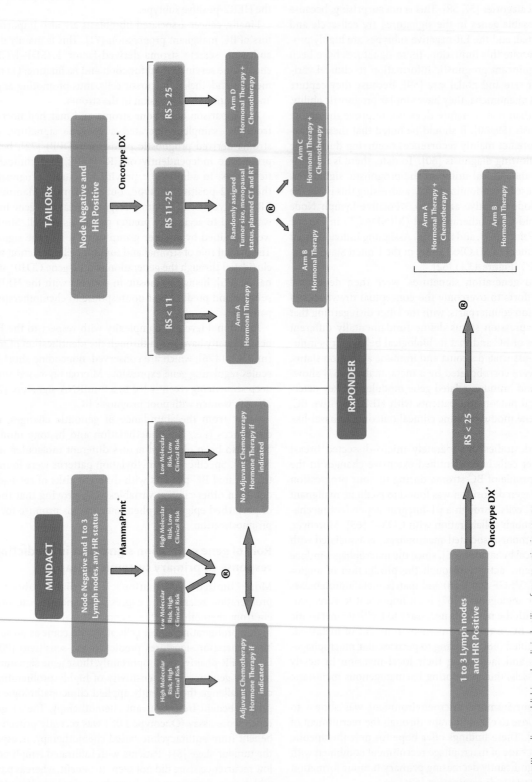

Fig. 43.1 Phase III studies establishing the clinical utility of prognostic signatures.

with node positive BC who have low to intermediate recurrence scores with Oncotype DX® (Figure 43.1).

Efforts to develop multigene classifiers that can predict sensitivity to specific therapeutic agents have also been presented, for example the 'anthracycline-based score (A-score)' predictive for response to anthracyclines [82]. The A-score—a combination of a topoisomerase IIα signature, a stroma signature and an immune-response signature—was found to have high negative predictive value for sensitivity to anthracyclines independently of HER2 expression status. Another approach for prediction of anthracycline resistance employed integrated genomics [83]. A small number of over-expressed and amplified genes from chromosome 8q22 were associated with early disease recurrence, despite anthracycline-based adjuvant chemotherapy. Overexpression of two of those genes, namely the antiapoptotic gene YWHAZ and the lysosomal gene LAPTM4B, was associated with poor tumour response to anthracyclines in the neoadjuvant setting, and thus appears to be a potential predictor of anthracycline resistance.

The prediction of response to endocrine treatment has also been pursued through gene expression profiling experiments, leading to the development of the sensitivity to endocrine therapy (SET) index comprising a set of 165 distinct genes co-regulated with the ESR1 gene [84]. The SET index was found to be predictive of response to any type of endocrine treatment, and it improved the predictive stratification when combined with existing clinicopathological standards. It was recently integrated into a predictive testing algorithm [85] together with newly developed predictive signatures for excellent pathologic response and for extensive residual disease in HER2-negative BC cases after sequentially administered taxane- and anthracycline-neoadjuvant chemotherapy. This combined predictive test was shown to add significantly to a multivariate clinicopathologic model assessing age, tumour size, nodal status, grade, ER status, and the type of taxane administered.

Lastly, attempts to predict sensitivity to specific therapeutic regimens through genetic testing of BC cells in vitro, with the implementation of functional testing (i.e., RNA interference) in some cases, have been presented [86]. However, the results from these experiments have failed to be reproduced robustly in humans, possibly because of the intrinsic limitations of using cultured cell lines as a model for human pharmacology.

Future directions

Accumulating molecular biology data has been critical, because it has helped us move away from the 'one-size-fits-all' paradigm in the clinical management of our BC patients. Identifying 'driver' mutational mechanisms through functional genomics and elucidating the molecular mechanisms that govern heterotypic signalling networks between BC cells and their surrounding microenvironment hold the promise for more efficient therapies. However, before the implementation of this new knowledge into clinical practice, it will be necessary to interpret all the information generated through deep genome, transcriptome- and epigenome-sequencing analyses of breast tumours, which poses a significant challenge. To address this challenge, it will be essential to make significant advances in bioinformatics, systems biology, statistics, and the systems architecture of information technology. Moreover, issues of intra-tumour heterogeneity still need to be addressed, as was recently emphasized by findings in support of the view that distinct aberrations

may vary between different biopsy samples of the very same tumour [87]. Ultimately, it will be necessary to conduct prospective clinical evaluations of new versus current classical approaches before we can change clinical practice.

In situ pathology of breast cancer

Until novel and more sophisticated approaches, for example serum proteomics or gene expression profiling of circulating tumour cells, will be readily available, the primary tumour of patients with breast cancer will remain the main source of information to assess the risk of disease recurrence and to inform the choice of the most appropriate systemic treatment. Accordingly, it is the main responsibility of pathologists to ensure that all the relevant information is derived from the primary tumour with the highest accuracy and reproducibility. Compliance with guidelines and recommendations issued by regulatory agencies and scientific bodies, as well as implementation and continuous participation in internal and external quality assurance program may assist the pathologists in coping with this unprecedented and very demanding task.

A comprehensive approach that includes the accurate evaluation of the morphological features of the tumour, with special reference to the histological type and grade, and the assessment of the main prognostic and predictive parameters should offer the patients and treating physicians a robust background upon which final therapeutic decisions can be safely taken. The robustness of this background, however, depends on the expertise and knowledge of pathologists, and on the accuracy and reproducibility of the assays for the assessment of relevant markers.

Classification of breast carcinoma

Breast cancer is unanimously considered a highly heterogeneous disease in several ways. Indeed, different tumour types exhibit variable histopathological and biological features, different clinical outcome, and different response to systemic interventions. Due to such a high degree of heterogeneity, breast cancer cannot be viewed as a single clinicopathological entity, but it must be necessarily dissected into a number of more homogeneous entities. Hence, there is a need for a classification that should be scientifically sound, clinically useful, easily applicable, and widely reproducible. Unfortunately, however, despite all the efforts in the past and in more recent years, the 'perfect' classification of breast cancer still has not been written.

The histopathological classification of breast carcinoma is based on the diversity of the morphological features of the tumours. In its current version, as endorsed by the WHO in 2003 [88], it includes some 20 major tumour types and 18 minor subtypes. This classification is adopted worldwide, it is reasonably reproducible, but has a major limitation. Indeed, some 70–80% of all breast cancers will eventually belong to either one of the two major histopathological classes, namely invasive ductal carcinoma not otherwise specified (IDC NOS) or invasive lobular carcinoma (ILC). This implies that the classification is unable to actually reflect the much wider heterogeneity of breast cancer with respect to the biological features, the clinical outcome, and the response to systemic therapy. It is also debatable whether the two major classes of breast cancer, ductal and lobular, do actually reflect clinical differences, and whether ILC per se constitutes a prognostically different group as compared to IDC [89, 90].

Interestingly, it is the correct identification of some minor tumour subtypes, the so-called 'special' tumour types, or of 'variants' of the main tumour types that may actually provide clinically useful information, because these tumours have distinct prognostic profiles. This is the case, for example, of the tubular and cribriform carcinomas, pursuing an almost indolent clinical course with an extremely good overall survival [91], and of the adenoid-cystic carcinomas, carrying a very favorable prognosis in the vast majority of the cases [92]. Conversely, other subtypes of breast cancer, like the metaplastic carcinomas, may have a significantly worse clinical outcome when compared with IDC NOS [93].

Another aspect of the WHO classification that has generated increasing debate is the appropriateness of using the term 'in situ carcinoma' for the non-invasive tumours of the duct and lobules (ductal carcinoma in situ or DCIS and lobular carcinoma in situ or LCIS). This terminology has been criticized for the dramatic psychological impact of the word 'carcinoma'. Indeed, in the understanding of patients 'carcinoma' often implies an incurable and life-threatening disease. It has been therefore suggested to replace the DCIS and LCIS terminology with the less frightening designation of 'ductal intraepithelial neoplasia (DIN)' and 'lobular intraepithelial neoplasia (LIN)' [94, 95].

The histopathological classification remains an essential component of the pathological report of breast cancer, despite its limited usefulness in assessing the prognosis of the disease, and in informing the choice of the systemic therapy.

Due to the limited prognostic and predictive power of the histopathological classification, at the beginning of this century new approaches have been taken to unveil the molecular basis for the heterogeneity of breast cancer. By using a hierarchical clustering analysis of gene expression profiling, Perou and colleagues were able to identify molecularly defined classes of breast cancer (luminal, HER2-enriched, basal-like and normal-like) with distinctive biological and clinical features [99–98]. This molecular classification has been shown to have prognostic value and also to be predictive of the response to chemotherapy [99].

The original molecular classification has been derived from investigations on fresh frozen tissue and it is not applicable to formalin-fixed and paraffin-embedded (FFPE) material. This jeopardized the wider application of the molecular classification in clinical practice. More recently, however, a gene expression assay using 50 genes (PAM50) has been developed for use on FFPE tissue. The assay, based on quantitative real time reverse transcription-PCR (qRT-PCR), accurately identifies the major molecular subtypes of breast cancer and generates risk-of-relapse scores [100]. Its prognostic value has been confirmed in several retrospective investigations using tumour samples of patients with long-term follow-up data and of patients enrolled in randomized clinical trials [101, 102].

Another attempt to bring the molecular classification of breast cancer into clinical practice has been to look for surrogate markers that would allow identifying the molecular subtypes using a more familiar immunohistochemical approach. Accordingly, the combined evaluation of oestrogen receptors (ER), progesterone receptors (PgR), HER2, and Ki67 immunoreactivity would approximate the molecular classification of luminal A, luminal B, HER2-enriched, and basal-like breast cancers [103]. It should be noted, however, that the immunohistochemically- and molecularly-defined classes do not overlap completely. As an example, some basal-like breast cancers (according to the molecular classification) will not show the expected triple-negative (ER-, PgR-, and HER2-negative) immunophenotype, and vice versa not all the immunohistochemically triple-negative breast cancer will be classified as basal-like by gene expression profiling [104].

Despite the lack of a complete overlap between the molecular classes and their immunohistochemical surrogates, the panellists of the 2011 St Gallen Consensus have endorsed the use of the immunohistochemical assays to identify breast cancer subtypes and to inform the choice of systemic treatments [105]. Interestingly, however, the panellists also stressed the fact that some 'special' types of breast cancer defined according to the more traditional histopathological classification, while belonging to one of the more recently defined classes, most likely could benefit from a different treatment approach.

The assessment of prognostic and predictive parameters

In the last decades, a major effort has been done to better inform the choice of systemic treatment for breast cancer patients. Risk assessment has been traditionally regarded as the main driver for the selection of the most appropriate therapy. Several histopathological parameters have been shown to correlate with the likelihood of tumour recurrence following local therapy of early breast cancer, including tumour size and grade, occurrence of peritumoral vascular invasion, extent of the intraductal component, and status of the regional lymph nodes. Some of these parameters may also be combined in prognostic scores such as the Nottingham Prognostic Index, constructed on tumour size, number of involved lymph nodes and tumour grade.

To reliably define the risk of tumour recurrence, all the above parameters should be assessed accurately, according to standardized protocols and recommendations, and eventually included into the final pathology report. The macroscopic size of the tumour should be confirmed histologically, to allow the measurement of the invasive component and the classification of the tumour according to the pT categories of the TNM classification [106]. Grading of breast cancer may be poorly reproducible and lose its prognostic significance if it is not performed strictly following the recommended thresholds for scoring the three parameters of the modified Bloom-Richardson-Elston grading system (also called the Nottingham system), namely tubule formation, nuclear atypia, and mitotic index [107, 108].

More recently, however, the concept of using risk assessment to inform systemic treatment has been challenged by the alternative option of relying on the expected responsiveness of the tumours to different therapeutic approaches, and then to fine-tune the treatment according to the patient's risk of relapse. This has been best exemplified at the 2009 St Gallen Consensus, with the panellists agreeing that the systemic therapy of early breast cancer is mainly informed by expression of hormone receptors and HER2 status [109].

It became, therefore, of primary importance for the optimal systemic therapy of patients with early breast cancer to ensure the most accurate assessment of these parameters in a reproducible and timely manner. The panellists of the 2009 St Gallen Consensus took the seminal decision of defining ER-positive and PgR-positive tumours as showing 1% or more immunoreactive cells [108]. This definition has been subsequently endorsed by the expert panel issuing the ASCO/CAP guideline recommendations for immuno-histochemical testing of ER and PgR in breast cancer [110]. In case of ER- or PgR-positive tumours, the actual percentage of neoplastic cells showing definite nuclear immunoreactivity must be reported, because the higher the number of positive cells, the larger is the expected benefit of endocrine therapies. Indeed, a higher expression (e.g.: >50% immunoreactive tumour cells) of ER correlates with a favorable outcome for patients treated with endocrine therapy, which cannot be significantly improved by the addition of chemotherapy, whereas patients with endocrine non-responsive tumours or lower expression of ER achieve the greatest benefit from systemic chemotherapy (with or without endocrine treatment) in both the neoadjuvant and the adjuvant settings [111–113].

In addition to the actual percentage of the positive cells, it is recommended to report on the average intensity of the staining, whereas the use of a combined scoring system (like the H score or the Allred score) [114, 115] is considered optional.

Guidelines and recommendations describing how to optimally perform the immunohistochemical and in situ hybridization assays for assessing HER2 status and evaluate and score the results have also been issued and recently updated [116, 117]. These assays have been clinically validated in several studies demonstrating the high predictive value of a HER2 positive status for the efficacy of HER2-targeted treatments. According to regulatory agencies world-wide and the trastuzumab package insert, only patients whose tumours over-express HER2 in more than 10% invasive tumour cells, or show HER2 gene amplification (four or more copies of the gene/cell, or a ratio ≥2 between the gene copy number and the chromosome 17 centromeres) are candidates for trastuzumab treatment.

Tumour proliferation is one of the most important prognostic parameters in breast cancer. In clinical practice, the evaluation of the tumour proliferative fraction is most commonly performed by the immunohistochemical staining of the Ki67 antigen [118]. The use of Ki67 immunolabelling as a prognostic and predictive marker has been extensively investigated in both the neoadjuvant and adjuvant settings [119–121]. The panellists of the 2009 St Gallen Consensus have included the assessment of Ki67 among the useful parameters to inform the choice of adding chemotherapy to endocrine therapies for patients with ER-positive and HER2-negative disease. Recognizing the relatively poor standardization and reproducibility of Ki67 evaluation, an ad hoc committee (the International Ki67 in Breast Cancer Working Group) has issued recommendations for optimal testing [122].

Predicting the response of patients with breast cancer to the different therapeutic options remains one of the most challenging tasks for translational and clinical researchers. Traditional markers play a major role in the selection of candidate patients to systemic interventions, but they are of limited value in predicting the actual response of the patients to different treatments, especially when these markers are evaluated individually. Future investigations will have to exploit the predictive value of the traditional markers when used in combination, so to offer a more comprehensive assessment of the biological features of the tumour cells [123]. More sophisticated molecular assays, based on gene expression profiling, are already available to complement the information provided by established markers [124]. The combined evaluation of clinical features, of established pathological markers and of gene expression profiles will eventually lead to more personalized treatment of patients with breast cancer.

In situ surgical management of breast cancer

Surgery for breast cancer has changed gradually over the past 30 years. For many decades, radical mastectomy was the only treatment for all types of cancer. Loco-regional surgery has evolved to a far less mutilating approach, while improving local control rates. These include breast-conserving therapy (BCT) with whole breast irradiation (WBI), mastectomy with immediate reconstruction, skin-sparing mastectomy with or without nipple preservation, and neoadjuvant chemotherapy followed by breast conservation. Treatment selection is nowadays based on the combination of extent of disease, the different surgical possibilities and patient preference [125]. More recently, axillary clearance as a staging procedure has largely been replaced by the sentinel node (SN) procedure, leaving axillary lymph node clearance only for those patients with a positive SN. The limited role of surgery is further evolving by the omission of axillary dissection in some node-positive women and preservation of the nipple areolar complex (NAC).

To obtain a high surgical standard proper training in breast surgery is mandatory, followed by protocolized surgical procedures in general practice and a sufficient caseload per surgeon. The most important determinant for high standard surgical cancer care is, however, a skilled surgeon who is very much interested in and dedicated to breast cancer, working in the setting of a structured breast clinic within a multidisciplinary breast team [126–128].

An optimal surgical technique provides for:

◆ The least possible mutilation with the best possible cosmetic result.

◆ The least possible complication rate.

◆ Conditions for the best locoregional control.

◆ Optimal information on the nature and extent of the disease locally and regionally.

The surgeon is the key to the information on local extent of the tumour (particularly in breast conservation) and regional-axillary-dissemination, which information influences adjuvant treatment, including radiotherapy and/or systemic therapy [129]. Lymphatic mapping followed by SN biopsy according to established procedures represents an important instrument to this aim.

Diagnosis and staging of breast cancer

In 2010, almost 50 000 new cases of invasive and almost 6000 new cases of non-invasive breast cancer were diagnosed in the United Kingdom. Approximately one-third of these were screen-detected cancers and two-thirds were diagnosed as a result of a symptomatic presentation. Of the screen-detected cancers, 80% were invasive cancer and 20% were non-invasive cancer [130].

Breast cancer is diagnosed through triple assessment, incorporating physical examination, radiological evaluation, and tissue diagnosis. Each element is scored (1–5) according to the degree of suspicion for the presence of cancer. Where there is concordance between the three elements, the diagnostic accuracy of triple assessment is around 99% [131].

Breast cancer staging is based on the TNM classification for solid tumours, taking into account the tumour size or extent (T), number of loco-regional nodes involved (N), and the absence or presence of distant metastasis (M). Staging is largely either clinical or pathological. The clinical staging (cTNM) is based on information gathered through clinical and radiological assessment prior to any treatment. The pathological staging (pTNM) is given after pathological assessment of a surgical specimen. Other prefixes include 'y' (yTNM) to indicate that the stage was assessed after neoadjuvant treatment (usually chemotherapy). Using the TNM classification, patients can be assigned to a stage which can give an idea of overall prognosis. Early breast cancer is considered to be stage 1 and 2, stage 3 represents locally advanced breast cancer, and stage 4 is metastatic breast cancer. A full explanation of the TNM staging for breast cancer is available on the website of the American Cancer Society: <http://www.cancer.org/cancer/breastcancer/detailedguide/breast-cancer-staging>.

Preventative surgery

Since 1994, human genes BRCA1 and BRCA2 have been discovered with, when mutated, an estimated lifetime risk of up to 85% of developing breast cancer [132, 133]. To reduce their increased risk from dying of breast cancer carriers of BRCA1 and BRCA2 mutations may consider (bilateral) salpingo-oophorectomy and/or prophylactic mastectomy as an alternative to intensive surveillance. A limitation of the surgical procedure is the possibility of incomplete removal of all glandular tissue, leaving a small risk of developing breast cancer. Thus, clinicians may be inclined to continue to follow the women with routine imaging after preventive surgery. However, in clinical practice, the risk of developing breast cancer after risk-reducing surgery appears extremely low at less than 1% at ten years [134–137]. This very low risk does not warrant surveillance for breast cancer after preventive surgery [137]. Further, given the very low risk of invasive cancer at the time of preventive surgery, a SN procedure during preventive bilateral mastectomy is not indicated [137].

Not only do asymptomatic carriers benefit from the risk-reducing procedure, also carriers who have developed breast cancer may benefit from secondary prophylactic measures. A number of studies found a substantial risk reduction from contralateral prophylactic mastectomy, even suggesting survival benefit [138–140].

If a breast cancer gene carrier chooses preventive mastectomy, such a procedure should be performed within the framework of psychosocial support, the availability of a plastic-reconstructive surgeon for immediate reconstruction, and a surgical oncologist to explain all pros and cons of such a procedure. Preferably, such women are treated in specialized centres.

In situ carcinoma

With increasing screening activities, in situ carcinoma of the breast is more frequently diagnosed. About 15% of all screen-detected malignancies appear to be in situ carcinoma [141].

Lobular carcinoma in situ is usually an incidental finding in a breast biopsy and can be considered as a marker lesion for the development of breast cancer. In these patients a wait-and-see policy with intensive surveillance is advocated [142].

Ductal carcinoma in situ is essentially a uni-segmental disease, originated within a specific part of the gallactoforic tree. DCIS consists of a wide range of different lesions defined by the nuclear grade of the tumour cells, the amount of necrosis, the architectural display, etc. Well-, intermediate-, and poorly-differentiated subtypes can be classified histologically. Diagnosis is preferably established by image- guided (ultrasound or stereotactic) biopsies. Diagnosis by core biopsies may underestimate, however, the risk of invasive breast cancer; in 15–20% of patients invasive cancer at excisional biopsy or mastectomy is seen [141].

DCIS is essentially treated by complete excision. In case of non-palpable lesions excision is performed after localizing the tumour with some form of localization technique, such as guide wire, ROLL technique, and Iodine-125 seed. The ROLL technique (radioguided occult lesion localization) is done with an image-directed (ultrasound- or stereotactic-guided) injection of a radioactive tracer (for instance Tc99 labelled albumin colloid). The excision is directed using the gammaprobe.

As the breast is not divided in anatomically recognizable segments, and DCIS is essentially a microscopic disease, the surgeon is not able to define the complete local excision clinically. Depending on the extent of the micro-calcifications, a treatment plan should be drawn with a wide local excision or an ablative procedure, preferably offered with an immediate breast reconstruction. A complete local excision with good cosmetic outcome can be facilitated with oncoplastic procedures [143]. Free margins of 1–2 mm are sufficient; wider margins hardly improve local control rates [144]. Axillary dissection is not indicated. In patients with extensive lesions diagnosed as DCIS by core biopsies (and thus limited sampling, insufficient to exclude invasive cancer), and for whom ablative surgery is the preferred treatment option, a SN procedure is reasonable. Further, since the risk of invasion is larger in patients with a palpable lesion, in DCIS grade III and in patients younger than 55 years of age, a SN procedure can also be performed [145].

Preoperative workup

Breast-conserving therapy now is widely accepted as a result of the convincing data generated by randomized studies [146]. The recent long-term outcomes from the EORTC trial 10801 show that also for larger tumours the results are equivalent to those of mastectomy [147]. Since breast-conserving therapy always involves wide local excision with a minimal macroscopic circumferential margin of 0.5–1 cm, in many instances the size of the lump will affect cosmesis. Therefore, one important consideration is the size of the tumour in relation to the size of the breast. The size of the tumour has to be judged on clinical grounds and the appearance on mammography and/or ultrasound. If there is doubt on the extent of the tumour and consequently the feasibility of breast conservation, MRI can be a helpful tool [148]. Further, to improve complete excision and cosmetic outcome, oncoplastic techniques should be applied.

If histology does not reveal risk factors for local recurrence (grossly incomplete excised invasive cancer, incomplete excised ductal carcinoma in situ (DCIS), extensive vascular invasion of the tumour, young age of the patient <35 yrs) breast conservation can safely be performed with good local control rates [129, 146]. Margins should be clear of invasive and of in situ cancer [149]. A specific 'safe' margin width cannot be given [150]. If the breast cancer involved area is too extensive to allow for a good cosmetic outcome and local control, a mastectomy is indicated, again preferably with the possibility of immediate reconstruction.

In selected cases, nipple-sparing procedures will result in good cosmetic results and local control rates [151]. It should be noted that a significant minority of the well-informed patients who are good candidates for breast conservation choose mastectomy [152, 153].

The management of the axilla

The knowledge whether regional and axillary lymph nodes contain metastatic disease is important for two reasons:

1. It provides prognostic information: should the patient receive adjuvant systemic treatments? It should be kept in mind that nowadays important prognostic information can also be gathered from the primary tumour: grade, lymphatic invasion, size, and gene expression arrays. It can be foreseen that in the near future lymph node status will become far less important as a prognosticator.

2. To guide elective treatment in case of metastasis in the lymph nodes: axillary lymph node dissection or radiotherapy to the axilla or to the other regional lymph node basins.

Involvement of regional lymph nodes can be detected by ultrasound of the axilla and guided FNA cytology or core biopsy of suspicious nodes, axillary lymph node dissection, the sentinel node procedure or PET/CT scanning [154]. US of the axilla is a cheap, simple and helpful tool to detect larger metastasis, and thus may spare an unnecessary SN procedure in 10–20% of patients with clinically negative nodes [155].

From the ever-growing published experience on the SN procedure in breast cancer, it is clear that this procedure is standard of care for those patients with clinically or ultrasound unsuspicious axillary lymph nodes. In experienced hands, the SN procedure offers the same staging opportunities as a full axillary clearance [156]. Two large European multicentre studies [157, 158] show a high SN identification rate. Both trials had an intensive audit and quality control program, which has led to these satisfactory figures. The same is seen in the NSABP B-32 trial, where also, even more importantly, no differences in axillary relapse and survival rates are observed [159].

Unless ultrasound of the axilla is negative, SN procedure is reliable in almost every clinical situation:

♦ Larger cancers (up to 5 cm); cancers at any location in the breast.

♦ Multifocal cancers.

♦ Before or after neoadjuvant chemotherapy; both have advantages and limitations.

♦ In pregnancy.

♦ In male breast cancer.

♦ In DCIS diagnosed on core biopsy where there is some risk of missed invasive cancer.

♦ After previous surgical procedures in the breast.

♦ In cases of breast relapse after breast conservation.

If the quality criteria are met, the clinical false-positive rate, i.e., the number patients with axillary lymph node metastases after a negative SN procedure, is low: approximately 0.3% after an average of three to five years of follow-up [156, 159]. Taking into account a SN false negative rate of 5–10% and an axillary recurrence rate of 0.3%, fewer than 6% of patients with microscopic residual disease will have clinical manifestation. This low rate of clinical manifestation is confirmed by five small series of patients with positive SNs who declined axillary dissection. If not treated, the two- to three-year risk of an axillary 'relapse' in these series is 0–1.4% [160–164]. These findings were confirmed in a prospective trial examining outcome of patients with SN metastases, the American College of Surgeons Oncology Group Z0011 trial. Patients with tumour-positive SN detected by standard H and E were randomized to undergo ALND after SLND (445 patients) versus SLND alone (446 patients) without specific axillary treatment. Loco-regional recurrence was evaluated. Patients in the two groups were similar with respect to age, Bloom-Richardson score, oestrogen receptor status, use of adjuvant systemic therapy, tumour type, grading, and tumour size. Patients randomized to SLND+ALND had a median of 17 axillary nodes removed compared with a median of only two SN removed with SLND alone (P <0.001). ALND also removed more positive lymph nodes (P < 0.001). At a median follow-up time of 6.3 years, there were no statistically significant differences in local recurrence (P = 0.11) or regional recurrence (P = 0.45) between the two groups. Regional lymph node relapse after SLND only was observed in four patients (0.9% and after SLND+ALND in two (0.5%). The conclusion of Giuliano et al. was that, despite the potential for residual axillary disease after SLND, SLND without ALND can offer excellent regional control and may be reasonable management for selected patients with early stage breast cancer treated with breast conserving therapy and adjuvant systemic therapy [165].

Two limitations of this clinical trial include: (1) the fact that it did not complete its planned accrual, and (2) the uncertainty of generalizing its results to all breast cancer subtypes or to patients who underwent a mastectomy (all patients in the 2011 trial received radiotherapy to the breast and lower axilla).

Take home messages for the surgical management of the axilla

♦ SN procedure is standard of care in all patients with invasive breast cancer and clinically and ultrasound unsuspicious axillary lymph nodes.

♦ No axillary treatment is indicated in patients with a negative SN, including those with small metastases <0.2 mm.

♦ Axillary clearance is indicated in patients with proven macrometastases in the axilla (by US and FNAC).

♦ In patients with limited cancer involvement of the removed SN and who will receive adjuvant systemic treatment and whole breast irradiation, axillary clearance can be omitted.

♦ Patients with higher risk of further axillary lymph node metastases after SN biopsy, ALND is still standard of care, and radiotherapy to the axilla can be considered as alternative.

Neoadjuvant chemotherapy and surgery

The use of primary systemic therapy, or neoadjuvant chemotherapy, has gained an important role in the treatment of breast cancer. Firstly, the rate of breast-conserving surgery can be increased due to primary systemic therapy, because of reduction of tumour load. In a recent meta-analysis, Mieog et al. describe an increase in breast-conserving surgery of 18% [166]. The efficacy of primary systemic therapy to this end can further be improved by tailoring the regimen to tumour characteristics and by switching regimen based on interim evaluation. Applying these strategies, adequate breast conservation can be achieved in about 40% of patients who were otherwise candidates for mastectomy [167]. It is imperative to mark the cancer in the breast before the start of chemotherapy to facilitate optimal local excision in case of a very good partial or complete remission.

In case of primary systemic therapy, the type of surgery of the breast, breast-conserving or mastectomy, is dependent on clinical tumour response and imaging, where MRI of the breast appears the most helpful tool [168–170]. In general, the same rules as in primary breast conserving apply: to obtain clear margins after local excision and adequate radiotherapy. For staging purposes, extra-axillary lymph node metastases and distant metastases, new generation 18F-FDG PET/CT scanning appears to outperform conventional imaging techniques, and will have impact on patient management [171].

Radiotherapy in breast cancer

Indications and prediction of outcome

Applied to the majority of patients, radiotherapy is today one of the mainstays of breast cancer treatment. As a part of combined treatment schedules, its aim is to improve local tumour control and hereby to increase survival. Breast-conserving surgery of invasive breast cancer followed by radiotherapy yields similar local control and survival rates compared to mastectomy [172]. Loco-regional tumour control rates range today between 70 and 95% after 10 years [173, 174]. The risk of loco-regional recurrence highly depends on patient age with young patients being at highest risk. Histopathologic risk factors include extensive ductal carcinoma in situ, vascular invasion, tumour size, or multicentricity and nodal involvement [175]. Attempts to classify patients into risk groups for local recurrence according to tumour gene expression profiles have been unsuccessful so far since they did not yield independent additive predictive value for treatment decisions [176]. There is currently no patient group in whom adjuvant radiotherapy can be safely omitted after BCS, while after mastectomy radiotherapy is only applied in high-risk patients (see below).

Radiotherapy after breast conserving surgery of invasive breast cancer

Whole breast radiotherapy

Radiotherapy of the whole breast improves local tumour control after breast-conserving surgery of invasive breast cancer. Independent on tumour stage, the advantage seems to be a reduction of local recurrences by ~50% and a reduction of the risk of death by about a sixth. One breast cancer death within 15 years of follow-up can be avoided by four recurrences avoided within 10 years of follow-up [174]. The absolute benefit of radiotherapy is higher in patients who express a high baseline risk of recurrence. A meta-analysis of individual data from >10 000 women in 17 randomized trials yielded absolute risk reductions for local recurrence in patients without nodal involvement between <10 and >20% dependent on age, grade, oestrogen-receptor status, tamoxifen use, and extent of surgery. Corresponding reductions in the risk of breast cancer death varied between 0.1% and 8% [174].

The standard radiotherapy treatment schedule for whole breast irradiation consists of a total dose of 45 to 50 Gy to the whole breast with a dose per fraction of 1.8 to 2.0 Gy (conventional fractionation). The long-term experience described above is mainly based on conventionally fractionated schedules. Applying this schedule for whole breast radiotherapy is a safe and effective treatment. Recent clinical trials have established alternative fractionation schedules, namely hypofractionated radiotherapy for breast cancer treatment. Here, total doses of 40 to 42 Gy are applied with doses per fraction of 2.67 to 3.2 Gy. In randomized trials, hypofractionated radiotherapy has been shown to be equally effective as compared to conventional fractionation [177–179]. Hypofractionated irradiation schedules are based on the evidence of a relatively high fractionation sensitivity of breast cancer, i.e., a high recovery between irradiation fractions. Thus, applying fewer fractions with higher dose per fraction allows reduction of the total dose without affecting the tumour control probability. It has to be mentioned that this fractionation sensitivity of the surrounding normal tissues like lung, heart or soft tissue lies in the same range (α/β-value 3–4 Gy), so that the therapeutic window, i.e., the ratio between tumour control probability and risk of severe late toxicity, is not expected to be improved. Although there is sufficient evidence for an equal efficacy and toxicity of hypofractionated schedules for patients in lower risk groups, i.e., aged ≥50 years, disease stage pT1-2 pN0, patients who did not receive chemotherapy, and who were treated with a high radiation dose homogeneity [180], follow-up of the trials is still not long enough to safely conclude on very late toxicity, in particular cardiotoxicity. Caution is necessary when applying hypofractionated schedules to patient groups that were not adequately represented in the trials and that may have a different tumour biology like very young patients, patients with locally advanced tumours or patients with indications for regional radiotherapy [180]. Regarding regional radiotherapy, the possibly very high fractionation sensitivity of the neural tissue (plexus brachialis) has to be kept in mind [181, 182].

Boost to the tumour bed

Boosting the tumour bed by an additional dose of 16 Gy further improves local tumour control by another 40–50% in all age groups, without further improving survival. The absolute benefit is highest in young patients below the age of 40 (14% local recurrences instead of 24% within 10 years) [173]. Other studies with shorter follow-up have shown a similar efficacy when using 10 Gy as boost dose [183]. Between 10 and 26 Gy boost dose, no further increase in local tumour control could be documented in patients with microscopic residual tumour [184]. Boost application has become standard for patients with invasive breast cancer after breast conserving radiotherapy. However, as boost irradiation also increases fibrosis, definition of subgroups of patients with a very low absolute benefit from the boost application can be a helpful tool for clinical decisions [185].

Partial breast irradiation

Recent research strategies aim at lowering the risk of chronic side effects by reducing the irradiated volume. Several clinical trials were performed to compare standard whole breast irradiation with partial breast irradiation using external beam or brachytherapy approaches. So far, equal efficacy of both approaches is not proven for any patient group by results of large-scale randomized clinical trials. However, patients with very low risk of local recurrence may be the best candidates for partial breast irradiation [186, 180]. In contrast to the first publication [187], a recent update of a randomized trial has shown significantly more recurrences after intraoperative radiotherapy (IORT) by kV x-rays versus whole breast

Table 43.1 Published and ongoing clinical trials on partial breast irradiation

Protocol	Conventional arm	Experimental arm	Result	Remark
TARGIT	Adjuvant whole breast radiotherapy	IORT (kV X-rays)	LR 0.95% (whole breast) vs 1.2% (IORT) at 4 years, average follow up 2 years (ns)	14% of patients in the IORT arm received additional whole breast radiotherapy
ELIOT	Adjuvant whole breast radiotherapy	IORT (electrons)		Closed, data not finally published
IMPORT-LOW (UK)	Adjuvant hypofractionated whole breast radiotherapy	Adjuvant dose-modified whole breast radiotherapy or partial breast irradiation		Closed, awaiting results
RAPID/Ontario Clinical Oncology Group	Adjuvant hypo- or normofractionated whole breast radiotherapy vs	Adjuvant hypofractionated partial breast irradiation		Closed, awaiting results
NSABP-B-39, RTOG-0413, SWOG-NSABP-B-39, NCT00103181	Adjuvant whole breast radiotherapy	Adjuvant partial breast irradiation		Ongoing
CDR0000629768 ICR-IMPORT-LOW, ICR-CTSU/2006/10001, ISRCTN12852634, EU-20896, IMPORT LOW, NCT00814567	Adjuvant hypofractionated whole breast radiotherapy	Reduced whole breast or partial breast irradiation		Ongoing
ISRCTN 34086741, MREC No. 99/0307, UKCRN ID 7265, NCT00983684	Adjuvant whole breast radiotherapy	IORT (kV X-rays)		Ongoing
RTS02-SHARE AFSSAPS, NCT01247233	Adjuvant normo- or hypofractionated whole breast radiotherapy	Adjuvant Accelerated partial breast irradiation		Ongoing
GEC-ESTRO	Adjuvant whole breast radiotherapy	Adjuvant partial breast irradiation using interstitial brachytherapy		Ongoing

IORT, intraoperative radiotherapy; ns, not significant.

radiotherapy in low-risk patients, although the current difference of 2% is still below the predefined criteria for non-interiority [188]. Beside the still short follow-up (mean < 5years), interpretation of the data is limited mainly by the fact that some patients in the IORT arm got additional whole breast radiotherapy. The data of this trial are still in line with the improvement of local tumour control by 50% after adjuvant radiotherapy compared to no adjuvant radiotherapy [189, 190]. Although the dose distribution of electrons is much more favourable a as compared to low-energy photons, another randomized phase III trial on intraoperative partial breast irradiation using electrons compared to whole breast irradiation showed higher recurrence rates in the IORT arm (ELIOT, data presented, not published so far). Further randomized trials are ongoing (see Table 43.1).

Radiotherapy treatment planning and technique

For whole breast radiotherapy, the clinical target volume (CTV) consists of the whole gland of the breast. The boost CTV includes the surgical cavity, which should intraoperatively be marked with surgical clips (Figure 43.2A). Ideally, up to six clips (e.g., titanium) are placed at all margins of the surgical cavity and positions of the clips are described in the surgical report. Correct placement has to be checked by the radiation oncologist by comparing the planning-CT with information from pretreatment imaging and the

surgical report. Determining the boost volume without clips by the visible tissue changes after surgery and the pretreatment imaging information is especially error prone after oncoplastic surgery, in patients with a dense breast, or after a long time interval between surgery and radiotherapy.

Standard radiation treatment is a 3D-conformal, CT-planned radiotherapy (Figure 43.2B). Photon treatment technique consists of tangential fields including a modification for different body diameters (wedges or field-in-field). To prevent under- and over-dosage, often more than two fields are applied today (Figure 43.2B–E). For boost or partial breast radiotherapy, electron or multifield photon techniques are used or radiotherapy is applied by brachytherapy techniques. The latter is expected to be advantageous especially in patients with large breasts and deep seated tumours closed to organs at risk like heart or lung. Novel radiotherapy techniques that may in the future reduce late toxicity to the normal tissue include deep-inspiration breath hold radiotherapy for left-sided breast cancer, aiming to separate the heart from the target volume, thereby reducing the heart dose [191].

Radiotherapy after mastectomy

After mastectomy, radiotherapy of the chest wall is given to patients with a high risk of local or regional recurrence. Indications are a large primary tumour size, incomplete resection, or very close

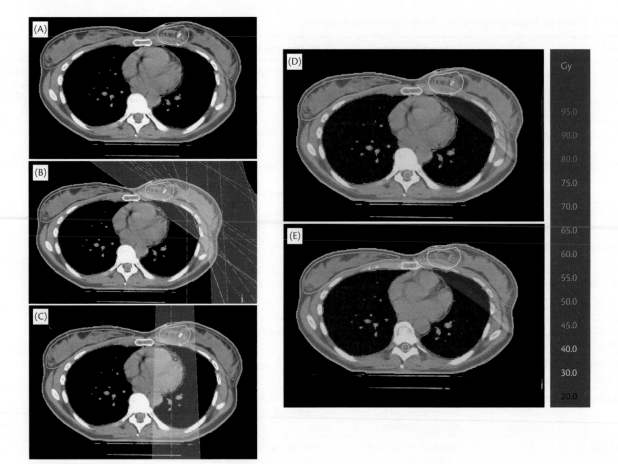

Fig. 43.2 Radiotherapy treatment planning and technique. (A) Contoured whole breast CTV/PTV (pink, orange), boost CTV/PTV (pink/yellow), and normal tissues (lungs, heart, left anterior descending artery, contralateral breast). A surgical clip is visible inside the boost CTV as well as a skin mark for the scar. In this case, no clear surgery-related tissue changes are visible, so that for the safety of the definition of the boost CTV the surgical clips are of high importance. (B) Tangential field arrangement for whole breast radiotherapy, here with nine fields coming four angles (field-in-field). (C) Single electron beam for boost irradiation. (D) Homogeneous dose distribution for whole breast irradiation. (E) Cumulative dose distribution for whole breast and boost irradiation.

surgical margins, or patients with four or more involved lymph nodes. However, also for patients at medium risk, i.e., with up to three positive lymph nodes, radiotherapy has been shown to improve loco-regional tumour control and should therefore be strongly considered [192, 193]. Subgroup analysis of the randomized DBCG 82 b&c trials revealed an even higher advantage for the group with up to three positive lymph nodes on survival as compared to the high-risk group with more than three lymph nodes, while both groups expressed a clearly lower loco-regional recurrence rate after post-mastectomy radiotherapy [194]. A likely reason is the lower risk of distant metastases in this group.

Radiotherapy to the chest wall is performed using conventional treatment schedules with a total dose of ~50 Gy and doses per fraction of 1.8 to 2 Gy. Hypofractionated schedules are not established for this indication, as this group of patients was underrepresented in the trials.

Radiotherapy treatment planning and technique

CTV is the soft tissue in the former area of the breast gland. The skin needs to be included if it was involved (e.g., inflammatory breast cancer or exulceration). Treatment technique is similar to the one applied to patients after breast-conserving radiotherapy. Electron beams can be used if feasible.

Regional radiotherapy

There are currently no randomized data with sufficient follow-up on the use of regional radiotherapy vs local radiotherapy alone. For patients with negative sentinel lymph node, the risk of regional recurrence is low and regional radiotherapy is therefore not recommended [192, 195, 196]. Regional radiotherapy of the supra/infra-clavicular region is recommended for patients with four or more involved axillary lymph nodes and should be strongly considered for patients with up to three involved lymph nodes [192]. Axillary radiotherapy is recommended if there was no adequate axillary surgery or if there is residual tumour in the axilla. Individual decisions for axillary radiotherapy may be made in cases of massive axillary involvement [197]. Internal mammary nodes are to be irradiated if they are clinically involved. For all other patients there is currently not enough evidence for a strong recommendation. Inclusion of clinically non-involved internal mammary nodes is controversial and not done on a routine basis, because late toxicity (especially heart in left-sided cancer) may be higher due to the depth of the irradiated volume and the clinical advantage is not proven so far. Randomized trials on this question have been performed or are underway, with final publications awaited within the next few years (CAN-NCIC-MA20 [NCT00005957], NCIC-CTG MA.20, EORTC

22922/10925). Early data from one randomized clinical trial support the use of regional radiotherapy at least for patients with risk factors [198].

Radiotherapy treatment planning and technique

CTV includes the lymph node areas that were not treated with axillary dissection by the surgeon previously, i.e., level III of the axilla, supra- and infraclavicular lymph node areas and, if indicated, internal mammary lymph nodes.

Male breast cancer

Because of the rarity of this disease, no randomized trials are available for radiotherapy of male breast cancer. As a mastectomy is usually the surgical treatment of choice, the indications for adjuvant radiotherapy as well as the techniques should be applied similarly to the post-mastectomy situation for females. Small datasets support the improvement of loco-regional tumour control when radiotherapy is applied in high-risk patients with positive lymph nodes, insufficient resection margins or locally advanced tumours [199, 200]. The use of alternative fractionation schedules cannot be recommended, as the biology of such tumours may be different and male patients were not included in the respective clinical trials.

Radiotherapy after neoadjuvant chemotherapy

As is done for patients receiving adjuvant chemotherapy, the tumour staging before chemotherapy, i.e., the initial clinical staging, needs to be considered for radiotherapy treatment decisions. The uncertainty of this staging can be reduced by performing the sentinel lymphadenectomy in patients without enlarged lymph nodes before the start of chemotherapy.

Ductal carcinoma in situ

The aim of radiotherapy in patients with ductal carcinoma in situ (DCIS) is to prevent local invasive or non-invasive recurrences. The relative rate of in-breast events (ipsilateral recurrence of DCIS or invasive breast cancer) is reduced on average by ~50% with radiotherapy [201, 202]. The absolute reduction is ~15% (28% without radiotherapy versus 13% with radiotherapy) [201]. This improvement is evident in all patient groups. By the nature of the disease, the reduction of ipsilateral in-breast events does not translate into a reduced rate of breast cancer death within 10 years of follow-up [201]. Radiotherapy is indicated in all patients after breast-conserving surgery. Exceptions include elderly patients and low-grade tumours with wide surgical margins, after discussion with the patient [203]. After mastectomy with sufficient surgical margins, there is no proof of an advantage from post-operative radiotherapy. Treatment fractionation, planning, and technique are similar to those applied for invasive breast cancer with the difference that there is no indication for boost irradiation.

Time interval between surgery and radiotherapy and sequencing of radiotherapy and systemic treatment modalities

Scheduling of radiotherapy and chemotherapy

If there is an indication for adjuvant chemotherapy and for radiotherapy, chemotherapy is mostly applied before radiotherapy. A simultaneous approach may slightly increase anti-tumour efficacy but also increases toxicity [204]. Comparing sequential schedules, there seems to be no major difference between the efficacy of adjuvant chemotherapy followed by radiotherapy or radiotherapy followed by chemotherapy [205]. However, prolonging the time interval between surgery and the start of radiotherapy can increase the risk of local recurrence, a factor that is especially important for higher-risk patients [206, 207]. The prolongation of the time interval before radiotherapy by the administration of adjuvant chemotherapy is in most cases justified, as for the respective patient group the risk of distant metastases is relatively high, calling for an early start of systemic treatment. If in individual patients the risk of local recurrence appears to be more important, radiotherapy can be performed before the start of chemotherapy.

Radiotherapy and anti-HER2 therapy

Simultaneous radiotherapy and trastuzumab does not seem to increase cardiac toxicity of trastuzumab in clinical trials and is therefore adopted in clinical practice for patients with HER2 amplified tumours [208]. However, whether very late radiation-induced cardiac toxicity is increased can only be clarified after long-term follow-up.

Radiotherapy and anti-hormonal treatment

Anti-hormonal treatment is started either during or after the end of radiotherapy. Both tamoxifen and aromatase inhibitors do not compromise tumour response to radiotherapy in vivo, but there is some evidence that tamoxifen can increase radiation-induced lung disease (RILD) [209, 210]. However, as the overall rates of symptomatic RILD are very low after breast cancer radiotherapy, this fact should not be seen as a contraindication for simultaneous application of both treatments. Instead, the therapeutic advantage has to be weighed against the potential risk of toxicity. Postponing the start of tamoxifen treatment should especially be discussed for patients with other risk factors for RILD, like a high radiation dose to the lung.

Radiotherapy of in-breast recurrences

Without pre-irradiation, the indications for radiotherapy are similar to the primary situation. After whole breast pre-irradiation, mastectomy is standard of care. Breast-conserving surgery followed by re-irradiation is not supported by prospective trials. However, there is experience from small series of patients where re-irradiation was performed as an individualized treatment in selected low-risk patients [211, 212, 213, 214, 215]. Such re-irradiation should be performed in experienced centres. It has to be considered that late toxicity, especially fibrosis and changes in breast appearance, is increased after re-irradiation. Radiotherapy should be preferentially performed as brachytherapy with the aim of reducing the non-involved irradiated volume. Also, external beam radiotherapy is possible, namely for tumours that are not suitable for brachytherapy.

Radiotherapy in the context of metastatic breast cancer

Palliative radiotherapy for multiple metastases

Palliative radiotherapy of distant metastases aims to reduce or prevent symptoms that affect quality of life without inducing a high risk of treatment-related toxicity. Typical indications are painful metastases, e.g., those affecting the skeleton, beginning or imminent paralysis through metastases of the spine, or brain metastases that are usually not sufficiently treated by systemic drugs. In all cases, short radiation treatment schedules between one and ten fractions are routinely used.

High-dose radiotherapy to single or oligo-metastases

In selected cases of distant metastases, high-dose radiotherapy may be indicated with the aim to inactivate the tumour manifestations. This applies to solitary or oligometastases appearing in patients in good overall condition who are expected to have a decent survival. Small metastases, e.g., in the brain, can be treated successfully by single-dose stereotactic radiotherapy (radiosurgery) with or without combined whole brain irradiation, a procedure that leads to similar local control rates as compared to surgery [216]. At other sites, e.g., solitary bone metastases, fractionated radiation treatment with doses of 50 Gy or higher as well as hypofractionated or single-dose stereotactic radiotherapy are used to induce a longer-term freedom of progression.

Acute toxicity of radiotherapy

Severe acute toxicity is a rare event in breast cancer radiotherapy, except in the context of a few known genetic diseases. Factors determining a relatively higher risk of toxicity are chemotherapy applied before or during radiotherapy, large breast size for skin reactions, or pre-existing cardiac diseases for cardiac side effects. The most frequent acute side effect is dermatitis within the irradiated area. Radiation pneumonitis is relatively frequent when radiographic changes are evaluated; however, only few patients (~1%) develop symptoms and therefore require treatment. Other rare events are esophagitis if supra/infraclavicular lymph nodes are irradiated or arrhythmia in patients with a previous medical history.

Late toxicity of radiotherapy

Fibrosis of the irradiated tissue is a common late toxicity after radiotherapy. After breast-conserving treatment, 15–30% of the patients develop fibrosis that impacts the cosmetic outcome. The likelihood increases with dose, boost application, infections, haematoma, and seroma after surgery. With modern techniques, teleangiectasia has become a rare event. Oedema of the breast often occurs transiently during irradiation. Chronically, oedema of the breast or arm can be caused by the sum of treatment, i.e., surgery and radiotherapy. The likelihood increases with the extent of treatment and is highest after axillary dissection followed by regional radiotherapy. Chronic fibrosis of the lung can develop from a pneumonitis; however, symptomatic chronic pneumopathy is a rare event. Cardiac side effects like myocardial fibrosis, sclerosis of the coronary vessels or cardiomyopathy are of importance especially for patients with a good prognosis and a long life expectancy. A measurable increase of the risk of cardiac-related death in the treated population occurs beyond 10–15 years [217]. Using modern techniques, the dose to the heart can today be considerably reduced in comparison to the one applied in patients for whom long-term follow-up data are available [217], however, more time is needed before one can prove reduction of late toxicity. Other rare late effects are osteoradionecrosis of the ribs or lesions of the plexus brachialis. Secondary cancers, e.g., of the contralateral breast, lung, oesophagus, or soft tissue, increase decades after radiotherapy, thus mainly affecting patients at younger age during radiotherapy. However, this risk is smaller than the survival benefit from radiotherapy [218].

Medical management of breast cancers

Four families of medical treatments have been shown to provide benefit in patients with breast cancer: (i) chemotherapy, (ii) endocrine therapy, (iii) targeted therapy, and (iv) bone-modifying agents. The primary aim of medical treatments for patients with non-metastatic breast cancers is to avoid metastatic relapse and eventually to cure patients. In the metastatic setting, the primary aim is to prolong survival while preserving quality of life. The major question for patients with breast cancer relates to the optimal definition of who should receive which treatment, and at which moment during the natural history of the disease.

Chemotherapy for breast cancer patients

Adjuvant and neoadjuvant chemotherapy

Adjuvant chemotherapy is defined as the post-operative administration of chemotherapy, while neoadjuvant chemotherapy is administered before the surgical procedure. A meta-analysis that included more than 100 000 women indicated that the administration of post-operative chemotherapy improves survival of patients with early breast cancer [219]. It is estimated that the administration of chemotherapy reduces the relative risk of mortality by about one-third. Although these numbers appear impressive, they must be interpreted in the context of absolute risks of death. As illustration, in the same meta-analysis, the average absolute gain in mortality was 5% for patients treated with a second-generation chemotherapy schedule as compared to no chemotherapy, suggesting that there is no or minimal benefit from chemotherapy for a significant number of patients.

The oncologist faces three sets of decisions in relation to chemotherapy: (i) Should my patient receive chemotherapy? (ii) Which regimen? (iii) Should the chemotherapy be given preoperatively?

Indications for adjuvant chemotherapy

To obtain benefit from adjuvant chemotherapy, a patient must present with both a significant risk of relapse and also to be sensitive to chemotherapy. The tumour staging (tumour size and lymph node involvement) and the standard pathological parameters (oestrogen receptor expression, tumour grade) remain important decision criteria. These parameters are integrated in the web-based tool Adjuvant! Online [220]. These criteria, that roughly evaluate tumour burden and aggressiveness, could represent the starting point to evaluate the risk of breast cancer death. Several tools have become recently available that improve the performance of Adjuvant! in evaluating which patient harbours a low risk of relapse and could therefore avoid adjuvant chemotherapy.

First, the use of molecular classification defined by immunohistochemistry (IHC) could allow the identification of a group of patients with very good prognosis. This classification includes expression oestrogen receptor (ER), status of human epidermal growth factor receptor-2 (HER2) and Ki67 determination [221]. Since HER2 overexpression has been shown to be associated with poor outcome in breast cancer patients [222] and could also define a subset of patients who are highly sensitive to chemotherapy [223, 224], it is therefore considered that HER2-overexpressing breast cancer patients with a tumour size above 5 mm should receive chemotherapy (<http://www.nccn.org/professionals/physician_gls/f_guidelines.asp#breast>, last accessed 23 April 2012). Patients with a triple negative breast cancer (absence of expression of ER and PgR and lack of overexpression of HER2 [225]) are also eligible for adjuvant chemotherapy [225, 226].

The controversies about who should receive adjuvant chemotherapy are mainly focused on patients with ER+/HER2-negative breast cancers. It has been proposed to divide this group of patients in two different categories (luminal A and luminal B) according to tumour grade and level of Ki67 expression. The luminal A breast cancers are characterised by low tumour grade and/or low Ki67 expression (<14% staining) and confer a better prognosis [227, 228, 229]. Immunohistochemistry could be used to identify patients with good prognosis if the other parameters do not indicate a large tumour burden. The problem here, however, resides in the poor standardization and evaluation of Ki67 staining (reviewed in [228]).

Genomic tests could also improve the prediction of outcome usually determined by clinical and pathological staging. Several genomic signatures have been developed to address this question (reviewed in [230]). The vast majority of these signatures only apply to patients with ER+/HER2-negative breast cancers. The recurrence score (Oncotype DX®) is a 21-gene signature assessed by RT-PCR on paraffin-embedded samples [231]. This signature has been consistently reported to identify a population of patients who presents a low risk of metastatic relapse [230]. Interestingly, this recurrence score has also been reported as predictor of the relative efficacy of chemotherapy in two retrospective studies [232, 233]. Two prospective studies are currently ongoing to evaluate the medical usefulness of the recurrence score (<http://www.clinicaltrials.gov>, NCT 00310180 and NCT01446185). The 70 genes signature from Amsterdam (Mammaprint©, Agendia) is the second most investigated gene signature for outcome prediction [230]. This signature has been validated in retrospective studies, and is currently being prospectively validated in the large randomized MINDACT trial [234]. Other gene signatures are being investigated, including the genomic grade (Mapquant®) and the breast cancer index [230].

Overall, considering the amount of consistent data obtained with samples from randomized trials, several national or international guidelines propose to include the recurrence score as a tool for decision about the indication of adjuvant chemotherapy (<http://www.nccn.org/professionals/physician_gls/f_guidelines.asp#breast>, last accessed 23 April 2012) [221].

The definite proof of the clinical utility of the various genomic signatures will hopefully emerge from the results of the already completed studies—mainly TailorX and MINDACT. These trials will generate greater confidence that a subgroup of women with ER positive, low proliferative tumours can be spared adjuvant chemotherapy. Additional molecular, non-genomic tests include UPA (Urokinase-type plasminogen activator)/PA1 assay [235]. This biomarker has been validated in a large meta-analysis and is now considered level I evidence for clinical use in several recommendations [236].

The other situation where chemotherapy could be spared is in the group of patients who present a significant risk of relapse, but whose tumours are resistant to treatment. Several attempts have been made in order to identify those patients whose tumours are insensitive to adjuvant chemotherapy. As mentioned before, the recurrence score has been suggested to be associated with resistance to chemotherapy in two small retrospective studies [232, 233]. Currently, though, the amount of evidence is not yet strong enough

to use these results in patients with a high risk of relapse. Ki67 has also been reported to be associated with resistance to treatment with docetaxel [237]. Nevertheless, other groups have found this biomarker as not predictive of benefit from CMF [238] and FAC [239] treatments. Overall, it is considered that, although its prognostic value is well documented, there is not enough data to consider Ki67 as a predictive biomarker for the resistance to adjuvant chemotherapy [229].

Which regimen should be used?

Chemotherapy schedules using anthracyclines, cyclophosphamide, and taxanes have been reported to improve outcome as compared to anthracycline-alone based chemotherapy [219]. Several different regimens are considered as optimal third generation chemotherapy. These include the sequential use of anthracyclines and cyclophosphamide, followed by three weekly docetaxel or weekly paclitaxel for a total of six to eight cycles [240]. Taxanes have been shown to be effective both in node-positive and node-negative [241] breast cancer.

Several other regimens have been evaluated. The administration of four cycles of docetaxel and cyclophosphamide was less effective than sequential use of anthracyclines and taxanes [242], but could be acceptable in selected cases where the absolute expected benefit from chemotherapy is low.

The concomitant use of anthracyclines, docetaxel, and cyclophosphamide seems to be more toxic than their sequential use. Finally, anthracycline-free regimens have shown good results in patients with HER2-overexpressing breast cancer [243].

When to use chemotherapy in the preoperative setting?

The use of neoadjuvant chemotherapy is usually recommended when a conservative surgery is not feasible and the tumour presents some features of chemosensitivity (ER-negativity, high grade, HER2 overexpression). The tumour shrinkage induced by chemotherapy allows breast conservation in a significant number of patients [244]. Several studies have compared the preoperative versus postoperative administration of chemotherapy and concluded that the timing of chemotherapy does not matter in terms of breast cancer mortality [245]. The residual disease after neoadjuvant chemotherapy is a robust prognostic indicator [246].

Chemotherapy in the metastatic setting

In the metastatic setting, the decision to administer chemotherapy, together with the choice of the drugs, is driven by the tumour biology (ER, HER2, grade), the resistance to the chemotherapy regimens administered in the adjuvant setting and the presence of symptoms that might require rapid tumour response. Overall, the recent guidelines recommend the use of chemotherapy as first-line treatment in patients with triple-negative breast cancer (TNBC) or in HER2-overexpressing breast cancer. In patients with ER-positive breast cancer, it is usual to administer endocrine therapy and to switch to chemotherapy at the acquisition of endocrine resistance. This rule does not apply for patients with aggressive ER-positive disease, for which cytotoxic regimens are used front line.

Both taxanes and anthracyclines have been shown to be effective in the metastatic setting [247, 248]. Nevertheless, their use is limited by the fact that most patients in Europe and the US have received these agents as adjuvant treatment. The use of these drugs is therefore limited to patients who present with stage IV disease at diagnosis or in case of long interval between adjuvant chemotherapy and metastatic relapse (at least two years).

A large number of cytotoxic agents have been shown to be active in patients with metastatic breast cancer previously treated with anthracyclines and taxanes [249]. Overall, current recommendations favour a sequential use of these drugs, with the exception of patients presenting with a very aggressive disease where a rapid response is required [250]. In these latter patients, a combination strategy could be indicated.

Capecitabine is approved in most of the countries and is a treatment of choice in patients who are resistant to anthracyclines and taxanes. Ixabepilone (Ixempra®, Bristol-Myers Squibb Company, Princeton, NJ) and nab-paclitaxel (Abraxane®, Abraxis Bioscience, Celgene Corporation, NJ) have been shown to improve progression-free survival in patients who are resistant to anthracyclines and taxanes [251, 252].

Until recently [253], there has not been any level I evidence that adding a new line of chemotherapy after two previous regimens was associated with survival improvement. Eribulin is the first agent shown to improve survival in patients previously treated with at least two different chemotherapy treatments in the metastatic setting [253].

Finally, other drugs are commonly used in this indication, including gemcitabine and vinorelbine [249].

A specific case is represented by cisplatin. Although there is no evidence that cisplatin improves outcome in patients with metastatic breast cancers, some data from small studies suggest that this drug could be effective in patients who present lack of BRCA1 function [254]. Ongoing randomized trials are evaluating this hypothesis.

Endocrine therapy

Adjuvant endocrine therapy

Endocrine therapy is the treatment of choice in patients with ER-positive tumours. A meta-analysis has shown that tamoxifen treatment when administered in the adjuvant setting could reduce the absolute risk of breast cancer death by around 10% [255]. This effect is observed specifically in patients with ER-expressing tumours. Based on the strong magnitude of the effect, it is recommended that endocrine therapy be given to all patients with invasive breast cancer that expresses ER.

The oncologist faces several additional questions in daily clinical practice. First: which endocrine therapy should be proposed? Second, what is the optimal duration for endocrine therapy?

As previously mentioned, tamoxifen is the cornerstone treatment in premenopausal women. In postmenopausal women, aromatase inhibitors have been shown to improve disease-free survival (DFS) as compared to tamoxifen in a meta-analysis. In the same meta-analysis, aromatase inhibitors marginally improved overall survival (absolute difference: 0.7%) [256, 257]. The BIG1.98 has explored whether letrozole should be administered frontline or after tamoxifen, and to what extent this drug can be safely switched to tamoxifen after two to three years. Results have shown that starting with aromatase inhibitors improves DFS as compared to starting with tamoxifen then switching to letrozole [257]. This effect was more pronounced in patients with node-positive disease. Interestingly, no difference was observed between five years of letrozole and two to three years of letrozole followed by tamoxifen. Overall, recent recommendations propose initial treatment in postmenopausal women with an aromatase inhibitor. If the treatment is not well tolerated, it is reasonable to propose a switch to tamoxifen after a two to three year exposure, especially if the risk of relapse is low.

The optimal duration of endocrine therapy is still in debate. This is due to the occurrence of late relapses in the population of patients with ER-positive breast cancer. Randomized trials have compared five to two years tamoxifen and could not provide evidence for an improved outcome [258]. One trial compared five years of tamoxifen followed by two to four years of letrozole to five years of tamoxifen alone and reported an improved outcome for the switch to letrozole, especially in node-positive disease [259]. For patients with low/intermediate risk recurrence, it seems reasonable today to propose a total of five years of endocrine therapy. For patients with high-risk breast cancer, the optimal duration is a matter of controversies, but there is an increased trend for using seven to ten years of endocrine therapy in this latter population.

Endocrine therapy for metastatic breast cancer patients

It is usually recommended to treat metastatic ER-positive breast cancer patients first with endocrine therapy. However, in some patients presenting with significant visceral involvement and/or highly aggressive disease, the treatment should start with chemotherapy.

Two different situations are being faced in the clinical practice. On one hand there are patients who are endocrine-naïve (stage IV) or relapse a long time after the end of adjuvant endocrine therapy. On the other hand, another group of patients will present a metastatic relapse while being treated with endocrine therapy in the adjuvant setting. For postmenopausal women, endocrine-naive (or long-term relapse) patients, there is a large body of evidence suggesting that aromatase inhibitors (AI) improve outcome as compared to tamoxifen in the metastatic setting [260]. After failure of a first line of endocrine therapy, it is usual, to start a second-line endocrine therapy especially in those patients who experienced prolonged (>12 months) disease control under first-line hormonal treatment. Several options are available in postmenopausal, metastatic breast cancer resistant to non-steroidal AI. The first one is the use of the steroidal AI, exemestane [261]. However, a more recent large trial [262] suggests that this approach is suboptimal. The second option is the use of fulvestrant. Initially, low-dose fulvestrant did not show benefit over exemestane in patients who present with non-steroidal aromatase inhibitor failure [263]. Nevertheless, recent data suggest that high-dose fulvestrant (500 mg/month) is more effective than the lower dose used in previous studies (250mg/month) [264, 265].

Overall, for patients who present with an endocrine sensitive disease defined by ER-positivity combined with a low aggressiveness, a sequential use of endocrine therapies is recommended before concluding about endocrine resistance and switching to chemotherapy.

Targeted agents

Four families of targeted agents have shown efficacy in patients with breast cancer. They include HER2-inhibitors, mTOR (mammalian target of rapamicin) inhibitors, angiogenesis inhibitors and Poly (adenosine diphosphate-ribose) polymerases (PARP) inhibitors.

HER2-inhibitors

HER2 is a transmembrane tyrosine kinase receptor encoded by the ERBB2 gene that mediates oncogenesis. Around 10–15% of breast cancer present with an amplification of ERBB2 that leads to HER2 receptor overexpression. Trastuzumab (Herceptin®, Genentech Inc, South San Francisco, CA) is a monoclonal antibody that targets HER2. Trastuzumab, in combination with chemotherapy, has been shown to improve survival in two randomized trials that included patients with metastatic, HER2-overexpressing breast cancer [266, 267]. Given these two pivotal trials, trastuzumab is considered as the cornerstone treatment of patients with HER2-positive breast cancer. Since HER2-overexpressing breast cancers present aggressive features, it is usually recommended to use trastuzumab in combination with chemotherapy (except anthracyclines). Nevertheless, several studies have shown that HER2 inhibitors can improve outcome when combined with endocrine therapy in the small subset of patients presenting HER2-overexpressing breast cancer without aggressive features [268, 269].

Six randomized trials have evaluated the efficacy of trastuzumab in the adjuvant setting [270]. All but one have concluded that the addition of trastuzumab to standard treatment is associated with improved outcome. Trastuzumab is therefore recommended in all HER2-over-expressing breast cancer patients presenting with a tumour size above 5 mm. Several questions remain open regarding the optimal use of adjuvant trastuzumab: (i) should trastuzumab be used concomitantly or sequentially with chemotherapy, and (ii) what is the optimal duration of trastuzumab?

The randomized trial NCCTG N9831 compared trastuzumab administered concomitantly with taxanes versus a sequential administration of trastuzumab [271]. This trial has reported that the concomitant administration of trastuzumab and taxanes was superior to sequential use. Based on this study, and some other indirect arguments [270], oncologists favour the administration of trastuzumab concomitantly with chemotherapy but formal statistical significance has not been tested.

Although most of the trials reported to date have evaluated a one year administration, there is controversy about whether shorter duration could be as effective as long duration. This originated from a small Finnish trial showing that shorter treatment could improve outcome. Several clinical trials are currently addressing the hypothesis that trastuzumab could safely be administered for a shorter period of time [272]. Only one trial—the HERA trial—has evaluated a longer administration of trastuzumab [273] (e.g., two years). Until the results of these comparisons become available, the actual recommendation is to administer adjuvant trastuzumab for one year.

More recently, combinations of HER2 inhibitors have been developed:

- Lapatinib is a tyrosine kinase inhibitor targeting HER2 and EGFR. This drug has been shown to improve progression-free survival when used in combination with capecitabine [274], in trastuzumab-resistant patients. Interestingly, the combination between lapatinib and trastuzumab has been shown to improve efficacy endpoints both in the neoadjuvant [275] and in the metastatic setting [276]. This combination is being evaluated in the large ALTTO trial in the adjuvant setting (<http://www.clinical-trials.gov>, NCT00490139).

- Pertuzumab (Omnitarg®, 2C4, Genentech, San Francisco, CA) is a monoclonal antibody that inhibits heterodimerization between HER2 and HER3. The concomitant administration of pertuzumab and trastuzumab has been shown to improve outcome in the context of a phase III randomized trial in the metastatic

setting [277]. These results confirmed previous findings from a phase II randomized trial performed in the neoadjuvant setting [278].

- Finally, other new compounds are being developed in order to improve efficacy over trastuzumab. As illustration, several phase II trials have suggested that TDM1 (trastuzumab-emtansine, Genentech, San Francisco, CA) an immunoconjugate between trastuzumab and emtansine (cytotoxic anti-microtubule agent) could reverse resistance to trastuzumab [279].

Other targeted agents

The development of new targeted agents is the focus of most of the current efforts in the breast cancer field. mTOR inhibitors have been developed with the aim of reversing the resistance to conventional treatment (endocrine therapy and trastuzumab). mTOR is a serine threonine kinase that mediates protein translation, metabolism and that induces phosphorylation of oestrogen receptor [280]. Several mTOR inhibitors are being developed in the field of breast cancer. Everolimus, a rapalog, has been shown to markedly improve progression-free survival in patients with ER-positive metastatic breast cancer who are resistant to NSAI [262]. This finding is consistent with two previous phase II randomized trials [278, 281] and opens new avenues in the field of targeted agents for ER-positive breast cancer.

Several others targeted agents have been assessed in breast cancer including bevacizumab and PARP inhibitors. Bevacizumab has been associated with improved outcomes in randomized trials [282]. Nevertheless, the magnitude of this efficacy was modest in most trials and no impact on overall survival was observed even in a pooled analysis of the randomized clinical trials. New research on biomarkers could allow the identification of the small subset of patients who derive clear benefit from this drug [283].

PARP1 is a protein involved in DNA repair. Preclinical studies have shown that PARP inhibition could lead to tumour cell death when BRCA1 or 2 is deficient [284]. In a phase II trial [285], the PARP1 inhibitor olaparib has shown major clinical efficacy in patients with BRCA1/2 mutations. Nevertheless, whether this drug improves outcome as compared to the standard of care still needs to be determined.

Bone-modifying agents

Zoledronic acid is a bisphosphonate that has initially been suggested to reduce the incidence of skeletal-related events (SRE) in patients with metastatic breast cancer with bone lesions [286]. The drug has then been developed in patients with early breast cancer. In this setting, zoledronic acid decreases the incidence of osteoporosis both during treatment with aromatase inhibitors [287] and after chemotherapy [288] (premenopausal women). Interestingly, in one trial, zoledronic acid has also been shown to improve DFS [289]. These latter data still need confirmation since results are not consistent across trials [290, 291].

More recently, antibodies directed against RANK ligands (denosumab) have been developed. One study suggests that denosumab could delay the onset of SRE as compared to zoledronic acid in patients with metastatic breast cancer [292]. This drug is now being evaluated in the adjuvant setting (D-CARE trial).

Overall, ASCO recommends the use of bone-modifying agents in patients with metastatic breast cancer with bone lesions [293]. Nevertheless, these guidelines do not make a recommendation between zoledronic acid and denosumab. Finally, more data, including biomarkers, are needed to have a clearer picture of the efficacy of bone-modifying agents in early breast cancer.

Summary of medical management of chemotherapy

The implementation of adjuvant chemotherapy and endocrine therapy has led to a dramatic improvement of breast cancer survival in the last three decades. In recent years, the most striking advance has been the development of trastuzumab along with efforts directed at high quality HER2 testing in order to select the right patients for this targeted therapy. The next decade will certainly be dedicated to the development of new targeted agents and their companion diagnostic tests with the aim of improving survival, and decreasing side effects of current conventional treatments.

Multidisciplinary management of complex cases

Clinical case study 1

In a small hospital, a 63-year-old postmenopausal patient was treated for an infiltrating ductal cancer of the left breast.

Tumour characteristics were as follows:

- Size: 1.7 cm
- Pathology: poorly differentiated (grade 3)
- ER: 0% cells positive
- PR: 0% cells positive
- HER2: IHC 1+ out of 3+
- Axillary nodes: 1/15 positive

She was initially treated with a lumpectomy, axillary lymphadenectomy, FEC-100 × 6 cycles, and radiation therapy.

Two and a half years later, she began complaining of fatigue. Her ECOG performance status was 1. A CT of the abdomen showed three nodules (less than 2 cm in size) in the liver. All other workup exams were normal.

The patient sought a second opinion.

> **What would you propose as the next step?**
> 1. A systemic treatment?
> 2. A liver biopsy?
> 3. Other?

Discussion—clinical case study 1

For over 30 years, researchers have investigated the extent to which expression of tumour receptors in the primary tumour are consistent with those in metastases, due to possible implications in clinical practice [294].

A meta-analysis of 62 studies comparing HER2 expression in matched primary and distant metastatic tumours estimated a discordance of 23% (95% CI 16–28%) between negative HER2 in the primary tumours to positive HER2 in the metastases. The discordance from positive HER2 in the primary tumours to negative HER2 in the metastases was 4% (95% CI 0–6%). This study reveals that if no biopsy of the metastatic site is done, nearly a quarter of patients may be denied the benefit of a HER2-targeted therapy [295].

Optimal testing for HER2 and HR remains challenging across different laboratories, as shown in a large clinical trial with central pathology review. Discordances are seen in up 12.1% of the cases for ER and 14.5% for HER2 [296]. There is, therefore, a rational for retesting the receptor expression in the present case. Biopsies of metastatic sites can provide valuable information for making treatment decisions; therefore, it is recommended to biopsy such sites if feasible and safe.

Follow-up—clinical case study 1

The patient underwent a liver biopsy. Her pathology revealed adenocarcinoma with the receptor expression as follows:

ER7/8, PgR-negative

HER2+++, FISH+

> **What treatment regimen would you have recommended to this patient?**
> 1. Trastuzumab + taxane or vinorelbine
> 2. Lapatinib + taxane
> 3. Docetaxel + trastuzumab + bevacizumab
> 4. Trastuzumab + pertuzumab + docetaxel
> 5. Letrozole + lapatinib
> 6. A clinical trial (with an investigational anti-HER2 therapy)
> 7. Other options

Treatment—clinical case study 1

An increasing body of evidence from clinical trials conducted in the neoadjuvant and metastatic settings suggests that dual HER2 blockade offers a significant advantage over single blockade for patients whose tumours overexpress the HER2 receptor.

In the neoadjuvant setting, a recent study of trastuzumab combined with lapatinib showed such benefit. The NeoALTTO trial randomized 455 patients to receive, prior to surgery, either trastuzumab, lapatinib, or the combination of both drugs, with weekly paclitaxel in all three study arms. The rate of pathological complete response (pCR) was 51.3% for the combination, 29.5% for trastuzumab alone, and 24.7% for lapatinib alone [297]. The NeoSphere trial randomized 417 patients to four treatment arms to receive preoperative trastuzumab and docetaxel, pertuzumab and docetaxel, the combination of trastuzumab and pertuzumab without cytotoxic chemotherapy, or the combination with docetaxel. Patients receiving the combination of pertuzumab and trastuzumab with docetaxel showed significant improvement in the pCR rate (45.8%) when compared to those who received trastuzumab plus docetaxel (29%), pertuzumab plus docetaxel (24%), or pertuzumab plus trastuzumab (17%) [298].

In the metastatic setting, Blackwell et al. tested the combination of lapatinib and trastuzumab in patients whose cancer progressed after a trastuzumab-containing treatment. The 296 patients included in the study had previously received a median of three trastuzumab-containing regimens. They were randomized to receive either lapatinib alone or trastuzumab combined with lapatinib. Patients receiving the combination had a superior median progression-free survival (12 weeks vs 8.1 weeks) and showed a trend towards better overall survival (51.6 weeks vs 39 weeks, HR = 0.75; CI 0.53 to 1.07; p = .106); however, their treatment was associated with a moderate increase of toxicity [299].

In another study for advanced breast cancer, CLEOPATRA, a dual HER2 blockade with pertuzumab and trastuzumab plus docetaxel was tested against trastuzumab, docetaxel and placebo, in the first-line metastatic setting. A clinically and statistically significant improvement of six months was observed in patients receiving the dual blockade (18.5 months vs 12.4 months). The cardiac safety profile was similar for both regimens, an increase of grade 3 neutropenia and diarrhea was observed in the dual HER2 blockade arm. There was a trend towards improved overall survival for patients receiving the dual blockade, but this analysis is still immature and requires more events [300]. In the light of these data, we consider that the combination of pertuzumab and trastuzumab with docetaxel is likely to become the reference first-line treatment for patients with HER2-positive metastatic breast cancer.

Another acceptable approach is to propose a clinical trial testing novel anti-HER2 drugs or their combinations. Trastuzumab-emtansine (TDM1) is an antibody drug conjugate that consists of a potent cytotoxic drug inhibiting microtubule polymerization coupled with trastuzumab [301]. In preclinical models exploring resistance to trastuzumab and lapatinib, TDM1 was shown to have antitumour activity [302, 303]. Trials testing the effectiveness of this target cytotoxic alone and in combination with pertuzumab are already in phase 3 (NCT00829166, NCT01419197, NCT01120184).

Treatment follow-up—clinical case study 1

With pertuzumab and trastuzumab given as 'maintenance' therapy, the patient enjoyed a long period of disease control (14 months). Upon complaint of a slight persistent headache, however, a brain MRI was performed and revealed two small brain lesions (3 and 4 mm).

What would you have recommended to the patient at this point in time?

1. Whole brain radiotherapy
2. Stereotaxic radiosurgery (Gamma Knife®)
3. Capecitabine + lapatinib

Whole brain radiotherapy (WBRT) is an effective treatment modality for controlling symptoms and improving survival in breast cancer patients with brain metastasis [304, 305]. However, it is associated with late neurological toxicity, leading to decreased neurocognitive function and quality of life [306].

An alternative to WBRT for patients with small lesions in the brain is stereotaxic radiosurgery (SRS), the so-called Gamma Knife®. It delivers a limited number of high-dose beams to a specific region of the brain, sparing normal cerebral tissue from radiation and, thereby, reducing neurologic toxicity [307]. There are no prospective data available comparing the efficacy of WBRT to SRS; however, retrospective studies suggest an improvement in outcome in favour of SRS alone [308, 309]. In retrospective and uncontrolled studies, SRS seems to be as effective as brain surgery with respect to metastasis control rate and survival [310, 311]. The addition of WBRT after definitive SRS was tested in a prospective study including multiple tumour types. Although it reduced the number of local relapses, the addition of WBRT failed to improve performance status and overall survival [312]. If a radiotherapeutic approach is chosen, SRS without WBRT is generally recommended.

For patients with HER2-positive breast cancer, an alternative is to start the treatment of brain metastases by administering lapatinib combined with capecitabine, postponing the radiotherapy approach. A single-arm phase II study evaluated this combination as upfront treatment before WBRT. 90% of the women included in the study had been previously treated with trastuzumab and more than 90% had PS 0 or 1 with minimal symptoms. In the preliminary analysis, progression-free survival was 5.5 months, and the time elapsed prior to WBRT was 8.3 months [305]. This treatment option makes it possible to delay brain irradiation and its adverse effects in a selected group of patients.

For HER2-positive disease treated with SRS where the systemic disease is under control with use of chemotherapy and a monoclonal antibody such as trastuzumab, it is recommended to continue with this same treatment. Monoclonal antibodies and most of the cytotoxic agents cannot pass through the intact blood-brain barrier. In the absence of systemic progression, it is likely that the treatment is still active against the disease elsewhere in the body.

Final remarks

Clinical cases illustrate some of the challenges of breast cancer management in daily practice. Each patient's case is unique, and the main objective of the attending multidisciplinary team is to offer the best possible treatment based on the best scientific data available and to always examine all suitable treatment modalities for each specific situation, whether clinical, surgical, or radiotherapeutic. However, there are situations for which strong evidence-based data is not available (and perhaps never will be). In these situations, good clinical judgment is crucial.

Online materials

Additional online materials for this chapter are available online at http://www.oxfordmedicine.com.

Further reading

Collaborative Group on Hormonal Factors in Breast Cancer. Menarche, menopause and breast cancer risk: individual participant meta-analysis including 118964 women with breast cancer from 117 epidemiological studies. Lancet Oncology 2012; 13: 1141–1151.

Collaborative Group on Hormonal Factors in Breast Cancer. Breast cancer and breastfeeding: collaborative reanalysis of individual data from 47 epidemiological studies in 30 countries, including 50302 women with breast cancer and 96973 women without the disease. Lancet 2002; 360(9328): 187–195.

Collaborative Group on Hormonal Factors in Breast Cancer. Breast cancer and hormonal contraceptives: collaborative reanalysis of individual data on 53 297 women with breast cancer and 100 239 women without breast cancer from 54 epidemiological studies. Lancet 1996; 347(9017): 1713–1727.

Collaborative Group on Hormonal Factors in Breast Cancer. Alcohol, tobacco and breast cancer—collaborative reanalysis of individual data from 53 epidemiological studies, including 58,515 women with breast cancer and 95,067 women without the disease. British Journal of Cancer 2002; 87(11): 1234–1245.

The Collaborative Group on Hormonal Factors in Breast Cancer. Familial Breast Cancer: collaborative reanalysis of individual data from 52 epidemiological studies including 58209 women with breast cancer and 101986 women without the disease. Lancet 2001; 358: 1389–1399.

Sotiriou C, Pusztai L. Gene-expression signatures in breast cancer. New England Journal of Medicine 2009; 360(8): 790–800.

Sotiriou C, Piccart MJ. Taking gene-expression profiling to the clinic: when will molecular signatures become relevant to patient care? Nature Reviews Cancer 2007; 7(7): 545–53.

Haibe-Kains B, Desmedt C, Loi S, Culhane AC, Bontempi G et al. A three-gene model to robustly identify breast cancer molecular subtypes. Journal of the National Cancer Institute 2012; 104(4): 311–25.

Curtis C, Shah SP, Chin S-F, Turashvili G, Rueda OM et al. The genomic and transcriptomic architecture of 2,000 breast tumours reveals novel subgroups. Nature [Online]. 18 April 2012 [cited 23 April 2012]. Available from: <http://www.nature.com/doifinder/10.1038/nature10983>.

Shah SP, Morin RD, Khattra J, Prentice L, Pugh T et al. Mutational evolution in a lobular breast tumour profiled at single nucleotide resolution. Nature 2009; 461(7265): 809–813.

Stephens PJ, McBride DJ, Lin M-L, Varela I, Pleasance ED et al. Complex landscapes of somatic rearrangement in human breast cancer genomes. Nature 2009; 462(7276): 1005–1010.

Ding L, Ellis MJ, Li S, Larson DE, Chen K et al. Genome remodelling in a basal-like breast cancer metastasis and xenograft. Nature 2010; 464(7291): 999–1005.

Desmedt C, Haibe-Kains B, Wirapati P, Buyse M, Larsimont D et al. Biological processes associated with breast cancer clinical outcome depend on the molecular subtypes. Clinical Cancer Research 2008; 14(16): 5158–5165.

Wirapati P, Sotiriou C, Kunkel S, Farmer P, Pradervand S et al. Meta-analysis of gene expression profiles in breast cancer: toward a unified understanding of breast cancer subtyping and prognosis signatures. Breast Cancer Research 2008; 10(4): R65.

Iwamoto T, Bianchini G, Booser D, Qi Y, Coutant C et al. Gene pathways associated with prognosis and chemotherapy sensitivity in molecular subtypes of breast cancer. Journal of the National Cancer Institute 2011; 103(3): 264–272.

Parker JS, Mullins M, Cheang MC, et al. Supervised risk predictor of breast cancer based on intrinsic subtypes. Journal of Clinical Oncology 2009; 27: 1160–1167.

Nielsen TO, Parker JS, Leung S et al. A comparison of PAM50 intrinsic subtyping with immunohistochemistry and clinical prognostic factors in tamoxifen-treated estrogen receptor-positive breast cancer. Clinical Cancer Research 2010; 16: 5222–5232.

Hugh J, Hanson J, Cheang MC et al. Breast cancer subtypes and response to docetaxel in node-positive breast cancer: use of an immunohistochemical definition in the BCIRG 001 trial. Journal of Clincal Oncology 2009; 27: 1168–1176.

Hammond ME, Hayes DF, Dowsett M et al. American Society of Clinical Oncology/College of American Pathologists guideline recommendations for immunohistochemical testing of estrogen and progesterone receptors in breast cancer. Journal of Clinical Oncology 2010; 28: 2784–2795.

Colleoni M, Bagnardi V, Rotmensz N, et al. Increasing steroid hormone receptors expression defines breast cancer subtypes non responsive to preoperative chemotherapy. Breast Cancer Research and Treatment 2009; 116: 359–369.

de Azambuja E, Cardoso F, de Castro G Jr, Colozza M, Mano MS et al. Ki-67 as prognostic marker in early breast cancer: a meta-analysis of published studies involving 12 155 patients. British Journal of Cancer 2007; 96: 1504–1513.

Dowsett M, Nielsen TO, Ahern R, et al. Assessment of Ki67 in Breast Cancer: recommendations from the International Ki67 in Breast Cancer Working Group. Journal of the National Cancer Institute 2011; 103: 1656–1664.

Ho A, Morrow M. The evolution of the locoregional therapy of breast cancer. Oncologist 2011; 16(10): 1367–1379.

Dunne C, Burke JP, Morrow M, Kell MR. Effect of margin status on local recurrence after breast conservation and radiation therapy for ductal carcinoma in situ. Journal of Clinical Oncology 2009; 27(10): 1615–1620.

Early Breast Cancer Trialists' Collaborative Group (EBCTCG), Darby S, McGale P, Correa C, et al. Effect of radiotherapy after breast-conserving surgery on 10-year recurrence and 15-year breast cancer death: meta-analysis of individual patient data for 10,801 women in 17 randomised trials. Lancet 2011; 378(9804): 1707–1716.

Litiere S, Werutsky G, Fentiman IS, et al. Breast conserving therapy versus mastectomy for stage I-II breast cancer: 20 year follow-up of the EORTC 10801 phase 3 randomised trial. Lancet Oncology 2012; 13(4): 412–419.

Sardanelli F, Boetes C, Borisch B, et al. Magnetic resonance imaging of the breast: recommendations from the EUSOMA working group. European Journal of Cancer 2010; 46(8): 1296–1316.

Krag DN, Anderson SJ, Julian TB et al. Sentinel-lymph-node resection compared with conventional axillary-lymph-node dissection in clinically node-negative patients with breast cancer: overall survival findings from the NSABP B-32 randomised phase 3 trial. Lancet Oncology 2010; 11(10): 927–933.

Giuliano AE, McCall L, Beitsch P et al. Locoregional recurrence after sentinel lymph node dissection with or without axillary dissection in patients with sentinel lymph node metastases: the American College of Surgeons Oncology Group Z0011 randomized trial. Annals of Surgery 2010; 252(3): 426–432.

Mieog JS, van der Hage JA, van de Velde CJ. Neoadjuvant chemotherapy for operable breast cancer. British Journal of Surgery 2007; 94(10): 1189–1200.

Kaufmann M, von Minckwitz G, Mamounas EP, et al. Recommendations from an international consensus conference on the current status and future of neoadjuvant systemic therapy in primary breast cancer. Annals of Surgical Oncology 2012; 19(5): 1508–1516.

Bartelink H, Horiot JC, Poortmans PM, et al. Impact of a higher radiation dose on local control and survival in breast-conserving therapy of early breast cancer: 10-year results of the randomized boost versus no boost EORTC 22881-10882 trial. Journal of Clinical Oncology 2007; 25: 3259–3265.

Correa C, McGale P, Taylor C, et al. Overview of the randomized trials of radiotherapy in ductal carcinoma in situ of the breast. Journal of the National Cancer Institute Monograph 2010: 162–177.

Darby S, McGale P, Correa C, et al. Effect of radiotherapy after breast-conserving surgery on 10-year recurrence and 15-year breast cancer death: meta-analysis of individual patient data for 10,801 women in 17 randomised trials. Lancet 2011; 378: 1707–1716.

Kyndi M, Overgaard M, Nielsen HM, Sorensen FB, Knudsen H et al. High local recurrence risk is not associated with large survival reduction after postmastectomy radiotherapy in high-risk breast cancer: a subgroup analysis of DBCG 82 b&c. Radiotherapy Oncology 2009; 90: 74–79.

Peto R, Davies C, Godwin J, Gray R, Pan HC et al. Comparisons between different polychemotherapy regimens for early breast cancer: meta-analyses of long-term outcome among 100,000 women in 123 randomised trials. Lancet 2012; 379: 432–444.

Paik S, Shak S, Tang G, Kim C, Baker J et al. A multigene assay to predict recurrence of tamoxifen-treated, node-negative breast cancer. New England Journal of Medicine 2004; 351: 2817–2826.

Martin M, Segui MA, Anton A, Ruiz A, Ramos M et al. Adjuvant docetaxel for high-risk, node-negative breast cancer. New England Journal of Medicine 2010; 363: 2200–2210.

Yin W, Jiang Y, Shen Z, Shao Z, Lu J. Trastuzumab in the adjuvant treatment of HER2-positive early breast cancer patients: a meta-analysis of published randomized controlled trials. PLoS One 2011; 6: e21030.

Curigliano G et al. Should liver metastases of breast cancer be biopsied to improve treatment choice? Annals of Oncology 2011; 22: 2227–2233.

Amir E et al. Prospective study evaluating the impact of tissue confirmation of metastatic disease in patients with breast cancer. Journal of Clinical Oncology 2012; 30: 587–592.

Curigliano G. New drugs for breast cancer subtypes: targeting driver pathways to overcome resistance. Cancer Treatment Reviews 2012: 38: 303–310.

Wilcken N, Hornbuckle J, Ghersi D. Chemotherapy alone versus endocrine therapy alone for metastatic breast cancer. Cochrane Database Systematic Reviews CD002747, 2003. doi:10.1002/14651858. CD002747

Boccardo F et al. Ovarian ablation versus goserelin with or without tamoxifen in pre-perimenopausal patients with advanced breast cancer: results of a multicentric Italian study. Annals of Oncology 1994; 5: 337–342.

Klijn JG et al. Combined treatment with buserelin and tamoxifen in premenopausal metastatic breast cancer: a randomized study. Journal of the National Cancer Institute 2000; 92: 903–911.

Perou CM et al. Molecular portraits of human breast tumours. Nature 2000; 406: 747–752.

Brennan MJ, Donegan WL, Appleby DE. The variability of estrogen receptors in metastatic breast cancer. American Journal of Surgery 1979; 137: 260–262.

Richter S, Zandvakili A. Meta Analysis of Discordant HER2 Status in Matched Primary and Metastatic Breast Cancer. SABCS 2011 PD05-05,

McCullough A et al. Abstract P3-10-36: Concordance of HER2 Central Assessment by Two International Central Laboratories: a Ring Study within the Framework of the Adjuvant HER2-Positive ALTTO Trial (BIG2-06/N063D/EGF106708). Cancer Research 2011; 70: P3-10-36–P3-10-36.

References

1. Globocan 2008. *Breast Cancer Incidence and Mortality Worldwide in 2008: Summary.* IARC.Section of Cancer Information (27/4/10).

2. Collaborative Group on Hormonal Factors in Breast Cancer. Menarche, menopause and breast cancer risk: individual participant meta-analysis including 118964 women with breast cancer from 117 epidemiological studies. Lancet Oncology 2012; 13: 1141–1151.

3. Collaborative Group on Hormonal Factors in Breast Cancer. Breast cancer and breastfeeding: collaborative reanalysis of individual data from 47 epidemiological studies in 30 countries, including 50302 women with breast cancer and 96973 women without the disease. Lancet 2002; 360(9328): 187–195.

4. Beral V, Bull D, Doll R, Peto R, Reeves G, Collaborative Group on Hormonal Factors in Breast Cancer. Breast cancer and abortion: collaborative reanalysis of data from 53 epidemiological studies, including 83000 women with breast cancer from 16 countries. Lancet 2004; 363(9414): 1007–1016.

5. Collaborative Group on Hormonal Factors in Breast Cancer. Breast cancer and hormonal contraceptives: collaborative reanalysis of individual data on 53 297 women with breast cancer and 100 239 women without breast cancer from 54 epidemiological studies. Lancet 1996; 347(9017): 1713–1727.

6. The Million Women Study Collaborators. Breast cancer and hormone replacement therapy in the Million Women Study. Lancet 2003; 362: 419–427.

7. Cancer Research UK. Breast Cancer Incidence Statistics. <http://www.infocancerresearchukorg. 2009>.

8. Key T, Appleby P, Barnes I, Reeves G. Endogenous sex hormones and breast cancer in postmenopausal women: reanalysis of nine prospective studies. Journal of the National Cancer Institute 2002; 94: 606–616.

9. Green J, Cairns BJ, Cassabonne D, Wright FL, Reeves G et al. Height and cancer incidence in the Milllion Women Study: prospective cohort, and meta-analysis of prospective studies for height and total cancer risk. Lancet Oncology 2011; 12(8): 785–794.

10. Travis R, Allen N, Appleby P, Spencer E, Roddam A et al. Prospective study of vegetarianism and isoflavone intake in relation to breast cancer risk in British women. International Journal of Cancer 2007; 122: 705–710.

11. Key T, Appleby P, Rosell M. Health effects of vegetarian and vegan diets. Proceedings of the Nutrition Society 2006; 65: 35–41.

12. Collaborative Group on Hormonal Factors in Breast Cancer. Alcohol, tobacco and breast cancer—collaborative reanalysis of individual data from 53 epidemiological studies, including 58,515 women with breast cancer and 95,067 women without the disease. British Journal of Cancer 2002; 87(11): 1234–1245.

13. Peto J, Collins N, Barfoot R, Seal S, Warren W et al. Prevalence of BRCA1 and BRCA2 gene mutations in patients with early-onset breast cancer. Journal of the National Cancer Institute 1999; 91(11): 943–949.

14. Key T, Verkasalo P, Banks E. Epidemiology of breast cancer. Lancet Oncology 2001; 2: 133–140.

15. The Collaborative Group on Hormonal Factors in Breast Cancer. Familial Breast Cancer: collaborative reanalysis of individual data from 52 epidemiological studies including 58209 women with breast cancer and 101986 women without the disease. Lancet 2001; 358: 1389–1399.

16. Nowell PC. The clonal evolution of tumor cell populations. Science 1976; 194(4260): 23–28.

17. Sotiriou C, Pusztai L. Gene-expression signatures in breast cancer. New England Journal of Medicine 2009; 360(8): 790–800.

18. Sotiriou C, Piccart MJ. Taking gene-expression profiling to the clinic: when will molecular signatures become relevant to patient care? Nature Reviews Cancer 2007; 7(7): 545–553.

19. Cheang MCU, Chia SK, Voduc D, Gao D, Leung S et al. Ki67 index, HER2 status, and prognosis of patients with luminal B breast cancer. Journal of the National Cancer Institute 2009; 101(10): 736–750.

20. Prat A, Perou CM. Deconstructing the molecular portraits of breast cancer. Molecular Oncology 2011; 5(1): 5–23.

21. Kreike B, Van Kouwenhove M, Horlings H, Weigelt B, Peterse H et al. Gene expression profiling and histopathological characterization of triple-negative/basal-like breast carcinomas. Breast Cancer Research 2007; 9(5): R65.

22. Prat A, Parker JS, Karginova O, Fan C, Livasy C et al. Phenotypic and molecular characterization of the claudin-low intrinsic subtype of breast cancer. Breast Cancer Research 2010; 12(5): R68.

23. Gucalp A, Traina TA. Triple-negative breast cancer: role of the androgen receptor. Cancer 2010; 16(1): 62–65.

24. Lehmann BD, Bauer JA, Chen X, Sanders ME, Chakravarthy AB et al. Identification of human triple-negative breast cancer subtypes and preclinical models for selection of targeted therapies. Journal of Clinical Investigation 2011; 121(7): 2750–2767.

25. Weigelt B, Mackay A, A'hern R, Natrajan R, Tan DSP et al. Breast cancer molecular profiling with single sample predictors: a retrospective analysis. Lancet Oncology 2010; 11(4): 339–349.

26. Haibe-Kains B, Desmedt C, Loi S, Culhane AC, Bontempi G et al. A three-gene model to robustly identify breast cancer molecular subtypes. Journal of the National Cancer Institute 2012; 104(4): 311–325.

27. Curtis C, Shah SP, Chin S-F, Turashvili G, Rueda OM et al. The genomic and transcriptomic architecture of 2,000 breast tumours reveals novel subgroups. Nature [online] 18 April 2012 [cited 23 April 2012]. Available from: <http://www.nature.com/doifinder/10.1038/nature10983>.

28. Law JH, Habibi G, Hu K, Masoudi H, Wang MYC et al. Phosphorylated insulin-like growth factor-i/insulin receptor is present in all breast cancer subtypes and is related to poor survival. Cancer Research 2008; 68(24): 10238–10246.

29. Creighton CJ, Casa A, Lazard Z, Huang S, Tsimelzon A et al. Insulin-like growth factor-I activates gene transcription programs strongly associated with poor breast cancer prognosis. Journal of Clinical Oncology 2008; 26(25): 4078–4085.

30. Turner N, Grose R. Fibroblast growth factor signalling: from development to cancer. Nature Reviews Cancer 2010; 10(2): 116–129.

31. Turner N, Pearson A, Sharpe R, Lambros M, Geyer F et al. FGFR1 amplification drives endocrine therapy resistance and is a therapeutic target in breast cancer. Cancer Research 2010; 70(5): 2085–2094.

32. Liu P, Cheng H, Roberts TM, Zhao JJ. Targeting the phosphoinositide 3-kinase pathway in cancer. Nature Reviews Drug Discovery 2009; 8(8): 627–644.

33. Miller TW, Hennessy BT, González-Angulo AM, Fox EM, Mills GB et al. Hyperactivation of phosphatidylinositol-3 kinase promotes escape from hormone dependence in estrogen receptor-positive human breast cancer. Journal of Clinical Investigation 2010; 120(7): 2406–2413.

34. Loi S, Haibe-Kains B, Majjaj S, Lallemand F, Durbecq V et al. PIK3CA mutations associated with gene signature of low mTORC1 signaling and better outcomes in estrogen receptor-positive breast cancer. Proceedings of the National Academy of Sciences USA 2010; 107(22): 10208–10213.

35. Baselga J, Swain SM. Novel anticancer targets: revisiting ERBB2 and discovering ERBB3. Nature Reviews Cancer 2009; 9(7): 463–475.

36. Garrett JT, Arteaga CL. Resistance to HER2-directed antibodies and tyrosine kinase inhibitors: mechanisms and clinical implications. Cancer Biology and Therapy 2011; 11(9): 793–800.

37. Berns K, Horlings HM, Hennessy BT, Madiredjo M, Hijmans EM et al. A functional genetic approach identifies the PI3K pathway as a major determinant of trastuzumab resistance in breast cancer. Cancer Cell 2007; 12(4): 395–402.

38. Zagozdzon R, Gallagher WM, Crown J. Truncated HER2: implications for HER2-targeted therapeutics. Drug Discovery Today 2011; 16(17–18): 810–816.

39. Arpino G, Wiechmann L, Osborne CK, Schiff R. Crosstalk between the estrogen receptor and the HER tyrosine kinase receptor family: molecular mechanism and clinical implications for endocrine therapy resistance. Endocrinology Reviews 2008; 29(2): 217–233.

40. Azim HA Jr, Piccart MJ. Simultaneous targeting of estrogen receptor and HER2 in breast cancer. Expert Review of Anticancer Therapy 2010; 10(8): 1255–1263.

41. Marchiò C, Natrajan R, Shiu KK, Lambros MBK, Rodriguez-Pinilla SM et al. The genomic profile of HER2-amplified breast cancers: the influence of ER status. Journal of Pathology 2008; 216(4): 399–407.

42. Rios J, Puhalla S. PARP inhibitors in breast cancer: BRCA and beyond. Oncology 2011; 25(11): 1014–1025.

43. Shien T, Tashiro T, Omatsu M, Masuda T, Furuta K et al. Frequent overexpression of epidermal growth factor receptor (EGFR) in mammary high grade ductal carcinomas with myoepithelial differentiation. Journal of Clinical Pathology 2005; 58(12): 1299–1304.

44. Saal LH, Gruvberger-Saal SK, Persson C, Lövgren K, Jumppanen M et al. Recurrent gross mutations of the PTEN tumor suppressor gene in breast cancers with deficient DSB repair. Nature Genetics 2008; 40(1): 102–107.

45. Shin BK, Lee Y, Lee JB, Kim HK, Lee JB et al. Breast carcinomas expressing basal markers have poor clinical outcome regardless of estrogen receptor status. Oncology Reports 2008; 19(3): 617–625.

46. Lim E, Vaillant F, Wu D, Forrest NC, Pal B et al. Aberrant luminal progenitors as the candidate target population for basal tumor development in BRCA1 mutation carriers. Nature Medicine 2009; 15(8): 907–913.

47. Holstege H, Horlings HM, Velds A, Langerød A, Børresen-Dale A-L et al. BRCA1-mutated and basal-like breast cancers have similar aCGH profiles and a high incidence of protein truncating TP53 mutations. BMC Cancer 2010; 10: 654.

48. Han W, Jung E-M, Cho J, Lee JW, Hwang K-T et al. DNA copy number alterations and expression of relevant genes in triple-negative breast cancer. Genes Chromosomes Cancer 2008; 47(6): 490–499.

49. Aparicio SA, Huntsman DG. Does massively parallel DNA resequencing signify the end of histopathology as we know it? Journal of Pathology 2010; 220(2): 307–315.

50. Greenman C, Stephens P, Smith R, Dalgliesh GL, Hunter C et al. Patterns of somatic mutation in human cancer genomes. Nature 2007; 446(7132): 153–158.

51. Shah SP, Morin RD, Khattra J, Prentice L, Pugh T et al. Mutational evolution in a lobular breast tumour profiled at single nucleotide resolution. Nature 2009; 461(7265): 809–813.

52. Stephens PJ, McBride DJ, Lin M-L, Varela I, Pleasance ED et al. Complex landscapes of somatic rearrangement in human breast cancer genomes. Nature 2009; 462(7276): 1005–1010.

53. Ellis MJ. Analysis of luminal-type breast cancer by massively parallel sequencing. Proceedings of the American Association of Cancer Research 2011 (abstr LB87).

54. Ding L, Ellis MJ, Li S, Larson DE, Chen K et al. Genome remodelling in a basal-like breast cancer metastasis and xenograft. Nature 2010; 464(7291): 999–1005.

55. Beck J, Urnovitz HB, Mitchell WM, Schütz E. Next generation sequencing of serum circulating nucleic acids from patients with invasive ductal breast cancer reveals differences to healthy and nonmalignant controls. Molecular Cancer Research 2010; 8(3): 335–342.

56. Leary RJ, Kinde I, Diehl F, Schmidt K, Clouser C et al. Development of personalized tumor biomarkers using massively parallel sequencing. Science Translational Medicine 2010; 2(20): 20ra14.

57. Desmedt C, Haibe-Kains B, Wirapati P, Buyse M, Larsimont D et al. Biological processes associated with breast cancer clinical outcome depend on the molecular subtypes. Clinical Cancer Research 2008; 14(16): 5158–5165.

58. Reis-Filho JS, Weigelt B, Fumagalli D, Sotiriou C. Molecular profiling: moving away from tumor philately. Science Translational Medicine 2010; 2(47): 47ps43.

59. Wirapati P, Sotiriou C, Kunkel S, Farmer P, Pradervand S et al. Meta-analysis of gene expression profiles in breast cancer: toward a unified understanding of breast cancer subtyping and prognosis signatures. Breast Cancer Research 2008; 10(4): R65.

60. Desmedt C, Piette F, Loi S, Wang Y, Lallemand F et al. Strong time dependence of the 76-gene prognostic signature for node-negative breast cancer patients in the TRANSBIG multicenter independent validation series. Clinical Cancer Research 2007; 13(11): 3207–3214.

61. Cardoso F, Van't Veer L, Rutgers E, Loi S, Mook S et al. Clinical application of the 70-gene profile: the MINDACT trial. Journal of Clinical Oncology 2008; 26(5): 729–735.

62. Sparano JA, Paik S. Development of the 21-gene assay and its application in clinical practice and clinical trials. Journal of Clinical Oncology 2008; 26(5): 721–728.

63. Ma X-J, Dahiya S, Richardson E, Erlander M, Sgroi DC. Gene expression profiling of the tumor microenvironment during breast cancer progression. Breast Cancer Research 2009; 11(1): R7.

64. White DE, Kurpios NA, Zuo D, Hassell JA, Blaess S et al. Targeted disruption of beta1-integrin in a transgenic mouse model of human breast cancer reveals an essential role in mammary tumor induction. Cancer Cell 2004; 6(2): 159–170.

65. Lyons TR, O'Brien J, Borges VF, Conklin MW, Keely PJ et al. Postpartum mammary gland involution drives progression of ductal carcinoma in situ through collagen and COX-2. Nature Medicine 2011; 17(9): 1109–1115.

66. Joyce JA, Pollard JW. Microenvironmental regulation of metastasis. Nature Reviews Cancer 2009; 9(4): 239–252.

67. Weis SM, Cheresh DA. Tumor angiogenesis: molecular pathways and therapeutic targets. Nature Medicine 2011; 17(11): 1359–1370.

68. Robinson BD, Sica GL, Liu Y-F, Rohan TE, Gertler FB et al. Tumor microenvironment of metastasis in human breast carcinoma: a potential prognostic marker linked to hematogenous dissemination. Clinical Cancer Research 2009; 15(7): 2433–2441.

69. Denardo DG, Brennan DJ, Rexhepaj E, Ruffell B, Shiao SL et al. Leukocyte Complexity Predicts Breast Cancer Survival and Functionally Regulates Response to Chemotherapy. Cancer Discovery 2011; 1: 54–67.

70. Ignatiadis M, Singhal SK, Desmedt C, Haibe-Kains B, Criscitiello C et al. Gene modules and response to neoadjuvant chemotherapy in breast cancer subtypes: a pooled analysis. Journal of Clinical Oncology [online] 16 April 2012 [cited 23 April 2012]. Available from: <http://www.ncbi.nlm.nih.gov/pubmed/22508827>.

71. Gonda TA, Varro A, Wang TC, Tycko B. Molecular biology of cancer-associated fibroblasts: can these cells be targeted in anti-cancer therapy? Seminars in Cell and Developmental Biology 2010; 21(1): 2–10.

72. Finak G, Bertos N, Pepin F, Sadekova S, Souleimanova M et al. Stromal gene expression predicts clinical outcome in breast cancer. Nature Medicine 2008; 14(5): 518–527.

73. Teschendorff AE, Miremadi A, Pinder SE, Ellis IO, Caldas C. An immune response gene expression module identifies a good prognosis subtype in estrogen receptor negative breast cancer. Genome Biology 2007; 8(8): R157.

74. Yau C, Esserman L, Moore DH, Waldman F, Sninsky J et al. A multigene predictor of metastatic outcome in early stage hormone receptor-negative and triple-negative breast cancer. Breast Cancer Research 2010; 12(5): R85.

75. Desmedt C, Majjaj S, Kheddoumi N, Singhal SK, Haibe-Kains B et al. Characterization and clinical evaluation of CD10+ stroma cells in the breast cancer microenvironment. Clinical Cancer Research 2012; 18(4): 1004–1014.

76. Herschkowitz JI, Fu X. MicroRNAs add an additional layer to the complexity of cell signaling. Science Signalling 2011; 4(184): jc5.

77. Volinia S, Galasso M, Sana ME, Wise TF, Palatini J et al. Breast cancer signatures for invasiveness and prognosis defined by deep sequencing of microRNA. Proceedings of the National Academy of Science USA 2012; 109(8): 3024–3029.

78. Dedeurwaerder S, Desmedt C, Calonne E, Singhal SK, Haibe-Kains B et al. DNA methylation profiling reveals a predominant immune component in breast cancers. EMBO Molecular Medicine 2011; 3(12): 726–741.

79. Rønneberg JA, Fleischer T, Solvang HK, Nordgard SH, Edvardsen H et al. Methylation profiling with a panel of cancer related genes: association with estrogen receptor, TP53 mutation status and expression subtypes in sporadic breast cancer. Molecular Oncology 2011; 5(1): 61–76.

80. Iwamoto T, Bianchini G, Booser D, Qi Y, Coutant C et al. Gene pathways associated with prognosis and chemotherapy sensitivity in molecular subtypes of breast cancer. Journal of the National Cancer Institute 2011; 103(3): 264–272.

81. Albain KS, Barlow WE, Shak S, Hortobagyi GN, Livingston RB et al. Prognostic and predictive value of the 21-gene recurrence score assay in postmenopausal women with node-positive, oestrogen-receptor-positive breast cancer on chemotherapy: a retrospective analysis of a randomised trial. Lancet Oncology 2010; 11(1): 55–65.

82. Desmedt C, Di Leo A, De Azambuja E, Larsimont D, Haibe-Kains B et al. Multifactorial approach to predicting resistance to anthracyclines. Journal of Clinical Oncology 2011; 29(12): 1578–1586.

83. Li Y, Zou L, Li Q, Haibe-Kains B, Tian R et al. Amplification of LAPTM4B and YWHAZ contributes to chemotherapy resistance and recurrence of breast cancer. Nature Medicine 2010; 16(2): 214–218.

84. Symmans WF, Hatzis C, Sotiriou C, Andre F, Peintinger F et al. Genomic index of sensitivity to endocrine therapy for breast cancer. Journal of Clinical Oncology 2010; 28(27): 4111–4119.

85. Hatzis C, Pusztai L, Valero V, Booser DJ, Esserman L et al. A genomic predictor of response and survival following taxane-anthracycline chemotherapy for invasive breast cancer. JAMA. 2011; 305(18): 1873–1881.

86. Juul N, Szallasi Z, Eklund AC, Li Q, Burrell RA et al. Assessment of an RNA interference screen-derived mitotic and ceramide pathway metagene as a predictor of response to neoadjuvant paclitaxel for primary triple-negative breast cancer: a retrospective analysis of five clinical trials. Lancet Oncology 2010; 11(4): 358–365.

87. Gerlinger M, Rowan AJ, Horswell S, Larkin J, Endesfelder D, Gronroos E, et al. Intratumor heterogeneity and branched evolution revealed by multiregion sequencing. New England Journal of Medicine 2012; 366(10): 883–892.

88. Ellis IO, Schnitt SJ, Sastre-garau X, et al. Invasive breast carcinoma. In: Tavassoli FA and Devilee P eds. Tumours of the Breast and Female Genital Organs. Lyon: IARC Press, 2003, 9–110.

89. Pestalozzi BC, Zahrieh D, Mallon E et al. Distinct clinical and prognostic features of infiltrating lobular carcinoma of the breast: combined results of 15 International Breast Cancer Study Group clinical trials. Journal of Clinical Oncology 2008; 26: 3006–3014.

90. Viale G, Rotmensz N, Maisonneuve P et al. Lack of prognostic significance of 'classic' lobular breast carcinoma: a matched, single institution series. Breast Cancer Research and Treatment 2009; 117: 211–214.

91. Colleoni M, Rotmensz N, Maisonneuve P, Mastropasqua MG, Luini A et al. Outcome of special types of breast cancer. Annals of Oncology 2012 Jun; 23(6):1428–1436.

92. Arpino G, Clark GM, Mohsin S, et al. Adenoid cystic carcinoma of the breast: molecular markers, treatment, and clinical outcome. Cancer 2000; 94: 2119–2127.

93. Leibl S, Gogg-Kammerer M, Sommersacher A, et al. Metaplastic breast carcinomas: are they of myoepithelial differentiation? Immunohistochemical profile of the sarcomatoid subtype using novel myoepithelial markers. American Journal of Surgical Pathology 2005; 29, 347–353.

94. Tavassoli FA. Ductal carcinoma in situ: introduction of the concept of ductal intraepithelial neoplasia. Modern Pathology 1998; 11: 140–154

95. Veronesi U, Viale G, Rotmensz N, Goldhirsch A. Rethinking TNM: breast cancer TNM classification for treatment decision-making and research. Breast 2006; 15: 3–8.

96. Perou CM, Sorlie T, Eisen MB et al. Molecular portraits of human breast tumours. Nature 2000; 406: 747–752.

97. Sorlie T, Perou CM, Tibshirani R et al. Gene expression patterns of breast carcinomas distinguish tumor subclasses with clinical implications. Proceedings of the National Academy of Science USA 2001; 98: 10869–10874.

98. Sorlie T, Tibshirani R, Parker J et al. Repeated observation of breast tumor subtypes in independent gene expression data sets. Proceedings of the National Academy of Science USA 2003; 100: 8418–8423.

99. Rouzier R, Perou CM, Symmans WF et al. Breast cancer molecular subtypes respond differently to preoperative chemotherapy. Clinical Cancer Research 2005; 11: 5678–5685.

100. Parker JS, Mullins M, Cheang MC, et al. Supervised risk predictor of breast cancer based on intrinsic subtypes. Journal of Clinical Oncology 2009; 27: 1160–1167.

101. Nielsen TO, Parker JS, Leung S et al. A comparison of PAM50 intrinsic subtyping with immunohistochemistry and clinical prognostic factors in tamoxifen-treated estrogen receptor-positive breast cancer. Clinical Cancer Research 2010; 16: 5222–5232.

102. Ellis MJ, Suman VJ, Hoog J et al. Randomized phase II neoadjuvant comparison between letrozole, anastrozole, and exemestane for postmenopausal women with estrogen receptor-rich stage 2 to 3 breast cancer: clinical and biomarker outcomes and predictive value of the baseline PAM50-based intrinsic subtype—ACOSOG Z1031. Journal of Clinical Oncology 2011; 29: 2342–2349.

103. Hugh J, Hanson J, Cheang MC et al. Breast cancer subtypes and response to docetaxel in node-positive breast cancer: use of an immunohistochemical definition in the BCIRG 001 trial. Journal of Clinical Oncology 2009; 27: 1168–1176.

104. Carey L, Winer E, Viale G, Cameron D, Gianni L. Triple-negative breast cancer: disease entity or title of convenience? Nature Reviews Clinical Oncology 2010; 7: 683–692.

105. Goldhirsch A, Wood WC, Coates AS, et al. Strategies for subtypes—dealing with the diversity of breast cancer: highlights of the St. Gallen International Expert Consensus on the Primary Therapy of Early Breast Cancer 2011. Annals of Oncology 2011; 22: 1736–1747.

106. Sobin LH, Gospodarowicz MK, Wittekind CH eds. TNM Classification of Malignant Tumors, 7th ed. Oxford: Wiley-Blackwell, 2009.

107. Bloom HJ, Richardson WW. Histological grading and prognosis in breast cancer; a study of 1409 cases of which 359 have been followed for 15 years. British Journal of Cancer 1957; 11: 359–377.

108. Elston CW, Ellis IO. Pathologic prognostic factors in breast cancer. I. The value of histological grades in breast cancer. Experience from a large study with long-term follow-up. Histopathology 1991; 19: 403–410.

109. Goldhirsch A, Ingle JN, Gelber RD et al. Thresholds for therapies: highlights of the St Gallen International Expert Consensus on the primary therapy of early breast cancer 2009. Annals of Oncology 2009; 20: 1319–1329.

110. Hammond ME, Hayes DF, Dowsett M et al. American Society of Clinical Oncology/College of American Pathologists guideline recommendations for immunohistochemical testing of estrogen and progesterone receptors in breast cancer. Journal of Clinical Oncology 2010; 28: 2784–2795.

111. Colleoni M, Viale G, Goldhirsch A. Lessons on responsiveness to adjuvant systemic therapies learned from the neoadjuvant setting. Breast 2009; 18: S137–140.

112. Colleoni M, Bagnardi V, Rotmensz N et al. Increasing steroid hormone receptors expression defines breast cancer subtypes non responsive to preoperative chemotherapy. Breast Cancer Research and Treatment 2009; 116: 359–369.

113. Pagani O, Gelber S, Simoncini E et al. Is adjuvant chemotherapy of benefit for postmenopausal women who receive endocrine treatment for highly endocrine-responsive, node-positive breast cancer? International Breast Cancer Study Group Trials VII and 12–93. Breast Cancer Research and Treatment 2009; 116: 491–500.

114. Allred DC, Harvey JM, Berardo M, Clark GM. Prognostic and predictive factors in breast cancer by immunohistochemical analysis. Modern Pathology 1998; 11: 155–168.

115. Harvey JM, Clark GM, Osborne CK, Allred DC. Estrogen receptor status by immunohistochemistry is superior to the ligand-binding assay for predicting response to adjuvant endocrine therapy in breast cancer. Journal of Clinical Oncology 1999; 17: 1474–1481.

116. Carlson RW, Moench SJ, Hammond ME et al. NCCN HER2 Testing in Breast Cancer Task Force. HER2 testing in breast cancer: NCCN Task Force report and recommendations. Journal of the National Comprehensive Cancer Network 2006; 4(Suppl 3): S1–22.

117. Wolff AC, Hammond ME, Schwartz JN et al. American Society of Clinical Oncology/College of American Pathologists guideline recommendations for human epidermal growth factor receptor 2 testing in breast cancer. Journal of Clinical Oncology 2007; 251: 118–145.

118. Gerdes J, Schwab U, Lemke H, Stein H. Production of a mouse monoclonal antibody reactive with a human nuclear antigen associated with cell proliferation. International Journal of Cancer 1983; 31: 13–20.

119. Thor AD, Liu S, Moore DH, Edgerton SM. Comparison of mitotic index, in vitro bromodeoxyuridine labeling, and MIB-1 assays to quantitate proliferation in breast cancer. Journal of Clinical Oncology 1999; 17: 470–477.

120. de Azambuja E., Cardoso F, de Castro G Jr, Colozza M, Mano MS et al. Ki-67 as prognostic marker in early breast cancer: a meta-analysis of published studies involving 12 155 patients. British Journal of Cancer 2007; 96: 1504–1513.

121. Jonat W, Arnold N. Is the Ki-67 labelling index ready for clinical use? Annals of Oncology 2011; 22: 500–502.

122. Dowsett M, Nielsen TO, A'hern R et al. Assessment of Ki67 in Breast Cancer: recommendations from the International Ki67 in Breast Cancer Working Group. Journal of the National Cancer Institute 2011; 103: 1656–1664.

123. Millar EK, Graham PH, O'Toole SA et al. Prediction of local recurrence, distant metastases, and death after breast-conserving therapy in early-stage invasive breast cancer using a five-biomarker panel. Journal of Clinical Oncology 2009; 27: 4701–4708.

124. Albain KS, Paik S, van't Veer L. Prediction of adjuvant chemotherapy benefit in endocrine responsive, early breast cancer using multigene assays. Breast 2009; 18: S141–145.

125. Ho A, Morrow M. The evolution of the locoregional therapy of breast cancer. Oncologist 2011; 16(10): 1367–1379.

126. Cataliotti L, De Wolf C, Holland R, et al. EUSOMA. Guidelines on the standards for the training of specialised health professionals dealing with breast cancer. European Journal of Cancer 2007; 43(4): 660–675.

127. Perry NM. EUSOMA Working Party. Quality assurance in the diagnosis of breast disease. EUSOMA Working Party. European Journal of Cancer 2001; 37(2): 159–172.

128. Houssami N, Sainsbury R. Breast cancer: multidisciplinary care and clinical outcomes. European Journal of Cancer 2006; 42(15): 2480–2491.

129. Rutgers EJ. EUSOMA Consensus Group. Quality control in the locoregional treatment of breast cancer. European Journal of Cancer 2001; 37(4): 447–453.

130. Cancer Research UK. Breast Cancer Key Facts. Cancer Research UK Publications [online], 2012. <http://www.cancerresearchuk.org/cancer-info/cancerstats/keyfacts/breast-cancer/>.

131. Britton P et al. One-stop diagnostic breast clinics: how often are breast cancers missed? British Journal of Cancer 2009; 100(12): 1873–1878.

132. Ford D, Easton DF, Bishop DT et al; Breast Cancer Linkage Consortium. Risks of cancer in BRCA1 mutation carriers. Lancet 1994; 343: 692–695.

133. Ford D, Easton DF, Stratton M et al. Genetic heterogeneity and penetrance analysis of the BRCA1 and BRCA2 genes in breast cancer families. American Journal of Human Genetics 1998; 62: 676–689.

134. Rebbeck TR, Friebel T, Lynch HT et al. Bilateral prophylactic mastectomy reduces breast cancer risk in BRCA1 and BRCA2 mutation carriers: the PROSE study group. Journal of Clinical Oncology 2004; 22: 1055–1062.

135. Heemskerk-Gerritsen BA, Brekelmans CT, Menke-Pluymers MB et al. Prophylactic mastectomy in BRCA1/2 mutation carriers and women at risk of hereditary breast cancer: long term experiences at the Rotterdam Family Cancer Clinic. Annals of Surgical Oncology 2007; 14: 3335–3344.

136. Hartmann LC, Sellers TA, Schaid DJ et al. Efficacy of bilateral prophylactic mastectomy in BRCA1 and BRCA2 gene mutation carriers. Journal of the National Cancer Institute 2001; 93: 1633–1637.

137. Kaas R, Verhoef S, Wesseling J, Rookus MA, Oldenburg HS et al. Prophylactic mastectomy in BRCA1 and BRCA2 mutation carriers: very low risk for subsequent breast cancer. Annals of Surgery 2010; 251(3): 488–492.

138. Sprundel TC van, Schmidt MK, Rookus MA et al. Risk reduction of contralateral prophylactic mastectomy in BRCA1 and BRCA2 mutation carriers. British Journal of Cancer 2005; 93: 287–292.

139. Herrinton LJ, Barlow WE, Yu O et al. Efficacy of prophylactic mastectomy in women with unilateral breast cancer: a cancer research network project. Journal of Clinical Oncology 2005; 23: 4275–4286.

140. McDonnell SK, Schaid DJ, Myers JL et al. Efficacy of contralateral prophylactic mastectomy in women with a personal and family history of breast cancer. Journal of Clinical Oncology 2001; 19: 3938–3943.

141. Virnig BA, Tuttle TM, Shamliyan T, Kane RL. Ductal carcinoma in situ of the breast: a systematic review of incidence, treatment, and outcomes. Journal of the National Cancer Institute 2010; 102(3): 170–178.

142. Lakhani SR, Audretsch W, Cleton-Jensen AM et al. EUSOMA. The management of lobular carcinoma in situ (LCIS). Is LCIS the same as ductal carcinoma in situ (DCIS)? European Journal of Cancer 2006; 42(14): 2205–2211.

143. Song HM, Styblo TM, Carlson GW, Losken A. The use of oncoplastic reduction techniques to reconstruct partial mastectomy defects in women with ductal carcinoma in situ. Breast 2010; 16(2): 141–146.

144. Dunne C, Burke JP, Morrow M, Kell MR. Effect of margin status on local recurrence after breast conservation and radiation therapy for ductal carcinoma in situ. Journal of Clinical Oncology 2009; 27(10): 1615–1620

145. Meijnen P, Oldenburg HS, Loo CE, Nieweg OE, Peterse JL et al. Risk of invasion and axillary lymph node metastasis in ductal carcinoma in situ diagnosed by core-needle biopsy. British Journal of Surgery 2007; 94(8): 952–956.

146. Early Breast Cancer Trialists' Collaborative Group (EBCTCG), Darby S, McGale P, Correa C et al. Effect of radiotherapy after breast-conserving surgery on 10-year recurrence and 15-year breast

cancer death: meta-analysis of individual patient data for 10,801 women in 17 randomised trials. Lancet 2011; 378(9804): 1707–1716.

147. Litiere S, Werutsky G, Fentiman IS et al. Breast conserving therapy versus mastectomy for stage I-II breast cancer: 20 year follow-up of the EORTC 10801 phase 3 randomised trial. Lancet Oncology 2012; 13(4): 412–419.

148. Sardanelli F, Boetes C, Borisch B, et al. Magnetic resonance imaging of the breast: recommendations from the EUSOMA working group. European Journal of Cancer 2010; 46(8): 1296–1316.

149. Kaufmann M, Morrow M, von Minckwitz G, Harris JR. Biedenkopf Expert Panel Members. Locoregional treatment of primary breast cancer: consensus recommendations from an International Expert Panel. Cancer 2010; 116(5): 1184–1191.

150. Azu M, Abrahamse P, Katz SJ, Jagsi R, Morrow M. What is an adequate margin for breast-conserving surgery? Surgeon attitudes and correlates. Annals of Surgical Oncology 2010; 17(2): 558–563.

151. de Alcantara Filho P, Capko D, Barry JM, Morrow M, Pusic A et al. Nipple-sparing mastectomy for breast cancer and risk-reducing surgery: the Memorial Sloan-Kettering Cancer Center experience. Annals of Surgical Oncology 2011; 18(11): 3117–3122.

152. Collins ED, Moore CP, Clay KF et al. Can women with early-stage breast cancer make an informed decision for mastectomy? Journal of Clinical Oncology 2009; 27(4): 519–525.

153. Molenaar S, Sprangers MA, Rutgers EJ et al. Decision support for patients with early-stage breast cancer: effects of an interactive breast cancer CDROM on treatment decision, satisfaction, and quality of life. Journal of Clinical Oncology 2001; 19(6): 1676–1687.

154. Cooper KL, Harnan S, Meng Y et al. Positron emission tomography (PET) for assessment of axillary lymph node status in early breast cancer: a systematic review and meta-analysis. European Journal of Surgical Oncology 2011; 37(3): 187–198.

155. Mainiero MB. Regional lymph node staging in breast cancer: the increasing role of imaging and ultrasound-guided axillary lymph node fine needle aspiration.Radiologic Clinics of North America 2010; 48(5): 989–997.

156. van der Ploeg IM, Nieweg OE, van Rijk MC, Valdos Olmos RA, Kroon BB. Axillary recurrence after a tumour-negative sentinel node biopsy in breast cancer patients: a systematic review and meta-analysis of the literature. European Journal of Surgical Oncology 2008; 34(12): 1277–1284.

157. Straver ME, Meijnen P, van Tienhoven G et al. Sentinel node identification rate and nodal involvement in the EORTC 10981-22023 AMAROS trial. Annals of Surgical Oncology 2010; 17(7): 1854–1861.

158. Mansel RE, Fallowfield L, Kissin M et al. Randomized multicenter trial of sentinel node biopsy versus standard axillary treatment in operable breast cancer: the ALMANAC Trial. Journal of the National Cancer Institute 2006; 98(9): 599–609.

159. Krag DN, Anderson SJ, Julian TB et al. Sentinel-lymph-node resection compared with conventional axillary-lymph-node dissection in clinically node-negative patients with breast cancer: overall survival findings from the NSABP B-32 randomised phase 3 trial. Lancet Oncology 2010; 11(10): 927–933.

160. Naik AM, Fey J, Gemignani M et al. The risk of axillary relapse after sentinel lymph node biopsy for breast cancer is comparable with that of axillary lymph node dissection: a follow-up study of 4008 procedures. Annals of Surgery 2004; 240: 462–468.

161. Jeruss JS, Winchester DJ, Sener SF et al. Axillary recurrence after sentinel node biopsy. Annals of Surgical Oncology 2005; 12:34–40.

162. Hwang RF, Gonzalez-Angulo AM, Yi M et al. Low locoregional failure rates in selected breast cancer patients with tumor-positive sentinel lymph nodes who do not undergo completion axillary dissection. Cancer 2007; 110: 723–730.

163. Guenther JM, Hansen NM, DiFronzo LA et al. Axillary dissection is not required for all patients with breast cancer and positive sentinel nodes. Archives of Surgery 2003; 138:52–56.

164. Fant JS, Grant MD, Knox SM et al. Preliminary outcome analysis in patients with breast cancer and a positive sentinel lymph node who declined axillary dissection. Annals of Surgical Oncology 2003; 10: 126–130.

165. Giuliano AE, McCall L, Beitsch P et al. Locoregional recurrence after sentinel lymph node dissection with or without axillary dissection in patients with sentinel lymph node metastases: the American College of Surgeons Oncology Group Z0011 randomized trial. Annals of Surgery 2010; 252(3): 426–432.

166. Mieog JS, van der Hage JA, van de Velde CJ. Neoadjuvant chemotherapy for operable breast cancer. British Journal of Surgery 2007; 94(10): 1189–1200.

167. Straver ME, Rutgers EJ, Rodenhuis S et al. The relevance of breast cancer subtypes in the outcome of neoadjuvant chemotherapy. Annals of Surgical Oncology 2010; 17(9): 2411–2418.

168. Kaufmann M, von Minckwitz G, Mamounas EP et al. Recommendations from an international consensus conference on the current status and future of neoadjuvant systemic therapy in primary breast cancer. Annals of Surgical Oncology 2012; 19(5): 1508–1516.

169. Straver ME, Loo CE, Rutgers EJ, Oldenburg HS, Wesseling J et al. MRI-model to guide the surgical treatment in breast cancer patients after neoadjuvant chemotherapy. Annals of Surgery 2010; 251(4): 701–707.

170. Loo CE, Straver ME, Rodenhuis S et al. Magnetic resonance imaging response monitoring of breast cancer during neoadjuvant chemotherapy: relevance of breast cancer subtype. Journal of Clinical Oncology 2011; 29(6): 660–666.

171. Koolen BB, Vrancken Peeters MJ, Aukema TS et al. 18F-FDG PET/CT as a staging procedure in primary stage II and III breast cancer: comparison with conventional imaging techniques. Breast Cancer Research and Treatment 2012; 131(1): 117–126.

172. Fisher B, Anderson S, Bryant J et al. Twenty-year follow-up of a randomized trial comparing total mastectomy, lumpectomy, and lumpectomy plus irradiation for the treatment of invasive breast cancer. New England Journal of Medicine 2002; 347: 1233–1241.

173. Bartelink H, Horiot JC, Poortmans PM et al. Impact of a higher radiation dose on local control and survival in breast-conserving therapy of early breast cancer: 10-year results of the randomized boost versus no boost EORTC 22881-10882 trial. Journal of Clinical Oncology 2007; 25: 3259–3265.

174. Darby S, McGale P, Correa C et al. Effect of radiotherapy after breast-conserving surgery on 10-year recurrence and 15-year breast cancer death: meta-analysis of individual patient data for 10,801 women in 17 randomised trials. Lancet 2011; 378: 1707–1716.

175. van der Leij F, Elkhuizen PH, Bartelink H van de Vijver MJ. Predictive factors for local recurrence in breast cancer. Seminars in Radiation Oncology 2012; 22: 100–107.

176. Kreike B, Halfwerk H, Armstrong N et al. Local recurrence after breast-conserving therapy in relation to gene expression patterns in a large series of patients. Clinical Cancer Research 2009; 15: 4181–4190.

177. Bentzen SM, Agrawal RK, Aird EG et al. The UK Standardisation of Breast Radiotherapy (START) Trial A of radiotherapy hypofractionation for treatment of early breast cancer: a randomised trial. Lancet Oncology 2008; 9: 331–341.

178. Bentzen SM, Agrawal RK, Aird EG et al. The UK Standardisation of Breast Radiotherapy (START) Trial B of radiotherapy hypofractionation for treatment of early breast cancer: a randomised trial. Lancet 2008; 371: 1098–1107.

179. Whelan TJ, Pignol JP, Levine MN et al. Long-term results of hypofractionated radiation therapy for breast cancer. New England Journal of Medicine 2010; 362: 513–520.

180. Smith BD, Bentzen SM, Correa CR et al. Fractionation for whole breast irradiation: an American Society for Radiation Oncology (ASTRO) evidence-based guideline. Int Journal of Radiation Oncology Biology Physics 2011; 81: 59–68.

181. Galecki J, Hicer-Grzenkowicz J, Grudzien-Kowalska M, Michalska T, Zalucki W. Radiation-induced brachial plexopathy and hypofractionated regimens in adjuvant irradiation of patients with breast cancer—a review. Acta Oncologica 2006; 45: 280–284.

182. Powell S, Cooke J, Parsons C. Radiation-induced brachial plexus injury: follow-up of two different fractionation schedules. Radiotherapy and Oncology 1990; 18: 213–220.

183. Romestaing P, Lehingue Y, Carrie C, et al. Role of a 10-Gy boost in the conservative treatment of early breast cancer: results of a randomized clinical trial in Lyon, France. Journal of Clinical Oncology 1997; 15: 963–968.

184. Poortmans PM, Collette L, Horiot JC et al. Impact of the boost dose of 10 Gy versus 26 Gy in patients with early stage breast cancer after a microscopically incomplete lumpectomy: 10-year results of the randomised EORTC boost trial. Radiotherapy and Oncology 2009; 90: 80–85.

185. Werkhoven E, Hart G, Tinteren H et al. Nomogram to predict ipsilateral breast relapse based on pathology review from the EORTC 22881-10882 boost versus no boost trial. Radiotherapy and Oncology 2011; 100: 101–107.

186. Polgar C, Van Limbergen E, Potter R, et al. Patient selection for accelerated partial-breast irradiation (APBI) after breast-conserving surgery: recommendations of the Groupe Europeen de Curietherapie-European Society for Therapeutic Radiology and Oncology (GEC-ESTRO) breast cancer working group based on clinical evidence (2009). Radiotherapy and Oncology 2010; 94: 264–273.

187. Vaidya JS, Joseph DJ, Tobias JS et al. Targeted intraoperative radiotherapy versus whole breast radiotherapy for breast cancer (TARGIT-A trial): an international, prospective, randomised, non-inferiority phase 3 trial. Lancet 2010; 376: 91–102.

188. Vaidya JS, Wenz F, Bulsara M et al. Targeted intraoperative radiotherapy for early breast cancer: TARGIT-A trial- updated analysis of local recurrence and first analysis of survival CTRC-AACR San Antonio Breast Cancer conference, San Antonio 2012; abstr S4-2.

189. Cameron D, Kunkler I, Dixon M, Jack W, Thomas J et al. Intraoperative radiotherapy for early breast cancer. Lancet 2010; 376: 1142; author reply 1143–1144.

190. Haviland JS, A'Hern R, Bliss JM. Intraoperative radiotherapy for early breast cancer. Lancet 2010; 376: 1142; author reply 1143–1144.

191. Vikstrom J, Hjelstuen MH, Mjaaland I, Dybvik KI. Cardiac and pulmonary dose reduction for tangentially irradiated breast cancer, utilizing deep inspiration breath-hold with audio-visual guidance, without compromising target coverage. Acta Oncologica 2011; 50: 42–50.

192. NCCN clinical practice guidelines in oncology. Breast Cancer 2012; vol. version 1.

193. Truong PT, Olivotto IA, Kader HA, Panades M, Speers CH et al. Selecting breast cancer patients with T1-T2 tumors and one to three positive axillary nodes at high postmastectomy locoregional recurrence risk for adjuvant radiotherapy. International Journal of Radiation Oncology Biology Physics 2005; 61: 1337–1347.

194. Kyndi M, Overgaard M, Nielsen HM, Sorensen FB, Knudsen H et al. High local recurrence risk is not associated with large survival reduction after postmastectomy radiotherapy in high-risk breast cancer: a subgroup analysis of DBCG 82 b&c. Radiotherapy Oncology 2009; 90: 74–79.

195. Veronesi U, Galimberti V, Mariani L et al. Sentinel node biopsy in breast cancer: early results in 953 patients with negative sentinel node biopsy and no axillary dissection. European Journal of Cancer 2005; 41: 231–237.

196. Veronesi U, Orecchia R, Zurrida S et al. Avoiding axillary dissection in breast cancer surgery: a randomized trial to assess the role of axillary radiotherapy. Annals of Oncology 2005; 16: 383–388.

197. Chang DT, Feigenberg SJ, Indelicato DJ et al. Long-term outcomes in breast cancer patients with ten or more positive axillary nodes treated with combined-modality therapy: the importance of radiation field selection. International Journal of Radiation Oncology Biology Physics 2007; 67: 1043–1051.

198. Whelan T, Olivotto I, Ackerman I, et al. NCIC-CTG MA.20: an intergroup trial of regional nodal irradiation in early breast cancer. ASCO annual meeting. Journal of Clinical Oncology 2011; 29: abstr LBA1003.

199. Cutuli B, Lacroze M, Dilhuydy JM et al. Male breast cancer: results of the treatments and prognostic factors in 397 cases. European Journal of Cancer 1995; 31A: 1960–1964.

200. Yu E, Suzuki H, Younus J et al. The impact of post-mastectomy radiation therapy on male breast cancer patients—a case series. International Journal of Radiation Oncology Biology Physics 2012; 82: 696–700.

201. Correa C, McGale P, Taylor C et al. Overview of the randomized trials of radiotherapy in ductal carcinoma in situ of the breast. Journal of the National Cancer Institute Monograph 2010: 162–177.

202. Goodwin A, Parker S, Ghersi D, Wilcken N. Post-operative radiotherapy for ductal carcinoma in situ of the breast—a systematic review of the randomised trials. Breast 2009; 18: 143–149.

203. Hughes LL, Wang M, Page DL et al. Local excision alone without irradiation for ductal carcinoma in situ of the breast: a trial of the Eastern Cooperative Oncology Group. Journal of Clinical Oncology 2009; 27: 5319–5324.

204. Bowden SJ, Fernando IN, Burton A. Delaying radiotherapy for the delivery of adjuvant chemotherapy in the combined modality treatment of early breast cancer: is it disadvantageous and could combined treatment be the answer? Clinical Oncology (Royal College of Radiology) 2006; 18: 247–256.

205. Hickey BE, Francis D, Lehman MH. Sequencing of chemotherapy and radiation therapy for early breast cancer. Cochrane Database Systematic Reviews 2006: CD005212.

206. Chen Z, King W, Pearcey R, Kerba M, Mackillop WJ. The relationship between waiting time for radiotherapy and clinical outcomes: a systematic review of the literature. Radiotherapy Oncololgy 2008; 87: 3–16.

207. Huang J, Barbera L, Brouwers M, Browman G, Mackillop WJ. Does delay in starting treatment affect the outcomes of radiotherapy? A systematic review. Journal of Clinical Oncology 2003; 21: 555–563.

208. Halyard MY, Pisansky TM, Dueck AC et al. Radiotherapy and adjuvant trastuzumab in operable breast cancer: tolerability and adverse event data from the NCCTG Phase III Trial N9831. Journal of Clinical Oncology 2009; 27: 2638–2644.

209. Chargari C, Toillon RA, Macdermed D, Castadot P, Magne N. Concurrent hormone and radiation therapy in patients with breast cancer: what is the rationale? Lancet Oncology 2009; 10: 53–60.

210. Varga Z, Cserhati A, Kelemen G, Boda K, Thurzo L et al. Role of systemic therapy in the development of lung sequelae after conformal radiotherapy in breast cancer patients. International Journal of Radiation Oncology Biology Physics 2011; 80: 1109–1116.

211. Adkison JB, Kuske RR, Patel RR. Breast conserving surgery and accelerated partial breast irradiation after prior breast radiation therapy. American Journal of Clinical Oncology 2010; 33: 427–431.

212. Deutsch M. Repeat high-dose external beam irradiation for in-breast tumor recurrence after previous lumpectomy and whole breast irradiation. International Journal of Radiation Oncology Biology Physics 2002; 53: 687–691.

213. Kauer-Dorner D, Potter R, Resch A et al. Partial breast irradiation for locally recurrent breast cancer within a second breast conserving treatment: alternative to mastectomy? Results from a prospective trial. Radiotherapy Oncology 2012; 102: 96–101.

214. Niehoff P, Dietrich J, Ostertag H, et al. High-dose-rate (HDR) or pulsed-dose-rate (PDR) perioperative interstitial intensity-modulated brachytherapy (IMBT) for local recurrences of previously irradiated breast or thoracic wall following breast cancer. Strahlentherapie und Onkologie 2006; 182: 102–107.

215. Wahl AO, Rademaker A, Kiel KD et al. Multi-institutional review of repeat irradiation of chest wall and breast for recurrent breast cancer. International Journal of Radiation Oncology Biology Physics 2008; 70: 477–484.

216. Muacevic A, Wowra B, Siefert A, Tonn JC, Steiger HJ et al. Microsurgery plus whole brain irradiation versus Gamma Knife surgery alone for treatment of single metastases to the brain: a randomized controlled multicentre phase III trial. Journal of Neurooncology 2008; 87: 299–307.

217. Darby SC, McGale P, Taylor CW, Peto R. Long-term mortality from heart disease and lung cancer after radiotherapy for early breast cancer: prospective cohort study of about 300,000 women in US SEER cancer registries. Lancet Oncology 2005; 6: 557–565.

218. Clarke M, Collins R, Darby S et al. Effects of radiotherapy and of differences in the extent of surgery for early breast cancer on local recurrence and 15-year survival: an overview of the randomised trials. Lancet 2005; 366: 2087–2106.

219. Peto R, Davies C, Godwin J, Gray R, Pan HC et al. Comparisons between different polychemotherapy regimens for early breast cancer: meta-analyses of long-term outcome among 100,000 women in 123 randomised trials. Lancet 2012; 379: 432–444.

220. Olivotto IA, Bajdik CD, Ravdin PM, Speers CH, Coldman AJ et al. Population-based validation of the prognostic model ADJUVANT! for early breast cancer. Journal of Clinical Oncology 2005; 23: 2716–2725.

221. Goldhirsch A, Wood WC, Coates AS, Gelber RD, Thurlimann B et al. Strategies for subtypes—dealing with the diversity of breast cancer: highlights of the St. Gallen International Expert Consensus on the Primary Therapy of Early Breast Cancer 2011. Annals of Oncology 2011; 22: 1736–1747.

222. Slamon DJ, Clark GM, Wong SG, Levin WJ, Ullrich A et al. Human breast cancer: correlation of relapse and survival with amplification of the HER-2/neu oncogene. Science 1987; 235: 177–182.

223. Hayes DF, Thor AD, Dressler LG, Weaver D, Edgerton S et al. HER2 and response to paclitaxel in node-positive breast cancer. New England Journal of Medicine 2007; 357: 1496–1506.

224. Gennari A, Sormani MP, Pronzato P, Puntoni M, Colozza M et al. HER2 status and efficacy of adjuvant anthracyclines in early breast cancer: a pooled analysis of randomized trials. Journal of the National Cancer Institute 2008; 100: 14–20.

225. Dent R, Trudeau M, Pritchard KI, Hanna WM, Kahn HK et al. Triple-negative breast cancer: clinical features and patterns of recurrence. Clinical Cancer Research 2007; 13: 4429–4434.

226. Rouzier R, Perou CM, Symmans WF, Ibrahim N, Cristofanilli M et al. Breast cancer molecular subtypes respond differently to preoperative chemotherapy. Clinical Cancer Research 2005; 11: 5678–5685.

227. Cheang MC, Chia SK, Voduc D, Gao D, Leung S et al. Ki67 index, HER2 status, and prognosis of patients with luminal B breast cancer. Journal of the National Cancer Institute 2009; 101: 736–750.

228. Viale G, Giobbie-Hurder A, Regan MM, Coates AS, Mastropasqua MG et al. Prognostic and predictive value of centrally reviewed Ki-67 labeling index in postmenopausal women with endocrine-responsive breast cancer: results from Breast International Group Trial 1-98 comparing adjuvant tamoxifen with letrozole. Journal of Clinical Oncology 2008; 26: 5569–5575.

229. Yerushalmi R, Woods R, Ravdin PM, Hayes MM, Gelmon KA. Ki67 in breast cancer: prognostic and predictive potential. Lancet Oncology 2010; 11: 174–183.

230. Sotiriou C, Pusztai L. Gene-expression signatures in breast cancer. New England Journal of Medicine 2009; 360: 790–800.

231. Paik S, Shak S, Tang G, Kim C, Baker J et al. A multigene assay to predict recurrence of tamoxifen-treated, node-negative breast cancer. New England Journal of Medicine 2004; 351: 2817–2826.

232. Paik S, Tang G, Shak S, Kim C, Baker J et al. Gene expression and benefit of chemotherapy in women with node-negative, estrogen receptor-positive breast cancer. Journal of Clinical Oncology 2006; 24: 3726–3734.

233. Albain KS, Barlow WE, Shak S, Hortobagyi GN, Livingston RB et al. Prognostic and predictive value of the 21-gene recurrence score assay in postmenopausal women with node-positive, oestrogen-receptor-positive breast cancer on chemotherapy: a retrospective analysis of a randomised trial. Lancet Oncology 2010; 11: 55–65.

234. Piccart M, Bogaerts J, Cardoso F, Werutsky G, Delaloge S et al. The EORTC 10041/BIG 03–04 MINDACT (Microarray in Node Negative and 1 to 3 Positive Lymph Node Disease May Avoid ChemoTherapy) Trial: Patients' Baseline Characteristics and Logistics Aspects After a Successful Accrual. European Journal of Cancer 2011; 47.

235. Duffy MJ. Urokinase plasminogen activator and its inhibitor, PAI-1, as prognostic markers in breast cancer: from pilot to level 1 evidence studies. Clinical Chemistry 2002; 48: 1194–1197.

236. Thomssen C, Scharl A, Harbeck N. AGO Recommendations for Diagnosis and Treatment of Patients with Primary and Metastatic Breast Cancer. Update 2011. Breast Care (Basel) 2011; 6: 299–313.

237. Penault-Llorca F, Andre F, Sagan C, Lacroix-Triki M, Denoux Y et al. Ki67 expression and docetaxel efficacy in patients with estrogen receptor-positive breast cancer. Journal of Clinical Oncology 2009; 27: 2809–2815.

238. Bottini A, Berruti A, Bersiga A, Brizzi MP, Bruzzi P et al. Relationship between tumour shrinkage and reduction in Ki67 expression after primary chemotherapy in human breast cancer. British Journal of Cancer 2001; 85: 1106–1112.

239. Bartlett JM, Munro AF, Dunn JA, McConkey C, Jordan S et al. Predictive markers of anthracycline benefit: a prospectively planned analysis of the UK National Epirubicin Adjuvant Trial (NEAT/BR9601). Lancet Oncology 2010; 11: 266–274.

240. Roche H, Fumoleau P, Spielmann M, Canon JL, Delozier T et al. Sequential adjuvant epirubicin-based and docetaxel chemotherapy for node-positive breast cancer patients: the FNCLCC PACS 01 Trial. Journal of Clinical Oncology 2006; 24: 5664–5671.

241. Martin M, Segui MA, Anton A, Ruiz A, Ramos M et al. Adjuvant docetaxel for high-risk, node-negative breast cancer. New England Journal of Medicine 2010 ;363: 2200–2210.

242. Swain SM, Jeong JH, Geyer CE, Jr, Costantino JP, Pajon ER et al. Longer therapy, iatrogenic amenorrhea, and survival in early breast cancer. New England Journal of Medicine 2010; 362: 2053–2065.

243. Slamon D, Eiermann W, Robert N, Pienkowski T, Martin M et al. Adjuvant trastuzumab in HER2-positive breast cancer. New England Journal of Medicine 2011; 365: 1273–1283.

244. Jinno H, Sakata M, Hayashida T, Takahashi M, Sato T et al. Primary systemic chemotherapy of breast cancer: indication and predictive factors. Breast Cancer 2011; 18: 74–79.

245. Mauri D, Pavlidis N, Ioannidis JP. Neoadjuvant versus adjuvant systemic treatment in breast cancer: a meta-analysis. Journal of the National Cancer Institute 2005; 97: 188–194.

246. Liedtke C, Mazouni C, Hess KR, Andre F, Tordai A et al. Response to neoadjuvant therapy and long-term survival in patients with triple-negative breast cancer. Journal of Clinical Oncology 2008; 26: 1275–1281.

247. Jones SE, Erban J, Overmoyer B, Budd GT, Hutchins L et al. Randomized phase III study of docetaxel compared with paclitaxel in metastatic breast cancer. Journal of Clinical Oncology 2005; 23: 5542–5551.

248. Paridaens R, Biganzoli L, Bruning P, Klijn JG, Gamucci T et al. Paclitaxel versus doxorubicin as first-line single-agent chemotherapy for metastatic breast cancer: a European Organization for Research and Treatment of Cancer Randomized Study with cross-over. Journal of Clinical Oncology 2000; 18: 724–733.

249. De Mattos-Arruda L, Cortes J. Advances in First-Line Treatment for Patients with HER-2+ Metastatic Breast Cancer. Oncologist 2012.

250. Miles D, von Minckwitz G, Seidman AD. Combination versus sequential single-agent therapy in metastatic breast cancer. Oncologist 2002; 7 Suppl 6: 13–19.

251. Sparano JA, Vrdoljak E, Rixe O, Xu B, Manikhas A et al. Randomized phase III trial of ixabepilone plus capecitabine versus capecitabine in patients with metastatic breast cancer previously treated with an anthracycline and a taxane. Journal of Clinical Oncology 2010; 28: 3256–3263.

252. Ibrahim NK, Samuels B, Page R, Doval D, Patel KM et al. Multicenter phase II trial of ABI-007, an albumin-bound paclitaxel, in women with metastatic breast cancer. Journal of Clinical Oncology 2005; 23: 6019–6026.

253. Cortes J, O'Shaughnessy J, Loesch D, Blum JL, Vahdat LT et al. Eribulin monotherapy versus treatment of physician's choice in patients with metastatic breast cancer (EMBRACE): a phase 3 open-label randomised study. Lancet 2011; 377: 914–923.

254. Byrski T, Gronwald J, Huzarski T, Grzybowska E, Budryk M et al. Pathologic complete response rates in young women with BRCA1-positive breast cancers after neoadjuvant chemotherapy. Journal of Clinical Oncology 2010; 28: 375–379.

256. Effects of chemotherapy and hormonal therapy for early breast cancer on recurrence and 15-year survival: an overview of the randomised trials. Lancet 2005; 365: 1687–1717.

257. Baum M, Budzar AU, Cuzick J, Forbes J, Houghton JH et al. Anastrozole alone or in combination with tamoxifen versus tamoxifen alone for adjuvant treatment of postmenopausal women with early breast cancer: first results of the ATAC randomised trial. Lancet 2002; 359: 2131–2139.

258. Thurlimann B, Keshaviah A, Coates AS, Mouridsen H, Mauriac L et al. A comparison of letrozole and tamoxifen in postmenopausal women with early breast cancer. New England Journal of Medicine 2005; 353: 2747–2757.

259. Fisher B, Dignam J, Bryant J, Wolmark N. Five versus more than five years of tamoxifen for lymph node-negative breast cancer: updated findings from the National Surgical Adjuvant Breast and Bowel Project B-14 randomized trial. Journal of the National Cancer Institute 2001; 93: 684–690.

259. Goss PE, Ingle JN, Martino S, Robert NJ, Muss HB et al. A randomized trial of letrozole in postmenopausal women after five years of tamoxifen therapy for early-stage breast cancer. New England Journal of Medicine 2003; 349: 1793–1802.

260. Mouridsen H, Gershanovich M, Sun Y, Perez-Carrion R, Boni C et al. Superior efficacy of letrozole versus tamoxifen as first-line therapy for postmenopausal women with advanced breast cancer: results of a phase III study of the International Letrozole Breast Cancer Group. Journal of Clinical Oncology 2001; 19: 2596–2606.

261. Jones S, Vogel C, Arkhipov A, Fehrenbacher L, Eisenberg P et al. Multicenter, phase II trial of exemestane as third-line hormonal therapy of postmenopausal women with metastatic breast cancer. Aromasin Study Group. Journal of Clinical Oncology 1999; 17: 3418–3425.

262. Baselga J, Campone M, Piccart M, Burris HA, 3rd, Rugo HS et al. Everolimus in postmenopausal hormone-receptor-positive advanced breast cancer. New England Journal of Medicine 2012; 366: 520–529.

263. Chia S, Gradishar W, Mauriac L, Bines J, Amant F et al. Double-blind, randomized placebo controlled trial of fulvestrant compared with exemestane after prior nonsteroidal aromatase inhibitor therapy in postmenopausal women with hormone receptor-positive, advanced breast cancer: results from EFECT. Journal of Clinical Oncology 2008; 26: 1664–1670.

264. Di Leo A, Jerusalem G, Petruzelka L, Torres R, Bondarenko IN et al. Results of the CONFIRM phase III trial comparing fulvestrant 250 mg with fulvestrant 500 mg in postmenopausal women with estrogen receptor-positive advanced breast cancer. Journal of Clinical Oncology 2010; 28: 4594–4600.

265. Robertson JF, Llombart-Cussac A, Rolski J, Feltl D, Dewar J, et al. Activity of fulvestrant 500 mg versus anastrozole 1 mg as first-line treatment for advanced breast cancer: results from the FIRST study. Journal of Clinical Oncology 2009; 27: 4530–4535.

266. Slamon DJ, Leyland-Jones B, Shak S, Fuchs H, Paton V et al. Use of chemotherapy plus a monoclonal antibody against HER2 for metastatic breast cancer that overexpresses HER2. New England Journal of Medicine 2001; 344: 783–792.

267. Marty M, Cognetti F, Maraninchi D, Snyder R, Mauriac L et al. Randomized phase II trial of the efficacy and safety of trastuzumab combined with docetaxel in patients with human epidermal growth factor receptor 2-positive metastatic breast cancer administered as first-line treatment: the M77001 study group. Journal of Clinical Oncology 2005; 23: 4265–4274.

268. Kaufman B, Mackey JR, Clemens MR, Bapsy PP, Vaid A et al. Trastuzumab plus anastrozole versus anastrozole alone for the treatment of postmenopausal women with human epidermal growth factor receptor 2-positive, hormone receptor-positive metastatic breast cancer: results from the randomized phase III TAnDEM study. Journal of Clinical Oncology 2009; 27: 5529–5537.

269. Johnston S, Pippen J, Jr., Pivot X, Lichinitser M, Sadeghi S et al. Lapatinib combined with letrozole versus letrozole and placebo as first-line therapy for postmenopausal hormone receptor-positive metastatic breast cancer. Journal of Clinical Oncology 2009; 27: 5538–5546.

270. Yin W, Jiang Y, Shen Z, Shao Z, Lu J. Trastuzumab in the adjuvant treatment of HER2-positive early breast cancer patients: a meta-analysis of published randomized controlled trials. PLoS One 2011; 6: e21030.

271. Perez EA, Romond EH, Suman VJ, Jeong JH, Davidson NE et al. Four-year follow-up of trastuzumab plus adjuvant chemotherapy for operable human epidermal growth factor receptor 2-positive breast cancer: joint analysis of data from NCCTG N9831 and NSABP B-31. Journal of Clinical Oncology 2011; 29: 3366–3373.

272. Joensuu H, Bono P, Kataja V, Alanko T, Kokko R et al. Fluorouracil, epirubicin, and cyclophosphamide with either docetaxel or vinorelbine, with or without trastuzumab, as adjuvant treatments of breast cancer: final results of the FinHer Trial. Journal of Clinical Oncology 2009; 27: 5685–5692.

273. Smith I, Procter M, Gelber RD, Guillaume S, Feyereislova A et al. 2-year follow-up of trastuzumab after adjuvant chemotherapy in HER2-positive breast cancer: a randomised controlled trial. Lancet 2007; 369: 29–36.

274. Geyer CE, Forster J, Lindquist D, Chan S, Romieu CG et al. Lapatinib plus capecitabine for HER2-positive advanced breast cancer. New England Journal of Medicine 2006; 355: 2733–2743.

275. Baselga J, Bradbury I, Eidtmann H, Di Cosimo S, de Azambuja E et al. Lapatinib with trastuzumab for HER2-positive early breast cancer (NeoALTTO): a randomised, open-label, multicentre, phase 3 trial. Lancet 2012; 379: 633–640.

276. Blackwell KL, Burstein HJ, Storniolo AM, Rugo H, Sledge G et al. Randomized study of Lapatinib alone or in combination with trastuzumab in women with ErbB2-positive, trastuzumab-refractory metastatic breast cancer. Journal of Clinical Oncology 2010; 28: 1124–1130.

277. Baselga J, Cortes J, Kim SB, Im SA, Hegg R et al. Pertuzumab plus trastuzumab plus docetaxel for metastatic breast cancer. New England Journal of Medicine 2012; 366: 109–119.

278. Baselga J, Gelmon KA, Verma S, Wardley A, Conte P et al. Phase II trial of pertuzumab and trastuzumab in patients with human epidermal growth factor receptor 2-positive metastatic breast cancer that progressed during prior trastuzumab therapy. Journal of Clinical Oncology 2010; 28: 1138–1144.

279. Burris HA, 3rd, Rugo HS, Vukelja SJ, Vogel CL, Borson RA et al. Phase II study of the antibody drug conjugate trastuzumab-DM1 for the treatment of human epidermal growth factor receptor 2 (HER2)-positive breast cancer after prior HER2-directed therapy. Journal of Clinical Oncology 2011; 29: 398–405.

280. Sabatini DM. mTOR and cancer: insights into a complex relationship. Nature Reviews Cancer 2006; 6: 729–734.

281. Bachelot T, Bourgier C, Cropet C, Guastalla J, Ferrero J et al. TAMRAD: a GINECO randomized phase II trial of everolimus in combination with tamoxifen versus tamoxifen alone in patients (pts) with hormone-receptor positive, HER2 negative metastatic breast cancer (MBC) with prior exposure to aromatase inhibitors (AI). Cancer Research 2010; 70: abstr S1–6.

282. Miles DW, Chan A, Dirix LY, Cortes J, Pivot X et al. Phase III study of bevacizumab plus docetaxel compared with placebo plus docetaxel for the first-line treatment of human epidermal growth factor receptor 2-negative metastatic breast cancer. Journal of Clinical Oncology 2010; 28: 3239–3247.

283. Jubb AM, Miller KD, Rugo HS, Harris AL, Chen D et al. Impact of exploratory biomarkers on the treatment effect of bevacizumab in metastatic breast cancer. Clinical Cancer Research 2011; 17: 372–381.

284. Bryant HE, Schultz N, Thomas HD, Parker KM, Flower D et al. Specific killing of BRCA2-deficient tumours with inhibitors of poly(ADP-ribose) polymerase. Nature 2005; 434: 913–917.

285. Tutt A, Robson M, Garber JE, Domchek SM, Audeh MW et al. Oral poly(ADP-ribose) polymerase inhibitor olaparib in patients with BRCA1 or BRCA2 mutations and advanced breast cancer: a proof-of-concept trial. Lancet 2010; 376: 235–244.

286. Berenson JR, Rosen LS, Howell A, Porter L, Coleman RE et al. Zoledronic acid reduces skeletal-related events in patients with osteolytic metastases. Cancer 2001; 91: 1191–1200.

287. Eidtmann H, de Boer R, Bundred N, Llombart-Cussac A, Davidson N et al. Efficacy of zoledronic acid in postmenopausal women with early breast cancer receiving adjuvant letrozole: 36-month results of the ZO-FAST Study. Annals of Oncology 2010; 21: 2188–2194.

288. Hershman DL, McMahon DJ, Crew KD, Cremers S, Irani D et al. Zoledronic acid prevents bone loss in premenopausal women undergoing adjuvant chemotherapy for early-stage breast cancer. Journal of Clinical Oncology 2008; 26: 4739–4745.

289. Gnant M, Mlineritsch B, Schippinger W, Luschin-Ebengreuth G, Pöstlberger S et al; ABCSG-12 Trial Investigators, Marth C. Endocrine therapy plus zoledronic acid in premenopausal breast cancer. New England Journal of Medicine 2009; 360: 679–691

290. Coleman RE, Marshall H, Cameron D, Dodwell D, Burkinshaw R et al. Breast cancer adjuvant therapy with zoledronic acid. New England Journal of Medicine 2011; 365: 1396–1405.

291. Yan T, Yin W, Zhou Q, Zhou L, Jiang Y et al. The efficacy of zoledronic acid in breast cancer adjuvant therapy: a meta-analysis of randomised controlled trials. European Journal of Cancer 2012; 48: 187–195.

292. Stopeck AT, Lipton A, Body JJ, Steger GG, Tonkin K et al. Denosumab compared with zoledronic acid for the treatment of bone metastases in patients with advanced breast cancer: a randomized, double-blind study. Journal of Clinical Oncology 2010; 28: 5132–5139.

293. Van Poznak CH, Temin S, Yee GC, Janjan NA, Barlow WE et al; American Society of Clinical Oncology. American Society of Clinical Oncology executive summary of the clinical practice guideline update on the role of bone-modifying agents in metastatic breast cancer. Journal of Clinical Oncology 2011; 29: 1221–1227.

294. Brennan MJ, Donegan WL, Appleby DE. The variability of estrogen receptors in metastatic breast cancer. American Journal of Surgery 1979; 137: 260–262.

295. Richter S, Zandvakili A. Meta analysis of discordant HER2 status in matched primary and metastatic breast cancer. SABCS 2011 PD05-05,

296. McCullough A et al. Abstract P3-10-36: Concordance of HER2 central assessment by two international central laboratories: a ring study within the framework of the adjuvant HER2-positive ALTTO trial (BIG2-06/N063D/EGF106708). Cancer Research 2011; 70: P3-10-36-P3-10-36.

297. Baselga, J et al. Lapatinib with trastuzumab for HER2-positive early breast cancer (NeoALTTO): a randomised, open-label, multicentre, phase 3 trial. Lancet 2012; 379: 633–640.

298. Gianni, L et al. Efficacy and safety of neoadjuvant pertuzumab and trastuzumab in women with locally advanced, inflammatory, or early HER2-positive breast cancer (NeoSphere): a randomised multicentre, open-label, phase 2 trial. Lancet Oncology 2012; 13: 25–32.

299. Blackwell KL et al. Randomized study of Lapatinib alone or in combination with trastuzumab in women with ErbB2-positive, trastuzumab-refractory metastatic breast cancer. Journal of Clinical Oncology 2010; 28: 1124–1130.

300. Baselga, J et al. Pertuzumab plus trastuzumab plus docetaxel for metastatic breast cancer. New England Journal of Medicine 2012; 366: 109–119.

301. LoRusso PM, Weiss D, Guardino E, Girish S, Sliwkowski MX. Trastuzumab emtansine: a unique antibody-drug conjugate in development for human epidermal growth factor receptor 2-positive cancer. Clinical Cancer Research 2011; 17: 6437–6447.

302. Lewis Phillips GD et al. Targeting HER2-positive breast cancer with trastuzumab-DM1, an antibody-cytotoxic drug conjugate. Cancer Research 2008; 68: 9280–9290.

303. Junttila TT, Li G, Parsons K, Phillips GL, Sliwkowski MX. Trastuzumab-DM1 (T-DM1) retains all the mechanisms of action of trastuzumab and efficiently inhibits growth of lapatinib insensitive breast cancer. Breast Cancer Research and Treatment 2011; 128: 347–356.

304. Borgelt B et al. The palliation of brain metastases: final results of the first two studies by the Radiation Therapy Oncology Group. International Journal of Radiation Oncology Biology Physics 1980; 6: 1–9.

305. Fokstuen T et al. Radiation therapy in the management of brain metastases from breast cancer. Breast Cancer Research and Treatment 2000; 62: 211–216.

306. Li J, Bentzen SM, Li J, Renschler M, Mehta MP. Relationship between neurocognitive function and quality of life after whole-brain radiotherapy in patients with brain metastasis. International Journal of Radiation Oncology Biology Physics 2008; 71: 64–70.

307. Chang EL et al. Neurocognition in patients with brain metastases treated with radiosurgery or radiosurgery plus whole-brain irradiation: a randomised controlled trial. Lancet Oncology 2010; 10, 1037–1044.

308. Akyurek S et al. Stereotactic radiosurgical treatment of cerebral metastases arising from breast cancer. American Journal of Clinical Oncology 2007; 30: 310–314.

309. Combs SE, Schulz-Ertner D, Thilmann C, Edler L, Debus J. Treatment of cerebral metastases from breast cancer with stereotactic radiosurgery. Strahlentherapie und Onkologie 2004; 180: 590–596.

310. Alexander E, Moriarty TM, Davis RB, Wen PY, Fine HA et al. Stereotactic radiosurgery for the definitive, noninvasive treatment of brain metastases. Journal of the National Cancer Institute 1995; 87: 34–40.

311. Flickinger JC, Kondziolka D, Lunsford LD, Coffey RJ, Goodman ML et al. A multi-institutional experience with stereotactic radiosurgery for solitary brain metastasis. International Journal of Radiation Oncology Biology Physics 1994; 28, 797–802.

312. Kocher M, Soffietti R, Abacioglu U, Villà S, Fauchon F et al. Adjuvant whole-brain radiotherapy versus observation after radiosurgery or surgical resection of one to three cerebral metastases: results of the EORTC 22952-26001 study. Journal of Clinical Oncology 2011; 29: 134–141.

CHAPTER 44

Gynaecological cancers

Richard Pötter, Shujuan Liu, Bolin Liu,
Sebastien Gouy, Sigurd Lax, Eric Leblanc,
Philippe Morice, Fabrice Narducci,
Alexander Reinthaller, Maximilian Paul Schmid,
Catherine Uzan, and Pauline Wimberger

Epidemiology of gynaecological cancers

Gynaecological cancers affect the female reproductive system including the vulva, vagina, cervix uteri, corpus uteri, ovary, placenta, and other unspecified organs.

Cervical cancer

Worldwide, cervical cancer is the third most common cancer in women, accounting for an estimated 529,800 new cases of cancer and 275,100 deaths annually. In contrast with endometrial cancer, developing countries have much higher rates of cervical cancer than developed countries. It is a model of viral carcinogenesis: high-risk human papilloma virus (HPV) infection is the major cause of almost all cervical cancers. Other cofactors associated with increased risk of cervical cancer include smoking, sexual behaviour, oral contraceptive use, HIV/AIDS, and lower socio-economic status. The incidence and mortality rates of cervical cancer have been reduced considerably with screening programs, which in combination with HPV vaccination may offer a promising way to lower the global burden of this disease.

Endometrial cancer

Worldwide, there are more than 287,100 newly diagnosed cases of endometrial cancer and around 73,900 deaths annually. It is the most common cancer among women in the developed world, with an incidence double those of the less developed countries. Most of the established risk factors for endometrial cancer are associated with excessive unopposed estrogen stimulation on the endometrium, including hormone replacement therapy, tamoxifen use, nulliparity, obesity, and diabetes. Physical activity, use of combined oral contraceptives, pregnancy and childbirth reduce the risk. There is no evidence-supported screening test for endometrial cancer, as most cases (85%) are diagnosed at low stage because of early symptoms like postmenopausal bleeding and survival rates are high.

Ovarian cancer

Approximately 225,500 ovarian cancers are diagnosed annually worldwide. It is the leading cause of gynaecological cancer death (140,200 worldwide annually), which accounts for more deaths than all the other gynaecological cancers combined. Although the aetiology of ovarian cancer is not yet clear, the strongest known risk factors are increasing age and certain gene mutations such as BRCA1 and BRCA2. Pregnancy and use of oral contraceptives are established protective factors. Large-scale randomized controlled trials have been conducted to screen preclinical ovarian cancers with transvaginal ultrasound and CA125. Preliminary results show that population-based screening or screening in a high-risk population are not recommended because no effective detection of early stage ovarian cancer is present and therefore no mortality benefits could be demonstrated compared with usual care.

Vaginal and vulvar cancers

Each year in the UK, approximately 280 and 1200 women are diagnosed with vaginal and vulvar cancers, respectively. The associated mortality rates are 90 and 410, respectively. HPV infection is the primary risk factor for vaginal and vulvar cancers; others include non-HPV sexually transmitted infections, smoking, exposure to diethylstilbestrol (DES) in utero (only for vaginal cancer), and iatrogenic immunosuppression.

Molecular biology and pathology of gynaecological cancers

Gynaecologic cancer may basically occur at four major sites: the uterus (cervix and corpus uteri, the latter including endometrium and myometrium) and its adnexae (ovary and fallopian tube), the vagina, and the vulva. These cancers are histologically biologically different according to their site and tissue of origin and, in particular, based on their aetiology and molecular pathogenesis. The incidence of these neoplasms is strongly influenced by key pathogenetic factors, although the aetiology has not been unravelled for all of these tumours. In the industrialized countries with an aging population, the most frequent gynaecologic cancers are endometrial and ovarian carcinoma, whereas cervical carcinoma has become rare compared to most developing countries due to early detection of precursors by screening programs. Histologically, most cancer types are carcinomas, whereas sarcomas and haematological neoplasms are rare. Anatomic and molecular pathology does not only provide insight into the tumorigenesis of the various types of gynaecological cancers but is also strongly involved in the diagnostic procedure, which precedes and accompanies the therapeutic process.

Molecular biology of cervical cancer

Cervical carcinoma is a global burden, although it has become infrequent in most industrialized countries. In South-east Asia, Africa, and most parts of Latin America the incidence is six- to tenfold that of Europe, the US, Canada, and Australia. The incidence of cervical carcinoma is strongly associated with early detection of its precursors by screening programs and by the availability of efficient screening for the population, respectively. This is even reflected by a strikingly different incidence within the EU.

The development of cervical carcinoma and its precursors is strongly related to HPV since HPV DNA is found in almost all cervical carcinomas except for some rare histological subtypes. High-grade squamous intraepithelial lesion (SIL)/cervical intraepithelial neoplasia (CIN) and squamous cell carcinoma, as well as adenocarcinoma in situ (AIS) and adenocarcinoma are associated with high-risk HPV types, in particular HPV 16, 18 and 31, 33, 45, and some others. These HPV types harbour oncogenic potential by affecting crucial mechanisms of the host cell. In particular, two viral proteins, E6 and E7, bind to the regulatory proteins p53 and Rb, respectively, and further activate cyclins A and E and inhibit the cyclin dependent kinase inhibitors WAF-1 and p27. Constitutive over-expression of E6 and E7 due to chronic viral infection of the host cell finally results in a block of unrestricted cell proliferation as well as of the apoptotic pathway. These changes impair the infected cells to respond adequately to damage by oncogenic factors by apoptosis or DNA repair after cell cycle arrest. Loss of function of p53 and Rb by inactivation, therefore, leads to an accumulation of genetic alterations and increasing genomic instability. In particular, loss of 3q where the FHIT gene is located is considered a frequent genetic alteration in cervical squamous cell carcinoma. Mutations of p53 and K-Ras are rare in cervical carcinoma. It is assumed that the basal cells of the cervical mucosa are infected by HPV after microabrasions. Proliferation of these transformed basal cells leads to an architectural change of the squamous epithelium that subsequently, in the setting of high-grade SIL, is completely composed of atypical basal cells and lacks terminal differentiation. In contrast to low-grade SIL, HPV DNA is integrated in the genome of the host cells of high-grade SIL/CIN and invasive squamous carcinoma as well as AIS and invasive adenocarcinoma. In this pathogenetic concept, HPV is considered the key factor that is able to infect and even transform cells but needs cofactors in particular for the development of invasive carcinoma. Immunosuppression, in particular by co-infection, cigarette smoking, use of oral contraceptives, and dietary factors are considered relevant cofactors for the development of cervical carcinoma. Nevertheless, only one-third of HPV-positive women show cytological abnormalities and viral clearance is supposed to occur in more than 90% of infections. Currently, persistence of infections by high-risk HPV for more than two years is currently considered the greatest risk for the development of cervical carcinoma.

Pathology of cervical cancer

Grossly, cervical cancer presents as enlargement of the cervix by tumour tissue, often with ulceration. It needs to be emphasized that small carcinomas, in particular microinvasive carcinomas, may present without grossly visible tumour. Histologically, the most frequent tumour type is squamous cell carcinoma, which may show keratinization. Adenocarcinoma with several variants is another major histological type. Rare histological type include neuroendocrine tumours (including small cell carcinoma), glassy cell carcinoma, adenosquamous carcinoma, adenoid cystic, and adenoid basal cell carcinoma. The latter type does not seem to be related to HPV. Based on data from the US and other countries, the percentage of adenocarcinoma has increased in relation to squamous cell carcinoma during the last three decades although the total number of cervical cancer cases has decreased. This may be due to the fact that early detection of adenocarcinoma and AIS by cytological screening may be more difficult compared to high-grade SIL. About 75% of endocervical adenocarcinoma reveal a similar histological pattern and are therefore named 'usual type'. The mucin content of endocervical adenocarcinoma cells may be sparse and may lead to the misconception of endometrioid carcinoma, which infrequently occurs in the cervix as a primary site. Other histological types, such as serous and clear cell carcinoma, are rare. Since tumour volume is an important parameter for the clinical course, early carcinoma stages have been designated as microinvasive carcinoma (MIC). By definition, MIC is limited to a horizontal tumour spread of 7mm and a depth of invasion of 3mm (pT1a1/FIGO stage IA1) and 5 mm (pT1a2/FIGO stage IA2), respectively. Microinvasive squamous cell carcinoma is associated with a very low frequency of lymph node metastases (less than 3% at stage IA1 and less than 8% at stage IA2), which also implicates a different therapeutic strategy. The role of lymphovascular space involvement (LVSI) as a predictor of lymph node metastases in MIC is, so far, unclear and has been controversial. However, most studies have shown that LVSI is an adverse prognostic factor and may be able to predict recurrence after cone biopsy and residual carcinoma within the hysterectomy specimen. Microinvasive adenocarcinoma is less well studied with respect to behaviour than squamous MIC and may be difficult to assess, in particular if it is associated with extensive AIS. The presence of AIS at the surgical margins is more problematic with respect to residual tumour compared to high-grade SIL/CIN3. Extension of cervical carcinoma involves the vagina (pT2a and 3a/FIGO stages IIA and IIIA), the parametria (pT2b and 3b/FIGO stages IIB and IIIB), the urinary bladder, and the rectum (pT4/FIGO stage IVA). Involvement of the uterine corpus does not affect stage and metastases to the adnexae are rare (less than 1%), but somewhat higher in the case of adenocarcinomas. Infiltration of the cervix by malignant lymphoma is unusual but needs to be recognized in cervical biopsy. Immunohistochemistry may be important for the distinction of lymphoma from other undifferentiated neoplasms and in some cases for the distinction between primary endometrial and cervical carcinoma.

Molecular biology of endometrial cancer

Endometrial carcinoma is the most frequent malignancy of the uterine corpus. In contrast to cervical carcinoma it is more frequent in the industrialized countries (except for Japan) compared to developing countries. This is most likely related to several factors such as higher age of the population, use of hormone replacement therapy, higher body mass index and others. One of the most important risk factors for endometrial carcinoma is unopposed oestrogen stimulation of the endometrium, which may not only be caused by exogenous oestrogen (e.g., for hormone replacement therapy) but also by endogenous factors such as non-ovulatory cycles, polycystic ovary syndrome, high BMI with conversion of DHEA to oestrogens by aromatase in the adipose tissue and oestrogens producing neoplasms such as granulosa cell tumour. However, about 15–20% of endometrial carcinomas do not seem to be oestrogen-related. Therefore, endometrial carcinoma is roughly divided into two biologically distinctive types, which can also be separated on the molecular genetic level. Type 1 carcinomas, at 80% the great majority, are related to oestrogen, which present at low stage and show a favourable clinical course. Histologically, they mostly represent low-grade (FIGO grade 1 and 2) endometrioid adenocarcinomas and its variants. They develop through atypical endometrial hyperplasia following an adenoma-carcinoma pathway. In contrast, the non-oestrogen-related type 2 carcinomas are frequently diagnosed at high stages, often with extensive extrauterine disease and/or distant metastases, and are typically associated with poor clinical outcome. The histological prototype, which is best studied, is serous carcinoma but also clear cell carcinomas, undifferentiated carcinomas, high-grade/FIGO grade 3 endometrioid carcinomas, carcinosarcomas, or mixed malignant Müllerian tumours (MMMT) are encountered among type 2 cancers. For serous carcinoma, a flat precursor lesion has been characterized and named serous endometrial intraepithelial carcinoma (SEIC); for the other histological types no precursors have been defined. It is likely that some type 2 carcinomas develop through low-grade type 1 carcinomas by tumour progression. Type 1 and type 2 endometrial carcinomas are also distinctive on the molecular level. Type 1 carcinomas show an adenoma-carcinoma sequence with a stepwise accumulation of molecular alterations comparable to colorectal carcinoma. Mutations in PTEN, K-Ras, ß-catenin, and PIK3CA as well as inactivation of Pax-2 occur in atypical hyperplasia and/or in low-grade endometrioid carcinoma and, therefore, are considered early events. In contrast, p53 mutations are typically found in high-grade endometrioid carcinoma, which suggests a late event

during tumour progression. Some of the abnormally expressed genes in type 1 carcinomas such as PIK3CA are related to endometrial homeostasis and regulated during menstrual cycle, in particular, by a link to ER expression. A subset of about 25–40% of type 1 carcinomas reveal a mutator phenotype which is characterized by a high degree of microsatellite instability (MSI). In sporadic endometrioid carcinoma, MSI is most frequently caused by inactivation of the mismatch repair protein MLH1 by methylation. Less than 5% of endometrial carcinoma is considered hereditary, most of which is associated with hereditary non-polyposis colorectal cancer (HNPCC, Lynch syndrome) and typically associated with germline mutation of one of the mismatch repair proteins MSH2, MLH1, or MSH6. Type 2 endometrial carcinomas are characterized by a high degree of genomic instability. The most frequent molecular alteration is p53 mutation, which affects more than 80% of serous carcinomas and leads to accumulation of inactive p53 in the nucleus. Over-expression of p53 can be demonstrated by immunohistochemistry and may show two different immunoreactive patterns: either intensely diffuse or less frequently flat negative. Recent studies using next generation sequencing have confirmed the high frequency of p53 mutations in endometrial serous carcinomas and found novel mutations in the genes FBXW7, PIK3CA, and PPP2R1A occurring in about 18–23% of endometrial serous carcinoma. Altered FBXW7 leads to overexpression of cyclin E1 in a subset of SEIC and serous carcinoma. Recently, the TCGA Research Network tried to characterize four different groups of endometrial carcinoma based on the amount of copy number alterations and was able to stratify them for overall survival. A subgroup with excellent prognosis characterized by mutations in the novel gene POLE was found. The molecular alterations in other type 2 carcinomas are less well defined. p53 mutations are found in about 30–40% and PTEN mutations in about 10–20% of clear cell carcinomas (see Figure 44.1).

Pathology of endometrial cancer

The various histological types of endometrial carcinoma are typically adenocarcinomas with distinctive features. Endometrioid carcinoma usually consists of well-preserved glands with straight luminal borders that more or less resemble proliferating

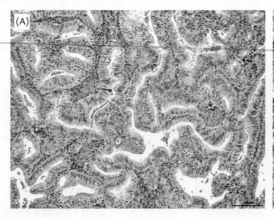
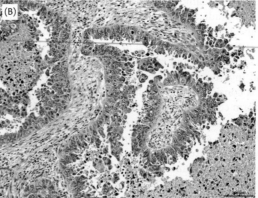

Fig. 44.1 The two major types of endometrial carcinoma, endometrioid (A) and serous (B) adenocarcinoma. Endometrioid adenocarcinoma, if well differentiated forms well preserved glands and shows mild to moderate nuclear atypia, whereas serous adenocarcinoma is characterized by highly atypical nuclei, detachment of tumour cells, and tumour cell necrosis. HE, 100 ×.

endometrium and, if poorly differentiated, reveals a predominantly solid pattern. FIGO grading of endometrioid carcinoma is based on its amount of solid, non-squamous growth. Grade 1 carcinomas contain 5% or less; grade 2, 6–50%; and grade 3 carcinomas more than 50% of a solid, non-squamous growth pattern. Variants of endometrioid carcinoma may show various histological patterns of differentiation such as squamous, secretory, mucinous, and ciliated type. Rarely, pure mucinous carcinoma may occur in the endometrium, which is biologically encountered among type 1 cancers. One hallmark of serous carcinoma is the combination of a well-differentiated architecture and a high degree of nuclear atypia. It is furthermore important to emphasize that not all serous carcinomas show a papillary pattern but may reveal glandular or even solid growth. In contrast to endometrioid carcinoma, the cells of serous carcinoma form buds and are frequently detached. Serous carcinoma may be confused with the villoglandular variant of endometrioid carcinoma which is typically composed of delicate papillae covered by pseudostratified endometrioid type epithelium with low to moderate degree of nuclear atypia. Clear cell carcinoma is composed of hobnail shaped or polygonal cells with clear or less frequently eosinophilic cytoplasm arranged in a tubule-cystic, solid, or papillary pattern. The secretory variant of endometrioid carcinoma should not be confused with clear cell carcinoma because of its better prognosis. Mixed malignant Müllerian tumours (MMMT, carcinosarcoma) are considered carcinomas with a sarcoma-like component. Recently, a group of carcinomas composed of a well-differentiated and an undifferentiated component was named dedifferentiated carcinoma. For optimal therapeutic management histological typing and grading needs to be performed on curettage specimen. Immunohistochemistry including a panel of p53, ER, Ki67, PTEN, and p16 may be helpful for typing. It needs be emphasized that diffuse p16 immunoreactivity is not only typical for the majority of serous carcinomas but also for mucinous carcinomas. For the extent of surgery in low-grade endometrioid carcinomas the intraoperative assessment of myometrial invasion by frozen section may be important. Usually, preoperative ultrasound gives an impression if T1 or T2 tumours are present. If it is not clear in the first procedure, laparoscopic total hysterectomy and bilateral oophorectomy is performed. If, in the final histology report, pT1b is documented a second surgery with pelvic and para-aortic lymphadenectomy is necessary. The determination of early myometrial invasion may be difficult, in particular if the endo-myometrial junction is extensively involved but does not affect pathological stage in the 2009 FIGO/UICC staging system. Tumours with infiltration of adenomyosis without invasion of the surrounding myometrium should be staged as tumours confined to the endometrium. LVSI is of prognostic value and needs to be recognized. Positive peritoneal cytology is an adverse prognostic factor although it is not included in FIGO staging. Several parameters and models have been tested for the prediction of prognosis. So far, histological type and grade, depth of myometrial invasion, and vascular space involvement are the strongest predictors of prognosis. Among molecular factors, a combination of p53 and p16 positivity has been demonstrated to detect tumours with poor prognosis.

Molecular biology of ovarian carcinoma

During the recent years new concepts for ovarian tumorigenesis have been introduced. Currently, two major pathways are distinguished for ovarian carcinoma comparable to that of endometrial carcinomas. Type 1 carcinomas, including low-grade serous, mucinous, endometrioid, and transitional cell carcinomas (malignant Brenner tumours) develop through the stage of a borderline tumour which can be considered an adenoma-carcinoma sequence. They are mostly slow-growing neoplasms that are frequently diagnosed at low stage and are associated with good prognosis. In contrast, type 2 carcinomas, to which high-grade serous and high-grade endometrioid carcinomas are encountered, seem to develop without an adenoma or borderline tumour stage. They are typically diagnosed at high stage and usually show rapid growth and poor outcome. MMMT (carcinosarcomas) and undifferentiated carcinomas are further included within the type 2 ovarian carcinoma category. There is strong evidence that the fallopian tube is strongly involved in the development of at least a subset of high-grade serous carcinomas, which seem to arise from a highly atypical precursor in the fimbria, named serous tubal intraepithelial carcinoma (STIC). The progression of STIC into high-grade serous carcinoma may lead to ovarian carcinomas with prominent surface involvement and early spread to the peritoneum. Furthermore, it has been demonstrated that serous inclusions are derived from the fallopian tube epithelium rather than from the ovarian surface. The development of ovarian inclusion cysts seems to be related to ovulation, which may explain the hypothesized association between the frequency of ovulation and the incidence of ovarian carcinoma. This may further explain the decreased ovarian carcinoma incidence with oral contraceptive use. Ovarian inclusion cysts are the origin of cystadenomas and borderline tumours and, therefore, most likely the origin for the type 1 carcinoma pathway, particular for low-grade serous carcinomas. Mucinous neoplasms are supposed to develop through mucinous metaplasia in inclusion cysts but may less frequently arise from mucinous cysts in teratomas. Endometrioid and clear cell carcinomas are frequently associated with ovarian endometrioisis which may be caused by retrograde menstruation. Brenner tumours seem to develop from Walthardt nests. The molecular alterations in type 1 and type 2 ovarian carcinomas are significantly different and can be compared to the dualistic model of endometrial carcinoma. Low-grade serous carcinomas frequently harbour mutations of K-ras and B-raf and partially show a mutator phenotype with a high frequency of MSI, whereas low-grade mucinous carcinomas frequently harbour K-ras mutations. P53 mutations seem to occur late, when low-grade serous and mucinous carcinoma progress into high-grade carcinomas. In contrast, high-grade serous carcinomas show frequent p53 mutations which are also present in STIC and, therefore, are considered an early event. Low-grade endometrioid carcinomas are characterized by mutations of ß-catenin, PTEN, and ARID1A, whereas clear cell carcinomas show frequent PIK3CA mutations. The degree of chromosomal instability is low in type 1 carcinomas and high in type 2 carcinomas. Ongoing research is particularly focused on type 2 carcinomas with its poor prognosis. Recently, a model for the prognostic stratification of high-grade serous carcinoma based on the expression profile of 879 genes has been proposed by the TCGA Network. A Japanese/US group showed that expression of the gene FNB1 is associated with early recurrence of high-grade serous carcinoma.

Pathology of ovarian carcinoma

See Figure 44.2. Histologically, almost all ovarian carcinomas are adenocarcinomas with a spectrum of differentiation similar to

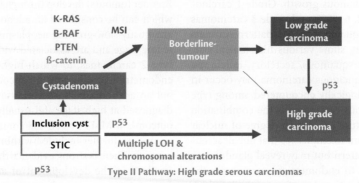

Fig. 44.2 Pathogenesis of ovarian carcinoma: currently, two major pathways are considered for the development of ovarian carcinoma. Type 1 carcinomas typically develop from an adenoma through a borderline tumour to a low-grade carcinoma following an adenoma-carcinoma sequence whereas type 2 carcinomas seem to occur de novo from an inclusion cyst or a high-grade intraepithelial lesion deriving from the fallopian tube (STIC).

the uterine corpus. The most frequent histological type is serous carcinoma which most closely resembles the fallopian tube epithelium. Serous carcinomas are characterized by a frequent, but not exclusive, papillary architecture and by budding and detachment of the tumour cells. A glandular or solid growth pattern may also be found. Traditionally, serous carcinoma have been graded by a 3-tiered system, which was recently changed into a 2-tiered system (low- vs high-grade) based on nuclear atypia and the number of mitosis. Mucinous carcinomas are mostly low grade, typically show a glandular or papillary architecture and consist of mucin-producing cells. Endometrioid and clear cell carcinomas closely resemble their counterparts within the endometrium and are typically associated with endometriosis. Malignant Brenner tumours usually reveal the histological features of transitional cell carcinomas of the urinary tract. Grading of mucinous and endometrioid carcinomas follows the rules for endometrial endometrioid carcinoma. For clear cell carcinomas, nuclear grading is used. Since some ovarian carcinomas may be heterogenous and may be associated with borderline tumours, careful gross inspection and adequate sampling is necessary. In difficult cases, immunohistochemistry may be helpful for differential diagnosis using a panel of several antibodies, in particular for p53, ER, WT1, ß-catenin, p16, vimentin, PTEN, and HNF1. In particular, WT1 positivity is typical for extrauterine serous carcinomas and not found in the other histological types. However, most serous carcinomas originating from the endometrium are also WT1 negative. High-grade serous carcinomas are further diffusely positive for p16, positive for ER, CA125 and PTEN and lack vimentin and nuclear ß-catenin staining. Mucinous carcinomas are negative for ER, PR, and CA125and can be focally positive for p16. Endometrioid carcinomas are positive for ER and frequently show nuclear ß-catenin staining and lack of PTEN and WT1, clear cell carcinomas are ER, WT1, and HNF1 negative. Mucinous neoplasms in the ovary may be in fact metastases from the gastrointestinal tract and mimic mucinous borderline tumours or carcinomas. Basically, metastases are more frequently bilateral and usually smaller, often less than 10 cm in diameter. They often show a nodular growth pattern, involvement of the ovarian surface, and pseudomyxoma peritonei and ovarii, which means mucin on the ovarian surface and within the peritoneal cavity and within the ovarian stroma, respectively. For differential diagnosis of primary ovarian and metastatic mucinous neoplasms, a panel

of CK7, CK20, and cdx2 may be useful only for a subset of cases. Metastatic neoplasms from the pancreatobiliary system may show the same immunoprofile as ovarian mucinous neoplasms and ovarian mucinous neoplasms derived from teratomas and may show the same immunoprofile as metastatic neoplasms from the colon. Thus, clinical and radiological information is very important for the pathologist. Metastatic colorectal carcinomas may also mimic endometrioid neoplasms. In this setting, immunohistochemistry is more reliable for differential diagnosis and may include oestrogen receptors in addition to CK7, CK20, and cdx2.

Since preoperative histological diagnosis of ovarian carcinoma is not possible except for cases with extensive peritoneal disease, intraoperative frozen section plays an important role for the therapeutical strategy. The sensitivity of frozen section is excellent for the typical, mostly high-grade serous carcinoma (more than 90%) but less good for borderline tumours (60–70%), and poor for metastases (less than 50%). In particular, the recognition of metastatic colorectal carcinoma is important since it changes the surgical procedure significantly. The most important prognostic factors are stage, residual tumour after surgery, histological type and grade. Currently, prognostic molecular markers are under development.

Molecular biology of vaginal carcinoma

Most women with vaginal carcinoma have associated carcinomas and/or intraepithelial neoplasias of cervix or vulva. A potential field effect has been discussed. It has been observed that radiation therapy of cervical carcinoma predisposes to subsequent HPV-related lesions in the vagina. Although the data are limited, the same molecular pathogenesis can be assumed as for HPV-related neoplasms of cervix and vulva.

Pathology of vaginal carcinoma

In contrast to carcinomas of the cervix and the vulva, vaginal carcinoma is rare. Histologically, it is typically a squamous cell carcinoma. It is very frequently associated with or preceded by vaginal intraepithelial neoplasia (VAIN). For the definition of primary vaginal carcinoma the tumour must be located in the vagina without involvement of cervix or vulva, which excludes bulky tumours of the upper vagina with infiltration of the cervix. Due to the thin wall of the vagina the tumours spread early to other pelvic tissues and structures. Microinvasive carcinoma is not separately defined but carcinomas with less than 3 mm of invasion show a low frequency of lymph node metastases. As with vulvar cancers, verrucous carcinoma is associated with excellent prognosis. A recently described type of vaginal cancer, with controversial prognosis and similarity to transitional cell carcinomas, is papillary squamotransitional carcinoma. Clear cell adenocarcinoma has been associated with exposure to diethylstilbestrol (DES) but may also occur unrelated to DES in the postmenopausal setting. It shows a tubule-cystic or solid pattern and spreads locally via lymphatics and even to the peritoneum. However, its general prognosis is favourable, particularly after DES exposure.

Molecular biology of vulvar carcinoma

Two molecular pathways are distinguished for vulvar carcinoma, one HPV-related, the other non-HPV-related. The HPV-related type is associated high-risk HPV, develops through warty or basaloid vulvar intraepithelial neoplasia (VIN) and occurs in women of middle age (mean age 50 years). These patients may further show other HPV-related lesions, e.g., in the vagina or cervix. Heavy cigarette smoking and chronic immunosuppression are further risk factors. The non-HPV-related type occurs in the postmenopausal age group (mean age 77 years) and is frequently associated with lichen sclerosus or rarely other chronic skin diseases such as granulomatoses. Differentiated VIN is considered a potential precursor of the latter type of vulvar carcinoma. P53 over-expression and mutation, respectively, may occur both in differentiated VIN and non-HPV-related invasive squamous cell carcinoma as well as overexpression of TGF-ß. If stratified by age, the older age group is rarely associated with HPV, while the younger age group is mostly HPV-related.

Pathology of vulvar carcinoma

The major histological type is squamous cell carcinoma of which several subtypes are distinguished. For therapy, tumour stage is important, which includes the tumour size as determined by the maximum diameter and the depth of invasion. An invasion of 1mm or less is considered most favourable for outcome. In addition, tumour thickness and the presence or absence of vascular space involvement needs to be included in the pathology report. Between 1 and 2 mm of invasion, the frequency of lymph node metastases rises from 0 to 12%. Verrucous carcinoma is a rare variant with pushing borders, rare lymph node metastases, and excellent prognosis if complete excision is possible. Adenocarcinoma of the vulva is very unusual. Sentinel lymph node biopsy has become a standard procedure for vulvar carcinoma.

Surgical management of gynaecological cancers

Surgical management of gynaecological tumours remains a cornerstone of the treatment of these tumours. Therefore, surgical intervention has diagnostic, staging, and therapeutic value. Surgical management at each location encompasses treatment of the initial tumour and lymph nodes, which remain the first site of spread.

Cervical cancer

Cervix cancer is the second cause of female cancer worldwide. Although surgery is particularly indicated at early stages of the disease, it can be selectively indicated after shrinkage of the tumour burden with chemotherapy or chemoradiation or in case of a local recurrence. Its unique HPV aetiology has prompted the development of efficient vaccines that, combined with an organized screening policy, should eradicate this disease over time.

Diagnosis and staging

Although ultrasound can be used, MRI is now recognized as the best imaging method for the assessment of local disease parameters such as the tumour size, paracervical extent, and to a lesser degree node involvement [1]. Hybrid 18-FDG PET CT is better indicated for assessing the extent of advanced disease or recurrence and/or to plan chemoradiation therapy [2]. However, the detection limits of functional imaging explain why diagnostic surgery may still play a role at any stage of the disease [3].

Principles of surgery

Surgical management of cervical carcinomas can be differentiated in three directions: diagnostic surgery to adapt the future treatment, radical surgery to cure patients, and preventive surgery to avoid morbidity and complications related to other treatments (especially radiation therapy).

Diagnostic and therapeutic surgery
Conization

Conization aims to remove the squamo-glandular junction in the cervix, better known as the transformation zone where cancer begins. This resection can be diagnostic or therapeutic provided all intraepithelial neoplasia has been excised with free margins. The use of a large electrical loop to excise the transformation zone has now systematically replaced the cold knife or CO2 laser conization, both of which gave rise to a higher rate of post-operative morbidity [4] or difficulties during specimen examination. However, cervix stenosis or obstetrical morbidities do not seem to be significantly different whatever the conization method [5]. But the rate of cervical insufficiency is less in the case of loop excision in comparison to cold knife excision.

Lymphadenectomies

Due to its prognostic and management impact, nodal involvement is an important event in the evolution of cervical cancer. As underlined above, the accuracy of either morphologic (MRI, CT) or functional (PET/CT) imaging techniques is not reliable enough for planning adequate treatment although improvements are in the pipeline. Surgery, including lymphadenectomies, is the gold standard method for achieving a reliable result. Anatomical principles for a comprehensive dissection have been studied [6], which have led to a clarified definition of the different levels of node resection [7].

Pelvic lymphadenectomy

The goal is to remove all nodes around the iliac pedicles down to the level of the obturator and ilio-lumbar nerves, from the obturator foramen caudally, up to the aorto-caval bifurcation cranially [8]. If dissection via laparotomy was the first and reference approach, laparoscopic dissection was subsequently introduced in the early 90s. No significant technical modifications have occurred since the first publication on the technique. Results compare favourably with the open trans- and extraperitoneal approaches in terms of the number of nodes, morbidity, and quality of life. Indeed, since the pioneer series, perioperative morbidity of laparoscopic lymphadenectomy is very low, especially after fulfilling learning curve requirements. Although infrequent, leg oedema remains the most debilitating distant complications [9].

Para-aortic lymphadenectomy

Due to a stepwise spread of nodal disease from the pelvis to the subclavicular area, the detection of para-aortic nodal disease can alter patient management. Indeed, para-aortic nodal disease is effectively treated with extended-field chemoradiation, but with significant haematological and digestive toxicity [10]. This drawback justifies reserving this treatment for patients with proven para-aortic nodal involvement. PET scanning has been suggested for the detection of para-aortic nodal disease; unfortunately, the results are disappointing in case of microscopic involvement [3].

Surgical staging is a good way to assess both the presence of intraperitoneal disease as well as nodal disease, especially at the para-aortic level, but is confounded by significant morbidity. However, among experienced teams, the laparoscopic para-aortic node dissection results in less morbidity, especially when radiation therapy is considered. As for laparotomy, Dargent's extraperitoneal laparoscopic approach seems to be superior to its transperitoneal counterpart for this indication [11].

In early-stage disease with positive pelvic nodes, the rate of para-aortic involvement attains 15%. Although this rate approaches 20%, the therapeutic value of this exploration in locally advanced cervical carcinomas is more questionable. Although a randomized study published in 2003 did not demonstrate any advantage of pretherapeutic surgical staging [12], more recent results seem to show a survival advantage of resecting microscopic nodal disease that is undetectable by PET scan [13]. Only a randomized trial, incorporating PET imaging, could address this important issue regarding the possible advantage of pretherapeutic surgical para-aortic staging in locally advanced disease (tumour size >4 cm).

Sentinel node

In order to limit the morbidity of extensive lymph node dissections and to improve the detection of nodal disease, the sentinel node concept, already validated for breast cancers, was recently implemented in cervical cancer. A recent prospective study compared the results of sentinel node resection, systematically followed by the comprehensive dissection of each hemi-pelvis. In addition to 15% of uncommon sentinel node sites, this study showed that nodal detection and examination had an overall sensitivity rate of 92% and a negative predictive value of 98.2%. If sentinel node detection is bilateral, the negative predictive value approaches 100% [14]. These results prompted a randomized study comparing sentinel node detection alone versus a full pelvic dissection; the study is currently accruing patients.

Radical surgery

Radical hysterectomy and trachelectomy

According to the pattern of spread of cervical cancer, a radical hysterectomy aims to remove the uterus and the tubes, with or without the ovaries (according to the patient's age), the upper part of the vagina, and a variable proportion of the paracervical tissues. A new classification of radical hysterectomies, based on internationally recognized anatomical landmarks, is attempting to clarify the different procedures and their indications [7, 15].

For young patients who wish to preserve their fertility, and fulfilling all criteria, a radical operation limited to the cervix and preserving the corpus is feasible and is called a radical trachelectomy or Dargent's operation, a radical vaginal trachelectomy [16].

Regarding lymphadenectomies, different approaches are available when performing a radical hysterectomy (or trachelectomy): abdominal (Wertheim-Meigs-Okabayashi operation), vaginal (Shauta-Amreich or Schauta-Stöckel operation), laparoscopic with (coelio-Schauta) or without (coelio-Wertheim) vaginal assistance, or robotic surgery have been extensively described by the authors and recently reviewed [17, 18].

Eventually, in the absence of a randomized comparative study, the choice of the type and approach for a radical operation will be based on patient and tumour characteristics as well as on hospital facilities and the surgeon's own experience!

Nowadays, the mortality of these operations is regularly less than 2%, and perioperative morbidity is directly related to the extent of the radicality of the procedure: haemorrhage, fistulas, and ureteral stenosis, ranging from 5–15%. By contrast, the rate of functional sequelae remains significant: almost 20% of patients suffer from urinary voiding disorders, sexual disturbances, or severe constipation. Most of these adverse effects can be limited by a more precise pelvic dissection, especially preserving, whenever possible, the autonomous pelvic nerves [19, 20]. An innovative new therapeutic surgical concept is the total mesometrial resection (TMMR) with resection of the embryologically-defined uterovaginal (Müllerian) compartment and therapeutic lymphadenectomy for higher local control and avoidance of adjuvant radiotherapy even in case of risk factors. In this case, the vascular and the ligamentous mesometrium will be resected and the uterus and tubes and part of the vagina, but sparing the nerves [21].

Exenteration

In selected locally advanced cervix tumours or recurrences, an exenterative procedure may be required. It consists of the removal of at least two pelvic organs: anterior (bladder and uterus); posterior (uterus and rectum); total (both compartments). Another classification has been suggested according to the height of the resection from the levator ani [22]. Reconstruction of the pelvic floor, by means of musculo-cutaneous, omental flaps, or human cellular dermal matrix [23], with or without a colpoplasty, is important to fill the empty pelvis and prevent bowel occlusion or fistulas. In the case of a latero-pelvic recurrence, a laterally-extended endopelvic resection can be successfully performed with acceptable morbidity and promising survival results [24]. Although the mortality engendered by the procedure has been reduced to less than 5% through improvements in intra- and perioperative care, morbidity remains high, especially if patients have previously received high-dose radiation therapy [25].

Surgery to reduce treatment-related morbidity

This concept aims to reduce the effects of post-operative radiation therapy.

Ovary or adnexal transposition

This procedure, initiated by Lerue Charlus, consists in disconnecting one or both adnexae from the uterus and mobilizing them along with their pedicle outside the future pelvic radiation field. They are transposed and secured high in the paracolic gutters, directly or through the prior extraperitonization of their vascular pedicle. The procedure can be performed by laparoscopy. Preservation of hormonal function can be obtained in more than 50% of cases [26]. Indications for this procedure are limited to patients devoid of risk or at a low risk of ovarian spread (stage IB1, squamous tumour without extracervical spread).

Pelvic exclusion prior to radiation therapy

The goal is to prevent radio-induced bowel damage by installing a mesh (resorbable or omental mesh) around the pelvic sling or placing a temporary breast implant [27].

Endometrial cancer

Due to early symptoms, the diagnosis of endometrial cancer (EC) is often made at an early stage and the prognosis is generally good. Major advances in recent years have been achieved in the knowledge of pathology. A new molecular classification defined two different molecular pathways of carcinogenesis [28]. Type I endometrioid tumours are oestrogen-related lesions. They occur more frequently in overweight patients, grow indolently, and, overall, carry a better prognosis. This group comprises hereditary tumours, especially those related to the hereditary non-polyposis colon cancer (HNPCC, Lynch) syndrome. This discovery, concerning 5% of endometrial cancer patients, should trigger genetic counselling and specific surveillance for colorectal cancer. By contrast, type II tumours consist of more aggressive subtypes such as papillary serous, clear cell, and carcinosarcomas. They are hormone-independent and are found in generally older and non-overweight postmenopausal women. Evolving more rapidly, they carry a worse prognosis than type I tumours.

In addition, the FIGO classification of endometrial cancer, based on thorough pathological staging, was updated in 2009 [29]. Surgery is the first treatment of endometrial cancer in most cases. Its extent is based on both pre- and intraoperative explorations. According to the FIGO stage, radiation therapy may or may not be used as adjuvant treatment. Medical treatments are currently reserved for patients with advanced disease, but are currently being investigated in early stage high-risk tumours.

Principles of the workup for endometrial cancer

Gynaecological bleeding in a postmenopausal woman, whatever the degree, is a uterine cancer until proven otherwise. After a complete general and gynaecological clinical examination, imaging is indicated. Pathological proof is necessary which can be obtained by biopsy or after a hysteroscopy-dilatation-curettage, especially if a biopsy is not possible or informative.

The imaging workup is useful to precisely define the disease extent. Due to its simplicity and reproducibility, ultrasound is usually the first examination performed if there is any suspicion of endometrial cancer. However, its accuracy is examiner-dependent. If MRI is currently the best morphological imaging method for precisely defining the intrauterine extent of disease, it is less accurate for the diagnosis of minimal node disease. Although results have improved through the use of nanoparticles of iron oxide, this procedure is not routinely performed and has not replaced surgery. Due to their propensity for distant spread, PET scan imaging may be useful for staging type 2 tumours in locally advanced or recurrent disease [30].

Principles of surgical treatment: diagnosis, staging, treatment

The results of peritoneal cytology, due to its controversial prognostic value, are no longer part of the new FIGO staging system. Total hysterectomy is the standard of care for clinical stage I endometrial cancer since occult cervical disease may exist in spite of a normal MRI or negative endocervical curettage. The question as to whether an intra- or extra-fascial hysterectomy is the most adequate has not been properly answered so far. If a systematic radical hysterectomy is not appropriate in stage I patients (less than 1% of positive parametrial involvement), it seems a logical indication in clinical stage II tumours but it must be balanced with the patient's general status [31]. Similarly, the role of the upper colpectomy is discussed and balanced with the simplicity and efficacy of post-operative vaginal high-dose rate brachytherapy. Bilateral adnexectomy is mandatory due to the rate (1–2%) of occult ovarian metastasis. In addition, patients are at an age of onset of ovarian cancer and bilateral adnexectomy may prevent this pathology.

A lymphadenectomy is the main controversial issue. Nodal involvement does indeed justify radiation therapy and adjuvant chemotherapy. Two recent randomized trials confirmed that systematic pelvic lymphadenectomy does not afford a survival advantage in early-stage well-differentiated endometrioid tumours, but increases morbidity [32, 33]. Adding a para-aortic node dissection was assessed in a recent controlled study. Only patients at intermediate or high risk of recurrence (IB grade 3 or type 2 tumours) benefited from a survival advantage of the combined procedure over a pelvic dissection alone [34]. If a para-aortic dissection is indicated, it should be performed bilaterally and up to the renal vessels [35]. In these extensive nodal dissections, the general condition and tolerance of the patients should always be balanced, to avoid exposing them to excessive morbidity. The sentinel node technique has been suggested to address the question of assessing the nodal status in early endometrioid carcinomas [36]. However, so far the reliability of the procedure has not been sufficiently confirmed to include it in routine practice [37]. Other staging procedures such as peritoneal biopsies or an omentectomy can be associated, especially for type 2 tumours [38].

The surgical approach is to be discussed according the patients' status and wishes, as well as the characteristics of her tumour (type, local extent) and uterus (size, vaginal accessibility).

A laparotomy is the standard approach for any endometrial cancer, whatever the stage of the disease or the uterine volume. However, morbidity may be high, especially in the aged with frequent co-morbidities (obesity, numerous other medical disorders).

The vaginal approach was successfully used very early in the history of gynaecological oncology. But, as removing the adnexae proved difficult and it was impossible to perform adequate staging via the same route, the indication was restricted to medically-compromised patients with a small uterus and a good vaginal access. The results were not so poor in this context, which still deserves to be applied to selected patients with an early type 1 tumour that does not require extensive staging [39, 40].

Since the late 80s, other minimally invasive approaches have been developed. Childers first described the laparoscopic management of endometrial cancer in 1992 [41]. Since that date, experience has grown rapidly all over the world, and several randomised studies in Europe confirmed the advantages of this approach over laparotomy in terms of perioperative outcomes, quality of life, and survival rates in patients with early stage endometrial cancer [42]. Even the largest American randomized study (LAP2), on the same topic including type 2 tumours, confirmed the perioperative advantages of laparoscopy, in spite of a 23% conversion rate due to a high percentage of obese patients and mandatory systematic thorough staging [43]. The late results of this trial, recently published, seem to confirm the absence of a detrimental effect of laparoscopic surgery on survival rates, with a low 0.24% incidence of port site recurrences [44].

Recently introduced, robot-assisted laparoscopy offers the possibility for 'abdominalist' surgeons to provide minimally invasive surgery to a larger proportion of patients. Although the additional costs of robotic surgery may be an issue [45], this assistance seems particularly interesting in the case of morbid obesity [46]. Robotic assistance has been shown to enable the surgeon to perform adequate staging with a lower rate of conversion in this group of patients [47]. However, a longer follow-up is needed as well as the results of controlled studies to confirm the long-term effects of this approach. Pooled results of different series comparing laparotomy to either laparoscopy or robotics seem to confirm the advantage of both laparoscopy and robotics over laparotomy.

Fertility-preserving surgery

Although very rare, with an incidence of less than 5% before 40 years of age, endometrial cancer may occur in young patients who wish to preserve their fertility. If all criteria are fulfilled (well-differentiated endometrioid tumour, confined to the mucosa, with no evidence of nodal, ovarian, or peritoneal involvement at pretherapeutic surgical staging), conservative treatment may be offered. It should be based on thorough curettage followed by at least six months of progestin therapy [48]. However, the recurrence rate is high [49], and possibly lethal but successful pregnancies have been reported, naturally or after assisted procreation [50].

Vaginal cancer

Preoperative workup for vaginal cancer

Vaginal tumour extension requires a very careful gynaecological examination (potentially under general anaesthesia). FIGO staging (that has a clear influence on further treatment) is based on clinical data [52]. The primary vaginal cancer (PVC) is preferentially located within the upper third of the posterior part and the lower third of the anterior part of the vagina, and 40 to 50% of the tumours are multifocal.

Standard imaging, such as that used in uterine cancers, is based on MRI that identifies tumour dimensions, potential extension beyond the vagina (bladder, rectum), and documents enlarged pelvic and para-aortic nodes and metastases [53]. FDG-PET was found to be relevant for detecting primary disease in all cases and nodal disease twice as often as CT and physical examination [54].

Principles and indications for surgery for vaginal cancer

Two types of treatments have been reported in primary carcinoma of the vagina: surgery or radiation therapy but given the rarity of primary carcinoma of the vagina, no randomized trial has been performed, particularly to assess the respective role of surgery and radiation therapy [55–59].

Unlike in the case of other gynaecological malignancies, surgery has not yet been really well codified in PVC. Surgical treatment concerns the primary tumour and lymph node staging.

Surgical treatment of the primary tumour can be limited (simple and limited vaginal excision), total simple colpectomy or more radical, such as radical colpectomy or pelvic exenteration. Basically, in stage 0 (in situ disease), surgery, a simple excision, is the treatment of choice. In stage I disease, two treatments are proposed in the literature: surgery (partial or total radical colpectomy) vs radiation therapy. In stage II to IVA disease, most teams consider that radiation therapy is the treatment of choice. Concomitant chemoradiation therapy in these situations has probably a key place but very limited experience has been reported [60].

The comparison between surgery and radiation therapy (for stage I disease) remains difficult in the light of the literature analysis. Several studies have reported poorer survival in patients treated with radiation therapy compared to patients treated by surgery [51, 58, 61]. Nevertheless, this comparison is heavily biased because other factors such as age and the general status could play a role in the choice between surgery and radiation therapy and furthermore could also have an impact on survival in disfavour of radiation therapy [51]. As in cervical cancer, if surgery is performed it should be 'sufficiently' radical to reduce the risk of involved margins (which then require adjuvant radiation therapy with a higher risk of morbidity) to a minimum (ideally to 0). Consequently, even in stage I disease (or in patients with stage 0 (in situ) disease but affecting a large length of the vagina), such surgery could impose a total resection of the vagina with a clear impact on quality of life (particularly sexual activity) since 15% of patients with invasive carcinoma are <49 years [51]. Even if reconstructive surgery of the vagina is done, no publication has focused on the sexual quality of life after surgery in PVC. The use of radiation therapy does not exert the same anatomical (and functional) impact because the organ is not surgically resected. This point also explains why, even if surgery remains the treatment of choice of stage 0 (in situ) disease, brachytherapy could play a role in young patients with recurrent disease and a previous history of colpectomy or in lesions affecting a large length of the vagina and requiring a total colpectomy. A recent series reported excellent local control with this treatment in these particular indications [62]. Basically, the place of the surgery has decreased during the past four decades, particularly in Stage >I disease.

Concerning lymph node staging, lymphatic extension of vaginal tumours is complex and correlates with the double embryologic origin of the vagina: the upper two-thirds drain towards the iliac nodes while the lower third drains towards the hypogastric and inguinal nodes [60]. Drainage of the posterior septum is located in the haemorrhoidal and sacral nodes. Consequently, these nodes should be treated (surgically or included in the radiation therapy field) at the same time as the PVC. Nevertheless, the complexity of the lymphatic drainage also explains why nodal staging surgery is not really codified in this tumour. Most reports concerning the surgical treatment of PVC have a low proportion of patients who underwent comprehensive nodal surgery (pelvic, para-aortic, or inguino-femoral). In the series by Stock et al. concerning 100 patients with PVC (53 of whom were treated surgically), 40 underwent a lymph node dissection [63]. Patients with positive inguinal nodes had involvement of the lower third of the vagina [63]. In the series by Davis et al. among 48 patients undergoing pelvic and para-aortic node assessment for stage I/II PVC, only one patient with stage I disease (6%) had nodal involvement but eight (26%) had nodal spread in stage II disease (in the pelvic area in seven and para-aortic nodes in one) [64].

Two papers recently reported the authors' experience of the feasibility of the sentinel node procedure in primary (or recurrent) VC [65]. In the experience reported by Frumovitz et al. (using a combined technique with blue dye and radiocolloid), three out of nine patients treated initially with radiation therapy had their radiation field altered based on the results of lymphoscintigraphy findings [65].

Vulvar cancer

Surgery is the cornerstone of the management of vulvar tumours and is associated with a high cure rate. According to the disease extent or definitive pathological results, radiation therapy can be used as adjuvant therapy or, combined with cisplatin chemotherapy, as neoadjuvant treatment in locally advanced tumours [66].

Principles of surgery

Vulvar surgery

A radical vulvectomy is the gold standard of treatment of invasive carcinomas defined as a tumour invading the stroma beyond 1 mm of depth. Its aim is to remove the tumour along with a sufficient amount of healthy skin. The adequate free margin should be at least 8 mm after formalin treatment, which corresponds to at least 1 cm on the patient [67]. New data concerning the resection margins show that 3 mm in each direction seem to be sufficient [68]. The underlying fatty tissue is resected down to the urogenital diaphragm covered by the superficial perineal aponeurosis. Indicated for invasive tumours, cosmesis issues should not interfere with the mandatory oncological radicality. A skinning vulvectomy, indicated for non-invasive neoplasia, removes the tumour and 5 mm of free skin laterally and within the underlying tissue. Except when unavoidable, a total radical vulvectomy along with a bilateral inguinal lymphadenectomy is no longer performed through the classic Basset-Taussig butterfly incision. Separate incisions for the vulvectomy and the inguinal lymphadenectomies are now the rule [69]. The incision is drawn taking into account the need for 1 cm free margins.

Partial vulvectomy

It consists of the resection of only a part of the vulva including the tumour and the required free margins. It is indicated whenever the tumour is isolated, small, and at least 10 mm away from the midline. In the case of a median but small tumour, a partial anterior or posterior resection is also feasible.

Principles of inguinal dissections

The inguino-femoral lymphadenectomy removes all nodes between the superficial aponeurosis and the saphenous vein within the limits of the Scarpa triangle. In addition to all nodes located medially to the femoral vein, a deep inguinal lymphadenectomy removes tissue from the pectineus muscle up to the inguinal ligament. The Cloquet node is the upper lymphatic structure in this area.

Principles of reconstructions

Whatever the technique (primary closure or flap reconstruction), the surgeon must ensure that the urethra is kept in its normal position, to avoid any uncomfortable deviation of the urinary stream. If necessary, up to 1cm of the urethra can be resected without incontinence. The use of a graft/flap is discussed whenever the primary closure seems under tension, with a high risk of secondary wound breakdown and for sufficient cosmetic and functional reconstruction.

Principles of perioperative care

Post-operative care of vulvar cancer patients is of paramount importance, combining careful nursing of clean and dry sutures, good nutrition, and efficient postoperative analgesia. Indeed, the morbidity engendered by this surgery remains high. In the series of 101 patients reported by Gaarenstrom, complications were observed in 76% of cases, especially wound breakdown and/or infection (56%), lymphocysts (40%), and lymphoedema (28%) [73]. If vacuum-assisted therapy has improved the management of wound breakdowns, its efficacy has been shown to prevent secondary breakdowns in case of large defects [70].

Indications for treatments of vulvar carcinoma

For a unifocal stage 1 tumour (T1a N0 M0) in a healthy vulva, a partial resection (lateral hemivulvectomy or subtotal anterior or posterior vulvectomy) with a minimal 1 cm free margin around the tumour, is acceptable. However, in the case of skin abnormalities, a total radical vulvectomy will avoid contralateral recurrences. An inguinal node dissection via a separate incision will be unilateral in the case of a lateral tumour and bilateral for a lesion which is less than 10 mm from the midline. The extent of the lymphadenectomy can be based on the frozen section analysis of the resected superficial nodes, with a false negative rate of 5–7% [71]. Sentinel node detection after intradermal double labelling (by 99m Technetium and patent blue), along with the ultrastaging examination (serial sections of sentinel node[s] and conventional haematoxylin-eosin staining plus pancytokeratin immunohistochemistry), seems an efficient way to reduce the morbidity of lymph node dissection, without jeopardizing oncological outcomes, as demonstrated in a recent international comparative study [72].

In the case of a stage IB-II tumour (T1b-2 N0M0), a total radical vulvectomy, with or without a urethra/anal skin resection, is required along with a bilateral inguinal node dissection.

In advanced stage III tumours (T1-2, N1-2M0) and some stage IVA (T1-2, N3M0 or T3 any N, M0), a total radical vulvectomy, with or without a urethra/anal skin resection and a bilateral complete node dissection, is required.

For stage IVA tumours, definitive chemoradiation therapy or an exenterative procedure are discussed after a thorough clinical evaluation under general anaesthesia. Patients with stage IVB disease (any T or N but M1) are managed according to their general status, either with cisplatin-based chemotherapy or the best supportive care.

Ovarian cancer

Preoperative workup

Ovarian cancer is renowned for its capacity to disseminate intraperitoneally and via lymphatic spread. Thus, surgical staging (or surgical resection) of peritoneal sites and lymph nodes remain the two strategic steps in the surgical treatment of this tumour. The reference imaging technique used to evaluate the spread of this tumour before the surgical procedure is the thoraco-abdomino-pelvic CT scan.

Principles and indications for surgery

Surgery is a crucial part of the management and treatment of ovarian tumours. It allows the clinician to make the diagnosis, to determine disease spread (surgery remains the most accurate procedure for evaluating the level of spread of the tumour in the abdomen), and is the cornerstone treatment for removing the tumour. The surgical procedures required depend on the disease stage. Besides stage, the postoperative residual tumour is the most important risk factor [94].

Early stage (patients with disease macroscopically confined to the ovary)

The surgical procedures required are well-defined and codified. In patients older than 40 years, radical treatment based on a hysterectomy and bilateral salpingo-oophorectomy is the standard of care. The rationale behind the use of a hysterectomy is twofold: (1) the presence of synchronous endometrial carcinoma associated with the ovarian tumour (15% to 20% of the endometrioid subtype) and (2) the uterine serosa could harbour microscopic peritoneal spread undetectable to the naked eye. Those two reasons explain why the uterus should be removed in patients who do not desire to preserve their fertility. In young patients (<40 years) desiring the potential for pregnancy, a unilateral salpingo-oophorectomy with preservation of the uterus could be proposed and seems to be safe in selected patients with early-stage disease and excellent prognostic factors (conventional histological subtypes such as low-grade serous, mucinous, or endometrioid lesions; macroscopic and radiological unilateral tumour; and absence of macroscopic and microscopic histological or cytological peritoneal spread after a definitive analysis of the specimen removed during staging surgery [grade 1 or 2 disease]) [73]. In such cases, uterine curettage is then required to verify the absence of synchronous endometrial cancer [73].

Whatever the procedure used on the uterus and ovaries (conservative or radical), staging surgery is required to identify the precise stage of the disease, in order to guide postoperative management and indications for adjuvant chemotherapy. In fact, patients with stage IA or IB and grade 1 disease could be treated exclusively with surgery. In patients with advanced stages, or grade 3 disease (or a clear cell tumour), adjuvant chemotherapy should be used after the surgical procedure.

Staging surgery is then crucial to accurately identify the disease stage. This staging surgery is, according to the potential spread of the tumour, peritoneal and/or nodal staging [74]. Peritoneal staging is based on peritoneal cytology, omentectomy, multiple peritoneal biopsies and an appendectomy (the latter only in mucinous tumours or in the case of involvement [75]). If lesions look suspicious on the peritoneum, they should be removed. Patients are restaged based on microscopic involvement of at least one of these specimens in nearly a third of the cases without any macroscopic suspicious lesion on the peritoneum or omentum [74].

The interest of the lymph node staging is debated more extensively. Indeed, this procedure is extremely useful because nearly 15% of patients will exhibit nodal involvement. Furthermore, 12% of patients with no cytological or histological peritoneal spread were upstaged solely based on nodal involvement [76]. Some of them then receive adjuvant chemotherapy exclusively based on the detection of this nodal involvement and would not have received such therapy with peritoneal staging alone [77].

The distribution of nodal involvement is very ubiquitous between the pelvic and para-aortic area. Fifty percent of patients with nodal involvement will have metastases in these areas, 25% exclusively in pelvic nodes and 25% exclusively in para-aortic nodes [77]. The rate of contralateral nodal involvement in patients with a stage I unilateral ovarian tumour is nearly 16% (series are summarized in Table 44.1). Consequently, if a lymphadenectomy is carried out in epithelial ovarian cancer, it should include the removal of pelvic and para-aortic nodes, up to the level of the left renal vein (the most frequent site of nodal metastasis is the nodal group between the inferior mesenteric artery and the left renal vein) and bilaterally even in patients with a macroscopic unilateral tumour. The rate of nodal involvement is correlated with the tumour grade (higher risk with grade 3 lesions) and the histological subtype of the tumour.

The point most discussed currently is the real therapeutic impact (in terms of improving survival) of this nodal surgery in addition to peritoneal staging in advanced stages with macroscopic complete resection. Some authors who consider that this surgery should not be used argue that the only randomized trial on this topic failed to demonstrate an improvement of survival using complete

Table 44.1 Laterality of nodal spread in stage I epithelial ovarian cancer

Series years	Ipsilateral or bilateral	Contralateral
Onda 1996 (n = 9) [78]	8	1
Baiocchi 1998 (n = 11) [79]	8	3
Sakuragi 2000 (n = 9) [80]	9	0
Suzuki 2000 (n = 4) [81]	2	2
Cass 2001 (n = 10) [82]	7	3
Morice 2003 (n = 9) [83]	8	1
Nagishi 2004 (n = 8) [84]	8	0
Nomura 2010 (n = 9 but stage I/II) [85]	7	2
Powless 2011 (n = 10) [86]	9	1
Total (n = 79)	66	13 (16%)

lymphadenectomy [87]. Nevertheless, the conclusions of this trial continue to fuel debate, the authors themselves stating that the trial was probably underpowered due to the number of patients (nearly 135 patients in each arm) to attain statistical significance (there was a trend towards a difference in overall and event-free survival which was not statistically significant). Nevertheless, many teams and national guidelines consider that this procedure should be included in the standard of care of early-stage epithelial ovarian cancer. Those different staging procedures (peritoneal and nodal) should be performed laparotomically (in the hands of surgeons trained to perform this type of surgery) [88]. Rare data exist that laparoscopic approach could be somewhat less accurate for staging.

Advanced stage ovarian cancer (patients with extra-ovarian macroscopic disease)

In patients with abdominal peritoneal disease (stage >II), the strongest prognostic factors compared to the others is the size of the residual disease (measured as the largest size of the bulkiest residuum at the end of debulking surgery, if residual disease is left in place) [89]. This debulking surgery requires experienced gynaecologic oncologists and teams (to optimize peri- and post-operative care in order to reduce morbidity) for advanced surgery. As the rate of achieving optimal cytoreductive surgery is correlated with the surgeon's skills in this kind of surgery, ovarian cancer is the best example among solid tumours of the fact that the surgeon alone may be a prognostic factor in this disease.

Technical procedures required in advanced stage ovarian cancer (ASOC) are the most complex because, in addition to the previous procedures detailed in early-stage disease that are also required (hysterectomy, omentectomy, bilateral salpingo-oophorectomies), as peritoneal spread of the tumour is very frequent, large peritonectomies, diaphragmatic surgery, bowel resection, and a splenectomy are frequently needed to remove the complete tumour. Thus, this surgery is a pan-abdominal surgical intervention requiring gynaecologic oncologists who are skilled in all kinds of abdominal procedures that are mandatory in this context. For multivisceral surgeries an interdisciplinary team is recommended [90]. The most frequent site of the bowel resection required is the recto-sigmoid colon. En bloc resection with the removal of the uterus, ovaries and fallopian tubes, Douglas' pouch, and the peritoneum of the pelvic cavity exhibiting macroscopic disease could then be easily removed using an extraperitoneal approach such as that described by Hudson et al. [91]. Nevertheless, other types of bowel resection could then be needed: transverse, ileo-caecal, or a small bowel resection [90].

This type of surgical procedure, so-called 'debulking' surgery, has been 'historically' qualified as 'optimal' if the remaining residual disease is small (the size of this cut-off has evolved during the last three decades: 2, 1, and 'now' 0 cm) and 'suboptimal' when larger residual disease is left in place [89, 90, 92, 94]. In fact 'optimal' surgery involves 'complete' cytoreductive surgery with absence of macroscopic residual disease. There is a clear difference in terms of the survival between patients with complete cytoreductive surgery and patients with minimal residual disease (considered as having undergone optimal surgery) [93, 94]. Only patients submitted to complete macroscopic resection of peritoneal spread would then be considered as having undergone 'optimal' cytoreductive surgery [95, 96]. This should be the first goal and the standard management of debulking surgery in epithelial ovarian cancer. When macroscopic residual disease is left in place the surgical procedure would then be considered suboptimal, whatever the size of the residue. Thus, in patients with stage IIIC disease, this kind of debulking surgery could require six to eight hours. This operative time also explains why the management of these tumours requires not only experienced surgeons but also multidisciplinary teams: gynaecologic oncologists, abdominal surgeons, anaesthesiologists, nurses, and intensive care clinicians to undertake the most adequate peri- and post-operative management in order to reduce morbidities.

Nevertheless, this cytoreductive surgery has been exposed to a good deal of criticism because of the significant morbidity engendered, particularly in patients with residual disease at the end of the surgery [97]. Post-operative morbidities are dominated by septic complications, post-operative bleeding, and post-operative anastomotic leakage requiring a transient enterostomy. Such complications could then delay the initiation of the first course of post-operative chemotherapy, which also appears to be a prognostic factor in ovarian cancer. Neoadjuvant chemotherapy should be an exception with a maximum of three chemotherapy cycles before interval surgery, for example, in the case of acute myocardial infarction or acute lung embolism. A prospective randomized phase III trial has not demonstrated that by reducing the size of peritoneal spread, this neoadjuvant chemotherapy decreases the radicality of surgical procedure required to remove the entire tumour and therefore reduces morbidity [98]. But in addition, only the 19% that had a macroscopic complete resection within primary surgery had a significant improved survival of seven months in comparison to the 40% that got complete resection after neoadjuvant chemotherapy [98]; therefore, primary surgery is the gold standard. However, the use of such neoadjuvant chemotherapy should not be an excuse for 'poor surgery'. If it is possible to totally remove peritoneal spread initially during surgery, it should be done [95, 96]. If disease spread is too massive and residual disease of more than 1 cm would be present after primary surgery, then neoadjuvant chemotherapy could be considered followed by interval debulking surgery. In the case of FIGO IV, patients also have a benefit after macroscopic complete resection [99]. Neoadjuvant strategies could be used in patients with a medical or a nutritional status that is too poor to enable them to undergo such initial debulking surgery.

The last question concerning the surgical procedures in ASOC concerns the addition of pelvic and para-aortic node resection.

There are strong arguments in favour of its use because of, firstly, the high rate of nodal spread in stage III or IV disease (nearly half to two-thirds of the patients) and, secondly, the dogma regarding the need to achieve a complete macroscopic resection that is now considered the standard of surgical care in ASOC. Nevertheless, as we observed in early-stage disease, a phase III trial failed to demonstrate an improvement of overall survival using a complete lymphadenectomy (but event-free survival was enhanced) [100]. Nevertheless, a large recent analysis reporting on patients included in three different trials testing different chemotherapy regimens focused on the impact of nodal surgery on survival. This series demonstrated that this surgery is of interest to improve the survival of patients undergoing a complete removal of peritoneal disease [101]. If this intraperitoneal debulking surgery fails to remove all the disease, then retroperitoneal nodal surgery is pointless [101]. Two randomized trials are ongoing in France and Germany to test the therapeutic interest of the lymphadenectomy in ASOC. Fortunately, the German LION trial has completely recruited and we hopefully expect the final results of this prospective randomized trial in 2018.

Role of radiotherapy

Since the early days of radiotherapy more than a century ago, radiotherapy and especially brachytherapy (Radium) were successfully performed in various gynaecologic cancers. Nowadays, radiotherapy is well established as an essential part in modern multimodality treatment and is being used for primary, neoadjuvant, adjuvant, and palliative purposes.

Cervix cancer

Primary, neoadjuvant, and adjuvant radiochemotherapy have been described as treatment options for cervix cancer. Patient selection for the different treatment approaches is mainly based on the tumour stage (FIGO) and lymph node status. However, since prospective randomized controlled trials addressing the question of patient selection for different therapy options (surgery vs radiotherapy vs combined treatments) are limited, the decision which treatment modality is applied is still a matter of debate and varies between countries and institutions. But two major findings should be respected in this discussion: primary surgery in patients with (extensive) parametrial involvement leads to a high number of incomplete resections (and thus to local tumour progression), and the combination of surgery and radiotherapy leads to an increased morbidity in comparison to each treatment modality alone ([102–104]. Therefore, there has been a consensus that radiochemotherapy is the treatment of choice in locally advanced stages (≥FIGO stage IIB distal, >4cm and/or positive lymph nodes) [105], whereas in earlier stages both treatment strategies can be performed as single modalities with similar outcome. Pre-invasive stages and the FIGO stage IA are usually restricted to surgery. In consequence, precise staging including assessment of local tumour extension (gynaecologic examination, ultrasound, MRI), regional lymph node involvement (CT, MRI, PET CT, laparoscopic lymph node staging) and distant metastasis (CT, PET CT) is crucial.

Primary radiochemotherapy

Primary radiochemotherapy consists of external beam radiotherapy with concomitant delivery of chemotherapy and brachytherapy.

External beam radiotherapy aims for initial tumour shrinkage as well as for treatment of suspected regional microscopic or macroscopic lymph node involvement. The clinical target volume in external beam radiotherapy includes the primary tumour, the complete uterus, parametria, upper vagina (depending on the extent of vaginal infiltration), internal, external, and common iliac lymph node stations as well as the obturator and presacral lymph nodes [106]. Target definition and treatment planning is generally based on computed tomography. Currently, different treatment techniques in external beam radiotherapy are applied. Most commonly 3D conformal techniques with four fields ('four field box') are used, which allow for a homogeneous dose distribution within the pelvis. More advanced external beam radiotherapy techniques such as intensity modulated radiotherapy (IMRT), tomotherapy or particle therapy are being investigated and show more heterogeneous dose profiles leading to reduced (high-dose) irradiation of the surrounding organs at risk (urinary bladder, rectum, colon, small bowel, femoral heads). The standard prescription dose for the target volume varies between 45–50 Gy at a dose per fraction of 1.8–2 Gy. An additional local boost of approximately 10 Gy to bulky lymph nodes appears reasonable; however, definite evidence for benefit is lacking. Irradiation of the para-aortic region in case of lymph node involvement showed contradictive results but may be beneficial in selected cases at the sake of increased morbidity. Based on five randomized trials, concomitant chemotherapy (5–6 cycles cisplatin 40mg/m2 +/– 5 fluorouracil) has been integrated into primary radiotherapy since 1999 as standard of care. Radiochemotherapy significantly improved local tumour control and survival compared to radiotherapy alone. An absolute improvement of ~6% overall survival has been demonstrated in a meta-analysis with 10 year follow-up [107, 108]. Apart from the systemic effect, concomitant chemotherapy is mainly considered as a radiosensitizer. Tumour regression during external beam radiotherapy and concomitant chemotherapy may be up to ~75%. Tumour size, tumour volume, tumour stage, lymph node involvement, tumour hypoxia, and histology are discussed as prognostic parameters for response to radiotherapy. The residual tumour volume after external beam radiotherapy is then treated by brachytherapy. Brachytherapy is performed in an operation theatre, where an applicator system (tandem-ring, tandem-ovoid, etc.) is placed directly at the cervix and in the uterine cavity. The specific dosimetric characteristics of brachytherapy (high-dose at the source with sharp circular dose fall off in the periphery) allow for high-dose delivery at the residual tumour while sparing the surrounding organs at risk. The former application of radium sources has widely been replaced by the use of afterloading systems with high-dose rate or pulsed-dose rate schedules. Dose prescription is generally performed to predefined dose points ('2D brachytherapy') in relation to the applicator such as 'point A' or 'point B' and varies according to centres and traditions between 2–6 fractions of 4–8.5 Gy for high dose rate (HDR) and 1–2 fractions of 20–35 Gy for pulsed dose rate (PDR) schedules.

Primary radiotherapy leads to a complete remission rate of approximately 98%. The five-year local tumour control ranges between 81–97% for stage IB and IIA, 74–82% for stage IIB, 44–66% for stage III and 18–25% for stage IVA and the five-year overall survival ranges between 80–90% for stage IB and IIA, 65–75% for stage IIB, 30–50% for stage III, and 10–15% for stage IVA. Acute side effects imply mainly urogenital and gastrointestinal symptoms such as increased urinary frequency and diarrhoea. Late side effects range from vaginal dryness (frequently) to incontinence and fistula (rare). Recently, major improvements have been described in the field of image-guided adaptive brachytherapy ('3D brachytherapy'). In image-guided adaptive brachytherapy dwell point optimisation is performed based on the integration of modern imaging techniques (CT, PET/CT, mainly MRI) into the treatment planning process leading to individually adapted treatment plans with an increased dose to the primary tumour while simultaneously sparing the surrounding organs at risk. The treated volume may be increased and additionally shaped by the insertion of interstitial needles, if indicated. A prospective multicentre study demonstrated that with image-guided adaptive brachytherapy a reduction of severe side effects by 50% is achievable with a simultaneous improvement of local tumour control in comparison to the standard 2D approach [109]. Retrospective single-centre trials showed a local tumour control rate of >95% for all locally advanced stages and severe side effects for the gastrointestinal and urogenital tract <5% [110, 111]. Prospective trials are ongoing; in the future, efforts to reduce distant metastasis and further improve quality of life will be necessary [112].

Neoadjuvant and adjuvant radiochemotherapy

Neoadjuvant brachytherapy for FIGO stage IB1 tumours and neoadjuvant external beam radiotherapy with concomitant chemotherapy followed by brachytherapy for higher stages (and/or regional lymph node involvement) has been performed by many centres. However, it has been shown that the addition of surgery seems to increase the morbidity rate without any evidence of benefit in local tumour control, progression-free survival or overall survival in comparison to radiochemotherapy alone. In consequence, surgery should be limited in this cohort to patients with persistent local disease six to eight weeks after radiochemotherapy.

Adjuvant radiotherapy after surgery is indicated in case of R1 or R2 resections, lymph node involvement, microscopic parametrial infiltration, lymphangiosis, infiltration of vessels, G3, and tumour size >4cm with deep stromal invasion for improving local and regional tumour control [113]. The radiotherapy technique is similar to the primary treatment but with brachytherapy only in selected cases (e.g., close or positive resection margin in the vaginal vault, macroscopic residual tumour) [114]. The standard prescription dose is 50 Gy with 1.8–2 Gy in a single dose. Concomitant delivery of chemotherapy (cisplatin, 5-fluorouracil) is recommended. Adjuvant radiochemotherapy significantly improves progression-free survival and overall survival in early-stage cervix cancer with high-risk factors in comparison to radiotherapy alone, whereas adjuvant radiotherapy alone only demonstrated a decrease in local recurrences without a long-term survival benefit in comparison to no adjuvant radiotherapy [115].

Endometrial cancer

Treatment of endometrial cancer is a multimodality therapy tailored according to clearly defined risk factors, with surgery as the cornerstone. Radiotherapy is mainly indicated as adjuvant treatment. Several randomized controlled trials [116–119] defined the role of radiotherapy and redefined treatment concepts recently. Primary radiotherapy is limited to inoperable patients or patients treated in palliative intention.

Adjuvant radiotherapy

After primary surgery alone, up to 30% loco-regional recurrences have been reported. Therefore, adjuvant radiotherapy has been integrated into the treatment concept of endometrial cancer for improving local tumour control. Currently, adjuvant radiotherapy is performed dependent of the presence of major prognostic factors, which are FIGO stage, age, histology, grade, depth of myometrial invasion, and lymphovascular space invasion. Based on these prognostic factors patients are divided into three risk groups: low-, intermediate-, and high-risk group. Low risk is defined as FIGO stage IA (with <50% myometrial invasion), G1 or 2 with endometrioid histology. Patients are classified as intermediate risk in case of FIGO stage IB (>50% myometrial invasion) and G1 or 2, or FIGO stage 1A and G3. All patients with FIGO stage II, III and FIGO stage IB with grade 3 or with non-endometrioid histology are considered high risk (Figure 44.3).

Low-risk patients have an excellent outcome after surgery with 95% five-year relapse-free survival and adjuvant radiotherapy is not recommended. Patients in the intermediate risk group should receive adjuvant radiotherapy as vaginal vault brachytherapy. The rationale for this treatment concept is mainly based on the findings that in these patients: (1) loco-regional recurrences after surgery alone occur after five years in up to 15%, (2) loco-regional recurrences are located in 75% in the vagina, (3) adjuvant external beam radiotherapy significantly improved locoregional tumour control but did not show any survival benefit in these patients, and

(4) with vaginal vault brachytherapy similar local (vaginal) tumour control rates with significantly less morbidity and better quality of life is achievable in comparison to external beam radiotherapy [120–123]. External beam radiotherapy, however, may be used as an alternative. Vaginal vault brachytherapy is usually performed with vaginal cylinders as applicator systems, which are directly placed in the vagina. The target volume for vaginal vault brachytherapy should encompass the vaginal scar and the vaginal lymphatic drainage in 5 mm depth in the upper one-third to two-thirds of the vagina (approximately 3–5 cm). 30–50 Gy in four to five days for PDR schedules or 15–25 Gy in 3–4 fractions with 5–7 Gy HDR single dose prescribed at 5 mm depth from the applicator surface is recommended. Vaginal vault brachytherapy is well tolerated with generally only few (low grade) vaginal, urogenital, and intestinal side effects. Vaginal recurrences after vaginal vault brachytherapy occur in 1.6% after five years. Lymph node recurrences appear more frequently than with external beam radiotherapy, since vaginal vault brachytherapy does not allow for treatment of regional lymph nodes (2.1% vs 5.1% [120]). Adjuvant radiotherapy in high-risk patients is usually performed by a combination of external beam radiotherapy and brachytherapy. Treatment planning for external beam radiotherapy is performed on CT with 3D conformal or intensity modulated radiotherapy techniques. The target volume

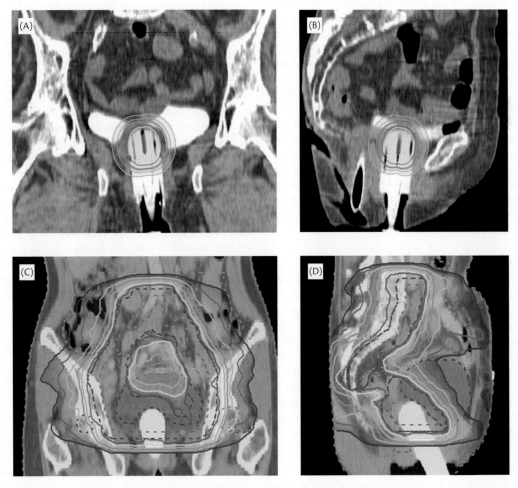

Fig. 44.3 CT images of a patient with intermediate-risk endometrial cancer (A) and high-risk endometrial cancer (B) in coronal (A and B) and sagittal (C and D, respectively) view. Note the difference in the treated volume of vaginal vault brachytherapy (C) and external beam radiotherapy by IMRT (D).

should include the complete uterus, parametria, upper vagina and the presacral, obturatrial, common, internal and external iliacal lymph node areas [114]. Dose prescription ranges from 45–50 Gy with 1.8–2 Gy in a single fraction. Brachytherapy follows the same principle as for intermediate-risk patients, but with a reduced dose scheme. In general, 11–15 Gy in 2–3 fractions (HDR) or 25 Gy over two days (PDR) are recommended. Side effects of combined external beam radiotherapy and brachytherapy are similar to primary radiotherapy in cervix cancer. Evidence for adjuvant radiotherapy in high-risk patients is limited, but in selected patients a survival benefit was shown in retrospective series. However, the high rate of distant metastases stresses the need for systemic treatment. Combined radiotherapy and chemotherapy is currently being investigated in prospective trials. First studies in this field demonstrated an increase in progression-free survival if chemotherapy is added (e.g., NSGO 9501/EORTC 55991: 79% vs 72% [124]).

Primary radiotherapy in endometrial cancer

Primary radiotherapy is indicated in inoperable patients or in patients treated in palliative intention. Literature for primary radiotherapy in endometrial cancer is limited. In patients with low-risk factors, brachytherapy can be performed as single modality, whereas in patients with higher-risk factors (G3, large tumour with deep myometrial infiltration) a combination of external beam radiotherapy and brachytherapy should be applied. Standard applicators for brachytherapy are the Heyman packing system or the Norman-Simon applicators. When using these applicator systems, small capsules, which are connected to the afterloader, are placed in the uterine cavity in an operation theatre. In stage I the target volume is the macroscopic tumour and the complete uterine corpus and in stage II the cervix is additionally included. Treatment planning should be preferably based on CT or MRI. The dose is prescribed to the uterine serosa. Typical fraction schedules are 6×7 Gy (HDR) for brachytherapy as a single modality or 3×7 Gy in case of a combined approach after 50 Gy external beam radiotherapy. External beam radiotherapy is performed in the same way as for adjuvant treatment. Treatment results are inferior to primarily surgically treated patients. In (clinical) stage IA, IB, and II, 86%, 68%, and 60%, respectively, can be locally controlled. Five-year overall survival ranges from 68–86% in stage I, ~60% in stage II, and 33–41% in stage III [125, 126].

Vaginal cancer

Primary vaginal cancer is a rare tumour site with subsequently only very limited data available. The direct proximity of vaginal cancer to surrounding organs as well as the submucosal tumour spread within the vagina impedes surgical procedures. Radical resections can often be reached only by complete colpectomy and/or pelvic exenteration. In contrast, primary radiotherapy offers the possibility of organ preservation. Therefore, primary radiotherapy in curative intent is the treatment method of choice in the majority of cases. Due to the similarity of cervix cancer and vaginal cancer (histology, pattern of tumour spread, topography, biology) experiences and treatment concepts from cervix cancer were mainly transferred and adapted for vaginal cancer.

Primary radiotherapy

Primary radiotherapy of locally advanced vaginal cancer consists usually of external beam radiotherapy and intravaginal

brachytherapy. In limited disease (FIGO Stage 0/I, superficial lesions with ≤5 mm invasion depth) brachytherapy can be performed as single modality. Brachytherapy is performed with a vaginal cylinder or with individually adapted applicators ('mould technique'). Usual dose prescription for brachytherapy only is 40–45 Gy in weekly fractions of 5–8 Gy (HDR) or 50–70 Gy for PDR brachytherapy prescribed in 5 mm depth. The dose may be increased in case of poor response. In advanced disease (≥FIGO II or involvement of regional lymph nodes) external beam radiotherapy allows for downsizing of the initial tumour volume and treatment of the pelvine lymph node areas. Target volume definition and the performance of external beam radiotherapy are similar to cervix cancer radiotherapy with 45–50 Gy in 1.8–2 Gy in a single fraction. In case of tumour involvement of the lower third of the vagina, the inguinal lymph node area should be included in the clinical target volume. Concomitant delivery of chemotherapy (cisplatin $40 mg/m^2$, 5–6 weekly doses) appears reasonable. After or in the end of external beam radiotherapy (+/– chemotherapy) the residual tumour volume should be treated by intravaginal brachytherapy. If the invasion depth of the residual tumour is ≥5 mm, a combined intravaginal and interstitial brachytherapy should be applied for better dose distribution. Interstitial needles are usually inserted via a perineal template in lithotomy position. It is recommended to apply 3–6 fractions of 5–8 Gy HDR brachytherapy or ~30–40 Gy PDR brachytherapy prescribed in 5mm from the applicator surface or as tumour encompassing reference isodose (in case of >5mm invasion). Due to the proximity to surrounding organs at risk, the larger therapeutic window of PDR schedules may be advantageous in comparison to HDR schedules. Excellent results have been achieved for small tumours (stage 0 + I) with 5-year disease-specific survival ranging from 83–100%. Locally advanced tumours (stage II–IVA), however, still represent a major therapeutic challenge. Local failures are the main site of recurrence. In locally advanced tumours, the 5-year local tumour control rate ranges from 68–84% for stage II, from 40–80% for stage III, and from 0–69% for stage IVA. Five-year overall survival ranges from 77–100%, 45–61%, 14–30%, and 0–18% for stages I, II, III, and IVA, respectively [127–133]. Acute side effects are mainly local inflammation, proctitis, and cystitis. Frequent late side effects are vaginal mucosal atrophy, vaginal shortening, narrowing, and vaginal fibrosis. Severe late side effects such as ulceration, necrosis, vesicovaginal or rectovaginal fistula are less frequent (~10% after five years), but mainly encountered in case of tumour involvement in the respective areas. Recently, in accordance with cervix cancer, image-guided adaptive brachytherapy was described as feasible for treatment of vaginal cancer. First retrospective studies demonstrated a local tumour control rate of >90% for all stages [134].

Adjuvant radiotherapy

Adjuvant radiotherapy in vaginal cancer may be indicated—depending on the localization of the primary tumour—in accordance to the procedures in cervical or vulvar cancer.

Vulvar cancer

Vulvar cancer is a rare disease with only very limited data available. In limited disease (T0, T1, T2) surgery is the therapy of choice, whereas in more advanced tumours individual treatment regimes are necessary with surgery, radiotherapy, and chemotherapy complementing one another. Outcome is highly dependent on the presence of lymph node metastasis. Inguinal lymph nodes are the first site of metastatic disease. If positive inguinal lymph nodes are detected, pelvic lymph node metastasis can be found in 20–30% [66].

Adjuvant radiotherapy

Adjuvant radiotherapy in vulvar cancer is mainly applied for treatment of regional lymph node areas and is adapted to the type of surgery and histopathologic findings. Adjuvant radiotherapy of the vulva is only indicated in case of positive or close resection margins (<3mm) [68] and if the primary tumour was infiltrating surrounding organs (T3, T4). Adjuvant radiotherapy of the inguinal lymph nodes is indicated (1) after lymph node debulking in c(p)N+ patients, or (2) after bilateral lymph node dissection if two or more lymph nodes were involved or if an extracapsular spread was detected [135], or (3) in cN+ patients if lymph node dissection could not be performed. Elective radiotherapy in cN0 patients without lymph node dissection and adjuvant radiotherapy in patients with one (intranodal) lymph node metastasis after lymph node dissection has to be discussed on an individual basis. Adjuvant radiotherapy of the inguinal lymph nodes may be only unilateral if the primary tumour as well as the suspected microscopic disease was/is strictly unilateral and was >10mm away from the midline. Adjuvant radiotherapy of the pelvic lymph nodes is only indicated in patients with positive inguinal lymph nodes. The role of adjuvant combined radiochemotherapy is currently unclear. Adjuvant radiotherapy is performed by external beam radiotherapy with the use of photon beams or a combination of photon and electron beams after CT-based treatment planning. The prescribed dose is usually 50 Gy with 1.8 Gy per fraction. A local boost up to a dose of at least 60 Gy is recommended in case of macroscopic residual tumour, positive resection margins, or (residual) macroscopic lymph node metastasis. Five-year survival is substantially influenced by the lymph node status and ranges from 25–41% and 70–93% in patients with and without inguinal lymph node metastasis, respectively. Adjuvant radiotherapy significantly reduces inguinal lymph node recurrences (24% vs 5%), significantly improves survival in patients with positive lymph nodes (68% vs 54%) and significantly reduces local recurrences in patients with close or positive resection margins (58% vs 16%) [136–138]. Side effects of adjuvant radiotherapy affect, apart from urogenital and gastrointestinal symptoms, mainly the vulvar and inguinal skin leading to local inflammation and desquamation and requiring local supportive measures. Late side effects of the skin include atrophy, telangiectasia, fibrosis, and pigmentary changes. The combination of lymph node dissection and radiotherapy has an increased risk for chronic lymphoedema.

Primary/neoadjuvant radiotherapy

Primary radiochemotherapy is indicated for locally advanced tumours, if surrounding organs are infiltrated and/or exenteration is necessary for achieving radical resection. In consequence, radiochemotherapy may be used for improving resectability or as single treatment. At first external beam radiotherapy is performed following the same principle as for adjuvant treatment. Primary radiotherapy is usually combined with concomitant chemotherapy. In accordance to the treatment of cervix or anal cancer, cisplatin, 5-FU, or mitomycin C is delivered. Depending on the localization of the primary tumour and the response to external beam radiotherapy and concomitant chemotherapy, interstitial (+/− intravaginal) brachytherapy should be considered for local dose escalation if surgery is not planned. The application technique has to be individually adapted using, e.g., flexible tubes for superficially located tumours or similar techniques as in vaginal cancer for deeper infiltrating tumours. PDR-schedules are recommended with 0.4–0.6 Gy per pulse up to a total (boost) dose of 14–24 Gy.

After (neoadjuvant) radiochemotherapy, operability can be achieved in 63–92% of the cases. A recent study demonstrated a complete clinical and pathological remission rate of ~50% and ~33%, respectively [139–142]. A Cochrane analysis between radiochemotherapy (primary or neoadjuvant) and primary surgery did not show a significant difference in overall survival or treatment-related side effects [143]. Primary radiochemotherapy with brachytherapy for limited stages achieves comparable results to surgery with 75–100% local tumour control. Side effects are similar to adjuvant radiotherapy and primary radiotherapy of vaginal cancer.

Ovarian cancer

Surgery and adjuvant chemotherapy are the cornerstones in primary treatment of ovarian cancer. Radiotherapy is currently not part of the primary treatment concept in the majority of cases. Historically, whole abdominal irradiation with 25–30 Gy in 1–1.5 Gy per fraction was performed due to the predominantly peritoneal tumour spread but was omitted because of advances in chemotherapy. However, radiotherapy is mainly applied in palliative intent for metastatic disease such as bone or brain metastasis and especially for inoperable isolated pelvic recurrences.

Medical management

Cervical cancer

This entity shows high sensitivity for radiotherapy. Combined radiochemotherapy with weekly 40 mg cisplatin in addition to radiotherapy led to an improved survival and apart from systemic effect chemotherapy is mainly considered as a radiosensitizer in this setting [107].

Neoadjuvant chemotherapy is an option in bulky disease with the aim of shrinkage of advanced disease. Neoadjuvant chemotherapy with dose dense weekly paclitaxel and carboplatin followed by standard combined radiochemotherapy is a feasible approach and is associated with a high response rate (67%) in locally advanced cervical cancer [144]. Another small study with neoadjuvant platinum-taxane based chemotherapy showed a response rate of 78.3% and the surgery completion rate was 78.3% [145].

In case of metastatic disease the combination chemotherapy with cisplatin and topotecan was the standard treatment since the randomized phase III GOG-179 trial cisplatin plus topotecan compared to cisplatin monotherapy showed a significantly prolonged progression-free survival (PFS) (4.6 vs 2.9 months, p = 0.014) and overall survival (OS) (9.4 vs 6.5 months, p = 0.017) [146]. These results led to the approval of the Food and Drug Administration (FDA) in 2006. The GOG-169 compared cisplatin/paclitaxel with cisplatin alone and showed only a significantly increased PFS, but no significant OS prolongation [147]. The ambitious phase III GOG-204 trial compared four different platinum-based doublets containing topotecan, paclitaxel, vinorelbine, and gemcitabine in advanced cervical cancer. No doublet was superior to cisplatin (50mg/m^2)/paclitaxel (135mg/m^2 over 24 h) in terms of OS. However, the trend in response rates, PFS, and OS favoured cisplatin/paclitaxel [148].

Kitagawa et al. recommended carboplatin/paclitaxel as the new standard treatment for stage IVB or recurrent cervical cancer. OS data showed no inferiority in comparison to cisplatin/paclitaxel, but milder toxicity profiles and quality of life [149].

For further chemotherapy lines, monotherapies with anthracyclines or taxane are recommended. Data of a phase III trial show an improved OS with bevacizumab in recurrent and metastatic disease [150].

Endometrial cancer

Endometrial cancer shows the highest incidence in gynaecologic malignancies. Early stages are most common due to early symptoms. Low-risk early stage endometrial cancer needs surgical treatment only and no adjuvant chemotherapy.

Chemotherapy has evolved into an important modality in high-risk early stage and advanced stage disease and in recurrent endometrial cancer. Multi-institutional trials are in progress to better define optimal adjuvant treatment for subsets of patients [151]. Type II endometrial cancers are very aggressive and behave like ovarian cancer and therefore should get adjuvant platinum/taxane-based chemotherapy.

The most active agents for chemotherapy-naïve patients in endometrial cancer are platinum agents, taxanes, and anthracyclines, all producing response rates of 20–30%. For patients able to tolerate aggressive therapy, multiagent chemotherapy produces higher response rates than single-agent therapy. A phase III study (GOG 209) is currently assessing carboplatin and paclitaxel versus cisplatin. Within a GOG trial in stage III or IV disease eight cycles of doxorubicin and cisplatin were compared to whole abdominal radiotherapy. A significant 5-year survival increase of 13% for patients was present for patients who got chemotherapy relative to the radiotherapy arm [152].

Meta-analysis of nine prospective, randomized trials with 2197 patients showed that adjuvant chemotherapy in high-risk endometrial carcinoma can decrease lethality by 25% [153]. The most favourable benefit/risk profile seems to have carboplatin/paclitaxel, but platinum/anthracycline and platinum/anthracycline/taxane combinations are effective also [154].

Hormonal therapy is standard treatment in metastatic hormonal receptor positive endometrial cancers, but not in the adjuvant setting. Hormonal therapy, primarily with progestins, is less toxic than chemotherapy and 20% response rates are seen in properly selected patients [155]. Tamoxifen shows modest response rates with 10% in phase II trials [156]. Limited phase II data are available for aromatase inhibitors with response rates from 9 to 11% [151].

For women with early stage, low-grade endometrial cancer that involves only endometrium and who declare a wish for fertility-preserving treatment, progestin, usually medroxyprogesterone acetate (100 to 800 mg/d for 4–14 months) is an option, but not a standard treatment with response rates of 57–76%. Control hysteroscopy and curettage is necessary and recommendation of hysterectomy and oophorectomy after childbearing [157].

For endometrial cancer, targeted agents including mammalian target of rapamycin (mTOR) inhibitors, have been discussed. Promising results of a phase II study of temsirolimus in patients with advanced endometrial cancer are documented. Although no correlation of molecular markers of the PI3K/AKT/mTOR pathway with the clinical outcomes were demonstrated, single-agent activity, especially in chemotherapy-naive patients, with 14% partial response and 69% stable disease was shown [158]. Promising data were documented in a phase II trial with an LHRH agonist treatment in LHRH positive tumours [159].

Vulvar cancer

Vulvar cancer is a rare disease, usually diagnosed in a stage still amenable to potentially curative treatments, including surgery and/or radiotherapy with or without chemotherapy. Prognosis of metastatic or recurrent disease not amenable to salvage surgery or radiotherapy is very poor. Evidence about the efficacy of chemotherapy in this setting is limited and its role still remains unclear. Combined radiochemotherapy with cisplatin can be used in the adjuvant setting as well as in the neoadjuvant setting in locally advanced tumours [66]. At present, patients with advanced vulvar carcinomas and patients with metastatic disease are usually treated with schedules adopted for chemoradiation or extrapolated from cervical cancer [160]. Criteria for the indication and performance of chemo/radiotherapy of the vulva, groins, and pelvis are still not fully established and vary between different countries and institutions due to the low level of evidence. Often an individualized therapeutic approach aside from guidelines is necessary to treat these patients adequately [66]. Most common applicated chemotherapy combination regimens in case of distant metastases are cisplatin/5-FU or a platinum/taxane-based chemotherapy.

Vaginal cancer

Vaginal cancer shows very low incidence and therefore phase III trials are missing. Current guidelines have been drawn on retrospective studies. The role of radiotherapy and concomitant chemotherapy with 5-FU and mitomycin C has shown good results in terms of local control [161]. In case of stage IV disease, the use of concomitant chemo-radiotherapy with agents such as 5-FU, mitomycin C, and cisplatin have shown promising results when combined with radiotherapy with complete response rates as high as 85%, but long-term results of such therapies have been variable [162, 60]. For distant metastases chemotherapy schedules similar to cervical cancer are applicable.

Ovarian cancer

For the past decade standard chemotherapy in advanced ovarian cancer was six cycles of carboplatin (AUC 5-6) and paclitaxel 175 mg/m2 q3w [163]. Adding a third cytotoxic drug failed to improve PFS or OS.

The addition of the monoclonal antibody bevacizumab, that inhibits the vascular endothelial growth factor (VEGF), showed a significantly prolonged PFS in first-line therapy [164, 165]. Burger et al. indicated that the use of bevacizumab up to ten months after carboplatin/paclitaxel prolonged the PFS by about four months and Perren et al. showed within the ICON-7 trial a prolongation of about two months with a maximum benefit at 12 months at the completion of planned bevacizumab treatment. PFS and OS were greater among patients at high risk for disease progression [164]. A phase III trial investigating the duration of bevacizumab treatment is ongoing (15 vs 30 months). In platinum-sensitive relapse the addition of bevacizumab to gemcitabine and carboplatin (GC) followed by bevacizumab until progression showed a significantly improved PFS of four months compared to GC plus placebo [166]. In platinum-resistant relapse situation a nearly doubling of PFS was present with addition of bevacizumab to non-platinum chemotherapy vs no bevacizumab (6.7 vs 3.4 months; HR 0.48) [167]. These data provide robust evidence for the important role of bevacizumab in ovarian cancer treatment.

Although intraperitoneal chemotherapy extended OS by 12 to 17 months [168], it is an option only for women in advanced ovarian cancer with a small amount residual disease after primary surgery and it is not widely used because of the very high toxicity. Therefore, it is recommended within clinical trials only.

Promising significant increased PFS and OS were presented from the Japanese Gynecologic Oncologic Group concerning dose-dense weekly paclitaxel in combination with carboplatin q3w [169]. Data from European clinical trials of dose-dense regimen with paclitaxel weekly could not confirm a survival benefit in comparison to standard treatment [170].

Neoadjuvant platinum/taxane-based chemotherapy in ovarian cancer is recommended only within clinical trials. Subgroup analysis of the neoadjuvant phase III trial of Vergote et al. documented that patients with primary surgery and macroscopic complete resection showed a significantly improved survival in comparison to all subgroups with neoadjuvant treatment [98]. Despite higher complete resection rates after neoadjuvant treatment, no improved survival was present and the documented extent of surgical management within this trial was very questionable [98]. If neoadjuvant chemotherapy was initiated because of contraindication for immediate radical surgery, interval debulking surgery should be performed after a maximum of two to three cycles because of the development of resistance mechanisms in case of later surgery [171].

About 50% of serous epithelial ovarian cancer might have disruption of the homologous recombination pathway—independently on BRCA-1 or BRCA-2 mutations—and be susceptible to PARP (poly adenosine diphosphate ribose polymerase) inhibitors like olaparib [172]. Maintenance therapy with olaparib significantly improved PFS in platinum-sensitive ovarian cancer relapse, but until now no OS benefit has been shown. A very mild toxicity profile was documented for maintenance therapy with olaparib [172].

The management of the very rare, but very aggressive small-cell carcinomas of the gynaecologic tract (cervix, ovary, uterus, vulva, and vagina) requires systemic chemotherapy with cisplatin and etoposide, both in the setting of early and advanced stage disease [173].

Multidisciplinary management of complex cases

Cervix cancer: Squamous cell carcinoma, FIGO IIIB, T3b, cN1 (CT/MRI), M0. Case report 1

A 45-year-old patient presented at the Department of Gynaecology with dyspareunia, vaginal bleeding, and persisting vaginal discharge for approximately three months. Gynaecologic examination revealed a 6cm × 5cm × 5cm (width, height, thickness) tumour located at the cervix uteri with infiltration of the right vaginal fornix, infiltration of the left proximal parametrium, and infiltration of the right parametrium up to the pelvic wall (see Figure 44.4).

General and surgical management

A biopsy was performed and histology showed invasive squamous cell carcinoma, grade 2. For further staging, FDG-PET CT and pelvic MRI were performed. PET CT showed a uterine cervical mass with an increased SUV uptake (SUV max 21), multiple enlarged pelvic lymph nodes but without any FDG uptake and no distant metastasis. T2-weighted MRI depicted a hyperintensive mass in the cervix uteri with infiltration of both parametria up to the pelvic wall and suspected infiltration of the posterior urinary bladder wall. Cystoscopy showed an intact urinary bladder mucosa and thus did not confirm bladder wall invasion. Stage was consequently FIGO IIIB (TNM: T3b, cN1 (CT/MRI), M0). The patient was presented at the gynaecological multidisciplinary tumour board. Due to advanced tumour stage with pelvic wall involvement and the presence of multiple enlarged lymph nodes without FDG uptake it was decided to perform laparoscopic lymph node staging for the assessment of regional and para-aortic lymph node status and resection of enlarged suspicious nodes followed by primary radiochemotherapy. After laparoscopic lymph node staging, 0 of 23 removed lymph nodes (12 pelvic, 11 para-aortic) showed malignant cells indicating a pN0 status.

Radiotherapy management

The patient was referred to the Department of Radiotherapy for initiation of primary radiochemotherapy consisting of external beam radiotherapy, concomitant chemotherapy, and image-guided adaptive brachytherapy. A CT, performed in supine position with maximum bladder filling, was used for target definition and treatment planning of external beam radiotherapy. The clinical tumour-related target volume included the whole uterus, the upper third of the vagina, the whole parametria and the (regional) lymph node areas up to the aortic bifurcation, internal/external/common iliac areas, para-rectal, and pre-sacral areas. An additional margin of 1 cm in all directions was applied to the clinical target volume (CTV) for defining the planning target volume (PTV) in order to adjust for setup errors and organ movement during EBRT. Contouring of organs at risk included rectum, sigmoid, bowel, urinary bladder. In total, 45 Gy in daily fractions of 1.8 Gy were delivered on working days to the PTV by 3D conformal EBRT using the 'four field-box-technique' within a time period of five weeks. Beginning with the first day of EBRT, cisplatin (40mg/m^2) was administered in weekly intervals. The fifth cycle of chemotherapy had to be delivered in reduced dosage due to impaired renal function. During EBRT and chemotherapy the patient developed a moderate increase in urinary and stool frequency (CTCV3.0 G1). In the last week of radiochemotherapy pelvic MRI and gynaecologic examination were re-performed for assessment of tumour regression and for brachytherapy pre-planning and revealed residual disease in the uterine cervix reaching up to the distal third of the right parametrium and the left parametrium and the vagina as tumour-free. Maximum asymmetrical tumour dimensions to the right were 5 cm × 3.5 cm × 4.3 cm. In week six, the first brachytherapy application was performed in an operation theatre under spinal anaesthesia. A tandem ring applicator was placed into the uterine cavity and ten interstitial needles were inserted through the ring (Vienna I/II) into the cervix and the right parametrium

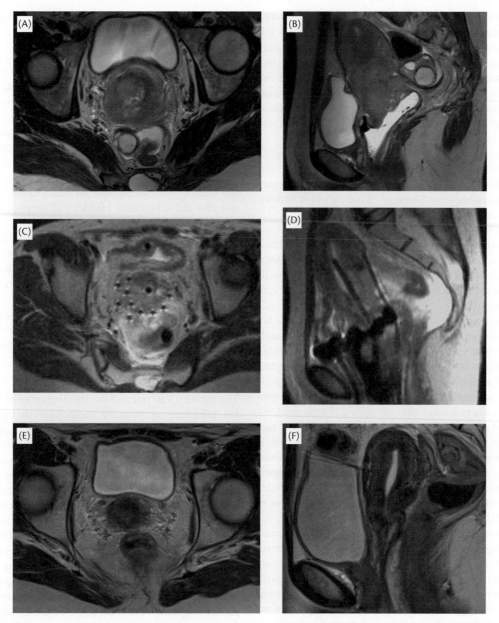

Fig. 44.4 T2-weighted MR images (A, C, E: transversal; B, D, F: sagittal) of a patient with locally advanced cervical cancer staged as FIGO IIIB cN1 treated with primary radiochemotherapy and image-guided adaptive brachytherapy. A, B: At the time of diagnosis: 6.8 × 5.2 × 4.1 cm hyperintensive mass at the uterine cervix with infiltration of both parametria. C, D: At the time of brachytherapy after 45 Gy of external beam radiotherapy and five cycles of chemotherapy: 5.5 × 4.2 × 3.0 cm residual tumour indicating poor response; a tandem ring applicator, and ten interstitial needles were inserted for image-guided adaptive brachytherapy. E, F: Complete remission six months after treatment.

under ultrasound guidance. T2 weighted pelvic MRI was performed with applicator and interstitial needles in place for treatment planning. Adaptive tumour-related CTVs were defined on MRI (high-risk CTV, intermediate-risk CTV) according to the Groupe Européen de Curiethérapie and the European SocieTy for Radiotherapy & Oncology (GEC-ESTRO) recommendations based on the residual tumour mass and the tumour regression pattern during EBRT and chemotherapy. The surrounding organs at risk (rectum, urinary bladder, sigmoid colon, and bowel) were delineated. An individual treatment plan was created allowing for high-dose delivery to the CTVs while simultaneously sparing the organs at risk (OARs). With this treatment plan two fractions of HDR brachytherapy were delivered with a 16 hour break in

between and afterwards the tandem ring applicator and the interstitial needles were removed. In week seven, the brachytherapy application, imaging, and treatment planning were repeated and two further fractions of HDR brachytherapy were applied. In total (EBRT + brachytherapy), an iso-effective dose (2 Gy fractions) of 92Gy (EQD2) was delivered to 90% the high-risk CTV (D90) and 85 Gy, 69 Gy, and 72 Gy (EQD2) to 2 cm^3 of the bladder, rectum, and sigmoid, respectively.

Follow-up
The patient achieved complete remission as assessed three months after completion of radiochemotherapy. Local treatment of the vagina with anti-inflammatory solution and vaginal dilation were

recommended and performed. Gynaecologic examination, MRI, and CT were regularly used for follow-up investigations. After 42 months, the patient is in continuous complete remission (MRI) and altogether well. Gynaecologic examination shows no evidence of disease and some vaginal shortening and narrowing in the upper third (G2). The patient reports vaginal dryness (G1) and occasional diarrhoea (G1). Rectosigmoidoscopy shows telangiectasia in the proximal anterior rectal wall but without any sign for bleeding.

Discussion

According to international and institutional guidelines based on clinical level 1 evidence this patient was treated with primary radiochemotherapy. Before initiation of radiochemotherapy laparoscopic lymph node staging was performed. The role of surgical lymph node staging is controversial. However, precise assessment of lymph node status is crucial for the definition of the lymph node target volume (pelvic vs pelvic + para-aortic). Furthermore, in lymph node positive patients, removal of bulky lymph nodes is assumed to be associated with a survival benefit.

Cisplatin-based chemotherapy was added to radiotherapy due to the significant overall survival benefit shown in randomized controlled trials. EBRT was performed as 3D conformal radiotherapy using a 'four-field-box technique' as the large bladder removed most of the bowel out of the treated pelvic region. Recent studies indicate that with the use of intensity-modulated radiotherapy (IMRT) acute gastrointestinal toxicity can be reduced by a reduction of high-dose delivery to significant parts of the bowel volume.

Image-guided adaptive brachytherapy (IGABT) using repetitive MRI is a novel treatment approach, which takes into account individual tumour spread, tumour remission, and changing pelvic topography. First studies on IGABT—including a prospective non-randomized multicentre study—indicate an improved therapeutic ratio compared to standard X-ray ('point A') based brachytherapy. The use of interstitial needles allows for significant dose escalation and increase of target dose coverage, if required by the individual tumour situation (e.g., asymmetrical tumour spread with residual parametrial disease as in this particular case) as shown by dosimetric comparisons. Due to these improvements and the resulting high local tumour control rate (~90–95% after three years) distant metastasis are becoming the predominant type of treatment failure. Patients with FIGO IIIB tumour stage, with and without lymph node metastasis, have a probability of approximately 40–60% to develop distant metastasis within five years of follow-up. Studies investigating the impact of additional adjuvant and/or intensified chemotherapy are currently ongoing.

Endometrium cancer: endometrioid adenocarcinoma G2, pT1b, pN0, pL0; FIGO stage IB. Case report 2

A seventy-one-year-old woman was referred by her gynaecologist because of recurrent vaginal bleeding since three months. The gynaecologist described a distinct endometrial hyperplasia diagnosed by vaginal ultrasound. She has three children and feels otherwise healthy. She has overweight with a body mass index of 37. She suffers from hypertension and type II diabetes mellitus. There are no other comorbidities. She has a sister who had breast cancer at the age of 62 years. There are no other malignant diseases in her close family.

The gynaecologic examination shows slight bleeding from the cervical canal. Vaginal ultrasound reveals a normal sized uterus and the endometrium is hyperplastic with a maximum thickness of 11 mm. Adnexal regions appear normal. The patient was scheduled for hysteroscopy and dilatation and curettage. Hysteroscopy showed a suspicious mass in the uterine cavity (fundus) with a diameter of approximately 2.5 cm. The cervical canal was visualized without suspicious findings and curettage was performed. Endometrial sampling revealed moderately differentiated (G2) endometrioid adenocarcinoma of the uterus. The pretherapeutic workup included a CT scan of the thorax and abdomen, a contrast-enhanced MRI of the pelvis and a referral to our pre-anaesthetic outpatient service regarding the planned surgery. CT of thorax and abdomen showed no signs of tumour spread beyond the uterus. Pelvic and peri-aortic lymph nodes appeared to be normal, MRI showed a myometrial tumour invasion of more than 50%.

Surgical management

Total laparoscopic hysterectomy with bilateral salpingo-oophorectomy with pelvic lymphadenectomy was performed. Frozen section analysis revealed a moderately-differentiated endometrioid adenocarcinoma and a myometrial tumour invasion of the outer half of the myometrium. Pelvic lymph nodes were negative. Because of the deep myometrial tumour invasion, the moderate tumour differentiation, and tumour size, peri-aortic lymph node dissection was performed. The histologic results were confirmed in the paraffin sections and all resected lymph nodes (n = 42) were found negative. Surgical-pathological (TNM) staging revealed a moderately differentiated (G2) endometrioid adenocarcinoma pT1b, pN0, pL0; stage IB according to the 2009 staging system of FIGO.

Adjuvant therapy

Based on clinical-pathological findings adjuvant radiotherapy was recommended. The patient received vaginal brachytherapy at a dose of 4 × 5/7 Gy at 5/0 mm corresponding to a total isoeffective dose of 30–40 Gy (EQD2).

Post-treatment surveillance

The patient was followed in our outpatient clinic with physical examination, vaginal vault cytology, abdominal ultrasound, and monitoring for symptoms. Three years after treatment she is free of disease.

Discussion

Treatment recommendations for endometrial cancer depend upon disease stage and additional factors that influence the risk of disease recurrence. Surgery performed as total hysterectomy with bilateral salpingo-oophorectomy, with or without lymphadenectomy, is usually curative for women who are at a low risk of disease recurrence. In patients with highly and moderately-differentiated endometrioid tumours that are confined to the endometrium or the inner half of the myometrium and a tumour size <2cm the risk of lymph node metastasis is less than 1% and lymphadenectomy is therefore not recommended. In patients with highly- and moderately-differentiated endometrioid tumours and deep myometrial infiltration (FIGO IB) or poorly-differentiated endometrioid tumours with an infiltration of the inner half of the myometrium and a tumour size <2cm the risk of lymph node metastasis is 9.3%. We recommend in these cases pelvic lymphadenectomy and frozen section. If pelvic lymph nodes are positive peri-aortic lymphadenectomy should be done.

In all other cases (FIGO IB G1 or G2 and tumour size >2cm, FIGO IB G3, serous-papillary, clear cell) pelvic and peri-aortic lymphadenectomy is recommended.

Patients who are at intermediate or high risk for disease recurrence are candidates for adjuvant therapy.

Based on clinical-pathological findings such as age (71 years), deep myometrial invasion, moderate tumour differentiation (G2), and large tumour size (>2.5cm) our patient was considered to be at intermediate risk of loco-regional recurrence. Therefore adjuvant brachytherapy was performed. Randomized controlled trials showed that vaginal brachytherapy is an adequate therapy for patients at intermediate risk of recurrence. Vaginal brachytherapy is associated with a more favourable toxicity profile (such as a lower rate of diarrhoea and other bowel symptoms) when compared with external beam radiation, resulting in equivalent loco-regional control rates. In addition, external beam radiation therapy seems to reduce long-term survival of patients less than 60 years of age at the time of treatment because of an increased risk of rectal and bladder malignancies. Patients with endometrial cancer at intermediate risk show five-year survival rates of more than 80% and a reduced risk of loco regional recurrences when vaginal brachytherapy is applied. External beam radiation should only be used in cases with lymph node metastasis or in advanced stage disease. The addition of chemotherapy in these cases should be considered.

Ovarian cancer: serous papillary adenocarcinoma G3, FIGO stage IIIC, T3b, N+, M0. Case report 3

A fifty-eight-year-old patient was referred with increasing abdominal pain and abdominal diameter. She had three children, no cases of malignant disease in her family and had been healthy. She had no obvious bowel dysfunction. She recognized that something did change in her abdomen about six months ago. Because of increasing complaints she saw her general practitioner who sent her to have an abdominal CT scan. The CT scan revealed a bilateral adnexal mass, ascites, and an enlarged omentum. CA 125 was elevated to 1.250 U/ml. Our pretherapeutic workup included a clinical gynaecologic examination, vaginal ultrasound, CT scan of the thorax, and a referral to our pre-anaesthetic outpatient service regarding the planned cyto-reductive surgery. We confirmed the already described lesions highly suspicious for ovarian cancer. The CT thorax showed no signs of tumour spread.

Surgical management

Subsequently the patient underwent explorative laparotomy. We found two litres of ascites, large bilateral adnexal masses, involving the complete pelvic peritoneum, uterus, and recto-sigmoid. Peritoneal carcinosis was present in both para-colic gutters, the right diaphragm, and in parts on the mesenterium of the small bowel. There was a solid tumour infiltration of the ileo-coecal region and an omental cake up to the transverse colon. Because of the good medical condition of the patient the tumour was assumed to be completely resectable. Frozen section revealed a high-grade serous papillary adenocarcinoma of the ovary.

We performed an en bloc resection with a complete pelvic peritoneumectomy and a recto-sigmoidal anastomosis, extensive peritoneumectomy in the described areas of tumour involvement, infra- and supra-colic omentectomy, and an ileo-coecal resection. Because there was no macroscopic intra-abdominal tumour left a systematic pelvic and peri-aortic lymphadenectomy was added. An intraperitoneal port system was placed during primary surgery.

The patient recovered well and the post-operative course was uneventful. The definitive histology described a high-grade serous papillary adenocarcinoma of the ovary in all described tumour locations. Four of 26 peri-aortic lymph nodes were positive, 38 pelvic lymph nodes were negative (FIGO stage IIIC).

Chemotherapy

The patient was given intraperitoneal (ip) chemotherapy with carbo-platinum AUC 6 ip and 175 mg/m^2 paclitaxel iv on day one and 60 mg/m^2 paclitaxel ip on day eight of a three week cycle. The patient underwent six cycles of chemotherapy. Chemotherapy was well tolerated. Pain episodes during intraperitoneal therapy were successfully managed by reducing the intraperitoneal infusion amount to 1500 ml and the prophylactic use of paracetamol. The patient developed peripheral neurotoxicity grade 2 in the last two cycles. No dose reduction or interval extension was required.

Follow-up

The patient was followed in our outpatient clinic. Three years after the termination of first-line chemotherapy CA 125 began to rise. The patient felt well and had no symptoms (performance status ECOG 0). The CA 125 continuously increased from normal levels (<10 U/ml) to 289 U/ml. At that point a PET/CT was performed showing a solitary lesion of approximately 6 cm in diameter adjacent to the descending colon. No other suspect lesions could be detected.

Management of recurrent disease

The patient underwent re-laparotomy and a complete tumour resection with segmental resection of the descending colon. No other malignant lesions could be detected after thorough abdominal inspection. After an uneventful post-operative course the patient received platinum-based re-induction chemotherapy with carboplatin AUC 4 iv on day one and gemcitabine 1000mg/m^2 iv on days one and eight of a three week cycle. Beginning with cycle two we added 15mg/kg of bevacizumab iv every three weeks. The patient is well and still on treatment with bevacizumab and there is no evidence of disease.

Discussion

Complete surgical tumour resection is still one of the most important prognostic factors in the therapy of advanced stage ovarian cancer. In centres capable of performing such complex surgical procedures 60 to 70% of patients with advanced stage disease can be debulked to no residual tumour rest. Neoadjuvant chemotherapy should not replace surgical skills. Complete cytoreduction may provide the patient with a median survival of 50 to 100 months, whereas interval cytoreduction after neoadjuvant chemotherapy is consistently associated with a median survival of only 30 to 36 months even if complete resection is attained in this setting.

In addition to optimal (R0) cytoreduction the application of platinum and taxane based chemotherapy is considered as gold standard in the therapy of advanced epithelial ovarian cancer. The use of intraperitoneal chemotherapy is discussed controversially. However, there are three randomized controlled trials showing an advantage of ip chemotherapy in progression free and overall survival.

Bevacizumab has been shown to be effective in the adjuvant treatment, as well as in the treatment of platinum sensitive and resistant disease. Proof of principle was demonstrated in four randomized controlled trials showing a significant improvement in progression-free survival.

In the management of platinum sensitive recurrent disease secondary cytoreduction is recommended if feasible. On the other hand, there are no RCTs supporting this approach. An international AGO trial (DESKTOP III) compares secondary cytoreduction followed by chemotherapy with chemotherapy alone in platinum-sensitive, recurrent epithelial ovarian cancer. This trial will probably define the role of secondary cytoreduction in this setting.

Further reading

Cancer Research UK, November 2013. <http://www.cancerresearchuk.org/cancer-info/cancerstats/keyfacts/vagina-and-vulva-cancer/>.

Cannistra SA. Cancer of the ovary. New England Journal of Medicine; 351: 2519–2529.

Carcangiu ML, Herrington S, Kurman RJ, Young RH (eds), Tumours of the Female Genital Tract, 4th ed. Lyon: International Agency for Research on Cancer, 2014.

Ferlay J, Shin HR, Bray F, Forman D, Mathers C et al. GLOBOCAN 2008 v1.2, Cancer Incidence and Mortality Worldwide. IARC Cancerbase No10 [online]. Lyon: International Agency for Research on Cancer, 2010. Available from: <http://globocan.iarc.fr>.

Jemal A, Bray F, Center MM, Ferlay J, Ward E, Forman D. Global cancer statistics. CA A Cancer Journal for Clinicians 2011; 61: 69–90.

Kurman RJ, Ellenson LH, Ronnett BM (eds), Blaustein's Pathology of the Female Genital Tract, 6th ed. Springer, 2011.

Panici PB, Plotti F, Zullo MA, et al. Pelvic lymphadenectomy for cervical carcinoma: laparotomy extraperitoneal, transperitoneal or laparoscopic approach? A randomized study. Gynecologic Oncology 2006; 103: 859–864.

References

1. Balleyguier C, Sala E, Da Cunha T, et al. Staging of uterine cervical cancer with MRI: guidelines of the European Society of Urogenital Radiology. European Journal of Radiology 2011; 21: 1102–1110.
2. Haie-Meder C, Mazeron R, Magne N. Clinical evidence on PET-CT for radiation therapy planning in cervix and endometrial cancers. Radiotherapy and Oncology 2010; 96: 351–355.
3. Leblanc E, Gauthier H, Querleu D, et al. Accuracy of 18-fluoro-2-deoxy-D-glucose positron emission tomography in the pretherapeutic detection of occult para-aortic node involvement in patients with a locally advanced cervical carcinoma. Annals of Surgical Oncology 2011; 18: 2302–2309.
4. Janthanaphan M, Wootipoom V, Tangsinmunkong K, Liabsuetrakul T. Comparison of success rate and complications of contour-loop excision of the transformation zone (C-LETZ) with cold knife conization (CKC) in high grade lesion (HGL) from colposcopic impression. Journal of the Medical Association of Thailand 2009; 92: 1573–1579.
5. Kyrgiou M, Koliopoulos G, Martin-Hirsch P, Arbyn M, Prendiville W et al. Obstetric outcomes after conservative treatment for intraepithelial or early invasive cervical lesions: systematic review and meta-analysis. Lancet 2006; 367: 489–498.
6. Michel G, Morice P, Castaigne D, Leblanc M, Rey A et al. Lymphatic spread in stage Ib and II cervical carcinoma: anatomy and surgical implications. Obstetrics and Gynecology 1998; 91: 360–363.
7. Querleu D, Morrow CP. Classification of radical hysterectomy. Lancet Oncology 2008; 9: 297–303.
8. Cibula D, Abu-Rustum NR. Pelvic lymphadenectomy in cervical cancer—surgical anatomy and proposal for a new classification system. Gynecologic Oncology 2010; 116: 33–37.
9. Querleu D, Leblanc E, Cartron G, Narducci F, Ferron G et al. Audit of preoperative and early complications of laparoscopic lymph node dissection in 1000 gynecologic cancer patients. American Journal of Obstetrics and Gynecology 2006; 195: 1287–1292.
10. Varia MA, Bundy BN, Deppe G et al. Cervical carcinoma metastatic to para-aortic nodes: extended field radiation therapy with concomitant 5-fluorouracil and cisplatin chemotherapy: a Gynecologic Oncology Group study. International Journal of Radiation Oncology Biology Physics 1998; 42: 1015–1023.
11. Dargent D, Ansquer Y, Mathevet P. Technical development and results of left extraperitoneal laparoscopic paraaortic lymphadenectomy for cervical cancer. Gynecologic Oncology 2000; 77: 87–92.
12. Lai CH, Huang KG, Hong JH et al. Randomized trial of surgical staging (extraperitoneal or laparoscopic) versus clinical staging in locally advanced cervical cancer. Gynecologic Oncology 2003; 89: 160–167.
13. Leblanc E, Narducci F, Frumovitz M et al. Therapeutic value of pretherapeutic extraperitoneal laparoscopic staging in locally advanced cervical carcinoma. Gynecologic Oncology 2007; 105: 304–311.
14. Lecuru F, Mathevet P, Querleu D et al. Bilateral negative sentinel nodes accurately predict absence of lymph node metastasis in early cervical cancer: results of the SENTICOL study. Journal of Clinical Oncology 2011; 29: 1686–1691.
15. Cibula D, Abu-Rustum NR, Benedetti-Panici P et al. New classification system of radical hysterectomy: emphasis on a three-dimensional anatomic template for parametrial resection. Gynecologic Oncology 2011; 122: 264–268.
16. Dargent D, Martin X, Sacchetoni A, Mathevet P. Laparoscopic vaginal radical trachelectomy: a treatment to preserve the fertility of cervical carcinoma patients. Cancer 2000; 88: 1877–1882.
17. Roy M, Plante M. Place of Schauta's radical vaginal hysterectomy. Best practice and research. Clinical Obstetrics and Gynecology 2011; 25: 227–237.
18. Sert BM, Abeler VM. Robotic-assisted laparoscopic radical hysterectomy (Piver type III) with pelvic node dissection—case report. European Journal of Gynaecological Oncology 2006; 27: 531–533.
19. Rob L, Holaska M, Robova H. Nerve-sparing and individually tailored surgery for cervical cancer. Lancet Oncology 2010; 11: 292–301.
20. Fujii S. Anatomic identification of nerve-sparing radical hysterectomy: a step-by-step procedure. Gynecologic Oncology 2008; 111(2 Suppl): S33–41.
21. Höckel M, Horn LC, Manthey N, Braumann UD, Wolf U, Teichmann G, Frauenschläger K, Dornhöfer N, Einenkel J. Resection of the embryologically defined uterovaginal (Müllerian) compartment and pelvic control in patients with cervical cancer: a prospective analysis. The Lancet Oncology 2009; 10(7): 683–92.
22. Magrina JF, Stanhope CR, Weaver AL. Pelvic exenterations: supralevator, infralevator, and with vulvectomy. Gynecologic Oncology 1997; 64: 130–135.
23. Momoh AO, Kamat AM, Butler CE. Reconstruction of the pelvic floor with human acellular dermal matrix and omental flap following anterior pelvic exenteration. Journal of Plastic, Reconstructive and Aesthetic Surgery 2010; 63: 2185–2187.
24. Hockel M. Laterally extended endopelvic resection (LEER)—principles and practice. Gynecologic Oncology 2008; 111(2 Suppl): S13–7.
25. De Wever I. Pelvic exenteration: surgical aspects and analysis of early and late morbidity in a series of 106 patients. Acta Chirugica Belgica 2011; 111: 273–281.
26. Morice P, Juncker L, Rey A, El-Hassan J, Haie-Meder C et al. Ovarian transposition for patients with cervical carcinoma treated by radiosurgical combination. Fertility and Sterility 2000; 74: 743–748.
27. Valle M, Federici O, Ialongo P, Graziano F, Garofalo A. Prevention of complications following pelvic exenteration with the use of mammary implants in the pelvic cavity: technique and results of 28 cases. Journal of Surgical Oncology 2011; 103: 34–38.
28. Wong YF, Cheung TH, Lo KW et al. Identification of molecular markers and signaling pathway in endometrial cancer in Hong Kong Chinese women by genome-wide gene expression profiling. Oncogene 2007; 26: 1971–1982.
29. Pecorelli S. Revised FIGO staging for carcinoma of the vulva, cervix, and endometrium. International Journal of Gynaecology and Obstetrics 2009; 105: 103–104.
30. Lee JH, Dubinsky T, Andreotti RF et al. Expert Panel on Women's Imaging and Radiation Oncology-Gynecology. ACR appropriateness

Criteria* pretreatment evaluation and follow-up of endometrial cancer of the uterus. Ultrasound Q 2011; 27: 139–145.

31. ASTEC study group, Kitchener H, Swart AM, Qian Q, Amos C, Parmar MK. Efficacy of systematic pelvic lymphadenectomy in endometrial cancer (MRC ASTEC trial): a randomised study. Lancet 2009; 373: 125–136.

32. Benedetti Panici P, Basille S, Maneshi F et al. Systematic pelvic lymphadenectomy vs. no lymphadenectomy in early-stage endometrial carcinoma: randomized clinical trial. Journal of the National Cancer Institute 2008; 100: 1707–1716.

33. Todo Y, Kato H, Kaneuchi M, Watari H, Takeda M et al. Survival effect of para-aortic lymphadenectomy in endometrial cancer (SEPAL study): a retrospective cohort analysis. Lancet 2010; 375: 1165–1172.

34. Mariani A, Dowdy SC, Cliby WA et al. Prospective assessment of lymphatic dissemination in endometrial cancer: a paradigm shift in surgical staging. Gynecologic Oncology 2008; 109: 11–18.

35. Ballester M, Dubernard G, Lécuru F et al. Detection rate and diagnostic accuracy of sentinel-node biopsy in early stage endometrial cancer: a prospective multicentre study (SENTI-ENDO). Lancet Oncology 2011; 12: 469–476.

36. Kang S, Yoo HJ, Hwang JH, Lim MC, Seo SS, Park SY. Sentinel lymph node biopsy in endometrial cancer: meta-analysis of 26 studies. Gynecologic Oncology 2011; 123: 522–527.

37. Greggi S, Mangili G, Scaffa C et al. Uterine papillary serous, clear cell, and poorly differentiated endometrioid carcinomas: a comparative study. International Journal of Gynecoloical Cancer 2011; 21: 661–667.

38. Chan JK, Lin YG, Monk BJ, Tewari K, Bloss JD et al. Vaginal hysterectomy as primary treatment of endometrial cancer in medically compromised women. Obstetrics and Gynecology 2001; 97(5 Pt 1): 707–711.

39. Moscarini M, Ricciardi E, Quarto A, Maniglio P, Caserta D. Vaginal treatment of endometrial cancer: role in the elderly. World Journal of Surgical Oncology 2011; 9: 74.

40. Childers JM, Surwit EA. Combined laparoscopic and vaginal surgery for the management of two cases of stage I endometrial cancer. Gynecologic Oncology 1992; 45: 46–51.

41. Palomba S, Ricciardi E, Quarto A, Maniglio P, Caserta D. Laparoscopic treatment for endometrial cancer: a meta-analysis of randomized controlled trials (RCTs). Gynecologic Oncology 2009; 112: 415–421.

42. Walker JL, Piedmonte MR, Spirtos NM et al. Laparoscopy compared with laparotomy for comprehensive surgical staging of uterine cancer: Gynecologic Oncology Group Study LAP2. Journal of Clinical Oncology 2009; 27: 5331–5336.

43. Walker JL, Piedmonte MR, Spirtos NM et al. Recurrence and Survival After Random Assignment to Laparoscopy Versus Laparotomy for Comprehensive Surgical Staging of Uterine Cancer: Gynecologic Oncology Group LAP2 Study. Journal of Clinical Oncology 2012; 30: 695–700.

44. Barnett J, Judd JP, Wu JM, Scales CD Jr, Myers ER et al. Cost comparisonamong robotic laparoscopic, and open hysterectomy for endometrial cancer. Obstetrics and Gynecology 2010; 116: 925–931.

45. Seamon LG, Bryant SA, Rheaume PS, Kimball KJ, Huh WK et al. Comprehensive surgical staging for endometrial cancer in obese patients: comparing robotics and laparotomy. Obstetrics and Gynecology 2009; 114: 16–21.

46. Seamon LG, Cohn DE, Henretta MS et al. Minimally invasive comprehensive surgical staging for endometrial cancer: robotics or laparoscopy? Gynecologic Oncology 2009; 113: 36–41.

47. Laurelli G, Di Vagno G, Scaffa C, Losito S, Del Giudice M et al. Conservative treatment of early endometrial cancer: preliminary results of a pilot study. Gynecologic Oncology 2011; 120: 43–46.

48. Kalogiannidis I, Agorastos T. Conservative management of young patients with endometrial highly-differentiated adenocarcinoma. Journal of Obstetrics and Gynaecology 2011; 31: 13–17.

49. Chao AS, Chao A, Wang CJ, Lai CH, Wang HS. Obstetric outcomes of pregnancy after conservative treatment of endometrial cancer: case series and literature review. Taiwanese Journal of Obstetrics and Gynecology 2011; 50: 62–66.

50. Zivanovic O, Carter J, Kauff ND, Barakat RR. A review of the challenges faced in the conservative treatment of young women with endometrial carcinoma and risk of ovarian cancer. Gynecologic Oncology 2009; 115: 504–509.

51. Creasman WT, Phillips JL, Menck HR. The national cancer data base report on cancer of the vagina. Cancer 1998; 83: 1033–1040.

52. Kottmeier HL. The classification and clinical staging of carcinoma of the uterus and vagina. Journal of the International Federation of Gynecology and Obstetrics 1963; 1: 83–93.

53. Taylor MB, Dugar N, Davidson SE et al. Magnetic resonance imaging of primary vaginal carcinoma. Clinical Radiology 2007; 62: 549–555.

54. Lamoreaux WT, Grigsby PW, Dehdashti F. FDG-PET evaluation of squamous cell carcinoma of the vagina. International Journal of Radiation Oncology Biology Physics 2005; 62: 138–147.

55. Frank SJ, Jhingran A, Levenback C et al. Definitive radiation therapy for squamous cell carcinoma of the vagina. International Journal of Radiation Oncology Biology Physics 2005; 62: 138–147.

56. De Crevoisier R, Sanfilippo N, Gerbaulet A et al. Exclusive radiotherapy for primary squamous cell carcinoma of the vagina. Radiotherapy and Oncology 2007; 85: 362–370.

57. Lee WR, Marcus RB Jr, Sombeck MD et al. Radiotherapy alone for carcinoma of the vagina: the importance of overall treatment time. International Journal of Radiation Oncology Biology Physics 1994; 29: 983–988.

58. Tjalma WA, Monaghan JM, de Barros Lopes A et al. The role of surgery in invasive squamous carcinoma of the vagina. Gynecologic Oncology 2001; 81: 360–365.

59. Perez C, Grigsby PW, Garipagaoglu M et al. Factors affecting long-term outcome of irradiation in carcinoma of the vagina. International Journal of Radiation Oncology Biology Physics 1999; 44: 37–45.

60. Nashiro T, Yagi C, Hirakawa M et al. Concurrent chemoradiation for locally advanced squamous cell carcinoma of the vagina: case series and literature review. International Journal of Clinical Oncology 2008; 13: 335–339.

61. Ball HG, Berman ML. Management of primary vaginal carcinoma. Gynecologic Oncology 1982; 14: 154–163.

62. Blanchard P, Monnier L, Dumas I et al. Low-dose-rate definitive brachytherapy for high-grade vaginal intraepithelial neoplasia. Oncologist 2011; 16: 182–188.

63. Stock RG, Chen AS, Seski J. A 30-year experience in the management of primary carcinoma of the vagina: analysis of prognostic factors and treatment modalities. Gynecologic Oncology 1995; 56: 45–52.

64. Davis KP, Stanhope CR, Garton GR, Atkinson EJ, O'Brien PC. Invasive vaginal carcinoma: analysis of early-stage disease. Gynecologic Oncology 1991; 42: 131–136.

65. Frumovitz M, Gayed IW, Jhingran A et al. Lymphatic mapping and sentinel lymph node detection in women with vaginal cancer. Gynecologic Oncology 2008; 108: 478–481.

66. Woelber L, Kock L, Gieseking F et al. Clinical management of primary vulvar cancer. European Journal of Cancer 2011; 47: 2315–2321.

67. De Hullu JA, Hollema H, Lolkema S et al. Vulvar carcinoma. The price of less radical surgery. Cancer 2002; 95: 2331–2338.

68. Wölber L, Choschzick M, Eulenburg C, Hager M, Jaenicke F, Gieseking F. Prognostic value of pathological resection margin distance in squamous cell cancer of the vulva. Annals of Surgical Oncology 2011; 18(13): 3811–3818. doi: 10.1245/s10434-011-1778-0. Epub 2011 May 19.

69. Gaarenstroom KN, Kenter GG, Trimbos JB et al. Postoperative complications after vulvectomy and inguinofemoral lymphadenectomy using separate groin incisions. International Journal of Gynecological Cancer 2003; 13: 522–527.

70. Narducci F, Samouelian V, Marchaudon V et al. Vacuum-assisted closure therapy in the management of patients undergoing vulvectomy. European Journal of Obstetrics and Gynecology and Reproductive Biology 2012.

71. Gordinier ME, Malpica A, Burke TW et al. Groin recurrence in patients with vulvar cancer with negative nodes on superficial inguinal lymphadenectomy. Gynecologic Oncology 2003; 90: 625–628.

72. Van Der Zee AG, Oonk MH, De Hullu JA et al. Sentinel node dissection is safe in the treatment of early-stage vulvar cancer. Journal of Clinical Oncology 2008; 26: 884–889.

73. Morice P, Denschlag D, Rodolakis A et al. Recommendations of the Fertility Task Force of the European Society of Gynecologic Oncology about the conservative management of ovarian malignant tumors. International Journal of Gynecological Cancer 2011; 21: 951–963.

74. Young RC, Decker DG, Wharton JT et al. Staging laparotomy in early ovarian cancer. Journal of the American Medical Association 1983; 250: 3072–3076.

75. Ramirez PT, Slomovitz BM, McQuinn L et al. Role of appendectomy at the time of primary surgery in patients with early-stage ovarian cancer. Gynecologic Oncology 2006; 103: 888–890.

76. Le T, Adolph A, Krepart GV et al. The benefits of comprehensive surgical staging in the management of early-stage epithelial ovarian carcinoma. Gynecologic Oncology 2002; 85: 351–355.

77. Morice P, Joulie F, Camatte S et al. Lymph node involvement in epithelial ovarian cancer: analysis of 276 pelvic and para-aortic lymphadenectomies and surgical implications. Journal of the American College of Surgeons 2003; 197: 198–205.

78. Onda T, Yoshikawa H, Yokota H, Yasugi T, Taketani Y. Assessment of metastases to aortic and pelvic lymph nodes in epithelial ovarian carcinoma. A proposal for essential sites for lymph node biopsy. Cancer 1996; 78(4): 803–808.

79. Baiocchi G, Raspagliesi F, Grosso G, Fontanelli R, Cobellis L et al. Early ovarian cancer: is there a role for systematic pelvis and para-aortic lymphadenectomy? International Journal of Gynecological Cancer 1998; 8: 103–108.

80. Sakuragi N, Takeda N, Hareyama H, Fujimoto T, Todo Y et al. A multivariate analysis of blood vessel and lymph vessel invasion as predictors of ovarian and lymph node metastases in patients with cervical carcinoma. Cancer 2000; 88(11): 2578–2583.

81. Suzuki M, Ohwada M, Yamada T, Kohno T, Sekiguchi I et al. Lymph node metastasis in stage I epithelial ovarian cancer. Gynecologic Oncology 2000; 79(2): 305–308.

82. Cass I, Baldwin RL, Varkey T, Moslehi R, Narod SA et al. Improved survival in women with BRCA-associated ovarian carcinoma. Cancer 2003; 97: 2187–2195. doi:10.1002/cncr.11310

83. Morice P, Joulie F, Camatte S, Atallah D, Rouzier R et al. Lymph node involvement in epithelial ovarian cancer: analysis of 276 pelvic and paraaortic lymphadenectomies and surgical implications. Journal of the American College of Surgeons 2003; 197(2): 198–205.

84. Nagishi H, Takeda M, Fujimoto T, Todo Y, Ebina Y et al. Lymphatic mapping and sentinel node identification as related to the primary sites of lymph node metastasis in early stage ovarian cancer. Gynecologic Oncology 2004; 94(1): 161–166.

85. Nomura DK1, Long JZ, Niessen S, Hoover HS, Ng SW et al. Monoacylglycerol lipase regulates a fatty acid network that promotes cancer pathogenesis. Cell 2010; 140(1): 49–61. doi:10.1016/j.cell.2009.11.027

86. Powless CA, Aletti GD, Bakkum-Gamez JN, Cliby WA. Risk factors for lymph node metastasis in apparent early-stage epithelial ovarian cancer: implications for surgical staging. Gynecologic Oncology 2011; 122(3): 536–540. doi:10.1016/j.ygyno.2011.05.001. Epub 1 June 2011.

87. Maggioni A, Benedetti Panici PL, Dell'Anna T et al. Randomised study of systematic lymphadenectomy in patients with epithelial ovarian cancer macroscopically confined to the pelvis. British Journal of Cancer 2006; 95: 699–704.

88. Leblanc E, Querleu D, Narducci F et al. Laparoscopic restaging of early stage invasive adnexal tumors: a 10-year experience. Gynecologic Oncology 2004; 94: 624–629.

89. Bristow RE, Tomacruz RS, Armstrong DK et al. Survival effect of maximal cytoreductive surgery for advanced ovarian carcinoma during the platinum era: a meta-analysis. Journal of Clinical Oncology 2002; 20: 1248–1259.

90. Eisenkop SM, Friedman RL, Wang HJ. Complete cytoreductive surgery is feasible and maximizes survival in patients with advanced epithelial ovarian cancer: a prospective study. Gynecologic Oncology 1998; 69: 103–108.

91. Hudson CN. A radical operation for fixed ovarian tumours. Journal of Obstetrics and Gynaecology of the British Commonwealth 1968; 75: 1155–1160.

92. Griffiths TC, Parker LM, Fuller AF. Role of cytoreductive surgical treatment in the management of advanced ovarian cancer. Cancer Treatment Reports 1979; 63: 235–240.

93. Chi DS, Franklin CC, Levine DA et al. Improved optimal cytoreduction rates for stages IIIC and IV epithelial ovarian, fallopian tube, and primary peritoneal cancer: a change in surgical approach. Gynecologic Oncology 2004; 94: 650–654.

94. du Bois A, Reuss A, Pujade-Lauraine E, Harter P, Ray-Coquard I et al. Role of surgical outcome as prognostic factor in advanced epithelial ovarian cancer: a combined exploratory analysis of 3 prospectively randomized phase 3 multicenter trials: by the Arbeitsgemeinschaft Gynaekologische Onkologie Studiengruppe Ovarialkarzinom (AGO-OVAR) and the Groupe d'Investigateurs Nationaux Pour les Etudes des Cancers de l'Ovaire (GINECO). Cancer 2009; 115: 1234–1244.

95. Stuart GC, Kitchener H, Bacon M et al. Participants of 4th Ovarian Cancer Consensus Conference (OCCC); Gynecologic Cancer Intergroup. 2010 Gynecologic Cancer InterGroup (GCIG) consensus statement on clinical trials in ovarian cancer: report from the Fourth Ovarian Cancer Consensus Conference. International Journal of Gynecological Cancer 2011; 21: 750–755.

96. Aebi S, Castiglione M. ESMO Guidelines Working Group. Epithelial ovarian carcinoma: ESMO clinical recommendations for diagnosis, treatment and follow-up. Annals of Oncology 2008; 19(Suppl 2): ii14–6.

97. Michel G, De Iaco P, Castaigne D et al. Extensive cytoreductive surgery in advanced ovarian carcinoma. European Journal of Gynaecological Cancer 1997; 18: 9–15.

98. Vergote I, Tropé CG, Amant F et al. Neoadjuvant chemotherapy or primary surgery in stage IIIC or IV ovarian cancer. New England Journal of Medicine 2010; 363: 943–953.

99. Wimberger P, Lehmann N, Kimmig R, Burges A, Meier W, Du Bois A. Prognostic factors for complete debulking in advanced ovarian cancer and its impact on survival. An exploratory analysis of a prospectively randomized phase III study of the Arbeitsgemeinschaft Gynaekologische Onkologie Ovarian Cancer Study Group (AGO-OVAR). Gynecologic Oncology 2007; 106(1): 69–74. Epub 2007 Mar 29.

100. Benedetti-Panici P, Maggioni A et al. Systematic aortic and pelvic lymphadenectomy versus resection of bulky nodes in optimally debulked advanced ovarian cancer: a randomized clinical trial. Journal of the National Cancer Institute 2005; 97: 560–566.

101. du Bois A, Reuss A, Harter P et al. Potential role of lymphadenectomy in advanced ovarian cancer: a combined exploratory analysis of three prospectively randomized phase III multicenter trials. Journal of Clinical Oncology 2010; 28: 1733–1739.

102. Landoni F, Maneo A, Colombo A et al. Randomized study of radical surgery versus radiotherapy for stage IB-IIA cervical cancer. Lancet 1997; 350: 535–540.

103. Morice P, Rouanet P, Rey A, Romestaing P, Houvenaeghel G, Boulanger JC et al. Results of the GYNECO 02 study, an FNCLCC phase III trial comparing hysterectomy with no hysterectomy in patients with a (clinical and radiological) complete response after chemoradiation therapy for stage IB2 or II cervical cancer. Oncologist 2012; 17(1): 64–71.

104. Keys HM, Bundy BN, Stehman FB et al. Radiation therapy with and without extrafascial hysterectomy for bulky stage IB cervical carcinoma: a randomized trial of the gynecologic oncology group. Gynecologic Oncology 2003; 89: 343–353.

105. Resbeut M, Fondrinier E, Fervers B et al. Carcinoma of the cervix. British Journal of Cancer 2001; 84: 24–30.

106. Lim K, Small W, Portelance L et al. Consensus guidelines for delineation of clinical target volume for intensity-modulated pelvic

radiotherapy for the definitive treatment of cervix cancer. International Journal of Radiation Oncology Biology Physics 2011; 79: 348–355.

107. Green JA, Kirwan JM, Tierney JF et al. Survival and recurrence after concomitant chemotherapy and radiotherapy for cancer of the uterine cervix: a systematic review and meta-analysis. Lancet 2001; 358: 781–786.

108. Vale C, Tierney JF, Stewart LA et al. Reducing uncertainties about the effects of chemoradiotherapy for cervical cancer: a systematic review and meta-analysis of individual patient data from 18 randomized trials. Journal of Clinical Oncology 2008; 26: 5802–5812.

109. Charra-Brunaud C, Harter V, Delannes M et al. Impact of 3D image-based PDR brachytherapy on outcome of patients treated for cervix carcinoma in France: results from the French STIC prospective study. Radiotherapy and Oncology 2012; 103: 305–313.

110. Pötter R, Dimopoulos J, Georg P et al. Clinical impact of MRI assisted dose volume adaptation and dose escalation in brachytherapy of locally advanced cervix cancer. Radiotherapy and Oncology 2007; 83: 148–155.

111. Pötter R, Georg P, Dimopoulos J et al. Clinical outcome of protocol based image (MRI) guided adaptive brachytherapy combined with 3D conformal radiotherapy with or without chemotherapy in patients with locally advanced cervical cancer. Radiotherapy and Oncology 2011; 100: 116–123.

112. Duenas-Gonzales A, Zarba JJ, Patel F et al. Phase III, open-label, randomized study comparing concurrent gemcitabine plus cisplatin and radiation followed by adjuvant gemcitabine and cisplatin versus concurrent cisplatin and radiation in patients with stage IIB to IVA carcinoma of the cervix. Journal of Clinical Oncology 2011; 29: 1678–1685.

113. Rotman M, Sedlis A, Piedmonte MR et al. A phase III randomized trial of postoperative pelvic irradiation in stage IB cervical carcinoma with poor prognostic features: follow-up of a gynecologic oncology group study. International Journal of Radiation Oncology Biology Physics 2006; 65: 169–176.

114. Small W Jr, Mell LK, Anderson P et al. Consensus guidelines for delineation of clinical target volume for intensity-modulated pelvic radiotherapy in postoperative treatment of endometrial and cervical cancer. International Journal of Radiation Oncology Biology Physics 2008; 71: 428–434.

115. Peters WA III, Liu PY, Barrett RJ II et al. Concurrent chemotherapy and pelvic radiation therapy compared with pelvic radiation therapy alone as adjuvant therapy after radical surgery in high-risk early-stage cancer of the cervix. Journal of Clinical Oncology 2000; 8: 1606–1613.

116. Creutzberg CL, van Putten WLJ, Koper PCM et al. Surgery and post-operative radiotherapy versus surgery alone for patients with stage-1 endometrial carcinoma: multicentre randomized trial. PORTEC study group. Lancet 2000; 355: 1404–1411.

117. Aalders J, Abeler V, Kolstad P et al. Postoperative external irradiation and prognostic parameters in stage I endometrial carcinoma: clinical and histopathologic study of 540 patients. Obstetrics & Gynecology 1980; 56: 419–427.

118. Keys HM, Roberts JA, Brunetto VL et al. A phase III trial of surgery with or without adjunctive external pelvic radiation therapy in intermediate risk endometrial adenocarcinoma: a Gynecologic Oncology Group study. Gynecologic Oncology 2004; 92: 744–751.

119. Blake P, Swart AM, Orton J et al. Adjuvant external beam radiotherapy in the treatment of endometrial cancer (MRC ASTEC and NCIC CTG EN.5 randomised trials): pooled trial results, systematic review, and meta-analysis. Lancet 2009; 373: 137–146.

120. Nout RA, Smit HBM, Putter H, Jürgenliemk-Schulz IM, Jobsen JJ et al. Vaginal brachytherapy versus pelvic external beam radiotherapy for patients with endometrial cancer of high-intermediate risk (PORTEC-2): an open-label, non-inferiority, randomised trial. Lancet 2010; 375: 816–823.

121. Nout RA, Putter H, Jürgenliemk-Schulz I et al. Quality of life after pelvic radiotherapy or vaginal brachytherapy for endometrial cancer: first results of the randomized PORTEC-2 Trial. Journal of Clinical Oncology 2009; 27: 3547–3556.

122. Nout RA, van de Poll-Franse LV, Lybeert ML et al. Long-term outcome and quality of life of patients with endometrial carcinoma treated with or without pelvic radiotherapy in the postoperative radiation therapy in endometrial carcinoma 1 (PORTEC-1) trial. Journal of Clinical Oncology 2011; 29: 1692–1700.

123. Nout RA, Putter H, Jürgenliemk-Schulz I et al. Five-year quality of life in endometrial cancer patients treated in the randomised Post Operative Radiation Therapy in Endometrial Cancer (PORTEC-2) trial and comparison with norm data. European Journal of Cancer 2012; 48: 1638–1648.

124. Hogberg T, Signorelli M, de Oliveira CF et al. Sequential adjuvant chemotherapy and radiotherapy in endometrial cancer—results from two randomised studies. European Journal of Cancer 2010; 46: 2422–2431.

125. Knocke TH, Kucera H, Weidinger B et al. Primary treatment of endometrial carcinoma with high-dose-rate brachytherapy: results of 12 years of experience with 280 patients. International Journal of Radiation Oncology Biology Physics 1997; 37: 359–365.

126. Weitmann HD, Pötter R, Waldhäusl C et al. Pilot study in the treatment of endometrial carcinoma with 3D image-based high-dose-rate brachytherapy using modified heyman packing: clinical experience and dose-volume histogram analysis. International Journal of Radiation Oncology Biology Physics 2005; 62: 468–478.

127. Frank SJ, Jhingran A, Levenback C, et al. Definitive radiation therapy for squamous cell carcinoma of the vagina. International Journal of Radiation Oncology Biology Physics 2005; 62: 138–147.

128. Chyle V, Zagars GK, Wheeler JA, et al. Definitive radiotherapy for carcinoma of the vagina: outcome and prognostic factors. International Journal of Radiation Oncology Biology Physics 1996; 35: 891–905.

129. Stock RG, Mychalczak B, Armstrong JG et al. The importance of brachytherapy technique in the management of primary carcinoma of the vagina. International Journal of Radiation Oncology Biology Physics 1992; 24: 747–753.

130. Perez CA, Camel HM, Galakatos AE et al. Definitive irradiation in carcinoma of the vagina: long-term evaluation of results. International Journal of Radiation Oncology Biology Physics 1988; 15: 1283–1290.

131. Samant R, Lau B, Choan E et al. Primary vaginal cancer treated with concurrent chemoradiation using cis-platinum. International Journal of Radiation Oncology Biology Physics 2007; 69: 746–775.

132. Mock U, Kucera H, Fellner C, et al. High-dose rate (HDR) brachytherapy with or without external beam radiotherapy in the treatment of primary vaginal carcinoma: long-term results and side effects. International Journal of Radiation Oncology Biology Physics 2003; 56: 950–957.

133. De Crevoisier R, Sanfilippo N, Gerbaulet A et al. Exclusive radiotherapy for primary squamous cell carcinoma of the vagina. Radiotherapy and Oncology 2007; 85: 362–370.

134. Dimopoulos JCA, Schmid MP, Fidarova E et al. Treatment of locally advanced vaginal cancer with radiochemotherapy and mr image-guided adaptive brachytherapy: dose volume parameters and first clinical results. International Journal of Radiation Oncology Biology Physics 2012; 82: 1880–1888.

135. Mahner S, Jueckstock J, Hilpert F, Neuser P, Harter P, de Gregorio N, Hasenburg A, Sehouli J, Habermann A, Hillemanns P, Fuerst S, Strauss HG, Baumann K, Thiel F, Mustea A, Meier W, du Bois A, Griebel LF, Woelber L; AGO-CaRE 1 investigators. Adjuvant therapy in lymph node-positive vulvar cancer: the AGO-CaRE-1 study. Journal of the National Cancer Institute 2015; 107(3).

136. Perez CA, Grigsby PW, Chao C et al. Irradiation in carcinoma of the vulva: factor affecting outcome. International Journal of Radiation Oncology Biology Physics 1992; 24: 335–344.

137. Homesley HD, Bundy BN, Sedlis A et al. Radiation therapy versus pelvic node resection for carcinoma of the vulva with positive groin nodes. Obstetrics & Gynecology 1986; 68: 733–740.

138. Stehman FB, Bundy BN, Thomas G et al. Groin dissection versus groin radiation in carcinoma of the vulva: a Gynecologic Oncology Group study. International Journal of Radiation Oncology Biology Physics 1992; 24: 389–396.

139. Van Doorn HC, Ansink A, Verhaar-Langerreis M et al. Neoadjuvant chemoradiation for advanced primary vulvar cancer. Cochrane Database of Systematic Reviews 2006; 3: DD003752.

140. Moore DH, Ali S, Koh WJ et al. A phase II trial of radiation therapy and weekly cisplatin chemotherapy for the treatment of locally advanced squamous cell carcinoma of the vulva: a Gynecologic Oncology Group study. Gynecologic Oncology 2012; 124: 529–533.

141. Montana GS, Thomas GM, Moore DH et al. Preoperative chemo-radiation for carcinoma of the vulva with N2/N3 nodes: a Gynecologic Oncology Group study. International Journal of Radiation Oncology Biology Physics 2000; 48: 1007–1013.

142. Moore DH, Thomas GM, Montana GS et al. Preoperative chemoradiation for advanced vulvar cancer: a phase II study of the Gynecologic Oncology Group. International Journal of Radiation Oncology Biology Physics 1998; 42: 79–85.

143. Shylasree TS, Bryant A, Howells RE. Chemoradiation for advanced primary vulvar cancer. Cochrane Database of Systematic Reviews 2011; 4: CD003752.

144. Singh RB, Chander S, Mohanti BK, Pathy S, Kumar S et al. Neoadjuvant chemotherapy with weekly paclitaxel and carboplatin followed by chemoradiation in locally advanced cervical cancer: a pilot study. Gynecologic Oncology 2013; Epub ahead.

145. Shoji T, Takatori E, Saito T, Omi H, Kagabu M et al. Neoadjuvant chemotherapy using platinum- and taxane-based regimens for bulky stage Ib2 to IIB non-squamous cell carcinoma of the uterine cervix. Cancer Chemotherapy and Pharmacology 2013; 71(3): 657–662.

146. Long HJ 3rd, Bundy BN, Grendys EC Jr. Randomized phase III trial of cisplatin with or without topotecan in carcinoma of the uterine cervix: a gynecologic Oncology Group study. Journal of Clinical Oncology 2005; 23(21): 4626–4633.

147. Moore DH, Blessing JA, McQuellon RP et al. Phase III study of cisplatin with or without paclitaxel in stage IVB, recurrent, or persistent squamous cell carcinoma of the cervix: a gynecologic oncology group study. Journal of Clinical Oncology 2004; 22(15): 3113–3119.

148. Monk BJ, Sill MW, McMeekin DS, et al. Phase III trial of four cisplatin containing doublet combinations in stage IVB, recurrent, or persistent cervical carcinoma: a Gynecologic Oncology Group study. Journal of Clinical Oncology 2009; 27: 4649–4655.

149. Kitagawa R, Katsumata N, Shibata T, Nakanishi T, Nishimura S et al. A randomized, phase III trial of paclitaxel plus carboplatin (TC) versus paclitaxel plus cisplatin (TP in stage IVb, persistent or recurrent cervical cancer: Japan Clinical Oncology Group study (JCOG 0505). Journal of Clinical Oncology 2012; 30: abstr 5006.

150. Tewari KS, Sill MW, Long HJ 3rd, Penson RT, Huang H. Improved survival with bevacizumab in advanced cervical cancer. The New England Journal of Medicine 2014; 370(8): 734–743. doi: 10.1056/NEJMoa1309748.

151. Tsikouras P, Bouchlariotou S, Vrachnis N, Dafopoulos A, Galazios G et al. Endometrial cancer: molecular and therapeutic aspects. European Journal of Obstetrics, Gynecology, and Reproductive Biology 2013. Epub ahead.

152. Randall ME, Filiaci VL, Muss H et al. Randomized phase III trial of whole-abdominal irradiation versus doxorubicin and cisplatin chemotherapy in advanced endometrial carcinoma: a Gynecologic Oncology Group study. Journal of Clinical Oncology 2006; 24: 36–44.

153. Johnson N, Bryant A, Miles T, Hogberg T, Cornes P. Adjuvant Chemotherapy for endometrial cancer after hysterectomy. Cochrane Database of Systematic Reviews 2011; 10: CD003175.

154. Hogberg T. What is the role of chemotherapy in endometrial cancer? Current Oncology Reports 2011; 13(6): 433–441.

155. Quinn MA. Hormonal treatment of endometrial cancer. Hematology/Oncology Clinics of North America 1999; 13: 163–187.

156. Thipgen T, Brady MF, Homesley HD et al. Tamoxifen in the treatment of advanced or recurrent endometrial carcinoma. A Gynecologic Oncology Group study. Journal of Clinical Oncology 2001; 19: 364–367.

157. Topuz S, Kalelioglu I, Iyibozkurt C, ergun B, Conservative management of a patient with endometrial carcinoma desiring fertility. How to inform? Eruopean Journal of Gynaecologic Oncology 2008; 29: 661–663

158. Oza, Elit L, Tsao MS, Kamel-Reid S, Biagi J, Provencner DM et al. Phase II study of temsirolimus in women with recurrent or metastatic endometrial cancer: a trial of the NCIC Clinical Trials Group. Journal of Clinical Oncology 2011; 29: 3278–3285.

159. Emons G, Gorchev G, Harter P, Wimberger P, Stähle A, Hanker L, Hilpert F, Beckmann MW, Dall P, Gründker C, Sindermann H, Sehouli J. Efficacy and safety of AEZS-108 (LHRH agonist linked to doxorubicin) in women with advanced or recurrent endometrial cancer expressing LHRH receptors: a multicenter phase 2 trial (AGO-GYN5). International Journal of Gynecological Cancer 2014; 24(2): 260–265.

160. Santeufemia DA, Capobianco G, Re GL, Miolo GM, Fadda GM. Cisplatin-gemcitabine as palliative chemotherapy in advanced squamous vulvar carcinoma: report of two cases. European Journal of Gynaecological Oncology 2012; 33(4): 421–422.

161. Kersh CR, Constable W, Spaulding C et al. A phase I-II trial of multimodality management of bulky gynecologic malignancy. Combined chemoradiosensitization and radiotherapy. Cancer 1990; 66: 30–34.

162. Roberts WS, Hoffman MS, Kavanagh JJ et al. Further experience with radiation therapy and concomitant intravenous chemotherapy in advanced carcinoma of the lower female genital tract. Gynecologic Oncology 1991; 43: 233–236.

163. Du Bois A, Lück HJ, Meier W, Adams HP, Möbus V et al. A randomized clinical trial of cisplatin/paclitaxel versus carboplatin/paclitaxel as first-line treatment of ovarian cancer. Journal of the National Cancer Institute 2003; 95(17): 1320–1329.

164. Perren TJ, Swart AM, Pfisterer J, Ledermann JA, Pujade-Lauraine E et al. A Phase 3 trial of bevacizumab in ovarian cancer. New England Journal of Medicine 2011; 365: 2484–2496.

165. Burger RA, Brady MF, Bookman MA, Fleming GF, Monk BJ et al. Incorporation of bevacizumab in the primary treatment of ovarian cancer. New England Journal of Medicine 2011; 365: 2473–2483.

166. Aghajanian C, Blank SV, Goff BA, Judson PL, Teneriello MG et al. OCEANS: a randomized, double-blind, placebo-controlled phase III trial of chemotherapy with or without bevacizumab in patients with platinum-sensitive recurrent epithelial ovarian, primary peritoneal, or fallopian tube cancer. Journal of Clinical Oncology 2012; 308: 2039–2045.

167. Pujade-Lauraine E, Hilpert F, Weber B, Reuss A, Poveda A et al. AURELIA: a randomized phase III trial evaluating bevacizumab (BEV) plus chemotherapy (CT) for platinum (PT)-resistant ovarian cancer (OC). Journal of Clinical Oncology 2012; 30: abstr LBA 5002.

168. Armstrong DK, Bundy B, Wenzel L, et al. Intraperitoneal cisplatin and paclitaxel in ovarian cancer. New England Journal of Medicine 2006; 354: 34–43.

169. Katsumata N, Yasuda M, Takahashi F, Isonishi S, Jobo T et al. Dose-dense paclitaxel once a week in combination with carboplatin every 3 weeks for advanced ovarian cancer: a phase 3, open-label, randomized controlled trial. Lancet 2009: 374(9698): 1331–1338.

170. van der Burg ME, Onstenk W, Boere IA, Look M, Ottevanger PB. Long-term results of a randomised phase III trial of weekly versus three-weekly paclitaxel/platinum induction therapy followed by standard or extended three-weekly paclitaxel/platinum in European patients with advanced epithelial ovarian cancer. European Journal of Cancer 2014; 50(15): 2592–2601. doi: 10.1016/j.ejca.2014.07.015. Epub 2014 Aug 2.

171. Pölcher M, Mahner S, Ortmann C, et al. Neoadjuvant chemotherapy with carboplatin and docetaxel in advanced ovarian cancer—a prospective multicenter phase II trial (PRIMOVAR). Oncology Reports 2009; 22(3): 605–613.

172. Ledermann J, Harter P, Gourley C, Friedlander M, Vergote I et al. Olaparib maintenance therapy in platinum-sensitive relapsed ovarian cancer. New England Journal of Medicine 2012; 366(15): 1382–1392.

173. Cohen JG, Chan JK, Kapp DS. The management of small-cell carcinomas of the gynecologic tract. Current Opinion in Oncology 2012; 24(5): 572–579.

CHAPTER 45

Genitourinary cancers

John Fitzpatrick, Asif Muneer, Jean de la Rosette, and Thomas Powles

Penile cancer

Introduction to penile care

Penile cancer is a rare malignancy and the diagnosis is often delayed due to patient embarrassment. Over the last 15 years, penile-preserving surgical techniques have been developed to preserve penile length without compromising local disease control. Despite improvements in the management of local disease, patients presenting with widespread metastatic disease continue to have a poor prognosis due to chemoresistance.

Incidence

Penile cancer is a rare malignancy, which in the UK accounts for <1% of all male malignancies. Cancer registries over a 30-year period from 1979 to 2009 in England have shown a 21% increase in the incidence of penile cancer from 1.10 to 1.33 per 100 000 [1]. This figure is similar to other Western European and North American countries, although in parts of Africa, Asia, and South America penile cancer has been reported to account for up to 20% of all male malignancies [2].

Pathology of penile cancer

The majority of tumours arise on the glans penis (80%) or the foreskin (15%). The vast majority are squamous cell carcinomas (SCC) and account for 95% of the tumours, with the remaining 5% comprising melanomas, sarcomas, and basal cell carcinomas. The SCC subtypes are listed in Table 45.1.

Pre-malignant penile lesions are often difficult to differentiate from benign genital dermatoses and often a biopsy is required in order to differentiate the two as there is a risk of progression to invasive disease if pre-malignant lesions are not diagnosed early. The current tumour-node-metastasis (TNM) staging for penile cancer was revised in 2009 and the grading, traditionally by Broder's system of well, moderate, and poorly-differentiated lesions [3], has recently been altered to adopt grades 1–4 with grade 4 being undifferentiated disease. The current TNM staging for penile cancer can be accessed at the website of the American Cancer Society: <http://www.cancer.org/cancer/penilecancer/detailedguide/penile-cancer-staging>.

Diagnosis of penile cancer

Penile SCC can appear as a nodular, ulcerative, or an erythematous lesion, with advanced cases being clinically obvious (Figure 45.1).

However, there is often a pathological phimosis covering the lesion which itself can only be palpated as a hard mass under the non-retractile foreskin. The diagnosis is confirmed by a penile biopsy and, where possible, additional imaging of the penis using MRI helps to define the extent of invasion of the tumour into the distal corpus cavernosum. Patients should also have their inguinal node status evaluated both clinically and using radiological imaging, most commonly CT. When there are palpable inguinal nodes, the risk of these harbouring metastatic disease is high and either an ultrasound guided fine needle aspiration cytology can be performed or an excisional biopsy of a palpable lymph node can be performed. Confirmation of metastatic disease within the inguinal lymph nodes will mean that the patient requires a radical inguinal lymphadenectomy. In situations where there are clinically impalpable inguinal nodes at presentation, the risk of micrometastatic disease in the inguinal nodes is approximately 20%; therefore, a risk-adapted approach is used to manage these patients in order to avoid overtreatment [4].

Management of the primary penile tumour

Up until the last two decades, the traditional treatment option for penile cancer has involved either a partial or total penectomy in order to ensure a 2 cm tumour-free margin. Although radical surgery undoubtedly provides excellent loco-regional control there is an impact on the urinary and sexual function together with the psychological impact of emasculinization [5]. Radical radiotherapy was previously used as an alternative option but the patient is often left with a disfigured penis, meatal stenosis, and even radionecrosis. Furthermore, local recurrence rates of up to 40% have been reported following radiotherapy and are deemed unacceptable.

Current practice utilizes penile-preserving techniques for distal penile tumours located on the glans penis which allows oncological control coupled with a reduction in the anatomical and functional morbidity. This approach stems from the realization that the requirement of a 2 cm margin is historical and cancer control can still be achieved with smaller margins. [6, 7]. In a further study, the resection margins in patients undergoing penile preserving surgery were reviewed together with the local recurrence rates. In this study, 48% had a surgical clearance of ≤10mm, whilst 90% had a clearance of ≤20mm. Local recurrence rates were reported at only 4%, with a mean follow-up time of 26 months. Furthermore, long-term survival does not appear to be compromised by local recurrence, as most cases are surgically salvageable [8].

Table 45.1 Pathologic subtypes of penile carcinoma

Squamous cell carcinoma	Squamous cell carcinoma, normal type
	Warty (condylomatous) carcinoma
	Verrucous carcinoma
	Papillary, not otherwise specified (NOS) carcinoma
	Basaloid carcinoma
	Sarcomatoid carcinoma
	Adenosquamous carcinoma
	Pseudoglandular (acantholytic, adenoid) carcinoma
	Carcinoma cuniculatum
	Mixed carcinoma
Other malignant epithelial tumours	Clear cell carcinoma
	Extramammary Paget's disease
	Malignant melanoma
Non-epithelial malignant tumours	Soft-tissue sarcomas (Kaposi's sarcoma, leiomyosarcoma, others)
	Malignant lymphoma

The treatment options available depend on the site and extent of disease and are reviewed below in the following section.

Carcinoma in situ and superficial verrucous carcinoma (Tis and Ta)

Topical therapy

Although carcinoma in situ (CIS) is not an invasive malignancy, it accounts for approximately 10% of penile lesions at diagnosis [9]. CIS may arise on the shaft of the penis, eponymously called Bowen's disease, or as one or multiple red, moist patches on the mucosal surfaces of the glans penis or inner prepuce, where it is known as erythroplasia of Queyrat (EQ). CIS can easily be misdiagnosed as a benign skin condition such as candidal balanitis, Zoon's balanitis, or lichen planus. It can also coexist with lichen sclerosus. If left untreated, the observed risk of progression to invasive SCC is 5–33% [10]. Provided that there is no evidence of invasive disease, first-line treatment for CIS uses topical 5% 5-fluorouracil (5-FU) cream. Whilst several regimes exist, the most popular is application

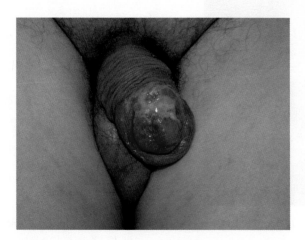

Fig. 45.1 A squamous cell carcinoma of the distal penis.
Image reproduced courtesy of Dr Alex Kirkham.

of 5-FU on alternate days for a four- to six-week period. Small studies (<10 patients) have shown excellent response rates approaching 100% at five years [11]. Patients not responding or relapsing can be offered further topical therapy using 5% imiquimod given in a similar regime. The success of this immune modulating cream has only been described in case reports [12].

Laser therapy

Laser therapy has been used in the treatment for both CIS and low-grade/stage invasive disease. Carbon dioxide (CO_2) and Neodymium:YAG (Nd:YAG) are the most commonly used lasers. A study of 19 patients, where eight were managed with CO_2 laser alone and 11 with both CO_2 and Nd:YAG, two recurrences (11%) were reported [13]. Shirahana and colleagues have demonstrated the importance of case selection for laser treatment [14]. Further studies have also used radiological assessment of the depth of tumour invasion; despite this long-term follow-up, a 48% risk of local recurrence has still been reported [15]. Overall, as with any topical therapy, local recurrences are higher than with conventional surgery and close follow-up is mandatory after treatment. The complications following laser therapy are reported in 1–7% of patients and include bleeding, moderate pain, and preputial lymphoedema [16–18].

Surgery for CIS—total glans resurfacing (TGR)

The use of topical therapy for carcinoma in situ requires well-motivated patients who will be compliant with the treatment regimen and close follow-up. Despite this there are still non-responders to topical treatment. The technique of total glans resurfacing (TGR) offers a surgical alternative for refractory disease or patients with recurrent CIS. Although TGR was initially described for the treatment of lichen sclerosus affecting the glans penis [19], it has recently also been used to manage CIS and stage Ta penile cancer [20]. The technique removes the glans epithelium and subepithelial tissues followed by coverage of the denuded corpus spongiosum using a split thickness skin graft harvested from the thigh. Published series have reported no evidence of disease recurrence at a median follow-up of 30 months (range 7–45) with all patients who were previously sexually active remaining sexually active within 3–5 months of surgery [20]. However, there has also been a report of a 28% positive surgical margin rate requiring further surgery [21].

T1 lesions confined to the prepuce

Circumcision/wide local excision

Circumcision is a common operation in the surgical management of penile cancer and is indicated for primary curative therapy when the tumour is confined to the prepuce [22]. If the lesion is more extensive, then a cuff can be taken from the penile shaft skin or the coronal sulcus as necessary [23, 24]. Recurrence rates of up to 30% have been reported following circumcision [25, 26], the majority of these occurring in the first two years following surgery [27]. Close post-operative surveillance is therefore essential, although if salvage surgery is required the long-term disease-specific survival remains unchanged [23, 28].

T1 lesions involving the glans penis

For these lesions, wide local excision (WLE) and primary closure may be possible if the lesion is discrete and not too close to the external meatus but recurrence rates of up to 50% have been reported, with most occurring in the first two post-operative years [29]. Recurrent disease can be managed successfully with further surgery in most cases without compromising overall survival [28, 30]. Again, close surveillance is essential for early detection of recurrence.

T2 lesions confined to the glans penis

T2 lesions confined to the glans penis are amenable to glansectomy [31]. The extent of tumour invasion can be assessed with preoperative gadolinium enhanced MRI imaging, with an artificial erection [32]. This is useful in assessing the location of the tumour and whether there is any invasion into the distal corpus cavernosum (Figure 45.2).

Total glansectomy

Total glansectomy (TG) involves the excision of the glans penis from the distal corporal heads. A split thickness skin graft is then used to cover the corporal heads and create a neo-glans (Figure 45.3) [27, 33]. A published series of 72 patients (65 new tumours and seven recurrences post-radiotherapy; 49% T1, 51% T2) undergoing glansectomy and reconstruction, 3 late recurrences (6%) with a mean follow-up of 27 months (range 4–68) have been reported [34].

Partial glansectomy for more proximal tumours has also been reported. The key advantage over total glansectomy is a reduction in spraying during micturition due to the preserved urethra [35, 36].

T2 tumours invading the corpora cavernosa

Distal corporectomy (partial penectomy) and split thickness skin grafting

This more extensive technique is required if there is evidence of corporal involvement either clinically or on MRI or if intraoperative frozen sections of the margins are positive (Figure 45.4). Penile

lengthening manoeuvres can be performed at the same time or at a later date to allow patients to engage in penetrative intercourse and to void standing up [37–39].

Salvage surgery post-radiotherapy

Approximately 40% of patients undergoing radical radiotherapy eventually require salvage surgery for local recurrence [40]. The chronic skin changes associated with radiotherapy make clinical detection of disease recurrence difficult. In a series of 17 patients undergoing post radiotherapy, at a mean follow-up of three years (range 1–6) found that 16 of 17 men were recurrence-free [39].

Management of inguinal lymph nodes

Lymph node metastasis remains the single most important prognostic factor for patients with penile cancer [41]. Over half of patients with SCC have clinically impalpable inguinal nodes at presentation, but up to 20% of these will harbour occult micrometastases (<2 mm) [42]. The currently available imaging modalities remain inaccurate for detecting micrometastases [43].

Although prophylactic bilateral inguinal lymph node dissection (ILND) is associated with high cure rates, the operation still has a morbidity rate of 30–50% and a mortality rate of up to 3% [44]. Moreover, up to 80% of patients will be found to have inguinal nodes without metastatic disease. A recent two-centre review of 342 patients with clinically impalpable inguinal nodes who underwent a sentinel lymph node biopsy (SLNB) concluded that 77% of men in the European Association of Urology (EAU) high-risk group for metastases would have had an unnecessary ILND [45].

Attempts have been made to identify subgroups of patients more likely to benefit from an ILND using predictive nomograms. Stage, grade of differentiation, depth of infiltration, and lymphovascular invasion of the primary tumour are known to be predictive factors for nodal metastasis, but relying solely on these factors still leads to unnecessary surgery [45–48].

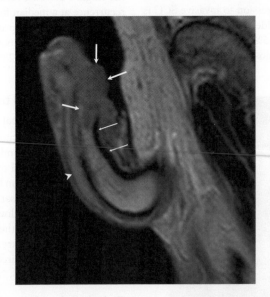

Fig. 45.2 MRI of a penile carcinoma showing absence of distal corpus cavernosum invasion (T2 sagittal). Thin arrow: tunica of corpus cavernosum; thick arrow: tumour; arrowhead: corpus spongiosum.

Image reproduced courtesy of Dr Alex Kirkham.

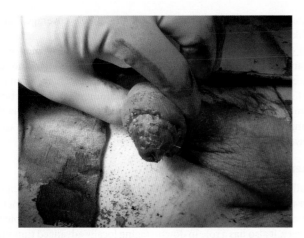

Fig. 45.3 Post-glansectomy appearance with application of a split thickness skin graft.

Image reproduced courtesy of Dr Alex Kirkham.

Development and use of dynamic sentinel lymph node biopsy in penile cancer

The concept of SLNB involves the identification and subsequent removal of specific lymph nodes where tumour cells will travel to first from the primary tumour. This was first proposed for penile cancer in 1977, where the sentinel lymph node (SLN) was identified wholly on anatomical landmarks [49]. This proved difficult to reproduce and the technique subsequently fell out of favour due to a high false-negative rate [50].

Throughout the 1990s, further developments have improved the detection of the SLN both before and during surgery. This focused on the use of radiolabelled nanocolloids and patent blue dye to aid detection. Excellent results achieved in patients with malignant melanoma and breast cancer have now seen the procedure introduced as routine practice in these conditions [51–53]. This led to renewed interest, particularly in penile cancer and other urological malignancies [54].

The Netherlands Cancer Institute (NKI) has pioneered the use of dynamic lymphoscintigraphy and SLNB in the treatment of penile cancer since 1994 [55]. In this centre over a ten-year period, SLNs were identified in 98% of 123 patients with ≥T2 tumours and clinically impalpable inguinal nodes, and 23% of excised nodes contained metastatic disease. The false-negative rate (FNR) amongst this cohort was initially unsatisfactory (18%) but the addition of preoperative ultrasonography, and more specific immunohistochemical staining and serial sectioning of excised specimens has reduced the FNR to ≈5% [56]. The technique is reproducible, with similar results reported in other centres worldwide [57, 58]. More importantly, improved survival has now been reported for patients undergoing immediate LND for occult lymph node metastases detected by SLN biopsy [59]. The disease-specific three-year survival of patients in this group was 84%, compared to 35% for patients with impalpable nodes following clinical surveillance.

A recent systematic review and meta-analysis of the accuracy of SLNB based on 19 studies found favourable pooled sensitivity (88% with 95% CI 83–92) and detection rates (90.1% with 95% CI 83.6–94.1) [60].

With the emergence of long-term data confirming SLNB safety and benefit in both reducing morbidity from unnecessary LND and improved five-year cancer specific survival, it is clear that SLNB has been a major advance for patients with penile cancer and the incorporation into standard management [58, 61, 62]. Modifications continue with the technique and recently co-localization with a hybrid fluorescent-radioactive tracer, indocyanine Green-99mTc-Nanocolloid has been used [63].

Survival following penile cancer

The majority of research regarding survival from penile cancer comprises of single centre studies with relatively low patient

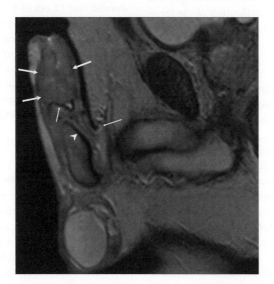

Fig. 45.4 MRI demonstrating an extensive tumour invading the corpus cavernosum (T2 sagittal). Thin arrow: surface of glans; thick arrow: tumour; arrowhead: tunica of corpus cavernosum.

Image reproduced courtesy of Dr Alex Kirkham.

numbers. However, Verhoeven and co-workers have examined the population-based survival of patients with penile cancer in Europe and the USA using data from registries contributing to the European Network for Indicators on Cancer (EUNICE) Survival Working Group and its American equivalent, the Surveillance, Epidemiology and End Results (SEER) program [64]. This incorporated data from 3297 European and 1820 American penile cancer patients, diagnosed with penile cancer from 1985–2007. In Europe, the overall five-year survival has increased marginally, but not to statistical significance, from 65% to 70% between 1990 and 2007. Within this group, a notable exception was Northern Europe, where an improvement from 63% to 77% was seen within the same time frame. Interestingly, the outlook was worse in the USA, with a statistically significant decrease in five-year survival from 72% to 63% from 1990 to 2007. Furthermore, there was no significant improvement in age-specific survival estimates during the period measured [64]. Further European data from the Surveillance of Rare Cancers in Europe (RARECARE) group, revealed a similar overall five-year survival rate of 69% in patients with penile cancer diagnosed from 1995 until 2002 [65]. Verhoeven's study showed a significant increased risk of mortality with increasing age in patients with penile cancer [64], which is broadly supported by Sant and co-workers who found that five-year survival after the age of 75 years was as low as 35% [66]. The reason behind this is unclear, as although there were insufficient data recorded in the EUNICE registries, there is no evidence for more advanced disease stage in penile cancer patients presenting later in life [64]. This is supported by Graafland and colleagues who carried out a study of 2000 patients diagnosed with penile cancer in the Netherlands between 1989 and 2006, and found that stage distribution did not vary significantly between age groups [67].

The reasons for the overall lack of improvement in survival is a matter for debate, and some authors postulate that it is simply because the impact of newer approaches such as SLNB have not had time to become apparent in the data. This may explain the emergence of more promising data from Northern Europe, as this region was the first to adopt the technique [64]. Other authors argue that the poor outcome data should prompt centralization of the treatment of penile cancer, only taking place in specialized units with a higher patient volume [65, 66].

Human papilloma virus

Several types of human papilloma virus (HPV) have been identified in pre-malignant penile lesions and around 50% of penile cancers express HPV types 16 or 18 [68, 69] with higher grade tumours being more likely to be HPV positive [70]. There are two vaccines available that protect against HPV: a bivalent vaccine that provides protection against HPV 16 and 18, and a quadrivalent vaccine that targets HPV 6, 11, 16, and 18. The latter is approved for preventing HPV-related disease in males [68] and both have been shown to be effective and safe [69]. In the UK, immunization with the bivalent vaccine has been in effect since 2008 for girls aged 12–13 years, with the aim of preventing cervical cancer, but no such scheme is in place for boys.

Marty and co-workers used a computer-based model to examine the incremental benefit of vaccinating boys and girls using the quadrivalent vaccine vs girls-only vaccination, looking for several diseases caused by HPV including penile cancer [68]. They found that vaccination of both girls and boys could reduce the incidence of penile cancer by 68% based on a figure of 70% coverage, but is unlikely to be cost-effective [69].

If one considers the overall benefits of vaccinating men with regards to preventing other diseases associated with HPV and the increased herd immunity, then an economic case can be made [71]. Indeed, the Advisory Committee on Immunizations Practices from the Centers for Disease Control and Prevention has recently changed its guidelines in favour of immunizing boys and men aged between 13 and 26 in the USA [72].

Chemotherapy

Penile cancers have a limited chemosensitivity. Systemic chemotherapy has been used mainly in the palliative setting, for metastatic and advanced loco-regional disease which is not amenable to surgery. It also has a role in down-staging locally advanced tumours prior to surgery.

Single chemotherapeutic agents in the 1970s were characterized by poor response rates and high levels of toxicity [73]. As a result, combination regimes have been used throughout the 1990s and, from these, cisplatin is a key chemotherapeutic agent in the treatment of SCC of the penis [74]. Taxane-based regimens then became more popular in the 2000s with three agent combinations dominating [75]. These included Dexeus' group's regimen consisting of cisplatin, methotrexate, and bleomycin [76]. Their initial study reported promising results with only moderate side effects, but with wider adoption of this protocol, poorer results and more severe side effects were seen [76]. More recent combination regimens comprising differing combinations of cisplatin, 5-FU, and paclitaxel have shown promise in the neoadjuvant treatment of penile cancer [77, 78].

Adjuvant and neoadjuvant treatment

The EAU guidelines recommend adjuvant chemotherapy for N2-3 disease. This is based on a study of 25 patients that revealed an 84% long-term disease-free survival rate [62].

In patients with palpable inguinal lymph nodes, neoadjuvant chemotherapy appears promising. In 2007, Lietje and colleagues showed that 12 out of 19 patients receiving five different neoadjuvant chemotherapy regimens showed a response, with eight achieving long-term disease-free survival after subsequent surgery [79].

Two further studies published in 2007 and 2010 reported up to a 50% response using paclitaxel, cisplatin and ifosfamide [77, 78]. The EAU guidelines therefore recommend neoadjuvant chemotherapy followed by lymph node dissection in patients with fixed or relapsed lymph node metastases [62].

Molecular biology of penile cancer and potential targeted therapy

Epidermal growth factor receptor

The cell-surface receptor epidermal growth factor receptor (EGFR) is involved in a key pathway that controls intracellular signalling [80]. Several types of ligands bind to this receptor to activate intracellular pathways that regulate processes such as cell proliferation, differentiation and apoptosis [81, 82]. This has been shown to be associated with uncontrolled cell division and proliferation of tumours by angiogenesis as well as protecting tumour cell from undergoing apoptosis.

Lavens and colleagues showed overexpression of EGFR in 17 patients diagnosed with penile SCC [81], and Di Lorenzo and co-workers found similar results in 30 patients, but were unable to identify specific mutations known to cause other tumours associated with EGFR over-expression [83]. A more recent study has demonstrated that the presence of cytosolic phosphorylated EGFR (p-EGFR) predicted recurrence and survival [84]. They therefore put the case forward for the use of p-EGFR status in informing the need for adjuvant therapy in patients with N0 and N1 disease.

Other mutations

Gou examined the expression of EGFR and RAS-association domain family 1A (RASSF1A) as well as mutation status of K-RAS and BRAF in 150 patients with penile SCC [85]. Once again, EGFR overexpression was found in all cases but only 3.42% expressed RASSF1A, one patient displayed the KRAS mutation and none expressed the BRAF mutation. This conflicts somewhat with a series of 28 cases from Spain where KRAS mutations were found in 22% of tumours [86]. Andersson also reported mutations in PIK3CA, HRAS and KRAS [87]. Stankiewicz and colleagues found HER-3 and -4 protein overexpression in penile SCC. Further analysis of their data revealed that HPV positive tumours were more associated with HER-2 expression and less associated with p-EGFR overexpression [88]. Additional work by this group showed HPV positivity was also associated with p16 and p21 expression and RB suppression in a series of 148 patients [89].

With regard to P53 mutations, some studies report an association with lymph node metastasis and poor survival, but others do not [90, 91]. Interestingly Golijanin and co-workers found that cyclooxygenase-2 (COX-2) and prostaglandin-E synthase 1 are highly expressed in dysplasia, penile intraepithelial neoplasia, and carcinoma [92]. This suggests a mechanism for inflammation in the pathogenesis of penile SCC as well raising the possibility of a therapeutic role for COX-2 inhibitors.

Targeted therapy

Given the key role that EGFR appears to play, several studies have examined the use of the monoclonal antibodies panitumumab and cetuximab in penile cancer. Carthorn and colleagues administered monoclonal antibodies together with differing combinations of platinum-based regimens to 13 patients with advanced penile SCC [93]. Median time to progression was 3.4 months and overall survival was 9.8 months, although four patients survived longer which compared favourably to results from chemotherapy [94].

Tyrosine kinase inhibitors may have an important role in targeting angiogenesis in penile SCC. Zhu and colleagues studied the effects of sorafenib and sunitinib on angiogenesis in six patients with penile SCC refractory to chemotherapy treatment [95]. One patient responded partially and four had stable disease; however, one patient died of sepsis and another suffered a ruptured femoral vein.

Conclusions

The last two decades has seen major advances for men diagnosed with penile cancer. Penile preserving techniques provide a surgical option with preservation of sexual and voiding function. The advent of SLNB has proved to be a safe and reproducible option for men with impalpable inguinal nodes. Furthermore, centralization of penile cancer patients to centres of excellence in both the UK and several European countries has allowed for greater experience to be gained by a few and improved research collaboration to take place.

Future challenges to improve survival and reduce morbidity from penile cancer will involve public and medical practitioner education and awareness of the disease. The introduction of a HPV vaccination in boys and girls may also have a beneficial effect on the disease incidence in the future.

Germ cell tumours

Most testicular cancers that arise are germ cell tumours; more rarely, other tumours may be found including lymphomas in more elderly patients (>60 years) and various sarcomas in the adolescent age group. The management of these will not be covered here. Germ cell tumours of the testis are the commonest malignant tumours of young adult males mostly occurring between the ages of 20–40. For therapeutic purposes they are split in to two groups—seminomas (SGCT) and non-seminomas (NSGCT). NSGCT comprise a large number of histological subtypes, such as embryonal carcinoma and choriocarcinoma. Overall, SGCT are slower growing and less likely to metastasize; they are also more susceptible to chemotherapy and radiotherapy. The management of metastatic germ cell tumours is often multidisciplinary and successful outcome may require more than one modality of therapy. Histological analysis is frequently complex particularly when looking at post-chemotherapy specimens and correct interpretation often requires an expert urological pathologist. Germ cell tumours overall have an excellent prognosis. Avoidance of overtreatment with the consequence of long-term side effects is important for the majority of patients currently predicted to have good prognosis.

Presentation

The most common presentation is that of a lump in the testis. This may be painful or painless; it may have grown rapidly (over a few days) or may have been present for many months. Any lump should be presumed to be malignant until proven otherwise. Sometimes patients will present with symptoms due to metastatic disease, with a tumour that may be detected in the testis but sometimes it will not be palpable. Examples of symptoms include the development of back pain due to para-aortic lymph node enlargement, cough, shortness of breath, or haemoptysis due to pulmonary metastases. Patients may rarely present with seizures, gynaecomastia, or infertility.

Diagnosis

The most usual way a diagnosis is made is from biopsy material, most commonly at orchiectomy. A proportion of these tumours produce tumour markers; they can be used alone to make a diagnosis in an emergency where they are elevated and no other cause exists. This can be very important in patients who are acutely ill as it allows the quick initiation of chemotherapy. Germ cell tumours produce hCG (chorionic gonadotropin), AFP (alphafetoprotein), and the non-specific marker LDH (lactate dehydrogenase). An elevated hCG may be detected rapidly by performing a pregnancy test [96].

Staging

The initial staging investigation will often be a testicular ultrasound—this will confirm the presence of a tumour. Both testes should be scanned as bilateral tumours do occur and small testes are more prone to be associated with infertility. The presence of microcalcification in a small contralateral testis may be an indication for a testicular biopsy [97].

It is often useful to scan the abdomen urgently at this point as it may reveal a large retroperitoneal mass with evidence of ureteric obstruction. In the absence of this or large volume pulmonary metastases seen on chest radiograph the next step is usually a radical inguinal orchiectomy. If time permits, preoperative sperm storage should be offered. Formal staging using CT should then be carried out of the chest, abdomen, and pelvis. Tumour markers should be measured both pre- and post-operatively. Staging using the TNM classification should be carried out and patients are placed into one of three prognostic groups. The prognostic group depends on the level of the markers and the sites of metastases. The outcome becomes less favourable as markers rise and documentation of adverse metastatic sites, placing patients in a poor prognosis group. The current International Germ Cell Consensus Classification (IGCCCG) categories recognize three prognostic groups [98]. Treatment and outcome is dependent on these groups.

If patients have low levels of tumour markers and no non-pulmonary visceral metastases (e.g., brain, bone, and liver) they belong to the good group with a five-year survival of 92%. These patients are treated with fewer cycles of combination chemotherapy than patients with more aggressive disease.

Patients with higher tumour markers but still no non-pulmonary visceral metastases fall into the intermediate group with a five-year survival of 75–80%. Those patients with either very high tumour markers or the presence of non-pulmonary visceral metastases fall into the poor prognosis group with a five-year survival as low as 47%. This data is now over 15 years old and newer data suggests that the outcome for this group is more favourable being in the region of 60%. SGCT are never classed as poor prognosis, instead only the presence of non-pulmonary visceral metastases can place them outside the good group in to the intermediate group (the level of tumour markers is not important). Patients who have symptoms suggesting central nervous system involvement or have very high tumour markers should have a magnetic resonance brain scan.

Treatment

For information on treatment please see Table 45.2.

Stage 1 seminoma germ cell tumour

This is disease confined to the testis. The outcome of patients with stage 1 disease is excellent with a survival of around 99%.

In all cases it is possible either to observe patients (surveillance) and only offer treatment on relapse or alternatively to offer adjuvant therapy (carboplatin AUC 7 X1 or radiotherapy to the para-aortic strip) which will reduce the relapse rate after orchiectomy, allowing a less intensive schedule of visits for blood tests and scans without an adverse affect on overall survival. Many now consider surveillance the preferable option [99]. The risk of recurrence after orchiectomy alone for patients with seminoma is between 11–30% [100]. Two risk factors have been identified: rete testis invasion and maximum tumour diameter of >40mm. If only one risk factor is present the recurrence rate is 18%. Following adjuvant therapy this falls to 4%. If adjuvant therapy is offered it is normally in the form of one cycle of carboplatin with dosing based on Calvert's formula. The dose depends on glomerular filtration and the optimal way of determining it is to perform an EDTA clearance; a single dose of carboplatin AUC7 will also reduce the risk of a contralateral tumour from 2–0.5% [101]. Radiotherapy is an alternative option although not widely given in Europe. In a randomized trial radiotherapy and single-agent carboplatin had a similar outcome. The long-term side effects of both radiotherapy and chemotherapy are undesirable and unquantified in this setting. There is also a lack of data on the optimal follow-up for surveillance. The majority of relapses occur in the first three years [102].

Stage 1 non-seminoma germ cell tumour

As with SGCT, surveillance is attractive in this disease, although adjuvant chemotherapy may be considered in patients with a high risk of relapse. The main risk factor for relapse is the presence of vascular invasion by the tumour or histology. If present the risk of recurrence is between 40–50%. The presence of embryonal carcinoma also raises the risk of recurrence to 25% otherwise it stands between 15–20% [103]. With adjuvant therapy the risk falls to around 4%. The use of one cycle of cisplatin, etoposide, and bleomycin (BEP) has been found to be effective in this situation [104]. The side effects of this therapy include nausea, vomiting, hearing damage, hair loss, ototoxicity, nephrotoxicity, and pulmonary toxicity. Whether long-term side effects may develop after only one cycle of therapy is currently unknown. One potential advantage of offering adjuvant therapy is the avoidance of potentially disruptive retroperitoneal surgery to remove residual nodes present post therapy for metastatic disease.

Table 45.2 Summary of management of patients with testis cancer after orchidectomy

	Stage I	Metastatic*		
IGCCCG risk	NA	Good	Intermediate	Poor
SGCT	Surveillance is preferable. Other options include carboplatin or RT	BEP (X3) combination chemotherapy	BEP (X4) combination chemotherapy	NA
NSGCT	Surveillance is preferable. Other options include BEP (x1)	BEP (X3) combination chemotherapy	BEP (X4) combination chemotherapy	BEP (X4) combination chemotherapy Consider other regimens

* Patients may require emergency chemotherapy prior to orchidectomy.

BEP, bleomycin, etoposide and cisplatin; SGCT, seminoma germ cell tumor; NSGCT, non-seminoma germ call tumor.

Management of metastatic disease

Metastatic disease is frequently managed with BEP chemotherapy. For patients with good prognosis disease three cycles is sufficient [105]. It is known that suboptimal dosing or drug reductions leads to inferior outcomes. The side effects have been described. The risk of infertility is less than 10% if the patient is already fertile. If the patient is infertile due to pre-existing testicular dysfunction or due to hormone imbalance secondary to the tumour then fertility may still recover following chemotherapy. Long-term side effects, namely hypertension and cardiovascular events, occur with an increased risk over time [106].

The risk of bleomycin-induced pneumonitis is low, but careful attention should be paid to patients developing respiratory symptoms. If bleomycin is contraindicated, e.g., because of poor existing lung function, then four cycles of cisplatin and etoposide may be considered [107]. Alternative treatments such as radiotherapy or single-agent carboplatin are given by some institution to patients SGCT with low-risk disease.

Patients who fall into the IGCCCG intermediate or poor prognostic groups are normally managed with four cycles of BEP. If bleomycin is contraindicated then ifosfamide may be substituted (VIP) [108]. Alternative regimens to standard BEP or VIP have not internationally established themselves in this setting. Particularly, high-dose therapy does not appear to have a role here (perhaps with the rare exception of mediastinal GCT). However, it may be possible to give one cycle of BEP and then depending on tumour marker decline reserve an intensive schedule for those whose response is unfavourable. This approach appears to be beneficial for these patients [109].

The role of surgery in GCTs

Following completion of chemotherapy patients may be left with residual masses on CT. If the markers have normalized this is not an indication for further chemotherapy but it is standard to consider surgical resection of residual masses (>3cm for SGCT and 1 cm for NSGCT [102]). The retroperitoneal lymph nodes are often removed first. The histology can be a guide as to what is likely to be found in other masses. The outcome is usually necrosis, viable cancer or mature teratoma. Mature teratoma has the propensity to de-differentiate many years later and is an indication for removal of other sites of disease. The presence of viable cancer indicates a higher risk of subsequent relapse although many patients who have less than 10% involvement are likely to remain disease free.

Managing relapse after chemotherapy

Patients may fail to enter remission (defined as normalization of tumour markers) or alternatively have rises in markers and/or develop new sites of disease following initial remission with chemotherapy. These patients can then be offered further therapy which may be curative. The chance of cure depends on the duration of the response to first-line therapy, tumour markers and the sites of subsequent relapse. Overall, between 25–60% may be cured with further therapy [110]. There is controversy regarding the use of high-dose therapy or conventional dose therapy in this setting. Standard conventional dose regimens include cisplatin and etoposide with either ifosfamide or paclitaxel [111, 112]. The most widely used high-dose therapy consists of high dose carboplatin and etoposide, although a paclitaxel-containing regimen also has

impressive data (TI-CE) [113, 114]. The mortality from high-dose chemotherapy ranges from 5–15%, with the risks being lower in patients who are fit and for whom the procedure is performed at first relapse.

Conclusion—germ cell tumours

Germ cell tumours form a curable group of metastatic cancers. The optimal use of currently available cytotoxic agents with appropriate surgery has led to an improving cure rate. The greater awareness of long-term side effects is likely to lead to attempts to reduce chemotherapy burden, particularly in patients who have low volume metastatic disease. To date the incorporation of targeted agents has failed to produce encouraging responses in this patient group.

Prostate cancer

Introduction to prostate cancer

Prostate cancer is the third most common neoplasm in men and second as far as cause of cancer death is concerned [115, 116]. In 2012, it was estimated that 92 247 men died in Europe from prostate cancer.

There were 399 964 new cases of prostate cancer in Europe in 2012 diagnosed mainly based on biopsy, which constituted 11.9% of total number of new cancer cases [116]. According to the American Cancer Society, approximately one million prostate biopsies are performed annually in the USA with an estimated 220 800 men diagnosed with prostate cancer in 2015, accounting for 26% of all male cancers.

Since there is a high incidence of prostate cancer in the Western world, screening has been proposed in order to reduce the mortality from prostate cancer death. Several screening studies have been executed in the last years in different parts of the world, but the most reliable data can be extracted from the European Randomized Screening Study for Prostate Cancer (ERSPC) [117, 118]. The most recent update with a median follow-up of 11 years demonstrated a relative reduction in prostate cancer death risk of 21% in the screened arm. However, still some questions have to be answered before a population-based screening programme can be introduced, e.g., influence on all-cause mortality, diagnosis of insignificant disease, impact on quality of life, and costs [119, 120]. Because of these uncertainties, the US preventive task services force advised against active screening and in most of the countries it is not advised to start population-based screening programmes, but asymptomatic patients who are well informed about the risks and benefits can be offered further investigations to detect or exclude the presence of prostate cancer [121].

Diagnosis

Medical history and symptoms

Age is one of the most important risk factors for prostate cancer and this is one of the reasons for the expected rising incidence for prostate cancer in the coming years. A second risk factor is a positive family history for prostate and breast cancer. This could be because of a higher awareness amongst family members, but also because DNA variants are being detected which increase the risk of prostate cancer development. Hopefully, this DNA research can identify high-risk groups of prostate cancer patients that need treatment [122]. There are no specific symptoms that are specific for the presence of prostate cancer. Only at a late stage, symptoms can be present when there is a large prostate cancer volume, e.g., voiding symptoms (irritative or obstructive), or obstruction of the ureter(s) resulting in hydronephrosis and/or uraemia, or when metastases are present, e.g., bone pain. In the majority of cases an elevated PSA (>3 ng/mL) is nowadays the reason for further investigations.

Digital rectal examination

The first step in the workup for prostate cancer is a digital rectal examination (DRE) although the positive predictive value is very low (33–83% in a screening population with a PSA ≥3 ng/mL) [123]. The reason to perform a DRE in a non-screening situation is the chance that high grade tumours can be missed if PSA is not elevated and it is also part of the TNM staging [124].

Prostate specific antigen and others

Prostate specific antigen (PSA) is a protein that is mainly produced by the prostate and as such *prostate tissue specific*, but not *prostate cancer specific*. Its function is to liquefy the semen, but due to disruption of the glandular structures in the prostate (e.g., prostatitis, biopsy), the serum level can be elevated. Also due to a prostatic enlargement the serum level can be increased. Because of these factors the specificity and sensitivity of an elevated PSA (>3 ng/mL) are rather low and only approximately 30% of patients with a PSA level between 3 and 10 ng/mL will show positive biopsies. Several methods have been explored to increase the sensitivity of PSA, e.g., PSA density (PSA level related to prostate volume), PSA velocity (increase of PSA over time), and looking at PSA isoforms, e.g., free PSA, complex PSA, pro PSA, PSA health index [125]. However, in the majority of cases the level of total PSA still determines the indication for further investigations. A relative new laboratory investigation is the PCA3 urinary test, which is a prostate cancer specific gene, which is over-expressed in 95% of prostate cancer cells, with a median 66-fold up-regulation compared to adjacent noncancerous prostate cells [126]. This urinary test is increasing the chance of finding a positive biopsy in case of an elevated PSA, but the test is now only approved in case of a first negative biopsy [127, 128]. The relation of PCA3 level and tumour aggressiveness has resulted in contradictory results and thus cannot be used to determine which patients with low volume disease need treatment or not [129].

Imaging

In case an elevated PSA or an abnormal DRE is found, the first imaging modality is a transrectal ultrasonography (TRUS) of the prostate. Again, the sensitivity and specificity of TRUS alone to demonstrate or exclude the presence of a malignancy is insufficient and nowadays TRUS is only used to aid guiding the biopsies of the prostate. Improvements in TRUS performance are sought by adding ultrasound contrast agents, looking at elastic properties of the prostate tissue (elastography) and using computer techniques to determine tissue characteristics (e.g., HistoScanning™) [130–132]. Multiparametric (mp)-MRI is one of the promising imaging modalities for prostate cancer detection; however, whether it can be applied for the determination to perform initial prostate biopsies in case of a suspicion of prostate cancer remains to be established. But if biopsies are negative there is a role for mp-MRI once the suspicion for prostate cancer remains [133, 134].

In case of a high suspicion for metastatic disease (PSA ≥20 ng/mL, locally advanced disease, Gleason score ≥8) bone scintigraphy is still the standard to exclude osteoblastic bone lesions. Axial skeletal MRI could replace bone scan in the future whereas the role of FDG-PET scan has not been established yet [135–137]. The precise identification of lymph node metastases is still a problem, because none of the imaging modalities are accurate to demonstrate or exclude positive nodes. The use of lymph node-specific contrast agents in combination with MRI improve the sensitivity, but this agent is not available in clinical practice [138, 139].

Biopsy and pathology

Once there is an indication for excluding or demonstrating the presence of a prostate cancer transrectal ultrasound-guided biopsies are performed. Since most of the tumours are not visible by TRUS, so-called random biopsies are taken, with the inherent risk of sampling error. Most of the tumours are located in the peripheral zone of the prostate and for this reason the biopsies are initially directed to this area of the prostate and in total a ten to twelve biopsies are obtained, but this depends also on the volume of the prostate [140]. In case the biopsies are found to be negative for prostate cancer and there remains a suspicion for the presence of prostate cancer, re-biopsies can be taken, because there is still a chance of between 20 to 35% that in these repeat biopsies prostate cancer can be detected [141]. Alternative strategies nowadays are the PCA3 test or mp-MRI investigations to determine the risk on finding cancer in a repeat biopsy session.

Before taking transrectal prostate biopsies a urinary tract infection should be excluded, the patient should receive prophylactic antibiotics and anticoagulation treatment should be interrupted. The complications of this diagnostic procedure are transient haematuria, haematospermia, rectal bleeding, urinary retention, and sepsis.

The biopsy specimens are sent in individual containers or in two containers (left and right) for histologic evaluation. The pathologist has to report the presence of an adenocarcinoma of the prostate and the Gleason grading [142]. The Gleason grading system is based on histological architectural patterns, e.g., tubular differentiation and pattern of stromal invasion [143]. Two dominant growth patterns determine the Gleason sum score (2 to 10) and the most dominant pattern is mentioned first, e.g., 3 + 4 or 4 + 3. Furthermore, the number of cores involved with prostate cancer and the percentage of tumour per core should be reported, because these have prognostic relevance [144].

Risk groups

Based on the diagnostic workup the risk group for the individual patient can be determined using DRE, PSA, and biopsy results. Several risk group determinations have been proposed; a commonly used one is that of the ESTRO/EAU/EORTC, as shown in Table 45.3 [145].

Based on the risk group classification the different treatment modalities are discussed with the patient.

Treatment

Low-risk localized prostate cancer

Since PSA is nowadays the main driving factor for the detection of prostate cancer, a great number of patients are diagnosed with low-risk, low-volume disease. It was shown in the screening studies

Table 45.3 Risk groups in prostate cancer

Low risk	T1c–T2a, Gleason score <7, iPSA <10 ng/mL
Intermediate risk	T2b–c, or Gleason score 7, or iPSA 10–20 ng/mL (in case of two factors high-risk)
High risk	T3, or Gleason score >7, or iPSA >20 ng/mL (one or more factors)

Reprinted from *Radiotherapy and Oncology*, Volume 57, Issue 3, Ash D et al., ESTRO/EAU/EORTC recommendations on permanent seed implantation for localized prostate cancer, pp. 315–321, Copyright © 2000 Elsevier Science Ireland Ltd., with permission from Elsevier, <http://www.sciencedirect.com/science/journal/01678140>

that these patients probably did not need active treatment in the majority of cases. The risk of dying from prostate cancer in this group of patients seems to be the same as for patients without detected prostate cancer in the same age group [146]. Recently, a randomized study comparing radical prostatectomy and observation did not show a benefit for the surgically treated low-risk patients [147]. These observations have led to the so-called active surveillance option for patients with low-risk prostate cancer, meaning that no immediate active treatment is offered to the patient, but observation and in case of demonstrated progression based on PSA or follow-up biopsies a treatment with curative intent is started [148]. This approach does not seem to have a negative impact on cancer-specific survival.

Intermediate-risk and high-risk localized prostate cancer

In these cases usually an active treatment is indicated unless the patient has such comorbidities that an active treatment for his prostate cancer will not be of benefit. In this case, a watchful waiting protocol can be discussed, meaning that palliative treatment will be started once symptoms occur. The treatment options are radical prostatectomy (open, laparoscopically, or robot-assisted laparoscopically) or radiotherapy (external beam or brachytherapy). Unfortunately, no randomized studies comparing these different treatment options have been performed. This means that patient preference is an important decisive factor based on the anticipated side effects that can occur with these treatments.

The results for radical prostatectomy seem not to differ between the three approaches once a sufficient number of surgical procedures are being done. Especially in the high-risk group an extended lymph node dissection is combined with the radical prostatectomy. The outcome is usually excellent with recurrence-free survival rates in the order of 75% [149]. Side effects of the surgical approach are erectile dysfunction and urinary incontinence. The incidence of these side effects depends on the extent of surgery (nerve-sparing or not), age of the patient, and pre-operative complaints, but erectile dysfunction is reported in the literature in the range of 13 to 78% and urinary incontinence in the range of 2 to 40% [150]. Nowadays, standard external beam radiotherapy uses dosage of 78 to 80 Gy given in a six- to eight-week period; for this, advanced radiation techniques are necessary, e.g., intensity modulated radiotherapy (IMRT) or image-guided radiotherapy. Using these techniques improved outcome has been reported for all risk groups [151, 152]. Side effects of external beam radiotherapy are erectile dysfunction (8–85%), voiding symptoms (2–6%), and bowel problems, e.g. blood, diarrhoea, soiling (15–30%) [153, 154]. In case of a high-risk tumour hormonal therapy is usually advised with radiotherapy.

Brachytherapy may be indicated in low-risk and intermediate-risk patients, but patients should not have voiding problems and the prostate volume should be <60 cc. The 10-year disease-free survival for low- and intermediate-risk prostate cancer ranges from 80–97% and 72–94%, respectively [155, 156]. Side effects of brachytherapy are erectile dysfunction (14–61%), urinary incontinence and retention (2–32%) [153, 154].

Experimental treatments

Several local thermal local treatments for localized prostate cancer have been explored over the past years. Cryosurgery aims to freeze the prostate introducing needles transperineally into the prostate. No randomized studies have been reported with this approach; progression-free survival rates of 36–92% have been reported, with a wide range demonstrating that patients with different disease characteristics have been treated [157]. This treatment should still be considered as an investigational approach.

High intensity focused ultrasound (HIFU) uses a transrectal approach where the ultrasound transducer emits focused ultrasound waves that generate heat and the tissue is destroyed by coagulative necrosis. No well-designed clinical trials have been reported, but progression-free survival has been published in the range of 63–87% [158]. The technique has improved over the years and seems to lead to improved outcome data, but evaluation parameters are different (PSA, biopsies) among the published studies [159, 160]. In case a small tumour is found, in the majority of cases not the whole organ is removed (cf. renal tumour, breast cancer) and this has led to the concept of focal therapy for prostate cancer. The prerequisite is that the dominant tumour can be identified with certainty and there is an effective treatment to focally treat the tumour. At present the use of laser alone or in combination with a sensitizer (TOOKAD), and irreversible electroporation (IRE) is being studied [161–163]. Imaging is improving and with mp-MRI there might be a modality to identify the aggressive lesion within the prostate and by using brachytherapy, cryotherapy, laser, and electroporation effective methods are now available to kill the tumour [164]. However, this concept has yet to be proven in prospective studies [165].

Locally advanced disease

Once there is evidence that the tumour has perforated the prostate capsule (T3a) or invaded the seminal vesicles (T3b) a metastatic workup is essential to exclude metastatic lesions. In case the patient is not a candidate for local treatment, watchful waiting should be discussed in case the PSA level is not too high (<50 ng/mL) and/or a PSA doubling time is longer than 12 months. It has been demonstrated that the risk of dying from prostate cancer was not worse if hormonal treatment was started at the time of symptomatic progression [166, 167].

Most studies have been performed using radiotherapy in this situation and it has been shown that the combination of radiotherapy plus hormonal therapy (at least two years) resulted in an improved overall survival (34–58% after 10 years) [168–170].

No prospective studies have been performed that evaluate radical prostatectomy in T3 disease. In patients with a 'small' T3 tumour, surgery is an option in combination with an extended lymph node dissection, because it was shown that pathological downstaging (pT2) is present in approximately 30% of cases. Surgery is, however, usually one step in the multimodal approach for this category of patients. If extensive capsular penetration is demonstrated on pathological examination the addition of adjuvant radiotherapy has shown to improve biochemical progression-free survival (74% versus 52.6% if no adjuvant therapy was given) [171]. The question at this moment is if all patients should receive immediate adjuvant radiotherapy if pT3 disease has been demonstrated or that early salvage radiotherapy should be given once a biochemical recurrence (PSA >0.2 ng/mL) has been shown, since this seems to give the same results [172].

Metastatic disease

Bone metastases are the most common metastatic sites and these are usually osteoblastic. In this case no curative options are available and palliative treatment can be offered. Nowadays, only a minority of patients present with symptomatic metastatic disease (bone pain, neurological symptoms). The common treatment is the induction of androgen deprivation, since androgens are the driving force in prostate cancer [173, 174]. Androgens are produced in the testes and the adrenals. Several approaches can lower the androgen serum levels (e.g., orchiectomy, GnRH analogues, LHRH antagonist, anti-androgens, oestrogens), and these approaches can induce palliation in the majority of patients, but there is no hard evidence that they leads to a longer survival.

If hormonal therapy is indicated, GnRH analogues are combined with an anti-androgen treatment in the first four weeks to prevent a flare reaction (initial rise of testosterone), especially in extensive metastatic disease. Since this can lead to serious complications (spinal cord lesion, hydronephrosis), this flare prevention is not necessary with orchiectomy or LHRH antagonists that induce an immediate testosterone decline. Combined androgen deprivation (blocking testosterone produced in the testes and adrenals) has been shown not to be of benefit [174]. Because of the lower testosterone levels several side effects can be expected, which can have a clear impact on the quality of life (erectile dysfunction, hot flashes, increase in weight, depression). It has been demonstrated that continuous lowered testosterone levels also influence the bone mineral density (osteopenia) and induce the metabolic syndrome (insulin intolerance, change in lipid profiles). Because of these side effects the timing of hormonal therapy and the scheme of hormonal therapy should be discussed with the patient. There is also a renewed interest in oestrogen therapy for prostate cancer, because this treatment has beneficial effects compared to the other treatments discussed, e.g., no effect on bone loss and preserves cognitive function. The negative effects of oestrogens (thromboembolic events) are absent if the oestrogens are given parenteral or transdermal [175, 176].

It is clear that symptomatic metastatic patients need immediate hormonal therapy, but in asymptomatic patients delay of start treatment should be discussed since this palliative treatment does induce side effects with a clear impact on the quality of life and some deleterious effects. Another approach is intermittent androgen deprivation treatment, where the start and stop of hormonal therapy is based on PSA levels, although different schedules are being used. Reported randomized studies did not show a clear difference between intermittent and continuous androgen deprivation therapy concerning survival, but improvement in quality of life parameters in the intermittent treatment group [177].

Castrate resistant prostate cancer

Androgen deprivation therapy is not a curative treatment and patients will show biochemical (PSA) or clinical progression after a variable period of time. The first step in case of a PSA rise could be to add an anti-androgen to the testosterone-lowering treatment, which can lead to a PSA decrease, but this combined treatment has not shown to influence survival. Once the patient develops again PSA progression with a demonstrated castration level of serum testosterone (<1.7 nmol/L) a castrate resistant prostate cancer (CRPC) is present. Until 2004, no effective agents were available to treat patients, but two studies showed a median survival benefit for docetaxel 75 mg/m^2 three-weekly combined with prednisone 5 mg bid of two to two and a half months [178, 179]. Recently, several new drugs have been introduced for the treatment of CRPC patients: (1) targeting the endocrine pathways (e.g., abiraterone, enzalutamide), (2) vaccine therapy (e.g., sipuleucel-T), (3) second-line chemotherapeutic approach (cabizataxel), (4) bone targeting approach (Radium ^{223}). These new agents have been evaluated pre- and post-docetaxel therapy.

Cabizataxel has been shown to result in an overall survival benefit post docetaxel of 2.4 months compared to mitoxantrone; this second-line chemotherapy did, however, have a number of grade 3/4 toxicities and experience is required to administer this treatment [180].

Abiraterone and enzalutamide have been tested in the pre- and post-docetaxel setting, where enzalutamide showed an overall survival benefit in both situations (pre-docetaxel: 4.8 months); the data pre-chemotherapy have not been published yet, but a 30% reduction in the risk of death was reported. Abiraterone showed also an overall survival benefit in the post-docetaxel setting (4.6 months compared to placebo), but only a radiological progression-free survival in the pre-docetaxel setting (47% reduction in the risk of progression) [181–183].

Sipuleucel-T has been tested in patients CRPC patients with minimal symptoms and it was for the first time that this immunotherapeutic approach showed a survival benefit (4.1 months compared to placebo) [184].

Bone targeting agents are used for painful metastases (e.g., Strontium^{89}, Samarium-153), but it was very surprising when the use of an alpha emitter (Radium^{223}) also showed a survival benefit as well in patients pretreated with docetaxel or not (3.6 months compared to placebo) [185].

With all these agents now available for patients with CRPC the challenge is to decide which treatment is indicated for which patient at which stage. There is no clear evidence for a single best approach and guidelines are contradictory. There are some indications that patients with aggressive disease would benefit from chemotherapy and those patients who had a long response to hormonal therapy might benefit from abiraterone or enzalutamide, but these suggestions have to be validated in prospective studies, where cross-resistance should also be evaluated.

Urothelial cell carcinoma

The urothelium is the epithelial layer that lines up the whole collecting system from renal papilla in the kidney to fossa navicularis in the urethra. It is composed of three to seven layers of cells and is also called transitional epithelium. Its surface is covered by protective glycoprotein plaques [186, 187].

Urothelial cell carcinoma is more often encountered in bladder (95%) than in the upper urinary tract (5%) [188]. This section will be divided according to the two main urothelial cell carcinoma topographies: bladder and upper urinary tract, comprising caliceal, pelvic, and ureter locations.

Bladder urothelial cell carcinoma

Epidemiology

With a worldwide incidence of 151/100 000 per year reported in 2012, bladder ranks ninth in terms of cancer location and ninth for mortality (52.4/100 000 per year). Males are more affected than females with a gender ratio of 3.6 [189]. Worldwide, 430 000 cases were diagnosed in 2012.

At initial presentation, 70–80% of cases are non-muscle invasive bladder carcinoma (NMIBC) [190]. At initial treatment, about 30% of patients treated for muscle invasive bladder carcinoma (MIBC) harbor detectable metastases [191, 192].

Some risk factors are clearly identified: tobacco is certainly the most important one, responsible for 50 to 60% of bladder cancers (BC) with a strong correlation between disease incidence and smoking exposure (years and total number of cigarettes) [193]. Occupational exposure concerns professions related to dyeing, fabrics, paints, metal, and petroleum industries. The chemical components incriminated are aromatic amines, polycyclic aromatic hydrocarbons, and chlorinated hydrocarbons. Authorities' regulations in Western countries have led to a decrease in the role of occupational hazards in BC for the past decades and it is currently believed to account for 10% of new cases [194–197]. Schistosomiasis has been related to squamous cell carcinoma of the bladder but there is no high level evidence connecting it to urothelial carcinoma [194].

Staging and grading

Like most solid malignant tumours, bladder cancer is staged according to the TNM classification. It was updated in 2009 (no change from 2002). Tumour stage is highly related to oncologic prognosis [198]. The TNM staging for bladder cancer can be accessed on the website of the American Cancer Society: <http://www.cancer.org/cancer/bladdercancer/detailedguide/bladder-cancer-staging>.

An important clinical boundary separates tumours confined to mucosa or submucosa: non-muscle invasive bladder carcinoma (NMIBC) (Tis, Ta, and T1) from tumours invading muscularis propria and beyond: muscle invasive bladder carcinoma (MIBC) (T2–T4).

For NMIBC, another important prognosis factor for recurrence or progression to MIBC is the grade, based on cytological and architectural criteria. Two grading systems are reported in daily clinical practices: the 1973 and 2004 World Health Organization (WHO) grading classifications. The 1973 classification separates NMIBC in 3 grades: 1 (well differentiated), 2 (moderately differentiated), and 3 (poorly differentiated). The 2004 grading is shown in Box 45.1.

Papillary urothelial neoplasm of low malignant potential (PUNLMP) is a lesion composed by normal urothelial cells in a papillar configuration without malignant cytological features. The risk of progression is negligible, although recurrences can occur. This lesion represents the lower spectrum of the NMIBC.

Most of the literature on urothelial bladder cancer grading is based on the 1973 classification and there is still no prognostic validation for the 2004 WHO classification. Therefore, the current guidelines recommend using both grading systems [199]. The two systems are compared in Table 45.4.

Box 45.1 2004 WHO grading of non-muscle invasive bladder carcinoma

- ◆ Flat lesions
  - Hyperplasia (flat lesion without atypia or papillary aspects)
  - Reactive atypia (flat lesion with atypia)
  - Atypia of unknown significance
  - Urothelial dysplasia
  - Urothelial carcinoma in situ
  - Papillary lesions
  - Urothelial papilloma (completely benign lesion)
  - Papillary urothelial neoplasm of low malignant potential (PUNLMP)
  - Low-grade papillary urothelial carcinoma
  - High-grade papillary urothelial carcinoma

Reproduced with permission from Miyamoto H et al., Non-invasive papillary urothelial neoplasms: The 2004 WHO/ISUP classification system, *Pathology International*, Volume 60, Issue 2, pp. 1–8, Copyright © 2009 The Authors. Journal compilation © 2009 Japanese Society of Pathology and Blackwell Publishing Asia Pty Ltd.

Diagnosis

Symptoms

Macroscopic haematuria constitutes the key symptom for urothelial carcinoma (bladder and upper urinary tract). When reported, cystoscopy and CT urography should be scheduled to confirm or rule it out. NMIBC is usually painless. Some less specific symptoms like refractory lower urinary tract symptoms (LUTS) without urinary infection should encourage investigations to rule out a carcinoma in situ (CIS).

Clinical examination

Clinical examination is nonspecific in urothelial carcinoma. However, a pelvic examination should be performed to detect gross lymph nodes. Clinical staging is unreliable [200] but pelvic fixation on digital rectal examination under anaesthesia presumes an inextirpable tumour in the setting of MIBC.

Cytology

Analyses of voided urine or bladder washout to look for exfoliated malignant cells from urinary tract presents high sensitivity

Table 45.4 Shifting from 1973 to 2004 WHO grading classification

WHO 1973	WHO 2004
	Urothelial papilloma
Grade 1 carcinoma	PUNLMP
	Low-grade carcinoma
Grade 2 carcinoma	Low-grade carcinoma
	High-grade carcinoma
Grade 3 carcinoma	High-grade carcinoma

NMIBC are divided into low- or high-grade in the last classification

MIBC are always high-grade

Source: data from Mostofi FK et al., Histological typing of urinary bladder tumours, *International Histological Classification of Tumours No. 10*, World Health Organization, Copyright © 1973; and Miyamoto H et al, Non-invasive papillary urothelial neoplasms: The 2004 WHO/ISUP classification system, *Pathology International*, Volume 60, Issue 2, pp. 1–8, Copyright © 2004.

Table 45.5 Risk group stratification according to 2011 EAU guidelines

Low-risk tumours	Primary, solitary, Ta, G1* (PUNLMP, LG), <3 cm, no CIS
Intermediate-risk tumours	All tumours not defined in the two adjacent categories (between the category of low and high risk)
High-risk tumours	Any of the following: ♦ T1 tumour ♦ G3** (high grade) tumour ♦ CIS ♦ Multiple, recurrent, and large (>3 cm) Ta G1G2 tumours (all conditions must be present in this point)

*low-grade is a mixture of G1 and G2.

**high-grade is a mixture of some G2 and all G3.

CIS, carcinoma in situ; HG, high-grade; LG, low-grade.

Reproduced with permission from Babjuk M et al., *Guidelines on Non-muscle-Invasive Bladder Cancer (Ta, T1, and CIS)*, European Society of Urology, Arnhem, The Netherlands, Copyright © 2015 European Society of Urology.

in the setting of high-grade carcinoma but sensitivity drops off for low-grade tumours. Thus, cytology is of interest in the follow-up of high-grade carcinoma or CIS.

Imaging

Trans-abdominal ultrasound (US) imaging can detect intraluminal tumours of the urinary tract. For bladder tumours, it can set transurethral resection of the tumour (TURT) indication, bypassing cystoscopic examination. At upper urinary tract level, US can detect tumours and hydronephrosis associated with obstruction. Although it cannot rule out an upper urinary tract tumour, it remains a useful tool in the setting of urothelial carcinoma diagnosis. Uro-CT, or in developing countries intravenous pyelography (IVP), can detect a defect in the upper urinary tract and should be performed at initial assessment of macroscopic haematuria to detect upper urinary tract tumours. For MIBC, contrast agent CT is also necessary to assess TNM staging. However, neither CT nor magnetic resonance imaging are reliable to differentiate bladder T stage under T3b (macroscopic extravesical extension) [201, 202] or N stage when lymph node enlargement is less than 8 mm [203, 204].

Cystoscopy

Cystoscopy is the best examination to identify bladder tumour. It can be performed at the office, under local anaesthesia, with a flexible cystoscope. It allows a thorough visualization of the whole bladder lining.

Markers

In the last few years, many attempts have been made to develop urinary markers that could potentially screen urothelial carcinoma with a less invasive procedure. Unfortunately, at the moment, none of these tests has reached an acceptable accuracy (sensitivity and sensibility) to be implemented in daily clinical practices [199].

Transurethral resection of tumour

TURT is performed under complete or regional anaesthesia, with an operative cystoscope incorporating a diathermic or bipolar loop (resectoscope). TURT is a diagnostic procedure allowing pathological confirmation of bladder urothelial carcinoma but it is also the

first step for NMIBC treatment. Pathological analyses confirm the diagnostic of urothelial carcinoma, grades the tumour and separates patient among two main prognostic groups that will determine the therapeutic strategy: MIBC or NMIBC. In the setting of NMIBC, recurrence and progression to MIBC can be predicted based on the EORTC scoring system and risk tables [205]. Risk factors for recurrence are the number of tumours, tumour diameter, prior recurrence rate, tumour stage (Ta or T1), presence of concurrent CIS and 1973 WHO tumour grade. Automatic calculators of risk groups predicting recurrence and progression at one and five years can be downloaded online on computers or smartphones for easier daily clinical use. (<http://www.eortc.be/tools/bladdercalculator/>). European guidelines panel recommends stratification of NMIBC patients in to three risk groups allowing adapted therapeutic strategies [199] (see Tables 45.4 and 45.6).

Treatment of non-muscle invasive bladder cancer

A complete TURT is the first step in NMIBC management. Since high incidence recurrence (30–60%) and progression (≈10%) is part of the disease natural history [205], adjuvant therapy is a valuable part of treatment.

Table 45.6 2015 European Guidelines treatment recommendations in TaT1 tumours according to risk stratifications

Risk category	Definition	Treatment recommendation
Low-risk tumours	Primary, solitary, Ta, LG/G1, <3 cm, no CIS	One immediate instillation of chemotherapy
Intermediate-risk tumours	All cases between categories of low and high risk	One immediate instillation of chemotherapy followed by further instillations, either chemotherapy for a maximum of one year or one year full-dose BCG
High-risk tumours	Any of the following: ♦ T1 tumours ♦ HG/G3 tumours ♦ CIS ♦ Multiple and recurrent and large (>3 cm) Ta G1G2 tumours (all these conditions must be presented)	Intravesical full-dose BCG instillations for 1–3 years or cystectomy (in highest-risk tumours)
Subgroup of highest-risk tumours	T1G3 associated with concurrent bladder CIS, multiple and/or large T1G3 and/or recurrent T1G3, T1G3 with CIS in prostatic urethra, unusual histology of urothelial carcinoma, LVI	Radical cystectomy should be considered in those who refuse RC, intravesical full-dose BCG installations for 1–3 years.
	BCG failures	Radical cystectomy is recommended

BCG, Bacillus Calmette-Guerin; CIS, carcinoma in situ; GR, grade of recommendation; HG, high-grade; LG, low-grade; LVI, lymphovascular invasion.

Reproduced with permission from Babjuk M et al., *Guidelines on Non-muscle-Invasive Bladder Cancer (Ta, T1, and CIS)*, European Society of Urology, Arnhem, The Netherlands, Copyright © 2015 European Society of Urology.

Immediate post-operative instillation of chemotherapy

A single instillation of mitomycin C (or epirubicin or doxorubicin) right after resection can decrease the recurrence rate of 11.7% when compared with resection alone [206]. Adjuvant chemotherapy seems more effective among single primary or small tumours groups. Those instillations are contraindicated if the bladder has been perforated during the TURT procedure [199].

Bacillus Calmette-Guérin intravesical immunotherapy

By sustaining patient's immune response against urothelial carcinoma, Bacillus Calmette-Guérin (BCG) therapy prevents recurrence [207, 208] and progression [209, 210] in NMIBC. It is more efficient in low- to intermediate-risk patients. It has been proven superior to intravesical chemotherapy [211]. The best BCG administration schedule is still under clinical trials scrutiny. It is usually delivered according to the original empirical six-weekly schedule introduced by Morales in 1976 [212]. Although it is a topical treatment, BCG-therapy presents toxicity and any clinician should be aware of its side effects ranging from local (cystitis, haematuria, symptomatic granulomatous prostatitis, epididymo-orchitis) to systemic adverse events (general malaise, fever, arthralgia, BCG sepsis, and allergic reactions).

BCG-therapy failure and recurrences after BCG

The aggressive nature of BCG therapy should not be underestimated. Cancer-specific mortality of this patient subgroup is important [213]. European guidelines recommend radical cystectomy as a standard treatment in case of BCG failure, see Table 45.6.

Treatment of muscle invasive bladder cancer

Radical surgery and urinary diversion

Radical cystectomy is standard of care in the setting of MIBC [192]. The surgical procedure includes the dissection of regional lymph nodes as part of the treatment but also to stage the cancer extension and thus, to select properly the candidates for adjuvant chemotherapy. An extended lymph node dissection is preferable and survival has been shown to increase with the number of lymph nodes dissected [214]. The procedure can be performed through a classical open approach, laparoscopically, or robot-assisted laparoscopy. After bladder removal, urinary diversion options are: abdominal diversion (urethrocutaneostomy, ileal, or colonic conduit and some forms of continent pouches), urethral diversion (orthotopic urinary diversion through intestinal neobladder pouches), or rectosigmoid diversion (uretero-rectostomy). The choice depends on predicted post-operative continence, comorbidities, cognitive functions, and life expectancy. Overall, radical cystectomy is a morbid procedure with estimated perioperative mortality of 3% and early complications (within three months of surgery) in up to 50–60% of cases [215]. Adverse events predictive factors are the surgeon and hospital volumes [216], patient's comorbidity, age, previous treatment, other pelvic disease, and type of urinary diversion [217].

Bladder-sparing multimodal therapy

Bladder-sparing multimodal therapy integrating radiotherapy and cisplatin-based chemotherapy can be offered as an alternative to surgical cystectomy for well-selected patients or when surgical extirpation cannot be performed [192]. In this setting, long-term oncologic outcomes are comparable to radical cystectomy [218].

Neoadjuvant chemotherapy

Neoadjuvant chemotherapy is recommended for T2-T4a, cN0M0 bladder cancer and should be a cisplatin-based combination therapy [192]. Several randomized controlled trials and meta-analyses reported an absolute benefit of 5–8% for neoadjuvant chemotherapy [219–221]. However, to date, there is no accurate marker to predict response to chemotherapy and thus, non-responders might lose chance of survival due to postponed surgery.

Metastatic disease

About 30% of patients initially diagnosed with MIBC present with a metastatic stage and about half of patients who underwent a radical cystectomy will eventually develop it during the follow-up. Cisplatin-based combination chemotherapy is the recommended first-line strategy [192]. Reported patients' median survival is of 14 months when they tolerate this treatment [222, 223].

Upper urinary tract urothelial cell carcinoma

Epidemiology

Primary upper tract urothelial cancer (UTUC) is rare and accounts for less than 5% of all urothelial tumours. Men are more affected than women with a gender ratio of 3:1 [224]. It often presents as multifocal and ≈60% of UTUCs are invasive at diagnostic [225]. Pyelocaliceal location is twice as frequent as ureter location [226]. During the three last decades, stage and grade migration have exhibit a trend towards more aggressive disease. However, cancer-specific mortality remains stable [227].

About 17% of UTUCs have concomitant bladder cancer at presentation [228] and 22–47% of patients with primary UTUC will develop tumours in the bladder during their follow-up [229, 230].

Unlike bladder carcinoma, genetic susceptibility for UTUC has been identified in families harbouring hereditary non-polyposis colorectal carcinoma (HNPCC; Lynch Syndrome) [231]. Clinicians should suspect a familial disease when a patient presents with UTUC at a young age, had previous HNPCC-related cancer or a family history of HNPCC-related cancer. In this setting, the family should undergo genetic counseling with DNA sequencing to search for HNPCC mutations [232].

Just like bladder carcinoma, tobacco and occupational exposure are the most important risk factors for UTUCs [233]. However, the Balkan endemic nephropathy is a UTUC's specific risk factor. It is associated with chronic exposure to aristolochic acid contained in *Aristolochia fangchi* and clematis, plants present abundantly in the Balkans or in Chinese herbs [234, 235].

Staging and grading

The grading system is the same as bladder carcinoma with the 1973 and 2004 WHO classifications. The staging classification is comparable and can be found in *AJCC Cancer Staging Manual*, Seventh Edition (2010) published by Springer-Verlag.

Diagnosis

Symptoms

Symptoms are rare in UTUC and when present they denote a locally advanced or systemic involvement. Haematuria with a normal cystoscopy should trigger suspicions of UTUC.

Imaging

Imaging of the upper urinary tract is usually performed after a negative cystoscopy. CT urography with a late post-injection phase

(10–15 minutes) is currently the gold standard (EAU guidelines recommendation grade A) to explore upper urinary tract in the setting of UTUC suspicion. The sensitivity and specificity are, respectively, 96% and 99%, and accuracy ranges from 59–88% [236]. In case of iodine allergy or renal insufficiency MRI is an acceptable alternative. MRI specificity remains high (97%) at a price of a lower sensitivity (≈70%) [236]. Accuracy decreases notably when the lesions are smaller than 1 cm with described sensitivities of 89% for lesions <5 mm and 40% for lesions <3 mm [236]. Retrograde ureteropyelography during cystoscopy can be an acceptable strategy to rule out an UTUC in the setting of positive cytology with no evidence of bladder tumour during the procedure [236]. A cystoscopy is anyway mandatory during diagnostic process of UTUC in order to exclude a concomitant bladder location [236].

Urinary cytology

Urinary cytology can be highly suggestive of UTUC when positive while no tumour had been found in the bladder (cystoscopy) and CIS had been ruled out in the lower urinary tract (bladder and urethra). However, sensitivity in upper urinary tract is not as good as in the bladder. It can be increased by gathering urine in situ (renal cavities with ureteral catheterization) [237].

Diagnostic ureteroscopy

Diagnostic ureteroscopy with a flexible device allows visualization and biopsies of the tumour all along the upper urinary tract. Biopsies tumour grading yield is around 90% [238]. However, undergrading occurs frequently, imposing a thorough follow-up after conservative strategies [239]. European guidelines recommend performing a ureteroscopy systematically (when available) before UTUC treatment [226].

Molecular markers

Several studies assessed the diagnostic value of markers related to molecular pathways involved in urothelial carcinoma pathogenesis (tumour cell adhesion, angiogenesis, proliferation, epithelial-mesenchymal transition, mitosis, and apoptosis among others) [240–243]. However, due to the low incidence of this disease, internal and external validation of such markers on large cohorts is challenging and none of these markers are currently approved in routine clinical practice [226].

Treatment of organ confined disease

Nephroureterectomy

Nephroureterectomy with excision of the bladder cuff is the gold standard treatment. Laparoscopic or open approach appeared to be equivalent based on a prospective study [244]. According to fundamental onco-surgery principles, the specimen has to be removed en bloc in order to prevent tumour seeding from the urinary tract [225]. The bladder cuff can be dissected through an open inguinal approach or cystoscopically with the resection of the distal ureter's intramural section [226]. Just like in MIBC, time from diagnosis to extirpative surgery is related to disease progression [245] and should ideally not exceed 45 days [226]. Lymph node dissection seems to present benefits in terms of oncologic outcomes although clear topographic patterns are still to be defined for each UTUC location (pyelocaliceal versus ureter) [226]. There is a high level of evidence (1b) that immediate postoperative single dose instillation of mitomycin C after nephroureterectomy prevents bladder recurrence [246] (European guidelines recommendation grade B).

Conservative treatment

Conservative treatment can be offered as an alternative to nephrourererectomy when renal function has to be preserved or in well-selected patients: unifocal tumour, less than 1cm, low-grade and non-invasive aspect on CT-urography. Prior histological confirmation of UTUC through a flexible ureteroscopy with biopsies is recommended and because of the significant risk of grade ≈ stage underestimation, a close and stringent follow-up is mandatory. Any recurrence should shift back the therapeutic strategy to the gold standard nephroureterectomy when possible. The different conservative approaches include resection or laser vaporization under flexible ureteroscopic approach, a percutaneous access (pyelocaliceal location) or a segmental ureteral resection with wide margins (ureteral location) [226].

Treatment of metastatic disease

A metastatic stage imposes a systemic treatment. Nephroureterectomy is no more relevant in this setting except for palliative indications (e.g., macroscopic haematuria). Although randomized control trials is still lacking, platinum-based chemotherapy seems to have similar effect as for bladder carcinoma [247].

Follow-up

Follow-up after initial UTUC management should rule out local recurrences, when conservative treatment applied, with ureteroscopy, bladder recurrence with cystoscopy and contralateral recurrence with CT-urography and cytology. CT scans will inform metastatic progression. Box 45.2 shows the 2013 European guidelines for post-UTUC treatment follow-up [226].

Renal cancer

Pathogenesis

Renal cell carcinoma (RCC) has a number of distinct pathological types. The commonest is clear cell histology which accounts for over 70% of renal malignancies. There are two grades of tumour (high and low). This has replaced the Furhman grading system. Clear cell renal cancer is intrinsically linked to von Hippel-Lindau (VHL) mutations and individuals with germ line mutations to VHL are predisposed to a number of vascular abnormalities as well as renal cancer.

Approximately 25–30% of people have metastatic spread by the time they are diagnosed with renal cell carcinoma [248]. The second commonest subtype is papillary renal cancer which is subdivided into types 1 and 2 which are associated with MET (cMET mutations) and FH (fumarate hydratase) mutations, respectively. Less common (and less malignant histological types) include oncocytoma and chromophore tumours.

At least four hereditary syndromes have been associated with renal cell carcinoma: von Hippel-Lindau (VHL) syndrome, hereditary papillary renal carcinoma (HPRC), familial renal oncocytoma (FRO) associated with Birt-Hogg-Dube syndrome (BHDS), and hereditary renal carcinoma (HRC) [249].

Renal cell carcinoma develops in nearly 40% of patients with VHL syndrome. Deletions of 3p occur commonly in renal cell carcinoma associated with VHL disease. The VHL gene is mutated in a high number of tumours with sporadic (non-hereditary) clear cell renal carcinoma. Mutations of the VHL gene result in the accumulation of hypoxia inducible factors (HIFs) that stimulate

---

Box 45.2 2013 European guidelines for post-UTUC treatment follow-up

After RNU, over at least five years

Non-invasive tumour

Cystoscopy/urinary cytology at three months and then yearly

CT every year

Invasive tumour

Cystoscopy/urinary cytology at three months and then yearly

CT urography every six months over two years and then yearly

After conservative management, over at least five years

Urinary cytology and CT urography at three and six months, and then yearly

Cystoscopy, ureteroscopy and cytology in situ at three and six months, and then every six months over two years, and then yearly

Reprinted from *European Urology*, Volume 63, Issue 6, Rouprêt M et al., European guidelines on upper tract urothelial carcinomas: 2013 update, pp. 1059–1071, Copyright © 2013 European Association of Urology, with permission from Elsevier, http://www.sciencedirect.com/science/journal/03022838

---

angiogenesis through vascular endothelial growth factor (VEGF) and its receptor (VEGFR) [250].

The risk of kidney cancer increases with age; other risk factors include smoking, obesity, hypertension, and the long-term use of non-steroidal anti-inflammatory drugs. Patients with end stage renal failure and tuberous sclerosis also have a higher chance of developing renal cell cancer [249].

Diagnosis

The application of ultrasound and cross-sectional imaging techniques in clinical practice has led to an increase in the detection of asymptomatic renal tumours and small renal masses. Approximately 50% of all kidney tumours are presently detected as incidental masses on non-invasive imaging and these findings by far supersede the classic triad of flank pain, haematuria, and a palpable mass [251]. Less common symptoms that may lead to the diagnosis of renal cell carcinoma are varicoceles, para-neoplastic syndromes as well as specific clinical signs following metastasis.

It is generally agreed that whole body CT imaging should be performed in patients with adequate renal function to assess local and systemic extent of the disease and aid in planning the therapeutic approach [251]. This includes a CT of the chest as the most accurate diagnostic tool to rule out pulmonary metastases. CT imaging sequences should be performed prior to and after injection of intravenous contrast medium. If required, ultrasound or magnetic resonance imaging can be supplemental, especially for visualization of vena cava involvement. There is an increasing role of pretherapeutic percutaneous renal biopsies. This is in part a consequence of the introduction of alternatives for surgical approaches for small renal masses, such as thermal ablation or active surveillance. In these situations, a proper histological diagnosis is desirable for risk assessment and tailoring follow-up. In metastatic disease a biopsy

may help to determine the subtype of RCC which has consequences for the selection of targeted therapy.

The most common subtype of RCC is clear cell carcinoma (75–85%) followed by papillary RCC (10–15%), chromophobe RCC (5%), and the rare collecting duct carcinoma (1%). As these subtypes differ in clinical course and response to therapy knowledge of the subtype may be of importance prior to planning therapy in certain clinical settings [252]. Approximately 30% of small renal masses are benign and a pretreatment biopsy may aid in selecting the best approach in patients with comorbidity or renal function impairment.

Following imaging RCC should be staged according to the 2009 UICC/TNM classification. The TNM staging for RCC can be accessed on the website of the American Cancer Society: <http://www.cancer.org/cancer/kidneycancer/detailedguide/kidney-cancer-adult-staging>.

Surgery

Surgical management of RCC is dependent on local and systemic extent of the disease [251]. Due to an increase in the diagnosis of small incidental renal masses nephron-sparing approaches for localized RCC are gaining ground. The role of active surveillance of small renal tumours is controversial and currently under investigation. It is of concern that even tumours smaller than 4 cm carry a risk of developing metastatic disease and the growth rate does not follow a linear pattern but instead may unpredictably increase in 20–25% of patients in active surveillance protocols. As a consequence, nephron-sparing surgery—or partial nephrectomy—is regarded the standard of care for renal tumours of ≥ 4 cm diameter. The surgical approach can be open, laparoscopic, or robot-assisted and will largely depend on the local surgical expertise and facilities. Although experienced single centres have demonstrated that laparoscopic partial nephrectomy can be performed safely with similar outcome in comparison to an open approach, retrospective multicentre data suggest that the surgical complication rate with laparoscopic partial nephrectomy is higher than with an open approach. Of additional concern is the longer warm ischemia time observed with laparoscopic partial nephrectomy that may have long term consequences for renal function. Robot-assisted laparoscopic partial nephrectomy may improve the laparoscopic approach but present data are premature to define the role of this technique. Guidelines, therefore, recommend the open approach as standard and the laparoscopic approaches as options in experienced hands [251].

A randomized trial for cT1a tumours has confirmed the oncological safety of partial nephrectomy in comparison to nephrectomy, and epidemiological data suggest that preservation of renal function is correlated to an improved overall survival independent of the diagnosis of RCC. The extent of the margin of renal tissue surrounding the tumour at surgery is not associated with local recurrence and there are reports suggesting that enucleation of the tumour and even positive surgical margins are without clinical consequences [253]. Increasing retrospective data suggest that it is not the size of the primary tumour but its location within the kidney which limits nephron-sparing surgery and case series report similar outcome and safety in ≥ cT1b RCC. Despite the recommendation of most guidelines that total nephrectomy should not be performed in patients with cT1a tumours it has to be recognized that the resection of some lesions is technically not feasible.

The surgical risk can be assessed prior to surgery with nephrometry scores. Epidemiological data on tumours of ≥ 4 cm show that partial nephrectomy is increasingly performed albeit still at a lower rate than total nephrectomy [254]. Patients with small renal masses can also be treated by thermal ablation such as radiofrequency or cryo-ablation (RFA and CA). The potential advantages of these minimal invasive approaches have led to initial experience in selected elderly and frail patients but more recent case series report safe oncological long-term outcome in general patient populations. Current data suggest that CA, which is often performed after laparoscopic exposition of the renal mass, yields better local control than the percutaneous RFA approach. Most critics of CA, however, argue that the laparoscopic approach abrogates its potential benefits over a laparoscopic partial nephrectomy. However, due to a lack of randomized studies the role of these techniques is ill-defined. Nephron-sparing surgery is the current standard of care but guidelines recognize ablation as a therapeutic option in selected patients [255].

Localized RCCs which are not suitable for partial nephrectomy due to either locally advanced tumour growth or an unfavourable location are best treated by laparoscopic or open nephrectomy. According to most international and national guidelines a laparoscopic nephrectomy should be favoured due to lower morbidity and faster recovery in comparison to open surgery for patients with cT1 and cT2 tumours in whom nephron sparing surgery is not feasible. Long-term follow-up has shown no difference in oncological outcome in comparison to open radical nephrectomy. Retrospective studies on volume and outcome association suggest that laparoscopic nephrectomy has a lower complication rate to open nephrectomy, which are more likely to be fatal [256–258].

Based on large retrospective data sets it is recommended that routine adrenalectomy is not indicated if presurgical cross-sectional imaging reveals no adrenal abnormalities [251].

The role of lymphadenectomy in RCC has been investigated in one single randomized phase III study (EORTC 30881) which failed to show a survival advantage of performing a complete lymph node dissection (LND) in patients with RCC [259]. Despite these results, the role of LND remains controversial since the definition of the extent of LND varies and the EORTC trial population predominantly included tumour stages with a low risk of occult lymph node metastasis. Only 4% of all patients in the LND arm revealed unsuspected lymph node metastases. Randomized trials with sufficient statistical power to specifically investigate the therapeutic or staging value in high risk patients are lacking. Currently, guidelines recommend for patients with clinically unsuspected lymph nodes on cross sectional imaging to perform standard LND for staging purposes only if indicated. However, suspicious nodes on preoperative imaging should be removed [260, 261].

In patients with renal or caval vein involvement without metastatic disease (cT3a-T3c) nephrectomy and thrombectomy can be curative and improve prognosis. To indicate the level of the tumour thrombus and assist in planning the surgical approach—which may be multidisciplinary—the thrombus can be staged as stage I (adjacent to the ostium of the renal vein), II (extending below the liver), III (involving the intrahepatic IVC but below the diaphragm and IV (extending above the diaphragm). While most surgeons would feel comfortable in performing a nephrectomy with thrombectomy in patients with level I or II as an open approach some centres have reported successful laparoscopic procedures. Due to the relative paucity of level III and IV thrombi and the need for potential cardiopulmonary bypasses it is recommended that these patients are treated in selected centres. Due to the unpredictable effect of targeted therapy on tumour thrombus downsizing primary surgical resection is favoured whenever feasible [262].

For patients with primary metastatic RCC and the tumour in situ, cytoreductive nephrectomy, with or without metastasectomy, is controversial. It is recognized that complete surgical removal of the primary tumour and metastases, if feasible, may cure selected patients. However, in the majority cytoreductive nephrectomy is part of a multimodality treatment including systemic therapy, and may at best lead to an improved overall survival. Alternatively, a complete surgical resection may lead to a delay starting systemic therapy, with its own adverse side effects.

Randomized phase III trials of interferon alpha with or without cytoreductive nephrectomy demonstrated a survival benefit of six months for surgery versus no surgery [263]. Currently, phase III trials investigating the role and sequence of cytoreductive nephrectomy are ongoing. Until these trials report it is generally recommended to perform cytoreductive nephrectomy in patients with oligometastatic disease and a good performance. For patients with metachronous metastasis following nephrectomy with curative intent, retrospective data suggest that complete metastasectomy of single, or oligometastases confers a survival benefit [264]. Due to the lack of randomized trials in this setting it still remains unclear in how far a selection of patients with a protracted course of the disease contributes to the beneficial outcome observed after metastasectomy [265].

Medical treatment of patients with metastatic or advanced disease

All randomized studies to date have focused on patients with clear cell renal cancer. A prognostic scoring system, developed out of the Memorial Sloan Kettering Cancer Center (MSKCC) has been widely used to stratify patients into good-, intermediate-, and poor-risk groups.

First-line treatment

Metastatic RCC is notoriously chemoresistant, and until recently, immunotherapy (in particular interferon-alpha) has represented the treatment of choice. However, this has proven to be largely ineffective and toxic, especially in patients with MSKCC intermediate- and poor-risk disease. There is still a role for high dose il-2 in a small subset of good-risk patients. Long-term remission has been extensively described in this group; however, this population is not well defined [266].

The increase in understanding of the biology of RCC has resulted in the development of targeted therapies including vascular endothelial growth factor multikinase inhibitors (VEGF TKIs) (sunitinib, sorafenib, axitinib, pazopanib), VEGF antibodies (bevacizumab), and mammalian target of rapamycin (mTOR) inhibitors (temsirolimus, everolimus) [266].

Both sunitinib and pazopanib are indicated for the first-line therapy of metastatic RCC as a consequence of a positive phase III trial versus interferon-alpha [267, 268]. Common toxicity includes hand-foot syndrome, hypertension, fatigue, and mucositis. Bevacizumab is also indicated in the first-line treatment of metastatic RCC given in combination with interferon-alpha as a consequence of two positive phase III trials [269]. Positive randomized data also exists for temsirolimus in patients with MSKCC poor-risk disease.

Two recent studies have compared sunitinib and pazopanib [269, 270]. Together, they showed that pazopanib was no less effective than sunitinib. However, symptomatic toxicity and patients preference favoured pazopanib. Liver toxicity was more common with pazopanib. The overall survival for these patients is in the region of 30 months, compared to 12 months in the pre-TKI era.

Second-line treatment

Sequential therapy is established in clear cell renal cancer. However, subsequent therapies follow a law of diminishing returns and cross resistance occurs. This includes VEFG and mTOR targets [271]. Second-line progression-free survival is between three and six months which is half that of first-line therapy. The median overall survival of patients who are resistant to first-line therapy is between one and two years.

Treatment after cytokine therapy

Sorafenib, pazopanib, and axitinib have positive randomized data in this area [270, 272, 273]. However, axitinib is superior to sorafenib in terms of progression-free survival and is therefore perhaps the optimal agent.

Treatment after VEGF-targeted agents

A phase III randomized double blind placebo controlled trial looked at the use of everolimus (mTOR inhibitor) in patients who developed progressive disease following the use of vascular endothelial growth factor targeted therapy. In this study, patients had progressed on sunitinib, sorafenib or both were randomized to receive either everolimus or placebo. Results showed there was an improved median progression-free survival in the everolimus arm (four months, 95% CI 3.7–5.5) compared to the placebo arm (1.9 months, 95% CI 1.8–1.9). The most commonly reported adverse events were stomatitis, fatigue, and rash [274]. Everolimus is therefore recommended in VEGF-refractory disease.

Recent results of the AXIS phase 3 trial demonstrated improved efficacy (progression-free survival) with second-line axitinib compared with sorafenib in patients who progressed on a variety of first-line targeted therapies, including sunitinib and interferon. Results showed that axitinib resulted in a longer progression-free survival compared to sorafenib: 6.7 months with axitinib compared to 4.7 months with sorafenib (hazard ratio 0.665; 95% CI 0.544–0.812; one-sided p <0.0001). The progression-free survival in the sunitinib-refractory patients was also superior for axitinib (4.6 months compared to 3.8 for sorafenib). However, there here was no overall survival difference. The most common side effects for axitinib were diarrhoea, hypertension, and fatigue [273].

In view of these findings, available clinical evidence, individual patient profile, and toxicity concerns should be carefully evaluated when deciding whether to administer everolimus or axitinib after progression on a first-line VEGF TKI.

Third-line treatment

The RECORD-1 study included patients who have failed multiple lines of VEFG-targeted therapy. Therefore, everolimus can be used third- or even fourth-line in VEGF-refractory disease [274]. There is no robust data for sunitinib, axitinib, or pazopanib in this setting.

Dovitinib has recent been tested in the third-line setting. It was compared to sorafenib in patients who had failed first-line VEFG TKI and second-line mTOR inhibitors. Dovitinib is a multitargeted receptor tyrosine kinase inhibitor that offers broader inhibition of the fibroblast growth factor receptor (FGFR) by binding FGFRS 1, 2, and 3. In addition, it also targets the platelet derived growth factor receptor (PDGFR), and VEGF receptors. The primary end-point was not met by the trial. The PFS was 3.7 and 3.6 months in the dovitinib and sorafenib arms, respectively (HR 0.86; p = 0.063). Median overall survival was also early the same at 11.1 months with dovitinib and 11.0 months in the sorafenib arm (HR 0.96; p = 0.357). The main side effects associated with dovitinib were diarrhoea, nausea, and vomiting [275].

Combination therapy

To date, no combination of targeted agents (including three randomized studies) has shown any benefit in combining any of the drugs mentioned above.

Biomarkers

No biomarkers exist to predict response to targeted therapy. Functional imaging has also proven ineffective. Radiological response to treatment and progression on cross-sectional imaging are widely used to determine staring and switching therapy.

Protein, gene, and DNA biomarkers have not been widely explored in this setting. What data is available is largely unhelpful. It appears that baseline angiogenic biomarkers such as VEGF ligand and receptor expression do not predict outcome [276].

Carbonic anhydrase IX (CAIX) was investigated as a predictive marker in patients with metastatic clear cell renal cell carcinoma (CCRCC) receiving high dose interleukin-2. Despite promising preliminary data, prospective data show no predictive effect [277].

References

1. Arya M, Li R, Pegler K, Sangar V, Kelly JD et al. Long-term trends in incidence, survival and mortality of primary penile cancer in England. Cancer Causes Control 2013; 24(12): 2169–2176.
2. Pow Sang MR, Benavente V, Pow Sang JE et al. Cancer of the penis. Cancer Control 2002; 9: 305–314.
3. Broders AC. Squamous cell epithelioma of the skin. Annals of Surgery 1921: 73: 141.
4. Pizzacaro G, Algaba F, Horenblas S et al. EAU Penile Cancer Guidelines 2009. European Urology 2010; 57: 1002–1012.
5. Opjordsmoen S, Fossa SD. Quality of life in patients treated for penile cancer. A follow-up study. British Journal of Urology 1994; 74(5): 652–657.
6. Agrawal A, Pai D, et al. The histological extent of the local spread of carcinoma of the penis and its therapeutic implications. British Journal of Urology International 2000; 85(2): 299–301.
7. Hoffman M, Renshaw A, Loughlin KR. Squamous cell carcinoma of the penis and microscopic pathologic margins. How much margin is needed for local cure? Cancer 1999; 85(7): 1565–1568.
8. Minhas S, Kayes O, Hegarty P et al. What surgical resection margins are required to achieve oncological control in men with primary penile cancer? British Journal of Urology International 2005; 96(7): 1040–1043.
9. Tercedor J, Lopez Hernandez B. Papilomavirus humanos y carcinoma epidermoide cutaneo-mucoso. Piel 1991; 6: 470–471.
10. Malek RS. Laser treatment of premalignant and squamous cell lesions of the penis. Lasers in Surgery and Medicine 1992;12: 246–253.
11. Goette DK, Elgart M, DeVillez RL. Erythroplasia of Queyrat. Treatment with topically applied fluorouracil. Journal of the American Medical Association 1975; 232(9): 934–937.

12. Micali G, Nasca MR, Tedeschi A. Topical treatment of intraepithelial penile carcinoma with imiquimod. Clinical and Experimental Dermatology 2003; 28(Suppl 1): 4–6.

13. Windhal T, Hellsten S. Laser treatment of localised squamous cell carcinoma of the penis. Journal of Urology 1995; 154: 1020–1023.

14. Shirahama T, Takemoto M, Nishiyama K et al. A new treatment for penile conservation in penile carcinoma: a preliminary study of combined laser hyperthermia, radiation and chemotherapy. British Journal of Urology 1998; 82: 687–693.

15. Meijer RP, Boon TA, van Venrooij GE, Wijburg CJ. Longterm follow-up after laser therapy for penile carcinoma. Urology 2007; 69(4): 759–762.

16. Windahl T, Anderson SO. Combined laser treatment for penile carcinoma: results after long-term follow up. Journal of Urology 2003; 169(6): 2118–2121.

17. Tietjen DN, Malek RS. Laser therapy of squamous cell dysplasia and carcinoma of the penis. Urology 1998; 52(4): 559–565.

18. Bandieramonte G, Colecchia M, Mariani L et al. Peniscopically controlled CO2 laser excision for conservative treatment of in situ and T1 penile carcinoma: report of 224 patients. European Urology 2008; 54(4): 875–882.

19. Depasquale I, Park AJ, Bracka A. The treatment of balanitis xerotica obliterans. British Journal of Urology International 2000; 86(4): 459–465.

20. Hadway P, Corbishley CM, Watkin NA. Total glans resurfacing for premalignant lesions of the penis: initial outcome data. British Journal of Urology International 2006; 98(3): 532–536.

21. Shabbir M, Muneer A, Kalsi J, Shukla CJ, Zacharakis E et al. Glans resurfacing for the treatment of carcinoma in situ of the penis: surgical technique and outcomes. European Urology 2011; 59(1): 142–147.

22. Bissada NK. Conservative extirpative treatment of cancer of the penis. Urologic Clinics of North America 1992; 19(2): 283–292.

23. McDougall WS, Kirchner FK, Edward RH, Killian LT. Treatment of carcinoma of the penis: the case of primary lymphadenectomy. Journal of Urology 1986; 136: 38–41.

24. Das S. Penile amputation for the management of primary carcinoma of the penis. Urologic Clinics of North America 1992; 19(2): 277–282.

25. Pizzocaro G, Piva L, Tana S. Up-to-date management of carcinoma of the penis. European Urology 1997; 32: 5–15.

26. Colberg JW, Andriloe GL, et al. Surgical management of penile cancer. In Vogelzang NJ, Scardino PT, Shipley WU et al. eds. Comprehensive Textbook of Genitourinary Oncology. Baltimore: Williams and Wilkins, 1999, 1103–1109.

27. Pietrzak P, Corbishley C, Watkin NA. Organ sparing surgery for invasive penile cancer. Early follow up data. British Journal of Urology International 2004; 94: 1253–1257.

28. Lindegaard JC, Nielsen OS, et al. A retrospective analysis of 82 cases of cancer of the penis. British Journal of Urology 1996; 77(6): 883–890.

29. Horenblas S, Van Tintern H. Squamous cell carcinoma of the penis. IV. Prognostic factors of survival: analysis of tumour, nodes, and metastatic classification system. Journal of Urology 151; 1239–1243.

30. Lont AP, Gallee MPW, Meinhardt W, van Tintern H, Horenblas S. Penis conserving treatment for T1 and T2 penile carcinoma: clinical implications of a local recurrence. Journal of Urology 2006; 176: 575–580.

31. Bracka A. Organerhaltende operationstechnik bei karzinomen der glans penis. Akt Urol 1996; 27: 1–V1.

32. Scardino E, Villa G, Bonomo G et al. Magnetic resonance imaging combined with artificial erection for local staging of penile cancer. Urology 2004; 63: 1158–1162.

33. Malone PR, Thomas JS, Blick C. A tie over dressing for graft application in distal penectomy and glans resurfacing: the TODGA technique. British Journal of Urology International 2011; 107(5): 836–840.

34. Smith Y, Hadway P, Biedrzcki O, Perry MJA, Corbishley C et al. Reconstructive surgery for invasive squamous carcinoma of the glans penis. European Urology 2007; 52(4): 1179–1185.

35. Brown CT, Minhas S, Ralph DJ. Conservative surgery for penile cancer: subtotal glans excision without grafting. British Journal of Urology International 2005; 96: 911–912.

36. Gulino G, Sasso F, Falabella R, et al. Distal urethral reconstruction of the glans for penile carcinoma: results of a novel technique at 1-year follow up. Journal of Urology 2007; 178(3): 941–944.

37. Smith Y, Hadway P, Ahmed S et al. Penile preserving surgery for male distal urethral carcinoma. British Journal of Urology International 2007; 100(1): 82–87.

38. Miranda-Sousa A, Keating M, Moreira S, Baker M, Carrion R. Concomitant ventral phalloplasty during penile implant surgery: a novel procedure that optimizes patient satisfaction and their perception of phallic length after penile implant surgery. Journal of Sexual Medicine 2007; 4: 1494–1499.

39. Shabbir M, Hughes BE, Swallow T, Corbishley C, Perry MJA et al. Management of chronic ulceration after radiotherapy for penile cancer. Journal of Urology 2008; 179(4): 785.

40. McLean M, Ahmed M, Warde P et al. The results of primary radiation therapy in the management of squamous cell carcinoma of the penis. International Journal of Radiation Oncology Biology Physics 1993; 25(4): 623–628.

41. Ornellas AA, Seixas AL, Marota A, Wisnescky A, Campos F et al. Surgical treatment of invasive squamous cell carcinoma of the penis: retrospective analysis of 350 cases. Journal of Urology 1994; 151: 1244–1249.

42. Abi-Aad AS, DeKernion JB. Controversies in ilioinguinal lymphadenectomy for cancer of the penis. Urologic Clinics of North America 1992; 19: 319–324.

43. Horenblas S, Van Tinteren H, Delemarre JF, Moonen LM, Lustig V et al. Squamous cell carcinoma of the penis: accuracy of tumour, nodes and metastasis classification system, and role of lymphangiography, computerized tomography scan and fine needle aspiration cytology. Journal of Urology 1991; 146: 1279–1283.

44. Bevan-Thomas R, Slaton JW, Pettaway CA. Contemporary morbidity from lymphadenectomy for penile squamous cell carcinoma: the M.D. Anderson Cancer Center Experience. Journal of Urology 2002; 167: 1638–1642.

45. Graafland NM, Lam W, Leijte JA, Yap T, Gallee MP et al. Prognostic factors for occult inguinal lymph node involvement in penile carcinoma and assessment of the high-risk EAU subgroup: a two-institution analysis of 342 clinically node-negative patients. European Urology 2010; 58(5): 742–747.

46. Solsona E, Iborra I, Rubio J, Casanova JL, Ricos JV et al. Prospective validation of the association of local tumour stage and grade as a predictive factor for occult lymph node micrometastasis in patients with penile carcinoma and clinically negative inguinal lymph nodes. Journal of Urology 2001; 165: 1506–1509.

47. Slaton JW, Morgenstern N, Levy DA et al. Tumour stage, vascular invasion and the percentage of poorly differentiated cancer: independent prognosticators for inguinal lymph node metastasis in penile squamous cancer. Journal of Urology 2001; 165: 1138–1142.

48. Solsona E, Iborra I, Ricos JV et al. Corpus cavernosum invasion and tumour grade in the prediction of lymph node condition in penile carcinoma. European Urology 1992; 22: 115–118.

49. Cabanas RM. An approach for the treatment of penile carcinoma. Cancer 1977; 39: 456–466.

50. Pettaway CA, Pisters LL, Dinney CP et al. Sentinel lymph node dissection for penile carcinoma: the M. D. Anderson Cancer Center experience. Journal of Urology 1995; 154: 1999–2003.

51. Mansel RE, Fallowfield L, Kissin M et al. Randomized multicentre trial of sentinel node biopsy versus standard axillary treatment in operable breast cancer: the ALMANAC trial. Journal of the National Cancer Institute 2006; 98: 599–609.

52. Veronesi U, Paganelli G, Viale G et al. A randomized comparison of sentinel node biopsy with routine axillary dissection in breast cancer. New England Journal of Medicine 2003; 349: 546–553.

53. Goyal A, Mansel R. Current status of sentinel lymph node biopsy in solid malignancies. World Journal of Surgical Oncology 2004; 2: 9.

54. Hadway P, Lynch M, Heenan S, Watkin NA. Current status of dynamic lymphoscintigraphy and sentinel lymph node biopsy in urological malignancies. British Journal of Urology International 2005; 96: 1235–1239.

55. Kroon BK, Horenblas S, Meinhardt W et al. Dynamic sentinel node biopsy in penile carcinoma. Evaluation of 10 years experience. European Urology 2005; 47: 601–606.

56. Leijte JAP, Kroon BK, Valdés Olmos RA, Nieweg OE, Horenblas S. Reliability and safety of current dynamic sentinel node biopsy for penile carcinoma. European Urology 2007; 52: 170–177.

57. Leijte JA, Hughes B, Graafland NM, et al. Two-center evaluation of dynamic sentinel node biopsy for squamous cell carcinoma of the penis. Journal of Clinical Oncology 2009; 27: 3325–3329.

58. Lam W, Alnajjar HM, La-Touche S, Perry M, Sharma D et al. Dynamic sentinel lymph node biopsy in patients with invasive squamous cell carcinoma of the penis: a prospective study of the long-term outcome of 500 inguinal basins assessed at a single institution. European Urology 2013; 63(4): 657–663.

59. Kroon BK, Horenblas S, Lont AP, Tanis PJ, Gallee MP et al. Patients with penile carcinoma benefit from immediate resection of clinically occult lymph node metastases. Journal of Urology 2005; 173: 816–819.

60. Sadeghi R, Gholami H, Zakavi SR, Kakhki VR, Tabasi KT et al. Accuracy of sentinel lymph node biopsy for inguinal lymph node staging of penile squamous cell carcinoma: systematic review and meta-analysis of the literature. Journal of Urology 2012; 187(1): 25–31.

61. Djajadiningrat RS, Graafland NM, van Werkhoven E, Meinhardt W, Bex A et al. Contemporary management of regional nodes in penile cancer: improvement of survival? Journal of Urology 2013; pii: S0022-5347(13)05054-4.

62. Pizzacaro G, Algaba F, Horenblas S, Solsona S, Tana S et al. EAU guidelines on Penile Cancer. European Urology 2010; 57: 1002–1012.

63. Brouwer OR, Buckle T, Vermeeren L, Klop WMC, Balm AJM et al. Comparing the hybrid fluorescent–radioactive tracer indocyanine green–99mTc-nanocolloid with 99mTc-nanocolloid for sentinel node identification: a validation study using lymphoscintigraphy and SPECT/CT. Journal of Nuclear Medicine 2012; 53: 1034–1040.

64. Verhoeven RHA, Janssen-Heijnen MLG, Saum KU, Zanetti R, Caldarella A et al. The EUNICE Survival Working Group. Population-based survival of penile cancer patients in Europe and the United States of America: no improvement since 1990. European Journal of Cancer 2013; 49: 1414–1442.

65. Visser O, Adolffson J, Rossi S, Verne J, Gatta G et al. Incidence and survival of rare urogenital cancers in Europe. European Journal of Cancer 2012; 48(4): 456–464.

66. Sant M, Allemani C, Santaquilani M, Knijn A, Marchesi F, Capocaccia R; EUROCARE Working Group. EUROCARE-4. Survival of cancer patients diagnosed in 1995–1999. Results and commentary. European Journal of Cancer 2009; 45(6): 931–991.

67. Graafland NM, Verhoeven RH, Coebergh JW, Horenblas S. Incidence trends and survival of penile squamous cell carcinoma in the Netherlands. International Journal of Cancer 2011; 128(2): 426–432.

68. Marty R, Roze S, Bresse X, Largeron N, Smith-Palmer J. Estimating the clinical benefits of vaccinating boys and girls against HPV-related diseases in Europe. BMC Cancer 2013; 13: 10.

69. Shabbir M, Barod R, Hegarty PK, Minhas S. Primary prevention and vaccination for penile cancer. Therapeutic Advances in Urology 2013; 5(3):161–169.

70. Cubilla AL, Lloveras B, Alejo M, Clavero O, Chaux A et al. The basaloid cell is the best tissue marker for human papillomavirus in invasive penile squamous cell carcinoma: a study of 202 cases from Paraguay. American Journal of Surgical Pathology 2010; 34(1): 104–114.

71. Eichler H, Kong S, Gerth W, Mavros P, Jönsson B. Use of cost-effectiveness analysis in health-care resource allocation decision-making: how are cost-effectiveness thresholds are expected to emerge? Value Health 2004; 7: 518–528

72. Centers for Disease Control and Prevention. Recommendations on the use of quadrivalent human papillomavirus vaccine in males—Advisory Committee on Immunization Practices (ACIP). Morbidity and Mortality Weekly Report 2011; 60: 1705–1708.

73. Protzel C, Hakenberg OW. Chemotherapy in patients with penile carcinoma. International Journal of Urology 2009; 82: 1–7.

74. Kattan J, Culine S, Droz JP, Fadel E, Court B et al. Penile cancer chemotherapy: twelve years' experience at Institut Gustave-Roussy. Urology 1993; 42: 559–562.

75. Hakenberg O, Protzel C. Chemotherapy in penile cancer. Therapeutic Advances in Urology 2012; 4(3): 133–138.

76. Dexeus FH, Logothetis CJ, Sella A, Amato R, Kilbourn R et al. Combination chemotherapy with methotrexate, bleomycin and cisplatin for advanced squamous cell carcinoma of the male genital tract. Journal of Urology 1991; 146: 1284–1287.

77. Pagliaro LC, Williams DL, Daliani D, Williams MB, Osai W et al. Neoadjuvant paclitaxel, ifosfamide, and cisplatin chemotherapy for metastatic penile cancer: a phase II study. Journal of Clinical Oncology 2010; 28: 3851–3857.

78. Bermejo C, Busby JE, Spiess PE, Heller L, Pagliaro LC et al. Neoadjuvant chemotherapy followed by aggressive surgical consolidation for metastatic penile squamous cell carcinoma. Journal of Urology 2007; 177: 1335–1338.

79. Leijte JA, Kerst JM, Bais E, Antonini N, Horenblas S. Neoadjuvant chemotherapy in advanced penile carcinoma. European Urology 2007; 52: 488–494.

80. Wells A. EGF receptor. International Journal of Biochemistry Cell Biology 1999; 31: 637–643.

81. Lavens N, Gupta R, Wood LA. EGFR overexpression in squamous cell carcinoma of the penis. Current Oncology 2010; 17(1): 4–6.

82. Salomon DS, Brandt R, Ciardiello F, Normanno N. Epidermal growth factor-related peptides and their receptors in human malignancies. Critical Reviews in Oncology/Hematology 1995; 19: 183–232.

83. Di Lorenzo G, Buonerba C, Gaudioso G, Gigantino V, Quarto G et al. EGFR mutational status in penile cancer. Expert Opinion on Therapeutic Targets 2013; 17(5): 501–505.

84. Di Lorenzo G, Perdonà S, Buonerba C, Sonpavde G, Gigantino V et al. Cytosolic phosphorylated EGFR is predictive of recurrence in early stage penile cancer patients: a retrospective study. Journal of Translational Medicine 2013; 11(1): 161.

85. Gou HF, Li X, Qiu M, Cheng K, Li LH et al. Epidermal growth factor receptor (EGFR)-RAS signaling pathway in penile squamous cell carcinoma. PLoS One 2013; 8(4): e62175.

86. Valverde CM, Hernandez-Losa J, Ferrandiz-Pulido C et al. BRAF and KRAS mutations in penile cancer and their correlation with clinical features. Journal of Clinical Oncology 2011; 29(Suppl 7) abstr 221.

87. Andersson P, Kolaric A, Windahl T, et al. PIK3CA, HRAS and KRAS gene mutations in human penile cancer. Journal of Urology 2008; 179: 2030–2034.

88. Stankiewicz E, Prowse DM, Ng M et al. Alternative HER/PTEN/Akt pathway activation in HPV positive and negative penile carcinomas. PLoS One 2011; 6(3): e17517.

89. Stankiewicz E, Prowse DM, Ktori E, et al. The retinoblastoma protein/p16 INK4A pathway but not p53 is disrupted by human papillomavirus in penile squamous cell carcinoma. Histopathology 2011; 58(3): 433–439.

90. Lopes A, Bezerra AL, Pinto CA, et al. p53 as a new prognostic factor for lymph node metastasis in penile carcinoma: analysis of 82 patients treated with amputation and bilateral lymphadenectomy. Journal of Urology 2002; 168: 81–86.

91. Poetsch M, Hemmerich M, Kakies C, et al. Alterations in the tumour suppressor gene p16 (INK4A) are associated with aggressive behavior of penile carcinomas. Virchows Archiv 2011; 458(2): 221–229.

92. Golijanin D, Tan JY, Kazior A, et al. Cyclooxygenase-2 and microsomal prostaglandin E synthase-1 are overexpressed in squamous cell carcinoma of the penis. Clinical Cancer Research 2004; 10: 1024–1031.

93. Carthon BC, Pettaway C, Pagliaro LC. Epidermal growth factor receptor (EGFR) targeted therapy in advanced metastatic squamous cell carcinoma (AMSCC) of the penis: updates and molecular analyses. Journal of Clinical Oncology 2010; 28(Suppl) abstr e15022.

94. Sonpavde G, Pagliaro LC, Buonerba C, Dorff TB, Lee RJ et al. Penile cancer: current therapy and future directions. Annals of Oncology 2013; 24(5): 1179–1189.

95. Zhu Y, Li H, Yao XD, et al. Feasibility and activity of sorafenib and sunitinib in advanced penile cancer: a preliminary report. International Journal of Urology 2010; 85: 334–340.

96. Caulfield MJ, Dilkes MG, Iles RK, Handel BT, Oliver RT. Rapid diagnosis of testicular choriocarcinoma by urinary pregnancy tests. Lancet 1990; 335(8699): 1230.

97. Heidenreich A, Moul JW. Contralateral testicular biopsy procedure in patients with unilateral testis cancer: is it indicated? Seminars in Urological Oncology 2002; 20(4): 234–238.

98. International Germ Cell Consensus Classification: a prognostic factor-based staging system for metastatic germ cell cancers. International Germ Cell Cancer Collaborative Group. Journal of Clinical Oncology 1997; 15(2): 594–603.

99. Nichols CR, Roth B, Albers P, Einhorn LH, Foster R et al. Active surveillance is the preferred approach to clinical stage I testicular cancer. Journal of Clinical Oncology 2013; 31(28): 3490–3493.

100. Warde P, Specht L, Horwich A, et al. Prognostic factors for relapse in stage I seminoma managed by surveillance: a pooled analysis. Journal of Clinical Oncology 2002; 20(22): 4448–4452.

101. Oliver RT, Mead GM, Rustin GJ, et al. Randomized trial of carboplatin versus radiotherapy for stage I seminoma: mature results on relapse and contralateral testis cancer rates in MRC TE19/EORTC 30982 study (ISRCTN27163214). Journal of Clinical Oncology 2011; 29(8): 957–962.

102. Schmoll HJ, Jordan K, Huddart R, Pes MP, Horwich A et al. ESMO Guidelines Working Group. Testicular seminoma: ESMO Clinical Practice Guidelines for diagnosis, treatment and follow-up. Annals of Oncology 2010; 21(Suppl 5): v140–6.

103. Cullen M. Surveillance or adjuvant treatments in stage 1 testis germ-cell tumours. Annals of Oncology 2012; 23(Suppl 10): x342–8.

104. Albers P, Siener R, Krege S, et al. Randomized phase III trial comparing retroperitoneal lymph node dissection with one course of bleomycin and etoposide plus cisplatin chemotherapy in the adjuvant treatment of clinical stage I Nonseminomatous testicular germ cell tumours: AUO trial AH 01/94 by the German Testicular Cancer Study Group. Journal of Clinical Oncology 2008; 26(18): 2966–2972.

105. de Wit R, Roberts JT, Wilkinson PM, de Mulder PH, Mead GM et al. Equivalence of three or four cycles of bleomycin, etoposide, and cisplatin chemotherapy and of a 3- or 5-day schedule in good-prognosis germ cell cancer: a randomized study of the European Organization for Research and Treatment of Cancer Genitourinary Tract Cancer Cooperative Group and the Medical Research Council. Journal of Clinical Oncology 2001; 19(6): 1629–1640.

106. Haugnes HS, Bosl GJ, Boer H, Gietema JA, Brydøy M et al. Long-term and late effects of germ cell testicular cancer treatment and implications for follow-up. Journal of Clinical Oncology 2012; 30(30): 3752–3763. doi:10.1200/JCO.2012.43.4431

107. Kondagunta GV, Bacik J, Bajorin D, et al. Etoposide and cisplatin chemotherapy for metastatic good-risk germ cell tumours. Journal of Clinical Oncology 2005; 23(36): 9290–9294.

108. Hinton S, Catalano PJ, Einhorn LH, Nichols CR, David Crawford E et al. Cisplatin, etoposide and either bleomycin or ifosfamide in the treatment of disseminated germ cell tumours: final analysis of an intergroup trial. Cancer 2003; 97(8): 1869–1875.

109. Fizazi K, Pagliaro L, Flechon A, Mardiak J, Geoffrois L et al. A phase III trial of personalized chemotherapy based on serum tumour marker decline in poor-prognosis germ-cell tumours: results of GETUG 13. ASCO 24 June 2013: LBA4500.

110. Lorch A, Beyer J, Bascoul-Mollevi C, Kramar A, Einhorn LH et al. Prognostic factors in patients with metastatic germ cell tumours who experienced treatment failure with cisplatin-based first-line chemotherapy. Journal of Clinical Oncology 2010; 28(33): 4906–4911.

111. Loehrer PJ Sr, Einhorn LH, Williams SD.VP-16 plus ifosfamide plus cisplatin as salvage therapy in refractory germ cell cancer. Journal of Clinical Oncology 1986; 4(4): 528–536.

112. Kondagunta GV, Bacik J, Donadio A, Bajorin D, Marion S et al. Combination of paclitaxel, ifosfamide, and cisplatin is an effective second-line therapy for patients with relapsed testicular germ cell tumours. Journal of Clinical Oncology 2005; 23(27): 6549–6555.

113. Einhorn LH, Williams SD, Chamness A, Brames MJ, Perkins SM et al. High-dose chemotherapy and stem-cell rescue for metastatic germ-cell tumours. New England Journal of Medicine 2007; 357(4): 340–348.

114. Feldman DR, Huddart R, Hall E, Beyer J, Powles T. Is high dose therapy superior to conventional dose therapy as initial treatment for relapsed germ cell tumours? The TIGER Trial. Journal of Cancer 2011; 2: 374–377.

115. Siegel R, Naishadham D, Jemal A. Cancer statistics, 2012. CA: A Cancer Journal for Clinicians 2012; 62: 10–29.

116. Ferlay J, Parkin DM, Steliarova-Foucher E. Estimates of cancer incidence and mortality in Europe in 2008. European Journal of Cancer 2010; 46: 765–781.

117. Andriole GL, Crawford ED, Grubb RL, et al. Prostate cancer screening in the randomized Prostate, Lung, Colorectal, and Ovarian cancer screening trial: mortality results after 13 years follow-up. Journal of the National Cancer Institute 2012; 104: 125–132.

118. Schröder FH, Hugosson J, Roobol MJ, et al. Prostate cancer mortality at 11 years of follow-up. New England Journal of Medicine 2012; 366: 981–990.

119. Klotz L. Cancer overdiagnosis and overtreatment. Current Opinions in Urology 2012; 22: 203–209.

120. Heijnsdijk EA, Wever EM, Auvinen A, et al. Quality-of-life effects of prostate-specific antigen screening. New England Journal of Medicine 2012; 367: 595–605.

121. Chou R, Croswell JM, Dana T, et al. Screening for prostate cancer: a review of the evidence for the U.S. Preventive Services Task Force. Annals of Internal Medicine 2011; 155: 762–771.

122. Kiemeney LA, Broeders MJ, Pelger M, et al. Screening for prostate cancer in Dutch hereditary prostate cancer families. International Journal of Cancer 2008; 122: 871–876.

123. Schröder FH, van der Maas P, Beemsterboer P, et al. Evaluation of the digital rectal examination as a screening test for prostate cancer. Rotterdam section of the European Randomized Study of Screening for prostate cancer. Journal of the National Cancer Institute 1998; 90: 1817–1823.

124. Borden LS Jr, Wright JL, Kim, J, Latchamsetty K, Porter CR. An abnormal digital rectal examination is an independent predictor of Gleason ≥7 prostate cancer in men undergoing initial prostate biopsy: a prospective study of 790 men. British Journal of Urology International 2007; 99: 559–563.

125. Loeb S, Sokoll LJ, Broyles DL, et al. Prospective multicentre evaluation of the Beckman Coulter Prostate Health Index using WHO calibration. Journal of Urology 2013; 189: 1702–1706.

126. Bussemakers MJ, van Bokhoven A, Verhaegh GW, et al. DD3: a new prostate-specific gene, highly overexpressed in prostate cancer. Cancer Research 1999; 59: 5975–5979.

127. de la Taille A, Irani J, Graefen M, et al. Clinical evaluation of the PCA3 assay in guiding initial biopsy decisions. Journal of Urology 2011; 185: 2119–2125.

128. Haese A, de la Taille A, van Poppel H, et al. Clinical utility of the PCA3 assay in European men scheduled for repeat biopsy. European Urology 2008; 54: 1081–1088.

129. Augustin H, Mayrhofer K, Pummer K, Mannweiler S. Relationship between prostate cancer gene 3 (PCA3) and characteristics of tumour aggressiveness. Prostate 2013; 73: 203–210.

130. Mitterberger M, Horninger W, Pelzer A, et al. A prospective randomized trial comparing contrast-enhanced targeted versus systematic ultrasound guided biopsies: impact on prostate cancer detection. Prostate 2007; 67: 1537–1542.

131. Pallwein L, Mitterberger M, Struve P, et al. Real-time elastography for detecting prostate cancer: preliminary experience. British Journal of Urology International 2007; 100: 42–46.

132. Simmons LA, Autier P Zat'ura F, et al. Detection, localisation and characterisation of prostate cancer by prostate HistoScanning™. British Journal of Urology International 2012; 110: 28–35.

133. Park BK, Park JW, Park SY, et al. Prospective evaluation of 3-T MRI performed before initial transrectal ultrasound-guided prostate biopsy in patients with high prostate-specific antigen and no previous biopsy. American Journal of Roentgenology 2011; 197: 876–881.

134. Hoeks CM, Schouten MG, Bomers JG, et al. Three-Tesla magnetic resonance-guided prostate biopsy in men with increased prostate-specific antigen and repeated, negative, random, systematic, transrectal ultrasound guided biopsies: detection of clinically significant prostate cancers. European Urology 2012; 62: 902–909.

135. Abuzallouf S, Daves I, Lukka H. Baseline staging of newly diagnosed prostate cancer: a summary of the literature. Journal of Urology 2004; 171: 2122–2127.

136. Lecouvet FE, El Mouedden J, Collette L, et al. Can whole-body magnetic resonance imaging with diffusion-weighted imaging replace Tc 99m bone scanning and computed tomography for single-step detection of metastases in patients with high-risk prostate cancer? European Urology 2012; 62: 68–75.

137. Picchio M, Spinapolice EG, Fallianca F, et al. [11C]Choline PET/CT detection of bone metastases in patients with PSA progression after primary treatment for prostate cancer: comparison with bone scintigraphy. European Journal of Nuclear Medicine and Molecular Imaging 2012; 39: 13–26.

138. Harisinganhi MG, Barentsz J, Hahn PF, et al. Noninvasive detection of clinically occult lymph-node metastases in prostate cancer. New England Journal of Medicine 2003; 348: 2491–2499.

139. Heesakkers RA, Hövels AM, Jager GJ, et al. MRI with lymph-node-specific contrast agent as an alternative to CT scan and lymph-node dissection in patients with prostate cancer: a prospective multicohort study. Lancet Oncology 2008; 9: 850–856.

140. Scattoni V, Zlotta A, Montironi R, Schulman C, Rigatti P et al. Extended and saturation prostatic biopsy in the diagnosis and characterisation of prostate cancer: a critical analysis of the literature. European Urology 2007; 52: 1309–1322.

141. Djavan B, Zlotta A, Remzi M, et al. Optimal predictors of prostate cancer on repeat biopsy: a prospective study of 1.051 men. Journal of Urology 2000; 163: 1144–1149.

142. Epstein JL, Alisbrook WC Jr, Amin MB, et al. The 2005 International Society of Urological Pathology (ISUP) consensus conference on Gleason grading of prostatic carcinoma. American Journal of Surgical Pathology 2005; 29: 128–142.

143. Gleason DF. Histologic grading in prostatic carcinoma. In Bostwick DG ed. Pathology of the Prostate. New York: Churchill Livingstone, 1990, 83–93.

144. Kattan MW, Eastham JA, Wheeler TM, et al. Counseling men with prostate cancer: a nomogram for predicting the presence of small, moderately differentiated, confined tumours. Journal of Urology 2003; 170: 1792–1797.

145. Ash D, Flynn A, Battermann J, et al. ESTRO/EAU/EORTC recommendations on permanent seed implantation for localized prostate cancer. Radiotherapy and Oncology 2000; 57: 315–321.

146. Albertsen PC, Hanley JA, Fine J. 20-year outcomes following conservative management of clinically localized prostate cancer. Journal of the American Medical Association 2005; 293: 2095–2101.

147. Wilt TJ, Brawer MK, Jones KM, et al. Radical prostatectomy versus observation for localized prostate cancer. New England Journal of Medicine 2012; 367: 203–213.

148. Klotz L. Active surveillance for favourable risk prostate cancer: rationale, risks, and results. Urologic Oncology 2007; 25: 505–509.

149. Han M, Partin AW, Pound CR, Epstein JI, Walsh PC. Long-term biochemical disease-free and cancer-specific survival following anatomic radical retropubic prostatectomy: the 15-year Johns Hopkins experience. Urologic Clinics of North America 2001; 28: 555–565.

150. Berryhill R Jr, Jhaveri J, Yadav R, et al. Robotic prostatectomy: a review of outcomes compared with laparoscopic and open approaches. Urology 2008; 72: 15–23.

151. Zietman AL, Bae K, Slater JD, et al. Randomized trial comparing conventional-dose with high-dose conformal radiation therapy in early-stage adenocarcinoma of the prostate: long-term results from proton radiation oncology group/American college of radiology 95-09. Journal of Clinical Oncology 2010; 28: 1106–1111.

152. Beckendorf V, Guerif S, Le Prisé E, et al. 70 Gy versus 80 Gy in localized prostate: 5-year results of GETUG 06 randomized trial. International Journal of Radiation Oncology Biology Physics 2011; 80: 1056–1063.

153. Wilt TJ, MacDonald R, Rutks I, Shamliyan TA, Taylor BC et al. Systematic review: comparative effectiveness and harms of treatments for clinically localized prostate cancer. Annals of Internal Medicine 2008; 148: 435–448.

154. Burnett AL, Aus G, Canby-Hagino ED, et al. Erectile function outcome reporting after clinically localized prostate cancer treatment. Journal of Urology 2007; 178: 597–601.

155. Henry AM, Al-Qaisieh B, Gould K, et al. Outcomes following iodine-125 monotherapy for localized prostate cancer: the results of Leeds 10-year single-centre brachytherapy experience. International Journal of Radiation Oncology Biology Physics 2010; 76: 50–56.

156. Morris WJ, Keyes M, Spadinger I, et al. Population-based 10-year oncologic outcomes after low-dose-rate brachytherapy for low-risk and intermediate-risk prostate cancer. Cancer 2013; 119: 1537–1546.

157. Bahn DK, Lee F, Badalament R, Kumar A, Greski J et al. Targeted cryoablation of the prostate: 7-year outcomes in the primary treatment of prostate cancer. Urology 2002; 60: 3–11.

158. Aus G. Current status of HIFU and cryotherapy in prostate cancer—a review. European Urology 2006; 50: 927–934.

159. Thüroff S, Chaussy C, Vallancien G, et al. High-intensity focused ultrasound and localized prostate cancer: efficacy results from the European multicentric study. Journal of Endourology 2003; 17: 673–677.

160. Cordeiro ER, Cathelineau X, Thüroff S, et al. High-intensity focused ultrasound (HIFU) for definitive treatment of prostate cancer. British Journal of Urology International 2012; 110: 1228–1242.

161. Eggener S, Salomon G, Scardino PT, de la Rosette J, Polascik TJ et al. Focal therapy for prostate cancer: possibilities and limitations. European Urology 2010; 58: 57–64.

162. Moore CM, Emberton M, Brown SG. Photodynamic therapy for prostate cancer—an emerging approach for organ-confined disease. Lasers in Surgery and Medicine 2011; 43: 768–775.

163. van den Bos W, Muller BG, de la Rosette JJ. A randomized controlled trial on focal therapy for localized prostate carcinoma: hemiablation versus complete ablation with irreversible electroporation. Journal of Endourology 2013; 27: 262–264.

164. Vos EK, Litjens GJ, Kobus T, et al. Assessment of prostate cancer aggressiveness using dynamic contrast-enhanced magnetic resonance imaging at 3 T. European Urology 2013; 64: 448–455.

165. Ahmed HU, Pendse D, Illing R, Allen C, van der Meulen JH et al. Will focal therapy become a standard of care for men with localized prostate cancer? Nature Clinical Practice Oncology 2007; 4: 632–642.

166. Studer UE, Whelan P, Albrecht W, et al. Immediate or deferred androgen deprivation for patients with prostate cancer not suitable for local treatment with curative intent: European Organisation for Research

and Treatment of Cancer (EORTC) Trial 30891. Journal of Clinical Oncology 2006; 24: 1868–1876.

167. Studer UE, Collette L, Whelan P, et al. Using PSA to guide timing of androgen deprivation in patients with T0-4 N0-2 M0 prostate cancer not suitable for local curative treatment (EORTC 30891). European Urology 2008; 53: 941–949.

168. Bolla M, Collette L, Blank L, et al. Long-term results with immediate androgen suppression and external irradiation in patients with locally advanced prostate cancer (an EORTC study): a phase III randomised trial. Lancet 2002; 360: 103–106.

169. Roach M 3rd, Bae K, Speight J, et al. Short-term neoadjuvant andro-gen deprivation therapy and external-beam radiotherapy for locally advanced prostate cancer: long-term results of RTOG 8610. Journal of Clinical Oncology 2008; 26: 585–591.

170. Bolla M, de Reijke TM, Van Tienhoven G, et al. Duration of androgen suppression in treatment of prostate cancer. New England Journal of Medicine 2009; 360: 2516–2527.

171. Bolla M, van Poppel H, Tombal B, Vekemans K, Da Pozzo L. Postoperative radiotherapy after radical prostatectomy for high-risk prostate cancer: long-term results of a randomised controlled trial (EORTC trial 22911). The Lancet 2012; 380(9858): 2018–2027. doi: 10.1016/S0140-6736(12)61253-7. Epub 2012 Oct 19.

172. Siegmann A, Bottke D, Faendrich J, et al. Salvage radiotherapy after prostatectomy—what is the best time to treat? Radiotherapy and Oncology 2012; 103: 239–243.

173. Huggins C. Effect of orchiectomy and irradiation on cancer of the prostate. Annals of Surgery 1942; 115: 1192–2000.

174. Eisenberger MA, Blumenstein BA, Crawford ED, et al. Bilateral orchi-ectomy with or without flutamide for metastatic prostate cancer. New England Journal of Medicine 1998; 339: 1036–1042.

175. Hedlund PO, Johansson R, Damber JE, et al. Significance of pretreat-ment cardiovascular morbidity as a risk factor during treatment with parenteral oestrogen or combined androgen deprivation of 915 patients with metastasized prostate cancer: evaluation of cardiovascu-lar events in a randomized trial. Scandinavian Journal of Urology and Nephrology 2011; 45: 346–353.

176. Ockrim JL, Lalani el-N, Kakkar AK, Abel P. Transdermal estradiol therapy for prostate cancer reduces thrombophilic activation and pro-tects against thromboembolism. Journal of Urology 2005; 174: 527–533.

177. Abrahamsson PA. Potential benefits of intermittent androgen suppres-sion therapy in the treatment of prostate cancer: a systematic review of the literature. European Urology 2010; 57: 49–59.

178. Petrylak DP, Tangen CM, Hussain MH, et al. Docetaxel and estra-mustine compared with mitoxantrone and prednisone for advanced refractory prostate cancer. New England Journal of Medicine 2004; 351: 1513–1520.

179. Tannock IF, de Wit R, Berry WR, et al. Docetaxel plus prednisone or mitoxantrone plus prednisone for advanced prostate cancer. New England Journal of Medicine 2004; 351: 1502–1512.

180. de Bono JS, Oudard S, Ozguroglu M, et al. Prednisone plus cabazi-taxel or mitoxantrone for metastatic castration-resistant prostate can-cer progressing after docetaxel treatment: a randomised open-label trial. Lancet 2010; 376: 1147–1154.

181. Scher HI, Fizazi K, Sad F, et al. Increased survival with enzalutamide in prostate cancer after chemotherapy. New England Journal of Medicine 2012; 367: 1187–1197.

182. Fizazi K, Scher HS, Molina A, et al. Abiraterone acetate for treat-ment of metastatic castration-resistant prostate cancer: final overall survival analysis of the COU-AA-301 randomised, double-blind, placebo-controlled phase 3 study. Lancet Oncology 2012; 13: 983–992.

183. Ryan CJ, Smith MR, de Bono JS, et al. Abiraterone in metastatic pros-tate cancer without previous chemotherapy. New England Journal of Medicine 2013; 368: 138–148.

184. Kantoff PW, Higano CS, Shore ND, et al. Sipuleucel-T immunother-apy for castration-resistant prostate cancer. New England Journal of Medicine 2010; 363: 411–422.

185. Parker C, Nilsson S, Heinrich D, et al. Alpha emitter radium-223 and survival in metastatic prostate cancer. New England Journal of Medicine 2013; 369: 213–223.

186. Jost SP, Gosling JA, Dixon JS. The morphology of normal human bladder urothelium. Journal of Anatomy 1989; 167: 103–115.

187. Cauberg ECC, Salomons MA, Kümmerlin IPED, de Reijke TM, Zwinderman AH et al. Trends in epidemiology and treatment of upper urinary tract tumours in the Netherlands 1995–2005: an analysis of PALGA, the Dutch national histopathology registry. British Journal of Urology International 2010; 105(7): 922–927.

188. Ploeg M, Aben KKH, Kiemeney LA. The present and future burden of urinary bladder cancer in the world. World Journal of Urology 2009; 27(3): 289–293.

189. Ferlay J, Steliarova-Foucher E, Lortet-Tieulent J, Rosso S, Coebergh JWW et al. Cancer incidence and mortality patterns in Europe: esti-mates for 40 countries in 2012. European Journal of Cancer 2013; 49(6): 1374–1403.

190. Vaidya A, Soloway MS, Hawke C, Tiguert R, Civantos F. De novo muscle invasive bladder cancer: is there a change in trend? Journal of Urology 2001; 165(1): 47–50; discussion 50.

191. Prout GR Jr, Griffin PP, Shipley WU. Bladder carcinoma as a systemic disease. Cancer 1979; 43(6): 2532–2539.

192. A Stenzl (chairman), JA Witjes (vice-chairman), NC Cowan, M De Santis, M Kuczyk et al. Guidelines on Bladder Cancer Muscle-Invasive and Metastatic. European Association of Urology 2011.

193. Brennan P, Bogillot O, Cordier S, Greiser E, Schill W et al. Cigarette smoking and bladder cancer in men: a pooled analysis of 11 case-control studies. International Journal of Cancer 2000; 86(2): 289–294.

194. Burger M, Catto JWF, Dalbagni G, Grossman HB, Herr H et al. Epidemiology and risk factors of urothelial bladder cancer. European Urology 2013; 63(2): 234–241.

195. Rushton L, Bagga S, Bevan R, Brown TP, Cherrie JW et al. Occupation and cancer in Britain. British Journal of Cancer 2010; 102(9): 1428–1437.

196. Rushton L, Hutchings SJ, Fortunato L, Young C, Evans GS et al. Occupational cancer burden in Great Britain. British Journal of Cancer 2012; 107(Suppl 1): S3–7.

197. Samanic CM, Kogevinas M, Silverman DT, Tardón A, Serra C et al. Occupation and bladder cancer in a hospital-based case-control study in Spain. Occupational and Environmental Medicine 2008; 65(5): 347–353.

198. Lynch CF, Davila JA, Platz CE. Cancer of the urinary bladder. In Ries LAG, Young JL, Keel GE, Eisner MP, Lin YD, Horner M-J, eds, SEER Survival Monograph: Cancer Survival Among Adults: U.S. SEER Program, 1988–2001, Patient and Tumour Characteristics. National Cancer Institute, SEER Program, NIH Pub. Bethesda, MD: NIH, 2007. Report No.: 07-6215.

199. Babjuk M, Oosterlinck W, Sylvester R, Kaasinen E, Böhle A et al. EAU guidelines on non-muscle-invasive urothelial carci-noma of the bladder, the 2011 update. European Urology 2011; 59(6): 997–1008.

200. Ploeg M, Kiemeney LALM, Smits GA, Vergunst H, Viddeleer AC et al. Discrepancy between clinical staging through bimanual palpa-tion and pathological staging after cystectomy. Urologic Oncology 2012; 30(3): 247–251.

201. Paik ML, Scolieri MJ, Brown SL, Spirnak JP, Resnick MI. Limitations of computerized tomography in staging invasive blad-der cancer before radical cystectomy. Journal of Urology 2000; 163(6): 1693–1696.

202. Barentsz JO, Jager GJ, Witjes JA, Ruijs JH. Primary staging of urinary bladder carcinoma: the role of MRI and a comparison with CT. European Radiology 1996; 6(2): 129–133.

203. Barentsz JO, Engelbrecht MR, Witjes JA, de la Rosette JJ, van der Graaf M. MR imaging of the male pelvis. European Radiology 1999; 9(9): 1722–1736.

204. Dorfman RE, Alpern MB, Gross BH, Sandler MA. Upper abdominal lymph nodes: criteria for normal size determined with CT. Radiology 1991; 180(2): 319–322.

205. Sylvester RJ, van der Meijden APM, Oosterlinck W, Witjes JA, Bouffioux C et al. Predicting recurrence and progression in individual patients with stage Ta T1 bladder cancer using EORTC risk tables: a combined analysis of 2596 patients from seven EORTC trials. European Urology 2006; 49(3): 466–465, discussion 475–477.

206. Sylvester RJ, Oosterlinck W, van der Meijden APM. A single immediate postoperative instillation of chemotherapy decreases the risk of recurrence in patients with stage Ta T1 bladder cancer: a meta-analysis of published results of randomized clinical trials. Journal of Urology 2004; 171(6 Pt 1): 2186–2190, quiz 2435.

207. Shelley MD, Kynaston H, Court J, Wilt TJ, Coles B et al. A systematic review of intravesical bacillus Calmette-Guérin plus transurethral resection vs transurethral resection alone in Ta and T1 bladder cancer. British Journal of Urology International 2001; 88(3): 209–216.

208. Han RF, Pan JG. Can intravesical bacillus Calmette-Guérin reduce recurrence in patients with superficial bladder cancer? A meta-analysis of randomized trials. Urology 2006; 67(6): 1216–1223.

209. Böhle A, Bock PR. Intravesical bacille Calmette-Guérin versus mitomycin C in superficial bladder cancer: formal meta-analysis of comparative studies on tumour progression. Urology 2004; 63(4): 682–686, discussion 686–687.

210. Sylvester RJ, van der Meijden APM, Lamm DL. Intravesical bacillus Calmette-Guerin reduces the risk of progression in patients with superficial bladder cancer: a meta-analysis of the published results of randomized clinical trials. Journal of Urology 2002; 168(5): 1964–1970.

211. Järvinen R, Kaasinen E, Sankila A, Rintala E. Long-term efficacy of maintenance bacillus Calmette-Guérin versus maintenance mitomycin C instillation therapy in frequently recurrent TaT1 tumours without carcinoma in situ: a subgroup analysis of the prospective, randomised FinnBladder I study with a 20-year follow-up. European Urology 2009; 56(2): 260–265.

212. Morales A, Eidinger D, Bruce AW. Intracavitary Bacillus Calmette-Guerin in the treatment of superficial bladder tumours. Journal of Urology 1976; 116(2): 180–183.

213. Davis JW, Sheth SI, Doviak MJ, Schellhammer PF. Superficial bladder carcinoma treated with bacillus Calmette-Guerin: progression-free and disease specific survival with minimum 10-year followup. Journal of Urology 2002; 167(2 Pt 1): 494–500, discussion 501.

214. Koppie TM, Vickers AJ, Vora K, Dalbagni G, Bochner BH. Standardization of pelvic lymphadenectomy performed at radical cystectomy: can we establish a minimum number of lymph nodes that should be removed? Cancer 2006; 107(10): 2368–2374.

215. Stein JP, Skinner DG. Radical cystectomy for invasive bladder cancer: long-term results of a standard procedure. World Journal of Urology 2006; 24(3): 296–304.

216. Eastham JA. Do high-volume hospitals and surgeons provide better care in urologic oncology? Urology and Oncology 2009; 27(4): 417–421.

217. Lawrentschuk N, Colombo R, Hakenberg OW, Lerner SP, Månsson W et al. Prevention and management of complications following radical cystectomy for bladder cancer. European Urology 2010; 57(6): 983–1001.

218. Caffo O, Fellin G, Graffer U, Mussari S, Tomio L et al. Gemcitabine and radiotherapy plus cisplatin after transurethral resection as conservative treatment for infiltrating bladder cancer: long-term cumulative results of 2 prospective single-institution studies. Cancer 2011; 117(6): 1190–1196.

219. Advanced Bladder Cancer Meta-analysis Collaboration. Neoadjuvant chemotherapy in invasive bladder cancer: a systematic review and meta-analysis. Lancet 2003; 361(9373): 1927–1934.

220. Winquist E, Kirchner TS, Segal R, Chin J, Lukka H. Neoadjuvant chemotherapy for transitional cell carcinoma of the bladder: a systematic review and meta-analysis. Journal of Urology 2004; 171(2 Pt 1): 561–569.

221. Advanced Bladder Cancer (ABC) Meta-analysis Collaboration. Neoadjuvant chemotherapy in invasive bladder cancer: update of a systematic review and meta-analysis of individual patient data advanced bladder cancer (ABC) meta-analysis collaboration. European Urology 2005; 48(2): 202–205, discussion 205–206.

222. Sternberg CN, Yagoda A, Scher HI, Watson RC, Geller N et al. Methotrexate, vinblastine, doxorubicin, and cisplatin for advanced transitional cell carcinoma of the urothelium. Efficacy and patterns of response and relapse. Cancer 1989; 64(12): 2448–2458.

223. Von der Maase H, Hansen SW, Roberts JT, Dogliotti L, Oliver T et al. Gemcitabine and cisplatin versus methotrexate, vinblastine, doxorubicin, and cisplatin in advanced or metastatic bladder cancer: results of a large, randomized, multinational, multicenter, phase III study. Journal of Clinical Oncology Journal of the American Society of Clinical Oncologists 2000; 18(17): 3068–3077.

224. Shariat SF, Favaretto RL, Gupta A, Fritsche H-M, Matsumoto K et al. Gender differences in radical nephroureterectomy for upper tract urothelial carcinoma. World Journal of Urology 2011; 29(4): 481–486.

225. Margulis V, Shariat SF, Matin SF, Kamat AM, Zigeuner R et al. Outcomes of radical nephroureterectomy: a series from the Upper Tract Urothelial Carcinoma Collaboration. Cancer 2009; 115(6): 1224–1233.

226. Rouprêt M, Babjuk M, Compérat E, Zigeuner R, Sylvester R et al. European guidelines on upper tract urothelial carcinomas: 2013 update. European Urology 2013; 63(6): 1059–1071.

227. Lughezzani G, Jeldres C, Isbarn H, Sun M, Shariat SF et al. Temporal stage and grade migration in surgically treated patients with upper tract urothelial carcinoma. British Journal of Urology International 2010; 105(6): 799–804.

228. Cosentino M, Palou J, Gaya JM, Breda A, Rodriguez-Faba O et al. Upper urinary tract urothelial cell carcinoma: location as a predictive factor for concomitant bladder carcinoma. World Journal of Urology 2013; 31(1): 141–145.

229. Zigeuner RE, Hutterer G, Chromecki T, Rehak P, Langner C. Bladder tumour development after urothelial carcinoma of the upper urinary tract is related to primary tumour location. British Journal of Urology International 2006; 98(6): 1181–1186.

230. Novara G, De Marco V, Dalpiaz O, Gottardo F, Bouygues V et al. Independent predictors of metachronous bladder transitional cell carcinoma (TCC) after nephroureterectomy for TCC of the upper urinary tract. British Journal of Urology International 2008; 101(11): 1368–1374.

231. Audenet F, Colin P, Yates DR, Ouzzane A, Pignot G et al. A proportion of hereditary upper urinary tract urothelial carcinomas are misclassified as sporadic according to a multi-institutional database analysis: proposal of patient-specific risk identification tool. British Journal of Urology International 2012; 110(11 Pt B): E583–589.

232. Acher P, Kiela G, Thomas K, O'Brien T. Towards a rational strategy for the surveillance of patients with Lynch syndrome (hereditary non-polyposis colon cancer) for upper tract transitional cell carcinoma. British Journal of Urology International 2010; 106(3): 300–302.

233. Colin P, Koenig P, Ouzzane A, Berthon N, Villers A et al. Environmental factors involved in carcinogenesis of urothelial cell carcinomas of the upper urinary tract. British Journal of Urology International 2009; 104(10): 1436–1440.

234. Chen C-H, Dickman KG, Moriya M, Zavadil J, Sidorenko VS et al. Aristolochic acid-associated urothelial cancer in Taiwan. Proceedings of the National Academy Sciences USA 2012; 109(21): 8241–8246.

235. Grollman AP, Shibutani S, Moriya M, Miller F, Wu L et al. Aristolochic acid and the etiology of endemic (Balkan) nephropathy. Proceedings of the National Academy Sciences USA 2007; 104(29): 12129–12134.

236. Razavi SA, Sadigh G, Kelly AM, Cronin P. Comparative effectiveness of imaging modalities for the diagnosis of upper and lower urinary tract malignancy: a critically appraised topic. Academic Radiology 2012; 19(9): 1134–1140.

237. Messer J, Shariat SF, Brien JC, Herman MP, Ng CK et al. Urinary cytology has a poor performance for predicting invasive or high-grade upper-tract urothelial carcinoma. British Journal of Urology International 2011; 108(5): 701–705.

238. Rojas CP, Castle SM, Llanos CA, Santos Cortes JA, Bird V et al. Low biopsy volume in ureteroscopy does not affect tumour biopsy grading in upper tract urothelial carcinoma. Urology and Oncology 2013; 31(8): 1696–1700.

239. Smith AK, Stephenson AJ, Lane BR, Larson BT, Thomas AA et al. Inadequacy of biopsy for diagnosis of upper tract urothelial carcinoma: implications for conservative management. Urology 2011; 78(1): 82–86.

240. Eltz S, Comperat E, Cussenot O, Rouprêt M. Molecular and histological markers in urothelial carcinomas of the upper urinary tract. British Journal of Urology International 2008; 102(5): 532–535.

241. Compérat E, Roupret M, Chartier-Kastler E, Bitker MO, Richard F et al. Prognostic value of MET, RON and histoprognostic factors for urothelial carcinoma in the upper urinary tract. Journal of Urology 2008; 179(3): 868–872, discussion 872.

242. Scarpini S, Rouprêt M, Renard-Penna R, Camparo P, Cussenot O et al. Impact of the expression of Aurora-A, p53, and MIB-1 on the prognosis of urothelial carcinomas of the upper urinary tract. Urology and Oncology 2012; 30(2): 182–187.

243. Kosaka T, Kikuchi E, Mikami S, Miyajima A, Shirotake S et al. Expression of snail in upper urinary tract urothelial carcinoma: prognostic significance and implications for tumour invasion. Clinical Cancer Research Journal of the American Association of Cancer Research 2010; 16(23): 5814–5823.

244. Simone G, Papalia R, Guaglianone S, Ferriero M, Leonardo C et al. Laparoscopic versus open nephroureterectomy: perioperative and oncologic outcomes from a randomised prospective study. European Urology 2009; 56(3): 520–526.

245. Sundi D, Svatek RS, Margulis V, Wood CG, Matin SF et al. Upper tract urothelial carcinoma: impact of time to surgery. Urology and Oncology 2012; 30(3): 266–272.

246. O'Brien T, Ray E, Singh R, Coker B, Beard R. British Association of Urological Surgeons Section of Oncology. Prevention of bladder tumours after nephroureterectomy for primary upper urinary tract urothelial carcinoma: a prospective, multicentre, randomised clinical trial of a single postoperative intravesical dose of mitomycin C (the ODMIT-C Trial). European Urology 2011; 60(4): 703–710.

247. Audenet F, Yates DR, Cussenot O, Rouprêt M. The role of chemotherapy in the treatment of urothelial cell carcinoma of the upper urinary tract (UUT-UCC). Urology and Oncology 2013; 31(4): 407–413.

248. Lam JS, Leppert JT, Belldegrun, AS, Figlin RA. Novel approaches in the therapy of metastatic renal cell carcinoma. World Journal of Urology 2005; 23(3): 202–212.

249. Bausch B, Jilg C, Glasker S, Vortmeyer A, Lutzen N et al. Renal cancer in von Hippel-Lindau disease and related syndromes. Nature Reviews Nephrology 2013; 9(9): 529–538.

250. Slevarajah J, Nathawat K, Moumen A, Ashcroft M, Carroll VA. Chemotherapy mediated p53 dependent DNA damage response in clear cell renal cell carcinoma: role of mTorc1/2 and hypoxia inducible factor pathways. Cell Death and Disease 2013; 4:e865. doi: 10.1038/cddis.2013.395.

251. Ljungberg B, Cowan NC, Hanbury DC, Hora M, Kuczyk MA et al. EAU guidelines on renal cell carcinoma: the 2010 update. European Urology 2010; 58(3): 398–406.

252. Pignot G, Elie C, Conquy S, Vieillefond A, Flam T et al. Survival analysis of 130 patients with papillary renal cell carcinoma: prognostic utility of type 1 and type 2 subclassification. Urology 2007; 69(2): 230–235.

253. Bensalah K, Pantuck AJ, Rioux-Leclercq N, Thuret R, Montorsi F et al. Positive surgical margin appears to have negligible impact on survival of renal cell carcinomas treated by nephron-sparing surgery. European Urology 2010; 57(3): 466–471.

254. Kummerlin IP, Ten Kate FJ, Wijkstra H, de la Rosette JJ, Laguna MP. Changes in the stage and surgical management of renal tumours during 1995–2005: an analysis of the Dutch national histopathology registry. British Journal of Urology International 2008; 102(8): 946–951.

255. Guillotreau J, Haber GP, Autorino R, Miocinovic R, Hillyer S et al. Robotic partial nephrectomy versus laparoscopic cryoablation for the small renal mass. European Urology 2012; 61(5): 899–904. doi: 10.1016/j.eururo.2012.01.007. Epub 2012 Jan 14.

256. Tan HJ, Wolf JS Jr, Ye Z, Wei JT, Miller DC. Complications and failure to rescue after laparoscopic versus open radical nephrectomy. Journal of Urology 2011; 186(4): 1254–1260.

257. Mitchell RE, Lee BT, Cookson MS, Barocas DA, Duke Herrell S et al. Radical nephrectomy surgical outcomes in the University HealthSystem Consortium Data Base: Impact of hospital case volume, hospital size, and geographic location on 40,000 patients. Cancer 2009; 115(11): 2447–2452.

258. Abouassaly R, Finelli A, Tomlinson GA, Urbach DR, Alibhai SM. Volume-outcome relationships in the treatment of renal tumours. Journal of Urology 2012; 187(6): 1984–1988.

259. Blom JH, Van Poppel H, Marechal JM, Jacqmin D, Schroder FH et al. Radical nephrectomy with and without lymph-node dissection: final results of European Organization for Research and Treatment of Cancer (EORTC) randomized phase 3 trial 30881. European Urology 2009; 55(1): 28–34.

260. Leibovich BC, Blute ML. Lymph node dissection in the management of renal cell carcinoma. Urologic Clinics of North America 2008; 35(4): 673–678.

261. Whitson JM, Harris CR, Reese AC, Meng MV. Lymphadenectomy improves survival of patients with renal cell carcinoma and nodal metastases. Journal of Urology 2011; 185(5): 1615–1620.

262. Bex A, van der Veldt AA, Blank C, Meijerink MR, Boven E. Progression of a caval vein thrombus in two patients with primary renal cell carcinoma on pretreatment with sunitinib. Acta Oncology 2010; 49(4): 520–523.

263. Flanigan RC, Mickisch G, Sylvester R, Tangen C, Van Poppel H et al. Cytoreductive nephrectomy in patients with metastatic renal cancer: a combined analysis. Journal of Urology 2004; 171(3): 1071–1076.

264. Alt AL, Boorjian SA, Lohse CM, Costello BA, Leibovich BC et al. Survival after complete surgical resection of multiple metastases from renal cell carcinoma. Cancer 2011; 117(13): 2873–2882.

265. Meimarakis G, Angele M, Staehler M, Clevert DA, Crispin A et al. Evaluation of a new prognostic score (Munich score) to predict long-term survival after resection of pulmonary renal cell carcinoma metastases. American Journal of Surgery 2011; 202(2): 158–167.

266. Powles T, Chowdhury S, Jones R, Mantle M, Nathan P et al. Sunitinib and other targeted therapies for renal cell carcinoma. British Journal of Cancer 2011; 104(5): 741–745.

267. Motzer RJ, Hutson TE, Tomczak P, et al. Sunitinib versus interferon alfa in metastatic renal-cell carcinoma. New England Journal of Medicine 2007; 356: 115–124.

268. Sternberg CN, Davis ID, Mardiak J, Szczylik C, Lee E et al. Pazopanib in locally advanced or metastatic renal cell carcinoma: results of a randomized phase III trial. Journal of Clinical Oncology 2010; 28(6): 1061–1068.

269. Motzer RJ, Hutson TE, Cella D, Reeves J, Hawkins R et al. Pazopanib versus sunitinib in metastatic renal-cell carcinoma. New England Journal of Medicine 2013; 369(8): 722–731.

270. Escudier B, Porta C, Bono P, De Giorgi U, Parikh O et al Patient preference between pazopanib (Paz) and sunitinib (Sun): results of a randomized double-blind, placebo-controlled, cross-over study in patients with metastatic renal cell carcinoma (mRCC)—PISCES study, NCT 01064310.

271. Bex A, Haanen J. Tilting the AXIS towards therapeutic limits in renal cancer. Lancet 2011; 378(9807): 1898–900.

272. Escudier B, Eisen T, Stadler WM, Szcylik C, Oudard S et al. Sorafenib for treatment of renal cell carcinoma: final efficacy and safety results of the phase III treatment approaches in renal cancer global evaluation trial. Journal of Clinical Oncology 2009; 27(20): 3312–3318.

273. Rini BI, Escudier B, Tomczak P, Kaprin A, Szczylik C et al. Comparative effectiveness of axitinib versus sorafenib in advanced renal cell carcinoma (AXIS): a randomised phase III study. Lancet 2011; 378(9807): 1931–1939.

274. Motzer RJ, Escudier B, Oudard S, Hutson TE, Porta C et al. RECORD-1 study group. Lancet 2008; 372(9637): 449–456.

275. Motzer R, Szczylik C, Sternberg C, Vogelzang N, Porta C et al. Dovitinib v.s. sorafenib as 3rd line therapy in metastatic clear cell renal cancer. ESMO 2013: Abstract E17–7035.

276. Rini BI, Michaelson MD, Rosenberg JE, Bukowski RM, Sosman JA et al. Antitumour activity and biomarker analysis of sunitinib in patients with bevacizumab-refractory metastatic renal cell carcinoma. Journal of Clinical Oncology 2008; 26(22): 3743–3748.

277. Choueiri TK, Regan MM, Rosenberg JE, Oh WK, Clement J et al. Carbonic anhydrase IX and pathological features as predictors of outcome in patients with metastatic clear-cell renal cell carcinoma receiving vascular endothelial growth factor-targeted therapy. British Journal of Urology International 2010; 106(6): 772–778.

CHAPTER 46

Lung cancer

Rafał Dziadziuszko, Michael Baumann,
Tetsuya Mitsudomi, Keith M. Kerr,
Solange Peters, and Stefan Zimmermann

Epidemiology and aetiology

Lung cancer remains the leading cause of cancer-related mortality globally with almost 1.6 million deaths worldwide each year. Estimates of 2008 lung cancer incidence and mortality in 40 European countries indicate 391 000 new cases (12.2% of all cancer diagnoses) and 342 000 deaths (19.9% of all cancer-related deaths) [1]. Lung cancer incidence is very variable across Europe with highest incidence in Central and Eastern European countries (Hungary and Poland) and lowest in Portugal and Sweden. The proportion of newly-diagnosed lung cancer patients in women is also highly variable—from approximately 10% in some Central and Eastern European countries to almost 50% in Denmark and Sweden, reflecting social differences in tobacco consumption. Lung cancer incidence and mortality figures show a stable decline in males in almost all countries, whereas the incidence and mortality in females is rising in majority of European countries except some high-risk countries showing stable or declining trends (Denmark, Iceland, UK). The incidence of lung cancer in never-smokers (persons who smoked less than 100 cigarettes in their life) is approximately two- to three-fold higher in females as compared to that in males [2]. Detailed data on trends in incidence of lung cancer in never-smokers are lacking, with some suggestions of slight increase over time.

It is estimated that almost 160 000 new lung cancer diagnoses occurred in the United States in 2013, with declining death rates in males for two decades and recently observed declining trends in death rates in females [3]. Global lung cancer burden is expected to rise as a consequence of increase in tobacco consumption, particularly in Asian countries. Lung cancer remains a devastating disease, with approximately 10–15% five-year survival rates in European countries and North America.

Active tobacco smoking is the prevailing risk factor for lung cancer development. It is estimated that cumulative lifetime lung cancer risk in heavy smokers may reach 30% as compared to less than 1% in never-smokers [4]. Globally, active smoking is responsible for approximately 50–90% of lung cancers in females and 80–95% of lung cancer in males with wide geographical variation. Passive tobacco inhalation is responsible for approximately 20–50% of lung cancer diagnoses in non-smokers. Tobacco smoke contains more than 50 identified carcinogens, including N-nitrosoamines, polycyclic aromatic hydrocarbons (PAHs), benzene, vinyl chloride, arsenic, and chromium [5]. Exposure of bronchial epithelium to these carcinogens leads to formation of DNA adducts and, if not repaired by DNA repair systems, permanent mutations. The spectrum of genetic and epigenetic changes in airway epithelium from smokers is very broad, including oncogene mutations, gene copy number changes, loss of tumour suppressors, and abnormal methylation pattern. Most of these abnormalities persist over time, explaining elevated risk of lung cancer in individuals who quit smoking. Lung cancer risk depends strongly on the duration of tobacco smoking and age of onset as well as on smoking intensity. Use of low tar and filtered cigarettes is not associated with lower lung cancer risk and contributes to observed phenomenon of increasing proportion of lung adenocarcinomas. Deeper inhalation, related to the need to deliver adequate nicotine amounts to nicotine-addicted individuals, leads to higher exposure of peripheral bronchi to smoke from these cigarettes. The risk of lung cancer gradually decreases after quitting smoking to the level of two- to three-fold of the risk of never-smokers. Other means of smoking tobacco, such as pipes or cigars, are also linked to elevated lung cancer risk, albeit this association appears less strong than for cigarettes—relative risks are within the range of two to five as compared to never-smokers.

Occupational carcinogens associated with lung cancer include asbestos, arsenic, beryllium, cadmium, chromium, nickel, silica, radon, vinyl chloride, and fumes from diesel fuels. Higher risk of lung cancer is also observed in individuals exposed to chest radiotherapy, such as survivors of breast cancer or lymphoma. Exposure to these agents is responsible for approximately 10% of lung cancers among males and 5% in females [6]. Chronic exposure to asbestos in industry workers (asbestos mining, construction, insulation, and shipbuilding industry) is associated with approximately 3–10 times the relative risk of lung cancer. The risk associated with asbestos is greatly increased with consumption of tobacco cigarettes. Exposure to radon (radioactive gas which is a decay product of radium 226 and uranium 238) is of a significant concern not only for mine workers but also for indoor air pollution at residential areas abundant in natural radium and uranium in the soil and rocks. While there is no discussion about the former as a risk factor, harmful effects of low-level radiation from indoor radon continue to be debated. Other occupational lung cancer carcinogens are related to a wide range of industries such as ceramics, glass, steel, mining, and chemical manufacturing.

Molecular biology

Genetic predisposition to lung cancer is highly complex with involvement of high-penetrance, low-frequency genes and genes with low penetrance occurring with higher frequencies. Lung cancer belongs to the spectrum of tumours found in patients with high-penetrance syndromes such as Li-Fraumeni (germline P53 mutations/deletions), Bloom (germline BLM mutations/deletions), Werner (germline WRN mutations/deletions), and BRCA (germline mutations/deletions of BRCA1 or BRCA2) syndromes. The precise risks of lung cancer development in careers of mutations or deletions in these genes are, however, difficult to estimate due to lack of large-scale molecular epidemiology studies. The majority of studies addressing low penetrance genetic predisposition focus on polymorphic variants of genes that encode enzymes mediating activation, detoxification, or repair of DNA damage caused by tobacco [7]. Most extensively studied phase I (oxidation, reduction, and hydrolysis) and phase II (conjugation) enzymes involved in the metabolism of tobacco carcinogens include CYP1A1, microsomal epoxide hydrolase-1 (mEH/EPHX1), myeloperoxidase (MPO), NAD(P)H quinone oxidoreductase-1 (NQO1), and glutathione S-transferases. Results of these studies revealed several candidate gene polymorphisms associated with significantly elevated or decreased risk of lung cancer with odds ratios typically in the range of 1.5–3, and suggesting important interactions among risk genotypes. Practical implementation of these associations into molecular tests that could be used to support selection of individuals into lung cancer screening programs remains difficult due to large heterogeneity among designs and results of these studies. Other candidate genetic markers of increased susceptibility to lung cancer include genes involved in inflammatory response and cell cycle control.

Intensive research performed during the last ten years with integrative molecular methods such as genome sequencing, comparative genomic hybridization, and transcriptome analysis led to accumulation of a large amount of data on the spectrum of molecular aberrations in lung cancer [8, 9]. Most of lung cancer genomes present hundreds of mutations, deletions/amplifications, gene rearrangements, and abnormal methylation patterns, a feature typical for cancers arising from exposure to tobacco-related carcinogens. Of those, only a few abnormalities lead to significant activation of cell signalling pathways leading to tumour growth, progression, and dissemination. Growth of lung adenocarcinomas may depend predominantly on a single molecular event, such as activating mutations in epidermal growth factor receptor (EGFR) gene, Kirsten ras sarcoma virus (KRAS) gene, ERBB2 (HER2) gene or rearrangements in ALK, ROS1, or RET oncogenes. These events are frequently non-overlapping and indicate different biological behaviour with distinct proliferation rate and chemo- and radio-sensitivity. For example, EGFR mutations indicate a more indolent course of the disease, substantial benefit from EGFR tyrosine kinase inhibitors, increased response rates to chemotherapy and increased radiosensitivity as compared to wild-type EGFR. Activating EGFR mutations and other above-mentioned molecular features fulfil the 'oncogene addiction' model and form the basis for the development of predictive molecular assays for particular targeted therapies, used either in clinical practice (EGFR and ALK inhibitors, briefly discussed below) or within clinical trials. These abnormalities are mainly confined to genes coding for growth factor receptors, intracellular pathway signaling proteins or transcription factors. The most extensively studied and the most frequent mutation of this type occurs in codons 12, 13, or 61 of the KRAS oncogene, which codes for a GTP-ase involved in signal transduction from tyrosine

kinase receptors. Most of the KRAS mutations are G to T transversions resulting in substitution of glycine by either cysteine or valine. KRAS mutations occur in approximately 10–25% of adenocarcinomas (less commonly in squamous cell carcinomas), are associated with smoking history, and are linked with slightly inferior survival or harbour no prognostic significance according to a number of studies performed in operable series of lung cancer patients [10]. With the exception of promising results of a small phase II study that combines the MEK inhibitor selumetinib with docetaxel as second-line therapy of advanced non-small cell lung carcinoma (NSCLC) with KRAS mutations [11], there is currently no effective targeted therapy for patients with tumours showing this mutation.

EGFR mutations are found in tumours from approximately 10–15% of unselected Western and 30–50% of Asian NSCLC patients, more frequently in never or light smokers. These mutations cluster in exon 18–21 of the gene, leading to conformal changes in the ATP-binding pocket of tyrosine kinase portion of the EGFR protein [12]. Most common mutations are small exon 19 deletions or exon 21 point mutations (L858R and L861X), linked with sensitivity to reversible EGFR tyrosine kinase inhibitors such as gefitinib or erlotinib. Rare exon 18 mutations are also associated with sensitivity, whereas exon 20 point mutations and small insertions are linked with resistance to EGFR inhibitors. Exon 20 T790M mutation is the most common mechanism of acquired resistance, which develops after a median of approximately ten months of gefitinib or erlotinib treatment. Clones of cells harboring T790M may be found by sensitive techniques in 30–50% of tumours prior to therapy with reversible EGFR inhibitors and expand during treatment through clonal selection. Current translational and clinical research efforts are directed towards breaking the mechanisms of acquired resistance with novel EGFR inhibitors or molecules aimed at other targets essential for abnormal cell growth.

ALK is a transmembrane protein of insulin-like growth factor receptor superfamily with tyrosine kinase activity. ALK gene rearrangement is found in approximately 3–5% of NSCLCs, almost exclusively in adenocarcinomas. Most frequently, an intracellular portion of ALK tyrosine kinase is fused with an N-terminal portion of microtubule-associated protein-like 4 (EML4), leading to constitutive activation of ALK. More than ten variants of ALK fusion genes have been identified in lung tumours, with EML4 being the most common and KIF5B, TFG, or KLC1less common fusion partners. ALK rearrangement can be detected in tumours by fluorescence in situ hybridization (FISH) break-apart assay or RT-PCR assay. In addition to these two tests, immunohistochemical staining for ALK protein with antibodies specifically validated for lung cancer appears very promising. The optimal testing methodology to define ALK-positive tumours remains to be established, although it should be noted that results of clinical trials with crizotinib, ALK, and MET inhibitor rely on patients with tumours defined as positive by the FISH assay. A testing strategy which relies on immunohistochemistry with specific anti-ALK antibodies followed by FISH break-apart assay in immunopositive cases is commonly adopted in many institutions. The less commonly rearranged ROS1 gene (approximately 1–2% of lung adenocarcinomas) codes for a protein of the same family as ALK, showing approximately 50% of amino acid sequence homology in the tyrosine kinase domain. At least ten fusion partners have been described for the ROS1 gene in lung cancer. Several publications suggest the clinical utility of immunohistochemistry to detect ROS1 protein and preselect tumours for FISH testing. Patients with ALK and ROS1 rearrangements are typically younger and tend to have no or limited tobacco smoking history. Both rearrangements are predictive for benefit from specific inhibitors, including crizotinib (approved in patients with ALK-positive NSCLC) and several other agents currently in clinical development.

Recent research on driving molecular aberrations in squamous cell carcinoma identified several candidate genes with mutations or amplifications leading to activation of downstream signalling. From a therapeutic perspective, most promising genetic changes include DDR2 and PIK3CA mutations or FGFR1, SOX2, or PIK3CA amplifications. Several clinical trials with inhibitors of the above targets are ongoing.

Dysregulation of tumour suppressor genes (TSGs) is a common finding in lung cancer. P53 gene mutations are almost universal in small-cell lung carcinoma (SCLC) and occur in approximately half of NSCLCs. P53 protein is involved in several cellular processes, such as DNA repair, cell-cycle and apoptosis control, autophagy, senescence, and ageing. Most P53 mutations are missense and cluster in the DNA-binding domain, resulting in the defective p53 protein not being able to transactivate target genes mediating the above processes. In addition, several P53 mutations are linked with gain-of-function properties typical for dominant oncogenes. Clinically, P53 mutations are associated with worse prognosis of surgically treated NSCLC patients and appear to associate with radio- and chemo-resistance. Several strategies to restore functional P53 pathway have been developed and tested in clinical trials. These strategies include retrovirus or adenovirus-mediated gene therapy with wild-type P53 [13], small molecule inhibitors of P53-MDM2 interaction [14], or mutation-specific P53-directed tumour vaccines [15].

Other important TSGs with a relatively high proportion of aberrations (mutations, allele losses, epigenetic modifications) in lung cancer include LKB1, NF1, PTEN, ATM, RB1, FHIT, and APC [8]. Other yet undefined suppressor genes are being unravelled through high-resolution genomic hybridization methods. The diagnostic and therapeutic significance of these abnormalities at present is unknown. Tumours with deleted TSGs may depend on activation of unsuppressed downstream pathways (e.g., loss of LKB1 results in mTOR activation; loss of NF1 results in RAS/RAF/MEK and/or mTOR activation). Inhibition of these pathways is currently explored in clinical trials.

Pathology

The pathology of lung cancer, like the molecular biology of this diverse group of malignant diseases, has become of even greater importance in the approach to diagnosis and treatment of this most common and fatal of malignancies. Traditional pathology is based upon haematoxylin and eosin (H&E)-stained section morphology, underpinning the WHO classification of lung tumours applied to resected cancer specimens. Most pathological tumour diagnosis is, however, made on small biopsy samples or cytology and increasingly, immunohistochemistry is used to resolve diagnostic problems (see below). Therapeutic choices for patients with lung cancer are based on detailed knowledge of tumour pathology, both in the advanced disease setting but also before, during, and after surgical resection. Choice of chemotherapy may be determined by

tumour cell type (small cell, squamous cell, and adenocarcinomas are treated differently) as may be genetic investigations to determine molecular targeted therapy. It is now no longer acceptable to classify lung cancer according to a simple dichotomy of small cell carcinoma; yes or no? The 'category of convenience' that was NSCLC comprises a number of biologically diverse malignant diseases which are treated in different ways. NSCLC should not be considered a single entity.

In the surgical setting, confirmation of malignancy in small samples is usually required before surgical resection. Intraoperative frozen section diagnosis may be used to inform surgical decision making but full diagnosis and classification of disease is made on the complete resection specimen. The 2015 WHO classification of lung tumours [16] is the standard used and names seven major subtypes of lung carcinoma: squamous cell, adenocarcinoma, large cell, sarcomatoid, adenosquamous, neuroendocrine, and salivary-type carcinomas. The pathology report of the resected tumour should subtype and pathologically stage the tumour according to the TNM system 7th edition [17]. Tumour stage is the major determinant of adjuvant therapy.

Adenocarcinoma

Adenocarcinoma is probably the most common type of lung cancer worldwide, although its dominance is less pronounced in Caucasian cohorts where smoking is the predominant aetiological factor. Most adenocarcinomas arise in the peripheral, parenchymal part of the lung, from precursor lesions of atypical adenomatous hyperplasia (AAH) and adenocarcinoma in situ (AIS—formerly known as pure non-mucinous brochioloalveolar carcinoma or BAC). These lesions arise from the peripheral lung epithelial compartment referred to as the terminal respiratory unit (TRU), characteristically expressing thyroid transcription factor 1 (TTF1).

Grossly these tumours show a wide range in size, and may be multifocal, either due to intrapulmonary spread or multiple synchronous primary lesions. A frequent mixed pattern of solid and 'ground glass' features on CT scans corresponds to peripheral parts of the tumour growing around alveolar walls without their destruction (lepidic growth), leading to the 'ground glass' appearance (Figure 46.1).

Relatively early spread to loco-regional lymph nodes is common and in advanced disease, lymphangitic spread in the lung

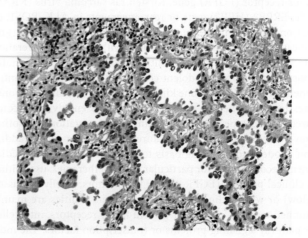

Fig. 46.1 Lepidic pattern adenocarcinoma which may represent adenocarcinoma in situ. Tumour cells grow around alveoli without destroying them (H&E × 200).

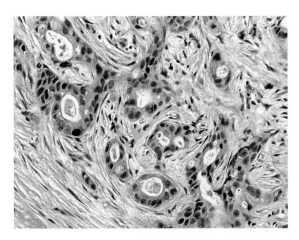

Fig. 46.2 Acinar pattern adenocarcinoma showing invasion of the fibrous stroma (H&E × 200).

is frequent. Their peripheral location and relative propensity for invasive growth, especially in the more aggressive subtypes, makes pleural invasion common.

Five main histological patterns of adenocarcinoma may be recognized: lepidic (formerly called bronchiolo-alveolar), acinar (Figure 46.2), papillary, micropapillary, and solid with mucin. Most lung adenocarcinomas comprise a mixture of two or more of these patterns. In resected cases, tumours which are predominantly of lepidic pattern have a relatively good prognosis and those which are predominantly micropapillary (Figure 46.3) or solid show significantly shorter post-operative survival with greater risk of relapse. By definition, all adenocarcinomas show glandular cells and architecture, and some cases show large amounts of mucin production and mucigenic tumour cells. Some mucinous adenocarcinomas of the lung show a tendency to spread within the lung, with or without tissue destruction, with less of a tendency to distant metastases. These cases were formerly classified as 'mucinous BAC' and often bear KRAS gene mutations. Adenocarcinomas, especially those arising in non-smokers, often bear a particular oncogene mutation. Many of these mutations appear to be mutually exclusive of each other (EGFR, KRAS, BRAF and HER2 mutations, and ALK gene rearrangements), implying biological significance and suggesting

so-called oncogene addiction. The therapeutic importance of these mutations is discussed above. Some of these mutations are associated with particular adenocarcinoma histological features.

Squamous cell carcinoma

In general, this type of lung cancer is the second most prevalent, after adenocarcinoma, though where smoking-induced cancers predominate it may remain the most common type. The archetypal form of the so-called bronchogenic lung carcinoma most commonly arises from the epithelium of central large bronchi, transformed by tobacco carcinogens. Progenitor lesions are well recognized; basal cell hyperplasia/squamous metaplasia gives rise to squamous dysplasia and squamous carcinoma in situ, wherein invasive disease develops. Most squamous cell carcinomas (SCC) are destructive growths which cause early bronchial obstruction and various degrees of obstructive pneumonia. Squamous cell carcinomas arising from smaller, more peripheral airways may be becoming more prevalent, presenting as peripheral solitary nodules akin to adenocarcinoma.

Histologically, these tumours are defined by the presence of squamous differentiation (keratin or intercellular bridge formation) (Figure 46.4) and most cases are relatively poorly differentiated. Invasive growth is often accompanied by a fibrous stroma and inflammation is variable. Endobronchial growth may have a papillary architecture whilst some peripheral SCCs grow within alveolar air spaces causing relatively little tissue destruction. Some SCCs show areas of tumour with smaller densely packed cells of basaloid morphology—this basaloid variant of SCC (basaloid carcinoma) is a relatively aggressive tumour. Necrosis is common and this may lead to tumour cavitation, although this process is not the preserve of squamous tumours. In general, spread to lymph nodes is a relatively late phenomenon, but these tumours can be extremely aggressive. The frequent association with obstructive pneumonia should demand caution in assuming that lymphadenopathy is malignant, as opposed to reactive, in a case of SCC.

Malignant neuroendocrine tumours

By far, the most important tumour in this category is small cell lung carcinoma (SCLC). In many countries this tumour is, like squamous cell carcinoma, declining in incidence, probably due to

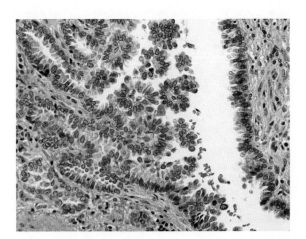

Fig. 46.3 A surgically resected adenocarcinoma showing predominance of this micropapillary pattern has a relatively poor post-operative survival (H&E × 200).

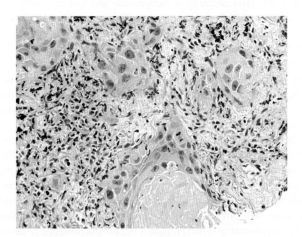

Fig. 46.4 Squamous cell carcinoma in a lung core biopsy. Keratinization and intercellular bridges are evident so a confident diagnosis can be made (H&E × 200).

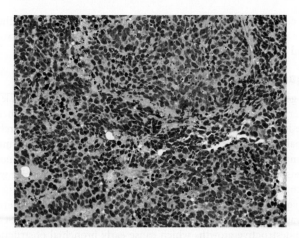

Fig. 46.5 Small cell lung carcinoma in a core biopsy of a paraspinal metastatic deposit (H&E × 200).

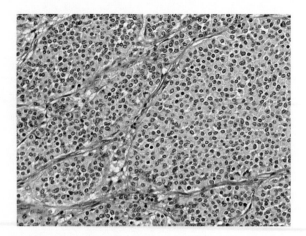

Fig. 46.6 Typical carcinoid tumour showing regular islands of small cells and abundant cytoplasm. (H&E × 200).

a fall in tobacco consumption, but where smoking remains common, SCLC still accounts for 15–20% of all lung cancers. SCLC tends to be a central, bronchogenic tumour which often presents with bulky central disease, contiguous with hilar and mediastinal lymph node metastases and direct spread into the mediastinum. Peripherally located, small tumours are uncommon, but may account for those rare cases which present with localized, surgically resectable disease. The vast majority of SCLC is stage 4 at presentation. Consequently, most contemporary pathological experience of SCLC is in small biopsy or cytopathology diagnosis.

These tumours comprise sheets of highly invasive, relatively small malignant cells whose nuclear features (stippled chromatin, moulding) are key to diagnosis. Necrosis, apoptosis, and mitotic activity are all abundant (Figure 46.5). Diagnosis is usually easy by H&E stains and immunohistochemical evidence of neuroendocrine differentiation is not a prerequisite. Sometimes, SCLC may coexist with other forms of NSCLC in the same lesion where, regardless of the amount of SCLC, a diagnosis of combined SCLC is made, and should be treated as SCLC.

Other forms of malignant neuroendocrine tumour (NET) of the lung are much less common than SCLC. Large cell neuroendocrine carcinoma (LCNEC) is another high-grade, aggressive tumour which may arise centrally or peripherally and has an equally poor prognosis to SCLC, at least in surgically resected series. This is a difficult diagnosis to confirm in small diagnostic samples, so the behaviour of LCNEC in the advanced disease setting is not clear. Many cases may be diagnosed as SCLC in small samples but awareness of this tumour type is increasing. Lesions comprise large tumour cells in prominent 'organoid' or 'neuroendocrine' architecture. Unlike SCLC, tumour cells usually have large, obvious nucleoli and abundant cytoplasm.

Carcinoid tumours are rare malignant neuroendocrine tumours which most often arise in central bronchi, grow slowly and often present with obstructive bronchial symptoms. Most are low-grade, so-called typical carcinoid tumours (Figure 46.6). Regional lymph node metastases are found in around 10% of cases; distant metastases are very rare. Atypical carcinoid tumours are morphologically very similar to typical tumours but for the presence of tumour necrosis and/or a slightly higher mitotic rate (between 2–10 mitoses per 2 mm² tumour). These are extremely rare tumours with a biological behaviour and post-surgical prognosis similar to SCC.

Typical carcinoid tumours with spindle cell morphology may arise in the lung periphery.

Large cell carcinomas

With the revision of definitions under the 2015 WHO classification, large cell carcinomas (LCC) account for around 4% of resected lung cancers and are defined by the absence of differentiated histological features (squamous or adenocarcinoma) anywhere in the tumours, and a lack of immunohistochemical features which may be associated with SCC or adenocarcinoma (Figure 46.7). This definition is important since it determines the fact that this tumour type can only be diagnosed in the surgical resection setting, when the whole lesion may be examined to exclude squamous or glandular differentiation somewhere in the lesion. These may be central or peripheral tumours, are generally aggressive, invasive, and molecular evidence supports that at least a proportion represents de-differentiated squamous cell or adenocarcinomas.

Sarcomatoid carcinomas

These tumours are diagnosed with certainty only in the surgically resected specimens, when more than 10% of the lesion shows spindle, pleomorphic, or tumour giant cells (Figure 46.8). The

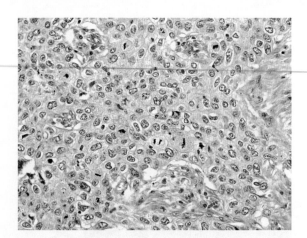

Fig. 46.7 This resected lung carcinoma shows large undifferentiated cells and abundant mitoses. In the absence of morphological differentiation, a diagnosis of large cell carcinoma is appropriate (H&E × 200).

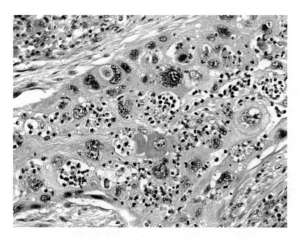

Fig. 46.8 This resected lung carcinoma showed evidence of squamous cell carcinoma but also, over 10% of the lesion showed these pleomorphic tumour giant cells, mandating a diagnosis of sarcomatoid carcinoma (H&E × 200).

remainder of the tumour may be undifferentiated or show squamous cell or adenocarcinoma. Extremely aggressive and invasive, such histological features may be recognized and at least described in small sample diagnosis.

Adenosquamous and other mixed tumours

Tumours showing at least 10% of each lesion as clear-cut squamous cell and adenocarcinoma are diagnosed as adenosquamous carcinoma. This is the best known of the combined lung cancer subtypes but is actually quite rare, if diagnostic criteria are strictly followed. They are usually peripherally located and may carry a relatively poor prognosis and represent another diagnosis that should only be offered in surgically resected cases. Other combinations may be encountered; adenocarcinoma with LCNEC is worthy of mention.

Salivary type carcinomas

These are extremely uncommon, and are found mostly in the trachea and main bronchi. They are the histological counterparts of adenoid cystic and mucoepidermoid carcinomas better known in the salivary glands and probably arise in the large airway seromucous glands.

Small biopsy and cytology sample diagnosis

Most patients with lung cancer present with advanced disease and never have their tumour resected. The only material available for diagnosis, tumour subtyping, and increasingly, for molecular analysis, is a small biopsy or cytology sample (Figure 46.9). Tumour subtyping may be difficult and inaccurate in this situation since most lung cancers comprise significant areas of undifferentiated tumour, which do not reflect the differentiated features present in other parts, which would determine the final, overall diagnosis if these were sampled, or if the whole lesion could be examined.

SCLC is reliably, consistently, and accurately diagnosed in small samples, but diagnosis of squamous cell and adenocarcinoma by H&E morphology alone can be inaccurate and inconsistent. Large cell, sarcomatoid, and mixed carcinomas, by definition, cannot be diagnosed consistently and accurately on such material. Carcinoid tumours should be recognized but usually cannot be ascribed to typical or atypical categories, whilst salivary type tumours may be recognized in good specimens.

Problems in recognizing a proportion of squamous cell and adenocarcinomas in small diagnostic samples led to the reasonable practice of diagnosing those cases where only undifferentiated carcinoma has been sampled as NSCLC not otherwise specified (NSCLC-NOS). This diagnosis may account for 20–40% of cases, depending on case mix, sample type, and pathologist experience or bias. The majority of NSCLC-NOS specimens are derived from differentiated tumours which have been poorly sampled; mostly adenocarcinomas. The need for more accurate subtyping has driven the use of immunohistochemistry (IHC) to predict the tumour subtype (IHC positive for p63, cytokeratin 5/6 or p40 predicts squamous cell carcinoma, TTF1 predicts adenocarcinoma) (Figure 46.10). This approach can accurately predict subtype in over 80% of cases, reducing the NSCLC-NOS rate to below 10%, a figure which cannot be reduced further, given the prevalence of large cell and sarcomatoid carcinomas in an unselected lung cancer population.

Symptoms

Increasing number of asymptomatic lung cancer patients are diagnosed with modern imaging techniques performed due to other indications. Typical symptoms from centrally located lung cancer include haemoptysis, cough, wheezing, dyspnoea, chest pain, and

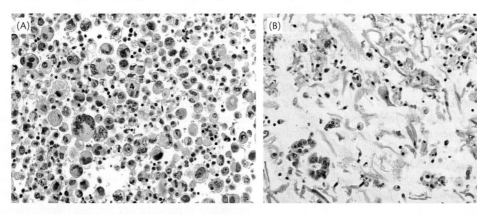

Fig. 46.9 (A) This cytology cell block of a pleural fluid shows abundant, large cells of metastatic lung adenocarcinoma. These are in a clear majority of the cells in the fluid and numerous—adequate for molecular testing (H&E × 200). (B) This sample of bronchial washings shows a lot of debris, inflammatory cells but only a tiny cluster of tumour cells (bottom left). These were TTF1 positive but molecular testing would be very problematic on a sample like this (H&E × 200).

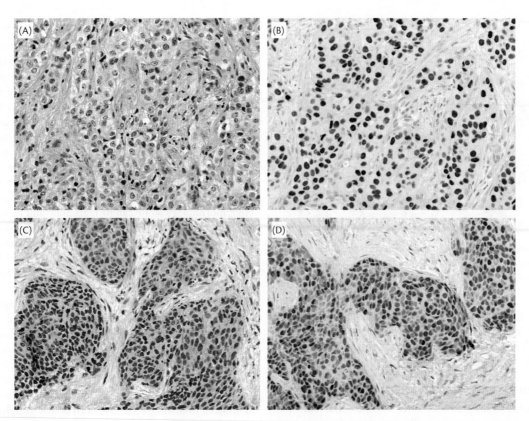

Fig. 46.10 (A) Mediastinal lymph node biopsy showing undifferentiated carcinoma lacking features to diagnose squamous cell or adenocarcinoma. This is NSCLC-NOS. Immunohistochemistry (B) shows strong TTF1 positivity so the diagnosis may be refined to 'NSCLC, probably adenocarcinoma' (× 200). (C) Lung core biopsy showing undifferentiated carcinoma lacking features to diagnose squamous cell or adenocarcinoma. This is NSCLC-NOS. Immunohistochemistry (D) shows strong p63 staining so the diagnosis may be refined to 'NSCLC, probably squamous cell carcinoma' (× 200).

frequent lung infections due to atelectasis. Peripheral lesion may be manifested by cough, pain due to invasion of chest wall, and dyspnoea. Tumours located in the superior sulcus are frequently associated with shoulder pain irradiating to forearm, fourth, and fifth fingers. Involvement of the lower brachial plexus is sometimes present with various degrees of neurological deficit. Horner's syndrome (myosis, ptosis, enophthalmos, and anhydrosis) is due to direct involvement of sympathetic chain. Mediastinal invasion may cause superior vena cava syndrome (SVCS) [18], dysphagia due to oesophageal compression or phrenic nerve palsy. Tumours or lymph nodes located at the aorto-pulmonary window typically result in hoarseness of voice due to recurrent laryngeal nerve palsy. Pleural involvement frequently results in accumulation of pleural fluid and dyspnoea. Occasionally, no primary tumour is present in radiological examinations of these patients, mimicking a clinical picture of mesothelioma. Pericardial involvement is a relatively infrequent but important cause of dyspnoea and other symptoms of cardiac tamponade. These two latter presentations are more frequent in patients with tumours harbouring ALK translocations [19].

A proportion of patients presents with symptoms resulting from metastatic spread. Brain metastases may lead to symptoms of increased intracranial pressure, seizures, or focal neurologic deficits. Bone metastases may cause pain and pathological fractures. An adrenal mass may occasionally be misdiagnosed as primary adrenal gland malignancy.

Lung cancer is relatively frequently associated with paraneoplastic syndromes [20]. Most common syndromes include syndrome of inappropriate antidiuretic hormone (ADH) excretion (SIADH), Cushing syndrome, hypercalcaemia due to production of parathyroid hormone-related protein (PTH-rp), carcinoid syndrome, neurological syndromes, hypertrophic pulmonary osteoarthropathy, and venous thromboembolism.

Diagnosis and staging

Diagnostic workup of patients with suspected lung cancer should include chest radiograms and computed tomography scans of the chest and upper abdomen. Pathological diagnosis remains the cornerstone of lung cancer management in all stages. For centrally located lesions, fibreoptic bronchoscopy (FOB) with forceps biopsy and brush cytology is recommended as a first step to establish tissue diagnosis. Careful description of bronchoscopic findings is essential for consideration of future surgery or definitive radiotherapy. Cytological examination of sputum is currently less frequently performed due to relatively low diagnostic accuracy. Peripheral lesions are accessible through fine needle aspiration, core needle biopsy, or video-assisted thoracic surgery (VATS), which should establish the diagnosis in 90–95% of cases in experienced hands. Although cytological diagnosis remains a valid proof of malignancy, histological diagnosis should be obtained whenever possible to ascertain precise histological subtyping. In patients with pleural effusions, inspection of pleural space through videothoracoscopy with biopsies of suspected lesions and cytological examination of pleural fluid should be performed. This procedure is often combined with pleurodesis to prevent further episodes of symptomatic accumulation of fluid in the pleural cavity.

Use of 18-fluorodeoxyglucose (FDG) positron emission tomography integrated with computed tomography (FDG PET/CT) has changed the paradigm of lung cancer staging. FDG PET/CT is currently indicated in all lung cancer patients with no overt dissemination, who are potential candidates for treatment with curative intent—surgery, radiotherapy, or combined chemoradiation. In a randomized clinical trial of FDG PET/CT versus conventional staging, a significant reduction of futile thoracotomies of about 20% was observed [21]. FDG PET is sensitive, but not very specific, for determination of the malignant nature of the primary lesion. According to two meta-analyses, sensitivity and specificity of FDG PET is around 95% and 80%, respectively [22, 23]. Adenocarcinomas with bronchioalveolar component, carcinoids, and salivary gland carcinomas may show low tracer uptake, whereas squamous cell carcinomas are characterized by relatively high standardized uptake values (SUVs) [24]. Tumours less than 1 cm in diameter may show low FDG uptake due to the effect of respiratory motion and low PET spatial resolution.

FDG PET/CT is particularly useful for nodal staging and outperforms conventional CT in terms of diagnostic accuracy. Recent systematic review and meta-analysis of FDG PET/CT for mediastinal lymph node staging indicated pooled sensitivity of 76% and specificity of 88% (patient-based data) [25], which is higher than those formerly reported for conventional CT. High negative predictive value (NPV) of FDG PET/CT exceeding 90% for mediastinal lymph node involvement in most reports indicate that stage I patients with negative mediastinal scan results do not need to undergo invasive mediastinal staging. Due to the relatively high rate of false-positive FDG PET/CT, results of approximately 10–20%, endoscopic biopsies or mediastinoscopy should be undertaken to confirm N2 or N3 disease with the exception of large, radiologically evident metastatic lymph nodes present on CT scans.

Mediastinoscopy, a short surgical procedure done under general anaesthesia, remains standard to assess paratracheal and subcarinal lymph node stations (stations 2–4 and 7 according to International Association for the Study of Lung Cancer (IASLC) nodal classification) [26]. At present, endobronchial ultrasound-guided fine needle aspiration (EBUS-FNA) and transoesophageal endoscopic ultrasound-guided fine needle aspiration (EUS-FNA) have largely replaced mediastinoscopy for initial staging of the mediastinum in lung cancer patients and are considered appropriate for invasive staging of the mediastinum. These techniques can assess a wider range of lymph node stations than mediastinoscopy (EBUS: stations 2–4, 7, 10–12; EUS: stations 2L, 4L, 5, 7, 8, and 9). In the largest randomized trial [27] that compared endoscopic staging with mediastinoscopy, sensitivity to detect lymph node metastases was 79% and 85%, respectively (P = 0.47). In patients with mediastinal lymph node involvement who are candidates for radical surgery after induction treatment, mediastinoscopy should be reserved for assessment of lymph node status after initial staging with endoscopic techniques.

The currently used 7th edition of NSCLC TNM staging system was developed by the IASLC based on the database comprising 46 series of patients from collaborative groups and single institutions (a complete dataset of approximately 67 000 subjects) from more than 20 countries worldwide [28]. The staging classification was endorsed by the International Union against Cancer (IUCC) and

the American Join Committee on Cancer (AJCC). The T category is subdivided into four subsets (T1–T4) according to tumour size, relationship to anatomical structures in the thorax, occurrence of satellite nodules, and presence of atelectasis (Table 46.1). Regional lymph node metastatic involvement may include N1 (bronchiopulmonary), N2 (ipsilateral mediastinal), or N3 (contralateral hilar, contralateral mediastinal, or supraclavicular) lymph node groups (Table 46.1). A revised map of thoracic lymph node stations was proposed and should be routinely used by pneumonologists, radiologists, thoracic surgeons, radiation oncologists, and all other health care professionals involved in the care of lung cancer patients (Figure 46.11) [29]. The M category is subdivided into M0 (no distant metastases), M1a (satellite lesions in contralateral lung or pleural involvement), or M1b (distant metastases).

Lung cancer stage definitions according to particular T, N, and M categories are shown in Table 46.2. Compared to previous staging system, approximately 15% of patients are placed into different stage categories leading to more accurate associations with outcome [28]. Most notable changes include shift of T3N0 category from previous IIIA to IIB stage group, distinction of satellite nodules in the same lobe as T3 category, in different ipsilateral lobe as T4 category, in the contralateral lobe as M1a category, and shift of pleural involvement from T4 category into M1a category, resulting in a shift of previous stage IIIB patients with this feature into current stage IV. The proportion of NSCLC patients surviving five years from diagnosis according to pathological stage is approximately 60–80% for stage I, 30–50% for stage II, 15–25% for stage III, and below 10% for stage IV, depending on published series.

Management of early stage non-small cell lung carcinoma

Surgery

Surgical resection of the lung remains the best treatment for patients with lung cancer whose extension is limited to the primary lesion or to the hilar lymph nodes, provided that the patient has good functional reserve. These patients belong to stage IA, IB, IIA, and IIB. Since the stage IIIA is very heterogeneous, surgery for patients with stage IIIA disease is sometimes controversial. A patient with IIIA disease without mediastinal lymph node involvement (T3N1, T4N0–1) can be considered as a surgical candidate usually in combination with chemo- or radiochemotherapy. It should be noted that chemotherapy adds significant, albeit modest, survival benefit. The T4 category ranges from invasion of mediastinal fat tissue to direct invasion to the aorta, or the heart itself. Combined resection of the superior vena cava or left atrium is usually feasible without the aid of cardiopulmonary bypass and sometimes is performed in combination with other modalities of therapy. Resections that require cardiopulmonary bypass are considered to be highly experimental.

Treatment for tumours with mediastinal lymph node involvement (N2 disease) is even more controversial. N2 disease is again heterogeneous in clinical outcome when treated by primary surgery. According to Andre et al., five-year survival rate for N2 diseases that were not detected preoperatively involving one lymph node level ('incidental' N2) was 34% and those with multiple level involvement was 11%, whereas those that were detected preoperatively with one level involvement was 8% and those with multiple level involvement was 3% [30]. Therefore, single station N2 disease candidates are often considered for surgery, usually combined with chemo/

Table 46.1 Definitions of T, N, and M descriptors of 7th TNM classification of lung cancer

T (primary tumour)	
Tx	Primary tumour cannot be assessed, or tumour proven by the presence of malignant cells in sputum or bronchial washings but not visualized by imaging or bronchoscopy
T0	No evidence of primary tumour
Tis	Carcinoma in situ
T1	Tumour ≤3 cm, surrounded by lung or visceral pleura, not more proximal than the lobar bronchus[a]
T1a	Tumour ≤2 cm in greatest dimension
T1b	Tumour >2 but ≤3 cm in greatest dimension
T2	Tumour >3 cm but ≤7 cm or tumour with any of the following features (T2 tumours with these features are classified T2a if ≤5 cm): - Involves main bronchus, ≥2 cm distal to the carina - Invades visceral pleura - Associated with atelectasis or obstructive pneumonitis that extends to the hilar region but does not involve the entire lung
T2a	Tumour >3 but ≤5 cm in greatest dimension
T2b	Tumour >5 but ≤7 cm in greatest dimension
T3	Tumour >7 cm or one that directly invades any of the following: chest wall (including superior sulcus tumours), diaphragm, phrenic nerve, mediastinal pleura, parietal pericardium; or tumour in the main bronchus <2 cm distal to the carina[a] but without involvement of the carina; or associated atelectasis or obstructive pneumonitis of the entire lung or separate tumour nodule(s) in the same lobe
T4	Tumour of any size that invades any of the following: mediastinum, heart, great vessels, trachea, recurrent laryngeal nerve, oesophagus, vertebral body, carina; separate tumour nodule(s) in a different ipsilateral lobe
N (regional lymph nodes)	
NX	Regional lymph nodes cannot be assessed
N0	No regional node metastasis
N1	Metastasis in ipsilateral peribronchial and/or ipsilateral hilar lymph nodes and intrapulmonary nodes, including involvement by direct extension
N2	Metastasis in ipsilateral mediastinal and/or subcarinal lymph node(s)
N3	Metastasis in contralateral mediastinal, contralateral hilar, ipsilateral or contralateral scalene, or supraclavicular lymph node(s)
M (distant metastasis)	
MX	Distant metastasis cannot be assessed
M0	No distant metastasis
M1a	Separate tumour nodule(s) in a contralateral lobe; tumour with pleural nodules or malignant pleural (or pericardial) effusion[b]
M1b	Distant metastasis

[a] The uncommon superficial spreading tumour of any size with its invasive component limited to the bronchial wall, which may extend proximally to the main bronchus, is also classified as T1.

[b] Most pleural (and pericardial) effusions with lung cancer are due to tumour. In a few patients, however, multiple cytopathologic examinations of pleural (pericardial) fluid are negative for tumour, and the fluid is nonbloody and is not an exudate. Where these elements and clinical judgment dictate that the effusion is not related to the tumour, the effusion should be excluded as a staging element and the patient should be classified as T1, T2, T3, or T4.

Reproduced from Goldstraw P et al., The IASLC Lung Cancer Staging Project: proposals for the revision of the TNM stage groupings in the forthcoming (7th) edition of the TNM classification of malignant tumours, *Journal of Thoracic Oncology*, Volume 2, Number 8, pp. 706–714, Copyright © 2007 International Association for the Study of Lung Cancer, with permission from Lippincott Williams and Wilkins/Wolters Kluwer Health.

radiotherapy in clinical practice. As discussed later, it is clear that post-operative adjuvant chemotherapy adds significant and modest survival benefit to stage III patients. However, for patients with N2 disease that were preoperatively diagnosed, there have been no clinical trials that clearly proved the role of pulmonary resection.

Removal of the affected pulmonary lobe (lobectomy) with mediastinal and hilar lymph node dissection remains a standard procedure. The extent of pulmonary resection is primarily based on the results of randomized trial performed by Lung Cancer Study Group reported in 1995 comparing standard lobectomy with limited

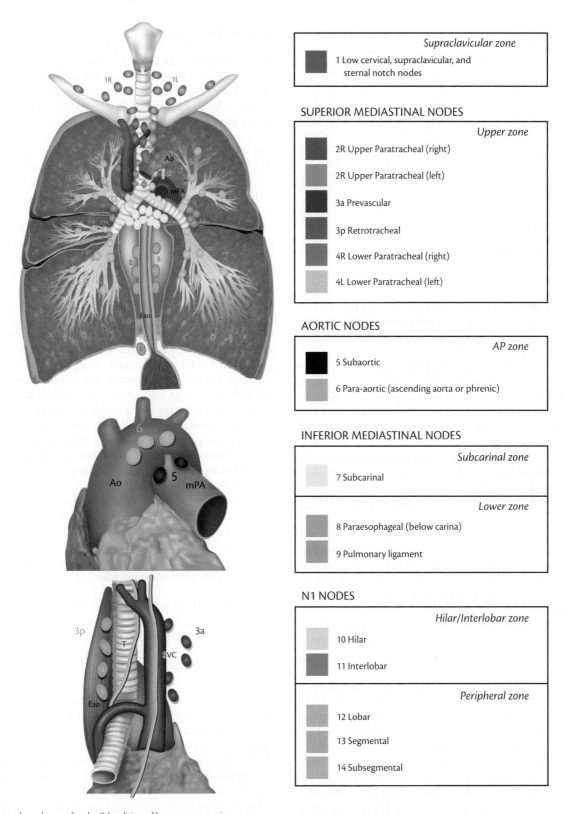

Fig. 46.11 Lymph node map for the 7th edition of lung cancer staging system.

Reproduced from Rusch VW et al., The IASLC lung cancer staging project: a proposal for a new international lymph node map in the forthcoming 7th edition of the TNM classification for lung cancer, *Journal of Thoracic Oncology*, Volume 4, Issue 5, pp. 568–570, Copyright © 2009 International Association for the Study of Lung Cancer, with permission from Lippincott Williams and Wilkins/Wolters Kluwer Health.

Table 46.2 Stage categories according to T, N, and M descriptors of 7th TNM classification of lung cancer

T/M	Subgroups	N0	N1	N2	N3
T1	T1a	IA	IIA	IIIA	IIIB
	T1b	IA	IIA	IIIA	IIIB
T2	T2a	IB	IIA	IIIA	IIIB
	T2b	IIA	IIB	IIIA	IIIB
T3	T3	IIB	IIIA	IIIA	IIIB
T4	T4	IIIA	IIIA	IIIB	IIIB
M1	M1a	IV	IV	IV	IV
	M1b	IV	IV	IV	IV

Reproduced from Goldstraw P et al., The IASLC Lung Cancer Staging Project: proposals for the revision of the TNM stage groupings in the forthcoming (7th) edition of the TNM classification of malignant tumours, *Journal of Thoracic Oncology*, Volume 2, Number 8, pp. 706–714, Copyright © 2007 International Association for the Study of Lung Cancer, with permission from Lippincott Williams and Wilkins/Wolters Kluwer Health.

resections (segmentectomy or wedge resection) for patients with tumours ≤3cm and no lymph node involvement [31]. This trial showed a trend toward worse outcomes in the patients with limited resection (one sided P = 0.062) [31].

Lymph node dissection is aimed to provide accurate lymph node staging and possibly therapeutic benefit. Although there is no doubt that lymph node dissection provides best staging, the therapeutic role of lymph node dissection is not clear as there have been limited numbers of phase III trials asking this question and their results have been inconsistent.

Recently, the American College of Surgeons has performed a randomized trial of mediastinal lymph node sampling vs lymph node dissection during pulmonary resection in patients with N0 or N1 non-small cell lung carcinoma [32]. In this trial, 2R, 4R, 7, and 10R lymph nodes for right-sided tumours and 5, 6, 7, and 10L for left-sided tumours were sampled, and when all these nodes were negative, patients were randomized either to perform complete lymph node dissection (dissection group) or to no further sampling (sampling group) [32]. There was no survival difference between two arms; the median survival was 8.1 years for the sampling group and 8.5 years for dissection (P = 0.25) [32]. The extensive sampling procedure makes the interpretation of the results difficult. The authors offered the caveats that these results are not generalizable to patients staged radiographically or those with higher stage tumours [32].

When the tumour is large and is located close to pulmonary hilus, it is not possible to remove the tumour by lobectomy. If surgery is indicated in such cases at all, pneumonectomy needs to be performed. Such indication should be carefully assessed and weighted against radical radiochemotherapy by experienced surgeon in a multidisciplinary team, because pneumonectomy (especially right-sided) may potentially cause significant morbidity and mortality. It is not always possible, but in some cases bronchoplastic procedure such as sleeve lobectomy can replace pneumonectomy without deterioration of long-term survival. For patients with poor pulmonary reserve or those with tumours with a supposedly benign nature, segmentectomy or wedge resection may be selected depending on tumour size, location, malignant potential, and patients' physiological condition.

Although limited resection is inferior to standard lobectomy, recent innovation of diagnostic imaging has made it possible to diagnose tumours of smaller size and with less opaque (ground glass-like) shadow. For these types of tumours, limited resection may be sufficient. The Japan Clinical Oncology Group prospectively evaluated preoperative thin-section computed tomography for its ability of prediction of non-invasiveness in clinical T1N0M0 peripheral lung tumours [33]. In a group of 545 patients, they concluded that radiological non-invasive peripheral lung adenocarcinoma could be defined as an adenocarcinoma ≤2.0 cm in diameter with ≤0.25 cm consolidation to the maximum tumour diameter [33]. Several clinical trials validating limited resection strategies for patients with tumours measuring less than 2 cm are underway.

There are several ways to access the lung during surgery. Posterolateral thoracotomy has been the standard for pulmonary resection in which the incision is about 30 cm in length and it starts at point midway between the medial border of the scapula and the thoracic spine, then it curves a little below the tip of the scapula and turns to run parallel with the ribs and extends to the submammary crease, usually dissecting latissimus and anterior serratus muscle. Recently, some surgeons prefer to use muscle-sparing thoracotomy in which division of latissimus or anterior serratus muscle is avoided. This thoracotomy can be used for most pulmonary surgeries including pneumonectomies or bronchoplastic procedures.

With the advent of appropriate imaging technology, VATS is becoming popular. It is expected that less invasion to the chest wall will result in less pain, shorter hospital stay, and less morbidity. However, recent systematic review evaluating two randomized and 19 non-randomized trials that compared VATS lobectomy with open lobectomy (most of them are through posterolateral thoracotomy) suggested that there was no statistically significant difference between two groups in terms of prolonged air leak, arrhythmia, pneumonia, or mortality [34].

In general, pulmonary resection has become a safe procedure with 30-day mortality below 3%. For example, in 11 663 pulmonary resections performed in Japan in 2004, grade >3 post-operative complication occurred in 523 (4.5%) and 30-day mortality was 0.4% [35]. Complications after lung cancer surgery are mostly related to cardiopulmonary sequelae.

Adjuvant post-operative chemotherapy

Results of meta-analysis of adjuvant chemotherapy trials in resected NSCLC published in 1995 provided the first unequivocal evidence favoring such treatment (5% survival improvement) [36]. Since then, several randomized trials have been conducted [37–42]. Most of the trials, summarized in Table 46.3, used cisplatin or carboplatin with new generation cytotoxic agents. In two meta-analyses that included recent adjuvant studies, an approximate 5% absolute survival improvement was indeed observed [43, 44]. The benefit was confined to patients with stage II and stage III disease. In stage IB, only patients with tumours larger than 4 cm appeared to benefit, whereas stage IA patients tended to have worse outcomes with adjuvant treatment. A performance status of 2 was associated with no benefit from adjuvant therapy. Current indications for adjuvant chemotherapy include pathological stage II and III NSCLC patients with complete postsurgical recovery and no contraindications to this therapy due to comorbidities. The use of adjuvant treatment in stage IB patients with larger tumours remains controversial. The benefit is observed irrespectively of gender, age, and histological

Table 46.3 Selected large clinical trials with adjuvant chemotherapy in non-small cell lung cancer

Trial [ref]	Number of patients	Chemotherapy agents (number of cycles)	Pathological stage	Survival probability at 5 years (experimental vs control group)	Survival hazard ratio (95% CI)	P value
IALT [36]	1865	Cisplatin/etoposide (3–4) Cisplatin/vinorelbine (3–4) Cisplatin/ vinblastine (3–4) Cisplatin/vindesine (3–4)	I–III	44–5% vs 40–4%	0.86 (0.76–0.98)	<0.03
ALPI [38]	1209	Mitomycin C/vindesine/cisplatin (3)	I–III	NR (1% absolute benefit)	0.96 (0.81–1.13)	0.96
CALGB 9633 [39]	344	Carboplatin/paclitaxel (4)	IB	59% vs 57%	0.83 (0.64–1.08)	0.10
BR.10 [41]	482	Cisplatin/vinorelbine (4)	IB–II	69% vs 54%	0.69 (0.52–0.91)	0.009
ANITA [37]	840	Cisplatin/vinorelbine (4)	IB–III	NR	0.80 (0.66–0.96)	0.017
Japan Lung Cancer Research Group [40]	979	Uracil-tegafur (2 years)	I	88% vs 85%	0.72 (0.53–1.00)	0.047

NR, not reported.

subtype. Since most of the adjuvant chemotherapy trials used platinum doublets with either vinorelbine or paclitaxel, these agents are commonly used in practice. Survival gain from adjuvant treatment appears to be less pronounced after longer observation in some, but not all, clinical trials, indicating possible impact of long-term toxicities from chemotherapy.

Based on the analyses of tumour tissue material from adjuvant chemotherapy trials, several biomarkers were proposed to associate with improved outcomes. Immunohistochemical expression of excision-repair cross-complementary 1 protein (ERCC1, a protein involved in the nucleotide excision repair pathway of DNA damage) appeared most promising for application in routine practice to select patients for adjuvant treatment. High ERCC1 expression was thought to be associated with lack of benefit from (platinum-based) adjuvant chemotherapy. A large validation study performed in the cohort of participant of the IALT adjuvant chemotherapy trial did not confirm the previous observations. No biomarker is currently recommended for use for selection of NSCLC patients to adjuvant therapy outside of clinical trials.

Current clinical research strategies to improve outcomes of NSCLC patients with post-operative adjuvant treatments include the use of targeted therapies in molecularly-selected subsets of patients, use of anti-angiogenic agents or immunotherapeutics, and selection of patients based on molecularly-defined risk scores. Until the results of clinical trials testing these strategies become available, they are not recommended for management of NSCLC patients outside of clinical trials.

Radical radiotherapy

The efficacy of modern conventional radiotherapy in patients with early-stage NSCLC is modest and most of the patients experience local relapse after treatment [45]. Most of the series exploring radical radiotherapy in early-stage NSCLC reported outcomes of those patients who were inoperable due to comorbidities or did not wish to undergo surgery. These patients remain at high risk of death due to other causes, such as chronic obstructive pulmonary disease (COPD) or cardiovascular disease. In patients with node-negative NSCLC, stereotactic radiotherapy (SBRT) is associated with

excellent long-term loco-regional control approaching surgical results of at least 70% and usually in the range of 80–95% [46]. The procedure is now widely used in developed countries and was demonstrated to impact on survival of early-stage NSCLC cohorts according to Dutch cancer registry data [47]. Main inclusion criteria for SBRT are pathological proof of malignancy (positive PET scan is acceptable only in patients for whom pathological confirmation is not possible) and outside of clinical trials size of less than 5 cm, location not adjacent to mediastinal structures or main bronchi and lymph node-negative disease as assessed by PET (mandatory). Strict radiotherapy quality control measures must be in place, including assessment of respiratory movement of the tumour during treatment planning and image-guided radiotherapy delivery. There is no universal agreement on the best fractionation schedule, but 54 Gy in three fractions, 55 Gy in five fractions or 60 Gy in eight fractions are commonly used in Europe and North America, or 48 Gy in four fractions in Japan. Current clinical studies are evaluating SBRT in larger or centrally located tumours. The use of sequential or concomitant chemotherapy or targeted agents in patients with early NSCLC treated with SBRT is not recommended. Patients with stage II disease who are not candidates for surgery should be managed outside of clinical trials with conventional definitive radiotherapy or radiochemotherapy, depending on comorbidities.

Management of locally advanced non-small cell lung carcinoma

Stage III NSCLC, according to the 7th edition of the AJCC TNM classification, describes a very heterogeneous group of different clinical entities, varying from the T3N1 category of patients to those with ipsilateral (N2) or contralateral (N3) mediastinal lymph node involvement. Management of patients with N2 or N3 lymph node stations involved by the tumour continues to be debated, mainly because of lack of sufficient evidence from randomized clinical trials regarding particular subsets. Several sub-classifications according to the extent of N2/N3 disease were proposed [48, 49] to formally address this need, yet none have been introduced into routine clinical practice. One of the proposals suggests describing N2/N3 nodal involvement as 'incidental' (i.e., unsuspected after careful nodal evaluation with PET and invasive staging), 'discrete', or 'minimal' when single or multiple normal or moderately enlarged lymph nodes are confirmed at staging and 'infiltrative' or 'bulky' when large nodes with possible mediastinal infiltration are present [49]. Other classifications emphasize single versus multiple nodal station involvement.

Historically, patients with 'resectable' stage IIIA N2 disease were treated with surgery and those with 'unresectable' IIIA and IIIB disease were treated with definitive radiotherapy. Results of both treatment modalities were unsatisfactory with five-year survival rates of approximately 5–15% [50, 51]. Patients with 'unsuspected' mediastinal nodal involvement discovered in post-operative pathological evaluation despite thorough preoperative staging according to current standards represent a relatively minor proportion, probably less than 10% of the operable NSCLC population. These patients should be treated with post-operative chemotherapy, with an expected absolute survival benefit of approximately 5% at five years [44]. The role of post-operative radiotherapy in pN2 patients with complete pathological resection (R0) remains unclear and should be a subject of individual risk/benefit evaluation. According to post-operative radiotherapy (PORT) meta-analysis on the role of adjuvant radiotherapy in surgically treated NSCLC [52, 53] patients with mediastinal nodal involvement had neither clear benefit nor detriment from radiation, whereas a survival detriment was clearly demonstrated for patients with pathological stage I and II. Post-operative radiotherapy resulted in improved local control in approximately half of the trials included in the PORT meta-analysis. Since the results of PORT meta-analysis are based on trials conducted more than two decades ago with outdated radiotherapy techniques, current evidence in support or against post-operative radiotherapy in patients with mediastinal nodal involvement remains weak. An ongoing phase III randomized study, Lung ART, should clarify the role of radiotherapy versus observation in patients with post-operative mediastinal nodal involvement. In the meantime, routine post-operative radiotherapy, typically in the dose of 54 Gy, is recommended in some centres in patients with a high risk of relapse (extracapsular extension or by individual assessment by surgeon), whereas other centres do not advocate this therapy. If chemotherapy and radiotherapy is indicated, chemotherapy should probably be administered sequentially to minimize toxicity [49], although no clear evidence exists regarding this strategy.

In patients who have pathologically proven 'potentially resectable' mediastinal lymph node involvement at presentation ('minimal N2') and in patients with unresectable stage III NSCLC ('infiltrative N2' and N3), the role of chemotherapy remains well established and optimal local treatment remains a matter of discussion. Based on two large randomized phase III trials, the role of surgery in both categories of patients appears minimal. The Integroup 0139 trial conducted in the United States randomly allocated patients with stages T1–3 N2 NSCLC to induction radiochemotherapy (radiation dose of 45 Gy with concurrent cisplatin 50mg/m^2 days 1, 8, 29, and 36 and etoposide 50mg/m^2 days 1–5 and 29–33) followed by surgery within three to five weeks in non-progressing patients or to definitive radiochemotherapy (radiation dose of 61 Gy, chemotherapy as above). Patients in both groups received two cycles of consolidation chemotherapy. The trial demonstrated no difference in overall survival (OS) (median of 23.6 months in group with surgery vs 22.2 months in group without surgery; HR = 0.87; P = 0.24). Progression-free survival was longer in patients randomized to surgery (median of 12.8 months vs 10.5 months; HR = 0.77; P = 0.017). Early mortality not attributable to lung cancer was higher in the surgical group (8% vs 2%, respectively), particularly after pneumonectomy. In an unplanned post hoc analysis of patients treated with lobectomy vs matched cohort receiving definitive chemoradiation, approximately 10% long-term survival advantage was noted. The authors concluded that potential benefit for patients treated with surgery was offset by increased complications and mortality from tri-modality treatment. The 08941 phase III trial by the EORTC Lung Cancer Group included patients with 'unresectable N2' NSCLC, a notable difference from the INT0139 trial discussed above. Patients were treated with three cycles of cisplatin or carboplatin induction chemotherapy doublet, most frequently with gemcitabine or a taxane, and then randomly allocated to surgery vs definitive radiotherapy (60–62.5 Gy to involved primary tumour and mediastinal lymph nodes and 40–46 Gy to uninvolved mediastinum). The response rate to induction treatment was 61%. Compliance with assigned treatment was high (92% and 93%, respectively). There was no survival difference for patients allocated to surgery (median of 16.4 months) as compared to radiotherapy (median of 17.5 months).

Based on the above trials, definitive radiochemotherapy is considered a standard treatment for most patients with stage III NSCLC. Given the subset results of INT 0139 and relative good long-term outcomes of some phase II trials [54], a few institutions continue to recommend surgery in very carefully selected patients with N2 disease after induction treatment (chemotherapy or concurrent chemoradiation). The decisions regarding the optimal choice and sequence of treatment must be taken by multidisciplinary teams of thoracic surgeons, radiation oncologists, medical oncologists, radiologists, pathologists, and pulmonologists. The additional value of radiotherapy added to chemotherapy in this setting is being uncertain and questioned [55]. Pneumonectomy after induction treatment should be avoided given high mortality rates of this procedure. Treatment should be given in high volume centres experienced in multimodality care.

Definitive radiochemotherapy should optimally consist of concurrent radiation and two cycles of cisplatin-based chemotherapy. Current radiotherapy recommendations in stage III NSCLC define target volumes around the tumour and involved nodal regions with appropriate margins, with no elective mediastinal irradiation [56, 57]. Technical advances in radiotherapy, such as PET-based treatment planning, control of respiratory motion by 4D CT, and image-guided radiotherapy delivery, are extremely important for achieving good outcomes. Radiotherapy plans should be qualitatively evaluated for dose distribution in critical organs, such as lung, oesophagus, spinal cord, heart, and brachial plexus to minimize radiation-induced toxicity. International guidelines are available to assist radiation oncologists in making appropriate choices based on dose distribution within organs at risk [58–60]. To select an optimal dose-distribution of a treatment plan, radiation oncologists should consider these guidelines within the context of the institutional experience and predefined quality control procedures. Minimal standards for definitive thoracic radiotherapy include 3D conformal radiotherapy planning and image-guided radiotherapy delivery according to the institutional protocol. Intensity modulated radiation therapy (IMRT) is commonly used in order to reduce radiation dose to the lung and oesophagus.

The value of concurrent vs sequential chemotherapy and radiotherapy in stage III NSCLC was tested in several clinical trials.

Meta-analysis of these trials [61] indicated an absolute benefit for concurrent treatment of 4.5% at five years (HR = 0.84, P = 0.004) at the expense of increased G3–4 acute esophageal toxicity (from 4–18%) with no difference regarding acute pulmonary toxicity. Cisplatin-etoposide (at full systemic doses) or cisplatin-vinorelbine (with decreased dose of vinorelbine) remain the most extensively studied regimens. Preliminary results of concurrent treatment with novel agents, such as pemetrexed or cetuximab, do not appear promising, although full results of several studies are awaited. The strategies of induction chemotherapy followed by concurrent radiochemotherapy [62] or concurrent radiochemotherapy followed by consolidation chemotherapy [63] have not led to improvement of survival in stage III NSCLC and are not recommended in a routine care.

In a preliminary report from RTOG 0617 phase III trial, conventionally-fractionated 60 Gy and 74 Gy radiotherapy doses were directly compared [64]. In this factorial design study, patients received concurrent chemotherapy (weekly doses of carboplatin and paclitaxel) and cetuximab or placebo, followed by consolidation treatment. Patients who received higher radiotherapy dose had significantly worse survival (median of 20.3 vs 28.7 months in the control group, P = 0.0007). No survival benefit was observed with the addition of cetuximab. In the RTOG 0617 trial, many centres included only few patients. Potential reasons for the unexpected results may lie in under-reported toxicity and in too-tight target volume margins in the high dose arm of the study. While full explanation of the results of RTOG 0617 awaits clarification, the dose of 60 Gy remains the standard of care with concurrent chemotherapy in stage III NSCLC in many institutions. A considerable number of institutions continue to use higher total radiotherapy doses of 66Gy, often exceeding 2 Gy per fraction (hypofractionation), sometimes with simultaneous integrated boost technique. In patients who are not eligible for concurrent radiochemotherapy due to age or comorbidities, sequential chemotherapy and radiation remains the best option. Those who are not eligible for chemotherapy should be treated with definitive radiotherapy alone.

Hyperfractionated and accelerated treatments were evaluated in a meta-analysis of several trials in non-metastatic NSCLC, most of which assessed different schedules of radiotherapy given alone or after induction chemotherapy. A small, but significant, advantage for accelerated schedules was observed with a 2.5% improvement in five-year survival (HR = 0.88, P = 0.009). Significantly better loco-regional outcomes were associated with highly accelerated schedules, emphasizing the importance of overall treatment time. The duration of definitive radiotherapy in stage III NSCLC should thus not be protracted (six weeks or even shorter whenever possible). Results of the CHARTWEL trial [65] indicate that the short overall time of radiotherapy delivery is particularly important in case of patients who received neoadjuvant chemotherapy (still significant proportion of patients treated worldwide) and for large tumours. Sequential schedules with highly accelerated radiotherapy are considered as important clinical research strategies to overcome the limitations of concurrent treatment.

Management of metastatic non-small cell lung carcinoma

More than half of NSCLC patients are diagnosed with metastatic disease; in addition, the majority of patients treated with curative intent for early or locally advanced disease will eventually relapse and develop metastatic disease. With the exception of a small proportion of patients presenting with oligometastatic disease, the prognosis of patients with stage IV NSCLC is fatal with a median survival of 9–15 months and a one-year survival of 30–58% [66, 67]. Systemic therapy is offered to patients with an Eastern Cooperative Oncology Group (ECOG) performance status (PS) of 0 to 2, aiming at prolongation of survival and maintaining quality of life. Therapy is individualized based on histological subtype, molecular pathology, age, comorbidities, expected toxicity, and patient preferences. Selected, practice-changing clinical trials addressing the role of chemotherapy in advanced NSCLC are summarized in Table 46.4.

Treatment for patients with metastatic NSCLC has historically consisted of systemic cytotoxic chemotherapy [68]. The identification of distinct subsets of NSCLC driven by specific genetic alterations, predicting for the benefit from targeted therapies, has substantially impacted on therapeutic strategies and improved outcome figures for molecularly-defined subsets of patients. Patients with tumours harbouring an activating mutation of the epidermal growth factor receptor (EGFR) or rearrangement of anaplastic lymphoma kinase (ALK) gene should be managed with an EGFR or ALK tyrosine kinase inhibitor (TKI), respectively. Other molecular aberrations, as for example HER2 and BRAF mutations, ROS1, and RET rearrangements, are amenable to targeted therapy and likely to influence lung cancer therapeutic portfolio in the very near future. For all other molecular subgroups representing the vast majority of NSCLC patients, cytotoxic chemotherapy remains the backbone of first-line treatment.

Management of patients with non-small cell lung carcinoma not characterized by a genetic driver alteration

First-line chemotherapy

Chemotherapy prolongs survival as compared to best supportive care, with a meta-analysis reporting a 27% relative reduction in the risk of death equivalent to a 10% improvement in one year survival [69, 70].

Platinum-based combination chemotherapy is considered the standard of care in first-line treatment for patients with good performance status. Third generation cytotoxic agents with documented single-agent activity in NSCLC include vinorelbine, gemcitabine, paclitaxel, docetaxel, irinotecan, and pemetrexed. The addition of a second drug to a single-agent regimen significantly increases the response rate (RR), one-year survival, and median overall survival at the expense of higher toxicity [71]. Three drug regimens further increase RR over two drug regimens, but fail to prolong survival, and are associated with increased toxicity [72].

Three meta-analyses evaluating the role of platinum-based vs platinum-free doublets reported a benefit in one-year survival in favour of platinum-based doublets, albeit of marginal statistical significance. This benefit was shown to be restricted to cisplatin in one analysis, and was absent when platinum-based doublet regimens were compared to third generation platinum-free doublets in another study. Platinum-based treatment was associated with a higher incidence of severe toxicity [73–75].

Three meta-analyses have shown a higher response rates for cisplatin when compared with carboplatin combinations. In the individual patient data meta-analysis of nine randomized trials with

Table 46.4 Selected large, practise-changing phase III trials of chemotherapy or immunotherapy (first-line, maintenance, and second-line) in advanced non-small cell lung cancer

Trial [ref] (setting)	Treatment arms	Number of patients	Median progression-free survival [months] (95% CI) Hazard ratio (95% CI; P-value)	Median survival [months] (95% CI) Hazard ratio (95% CI; P-value)
Big Lung Trial [68] (first-line)	Cisplatin-based chemotherapy vs best supportive care	725	NR	8.0 vs. 5.7 HR 0.77 (0.66–0.89; P = 0.0006)
Schiller et al. [66] (first-line)	Cisplatin and paclitaxel Cisplatin and gemcitabine Cisplatin and docetaxel Carboplatin and paclitaxel	1115	Time to progression 3.4 (2.8–3.9) 4.2 (3.7–4.8) 3.7 (2.9–4.2) 3.1 (2.8–3.9)	7.8 (7.0–8.9) 8.1 (7.2–9.4) 7.4 (6.6–8.8) 8.1 (7.0–9.5)
Scagliotti et al. [79] (first-line)	Cisplatin and pemetrexed vs cisplatin and gemcitabine	1725	Overall: 4.8 vs 5.1 HR = 1.04 (0.94–1.15)	Overall: 10.3 vs 10.3 HR = 0.94 (0.84 to 1.05) Squamous: 9.4 vs 10.8 HR = 1.23 (1.00–1.51, P = 0.05) Non-squamous: 11.8 vs 10.4 HR = 0.81 (0.70–0.94, P = 0.005)
PARAMOUNT [91] (maintenance)	Pemetrexed maintenance vs placebo (in patients non-progressive after 4 cycles cisplatin and pemetrexed, non-squamous tumours)	539	4.1 vs 2.8 HR = 0.62 (0.49–0.79, P<0.0001)	13.9 vs 11.0 HR = 0.78 (0.64–0.96, P = 0.0195)
Shepherd et al. [108] (second-line)	Docetaxel vs best supportive care	204	Time to progression 2.47 vs 1.56 (P <0.001)	7.0 vs 4.6 (P = 0.047)
Hanna et al. [109] (second-line)	Pemetrexed vs docetaxel	571	Overall: 2.9 vs 2.9 (P = not significant) Squamous: 2.3 vs 2.7 HR = 1.40 (1.01–1.96, P = 0.046) Non-squamous: 3.1 vs 3.0 HR = 0.82 (0.66–1.02, P = 0.076)	Overall: 8.3 vs 7.9 (P = not significant) Squamous: 6.2 vs 7.4 HR = 1.56 (1.08–2.26, P = 0.018) Non-squamous: 9.3 vs 8.0 HR = 0.78 (0.61–1.00, P = 0.048)
CheckMate057 [120] (second-line)	Nivolumab vs docetaxel	582 (non-squamous histology only)	2.3 vs 4.2 HR 0.92 (0.77–1.11, P = 0.3932)	12.2 vs 9.4 HR = 0.73 (0.59–0.89, P = 0015)
CheckMate017 [119] (second-line)	Nivolumab vs docetaxel	271 (squamous histology only)	3.5 vs 2.8 HR = 0.62 (0.47–0.81, P = 0.0004)	9.2 vs 6.0 HR = 0.59 (0.44–0.79, P = 0.00025)

NR, not reported.

Adapted with permission from Pallis AG et al., Chemotherapy of advanced non-small-cell lung cancer, *Clinical Investigation*, Volume 3, Issue 1, pp. 265–279, Copyright © 2013 Future Science.

almost 3000 patients [76], survival figures with cisplatin regimens were non-significantly better (median survival of 9.1 vs 8.4 months, respectively, P = 0.10). In the subset analysis, significantly superior efficacy was noted in the subgroup of non-squamous tumours and in patients treated with third generation cytotoxics. Cisplatin-based chemotherapy was associated with more nausea and vomiting as well as peripheral neuropathy and renal impairment, while haematological toxicity was higher with carboplatin [76–78].

No single regimen has clearly demonstrated superiority in unselected patients with advanced NSCLC. The largest trial comparing different platinum-based doublet regimens (cisplatin-paclitaxel, cisplatin-gemcitabine, cisplatin-docetaxel, carboplatin-paclitaxel) failed to demonstrate any difference in response or survival among the four arms [66]. Pemetrexed is preferred to gemcitabine in patients with non-squamous tumours based on a survival benefit demonstrated in a planned subgroup analysis of a randomized phase III first-line trial, whereas it was shown inferior in patients with tumours of squamous histology [79].

Maintenance therapy

Prolongation of the initial chemotherapy doublet from four to six cycles did not improve survival and resulted in substantial additional toxicity in a randomized phase III trial [80]. Prolongation of treatment beyond four to six cycles was associated with a statistically significant improvement in progression-free survival (PFS), and a modest but significant improvement in survival in one meta-analysis. Prolongation of treatment, however, was also associated with a higher rate of adverse events and possible impairments of health-related quality of life [81]. Two further meta-analyses evaluating the effects of prolonged first-line third generation platinum doublet chemotherapy beyond four cycles could not demonstrate any improvement in OS [82, 83], establishing the standard of frontline 4 cycles of platinum-based chemotherapy [83].

In clinical practice, only 50–60% of patients receive second-line treatment, with rapid disease progression being the main reason for not administering subsequent therapies. In an attempt to improve the results of first-line combination therapy administered for a standard number of cycles, several maintenance strategies have been tested, either continuing one agent previously administered as first-line (continuation maintenance) or commencing an agent with a different mechanism of action (switch maintenance). Maintenance therapy is given without treatment-free period after the completion of first-line chemotherapy. Numerous randomized trials have demonstrated that maintenance treatment is associated with an improvement of PFS, as well as OS to a variable extent depending on defined strategy [84].

Docetaxel switch maintenance improves PFS with a trend for OS improvement after four cycles of carboplatin and gemcitabine, with no detrimental effect in quality of life [85]. Erlotinib switch maintenance therapy improved PFS in two randomized trials. OS was prolonged with erlotinib in the largest, adequately powered trial to detect such differences, but this benefit was restricted to patients with stable disease after completion of first-line chemotherapy. This benefit was also seen in the patient subgroup without activating mutation of the EGFR gene [86, 87]. These results could not be reproduced with gefitinib switch maintenance [88]. Continuation maintenance with gemcitabine was tested in three randomized clinical trials, with improvement in time-to-treatment failure (TTF) or PFS in two, without improvement in survival, potentially because of sample size [87, 89]. Pemetrexed, either as switch maintenance or continuation maintenance, improves both PFS and OS, with no significant impact on quality of life [90, 91]. Its use should be restricted to patients with non-squamous tumours [92].

To date, there is no definite clinical parameter or biomarker helping to identify patients at risk of rapid progression that would potentially benefit more from a maintenance strategy. In addition, there is very limited comparative evidence among the different maintenance options, and maintenance decisions are currently often left to the physician's clinical judgment and subject to discussion with the patient.

Maintenance therapy should not be offered to patients with a performance status of 2 or greater or with persistent chemotherapy-induced toxicity. Furthermore, despite the low rate of grade 3 or 4 toxicities during maintenance treatment, the prolonged exposure of patients to grade 1 or 2 toxicities may be of significant concern.

Elderly patients and patients with poor performance status

Age and comorbidity may limit tolerance to chemotherapy. Single-agent chemotherapy offers a survival benefit compared to best supportive care in elderly NSCLC patients, where gemcitabine was shown similar activity to vinorelbine [93, 94]. The combination of monthly carboplatin with weekly paclitaxel in patients aged 70–89 years with PS 0–2 offers an advantage in PFS and survival over single-agent treatment with either vinorelbine or gemcitabine [95]. In patients with performance status of 2, combination therapy of carboplatin and pemetrexed offers a significant survival advantage over pemetrexed alone [96].

Addition of targeted agents to chemotherapy in first-line treatment

Bevacizumab, a monoclonal antibody against vascular endothelial growth factor (VEGF), improved survival when administered concurrently with paclitaxel and carboplatin and continued until disease progression in patients with non-squamous NSCLC [97]. Another large placebo-controlled randomized trial with two doses of bevacizumab combined with gemcitabine-cisplatin failed to demonstrate survival advantage [98], although PFS prolongation was observed. A meta-analysis of four randomized trials demonstrated a clinically marginal survival improvement with bevacizumab (HR = 0.90, P = 0.03) as compared with chemotherapy alone [99]. Bevacizumab treatment is associated with a higher risk of thrombosis, hypertension, bleeding, proteinuria, and pulmonary haemorrhage [100]. When considering bevacizumab therapy, an individualized risk-benefit assessment should be undertaken in all patients. Bevacizumab is contraindicated in patients with squamous NSCLC or history of haemoptysis, but can be used in patients with previously treated brain metastases and in patients with full anticoagulation [101].

Cetuximab, a monoclonal antibody against EGFR, has been tested in two first-line phase III trials in combination with cisplatin-vinorelbine or cisplatin-taxane [102, 103]. A modest survival prolongation was observed in the first trial only. EGFR protein expression intensity was retrospectively identified as a potential predictive biomarker of cetuximab efficacy. Due to conflicting results, cetuximab is no longer being developed in the indication of NSCLC. Necitumumab, another monoclonal antibody against EGFR, has been tested in two parallel first-line phase III trials in combinations with platinum-based chemotherapy. The first trial, comparing necitumumab plus pemetrexed and cisplatin with pemetrexed and cisplatin alone in patients with previously untreated non-squamous NSCLC was stopped early based on the absence of any difference in overall survival between treatment groups [104]. The second trial, focusing on squamous NSCLC patients using a gemcitabine and cisplatin chemotherapy backbone demonstrated a modest improvement in survival, with no improvement of the objective response rate or median PFS [105].

Second-line and subsequent lines of treatment

All patients inevitably develop progressive disease after first-line chemotherapy. Second-line treatment with either chemotherapy or EGFR TKI may provide symptom palliation and prolong survival. Combination regimens have failed to show any survival benefit over single-agent regimens in one meta-analysis [106]. Erlotinib was shown to improve survival in unselected second-line or third-line NSCLC patients not eligible for further chemotherapy with tumours of all histologies [107]. Docetaxel significantly improved survival compared with best supportive care [108]. Pemetrexed showed similar RR and survival in a comparison with docetaxel, with less toxicity [109]. Erlotinib was also shown to be of similar efficacy compared with docetaxel or pemetrexed in unselected patients refractory to first-line platinum-based chemotherapy [110]. Gefitinib was proven non-inferior to docetaxel [111]. Also in the second-line setting, afatinib, an irreversible second-generation pan-Her TKI inhibiting EGFR, HER2 and HER4, has demonstrated a modest median OS benefit when compared to erlotinib in patients with squamous cell carcinoma of the lung [112]. Median PFS, disease control rate, and global health status/quality of life were also improved, while toxicity was higher. It should be noted, however, that when NSCLC patients are selected by EGFR gene mutation status, those with tumours characterized by a wild-type EGFR demonstrate a better survival when treated with second-line docetaxel as compared to erlotinib [113–115] as shown by a randomized phase III trial and at least two meta-analyses. Thus, assessment of EGFR mutation status in tumours is mandatory for clinical decisions favouring EGFR TKIs or chemotherapy. In case of EGFR mutation-positive or negative NSCLC, EGFR TKIs are not considered an appropriate second-line treatment for patients considered fit to receive chemotherapy.

The addition of anti-angiogenic agents to docetaxel has been shown to improve its efficacy. Ramucirumab, a human monoclonal antibody against the extracellular domain of vascular endothelial growth factor receptor 2 (VEGFR-2), showed improved response rate, median PFS, and OS compared to docetaxel alone, in patients with both squamous and non-squamous histology [116]. The addition of nintedanib, an oral angiokinase inhibitor to VEGFR1-3, fibroblast growth factor receptors (FGFR) 1-3, and platelet-derived growth factor receptors (PDGFR) alpha and beta, showed a benefit in median PFS compared to docetaxel in patients with NSCLC, and a benefit in median OS compared to docetaxel but only restricted to the patients with adenocarcinoma, an effect also shown to be most prominent in those patients who had progressed within nine months after initiation of first-line therapy in a retrospective subgroup analysis [117].

Additional anticancer agents, including gemcitabine, paclitaxel, vinorelbine, topotecan, and irinotecan, show some activity in chemotherapy-pretreated patients, but have not been adequately evaluated in randomized clinical trials and thus are not routinely recommended. Efficacy of all agents in this setting is generally poor, with response rates below 10% and median survival around six months. Significant improvements in overall quality of life with second-line treatment are infrequent. Quality of life can nevertheless be maintained using single-agent docetaxel or pemetrexed [109, 118].

Recent data have shown that docetaxel second-line chemotherapy as a standard of care after platinum-based doublet chemotherapy has been supplanted by immunotherapeutics. Two phase III trials of nivolumab, a fully human programmed-death (PD)-1 immune checkpoint inhibitor, versus docetaxel conducted in squamous and non-squamous histologies, respectively, have demonstrated a superiority in median OS, median PFS, RR, and toxicity for nivolumab, with a hazard ratio for death of 0.57 in patients with squamous NSCLC, and 0.73 for non-squamous histology, while being considerably less toxic than docetaxel [119, 120]. Other promising checkpoint inhibitors are in late-phase clinical development and predictive factors for the benefit from these therapies, such as immunohistochemical evaluation of PDL-1 ligand in the tumour and stroma, are currently being evaluated. The exact sequence of immune checkpoint inhibitors and chemotherapy will be refined over the next years, evaluating first-line immunotherapy strategies as well as combination with chemotherapy or targeted therapies.

Patients progressing after second-line chemotherapy are sometimes considered for further chemotherapy therapy in clinical practice, depending on performance status and toxicities from previous treatments. However, the evidence favouring efficacy of third-line therapy is lacking, with the exception of erlotinib in patients not eligible for further chemotherapy [107]. Clinical trials should strongly be considered in this setting, particularly with designs based on selection of patients based on molecular predictive assays.

Management of patients with non-small cell lung carcinoma harbouring EGFR mutation or ALK rearrangement

EGFR mutations

Sensitizing mutations in the EGFR sequence coding for tyrosine kinase are observed in approximately 15% of lung adenocarcinomas in Caucasian populations. These aberrations occur more frequently in patients from the Far East, never or light smokers and females. Testing for EGFR mutations is not recommended in patients with a confident diagnosis of squamous cell carcinoma, except in never/former light smokers (<15 packs per year). The presence of an EGFR activating mutation confers a more favourable prognosis and is strongly predictive of sensitivity to EGFR TKI therapy. Several randomized studies confirmed the value of first-line reversible EGFR TKIs (gefitinib and erlotinib) as compared to chemotherapy [121–126]. Selected large trials addressing the role of EGFR tyrosine kinase inhibitors vs chemotherapy in patients with tumours harbouring EGFR mutations are summarized in Table 46.5. All but one of these phase III trials were conducted in Asian populations. Cross-study comparisons suggest that, although the incidence of EGFR mutations is lower in Caucasian populations, the response

Table 46.5 Selected trials comparing first-line EGFR tyrosine kinase inhibitor with chemotherapy in patients with an EGFR activation mutation

Study [ref]	Author	EGFR tyrosine kinase inhibitor	Control arm	Number of patients	Tumour response rate	Median progression-free survival [months] Hazard ratio (95% CI; P-value)	Median survival [months] (95% CI) Hazard ratio (95% CI; P-value)
IPASS [121]	Mok et al.	Gefitinib	Carboplatin / paclitaxel	261	71.2 vs 47.3	9.8 vs 6.4 HR = 0.48 (0.36–0.64, P < 0.001)	21.6 vs 21.9 HR = 1.00 (0.76–1.33, P = 0.99)
WJTOG 3405 [123]	Mitsudomi et al.	Gefitinib	Cisplatin / docetaxel	172	62.1 vs 32.2	9.6 vs 6.6 HR = 0.52 (0.38–0.72, P < 0.0001)	35.5 vs 38.8 HR = 1.18 (0.77–1.83)
NEJ002 [124]	Maemondo et al.	Gefitinib	Carboplatin / paclitaxel	228	73.7 vs 30.7	10.8 vs 5.4 HR = 0.32 (0.24–0.44, P < 0.001)	27.7 vs 26.6 HR = 1.04 (0.63–1.24, P = 0.31)
OPTIMAL [125]	Zhou et al.	Erlotinib	Carboplatin / gemcitabine	154	83.0 vs 36.0	13.7 vs 4.6 HR = 0.16 (0.11–0.26, P < 0.0001)	22.7 vs 28.9 HR = 1.04 (0.69–1.58)
EURTAC [126]	Rosell et al.	Erlotinib	Cisplatin or carboplatin / docetaxel Or Cisplatin or carboplatin / gemcitabine	173	58.1 vs 14.9	9.7 vs 5.2 HR = 0.37 (0.25–0.54, P < 0.0001)	19.3 vs 19.5 HR = 1.04 (0.65–1.68)
LUX-lung 3 [127]	Sequist et al.	Afatinib	Cisplatin / pemetrexed	345	56 vs 23	11.14 vs 6.90 HR = 0.58 P < 0.001	28.2 vs 28.2 HR = 0.88 (0.66–1.17)
LUX-Lung 6 [128]	Wu et al.	Afatinib	Cisplatin / gemcitabine	364	66.9 vs 28.0	11.0 vs 5.6 HR = 0.28 P < 0.0001	23.1 vs 23.5 HR = 0.93 (0.72–1.22)

NR, not reported.

rates and PFS are similar in Asian patients with EGFR mutations. All these studies consistently report superior response rates (58.1 to 84.6% vs 14.9 to 47.3%) and PFS (9.7 to 13.7 months vs 4.6 to 6.7 months) to EGFR TKI therapy as compared to standard chemotherapy, with more favourable toxicity profiles and improved quality of life. None of these studies could demonstrate an improvement of survival (median ranging from 19.3 to 30.1 months), probably because of intensive crossover from chemotherapy to EGFR TKI at disease progression in the control arms. The second generation irreversible EGFR TKI afatinib also showed a significant PFS benefit compared with cisplatin-pemetrexed, at the expense of higher incidence of skin rash, diarrhoea, and mucositis [127, 128]. No adequately powered trial has directly compared gefitinib, erlotinib, and afatinib. In a pooled analysis of two trials comparing afatinib with cisplatin-based doublet chemotherapy, overall survival was significantly longer for patients with del 19-positive tumours in the afatinib group than in the chemotherapy group, while there was no significant difference by treatment group for patients with point mutation EGFR Leu858Arg in exon 21 positive tumours. As with first-generation reversible EGFR TKIs, response rates and median PFS were greatly improved in the afatinib group as compared with the chemotherapy groups, in both del 19-positive tumours and

EGFR Leu858Arg-positive tumours [129]. The same observation about differential biology of del 19-positive tumours and EGFR Leu858Arg-positive tumours [129] when treated with EGFR TKI, in particular in terms of PFS, was confirmed in a subsequent meta-analysis [130].

Concurrent continuous administration of chemotherapy and EGFR TKI does not provide any response or survival advantage [131, 132]. EGFR tyrosine kinase inhibitors were also tested with pharmacodynamic separation, i.e., starting the EGFR inhibitor several days after cytotoxic agents and stopping before the next chemotherapy cycle ('intercalated schedules'). A phase III study testing intercalated erlotinib with gemcitabine-cisplatin resulted in improved PFS and survival in the subset of patients with EGFR-mutated tumours, despite extensive crossover to erlotinib in the control arm [133]. Further studies with intercalated schedules in patients with EGFR mutation-positive NSCLC are needed before this treatment strategy is introduced into routine practice. Continuation of gefitinib beyond progression in combination with cisplatin and pemetrexed in patients with acquired resistance to gefitinib does not improve outcome [134], as shown in a phase III randomized trial. Central nervous system penetration of erlotinib or gefitinib is limited (approximately 1–5% of plasma levels), but are, however, sufficient to obtain responses similar to extracranial disease [135]. Despite initial activity of EGFR TKIs, all patients eventually develop acquired resistance. The most common mechanism of resistance is the EGFR T790M secondary mutation, which accounts for 50–60% of cases, and prevents gefitinib or erlotinib from binding to the ATP-binding pocket of EGFR protein. Second generation EGFR TKIs are effective in preclinical gefitinib- and erlotinib-resistant EGFR T790M models, but their delivery in EGFR TKI resistant patients have shown modest activity to date in the clinic, with low response rates and side effects limiting the ability to administer doses that effectively inhibit T790M EGFR [136, 137]. Third-generation 'mutant-selective' irreversible EGFR TKIs specifically inhibit T790M and other activating EGFR mutations while sparing wild-type EGFR. Among these, mereletinib and rociletinib are in the late phase of their development [138, 139]. Other mechanisms of resistance include MET amplification, HER2 amplification, BRAF mutation, or histologic transformation to small-cell lung cancer [140].

ALK rearrangements

Translocations involving the ALK (anaplastic lymphoma kinase) tyrosine kinase are present in approximately 2–4% of lung adenocarcinomas in Caucasian populations, more frequently in younger patients and light or never-smokers. Patients with tumours harbouring ALK rearrangement more often present with brain and liver metastases as well as pleural and pericardial effusions. The presence of an ALK rearrangement is strongly predictive of sensitivity to ALK inhibitor therapy. Crizotinib, an oral ALK, MET and ROS1 inhibitor, provides increased response rates and PFS compared to either pemetrexed or docetaxel monotherapy, respectively, in the second-line setting [141] (median of 7.7 vs 4.2 vs 2.6 months). Because of significant crossover of patients from the chemotherapy arm at the time of progression, OS was not significantly different. In the first-line setting, crizotinib significantly improves response rate and PFS (median 10.9 vs 7.0 months) when compared to cisplatin or carboplatin plus pemetrexed, establishing crizotinib as the standard first-line treatment in this subgroup [142]. Crizotinib is generally well tolerated and is associated with gastrointestinal disturbance, visual changes, low testosterone levels, and elevated transaminases. Low penetration of crizotinib into the central nervous system might result in underexposure of brain metastases to the drug, leading to 'pharmacodynamic resistance', a phenomenon of exclusive progression in the brain while response in other tumour sites is maintained [143]. Several resistance mechanisms to crizotinib have been identified, including active ALK-dominant (resistance mutations and ALK copy number gain) and ALK non-dominant pathways (the outgrowth of clones containing a separate activated oncogene) [19]. Second-generation ALK inhibitors are more potent against ALK in vitro than crizotinib and can overcome selected ALK kinase domain mutations associated with resistance to crizotinib. Among these, ceritinib and alectinib are in the late phase of their development. Both drugs demonstrate activity against central nervous system disease [144], owing to their related better CNS penetration [145]. Ceritinib and alectinib have been approved in the setting of crizotinib resistance in some countries [146].

Other agents, including third generation ALK TKIs, are under development [147].

Management of oligometastatic disease

Stage IV NSCLC patients presenting with solitary metastases localized to brain, adrenals, or lung can be considered for treatment with curative intent after adequate staging workup has been conducted. Prognosis of patients with oligometastatic NSCLC is worse for synchronous metastases than for metachronous metastases. In the case of solitary brain metastasis, surgical resection, or stereotactic radiosurgery may be of benefit. The addition of whole brain radiotherapy (WBRT) after surgery or stereotactic radiotherapy was tested in a phase III trial in patients with one to three metastases from different primary sites, most commonly from NSCLC [148]. This study, conducted in 359 patients, demonstrated better local control after WBRT but no impact on survival. Five-year survival in patients in whom complete resection of metastases has been achieved ranges from approximately 10% to 30%. In the case of solitary adrenal metastasis, prolonged survival after resection of both primary tumour and adrenal has been suggested, with a five-year survival of 10–26% [149, 150]. There are no data regarding the role of adjuvant chemotherapy in patients who have undergone curative resection of a brain or adrenal metastasis, however most physicians use systemic treatment in this setting. A solitary pulmonary lesion in a different lobe, particularly in the absence of mediastinal lymph node involvement, should be considered as a synchronous second primary tumour and treated with curative intent. The survival of these patients is highly variable according to reported series, with five-year survival ranging from 0 to 50% according to patient selection criteria.

Management of small cell lung carcinoma and other neuroendocrine tumours

Small cell lung carcinoma

Until recently, SCLC has been classified into two stage categories: limited and extensive disease. This practical classification, introduced by the Veterans Administration Lung Cancer Study Group, was used in most clinical trials conducted in SCLC that provided evidence for present standards of care. According to the current 7th edition of the AJCC TNM classification, limited disease corresponds to T1-T4 N0-N3 M0 whereas extensive disease corresponds to any T/any N, M1a or M1b stage categories.

Early stage small cell lung carcinoma (T1-T4 N0-N3 M0)

Prognosis of patients diagnosed with early stage SCLC is characterized by median survival of approximately 16–24 months and five-year survival probability of approximately 20%. Extensive evidence supports chemoradiotherapy as the standard of care in fit early stage patients who are candidates for this treatment. Historically, the introduction of chemotherapy improved very poor outcomes of these patients, some of whom had been previously treated with surgery. Subsequent addition of chest radiotherapy increased three-year survival probability by 5.4% according to the meta-analysis of several trials [151]. Further trials focused on optimization of chemotherapy, optimization of radiotherapy, and better integration of these treatment modalities.

A combination of four to six cycles of cisplatin-etoposide is recommended for treatment of patients with early stage SCLC [152].

Although similar results are achieved with carboplatin-etoposide [153], small number of patients with limited disease in the meta-analysis precludes definitive conclusions regarding equivalence of both schedules. Anthracycline-based schedules are inferior to platinum-based chemotherapy in patients with early-stage SCLC [154] and are more toxic when combined with radiotherapy, and are therefore not recommended. No progress has been observed with other agents or strategies tested to improve systemic treatment results of early SCLC.

Optimal timing of chemotherapy and radiotherapy has been studied extensively in the past. Data from clinical trials and several meta-analyses [155, 156] have yielded conflicting results, with some studies suggesting the benefit from early (starting with the first or second chemotherapy cycle) vs late radiotherapy, whereas other trials did not confirm this finding. When analysis was limited to trials with radiotherapy combined with platinum-etoposide, the benefit from early concurrent treatment was observed, particularly in trials in which dose intensity of chemotherapy was maintained despite early administration of radiotherapy. Another meta-analysis of four randomized trials with platinum-etoposide chemotherapy indicated that time of start of any treatment to end of radiotherapy (SER) of less than 30 days was associated with significantly better five-year survival probabilities at the expense of higher severe esophagitis rates [157]. Thus, combined chemotherapy with early radiotherapy (starting with the first or second cycle) should be considered in fit patients with early stage SCLC. In practice, there are patients who are not candidates for early chemoradiation due to comorbidities or due to large tumour volume affecting planned dose-volume parameters to the extent precluding definitive treatment. In such patients, late or sequential radiotherapy should be considered. Post-chemotherapy target volumes for primary tumour are sufficient in treatment planning, but all initially affected lymph node stations should be included in the radiotherapy field.

Optimal chest radiotherapy dose and fractionation has also been studied extensively. Most radiotherapy departments recommend either a hyperfractionated accelerated schedule of 45 Gy delivered twice daily or a conventionally fractionated or slightly hypofractionated schedule of 54–66 Gy delivered every day. Dose and schedule of concurrent radiochemotherapy in SCLC is often considered individually taking into account planning target volumes and expected toxicity based on dose distribution in organs at risk, particularly lung and oesophagus. The rationale to use accelerated radiotherapy schedules stems from radiobiological data of increased SCLC radiosensitivity to low radiation doses. In the pivotal clinical trial that addressed the issue of accelerated hyperfractionation [158], long-term survival was significantly increased from 16% (standard arm, 45 Gy in 25 fractions once daily) to 26% (experimental arm, 45 in 30 fractions twice daily) at the expense of higher severe esophagitis rates (11% and 27%, respectively). Despite this evidence, recommended also in current European guidelines for management of SCLC [152], some radiation oncologists still use conventionally fractionated doses of 60 Gy or more arguing that radiation dose in the standard arm of the above-mentioned Intergroup study is inadequately low, twice daily radiotherapy is logistically difficult and associated with clinically problematic oesophageal toxicity. Two large clinical trials are ongoing to address the optimal radiotherapy dose and schedule in SCLC (CONVERT trial conducted in Europe and Canada, comparing 45 Gy in 30 fractions and 70 Gy in 35 fractions and the CALGB 30610/RTOG0538

trial conducted in the United States assessing three different fractionation schedules). Results of these trials should provide further evidence to guide clinical practice.

Prophylactic cranial irradiation (PCI) should be given to all patients who have responded to initial treatment. The main goal of this therapy is to reduce the incidence of brain metastases by approximately 50% and to increase long-term survival by approximately 5%, as evidenced by meta-analysis of individual data from seven randomized trials that included mostly patients with limited disease SCLC [159]. The optimal dose of PCI was analysed in the phase III Intergroup trial led by French investigators, in with patients were randomly allocated to 25 Gy or 36 Gy [160]. The incidence of brain metastases at two years, the primary study endpoint, was not significantly different between study arms (29% and 23%, respectively, P = 0.18). Worse survival was observed in the high PCI dose arm due to a higher number of cancer-related deaths (HR = 1.20, P = 0.05). Minor neurological decline in time was noted across both arms of the trial with no difference between radiation doses [161]. While this study established 25 Gy in 10 fractions as a standard dose for PCI in patients with SCLC, some centres continue to use the dose of 30 Gy in 15 fractions, which was not compared in clinical trials. The advantages of PCI may be offset by increased neurocognitive deficits in elderly patients with pre-existing dementia, mandating careful consideration of its use in this patient category.

The value of surgery is debated in very early SCLC with no nodal involvement. In this rare patient category, no comparative evidence-based data exist to guide management. Results of surgical treatment followed by adjuvant chemotherapy are relatively good with long-term survival in the order of 30–50% [162], prompting many physicians to recommend this strategy in highly-selected patients. If this approach is taken, prophylactic cranial irradiation should be also routinely performed and chest radiotherapy should be considered in patients with incomplete resections [152].

Metastatic small cell lung carcinoma (any T, any N, M1a, or M1b)

The first proof of benefit of cytotoxic agents in SCLC was demonstrated in the early 1970s when studies exploring cyclophosphamide demonstrated significant survival prolongation compared to best supportive care. Subsequently, a number of other agents and combination therapies were tested with anthracyclines, etoposide, and platinum compounds selected as the most active in this disease. Combination of cyclophosphamide, doxorubicin, and vincristine (CAV), cyclophosphamide, doxorubicin, and etoposide (CAE), or cyclophosphamide, doxorubicin, vincristine, and etoposide (CAVE) were shown to have similar efficacy to cisplatin-etoposide in patients with extensive SCLC, whereas cisplatin-etoposide was associated with better outcome and was less toxic when combined with thoracic radiotherapy in patients with limited SCLC. Platinum-etoposide is also associated with less myelosuppression as compared to anthracycline-based chemotherapy. The optimal duration of first-line chemotherapy was established to be four to six cycles. Several other strategies were tested in the last two decades in phase II or phase III clinical trials: alternating treatment with different schedules, maintenance treatment, chemotherapy dose intensification with or without hematopoietic growth factor support, addition of other cytotoxic agent to platinum-etoposide, use of targeted therapies, or immunotherapy. These strategies failed to improve clinically meaningful patient outcomes. Several clinical trials comparing cisplatin and carboplatin were summarized in a meta-analysis from individual data of 663 patients [153]. Median survival of patients treated with cisplatin-based chemotherapy was 9.6 months as compared to 9.4 months for carboplatin (HR = 1.08, P = 0.37). Use of carboplatin was associated with more haematological toxicities, whereas use of cisplatin was linked to higher likelihood of nausea/vomiting, peripheral neuropathy, and renal impairment. In the last decade, a set of studies was conducted with camphthotecin derivatives (topoisomerase I inhibitors: irinotecan and topotecan) and amrubicin, an anthracycline with favorable cardiac toxicity profile and high topoisomerase II inhibition potency. A phase II clinical trial conducted by the Japanese Clinical Oncology Group evaluated cisplatin-irinotecan combination versus cisplatin-etoposide as front-line therapy in patients with metastatic SCLC [163]. The trial was closed after interim analysis of 154 patients showed a significantly superior survival favouring irinotecan (median survival of 12.8 months vs 9.4 months, P = 0.002). Phase III trials with irinotecan [164–167] or topotecan [168] conducted in the United States or Europe have not confirmed the superiority of camphthotecins over platinum-etoposide, except for one trial in which relatively poor outcome of patients in a control group treated with carboplatin and oral etoposide was reported [165]. Amrubicin-cisplatin has shown similar efficacy to cisplatin-etoposide in one phase III first-line trial in metastatic SCLC [169]. In summary, four to six cycles of cisplatin-etoposide or carboplatin-etoposide combination are recommended in metastatic SCLC. In patients with SCLC who have contraindications to platinum compounds, anthracycline-based chemotherapy (CAE or CAV) should be considered as a reasonable alternative.

Reported response rates in patients with metastatic SCLC to first-line chemotherapy are in the order of 50–70%, median progression-free survival is approximately five months and OS is approximately 9–12 months. In patients who relapse, options for systemic treatment are limited and depend primarily on duration of response to first-line therapy, patient performance status, age, comorbidities, and toxicities from previous chemotherapy. Patients who respond to first-line chemotherapy and progress within three months of last chemotherapy administration are categorized as 'refractory' whereas those who have a longer relapse-free interval are categorized as 'sensitive'. In patients with refractory disease, oral topotecan, intravenous topotecan, anthracycline-based chemotherapy, or best supportive care should be considered. In this category, treatment outcome is poor with response rates of approximately 5–20%. Patients with sensitive disease should be treated with single-agent topotecan, anthracycline-based chemotherapy, or re-induction with platinum-etoposide, particularly if relapse-free period exceeds six months. Reported response rates in this category are typically between 20–40%. In patients who received anthracycline-based chemotherapy as front-line treatment, subsequent therapy with platinum-etoposide should be considered.

Prophylactic cranial irradiation was investigated in metastatic SCLC patients who have responded to first-line chemotherapy in a phase III clinical trial that aimed to demonstrate the reduction of proportion of patients who experience clinical progression in the brain. The trial met its primary endpoint, showing that PCI reduces the risk of brain metastases from 40.4% in the control arm to 14.6% in experimental arm at one year. This trial also showed that the use of PCI is associated with survival benefit (median of 6.7 vs 5.4 months, respectively; HR = 0.68, P = 0.003). Based on the above study, PCI is recommended in metastatic SCLC patients who had a response to initial chemotherapy. Treatment should start within five weeks after the last chemotherapy cycle. The dose of 25 Gy in 10 fractions is most commonly used.

Carcinoid tumours and large cell neuroendocrine carcinoma

The spectrum of neuroendocrine malignancies includes typical carcinoids (fewer than two mitoses per 2 mm^2 or ten high power fields), atypical carcinoids (more than two mitoses per 2 mm^2), large cell neuroendocrine carcinoma (LCNEC), and SCLC discussed above. Two former entities are low and intermediate grade whereas the two latter entities are high-grade neuroendocrine tumours. These two groups share neuroendocrine differentiation markers but have distinct molecular profiles and very different biological and clinical characteristics. Carcinoid syndrome, associated with serotonin and kallikrein secretion by the tumour, is manifested by flushing, diarrhoea, wheezing, and heart failure. Syndrome occurs in up to 3% of patients and is usually associated with a high tumour burden, and typically with liver metastases. Somatostatin receptors are present in the majority of neuroendocrine tumours and may be visualized by somatostatin scintigraphy (Octreoscan™) and indium-111 or gallium-68 radiolabelled PET tracers, used for the purpose of staging. Staging of carcinoids and LCNEC is performed according to current TNM classification. Due to low incidence, comparative evidence for management of carcinoids and LCNEC does not exist and most data are derived from single-arm trials or comparative trials in which pulmonary neuroendocrine tumours usually represent a minor proportion of patients.

Pulmonary carcinoids belong to the group of foregut neuroendocrine tumours, constitute up to 3% of lung malignancies and typically occur in the main bronchi. Peripheral carcinoids are observed in about 30% of cases. Ten-year survival probabilities for patients with typical and atypical carcinoids are approximately 90% and 50%, respectively. Distant metastases occur most commonly in the lungs, liver, and bones. Centrally located stage I and II carcinoids should be managed with lung parenchyma-sparing surgery and mediastinal lymph node dissection or sampling. Surgical margins may be minimal to avoid extensive resections. Atypical carcinoids are more likely to occur as peripheral lesions, hence a lobectomy is often considered in a patient with stage I or II disease and adequate pulmonary reserve, although limited resections may also be an option. Significant controversy exists regarding the optimal management of carcinoids with mediastinal lymph node involvement which is sometimes observed in the case of atypical tumours. In this setting, most physicians recommend a combined modality approach with aggressive surgery if technically feasible. Adjuvant chemotherapy or radiotherapy is not indicated for typical carcinoids and atypical carcinoids with no nodal involvement. Adjuvant chemotherapy is controversial in patients with atypical carcinoids and involved lymph nodes; prognosis of these patients is considerably worse, but there is no evidence of benefit from adjuvant treatment.

Several cytotoxic agents are used in the management of metastatic carcinoid tumours. These agents include cisplatin, carboplatin, etoposide, streptozocin, doxorubicin, and 5-fluorouracil. The response rates to platinum-etoposide or streptozocin-based regimens depends on tumour grade and is typically in the range of 10% for typical carcinoids and 20–50% for atypical carcinoids, with no clear evidence favouring any particular regimen. Somatostatin analogues, such as octreotide acetate long-acting repeatable (LAR) formulation, provide benefit to the majority of patients with hormone-related symptoms. Objective tumour responses to somatostatin analogues are infrequent (<10%), hence the direct anti-tumour effect of these agents have been debated. The PROMID trial, conducted in 85 patients with functionally active and inactive well-differentiated metastatic mid-gut neuroendocrine tumours, showed prolongation of time-to-progression in patients treated with long-acting octreotide as compared to placebo (median of 14.3 vs 6 months, HR = 0.34, P = 0.00072) [170]. Results of this study have been extrapolated to bronchiopulmonary carcinoids, although no clear evidence exists regarding survival benefit from the use of these agents. Radionuclide therapy with radiolabelled somatostatin analogues have been developed and tested in patients with positive diagnostic octreotide scintigraphy. In a phase II study, 90 patients with various carcinoid tumours refractory to octreotide therapy, received three doses of ^{90}Y-edotreotide every six weeks. Objective responses were observed in 4% of patients, disease control was noted in 74% of patients, and median progression-free and overall survival was 16.3 and 26.9 months, respectively [171].

Recent clinical studies have demonstrated prolongation of progression-free survival in patients with pancreatic neuroendocrine tumours when treated with octreotide LAR combined with everolimus (mammalian target of rapamycin, mTOR inhibitor) or with sunitinib [172, 173]. The impact of these agents on outcomes of metastatic lung carcinoid patients is unknown.

Diagnosis of LCNEC is difficult, particularly in small specimens. LCNEC is an aggressive malignancy, most often diagnosed in locally advanced or metastatic stage, with clinical behaviour and spectrum of molecular aberrations similar to SCLC. The optimal chemotherapy has not been established in comparative trials. A retrospective analysis of patients with pure pulmonary LCNES suggests that platinum-etoposide is more effective than chemotherapy schedules typically used in NSCLC, such as cisplatin-gemcitabine or cisplatin-paclitaxel [174]. A prospective phase II trial exploring the efficacy of platinum-etoposide in 42 LCNEC advanced patients reported median progression- free and overall survival of 5.2 and 7.7 months, respectively. Due to poor survival after surgery alone in stage I LCNEC, adjuvant chemotherapy is suggested similarly to SCLC.

References

1. Ferlay J, Parkin DM, Steliarova-Foucher E. Estimates of cancer incidence and mortality in Europe in 2008. European Journal of Cancer 2010; 46(4): 765–781.
2. Wakelee HA, Chang ET, Gomez SL et al. Lung cancer incidence in never smokers. Journal of Clinical Oncology 2007; 25(5): 472–478.
3. Siegel R, Naishadham D, Jemal A. Cancer statistics, 2013. CA A Cancer Journal for Clinicians 2013; 63(1): 11–30.
4. Mattson ME, Pollack ES, Cullen JW. What are the odds that smoking will kill you. American Journal of Public Health 1987; 77(4): 425–431.
5. Rodgman A, Smith CJ, Perfetti TA. The composition of cigarette smoke: a retrospective, with emphasis on polycyclic components. Human and Experimental Toxicology 2000; 19(10): 573–595.
6. Driscoll T, Nelson DI, Steenland K et al. The global burden of-disease due to occupational carcinogens. American Journal of Industrial Medicine 2005; 48(6): 419–431.
7. Schwartz AG, Prysak GM, Bock CH et al. The molecular epidemiology of lung cancer. Carcinogenesis 2007; 28(3): 507–518.
8. Ding L, Getz G, Wheeler DA et al. Somatic mutations affect key pathways in lung adenocarcinoma. Nature 2008; 455(7216): 1069–1075.
9. Cancer Genome Atlas Research Network. Comprehensive genomic characterization of squamous cell lung cancers The Cancer Genome Atlas Research Network (2012; 489, 519). Nature 2012; 491(7423): 288.
10. Nakamura H, Kawasaki N, Taguchi M, et al. Role of preoperative chemotherapy for non-small-cell lung cancer: a meta-analysis. Lung Cancer 2006; 54(3): 325–329.
11. Jaenne PA, Shaw AT, Pereira JR, et al. Selumetinib plus docetaxel for KRAS-mutant advanced non-small-cell lung cancer: a randomised, multicentre, placebo-controlled, phase 2 study. Lancet Oncology 2013; 14(1): 38–47.
12. Pao W, Miller VA. Epidermal growth factor receptor mutations, small-molecule kinase inhibitors, and non-small-cell lung cancer: current knowledge and future directions. Journal of Clinical Oncology 2005; 23(11): 2556–2568.
13. Soussi T, Wiman KG. Shaping genetic alterations in human cancer: the p53 mutation paradigm. Cancer Cell 2007; 12(4): 303–312.
14. Khan A, Lu H. Inhibition of MDM2-p53 feedback loop by various small molecules for potential cancer chemotherapy. Cancer Biology and Therapy 2008; 7(6): 853–855.
15. Carbone DP, Ciernik IF, Kelley MJ, et al. Immunization with mutant p53- and K-ras-derived peptides in cancer patients: immune response and clinical outcome. Journal of Clinical Oncology 2005; 23(22): 5099–5107.
16. Travis WD, Brambilla E, Burke AP, Marx A, Nicholson AG. WHO classification of tumours of the lung, pleura, thymus and heart. 4th ed. WHO press, Geneva, 2015.
17. Chansky K, Sculier JP, Crowley JJ, et al. The International Association for the Study of Lung Cancer Staging Project: prognostic factors and pathologic TNM stage in surgically managed non-small cell lung cancer. Journal of thoracic oncology: official publication of the International Association for the Study of Lung Cancer 2009; 4(7): 792–801.
18. Wilson LD, Detterbeck FC, Yahalom J. Superior vena cava syndrome with malignant causes. New England Journal of Medicine 2007; 356(18): 1862–1869.
19. Doebele RC, Pilling AB, Aisner DL, et al. Mechanisms of resistance to crizotinib in patients with ALK gene rearranged non-small cell lung cancer. Clinical Cancer Research 2012; 18(5): 1472–1482.
20. Yeung S-CJ, Habra MA, Thosani SN. Lung cancer-induced paraneoplastic syndromes. Current Opinion in Pulmonary Medicine 2011; 17(4): 260–268.
21. Fischer B, Lassen U, Mortensen J, et al. Preoperative staging of lung cancer with combined PET-CT. New England Journal of Medicine 2009; 361(1): 32–39.
22. Gould MK, Maclean CC, Kuschner WG, et al. Accuracy of positron emission tomography for diagnosis of pulmonary nodules and mass lesions—a meta-analysis. Journal of the American Medical Association 2001; 285(7): 914–924.
23. Hellwig D, Ukena D, Paulsen F, et al. Meta-analysis of the efficacy of positron emission tomography with F-18-fluorodeoxyglucose in lung tumors. Basis for discussion of the German Consensus Conference on PET in Oncology 2000. Pneumologie (Stuttgart, Germany) 2001; 55(8): 367–377.
24. Vesselle H, Salskov A, Turcotte E, et al. Relationship between non-small cell lung cancer FDG uptake at PET, tumor histology, and Ki-67 proliferation index. Journal of Thoracic Oncology 2008; 3(9): 971–978.
25. Lv Y-L, Yuan D-M, Wang K, et al. Diagnostic performance of integrated positron emission tomography/computed tomography for mediastinal lymph node staging in non-small cell lung cancer a bivariate systematic review and meta-analysis. Journal of Thoracic Oncology 2011; 6(8): 1350–1358.
26. Vallieres E, Shepherd FA, Crowley J, et al. The IASLC lung cancer staging project proposals regarding the relevance of TNM in the pathologic

staging of small cell lung cancer in the forthcoming (seventh) edition of the TNM classification for lung cancer. Journal of Thoracic Oncology 2009; 4(9): 1049–1059.

27. Annema JT, van Meerbeeck JP, Rintoul RC, et al. Mediastinoscopy vs endosonography for mediastinal nodal staging of lung cancer a randomized trial. Journal of the American Medical Association 2010; 304(20): 2245–2252.

28. Goldstraw P, Crowley J, Chansky K, et al. The IASLC Lung Cancer Staging Project: proposals for the revision of the TNM stage groupings in the forthcoming (seventh) edition of the TNM Classification of malignant tumours. Journal of thoracic oncology: official publication of the International Association for the Study of Lung Cancer 2007; 2(8): 706–714.

29. Rusch VW, Crowley J, Giroux DJ, et al. The IASLC Lung Cancer Staging Project: proposals for the revision of the N descriptors in the forthcoming seventh edition of the TNM classification for lung cancer. Journal of thoracic oncology: official publication of the International Association for the Study of Lung Cancer 2007; 2(7): 603–612.

30. Andre F, Grunenwald D, Pignon JP, et al. Survival of patients with resected N2 non-small-cell lung cancer: evidence for a subclassification and implications. Journal of Clinical Oncology 2000; 18(16): 2981–2989.

31. Ginsberg RJ, Rubinstein LV. Randomized trial of lobectomy versus limited resection for T1 N0 non-small cell lung cancer. Lung Cancer Study Group. Annals of Thoracic Surgery. 1995; 60(3): 615–622; discussion 622–613.

32. Darling GE, Allen MS, Decker PA, et al. Randomized trial of mediastinal lymph node sampling versus complete lymphadenectomy during pulmonary resection in the patient with N0 or N1 (less than hilar) non-small cell carcinoma: results of the American College of Surgery Oncology Group Z0030 Trial. Journal of Thoracic and Cardiovascular Surgery 2011; 141(3): 662–670.

33. Suzuki K, Koike T, Asakawa T, et al. A prospective radiological study of thin-section computed tomography to predict pathological noninvasiveness in peripheral clinical ia lung cancer (Japan Clinical Oncology Group 0201). Journal of Thoracic Oncology 2011; 6(4): 751–756.

34. Yan TD, Black D, Bannon PG, et al. Systematic review and meta-analysis of randomized and nonrandomized trials on safety and efficacy of video-assisted thoracic surgery lobectomy for early-stage non-small-cell lung cancer. Journal of Clinical Oncology 2009; 27(15): 2553–2562.

35. Sawabata N, Miyaoka E, Asamura H, et al. Japanese Lung Cancer Registry study of 11,663 surgical cases in 2004 demographic and prognosis changes over decade. Journal of Thoracic Oncology 2011; 6(7): 1229–1235.

36. Chemotherapy in non-small cell lung cancer: a meta-analysis using updated data on individual patients from 52 randomised clinical trials. Non-small Cell Lung Cancer Collaborative Group. British Medical Journal 1995; 311(7010): 899–909.

37. Douillard JY, Rosell R, De Lena M, et al. Adjuvant vinorelbine plus cisplatin versus observation in patients with completely resected stage IB-IIIA non-small-cell lung cancer (Adjuvant Navelbine International Trialist Association [ANITA]): a randomised controlled trial. Lancet Oncology 2006; 7(9): 719–727.

38. Scagliotti GV, Fossati R, Torri V, et al. Randomized study of adjuvant chemotherapy for completely resected stage I, II, or IIIA non-small-cell Lung cancer. Journal of the National Cancer Institute 2003; 95(19): 1453–1461.

39. Strauss GM, Herndon JE, 2nd, Maddaus MA, et al. Adjuvant paclitaxel plus carboplatin compared with observation in stage IB non-small-cell lung cancer: CALGB 9633 with the Cancer and Leukemia Group B, Radiation Therapy Oncology Group, and North Central Cancer Treatment Group Study Groups. Journal of Clinical Oncology 2008; 26(31): 5043–5051.

40. Kato H, Ichinose Y, Ohta M, et al. A randomized trial of adjuvant chemotherapy with uracil-tegafur for adenocarcinoma of the lung. New England Journal of Medicine 2004; 350(17): 1713–1721.

41. Winton T, Livingston R, Johnson D, et al. Vinorelbine plus cisplatin vs. observation in resected non-small-cell lung cancer. New England Journal of Medicine 2005; 352(25): 2589–2597.

42. Arriagada R, Bergman B, Dunant A, et al. Cisplatin-based adjuvant chemotherapy in patients with completely resected non-small-cell lung cancer. New England Journal of Medicine 2004; 350(4): 351–360.

43. Pignon JP, Tribodet H, Scagliotti GV, et al. Lung adjuvant cisplatin evaluation: a pooled analysis by the LACE Collaborative Group. Journal of Clinical Oncology 2008; 26(21): 3552–3559.

44. Auperin A, Le Chevalier T, Le Pechoux C, et al. Adjuvant chemotherapy, with or without postoperative radiotherapy, in operable non-small-cell lung cancer: two meta-analyses of individual patient data. Lancet 2010; 375(9722): 1267–1277.

45. Verstegen NE, Lagerwaard FJ, Senan S. Developments in early-stage NSCLC: advances in radiotherapy. Annals of Oncology 2012; 23: 46–51.

46. Senthi S, Lagerwaard FJ, Haasbeek CJA, et al. Patterns of disease recurrence after stereotactic ablative radiotherapy for early stage non-small-cell lung cancer: a retrospective analysis. Lancet Oncology 2012; 13(8): 802–809.

47. Palma D, Visser O, Lagerwaard FJ, et al. Impact of introducing stereotactic lung radiotherapy for elderly patients with stage I non-small-cell lung cancer: a population-based time-trend analysis. Journal of Clinical Oncology 2010; 28(35): 5153–5159.

48. Robinson LA, Ruckdeschel JC, Wagner H, Jr, et al. Treatment of non-small cell lung cancer-stage IIIA—ACCP evidence-based clinical practice guidelines (2nd edition). Chest 2007; 132(3): 243S–265S.

49. Ramnath N, Dilling TJ, Harris LJ, et al. Treatment of stage III non-small cell lung cancer: diagnosis and management of lung cancer, 3rd ed.: American College of Chest Physicians evidence-based clinical practice guidelines. Chest 2013; 143(5 Suppl): e314S–340S.

50. Jassem J. Combined chemotherapy and radiation in locally advanced non-small-cell lung cancer. Lancet Oncology 2001; 2(6): 335–342.

51. DeCamp MM, Ashiku S, Thurer R. The role of surgery in N2 non-small cell lung cancer. Clinical Cancer Research 2005; 11(13): 5033S–5037S.

52. PORT Meta-analysis Trialists Group. Postoperative radiotherapy in non-small-cell lung cancer: systematic review and meta-analysis of individual patient data from nine randomised controlled trials. Lancet 1998; 352(9124): 257–263.

53. Group PM-aT. Postoperative radiotherapy for non-small cell lung cancer. Cochrane Database Systematic Reviews 2005(2): CD002142.

54. Betticher DC, Hsu Schmitz SF, Totsch M, et al. Mediastinal lymph node clearance after docetaxel-cisplatin neoadjuvant chemotherapy is prognostic of survival in patients with stage IIIA pN2 non-small-cell lung cancer: a multicenter phase II trial. Journal of Clinical Oncology 2003; 21(9): 1752–1759.

55. Shah AA, Berry MF, Tzao C, et al. Induction chemoradiation is not superior to induction chemotherapy alone in stage IIIA lung cancer. Annals of Thoracic Surgery 2012; 93(6): 1807–1812.

56. De Ruysscher D, Faivre-Finn C, Nestle U, et al. European organisation for research and treatment of cancer recommendations for planning and delivery of high-dose, high-precision radiotherapy for lung cancer. Journal of Clinical Oncology 2010; 28(36): 5301–5310.

57. Yuan S, Sun X, Li M, et al. A randomized study of involved-field irradiation versus elective nodal irradiation in combination with concurrent chemotherapy for inoperable stage III nonsmall cell lung cancer. Journal of Clinical Oncology 2007; 30(3): 239–244.

58. Gagliardi G, Constine LS, Moiseenko V, et al. Radiation dose-volume effects in the heart. International Journal of Radiation Oncology Biology Physics 2010; 76(3 Suppl): S77–85.

59. Marks LB, Bentzen SM, Deasy JO, et al. Radiation dose-volume effects in the lung. International Journal of Radiation Oncology Biology Physics 2010; 76(3 Suppl): S70–76.

60. Werner-Wasik M, Yorke E, Deasy J, et al. Radiation dose-volume effects in the esophagus. International Journal of Radiation Oncology Biology Physics 2010; 76(3 Suppl): S86–93.

61. Auperin A, Le Pechoux C, Rolland E, et al. Meta-Analysis of concomitant versus sequential radiochemotherapy in locally advanced

non-small-cell lung cancer. Journal of Clinical Oncology 2010; 28(13): 2181–2190.

62. Vokes EE, Herndon JE, II, Kelley MJ, et al. Induction chemotherapy followed by chemoradiotherapy compared with chemoradiotherapy alone for regionally advanced unresectable stage III non-small-cell lung cancer: Cancer and Leukemia Group B. Journal of Clinical Oncology 2007; 25(13): 1698–1704.

63. Jalal SI, Riggs HD, Melnyk A, et al. Updated survival and outcomes for older adults with inoperable stage III non-small-cell lung cancer treated with cisplatin, etoposide, and concurrent chest radiation with or without consolidation docetaxel: analysis of a phase III trial from the Hoosier Oncology Group (HOG) and US Oncology. Annals of Oncology 2012; 23(7): 1730–1738.

64. Bradley JD, Paulus R, Komaki R et al. Standard-dose versus high-dose conformal radiotherapy with concurrent and consolidation carboplatin plus paclitaxel with or without cetuximab for patients with stage IIIA or IIIB non-small-cell lung cancer (RTOG 0617): a randomized, two-by-two factorial phase 3 study. Lancet Oncology 2015; 16: 187–199. PMID: 25601342.

65. Baumann M, Herrmann T, Koch R, et al. Final results of the randomized phase III CHARTWEL-trial (ARO 97–1) comparing hyperfractionated-accelerated versus conventionally fractionated radiotherapy in non-small cell lung cancer (NSCLC). Radiotherapy and Oncology 2011; 100(1): 76–85.

66. Schiller JH, Harrington D, Belani CP, et al. Comparison of four chemotherapy regimens for advanced non-small-cell lung cancer. New England Journal of Medicine 2002; 346(2): 92–98.

67. Scagliotti G, Hanna N, Fossella F, et al. The differential efficacy of pemetrexed according to NSCLC histology: a review of two phase iii studies. Oncologist 2009; 14(3): 253–263.

68. Spiro SG, Rudd RM, Souhami RL, et al. Chemotherapy versus supportive care in advanced non-small cell lung cancer: improved survival without detriment to quality of life. Thorax 2004; 59(10): 828–836.

69. Alberti W, Anderson G, Bartolucci A, et al. Chemotherapy in non-small-cell lung-cancer—a metaanalysis using updated data on individual patients from 52 randomized clinical-trials. British Medical Journal 1995; 311(7010): 899–909.

70. Burdett S, Stephens R, Stewart L, et al. Chemotherapy in addition to supportive care improves survival in advanced non-small-cell lung cancer: a systematic review and meta-analysis of individual patient data from 16 randomized controlled trials—NSCLC meta-analyses collaborative group. Journal of Clinical Oncology 2008; 26(28): 4617–4625.

71. Delbaldo C, Michiels S, Syz N, et al. Benefits of adding a drug to a single-agent or a 2-agent chemotherapy regimen in advanced non-small-cell lung cancer—a meta-analysis. Journal of the American Medical Association 2004; 292(4): 470–484.

72. Azim HA, Jr, Elattar I, Loberiza FR, Jr, et al. Third generation triplet cytotoxic chemotherapy in advanced non-small cell lung cancer: a systematic overview. Lung Cancer 2009; 64(2): 194–198.

73. Pujol JL, Barlesi F, Daures JP. Should chemotherapy combinations for advanced non-small cell lung cancer be platinum-based? A meta-analysis of phase III randomized trials. Lung Cancer 2006; 51(3): 335–345.

74. D'Addario G, Pintilie M, Leighl NB, et al. Platinum-based versus non-platinum-based chemotherapy in advanced non-small-cell lung cancer: a meta-analysis of the published literature. Journal of Clinical Oncology 2005; 23(13): 2926–2936.

75. Rajeswaran A, Trojan A, Burnand B, et al. Efficacy and side effects of cisplatin- and carboplatin-based doublet chemotherapeutic regimens versus non-platinum-based doublet chemotherapeutic regimens as first line treatment of metastatic non-small cell lung carcinoma: a systematic review of randomized controlled trials. Lung Cancer 2008; 59(1): 1–11.

76. Ardizzoni A, Boni L, Tiseo M, et al. Cisplatin-versus carboplatin-based chemotherapy in first-line treatment of advanced non-small-cell lung cancer: an individual patient data meta-analysis. Journal of the National Cancer Institute 2007; 99(11): 847–857.

77. Hotta K, Matsuo K, Ueoka H, et al. Meta-analysis of randomized clinical trials comparing cisplatin to carboplatin in patients with advanced non-small-cell lung cancer. Journal of Clinical Oncology 2004; 22(19): 3852–3859.

78. Jiang J, Liang X, Zhou X, et al. A meta-analysis of randomized controlled trials comparing carboplatin-based to cisplatin-based chemotherapy in advanced non-small cell lung cancer. Lung Cancer 2007; 57(3): 348–358.

79. Scagliotti GV, Parikh P, von Pawel J, et al. Phase III study comparing cisplatin plus gemcitabine with cisplatin plus pemetrexed in chemotherapy-naive patients with advanced-stage non-small-cell lung cancer. Journal of Clinical Oncology 2008; 26(21): 3543–3551.

80. Park JO, Kim S-W, Ahn JS, et al. Phase III trial of two versus four additional cycles in patients who are nonprogressive after two cycles of platinum-based chemotherapy in non-small-cell lung cancer. Journal of Clinical Oncology 2007; 25(33): 5233–5239.

81. Soon YY, Stockler MR, Askie LM, et al. Duration of chemotherapy for advanced non-small-cell lung cancer: a systematic review and meta-analysis of randomized trials. Journal of Clinical Oncology 2009; 27(20): 3277–3283.

82. da Silveira Nogueira Lima JP, dos Santos LV, Sasse EC, et al. Optimal duration of first-line chemotherapy for advanced non-small cell lung cancer: a systematic review with meta-analysis. European Journal of Cancer 2009; 45(4): 601–607.

83. Rossi et al. Six versus fewer planned cycles of first-line platinum-based chemotherapy for non-small-cell lung cancer: a systematic review and meta-analysis of individual patient data. Lancet Oncology 2014; 1254–1262. PMID: 25232001.

84. Zhang X, Zang J, Xu J, et al. Maintenance therapy with continuous or switch strategy in advanced non-small cell lung cancer a systematic review and meta-analysis. Chest 2011; 140(1): 117–126.

85. Fidias PM, Dakhil SR, Lyss AP, et al. Phase III study of immediate compared with delayed docetaxel after front-line therapy with gemcitabine plus carboplatin in advanced non-small-cell lung cancer. Journal of Clinical Oncology 2009; 27(4): 591–598.

86. Cappuzzo F, Ciuleanu T, Stelmakh L, et al. Erlotinib as maintenance treatment in advanced non-small-cell lung cancer: a multicentre, randomised, placebo-controlled phase 3 study. Lancet Oncology 2010; 11(6): 521–529.

87. Perol M, Chouaid C, Perol D, et al. Randomized, Phase III study of gemcitabine or erlotinib maintenance therapy versus observation, with predefined second-line treatment, after cisplatin-gemcitabine induction chemotherapy in advanced non-small-cell lung cancer. Journal of Clinical Oncology 2012; 30(28): 3516–3524.

88. Zhang L, Ma S, Song X, et al. Gefitinib versus placebo as maintenance therapy in patients with locally advanced or metastatic non-small-cell lung cancer (INFORM; C-TONG 0804): a multicentre, double-blind randomised phase 3 trial. Lancet Oncology 2012; 13(5): 466–475.

89. Brodowicz T, Krzakowski M, Zwitter M, et al. Cisplatin and gemcitabine first-line chemotherapy followed by maintenance gemcitabine or best supportive care in advanced non-small cell lung cancer: a phase III trial. Lung Cancer 2006; 52(2): 155–163.

90. Ciuleanu T, Brodowicz T, Zielinski C, et al. Maintenance pemetrexed plus best supportive care versus placebo plus best supportive care for non-small-cell lung cancer: a randomised, double-blind, phase 3 study. Lancet 2009; 374(9699): 1432–1440.

91. Paz-Ares L, de Marinis F, Dediu M, et al. Maintenance therapy with pemetrexed plus best supportive care versus placebo plus best supportive care after induction therapy with pemetrexed plus cisplatin for advanced non-squamous non-small-cell lung cancer (PARAMOUNT): a double-blind, phase 3, randomised controlled trial. Lancet Oncology 2012; 13(3): 247–255.

92. Scagliotti G, Brodowicz T, Shepherd FA, Zielinski C, Vansteenkiste J et al. Treatment-by-histology interaction analyses in three phase III trials show superiority of pemetrexed in nonsquamous non-small cell lung cancer. Journal of Thoracic Oncology 2011; 6(1): 64–70. doi: 10.1097/JTO.0b013e3181f7c6d4.

93. Effects of vinorelbine on quality of life and survival of elderly patients with advanced non-small-cell lung cancer. The Elderly Lung Cancer Vinorelbine Italian Study Group. Journal of the National Cancer Institute 1999; 91(1): 66–72.

94. Gridelli C, Perrone F, Gallo C, et al. Chemotherapy for elderly patients with advanced non-small-cell lung cancer: the Multicenter Italian Lung Cancer in the Elderly Study (MILES) phase III randomized trial. Journal of the National Cancer Institute 2003; 95(5): 362–372.

95. Quoix E, Zalcman G, Oster J-P, et al. Carboplatin and weekly paclitaxel doublet chemotherapy compared with monotherapy in elderly patients with advanced non-small-cell lung cancer: IFCT-0501 randomised, phase 3 trial. Lancet 2011; 378(9796): 1079–1088.

96. Zukin M, Barrios CH, Rodrigues Pereira J, et al. Randomized phase III trial of single-agent pemetrexed versus carboplatin and pemetrexed in patients with advanced non-small-cell lung cancer and eastern cooperative oncology group performance status of 2. Journal of Clinical Oncology 2013.

97. Sandler A, Gray R, Perry MC, et al. Paclitaxel-carboplatin alone or with bevacizumab for non-small-cell lung cancer. New England Journal of Medicine 2006; 355(24): 2542–2550.

98. Reck M, von Pawel J, Zatloukal P, et al. Overall survival with cisplatin-gemcitabine and bevacizumab or placebo as first-line therapy for nonsquamous non-small-cell lung cancer: results from a randomised phase III trial (AVAiL). Annals of Oncology 2010; 21(9): 1804–1809.

99. Soria JC, Mauguen A, Reck M, et al. Systematic review and meta-analysis of randomised, phase II/III trials adding bevacizumab to platinum-based chemotherapy as first-line treatment in patients with advanced non-small-cell lung cancer. Annals of Oncology 2013; 24(1): 20–30.

100. Crino L, Dansin E, Garrido P, et al. Safety and efficacy of first-line bevacizumab-based therapy in advanced non-squamous non-small-cell lung cancer (SAiL, MO19390): a phase 4 study. Lancet Oncology 2010; 11(8): 733–740.

101. Reck M, Barlesi F, Crino L, et al. Predicting and managing the risk of pulmonary haemorrhage in patients with NSCLC treated with bevacizumab: a consensus report from a panel of experts. Annals of Oncology 2012; 23(5): 1111–1120.

102. Pirker R, Pereira JR, Szczesna A, et al. Cetuximab plus chemotherapy in patients with advanced non-small-cell lung cancer (FLEX): an open-label randomised phase III trial. Lancet 2009; 373(9674): 1525–1531.

103. Lynch TJ, Patel T, Dreisbach L, et al. Cetuximab and first-line taxane/carboplatin chemotherapy in advanced non-small-cell lung cancer: results of the randomized multicenter phase III trial BMS099. Journal of Clinical Oncology 2010; 28(6): 911–917.

104. Paz-Ares L, Mezger J, Ciuleanu TE, Fischer JR, von Pawel J et al. INSPIRE investigators. Necitumumab plus pemetrexed and cisplatin as first-line therapy in patients with stage IV non-squamous non-small-cell lung cancer (INSPIRE): an open-label, randomised, controlled phase 3 study. Lancet Oncology 2015; 16(3): 328–337. doi: 10.1016/S1470-2045(15)70046-X. Epub 18 February 2015.

105. Thatcher et al. A randomized, multicenter, open-label, phase III study of gemcitabine-cisplatin (GC) chemotherapy plus necitumumab (IMC-11F8/LY3012211) versus GC alone in the first-line treatment of patients (pts) with stage IV squamous non-small cell lung cancer (sq-NSCLC). ASCO Annual Meeting 2014.

106. Di Maio M, Chiodini P, Georgoulias V, et al. Meta-analysis of single-agent chemotherapy compared with combination chemotherapy as second-line treatment of advanced non-small-cell lung cancer. Journal of Clinical Oncology 2009; 27(11): 1836–1843.

107. Shepherd FA, Pereira JR, Ciuleanu T, et al. Erlotinib in previously treated non-small-cell lung cancer. New England Journal of Medicine 2005; 353(2): 123–132.

108. Shepherd FA, Dancey J, Ramlau R, et al. Prospective randomized trial of docetaxel versus best supportive care in patients with non-small-cell lung cancer previously treated with platinum-based chemotherapy. Journal of Clinical Oncology 2000; 18(10): 2095–2103.

109. Hanna N, Shepherd FA, Fossella FV, et al. Randomized phase III trial of pemetrexed versus docetaxel in patients with non-small-cell lung cancer previously treated with chemotherapy. Journal of Clinical Oncology 2004; 22(9): 1589–1597.

110. Ciuleanu T, Stelmakh L, Cicenas S, et al. Efficacy and safety of erlotinib versus chemotherapy in second-line treatment of patients with advanced, non-small-cell lung cancer with poor prognosis (TITAN): a randomised multicentre, open-label, phase 3 study. Lancet Oncology 2012; 13(3): 300–308.

111. Kim ES, Hirsh V, Mok T, et al. Gefitinib versus docetaxel in previously treated non-small-cell lung cancer (INTEREST): a randomised phase III trial. Lancet 2008; 372(9652): 1809–1818.

112. Soria et al. Afatinib (A) vs erlotinib (E) as second-line therapy of patients (pts) with advanced squamous cell carcinoma (SCC) of the lung following platinum-based chemotherapy: overall survival (OS) analysis from the global phase III trial LUX-Lung 8 (LL8). ASCO Annual Meeting 2015. Journal of Clinical Oncology 2015; 33: (suppl; abstr 8002).

113. Torri et al. Individual patients data analysis (IPD) of three randomized studies comparing erlotinib (E) with chemotherapy (CT) in patients with advanced wild-type epidermal growth factor receptor (wtEGFR) non-small cell lung cancer (NSCLC). ASCO Annual Meeting 2015. Journal of Clinical Oncology 2015; 33(suppl; abstr 8048).

114. Garassino MC, Martelli O, Broggini M, Farina G, Veronese S et al.; TAILOR trialists. Erlotinib versus docetaxel as second-line treatment of patients with advanced non-small-cell lung cancer and wild-type EGFR tumours (TAILOR): a randomised controlled trial. Lancet Oncology 2013; 14(10): 981–988. doi: 10.1016/S1470-2045(13)70310-3. Epub 22 July 2013. PMID: 23883922.

115. Lee CK, Brown C, Gralla RJ, Hirsh V, Thongprasert S et al. Impact of EGFR inhibitor in non-small cell lung cancer on progression-free and overall survival: a meta-analysis. Journal of the National Cancer Institute 2013; 105(9): 595–605. doi: 10.1093/jnci/djt072. Epub 17 April 2013.

116. Garon et al. Ramucirumab plus docetaxel versus placebo plus docetaxel for second-line treatment of stage IV non-small-cell lung cancer after disease progression on platinum-based therapy (REVEL): a multicentre, double-blind, randomised phase 3 trial. Lancet 2014; 665–673. PMID: 24933332.

117. Reck et al. Docetaxel plus nintedanib versus docetaxel plus placebo in patients with previously treated non-small-cell lung cancer (LUME-Lung 1): a phase 3, double-blind, randomised controlled trial. Lancet Oncology 2014; 143–155. PMID: 24411639.

118. Dancey J, Shepherd FA, Gralla RJ, et al. Quality of life assessment of second-line docetaxel versus best supportive care in patients with non-small-cell lung cancer previously treated with platinum-based chemotherapy: results of a prospective, randomized phase III trial. Lung Cancer 2004; 43(2): 183–194.

119. Spigel et al. A phase III study (CheckMate 017) of nivolumab (NIVO; anti-programmed death-1 [PD-1]) vs docetaxel (DOC) in previously treated advanced or metastatic squamous (SQ) cell non-small cell lung cancer (NSCLC). ASCO Annual Meeting 2015.

120. Paz-Ares et al. Phase III, randomized trial (CheckMate 057) of nivolumab (NIVO) versus docetaxel (DOC) in advanced non-squamous cell (non-SQ) non-small cell lung cancer (NSCLC). ASCO Annual Meeting 2015.

121. Mok TS, Wu Y-L, Thongprasert S, et al. Gefitinib or carboplatin-paclitaxel in pulmonary adenocarcinoma. New England Journal of Medicine 2009; 361(10): 947–957.

122. Han J-Y, Park K, Kim S-W, et al. First-SIGNAL: first-line single-agent iressa versus gemcitabine and cisplatin trial in never-smokers with adenocarcinoma of the lung. Journal of Clinical Oncology 2012; 30(10): 1122–1128.

123. Mitsudomi T, Morita S, Yatabe Y, et al. Gefitinib versus cisplatin plus docetaxel in patients with non-small-cell lung cancer harbouring mutations of the epidermal growth factor receptor (WJTOG3405): an open label, randomised phase 3 trial. Lancet Oncology 2010; 11(2): 121–128.

124. Maemondo M, Inoue A, Kobayashi K, et al. Gefitinib or chemotherapy for non-small-cell lung cancer with mutated EGFR. New England Journal of Medicine 2010; 362(25): 2380–2388.

125. Zhou C, Wu Y-L, Chen G, et al. Erlotinib versus chemotherapy as first-line treatment for patients with advanced EGFR mutation-positive non-small-cell lung cancer (OPTIMAL, CTONG-0802): a multicentre, open-label, randomised, phase 3 study. Lancet Oncology 2011; 12(8): 735–742.

126. Rosell R, Carcereny E, Gervais R, et al. Erlotinib versus standard chemotherapy as first-line treatment for European patients with advanced EGFR mutation-positive non-small-cell lung cancer (EURTAC): a multicentre, open-label, randomised phase 3 trial. Lancet Oncology 2012; 13(3): 239–246.

127. Sequist LV, Yang JC, Yamamoto N, et al. Phase III study of afatinib or cisplatin plus pemetrexed in patients with metastatic lung adenocarcinoma with EGFR mutations. Journal of Clinical Oncology 2013; 31(27): 3327–3334. doi: 10.1200/JCO.2012.44.2806. Epub 1 July 2013. PMID: 23816960.

128. Wu et al. Afatinib versus cisplatin plus gemcitabine for first-line treatment of Asian patients with advanced non-small-cell lung cancer harbouring EGFR mutations (LUX-Lung 6): an open-label, randomised phase 3 trial. Lancet Oncology 2014; 15(2): 213–222. doi: 10.1016/S1470-2045(13)70604-1. Epub 15 January 2014. PMID: 24439929.

129. Yang et al. Afatinib versus cisplatin-based chemotherapy for EGFR mutation-positive lung adenocarcinoma (LUX-Lung 3 and LUX-Lung 6): analysis of overall survival data from two randomised, phase 3 trials. Lancet Oncology 2015; 16(2): 141–151. doi: 10.1016/S1470-2045(14)71173-8. Epub 12 January 2015. PMID: 25589191.

130. Lee CK, Wu YL, Ding PN, Lord SJ, Inoue A et al. Impact of specific epidermal growth factor receptor (EGFR) mutations and clinical characteristics on outcomes after treatment with EGFR tyrosine kinase inhibitors versus chemotherapy in EGFR-mutant lung cancer: a meta-analysis.

131. Herbst RS, Prager D, Hermann R, et al. TRIBUTE: a phase III trial of erlotinib hydrochloride (OSI-774) combined with carboplatin and paclitaxel chemotherapy in advanced non-small-cell lung cancer. Journal of Clinical Oncology 2005; 23(25): 5892–5899.

132. Gatzemeier U, Pluzanska A, Szczesna A, et al. Phase III study of erlotinib in combination with cisplatin and gemcitabine in advanced non-small-cell lung cancer: the Tarceva lung cancer investigation trial. Journal of Clinical Oncology 2007; 25(12): 1545–1552.

133. Mok TSK, Lee JS, Zhang L, et al. Biomarker analyses and overall survival (os) from the randomized, placebo-controlled, phase 3, fastact-2 study of intercalated erlotinib with first-line chemotherapy in advanced non-small-cell lung cancer (NSCLC). Annals of Oncology 2012; 23: 400–401.

134. Mok et al. Gefitinib/chemotherapy vs chemotherapy in epidermal growth factor receptor (EGFR) mutation-positive non-small-cell lung cancer (NSCLC) after progression on first-line gefitinib: the phase III, randomised impress study. ESMO Meeting 2014. Annals of Oncology 2014; 25 (Suppl 4). doi: 10.1093/annonc/mdu438.45.

135. Porta R, Sanchez-Torres JM, Paz-Ares L, et al. Brain metastases from lung cancer responding to erlotinib: the importance of EGFR mutation. European Respiratory Journal 2011; 37(3): 624–631.

136. Sequist LV, Besse B, Lynch TJ, et al. Neratinib, an irreversible pan-erbb receptor tyrosine kinase inhibitor: results of a phase II trial in patients with advanced non-small-cell lung cancer. Journal of Clinical Oncology 2010; 28(18): 3076–3083.

137. Miller VA, Hirsh V, Cadranel J, et al. Afatinib versus placebo for patients with advanced, metastatic non-small-cell lung cancer after failure of erlotinib, gefitinib, or both, and one or two lines of chemotherapy (LUX-Lung 1): a phase 2b/3 randomised trial. Lancet Oncology 2012; 13(5): 528–538.

138. Sequist LV, Soria JC, Goldman JW, Wakelee HA, Gadgeel SM et al. Rociletinib in EGFR-mutated non-small-cell lung cancer. New England Journal of Medicine 2015; 372(18): 1700–1709. doi: 10.1056/NEJMoa1413654.

139. Jänne PA, Yang JC, Kim DW, Planchard D, Ohe Y et al. AZD9291 in EGFR inhibitor-resistant non-small-cell lung cancer. New England Journal of Medicine 2015; 372(18): 1689–1699. doi: 10.1056/NEJMoa1411817.

140. Sequist LV, Waltman BA, Dias-Santagata D, et al. Genotypic and histologic evolution of lung cancers acquiring resistance to EGFR inhibitors. Science Translational Medicine 2011; 3(75).

141. Shaw AT, Kim DW, Nakagawa K, et al. Crizotinib versus chemotherapy in advanced ALK-positive lung cancer. New England Journal of Medicine 2013; 368(25): 2385–2394. doi: 10.1056/NEJMoa1214886. Epub 1 June 2013. PMID: 23724913.

142. Solomon et al. First-line crizotinib versus chemotherapy in ALK-positive lung cancer. New England Journal of Medicine 2014; 371(23): 2167–2177. doi: 10.1056/NEJMoa1408440. PMID: 25470694.

143. Costa DB, Kobayashi S, Pandya SS, et al. CSF Concentration of the anaplastic lymphoma kinase inhibitor crizotinib. Journal of Clinical Oncology 2011; 29(15): E443–E445.

144. Ou et al. Efficacy and safety of the ALK inhibitor alectinib in ALK+ non-small-cell lung cancer (NSCLC) patients who have failed prior crizotinib: an open-label, single-arm, global phase 2 study (NP28673). ASCO Annual Meeting 2015. Journal of Clinical Oncology 2015; 33(suppl; abstr 8008).

145. Shaw AT, Kim DW, Mehra R, Tan DS, Felip E et al. Ceritinib in ALK-rearranged non-small-cell lung cancer. New England Journal of Medicine 2014; 370(13): 1189–1197. doi: 10.1056/NEJMoa1311107.

146. Gadgeel SM, Gandhi L, Riely GJ, Chiappori AA, West HL et al. Safety and activity of alectinib against systemic disease and brain metastases in patients with crizotinib-resistant ALK-rearranged non-small-cell lung cancer (AF-002JG): results from the dose-finding portion of a phase 1/2 study. Lancet Oncology 2014; 15(10): 1119–1128. doi: 10.1016/S1470-2045(14)70362-6. Epub 18 August 2014. PMID: 25153538.

147. Zou HY, Li Q, Engstrom LD, West M, Appleman V et al. PF-06463922 is a potent and selective next-generation ROS1/ALK inhibitor capable of blocking crizotinib-resistant ROS1 mutations. Proceedings of the National Academy of Sciences of the United States of America 2015; 112(11): 3493–3498. doi: 10.1073/pnas.1420785112. Epub 2 March 2015. PMID: 25733882.

148. Kocher M, Soffietti R, Abacioglu U, et al. Adjuvant whole-brain radiotherapy versus observation after radiosurgery or surgical resection of one to three cerebral metastases: results of the EORTC 22952–26001 study. Journal of Clinical Oncology 2011; 29(2): 134–141.

149. Porte H, Siat J, Guibert B, et al. Resection of adrenal metastases from non-small cell lung cancer: a multicenter study. Annals of Thoracic Surgery 2001; 71(3): 981–985.

150. Pfannschmidt J, Dienemann H. Surgical treatment of oligometastatic non-small cell lung cancer. Lung Cancer 2010; 69(3): 251–258.

151. Pignon JP, Arriagada R, Ihde DC, et al. A meta-analysis of thoracic radiotherapy for small-cell lung cancer. New England Journal of Medicine 1992; 327(23): 1618–1624.

152. Fruh M, De Ruysscher D, Popat S, et al. Small-cell lung cancer (SCLC): ESMO Clinical Practice Guidelines for diagnosis, treatment and follow-up. Annals of Oncology 2013.

153. Rossi A, Di Maio M, Chiodini P, et al. Carboplatin- or cisplatin-based chemotherapy in first-line treatment of small-cell lung cancer: the COCIS meta-analysis of individual patient data. Journal of Clinical Oncology 2012; 30(14): 1692–1698.

154. Sundstrom S, Bremnes RM, Kaasa S, et al. Cisplatin and etoposide regimen is superior to cyclophosphamide, epirubicin, and vincristine regimen in small-cell lung cancer: results from a randomized phase

III trial with 5 years' follow-up. Journal of Clinical Oncology 2002; 20(24): 4665–4672.

155. Huncharek M, McGarry R. A meta-analysis of the timing of chest irradiation in the combined modality treatment of limited-stage small cell lung cancer. Oncologist 2004; 9(6): 665–672.

156. Spiro SG, James LE, Rudd RM, et al. Early compared with late radiotherapy in combined modality treatment for limited disease small-cell lung cancer: a London Lung Cancer Group multicenter randomized clinical trial and meta-analysis. Journal of Clinical Oncology 2006; 24(24): 3823–3830.

157. De Ruysscher D, Pijls-Johannesma M, Bentzen SM, et al. Time between the first day of chemotherapy and the last day of chest radiation is the most important predictor of survival in limited-disease small-cell lung cancer. Journal of Clinical Oncology 2006; 24(7): 1057–1063.

158. Turrisi AT, 3rd, Kim K, Blum R, et al. Twice-daily compared with once-daily thoracic radiotherapy in limited small-cell lung cancer treated concurrently with cisplatin and etoposide. New England Journal of Medicine 1999; 340(4): 265–271.

159. Auperin A, Arriagada R, Pignon JP, et al. Prophylactic cranial irradiation for patients with small-cell lung cancer in complete remission. Prophylactic Cranial Irradiation Overview Collaborative Group. New England Journal of Medicine 1999; 341(7): 476–484.

160. Le Pechoux C, Dunant A, Senan S, et al. Standard-dose versus higher-dose prophylactic cranial irradiation (PCI) in patients with limited-stage small-cell lung cancer in complete remission after chemotherapy and thoracic radiotherapy (PCI 99-01, EORTC 22003-08004, RTOG 0212, and IFCT 99-01): a randomised clinical trial. Lancet Oncology 2009; 10(5): 467–474.

161. Le Pechoux C, Laplanche A, Faivre-Finn C, et al. Clinical neurological outcome and quality of life among patients with limited small-cell cancer treated with two different doses of prophylactic cranial irradiation in the intergroup phase III trial (PCI99-01, EORTC 22003-08004, RTOG 0212 and IFCT 99-01). Annals of Oncology 2011; 22(5): 1154–1163.

162. Yu JB, Decker RH, Detterbeck FC, et al. Surveillance epidemiology and end results evaluation of the role of surgery for stage I small cell lung cancer. Journal of Thoracic Oncology 2010; 5(2): 215–219.

163. Noda K, Nishiwaki Y, Kawahara M, et al. Irinotecan plus cisplatin compared with etoposide plus cisplatin for extensive small-cell lung cancer. New England Journal of Medicine 2002; 346(2): 85–91.

164. Hanna N, Bunn PA, Jr, Langer C, et al. Randomized phase III trial comparing irinotecan/cisplatin with etoposide/cisplatin in patients with previously untreated extensive-stage disease small-cell lung cancer. Journal of Clinical Oncology 2006; 24(13): 2038–2043.

165. Hermes A, Bergman B, Bremnes R, et al. Irinotecan plus carboplatin versus oral etoposide plus carboplatin in extensive small-cell lung cancer: a randomized phase III trial. Journal of Clinical Oncology 2008; 26(26): 4261–4267.

166. Lara PN, Jr, Natale R, Crowley J, et al. Phase III trial of irinotecan/cisplatin compared with etoposide/cisplatin in extensive-stage small-cell lung cancer: clinical and pharmacogenomic results from SWOG S0124. Journal of Clinical Oncology 2009; 27(15): 2530–2535.

167. Schmittel A, Sebastian M, Fischer von Weikersthal L, et al. A German multicenter, randomized phase III trial comparing irinotecan-carboplatin with etoposide-carboplatin as first-line therapy for extensive-disease small-cell lung cancer. Annals of Oncology 2011; 22(8): 1798–1804.

168. Eckardt JR, von Pawel J, Papai Z, et al. Open-label, multicenter, randomized, phase III study comparing oral topotecan/cisplatin versus etoposide/cisplatin as treatment for chemotherapy-naive patients with extensive-disease small-cell lung cancer. Journal of Clinical Oncology 2006; 24(13): 2044–2051.

169. Sun Y, Cheng Y, Hao X, Wang J, Hu, C et al. Result of phase III trial of amrubicin/cisplatin versus etoposide/cisplatin as first-line treatment for extensive small cell lung cancer. Journal of Clinical Oncology 2003; 31(suppl; abstr 7507).

170. Rinke A, Muller HH, Schade-Brittinger C, et al. Placebo-controlled, double-blind, prospective, randomized study on the effect of octreotide LAR in the control of tumor growth in patients with metastatic neuroendocrine midgut tumors: a report from the PROMID Study Group. Journal of Clinical Oncology 2009; 27(28): 4656–4663.

171. Bushnell DL, Jr, O'Dorisio TM, O'Dorisio MS, et al. 90Y-edotreotide for metastatic carcinoid refractory to octreotide. Journal of Clinical Oncology 2010; 28(10): 1652–1659.

172. Pavel ME, Hainsworth JD, Baudin E, et al. Everolimus plus octreotide long-acting repeatable for the treatment of advanced neuroendocrine tumours associated with carcinoid syndrome (RADIANT-2): a randomised, placebo-controlled, phase 3 study. Lancet 2011; 378(9808): 2005–2012.

173. Raymond E, Dahan L, Raoul JL, et al. Sunitinib malate for the treatment of pancreatic neuroendocrine tumors. New England Journal of Medicine 2011; 364(6): 501–513.

174. Rossi G, Cavazza A, Marchioni A, et al. Role of chemotherapy and the receptor tyrosine kinases KIT, PDGFRalpha, PDGFRbeta, and Met in large-cell neuroendocrine carcinoma of the lung. Journal of Clinical Oncology 2005; 23(34): 8774–8785.

CHAPTER 47

Neoplasms of the thymus

Rebecca Bütof, Axel Denz, Gustavo Baretton,
Jan Stöhlmacher-Williams, and Michael Baumann

Epidemiology

The thymus is located in the anterior mediastinum and involutes during adulthood. The organ contains two types of cells: epithelial cells and lymphocytes. Thymic epithelial cells are the origin of two major groups of thymic malignancies: thymomas and thymic carcinomas. Thymomas are slow-growing, less invasive tumours whereas thymic carcinomas have higher metastatic capacity and local aggressiveness. Thymic tumours are rare, accounting for only 0.2% to 1.5% of all malignancies [1]. Overall, 90% of thymic neoplasms are thymomas with an overall incidence of approximately 0.13 cases per 100 000 persons per year [2, 3]. Thymomas can occur at any age but the frequency is highest within the 40–70 year age group. So far, the aetiology remains unclear and environmental risk factors are currently unknown. However, an association between Epstein–Barr virus infection and thymic malignancies has been discussed in the literature [4, 5].

Diagnosis and staging

In 30–50% of cases, patients have no symptoms at diagnosis. Therefore, thymomas are often detected during routine chest X-rays [1, 5]. A variety of clinical findings can be observed in symptomatic patients mostly depending on the histological subtype: thymic carcinomas may lead to chest pain, persistent coughing, dyspnoea, and superior vena cava syndrome; thymomas are often associated with paraneoplastic syndromes. Myasthenia gravis occurs in approximately 45% of patients with thymoma whereas 2–6% have red cell aplasia or hypogammaglobulinaemia [1]. Furthermore, patients with thymoma have an increased risk of a second synchronous or metachronous tumour. Therefore, lifelong follow-up is recommended.

For diagnosis, computerized tomography (CT) with intravenous contrast should be the first choice of imaging. MRI or 18-FDG-PET may be useful for specific questions as well as in case of contraindications against iodine contrast, or for detection of metastatic disease [1, 5]. Thymomas are mostly located in the anterior compartment of the mediastinum. Consequently, the potential differential diagnoses include lymphoma, germ cell tumours, metastases, or benign conditions (i.e., intrathoracic goitre, thymic cysts, aortic aneurysms). In order to achieve a definitive diagnosis and for determination of the histological subtype a biopsy is recommended (e.g., CT-guided core needle biopsy or open biopsy). Biopsy of a possible thymoma should avoid a transpleural approach. Further diagnostic procedures include blood tests (e.g., serum immunoglobulins, LDH, beta HCG, alpha fetoprotein), echocardiography, and tests for detection of autoimmune reactions [1].

Thymomas can be classified based on different histological subtypes according to the World Health Organization (see Table 47.1). This system takes into account the morphology of epithelial cells and the lymphocytic/epithelial ratio. Therefore, resulting subtypes A, AB, B1, B2, and B3 represent specific tumours [1, 3, 5]. One meta-analysis has shown significant differences in survival rates between A/AB/B1 vs B2 vs B3 categories [6, 7]. The thymic carcinoma group (type C thymoma) contains histologically and clinically diverse tumours.

In addition to this WHO classification, the Masaoka-Koga staging system has been developed and is commonly used (see Table 47.2). It is based on clinical and microscopic invasion of the tumour [8, 9]. Several studies have demonstrated a significant correlation between Masaoka-Koga stage and survival [5, 10]. For early-stage thymic malignancies, five-year overall survival rates of 80–95% and for locally advanced stages of 40–70% have been published. Although different TNM classifications have been proposed, they have not prevailed in routine clinical practice.

Treatment options

For treatment of thymomas the following methods are used: surgery, radiotherapy, chemotherapy, and targeted drugs. The optimal type of therapy depends on tumour stage, histological subtype, and general health condition of the patient.

Surgery

A complete surgical excision of the tumour with total thymectomy is the mainstay of therapy for all thymic malignancies. A large proportion of these tumours are resectable with an inverse correlation with the Masaoka-Koga stage at diagnosis (e.g., resectability of 100% in stage I and 29% in stage IV) [5, 11]. The completeness of resection is one of the most important prognostic factors for survival. Median sternotomy is used as the most common surgical approach. An en bloc resection is recommended by the International Thymic Malignancy Interest Group (ITMIG) and includes complete thymectomy with all surrounding mediastinal fatty tissue bordered laterally by the phrenic nerves and cranially by the cervical poles [12]. If the tumour invades adjacent structures like pleura, pericardium, lung, or major vascular structures, the resection has to be extended accordingly. Minimally invasive methods like video-assisted thoracoscopic resections, mini-sternotomy, or robotic surgery may be considered if all oncologic goals

Table 47.1 Histological WHO classification of neoplasms of the thymus

WHO type	Definition
A	Spindle cell, medullary thymoma
AB	Mixed thymoma
B1	Lymphocyte-rich, lymphocytic, or predominantly cortical thymoma
B2	Cortical thymoma
B3	Epithelial, atypical, squamoid thymoma, or well-differentiated thymic carcinoma
C	Heterogeneous thymic carcinoma

Reproduced from Springer, World Health Organization, *Histological Classification of Tumours of the Thymus, Second Edition*, Juan Rosai, Springer-Verlag, Berlin, Heidelberg, Copyright © 1999, with kind permission from Springer Science and Business Media.

can be achieved at the level of standard procedure [13]. For well-encapsulated tumours, local recurrence rate after surgery is less than 3% [14]. Surgical mortality rates of approximately 2.5% have been reported in the literature [1, 11].

Radiotherapy

Thymomas are generally classified as radiosensitive tumours; therefore, radiotherapy plays an important role in multimodal treatment approaches. Patients may receive irradiation in case of unresectable disease, preoperatively in order to improve resectability or post-operatively after incomplete resection. It has been shown that adjuvant radiotherapy increases disease-free survival in patients with R1 or R2 resection whereas in cases with limited stage and R0 resection and for thymomas type A, AB, and B1 no benefit could be detected [15]. In contrast, for R0 resected stage III or IV thymic malignancies adjuvant radio/chemotherapy is recommended [5, 14, 16, 17]. Radiotherapy doses and target volumes are not stated consistently in the literature. In the adjuvant situation doses range between 30–60 Gy with 1.8 to 2.0 Gy

Table 47.2 Masaoka-Koga staging system

Stage	Definition
I	Completely encapsulated tumour
IIa	Microscopic transcapsular invasion
IIb	Macroscopic invasion into thymic or surrounding fatty tissue or grossly adherent to but not breaking through mediastinal pleura or pericardium
IIIa	Macroscopic invasion into surrounding structures (i.e., pericardium, pleura, lung) without invasion of great vessels
IIIb	Macroscopic invasion into surrounding structures with invasion of great vessels
IVa	Distant pleural or pericardial metastases
IVb	Lymphogenous or haematogenous metastases

Reproduced from Masaoka et al., Follow-up study of thymomas with special reference to their clinical stages, *Cancer*, Volume 48, Issue 11, pp. 2485–2492, Copyright © 1981 American Cancer Society, with permission from John Wiley and Sons.

per fraction, depending on resection margins and performance status of the patient [14]. Clinical target volume concepts include mediastinal irradiation with involvement of the mediastinal pleura or alternatively limited radiotherapy of only upper and middle mediastinum. For primary radio/chemotherapy doses between 60–70 Gy are recommended. Most commonly used radiotherapy techniques are 3D conformal radiation therapy and intensity-modulated radiotherapy (IMRT). The role of proton therapy has not been sufficiently explored. In order to reduce side effects the dose to organs at risk, i.e. heart, lung, oesophagus, and spinal cord, should be minimized. Possible acute and late toxicities are pneumonitis, oesophagitis, pericarditis, pulmonary fibrosis, and coronary stenosis.

Chemotherapy

Chemotherapy can be used in various indications in the treatment of thymomas. The role of adjuvant chemotherapy alone is currently unknown [5]. In retrospective studies patients with type A, AB, and B1 thymomas or R0 resected stage II tumours do not benefit from systemic chemotherapy alone [5, 18]. In contrast, for incompletely resected tumours or R0 resected stage III thymic malignancies adjuvant chemoradiotherapy is increasingly administered [18]. For locally advanced disease induction chemotherapy might be an option in order to achieve complete resection. After re-evaluation with CT, simultaneous chemoradiotherapy is recommended for patients with incomplete response or inoperability due to poor performance status. Systemic chemotherapy should be the treatment of choice for patients with extensive metastatic disease. Ifosfamide and cisplatin have been applied as monotherapy. The treatment results for combined therapies of cisplatin, e.g., PAC (cyclophosphamide, doxorubicin, and cisplatin) or ADOC (cyclophosphamide, doxorubicin, vincristine, and cisplatin) regimes are better than monotherapy with reported remission rates of 30–100% [1, 3].

Targeted drugs and novel strategies

There is an emerging body of evidence for presence of specific genetic aberrations in thymic malignancies. During the last years targeted therapies have been investigated in order to improve treatment results. Some of the thymic tumours can be treated with octreotide because of their expression of somatostatin receptors. Also, combined therapies with corticosteroids have been shown to increase response rates.

Different molecular pathways are suitable as targets for novel therapeutic approaches. An over-expression of the receptor tyrosine kinase KIT was found in approximately 80% of thymic carcinomas and 2% of thymomas [5]. These patients might therefore benefit from treatment with tyrosine kinase inhibitors such as imatinib [19]. Although epidermal growth factor receptor (EGFR) over-expression is also a common phenomenon in thymomas and thymic carcinomas, response rates were poor after use of EGFR inhibitors [3, 5]. One possible explanation might be that EGFR mutations are extremely rare in thymic tumours. Further suitable targets might be vascular endothelial growth factor (VEGF) receptors and insulin-like growth factor-1 receptor [19]. Ongoing clinical trials will determine the efficacy of specific inhibitors of these targets. Furthermore some case reports about successful treatment with high-dose chemotherapy and peripheral blood stem cell transplantation have been published [1].

Multidisciplinary therapy according to the stage of disease

All patients with thymic tumours should be managed in a multidisciplinary team in order to determine the optimal management for each individual case.

Stage I

Standard treatment for stage I thymoma is surgery alone. There is no indication for adjuvant therapy after complete resection of a well-encapsulated tumour [1, 3]. In rare cases of positive resection margins (R1 or R2) adjuvant radiotherapy is recommended.

Stage II

For stage II thymic malignancies a complete resection should be treatment of choice. Radiotherapy or combined radiochemotherapy should be administered post-operatively for patients with incomplete resection or as primary treatment for unresectable tumours [14]. In cases with clear undisputed R0 resection and for thymomas type A, AB, and B1 adjuvant therapy seems not to be beneficial [1].

Stage III and IV

If feasible, surgical en bloc resection and adjuvant radio/chemotherapy should be performed in stage III or IVa disease [1, 5]. For unresectable tumours, induction chemotherapy might be an option in order to reduce tumour volume and achieve resectability. After re-evaluation, chemo/radiotherapy can be utilized for patients with progressive disease, incomplete response, or inoperability due to poor performance status. It has to be considered that induction chemotherapy has not been directly compared to neoadjuvant radiotherapy or radiochemotherapy. Therefore, the role of neoadjuvant treatment approaches is not yet clear. In some of these locally advanced stages surgery may not be possible, so that radiochemotherapy is the favourable treatment. Nevertheless the prognosis even for patients with partially resected thymoma is significantly better than for patients without surgery [1, 20]. Systemic chemotherapy should be treatment of choice for patients with stage IVb disease.

Recurrent disease

For advanced stage thymomas, and especially thymic carcinomas, high rates of recurrences up to 51% have been reported in the literature [5]. The average time to relapse of five years requires long follow-up care of all patients with thymic malignancies. The treatment option with highest efficacy for recurrent disease is repeated surgical resection, particularly for local relapses [12]. Post-operative radiotherapy is recommended in case of incomplete resection and only for selected patients after R0 resection of recurrent thymoma. For unresectable tumours neoadjuvant radiotherapy or therapy with corticosteroids or definitive radio/chemotherapy could be performed based on pretreatment.

Summary

Thymic tumours are among malignant diseases with very low incidence. Therefore, clinical research and development of new treatment options pose an ongoing challenge. A complete surgical resection is still the mainstay of therapy. For patients with incomplete resection or in locally advanced stages adjuvant radio/chemotherapy is recommended. Neoadjuvant treatment approaches and novel targeted therapies are under investigation. Life-long follow-up is recommended because of possible late recurrences.

Further reading

Koppitz H, Rockstroh JK, Schuller H, Standop J, Skowasch D et al. State-of-the-art classification and multimodality treatment of malignant thymoma. Cancer Treatment Reviews 2012; 38(5): 540–548. Epub 17 January 2012.

Lamarca A, Moreno V, Feliu J. Thymoma and thymic carcinoma in the target therapies era. Cancer Treatment Reviews 2013; 39(5): 413–420. Epub 25 December 2012.

Rashid OM, Cassano AD, Takabe K. Thymic neoplasm: a rare disease with a complex clinical presentation. Journal of Thoracic Disease 2013; 5(2): 173–183. Epub 16 April 2013.

Tsuchiya R, Koga K, Matsuno Y, Mukai K, Shimosato Y. Thymic carcinoma: proposal for pathological TNM and staging. Pathology International 1994; 44(7): 505–512. Epub 1 July 1994.

Yamakawa Y, Masaoka A, Hashimoto T, Niwa H, Mizuno T et al. A tentative tumor-node-metastasis classification of thymoma. Cancer 1991; 68(9): 1984–1987. Epub 1 November 1991.

<http://www.itmig.org>. 2013.

References

1. Koppitz H, Rockstroh JK, Schuller H, Standop J, Skowasch D et al. State-of-the-art classification and multimodality treatment of malignant thymoma. Cancer Treatment Reviews 2012; 38(5): 540–548. Epub 17 January 2012.
2. Engels EA. Epidemiology of thymoma and associated malignancies. Journal of Thoracic Oncology 2010; 5(10 Suppl 4): S260–S265. Epub 5 October 2010.
3. Rashid OM, Cassano AD, Takabe K. Thymic neoplasm: a rare disease with a complex clinical presentation. Journal of Thoracic Disease 2013; 5(2): 173–183. Epub 16 April 2013.
4. Chen PC, Pan CC, Yang AH, Wang LS, Chiang H. Detection of Epstein–Barr virus genome within thymic epithelial tumours in Taiwanese patients by nested PCR, PCR in situ hybridization, and RNA in situ hybridization. Journal of Pathology 2002; 197(5): 684–688. Epub 5 September 2002.
5. Lamarca A, Moreno V, Feliu J. Thymoma and thymic carcinoma in the target therapies era. Cancer Treatment Reviews 2013; 39(5): 413–420. Epub 25 December 2012.
6. Baas P, Rhodius R. Thymoma update 2011. European Journal of Cancer 2011; 47(Suppl 3): S315–S316. Epub 29 September 2011.
7. Korst RJ, Kansler AL, Christos PJ, Mandal S. Adjuvant radiotherapy for thymic epithelial tumors: a systematic review and meta-analysis. Annals of Thoracic Surgery 2009; 87(5): 1641–1647. Epub 22 April 2009.
8. Tsuchiya R, Koga K, Matsuno Y, Mukai K, Shimosato Y. Thymic carcinoma: proposal for pathological TNM and staging. Pathology International 1994; 44(7): 505–512. Epub 1 July 1994.
9. Yamakawa Y, Masaoka A, Hashimoto T, Niwa H, Mizuno T et al. A tentative tumor-node-metastasis classification of thymoma. Cancer 1991; 68(9): 1984–1987. Epub 1 November 1991.
10. Detterbeck FC, Nicholson AG, Kondo K, Van Schil P, Moran C. The Masaoka-Koga stage classification for thymic malignancies: clarification and definition of terms. Journal of Thoracic Oncology 2011; 6(7 Suppl 3): S1710–S176. Epub 29 September 2011.
11. Detterbeck FC, Parsons AM. Thymic tumors. Annals of Thoracic Surgery 2004; 77(5): 1860–1869. Epub 28 April 2004.
12. Available from: <http://www.itmig.org>. 2013.
13. Pennathur A, Qureshi I, Schuchert MJ, Dhupar R, Ferson PF et al. Comparison of surgical techniques for early-stage thymoma: feasibility

of minimally invasive thymectomy and comparison with open resection. Journal of Thoracic and Cardiovascular Surgery 2011; 141(3): 694–701. Epub 25 January 2011.

14. Fuller CD, Ramahi EH, Aherne N, Eng TY, Thomas CR, Jr. Radiotherapy for thymic neoplasms. Journal of Thoracic Oncology 2010; 5(10 Suppl 4): S327–S335. Epub 5 October 2010.

15. Utsumi T, Shiono H, Kadota Y, Matsumura A, Maeda H et al. Postoperative radiation therapy after complete resection of thymoma has little impact on survival. Cancer 2009; 115(23): 5413–5420. Epub 18 August 2009.

16. Chang JH, Kim HJ, Wu HG, Kim JH, Kim YT. Postoperative radiotherapy for completely resected stage II or III thymoma. Journal of Thoracic Oncology 2011; 6(7): 1282–1286. Epub 7 June 2011.

17. Weksler B, Shende M, Nason KS, Gallagher A, Ferson PF, Pennathur A. The role of adjuvant radiation therapy for resected stage III thymoma: a population-based study. Annals of Thoracic Surgery 2012; 93(6): 1822–1828; discussion, 8–9. Epub 4 May 2012.

18. Girard N, Lal R, Wakelee H, Riely GJ, Loehrer PJ. Chemotherapy definitions and policies for thymic malignancies. Journal of Thoracic Oncology 2011; 6(7 Suppl 3): S1749–S1755. Epub 24 August 2011.

19. Kelly RJ, Petrini I, Rajan A, Wang Y, Giaccone G. Thymic malignancies: from clinical management to targeted therapies. Journal of Clinical Oncology 2011; 29(36): 4820–4827. Epub 23 November 2011.

20. Kondo K, Monden Y. Therapy for thymic epithelial tumors: a clinical study of 1,320 patients from Japan. Annals of Thoracic Surgery 2003; 76(3): 878–885; discussion, 884–885. Epub 10 September 2003.

CHAPTER 48

Pleural mesothelioma

Andrea S. Wolf, Assunta de Rienzo, Raphael Bueno,
Lucian R. Chirieac, Joseph M. Corson,
Elizabeth H. Baldini, David Jackman,
Ritu Gill, Walter Weder, Isabelle Opitz,
Ann S. Adams, and David J. Sugarbaker

Introduction to pleural mesothelioma

Mesothelioma is an aggressive cancer of the pleura associated with asbestos exposure. The latency between exposure and expression of symptoms is long, typically lasting 20–40 years, as it requires decades for cumulative alterations in the cellular apparatus to incite a malignant transformation. Once the diagnosis is made, commonly in the sixth decade of life, patients generally succumb within months as the tumour grows, spreads, and encases the lung, restricting breathing. Median survival without treatment is seven months [1]. Early efforts to treat mesothelioma with single modality therapies, i.e., chemotherapy, radiation, and surgery alone produced dismal results, leading clinicians to add innovative multi-modality approaches to the treatment paradigm.

The current multimodality approach to malignant pleural mesothelioma (MPM) is defined as a macroscopic complete resection (MCR) [2] followed or preceded by some form of therapy for micrometastatic control. The latter usually consists of adjuvant or neoadjuvant chemotherapy and radiation (trimodal therapy), but novel approaches are also being investigated, such as heated intracavitary chemotherapy, photodynamic therapy, and novel radiation techniques. Concurrent developments in diagnostic procedures, histopathologic characterization of mesothelial cells, and staging have improved patient selection, but more research is needed to extend survival by limiting the micrometastatic spread of tumours. This chapter updates current trends in surgery-based multimodality management, with special emphasis on promising new strategies.

Epidemiology

Occupational and environmental exposure to asbestos is a global health problem that has reached epidemic proportion, raising the urgency of finding a cure [3–7]. The history of this cancer can be traced to the mining and manufacture of asbestos in the late 19th and 20th centuries. The association between asbestos and mesothelioma was first recognized in 1960 by Wagner et al. who reported the first series of cases in a mining community in North Western Cape Town Province, South Africa [8]. The association between asbestos and cancer was definitively established by Selikoff in the 1970s [9], prompting the first round of regulatory measures to be implemented in developed countries, beginning in the UK and shortly thereafter the US. As a result of this regulation, the incidence of new cases has stabilized in the US at about 2500 cases per year. However, incidence rates in European nations other than the UK have continued to rise, with peak incidences projected in 2020 and beyond [3]. Moreover, asbestos use continues unabated in many developing regions of the world ensuring that this epidemic will certainly continue for decades beyond current projections.

Molecular biology of pleural mesothelioma

Investigation of the molecular characteristics of malignant pleural mesothelioma continues to be an active area of research, since a standard treatment approach has not been defined. Asbestos is regarded as the primary factor in the pathogenesis of mesothelioma, with more than 80% of patients having a history of asbestos exposure at diagnosis [10]. How asbestos fibres confer key gene alterations and induce cellular transformation of normal mesothelial cells remains poorly understood. The remaining 20% of cases, which report no history of asbestos exposure, may be related to other factors. Several candidates have been investigated, including exposure to simian virus 40 (SV40), radiation, other mineral fibres, and the no-longer used contrast reagent Thorotrast [11]. Characterized by a very long latency, typically 20 to 40 years, many years pass before the malignant diagnosis is made. This suggests that multiple somatic genetic events are required for the tumorigenic conversion of mesothelial cells [12]. Genetic predisposition also has been implicated in a small number of cases [13].

The modified expression of several mitogen-activated protein kinases (MAPK) and receptor tyrosine kinases (RTKs), such as the epidermal growth factor receptor (EGFR), c-Met, and the insulin growth factor receptor has been demonstrated in several studies [14, 15]. Constitutive activation of these kinases results in deregulation of downstream signalling cascades, which disrupt the normal cell cycle, causing—among other effects—the inhibition of apoptosis (cell death). However, for the majority of cases no specific molecular aberration has been associated with deregulation of these cellular pathways. Epigenetic studies also have been conducted in MPM to investigate modifications in gene expression [16]. Although promoter methylation associated with changes in gene expression is a frequent event in MPM, no satisfactory bio-markers have been identified for diagnosis or prognosis.

Chromosomal aberrations

Karyotypic studies and comparative genomic hybridization (CGH) analyses performed on MPM specimens and cell lines have revealed the complexity of the genetic alterations involved in the pathogenesis of MPM. All chromosomes contribute to these numerical changes, with losses being more common than gains. In addition, all chromosomes except Y participate in these structural alterations. Although there is no specific chromosomal aberration common to all cases of malignant mesothelioma, several prominent sites of chromosome loss have been identified [11].

Next-generation sequencing studies

The past decade has seen a remarkable improvement in the application of automated high-throughput DNA sequencing. The new methods, known as next-generation sequencing (NGS), have revolutionized the genetic analysis of mesothelioma and other disease [17]. Transcriptome analyses of four MPM tumours and two controls resulted in the discovery of previously uncharacterized human cancer mutations [18]. These four MPMs displayed unique non-overlapping mutational profiles. Fifteen non-synonymous point mutations were discovered and three of them (COL5A2, UQCRC1, and MXRA5) were found to be present in 4–6% of a larger cohort of MPM tumours. A later study analysed the whole genome of a human primary MPM tumour and its matched normal using a combination of sequencing-by-synthesis and pyrosequencing methodologies [19]. This investigation confirmed that DNA rearrangements represent the dominant type of mutations in MPM. Many more tumour-specific rearrangements than point mutations were uncovered resulting in the discovery of novel, large-scale, inter- and intra-chromosomal deletions, inversions, and translocations. In particular, one large deletion within the DPP10 gene, mapping on chromosome 2q14.1, produced a truncated fusion transcript unique to the tumour's transcriptome. The analysis of 56 additional MPM samples showed this DPP10 transcript in 31 of 56 (55%) MPMs. Patients with tumours expressing DPP10 mRNA had statistically significant better overall survival than patients whose tumours lacked DPP10 expression. This study supported the potential role of chromosomal rearrangements as oncogenic driver mutations, therapeutic targets, and prognostic biomarkers in MPM.

Tumour suppressor genes

Genes, such as TP53, RAS, and RB, that are found to be mutated at high frequency in other tumours are rarely mutated in MPM. Only a few genes mapping in critical locations on chromosomes 22q, 9p, and 3p have shown a high mutation rate in this malignancy.

NF2

The tumour suppressor gene (TSG) merlin (NF2) is located on chromosome 22q12 and is responsible for the hereditary disease neurofibromatosis type 2 (NF2) characterized by nervous system and skin tumours, as well as ocular abnormalities [20]. NF2 protein interacts with cell-surface proteins, proteins involved in cytoskeletal dynamics, and proteins involved in regulating ion transport. Mutations in the NF2 gene, mostly related to frequent loss of part or all of chromosome 22, have been found in more than 40% of MPM cell lines [21–23]. A recent investigation has confirmed that the disruption of NF2 signalling occurs in most MPM tumour samples and that it is essential for the development of MPM [24].

CDKN2A

CDKN2A encodes, through alternative reading-frames, two important cell cycle regulatory proteins: p16 and p14^{ARF}. Homozygous deletion of 9p21 locus is found at high frequency in MPM cell lines and tumour specimens [22, 25–28]. p16 is a cyclin-dependent kinase inhibitor protein that functions in the retinoblastoma (Rb) pathway, regulating the cell cycle during the G1/S phase [29]. Cells lacking p16 lose their cell cycle control and undergo a neoplastic transformation. p14^{ARF} binds Mdm2, thus preventing the latter from binding p53 and targeting it for degradation [30]. Deletions at this locus are clinically very relevant in MPM, because they are negative prognostic factors, potential targets for gene therapy, and can be used as markers in body cavity effusions [31].

BAP1

In the last few years, two independent investigations have identified the gene encoding BRCA1 associated protein-1 (BAP1) as a TSG located in 3p21.1 in MPM [13, 32]. BAP1 encodes a ubiquitin COOH-terminal hydrolase originally identified through its interaction with BRCA1. BAP1 is believed to mediate its effects through chromatin modulation, transcriptional regulation, and possibly via the ubiquitin-proteasome system and the DNA damage response pathway [33]. Somatic BAP1 mutations have been identified in approximately 22% of sporadic MPM samples, whereas congenital BAP1 mutations were identified in sporadic and familiar MPMs [13]. Because several individuals carrying BAP1 mutations had been diagnosed with one or more additional tumours, the existence of a BAP1-related cancer syndrome characterized by mesothelioma, uveal melanoma, and possibly other cancer types has been suggested. It has been hypothesized that when individuals with BAP1 mutations are exposed to asbestos, mesothelioma predominates. Alternatively, BAP1 mutation, alone, may be sufficient to cause mesothelioma [13, 34].

Genetic tests

Microarray profiling technology permits simultaneous measurement of multiple levels of gene expression in a single experiment. It has been successfully applied to cancer research for the discovery of novel biomarkers [35]. Recently, a bioinformatic algorithm, called the 'gene expression ratio technique', was developed to translate comprehensive expression profiling data into simple molecular tests that are based on the expression levels of a relatively small number of genes [36]. This method has been used successfully to predict clinical parameters such as differential diagnosis and prognosis in MPM [37, 38]. This study has shown that a molecular test from tissue obtained using minimally invasive techniques can be performed before major surgical interventions to accurately predict post-surgical outcome. This is an important issue in mesothelioma since median survival in patients undergoing multimodality therapy is one to two years, whereas 20% of those patients can live disease-free for 3 to 15 years. The problem lies in the ability to predict which patients will survive with aggressive surgery-based therapy. The ability to predict post-surgical outcome using a simple genetic test based on microarray profiling technology would vastly improve patient selection for aggressive multimodality therapy.

Pathology of pleural mesothelioma

Pathology plays a critical role in the surgical treatment of MPM, from diagnosis and classification to prognosis and treatment planning. Making the correct diagnosis is challenging because the epithelioid type may be difficult to distinguish from adenocarcinoma or thymoma metastatic to the pleura, and the sarcomatoid type may be difficult to separate from other sarcomas or tumours with sarcomatoid histologies.

Diagnosis and preresection lymph node staging

While the initial diagnosis of MPM may be possible with pleural fluid cytology or fine needle aspiration, a core needle biopsy, thoracoscopic or small-incision open biopsy may be required to obtain adequate tissue for pathologic analysis, since multiple techniques are used in the differential analysis. First, there must be evidence of tumour invasion into parietal pleural fibrous tissue, extrapleural adipose tissue, or the chest wall soft tissues. The presence of proliferating mesothelial cells in an organizing fibrinous exudate that may mimic pleural tissue on intraoperative examination does not constitute invasion. In addition, the surgical biopsy should provide sufficient tumour for accurate classification of the histologic type (e.g., epithelioid, sarcomatoid, and biphasic or mixed). Accuracy in predicting cell type varies with the number of biopsy samples obtained, the heterogeneity of the tumour, and tumour histology [39]. As many as 20–25% of diffuse MPM patients with biopsy classified as epithelial on pathologic analysis have been reported to have mixed type on analysis of specimens obtained at surgical resection [39, 40]. This disparity often reflects the limited tissue present in biopsy specimens, particularly if tissue is obtained via closed core needle biopsy. It also emphasizes the importance of adequate biopsy sampling and the value of surgical resection for accurate classification of histologic type [40]. Lymph node status is critical to staging and prognosis for potential surgical candidates [41]. Mediastinoscopy with pathologic examination of lymph nodes in permanent sections remains the pre-resection gold standard for evaluating lymph node status.

Evaluation of surgical resection specimens

Additional specimens are often evaluated intraoperatively with frozen section examination. Although this examination accurately reports the presence of malignancy in most instances, it cannot be relied on for an accurate distinction from adenocarcinoma and the many other tumours that mimic diffuse MPM.

Extrapleural pneumonectomy

The most complete sampling for pathologic staging is provided by extrapleural pneumonectomy (EPP). In general, an EPP specimen contains the lung, surrounding visceral pleura, parietal pleura of the chest wall, diaphragm, mediastinum, ipsilateral hemidiaphragm, and a portion of the ipsilateral pericardium. The procedure for processing such specimens used by the Department of Pathology of the Brigham and Women's Hospital has been described [42]. The procedure includes weighing the specimen and recording its dimensions (total dimensions of the specimen and dimensions of the lung, diaphragm, pericardium, and bronchial margins), assessing areas of pleural involvement, and describing the range in size of the tumour nodules and the range in thickness of the fused and unfused pleura.

Gross examination of the surgical pathology resection specimen also involves the identification of lesions that may be difficult to distinguish from diffuse MPM on gross examination, such as pleural hyaline plaques, talc granulomata, and incidental adenocarcinomas or other tumours [43, 44]. Pleural hyaline plaques are discrete, white, firm-to-hard patches of thickened pleura (1–5 mm) that range in size from 1–10 cm or larger and are often focally calcified. Most occur in the parietal pleura and have shell-like margins unless fused with tumour. Talc deposits resulting from previous talc pleurodesis generate a granulomatous inflammatory response and fibrosis. These lead to the formation of nodular or plaque-like, tan-to-yellow areas that thicken the pleura (1–3 mm) and are recognized as granulomata.

During gross examination of the tumour, we also sample fresh tissue for other tests, including electron microscopy (EM), cytogenetic analysis, and molecular studies. After formalin fixation, approximately 5 cm^3 of fixed lung parenchyma is taken (with care to avoid tumour, hyaline pleural plaque, and talc granulomata) and submitted for asbestos analysis. Asbestos bodies comprise an asbestos fiber core and an iron protein coat. They are visible by light microscopy in H&E sections and may be quantified after digestion of lung parenchyma and filtration through a Millipore filter. Asbestos fibres are invisible by light microscopy but are detected by both scanning and transmission electron microscopy. Elevated asbestos body 'counts' or asbestos fiber levels in lung tissue indicate increased inhalation of asbestos fibres. They are used widely to establish causation in cases of diffuse MPM [45, 46]. Asbestos body and asbestos fiber levels in lung tissue are not reliable aids in establishing a pathologic diagnosis of diffuse MPM, because other tumours that mimic diffuse MPM may also occur in association with elevated asbestos bodies/levels. Conversely, diffuse MPM may occur in the absence of elevated asbestos bodies/fibre levels.

Pleurectomy/decortication

A pleurectomy/decortication (P/D) specimen usually consists of multiple fragments of pleura with tumour implants without identifiable normal structures. These specimens are approached by describing the components, overall dimensions, and weight of the specimen, and the dimensions and gross features of the various fragments of the pleura and tumour. It is important to search for additional structures, such as skeletal muscle, adipose tissue, and/or pericardium that may be invaded by tumour. Any attached normal lung tissue may be used for asbestos body counts.

Histologic features

MPM is classified by light microscopic examination into the following three types: epithelial (epithelioid), sarcomatous (sarcomatoid), and mixed (biphasic) types, with the desmoplastic variant categorized as a subtype of sarcomatous diffuse MPM [47]. The World Health Organization divides diffuse MPM into the four following types: epithelioid, sarcomatoid, biphasic, and desmoplastic [48]. Extensive sampling of resection specimens is necessary for accurate classification of histologic type [39].

Immunohistochemical staining

Immunohistochemistry (IHC) is now widely used by pathologists to distinguish diffuse MPM from its many histologic mimics [49–55]. The most common problem is separating diffuse MPM from metastatic adenocarcinomas. No single antibody has been identified that is specific for diffuse MPM or adenocarcinoma; therefore, panels of antibodies are used to make this distinction. A panel of four markers, two positive in diffuse MPM, but negative in adenocarcinoma, and two with the converse pattern of immunoreactivity, has demonstrated utility in making this distinction in most cases. We routinely use a panel of the four following antibodies: two that are positive markers for epithelial diffuse MPM: AE1/AE3 keratins, calretinin, WT-1 (nuclear staining), and D2-40 to distinguish diffuse MPM from other epithelioid malignancies. Two are negative markers: pCEA and TTF1. In contrast to its use in epithelial cell type, IHC is less helpful in the differential diagnosis of sarcomatoid diffuse MPM [56–59]. Antibodies that are positive in sarcomatoid diffuse MPM include keratin proteins, calretinin, WT-1, and D2-40, which identify podoplanin and antipodoplanin, but many pleural-based sarcomas and sarcomatoid carcinomas are also positive for these markers. The utility of panels comprising positive and negative (exclusionary) markers for sarcomatoid MPM remains to be determined [52, 53, 56–59].

Electron microscopy

Although immunohistochemistry has largely replaced electron microscopy (EM) in the diagnosis of MPM, it is advisable to take fresh tumour tissue for EM since, occasionally, the diagnosis is not resolved by light microscopy.

Pathologic staging

Only a fraction of patients with diffuse MPM undergo surgical resection. Surgical series large enough to inform staging have generally been retrospective studies from single institutions. Differing degrees of resection, failing to distinguish histological subtypes, variable application of non-surgical therapies, and treatment-related morbidity and mortality—each of which may influence outcome independent of stage—have hampered attempts to elucidate more subtle influences of staging criteria on patient prognosis. These factors have led to the proposal over the past several decades of a number of independent staging systems that differ in the significance attributed to specific classification criteria [60].

All proposed staging systems have been derived from and are primarily applicable to the subset of patients undergoing surgery, which represents the minority of MPM patients. There has been at best modest correlation between these staging systems and patient outcome. Close apposition of multiple vital structures to pleural surfaces does not permit wide surgical margins in surgery for MPM, and this leads to probable underestimation of involvement of adjacent structures in determining pathologic stage. Furthermore, there is poor correspondence between preoperative clinical stage and final pathological stage. In part, this results from the unique morphology and growth pattern of the primary tumour which limits radiographic assessment. The accuracy of clinical staging for the majority of MPM patients who are not treated surgically cannot be directly evaluated, but is likely to be similarly low unless there is unambiguous evidence of metastatic disease.

Surgical management of pleural mesothelioma

Surgery-based multimodality management offers the best chance for extended survival. Several multimodality strategies are being actively explored, and these are discussed under 'Multidisciplinary management of potentially resectable mesothelioma'.

Surgery in malignant pleural mesothelioma: macroscopic complete resection (MCR)

The goal of surgery in MPM is MCR [2]. This entails the complete removal of all grossly visible tumour. Unlike other solid tumours, complete eradication of the tumour with negative surgical margins (R0 resection) is frequently not possible with MPM because of the irregular anatomy of the pleura and close proximity to vital structures which creates a tendency for local invasion of the diaphragm, pericardium, chest wall, and mediastinum. Consequently, foci of microscopic disease often persist at the surgical margins, and patients are treated with adjuvant or neoadjuvant therapies to prevent local recurrence and/or metastases. Despite these limitations, MCR offers the fastest, least morbid, and often only method of cytoreduction to microscopic levels in surgery for mesothelioma.

Two operations have been developed for surgical resection. These are extrapleural pneumonectomy (EPP) and radical pleurectomy/decortication (P/D) (Figure 48.1). EPP is suitable for tumours that invade the lung parenchyma, while P/D is appropriate when the lung parenchyma is spared. The decision hinges on whether or not a macroscopic complete resection can be achieved. Partial pleurectomy is a different operation that is performed in the palliative setting to treat recurrent pleural effusion or to obtain extensive tissue for biopsy and further testing.

Preoperative assessment

The preoperative evaluation for EPP or radical P/D is identical as the decision to proceed with one or the other operation is occasionally made pending intraoperative findings. All patients undergo pulmonary function tests (including spirometry and diffusion lung capacity) and imaging (described below). All patients undergo transthoracic echocardiogram to assess global ventricular function, valvular disease, and, in particular, when EPP is being considered, to evaluate pulmonary artery pressure because of the potential for pulmonary hypertension and right heart strain induced by pneumonectomy. Duplex studies of the lower extremity veins also are done because mesothelioma patients represent one of the highest risk groups for venous thromboembolism. Treatment of deep vein thrombosis (DVT) with anticoagulation (and, if appropriate, inferior vena cava filter) prior to surgery is thought to reduce the risk of life-threatening pulmonary embolus after pneumonectomy.

Surgical patients should have a Karnofsky performance status of greater than 70 [61], normal liver and renal function tests, and normal room air oxygen saturation [62]. While a forced expiratory volume in 1 second (FEV_1) of greater than 2 L is generally adequate for pneumonectomy, quantitative ventilation/perfusion scanning is performed in all patients. The product of the perfusion to the unaffected lung and the preoperative FEV_1 yields the predicted postoperative (PPO) FEV_1. While this value ideally exceeds 1.2 L, patients with a PPO-FEV_1 greater than 800 cc are acceptable candidates for EPP depending on their body mass. Patients with ppo-FEV_1 of less than 800 cc may be considered for P/D if appropriate.

The presence of extensive pain, consumption of high-dose narcotics preoperatively, and/or a contracted hemithorax are clinical indicators of extensive chest wall invasion and the patient is likely unresectable. While chest radiography may suggest invasion, often the resectability of a tumour is not known until surgery. In fact, in

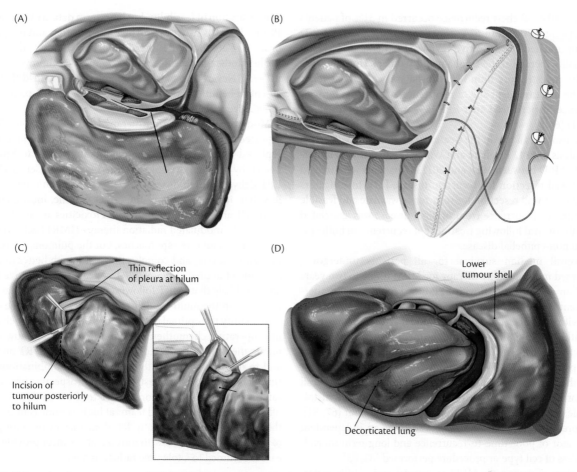

(A)

(B)

(C)

Thin reflection
of pleura at hilum

Incision of
tumour posteriorly
to hilum

(D)

Lower
tumour shell

Decorticated lung

Fig. 48.1 (A, B) Extrapleural pneumonectomy (EPP). (C, D) Pleurectomy/decortication (P/D).
Reproduced by permission of the illustrator Marcia Williams, Copyright © Marcia Williams.

25% of cases, resectability of tumour cannot be determined preoperatively, and if critical mediastinal structures (e.g., aorta, oesophagus, vertebral bodies) are found to be involved at thoracotomy, the tumour is classified as T4, extensive resection is not recommended, and the operation does not proceed. The differentiation between radiographic evidence for the displacement (versus invasion) of mediastinal structures is a critical distinction, as many patients have been erroneously denied surgery based on displacement of mediastinal structures by resectable tumour. Similarly, imaging has limited value in distinguishing compression of tumour on the diaphragm from transdiaphragmatic abdominal invasion. If imaging suggests transdiaphragmatic extension, intra-abdominal tumour, or ascites, staging laparoscopy should be performed to evaluate the peritoneum prior to potential thoracic resection. Finally, patients with limited chest wall invasion on imaging without evidence of locally advanced invasive disease or metastases may be amenable to a surgical resection, and these patients should be considered for exploratory thoracotomy.

Histologic diagnosis is accomplished by thoracoscopic pleural biopsy via a single port placed in the location of a future thoracotomy (such that this can be excised at the time of future resection). We recommend staging cervical mediastinoscopy to rule out involvement of the mediastinal nodes, although there are limitations of this modality in diagnosing most extrapleural nodal disease. Patients who have mediastinal lymph node involvement are

offered induction chemotherapy and reassessment for surgery after two to four cycles of chemotherapy.

Outcomes for surgery

EPP and P/D result in distinctly different amounts of residual tissue previously associated with tumour. This impacts the biology and patterns of recurrence in MPM. With EPP, these potential sites for recurrence are limited to the resection margins of the diaphragm and pericardium, the lateral anterior and posterior chest walls, and the upper mediastinum and apex. With radical P/D, the surface area also includes all lung surfaces, leaving a much broader field for potential recurrence, although the benefit of sparing the lung from removal may offset this disadvantage. The appropriate operation depends on the characteristics of the individual tumour, whether the patient can tolerate the surgery, and which procedure can deliver MCR.

MPM has a distinct pattern of failure [63]. Unlike other solid tumours, in which haematogenous and lymphangitic metastases are the common sources of recurrence, the majority of patients with mesothelioma recur locally. The abdomen is the most common site and most likely represents regional spread by local invasion. It is rare for the tumour to metastasize via haematogenous spread to the contralateral chest. The patterns of recurrence differ between EPP and P/D. In a multicentre study of 663 consecutive patients who underwent surgery for mesothelioma, Flores and colleagues found that ipsilateral chest recurrence occurred in 31% of patients who underwent EPP and in 63% of patients who underwent P/D [64]. In an updated retrospective review of patients undergoing multimodality therapy at the Brigham and Women's Hospital from 2001–2010, investigators found that ipsilateral chest recurrence was still the most frequent site of recurrence, accounting for 69% of recurrences experienced after EPP [65] and 95% of those after radical P/D [66].

Surgery also plays a role in the treatment of recurrent MPM. In a recent analysis of 1142 Brigham and Women's patients who underwent EPP or P/D between 1988 and 2011, 47 patients were treated with chest wall resection for recurrent disease [67]. Investigators found that chest wall resection for recurrence was safe and feasible and that time-to-recurrence from original disease was associated with overall survival following treatment of recurrence in both epithelial and non-epithelial disease.

The overall median survival for all patients undergoing surgery-based multimodality therapy for MPM is one to two years [41]. Median overall survival with EPP-based multimodality therapy in recent studies has been 10–35 months [63, 68–73]. Median survival with radical P/D-based multimodality therapy has been 8–22 months [64, 73–78]. In contrast, the median survival range for patients who receive cisplatin chemotherapy alone or in combination with pemetrexed is 9.3–13.3 months, respectively [79], and for palliative therapy, seven months [1, 80]. Predictors of longer overall survival for patients treated with surgery include epithelial histology, female gender, young age, and normal haemoglobin [67, 81]. Notably, preoperative anaemia has proved to be an independent prognosticator of poor time-to-recurrence and long-term mortality, regardless of cell type or procedure performed [82, 83].

While critics of surgery for MPM, in general, and of EPP, in particular, have claimed the risks of these procedures outweigh unclear survival benefit, attempts to randomize patients to surgery vs no surgery have not met with success. The Mesothelioma and Radical Surgery (MARS) trial was conceived to evaluate the role of EPP in treating MPM, but its design did not demonstrate feasibility, and exploratory analyses of data derived were performed with inadequate power to draw meaningful conclusions [84–86]. A recent multidisciplinary consensus opinion of surgeons, medical oncologists, and radiation oncologists formulated at the International Mesothelioma Interest Group Meeting (IMIG) in 2012 emphatically supported the role of either EPP or P/D, depending on tumour characteristics and surgeon experience, in the multimodality treatment of MPM [87].

Role of radiation therapy

Designing treatment plans for radiation therapy (RT) in MPM is challenging because of the large size and irregular architecture of the hemithorax, as well as the problematic presence of several normal structures with low tolerance to radiation within or adjacent to the treatment volume. The difficulty lies in devising a plan that can deliver sufficiently high doses of RT to the complex target while maintaining minimal doses to radiosensitive normal organs.

The role of RT in the curative treatment of MPM remains undefined. Published data do not support a role for RT as a single modality for curative treatment of unresected mesothelioma. Intensity-modulated radiation therapy (IMRT) to the circumferential pleural envelope following P/D has theoretical appeal and early demonstration of feasibility, but long-term data are lacking [88–90]. Pleural IMRT is worthy of further investigation and is a potentially promising approach. RT after EPP is the best studied and perhaps the best indication for RT, and does appear to improve local control [91–93]. Nevertheless, delivering radiation to a field that includes an entire hemithorax with adequate dosing in the pleural recesses remains very challenging.

Moderate-dose radiation therapy (MDRT) (i.e., 30–40 Gy) has reported only fair results. Accordingly, this technique has been replaced by the electron-photon therapy (EPT) technique pioneered by the Memorial Sloan Kettering Cancer Center (MSKCC). EPT delivers a high dose of RT (54 Gy), and although it achieves less than ideal coverage of the target volume, local control rates with EPT are superior to MDRT and toxicities are low [94].

Intensity-modulated radiation therapy (IMRT) achieves the best dosimetry of all three approaches, but the pulmonary toxicity profile can be severe, and complications, although better understood, are difficult to predict [95–97]. RT appears to be effective for MPM and it is likely that IMRT following P/D and EPP will have an ultimate role in the multi-modality treatment of MPM. The challenge is to identify the optimal combinations of modalities such as heated intraoperative chemotherapy, systemic chemotherapy, photodynamic therapy, and targeted agents in addition to RT and surgery and to do this safely. For this reason, new combinations of multimodality therapies are best tested on prospective protocols with safety oversight. Furthermore, IMRT to the hemithorax should be offered only by experienced teams at high-volume centres until further data are acquired. Finally, RT alone may be used for palliation of symptoms in patients with unresectable cancer provided the disease is confined to a tolerable radiation field.

Systemic chemotherapy

Systemic chemotherapy for malignant mesothelioma remains a central component of treatment for most patients with the disease. There are several specific challenges to the development of new agents in mesothelioma. First and foremost is the low incidence of malignant pleural mesothelioma in all countries (e.g., 3300 cases per year in the US) [98]. Owing in part to this low incidence, much of the published literature in mesothelioma consists of single-institution case series or small, single-arm trials. Another obstacle to determining treatment efficacy in mesothelioma is the assessment of tumour response; the applicability of standard Response Evaluation Criteria in Solid Tumours (RECIST) has been limited in mesothelioma, particularly with respect to serial assessments of the pleural rind.

First-line chemotherapy for unresectable disease

The standard first-line therapy for patients with unresectable mesothelioma is cisplatin plus the antifolate agent pemetrexed. In a phase III trial, the addition of pemetrexed to cisplatin was generally well-tolerated by patients and led to measurable improvements in tumour response (41.3% vs 16.7%, p <0.0001), median time-to-progression (TTP) (5.7 vs 3.9 months, p = 0.002), and median overall survival (OS) (12.1 vs 9.3 months, p = 0.02). When poor performance status and/or presence of medical comorbidities preclude patients from receiving cisplatin-based therapy, treatment with pemetrexed plus carboplatin or pemetrexed monotherapy can be considered. The optimal duration of first-line therapy with platinum-pemetrexed combination chemotherapy has not been firmly established. In the registrational phase III trial, there was no limit to the number of cycles administered. In that study, the range was 1–12 cycles, with a median of six cycles [79]. In practice, physicians often stop after four to six cycles.

Pemetrexed as maintenance therapy or second-line therapy

For patients who do not receive pemetrexed in the first-line setting, use of this agent as a second-line treatment is warranted [99, 100]. Furthermore, for patients who receive pemetrexed in the first-line setting and who do not progress during or shortly after receiving such treatment, consideration should be given to re-initiation of pemetrexed at the time of subsequent progression.

Additionally, both gemcitabine and vinorelbine have demonstrated activity in this disease and could be considered in patients who have progressed after pemetrexed-based regimens.

Trends in radiology

Preoperative evaluation

Accurate preoperative determination of resectability by imaging allows appropriate treatment planning. The initial presentation of MPM is generally heralded by the presence of pleural effusion and other nonspecific signs of pleural disease on plain chest radiographs, but CT continues to be the mainstay of the radiologic analysis of MPM and the primary modality for diagnosis [101]. The constellation of imaging findings include, but are not limited to, unilateral pleural effusion, circumferential nodular pleural thickening, pleural masses, and contraction of the involved hemithorax. Invasion of adjacent structures, adenopathy, and presence of osseous, pulmonary, and distant metastases are more commonly observed in advanced disease [41, 102]. Detecting chest wall invasion, transdiaphragmatic spread, peritoneal involvement, and lymph node metastases, particularly N2 disease, carries a poor prognosis [103] and continues to be challenging by CT alone (see Figures 48.2 and 48.3), and can be enhanced with a multi-modality approach with complementary information derived from MRI and FDG PET-CT.

Newer and innovative techniques such as tumour volumetric analysis, DCE-MRI (dynamic contrast enhanced MRI), DWI (diffusion weighted imaging), and newer PET tracers can help optimize management strategies.

Multidisciplinary management of potentially resectable mesothelioma

The concept of MCR by EPP and P/D has been described under 'Surgical management of pleural mesothelioma' [2]. Here we discuss four well-documented multimodality strategies.

Extrapleural pneumonectomy followed by chemoradiotherapy

The largest published series to date involving EPP in a multimodality setting with adjuvant chemotherapy and radiotherapy is that of Sugarbaker and the group from Brigham and Women's Hospital in Boston (US) [104–106]. In 1999, they reported 176 patients with

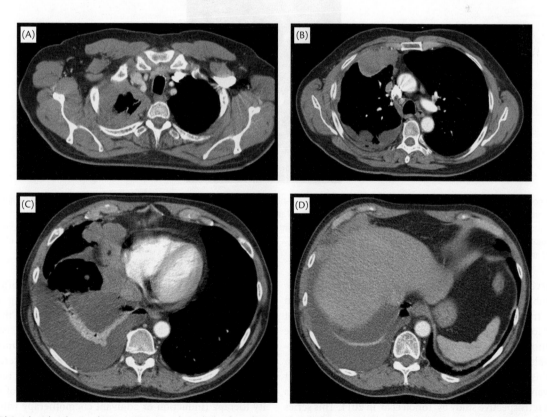

Fig. 48.2 (A–D) Serial axial and coronal images CT images through the chest showing pleural rind encasing the right hemithorax, most marked along the upper chest. There is a small volume right pleural effusion as well. No evidence of chest wall invasion, or contra-, lateral, or intra-abdominal disease.

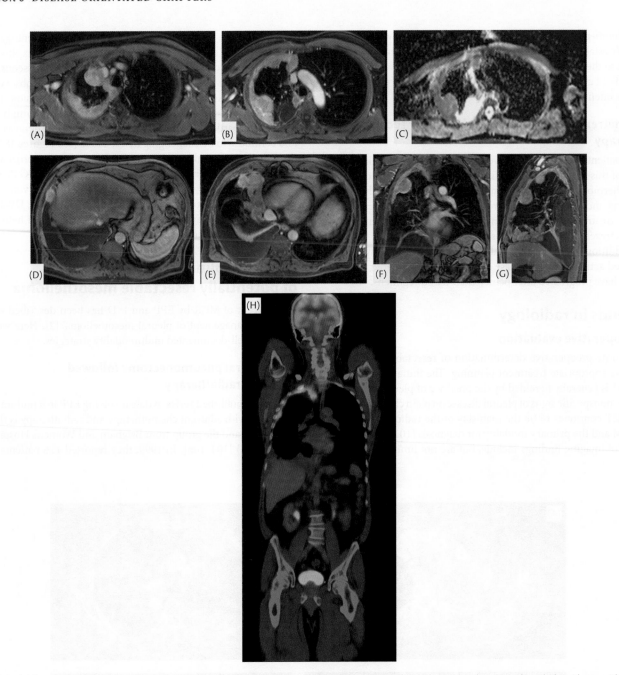

Fig. 48.3 Axial, coronal and sagittal post contrast MR images (VIBE) (A, B, D–G) showing enhancing circumferential pleural rind encasing the right hemithorax with the bulk of the tumour in the upper hemithorax; there is a moderate right pleural effusion. No evidence of mediastinal invasion, chest wall invasion, transdiaphragmatic spread, or contralateral disease. (C) The tumour has restricted diffusion on DWI with an apparent diffusion coefficient (ADC) value of 1.10 (±0.16) x 10^{-3} mm^2/s which is suggestive of biphasic mesothelioma. (H) Coronal fused PET-CT image showing a right mesothelioma confined to the right hemithorax, no evidence of distant metastasis. The patient underwent an extrapleural pneumonectomy.

a median survival of 19 months and operative mortality of 3.8%. An update published in 2004 reported 183 patients with intention to treat by a trimodality approach and an operative mortality of 3.4%, similar to mortality rates reported for pneumonectomy alone without additional treatments [41]. The Mayo Clinic reported a retrospective evaluation of EPP with adjuvant chemotherapy. Median survival in this series was 16 months (n = 73) with neoadjuvant and/or adjuvant radiotherapy [75]. To date, the best survival was reported in a retrospective study by Tonoli et al. in 2011. This series demonstrated a median survival of four years (four-year survival of 50% with SD +/- 9) in 56 patients treated with EPP followed

by various methods of radiation (mostly IMRT) with chemotherapy (generally cisplatin-pemetrexed) given before or after surgery [107]. These results were more promising even than those reported by Aziz et al. in 2002, in which EPP followed by cisplatin-based systemic chemotherapy was associated with a 35-month median survival [73]. Table 48.1 summarizes the reported literature on EPP with adjuvant chemotherapy. Cao et al. report their recent systematic review of the literature on EPP in the context of multimodality therapy (induction or adjuvant chemotherapy with or without adjuvant radiotherapy) [108]. The authors' summary of perioperative outcomes in the 16 studies included in the summary report

Table 48.1 Current data for extrapleural pneumonectomy plus adjuvant therapy

Author	Study design	EPP (n)	Modalities	Mortality (%)	Median OS (months)
Branscheid et al. (1991) [120]	Retrospective	76	Adjuvant CTX	11.8	9.3
Allen et al. (1994) [121]	Retrospective	40	Adjuvant CTX + RT	7.5	13.3
Baldini et al. (1997) [63]	Retrospective	49	Adjuvant CTX + RT	4	22
Sugarbaker et al. (1999) [41]	Retrospective	183	Adjuvant CTX + RT	3.8	19
Rusch et al. (1999) [71]	Prospective	115	Adjuvant CTX + /RT	5	14.7
Maggi et al. (2001) [72]	Prospective	23	Adjuvant CTX +/ RT	6	9.5
Rusch et al. (2001) [122]	Prospective	62	Adjuvant RT	11	17
Aziz et al. (2002) [73]	Retrospective	64	Adjuvant CTX	9	35
Rosenzweig et al. (2005) [123]	Prospective	7	HDR-IORT	14.3	Study closed
Pagan et al. (2006) [124]	Retrospective	44	Adjuvant CTX +/RT	4.5	20
Rice et al. (2007) [125]	Prospective	37	Neo(adj.) CTX + adjuvant IMRT	8	10.2
		EPP + IMRT 63			14.2
Schipper et al. (2008) [75]	Retrospective	73	Neo/adjuvant CTX + /adjuvant RT	8.2	16
Flores et al. (2008) [64]	Retrospective	385	Adjuvant CTX +/ RT	7	12
Batirel et al. (2008) [126]	Prospective	16	Adjuvant CTX + RT	5	17
Luckraz et al. (2010) [127]	Retrospective	49	Adjuvant CTX +/RT	8.2	19.5[a]
Tonoli et al. (2011) [107]	Retrospective	56	Adjuvant CTX + RT	NR	46.9[a]
Rena et al. (2012) [128]	Retrospective	40	Adjuvant CTX + RT	5	20
Patel et al. (2012) [129]	Retrospective	30	Adjuvant CTX + RT	NR	23.2[a]
Ambrogi et al. (2012) [130]	Retrospective	29	Adjuvant CTX +/RT	3.4	19.5[a]

CTX, chemotherapy; RT, radiotherapy; HDR-IORT, high-dose rate intraoperative radiotherapy; IMRT, intensity-modulated radiation therapy; OS, overall survival; NR, not reported.
[a]date of surgery.

perioperative mortality ranging from 0–12.5% and overall morbidity of 50–83%, with major perioperative complications occurring in 24–54% of patients.

Extrapleural pneumonectomy or radical pleurectomy/decortication with heated intraoperative chemotherapy

In addition to trimodality therapy, Sugarbaker and colleagues have evaluated the concept of heated intraoperative chemotherapy (HIOC) after macroscopic complete surgical resection as a means of local disease control, under the theory that local recurrence limits survival in this disease. The protocol for HIOC has been previously described [109–111]. The rationale for bathing the empty thorax with a heated solution of chemotherapy after the surgical specimen has been removed is based on sound pharmacological principles. Hyperthermia increases the cytotoxicity of the compound and systemic toxicity is spared because the majority of drug is delivered locally enabling larger dose delivery to surgical margins. This technique also has been successfully applied to the peritoneum in malignant peritoneal mesothelioma [112]. After testing several protocols to determine the maximum tolerated dose and feasibility of this treatment, the protocol was refined by the addition of chemical agents for organ protection. The results of this multimodality approach have been published in a series of

papers. Most recently, Sugarbaker et al. reported extended interval to recurrence (27.1 vs 12.8 months) and overall survival (35.3 vs 22.8 months) in a group of low-risk patients (n = 72) with epithelial histopathology and other favourable prognostic factors (tumour volume ≤500 cm (3); male gender with a haemoglobin level of ≥13 g/dL; or female) compared with controls (n = 31). The findings were particularly evident among subgroups that did not receive hemithoracic radiotherapy and/or had pathologic stage N1 or N2 lymph node metastases [111].

Extrapleural pneumonectomy after neoadjuvant chemotherapy

The rationale for administering chemotherapy prior to radical resection in MPM is several fold. The primary objective is to downstage the tumour or eradicate the outer tumour layer for better resectability [106]. This concept was prompted by the positive experience with neoadjuvant therapy in patients with stage IIIA NSCLC (non-small cell lung cancer). Further justification for sequencing chemotherapy before surgery is the patient's ability to tolerate the recommended chemotherapeutic regimen. Patients have difficulty complying with the rigours of post-operative chemotherapy after a major resection and often are unable to tolerate the recommended dose and/or complete the recommended cycle. This has been supported in a study of pemetrexed plus cisplatin in NSCLC where

Table 48.2 Current data for neoadjuvant chemotherapy plus extrapleural pneumonectomy

Author	Study design	EPP (n)	Modalities	Mortality (%)	Median OS (months)
Weder et al. (2004) [115]	Prospective	19	Neoadjuvant CTX + adjuvant RT	0	23
Flores et al. (2006) [74]	Prospective	8	Neoadjuvant CTX + adjuvant RT	0	33.5
Weder et al. (2007) [69]	Prospective	61	Neoadjuvant CTX + /adjuvant RT	2.2	23
Rea et al. (2007) [131]	Prospective	21	Neoadjuvant CTX + /adjuvant RT	0	25.5
de Perrot et al. (2009) [132]	Retrospective	45	Neoadjuvant CTX + /adjuvant RT	6.7	59[a]
Krug et al. (2009) [70]	Retrospective	54	Neoadjuvant CTX + /adjuvant RT	3.7	29.1
Buduhan et al. (2009) [133]	Retrospective	46	Neoadjuvant CTX + /adjuvant RT	4.3	25
Van Schil et al. (2010) [134]	Prospective	58	Neoadjuvant CTX + /adjuvant RT	6.5	18.4[b]
Treasure et al. (2011) [84]	RCT	19	Neoadjuvant CTX + /adjuvant RT	12.5	14.4
Lang-Lazdunski et al. (2012) [135]	Retrospective	22	Neoadjuvant CTX + /adjuvant RT	4.5	12.8

[a]Patients with completed trimodality treatment and without mediastinal lymph node involvement, [b]Intention-to-treat.

RCT, randomized controlled trial; CTX, chemotherapy; RT, radiotherapy; OS, overall survival.

Table 48.3 Current data for radical pleurectomy/decortication plus adjuvant therapy

Author	Study design	P/D (n)	Modalities	Mortality (%)	Median OS (months)
Chailleux et al. (1988) [136]	Retrospective	14	Adjuvant CTX +/RT	NR	13
Achatzy et al. (1989) [137]	Retrospective	Radical P/D 46	Adjuvant CTX + RT	4.3	9.2
		Pall. P/D 72		11.1	
Ruffie et al. (1989) [138]	Retrospective	63	Adjuvant CTX + RT	NR	9.8
Branscheid et al. (1991) [120]	Retrospective	82	Adjuvant CTX	2.7	10.4
Allen et al. (1994) [121]	Retrospective	56	Adjuvant CTX + RT	5.4	9
Pass et al. (1997) [76]	Prospective	39	PDT/CTX	2	14.5
Pass et al. (1998) [77]	Prospective	23	PDT/ICTX	2.1	22
Moskal et al. (1998) [78]	Prospective	28	PDT	0	15
Rusch et al. (1999) [71]	Prospective	59	Adjuvant CTX + /RT	3	18.5
Aziz et al. (2002) [73]	Retrospective	47	Adjuvant CTX	0	14
de Vries et al. (2003) [139]	Retrospective	29	Adjuvant CTX + /RT	3.8	9
Schipper et al. (2008) [75]	Retrospective	Sub tot. P/D 34	Neo/ adjuvant CTX +/ adjuvant RT	2.9	8
		Radical P/D 10		0	17.2
Flores et al. (2008) [64]	Retrospective	278	Adjuvant CTX + /RT	4	16
Nakas et al. (2008) [140]	Retrospective age 65 years	P/D 8	Adjuvant CTX + /RT	12.5	12.4
		VATS P/D Pall. 42		7.1	14
Bolukbas et al. (2011) [141]	Prospective	35	Adjuvant CTX + RT	2.9	30
Rena et al. (2012) [128]	Prospective	37	Neo- (adjuvant CTX) + RT	0	25
Nakas et al. (2012) [142]	Prospective	67	Neo- (adjuvant CTX)	3	13.4
Rosenzweig et al. (2012) [143]	Retrospective	20	Neoadjuvant CTX + IMRT	NR	26
Friedberg et al. (2012) [119]	Retrospective	38	Neo- (adjuvant CTX) + intraoperative PDT	2.6	31.7
Lang-Lazdunski et al. (2012) [135]	Prospective	54	Adjuvant CTX + RT HPL	0	23

CTX, chemotherapy; RT, radiotherapy; ICTX, immunochemotherapy; ITX, immunotherapy; PDT, photodynamic therapy; ip, intrapleural; HPL, hyperthermic pleural lavage; NR, not reported; OS, overall survival.

patients who received neoadjuvant chemotherapy were more likely to complete the recommended dose and cycle [113, 114]. Another value to neoadjuvant therapy was demonstrated in a multicentre phase II trial suggesting that initial response to neoadjuvant chemotherapy may have prognostic significance for extended survival in patients undergoing trimodality therapy [70].

The strategy of using neoadjuvant chemotherapy followed by EPP to treat patients with resectable MPM was pioneered by Weder et al. in a pilot study of 19 patients with MPM who underwent extrapleural pneumonectomy after neoadjuvant cisplatin plus gemcitabine [115]. The study was conducted at the University Hospital of Zurich, Switzerland, and yielded a response rate of 31%. Sixteen patients underwent EPP with no perioperative mortality. Median survival was 23 months and two patients remained disease-free six years after surgery. Table 48.2 summarizes the experience with neoadjuvant chemotherapy and EPP or P/D.

Recent reviews confirm that pemetrexed and cisplatin combination produces the best overall survival and quality of life for patients. Four to six weeks is considered the optimal timing after the last cycle of neoadjuvant chemotherapy has been completed for surgical resection.

The choice of operation (EPP or P/D) remains undefined. A large multicentre retrospective review of 663 cases combining the experience of three large centres in the US experienced in EPP and P/D emphasized similarities in outcome irrespective of procedure, although there is a bias in selection and the local recurrence rate for P/D is higher [64]. Conversely, initial analysis of the International Association for the Study of Lung Cancer (IASLC) reported a survival advantage in patients undergoing EPP [116]. Currently, there are no data in the literature that clearly support one or the other procedure, and the only clear indication is for P/D in patients with cardiac or other comorbidities who are physically unable to tolerate EPP.

Extrapleural pneumonectomy plus chemoradiotherapy

As described above, the role of radiotherapy in MPM remains undefined. However, the risk of disease recurrence in the ipsilateral chest is not unforeseen given that EPP is an R1 resection by definition. In 1997, Baldini et al. reported a 35% rate of recurrence in patients undergoing EPP [63]. This experience prompted the investigation of adjuvant radiotherapy in surgically resected patients. The clinical investigation of adjuvant chemotherapy has been adequately described under 'Systemic chemotherapy'.

Pleurectomy/decortication and adjuvant therapy

A variety of adjuvant treatments have been applied in patients undergoing P/D. These studies include chemotherapy, radiotherapy, intrapleural therapy, hyperthermic intracavitary chemotherapy, and photodynamic therapy (Table 48.3).

Photodynamic therapy is a light-based treatment that requires a non-toxic photosensitizing compound, oxygen, and visible light. The treatment is delivered into the empty hemithoracic cavity. The therapeutic principles are similar to HIOC, to control local spread of tumour by achieving greater penetration of tissues at the surgical margins [117–119]. In addition, photodynamic therapy is thought to stimulate immunologic events that boost healing.

The real success in mesothelioma can be found in series that follow a strict paradigm of surgical cytoreduction followed or preceded by adjuvant treatment. Further advances will come with greater understanding of the biology and genetics of the disease and with the use of additional targeted biologic therapies.

References

1. Merritt N, Blewett CJ, Miller JD, Bennett WF, Young JE et al. Survival after conservative (palliative) management of pleural malignant mesothelioma. Journal of Surgical Oncology 2001; 78: 171–174.
2. Sugarbaker DJ. Macroscopic complete resection: the goal of primary surgery in multimodality therapy for pleural mesothelioma. Journal of Thoracic Oncology 2006; 1: 175–176.
3. Peto J, Decarli A, La Vecchia C, Levi F, Negri E. The European mesothelioma epidemic. British Journal of Cancer 1999; 79: 666–672.
4. Robinson BW, Lake RA. Advances in malignant mesothelioma. New England Journal of Medicine 2005; 353: 1591–1603.
5. Nowak AK, Byrne MJ, Williamson R, Ryan G, Segal A, et al. A multicentre phase II study of cisplatin and gemcitabine for malignant mesothelioma. British Journal of Cancer 2002; 87: 491–496.
6. Baris YI, Artvinli M, Sahin AA. Environmental mesothelioma in Turkey. Annals of the New York Academy of Sciences 1979; 330: 423–432.
7. Roushdy-Hammady I, Siegel J, Emri S, Testa JR, Carbone M. Genetic-susceptibility factor and malignant mesothelioma in the Cappadocian region of Turkey. Lancet 2001; 357: 444–445.
8. Wagner JC, Sleggs CA, Marchand P. Diffuse pleural mesothelioma and asbestos exposure in the North Western Cape Province. British Journal of Industrial Medicine 1960; 17: 260–271.
9. Selikoff IJ. Lung cancer and mesothelioma during prospective surveillance of 1249 asbestos insulation workers, 1963–1974. Annals of the New York Academy of Sciences 1976; 271: 448–456.
10. Prazakova S, Thomas PS, Sandrini A, Yates DH. Asbestos and the lung in the 21st century: an update. Clinical Respiratory Journal 2013.
11. Carbone M, Kratzke RA, Testa JR. The pathogenesis of mesothelioma. Seminars in Oncology 2002; 29: 2–17.
12. Sekido Y. Molecular biology of malignant mesothelioma. Environmental Health and Preventive Medicine 2008; 13: 65–70.
13. Testa JR, Cheung M, Pei J, Below JE, Tan Y, et al. Germline BAP1 mutations predispose to malignant mesothelioma. Nature Genetics 2011; 43: 1022–1025.
14. Jean D, Daubriac J, Le Pimpec-Barthes F, Galateau-Salle F, Jaurand MC. Molecular changes in mesothelioma with an impact on prognosis and treatment. Archives of Pathology and Laboratory Medicine 2012; 136: 277–293.
15. Pisick E, Salgia R. Molecular biology of malignant mesothelioma: a review. Hematology/Oncology Clinics of North America 2005; 19: 997–1023, v.
16. Vandermeers F, Neelature Sriramareddy S, Costa C, Hubaux R, Cosse JP et al. The role of epigenetics in malignant pleural mesothelioma. Lung Cancer 2013; 81: 311–318.
17. Biesecker LG. Hypothesis-generating research and predictive medicine. Genome Research 2013; 23: 1051–1053.
18. Sugarbaker DJ, Richards WG, Gordon GJ, Dong L, De Rienzo A, et al. Transcriptome sequencing of malignant pleural mesothelioma tumors. Proceedings of the National Academy of Sciences USA 2008; 105: 3521–3526.
19. Bueno R, De Rienzo A, Dong L, Gordon GJ, Hercus CF et al. Second generation sequencing of the mesothelioma tumor genome. PLoS One 2010; 5: e10612.
20. Beltrami S, Kim R, Gordon J. Neurofibromatosis type 2 protein, NF2: an uncoventional cell cycle regulator. Anticancer Research 2013; 33: 1–11.
21. Sekido Y, Pass HI, Bader S, Mew DJ, Christman MF et al. Neurofibromatosis type 2 (NF2) gene is somatically mutated in mesothelioma but not in lung cancer. Cancer Research 1995; 55: 1227–1231.

22. Bianchi AB, Mitsunaga SI, Cheng JQ, Klein WM, Jhanwar SC et al. High frequency of inactivating mutations in the neurofibromatosis type 2 gene (NF2) in primary malignant mesotheliomas. Proceedings of the National Academy of Sciences USA 1995; 92: 10854–10858.

23. Deguen B, Goutebroze L, Giovannini M, Boisson C, van der Neut et al. Heterogeneity of mesothelioma cell lines as defined by altered genomic structure and expression of the NF2 gene. International Journal of Cancer 1998; 77: 554–560.

24. Thurneysen C, Opitz I, Kurtz S, Weder W, Stahel RA et al. Functional inactivation of NF2/merlin in human mesothelioma. Lung Cancer 2009; 64: 140–147.

25. Illei PB, Ladanyi M, Rusch VW, Zakowski MF. The use of CDKN2A deletion as a diagnostic marker for malignant mesothelioma in body cavity effusions. Cancer 2003; 99: 51–56.

26. Ladanyi M. Implications of P16/CDKN2A deletion in pleural mesotheliomas. Lung Cancer 2005; 49(Suppl 1): S95–S98.

27. Wong L, Zhou J, Anderson D, Kratzke RA. Inactivation of p16INK4a expression in malignant mesothelioma by methylation. Lung Cancer 2002; 38: 131–136.

28. Xio S, Li D, Vijg J, Sugarbaker DJ, Corson JM et al. Codeletion of p15 and p16 in primary malignant mesothelioma. Oncogene 1995; 11: 511–515.

29. Romagosa C, Simonetti S, López-Vicente L, Mazo A, Lleonart ME et al. p16(Ink4a) overexpression in cancer: a tumor suppressor gene associated with senescence and high-grade tumors. Oncogene 2011; 30: 2087–2097.

30. Sherr CJ. The INK4a/ARF network in tumour suppression. Nature Reviews Molecular Cell Biology 2001; 2: 731–737.

31. Musti M, Kettunen E, Dragonieri S, Lindholm P, Cavone D, et al. Cytogenetic and molecular genetic changes in malignant mesothelioma. Cancer Genetics and Cytogenetics 2006; 170: 9–15.

32. Bott M, Brevet M, Taylor BS, Shimizu S, Ito T, Wang L, et al. The nuclear deubiquitinase BAP1 is commonly inactivated by somatic mutations and 3p21.1 losses in malignant pleural mesothelioma. Nature Genetics 2011; 43: 668–672.

33. Murali R, Wiesner T, Scolyer RA. Tumours associated with BAP1 mutations. Pathology 2013; 45: 116–126.

34. Carbone M, Yang H, Pass HI, Krausz T, Testa JR, Gaudino G. BAP1 and cancer. Nature Reviews Cancer 2013; 13: 153–159.

35. Quackenbush J. Microarray analysis and tumor classification. New England Journal of Medicine 2006; 354: 2463–2472.

36. Gordon GJ, Jensen RV, Hsiao LL, Gullans SR, Blumenstock JE et al. Translation of microarray data into clinically relevant cancer diagnostic tests using gene expression ratios in lung cancer and mesothelioma. Cancer Research 2002; 62: 4963–4967.

37. Bueno R, Gordon GJ. Genetics of malignant pleural mesothelioma: molecular markers and biologic targets. Thoracic Surgery Clinics 2004; 14: 461–468.

38. De Rienzo A, Richards WG, Yeap BY, Coleman MH, Sugarbaker PE et al. Sequential binary gene ratio tests define a novel molecular diagnostic strategy for malignant pleural mesothelioma. Clinical Cancer Research 2013; 19: 2493–2502.

39. Bueno R, Reblando J, Glickman J, Jaklitsch MT, Lukanich JM et al. Pleural biopsy: a reliable method for determining the diagnosis but not subtype in mesothelioma. Annals of Thoracic Surgery 2004; 78: 1774–1776.

40. Foo W, Hofer M, Sugarbaker D. The accuracy of pretreatment biopsy of pleural malignant mesothelioma in predicting histopathologic type in extrapleural pneumonectomy. Laboratory Investigation 2008; 88: 341A–342A.

41. Sugarbaker DJ, Flores RM, Jaklitsch MT, Richards WG, Strauss GM et al. Resection margins, extrapleural nodal status, and cell type determine postoperative long-term survival in trimodality therapy of malignant pleural mesothelioma: results in 183 patients. Journal of Thoracic and Cardiovascular Surgery 1999; 117: 54–63; discussion, 5.

42. Lester S. Manual of Surgical Pathology, 2nd ed. Edinburgh/ New York: Elsevier Churchill Livingstone, 2006.

43. Cagle PT, Wessels R, Greenberg SD. Concurrent mesothelioma and adenocarcinoma of the lung in a patient with asbestosis. Modern Pathology 1993; 6: 438–441.

44. Cagle PT. Correspondence re: Philip T. Cagle, Robert Wessels, and S. Donald Greenberg. Concurrent mesothelioma and adenocarcinoma of the lung in a patient with asbestosis. Modern Pathology 1993; 6: 438. Modern Pathology 1994; 7: 148–149.

45. Roggli VL, Vollmer RT. Twenty-five years of fiber analysis: what have we learned? Human Pathology 2008; 39: 307–315.

46. Dodson R, Hammar S. Asbestos: Risk Assessment, Epidemiology, and Health Effects. Boca Raton: Taylor & Francis, 2006.

47. Chirieac LR, Corson JM. Pathologic evaluation of malignant pleural mesothelioma. Seminars in Thoracic and Cardiovascular Surgery 2009; 21: 121–124.

48. Travis W, ed. Histological Typing of Lung and Pleural Tumours, 3rd ed. Berlin/New York: Springer-Verlag, 1999.

49. Hammar SP. Macroscopic, histologic, histochemical, immunohistochemical, and ultrastructural features of mesothelioma. Ultrastructural Pathology 2006; 30: 3–17.

50. Allen TC. Recognition of histopathologic patterns of diffuse malignant mesothelioma in differential diagnosis of pleural biopsies. Archives of Pathology and Laboratory Medicine 2005; 129: 1415–1420.

51. Litzky LA. Pulmonary sarcomatous tumors. Archives of Pathology and Laboratory Medicine 2008; 132: 1104–1117.

52. Marchevsky AM. Application of immunohistochemistry to the diagnosis of malignant mesothelioma. Archives of Pathology and Laboratory Medicine 2008; 132: 397–401.

53. Suster S, Moran CA. Applications and limitations of immunohistochemistry in the diagnosis of malignant mesothelioma. Advances in Anatomic Pathology 2006; 13: 316–329.

54. Ordonez NG. What are the current best immunohistochemical markers for the diagnosis of epithelioid mesothelioma? A review and update. Human Pathology 2007; 38: 1–16.

55. Granville L, Laga AC, Allen TC, Dishop M, Roggli VL, Churg A et al. Review and update of uncommon primary pleural tumors: a practical approach to diagnosis. Archives of Pathology and Laboratory Medicine 2005; 129: 1428–1443.

56. Attanoos RL, Dojcinov SD, Webb R, Gibbs AR. Anti-mesothelial markers in sarcomatoid mesothelioma and other spindle cell neoplasms. Histopathology 2000; 37: 224–231.

57. Chirieac L, Pinkus G, Pinkus J. Sarcomatoid malignant mesothelioma: immunohistochemical characteristics of 24 cases. Laboratory Investigation 2006; 86: 305A.

58. Lucas DR, Pass HI, Madan SK, Adsay NV, Wali A et al. Sarcomatoid mesothelioma and its histological mimics: a comparative immunohistochemical study. Histopathology 2003; 42: 270–279.

59. Padgett DM, Cathro HP, Wick MR, Mills SE. Podoplanin is a better immunohistochemical marker for sarcomatoid mesothelioma than calretinin. American Journal of Surgical Pathology 2008; 32: 123–127.

60. Copeland MM. American Joint Committee on cancer staging and end results reporting. Objectives and progress. Cancer 1965; 18: 1637–1640.

61. Karnofsky D, Burchenal J, eds. The Clinical Evaluation of Chemotherapeutic Agents in Cancer. New York: Columbia University Press, 1949.

62. Wolf AS, Daniel J, Sugarbaker DJ. Surgical techniques for multimodality treatment of malignant pleural mesothelioma: extrapleural pneumonectomy and pleurectomy/decortication. Seminars in Thoracic and Cardiovascular Surgery 2009; 21: 132–148.

63. Baldini EH, Recht A, Strauss GM, DeCamp MM Jr, Swanson SJ et al. Patterns of failure after trimodality therapy for malignant pleural mesothelioma. Annals of Thoracic Surgery 1997; 63: 334–338.

64. Flores RM, Pass HI, Seshan VE, Dycoco J, Zakowski M et al. Extrapleural pneumonectomy versus pleurectomy/decortication in the surgical management of malignant pleural mesothelioma: results in 663 patients. Journal of Thoracic and Cardiovascular Surgery 2008; 135: 620–626, 6 e1–3.

65. Baldini EH, Richards WG, Gill RR, Goodman BM, Gill RR, Winfrey OK, et al. Patterns of recurrence following extrapleural pneumonectomy (EPP) for malignant pleural mesothelioma (MPM). In: International Mesothelioma Interest Group, September 11–4, 2012. Boston, MA, 2013.

66. Sugarbaker DJ, Gill RR, Yeap BY, Wolf AS, DaSilva MC et al. Patterns of recurrence following pleurectomy/decortication for malignant pleural mesothelioma. In: International Mesothelioma Interest Group, September 11–14, 2012. Boston, MA, 2013.

67. Burt BM, Ali SO, DaSilva MC, Yeap BY, Richards WG et al. Clinical indications and results after chest wall resection for recurrent mesothelioma. Journal of Thoracic and Cardiovascular Surgery 2013; 146: 1373–1379; discussion, 9–80.

68. Yan TD, Boyer M, Tin MM, Wong D, Kennedy C et al. Extrapleural pneumonectomy for malignant pleural mesothelioma: outcomes of treatment and prognostic factors. Journal of Thoracic and Cardiovascular Surgery 2009; 138: 619–624.

69. Weder W, Stahel RA, Bernhard J, Bodis S, Vogt P et al. Multicenter trial of neo-adjuvant chemotherapy followed by extrapleural pneumonectomy in malignant pleural mesothelioma. Annals of Oncology 2007; 18: 1196–1202.

70. Krug LM, Pass HI, Rusch VW, Sugarbaker DJ, et al. Multicenter phase II trial of neoadjuvant pemetrexed plus cisplatin followed by extrapleural pneumonectomy and radiation for malignant pleural mesothelioma. Journal of Clinical Oncology 2009; 27: 3007–3013.

71. Rusch VW, Venkatraman ES. Important prognostic factors in patients with malignant pleural mesothelioma, managed surgically. Annals of Thoracic Surgery1999; 68: 1799–1804.

72. Maggi G, Casadio C, Cianci R, Rena O, Ruffini E. Trimodality management of malignant pleural mesothelioma. European Journal of Cardiothoracic Surgery 2001; 19: 346–350.

73. Aziz T, Jilaihawi A, Prakash D. The management of malignant pleural mesothelioma; single centre experience in 10 years. European Journal of Cardiothoracic Surgery 2002; 22: 298–305.

74. Flores RM, Akhurst T, Gonen M, Zakowski M, Dycoco J et al. Positron emission tomography predicts survival in malignant pleural mesothelioma. Journal of Thoracic and Cardiovascular Surgery 2006; 132: 763–768.

75. Schipper PH, Nichols FC, Thomse KM, Deschamps C, Cassivi SD, et al. Malignant pleural mesothelioma: surgical management in 285 patients. Annals of Thoracic Surgery 2008; 85: 257–264; discussion, 64.

76. Pass HI, Temeck BK, Kranda K, Thomas G, Russo A et al. Phase III randomized trial of surgery with or without intraoperative photodynamic therapy and postoperative immunochemotherapy for malignant pleural mesothelioma. Annals of Surgical Oncology 1997; 4: 628–633.

77. Pass HI, Temeck BK, Kranda K, Steinberg SM, Feuerstein IR. Preoperative tumor volume is associated with outcome in malignant pleural mesothelioma. Journal of Thoracic and Cardiovascular Surgery 1998; 115: 310–317; discussion, 7–8.

78. Moskal TL, Urschel JD, Anderson TM, Antkowiak JG, Takita H. Malignant pleural mesothelioma: a problematic review. Surgical Oncology 1998; 7: 5–12.

79. Vogelzang NJ, Rusthoven JJ, Symanowski J, Denham C, Kaukel E et al. Phase III study of pemetrexed in combination with cisplatin versus cisplatin alone in patients with malignant pleural mesothelioma. Journal of Clinical Oncology 2003; 21: 2636–2644.

80. Calavrezis A, Koschel G, Husselmann H. Malignant mesothelioma of the pleura. A prospective therapeutic study of 132 patients from 1981–1985. Wiener Klinische Wochenschrift1988; 66: 607–613.

81. Sugarbaker DJ, Wolf AS, Chirieac LR, Godleski JJ, Tilleman TR et al. Clinical and pathological features of three-year survivors of malignant pleural mesothelioma following extrapleural pneumonectomy. European Journal of Cardiothoracic Surgery 2011; 40: 298–303.

82. Baldini EH, Gill R, Wolf AS, Yeap BY, DaSilva MC et al. Preoperative anemia as a prognostic biomarker for time to recurrence (TTR) and overall survival (OS) following extra-pleural pneumonectomy (EPP) and pleurectomy/decortication (PD) for malignant pleural mesothelioma (MPM). In: International Mesothelioma Interest Group, September 11 –14, 2012. Boston, MA: iMig; 2013.

83. Richards WG, Gill RR, Baldini EH, Yeap BY, Wolf AS et al. Impact of incorporating hemoglobin level on the accuracy of clinical lymph node staging in malignant pleural mesothelioma (MPM). In: International Mesothelioma Interest Group, September 11–14, 2012. Boston, MA: iMig; 2013.

84. Treasure T, Lang-Lazdunski L, Waller D, Bliss JM, Tan C et al. Extra-pleural pneumonectomy versus no extra-pleural pneumonectomy for patients with malignant pleural mesothelioma: clinical outcomes of the Mesothelioma and Radical Surgery (MARS) randomised feasibility study. Lancet Oncology 2011; 12: 763–772.

85. Frauenfelder T, Tutic M, Weder W, Götti RP, Stahel RA, et al. Volumetry: an alternative to assess therapy response for malignant pleural mesothelioma? European Respiratory Journal 2011; 38: 162–168.

86. Weder W, Stahel RA, Baas P, Dafni U, de Perrot M et al. The MARS feasibility trial: conclusions not supported by data. Lancet Oncology 2011; 12: 1093–1094; author reply, 4–5.

87. Rusch V, Baldini EH, Bueno R, De Perrot M, Flores R, et al. The role of surgical cytoreduction in the treatment of malignant pleural mesothelioma: meeting summary of the International Mesothelioma Interest Group Congress, September 11–14, 2012, Boston, Mass. Journal of Thoracic and Cardiovascular Surgery 2013; 145: 909–910.

88. Tobler M, Watson G, Leavitt DD. Intensity-modulated photon arc therapy for treatment of pleural mesothelioma. Medical Dosimetry 2002; 27: 255–259.

89. Rosenzweig KE, Zauderer MG, Laser B, Krug L M, Yorke E et al. Pleural intensity-modulated radiotherapy for malignant pleural mesothelioma. International Journal of Radiation Oncology Biology Physics 2012; 83: 1278–1283.

90. Minatel E, Trovo M, Polesel J, Baresic T, Bearz A et al. Radical pleurectomy/decortication followed by high dose of radiation therapy for malignant pleural mesothelioma. Final results with long-term follow-up. Lung Cancer 2014; 83: 78–82.

91. Ahamad A, Stevens CW, Smythe WR, Vaporciyan AA, Komaki R et al. Intensity-modulated radiation therapy: a novel approach to the management of malignant pleural mesothelioma. International Journal of Radiation Oncology Biology Physics 2003; 55: 768–775.

92. Gomez DR, Hong DS, Allen PK, Welsh JS, Mehran RJ et al. Patterns of failure, toxicity, and survival after extrapleural pneumonectomy and hemithoracic intensity-modulated radiation therapy for malignant pleural mesothelioma. Journal of Thoracic Oncology 2013; 8: 238–245.

93. Giraud P, Sylvestre A, Zefkili S, Lisbona A, Bonnette P et al. Helical tomotherapy for resected malignant pleural mesothelioma: dosimetric evaluation and toxicity. Radiotherapy Oncology 2011; 101: 303–306.

94. Yajnik S, Rosenzweig KE, Mychalczak B, Krug L, Flores R et al. Hemithoracic radiation after extrapleural pneumonectomy for malignant pleural mesothelioma. International Journal of Radiation Oncology Biology Physics 2003; 56: 1319–1326.

95. Rice DC, Smythe WR, Liao Z, Guerrero T, Chang JY et al. Dose-dependent pulmonary toxicity after postoperative intensity-modulated radiotherapy for malignant pleural mesothelioma. International Journal of Radiation Oncology Biology Physics 2007; 69: 350–357.

96. Allen AM, Czerminska M, Janne PA, Sugarbaker DJ, Bueno R et al. Fatal pneumonitis associated with intensity-modulated radiation therapy for mesothelioma. International Journal of Radiation Oncology Biology Physics 2006; 65: 640–645.

97. Miles EF, Larrier NA, Kelsey CR, Hubbs JL, Ma J et al. Intensity-modulated radiotherapy for resected mesothelioma: the Duke experience. International Journal of Radiation Oncology Biology Physics 2008; 71: 1143–1150.

98. Teta MJ, Mink PJ, Lau E, Sceurman BK, Foster ED. US mesothelioma patterns 1973–2002: indicators of change and insights into

background rates. European Journal of Cancer Prevention 2008; 17: 525–534.

99. Janne PA, Wozniak AJ, Belani CP, Keohan ML, Ross HJ et al. Pemetrexed alone or in combination with cisplatin in previously treated malignant pleural mesothelioma: outcomes from a phase IIIB expanded access program. Journal of Thoracic Oncology 2006; 1: 506–512.

100. Jassem J, Ramlau R, Santoro A, Schuette W, Chemaissani A et al. Phase III trial of pemetrexed plus best supportive care compared with best supportive care in previously treated patients with advanced malignant pleural mesothelioma. Journal of Clinical Oncology 2008; 26: 1698–1704.

101. Patz EF Jr, Shaffer K, Piwnica-Worms DR, Jochelson M, Sarin M, et al. Malignant pleural mesothelioma: value of CT and MR imaging in predicting resectability. American Journal of Roentgenology 1992; 159: 961–966.

102. Wang ZJ, Reddy GP, Gotway MB, Higgins CB, Jablons DM et al. Malignant pleural mesothelioma: evaluation with CT, MR imaging, and PET. Radiographics 2004; 24: 105–119.

103. Gill RR. Imaging of mesothelioma. Recent Results in Cancer Research 2011; 189: 27–43.

104. Sugarbaker DJ, Strauss GM, Lynch TJ, Richards W, Mentzer SJ et al. Node status has prognostic significance in the multimodality therapy of diffuse, malignant mesothelioma. Journal of Clinical Oncology 1993; 11: 1172–1178.

105. Sugarbaker DJ, Garcia JP, Richards WG, Harpole DH Jr, Healy-Baldini E et al. Extrapleural pneumonectomy in the multimodality therapy of malignant pleural mesothelioma. Results in 120 consecutive patients. Annals of Surgery 1996; 224: 288–294; discussion, 94–96.

106. Sugarbaker DJ, Garcia JP. Multimodality therapy for malignant pleural mesothelioma. Chest 1997; 112: 272S–275S.

107. Tonoli S, Vitali P, Scotti V, Bertoni F, Spiazzi L, et al. Adjuvant radiotherapy after extrapleural pneumonectomy for mesothelioma. Prospective analysis of a multi-institutional series. Radiotherapy and Oncology 2011; 101: 311–315.

108. Cao C, Yan TD, Bannon PG, McCaughan BC. Summary of prognostic factors and patient selection for extrapleural pneumonectomy in the treatment of malignant pleural mesothelioma. Annals of Surgical Oncology 2011; 18: 2973–2979.

109. Tilleman TR, Richards WG, Zellos L, Johnson BE, Jaklitsch MT, et al. Extrapleural pneumonectomy followed by intracavitary intraoperative hyperthermic cisplatin with pharmacologic cytoprotection for treatment of malignant pleural mesothelioma: a phase II prospective study. Journal of Thoracic and Cardiovascular Surgery 2009; 138: 405–411.

110. Richards WG, Zellos L, Bueno R, Jaklitsch MT, Jänne PA et al. Phase I to II study of pleurectomy/decortication and intraoperative intracavitary hyperthermic cisplatin lavage for mesothelioma. Journal of Clinical Oncology 2006; 24: 1561–1567.

111. Sugarbaker DJ, Gill RR, Yeap BY, Wolf AS, DaSilva MC et al. Hyperthermic intraoperative pleural cisplatin chemotherapy extends interval to recurrence and survival among low-risk patients with malignant pleural mesothelioma undergoing surgical macroscopic complete resection. Journal of Thoracic and Cardiovascular Surgery 2013; 145: 955–963.

112. Sugarbaker PH. Comprehensive management of peritoneal surface malignancy using cytoreductive surgery and perioperative intraperitoneal chemotherapy: the Washington Cancer Institute approach. Expert Opinion on Pharmacotherapy 2009; 10: 1965–1977.

113. Felip E, Rosell R, Maestre JA, Rodríguez-Paniagua JM, Morán T, et al. Preoperative chemotherapy plus surgery versus surgery plus adjuvant chemotherapy versus surgery alone in early-stage non-small-cell lung cancer. Journal of Clinical Oncology 2010; 28: 3138–3145.

114. Girard N1, Mornex F, Douillard JY, Bossard N, Quoix E, et al. Is neoadjuvant chemoradiotherapy a feasible strategy for stage IIIA-N2 non-small cell lung cancer? Mature results of the randomized IFCT-0101 phase II trial. Lung Cancer 2010; 69: 86–93.

115. Weder W, Kestenholz P, Taverna C, Bodis S, Lardinois D, et al. Neoadjuvant chemotherapy followed by extrapleural pneumonectomy in malignant pleural mesothelioma. Journal of Clinical Oncology 2004; 22: 3451–3457.

116. Rusch VW, Giroux D, Kennedy C, Ruffini E, Cangir AK et al. Initial analysis of the international association for the study of lung cancer mesothelioma database. Journal of Thoracic Oncology 2012; 7: 1631–1639.

117. Friedberg JS, Mick R, Stevenson J, Metz J, Zhu T et al. A phase I study of Foscan-mediated photodynamic therapy and surgery in patients with mesothelioma. Annals of Thoracic Surgery 2003; 75: 952–959.

118. Friedberg JS1, Mick R, Stevenson JP, Zhu T, Busch TM, et al. Phase II trial of pleural photodynamic therapy and surgery for patients with non-small-cell lung cancer with pleural spread. Journal of Clinical Oncology 2004; 22: 2192–2201.

119. Friedberg JS, Culligan MJ, Mick R, Stevenson J, Hahn SM, et al. Radical pleurectomy and intraoperative photodynamic therapy for malignant pleural mesothelioma. Annals of Thoracic Surgery 2012; 93: 1658–1665; discussion, 65–67.

120. Branscheid D, Krysa S, Bauer E, Bulzebruck H, Schirren J. Diagnostic and therapeutic strategy in malignant pleural mesothelioma. European Journal of Cardiothoracic Surgery 1991; 5: 466–472; discussion, 73.

121. Allen KB, Faber LP, Warren WH. Malignant pleural mesothelioma. Extrapleural pneumonectomy and pleurectomy. Chest Surgery Clinics of North America 1994; 4: 113–126.

122. Rusch VW, Rosenzweig K, Venkatraman E, Leon L, Raben A et al. A phase II trial of surgical resection and adjuvant high-dose hemithoracic radiation for malignant pleural mesothelioma. Journal of Thoracic and Cardiovascular Surgery 2001; 122: 788–795.

123. Rosenzweig KE, Fox JL, Zelefsky MJ, Raben A, Harrison LB et al. A pilot trial of high-dose-rate intraoperative radiation therapy for malignant pleural mesothelioma. Brachytherapy 2005; 4: 30–33.

124. Pagan V, Ceron L, Paccagnella A, Pizzi G. 5-year prospective results of trimodality treatment for malignant pleural mesothelioma. Journal of Cardiovascular Surgery (Torino) 2006; 47: 595–601.

125. Rice DC, Stevens CW, Correa AM, Vaporciyan AA, Tsao A et al. Outcomes after extrapleural pneumonectomy and intensity-modulated radiation therapy for malignant pleural mesothelioma. Annals of Thoracic Surgery 2007; 84: 1685–1692; discussion, 92–93.

126. Batirel HF, Metintas M, Caglar HB, Yildizeli B, Lacin T, et al. Trimodality treatment of malignant pleural mesothelioma. Journal of Thoracic Oncology 2008; 3: 499–504.

127. Luckraz H, Rahman M, Patel N, Szafranek A, Gibbs AR, Butchart EG. Three decades of experience in the surgical multi-modality management of pleural mesothelioma. European Journal of Cardiothoracic Surgery 2010; 37: 552–556.

128. Rena O, Casadio C. Extrapleural pneumonectomy for early stage malignant pleural mesothelioma: a harmful procedure. Lung Cancer 2012; 77: 151–155.

129. Patel PR, Yoo S, Broadwater G, Marks LB, Miles EF, et al. Effect of increasing experience on dosimetric and clinical outcomes in the management of malignant pleural mesothelioma with intensity-modulated radiation therapy. International Journal of Radiation Oncology Biology Physics 2012; 83: 362–368.

130. Ambrogi V, Baldi A, Schillaci O, Mineo TC. Clinical impact of extrapleural pneumonectomy for malignant pleural mesothelioma. Annals of Surgical Oncology 2012; 19: 1692–1699.

131. Rea F, Marulli G, Bortolotti L, Breda C, Favaretto AG et al. Induction chemotherapy, extrapleural pneumonectomy (EPP) and adjuvant hemi-thoracic radiation in malignant pleural mesothelioma (MPM): feasibility and results. Lung Cancer 2007; 57: 89–95.

132. de Perrot M, Feld R, Cho BC, Bezjak A, Anraku M, et al. Trimodality therapy with induction chemotherapy followed by extrapleural pneumonectomy and adjuvant high-dose hemithoracic radiation for malignant pleural mesothelioma. Journal of Clinical Oncology 2009; 27: 1413–1418.

133. Buduhan G, Menon S, Aye R, Louie B, Mehta V, Vallières E. Trimodality therapy for malignant pleural mesothelioma. The Annals of Thoracic Surgery 2009; 88(3): 870–875.

134. Van Schil PE, Baas P, Gaafar R, Maat AP, Van de Pol M, et al. Trimodality therapy for malignant pleural mesothelioma: results from an EORTC phase II multicentre trial. European Respiratory Journal 2010; 36: 1362–1369.

135. Lang-Lazdunski L, Bille A, Lal R, Cane P, McLean E et al. Pleurectomy/decortication is superior to extrapleural pneumonectomy in the multimodality management of patients with malignant pleural mesothelioma. Journal of Thoracic Oncology 2012; 7: 737–743.

136. Chailleux E, Dabouis G, Pioche D, de Lajartre M, de Lajartre AY et al. Prognostic factors in diffuse malignant pleural mesothelioma. A study of 167 patients. Chest 1988; 93: 159–162.

137. Achatzy R1, Beba W, Ritschler R, Wörn H, Wahlers B et al. The diagnosis, therapy and prognosis of diffuse malignant mesothelioma. European Journal of Cardiothoracic Surgery 1989; 3: 445–447; discussion, 8.

138. Ruffie P, Feld R, Minkin S, Cormier Y, Boutan-Laroze A et al. Diffuse malignant mesothelioma of the pleura in Ontario and Quebec: a retrospective study of 332 patients. Journal of Clinical Oncology 1989; 7: 1157–1168.

139. de Vries WJ, Long MA. Treatment of mesothelioma in Bloemfontein, South Africa. European Journal of Cardiothoracic Surgery 2003; 24: 434–440.

140. Nakas A, Martin Ucar AE, Edwards JG, Waller DA. The role of video assisted thoracoscopic pleurectomy/decortication in the therapeutic management of malignant pleural mesothelioma. European Journal of Cardiothoracic Surgery 2008; 33: 83–88.

141. Bolukbas S, Manegold C, Eberlein M, Bergmann T, Fisseler-Eckhoff A, Schirren J. Survival after trimodality therapy for malignant pleural mesothelioma: radical pleurectomy, chemotherapy with cisplatin/pemetrexed and radiotherapy. Lung Cancer 2011; 71: 75–81.

142. Nakas A, von Meyenfeldt E, Lau K, Muller S, Waller D. Long-term survival after lung-sparing total pleurectomy for locally advanced (International Mesothelioma Interest Group Stage T3-T4) non-sarcomatoid malignant pleural mesothelioma. European Journal of Cardiothoracic Surgery 2012; 41: 1031–1036.

143. Rosenzweig KE, Zauderer MG, Laser B, Krug LM, Yorke E, et al. Pleural intensity-modulated radiotherapy for malignant pleural mesothelioma. International Journal of Radiation Oncology Biology Physics 2012; 83: 1278–1283.

CHAPTER 49

Skin cancer: melanoma

John F. Thompson, Richard A. Scolyer,
and Richard F. Kefford

Introduction to melanoma

Melanoma is a malignant, often aggressive, potentially fatal tumour that develops when genetic and metabolic abnormalities occur in melanocytes. The latter are pigment-producing cells that originate in the neural crest and migrate to the skin and other body sites during embryonic development. Because most melanocytes are found in the skin, the majority of melanomas are cutaneous in origin and this chapter will deal principally with cutaneous melanoma. However, melanoma can also arise from melanocytes at non-cutaneous sites. The clinical features and management of mucosal melanomas will be discussed briefly, but ocular melanomas will be considered separately (see Chapter 57, Tumours of the eye and orbit).

Cutaneous melanoma is a steadily increasing health problem in developed countries with mainly fair-skinned populations, and the rate of increase in its incidence is greater than that of any other solid tumour type. Until recently, the treatment of all forms of melanoma was primarily surgical. However, recent advances in knowledge of molecular biology and the recognition that melanoma develops as a result of the accumulation of multiple genetic abnormalities within melanocytes, together with improved understanding of the role of the immune system in regulating melanoma, have led to much more effective medical therapies than were previously available. Fortunately, the great majority of patients who develop melanoma present at a stage when cure can be achieved by relatively simple surgery. Nevertheless, 10–15% of those who present with a primary cutaneous melanoma will eventually develop distant metastases; at the present time in almost all these patients the disease will ultimately prove fatal. Medical therapy for advanced melanoma is, however, a rapidly evolving field, and there are grounds for considerable optimism that within the next few years new systemic treatments will achieve good long-term control and possibly even elimination of metastatic melanoma at distant sites.

Molecular biology and pathogenesis

Sun exposure is calculated to be involved in the causation of more than 80% of cutaneous melanomas. Ultraviolet (UV) radiation induces pyrimidine dimer mutations in DNA, resulting in a characteristic profile of UV-induced damage on whole exome sequencing of melanomas. UV radiation also promotes the production of growth factors from keratinocytes and other skin cells, and suppresses T cell-mediated cutaneous immune defences. The stimulation of melanin production by UV radiation produces reactive oxygen species of melanin that cause DNA damage and suppress apoptotic mechanisms. Melanoma forms as the result of accumulated abnormalities in genetic pathways within the melanocyte that promote cell proliferation and prevent normal pathways of cell death in response to DNA damage. The genetically unstable melanocyte is thereby predisposed to accumulate successive DNA damage. This results in the rapid selection for genetic mutations that permit and promote angiogenesis and evasion of the immune response and allows rapid selection of variants capable of invasion and metastasis. Melanoma cells display resistance to cellular death mechanisms at multiple levels; this probably explains much of the observed resistance of melanoma cells to cytotoxic attack using chemotherapy, radiotherapy, or immunotherapy.

Benign proliferations of melanocytes (naevi) frequently carry mutations in the BRAF oncogene, but are arrested through protective triggering of senescence. Melanomas may arise in naevus precursors when naevus cells escape senescence, although the mechanisms of this remain controversial. The primary somatic genetic mutations in melanoma are unknown, but tumour progression usually involves activation of the mitogen-activated protein kinase (MAPK) pathway by acquisition of mutations in BRAF (50%), NRAS (20%), EGFR (10%), or other mechanisms. One of the principal downstream targets of the MAPK pathway is the master melanocyte-regulator, micropthalmia transcription factor (MITF), which is also mutated in 10% of melanomas. MITF regulates a suite of genes governing cellular proliferation, survival, and invasion. Genes frequently disregulated in melanoma are shown in Table 49.1.

Controversy continues over the role of stem cells in melanoma but the demonstration that the majority of cells within an established melanoma are capable of stem-like behaviour encourages a concept of plasticity in melanoma ontogeny, rather than the classical hierarchical pattern familiar from haematology.

Genetic predisposition to melanoma

Melanoma risk is substantially increased in those with a family history of melanoma. The presence of one affected first-degree relative doubles risk, and risk further escalates with additional affected close relatives, relatives with multiple primary melanomas, and relatives affected at younger ages.

Around 2% of all melanomas are due to identifiable, heritable mutations in highly-penetrant genes, including CDKN2A and, very rarely, CDK4, and BAP1 (Table 49.2). Some, but not all, of these families also display the phenotype of multiple atypical naevi,

Table 49.1 Genes frequently altered somatically in melanoma

Gene	Full name	Function
MITF	MIcropthalmia Transcription Factor	Master melanocyte transcription factor
BRAF	B-Rapidly Accelerated Fibrosarcoma gene	Growth factor signalling
NRAS	N-RAt Sarcoma protein	Growth factor signalling
EGFR	Epidermal Growth Factor Receptor	Growth factor signalling
TERT	TElomerase Reverse Transcriptase	Regeneration of telomeres evading cell death
CDKN2A	Cyclin Dependent Kinase iNhibitor 2A	Cell cycle control
PTEN	Phosphatase and TENsin homologue	Regulation of growth factor signalling
PREX2	Phosphatidylinositol-3,4,5-trisphosphate-dependent Rac EXchange factor 2	Regulation of growth factor signalling

including polypoid atypical Spitz naevi in those with BAP1 germline mutations. The presence of multiple naevi in an individual, whether atypical or not, is a strong marker for melanoma risk irrespective of family history. The presence of naevi alone cannot be used to predict the presence of CDKN2A germline mutations. Certain families with inherited CDKN2A mutations also have an increased risk of pancreatic cancer. Carriers of inactivating mutations in the gene display a risk of melanoma of between 50% and 90% by the age of 80. Inherited mutations in this gene are found in 30–40% of families with three or more melanoma-affected close relatives.

Cancer genetics consultation should be considered according to the 'rule of threes': (1) patients with three or more melanomas in first-degree or second-degree relatives on the same side of family; (2) families with three or more cases of melanoma or pancreatic cancer on the same side of the family; or (3) in lower incidence countries, like Northern Europe, individuals with three or more primary melanomas.

Certain inherited variants of the melanocortin-1 receptor (MC1R) gene confer increased UV-sensitivity and a two- to four-fold elevation in melanoma risk. Alterations in other genes associated with skin pigmentation also confer small elevations in risk (Table 49.2).

Epidemiology and prevention

Cutaneous melanoma is a malignancy that mainly affects fair-skinned people, particularly those with Celtic ancestry. It occurs most frequently when such individuals are exposed to high levels of solar UV radiation, especially when sun exposure is intense and intermittent, particularly during childhood. Other factors associated with melanoma are the presence of many naevi, particularly atypical (dysplastic) naevi, and higher socio-economic status. Individuals with a past history of melanoma are at higher risk, as are those with a history of non-melanoma skin cancer and those with a family history of melanoma.

Worldwide, the incidence of cutaneous melanoma has been increasing steadily for several decades. It now represents a major health problem for many developed nations, with incidence figures already approaching those of lung cancer, breast cancer, prostate cancer, and bowel cancer in countries such as Australia and New Zealand where the majority of the population is fair-skinned

Table 49.2 Genes associated with inherited melanoma risk

	Chromosome	Protein	Function	Penetrance	Population frequency of mutations/variants	Predictive gene testing
High risk						
CDKN2A	9p21	p16^{INK4A}, p14ARF	Cell-cycle regulation, apoptosis	High	Low	Consider, by rule of threes
CDK4	12q14	Cyclin-dependent kinase 4	Cell-cycle regulation	High	Low	Very rarely in specific families
BAP1	3p21	BRCA1-Associated Protein 1	Chromatin modulation, transcriptional regulation, ubiquitin-proteasome system	High	Low	Very rarely in specific families
Low risk						
MC1R	16q24	Melanocortin 1 receptor	Pigmentation	Low	High	No
ASIP	20q11	Agouti signalling protein	Pigmentation	Low	High	No
TYR	11q14	Tyrosinase	Pigmentation	Low	High	No
TYRP1	9p23	Tyrosinase-related protein 1	Pigmentation	Low	High	No
MITF	14q32	Micropthalmia-associated transcription factor	Regulation of melanocyte differentiation and stemness	Medium	Low	No
Unknown	1q21	N/A	N/A	N/A	N/A	No

Table 49.3 Melanoma incidence rates for Australia, the USA, the Netherlands, and the UK

	Age-standardized incidence (10⁵/year)	Lifetime risk (incidence)	Incidence trend over 10 years	Mortality trend	Age-standardized mortality (10⁵ year)	National Cancer Frequency (ranking)
Australia (2009/2010)						
Men	61.7	1 in 14	42% increase (1991–2009)	No significant increase or decrease (1991–2009)	8.9	3rd
Women	40	1 in 23	18% increase (1991–2009)	No significant increase or decrease (1991–2009)	3.5	3rd
USA (2009/2010)						
Men (whites only)	31.9	1 in 41	19% increase (2000–2009)	11% increase (2000–2009)	4.6	5th
Women (whites only)	20	1 in 61	20% increase (2000–2009)	No significant increase or decrease (2000–2009)	2.0	6th
The Netherlands (2008)						
Men	14.7	1 in 71*	45% increase (1989–2008)	64% increase (2002–2011)	3.0	12th
Women	18.8	1 in 59*	37% increase (1989–2008)	52% increase (2002–2011)	2.0	12th
UK (2010)						
Men	17.2	1 in 55	63% increase (2000–2010)	82% increase (2000–2010)	3.1	6th
Women	17.3	1 in 56	67% increase (2000–2010)	90% increase (2000–2010)	1.8	6th

*Only 2006 estimates of lifetime risk available.

Source: data from Australian Institute of Health and Welfare, *Cancer in Australia: An overview, 2012*, Australian Institute of Health, and Welfare and Australasian Association of Cancer Registries, Canberra, Australia, Copyright © 2012; National Cancer Institute, *SEER Stat Fact Sheets: Melanoma of the Skin*, Copyright © 2013, available from <http://seer.cancer.gov/statfacts/html/melan.html>; Jemal A. et al. Annual Report to the Nation on the Status of Cancer, 1975–2009, featuring the burden and trends in human papillomavirus(HPV)-associated cancers and HPV vaccination coverage levels, *Journal of National Cancer Institute*, Volume 105, Issue 3, pp. 175–201, Copyright © 2013; International Agency for Research on Cancer (IARC), *EUCAN Factsheets, The Netherlands*, Copyright © IARC 2012, available from <http://eu-cancer.iarc.fr/EUCAN/Default.aspx>; Hollestein LM et al., Trends of cutaneous melanoma in The Netherlands: increasing incidence rates among all Breslow thickness categories and rising mortality rates since 1989, *Annals of Oncology*, Volume 23, Issue 2, pp. 524–530, Copyright © 2012; The Netherlands Cancer Registry, Centers AoCC, *Cancer in Figures*, Utrecht, The Netherlands, Copyright © 2009, <http://www.cijfersoverkanker.nl/?language=en>; and Cancer Research UK, *Skin cancer incidence statistics*, Copyright © 2013, available from <http://www.cancerresearchuk.org/cancer-info/cancerstats/types/skin/incidence/uk-skin-cancer-incidence-statistics>.

and exposed to high levels of solar UV radiation. Melanoma incidence rates for Australia, the USA, the Netherlands, and the UK are shown in Table 49.3. The table shows that melanoma incidence continues to increase at an alarming rate around the world. In the Netherlands and the UK, melanoma mortality rates continue to rise, but in Australia and the US mortality rates appear to have stabilized since the turn of the century.

The mutagenic effect of UV light, particularly UVB, on melanocytes has been clearly established, and sun-protection education programs are now conducted in many countries where the incidence of melanoma is high. There are some early indications that attempts to reduce the incidence of melanoma through these programs are proving effective, but because the latent period for melanoma development following UV-induced initiation may be several decades, further time will need to elapse before their value can be fully assessed. The dangers of UV exposure through sunbed use, particularly in teenagers and young adults, have also been recognized and for this form of cutaneous UV exposure the latent period for melanoma development may be short.

Clinical diagnosis and biopsy confirmation of diagnosis

The diagnosis of cutaneous melanoma is normally straightforward. However, even for experienced dermatologists it can sometimes be challenging to differentiate an early invasive melanoma from a benign naevus, and the clinical differentiation between a dysplastic naevus and an in situ melanoma can also be extremely difficult. Furthermore, up to 10% of melanomas do not have the typical dark pigmentation but are non-pigmented, often pink lesions when examined with the naked eye; these are termed amelanotic melanomas, and they may be confused with non-melanocytic skin cancers such as squamous cell carcinomas or basal cell carcinomas.

The classical diagnostic features of a melanoma, whether it presents as a change in a pre-existing pigmented lesion on the skin or as a new pigmented lesion, are asymmetry, border irregularity, and colour variegation. Transformation of a previously flat lesion into one that is elevated and palpable should always also arouse suspicion, and a larger lesion (more than 6 mm in diameter) is more likely to be a melanoma than a smaller lesion. To aid diagnosis, these features have been fitted into an ABCDE system (Asymmetry, Border irregularity, Colour variegation, Diameter >6mm, and Elevation). Some have suggested that 'E' might also be used for Evolution, i.e., change in appearance. When assessing suspicious skin lesions it must always be borne in mind that up to 50% of cutaneous melanomas do not arise in pre-existing naevi but in apparently normal skin.

Critical to the proper assessment of pigmented skin lesions and the diagnosis of melanomas is careful examination with good lighting, preferably with a magnifying device. A hand-held dermatoscope allows suspicious lesions to be assessed in more detail. Dermoscopy has been shown in several large, carefully conducted studies to improve diagnostic accuracy considerably, particularly for clinicians who are not dermatologists. The technique not only provides the requisite magnification and good lighting but additionally it uses epiluminescence microscopy to assist in differentiating benign from malignant melanocytic lesions. Also useful in melanoma diagnosis is computerized imaging, which if repeated can allow suspicious lesions to be monitored carefully and changes identified. High quality whole-body digital photography is another technology that is useful for monitoring. Careful serial assessment of lesions with photography or computerized imaging has been shown to be of value in patients with many lesions, particularly those with numerous atypical (dysplastic) naevi (the 'dysplastic naevus syndrome'). An evolving technique for melanoma diagnosis is reflectance confocal laser microscopy, which allows in vivo microscopic examination in a horizontal plane. Confocal microscopy is particularly useful for defining the extent of in situ melanomas. A detailed description of diagnostic techniques for melanoma is beyond the scope of this chapter, but well-illustrated guides are available in both printed and electronic forms.

When careful clinical examination with use of relevant technological aids indicates that a lesion might be a melanoma, a surgical biopsy should be performed. Complete excisional biopsy with 2 mm clearance margins is preferred, and gives the reporting histopathologist the best opportunity to provide an accurate diagnosis. Incision biopsies and shave biopsies often make interpretation difficult for the pathologist, and it is important to note that the majority of cases of litigation related to misdiagnosis of melanomas involve the use of partial biopsies.

The importance of clinical history in melanoma diagnosis cannot be over-emphasized, and if a patient reports that a lesion has appeared only recently, has become larger, itches or has begun to bleed intermittently, the clinician's level of suspicion must be high and a biopsy performed unless a very confident diagnosis of a benign lesion can be made.

Histopathological features and reporting of cutaneous melanoma, and histological classification

Pathological diagnosis of melanoma

To determine whether a pigmented lesion is a melanoma or a benign naevus, the pathologist must assess a range of microscopic features and correlate these with clinical information, including the anatomical site of the lesion, the patient's age, and more specific details about the lesion such as a history of change or prior trauma. If the clinical features do not correlate with the pathological interpretation, it is usually prudent to review the pathology in the clinical context and, if a partial biopsy has been performed, consider performing a further biopsy of the lesion (preferably complete excision biopsy).

Histologically ambiguous tumours ('melanocytic tumours of uncertain malignant potential')

Whilst the vast majority of melanocytic tumours can be rapidly and accurately classified as naevi or melanomas by routine pathological assessment, it is now well recognized that there exists a small subset of cases which display some benign features and other features suggestive of melanoma. Such lesions have been described using a variety of terms including 'melanocytic tumour of uncertain malignant potential' (MelTUMP), histologically ambiguous melanocytic tumour, or borderline melanoma. These terms should not be regarded as specific diagnoses but rather as a means of communicating uncertainty regarding their biological potential. For such problematic tumours, it is now well-documented that the interobserver reproducibility for their pathological classification is poor, and even tumours regarded as benign by a majority of acknowledged experts may on occasion prove lethal.

There is increasing recognition of the likely existence of a poorly-defined intermediate grade of melanocytic neoplasms with low-grade malignant potential that show frequent involvement of sentinel lymph nodes but infrequent spread beyond the regional lymph nodes to distant metastatic sites. The assessment of risk and prognostic factors (and as a consequence, management decisions) for such tumours remains problematic. In recent years, there have been concerted efforts to develop adjunctive diagnostic techniques, particularly molecular techniques that may assist in the more accurate classification of such tumours.

Molecular assessment of primary melanocytic tumours

Molecular studies have demonstrated that melanomas are characterized by the presence of numerous chromosomal copy number gains and losses and that in most naevi (apart from Spitz naevi, which may occasionally show chromosomal gains in 11p or 7q) such aberrations are not observed. The classification of difficult melanocytic tumours, in which accurate characterization of the tumour as benign or malignant is difficult based on routine histopathology, may be assisted by assessment for the presence of chromosomal copy number aberrations.

Comparative genomic hybridization

Comparative genomic hybridization (CGH) can be used to detect chromosomal copy number aberrations in formalin-fixed, paraffin-embedded tissue. Although this technique has the advantage of being able to detect any aberrations occurring in the genome, there are a number of technical and practical reasons why it is often not an appropriate adjunct to pathological diagnosis in routine clinical practice.

Fluorescence in situ hybridization

Fluorescence in situ hybridization (FISH) is a technique that can be utilized to directly visualize specific chromosomal copy number changes within individual tumour cells. While it has the limitation of being able to test for only a limited number of changes (compared to CGH, which tests for chromosomal aberrations in the entire genome), FISH is more easily applied in routine clinical practice and can be successfully performed on small tumour samples.

Classification of melanoma

It has long been recognized that melanoma is not a single disease entity but consists of a number of disease subtypes. The traditional clinicopathological classification scheme for melanoma, based on the pioneering work of Clark, McGovern, and others in the late 1960s and the 1970s, includes four main subtypes: superficial spreading melanoma, nodular melanoma, lentigo maligna melanoma, and acral lentiginous melanoma. Other less common melanoma subtypes such as desmoplastic melanoma and naevoid melanoma have been recognized and characterized more recently.

From a clinical perspective, the major importance of the traditional Clark-McGovern melanoma classification scheme is that it highlights the various clinical and histological appearances of melanoma that must be recognized by clinicians and pathologists in order to avoid misdiagnosis. As detailed below, the prognosis for a patient with apparently localized primary cutaneous melanoma is principally determined by tumour thickness [1], and the melanoma subtype does not have independent prognostic significance.

Molecular classification of melanoma

In the past decade, critical molecular alterations in melanomas have been identified, as previously discussed. A comparison of the traditional clinicopathological melanoma classification with a classification based on the somatic mutation status reveals remarkable similarities. For example, melanomas associated with prominent solar damage (lentigo maligna melanomas) commonly have NRAS and sometimes KIT mutations, while superficial spreading melanomas that arise in the skin of intermittently sun-exposed areas often have BRAF mutations. BRAF mutant melanoma is also associated with younger patient age, lack of cumulative sun-induced damage at the primary site, truncal location, and a high body naevus count. A recent study reported that of patients with a BRAF mutation, 73% were V600E, 19% V600K, and 8% other genotypes. There was an inverse relationship between BRAF mutation prevalence and age. All patients <30 years and only 25% of patients ≥70 years had BRAF-mutant melanoma. Amongst BRAF-mutant melanoma, the frequency of non-V600E genotypes (including V600K) increased with increasing age.

The melanoma pathology report

Pathological features of the primary melanoma are strong predictors of outcome for patients with clinically localized primary cutaneous melanomas [2]. Numerous studies have shown that tumour thickness (measured using the method described by Breslow) is the strongest prognostic factor. Multiple recent studies have demonstrated that the mitotic rate of the dermal component of a melanoma is also a strong prognostic factor, as is ulceration.

It has been demonstrated that a structured or 'synoptic' format can facilitate the reporting of all relevant histological features in the pathology report, allowing formulation of an appropriate management plan and an accurate estimation of prognosis (Table 49.4).

Various pathological features and their significance

Breslow thickness

Breslow thickness is the single most important prognostic factor for patients with clinically localized primary melanoma who have

Table 49.4 Example of a structured (synoptic) pathology report format for a primary cutaneous melanoma

Specimen type	Excision
Site	Left thigh
Diagnosis	Primary cutaneous melanoma
Classification/main pattern	Superficial spreading
Breslow thickness	2.7 mm
Clark level	IV
Ulceration	Present
Diameter of ulcer	5.5 mm
% of dermal invasive tumour width	60%
Dermal mitotic rate	12/mm^2
Predominant cell type	Epithelioid
Intravascular/intralymphatic invasion	Absent
Neurotropism	Present (perineural)
Satellites	Absent
Desmoplastic component	Absent
Features of regression	
Early (TILs)	Grade 1 (Focal and mild)
Intermediate	Absent
Late (fibrosis and loss of rete ridges)	Absent
Associated naevus (type)	Dysplastic compound
Actinic/Solar elastosis	Moderate
Margins	
In situ component—nearest peripheral	3.2 mm clear of inferior margin
Invasive component—nearest peripheral	5.2 mm clear of inferior margin
Invasive component—nearest deep	4.4 mm

not had pathological regional node staging. Breslow thickness is measured from the top of the granular layer of the epidermis (or, if the surface is ulcerated, from the base of the ulcer) to the deepest invasive cell.

Ulceration

Ulceration is an integral component of the American Joint Committee on Cancer (AJCC)/International Union Against Cancer (UICC) staging system and an independent predictor of outcome in patients with clinically localized primary cutaneous melanoma. The extent of ulceration (measured either as diameter or percentage of tumour width) provides more accurate prognostic information than the mere presence of ulceration.

Mitotic rate

Multiple recent studies have demonstrated that mitotic rate (of the invasive component of a melanoma) is an important prognostic factor for clinically localized primary melanomas and its routine reporting is recommended by the AJCC (Figure 49.1). Furthermore, the presence or absence of mitotic figures in non-ulcerated thin (≤1.0 mm) melanomas is utilized in the seventh (2010) edition of

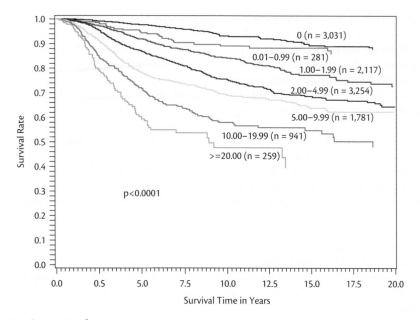

Fig. 49.1 Survival curves by number of mitoses/mm².

the AJCC Staging System for Melanoma for separating pT1a and pT1b tumours. For consistency and reproducibility, a standardized method for determining the mitotic rate must be used.

Other factors

Other pathological features of the primary melanoma that influence prognosis include the presence of lymphatic or blood vessel invasion, Clark level of invasion, tumour-infiltrating lymphocytes, tumour regression, and the presence of a desmoplastic melanoma component.

Satellites

Up to 13% of melanoma patients (with or without a positive sentinel lymph node [SLN]) develop recurrence between the primary tumour site and regional lymph nodes. Depending on their proximity to the primary tumour site, such recurrences have been termed local recurrences, satellites, and intransit metastases (although the definitions used by different investigators have not been consistent). Apart from true local recurrences due to incompletely excised primary melanomas (persistent primary melanomas), all of these terms represent a biologically similar phenomenon (i.e., local metastasis) and the definitions used for them are therefore somewhat arbitrary The presence of satellites or intransit metastases has serious adverse prognostic impact and, in the absence of synchronous nodal metastases, such patients are included in the same prognostic group as those with nodal metastases (N2c) in the seventh (2010) edition of the AJCC Staging System [1].

Pathology of sentinel lymph nodes

A SLN can be defined as any lymph node that receives direct lymphatic drainage from the primary tumour site. At the present time, although the optimal methodology for SLN pathological examination is not uniformly agreed, there is general consensus that both haematoxylin-eosin stained sections and sections stained

immunohistochemically for various melanoma-associated antigens (such as S-100 protein, HMB-45, and MelanA/MART1) should be examined.

Multiple recent studies have demonstrated that both the location and extent of tumour deposits within SLNs are not only strong predictors of the presence of positive non-SLNs in completion lymph node dissection (CLND) specimens but also provide important prognostic information. For example, if there are only a few metastatic tumour cells in the SLN subcapsular sinus, the probability of finding additional metastatic disease in a CLND specimen is extremely small and the patient's prognosis is very good. In contrast, if there are multiple large metastatic foci and the tumour cells extend deeply into the central part of the SLN, the chance of finding metastases in non-SLNs in a CLND specimen is much higher and the prognosis is much worse.

Molecular pathology mutation testing

Molecular genetic testing of melanocytic tumours has the potential to identify subgroups of tumours with specific genetic signatures that may accurately predict their likely clinical course and/or response to treatment. It is usually performed in the context of patients with advanced stage metastatic disease who are being considered for targeted therapies. Mutation testing can be performed on routinely collected archival formalin-fixed, paraffin-embedded tissue. It can also be performed on fresh tissue, but this is not essential. Specimens containing a high percentage of viable tumour cells are the most suitable (thus SLNs containing micrometastases admixed with numerous lymphocytes are often unsatisfactory). Nevertheless, core biopsies and cell blocks made from fine-needle biopsy cytology specimens can often yield diagnostic results.

An important issue to consider when ordering mutation testing is which is the most appropriate specimen to test. At the current time, only limited data are available regarding the concordance of BRAF and NRAS mutation status between primary and metastatic melanomas from individual patients. In one recent study, the concordance rates ranged from 75–96% in metastases from different locations. Therefore, it would appear most appropriate to perform mutation testing on the most recent distant metastatic melanoma specimen provided sufficient viable tumour cells with minimal admixed non-tumour cells is available. If this is not available, testing of locoregional/in-transit metastases is preferred to testing of the primary melanoma.

Mutation testing assays currently in widespread use in clinical practice include traditional Sanger sequencing, allele-specific reverse transcriptase-polymerase chain reaction (RT-PCR), mass spectroscopy/multiplex assays, and pyrosequencing. Each of these techniques has some advantages and disadvantages, and as a consequence no single testing methodology is ideal. Sanger sequencing, usually supplemented by pre-screening with high-resolution melting curve analysis to select only abnormal specimens for further analysis, has traditionally been considered the gold standard. While it detects all known and new mutations (i.e., it is comprehensive), it has only moderate technical sensitivity (about 25%). Hence, careful macrodissection by pathologists to enrich for tumour cells is an important pre-analytical step with this technique. Allele-specific RT-PCR tests (e.g., the Roche cobas 4800 BRAF V600 mutation test) offer high sensitivity but will only detect specific targeted mutations. For example, the Roche cobas test was designed to detect $BRAF^{V600E}$ mutations and does not detect other BRAF mutations (including a significant proportion of $BRAF^{V600K}$ mutations). This may have important clinical consequences because $BRAF^{V600K}$ mutations have been reported to occur in 19–30% of BRAF-mutant melanomas and may not be identified using some testing methodologies. Pyrosequencing and mass spectroscopy assays offer high sensitivity and the ability to test for the presence of a range of mutations in a single test.

Immunohistochemistry (IHC) may also be used for molecular testing. Recent studies showed high correlation of IHC expression of the $BRAF^{V600E}$-specific antibody VE1 with the presence of the $BRAF^{V600E}$ mutation and, in fact, appeared to be more accurate than testing with traditional molecular techniques in one study. The ability to detect mutations by immunochemistry has a number of potential advantages over traditional molecular techniques including faster turnaround times, cost savings, and availability in most pathology laboratories. Potentially, this may facilitate the rapid triage of patients into appropriate treatment pathways at a time when a delay in initiating treatment may result in an adverse outcome.

Melanoma staging and prognosis

The earliest melanoma staging system had three stages, based on each patient's primary tumour (T stage), regional lymph node status (N stage), and the presence or absence of distant metastases (M stage). This staging system, however, was primarily clinical and did not involve microstaging, and it was not until the AJCC Staging System was published in 1977 and 1978 that microstaging was integrated into the staging system for cutaneous melanoma. The AJCC Melanoma Staging System has since been reviewed and updated several times, most recently in 2009 [1]. The current AJCC Staging System, also used by the European-based UICC, is based on assessment of the primary tumour (with Breslow thickness, ulceration, and mitotic rate as the major prognostic factors), evaluation of the regional lymph nodes (with size of metastatic deposits and number

of involved nodes having prognostic significance) and evaluation of distant metastatic sites as well as serum lactose dehydrogenase (LDH) levels. Based on the large AJCC melanoma database, prognostic models were able to be developed by the Melanoma Staging Committee of the AJCC and clear differences in survival outcome based on AJCC staging and substaging were demonstrated (see Figure 49.2). Electronic tools that provide prognostic estimates for individual patients are now available and are often helpful both to patients and to their treating clinicians.

Initial investigations

For patients who present with a primary cutaneous melanoma of any thickness and who have no clinical evidence of regional node metastasis, there is no evidence that investigations such as blood tests, X-rays, or scans are of benefit. For patients found to have micrometastatic disease in regional lymph nodes on SLN biopsy (i.e., with Stage IIIA disease), there is likewise currently no evidence that staging with blood tests, X-rays, or scans is of value. For patients first presenting with Stage IV disease, however, it is appropriate to perform full staging with either whole body CT scans or a PET/CT scan and a CT or MRI scan of the brain. Serum LDH should be checked in those with Stage IIB, Stage IIIC, or Stage IV disease, and if systemic therapy is contemplated the presence or absence of a BRAF mutation in the patient's melanoma should be determined.

Surgical management of the primary melanoma

Any lesion thought to be a primary cutaneous melanoma is best removed by complete excision-biopsy in the first instance, with 2 mm clearance margins, as previously discussed. This allows full histological assessment and rational treatment planning. Immediate performance of a wide excision is not recommended, even if a confident diagnosis of melanoma is made, because clinical estimates of Breslow thickness are notoriously unreliable. If an immediate wide excision is performed, not only might an inappropriate wide excision margin be taken but the opportunity to perform accurate lymphatic mapping and a SLN biopsy (SLNB) procedure might be lost if the melanoma proves to be thicker than anticipated or to have adverse features such as a high mitotic rate.

Wide excision margins

Having established a diagnosis of primary cutaneous melanoma, definitive treatment can be planned. Currently recommended excision margins for primary melanomas are shown in Table 49.5. They are based on the results of a number of prospective randomized trials.

Management of the regional lymph nodes

It is well established that the presence or absence of metastatic disease in regional lymph nodes is the most significant prognostic factor in patients with clinically localized cutaneous melanoma. In the late nineteenth century, Snow advocated routine prophylactic CLND for all patients with cutaneous melanoma who had no clinical evidence of metastatic disease in their regional lymph nodes. The rationale was to remove clinically occult metastatic disease in the regional nodes before spread to distant sites occurred.

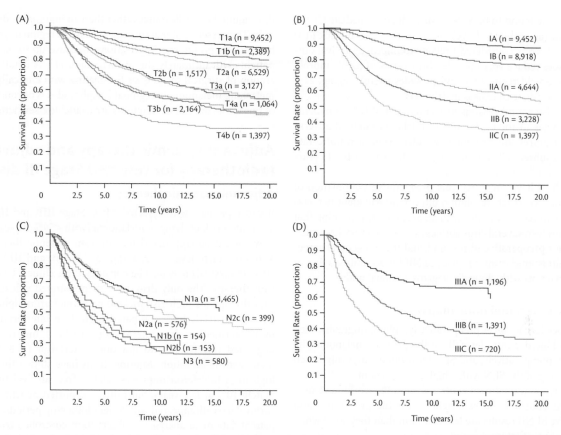

Fig. 49.2 Survival curves from the American Joint Committee on Cancer Melanoma Staging Database comparing (A) the different T categories and (B) the stage groupings for Stages I and II melanoma. For patients with Stage III disease, survival curves are shown comparing (C) the different N categories and (D) the stage groupings.

However, no prospective randomized trial has shown a convincing overall survival benefit for elective lymph node dissection (ELND), although some studies have suggested a benefit for patients with intermediate thickness melanomas.

Sentinel lymph node biopsy

In the early 1990s, Morton et al. introduced the concept of lymphatic mapping and SLNB as a minimally invasive alternative to ELND [3]. The SLNB concept was simple. Lymphatic drainage from a primary melanoma site is initially to a sentinel lymph node in the regional node field, with subsequent onward passage of lymph to other nodes in that field. If melanoma cells spread via

Table 49.5 Surgical excision margins (as recommended in most national guidelines)

T stage	Breslow thickness of melanoma	Excision margin recommended
pTis	in situ only	5 mm
pT1	<1 mm	1 cm
pT2	1.0–2 mm	1–2 cm
pT3	2.0–4.0 mm	2 cm
pT4	>4.0 mm	2–3 cm

lymphatics to the regional lymph node field, they will lodge initially in the sentinel lymph node. Thus, if this node can be identified and removed, which is possible using preoperative lymphoscintigraphy and intraoperative localization with blue dye and a gamma probe, the presence or absence of metastatic disease in the regional lymph node field can be determined with very great accuracy. After the initial report by Morton et al., several validation studies confirmed that this hypothesis was correct.

The common practice of sentinel lymph node (SLN) biopsy in patients with melanoma does not improve their long-term survival, according to the final results of a landmark international trial published in the *New England Journal of Medicine* [4]. The investigators of the Multicenter Selective Lymphadenectomy (MSLT-I) trial compared SLN biopsy with a watch-and-wait approach (only removing nodes once palpable) in melanoma. The 10-year, disease-specific survival in the overall study population was the primary outcome and was not significantly different between the biopsy and observation arms (81.4% vs 78.3%; p = .18).

Today, SLNB is a standard staging procedure in most melanoma treatment centres around the world; in 2012, an evidence-based guideline produced by the American Society of Clinical Oncology and the Society of Surgical Oncology recommended its use in all patients with intermediate thickness melanomas. SLNB allows these patients to be accurately staged according to the AJCC/UICC staging system. As well, it appears to provide a substantial survival benefit for those found to be SLN-positive, if an immediate CLND is performed (as outlined above) [5]. In patients with thick (T4) melanomas SLNB is considered unlikely to improve survival outcome, but does reduce very considerably the risk of highly morbid regional node field recurrence and provides useful staging, as it does for intermediate thickness melanomas.

There are also sound reasons to recommend SLNB for patients with melanomas in the 0.75–1.0 mm thickness range, if adverse prognostic features are present (e.g., ulceration, a mitotic rate >1/mm^2 in a subset of T1b tumours), or if the patient is <45 years of age.

Some authors have suggested that preoperative examination of regional nodes with high-resolution ultrasound will identify metastatic disease in regional nodes with an accuracy approaching that of SLNB. However, several large studies have shown very low sensitivity rates for preoperative ultrasound, and there is general agreement that ultrasound cannot replace SLNB for accurate staging of melanoma patients with clinically negative regional nodes.

Technique of sentinel node biopsy

A SLNB procedure involves preoperative lymphoscintigraphy, then injection of blue dye intradermally at the primary melanoma site immediately preoperatively, and SLN localization surgically-based on blue staining of the SLN with a high gamma count.

Major melanoma treatment centres around the world have now accumulated considerable experience with the procedure, and false-negative SLNB results are less common than they were when the technique was first introduced.

Management of positive sentinel lymph nodes

The standard treatment recommendation for patients found to have metastatic disease in a SLN is an immediate CLND, but whether this is always necessary is being tested in a second Multicenter Selective Lymphadenectomy Trial (MSLT-II). In this trial, patients found to be SLN-positive are randomized either to have a CLND or to have the residual nodes in the regional node field monitored carefully using regular high-resolution ultrasound, with CLND only if metastatic disease in a node field becomes apparent (ClinicalTrials. gov Identifier: NCT00297895). A registration trial in Europe (the MINITUB study) is also examining this question in a prospective fashion. However, it will be several years before the results of these studies are available, and until then CLND must remain the standard therapy for patients found to be SLN-positive.

Management of clinically involved regional lymph nodes

Standard management of patients with clinically involved regional lymph nodes involves full regional lymph node dissection. For the axilla this means complete clearance of lymph node levels I, II, and III. For the neck, however, selective node dissections may be performed, depending on the site of the primary tumour. For involved groin lymph nodes, a complete clearance of nodes in the femoral triangle (i.e., below the level of the inguinal ligament) is standard, but whether pelvic nodes need clearance is a matter of ongoing debate. In most centres, an iliac and obturator node clearance is recommended if there are multiple involved nodes below the inguinal ligament, or if these nodes are large. Involvement of Cloquet's node is also regarded by many as an indication to perform an ilio-inguinal node clearance rather than an inguinal node clearance only. The presence of macroscopic disease in regional lymph nodes has serious prognostic implications, because up to 50% of these patients will ultimately die of melanoma [1]. A detailed consideration of surgical techniques for dealing with clinically apparent metastatic melanoma in regional lymph nodes is beyond the scope of this book, but full descriptions are available elsewhere.

Adjuvant systemic therapy and adjuvant radiotherapy for resected Stage III disease

Adjuvant systemic therapy

Because patients with resected AJCC Stage IIIB and IIIC disease are at high risk of dying of melanoma (with <50% 10-year survival) they should be considered for adjuvant systemic therapy. Those at intermediate levels of risk (Stage IIA, IIB, and IIIA) (51–64% 10-year survival) may also be considered for clinical trials of adjuvant therapy. The only drug with demonstrated efficacy as adjuvant therapy for high-risk melanoma is interferon-alpha2b. Phase III clinical trials have compared high-dose interferon (20 MU/m2), intermediate-dose interferon (5–10 MU), intermediate-dose pegylated interferon, and low-dose interferon (1–3 MU) regimens with observation. Multiple trials have shown that adjuvant high-dose interferon improves relapse-free survival by approximately 10% at five years, but initially reported benefits in overall survival have disappeared with longer follow-up periods. Individual patient data meta-analyses of observation-controlled trials of various dosing regimens showed a statistically significant benefit of interferon for event-free survival, and an absolute overall survival benefit of 3% (CI 1–5%) at five years. There was no evidence of any difference according to dose or duration of therapy. Individual Phase III trials of intermediate- and low-dose interferon have not shown a clear advantage for interferon over observation. Long-term pegylated interferon improved four-year relapse-free survival by 7% but had no effect on distant metastasis-free survival or overall survival. High-dose interferon-alpha remains the only FDA-approved systemic adjuvant therapy for melanoma. The toxicity of high-dose interferon-alpha is substantial but reversible and requires experienced medical oncology management, aggressive supportive measures including the use of prophylactic antidepressants, and careful monitoring and dose-reduction strategies, particularly for hepatotoxicity. Because of the toxicity of high-dose interferon and the uncertain benefits of lower dosing regimens, patient participation in clinical trials of new adjuvant therapies is strongly encouraged and observation remains an appropriate comparator in Phase III trials. Experimental approaches undergoing current investigation with prospective randomized placebo-controlled double-blind clinical trials include immunotherapy with anti-MAGE-A3 vaccine, ipilimumab, or PEG-interferon (in patients with ulcerated primary melanomas and microscopic lymph node involvement). Drugs targeting the MAP kinase pathway are also in placebo-controlled adjuvant clinical trials using vemurafenib (GO27826, 'BRIM-8') or the combination of dabrafenib and trametinib (BRF115532, 'Combi-AD').

Adjuvant radiotherapy

Following surgical clearance of macroscopic (clinically detectable) disease in regional lymph nodes, recurrence in the node field is most common when at least one involved node is large (>3 cm), where multiple nodes are involved, or if there is histological evidence of extranodal spread. To reduce this risk of node field recurrence, adjuvant postoperative radiotherapy to the node field may be given. In the only large prospective trial that has examined the value of this adjuvant radiotherapy following regional node clearance in high-risk melanoma patients, the rate of node field recurrence was 33% in the control group and 18% in the group that received adjuvant radiotherapy, with acceptably low morbidity.

Local and transit recurrences

True local recurrence of a primary melanoma, i.e., within a previous wide excision scar, is rare if adequate margins are achieved. Thus most recurrences adjacent to a previous melanoma wide excision site, like in transit metastases that occur between the primary site and the draining regional lymph node field, are probably due to intralymphatic metastasis. The term 'satellitosis' is frequently used for microscopic or macroscopic recurrences that are within a few centimetres of the primary site. These, too, are likely to be due to the same pathophysiological process, i.e., intralymphatic metastasis.

When local or in transit metastasis occurs, the patient's prognosis becomes much worse. Up to 50% of patients who develop even a single local or in transit metastasis ultimately die of melanoma. The treatment modality employed to deal with local and in transit metastases does not appear to have any effect on ultimate outcome, and the goal of treatment is therefore to deal with the problem of loco-regional disease in the most efficient but least invasive and least morbid way possible. The recent introduction of effective forms of systemic therapy may improve the outcome for patients with in transit metastases not able to be treated by any of the methods outlined below.

Simple excision, ablative techniques, intralesional, and topical therapies

If local or in transit metastases are small and few in number, simple surgical excision is the best treatment option. If the disease is superficial but more extensive, simple ablative techniques such as diathermy-fulguration or CO2 laser ablation are effective. When the disease is unable to be controlled by simple measures such as those just outlined, consideration may need to be given to intralesional therapy (e.g., with BCG, IL-2 or Rose Bengal) and radiotherapy may also be employed if the disease is localized.

Extensive but superficial disease can also be treated with topical agents. One of the most promising of these is topical diphencyprone, which enhances local skin immunity and leads to tumour involution in many patients, even after other forms of treatment, including surgery and radiotherapy, have failed.

Isolated limb perfusion and isolated limb infusion with cytotoxic drugs

When locally recurrent or in transit disease is not suitable for treatment with any of the modalities described above and the disease is confined to a limb, regional chemotherapy with vascular isolation, using the techniques of isolated limb perfusion (ILP) or isolated limb infusion (ILI), is often effective. Both these techniques involve the administration of high-dose chemotherapy to a limb when its blood supply is isolated from the general circulation with a tourniquet. Isolated limb perfusion has been used for more than 50 years, and was developed shortly after the technique of cardiopulmonary bypass was introduced,

using similar equipment and based on similar principles. Large bore cannulas are placed by open operation into the major vein and artery of the affected limb, and the cannulas are connected to an extracorporeal circuit through which circulation is maintained with a pump that incorporates an oxygenator and a heat exchanger, as for cardiopulmonary bypass. The limb is isolated from the vasculature of the body by placing a tourniquet around the root of the limb to occlude all blood vessels, and high-dose cytotoxic agents are perfused through the limb, usually for a period of 60–90 minutes. The drug most commonly used is melphalan, and its efficacy is enhanced by adjusting the temperature in the perfusion circuit so that mild to moderately hyperthermic limb temperatures (39–41°C) are achieved.

Even for patients with extensive in transit disease in a limb, complete response rates of 40–50% are reported after ILP and partial response rates of 30–40%, resulting in good disease control in 80–90% of patients who are treated in this way. Better results for patients with very bulky disease have been reported when TNF has been used with melphalan, but there are significant risks associated with systemic leakage of the TNF, and there has been no clinical trial evidence of superior efficacy of ILP with melphalan and TNF over ILP with melphalan alone.

An alternative but much simpler technique of regional chemotherapy with vascular isolation is isolated limb infusion. This technique was conceived as a method of achieving the benefits of ILP more simply and more safely. In a large experience of the ILI technique in Sydney, where it was developed, complete response rates of 38% and partial response rates of 46% were achieved. An ILI procedure is performed via small calibre catheters that are inserted percutaneously by a radiologist into the axial vessels of the affected limb via the opposite groin. Having applied a pneumatic tourniquet to the root of the limb, cytotoxic drugs in high concentration (normally melphalan and actinomycin D) are infused and circulated in the limb using a hand-held syringe via a three way stopcock in the external circuit (which also contains a blood warmer) for a period of 30 minutes. At the end of this time the limb vasculature is flushed with an electrolyte solution, the venous effluent is discarded, the tourniquet is deflated and the catheters are withdrawn.

Both ILP and ILI inevitably produce an inflammatory reaction in the normal tissues of the treated limb, and occasionally more severe reactions in the limb can occur, with skin and muscle necrosis. The tumour deposits in the limb usually begin to undergo involution within a week of the procedure, but the full effect of the treatment may not be apparent for up to three months.

Limb amputation

When all the above forms of treatment fail to control disease in a limb, amputation is very occasionally required. Even when this is necessary, some patients remain disease-free indefinitely, although the majority go on to develop systemic metastases and eventually die of melanoma.

Follow-up and surveillance for new melanomas and metastatic disease

There are two distinctly separate reasons for periodic review of patients with melanoma. The first is to identify recurrent disease and the second is to diagnose new primary melanomas at an early stage. It is well documented that any patient who has had a primary melanoma is at greatly increased risk of developing another primary melanoma in the future. The risk of recurrence of the original primary depends on its thickness and other histological features (such as ulceration and mitotic rate). This means that more intensive follow-up schedules are usually recommended for patients with thick melanomas and less intensive schedules for those with thin melanomas. There are, however, no good prospective clinical trial data to indicate the optimal frequency of follow-up visits, and most follow-up schedules are based on very low level evidence. Nevertheless, it is commonly recommended that patients with thin (<1 mm) melanomas be checked at least annually following their definitive melanoma treatment, while patients with intermediate thickness (1–4 mm) and thick (>4 mm) melanomas be checked every three to four months for the first two years, and less frequently thereafter.

In considering follow-up strategies, however, it must be borne in mind that the great majority of melanoma recurrences and new primary melanomas are detected not by doctors at routine visits but by the patient or their partner. In most series where this has been examined, no more than 15–20% of recurrences and new primary melanomas have been detected by doctors at routine visits. A very useful part of melanoma patient care is, therefore, to provide adequate education which will help early recognition of recurrent disease or new primary tumours. Such programs already exist in many major melanoma treatment centres.

The value of routine follow-up blood tests, X-rays, and scans is controversial. Until recently, many clinicians involved in the care of patients with melanoma considered that early diagnosis of systemic metastatic disease in asymptomatic patients was of little benefit because there was no effective therapy. The advent of systemic agents that are effective, at least in the short- to medium-term, means that this nihilistic approach to follow-up investigations may need to be reappraised. With the ready availability of CT and PET/CT scanning in most countries where melanoma incidence is high, it would seem reasonable to offer whole body imaging (either CT or PET/CT scans) at least annually to patients considered to be at high risk of systemic metastasis (e.g., those with treated Stage IIC, IIIA, IIIB, and IIIC disease, as well as those with Stage IV disease following apparently successful surgical treatment).

Surgical treatment of American Joint Committee on Cancer Stage IV disease

For patients with AJCC Stage I, Stage II, and Stage III melanoma, surgery is the standard treatment. For patients with Stage IV disease, however, the role of surgery is less well defined. Resection of metastatic melanoma at distant sites may be considered appropriate if complete removal of all identifiable disease appears to be possible, with potentially curative intent. It may also be considered for patients with resectable disease that is causing troublesome symptoms, or is considered likely to cause troublesome symptoms before the patient dies of the disease. In each patient, the potential benefits of the proposed surgery should outweigh the risks. If surgical excision of metastases can be accomplished with low morbidity, quick and effective palliation (or expectant palliation) is possible.

Surgery with curative intent for patients with Stage IV melanoma

Many studies have demonstrated that complete surgical resection of metastatic disease gives patients the greatest chance of prolonged survival with a good quality of life. Five-year survival rates of 20–30% are reported after complete surgical resection of visceral metastases, compared with five-year survival rates of around 10% in patients treated with the best available systemic therapies. In assessing the results of surgical treatment for distant metastatic disease, it must be borne in mind that the outlook for patients with involvement of distant skin, subcutaneous tissues, or distant lymph nodes is substantially better than the outlook for patients with metastatic disease at visceral sites (see Figure 49.3).

With present day sophisticated imaging techniques, particularly PET/CT and MRI scanning, the identification of patients with metastatic disease that is completely resectable has become easier and more reliable. Even if there is residual metastatic melanoma in the body, not detected by conventional imaging techniques, there is some evidence that the cytoreductive surgery may allow the patient's cellular and/or humoral immunity to more effectively control the growth of residual occult tumour cells. Even when further distant metastases become apparent following previous surgical

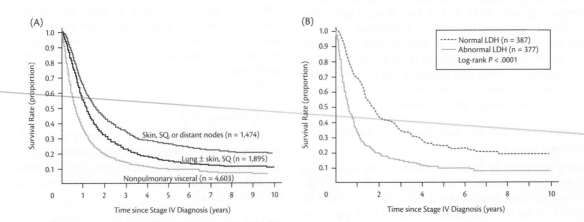

Fig. 49.3 Survival curves of 7635 patients with metastatic melanomas at distant sites (Stage IV) grouped by (A) the site of metastatic disease and (B) serum lactose dehydrogenase (LDH) levels. LDH values are not used to stratify patients. Curves in (A) are based only on site of metastasis. The number of patients is shown in parenthesis.

SQ, subcutaneous.

excision of apparently isolated distant melanoma metastases, salvage by repeated surgical excision may be possible. In one study, a 90% five-year survival rate was reported after complete resection for recurrence after initial metastasectomy.

Outcomes after resection of melanoma metastases at specific sites

Skin, subcutaneous tissue, and lymph nodes

These are the most common sites for non-loco-regional metastatic melanoma. When only a few lesions exist in distant skin, subcutaneous tissues, or lymph nodes, excellent results have been reported after surgical excision. Repeated excisions are often necessary, but appear to be worthwhile if there is no evidence of visceral disease. There is no evidence that excision of metastatic disease at these sites with very wide margins is necessary, but it is clearly important that they be removed with a cuff of apparently normal tissue so that histologically clear margins are achieved.

Lung

Melanoma metastases in the lung are diagnosed more frequently than metastases at other visceral sites, perhaps because they are more readily identified with modern imaging techniques than metastases elsewhere. The lung metastases are usually asymptomatic, and they are associated with longer survival (median 10–11 months) than metastases in other viscera. Reports from a number of single institutions and the International Registry of Lung Metastases have demonstrated prolonged survival in appropriately selected patients who have had lung metastases resected. As is the case for patients with melanoma metastases in other viscera, patients with lung metastases are likely to have the best outcome if there is no evidence of metastatic disease at any other site.

Brain

Cerebral metastases account for 20–54% of deaths from melanoma, and post-mortem studies have shown that the great majority of patients who die of melanoma have brain metastases. Without treatment, the median survival for a patient with a symptomatic brain metastasis is only approximately one month without treatment and two months with palliative corticosteroid therapy alone. In the past, the active treatment options for patients with brain metastases were surgical resection or whole brain radiotherapy (WBRT). In more recent times stereotactic radiotherapy has been shown to have similar efficacy to surgery, and is particularly appropriate when multiple lesions require treatment. Several studies have shown that symptoms are relieved and survival times are increased in the great majority of patients whose cerebral melanoma metastases are treated. Symptoms due to cerebral metastases are improved in more than two-thirds of melanoma patients treated with WBRT; however, the median survival after WBRT alone is only 3.5 months. The role of WBRT after surgical resection of cerebral metastases has been controversial.

Gastrointestinal tract

Melanoma metastases in the gastrointestinal tract are also very common in post-mortem studies, but are less frequently symptomatic during life. The most common symptoms are abdominal pain, bleeding (and associated anaemia), and bowel obstruction. In any patient with a history of melanoma who presents with anaemia, the possibility of one or more metastases in the gastrointestinal tract, most commonly small bowel, must be considered. Melanoma metastases in the oesophagus and stomach are best treated by surgical resection if they isolated; as well as achieving good relief of symptoms, long-term survival is sometimes achieved. Patients with small bowel metastases often present with small bowel obstruction due to intussusception. Even when there is disease at other sites, surgery to resect the segment of small bowel containing the intussuscepting metastasis is worthwhile, as it produces immediate relief of symptoms, restores good quality of life, and often extends survival considerably.

Liver and biliary tract

Patients with melanoma metastases in their liver generally have a very short life expectancy (2–4 months). However, patients who have apparently isolated liver metastases that are able to be resected surgically occasionally achieve long-term survival. In recent times, ablative techniques for multiple liver metastases have been introduced, such as cryotherapy and radiofrequency ablation. These have extended the therapeutic options for patients who have multiple hepatic metastases. Regional therapy via the hepatic artery (using agents such as fotemustine and radioactive spheres) is now quite widely used with palliative intent, but has not been shown in clinical trials to improve survival outcome.

Spleen

Isolated melanoma metastases in the spleen are uncommon, and there are usually synchronous metastases at other intra-abdominal sites. For patients in whom the splenic disease is apparently isolated or symptomatic, however, surgery should be considered.

Bone

It is unusual for patients to have melanoma bone metastases without metastatic disease at other sites, and the main role of surgery is to prevent or relieve symptoms. This may involve bone resection, enucleation of the tumour (then filling the resulting cavity with bone cement), joint replacement, operative bone fixation, or the use of external braces or a cast. Many bone metastases can be treated effectively with radiotherapy, and radiation is often given as adjuvant therapy following a surgical procedure for a bone metastasis. Metastases involving the spinal vertebrae have potentially serious implications, because pathological fractures or tumour expansion may cause spinal cord compression. When this occurs, urgent decompressive laminectomy may be required with adjuvant postoperative radiotherapy. If there is judged to be no imminent risk of spinal cord compression, most vertebral metastases can be treated effectively with external beam radiotherapy.

Systemic therapy for Stage IV disease

Targeted drugs

BRAF inhibitors

The MAPK pathway is strongly activated in 90% of melanomas. In approximately 50% of cases this is caused by activating mutations in BRAF; the most common of these is substitution of glutamic acid for valine at amino acid position 600 (V600E), which locks the kinase in activated conformation. Other activating mutations also occur, including V600K, V600D, and V600R. Vemurafenib and dabrafenib are potent and selective inhibitors of mutant BRAF. They induce tumour regression in the majority of patients who have V600-mutant BRAF melanoma, with overall response rates of 50–60%. Responses occur in all sites, including brain. In a Phase 3 trial of vemurafenib in treatment-naive patients there was a statistically significant improvement in overall survival from 9.6 months with the standard comparator, dacarbazine (DTIC), to 13.2 months with vemurafenib. The true benefit of vemurafenib was underestimated in this trial, however, because 50 dacarbazine-treated patients crossed over to receive vemurafenib 12 months after trial commencement when the clear benefits of the test drug became obvious at interim data monitoring. Vemurafenib and dabrafenib have both been approved by the FDA for treatment of V600-mutant BRAF melanoma.

Median progression-free survival with vemurafenib and dabrafenib is 5–6 months, and this has prompted vigorous examination of mechanisms of emergent resistance to therapy with BRAF inhibitors [6]. Most clinically relevant mechanisms involve reactivation of the MAPK pathway by upstream activation, including NRAS mutation and RTK over-expression, amplification of mutant BRAF, and emergence of active splice variants of BRAF which are unaffected by BRAF inhibitors. Approaches to overcome resistance to BRAF inhibitors include combining BRAF and MEK inhibitors (see below), adaptive trial design using other combinations of targeted drugs, and the use of pulsed therapy, which has shown remarkable efficacy in an animal model.

BRAF inhibitors are well tolerated. The most common side effects are skin rashes, including Grover's disease, papillomas and verrucas, and other keratopathies. Vemurafenib, but not dabrafenib, is severely photosensitizing, an effect unrelated to BRAF inhibition. Paradoxical activation of the MAPK pathway may occur in keratinocytes carrying upstream activators like RAS mutations. In the presence of BRAF inhibition this results in heterodimer formation between RAF family members and downstream MAPK stimulation. In 10–20% of treated patients this may result in the formation of keratoacanthomas or squamous cell carcinomas. These are readily treated by surgical excision, but regular skin surveillance is essential for patients on BRAF inhibitors. This paradoxical oncogenesis has also been associated with an increased incidence of second primary melanomas and induction of acute leukaemia.

MEK inhibitors

MEK inhibitors are active in patients with mutant BRAF melanoma, presumably because of the high level of stimulation of the pathway downstream of BRAF in these tumours. A number of drugs in this class are undergoing clinical development. Trametinib confers benefits in both progression-free and overall survival compared to standard chemotherapy, with an overall response rate of 22%. Some MEK inhibitors such as MEK162 show some evidence of activity in mutant NRAS melanoma, for which there are currently no other established targeted systemic treatment options, and clinical trials are proceeding with these drugs.

The dominant toxicities of MEK inhibitors are acneiform rashes, diarrhoea, nausea, oedema, and fatigue. Central serous retinopathy and retinal vein occlusion are rare side effects which mandate careful ophthalmological monitoring of all patients treated with these agents.

Combined BRAF and MEK inhibition

The demonstration that MAPK reactivation was responsible for most cases of emergent resistance to BRAF inhibition, together with in vitro demonstrations of synergy and reduced toxicity, led to clinical trials of combined BRAF and MEK inhibition. In a randomized Phase 2 study the combination of dabrafenib plus trametinib in patients naïve to BRAF inhibitors showed an overall response rate of 63% in the maximally dosed cohort, with a median progression-free survival of 9.4 months compared with 5.8 months in the single-agent dabrafenib arm and 12-month progression-free survival of 41% vs 9%. The combination also rescued some patients refractory to BRAF inhibitors, with an overall response rate of 19% and median progression-free survival of 3.6 months. Phase 3 trials have commenced comparing the doublet with single-agent dabrafenib or vemurafenib, but these early results suggest that dual MAPK blockade with BRAF and MEK inhibitors is likely to become standard therapy for BRAF-mutant melanoma. The impressive activity of this combination has led to the dabrafenib/trametinib doublet being tested in the adjuvant setting in the 'Combi-AD' trial.

Some of the more notable toxicities of the MAPK inhibitors cancel each other out when used in combination. The presence of a MEK inhibitor appears to block paradoxical MAPK activation in keratinocytes, reducing SCC incidence to near-background levels, and BRAF inhibition appears to block the acneiform rash of MEK inhibitors. Drug-induced fever occurs, however, in more than 50% of patients on the dabrafenib/trametinib combination.

Other BRAF/MEK inhibitor combinations being assessed in early clinical trials include LGX818/MEK162 and vemurafenib/cobimetinib.

KIT inhibition

A small subset of mucosal, acral, and chronic sun-damaged skin melanomas carry activating mutations in the KIT oncogene. Some, but not all, of these mutations are sensitive to inhibition with imatinib, sunitinib, or nilotinib. The likelihood of response correlates with the ratio of mutated:wild-type KIT alleles in the melanoma cell. Response duration is generally measured in months.

Other molecular targets

Approximately 20% of cutaneous melanomas carry NRAS mutations. These are nearly always reciprocal to BRAF mutations, unless the tumour has been previously exposed to the selective environment of BRAF inhibition. NRAS is a difficult target for designing small molecule inhibitors, and preclinical and early clinical focus is on downstream effectors including MEK and PI3K.

There is evidence for activation of the AKT/PI3K pathway in many melanomas, and in a subset of tumours resistant to BRAF inhibitors. Multiple PI3K inhibitors are being assessed in clinical trials both as single agents and in combination with MAPK inhibitors.

The high frequency of CDKN2A/p16 alterations in melanoma and amplification of cyclin D1 both point to the importance of this for regulation of the melanoma cell cycle, and drugs targeting this axis are in early clinical development.

Immunotherapy

Vaccines

Despite the presence of detectable immune responses in 30–60% of patients, tumour regression occurs in only a minority of vaccine-treated metastatic melanoma patients. Vaccine therapy remains under intense investigation in the adjuvant setting, and may have a role in combination with other immunotherapies in metastatic disease.

Adoptive immunotherapy

In carefully selected patients, high rates of disease control are reported with adoptive immunotherapy programs. These involve harvesting, then ex vivo expansion and sometimes genetic manipulation, of tumour infiltrating lymphocytes (TIL). Typically, patients are conditioned with lymphodepleting cytotoxic chemotherapy, with or without cytokines and whole body radiotherapy, before reinfusion of expanded TIL. The best series response rates were 50–70%, with small numbers of patients remaining disease-free at over four years. Inpatient support is required following immuno-conditioning and toxicity includes febrile neutropaenia in 12–16% of patients. Several centres internationally are developing simplified and less toxic protocols of adoptive immunotherapy, including the use of genetically-engineered T cells expressing chimeric antigen receptors (CAR-T cells).

Interleukin-2 and interferon-alpha

Interleukin-2 (IL-2) is FDA-approved for treating metastatic melanoma based on a retrospective series showing sustained disease control in a small subset of treated patients. Although the overall response rate was just 16%, one quarter of responding patients had sustained disease control, most beyond five years. Gene expression profiles may assist in identifying those who may benefit from IL-2. The toxicity of IL-2 therapy is high and includes hypotension in 64% of patients and treatment-related mortality in 2.2%.

Single agent interferon-alpha has a response rate of approximately 20% in metastatic melanoma in Phase 2 trials but response duration is brief and use is restricted by the high incidence of influenza-like toxicity including fatigue and fever. Routine use is not recommended by most international guidelines except in the adjuvant setting and in clinical trials.

Immune check-point regulators

Activation of the immune response is kept in check at both induction and effector phases by complex molecular interactions inducing feedback inhibition of T cell proliferation and cytokine release to dampen down the immune response and prevent autoimmunity. Melanoma cells subvert this system to induce immunological tolerance. Molecules which target check-point regulation induce potent immune responses against melanoma cells and are active in the treatment of metastatic disease.

CTLA4 inhibitors

Ipilimumab is a monoclonal antibody which binds to CTLA4 on regulatory T cells, inhibiting its interaction with B7 on antigen-expressing cells, and removing a regulatory brake on T cell activation. In a phase 3 clinical trial of metastatic melanoma patients refractory to prior systemic therapy, ipilimumab (3 mg/kg) with or without a gp100 vaccine proved superior to vaccine control in overall survival. In first-line therapy of metastatic melanoma, the combination of ipilimumab (10 mg/kg) with the cytotoxic drug dacarbazine proved superior in overall survival to dacarbazine/placebo control. Notable in this trial was a 10% improvement in landmark absolute overall survival benefit at two years (28.5% vs 17.9%) and three years (20.8% vs 12.2%).

Tumour response rates to ipilimumab are low (~10%), and grade 3–4 autoimmune toxicity occurs in more than one half of all treated patients. Dermatitis and colitis are the most common toxicities, but are readily reversible with corticosteroids. Biopredictors of the subgroup of metastatic melanoma patients who respond to CTLA4 inhibition are eagerly sought, as they are for all forms of immunotherapy of this disease. Ipilimumab is FDA approved for the treatment of metastatic melanoma.

A second anti-CTLA4 monoclonal antibody, tremelimumab, showed similar promise to ipilimumab in Phase 2 clinical trials, but failed to show superiority over chemotherapy as first-line therapy. The reasons for the failure of tremelimumab to replicate the benefits of ipilimumab are not clear but may relate to dosage schedules or pharmacokinetic and pharmacodynamic factors.

Drugs targeting PD-1 and PD-1 ligand

Pro-death receptor-1 ligand 1 (PD-L1) is expressed on many melanoma cells. PD-1 is an immune check-point regulator expressed on cytotoxic T lymphocytes which dampens the immune response and induces immune tolerance. Phase I trials of the monoclonal antibodies nivolumab and lambrolizumab, which target the interaction between PD-1 and its ligand, show promising activity with remissions in around 20–50% of patients. Autoimmune toxicity seems much lower than that seen with ipilimumab. Expression of PD-L1 on tumour and stromal tissue is being investigated as a possible biomarker predicting response to anti-PD-1 therapy. Monoclonal antibodies against PD-L1 also have activity against metastatic melanoma and are in clinical trials.

Combined use of nivolumab with ipilimumab provides synergistic benefit in patients with metastatic melanoma, with tumour remissions that are frequent, rapid and durable, with median two-yearly survival close to 80% and with manageable toxicity [7].

Chemotherapy

Melanoma has formidable defences against the induction of apoptosis and this probably accounts for its relative resistance to cytotoxic chemotherapy. Single-agent dacarbazine (DTIC), temozolamide, and fotemustine are used as systemic therapy of metastatic melanoma because of their relatively low toxicity and simplicity of administration, and because of the failure of more toxic combination therapies to show superiority in terms of survival outcomes. However, response rates to dacarbazine and temozolamide in recent randomized trials have been less than 10%, the median duration of response is brief, and the median overall survival nine months. The small group of patients who benefit cannot be reliably predicted by tumour biomarkers. Chemotherapy response is more likely in subcutaneous, lymph node, and pulmonary metastases than in other visceral sites, and in those with better performance status. A Phase III Trial of three-agent chemotherapy versus the same drugs plus interferon-alpha and interleukin-2 ('biochemotherapy') produced a slightly higher response rate and progression-free survival for biochemotherapy, but this was not associated with either improved quality of response or better overall survival. NAB-paclitaxel shows improved progression-free survival over dacarbazine and the combination of paclitaxel and carboplatin also produces slightly higher response rates (18%). However, these small gains are not matched by overall survival benefits and are only achieved at the cost of higher haematological and neural toxicities.

The role of radiotherapy for Stage IIIC and Stage IV melanoma

Sixty years ago it was suggested that melanoma was a tumour type that was particularly resistant to radiation therapy. However, this perception was based on the results of radiotherapy techniques that have long since been superseded.

Today radiation therapy is widely used to treat metastatic melanoma at distant sites. It is usually given with palliative intent, and in some patients prolonged disease control is achieved. A detailed consideration of the clinical radiobiology of melanoma is beyond the scope of this chapter, but is discussed in detail elsewhere.

Cutaneous and subcutaneous metastases

When surgical excision of troublesome cutaneous or subcutaneous metastases at distant sites is not possible, radiotherapy may be an effective treatment option.

Lymph node metastases

Extensive metastatic lymph node disease that is not amenable to surgical treatment and has failed to respond to systemic therapy can often be effectively palliated with radiotherapy. A commonly used treatment schedule involves the administration of 20 Gy in five daily fractions. A bolus dose may be required for nodal masses that have fungated.

Cerebral metastases

Cerebral metastases frequently cause significant morbidity and without treatment the prognosis of patients who develop cerebral metastases is bleak; their median survival is only three to four months, and up to 95% of them die as a direct result of their brain metastases. Although it is difficult to separate out the effects of case selection, there is persuasive evidence that treatment involving surgery and/or radiotherapy can extend survival times considerably. There is also evidence that stereotactic radiosurgery (SRS) is as effective as surgical excision of single brain metastases, but several metastases may be readily treated by SRS, whereas surgery is rarely considered feasible under these circumstances. Control rates reported after SRS for the treatment of melanoma metastases in the brain are high, with individual treatment centres reporting local control rates of 80–90%.

The role of WBRT after surgical resection of cerebral metastases or following their treatment with SRS remains controversial. The main deterrent to the use of WBRT has been the perception that there is a treatment-related decline in neurocognitive function following its use. A large prospective, multicentre randomized trial assessing the value of WBRT following treatment of melanoma cerebral metastases by surgery or SRS is currently in progress.

Spinal cord compression due to melanoma metastases

This problem usually arises as a result of extra-dural compression from an expanding vertebral metastasis. Occasionally, however, the compression arises from a metastasis within the spinal cord itself or as a result of diffuse meningeal involvement. The classical clinical picture is of progressively severe back pain in a patient known to have disseminated melanoma. This is followed by the typical clinical signs and symptoms of spinal cord compression, with loss of bladder and bowel control, loss of strength in the lower limbs, with paresthesiae or numbness, and ultimately paraplegia. Malignant spinal cord compression constitutes an oncological emergency. The definitive investigation is an MRI scan of the spine, and high-dose corticosteroids should be commenced immediately if the condition is suspected. Treatment options are surgical decompression or urgent radiotherapy. A decision about which treatment to offer the patient depends on numerous factors, not only the location and extent of the metastasis that is causing the problem, but also the patient's general condition, the presence of systemic metastases at other sites, and the extent of spinal involvement. There is general consensus that patients with isolated vertebral lesions causing spinal cord compression who are considered to have a reasonable life expectancy should be offered decompressive surgery followed by post-operative radiotherapy. In patients who are not considered to require urgent surgery, radiotherapy should be offered. Steroid therapy is continued throughout the treatment course and then slowly tapered when it is complete. If neurological deterioration is observed during the course of palliative radiotherapy to the spine, urgent surgical decompression must be considered to avoid paraplegia. However, relief of symptoms after palliative radiotherapy for threatened spinal cord compression has been reported in two-thirds of patients.

Bone metastases

Metastases involving bone (other than the vertebral column) are a common problem in patients with disseminated melanoma. Patients with bone metastases typically present with pain, with progression to pathological fracture of the involved bone in many cases if the lesion is not treated. Bone metastases frequently extend into the surrounding tissues, a situation that may be apparent on CT or MRI scans. Bone metastases are often well managed by palliative radiotherapy, which provides relief of pain in over 65% of cases. Threatened or actual pathological fractures require internal fixation, followed by post-operative radiotherapy.

Other sites that may be treated with radiotherapy

Other indications for the treatment of metastatic melanoma with radiotherapy include metastases in soft tissues that are causing pain as a result of local invasion, lesions that are causing blood loss, e.g., in the bronchial tree, and lesions that are causing obstructive symptoms, e.g., metastatic nodes in the mediastinum or metastatic deposits in the oropharynx, pharynx, trachea, or the bronchial tree. Another situation where radiotherapy is sometimes useful is when there is metastatic disease in the orbit, causing proptosis, diplopia, and impaired visual acuity.

Metastatic melanoma from an unknown primary site

In approximately 10% of patients in whom metastatic melanoma is diagnosed in lymph nodes, there is neither evidence of nor any prior history of a primary melanoma. This phenomenon is attributed either to complete regression of a previously existing unrecognized primary melanoma, or to de novo development of melanoma in naevus cells within a lymph node (which are commonly observed). Whatever the aetiology of the condition, the prognosis for the patient is somewhat better than for a patient with equivalent nodal disease from a known primary site. Much less frequently, systemic metastases are diagnosed when there is no known primary melanoma site. In both situations, treatment should be the same as for metastatic disease from a known primary site.

Non-cutaneous melanoma

Although the majority of melanomas arise in the skin, melanomas can also develop at mucosal sites. Ocular melanomas are considered in Chapter 57, Tumours of the eye and orbit. Mucosal melanomas are rare. Sites at which they can develop include the oropharynx, oesophagus, lung, stomach, gall bladder, small bowel, large bowel, rectum, anus, urethra, vagina, and cervix. The principles of treatment for primary melanomas arising in all of these sites are similar, i.e., by complete surgical excision whenever possible. There may be a role for radiotherapy as definitive therapy in the management of mucosal melanoma.

Guidelines for the management of melanoma and the importance of multidisciplinary care

Over the past twenty years, the surgical management of primary cutaneous melanoma has changed substantially. Whereas elective dissection of regional lymph node fields was routine in many melanoma treatment centres until the early 1990s, the introduction of SLNB has meant that the great majority of patients have been spared the morbidity of that approach, and only those found to have metastatic disease in a SLN (around 20% of those with melanoma >1mm in thickness) are subjected to CLND. The recommended width of excision for a primary cutaneous melanoma has reduced progressively, after clinical trials indicated that 1–2cm margins were adequate for most patients, with very low rates of local recurrence and no adverse effect on melanoma-specific survival compared with wider excision margins. More recently, the introduction of several forms of effective systemic therapy has changed management strategies for patients with Stage IV disease; these may be quite complex, depending on drug availability and eligibility for clinical trials. What this proliferation of treatment options means for patients with Stage III and Stage IV disease is that he or she is best served if a management plan is discussed by a multidisciplinary team. This approach will ensure that all treatment options are canvassed, and an appropriate management strategy devised for each patient. It is also important for patients to be offered participation in clinical trials whenever possible, so that new options for adjuvant therapy (in patients with surgically resected Stage III and Stage IV disease) and for definitive therapy (in patients with unresectable Stage IV disease) can be properly assessed and outcomes further improved. A particular multidisciplinary challenge is posed by brain metastases. Targeted drugs and immunotherapy have activity in brain metastases, so careful clinical planning is required, involving neurosurgeons, radiation oncologists, and medical oncologists. For patients with straightforward Stage I and Stage II disease, management according to nationally-agreed guidelines will ensure that optimal treatment outcomes are achieved.

References

1. Balch CM, Gershenwald JE, Soong SJ, Thompson JF, Atkins MB et al. Final version of 2009 AJCC melanoma staging and classification. Journal of Clinical Oncology 2009; 27(36): 6199–6206.
2. Scolyer RA, Judge MJ, Evans A, Frishberg DP, Prieto VG et al. Data set for pathology reporting of cutaneous invasive melanoma: recommendations from the International Collaboration on Cancer Reporting (ICCR). American Journal of Surgical Pathology 2013 (December); 37(12): 1797–1814. doi: 10.1097/PAS.0b013e31829d7f35.
3. Morton DL, Wen DR, Wong JH, Economou JS, Cagle LA et al. Technical details of intraoperative lymphatic mapping for early stage melanoma. Archives of Surgery 1992; 127(4): 392–399.
4. Morton DL, Thompson JF, Cochran AJ, Mozzillo N, Nieweg OE et al. for the MSLT Group. Final trial report of sentinel-node biopsy versus nodal observation in melanoma. New England Journal of Medicine 2014; 370: 599–609.
5. Morton DL, Thompson JF, Cochran AJ, Mozzillo N, Elashoff R et al. Sentinel-node biopsy or nodal observation in melanoma. New England Journal of Medicine 2006; 355(13): 1307–1317.
6. Ribas A, Flaherty KT. BRAF targeted therapy changes the treatment paradigm in melanoma. Nature Reviews Clinical Oncology 2011; 8(7): 426–433.
7. Wolchok JD, Kluger H, Callahan MK, Postow MA, Rizvi NA et al. Nivolumab plus ipilimumab in advanced melanoma. New England Journal of Medicine 2013; 369(2): 122–133.

CHAPTER 50

Skin cancer: non-melanoma

Diona L. Damian, Richard A. Scolyer, Graham Stevens, Alexander M. Menzies, and John F. Thompson

Non-melanoma skin cancer and the oncologist

Non-melanoma skin cancer (NMSC) is the most common malignancy in fair-skinned populations. In areas with high solar ultraviolet (UV) irradiance such as Australia, NMSC is more than four times as common as all other cancers combined. In Australia, the annual incidence of NMSC is ~1000 per 100 000 person-years, which is ten times that in the United Kingdom, a country with lower solar exposure. The vast majority of NMSC are basal cell carcinomas (BCCs), which rarely metastasize, or squamous cell carcinomas (SCCs), which do have metastatic potential, especially in immune-suppressed individuals. Because of their high frequency in the general population, particularly in older people, NMSCs are likely to occur in many general oncology patients. Skin cancer risk can be additionally increased in oncology patients as a result of disease-induced immune suppression (e.g., non-Hodgkin lymphoma) or by a range of cancer treatments including iatrogenic immune suppression, radiation therapy, arsenic, and BRAF inhibitors. Chronic stress suppresses skin immune responses and increases susceptibility to UV-induced SCC in murine models.

Aetiology

UV radiation reaching the earth's surface at sea level comprises UVB (wavelength 290–320 nm), which causes sunburn, and longer-wave UVA (320–400 nm). UV exposure is estimated to cause 95% of NMSC. Even at very low exposure doses, well below the sunburn threshold, both UVB and UVA can cause genetic damage in the skin and can profoundly suppress the skin's anti-tumour immune defences.

Skin tumours are generally more antigenic than internal malignancies, and hence immune suppression is a potent enhancer of skin cancer development. Chronically immune-suppressed organ transplant recipients have rates of SCC 80-fold higher than immune competent controls, whilst rates of BCC are ~fivefold higher in transplant recipients. The incidence of Merkel cell carcinoma has also been reported as increased 70-fold in this population. Tumours developing in immune-suppressed individuals tend to be more aggressive as well as more plentiful, with skin cancer the main cause of death in cardiac transplant recipients at ten years post-grafting in Australia.

Other causes of immune suppression are also linked with increased skin cancer risk, including HIV infection and chronic haematological malignancies such as chronic lymphocytic leukaemia (CLL). Patients with CLL have greatly elevated risks of developing both primary NMSC (including a 16-fold increase in Merkel cell carcinoma and increases in adnexal carcinomas and atypical fibroxanthomas as well as BCC and SCC) and also metastatic SCC. Tumours in these patients tend to exhibit peritumoral infiltrates of immune suppressive leukaemic B cells, and extend histologically further beyond their clinically apparent edge than comparable tumours in immune competent individuals. The mortality rate from cutaneous SCC in CLL patients with these lesions is more than 10%, whereas SCC-related deaths in the immune competent population are rare.

Ionizing radiation exposure can cause a two- to three-fold increase in risk of BCC and smaller increases in cutaneous SCC, with a latency of many years to decades after radiation exposure. The use of ionizing radiation in the past as a treatment for acne in young patients has been especially associated with increases in BCC incidence. Exposure to more than 350 treatments with psoralens and UVA (PUVA) for the treatment of psoriasis is associated with a sixfold increase in cutaneous SCC, but with only modest increases in BCC. Chronic inflammation within burns scars or other chronic wounds can also give rise to highly aggressive SCCs with greatly elevated metastatic risk ('Marjolin's ulcer').

Arsenic acts as a co-carcinogen with UV radiation, causing arsenical keratoses and NMSC. Arsenic contamination of drinking water from tube wells causes high rates of NMSC in populations in West Bengal and Bangladesh, whilst arsenical cancers are still observed in elderly patients given Fowler's solution (arsenic trioxide) as a treatment in the 1950s for conditions such as psoriasis and asthma. Arsenic trioxide is in current use for acute promyelocytic leukaemia, and probably increases skin cancer risk in this setting also.

A variety of rare genetic syndromes are associated with increased NMSC risk. Gorlin's syndrome (basal cell naevus syndrome; autosomal dominant) results from a mutation in the PTCH1 gene at 9q22-31 and is associated with multiple BCCs, developing from childhood or early adolescence. Other features of Gorlin's syndrome include macrocephaly, falx calcification, bifid ribs, palmo-plantar pits, odontogenic keratocysts, medulloblastoma, cardiac and ovarian fibromas, foetal rhabdomyoma, and ovarian fibrosarcoma. These patients must not be treated with ionizing radiation, as this results in even greater numbers of BCCs.

Xeroderma pigmentosum (XP) is an autosomal recessive disorder of nucleotide excision repair. These patients can display extreme sensitivity to sunburn and UV-induced immune suppression, neurodegeneration, central nervous system tumours, and genomic instability, as well as a 10 000-fold increase in the risk of skin cancers, which often develop in patients younger than 20 years old if rigorous sun protection is not practised. The average age of onset of NMSC in XP patients is less than ten years, compared to ~22 years for onset of melanoma, highlighting the importance of DNA repair in protection from NMSC.

Epidermolysis bullosa (EB) comprises a heterogeneous group of genodermatoses characterized by skin fragility and blisters, reflecting mutations in ten different basement membrane genes. More than 90% of patients with recessive dystrophic EB (mutation in type VII collagen) develop cutaneous SCC by 55 years of age at sites of chronic skin erosion, with a greater than 85% risk of death by age 45 due to metastatic SCC. Risk of metastasis does not correlate with tumour grade, and even apparently well-differentiated SCCs can prove fatal. There is also an increased SCC risk, although with later age of onset, in patients with junctional EB (mutations in laminin 5 or type XVII collagen).

Basal cell carcinoma

Basal cell carcinoma (BCC) is the most common malignancy in Caucasian populations, and in immune-competent individuals BCC is three to four times as common as SCC. Dysregulation of the hedgehog pathway (for example by deletion of PTCH1 or overactivation of Smoothened) is central in the pathogenesis of BCCs, which are currently thought to derive mainly from hair follicle bulge stem cells, but which might also originate from other epidermal locations under conditions such as wounding. BCC is associated with patterns of intermittent, recreational sun exposure; the use of artificial UV tanning devices has also been associated with an increased risk (odds ratio 1:5) for this tumour. BCCs tend to be slowly growing (over months to years), and whilst locally invasive, they rarely metastasize.

BCCs occur in a range of subtypes, which determine treatment options and predict tumour behaviour (Figure 50.1). Superficial and nodular BCCs are the most common subtypes. Superficial BCCs (sBCCs) are erythematous, slighty pearly patches or plaques, which may be multifocal. Nodular BCCs (nBCCs) are clinically thicker and present clinically as papules, nodules, or plaques, are generally pearly and often display surface telangiectases. Nodular BCCs may be flesh-coloured or pigmented and are characterized histologically by round lobules of tumour cells with peripheral palisading (Figure 50.2). Micronodular BCCs, which have small tumour islands less than 0.15mm in diameter, tend to have higher rates of recurrence and greater subclinical extension, leading to higher recurrence rates. Tumour cell aggregates in infiltrating BCCs extend irregularly and widely through the dermis, making clinical detection of these subtle lesions difficult and preventing accurate clinical distinction of tumour margins. Morphoeic BCCs, which have a dense fibrotic stromal reaction compressing the tumour islands into narrow strands, are also very difficult to delineate clinically and have higher rates of recurrence than superficial or nodular BCCs. Micronodular, morphoeic, and infiltrating BCCs often exhibit substantial subclinical tumour extension (Figure 50.1).

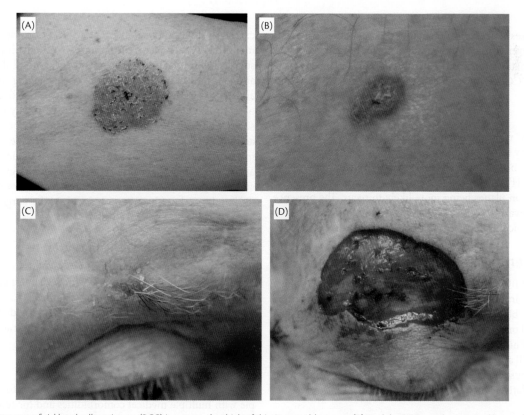

Fig. 50.1 (A) A large superficial basal cell carcinoma (BCC) is seen on the thigh of this 60-year-old woman. (B) Nodular BCCs are characterized by an often rolled, pearly edge and surface telangiectases. (C) Infiltrating BCCs are often clinically subtle, in this case presenting as scar-like changes and central erosion. These tumours can exhibit wide subclinical extension, as revealed during microscopically controlled excision. (D) This patient had substantial perineural involvement.
Figures 50.1 (c,d) reproduced courtesy of Dr Andrew Satchell.

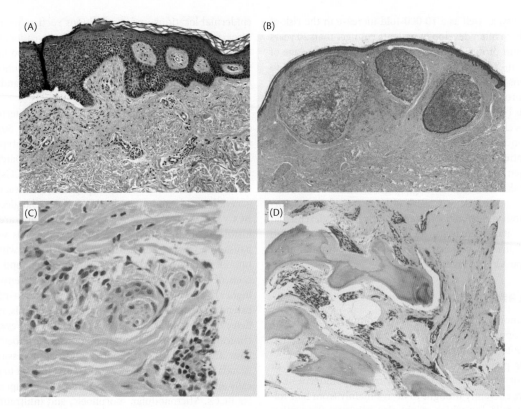

Fig. 50.2 Basal cell carcinoma (BCC) histological subtypes: (A) superficial BCC; (B) nodular BCC; (C) infiltrating BCC with perineural involvement; (D) metastatic BCC involving bone.

BCCs may also exhibit atypical squamous differentiation; when it is moderate or severe this can predict higher rates of recurrence and occasionally metastatic spread ('basosquamous' or 'metatypical' BCC'). Many BCCs do however contain multiple growth patterns.

Prognosis

The risk of BCC recurrence is influenced not only by tumour subtype, but also by tumour size, with larger diameter tumours more prone to recurrence. Tumour site is also a determinant, with lesions located in the 'H' zone of the face (ears, periocular) and those at embryonal fusion planes being more likely to recur. The presence of perineural invasion on histopathology indicates a greater risk of tumour recurrence, as does host immune suppression.

Management of basal cell carcinoma

Although most BCCs can be diagnosed clinically, tissue pathology diagnosis is desirable whenever possible. This can be achieved by punch or shave biopsy as well as by complete lesion excision. Such procedures will provide confirmation that the lesion is indeed BCC (and exclude clinical differential diagnoses such as amelanotic melanoma) and will also provide information on BCC subtype. This is important because many treatment options suitable for superficial BCC will be relatively ineffective for other BCC subtypes.

Surgery

Standard excision with 3 mm clinical margins enables histological clearance in ~85% of primary BCCs, whilst use of 4 mm margins

extends histological clearance rates to 98%. Cure rates for all modalities are lower for recurrent tumours. For difficult primary BCCs, such as infiltrating or morphoeic subtypes with ill-defined borders, and for nodular BCCs at cosmetically challenging sites where large arbitrary margins will compromise cosmetic outcomes (such as the nasal tip) and for recurrent BCCs, microscopically-controlled excision (Mohs' surgery) enables both the highest possibility of cure and also maximal conservation of normal tissue. This technique involves histological examination of excised tissue margin en face as frozen sections, so that the entire excision margin, both laterally and at depth, can be examined for residual tumour. Cure rates of 99% and 96% have been reported with Mohs' surgery for primary and recurrent BCCs, respectively.

Cryotherapy, curettage, and cautery

Cryotherapy with liquid nitrogen (30 second double freeze-thaw cycle) can also be used for some primary superficial BCCs, with long-term cure rates of ~90%. Some superficial BCCs may be suited to shave, curettage, and cautery, which can provide both diagnosis and treatment in a single procedure, with cure rates of ~80–90% depending on tumour site and diameter.

Radiotherapy

Radiotherapy is a valuable non-surgical option for BCCs in people with multiple medical comorbidities and for tumours at surgically difficult or cosmetically sensitive sites particularly in elderly patients. BCCs, with a 5–10 mm margin, can be effectively treated with fractionated courses of superficial X-rays or electron beams, with careful attention to ensure adequate dose at the depth of the tumour. BCCs can be effectively treated with superficial X-rays or electron beams, with a 5–10 mm margin. Long-term BCC cure rates with radiotherapy are >90%. Adjunctive radiotherapy also has a valuable role in reducing the risk of recurrence in high-risk BCCs, such as lesions demonstrating significant perineural invasion or lesions with positive margins after surgery. Radiation therapy also has a role in the palliation of inoperable tumours.

Imiquimod

Imiquimod is a topical immune response modifier and toll-like receptor 7 agonist. It is applied to the BCC with a 5 mm margin of surrounding normal skin five to seven nights per week for six weeks. An inflammatory reaction is generated at the treatment site, which may develop crusting or ulceration if inflammation is severe. Patients treating larger surface areas with imiquimod may report flu-like symptoms of myalgia, fatigue, and malaise, reflecting imiquimod-induced production of α-interferon (intralesional injection of α-interferon was previously used for treatment of nodular BCC). Five-year clearance rates with imiquimod are approximately 80% for superficial BCC and 40–75% for primary nodular BCC. Imiquimod is less effective against recurrent tumours and is not suitable for micronodular, infiltrating, morphoeic, or metatypical BCCs.

Topical photodynamic therapy

In topical photodynamic therapy (PDT), haeme precursors such as aminolaevulinic acid (ALA) and its esters are applied to skin lesions under occlusion for three to six hours. During this time, the haeme precursors are preferentially taken up by tumour cells and converted to the photosensitizer protoporphyrin IX, which accumulates in dysplastic and neoplastic tissue with an absorption peak at 633 nm (red light used to irradiate the photosensitizer-treated tumour). As well as causing direct necrosis and apoptosis of tumour cells mediated via reactive oxygen species generation and mitochondrial damage, PDT can also cause vascular shutdown around tumours. Topical PDT is especially useful for tumours involving cosmetically sensitive sites and is a relatively non-invasive treatment for frail or elderly patients, for tumours at sites prone to poor healing such as the lower legs, and for patients with huge numbers of NMSC where surgery is not feasible. PDT is best suited to primary superficial BCCs where it offers cure rates of ~80%. Cure rates for PDT in nodular BCC are ~70–75%. PDT is not a suitable treatment for recurrent BCC, or for infiltrating, morphoeic, or micronodular BCC.

Metastatic and unresectable BCC

Metastatic BCC is rare. When it does occur, metastasis is mainly to regional lymph nodes, with pulmonary, bony, and distant skin the next most frequent sites, respectively. The rate of metastasis is estimated to be ~0.03 to 0.1%, with 85% of metastatic cases originating from primary head and neck BCCs. The median age of these patients is 45 years. Risk factors for metastasis include multi-recurrent lesions, large primary size, male gender, and immunosuppression. Five-year survival in patients with metastatic BCC is ~10%, with a median survival of 13.6 years for nodal metastases and eight months in patients with distant disease.

Regional nodal metastases are managed by surgical dissection if operable, either alone or followed by adjuvant radiation therapy, depending on the pathological findings. The true benefit of chemotherapy for metastatic BCC has not been proven with clinical trials, but review of case reports in the literature has suggested response rates of up to 83%, including 37% complete response rates, in metastatic BCC treated with cisplatin-containing regimens. This agent has been used alone and also in combination with doxorubicin, bleomycin, 5-fluorouracil, methotrexate, and paclitaxel. Almost 40% of BCCs show strong expression of epidermal growth factor receptor (EGFR), and there have been isolated case reports of the effectiveness of the anti-EGFR antibody cetuximab for metastatic BCC patients.

Abnormal signalling in the hedgehog/glioma-associated oncogene pathway is a central feature of BCC pathogenesis; all sporadic BCCs have upregulated hedgehog signalling, often associated with mutations in the tumour suppressor gene PTCH1. This results in disinhibition of Smoothened, which then activates glioma-associated oncogene proteins. The Smoothened inhibitor vismodegib has been used orally in a Phase II clinical trial setting in 33 patients with metastatic BCC, with a response rate of 30% and median response duration of 7.6 months. A further 63 patients with locally advanced, unresectable BCC demonstrated a response rate of 43% and similar response duration. Adverse events were reported in 30% of patients, including weight loss, fatigue, muscle spasms, and taste disturbance. This agent and sonidegib, another inhibitor of the hedgehog signalling pathway, are now FDA-approved.

Follow-up

Patients with BCC should have regular follow-up after treatment, especially after non-surgical treatments, both to check for recurrence and for new primary skin cancers. The risk of subsequent NMSC is proportional to the number of previously diagnosed skin cancers; in a US study, the 5-year risk of developing another skin cancer was estimated at >60% for individuals with two previous BCCs and at >90% for individuals with four or five previous BCCs; a third of this group developed new skin cancers within 12 months.

Squamous cell carcinoma

Cutaneous SCCs are ~four times less common than BCCs in immune-competent individuals, with SCC risk tending to reflect recent, chronic sun exposure rather than intermittent, recreational exposure. There is also a 50% increase in cutaneous SCC incidence in smokers, which is not seen for BCC. UV-induced mutations of the gene for Tp53, which is centrally involved in cellular apoptosis, proliferation, and DNA repair are present in a high proportion of SCCs, but also in premalignant actinic keratoses (AKs) and normal skin. Activating RAS mutations are also found in 10–30% of cutaneous SCCs, whilst RAS overactivation has been observed in the majority of both SCCs and AKs. RAS mutations are frequent in SCCs in melanoma patients receiving treatment with the BRAF inhibitors vemurafenib and dabrafenib. In this setting, SCCs tend to have higher rates of RAS mutation than sporadic SCCs, and can develop—often from verrucal keratosis—within weeks of commencing treatment with BRAF inhibitors. Human papilloma virus is also believed to be contributory to cutaneous SCC development, especially in immune-compromised individuals.

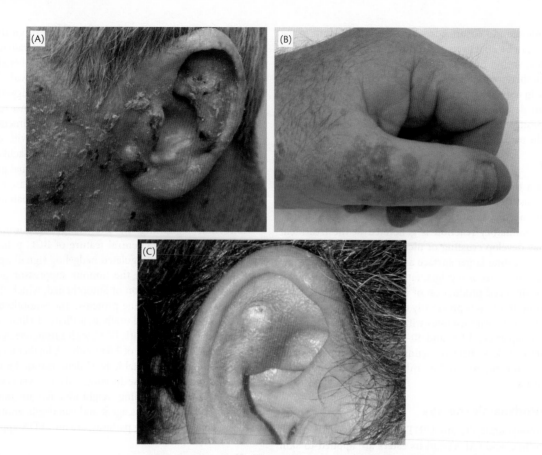

Fig. 50.3 (A) The spectrum of squamous lesions includes premalignant actinic keratoses (AKs), which in this elderly man are accompanied by a preauricular invasive squamous cell carcinoma (SCC). (B) SCC in situ (Bowen's disease), presents as a scaling plaque which may be clinically difficult to differentiate from superficial basal cell carcinoma. (C) This lesion was one of dozens of SCCs developing in a patient receiving the BRAF inhibitor vemurafenib for metastatic melanoma.

Actinic keratoses (Figure 50.3) are scaling, erythematous lesions which occur mainly on chronically sun-exposed skin, and which affect more than 60% of the >40 years of age population in Australia. AKs may progress to SCC, at an estimated rate of ~1 in 1000 to one in 10 000 lesions, with progression often heralded by an increase in tenderness of the lesion. AKs may also remain stable, and often spontaneously regress. This presumably immune-mediated regression is observed particularly during the winter months, when reductions in AK counts of up to 25% have been reported. Histologically, AKs are characterized by basal rather than full-thickness epidermal keratinocyte atypia.

Squamous lesions composed of dysplastic squamous cells filling the entire epidermal thickness are referred to as SCC in situ (Bowen's disease; Figures 50.3 and 50.4). Bowen's disease can present as indolent, scaling erythematous plaques which may remain essentially static for many years. These lesions can sometimes be clinically indistinguishable from superficial BCC. Approximately 3–5% of Bowen's disease lesions are thought to progress to invasive SCC. Keratoacanthomas (KAs) are considered a well-differentiated SCC variant, which demonstrate spontaneous regression usually starting six to eight weeks after first appearance. Mature keratoacanthomas have a characteristic central keratin-filled crater. In many instances, confident histological distinction between keratoacanthoma and SCC is not possible. Keratoacanthomas are generally treated in the same way as invasive SCCs.

Invasive SCC (Figure 50.3) usually presents as a rapidly growing nodular lesion, which may develop within weeks to months. There

are a range of SCC subtypes and grades of differentiation which strongly influence tumour treatment and outcome (Figure 50.4). SCC can be both locally invasive and metastatic. More than 80% of SCC metastases occur in draining lymph nodes, with subcutaneous metastases the next most common site. Pulmonary and bone metastases are also seen.

Management of squamous cancers and precancers

Actinic keratoses

AKs can be reduced by 30–40% by daily use of a broad-spectrum, high sun protection factor (SPF) sunscreen, often within a few months of commencing sunscreen use. Hence, sunscreen should be considered an active treatment for patients with multiple AKs, and not only a preventive measure. Patients with only a limited number of AKs may have lesions treated successfully with cryotherapy. More extensive lesions are better treated with field therapies such as topical 5-fluorouracil (5-FU), which is applied by patients twice daily, usually for two to three weeks, until a brisk level of inflammation in the AKs is observed (Figure 50.5). AKs on the hands and arms can also be treated with 5-FU, but a longer treatment duration (usually four to eight weeks) is required for these sites. For facial AKs, 5-FU can clear >90% of lesions, with most patients not needing further 5-FU for many years. Sun-damaged patients receiving systemic 5-FU for internal malignancies may also experience dramatic inflammation within their AKs.

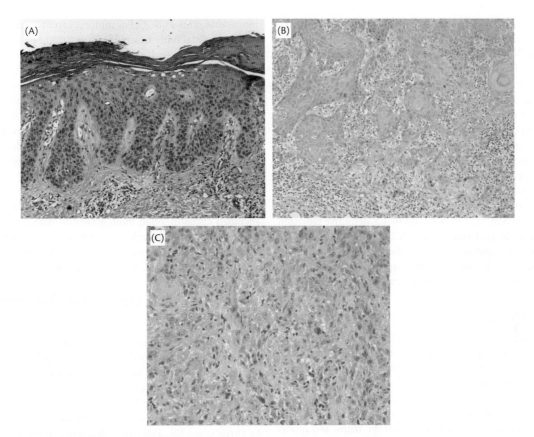

Fig. 50.4 (A) Bowen's disease is characterized pathologically by full-thickness epidermal dysplasia with no invasion of the underlying dermis. (B) In contrast, this well-differentiated invasive SCC has squamous cells irregularly infiltrating the dermis associated with a reactive fibroinflammatory response, with well-formed intercellular bridges and keratin formation (hallmarks of squamous differentiation). (C) This poorly-differentiated SCC shows a much greater degree of cellular atypia, and metastasized to bone within a few months of diagnosis.

Other treatment options for multiple AKs include topical imiquimod (usually three times per week for two to four weeks) with reported clearance rates of 50–60%, and topical diclofenac, which requires three months of twice daily treatment and can reduce AKs by ~60%. Topical photodynamic therapy has also been used for AKs, but can be exceptionally painful for patients with sun-damaged skin and multiple AKs.

SCC in situ (Bowen's disease)

In very elderly or frail patients, observation may be the only appropriate management option. Active therapies for Bowen's disease include excision, curettage and cautery, or cryotherapy. These lesions may also be effectively treated with topical imiquimod, which produces clearance rates of ~75% for Bowen's disease, topical 5-FU, or topical PDT, which produces long-term clearance in ~66–80% of lesions.

Keratoacanthoma and invasive SCC

Keratoacanthomas are usually excised, but can sometimes be treated with intralesional agents such as bleomycin, methotrexate, or 5-FU. Invasive SCC is best treated surgically whenever possible. Mohs surgery is sometimes helpful for clinically more subtle

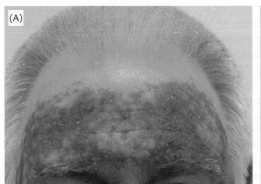

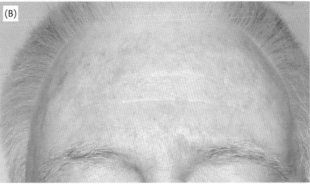

Fig. 50.5 Multiple actinic keratoses can be effectively treated with topical 5-fluorouracil, which causes inflammation within areas of dysplastic skin, whilst normal skin is unaffected. (A) Most patients achieve a suitable level of inflammation about two weeks into treatment. (B) 5-fluorouracil is then ceased, with both inflammation and AKs resolving over the next one to three weeks.

lesions, and especially for infiltrating SCC, at cosmetically sensitive sites. The role of sentinel node biopsy in SCC is still unclear, but may be indicated for very high-risk head and neck lesions, such as those with poor differentiation, large tumour diameter and thickness, host immune suppression, and where there is perineural and/or lymphovascular invasion. Post-operative radiotherapy to the tumour bed may be indicated for SCC at high risk of recurrence, including tumours with lymphovascular or perineural invasion and close (or positive) margins. Radiation doses to 60 Gy are required to reduce risk of recurrence. For perineural infiltration of large nerves, particularly cranial nerves or their major branches, the radiation fields should include the entire course of the nerve.

Radiation treatment planning is complex, requiring CT and/or MRI image acquisition. In common with BCCs, definitive radiation therapy (RT) may be preferred to treat SCCs in the elderly in sites requiring difficult reconstruction, particularly around the nose and eyes. Short courses of hypofractionated superficial or electron RT with custom lead cutouts result in high local control rates.

Prognosis in SCC

Factors influencing the risk of SCC recurrence and metastasis include tumour size, differentiation, infiltration, perineural invasion, and lymphovascular invasion. Host immune suppression is a critical determinant of SCC outcome, with metastatic risk dramatically elevated in chronically immune-suppressed individuals. Head and neck SCCs, especially at vascular sites such as lip and ear, have higher rates of metastasis than tumours on the trunk and limbs; overall, the risk of metastasis from cutaneous SCC is ~2–2.5%, with reported rates of metastasis from lesions >2cm in diameter rising to almost 6%. Almost 95% of SCC metastases occur within five years of the primary tumour diagnosis, with an average interval to metastasis of ~two years.

Unresectable and metastatic squamous cell carcinoma

Unresectable SCC, or primary tumours where only partial surgical clearance is possible, may be suitable for radiation therapy. Tumours with perineural or local bony invasion should also be considered for postoperative adjuvant radiotherapy [1], as should nodal basins harbouring multiple involved lymph nodes and/or extranodal disease. Radiotherapy is also valuable for palliative treatment of locally-advanced SCC.

A range of systemic therapies has been used for unresectable primary SCC, including oral retinoids such as isotretinoin and etretinate, sometimes in combination with interferon, the EGFR inhibitor cetuximab and the oral 5-FU prodrug capecitabine. Occasionally, patients with extreme numbers of high-risk primary lesions may need systemic therapy. Capecitabine was used in three organ transplant recipients with multiple primary SCCs, with reduction in numbers of new tumours from a baseline of 35 cancers in the six months prior to capecitabine, compared to one cancer in six months after commencing treatment [2].

Intravenous agents such as platinum compounds, sometimes in combination with doxorubicin, 5-FU, or paclitaxel, have also achieved some rapid responses in unresectable disease, maintained for up to three years. Bleomycin, vincristine, cyclophosphamide, methotrexate, and 5-FU have also been used intravenously for inoperable primary SCC. For multirecurrent or inoperable primary SCC on a distal limb, isolated limb perfusion or isolated limb infusion with agents such as melphalan, bleomycin, vincristine, and actinomycin have been effective.

Suspected nodal disease may be initially investigated with fine needle biopsy, ideally under ultrasound guidance so that nodal morphology can be assessed and the most abnormal area(s) targeted for biopsy. Staging of patients with known metastatic disease can be done using computed tomography; fluorodeoxyglucose positron emission tomography (PET) may also be useful in metastatic SCC, whilst magnetic resonance imaging (MRI) can provide the best definition of perineural invasion.

Systemic therapies for metastatic SCC have most commonly included cisplatin, often in combination with doxorubicin. Other reported agents include 5-FU, methotrexate, bleomycin, and vindesine. Complete response rates of ~30%, and overall response rates of more than 80%, have been reported in this setting [3].

Follow-up after cutaneous squamous cell carcinoma

Frequency and duration of follow-up after treatment of squamous lesions is determined by the nature of the primary lesion, the type of treatment given and host immune status. Non-invasive lesions such as Bowen's disease, treated non-surgically with agents such as PDT, imiquimod, or 5-FU, should be reviewed ~three months after therapy and then twice-yearly follow-up considered for two to three years [3]. Following diagnosis of an invasive SCC, the three-year cumulative risk of subsequent primary SCC has been estimated at 18%, providing additional reason to maintain close surveillance [3]. Immune-suppressed patients with large numbers of aggressive SCCs, such as organ transplant recipients, may need follow-up every two to three months indefinitely.

Merkel cell carcinoma

Merkel cell carcinoma (MCC) is a rare aggressive cutaneous neuroendocrine tumour, with an estimated incidence of 0.44 per 100 000 people, although this rate is increasing. It usually develops at chronically sun-exposed sites (predominantly the head and neck) in elderly individuals; mean age at diagnosis is 69 years and 95% of patients are fair-skinned [4]. Merkel cell carcinoma is more common in men [4]. Clonally-integrated Merkel cell polyomavirus is found in the genomes of ~80% of MCCs suggesting that it is aetiologically implicated in MCC pathogenesis, and a greatly increased incidence of MCC is observed in the setting of chronic immune suppression.

Clinically, MCC may present as a rapidly growing violaceous or erythematous nodule; erosion is frequent and tumours can double in size within a week, although spontaneous regression is occasionally observed [4]. Histologically, MCC is characterized by monomorphous sheets of cells with neuroendocrine nuclear characteristics (granular chromatin, inconspicuous nucleoli) and minimal cytoplasm. The cells stain positive for various cytokeratins (CK) including CK20 in 95% of cases, and for one or more neuroendocrine markers (such as chromogranin, synaptophysin, neuron specific enolase, and CD57; Figure 50.6). Primary tumour thickness and lymphovascular invasion are predictors of recurrence and survival in clinically localized MCC patients. Lymphatic

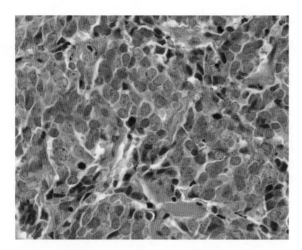

Fig. 50.6 Merkel cell carcinoma. Cohesive clusters of mitotically active tumour cells with granular chromatin, inconspicuous nucleoli and minimal cytoplasm are infiltrating between dermal collagen bundles.

invasion tends to occur early, with a local recurrence rate of ~30%; nodal involvement is present in 30% of patients at the time of presentation, ultimately affecting 50% of all patients [4]. Hence, staging investigations, such as PET-CT, should be considered at the time of initial diagnosis.

Primary MCC is usually treated with wide excision, usually with 2–3 cm margins if surgically feasible. MCCs are, however, highly radiosensitive and radiation therapy alone, generally at doses of 50–55 Gy in 20–25 fractions, may also achieve local control, with in-field control rates of 75% reported. Adjuvant irradiation of regional node fields has been reported to reduce the risk of nodal recurrence, although without impact on overall survival. If radiation therapy is considered appropriate, it should be delivered as promptly as possible, as higher rates of disease progression are seen in patients whose radiation therapy is delayed by more than 24 days. Alternatively, sentinel node biopsy may be offered in MCC at the time of local wide excision, although a greater SNB false negative rate has been reported for MCC compared to melanoma and surgical patients may experience greater delays in receiving radiotherapy.

Distant metastasis to sites such as bone, lung, skin, brain, and liver, is associated with a median survival of nine months. MCC is often initially (although not durably) chemosensitive, and systemic agents such as cisplatin, carboplatin, and etoposide have been used in an adjuvant setting as well as for treatment of known metastatic disease [4]. The use of systemic agents may also enhance the efficacy of concurrent radiation.

Atypical fibroxanthoma

Atypical fibroxanthoma (AFX) is an uncommon cutaneous tumour that appears malignant histologically but paradoxically is associated with benign clinical behaviour. It usually presents as a rapidly-growing nodule in chronically sun-damaged skin of elderly men (male:female ratio of 7:1), with a predilection for head and neck sites (75%) compared to trunk and limbs. AFX is now generally regarded as a superficial counterpart of an undifferentiated pleomorphic sarcoma (so-called malignant fibrous histiocytoma; MFH). Its excellent prognosis is a consequence of its smaller size,

superficial location, and amenability to complete excision. Because a histologically identical tumour would be diagnosed as MFH if it extended into the subcutis or exhibited lymphovascular invasion, necrosis or diameter >2cm, a definitive diagnosis of AFX cannot be made on the basis of an incomplete biopsy. AFX has been reported in younger patients with XP. AFX are comprised of atypical spindle cells, often with frequent mitoses, within a fibrous stroma. Other malignant tumours, including sarcomatoid (spindle cell) SCC and spindle cell melanoma, can be histologically indistinguishable from AFX on haematoxylin-eosin stained sections. Therefore, a diagnosis of AFX requires exclusion of such possibilities and immunochemical stains are mandatory in the pathological work up. There are no currently known specific immunochemical markers diagnostic of AFX, which remains a diagnosis of exclusion. Hence S100, HMB45, and MelanA should be used to exclude melanoma as well as high molecular weight keratin stains (such as CK5/6, 34BE12, and MNF116) to rule out SCC.

AFX is regarded as a tumour with little metastatic potential, particularly if strict diagnostic criteria are applied. Treatment is by surgical excision with clear margins. Recurrence is reported to occur in approximately 5% of cases, but in most instances this is due to incomplete removal. Mohs' micrographic surgery may yield a higher cure rate than standard excision, but all patients should have close follow-up, at least six monthly, for recurrence as well as for other NMSC, which are very common in AFX patients. The risk of metastatic spread, almost always to regional nodes, is ~1%. Risk factors for metastasis include immune suppression, subcutaneous tumour extension, and tumours arising in previously irradiated skin.

Skin cancer prevention

Sun minimization and use of appropriate clothing, hats, and sunglasses are essential to reduce NMSC risk, especially in high-risk individuals. Sunscreens can reduce both the DNA-damaging and also the immune suppressive effects of UV exposure. Daily use of broad-spectrum sunscreens, which reduce exposure to both UVB and UVA, can reduce numbers of premalignant AKs by up to 40% within a few months and have been shown to reduce SCC incidence by a similar proportion within two years of follow-up. There is some evidence suggesting that reductions in BCC risk (and in melanoma) may occur with follow-up extending beyond eight years.

Individuals with large numbers of NMSC may benefit from systemic chemoprevention. Retinoids such as acitretin can modulate keratinocyte growth, differentiation, and apoptosis and have been found to reduce numbers of SCCs and sometimes BCCs in both immune-competent and immune-suppressed patients, and in patients with XP. Skin cancer incidence in patients taking retinoids does tend to return to baseline levels upon drug discontinuation. Side effects of oral retinoids include cheilitis, dry eyes, skin fragility, hair loss, liver function abnormalities, increased serum lipids, and teratogenicity, whilst very long-term use can cause osteoporosis.

The enzyme cyclo-oxygenase 2 plays a key role in skin carcinogenesis, and population-based case-control studies have found that use of nonsteroidal anti-inflammatory drugs (NSAIDs) is associated with a reduced risk of SCC but not BCC. The COX2 inhibitor celecoxib reduced numbers of new NMSCs, but not AKs, within 11 months compared to placebo in 240 patients presenting with actinic keratoses (RR 0.43). NSAIDs do, however, carry risks of gastric bleeding and irritation, renal impairment, and hypertension, and may not be suitable for long-term use in many patients.

Nicotinamide (vitamin B3) is a precursor of NAD+, and replenishes cellular energy levels, which are depleted after UV exposure. Nicotinamide prevents UV-induced immunosuppression and carcinogenesis in mice, and prevents UV immunosuppression in humans. This agent has an established safety profile, without the vasodilatory effects of nicotinic acid. In Phase 2 studies, nicotinamide reduced AKs by 30% compared to placebo and also reduced incidence of new NMSCs in heavily sun-damaged Australian patients. Nicotinamide may provide an inexpensive, non-toxic approach to systemic skin cancer chemoprevention and Phase 3 studies of this agent are currently underway.

References

1. Hulyalkar R, Rakkhit, Garcia-Zuazaga J. The role of radiation therapy in the management of skin cancers. Dermatology Clinics 2011; 29: 287–296.
2. Endrizzi BT, Lee PK. Management of carcinoma of the skin in solid organ transplant recipients. Dermatologic Surgery 2009; 35: 1567–1572.
3. Basal Cell Carcinoma, Squamous Cell Carcinoma (and Related Lesions)—a Guide to Clinical Management in Australia. Cancer Council Australia and Australian Cancer Network Sydney, 2008.
4. Swann MH, Yoon J. Merkel cell carcinoma. Seminars in Oncology 2007; 34: 51–56.

CHAPTER 51

Acute leukaemias

Adele K. Fielding, Charles G. Mullighan, Dieter Hoelzer, Eytan M. Stein, Ghada Zakout, Martin S. Tallman, Yishai Ofran, Jacob M. Rowe, and Ross L. Levine

Prognostic factors in acute myeloid leukaemia

Although the majority of patients with acute myeloid leukaemia (AML) achieve complete remission with induction chemotherapy, relapse after achievement of clinical remission remains the most critical clinical challenge facing AML patients and clinicians today. Although consolidation with high-dose cytarabine or stem cell transplantation reduces relapse rates and offers the possibility of cure to a subset of AML patients, the majority of AML patients suffer relapsed disease. Notably, outcomes in AML remain highly heterogeneous, such that some patients achieve cure with existing therapies and other patients relapse, despite presenting with similar clinical, pathologic, and flow cytometric characteristics. There is therefore a pressing need to improve prognostication in AML.

Current standard of care for molecular prognostication in acute myeloid leukaemia

In the current clinical setting, chromosomal translocations—specifically CBF translocations and *PML-RARA*—predict for favourable outcome and, in the case of *PML-RARA*-positive APL, confer sensitivity to all-trans retinoic acid (ATRA) and arsenic trioxide. However, the field of prognostication in AML, and the utility of molecular markers to inform prognosis and outcome in AML, changed with a seminal study by Schlenck et al. [1]. They performed targeted mutational analysis of more than 800 patients with cytogenetically normal AML. In their study, normal karyotype-AML patients with *CEBPa* mutations, or with NPM1 mutations without co-occurring *FLT3-ITD* mutations, had an improved outcome. By contrast, patients with *FLT3-ITD*, or who were negative for mutations in *NPM1, FLT3,* and *CEBPa*, had a significantly worse outcome. These data demonstrated, for the first time, that mutational profiling could be used to inform prognostication in AML, particularly in patients with cytogenetically-defined, intermediate-risk disease.

However, this study had a second, equally important, observation. Given that patients in the trial cohort were assigned to receive consolidation alone or to receive allogeneic stem cell transplantation (ASCT) based on donor availability, the authors were able to determine if different genetically-defined subsets of AML patients derived benefit from allograft. Specifically, this allowed them to demonstrate that allogeneic transplantation improved outcomes in patients with *FLT3-ITD* mutations and in patients without mutations in *NPM1, FLT3,* and *CEBPa*, but not in normal karyotype-AML patients with *CEBPa* mutations, or with NPM1 mutations without co-occurring *FLT3-ITD* mutations.

This study represented the first demonstration of how mutational profiling can inform AML biology and prognosis, and led to the incorporation of testing for *CEBPa, NPM1,* and *FLT3-ITD* into the routine clinical care for AML patients who are less than 60–65 years of age. However, there are several important caveats to this study, particularly with regard to its relevance to the clinical setting. First, the data have not been robustly validated in an independent cohort. Second, although the findings relating to outcome and response to allogeneic transplantation were statistically and clinically significant, the numbers of patients in specific subgroups (e.g., patients with *CEBPa* mutations) were quite small, such that one might well base important therapeutic decisions in the clinical setting on a single study cohort with less than 20 patients. Third, and most importantly, since this study a series of novel disease alleles have been identified in AML patients, such that an updated molecular prognostic schema is needed to further refine our ability to predict outcome in AML. Nonetheless, this study established the need for real-time genotyping of AML patients for specific somatic mutations and paved the way for subsequent studies investigating prognosis in AML (Figure 51.1).

Role of novel acute myeloid leukaemia disease alleles in predicting outcome

Our understanding of the molecular pathogenesis of AML has been markedly improved by a series of recent discoveries of novel, recurrent, prognostically significant disease alleles in AML patient samples. The first study to use whole-genome sequencing to elucidate the somatic mutational spectrum in AML, or in any malignancy, was reported by Ley and colleagues [2] who performed whole-genome sequencing of a patient who presented with normal karyotype AML. Whole-genome sequencing and detailed bioinformatics analysis identified somatic mutations in *NPM1* and the *FLT3-ITD* allele as well as a small set (eight in total) of novel mutations which were not observed in other patients in detailed recurrence testing. Although this first study did not identify novel recurrent disease alleles of biologic or clinical relevance, it opened the way to a series of studies using whole-genome and whole-exome sequencing to identify mutations in IDH1 [3], *DNMT3a* [4, 5], and mutations

Revised Risk Stratification

Cytogenetic Classification	Mutations		Overall Risk Profile
Favourable	Any		Favourable
Normal karyo-type or inter-mediate-risk ctyogenetic lesions	FLT3-ITD-negative	Mutant NPM1 and IDH1 or IDH2	
	FLT3-ITD-negative	Wild-type ASXL1, MLL-PTD, PHF6, and TET2	Intermediate
	FLT3-ITD-negative or positive	Mutant CEBPA	
	FLT3-ITD-positive	Wild-type MLL-PTD, TET2, and DNMT3A and trisomy 8–negative	
	FLT3-ITD-negative	Mutant TET2, MLL-PTD, ASXL1, or PHF6	
	FLT3-ITD-positive	Mutant TET2, MLL-PTD, DNMT3A, or trisomy 8, without mutant CEBPA	Unfavourable
Unfavourable	Any		

Test Cohort

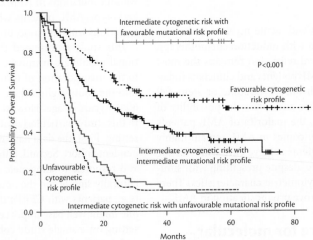

Effect of Mutational Profiling

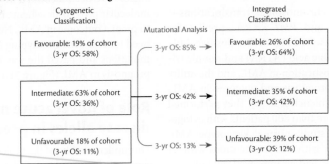

Fig. 51.1 Revised risk stratification of patients with AML on the basis of integrated genetic analysis, showing prognostic algorithm and survival curves with integrated mutational profiling.

From *New England Journal of Medicine*, Patel JP et al., Prognostic relevance of integrated genetic profiling in acute myeloid leukemia, Volume 366, Number 12, pp. 1079–1089, Copyright © 2012 Massachussetts Medical Society. Reprinted with permission from Massachussetts Medical Society.

in the cohesin complex [6]. Moreover, copy number analyses and candidate gene studies have identified additional recurrent somatic mutations in AML patients including in *TET2* [7, 8], *ASXL1* [9, 10], *IDH2* [11, 12], and *PHF6* [13]. The critical question, though, is how these seminal discoveries improve prognostication in AML and whether mutational profiling can be used to inform outcome and therapy in AML.

IDH1, IDH2, and TET2 mutations in acute myeloid leukaemia

IDH1 mutations were first identified in exome sequencing studies of malignant glioma [14, 15]. The first study identified *IDH1* mutations in patients with glioblastoma multiforme (GBM), and subsequently mutations in *IDH1* and in *IDH2* were found to occur most commonly in patients with lower-grade astrocytic neoplasms that subsequently progress to GBM. Ley and colleagues used whole-genome sequencing to identify recurrent *IDH1* mutations in AML [16]. Subsequent studies identified recurrent *IDH2* mutations in AML [11, 12], including mutations at residue R140, which are seen in leukaemias but not in epithelial malignancies.

In 2009, microdeletions and copy neutral loss of heterozygosity on chromosome 4q24 were used to identify recurrent somatic mutations in *TET2* in patients with myelodysplastic syndromes (MDS) and with myeloproliferative neoplasms (MPN) [7, 17]. *TET2* mutations occur in 10% of AML patients [8]. *TET2* is a member of the TET family of proteins that catalyze conversion of 5-methylcytosine (5-mC) to 5-hydroxymethylcytosine (5-hmC) [18]. 5-hmC placement leads to subsequent DNA demethylation; TET2-mutant AML patients are characterized by loss of 5-hmC and by and increased promoter methylation [19]. Of note, murine conditional targeting studies indicate loss of TET2 results in increased self-renewal and in myeloid transformation in vivo [20–23].

IDH1 and IDH2 are enzymes critical in the Krebs cycle that normally convert isocitrate to alpha-ketoglutarate in an NADP+ dependent manner. Biochemical studies have shown that mutant IDH proteins have neomorphic enzymatic activity and convert alpha-ketoglutarate to 2-hydroxyglutarate (2-HG) [24]. Notably, 2-HG can be detected in vast excess in the serum of AML patients with *IDH1/2* mutations [12, 25], suggesting 2-HG may serve as an effective biomarker for minimal residual disease and as a method to prospectively track leukaemic disease burden. Notably, the observation that mutations in *IDH1/2* and *TET2* do not co-occur in the same patients suggested functional convergence by these disease alleles. Indeed, IDH-mutant mediated 2-HG production inhibits TET2 function and promotes hypermethylation [19].

ASXL1

Targeted genomic studies aimed at identifying mutations in epigenetic modifiers led to the discovery of mutations in *ASXL1* in MDS and AML patients [9]. *ASXL1* mutations occur in MPN, MDS, AML and chronic myelomonocytic leukaemia (CMML) and are associated with a poor outcome in all myeloid malignancies studied to date [9, 26]. *ASXL1* mutations are uncommon in younger patients with AML (3–5%) [27], but increase in prevalence with increasing age [28]. Given that the majority of *ASXL1* mutations are somatic nonsense or frameshift mutations, *ASXL1* mutations likely result in loss of ASXL1 function. Recent work suggests ASXL1 loss results in loss of histone H3 lysine 27 methylation, a histone mark associated with transcriptional repression, and with diminished recruitment of the polycomb repressive complex 2 (PRC2) to specific target loci [29].

DNMT3A

Next-generation sequencing of a set of genes involved in haematopoietic development led to the discovery of mutations at the highly conserved R882 residue in *DNMT3A* [30]. Subsequent genome/exome sequencing identified *DNMT3A* mutations at a high frequency in AML [5, 31]. *DNMT3A* mutations occur in more than 20% of de novo AML patients. *DNMT3A* functions as a de novo methyltransferase; however, the specific role of *DNMT3A* mutations in altering epigenetic patterning and in AML pathogenesis has not been conclusively delineated. Importantly, approximately 50% of AML patients present with mutations at codon R882 while retaining the second, wild-type *DNMT3A* allele consistent either with a novel oncogenic or dominant negative function.

Recently identified acute myeloid leukaemia disease alleles

More recent studies have identified additional disease alleles in AML patients. Welch and colleagues performed whole genome sequencing of 24 patients with AML [6]. In addition to previously described disease alleles, they identified mutations in members of the cohesin complex in AML, including in *SMC1A* and *SMC3*. Majeti and colleagues performed exome sequencing of purified leukaemia stem cells to profile the complement of somatic mutations in leukaemia initiating cells and identified mutations in the cohesin complex in AML [32]. More recently, mutations in the splicesome complex [33–35], and in the BCOR/BCORL1 complex [36, 37], have been identified in patients with myeloid malignancies, including AML. The prognostic and therapeutic relevance of these recently-identified disease alleles remains unknown, but we would predict that these disease alleles would allow us to better discriminate outcome and therapeutic response in AML.

Prognostic relevance of newly identified genes

We now have an ever-increasing set of mutations and over-expressed genes with prognostic relevance in AML. However, few of these biomarkers have been adopted into clinical practice. The relative paucity of clinically-utilized biomarkers is due to several factors. Many biomarker studies focus on a specific genetic lesion and its prognostic relevance, without assessing whether specific mutations independently predict outcome in AML in multivariate analysis compared to all known clinical/molecular biomarkers. In addition, most correlative studies are performed in small, retrospective single-institution cohorts such that the effects of treatment on outcome cannot be controlled and investigated. Finally and most importantly, most studies have not validated their prognostic schema in independent sample sets, which is needed to demonstrate robustness of the clinical predictor and to conclusively demonstrate a specific biomarker or molecular classifier is sufficiently valid for use in the clinical setting.

In an effort to determine if a larger set of mutant disease alleles can inform outcome in AML, we recently performed mutational profiling of all known AML disease alleles from a large set of patients enrolled in a single phase III trial cohort of AML patients younger than 60 years of age [38]. This seminal clinical trial evaluated the use of anthracycline dose intensification during induction therapy. At enrollment, patients were randomized to receive standard induction with 45 mg/m² of daunorubicin plus cytarabine or to receive dose-intensive induction with 90 mg/m² of daunorubicin plus cytarabine. This allowed us to perform extensive mutational profiling from diagnostic samples and to correlate molecular data with outcome including disease-free and overall survival and response to induction therapy.

Given the established importance of the three broad cytogenetic risk categories in AML, it is therefore important to determine if mutational status for specific mutations or for combinations of mutations have an impact on the outcome in different cytogenetic risk categories. As discussed previously, mutational analysis of *CEBPA*, *NPM1*, and *FLT3*-ITD can risk-stratify intermediate-risk AML patients [1]. By contrast, more detailed mutational analysis better discriminates intermediate-risk AML patients into distinct risk groups. In the subset of patients with *FLT3*-ITD-negative intermediate-risk AML, *FLT3*-ITD-negative, *NPM1/IDH* mutant patients had a more favourable outcome than patients with inv(16) or t(8;21)-positive AML. *FLT3*-ITD-negative *NPM1*-mutant patients without concurrent *IDH* mutations had a much less favourable outcome. In addition, mutations in *ASXL1*, *PHF6*, and/or *MLL*-PTD conferred adverse overall survival for *FLT3*-ITD wild-type, intermediate-risk patients. Patients with *FLT3*-ITD mutations and co-occurring mutations in *TET2*, *DNMT3A*, *MLL*-PTD, or trisomy(8) also had very poor outcome.

These data suggest that mutational profiling can be used to improve prognostication in AML, such that intermediate-risk patients can be reclassified as having favourable, intermediate, or poor risk based on the mutational status of nine genes. Most importantly, patients with mutationally-defined adverse-risk AML have an outcome similar to patients with adverse karyotypic risk, such that standard therapies are not sufficient to offer a chance of cure to patients with these poor-risk molecular lesions. We believe clinical trials should aim to identify genetically-defined high-risk patients and to offer these patients novel therapies early in their disease course, in an effort to reduce relapse and increase cure.

Although studies suggest mutational profiling offers significant added value to prognostication in AML, validation of these findings in other large, homogeneously treated patient cohorts should remain the highest priority. As such, subsequent biomarker efforts should determine if different mutational genotypes predict outcome in large cohorts of younger and older adults treated with different AML therapies. Moreover, we need to incorporate additional, recently defined molecular lesions, including *BCOR/BCORL1* mutations, cohesin mutations, spliceosome mutations, and epigenetic/microRNA alterations, into our biomarker studies and into our integrative analyses, to determine which molecular lesions are independently predictive of favourable/unfavourable outcomes in large AML patient cohorts.

Anthracycline dose intensification for induction therapy in acute myeloid leukaemia

The ECOG E1900 trial evaluated the use of anthracycline dose intensification during induction therapy by comparing the efficacy of induction with 45 mg/m^2 of daunorubicin or a higher dose of 90 mg/m^2. The higher dose cohort was associated with a significant, albeit modest, improvement in overall survival. Post hoc analysis revealed that high-dose daunorubicin markedly improved outcomes for patients with *DNMT3A* mutations [27], *MLL* fusions or with *NPM1* mutations, but not in patients wild-type for these genes (Figure 51.2). Although these findings need to be further validated in a prospective clinical trial, these data suggest specific molecularly defined subsets of AML patients benefit from dose-intense induction chemotherapy, and demonstrate how genomic studies can inform prognosis and therapeutic decisions.

Translating novel genetic findings to the clinic

With the discovery of novel genes associated with AML pathogenesis, the challenge is to integrate this knowledge into the clinical context. Although whole-genome and whole-exome sequencing have been critical technologies in cancer discovery efforts, their applicability to the clinic today presents several challenges in the wider clinical setting. Welch et al. [39] used whole-genome sequencing to identify a cryptic *PML-RARA* translocation in a patient with M3-AML who had negative FISH analysis for PML-RARA. Whole-genome sequencing may become part of the standard diagnostic evaluation within the next few years; however, the cost, turnaround time, and bioinformatics challenges limit the use of genome and exome sequencing in the current clinical context. We would contend that targeted next-generation sequencing may represent the best option for clinical utilization of molecular genetic information in the near-term. Newer sequencing technologies will allow for rapid, higher throughput, mutational studies in the clinical setting such that this data can used to inform induction and post-remission therapies in AML.

However, there remains a second, equally important challenge: the lack of robust data for novel disease alleles on clinically annotated, homogeneously treated patient cohorts. We would predict that the continued development and implementation of cost-effective genomic profiling platforms will empower collaborative efforts to evaluate novel biomarkers for clinical utility in AML. This will require use of large patient datasets with high quality material and clinical annotation and validation studies to determine which molecular lesions are most useful in the near-term clinical setting. While functional studies of novel disease alleles will lead to a greater understanding of AML pathogenesis, we believe the incorporation of novel biomarkers into the clinical setting is the most important short-term goal facing AML patients and clinicians today.

Basic biology of acute myeloid leukaemia

AML is a clonal haematopoietic malignancy characterized by differentiation block and proliferation of immature myeloid cells (myeloblasts) that leads to peripheral blood cytopenias, and eventual bone marrow (BM) failure. Without treatment and in the face of treatment resistance, patients succumb to the complications of anaemia, thrombocytopenia, and neutropenia and/or the effects of hyperleukocytosis. In this section, we discuss the basic epidemiology, aetiology, clinical presentation, and diagnosis of AML.

Epidemiology

20,830 people are estimated to be diagnosed with AML in 2015 in the US [40]. Of these, 12,730 are estimated to be men and 8100 are estimated to be women, resulting in 10,460 deaths. Although AML is diagnosed in patients of all age groups (including children) it is primarily a disease of older adults with a median age at diagnosis of 72 years [41]. Unfortunately, the outcomes of older adults diagnosed with AML have remained stagnant since the 1970s, both in Europe and the US. Burnett and colleagues collected outcome data from patients over the age of 60 treated on European clinical trials between 1970 and 2009 [42]. According to these data, five-year

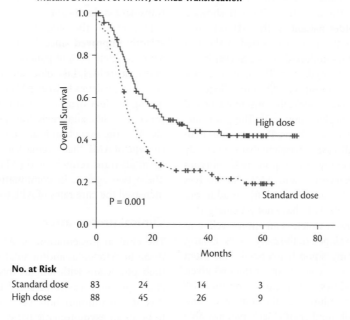

Mutant *DNMT3A* or *NPM1*, or *MLL* Translocation

No. at Risk				
Standard dose	83	24	14	3
High dose	88	45	26	9

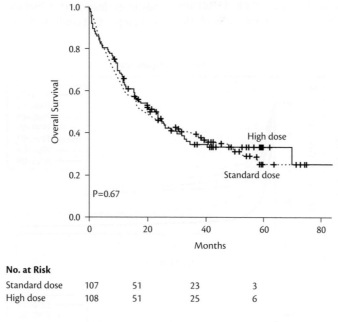

Wild-type *DNMT3A* and *NPM1* and *MLL* Translocation

No. at Risk				
Standard dose	107	51	23	3
High dose	108	51	25	6

Outcomes with High-Dose vs. Low-Dose Induction

	Mutant *DNMT3A* or *NPM1*, or *MLL* Translocation	All Other Genotypes
High Dose	3-yr OS: 44%	3-yr OS: 35%
Standard Dose	3-yr OS: 25%	3-yr OS: 39%

Fig. 51.2 Molecular determinants of response to high-dose daunorubicin induction chemotherapy. Shows benefit of high-dose vs standard-dose daunorubicin in patients with *NPM1/DNMT3A* mutations or with MLL translocations vs those wild-type for all three AML disease alleles.

From *New England Journal of Medicine*, Patel JP et al., Prognostic relevance of integrated genetic profiling in acute myeloid leukemia, Volume 366, Number 12, pp. 1079–1089, Copyright © 2012 Massachussetts Medical Society. Reprinted with permission from Massachusetts Medical Society.

survival rates in older adults remained below 10% between 1970 and 2004 (Figure 51.3). While the data from Burnett shows a slight increase in survival for older patients with AML on clinical trials between 2005 and 2009, this is not supported by the 'real world' population-based outcomes collected in the Surveillance, Epidemiology, and End Results (SEER) dataset. This may be attributable to the adoption of reduced-intensity conditioning allogeneic transplantation in patients who were historically considered too old to endure the rigours of BM transplantation [40]. The poor outcome of older adults has multiple explanations. Patients older than 60 often present with poor-risk disease at baseline that is relatively resistant to induction chemotherapy. These poor-risk subtypes include AML with a complex karyotype and AML that evolves from an antecedent haematologic disorder [43–46]. In addition, new drugs that are more effective for AML have not yet emerged to supplant primary induction therapy, which is an anthracycline in combination with cytarabine, developed in the early 1970s. Finally, traditional induction chemotherapy is poorly tolerated—and often not able to be offered at all—among patients older than 60 given the presence of medical comorbidities such as cardiac dysfunction (ischaemic heart disease or heart failure), renal insufficiency, and liver abnormalities. For the small number of elderly patients able to tolerate induction chemotherapy and who achieve a complete remission (CR), strategies for consolidation are limited. Patients older than 60 do not tolerate high-dose cytarabine, and the

morbidity and mortality from even a reduced intensity allogeneic transplant is significant.

In contrast, the outcomes for patients younger than 60 have steadily improved since 1970 both in the US and Europe, with approximately 50% of patients surviving five years from the time of diagnosis [42]. Like older adults, this improved survival is unrelated to new drugs to treat AML, but rather due to modifications of dosing of older drugs, such as intensified dose daunorubicin, and procedures like allogeneic transplantation and better antimicrobials [47]. The exception is acute promyelocytic leukaemia (APL), a subtype of AML that is remarkably responsive to the differentiating agent all-trans retinoic acid (ATRA) and arsenic trioxide (ATO). These two agents, in combination with an anthracycline, have increased the cure rates of APL to well above 80% [48–50].

Clinical presentation

The clinical presentation of AML is often related to anaemia, thrombocytopenia, and/or neutropenia. Patients may present to their physicians with fatigue, dyspnoea on exertion, pallor, petechiae, purpura, gastrointestinal bleeding, or frequent infections. It is not uncommon, however, for the initial presentation of AML to be in an asymptomatic patient who is noted on routine blood counts to have a mild cytopenia. This inevitably leads to a diagnostic evaluation that includes a bone marrow (BM) aspiration and biopsy that confirms the diagnosis of AML. Patients with APL

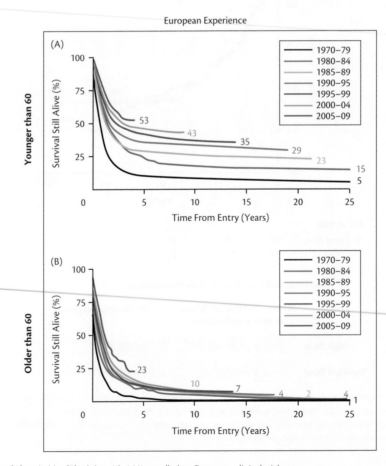

Fig. 51.3 Survival rates for younger (A) and older (B) adults with AML enrolled on European clinical trials.

commonly present with bleeding, usually subcutaneous, in the central nervous system, or in the gastrointestinal tract, which can be life-threatening and may be catastrophic.

Diagnosis

The diagnostic criteria for AML require the demonstration of a block in myeloid differentiation and proliferation of immature myeloblasts. The presence of 20% or greater myeloblasts in the peripheral blood or BM is sufficient to establish a diagnosis of AML. Patients with an elevated myeloblast percentage that is less than 20% are said to have a myelodysplastic syndrome. Of course, progression from MDS to AML is a continuum, and whether patients with 19% myeloblasts behave clinically in a way that is different than those with 21% myeloblasts is doubtful. An exception to the '20% rule' is made for AML with recurrent cytogenetic abnormalities such as t(15;17) and the so-called core binding factor leukaemias [inv(16), t(8;21)], where the presence of characteristic cytogenetic abnormalities is sufficient to make a diagnosis of AML, even in the absence of the threshold 20% blast percentage.

Initially, a BM aspirate and biopsy is performed and the clinician will estimate a percentage of blasts from the aspirate smear. Wherever possible, a trephine biopsy should be obtained with the aspirate both to confirm the percentage of blasts seen in the aspirate, to assess the overall architecture of the BM, and to perform immunohistochemical testing to establish blast lineage. The initial designation of blast lineage—whether myeloid or lymphoid—is crucial, as patients with elevated lymphoblasts have acute lymphoblastic rather than acute myeloid leukaemia, leading to significant changes in the diagnostic evaluation, treatment, and prognosis. Myeloblasts can be distinguished from lymphoblasts morphologically by the presence of prominent nucleoli, relatively open nuclear chromatin, and cytoplasmic granulation. In some cases, cytoplasmic granules coalesce to rod-like structures called Auer Rods in AML (Figure 51.4). Although immunohistochemical stains can help confirm the blast lineage, in all cases the BM aspirate should be sent for immunophenotyping by flow cytometry to confirm the myeloid lineage. Myeloblasts typically express CD33, CD34, CD117 and myeloperoxidase, although aberrant expression of a lymphoid marker is not uncommon. However, the percentage of blasts should not be routinely based on flow cytometric findings (e.g., percentage of CD34+ cells) as some myeloblasts do not express CD34 and

haemodilution during processing can produce falsely low estimates of the myeloblast percentage. The diagnosis of highly undifferentiated AML (M0 in the French American British classification system) can only be established by immunophenotyping.

In some cases, the blast lineage is ambiguous, with two separate populations of cells, one expressing myeloid markers and one expressing lymphoid markers or the co-expression of myeloid and lymphoid markers on the same cell. The World Health Organization (WHO) classifies this subtype of leukaemia as acute leukaemia of ambiguous lineage. This diagnosis should be confirmed at a centre with experienced haematopathologists. Whether to treat acute leukaemia of ambiguous lineage with regimens for AML or acute lymphoblastic leukaemia (ALL) should be made in consultation with an experienced leukaemia physician at a tertiary referral centre.

Once the blast lineage has been established, AML is grouped into specific subtypes. Historically, the French, American, and British (FAB) classification was used and based on morphology and cytochemical stains alone. Currently, the most accepted classification system is that devised by the WHO and is based on morphology, cytochemistry, immunophenotype, cytogenetics, and molecular genetics of the abnormal myeloblasts. Practically, these classifications allow better prognostication of expected responses to therapy and the determination of whether patients should proceed to consolidation with an allogeneic transplant or high-dose chemotherapy once they have reached a complete remission after induction chemotherapy. The exception to this rule is APL, which has a specific morphologic appearance (differentiation block at the promyelocyte stage) and a recurrent reciprocal balanced translocation involving chromosomes 15 and 17. As mentioned earlier, APL is treated differently from other forms of AML and incorporates the use of the differentiating agent ATRA.

Pathophysiology

The development of AML is surmised to result from a genetic event in a putative leukaemic stem cell. This cell, relatively resistant to the effects of chemotherapy, gives birth to the abnormal clone of myeloblasts that cannot differentiate, but can proliferate. A model proposed by Gilliland and colleagues suggests a two-hit model of AML pathogenesis: the first hit is a mutational event in a gene related to differentiation and the second hit is a mutational event in a gene related to proliferation [51]. In recent years, it has become apparent that this model should be expanded, as many mutations have been discovered in genes that encode epigenetic modifications that activate or suppress gene transcription. These epigenetic genes include *IDH 1* and *IDH2, ASXL1* and *DNMT3A*, among others [52–55].

Much has been written about the leukaemic stem cell, a cell that acquires the genetic or epigenetic aberrations that leads to the development of AML and is relatively resistant to the effects of chemotherapy [56]. While the leukaemic stem cell may initiate the disease and its progression, the cytopaenias and BM failure that are characteristic of AML may not be related to 'crowding out' of the marrow by proliferating myeloblasts. This is evident in routine clinical evaluations, as the percentage of myeloblasts does not always correlate with the degree of cytopenia. It is likely that changes in the BM environment induced by the abnormal myeloblasts, rather than proliferation, is the cause of the cytopenias seen in the disease.

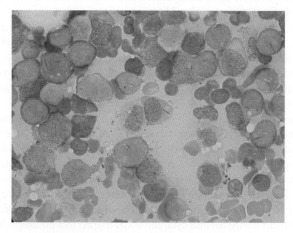

Fig. 51.4 Myeloblasts with auer rods.

Aetiology

Aside from a few well-known environmental factors and genetic syndromes, the causes of the genetic and epigenetic changes that lead to AML in most patients are poorly understood. Of the few known genetic and environmental risk factors for AML, syndromes such as Down syndrome and Fanconi anaemia, exposure to ionizing radiation, prior cytotoxic chemotherapy, and benzene exposure all increase the risk of developing AML [57–59].

Benzene exposure

It is well known that benzene is a potent carcinogen that can lead to the development of AML. Less appreciated is that exposure to even low levels of benzene, either by accidental environmental exposure or through the inhalation of byproducts of cigarette smoke, can also lead to the development of AML [60–63].

Cytotoxic chemotherapy

It is well established that cytotoxic chemotherapy itself, given for other malignancies, can induce changes in DNA that promote leukaemogenesis [64–66]. The most common agents implicated in the development of therapy-related AML are alkylating agents like cyclophosphamide, topoisomerase II inhibitors such as etoposide, and anthracyclines. These agents produce characteristic patterns of AML with alkylating agents most often inducing changes in chromosomes 5 and 7 approximately five years after administration and topoisomerase II inhibitors causing abnormalities of chromosome 11 at position 11q23. Therapy-related AML developing after exposure to alkylating agents typically has a relatively long latency and often an antecedent myelodysplastic syndrome phase. In contrast, those arising after exposure to the epipodophyllotoxins and anthracyclines usually have a shorter latency period, no period of myelodysplasia, and monocytic morphology.

Ionizing radiation

The survivors of the atomic bombings at Hiroshima and Nagasaki, as well as individuals exposed to large doses of radiation after the Chernobyl nuclear accident, have increased risks of developing AML. The effect of exposure to low levels of radiation over a lifetime, from medical radiological imaging, radon, and frequent travel in airplanes, is unknown [67, 68].

Management of acute myeloid leukaemia

Evaluation and general consideration

Acute myeloid leukaemia (AML) is the most common acute leukaemia in adults. Survival of AML patients is continuously improving, especially among younger patients [69]. Nevertheless, only 35–40% of newly diagnosed AML patient younger than 60 years are cured of their disease (Figure 51.5) [70, 71, 151, 152]. Treating an AML patient with curative intent requires inducing the most durable remission and prescribing some form of post-remission therapy. During evaluation and therapy initiation, infectious complications, tumour lysis syndrome (TLS), hyperleukocytosis, and disseminated intravascular coagulation (DIC) are common and require special attention and treatment [72]. Active infection and occult bleeding should be ruled out and chest radiography, complete blood count, blood chemistry studies and coagulation panel, including fibrinogen, are indicated.

Adequate hydration to maintain high urinary flow and rapid response to any signs or symptoms of infection are mandatory.

Daily biochemistry studies are recommended and, in some rapidly proliferative conditions, pseudohypoxaemia or pseudohyperkalaemia may be observed [73]. A 25% rise from baseline of two or more of LDH, uric acid, potassium, creatinine, BUN, and phosphorus, or a decrease in calcium level, is suggestive of tumour lysis syndrome [74]. Hyperuricaemia is common, and allopurinol—or in patients presenting with severe renal failure, at least a single dose of recombinant urate oxidase (rasburicase)—should be prescribed [75]. Dyspnoea and stupor, ischaemic symptoms of heart, kidneys, distal extremities, or priapism, in the absence of alternative aetiology, may suggest hyperleukocytosis and leukopheresis should be considered [76]. Fundoscopy is indicated whenever the white blood cell count is >100 000 cells/μl.

Extramedullary leukaemic infiltration may exist but no routine evaluation or imaging is required. Brain imaging and lumbar puncture are indicated only when clinical symptoms are suspicious for central nervous system involvement [77]. It may also be justified in patients presenting with very high counts, but should be delayed until blasts are eradicated from peripheral blood. Blood products should be used punctiliously. Prophylactic transfusion are indicated when the platelet count is lower than 10 000/μl. There is no numerical cut-off for obligatory red cell transfusion. Irradiated and leukodepleted blood products are recommended to prevent transfusion-related graft-versus-host-disease (GVHD) and allo-immunization, especially in patients who may be candidates for allogeneic stem cell transplantation (allo-SCT). Of all cancers, acute leukaemias are particularly recognized for a very rapid progression from diagnosis to initiation of therapy.

Induction

Achievement of complete remission (CR) is the sine qua non for cure of AML. Of long-term AML survivors, 91% attain CR [78]. In recent years, multiple ways of intensifying the traditional protocol of three daily doses of anthracycline and a week-long continuous infusion of cytarabine (3 + 7) have been tested. Doubling daunorubicin doses from 45 to 90 mg/m^2 yielded a significantly higher CR rate (70.6% vs 57.3%) with no increase in adverse event rate [79]. However, intensifying induction by administering 50 mg/m^2 of daunorubicin for five days failed to improve patient outcome [80]. It may well be that achievement of high peak plasma levels is more important than the total daunorubicin administrated dose. The ongoing Medical Research Council (MRC) AML17 trial is prospectively comparing daunorubicin doses of 60 and 90mg/m^2; doses of 45 mg/m^2 should no longer be considered appropriate [81]. Escalated doses of cytarabine (1 g/m^2 every 12 hours for five days) in combination of idarubicin failed to improve CR rate [82]. The addition of cladribine 5 mg/m^2, administered in a three-hour infusion on days one to five, to a standard 3 + 7 protocol improved CR and overall survival (OS) rates in a prospective phase III randomized trial [83].

Induction intensification by prescribing an additional intensive chemotherapy cycle between days 20–22 of therapy to all patients, regardless of the results of the first induction course, is known as a double induction approach. Several double induction protocols exist but only few have been compared to a regular 3 + 7 protocol. The Acute Leukemia French Association (ALFA) conducted a three-arm prospective randomized trial comparing 3 + 7 with daunorubicin 80 mg/m^2 and cytarabine 200 mg/m^2 to a double induction with identical 3 + 7 followed by mitoxantrone and cytarabine

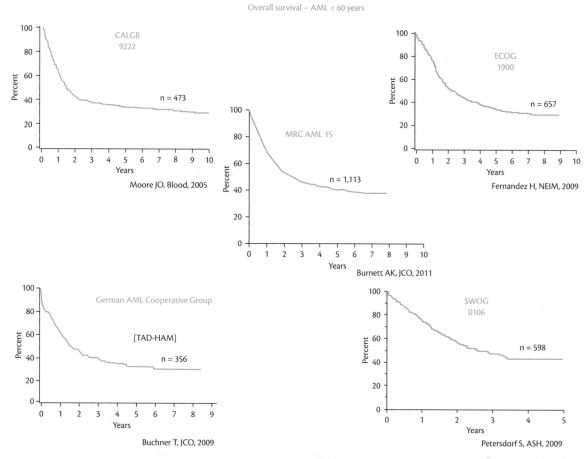

Fig. 51.5 Overall survival from diagnosis of patients younger than 60 years with acute myeloid leukaemia. Virtually identical survival curves from major co-operative groups, despite varying treatment regimens, population size, and countries.

Abbreviations: AML, acute myeloid leukaemia; CALGB, Cancer and Leukemia Group B; ECOG, Eastern Cooperative Oncology Group; SWOG, Southwest Oncology Group.

Source: data from Fernandez HF et al., Anthracycline dose intensification in acute myeloid leukemia, *New England Jouranl of Medicine*, Volume 361, Number 13, pp. 1249–1259, Copyright © 2009 Massachussetts Medical Society; Burnett AK et al., Identification of patients with acute myeloblastic leukemia who benefit from the addition of gemtuzumab ozogamicin: Results of the MRC AML15 trial, *Journal of Clinical Oncology*, Volume 29, Issue 4, pp. 369–377, Copyright © 2011 American Society of Clinical Oncology; Moore JO et al., Sequential multiagent chemotherapy is not superior to high-dose cytarabine alone as postremission intensification therapy for acute myeloid leukemia in adults under 60 years of age: Cancer and Leukemia Group B Study 9222, *Blood*, Volume 105, Issue 9, pp. 3420–3427, Copyright © 2005 by American Society of Hematology; Buchner T et al., Age-related risk profile and chemotherapy dose response in acute myeloid leukemia: a study by the German Acute Myeloid Leukemia Cooperative Group, *Journal of Clinical Oncology*, Volume 27, Issue 1, pp. 61–69, Copyright © 2009 American Society of Clinical Oncology; Petersdorf S et al., Preliminary Results of Southwest Oncology Group Study S0106: An International Intergroup Phase 3 Randomized Trial Comparing the Addition of Gemtuzumab Ozogamicin to Standard Induction Therapy Versus Standard Induction Therapy Followed by a Second Randomization to Post-Consolidation Gemtuzumab Ozogamicin Versus No Additional Therapy for Previously Untreated Acute Myeloid Leukemia, *Blood*, Volume 114, 790a, Copyright © 2009 by American Society of Hematology.

on day 20 or to a timed-sequential protocol [84]. The CR rate, duration, and adverse event rate were identical for all three arms. In the MRC AML15 study [85], 1113 patients younger than 60 were randomized to either receive or not receive a CD33-targeted therapy, gemtuzumab ozogamicin (GO, Mylotarg®), in addition to induction. Surprisingly, the survival benefit of GO was not associated with the expression of CD33 on myeloid blasts with favourable cytogenetics. For patients presenting with intermediate-risk cytogenetics, a multivariable model was in favour of GO administration with the exception of those with a low-performance status and older age. Similar results were observed in a French randomized, open-label, phase III study (ALFA 0701) [86]. Currently GO is not commercially available, but since the effect of GO was not CD33-related and daunorubicin doses used in those trials were 50 and 60 mg/m², it might resemble the effect of other induction intensification. Similarly, with high daunorubicin doses the median

survival of patients with favourable or intermediate cytogenetic profile has been significantly improved (from 20.7 to 34.3 months) but not in patients with unfavourable cytogenetics [79], although the number of patients (n = 5a) in this cohort was relatively small (Figure 51.6).

Considering the dismal prognosis of patients who experience induction failure, early identification of resistant disease is warranted. In typical US cooperative group prospective studies, the presence of >10% blasts in a non-hypoplastic BM at day 12–14 of induction calls for re-induction. Data from 1980 patients who participated in six different Eastern Cooperative Oncology Group (ECOG) protocols demonstrated that the long-term outcome of patients who attained CR following re-induction at day 14 is identical to those who entered CR following a single induction [87]. Such data were derived, as the post-remission therapy in these studies was not altered by the number of cycles needed to achieve

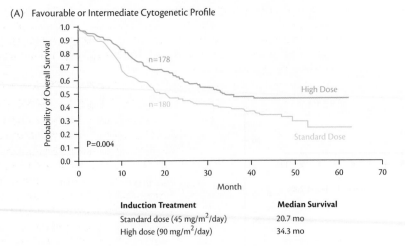

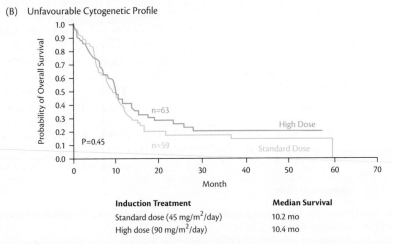

Fig. 51.6 Effect of induction with intensified daunorubicin dose on overall survival. Intensifying induction by doubling daunorubicin dose improves OS in patients with favourable and intermediate cytogenetics (A). Such a difference could not be demonstrated, in smaller numbers, among patients with unfavourable cytogenetics (B).
From *New England Journal of Medicine*, Fernandez HF et al., Anthracycline dose intensification in acute myeloid leukemia, Volume 361, Number 13, pp. 1249–1259, Copyright © 2009 Massachussetts Medical Society. Reprinted with permission from Massachussetts Medical Society.

CR. Unfortunately, the positive and negative predictive value of BM examinations on either day 14 or 21 are low [88].

Discriminating patients who are likely to achieve CR with current protocols from those who are in need of novel therapies is a challenge. High doses of anthracyclines are safe and, although less beneficial for those with adverse cytogenetics, the 3 + 7 regimen remains the gold standard for all patients with AML.

Induction in older patients

Age is a prominent independent prognostic factor in AML, with adverse genetic profiles more prevalent in the elderly. Yet, in patients older than 60 who present with a favourable cytogenetic or genotype, CR rate has been reported to be as high as 80% following intensive induction [89]. Unfortunately, partly due to the inability to deliver maximal post-remission therapy, relapse rates are higher in older patients and only a small portion of patients can be cured.

The decision regarding a patient's fitness for intensive induction depends very much on the doctor's clinical impression and the patient's preference. The following data should guide physicians in their judgement and must be carefully explained to patients. Mortality rate during the first month following intensive induction protocol is 10% in patients over 60 years, compared to 5% in younger patients. However, early deaths are mainly attributed to leukaemia and not to therapy. This is intuitively understandable when death is due to hyperleukocytosis or tumour lysis syndrome, but is also true in cases of fatal infections or bleeding which have similar prevalence among patients treated with palliative care only [90]. Comorbidities and performance status—but not age alone—are predictive parameters for early death [90]. In older adults, intensifying induction with high daunorubicin dose of 90 mg/m² is safe, induces more remissions, and may also provide a survival advantage for some patients over 60 [91]. Moreover, the addition of gemtuzumab ozogamicin 3mg/m² to induction with daunorubicin 50 mg/m² plus either cytarabine or clofarabine reduced relapse rate and improved OS [92]. However, there is no reason to believe that the same results could not have been achieved using a higher anthracycline dose. Thus, attenuating standard induction for older adults should be discouraged. Low-intensity induction protocols may have fewer side effects but are much less effective in inducing complete remission [93]. Data from Swedish and Swiss registries suggest that older patients, even those with poorer performance status, do better with intensive induction than with best supportive care only [90] (Table 51.1).

Table 51.1 Outcome with different first line approaches in older AML patients

Approach	CR rate	Early death	2–3-year OS	References
7 + 3*	54%	12%	26%	Lowenberg et al. [91])
	58%	8%	20%	Burnett et al. [92]
	57%	10%	27%	Gardin et al. [136]
	53%	15.5%	---(<20%)	Roboz et al. [93]
	61%	3%	38%	Pautas et al. [153]
	52%	31%	---(30%)	Tilly et al. [96]
Intensified 7 + 3#	64%	11%	31%	Lowenberg et al. [91]
	62%	9%	25%	Burnett et al. [92]
	70%	7%	38%	Pautas et al. [153]
Low-dose Ara-C	18%	26%	8%	Burnett et al. [97]
	7.8%	8%	<5%	Kantarjian et al. [99]
	23%	9.7%	--(<20%)	Roboz et al. [93]
	32%	10%	--(<20%)	Tilly et al. [96]
Hypomethylation	24%	7%	<8%	Cashen et al. [100]
	17.8%	9%	<5	Kantarjian et al. [99]
Supportive care	1%	26%	0%	Burnett et al. [97]

A summary of outcome results of prospective studies of different first line approaches designed for older patients with AML. The cited CR rate is the rate achieved by a single induction cycle not including patients who went into remission following a second induction or salvage protocols. Early death is the mortality rate from all causes within the first 30 days of therapy. OS is for two or three years depending on the period reported in each study.

* Studies that used 7 + 3 regimen with daunorubicin at a dose of 60 mg/m^2 or lower.

Studies that used 7 + 3 regimen with daunorubicin doses higher than 60 mg/m^2

CR, complete remission; OS, overall survival.

Alternative induction regimens for older patients have been suggested. Phase II studies of intravenous clofarabine at 30 mg/m^2/day for five days as monotherapy reported a CR rate of 32–38% in high-risk patients [94]. The addition of daily 20 mg/m^2 cytarabine subcutaneously for 14 days to clofarabine improved remission rate to 63%, but with a price of increased induction mortality [95]. Overall survival following clofarabine induction and consolidation was 10–12 months in all reported studies. However, a phase III ECOG study in older adults (E2906), comparing induction with clofarabine 40 mg/m^2/day for five days to a standard 3 + 7 regimen (with 60 mg/m^2 of daunorubicin) was suspended in early 2015 due to differences in survival rates favouring standard induction and consolidation compared to clofarabine induction and consolidation.

The role of low-dose cytarabine and hypomethylating agents

Cytarabine has been used in AML therapy for nearly 40 years. In 1990, Tilly et al. randomized 87 patients older than 65 to receive either low-dose cytarabine or intensive induction and reported a lower number of early deaths but also lower CR with the low-dose cytarabine arm [96]. OS was similar in both arms. Currently, low-dose cytarabine (s.c. 10 mg/m^2 bid for 10–14 days) is reserved

for patients considered unfit for intensive induction. A randomized study conducted by the MRC established the superiority of low-dose cytarabine over hydroxyurea in this palliative setting [97].

Azacitidine and decitabine are cytidine nucleoside analogs which are incorporated into DNA, inhibit DNA methyltransferase, and thus induce DNA damage and hypomethylation. Azacitidine activity in AML was shown in a sublet analysis of a phase III study. In this study, patients with myelodysplastic syndrome (MDS) were randomized to azacitidine or to one of three alternative predetermined physician-chosen therapies (intensive chemotherapy, low-dose cytarabine, and best supportive care). Analyzing outcome of 113 MDS patients who presented with >20% blasts, and therefore regarded as AML, demonstrated a superior two-year OS (50% vs 16%, p = 0.001) with azacitidine [98]. However, great caution is indicated in interpreting these data. Only 63 (56%) patients were randomized to best supportive care and the number of patients randomized to low-dose cytarabine and intensive chemotherapy was also small. Decitabine was prospectively compared in AML patients older than 65 years of age in a study of a similar design [99]. For patients randomized to not receive decitabine, low-dose cytarabine was offered to 88% and only 12% of patients were assigned to supportive care. No clinically significant effect was demonstrated with decitabine. Several studies of AML patients treated with azacitidine and decitabine [98–100] have reported low CR and early mortality rates (13–24% and 7–12%, respectively) that are similar to results with low-dose cytarabine but inferior to reported rates in fit patients treated with intensive chemotherapy. Therefore, azacitidine or decitabine, though they may prolong survival of some patients, should not be a substitute for intensive chemotherapy in patients who can tolerate it (Table 51.1). The OS advantage with azacitidine that was demonstrated in patients with low blast count [98] suggested that benefit of hypomethylating agents is most pronounced in low-proliferative diseases.

Post-remission therapy

The importance of post-remission therapy in AML is well recognized. A three-arm study that compared intensive consolidation, low-dose protracted maintenance, or no further therapy for AML patients in first complete response was interrupted following interim monitoring. The non-treatment control arm was terminated due to a significantly shorter remissions and higher relapse rates [101]. Eventually, all patients who received no post-remission therapy relapsed. This study also demonstrated that a single intensive consolidation cycle of IV cytarabine 3 g/m^2 over one hour every 12 hours for 12 doses followed by amsacrine 100 mg/m^2/d for three days is superior to maintenance with oral thioguanine and subcutaneous cytarabine for two years [102]. Retrospective analysis of 1414 patients from six different ECOG protocols demonstrated a survival benefit with escalation of post-remission intensity [103]. In a landmark study by the Cancer and Leukemia Group B (CALGB), consolidation with four cycles of twice daily cytarabine 3 g/m^2 in a three-hour infusion on days one, three, and five, significantly prolonged OS compared to lower cytarabine doses when followed by four cycles of maintenance therapy—a point largely ignored by the community at large [104]. In this study, a four-year disease-free survival (DFS) of 44% and an OS of 52% were reported; thus this consolidation protocol was adopted by many centres, even though no evidence is provided that four cycles of high-dose cytarabine are needed [105].

There were several attempts to further improve long-term results using different consolidation protocols. Intensifying cytarabine dose, up to 3 g/m^2 twice daily for six consecutive days in combination with mitoxantrone failed to improve outcome; five-year DFS and OS rates of 33% and 38%, respectively, were reported [106]. When prospectively compared, three cycles of sequential multiagent chemotherapy were equal to three cycles of high-doses cytarabine (HIDAC) [107]. In larger studies that also included patients with intermediate-risk cytogenetics, DFS and OS following three or four HIDAC courses did not improve outcome even with the addition of up to eight consolidation courses or with concurrent administration of multiple chemotherapy agents [108–110].

Post-remission therapy in older patients

Unlike in younger adults, there is no unequivocal evidence that any form of post-remission therapy changes the long-term outcome in older patients [105]. Nevertheless, virtually every major study in older adults includes some form of post-remission therapy.

The question of the optimal number of consolidation cycles in older patients was addressed by the MRC11 trial [111]. The reported results of comparable long-term outcome with either one or three consolidation cycles following double induction should be carefully interpreted. While some young adults in first complete response (CR1) can be cured by repetitive consolidations, for older patients in CR1, the lifelong relapse rate following identical regimen can reach 80%. In addition, the toxicity and mortality with each consolidation cycle is age-dependent. Mortality, mostly due to infection, after a single consolidation cycle, was reported to be 1–2% in younger but 5–10% in older patients. Thus, the cumulative mortality risk related to the administration of three to four cycles can reach 5% in younger and 30% in older adults.

Thus, for patients in CR1 in a non-transplant setting, data support the administration of at least one course of intensive consolidation. However, only in young adults do the benefits of repetitive consolidations outweigh toxicity. There is no agreement regarding the number, drug combination, or doses of consolidation cycles. The common practice of administrating multiple courses is based on retrospective data and, except for patients with favourable cytogenetics, a considerable relapse risk should be expected [112]. For most AML patients, if cure is desired, alternative post-remission modalities should be considered.

The role of autologous stem cell transplantation in first complete response

Autologous stem cell transplantation (auto-SCT) augments the anti-leukaemic activity of chemotherapy by significant dose intensification. Indeed, in multiple studies, auto-SCT during CR1 was followed by a lower relapse rate. Results of auto-SCT reported decades ago were characterized by a relatively high treatment-associated mortality rate. With improvement of supportive care, mortality has decreased and is now predicted as low as 0–4% [113, 114]. As a result, the 2010 LeukemiaNet expert panel recommended that, in patients with favourable- and intermediate-risk cytogenetics, auto-SCT is at least as good as repetitive chemotherapy cycles [77]. Recently, younger adults in CR1 were prospectively randomized in a phase III study between auto-SCT and intensive chemotherapy. Auto-SCT was found to be associated with a lower relapse rate (58% vs 70%, p = .02). However, five-year OS was similar (44% vs 41%) because patients relapsing on the chemotherapy arm had

more salvage opportunities [115]. Promising results with auto-SCT were also reported by a similarly large ECOG trial [114].

Allogeneic stem cell therapy in first complete response and patients' assignment for transplantation

Of all post-remission strategies, the most prominent anti-leukaemic effect leading to the lowest relapse rates is provided by allogeneic stem cell transplantation (allo-SCT) [116–118]. Some retrospective studies suggest that if allo-SCT is performed shortly after completion of induction, the single high-dose consolidation course that is usually advised can be spared [119, 120]. With the introduction of high-resolution tissue typing and the availability of large international donor repositories, allo-SCT should be considered for a significant portion of AML patients [121]. Nevertheless, since allo-SCT is associated with considerable non-relapse mortality and morbidity, doctors and patients alike often hesitate to elect an allo-SCT while in CR1. A prospective trial and meta-analysis of three additional studies, demonstrated an OS benefit of 12% for allo-SCT over repetitive consolidations for all AML patients except those with favourable cytogenetics [116]. Allo-SCT is therefore a reasonable option for most AML patients in CR1 [112]. However, more definitive indications for all SCT are required. Improvement in conditioning protocols and in supportive care to reduce transplant-related toxicity will hopefully crystallize the indications of an allo-SCT. In addition, with novel genetic prognostication, a more accurate prediction of relapse risk will enable a more personalized allo-SCT indication.

The European LeukemiaNet AML Working Party has recently published a consensus statement on the usage of allo-SCT in CR1 [122]. In this statement, an integrated risk-adapted approach is suggested. The benefit from allo-SCT, calculated as the actual reduction in relapse risk, is predicted for each individual patient weighed against the predicted transplant-related mortality risk. Allo-SCT in CR1 is only indicated when transplant is predicted to more likely prevent a leukaemic relapse than the likelihood of an adverse transplant-related outcome. In general, the relative reduction in relapse risk following an allo-SCT is around 50% across most AML risk categories [116, 123]. For patients presenting with a 'favourable' genetic characterization, a relative reduction of 50% from the projected relapse risk of 35% with repetitive chemotherapy courses, will translate into 20% actual risk reduction. Non-relapse mortality (NRM) rate following allo-SCT is higher than 20%, even in young patients with no other co-morbidities who are being transplanted from a fully matched donor in optimal conditions. Thus, although allo-SCT in 'favourable' risk AML can prevent a relapse in one out of five patients, the transplant-related risk outweighs its benefit; until the NRM is reduced it should not be recommended. At the other end of the spectrum, data from allo-SCT in patients with monosomal karyotype suggest that, in this very poor risk group, allo-SCT prevents much less than 50% of relapses [124–126]. However, for patients presenting with a monosomal karyotype who enter CR1, the unsatisfying results with allo-SCT are still the best available compared to the ultimate risk of relapse with any other modality. Thus, allo-SCT is currently indicated in patients with very poor risk AML.

The vast majority of AML patients present within a wide intermediate-risk zone. Cytogenetics was traditionally the sole molecular parameter that served as an indication for allo-SCT in AML patients in CR1 [127]. With the growing number of mutations identified with additive prognostic value to cytogenetics, the traditional discrimination between 'favourable' or 'unfavourable' cytogenetics is now being replaced by more complex genetic profiles [128, 129]. Progress in genetic risk classification allows a more accurate prediction of relapse risk [130, 131] significantly decreasing the number of patients in CR1 in whom the predicted relapse rate is moderated within a wide range.

Transplant-related mortality risk is also individualized. Three general transplant-related risk score systems were suggested based on retrospective data from the European Group for Blood and Marrow Transplantation (EBMT) [132], the Dana Farber Cancer Institute (DFCI) [133], and the University of Washington [134]. When discussing allo-SCT as a therapeutic option for an AML patient in CR1, the risk of disease relapse and the safety of allo-SCT should be weighed. The more likely the risk of relapse and the safer the transplant, the stronger the indication for allo-SCT. Table 51.2 summarizes the allo-SCT recommendation along the integration of both AML relapse risk and mortality risk.

Patients with high-risk acute myeloid leukaemia or high transplant-related risk

The most challenging clinical situations are patients in CR1, in whom the probability of relapse is high but there is also risk from allo-SCT. Such clinical scenarios are common, especially in older patients where unfavourable genetics are frequent and the probabilities for transplant-related complications are high. Two main paths of therapy exist in such conditions but it must be recognized that they are directed at different goals. The first, aiming for cure, requires allo-SCT. For a patient considered unfit for full myeloablative allo-SCT, a reduced-intensity condition (RIC-allo-SCT)

is an option. The effectiveness of RIC-allo-SCT in AML has been reported in retrospective studies to be comparable to traditional full myeloablative allo-SCT. RIC-allo-SCT was associated with a lower early death rate but with a higher risk of leukaemic relapses, with OS similar to that anticipated with a full myeloablative conditioning. To better address this issue, a German intergroup study prospectively randomized AML patients in CR1 between full- and reduced-intensity conditioning protocols. The study was stopped due to slow accrual but results from randomization of 195 patients were recently published [135]. With a median follow-up of 27 months, no difference was detected in non-relapse mortality, relapse rate, and OS. Thus, RIC-allo-SCT is an option for elderly patients and cure may be achieved, but morbidity and mortality remain high.

Alternative strategies for high-risk patients not considered candidates for any kind of allo-SCT is administration of at least one high-dose consolidation cycle followed by either observation or some maintenance therapy. Since ultimate relapse is predicted, the main goal of such therapy is prolonging life with the best quality. A French study suggested that in older patients, prolonged less intensive consolidation protocol is associated with higher two-year OS rates [136].

Maintenance therapy in acute myeloid leukaemia

In the well-cited CALGB study that confirmed the value of high-dose cytarabine as post-remission therapy, both arms received four cycles of maintenance therapy but its value has never been reassessed [104]. A large Japanese study demonstrated that for patients receiving three intensive consolidation courses, the addition of maintenance improved outcome no better than a shorter

Table 51.2 Risk-adapted approach recommendation for allo-SCT in CR1

AML risk group	AML risk assessment*	Risk of relapse following consolidation approach (%)		Allo-SCT is indicated only if	
		Chemotherapy or Auto SCT	Allo-SCT	Predicted NRM is less than (%)	Risk score is
Good	t(8;21) with WBC ≤20 Inv(16)/t(16;16) Mutated CEBPA (double allelic) Mutated NPM1 (no FLT3–ITD mutation) Early first complete remission and no MRD	35–40	15–20	15	None
Intermediate	t(8;21) with WBC >20 Cytogenetically normal (or with loss of X and Y chromosomes), WBC count ≤100 and early first complete remission (after first cycle of chemotherapy)	50–55	20–25	25	EBMT score ≤2 HCT-CI score ≤2
Poor	Otherwise good or intermediate, but no complete remission after first cycle of chemotherapy Cytogenetically normal and WBC >100 Cytogenetically abnormal	70–80	30–40	30	EBMT score ≤3 HCT-CI score ≤3
Very poor	Monosomal karyotype Abn3q26 Enhanced Evi-1 expression	>90	40–50	40	EBMT score ≤5 HCT-CI score ≤5

The European LeukemiaNet AML Working Party consensus statement suggested that allogeneic-HSCT should be indicated only if the disease-free survival benefit of transplant exceeds 10% for an individual patient compared with consolidation by a nonallogeneic-HSCT approach.

*Includes response to first induction. Categorization requires one of the parameters indicated.

Abbreviations: AML, acute myeloid leukaemia; EBMT, European Group For Blood and Marrow Transplantation; Evi-1, Ecotropic viral integration site 1, HCT-CI, haematopoietic cell transplantation comorbidity index; HSCT, haematopoietic stem cell transplantation; CEBPA, gene encoding CCAAT enhancer-binding protein α; FLT3, gene encoding fms-like tyrosine kinase receptor-3; ITD, internal tandem duplication; NA, not advocated; NMP1, gene encoding nuclear matrix protein; MRD, minimal residual disease; WBC, white blood cell count; NRM, non-relapse mortality.

Adapted by permission from Macmillan Publishers Ltd: *Nature Reviews Clinical Oncology*, Cornelissen JJ et al., The European LeukemiaNet AML Working Party consensus statement on allogeneic HSCT for patients with AML in remission: an integrated-risk adapted approach, Volume 9, Issue 10, pp. 579–590, Copyright © 2012 Rights Managed by Nature Publishing Group.

protocol with four high-dose courses [137]. Reducing relapse risk and prolonging survival were demonstrated with maintenance of histamine dihydrochloride and interleukin-2 [138] and with azacitidine post-allo-SCT for patients with early signs predicting for relapse [139]. Thus, maintenance protocols that carry a low risk may be justified during CR1 in patients with a high risk of imminent relapse who are not candidates for allo-SCT. It seems that this modality has not been adequately studied in large prospective trials, including maintenance for young adults after intensive chemotherapy, autologous transplant, or even allogeneic transplant.

Incorporating minimal residual disease monitoring into clinical decisions

The role of minimal residual disease (MRD) monitoring in ALL is well established. It has been suggested that in the future quantifying of MRD may guide post-remission therapy in AML. Support for such approach was demonstrated in a paediatric population using multi-parameter flow-cytometry [140].

Immunophenotyping has been traditionally accepted as the backbone of MRD measurement and efforts have been made towards standardization of measurement techniques [141]. In addition, some molecular aberrations can serve as sensitive markers for imminent relapse [142]. It should be emphasized that large-scale observational studies are required for assessing a specific laboratory component as sufficient for a change in treatment plan, especially if allo-SCT is considered.

The role of targeted and adoptive therapy

Currently there is no 'imatinib-like' magic bullet in AML. FLT3 inhibitors are in clinical trials; quizartinib and sorafenib are the most promising. Acquired point mutations in FLT3 gene are common and contribute to resistance to the targeted agent [143]. Excluding donor lymphocyte infusion post-allo-SCT, adoptive therapy is still an experimental therapy in AML. Recently, a Chinese group demonstrated that infusion of HLA-mismatched peripheral blood stem cells concurrent with induction improved long-term outcome [144]. These investigators have further shown that repetitive infusions of G-CSF mobilized HLA-mismatched cells following each of three consolidation cycles yielded a promising six-year leukaemia-free survival [145]. A measurable anti-leukaemic T-cell response was demonstrated, with no signs or symptoms of GVHD.

Treatment of relapsed/refractory disease

In relapsed/refractory AML, allo-SCT is the only curative modality. Retrospective observations of different large cohorts identified early relapse (<one year), poor cytogenetics, and FLT3-ITD (FLT3-internal tandem duplication) as poor prognostic factors in relapsed disease [146]. Multiple novel agents have been studied with various promising results, however, these agents can only serve as a bridge to transplantation. If allo-SCT is not an option, therapy should focus on prolongation of the patient's life with the best possible quality. Intensive chemotherapy aiming at second remission is appropriate in patients with late relapse and no adverse factors. For patients with poor prognosis for relapse, however, the chance of entering second remission with intensive chemotherapy is as low as 20% [147] and mortality rate from induction therapy is as high as 20% [148]. Therefore, in these patients, intensive chemotherapy targeting second remission may be considered futile. If a donor is available, such patients may be candidates for cytoreductive chemotherapy followed by RIC-allo-SCT and prophylactic transfusion of donor lymphocytes [149]. The role of azacitidine or lenalinomide in relapsed AML has yet to be determined. Preliminary data suggest that given with first signs of molecular relapse, they may delay relapse and may serve as a bridge to allo-SCT [139, 150].

Prognostic factors in acute lymphoblastic leukaemia

The survival rate for ALL in the 1970s was only about 10%, and a variety of single prognostic factors had been found to have an influence on treatment outcome. However, such factors became relevant only with uniform treatment strategies and larger patient numbers from prospective multicentre trials. The first described prognostic factors for remission duration and OS were age, white blood cell count, and time to achieve complete remission [154].These prognostic factors, still used in most studies, were later extended to immunophenotypes, cytogenetic and genetic alterations [155, 156]. The aim of evaluating prognostic factors in acute lymphoblastic leukaemia is to stratify patients into good- and poor-risk groups and to adapt different treatment strategies accordingly. There are principally two phases where prognostic factors are evaluated; the first is the patient characteristics at diagnosis and the second is the response to treatment.

Pretherapeutic prognostic factors

The most important prognostic factors evaluated at diagnosis are given in Table 51.3.

Age

Increasing age is associated with poorer outcome. The age cutpoint at 35 years was the best separation in the survival curve, and was considered the age-limit for allo-SCT [154]. This age-limit is still of relevance since recently-applied paediatric-inspired protocols for adolescents and young adults (AYA) were applicable up to an age of 35–40 years. Patients above this age-limit have a poorer outcome [155, 156] and an increasing incidence of adverse risk factors.

White blood cell count

An increased WBC, reflecting a large leukaemic tumour mass, has been shown to be an adverse influence in nearly all studies. In most

Table 51.3 Major adverse prognostic factors in adult ALL

Factor	
Age	Worse outcome with advancing age
White blood cell count	B-lineage: >30 x 10^9/L T-lineage: >100 x 10^9/L
Immunological subtype	Pro-B ALL vs Pre/Common B-ALL Early T-ALL/Mature T-ALL vs Thymic T-ALL
Cytogenetic markers	t(9;22)/BCR-ABL t(4;11)/MLL-AF4 t(8;14) t(1;19) Complex karyotype
Molecular markers	ERG/BALLC expression NOTCH1 mutations IKAROS deletions/sequence mutations CRLF2 over-expression CEBPalpha FLIT3

studies, a >30 × 10⁹/L for B-cell lineage ALL and >100 × 10⁹/L for T-cell ALL is considered a poor prognostic factor [154–156].

Immunophenotype

The earlier observed adverse prognostic impact of T-lineage ALL compared to B-lineage ALL has disappeared. There are, however, differences within the immunophenotypically-defined ALL subgroups.

- In *B-lineage ALL* patients, those with a pro-B ALL, defined as CD10-negative—mostly associated with the cytogenetic aberration t(4;11)—have an inferior outcome compared to pre-B and common ALL, but benefit from an allo-SCT in CR1 [157].

- In *T-lineage ALL* there is a strong correlation of outcome to the subtypes cortical/thymic T-ALL vs early T-ALL or mature T-ALL. Thymic T-ALL is CD1a-positive and constitutes about half of adult T-ALL patients; their survival at five years is >50–60% [158]. The subtypes, early-T-ALL and mature T-ALL, have a lower rate of CR and a poorer survival; both subtypes profit from an allo-SCT in CR1. Early T precursor (ETP), a recently genetically defined subgroup, confirms this poor prognosis. Recently, the prognostic impact of genetically defined T-ALL subgroups was retrospectively analysed [159, 160] but implications for prospective risk classification in trials are limited.

- *Antigen-expression as a prognostic marker.* With emerging targeted monoclonal therapies directed against surface antigens, e.g., CD20, CD19, CD22 [161–164], the question arises whether antigen expression itself is a prognostic marker. CD20 expression, observed in ~40% of adult pre-B/common B ALL, seems to have an adverse impact, but the data are controversial [161], and was recently shown not to have an adverse impact in childhood ALL. Also, the improved outcome of CD20+ B-lineage ALL receiving anti-CD20 monoclonal antibody (rituximab) has already abolished the potential adverse influence [162, 163].

- *Cytogenetics.* The most frequent cytogenetic abnormality in adults is the Philadelphia chromosome, which accounts for 25% of all adult B-lineage ALLs. There is a strong age-related incidence on Ph-positivity, increasing from <3% in children up to 40-50% in adults aged >50–60. Ph+ ALL is the poorest ALL subtype with a CR rate of ~70%, a survival at five years of <10% with chemotherapy, and <30% with allo-SCT. Targeted therapy with tyrosine kinase inhibitors (TKIs) directed against the BCR-ABL fusion transcript has changed prognosis completely; CR rates are now >90% and survival >50%. Several other cytogenetic abnormalities (Table 51.3) are also associated with a poor outcome [155, 156]. In addition, there are a large number of other chromosomal aberrations in ALL, but with a low frequency and with undetermined prognostic impact [155, 156].

- *Molecular genetics.* There is an increasing number of well-defined genetic alterations in ALL (Table 51.3). Their prognostic impact often remains uncertain and they are not always included in prospective trials. However, they have the great therapeutic potential for new targeted therapies, e.g., inhibitors of BCR-ABL, NOTCH1, or FLT3.

Response measures

Response measures after induction therapy are most predictive for outcome of a patient with an ALL, such as time to achieve a CR within three to four weeks [154–156]. The rate of CR is prognostically less relevant, since >95% of children and >90% of adults achieve a CR. Although CR rates are high, 40–50% of adult patients eventually relapse. One reason is the limited sensitivity to measure the cell reduction by cytomorphology, with potentially 1–5% leukaemic cells in the bone marrow. There are more sensitive methods that detect leukaemic cells on a molecular level to identify minimal residual disease (MRD); standardized methods for MRD are well defined [165, 166].

Stratification into risk groups

Pretherapeutic prognostic factors and response parameters, now preferably MRD, are used to define risk groups. Standard-risk (SR) patients are defined as those without any of the previously described risk factors, whereas high-risk (HR) patients have one or more risk factors. Several large adult ALL study groups have similarly-defined risk groups [155, 156]. The aim of these prognostic models is to identify a SR group with a good outcome, e.g., with an expected >50% survival probability at five years in adults, and the HR patient group with a less favourable outcome. HR patients are generally candidates for an immediate SCT in CR1, whereas SR patients in most studies continue with consolidation cycles ± reduction and maintenance therapy.

Will minimal residual disease evaluation replace pretherapeutic risk factors?

Questions arise as to whether the evaluation of MRD overcomes all the pretherapeutic risk factors, whether it should be combined with the pretherapeutic risk factors, or whether it should remain as the only stratification criterion [167, 168].

The following risk model (Figure 51.7) used in the risk stratification of the GMALL studies (German Multicenter Study Group for Adult Acute Lymphoblastic Leukemia) is a practical approach to bring the conventional prognostic factors and MRD into a decision algorithm. At diagnosis, patients are stratified into SR or HR patients. Since HR patients are candidates for a SCT in CR1 after induction and consolidation therapy, the optimal time point for the donor search is immediately after diagnosis. By this, a suitable HLA-matched, mostly unrelated, donor will be found within the period of ~three months to guarantee a SCT rate of 79–80%. Initial diagnosis also identifies the patients who are candidates for a targeted therapy; e.g., Ph/bcrabl-positive patients for tyrosine kinase inhibitors or those with specific surface antigens for a treatment with monoclonal antibodies, e.g., CD20 + B-lineage patients for anti-CD20 rituximab.

Minimal residual disease response after induction therapy and impact on outcome

Achievement of molecular remission after induction therapy is the most relevant independent prognostic factor associated with better outcome in several recent trials [167, 169]. The molecular CR rate in relation to cytologic CR rate is given in Table 51.4. Albeit MRD is the most relevant independent prognostic factor, other high-risk features such as age or WBC still has prognostic impact in some, but not in other, studies. If there is no opportunity to evaluate MRD, patients should be stratified according to their conventional risk factors.

Patients with molecular failure after induction therapy have the worst outcome of all ALL subgroups and are candidates for a SCT. In a Northern Italy Leukemia Group study [170] the probability for DFS at four years in patients with SCT was 0.33 vs 0 for those with chemotherapy. In a GMALL study [169], there was also a substantial benefit for SR patients with molecular failure receiving SCT, with a probability

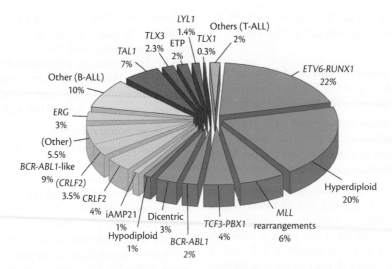

Fig. 51.7 Subclassification of childhood ALL. Blue wedges refer to B-progenitor ALL, yellow to recently identified subtypes of B-ALL, and red wedges to T-lineage ALL.

Table 51.4 Cytologic and molecular response rates after induction (day 71) in correlation to prognostic factors

	Cytologic CR rate N = 1648		Molecular CR rate N = 580	
Overall	89%		70%	
Age				
15–35 years	91%	0.1	71%	NS
35–55 years	87%		69%	
Leukocyte count				
B-lineage				
<30 000 µL	90%	NS	68%	0.6
>30 000 µL	87%		56%	
T-lineage				
<100 000 µL	89%	NS	81%	NS
>100 000 µL	87%		71%	
Immunophenotype				
B lineage	89%	NS	69%	.001
T lineage	89%	NS	79%	.001
c-ALL	89%	.0009	67%	<.0001
Pro-B-ALL	90%	.0009	48%	<.0001
Early T-ALL	85%	.0009	45%	<.0001
Mature T-ALL	78%	.0009	39%	<.0001
Thymic T-ALL	93%	.0009	89%	<.0001
Risk groups				
Standard risk	92%	.0001	77%	<.0001
High risk	85%		51%	

The data are from the largest prospective trial (GMALL07/2003) with MRD evaluation and demonstrate the relation of Cytologic CR rate and Molecular CR rate; with an implication on outcome. SR patients with a molCR at week 16 had an five-year OS of 81% ± 3% compared to 43% ± 6% for SR patients with molecular failure (p <0.0001).

Source: data from Gökbuget N et al., German Multicenter Study Group for Adult Acute Lymphoblastic Leukemia: Adult patients with acute lymphoblastic leukemia and molecular failure display a poor prognosis and are candidates for stem cell transplantation and targeted therapies, *Blood*, Volume 120, Issue 9, pp. 1868–1876, Copyright © 2012 by American Society of Hematology.

of complete cytogenetic response (CCR) after five years of 66% vs 12% for non-SCT patients (p < 0.001). MRD evaluation may also become relevant for autologous SCT. A retrospective analysis showed a significant survival benefit for auto-SCT in patients who were MRD-negative at time of transplant [171], with no residual disease in the patients or in the stem cell harvests. With an increasing fraction of patients achieving MRD-negative status, partly due to the addition of targeted therapy, prospective trials are ongoing to prove this concept.

MRD is also an efficacy parameter for other targeted therapies. In several studies with antibody therapy, e.g., directed against CD20, CD22, or CD19, within the patients achieving a CR the rate of molecular remission was high [161].

Prognostic impact of targeted therapies on minimal residual disease

When the tyrosine kinase inhibitor (TKI) imatinib (IM) became available, most multicentre adult ALL trials added IM to intensive induction chemotherapy in Ph + ALL. The molecular CR rate (bcr-abl negativity) increased from ~5% to 50–80%, translating to substantially better outcome. Maintenance with IM after SCT can substantially reduce the negative impact of MRD positivity before or after SCT [172].

Minimal residual disease conversion as a new study endpoint for clinical trials

Patients with a molecular relapse have a poor outcome since it precedes clinical relapse by several months. Conversion of MRD positivity to MRD negativity is therefore a reasonable clinical endpoint. Thus, in a study of B-lineage adult ALL patients who were MRD refractory or relapsed received the bispecific (CD3/CD19) antibody, with a conversion rate to MRD negativity of 80% and promising survival, with or without SCT [173]. The question arises as to whether patients with a molecular relapse profit from earlier therapy compared to patients treated later at relapse. Although there is no randomized study to compare these approaches, there is some evidence that earlier intervention is of benefit.

Pitfalls of minimal residual disease prediction

Unfortunately, 20–30% of adult ALL patients with MRD negativity after induction therapy will experience relapse. There are several potential reasons for failure to predict relapse by MRD. The first is sensitivity: MRD negativity is consensus-defined as $<1 \times 10^{-4}$ leukaemic cells. However, the biologically relevant MRD level may vary for different ALL subtypes, e.g., in bcr-abl positive ALL a positive signal at the level of 10^{-5} is highly predictive for relapse. Second, for various genetic aberrations, the molecular CR rate is different [165], but it is noteworthy that in larger multicentre trials MRD is measured by flow cytometry or PCR for Ig/TCR and not for the specific genetic aberration. Third, clonal evolution of leukaemic subclones is a further reason for failure to predict relapse by MRD, since it detects the major clone but the number of potentially emerging subclones is much larger than expected [174]. Next generation sequencing (NGS), based on high-throughput sequencing that universally amplifies antigen-receptor gene segments and identifies all clonal gene rearrangements at diagnosis, may be a new technical tool to increase sensitivity and to explore different relevant MRD levels for ALL subtypes [175].

Conclusion

MRD evaluation has emerged as the most important prognostic marker in childhood and adult ALL for treatment decisions and is now an integral part of most prospective trials. Other pretherapeutic markers and patient characteristics at diagnosis are, however, still relevant. Patients with molecular failure after induction reflect refractoriness to chemotherapy ± targeted therapy and are now the most poor prognosis ALL subgroup, and are thus candidates for an experimental treatment approach or immediate SCT. MRD conversion from positive to negative status will most likely be a new endpoint accepted for clinical studies in the near future, with the advantage of being better quantified and allowing a shorter follow-up. The future goal is to identify within the MRD negative group the 20–30% patients relapsing despite a MRD 'remission'; with new methods, their residual leukaemic cells will hopefully be detected.

Basic biology of acute lymphoblastic leukaemia

ALL is a neoplasm of immature lymphoid cells, termed leukaemic blasts, that infiltrate the bone marrow, blood, and extramedullary sites, notably the central nervous system. ALL may be of either B-progenitor or less commonly, T-cell lineage. ALL is the most common childhood malignancy, with an incidence of approximately three to four cases per 100 000 per year, and a peak incidence at 2–5 years of age. Progressive refinements in combination chemotherapy and central nervous system prophylaxis have witnessed increases in long-term disease-free survival rates to over 80% in developed countries. However, relapse occurs in approximately 20% of patients with ALL, and is associated with low cure rates. As discussed in the section on chromosomal aberrations, ALL comprises a number of subtypes characterized by constellations of gross and submicroscopic structural DNA alterations and sequence mutations; specific subtypes are associated with relapse risk [176, 177]. However, relapse occurs across the spectrum of ALL subtypes, and there is consequently great interest in defining the genetic basis of ALL and identifying genetic alterations that may serve as new diagnostic and therapeutic targets. While ALL is less frequent in adults, the outcome is inferior to that in children. Chromosomal alterations associated with

favourable outcome in childhood ALL (e.g., *ETV6-RUNX1* rearrangement and high hyperdiploidy) are less common, and unfavourable alterations (e.g., *BCR-ABL1* and *MLL* rearrangement) are more common, but these do not fully explain the poor outcome of adult ALL.

ALL is one of the most comprehensively studied neoplasms at the genetic level. The first chromosomal rearrangement identified in cancer—the 'Philadelphia' chromosome—was first identified in chronic myeloid leukaemia (CML) and subsequently in ALL, and was subsequently shown to be a reciprocal chromosomal translocation between chromosomes 9 and 22 t(9;22)(q34;q11) [178]. Over 10 years later, it was shown that this rearrangement led to the fusion of the *BCR* gene at 22q11 to the *ABL1* gene at 9q34. This results in a chimeric *BCR-ABL1* fusion gene that induces CML in experimental models and is a founding lesion of *BCR-ABL1* positive ALL [179–183]. Subsequently, multiple recurring chromosomal alterations have been identified in ALL, including aneuploidy (high hyperdiploidy and hypodiploidy) and additional rearrangements, shown to be the initiating lesions in leukaemogenesis.

Chromosomal translocations are the result of an exchange of genetic material between two chromosomes, and resulting in either the juxtaposition of an oncogene to the vicinity of strong promoter elements from the immunoglobulin heavy genes (*IGH*) or the T-cell receptor genes (*TCR*). This leads to aberrant expression of the oncogene or, more commonly, the disruption of two genes and subsequent re-joining of coding sequences from the two genes and creation of a chimeric fusion gene. Typically, the genes rearranged by the latter mechanism encode transcription factors that are important regulators of normal haematopoiesis. By dysregulating or encoding chimeric fusion genes, the chromosomal rearrangements in ALL commonly deregulate the function of the rearranged transcription factor, resulting in excessive activity or acquisition of functions not otherwise observed in normal haematopoiesis [184].

Several observations indicate that additional genetic changes are required for the development of clinically manifest leukaemia. Commonly, expression of the chimeric fusion genes encoded by the chromosomal rearrangements fails to induce leukaemia alone in experimental models. Several chromosomal rearrangements, such as *ETV6-RUNX1*, arise in utero but leukaemia does not manifest for several years [185, 186]. Together, these observations suggest that additional genetic changes not evident on conventional cytogenetic analysis, including submicroscopic deletions and gains (amplification) of DNA and sequence mutations or epigenetic changes are also required for leukaemogenesis. In support of this, low-resolution genomic profiling studies and sequencing of individual genes have identified recurring genetic changes in genes encoding tumour suppressors and cell cycle regulators (e.g., *TP53* [p53] and *CDKN2A/CDKN2B* [INK4A/ARF]) and Ras signalling genes (*NRAS* and *KRAS*).

Our understanding of the genetic basis of ALL has been transformed in the last decade by the advent of high-resolution genome-wide approaches to identify alterations in the genome, transcriptome, and epigenome. These findings have been extended in the last few years by the availability of high-throughput NGS, including whole-exome and whole-genome sequencing and sequencing of the expressed genome (transcriptome sequencing, or RNA-seq) [187]. Although the individual targets of mutation vary between ALL subtypes, several pathways are frequently mutated, including loss-of-function mutations targeting transcriptional regulation of lymphoid development; activating mutations driving cytokine receptor, tyrosine kinase, and Ras signalling; mutations disrupting tumour suppressors; and regulators of cell cycle; and epigenetic modifiers [188, 189]. It is likely that the majority of ALL cases require alterations perturbing several or all of these pathways. In addition, there is growing evidence of clonal heterogeneity in ALL, and the nature of genetic alterations that drive resistance to therapy and disease relapse. While much effort has focused on cataloguing somatic (tumour-acquired) genetic alterations, inherited or germline genetic variations are also important determinants of population-based risk of ALL, and also in promoting the development of familial ALL. Genome-wide studies of epigenetic alterations are less mature than studies profiling structural genetic alterations, but emerging data are identifying subtype-specific epigenetic alterations, and also illustrating the complex but important interrelationship between structural genetic alterations, epigenetic alterations, and the leukaemic transcriptome.

Chromosomal aberrations in paediatric B-cell precursor (BCP)-acute lymphoblastic leukaemia

Gross chromosomal alterations including aneuploidy and chromosomal translocations are present in the leukaemic cells of approximately three-quarters of childhood ALL cases, and are important for diagnosis and risk stratification (Table 51.5, Figure 51.8). The key genetic and biologic features of some important subtypes are reviewed in the following section; more detailed features are included in the tables and figures.

High hyperdiploid acute lymphoblastic leukemia

High hyperdiploid ALL (51-67 chromosomes) is identified in about 25–30% of BCP-ALL cases and is characterized by recurring, non-random gain of at least five chromosomes, most commonly X, 4, 6, 8, 10, 14, 17, 18, and 21. High hyperdiploidy is associated with a favourable prognosis with an overall survival of about 90%; however, 15–20% of cases relapse [190, 191]. High hyperdiploidy is strongly associated with BCP-ALL and is less common in adult ALL and rare in T-cell leukaemia. There is a pronounced age peak at 2–4 years of age with a median age of 3.7 years. Attempts have been made to identify cytogenetic subtypes among high hyperdiploid ALL that correlate with outcome, suggesting that gain of chromosomes 4, 10, 17, and 18 are associated with a favourable prognosis [190, 192]. About 50% of cases contain a structural variation in addition to the high hyperdiploidy; most commonly, the structural variants are unbalanced changes and include partial gains if 1q, deletions of 6q, and isochromosome 7q or 17q. Balanced translocations are rarely seen [193].

The mechanisms leading to the generation of hyperdiploidy, and its contribution to leukaemogenesis, are poorly understood. The highly stereotyped patterns of chromosomal gain and copy-neutral loss-of-heterozygosity of non-triplicated chromosomes suggests an early catastrophic chromosomal loss and reduplication event leading to hyperdiploidy, rather than the ongoing chromosomal aberrations characteristic of aneuploid solid tumours. The molecular evidence behind the formation of high hyperdiploidy points towards two major routes, with the most common (70%) being a simultaneous gain in one single abnormal cell division and less common (30%) initial tetraploidy with subsequent loss of chromosomes [193]. It has been suggested that overexpression of genes on the gained chromosomes is important. Microarray gene expression profiling has shown that the majority of genes on the triplicated chromosomes exhibit increased expression, with a minority showing no increase or absent expression. This suggests alternate mechanisms of regulation of gene expression, such as epigenetic changes deregulating gene expression [194, 195]. Consistent with this notion, genome-wide studies of cytosine methylation in ALL have shown that a substantial proportion of genes on triploid chromosomes that do not show increased expression are subject to methylation-induced silencing [196].

Co-operating mutations in high hyperdiploid ALL include activating mutations in the receptor tyrosine kinase/Ras pathway in approximately one-third of cases: *FLT3* in 10–25%, *KRAS/NRAS* in 15–30%, and *PTPN11* in 10–15% [197]. These mutations appear to be mutually exclusive suggesting that activation of the RAS pathway or kinase signalling is an important co-operating event in this ALL subtype. Mutations of *CREBBP*, encoding in the *CREB*-binding protein (also known as CBP) are present in two-thirds of relapsed high hyperdiploid ALL cases [198]. *CREBBP* mutations are also common in other BCP and T-lineage ALL cases that relapse [199]. CREBBP acetylates both histone and non-histone targets, and has a role in regulating the transcriptional response to glucocorticoid therapy. Glucocorticoids such as prednisolone and dexamethasone are key agents in ALL therapy, and poor responsiveness to initial steroid treatment predicts a high risk of relapse. These findings suggest that *CREBBP* alterations confer resistance to glucocorticoids and promote the emergence of steroid resistance subclones.

Hypodiploid acute lymphoblastic leukemia

Hypodiploid ALL with less than 46 chromosomes comprises 5% of BCP-ALL, with the majority having 45 chromosomes [200, 201]. Hypodiploid ALL can be divided into three genetic subtypes: near-haploidy (24-31 chromosomes), low hypodiploidy (32-39 chromosomes), and high hypodiploidy (40-45 chromosomes) [200, 202]. Near-haploid cases tend to be younger with a median age of 7 years [200, 203–205]. The prognosis is poor with a three-year event-free survival of 29%. Low hypodiploid (33-39 chromosomes) patients tend to be older than the near-haploid cases, with most being ten years or older and a median age of 15, and also have poor outcome [200, 205, 206].

High hypodiploidy (42-45 chromosomes), accounts for the majority of hypodiploid cases with a modal number of 45 being by far the most common. Common alterations in cases with a modal number of 45 are loss of a sex chromosome and the presence of dicentric or isochromosomes, most commonly involving chromosomes 7, 9, 12, and 20 [200, 202].

Until recently, little was known regarding the additional, submicroscopic genetic alterations and mutations underlying the pathogenesis and poor prognosis of hypodiploid ALL with less than 44 chromosomes. Genomic hypodiploid ALL cases, using single nucleotide polymorphism (SNP) and gene expression

Table 51.5 Key cytogenetic subtypes of ALL

Subtype	Frequency (%)	Comment
B cell precursor		
Hyperdiploidy with more than 50 chromosomes	20–30	Excellent prognosis with antimetabolite-based therapy
Hypodiploidy <44 chromosomes	1–2	Poor prognosis, high frequency of Ras pathway and IKAROS gene family mutations
t(12;21)(p13;q22) *ETV6-RUNX1*	15–25	Expression of myeloid antigens, excellent outcome
t(1;19)(q23;p13) *TCF3-PBX1*	2–6	Increased incidence in blacks, generally excellent prognosis, association with CNS relapse
t(9;22)(q34;q11.2) *BCR-ABL1*	2–4	Historically dismal outcome, improved with addition of imatinib to intensive chemotherapy
PAX5 rearrangement	~2%	Multiple partners, commonly from dic(7;9), dic/t(9;12) and dic(9;20), outcome unknown
ABL1, PDGFRB, JAK2 rearrangements	2–5	Multiple rearrangements encoding chimeric proteins fusing 5' partners with 3' kinase domains. Associated with *IKZF1* alteration and very high leukocyte count, potentially amenable to tyrosine kinase inhibitor therapy
t(4;11)(q21;q23) *MLL-AF4*	1–2	Common in infant ALL (especially <6 months of age), poor prognosis
t(8;14)(q24;q32), t(2;8)(q12;q24), t(2;8)(q12;q24); *MYC* rearrangement	2	Favourable prognosis with short term high-dose chemotherapy
CRLF2 rearrangement (*IGH-CRLF2*; PAR1 deletion and *P2RY8-CRLF2*)	5–7	Extremely common in Down syndrome ALL (55%); association with *IKZF1* deletion/mutation and *JAK1/2* mutation and poor prognosis in non-Down syndrome ALL
ERG deletion	7	Defines a novel subtype of B-ALL with distinct gene expression profile; favourable outcome
T-lineage ALL		
t(1;7)(p32;q35), t(1;14)(p32;q11) and interstitial 1p32 deletion *TAL1* dysregulation	15–18	Generally favourable outcome
t(11;14)(p15;q11) and 5' *LMO2* deletion; LMO2 dysregulation	10	Generally favourable outcome
t(10;14)(q24;q11) and t(7;10)(q35;q24); *TLX1 [HOX11]* dysregulation	7	Good prognosis
t(5;14)(q35;q32); *TLX3*	20	Commonly fused to *BCL11B*, also a target of deletion/mutation in T-ALL. Poor prognosis
t(10;11)(p13;q14); *PICALM-MLLT10 [CALM-AF10]*	10	May have poor outcome
MLL-MLLT1 [MLL-ENL]	2–3	Superior prognosis to other *MLL*-rearranged leukaemias
NUP214-ABL1	6	Potentially amenable to tyrosine kinase inhibitors, also identified in high-risk B-ALL; other kinase fusions identified in T-ALL include *EML1-ABL1, ETV6-JAK2, ETV6-AL1*
t(7;9)(q34;q34)	<1%	Rearrangement of *NOTCH1*, mutated in >50% T-ALL
Early T-cell precursor	12	Immature immunophenotype, expression of myeloid and/or stem cell markers, very poor outcome. Underlying genetic alterations unknown; *MEF2C* dysregulation.

microarray analysis and second-generation sequencing (whole genome, exome, and transcriptome sequencing) demonstrated that near haploid and low hypodiploid ALL have distinct transcriptomic signatures and submicroscopic DNA copy number alterations and sequence mutations differ from other B-ALL subtypes [207]. Hypodiploid cells from both near-haploid and low hypodiploid cases exhibit activation of Ras-Raf-MEK-ERK and phosphatidylinositol-3-OH kinase (PI3K) signalling that is sensitive to PI3K and PI3K/mTOR inhibitors, suggesting that PI3K inhibition represents a therapeutic approach. An unexpected finding was that the *TP53* sequence mutations identified in low hypodiploid ALL are commonly present in matched non-tumour cells, suggesting germline inheritance. This has been confirmed in a limited number of kindreds, indicating that low hypodiploid ALL is a manifestation of Li-Fraumeni syndrome [207, 208]. Additional deleterious germline mutations were identified in other hypodiploid ALL cases, including activating mutations of *NRAS* and *PTPN11*.

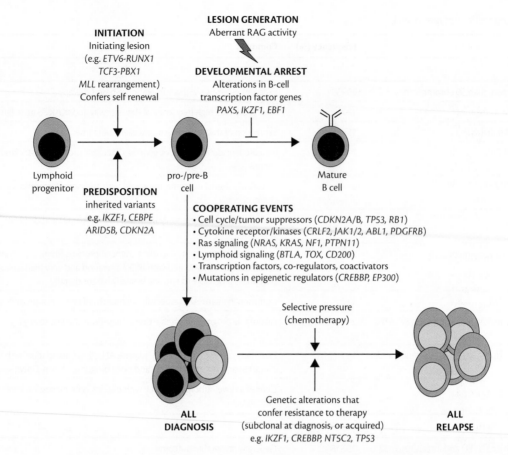

Fig. 51.8 Schema for the nature and timing of acquisitions of genetic alterations in the pathogenesis of B-ALL. Chromosomal rearrangements are acquired early in leukaemogenesis, and drive transcriptional and epigenetic dysregulation and aberrant self-renewal. These lesions and/or secondary genetic alterations disrupt lymphoid development and result in an arrest in maturation. Additional genetic alterations target cellular pathways including cell cycle regulation, tumour suppression, cytokine receptor and kinase signalling, and chromatin modification. Diagnosis ALL samples are commonly clonally heterogeneous, and genetic alterations in minor clones may confer resistance to therapy and promote relapse. A similar schema can be proposed for T-ALL, where lesions targeting lymphoid development, self-renewal, and kinase signalling are also observed; and in which there are multiple targets of mutation of unknown role in leukemogenesis (e.g., PHF6, WT1).

t(12;21)(p13;q22) *ETV6-RUNX1* acute lymphoblastic leukemia

The t(12;21)(p13;q22) rearrangement is identified in about 25–30% of childhood BCP-ALL cases [209–211], but is uncommon in adults with ALL (1–4%) [212–215]. The t(12;21) is usually cryptic on cytogenetic analysis and may be identified by fluorescence in situ hybridization (FISH) or molecular assays [216]. This translocation fuses the *ETV6* gene (encoding ETS variant 6, or TEL) at 12p13 to the runt-related transcription factor 1 (*RUNX1*, formerly *AML1*) gene at 21q22, resulting in expression of the *ETV6-RUNX1* chimeric fusion [217, 218]. *ETV6-RUNX1* positive childhood ALL has a favourable outcome, with overall survival of approximately 88% [209, 210, 225, 226]. Recent data indicates that relapse is rare with contemporary risk-directed therapy [226]. The rearrangement commonly arises in utero [227–229], but the prolonged latency to overt leukaemia [219–224] together with twin studies [229] suggest that additional genetic events are needed for the development of overt leukaemia. In addition, screening of normal cord blood has shown that the *ETV6-RUNX1* fusion gene is present at up to a 100-fold higher incidence than the corresponding risk of the leukaemia [230], although the exact frequency of this fusion in neonatal studies has varied among studies [231]. Taken together, these data suggest that additional secondary genetic events are required for the development of leukaemia [232–246].

t(1;19)(p13;q22) [*TCF3-PBX1*]

The t(1;19)(p13;q22) results in the *TCF3-PBX1* fusion gene that is present in about 5% of childhood and about 3–6% of adult ALL cases, with a higher incidence in younger adults and African-American ancestry [247– 249]. *TCF3-PBX1* ALL was originally considered a high-risk leukaemia that often presented with central nervous system involvement and an increased risk of relapse [250–254]. With intensified protocols, the presence of a *TCF3-PBX1* fusion gene stratifies the patient to a standard-risk protocol, but the presence of the *TCF3/PBX1* fusion gene is still an independent risk factor for CNS relapse [255, 256].

11q23/*MLL* gene rearrangements

Rearrangements of the mixed lineage leukaemia (or myeloid lymphoid leukaemia; *MLL*) gene at chromosome band 11q23 are common in acute leukaemia, in particular among infants where >70% carry a rearrangement of the *MLL* gene [257–259]. *MLL* rearrangements are seen in all ages and in both lymphoid and myeloid leukaemias and are present in 1–3% of childhood ALL [260–262], 15–20% of childhood AML cases [263–265], and in 4–9% of adult leukaemia cases [266–269]. In addition, *MLL* rearrangements are associated with secondary leukaemias in patients previously treated with topoisomerase inhibitors [270–272]. The prognosis of *MLL*-rearranged infant leukaemia is poor with an event-free survival of only 22–48% [273–276]. Among older children with ALL, the event-free survival is 42–65%, with the t(4;11) and t(9;11) being associated with a worse prognosis [273, 277–284]. Over 121 fusion partners of *MLL* have been reported [285], however five account for around 80% of the *MLL* leukaemias, including t(4;11)(q21;q23) (*MLL-AFF1* (*MLL-AF4*)), t(9;11)(p22;q23) (*MLL-MLLT3* (*MLL-AF9*)), t(11;19)(q23;p13.3) (*MLL-MLLT1* (*MLL-ENL*)), t(10;11)(p12;q23) (*MLL-MLLT10* (*MLL-AF10*)), and t(6;11)(q27;q23) (*MLL-MLLT4* (*MLL-AF6*)). For accurate diagnosis of *MLL*-rearrangements, a combination of genetic and molecular genetic analyses is needed and includes cytogenetic analysis, FISH, Southern blot, and/or RT-PCR for specific fusion genes.

MLL-rearranged childhood leukaemias are characterized by early acquisition of *MLL* rearrangement (in utero for most childhood cases), lymphoid and myeloid features, and poor outcome. *MLL*-rearranged leukaemias are also exceptional in the spectrum of childhood ALL cases for the paucity of additional DNA copy number alterations and sequence mutations, with the exception of Ras mutations [188, 286–319]. New and targeted therapies for *MLL*-rearranged leukaemias are being actively pursued due to the aggressiveness of this form of leukaemia. One promising target is the methyltransferase DOT1L which interacts directly or indirectly with several of the *MLL* fusion partners [320–324]. Selective killing of *MLL*-rearranged leukaemic cells on exposure to a potent DOT1L inhibitor was recently shown [325]. DOT1L is required for successful transformation and maintenance of *MLL-MLLT3* (*AF9*) leukaemia in vivo [326]. In addition, inhibitors towards the protein-protein interaction between MLL fusion proteins and menin show promising result with reversal of the oncogenic activity of *MLL*-rearranged leukaemias [327].

t(9;22)(q34;q11.1) [*BCR-ABL1*] acute lymphoblastic leukemia

The t(9;22)(q34;q11.1) rearrangement results in the formation of the Philadelphia chromosome and is seen in most cases of CML, in 25% of adult ALL and in 3–5% of paediatric ALL [213, 328–331]. The Philadelphia (Ph) chromosome was first identified by Nowell and Hungerford in 1960, and was subsequently shown by Janet Rowley in 1973 to be the product of a reciprocal chromosomal translocation between chromosome 9 and 22 [178]. This rearrangement results in fusion of the human homolog of the Abelson murine leukaemia virus, *ABL1*, at 9q34 to a 5.8kb region of the Breakpoint Cluster Region (*BCR*) gene at 22q11 [332–334]. The *BCR* gene encodes a serine/threonine kinase and *ABL1* encodes a protein structurally similar to the Src family of kinases. The leukemogenic properties of BCR-ABL1 are dependent upon the constitutive activity of ABL1. Multiple signalling pathways have been shown to become activated upon transformation by BCR-ABL1 including RAS/MAPK, STAT, PI3K, JNK/SAPK, and NF-κB [335]. In addition, BCR-ABL1 results in deregulation of apoptosis, differentiation, and cell adhesion.

The majority of Ph+ALL cases have additional secondary aberrations present at diagnosis including gain of a second copy of the Ph chromosome, a hyperdiploid karyotype, or −7/7q- [336]. Thus, in cases with a hyperdiploid karyotype it is important to identify the Ph chromosome so the patient receives appropriate treatment with tyrosine kinase inhibitors. The *BCR-ABL1* fusion gene is present in 3–5% of paediatric ALL and is associated with and older age (median age of about eight years), a high incidence of CNS involvement at diagnosis, a high leukocyte count, a pseudodiploid karyotype, resistance to therapy, and adverse outcome [328, 329]. Prior to the advent of tyrosine kinase inhibitor therapy, the outcome of *BCR-ABL1*-positive leukaemia was poor with a three-year event-free survival of about 25–30% [328–330, 337–342]. However, the introduction of imatinib mesylate [343] has transformed the prognosis of this leukaemia. The combination of intensive chemotherapy and imatinib resulted in improved event-free survival of 80% [344]. More potent second generation kinase inhibitors such as dasatinib and nilotinib may potentially further improve outcomes [345, 346].

CRLF2 rearrangements and Janus kinase mutations in acute lymphoblastic leukaemia

The cytokine receptor gene *CRLF2* is rearranged or mutated in approximately 7% of childhood B-ALL (Figure 51.8), and 50% of cases are associated with Down's syndrome (DS-ALL) [347–350]. *CRLF2* is located in the pseudoautosomal region (PAR1) at Xp22.3/Yp11.3 and encodes cytokine receptor-like factor 2 (also known as thymic stromal lymphopoietin receptor, TSLPR). With the interleukin-7 receptor alpha peptide, CRLF2 forms a heterodimeric receptor for TSLP (thymic stromal lymphopoietin). CRLF2 is rearranged by translocation into the immunoglobulin heavy chain locus (*IGH-CRLF2*), or by a focal deletion upstream of *CRLF2* that result in expression of *P2RY8-CRLF2* that encodes full-length CRLF2. Both rearrangements result in aberrant over-expression of CRLF2 on the cell surface of leukaemic lymphoblasts that may be detected by immunophenotyping [349].

Approximately half of *CRLF2*-rearranged ALL cases harbour activating mutations of the Janus kinase genes *JAK1* or *JAK2* [348, 349, 351], which with the exception of T-lineage ALL are otherwise uncommon in ALL [352, 353]. The JAK mutations are most commonly missense mutations at or near p.Arg683 in the pseudokinase domain of JAK2. *CRLF2*-rearranged leukemic cells exhibit activation of JAK-STAT and PI3K/mTOR pathways, and are sensitive to JAK and mTOR inhibitors in vitro and in vivo [354–360]. The activity of the JAK inhibitor ruxolitinib in childhood B-ALL cases with JAK-STAT activating lesions, including *CRLF2*-rearrangements, is being evaluated in clinical trials.

In non-DS ALL, *CRLF2* alterations and JAK mutations are associated with *IKZF1* deletion/mutation and poor outcome, particularly in cohorts of high-risk B-ALL [361–364]. *CRLF2* and *IKZF1* alterations are associated with inferior outcome in multiple cohorts, and elevated *CRLF2* expression in the absence of rearrangement is also an adverse prognostic feature [365].

'BCR-ABL1-like' or 'Ph-like' acute lymphoblastic leukaemia

Recently, a new subtype of B-ALL has been described in which leukemic cells lack expression of BCR-ABL1, but exhibits a leukaemic cell gene expression profile similar to Ph-positive ALL and like Ph-positive ALL commonly harbours deletion or mutation of *IKZF1* [366, 367]. BCR-ABL1-like, or Ph-like ALL comprises up to 10–15% of childhood B-ALL, and up to one-third of B-ALL in adolescents and young adults, and is associated with poor outcome [368, 369]. Approximately half of BCR-ABL1-like ALL cases harbour *CRLF2* rearrangements and concomitant JAK1/2 mutations. Transcriptome and whole genome sequencing has shown that non-*CRLF2*-rearranged Ph-like ALL cases harbour a diverse range of genomic alterations that activate cytokine receptors and tyrosine kinases including *ABL1*, *ABL2*, *CSF1R*, *EPOR*, *JAK2* and *PDGFRB* [370]. These alterations are most commonly chromosomal rearrangements resulting in chimeric fusion genes deregulating tyrosine kinases (e.g. *NUP214-ABL1*, *ETV6-ABL1*, *RANBP2-ABL1*, *RCSD1-ABL1*, *BCR-JAK2*, *PAX5-JAK2*, *STRN3-JAK2* and *EBF1-PDGFRB*) and cytokine receptors (*IGH-EPOR*). Up to 20% of BCR-ABL1-like cases lack a chimeric fusion, and additional alterations activating kinase signalling, including activating mutations of *FLT3* and *IL7R*, and focal deletions of *SH2B3*, or LNK, which constrains JAK signalling [371], have been identified in fusion-negative cases. These diverse genetic alterations activate a limited number of signalling pathways, notably *ABL1* and *PDGFRB* and JAK-STAT signalling, and it is predicted that the majority of BCR-ABL-like ALL cases will be amenable to therapy with a limited number of tyrosine kinase inhibitors: imatinib-class TKIs for *ABL1*, *ABL2*, *CSF1R*, and *PDGFRB* rearrangements, and JAK inhibitors such as ruxolitinib for alterations activating JAK-STAT signalling (*EPOR*, *IL7R*, *JAK2*, and *SH2B3*). These rearrangements have been shown to activate signalling pathways in model cell lines and in primary leukaemic cells [360, 370], and xenografts of BCR-ABL1-like ALL are highly sensitive to TKIs in vivo. There are also multiple anecdotal reports of responsiveness of refractory BCR-ABL1-like ALL to appropriate TKI therapy, for example *EBF1-PDGFRB* ALL to imatinib [372, 373].

B-progenitor ALL with intrachromosomal amplification of chromosome 21 (iAMP21)

iAMP21 is characterized by gain of at least three copies of a (usually large) region of 21 that always includes *RUNX1* [374–376]. The presence of iAMP21 is generally associated with unfavourable outcome, although this is mitigated with intensive chemotherapy [377].

ERG-altered acute lymphoblastic leukaemia

While many of the recurrent focal deletions observed in ALL are observed in multiple ALL subtypes, a notable exception is alteration of the ETS-family transcription factor *ERG* (ETS-related gene), which occurs exclusively in cases lacking known chromosomal rearrangements and is a hallmark of a novel subtype of B-ALL with a distinct gene expression profile [378]. Such cases frequently express a truncated form of ERG. Notably, despite the presence of *IKZF1* alterations in a proportion of *ERG*-deregulated cases, the outcome of this subtype of ALL is favourable [362, 379, 380].

Submicroscopic genetic alterations in B-lineage acute lymphoblastic leukaemia

Microarray-based profiling of DNA copy number alterations permits the identification of DNA copy number alterations (deletions and gains) at sub-kilobase resolution. Widely-used platforms include single-nucleotide polymorphism microarrays that also permit interrogation of copy-neutral loss-of-heterozygosity (LOH, also known as acquired somatic uniparental disomy), and array-based comparative genomic hybridization (array-CGH) [381]. From 2007, microarray profiling studies, and subsequently, genome sequencing studies have shown that while ALL genomes typically harbour fewer structural alterations than many solid tumours, over 50 recurring deletions or amplifications have been identified many of which involve a single gene or few genes (details are included in Table 51.6 and Figure 51.8) [188, 382–384].

Many of the focal deletions in ALL genomes arise from aberrant activity of the recombinase activating gene (RAG) enzymes. The RAG enzymes normally mediate productive rearrangement of the lymphoid antigen receptors, and recognize conserved motifs (heptamers, spacers, and nonamers) in order to juxtapose members of the antigen receptor variable, diversity and joining (V, D, and J) gene families [385, 386]. The terminal deoxynucleotidyl transferase (TdT) enzyme adds additional nucleotides between the antigen receptor segments to further increase diversity. Sequencing of the genomic breakpoints of recurring deletions in ALL (e.g., *PAX5*, *BTG1*, *IKZF1*, and *NF1*) has demonstrated partly- or fully-conserved heptamer recognition sequences immediately within the deletion breakpoints, and additional non-template nucleotides between the flanking genomic regions [188, 207, 337, 387, 388]. Moreover, many of the targets of deletion in ALL are expressed during B lymphoid ontogeny. These observations, and high level of RAG gene expression in several subtypes of BCR-ALL, such as *ETV6-RUNX1* ALL, suggest that aberrant RAG-mediated deletion of developmentally regulated genes in B cell precursors confers a selective advantage to preleukaemic clones harboring founding translocations (such as *ETV6-RUNX1*, or *BCR-ABL1*) and are co-operating lesions in leukaemogenesis. Consistent with this notion, experimental BCP-ALL generated in *Rag* null mice exhibit a dearth of secondary focal genomic alterations [389]. This hypothesis provides a potential explanation for the observation that focal deletions are uncommon in subtypes of leukaemia that exhibit low RAG activity, such as *MLL*-rearranged leukaemia [286, 287, 390] and AML [391–393].

The nature and frequency of genetic lesions are subtype-dependent. *MLL*-rearranged leukaemias harbour very few additional structural or sequence alterations [188, 287, 390]. In contrast, the majority of non-*MLL* ALL cases harbour recurring submicroscopic deletions, for example at least six to eight per case in *ETV6-RUNX1* and *BCR-ABL1* ALL [188, 236, 337].

Alteration of transcription factor genes in B-lineage acute lymphoblastic leukaemia

Deletion, sequence mutation, or rearrangement of genes encoding transcriptional regulators of lymphoid development is a hallmark of B-ALL. Alteration of *PAX5* (~35%), *IKZF1* (~15%), and *EBF1* (~5%) are the most common alterations, with at least two-thirds of B-ALL cases harbouring one or more lesions in this pathway [188, 394]. These alterations are usually loss of function or dominant negative lesions that result in arrested lymphoid maturation, which is characteristic of leukaemic cells. Notably, while *PAX5* alterations are the most common genetic alteration in B-ALL, they are not associated with outcome [394, 395]. In contrast, alteration of *IKZF1* (IKAROS) is a hallmark of high-risk ALL, particularly BCR-ABL1-positive ALL [337, 338, 396], and BCR-ABL1-like (Ph-like) ALL [366, 367, 370]. *IKZF1* encodes IKAROS, the founding member of a family of zinc finger transcription factors that is required for the development of all lymphoid lineages [397]. The *IKZF1* alterations include focal or broad deletions that result in loss of expression of IKZF1, and deletions of coding exons 4–7 that remove the N-terminal DNA-binding zinc fingers, leading to expression of a dominant negative isoform, IK6. *IKZF1* alterations are present in over 70% of *BCR-ABL1* lymphoid leukaemia, including de novo ALL and CML at progression to lymphoid blast crisis [337], and are associated with poor outcome in both BCR-ABL1-positive ALL and BCR-ABL1-negative B-ALL [361, 365, 366, 396, 398–407]. Experimental data support a role of alterations of these B-lineage transcriptional factor alterations in leukaemogenesis. Deletion of *Pax5* and *Ikzf1* accelerates the onset of leukaemia in retroviral BM transplant and transgenic models of

Table 51.6 Key submicroscopic genetic alterations in ALL

Gene	Alteration	Frequency	Pathway and consequences of alteration	Clinical relevance	References
PAX5	Focal deletions, translocations, sequence mutations	31.7% of B-ALL	Transcription factor required for B-lymphoid development. Mutations impair DNA binding and transcriptional activation		[188, 337, 383]
IKZF1	Focal deletions or sequence mutations	15% of all paediatric B-ALL cases.	Transcription factor required for development of HSC to lymphoid precursor. Deletions and mutations result in loss of function or dominant negative isoforms		[188]
IKZF1		Over 80% BCR-ABL1 ALL and 66% CML in lymphoid blast crisis		Associated with poor outcome	[337, 338, 396]
IKZF1		One-third of high-risk BCR-ABL1 negative ALL		Tripling in CIR	[367, 394, 399]
IKZF1	Inherited variants			Increased risk of ALL	[539, 540]
JAK1/2	Pseudokinase and kinase domain mutations	18–35% DS-ALL and 10.7% High-risk BCR-ABL1-ALL	Constitutive JAK-STAT activation. Transforms mouse Ba/F3-EpoR lymphoid haematopoietic cell line.		[356–358]
CRLF2	Rearrangement as IGH-CRLF2 or P2RY8-CRLF2 resulting in over-expression	5–16% paediatric and adult B-ALL, and >50% DS-ALL 50% of BCR-ABL1-like ALL	Associated with mutant JAK in up to 50% of cases. CRLF2 mutations and JAK mutations cotransforming in Ba/F3 cells and results in constitutive STAT activation.		[348, 349, 351]
CRLF2		14% paediatric high-risk ALL	Associated with IKZF1 alteration and JAK mutations	Associated with poor outcome	[361, 363]
Kinase and signalling alterations	Rearrangements of ABL1, ABL2, CSF1R, EPOR, JAK2, PDGFRB; sequence mutations of IL7R and FLT3, deletions of SH2B3	10% childhood B-ALL, up to 30% ALL in adult ALL. Associated with BCR-ABL1-like gene expression profile.	Activate kinase signalling pathways and amenable to tyrosine kinase inhibitor therapy	Associated with high risk features and increased risk of relapse. Anecdotal reports of response to TKI therapy	[366, 368, 370, 372, 373]
CREBBP	Focal deletion and sequence mutations	19% of relapsed ALL. Also mutated in non-Hodgkin lymphoma	Mutations result in impaired histone acetylation and transcriptional regulation.	Mutations selected for at relapse, and associated with glucocorticoid resistance.	[199]
NT5C2	Focal mutations	Up to 20% relapsed mutation	Mutations confer resistance to nucleoside analogies	Mutations selected at relapse	[531, 532]
TP53	Deletions and focal mutations	Hallmark of low hypodiploid ALL at diagnosis; 50% of which are inherited. Otherwise uncommon in major clone at diagnosis. Associated with disease relapse			[522, 524, 525]

BCR-ABL1 ALL, and in chemical and retroviral models of leukaemia [408, 409].

Chromosomal rearrangements in T-lineage acute lymphoblastic leukaemia

T-ALL is characterized by an older age of onset than B-ALL, male sex preponderance, and inferior outcome in comparison to B-ALL [410]. Chromosomal abnormalities and rearrangements are evident on cytogenetic analysis in up to 70% of T-ALL cases, and commonly involve one of the T-cell antigen receptor loci, including TRA and TRD at 14q11, TRB at 7q34 and TRG at 7p14. These rearrangements occur in approximately one-third of T-ALL cases, but may be cryptic on cytogenetic analysis. These rearrangements may arise from aberrant antigen receptor gene recombination mistakes in the normal recombination process involved in the generation of functional antigen receptors [411]. The rearrangements in T-ALL commonly dysregulate transcription factor genes [412], including members of the bHLH family (MYC, TAL1, TAL2, LYL1, and BHLHB1) [413–419], genes encoding the LIM-only domain proteins (LMO1 and LMO2) [420–422], and homeodomain genes (HOX11, also known as

TLX1, and *HOX11L2*, also known as *TLX3*) [422–425]. Similar to BCP-ALL, T-ALL is also characterized by the presence of sub-microscopic deletions and sequence mutations, including activating mutations of *NOTCH1* [426], deletion/mutation of *PTEN* [427], *WT1* [428], *FBXW7* [429], and amplification of *MYB* [188, 430, 431].

TAL1 rearranged T-lineage acute lymphoblastic leukaemia

Alteration of *TAL1* (*SCL*, *TCL5*) at 1p32 is the most frequent transcription factor rearrangement in childhood T-ALL. This arises from either a t(1;14)(p32;q11) that occurs in 3% of cases and juxtaposes *TAL1* into the *TRA/TRD* locus [432–439], or the more frequent cryptic interstitial deletion at 1p32 that is present in approximately 15% of cases, and results in a chimeric *SIL-TAL1* fusion transcript [435, 439, 440]. Additional cases without these rearrangements express high *TAL1* mRNA levels [439, 441]. Less commonly, the *TAL2* gene is juxtaposed to the *TRB* locus as a result of a t(7;9)(q34;q32) rearrangement [417]. TAL1 and LYL1, over-expressed in T-cell leukaemias carrying the t(7;19), are members of the class II family of bHLH proteins and heterodimerize with class I bHLH proteins, such as TCF3 (E2A) [442, 443]. TAL1:TCF3 complexes have been detected in erythroid cells and T-cell leukaemias and bind DNA in a site-specific manner. Additional studies have shown that *Tal1* is required not only for erythropoiesis [444, 445], but also for the earliest steps in the lineage commitment of pluripotent embryonic haematopoietic stem cells [446, 447]. TAL1:TCF3 heterodimers are transcriptionally inactive [448, 449] and the observations that loss of TCF3 function induces T-cell leukaemia in mice [450, 451] and that the DNA-binding domain of TAL1 is dispensable for transformation support the notion that TAL1 mediates leukemogenesis through a dominant negative mechanism [452–460].

The homeobox family of transcription factors comprises two classes of genes. Class I HOX genes are in four clusters (*HOXA*, *HOXB*, *HOXC*, and *HOXD*), and class II genes are distributed throughout the genome. The HOX genes exert key roles in anteroposterior patterning, differentiation, and also regulation of haematopoiesis and leukaemogenesis [461–464]. Two HOX genes, *HOX11* and *HOX11L2*, are rearranged in T-ALL. Approximately 7% of childhood T-ALL cases have ectopic expression of *HOX11* arising from t(10;14)(q24;q11) and the variant t(7;10)(q35;q24) translocations that juxtaposes *HOX11* to the *TRA* or *TRB* loci [423, 424, 465, 466]. Approximately 20% of childhood T-ALL cases exhibit over-expression of *HOX11L2* [474–476], most commonly from a cryptic t(5;14)(q35;q32) rearrangement that juxtaposes *HOX11L2* to *BCL11B* (274), a zinc finger protein expressed during T-cell ontogeny, and recently identified as a target of deletion and somatic sequence mutation in T-ALL [467–473, 477–481]. *MLL* is rearranged in 4–8% of T-ALL cases, most commonly to *MLLT1* (*ENL*) [482]. This rearrangement is commonly observed in adolescents and has a superior prognosis to other *MLL*-rearranged leukaemias [483]. Other *MLL* fusions are occasionally seen. *MLL*-rearranged T-ALL represents a distinct biologic entity with a transcriptional profile that differs from other *MLL*-rearranged cases [441, 484].

The t(10;11)(p13;q14) rearrangement is observed in up to 10% of T-ALL cases, may be cytogenetically cryptic, and results in expression of the *PICALM-MLLT10* (*CALM-AF10*) fusion [485, 486]. Notably, both partner genes are infrequently fused to *MLL*, and like *MLL*-rearranged ALL, *PICALM-MLLT10* cases exhibit upregulation of *HOX* genes and *MEIS1*, suggesting common oncogenic pathways. This rearrangement is typically seen in γδT-ALL cases, either in immature or mature cells, and is associated with poor outcome [486–488]. Expression of the fusion in haematopoietic cells, either by retroviral transduction or as a transgene, results in the development of leukaemia, which is often myeloid in phenotype [489–491].

A substantial proportion of T-ALL lacks a known genetic alteration, and the genetic basis of these cases is poorly understood.

Early T-cell precursor acute lymphoblastic leukaemia

Early T-cell precursor (ETP) ALL is an aggressive subtype of immature leukaemia that is associated with very poor outcome [492–494]. Various laboratory criteria have been proposed to identify these immature cases, but the original definition utilized immunophenotypic criteria: the expression of T-lineage markers (e.g., cytoplasmic CD3) but lack of expression of markers otherwise characteristic of T-ALL, such as CD1a and CD8, weak or negative CD5 expression, and aberrant expression of myeloid and/or stem cell markers [492]. This pattern is reminiscent of the murine early T-cell precursor [495], the earliest stage of thymic T-cell maturation that retains lineage plasticity.

Whole genome sequencing (WGS) of tumour and matched non-tumour DNA of 12 ETP ALL cases, and mutation recurrence testing of selected genes in 94 additional ETP and non-ETP T-ALL cases, identified marked diversity in the frequency and nature of genetic alterations [353]. These included inactivating mutations targeting genes regulating hematopoietic and lymphoid development (e.g. *RUNX1*, *GATA3*), mutations activating cytokine receptor and kinase signaling (e.g. *IL7R*, *JAK1*, and *JAK3*), and loss of function mutations targeting epigenetic mutations, particularly genes encoding the polycomb repressor complex 2 (PRC2; *EZH2*, *SUZ12*, *EED*), that mediates histone 3 lysine 27 trimethylation [496–512].

Although similarly comprehensive studies of 'typical' T-ALL are awaited, recent studies have performed exome sequencing of T-ALL that have identified additional targets of mutation including *CNOT3*, a member of transcriptional regulatory complex, and ribosomal proteins [513]. To gain further insight into the male sex preponderance of T-ALL, Ferrando and colleagues performing targeted capture and sequencing of X chromosome genes, and identified sequence mutations and deletions of PHF6 in 16% and 38% of childhood and adult T-ALL, respectively [514]. The *PHF6* alterations result in loss of *PHF6* expression and are associated with *TLX1/3* and *TAL1* rearranged ALL [514, 515]. The role of PHF6 in leukaemogenesis is poorly understood, but has been shown to be a RNA-interacting protein and component of the nucleosome remodeling and deacetylation (NuRD) complex [516, 517]. Thus, PHF6 may have complex and multifactorial roles as a tumour suppressor.

Relapsed acute lymphoblastic leukaemia

Several chromosomal alterations such as *BCR-ABL1* and *MLL*-rearrangement are associated with a high risk of treatment failure; however, relapse occurs across the spectrum of ALL sub-types. It has also long been recognized that ALL genomes are not static but exhibit acquisition of chromosomal abnormalities over time [518]. There is thus great interest in genomic profiling of matched diagnosis and relapse samples to dissect the genetic basis of clonal heterogeneity in ALL, and the relationship of such heterogeneity to risk of relapse. SNP microarray profiling has demonstrated that the majority of ALL cases show changes in the patterns of structural genomic alterations from diagnosis to relapse [518–520], and that many relapse-acquired lesions, including *IKZF1* and *CDKN2A/B*, are present at low levels at diagnosis [519, 521].

Apart from low hypodiploid ALL, *TP53* mutations are uncommon in major clones at ALL diagnosis, but are associated with treatment failure and emerge in major clones at relapse [522–526]. Sequencing of 300 genes in matched diagnosis-relapse samples identified mutations in the transcriptional coactivator and histone and non-histone acetyl transferase CREBBP (CREB-binding protein, or CBP) as a relapse-acquired lesion in up to 20% of relapsed ALL samples [199, 527, 528]. CREBBP has an important role in mediating the transcriptional response to glucocorticoids [529, 530], and histone deacetylase inhibitors were active in steroid-resistant ALL cell lines [199]. Recently, two groups independently identified relapse-acquired mutations in the 5' nucleotidase gene *NT5C2* that confer increased resistance to purine analogues [531, 532]. Thus, mutations that confer resistance to drugs commonly used to treat ALL represent a key mechanism of treatment failure and resistance.

Germline genetic variation and acute lymphoblastic leukaemia risk

Inherited genetic variants are associated with the ALL, clinical features and outcome. These include common inherited polymorphisms that influence ALL risk. In addition [533, 534], several inherited germline mutations associated with segregation of ALL in kindreds have recently been reported [207, 535]. The risk to siblings of developing ALL is modest, and while the development of ALL in monozygotic twin pairs is well described, this may be explained by transmission of pre-leukaemic clones between twins rather than inherited predisposition [536]. A notable setting of increased risk of ALL is Down syndrome, which is associated with a markedly elevated risk of both ALL (~40-fold at age 0–4 years) and AML [537]. The reasons for this elevated risk are poorly understood, although somatic rearrangement of *CRLF2* is a hallmark of Down syndrome-associated ALL [349].

Multiple studies have used a case-control approach to associations between common inherited polymorphisms and ALL risk, initially with a candidate gene approach [538], and more recently with genome-wide association studies (GWAS) [534]. GWAS examine associations between hundreds of thousands to millions of inherited variants and a phenotype. Such studies typically examine hundreds to thousands of patients and ethnically-matched, require stringent p value thresholds to account for the large number of comparisons made, and verify findings by examining associated SNPs in one or more independent cohorts [539–546]. The associations between inherited single nucleotide variants and disease risk typically have modest effect sizes (odds rations of 1.5 or less), and it is likely that multiple variants together influence the risk of developing leukaemia. The most reproducible associations have been in four genes (*IKZF1*, *ARID5B*, *CEBPE*, and *CDKN2A*), three of which are involved by somatic genetic alterations in ALL (*IKZF1* by deletions and sequence mutations, *CEBPE* by rearrangement, and *CDKN2A/B* by deletion). IKZF1 and CEBPE are transcriptional regulators, and *CDKN2A/B* encodes the INK4/ARF family of tumour suppressors and cell cycle regulators, suggesting that the associated variants may influence gene expression and leukaemogenesis. In addition, specific variants are associated with ALL risk and outcome in specific ethnic groups (*ARID5B*) and with specific subtypes of ALL (*GATA3* and Ph-like ALL). Thus, it is likely that inherited genetic variants and somatic genetic alterations together drive leukaemogenesis.

Deleterious germline mutations are also implicated in both sporadic and familial ALL. Whole genome sequencing of hypodiploid ALL identified germline *TP53* mutations in approximately half of low hypodiploid ALL cases, as well as germline variants were identified in the Ras pathway genes *NRAS* and *PTPN11*. A number of additional novel variants were identified that were predicted to be deleterious and that involved key cellular pathways, particularly DNA damage and repair.

Familial ALL is uncommon, but such kindreds may be exceptionally informative in enabling the discovery of germline variations or mutations that influence the risk of developing ALL. A recent example is the identification of a novel *PAX5* sequence mutations, p.Gly183Ser in three unrelated kindreds with autosomal dominant ALL [535, 547]. Somatic *PAX5* sequence mutations are common in B-ALL, and typically involve the DNA-binding paired domain (and interfere with binding of PAX5 to its DNA targets) or the C-terminal transactivating domain. The Ser183 mutation is otherwise rare in ALL and involves the octapeptide domain. This mutation results in partial loss of transcriptional activation, and may act by impeding interaction between PAX5 and cofactors that enhance PAX5 activity. All patients with this mutation exhibited loss of the *PAX5* wild-type gene by deletion of chromosome 9p, indicating that transmission of this mutation is tolerable in the heterozygous state, but severe attenuation of PAX5 activity is required for leukemogenesis. Germline mutations in a second transcription factor gene, *ETV6*, have also been identified in several kindreds with familial ALL.

Management of acute lymphoblastic leukaemia, including transplantation

The outcome of therapy for ALL has improved over the past two decades, particularly in the paediatric population [548–556]. With the exception of those over 60 years, the reported survival rates from US registry data significantly improved over a twenty-year period [556]. The improvement in survival can be attributed to multiple factors: more precise risk stratification leading to risk-adapted therapeutic approaches, improved techniques for monitoring residual disease, better understanding of leukaemic and host cell pharmacokinetics and -genetics, improved supportive care, and the advent of some novel targeted treatment strategies. As a result, the current overall CR rate is about 95%, the estimated five-year OS rate is over 85% and the cure rate approaching 90% in paediatric ALL [548–558]. However, treating adults remains challenging with a greater frequency of higher-risk cytogenetic profiles, larger proportion of drug-resistant disease, and poorer tolerance of therapy.

Concepts of treatment

Leukaemic cell expansion adopts a Gompertzian growth curve with near exponential growth [559]. The primary aim of induction therapy is to induce cytological remission thereby allowing normal haematopoiesis with the least adverse events. The second aim is to offer adequate prophylactic therapy to sanctuary sites such as the central nervous system (CNS). Although specific treatment regimens, drug and dosing schedules, and treatment duration across different age groups and ALL subtypes differ, the basic principles are similar. The standard therapeutic approach for de novo ALL consists of an intensive chemotherapy framework starting with remission induction, followed by consolidation/

intensification, then maintenance. The majority of these treatment regimens are modifications of those originally developed by the Berlin-Frankfurt-Munster (BFM) Group for paediatric patients, later adopted in adults [559]. Although CR rates are similar, retrospective studies have consistently shown that event-free survival rates (EFS) among the adolescents and young adults (AYA) treated on paediatric protocols were substantially higher than those of the same age group treated according to adult protocols [560–568]. Comparative retrospective studies attributed this to earlier and more intensive CNS prophylaxis and/or higher cumulative doses of non-myelosuppressive agents in paediatric-inspired protocols [560, 562, 564] (Table 51.7). These findings partly explain the greatest statistically significant improvement in survival [553, 556] noted among such groups particularly the 15–19 years age bracket [556]. Hence, AYA ALL patients should be treated, at least initially, with intensive 'paediatric-inspired' regimens. The feasibility of the 'paediatric' approach in the 'older' adults remains to be determined. Poor tolerance and significant toxicities [562] result in both treatment delays and treatment-related deaths, both being major reasons for poor outcome in this age group [569]. In regimens designed specifically for older patients, the average CR rate

Table 51.7 Comparison of selected retrospective analytic studies involving AYA ALL patients

Study Group	N	Age (median)	Ph+ (%)	T-cell (%)	CR (%)	OS	EFS	Relapse rate (%)
CCG * vs	197	16–20	3	16	90	67% at 7 years	63% at 7 years	17.9 (1% for isolated CNS relapse)
CALGB [564]	124	16–20 (19)	6	25	90	46% at 7 years	34% at 7 years	N/S (11% for isolated CNS relapse)
MRC ALL97* vs	61	15–17	8	22	98	71% at 5 years	65% at 5 years	24.6
UKALLXII/ECOG 2993 [566]	67	15–17	3	11	94	56% at 5 years	49% at 5 years	28.4
FRALLE-93* vs	77	15–19.7 (15.9)	1.3	23	94	77% at 6 years	67% at 5 years	14.3
LALA-94 [560]	100	15.2–20 (17.9)	3	28	83	40% at 6 years	41% at 5 years	38
GRAALL-2003* vs	214	15–55 (31)	N/A	35	93.5	61% at 42 months	57% at 42 months	31 at 42 months
LALA-94 [562]	712	15–55 (29)	N/S	35	88	41% at 42 months	33% at 42 months	55 at 42 months
AIEOP* vs	150	14–17 (15)	1.3	22	97	81% at 2 years (77% at 10 years)[22]	78% at 2 years (75% at 10 years)[22]	16
GIMEMA [565]	92	14–17 (16)	4.3	25	89	71% at 2 years	47% at 2 years	43
NOPHO-92* vs	144	10–18 (13)	5	31	99	N/S	66% at 5 years	N/S
Swedish Adult ALL Group [567]	50	15–25 (21)	8	4	90	N/S	42% at 5 years	N/S
NOPHO* vs	128	10–17.7 (12.9)	N/S	16	96	77	67% at 5 years	26
Finnish Leukemia Group [568]	97	15.7–25.5 (18.9)	N/S	19	97	70	60% at 5 years	31

*denotes paediatric-inspired regimens.

Abbreviations: Ph+, Philadelphia chromosome-positive; CR, Complete remission; OS, overall survival; EFS, event-free survival; CCG, Children's Cancer Group; CALGB, Cancer and Leukemia Group B Study; MRC ALL97, Medical Research Council ALL 97; FRALLE-93, French Group for childhood ALL-93; LALA94, Leucémie Aiguë Lymphoblastique de l'Adulte 94; GRAALL, Group for Research on Adult Acute Lymphoblastic Leukemia; AIEOP, Italian Association of Pediatric Hematology and Oncology; GIMEMA, Gruppo Italiano Malattie Ematologiche dell'Adulto; NOPHO, Nordic Society of Pediatric Hematology and Oncology; N/A, not applicable; N/S, not stated; N, number of patients.

Table 51.8 Outcomes from prospective trials in Ph⁻older ALL patients

Study	N	Age (median)	CR (%)	Induction death (%)	Induction failure	EFS	OS	Relapse Rate
MRC UKALLXII/ ECOG2993 [571]	67	55–65	N/S	N/S	N/S	22% at 5 years	N/S	N/S
PETHEMA ALL-96 [572]	33	56–77 (65)	57.6	36.4	6	46% at 2 years	39% at 2 years	15
GMALL [573	146	55–81 (67)	73	18	8	N/S	24 at 4 years	N/S
EWALL [574]	54	56–73 (66)	85	0	15	N/S	61% at 1 year	20
GRAALL-SA1 [575]								
◆ Arm 1	31	55–77 (68)	90	7	3	35% at 2 years	35% at 2 years	45
◆ Arm 2	29	60–80 (66)	72	10	17	24% at 2 years	24% at 2 years	48

Abbreviations: MRC UKALL/ECOG2993, Medical Research Council UK ALL/Eastern Cooperative Oncology Group 2993; PETHEMA ALL-96, Programa para el Estudio de la Terape´utica en Hemopatia Maligna ALL-96; GMALL, German Multicenter ALL; EWALL, European Working Group on ALL; GRAALL-SA1, Group for Research on Adult Acute Lymphocytic Leukemia Study.

is 71% (43–90%) and survival rate is 33% (16–71%) [570–575]. Table 51.8 summarizes selected prospective trials for Philadelphia chromosome-negative (Ph⁻) older ALL patients.

Remission induction chemotherapy

The initial phase of therapy involves the administration of a multi-drug regimen typically based on a backbone of a steroid, vincristine, and an anthracycline, with or without asparaginase and/or cyclophosphamide [563, 576–579]. Whilst prednisolone was the 'traditional' steroid used, several randomized studies comparing it with dexamethasone as part of induction therapy, in paediatric ALL patients dexamethasone significantly decreased CNS relapse rate, improved EFS outcomes [580–582], significantly reduced risk of events (death from any cause, refractory or relapsed leukaemia, or second malignancy) [583], and improved overall outcome [584]. This is attributed, in part, to better CNS penetration of dexamethasone [585]. Anthracyclines have been an integral part of remission induction chemotherapy with CR rates and median remission duration superior in those receiving compared to those who did not [586, 587]. Whilst the most frequently used is daunorubicin, there is no difference in anthracycline dosing or schedule [587–589]. Attempts at dose escalation in adults were not associated with improved outcome [590] although in paediatric setting dose reduction was associated with improved outcome [591]. Another fundamental component of ALL induction and consolidation therapy is L-asparaginase (L-Asp), currently available in several formulations with different pharmacologic and immunogenic properties [592]. Increased dose intensity of L-Asp as opposed is associated with significant improvement in EFS and reduced risk of haematologic and CNS relapses in paediatric patients [593, 594]. Currently there is growing evidence supporting its potential for improved survival in adult patients [595, 596]. The pegylated form of Escherichia coli L-Asp (PEG-Asp) has widely replaced the native formulation due to its convenient administration route, less frequent dosing, and less immunogenicity [592, 597]; the latter may or may not (referred to as silent hypersensitivity and subsequent silent inactivation [598]) result in hypersensitivity reactions [592]. Cross-reactivity between anti-asparaginase neutralizing antibodies against the two E coli forms has been reported [597]. These can be clinically significant as they result not only in decreased asparaginase activity

[599] but also in higher dexamethasone clearance, which in turn was reported to be associated with higher risk of any relapse [600]. To overcome this, Erwinia L-Asp can be used as there is no cross-reactivity between antibodies [601] and its use did not negatively impact EFS outcome [602]. The most notable L-asp-related toxicities include hepatotoxicity, pancreatitis, and coagulopathy, particularly associated with a high rate of thrombosis. Adverse events can be severe (i.e., grade 3–4) [603], are more frequent in older patients [604, 605], and results in difficult decisions regarding the continuation of the drug. Management of thrombosis is difficult, but continuation of L-asp therapy with anticoagulation and antithrombin replacement is a reasonable strategy [606].

Consolidation/intensification chemotherapy

Consolidation/intensification, is aimed at eliminating any potential residual leukaemic cells. This, too, involves a combination of drugs fundamentally similar to those used during the induction phase, with one or two re-induction blocks but with the addition other agents including methotrexate, cytarabine, mercaptopurine, and high-dose L-asp given for an extended period. There is no consensus on the optimum regimen or duration. A number of therapeutic strategies however have been noted to impact either outcome measures or pharmacodynamic profiles. For example, altering the dose of dexamethasone during delayed intensification appeared to reduce the incidence of osteonecrosis in paediatric patients [607]. Paediatric patients with B cell ALL who received L-asp intensification had significantly higher EFS than those who did not (71% vs 31% at a median follow-up of 9.4 years) [608]. Higher doses of methotrexate appear to improve outcome of patient with T-cell ALL [609] and patients with TCF3-PBX1 fusion [610] as blast cells in these subtypes accumulate lower levels of methotrexate polyglutamates than B-cell ALL and those without the genetic abnormality, respectively [610].

Maintenance chemotherapy

The majority of maintenance regimens include a core of daily mercaptopurine and weekly low-dose methotrexate with periodic addition of steroids and vincristine for a total duration of two to three years. This phase is crucial—attempts at omitting or shortening it were associated with inferior outcome in B-ALL but it may be less significant in T-cell precursor ALL [611]. Dose adjustment to the limits of haematologic tolerance has been associated with improved outcome [612]. Polymorphisms in function and expression of drug metabolizing genes are well described and have influenced treatment responses [613]. One of the most widely studied is thiopurine methyltransferase (TPMT) gene polymorphism. TPMT is the enzyme that catalyzes S-methylation of thiopurines to its inactive forms. Patients with TPMT deficiency are at risk of thiopurine-induced haematologic toxicity and lately noted to be at higher risk of developing second malignant neoplasms [614]. Guidance on dose adjustments based on enzyme phenotype/genotype has been recently published aiming at reducing haematologic toxicity without compromising efficacy of ALL therapy [615].

Central nervous system-directed prophylaxis

CNS-directed prophylaxis has long been recognized as an integral aspect of ALL therapy to clear leukaemic cells at sites inaccessible by systemic chemotherapy to prevent CNS disease/relapse [589]. The five-year cumulative incidence of CNS relapse was 3–5% in paediatric [616, 617] and 2–6% in adult patients [618–621] who received intrathecal and/or intensive systemic chemotherapy for CNS prophylaxis. Most commonly used treatments include intrathecal chemotherapy, cranial irradiation, and high-dose blood-brain-barrier penetrating chemotherapy [563, 577, 585]. With the current combination of effective systemic and intrathecal chemotherapies and the devastating late-onset sequel of cranial radiotherapy [622, 623] (particularly in long-term survivors of paediatric ALL cranial irradiation) it is often omitted. Several studies in paediatric [554, 557, 623, 624] and adult [624, 625] age groups have shown omission is not associated with inferior outcomes or increased risk of CNS relapse. The optimum prophylactic intrathecal therapy has yet to be defined. Triple intrathecal therapy (methotrexate, cytarabine, and hydrocortisone) was associated with significantly lower incidence of CNS relapse than intrathecal methotrexate but with significantly more haematologic and testicular relapse resulting in significantly inferior survival [626]. However, a meta-analysis showed that intravenous methotrexate improved outcome when added to triple intrathecal therapy but had no significant benefit in those treated with intrathecal methotrexate [627].

Role of minimal residual disease monitoring in acute lymphoblastic leukaemia therapy

One of the major developments over the past two decades that defined ALL management is MRD evaluation. Its detection and quantification is now considered the most powerful independent predictor of EFS and OS for paediatric [628–635] and adult ALL patients [636–643]. Hence, it has become an integral part of treatment protocols employing its quantitative assays at specific protocol-defined informative time-points to risk-stratify and monitor therapy. A prospective study by the German Multicenter Study Group for Adult ALL (GMALL) has identified a subset of standard-risk ALL patients with molecular relapse who became MRD positive after an initial post-therapy documented negative result [643]. The median duration from molecular to clinical relapse was 9.5 months. This further underscores the highly predictive power of MRD monitoring, although what interventions would be appropriate in this situation remain unclear.

Several studies in paediatric and adult ALL patients observed that a difference may exist in leukaemic cell eradication kinetics between the two groups. By the end of initial induction therapy 60–75% of paediatric patients [628, 630, 631, 637] achieved MRD negativity versus only 30–50% of adults [640, 642]. The slower rate of leukaemic cell clearance in adults is at least in part related to differences in ALL pathobiology and therapeutic regimens.

Transplantation in acute lymphoblastic leukaemia

The role of allogeneic haematopoietic stem cell transplantation (allo-HSCT) for ALL patients in first CR (CR1) remains to be determined as non-transplant therapies evolve. The role of auto-HSCT was evaluated in a number of trials which revealed inferiority [644] or at best no difference in terms of outcome when compared to conventional consolidation/maintenance chemotherapy [645, 646]. Firm evidence of the donor T-cell-medicated graft-versus-leukaemia (GvL) effect [644, 647] in addition to the potential benefits of higher dose chemotherapy with total body irradiation have made allo-HSCT the 'ultimate' post-remission therapy. However, the high treatment-related mortality (TRM), particularly in adults, and morbidity from graft-versus-host disease (GvHD) in long-term survivors mandate prudence in patient selection.

Several trials [648–650], including a meta-analysis [646,] have confirmed the survival advantage in having a sibling donor. The largest, UKALLXII/US Eastern Cooperative Oncology Group (ECOG) 2993 [644] where the five-year OS of Ph− ALL patients with standard-risk disease who had such a donor was significantly better than those who did not (53% vs 45%; p = 0.01), associated with lower relapse rate risk [644] noted across all adult age groups. However, there was no advantage to having a donor in the high-risk group, attributed to the high non-relapse mortality (36% at two years vs 14%, respectively) of older patients in the high-risk category. PETHEMA ALL-93 [651] trials did not show inferior outcomes in those without a donor in this group. In standard-risk ALL, the evidence is less conclusive and is controversial. Similar results were reported by the HOVON co-operative group whereby the donor arm had a significantly higher five-year DFS rate and lower five-year cumulative incidence of relapse when compared to the no-donor arm (60% vs 42%, p < 0.01; 24% vs 55%, p < 0.001, respectively) [652]. The feasibility of using unrelated and alternative donors has been explored. Retrospective analysis of outcome data from the Center for International Blood and Marrow Transplant Research (CIBMTR) in unrelated donor transplants in Ph− ALL in CR1, the five-year TRM, relapse, and OS were 42%, 20%, and 39%, respectively [653]. Several retrospective studies have addressed the issue of donor type in ALL in CR1 using myeloablative conditioning and these showed no difference in TRM, relapse rate, or OS between related and unrelated donor transplants [654–656]. However, the TRM was higher with HLA-mismatched donors; with TRM the major cause of treatment failure, selecting closely HLA-matched unrelated donors should improve results [653]. With more resolute HLA-matching [657] and improved supportive care [658] this has mitigated the differences in outcome between the two groups [659–661]. Alternative donor transplantation has recently become a viable option for those lacking suitable donors with current experience showing reasonable OS rates [662–665] but with the disadvantage of significantly higher TRM, GvHD, and graft failure.

Reduced-intensity conditioned (RIC) allo-HSCT, using the principle of a conditioning regimen that promotes GvL effect and mitigates the acute associated transplant-related toxicities, is increasingly used in ALL. Current evidence on efficacy of RIC transplantation is based on retrospective data that includes small cohort of patients that are therefore subject to considerable bias, but encouraging results have been reported [666–668]. In a retrospective comparative study of patients receiving RIC or myeloablative conditioning, multivariate analysis showed that conditioning intensity did not affect TRM or relapse risk [669]. Data from the European Blood and Marrow Transplantation (EBMT) registry from 97 patients showed a two-year OS and leukaemia-free survival of 52% and 42% with RIC transplants in CR1, respectively, and non-relapse mortality of 18% [670]. The MRD status pre-transplant impacts the outcome of RIC transplants. A report from the Fred Hutchinson Cancer Research Center revealed that three-year OS rate in high-risk ALL patients using low-dose TBI approach was 62% in those with evidence of MRD vs 73% who did not [667]. The use of T-cell depletion (TCD) to lower risk of GvHD has been used with encouraging results though with the disadvantage of increased relapse risk. In a report from the British Society of Blood and Marrow Transplantation Registry (BSBMT), 96% of 48 adults with high-risk Ph- ALL reported a five-year OS, DFS, and relapse mortality of 61%, 59%, and 13% using in vivo TCD using alemtuzumab [671]. The incidences of acute grade II-IV GvHD and extensive chronic GvHD were 27% and 22%, respectively [671]. The encouraging results have made RIC transplantation in the 'older' ALL patient a more plausible option—this is currently subject to a prospective trial in the UK, UKALL14.

In summary, allo-HSCT is currently recommended for patients with high-risk disease in CR1 who have a reasonable performance status and a 'suitable' donor [644, 646, 672]. Patients with molecular failure defined as persistence of MRD at a protocol appropriate time point are also considered a high-risk group, relapsing after a median of 7.6 months with a five-year continuous CR and OS rate of 12% and 33%, respectively [673] if they do not receive HSCT in CR1. Table 51.9 summarizes the other high-risk criteria in Ph- ALL patients as defined by selected large international trials in whom allo-HSCT have been considered. With better understanding of disease pathobiology through high-resolution genome-wide analyses most of the patient demographic criteria are no longer as relevant as disease risk factors.

Treatment of Philadelphia chromosome-positive (Ph+) acute lymphoblastic leukaemia

Ph+ ALL, where BCR-ABL1 oncogenic protein is expressed as result of t(9;22), carries one of the worst prognosis amongst ALL subsets with a median survival of eight months [687]. With the advent of targeted therapy in the form of BCR-ABL specific tyrosine kinase inhibitors (TKIs) there has been a significant improvement in initial responses resulting in higher CR rates reaching to almost 95% [688–693] without additional toxicities. The most widely used TKI

is imatinib. Table 51.10 summarizes the outcome of selected studies in de novo Ph+ ALL.

Given the significant TKI-attributed improvement in CR rates, the plausibility of reducing or omitting chemotherapy from initial induction therapy was contemplated. However, despite several studies reporting an almost 100% CR rate with single-agent TKI or in combination with minimal chemotherapy [703, 705, 708] the long-term outcome of a chemotherapy-free/minimal chemotherapy approaches is not clear. Dasatinib, a second generation TKI that inhibits BCR-ABL and SRC family kinases, has a 325-fold greater potency in inhibiting in vitro growth of wild-type BCR-ABL cells than imatinib [709] and may theoretically hold more promise of long-term benefit than imatinib. Phase II and III dose comparison studies showed it to induce rapid haematologic and cytogenetic responses in imatinib-resistant or -intolerant adult patients [710–712]. Initial data of combinations with dasatinib with steroid or chemotherapy confers promising results with better OS rates in adults [702, 705, 708]. Unlike imatinib, which penetrates poorly the blood-brain-barrier with concentration around two logs lower in the cerebrospinal fluid (CSF) [713], dasatinib appears to exhibit activity against CNS leukaemia [714]. Nevertheless, results from studies to date (which include small numbers, relatively short follow-up duration, and lack of randomized controlled head-to-head comparisons with imatinib) cannot explicitly justify adding dasatinib to chemotherapy combinations for de novo Ph+ ALL therapy. Safety profile and tolerability of dasatinib are not as favourable as imatinib, with bleeding and pleural effusions being a concern [702].

Despite high CR rates, such response is short-lived and relapses are common [697, 715]. With virtually no alternative therapeutic modality to date that offers long-term survival, benefit allo-HSCT remains the mainstay of treatment for eligible patients although associated with significant toxicities. Outcome data from the UKALLXII/ECOG collaboration [706] showed the addition of imatinib to chemotherapy in the absence of allo-HSCT did not confer survival benefit even on excluding patients in remission who did not survive to allo-HSCT. A similar conclusion was reported by GMALL group [716]. Prospective data from the UKALLXII/ECOG 2993 trial showed the relevant three-year OS was 59% with combination of imatinib-based chemotherapy and myeloablative allo-HSCT despite the TRM [717]. Reported three-year OS by the GMALL group was 72% with myeloablative allo-HSCT when an imatinib-based induction was used [716]. The Japanese Adult Leukemia Study Group reported a three-year OS of 65% using the same approach [718]. In a recent retrospective analysis of long-term follow-up data from the American Society for Blood and Marrow Transplantation, TKI use pre- or post-HSCT did not significantly impact transplant outcomes [719]. Based on this evidence allo-HSCT is considered the standard of care for adult Ph+ ALL, but its role in paediatric patients is less clear, particularly in the TKI era. A retrospective study in paediatric Ph+ ALL who underwent allo-HSCT (aged 1–16 years) the addition of imatinib pre-and/or post-HSCT did not significantly improve outcomes (three-year DFS rate 62% vs 53% and three-year relapse rate 15% vs 26% for those who did not receive imatinib) [720]. A study from the Spanish Cooperative Group of outcomes of children up to the age of 15 years treated with imatinib-based chemotherapy followed by allo-HSCT showed significantly higher three-year EFS rate when compared to historical controls who did not receive imatinib (79% vs 30%)

Table 51.9 High-risk criteria in Ph⁻ ALL patients as defined by selected large international trials in whom allo-HSCT have been considered

Risk stratification criterion that defined HR	Risk subset	Study group(s)/data source	Outcome
At diagnosis			
Age	Advancing age	MRC UKALLXII/ECOG 2993 [717], CALGB [589], GMALL [674]	Worse outcome—no clear age cut-off in adults
Presenting WBC count	> 30x 109/l (B-cell ALL) >100 x 109/l (T-cell ALL)	MRC UKALLXII/ECOG 2993 [718], GMALL [674]	Inferior outcome measures—CR rates, OR, EFS, DFS
Immunophenotype	T-cell ALL vs B-cell ALL Blast expression of CD20	MRC UKALLXII/ECOG 2993 [718], GMALL [674]	In adults, T-ALL can have a better outcome than B-ALL Increased CD20 expression—inferior CR rates and OS
Cytogenetics	Poor: t(4;11)(q21;q23), t(8;14)(q24.1;q32), complex (>5 abnormalities), low hypodiploidy, near triploidy	MRC UKALL XII/ECOG 2993 [675], SWOG 9400 [676]	Inferior rates of DFS and OS when compared with other patients
Specific molecular abnormalities	CRLF2 +/- JAK1/2 sequence mutation 'BCR-ABL-like' gene with IZKF1 'BCR-ABL-like' gene lacking CRLF2 dysregulation IKZF1 deletions TP53	COG [677] Mulligan et al. [678] Den Boer et al. [679] MRC UKALLXII/ECOG 2993 [680], GRAALL [681] Hof et al. [682]	Poor outcome High relapse risk irrespective of age, WBC count, cytogenetics or MRD status post induction Inferior outcome Poor outcome
Response to Therapy			
Steroid responsiveness	Response to steroids has clear relationship with outcome in childhood ALL. Less well defined and tested in adult ALL	Schrappe et al. [683]	Poor OS
Speed of initial response	Rapid initial response	PALG [684]	CR within 4 weeks predicts better outcome. Not uniformly demonstrated
MRD	Clear relationship between MRD at protocol-specific time points and outcome irrespective of risk stratification at diagnosis 91, 94, 95	• MRC UKALLXII/ECOG 2993 [685] • GMALL [642, 673] • PETHEMA [686] • NILSG [636]	MRD −ve vs +ve: • 5-year DFS 74% vs 30% • SR: 5-year OS 67% vs 38% • HR: 5-year OS 66% vs 42% • 4-year DFS 54% vs 2-year DFS 31% • 5-year DFS 72% vs 14%

Abbreviations: MRC UKALL/ ECOG2993, Medical Research Council UK ALL/Eastern Cooperative Oncology Group 2993; CALGB, Cancer and Leukemia Group B Study; GMALL, German Multicenter ALL; MRC UKALL X and XA, Medical Research Council UKALL X and XA; SWOG 9400, South West Oncology Group 9400; COG, Children's Oncology Group; PETHEMA, Programa para el Estudio de la Terape´utica en Hemopatı´a Maligna; GRAALL, Group for Research on Adult Acute Lymphocytic Leukemia Study; NILSG, Northern Italian Leukemia Study Group; PALG, Polish Adult Leukemia Group; OS, overall survival; SR, standard risk; HR, high risk; DFS, disease- free survival; MRD, minimal residual disease.

[695]. A study by the Children's Oncology Group (COG) in Ph⁺ ALL patients up to the age of 21 years treated with imatinib-based intensive chemotherapy showed an improved three-year EFS rate of 80% +/- 11% among those who received continuous imatinib, more than twice historical controls with no appreciable increase in toxicity [694]. Three-year EFS rate was similar for patients treated with chemotherapy plus imatinib (88% +/−11%) or sibling donor HSCT (57% +/- 22%) [694]. Whilst such studies question the role of allo-HSCT in paediatric Ph⁺ ALL, these were not powered to address the dispensability of allo-HSCT; long-term follow-up data may answer this. Older patients unfit for myeloablative allo-HSCT, RIC-HSCT would be an alternative given its acceptable TRM. No optimal conditioning regimen has been described. Whether TKI

is needed post allo-HSCT is not clear. An ongoing German study randomizing patients to either starting imatinib three months post allo-HSCT versus only on BCR-ABL positivity has noted its poor tolerability [700].

BCR-ABL monitoring by real-time quantitative polymerase chain reaction (RQ-PCR) has been increasingly employed to assess MRD in Ph⁺ ALL. However, optimal practice, methodology standardization, and interpretation of results are unclear in addition to conflicting reports on its association with long-term outcome. In the pre-imatinib era good correlation between BCR-ABL transcript levels and outcome have been reported [721, 722]. Based on clinical trials that included TKIs, BCR-ABL transcript levels correlated with response [707] though there is no consensus on what constitutes

Table 51.10 Outcome of selected studies in de novo Ph$^+$ ALL where TKI was added concomitantly to induction therapy at various intensities, following induction or intermittently between cycles of chemotherapy across different age groups

Data source	Study group	TKI dose (mg)	N	CR (%)	Transplantation rate (%)	OS
Published studies						
◆ Paediatric						
Schultz et al. [694]	COG	Im 340/m^2	92	N/S	N/A	80% (EFS) at 36 mo
Rives et al. [695]	SHOP	Im 260/m^2	16	100	N/A	79% at 36 mo
◆ Adults						
Thomas et al. [696]	MD Anderson	Im 400	20	93	50	75% at 20 mo
Yanada et al. [697]	JALSG	Im 600	80	96	61	75% at 12 mo
Wassmann et al. [698]	GMALL	Im 400, Im 600	92	95	77	36% (alternating Im); 43% (concurrent Im at 24 mo)
DeLabarathe et al. [699]	GRAAPH	Im 600	45	96	48	65% at 18 mo
Ribera et al. [700]	PETHEMA	Im 400	30	90	70	30% at 48 mo
Stein et al. [701]	NILSG	Im 600	59	92	63	38% at 60 mo
Ravandi et al. [702]	MD Anderson	Das 50 bd (or 100 od)	35	94	N/A as not part of protocol	64% at 24 mo
Foà et al. [705]	GIMEMA LAL1205	Das 70 bd 12 weeks	53	100	N/A	69.2% at 20 mo
◆ 'Older' Adults						
Vignetti et al. [703]	GIMEMA	Im 800	30	100	N/A	74% at 12 mo
Ottman et al. [704]	GMALL	Im 600	55	96 (Im) 50 (chemo)	N/A	42% at 24 mo
Unpublished studies—All of these were in adults with the exception of Rousselot et al. study were patients were in 'older' patients only (over 70 years)						
Fielding et al. [706]	UK NCRI/ECOG	Im 600	145	95	44	43% at 36 mo
Chalandon et al. [707]	GRAALL	Im 800	188	100 (Im DIV) 96 (Im+Hyper-CVAD)	62	62% at 24 mo
Rousselot et al. [708]	EWALL	Das 140 od (100 od > 70yrs)	71	90	N/A	Median 27.1 mo

Abbreviations: COG, Children's Oncology Group; SHOP, Sociedad Española de Hematologia y Oncologia Pediátrica; JALSG, Japanese Adult Leukemia Study Group; NILSG, Northern Italian Leukemia Study Group; UK NCRI/ECOG, UK National Cancer Research Institute/Eastern Cooperative Oncology Group; Im, Imatinib; Das, Dasatinib; DIV, Dexamethasone, imatinib, vincristine; mo, months.

an optimal response. A recent study by Lee et al. [723] has shown a significant correlation between MRD kinetics and long-term HSCT outcome in adult Ph$^+$ ALL treated with imatinib-based chemotherapy before allo-HSCT. Intermediate and poor molecular responders had worse relapse and DFS rates in comparison to early molecular responders [723].

An emerging significant issue in Ph$^+$ ALL is resistance [696] to one or more TKIs developing during therapy [700] or resistance prior to therapy [712, 721, 724, 725] and carries a particularly poor prognosis. Unlike CML, these are less well studied and do not necessarily arise from the dominant tumour clone(s), the latter perhaps arising in response to TKI-driven selective pressure [724]. This explains why an initial reduction in BCR-ABL transcript level does not correlate with good long-term outcome [693, 704, 722, 726]. ABL-kinase domain point mutations [724, 726, 727] are one of the common causes of imatinib resistance and involve the following regions: ATP binding pocket (P-loop), catalytic domain (most often at the 'gate-keeper' residue threonine 315), and activation loop (A-loop) [724]. Less commonly are those involving alternative signalling pathways mediated by SRC family kinase (SH2 or SH3 contact) [727]. BCR-ABL mutations associated with relapse with imatinib are predominantly in the P-loop and T315I, whilst dasatinib is most frequently associated with T315I mutations. In patients receiving imatinib who are in complete haematologic remission an increase in BCR-ABL level should suggest mutational analysis.

Management of relapse/refractory disease

Despite the major advances in ALL therapy and high remission rates, 20% of paediatric [728, 729] and 50–60% [589, 618, 619, 730–733] of adult patients relapse following initial CR to first-line chemotherapy. The estimated incidence of primary refractory ALL is almost 2% in children and around 10% in adults. Management of relapsed/refractory ALL poses an extremely challenging problem with post relapse strategies rarely resulting in long-term survival [734–737]. Only 30% of paediatric ALL patients go on to achieve long-term remission with salvage therapy [738, 739]. Data from COG studies has shown that EFS and OS outcomes of relapsed paediatric ALL depended on timing and site of relapse with early (defined as within 18 months from diagnosis), with isolated bone marrow relapse having the worst prognosis [729, 740] where the five-year survival was only 11.5% [729]. Similarly, data from two of the largest series of adults with relapsed ALL have shown a median OS after relapse of 4.5–6 months and five-year OS rate of 7–10% [737, 741]. Less than 30% of patients achieve a second CR with salvage therapy [741]. CNS involvement and relapse within two years of diagnosis were the worst prognostic factors on multivariate analysis and initial therapy does not affect the outcome after relapse [737]. A recent report from the GMALL group identified relapse site, response to salvage, performance of allo-HSCT and age as prognostic factors for survival [742]. With currently available induction chemotherapy largely aimed at preventing relapse, and hence survival benefit, once relapse occurs subsequent cure becomes unlikely [737]. Furthermore, only a small proportion of patients who received chemotherapy alone are eligible for allo-HSCT and go on to achieve second CR. Much attention has now been directed towards novel, targeted therapeutic agents commonly delivered within prospective clinical trials. Clofarabine, a nucleoside analog, given as a single agent or in combination was noted to be active in relapsed/refractory ALL in paediatric [743, 744] and adult [745] patients. Reported CR rates are variable and reach 50% with OS of 18 months [743]. Nelarabine, another nucleoside analog with T-cell specific action recently approved for treatment of relapsed/refractory T-cell ALL achieved responses in 48% of adult [746] and 55% of paediatric patients following first relapse and 27% in second relapse [747]. Remissions were not durable with the only chance of cure being allo-HSCT. Blinatumomab, a T-cell engaging anti-CD3/CD19-bispecific monoclonal antibody has shown early promising results with 67% of patients with relapsed/refractory B-precursor ALL achieving CR [748]. Other targeted investigational agents developed following recent insights from genome-wide analyses include phosphorylase inhibitors; anti-CD22 monoclonal antibody/-drug conjugates; inhibitors of NOTCH1, histone deacetylase, proteosome, and DNA methyltransferase; and kinase-dependent signalling pathways [749].

Management of extramedullary disease

CNS involvement at diagnosis is uncommon, but over 50% of patients would eventually develop it if CNS-directed therapy were not given [563, 577]. Its presence at diagnosis in paediatric patients is associated with significantly decreased EFS rates [591, 617]. In adults, although the five-year DFS rates were no different when compared to those with no involvement at diagnosis, it was associated higher risk of CNS relapse [750, 751] and inferior OS [750]. CNS-directed therapy includes similar therapeutic options as the prophylactic approach. With more effective intrathecal and high-dose systemic chemotherapy regimens, the role of cranial irradiation is diminishing particularly given its association with neuro-cognitive dysfunctions and secondary malignancies [577, 585, 752]. Intrathecal chemotherapy needs to continue bi-weekly until resolution of CNS disease evidenced by clearance of blasts from the CSF. In T-cell ALL upregulation of the CCR7 gene via NOTCH signalling appears to be essential in directing ALL cells into the CNS, a finding that could be targeted with novel therapeutic approaches [753].

Testicular involvement, more commonly seen in T-cell ALL patients, should be treated with testicular irradiation if not fully resolved by the end of induction chemotherapy.

Late effects of therapy

With significant improvements in survival rates in the context of a disease most prevalent in paediatric age group more patients experience late adverse events [754]. Their occurrence depends on type, intensity, and age at which patients were exposed to therapy. For example, children under six years of age have the highest risk of neurocognitive impairment following cranial irradiation and intrathecal chemotherapy [622, 623]. High-dose cranial irradiation in children and adolescents also increases the risk of stroke, auditory-vestibular-visual deficits, seizures, coordination defects [623, 755], and reduced fertility [756]. Osteonecrosis is a well-recognized problem with steroids, most often affecting weight-bearing joints. Adolescents, rather than children or adults, appear to have the highest incidence of such complications [757–759]. Other than age, a lower albumin, high lipids, and dexamethasone exposure are associated with an increased risk of osteonecrosis [760]. Anthracycline-related cardiotoxicity [761] has become an infrequent late complication with current regimens that use these agents at lower doses. Second neoplasms, the most common being haematologic and brain malignancies [762, 763], are serious late effects in successfully treated ALL patients [764]. In one series, the overall cumulative risk of second neoplasms was 2.1% at five years, 4.9% at ten years and 9.4% at 15 years [765].

Therefore, given the risk of such late effects it is prudent that all survivors of ALL continue to be followed-up following completion of chemotherapy.

Further reading

Asnafi V, Buzyn A, Le Noir S, Baleydier F, Simon A et al. NOTCH1/FBXW7 mutation identifies a large subgroup with favorable outcome in adult T-cell acute lymphoblastic leukemia (T-ALL): a Group for Research on Adult Acute Lymphoblastic Leukemia (GRAALL) study. Blood 2009; 113(17): 3918–3924.

Bain G, Maandag EC, Izon DJ, Amsen D, Kruisbeek AM et al. E2A proteins are required for proper B cell development and initiation of immunoglobulin gene rearrangements. Cell 1994; 79(5): 885–892.

Bassan R, Hoelzer D. Modern therapy of acute lymphoblastic leukemia. Journal of Clinical Oncology 2011; 29(5): 532–543.

Bassan R, Spinelli O, Oldani E, Intermesoli T, Tosi M et al. Improved risk classification for risk-specific therapy based on the molecular study of minimal residual disease (MRD) in adult acute lymphoblastic leukemia (ALL). Blood 2009; 113(18): 4153–4162.

Bijl J, Sauvageau M, Thompson A, Sauvageau G. High incidence of proviral integrations in the Hoxa locus in a new model of E2a-PBX1-induced B-cell leukemia. Genes and Development 2005; 19(2): 224–233.

Brüggemann M, Schrauder A, Raff T, Pfeifer H, Dworzak M et al. European Working Group for Adult Acute Lymphoblastic Leukemia (EWALL); International Berlin-Frankfurt-Münster Study Group (I-BFM-SG). Standardized MRD quantification in European ALL trials: Proceedings of the Second International Symposium on MRD assessment in Kiel, Germany, 18–20 September 2008. Leukemia 2010; 24: 521–535.

Campana D. Minimal residual disease in acute lymphoblastic leukemia. Hematology—American Society of Hematology Education Program 2010: 7–12.

DiMartino JF, Selleri L, Traver D, Firpo MT, Rhee J et al. The Hox cofactor and proto-oncogene Pbx1 is required for maintenance of definitive hematopoiesis in the fetal liver. Blood 2001; 98(3): 618–626.

Felice MS, Gallego MS, Alonso CN, Alfaro EM, Guitter MR et al. Prognostic impact of t(1;19)/TCF3-PBX1 in childhood acute lymphoblastic leukemia in the context of Berlin-Frankfurt-Munster-based protocols. Leukemia Lymphoma 2011; 52(7): 1215–1221.

Giebel S, Stella-Holowiecka B, Krawczyk-Kulis M et al. Status of minimal residual disease determines outcome of autologous hematopoietic SCT in adult ALL. Bone Marrow Transplant 2009; 45:1095–1101.

Gökbuget N, Kneba M, Raff T, Trautmann H, Bartram CR et al. German Multicentre Study Group for Adult Acute Lymphoblastic Leukemia. Adult patients with acute lymphoblastic leukemia and molecular failure display a poor prognosis and are candidates for stem cell transplantation and targeted therapies. Blood 2012; 120(9): 1868–1876.

Hoelzer D, Gökbuget N. Chemoimmunotherapy in acute lymphoblastic leukemia. Blood Reviews 2012; 26(1): 25–32.

Hoelzer D, Huettmann A, Kaul F, Irmer SI, Jaeckel NJ et al. Immunochemotherapy with rituximab in adult CD20 B-precursor ALL improves molecular CR rate and outcome in standard risk (SR) as well as in high risk (HR) patients with SCT. Haematologica 2009; 94: abstr 481.

Hoelzer D, Thiel E, Löffler H, Büchner T, Ganser A et al. Prognostic factors in a multicenter study for treatment of acute lymphoblastic leukemia in adults. Blood 1988; 71(1): 123–131.

Kamps MP, Baltimore D. E2A-Pbx1, the t(1;19) translocation protein of human pre-B-cell acute lymphocytic leukemia, causes acute myeloid leukemia in mice. Molecular Cell Biology 1993; 13(1): 351–357.

Kee BL, Murre C. Induction of early B cell factor (EBF) and multiple B lineage genes by the basic helix-loop-helix transcription factor E12. Journal of Experimental Medicine 1998; 188(4): 699–713.

Lu Q, Kamps MP. Heterodimerization of Hox proteins with Pbx1 and oncoprotein E2a-Pbx1 generates unique DNA-binding specificities at nucleotides predicted to contact the N-terminal arm of the Hox homeodomain—demonstration of Hox-dependent targeting of E2a-Pbx1 in vivo. Oncogene 1997; 14(1): 75–83.

Patel B, Rai L, Buck G, Richards SM, Mortuza Y et al. Minimal residual disease is a significant predictor of treatment failure in non T-lineage adult acute lymphoblastic leukaemia: Final results of the international trial UKALLXII/ECOG2993. British Journal of Haematology 2010; 148: 80–89.

Pfeifer H, Wassmann B, Bethge W, Dengler J, Bornhauser M et al. Randomized comparison of prophylactic and minimal residual disease-triggered imatinib after allogeneic stem cell transplantation for BCR-ABL1 positive acute lymphoblastic leukaemia. Leukemia 2013: 27: 1254–1262.

Rowe JM. Prognostic factors in adult acute lymphoblastic leukaemia. British Journal of Haematology 2010; 150(4): 389–405.

Secker-Walker LM, Berger R, Fenaux P, Lai JL, Nelken B et al. Prognostic significance of the balanced t(1;19) and unbalanced der(19)t(1;19) translocations in acute lymphoblastic leukemia. Leukemia 1992; 6(5): 363–369.

Shanmugam K, Green NC, Rambaldi I, Saragovi HU, Featherstone MS. PBX and MEIS as non-DNA-binding partners in trimeric complexes with HOX proteins. Molecular Cell Biology 1999; 19(11): 7577–7588.

Sykes DB, Kamps MP. E2a/Pbx1 induces the rapid proliferation of stem cell factor-dependent murine pro-T cells that cause acute T-lymphoid or myeloid leukemias in mice. Molecular Cell Biology 2004; 24(3): 1256–1269.

Thomas DA, O'Brien S, Faderl S, Garcia-Manero G, Ferrajoli A et al. Chemoimmunotherapy with a modified hyper-CVAD and rituximab regimen improves outcome in de novo Philadelphia chromosome-negative precursor B-lineage acute lymphoblastic leukemia. Journal of Clinical Oncology 2010; 28(24): 3880–3889.

Topp MS, Kufer P, Gokbuget N, Goebeler M, Klinger M et al. Targeted therapy with the T-cell-engaging antibody blinatumomab of chemotherapy-refractory minimal residual disease in B-lineage acute lymphoblastic leukemia patients results in high response rate and prolonged leukemia-free survival. Journal of Clinical Oncology 2011; 29: 2493–2498.

Zhang MY, Churpek JE, Keel SB, Walsh T, Lee MK, et al. Germline ETV6 mutations in familial thrombocytopenia and hematologic malignancy. Nature Genetics 2015; 47(2): 180–185.

References

1. Schlenk RF, Dohner K, Krauter J et al. Mutations and treatment outcome in cytogenetically normal acute myeloid leukemia. New England Journal of Medicine 2008; 358: 1909–1918.

2. Ley TJ, Mardis ER, Ding L, et al. DNA sequencing of a cytogenetically normal acute myeloid leukaemia genome. Nature 2008; 456: 66–72.

3. Mardis ER, Ding L, Dooling DJ et al. Recurring mutations found by sequencing an acute myeloid leukemia genome. New England Journal of Medicine 2009; 361: 1058–1066.

4. Li Z, Huang H, Li Y et al. Up-regulation of a HOXA-PBX3 homeobox-gene signature following down-regulation of miR-181 is associated with adverse prognosis in patients with cytogenetically abnormal AML. Blood 2012; 119: 2314–2324.

5. Yan XJ, Xu J, Gu ZH et al. Exome sequencing identifies somatic mutations of DNA methyltransferase gene DNMT3A in acute monocytic leukemia. Nature Genetics 43: 309–315.

6. Welch JS, Ley TJ, Link DC et al. The origin and evolution of mutations in acute myeloid leukemia. Cell 2012; 150: 264–278.

7. Delhommeau F, Dupont S, Della Valle V et al. Mutation in TET2 in myeloid cancers. New England Journal of Medicine 2009; 360: 2289–2301.

8. Abdel-Wahab O, Mullally A, Hedvat C et al. Genetic characterization of TET1, TET2, and TET3 alterations in myeloid malignancies. Blood 2009; 114: 144–147.

9. Gelsi-Boyer V, Trouplin V, Adelaide J et al. Mutations of polycomb-associated gene ASXL1 in myelodysplastic syndromes and chronic myelomonocytic leukaemia. British Journal of Haematology 145: 788–800.

10. Abdel-Wahab O, Manshouri T, Patel J et al. Genetic analysis of transforming events that convert chronic myeloproliferative neoplasms to leukemias. Cancer Research 2010; 70: 447–452.

11. Kolitz JE, George SL, Marcucci G et al. P-glycoprotein inhibition using valspodar (PSC-833) does not improve outcomes for patients younger than age 60 years with newly diagnosed acute myeloid leukemia: Cancer and Leukemia Group B study 19808. Blood 2010; 116:1413–1421.

12. Ward PS, Patel J, Wise DR et al. The common feature of leukemia-associated IDH1 and IDH2 mutations is a neomorphic enzyme activity converting alpha-ketoglutarate to 2-hydroxyglutarate. Cancer Cell 2010; 17: 225–234.

13. Van Vlierberghe P, Patel J, Abdel-Wahab O et al. PHF6 mutations in adult acute myeloid leukemia. Leukemia 2011; 25: 130–134.

14. Parsons DW, Jones S, Zhang X et al. An integrated genomic analysis of human glioblastoma multiforme. Science 2008; 321: 1807–1812.

15. Yan H, Parsons DW, Jin G et al. IDH1 and IDH2 mutations in gliomas. New England Journal of Medicine 2009; 360:765–773.

16. Mardis ER, Ding L, Dooling DJ et al. Recurring mutations found by sequencing an acute myeloid leukemia genome. New England Journal of Medicine 2009; 361:1058–1066.

17. Langemeijer SM, Kuiper RP, Berends M et al. Acquired mutations in TET2 are common in myelodysplastic syndromes. Nature Genetics 2009; 41:838–842.

18. Tahiliani M, Koh KP, Shen Y et al. Conversion of 5-methylcytosine to 5-hydroxymethylcytosine in mammalian DNA by MLL partner TET1. Science 2009; 324: 930–935.

19. Figueroa ME, Abdel-Wahab O, Lu C et al. Leukemic IDH1 and IDH2 mutations result in a hypermethylation phenotype, disrupt TET2 function, and impair hematopoietic differentiation. Cancer Cell 2010; 18: 553–567.

20. Ko M, Bandukwala HS, An J et al. Ten-Eleven-Translocation 2 (TET2) negatively regulates homeostasis and differentiation of hematopoietic

stem cells in mice. Proceedings of the National Academy of Sciences USA 108: 14566–14571.

21. Moran-Crusio K, Reavie L, Shih A et al. Tet2 loss leads to increased hematopoietic stem cell self-renewal and myeloid transformation. Cancer Cell 2011; 20: 11–24.

22. Quivoron C, Couronne L, Della Valle V et al. TET2 inactivation results in pleiotropic hematopoietic abnormalities in mouse and is a recurrent event during human lymphomagenesis. Cancer Cell 2011; 20: 25–38.

23. Li Z, Cai X, Cai C et al. Deletion of Tet2 in mice leads to dysregulated hematopoietic stem cells and subsequent development of myeloid malignancies. Blood 2011; 118(17): 4509–4518.

24. Dang L, White DW, Gross S et al. Cancer-associated IDH1 mutations produce 2-hydroxyglutarate. Nature 2009; 462: 739–744.

25. Gross S, Cairns RA, Minden MD et al. Cancer-associated metabolite 2-hydroxyglutarate accumulates in acute myelogenous leukemia with isocitrate dehydrogenase 1 and 2 mutations. Journal of Experimental Medicine 2010; 207: 339–344.

26. Carbuccia N, Murati A, Trouplin V et al. Mutations of ASXL1 gene in myeloproliferative neoplasms. Leukemia 2009; 23: 2183–2186.

27. Patel JP, Gonen M, Figueroa ME et al. Prognostic relevance of integrated genetic profiling in acute myeloid leukemia. New England Journal of Medicine 2012;366: 1079–1089.

28. Metzeler KH, Becker H, Maharry K et al. ASXL1 mutations identify a high-risk subgroup of older patients with primary cytogenetically normal AML within the ELN Favorable genetic category. Blood 2011; 118: 6920–6929.

29. Abdel-Wahab O, Adli M, Lafave LM et al. ASXL1 Mutations Promote Myeloid Transformation through Loss of PRC2-Mediated Gene Repression. Cancer Cell 2012; 22: 180–193.

30. Yamashita Y, Yuan J, Suetake I et al. Array-based genomic resequencing of human leukemia. Oncogene 2010; 29: 3723–3731.

31. Ley TJ, Ding L, Walter MJ et al. DNMT3A mutations in acute myeloid leukemia. New England Journal of Medicine 2010; 363:2424–2433.

32. Jan M, Snyder TM, Corces-Zimmerman MR et al. Clonal evolution of preleukemic hematopoietic stem cells precedes human acute myeloid leukemia. Science Translational Medicine 2012; 4: 149ra118.

33. Graubert TA, Shen D, Ding L et al. Recurrent mutations in the U2AF1 splicing factor in myelodysplastic syndromes. Nature Genetics 2012; 44: 53–57.

34. Papaemmanuil E, Cazzola M, Boultwood J et al. Somatic SF3B1 mutation in myelodysplasia with ring sideroblasts. New England Journal of Medicine 2011; 365: 1384–1395.

35. Yoshida K, Sanada M, Shiraishi Y et al. Frequent pathway mutations of splicing machinery in myelodysplasia. Nature 2011; 478: 64–69.

36. Li M, Collins R, Jiao Y et al. Somatic mutations in the transcriptional corepressor gene BCORL1 in adult acute myelogenous leukemia. Blood 2011; 118: 5914–17.

37. Grossmann V, Tiacci E, Holmes AB, et al. Whole-exome sequencing identifies somatic mutations of BCOR in acute myeloid leukemia with normal karyotype. Blood 2011; 118: 6153–6163.

38. Patel JP, Gonen M, Figueroa ME et al. Prognostic Relevance of Integrated Genetic Profiling in Acute Myeloid Leukemia. New England Journal of Medicine 2012; 366: 1079–1089.

39. Welch JS, Westervelt P, Ding L et al. Use of whole-genome sequencing to diagnose a cryptic fusion oncogene. JAMA 2011; 305: 1577–1584.

40. <http://seer.cancer.gov/statfacts/html/amyl.html>.

41. Juliusson G, Antunovic P, Derolf A, Lehmann S, Mollgard L et al. Age and acute myeloid leukemia: Real world data on decision to treat and outcomes from the swedish acute leukemia registry. Blood 2009; 113: 4179–4187.

42. Burnett A, Wetzler M, Lowenberg B. Therapeutic advances in acute myeloid leukemia. Journal of Clinical Oncology 2011; 29: 487–494.

43. Breems DA, Van Putten WL, De Greef GE, Van Zelderen-Bhola SL, Gerssen-Schoorl KB et al. Monosomal karyotype in acute myeloid leukemia: A better indicator of poor prognosis than a complex karyotype. Journal of Clinical Oncology 2008; 26: 4791–4797.

44. Lugthart S, Groschel S, Beverloo HB, Kayser S, Valk PJ et al. Clinical, molecular, and prognostic significance of who type inv(3) (q21q26.2)/t(3;3)(q21;q26.2) and various other 3q abnormalities in acute myeloid leukemia. Journal of Clinical Oncology 2010; 28: 3890–3898.

45. Haferlach C, Alpermann T, Schnittger S, Kern W, Chromik J et al. Prognostic value of monosomal karyotype in comparison to complex aberrant karyotype in acute myeloid leukemia: A study on 824 cases with aberrant karyotype. Blood 2012; 119: 2122–2125.

46. Byrd JC, Mrozek K, Dodge RK, Carroll AJ, Edwards CG et al. Pretreatment cytogenetic abnormalities are predictive of induction success, cumulative incidence of relapse, and overall survival in adult patients with de novo acute myeloid leukemia: Results from cancer and leukemia group b (calgb 8461). Blood 2002; 100: 4325–4336.

47. Fernandez HF, Sun Z, Yao X, Litzow MR, Luger SM et al. Anthracycline dose intensification in acute myeloid leukemia. New England Journal of Medicine 2009; 361: 1249–1259.

48. Tallman MS, Andersen JW, Schiffer CA, Appelbaum FR, Feusner JH et al. All-trans-retinoic acid in acute promyelocytic leukemia. New England Journal of Medicine 1997; 337: 1021–1028.

49. Lo-Coco F, Avvisati G, Vignetti M, Breccia M, Gallo E et al. Front-line treatment of acute promyelocytic leukemia with aida induction followed by risk-adapted consolidation for adults younger than 61 years: Results of the aida-2000 trial of the gimema group. Blood 2010; 116: 3171–3179.

50. Ades L, Guerci A, Raffoux E, Sanz M, Chevallier P et al. Very long-term outcome of acute promyelocytic leukemia after treatment with all-trans retinoic acid and chemotherapy: The european apl group experience. Blood 2010; 115: 1690–1696.

51. Dash A, Gilliland DG. Molecular genetics of acute myeloid leukaemia. Best practice and Research Clinical Haematology 2001; 14: 49–64.

52. Ward PS, Patel J, Wise DR, Abdel-Wahab O, Bennett BD et al. The common feature of leukemia-associated idh1 and idh2 mutations is a neomorphic enzyme activity converting alpha-ketoglutarate to 2-hydroxyglutarate. Cancer Cell 2010; 17: 225–234.

53. Ley TJ, Ding L, Walter MJ, McLellan MD, Lamprecht T et al. Dnmt3a mutations in acute myeloid leukemia. New England Journal of Medicine 2010; 363: 2424–2433.

54. Metzeler KH, Becker H, Maharry K, Radmacher MD, Kohlschmidt J et al. Asxl1 mutations identify a high-risk subgroup of older patients with primary cytogenetically normal aml within the eln favorable genetic category. Blood 2011; 118: 6920–6929.

55. Abdel-Wahab O, Mullally A, Hedvat C, Garcia-Manero G, Patel J et al. Genetic characterization of tet1, tet2, and tet3 alterations in myeloid malignancies. Blood 2009; 114: 144–147.

56. Walter RB, Appelbaum FR, Estey EH, Bernstein ID. Acute myeloid leukemia stem cells and cd33-targeted immunotherapy. Blood 2012; 119: 6198–6208.

57. Soulier J. Fanconi anemia. Hematology/the Education Program of the American Society of Hematology. American Society of Hematology Education Program 2011; 492–497.

58. Xavier AC, Ge Y, Taub J. Unique clinical and biological features of leukemia in down syndrome children. Expert Review of Hematology 2010; 3: 175–186.

59. Khan I, Malinge S, Crispino J. Myeloid leukemia in down syndrome. Critical Reviews in Oncogenesis 2011; 16: 25–36.

60. Wong O. Risk of acute myeloid leukaemia and multiple myeloma in workers exposed to benzene. Occupational and Environmental Medicine 1995; 52: 380–384.

61. Korte JE, Hertz-Picciotto I, Schulz MR, Ball LM, Duell EJ. The contribution of benzene to smoking-induced leukemia. Environmental Health Perspectives 2000; 108: 333–339.

62. Jamall IS, Willhite CC. Is benzene exposure from gasoline carcinogenic? Journal of Environmental Monitoring 2008; 10: 176–187.

63. Sandler DP, Shore DL, Anderson JR, Davey FR, Arthur D et al. Cigarette smoking and risk of acute leukemia: Associations with morphology and cytogenetic abnormalities in bone marrow. Journal of the National Cancer Institute 1993; 85: 1994–2003.

64. Feldman EJ. Does therapy-related aml have a poor prognosis, independent of the cytogenetic/molecular determinants? Best Practice and Research Clinical Haematology 2011; 24: 523–526.

65. Armand P, Kim HT, DeAngelo DJ, Ho VT, Cutler CS et al. Impact of cytogenetics on outcome of *de novo* and therapy-related aml and mds after allogeneic transplantation. Journal of the American Society for Blood and Marrow Transplantation 2007; 13: 655–664.

66. Schoch C, Kern W, Schnittger S, Hiddemann W, Haferlach T. Karyotype is an independent prognostic parameter in therapy-related acute myeloid leukemia (t-aml): An analysis of 93 patients with t-aml in comparison to 1091 patients with *de novo* aml. Leukemia: Official Journal of the Leukemia Society of America, Leukemia Research Fund, UK 2004; 18: 120–125.

67. Tsushima H, Iwanaga M, Miyazaki Y. Late effect of atomic bomb radiation on myeloid disorders: Leukemia and myelodysplastic syndromes. International Journal of Hematology 2012; 95: 232–238.

68. Gundestrup M, Storm HH. Radiation-induced acute myeloid leukaemia and other cancers in commercial jet cockpit crew: A population-based cohort study. Lancet 1999; 354: 2029–2031.

69. Derolf AR, Kristinsson SY, Andersson TM, Landgren O, Dickman PW et al. Improved patient survival for acute myeloid leukemia: a population-based study of 9729 patients diagnosed in Sweden between 1973 and 2005. Blood 2009; 113(16): 3666–3672.

70. Rowe JM. Evaluation of prognostic factors in AML. Preface. Best Practice and Research in Clinical Haematology 2011; 24(4): 485–488.

71. Buchner T, Berdel WE, Haferlach C, Haferlach T, Schnittger S et al. Age-related risk profile and chemotherapy dose response in acute myeloid leukemia: a study by the German Acute Myeloid Leukemia Cooperative Group. Journal of Clinical Oncology [Randomized Controlled Trial Research Support, Non-U.S. Government] 2009; 27(1): 61–69.

72. Zuckerman T, Ganzel C, Tallman MS, Rowe JM. How I treat hematologic emergencies in adults with acute leukemia. Blood 2012; 120(10): 1993–2002.

73. Hess CE, Nichols AB, Hunt WB, Suratt PM. Pseudohypoxemia secondary to leukemia and thrombocytosis. New England Journal of Medicine 1979; 301(7): 361–363.

74. Tosi P, Barosi G, Lazzaro C, Liso V, Marchetti M et al. Consensus conference on the management of tumor lysis syndrome. Haematologica 2008; 93(12): 1877–1885.

75. Vadhan-Raj S, Fayad LE, Fanale MA, Pro B, Rodriguez A et al. A randomized trial of a single-dose rasburicase versus five-daily doses in patients at risk for tumor lysis syndrome. Annals of Oncology 2012; 23(6): 1640–1645.

76. Ganzel C, Becker J, Mintz PD, Lazarus HM, Rowe JM. Hyperleukocytosis, leukostasis and leukapheresis: practice management. Blood Reviews 2012; 26(3): 117–122.

77. Dohner H, Estey EH, Amadori S, Appelbaum FR, Buchner T et al. Diagnosis and management of acute myeloid leukemia in adults: recommendations from an international expert panel, on behalf of the European LeukemiaNet. Blood 2010; 115(3): 453–474.

78. Walter RB, Kantarjian HM, Huang X, Pierce SA, Sun Z et al. Effect of complete remission and responses less than complete remission on survival in acute myeloid leukemia: a combined Eastern Cooperative Oncology Group, Southwest Oncology Group, and M. D. Anderson Cancer Center Study. Journal of Clinical Oncology 2010; 28(10): 1766–1771.

79. Fernandez HF, Sun Z, Yao X, Litzow MR, Luger SM et al. Anthracycline dose intensification in acute myeloid leukemia. New England Journal of Medicine 2009; 361(13): 1249–1259.

80. Ohtake S, Miyawaki S, Fujita H, Kiyoi H, Shinagawa K et al. Randomized study of induction therapy comparing standard-dose idarubicin with high-dose daunorubicin in adult patients with previously untreated acute myeloid leukemia: the JALSG AML201 Study. Blood 2011; 117(8): 2358–2365.

81. Roboz GJ. Novel approaches to the treatment of acute myeloid leukemia. Hematology American Society of Hematology Education Program 2011: 43–50.

82. Lowenberg B, Pabst T, Vellenga E, van Putten W, Schouten HC et al. Cytarabine dose for acute myeloid leukemia. New England Journal of Medicine 2011; 364(11): 1027–1036.

83. Holowiecki J, Grosicki S, Giebel S, Robak T, Kyrcz-Krzemien S et al. Cladribine, but not fludarabine, added to daunorubicin and cytarabine during induction prolongs survival of patients with acute myeloid leukemia: a multicenter, randomized phase III study. Journal of Clinical Oncology 2012; 30(20): 2441–2448.

84. Castaigne S, Chevret S, Archimbaud E, Fenaux P, Bordessoule D et al. Randomized comparison of double induction and timed-sequential induction to a '3 + 7' induction in adults with AML: long-term analysis of the Acute Leukemia French Association (ALFA) 9000 study. Blood 2004; 104(8): 2467–2474.

85. Burnett AK, Hills RK, Milligan D, Kjeldsen L, Kell J et al. Identification of patients with acute myeloblastic leukemia who benefit from the addition of gemtuzumab ozogamicin: results of the MRC AML15 trial. Journal of Clinical Oncology 2011; 29(4): 369–377.

86. Castaigne S, Pautas C, Terre C, Raffoux E, Bordessoule D et al. Effect of gemtuzumab ozogamicin on survival of adult patients with *de-novo* acute myeloid leukaemia (ALFA-0701): a randomised, open-label, phase 3 study. Lancet 2012; 379(9825): 1508–1516.

87. Rowe JM, Kim HT, Cassileth PA, Lazarus HM, Litzow MR et al. Adult patients with acute myeloid leukemia who achieve complete remission after 1 or 2 cycles of induction have a similar prognosis: a report on 1980 patients registered to 6 studies conducted by the Eastern Cooperative Oncology Group. Cancer 2010; 116(21): 5012–5021.

88. Yanada M, Borthakur G, Ravandi F, Bueso-Ramos C, Kantarjian H et al. Kinetics of bone marrow blasts during induction and achievement of complete remission in acute myeloid leukemia. Haematologica 2008; 93(8): 1263–1265.

89. Becker H, Marcucci G, Maharry K, Radmacher MD, Mrozek K et al. Favorable prognostic impact of NPM1 mutations in older patients with cytogenetically normal *de novo* acute myeloid leukemia and associated gene- and microRNA-expression signatures: a Cancer and Leukemia Group B study. Journal of Clinical Oncology 2010; 28(4): 596–604.

90. Juliusson G, Antunovic P, Derolf A, Lehmann S, Mollgard L et al. Age and acute myeloid leukemia: real world data on decision to treat and outcomes from the Swedish Acute Leukemia Registry. Blood 2009; 113(18): 4179–4187.

91. Lowenberg B, Ossenkoppele GJ, van Putten W, Schouten HC, Graux C et al. High-dose daunorubicin in older patients with acute myeloid leukemia. New England Journal of Medicine 2009; 361(13): 1235–1248.

92. Burnett AK, Russell NH, Hills RK, Kell J, Freeman S et al. Addition of Gemtuzumab Ozogamicin to Induction Chemotherapy Improves Survival in Older Patients With Acute Myeloid Leukemia. Journal of Clinical Oncology 2012; 30(32): 3924–3931

93. Roboz GJ, Wissa U, Ritchie EK, Gergis U, Mayer S et al. Are low-intensity induction strategies better for older patients with acute myeloid leukemia? Leukemia Research 2012; 36(4): 407–412.

94. Burnett AK, Russell NH, Kell J, Dennis M, Milligan D et al. European development of clofarabine as treatment for older patients with acute myeloid leukemia considered unsuitable for intensive chemotherapy. Journal of Clinical Oncology 2010; 28(14): 2389–2395.

95. Faderl S, Ravandi F, Huang X, Garcia-Manero G, Ferrajoli A et al. A randomized study of clofarabine versus clofarabine plus low-dose cytarabine as front-line therapy for patients aged 60 years and older with acute myeloid leukemia and high-risk myelodysplastic syndrome. Blood 2008; 112(5): 1638–1645.

96. Tilly H, Castaigne S, Bordessoule D, Casassus P, Le Prise PY et al. Low-dose cytarabine versus intensive chemotherapy in the treatment of acute nonlymphocytic leukemia in the elderly. Journal of Clinical Oncology 1990; 8(2): 272–279.

97. Burnett AK, Milligan D, Prentice AG, Goldstone AH, McMullin MF et al. A comparison of low-dose cytarabine and hydroxyurea with

or without all-trans retinoic acid for acute myeloid leukemia and high-risk myelodysplastic syndrome in patients not considered fit for intensive treatment. Cancer 2007;109(6): 1114–1124.

98. Fenaux P, Mufti GJ, Hellstrom-Lindberg E, Santini V, Gattermann N et al. Azacitidine prolongs overall survival compared with conventional care regimens in elderly patients with low bone marrow blast count acute myeloid leukemia. Journal of Clinical Oncology 2010; 28(4): 562–569.

99. Kantarjian HM, Thomas XG, Dmoszynska A, Wierzbowska A, Mazur G et al. Multicenter, randomized, open-label, phase III trial of decitabine versus patient choice, with physician advice, of either supportive care or low-dose cytarabine for the treatment of older patients with newly diagnosed acute myeloid leukemia. Journal of Clinical Oncology 2012; 30(21): 2670–2677.

100. Cashen AF, Schiller GJ, O'Donnell MR, DiPersio JF. Multicenter, phase II study of decitabine for the first-line treatment of older patients with acute myeloid leukemia. Journal of Clinical Oncology 2010; 28(4): 556–561.

101. Cassileth PA, Harrington DP, Hines JD, Oken MM, Mazza JJ et al. Maintenance chemotherapy prolongs remission duration in adult acute nonlymphocytic leukemia. Journal of Clinical Oncology 1988; 6(4): 583–587.

102. Cassileth PA, Lynch E, Hines JD, Oken MM, Mazza JJ et al. Varying intensity of postremission therapy in acute myeloid leukemia. Blood 1992; 79(8): 1924–1930.

103. Bennett JM, Young ML, Andersen JW, Cassileth PA, Tallman MS et al. Long-term survival in acute myeloid leukemia: the Eastern Cooperative Oncology Group experience. Cancer 1997; 80(11 Suppl): 2205–2209.

104. Mayer RJ, Davis RB, Schiffer CA, Berg DT, Powell BL et al. Intensive postremission chemotherapy in adults with acute myeloid leukemia. Cancer and Leukemia Group B. New England Journal of Medicine 1994; 331(14): 896–903.

105. Rowe JM. Optimal induction and post-remission therapy for AML in first remission. Hematology American Society of Hematology Education Program 2009: 396–405.

106. Schaich M, Rollig C, Soucek S, Kramer M, Thiede C et al. Cytarabine dose of 36 g/m(2) compared with 12 g/m(2) within first consolidation in acute myeloid leukemia: results of patients enrolled onto the prospective randomized AML96 study. Journal of Clinical Oncology 2011; 29(19): 2696–2702.

107. Moore JO, George SL, Dodge RK, Amrein PC, Powell BL et al. Sequential multiagent chemotherapy is not superior to high-dose cytarabine alone as postremission intensification therapy for acute myeloid leukemia in adults under 60 years of age: Cancer and Leukemia Group B Study 9222. Blood 2005; 105(9): 3420–3427.

108. Elonen E, Almqvist A, Hanninen A, Jansson SE, Jarventie G et al. Comparison between four and eight cycles of intensive chemotherapy in adult acute myeloid leukemia: a randomized trial of the Finnish Leukemia Group. Leukemia 1998; 12(7): 1041–1048.

109. Burnett AK, Hills RK, Milligan DW, Goldstone AH, Prentice AG et al. Attempts to optimize induction and consolidation treatment in acute myeloid leukemia: results of the MRC AML12 trial. Journal of Clinical Oncology 2010; 28(4): 586–595.

110. Miyawaki S, Ohtake S, Fujisawa S, Kiyoi H, Shinagawa K et al. A randomized comparison of 4 courses of standard-dose multiagent chemotherapy versus 3 courses of high-dose cytarabine alone in postremission therapy for acute myeloid leukemia in adults: the JALSG AML201 Study. Blood 2011; 117(8): 2366–2372.

111. Goldstone AH, Burnett AK, Wheatley K, Smith AG, Hutchinson RM et al. Attempts to improve treatment outcomes in acute myeloid leukemia (AML) in older patients: the results of the United Kingdom Medical Research Council AML11 trial. Blood 2001; 98(5): 1302–1311.

112. Rowe JM, Tallman MS. How I treat acute myeloid leukemia. Blood 2010; 116(17): 3147–3156.

113. Cassileth PA, Lee SJ, Litzow MR, Miller KB, Stadtmauer EA et al. Intensified induction chemotherapy in adult acute myeloid leukemia followed by high-dose chemotherapy and autologous peripheral blood stem cell transplantation: an Eastern Cooperative Oncology Group trial (E4995). Leukemia Lymphoma 2005; 46(1): 55–61.

114. Fernandez HF, Sun Z, Litzow MR, Luger SM, Paietta EM et al. Autologous transplantation gives encouraging results for young adults with favorable-risk acute myeloid leukemia, but is not improved with gemtuzumab ozogamicin. Blood 2011; 117(20): 5306–5313.

115. Vellenga E, van Putten W, Ossenkoppele GJ, Verdonck LF, Theobald M et al. Autologous peripheral blood stem cell transplantation for acute myeloid leukemia. Blood 2011; 118(23): 6037–6042.

116. Cornelissen JJ, van Putten WL, Verdonck LF, Theobald M, Jacky E et al. Results of a HOVON/SAKK donor versus no-donor analysis of myeloablative HLA-identical sibling stem cell transplantation in first remission acute myeloid leukemia in young and middle-aged adults: benefits for whom? Blood 2007; 109(9): 3658–3666.

117. Suciu S, Mandelli F, de Witte T, Zittoun R, Gallo E et al. Allogeneic compared with autologous stem cell transplantation in the treatment of patients younger than 46 years with acute myeloid leukemia (AML) in first complete remission (CR1): an intention-to-treat analysis of the EORTC/GIMEMAAML-10 trial. Blood 2003; 102(4): 1232–1240.

118. Sakamaki H, Miyawaki S, Ohtake S, Emi N, Yagasaki F et al. Allogeneic stem cell transplantation versus chemotherapy as post-remission therapy for intermediate or poor risk adult acute myeloid leukemia: results of the JALSG AML97 study. International Journal of Hematology 2010; 91(2): 284–292.

119. Tallman MS, Rowlings PA, Milone G, Zhang MJ, Perez WS et al. Effect of postremission chemotherapy before human leukocyte antigen-identical sibling transplantation for acute myelogenous leukemia in first complete remission. Blood 2000; 96(4): 1254–1258.

120. Cahn JY, Labopin M, Sierra J, Blaise D, Reiffers J et al. No impact of high-dose cytarabine on the outcome of patients transplanted for acute myeloblastic leukaemia in first remission. Acute Leukaemia Working Party of the European Group for Blood and Marrow Transplantation (EBMT). British Journal of Haematology 2000; 110(2): 308–314.

121. Gupta V, Tallman MS, Weisdorf DJ. Allogeneic hematopoietic cell transplantation for adults with acute myeloid leukemia: myths, controversies, and unknowns. Blood 2011; 117(8): 2307–2318.

122. Cornelissen JJ, Gratwohl A, Schlenk RF, Sierra J, Bornhauser M et al. The European LeukemiaNet AML Working Party consensus statement on allogeneic HSCT for patients with AML in remission: an integrated-risk adapted approach. Nature Reviews Clinical Oncology 2012; 9(10): 579–590.

123. Koreth J, Schlenk R, Kopecky KJ, Honda S, Sierra J et al. Allogeneic stem cell transplantation for acute myeloid leukemia in first complete remission: systematic review and meta-analysis of prospective clinical trials. JAMA. 2009; 301(22): 2349–2361.

124. Kayser S, Zucknick M, Dohner K, Krauter J, Kohne CH et al. Monosomal karyotype in adult acute myeloid leukemia: prognostic impact and outcome after different treatment strategies. Blood 2012; 119(2): 551–558.

125. Fang M, Storer B, Estey E, Othus M, Zhang L et al. Outcome of patients with acute myeloid leukemia with monosomal karyotype who undergo hematopoietic cell transplantation. Blood 2011;118(6): 1490–1494.

126. Yanada M, Kurosawa S, Yamaguchi T, Yamashita T, Moriuchi Y et al. Prognosis of acute myeloid leukemia harboring monosomal karyotype in patients treated with or without allogeneic hematopoietic cell transplantation after achieving complete remission. Haematologica 2012; 97(6): 915–918.

127. Grimwade D, Hills RK, Moorman AV, Walker H, Chatters S et al. Refinement of cytogenetic classification in acute myeloid leukemia: determination of prognostic significance of rare recurring chromosomal abnormalities among 5876 younger adult patients treated in the United Kingdom Medical Research Council trials. Blood 2010; 116(3): 354–365.

128. Ganzel C, Rowe JM. Prognostic factors in adult acute leukemia. Hematology/Oncology Clinics of North America 2011; 25(6): 1163–1187.

129. Ofran Y, Rowe JM. Genetic profiling in acute myelogenous leukaemia—where are we and what is its role in patient management. British Journal of Haematology 2013; 160(3): 303–320.

130. Patel JP, Gonen M, Figueroa ME, Fernandez H, Sun Z et al. Prognostic relevance of integrated genetic profiling in acute myeloid leukemia. New England Journal of Medicine 2012; 366(12): 1079–1089.

131. Grossmann V, Schnittger S, Kohlmann A, Eder C, Roller A et al. A novel hierarchical prognostic model of AML solely based on molecular mutations. Blood 2012; 120(15): 2963–2972.

132. Gratwohl A. The EBMT risk score. Bone Marrow Transplant 2012; 47(6): 749–756.

133. Armand P, Gibson CJ, Cutler C, Ho VT, Koreth J, Alyea EP, et al. A disease risk index for patients undergoing allogeneic stem cell transplantation. Blood 2012; 120(4): 905–913.

134. Sorror ML, Giralt S, Sandmaier BM, De Lima M, Shahjahan M et al. Hematopoietic cell transplantation specific comorbidity index as an outcome predictor for patients with acute myeloid leukemia in first remission: combined FHCRC and MDACC experiences. Blood 2007; 110(13): 4606–4613.

135. Bornhauser M, Kienast J, Trenschel R, Burchert A, Hegenbart U et al. Reduced-intensity conditioning versus standard conditioning before allogeneic haemopoietic cell transplantation in patients with acute myeloid leukaemia in first complete remission: a prospective, open-label randomised phase 3 trial. Lancet Oncology 2012; 13(10): 1035–1044.

136. Gardin C, Turlure P, Fagot T, Thomas X, Terre C et al. Postremission treatment of elderly patients with acute myeloid leukemia in first complete remission after intensive induction chemotherapy: results of the multicenter randomized Acute Leukemia French Association (ALFA) 9803 trial. Blood 2007;109(12): 5129–5135.

137. Miyawaki S, Sakamaki H, Ohtake S, Emi N, Yagasaki F et al. A randomized, postremission comparison of four courses of standard-dose consolidation therapy without maintenance therapy versus three courses of standard-dose consolidation with maintenance therapy in adults with acute myeloid leukemia: the Japan Adult Leukemia Study Group AML 97 Study. Cancer 2005; 104(12): 2726–2734.

138. Brune M, Castaigne S, Catalano J, Gehlsen K, Ho AD et al. Improved leukemia-free survival after postconsolidation immunotherapy with histamine dihydrochloride and interleukin-2 in acute myeloid leukemia: results of a randomized phase 3 trial. Blood 2006; 108(1): 88–96.

139. Platzbecker U, Wermke M, Radke J, Oelschlaegel U, Seltmann F et al. Azacitidine for treatment of imminent relapse in MDS or AML patients after allogeneic HSCT: results of the RELAZA trial. Leukemia 2012; 26(3): 381–389.

140. Rubnitz JE, Inaba H, Dahl G, Ribeiro RC, Bowman WP et al. Minimal residual disease-directed therapy for childhood acute myeloid leukaemia: results of the AML02 multicentre trial. Lancet Oncology 2010; 11(6): 543–552.

141. van Dongen JJ, Orfao A. EuroFlow. Resetting leukemia and lymphoma immunophenotyping. Basis for companion diagnostics and personalized medicine. Leukemia 2012; 26(9): 1899–1907.

142. Liu Yin JA, O'Brien MA, Hills RK, Daly SB, Wheatley K et al. Minimal residual disease monitoring by RT-qPCR in core-binding factor AML allows risk-stratification and predicts relapse: results of the UK MRC AML-15 trial. Blood 2012; 120(14): 2826–2835.

143. Smith CC, Wang Q, Chin CS, Salerno S, Damon LE et al. Validation of ITD mutations in FLT3 as a therapeutic target in human acute myeloid leukaemia. Nature 2012; 485(7397): 260–263.

144. Guo M, Hu KX, Yu CL, Sun QY, Qiao JH et al. Infusion of HLA-mismatched peripheral blood stem cells improves the outcome of chemotherapy for acute myeloid leukemia in elderly patients. Blood 2011; 117(3): 936–941.

145. Guo M, Hu KX, Liu GX, Yu CL, Qiao JH et al. HLA-mismatched stem-cell microtransplantation as postremission therapy for acute myeloid leukemia: long-term follow-up. Journal of Clinical Oncology 2012; 30(33): 4084–4090.

146. Ofran Y, Rowe JM. Treatment for relapsed acute myeloid leukemia: what is new? Current Opinions in Hematology 2012; 19(2): 89–94.

147. Litzow MR, Othus M, Cripe LD, Gore SD, Lazarus HM et al. Failure of three novel regimens to improve outcome for patients with relapsed or refractory acute myeloid leukaemia: a report from the Eastern Cooperative Oncology Group. British Journal of Haematology 2010; 148(2): 217–225.

148. Estey EH. Treatment of relapsed and refractory acute myelogenous leukemia. Leukemia 2000; 14(3): 476–479.

149. Schmid C, Schleuning M, Schwerdtfeger R, Hertenstein B, Mischak-Weissinger E et al. Long-term survival in refractory acute myeloid leukemia after sequential treatment with chemotherapy and reduced-intensity conditioning for allogeneic stem cell transplantation. Blood 2006; 108(3): 1092–1099.

150. Blum W, Klisovic RB, Becker H, Yang X, Rozewski DM et al. Dose escalation of lenalidomide in relapsed or refractory acute leukemias. Journal of Clinical Oncology 2010; 28(33): 4919–4925.

151. Buchner T, Berdel WE, Haferlach C, Haferlach T, Schnittger S et al. Age-related risk profile and chemotherapy dose response in acute myeloid leukemia: a study by the German Acute Myeloid Leukemia Cooperative Group. Journal of Clinical Oncology 2009; 27(1): 61–69.

152. Petersdorf S, Kopecky K, Stuart RK, Larson RA, Nevill TJ et al. Preliminary results of Southwest Oncology Group Study S0106: an international intergroup phase 3 randomized trial comparing the addition of gemtuzumab ozogamicin to standard induction therapy versus standard induction therapy followed by a second randomization to post-consolidation gemtuzumab ozogamicin versus no additional therapy for previously untreated acute myeloid leukemia. Blood 2009; 114: 790a.

153. Pautas C, Merabet F, Thomas X, Raffoux E, Gardin C et al. Randomized study of intensified anthracycline doses for induction and recombinant interleukin-2 for maintenance in patients with acute myeloid leukemia age 50 to 70 years: results of the ALFA-9801 study. Journal of Clinical Oncology 2010; 28(5): 808–814.

154. Hoelzer D, Thiel E, Löffler H, Büchner T, Ganser A et al. Prognostic factors in a multicenter study for treatment of acute lymphoblastic leukemia in adults. Blood 1988; 71(1): 123–131.

155. Rowe JM. Prognostic factors in adult acute lymphoblastic leukaemia. British Journal of Haematology 2010; 150(4): 389–405.

156. Bassan R, Hoelzer D. Modern therapy of acute lymphoblastic leukemia. Journal of Clinical Oncology 2011; 29(5): 532–543.

157. Gökbuget N, Arnold R, Bohme A et al. Improved outcome in high risk and very high risk ALL by risk adapted SCT and in standard risk ALL by intensive chemotherapy in 713 adult ALL patients treated according to the prospective GMALL study 07/2003. Blood 2007; 110.

158. Hoelzer D, Thiel E, Arnold R et al. Successful subtype oriented treatment strategies in adult TALL: Results of 744 patients treated in three consecutive GMALL studies. Blood 2009; 114(abstr 324): 137.

159. Asnafi V, Buzyn A, Le Noir S, Baleydier F, Simon A et a. NOTCH1/FBXW7 mutation identifies a large subgroup with favorable outcome in adult T-cell acute lymphoblastic leukemia (T-ALL): a Group for Research on Adult Acute Lymphoblastic Leukemia (GRAALL) study. Blood 2009; 113(17): 3918–3924.

160. Patel B, Rai L, Buck G et al. Minimal residual disease is a significant predictor of treatment failure in non T-lineage adult acute lymphoblastic leukaemia: Final results of the international trial UKALLXII/ECOG2993. British Journal of Haematology 2010; 148: 80–89.

161. Hoelzer D, Gökbuget N. Chemoimmunotherapy in acute lymphoblastic leukemia. Blood Reviews 2012; 26(1): 25–32.

162. Hoelzer D, Huettmann A, Kaul F, Irmer SI, Jaeckel NJ et al. Immunochemotherapy with rituximab in adult CD20 B-precursor ALL improves molecular CR rate and outcome in standard risk (SR) as well as in high risk (HR) patients with SCT. Haematologica 2009; 94(abstr 481).

163. Thomas DA, O'Brien S, Faderl S, Garcia-Manero G, Ferrajoli A et al. Chemoimmunotherapy with a modified hyper-CVAD and rituximab regimen improves outcome in de novo Philadelphia chromosome-negative precursor B-lineage acute lymphoblastic leukemia. Journal of Clinical Oncology 2010; 28(24): 3880–3889.

164. Raetz EA, Cairo MS, Borowitz MJ, Blaney SM, Krailo MD et al. Chemoimmunotherapy reinduction with epratuzumab in children with acute lymphoblastic leukemia in marrow relapse: a Children's Oncology Group Pilot Study. Journal of Clinical Oncology 2008; 26: 3756–3762.

165. Campana D. Minimal residual disease in acute lymphoblastic leukemia. Hematology American Society Hematology Education Program 2010: 7–12.

166. Brüggemann M, Schrauder A, Raff T et al. European Working Group for Adult Acute Lymphoblastic Leukemia (EWALL); International Berlin-Frankfurt-Münster Study Group (I-BFM-SG). Standardized MRD quantification in European ALL trials: Proceedings of the Second International Symposium on MRD assessment in Kiel, Germany, 18–20 September 2008. Leukemia 2010; 24: 521–535.

167. Brüggemann M, Raff T, Kneba M. Has MRD monitoring superseded other prognostic factors in adult ALL? Blood 2012; 120(23): 4470–4481.

168. Hoelzer D, Gökbuget N. Change in prognostic factors. Leukemia Supplements August 2012; 1: 1–2.

169. Gökbuget N, Kneba M, Raff T, Trautmann H, Bartram CR et al. German Multicenter Study Group for Adult Acute Lymphoblastic Leukemia. Adult patients with acute lymphoblastic leukemia and molecular failure display a poor prognosis and are candidates for stem cell transplantation and targeted therapies.Blood 2012; 120(9): 1868–1876.

170. Bassan R, Spinelli O, Oldani E et al. Improved risk classification for risk-specific therapy based on the molecular study of minimal residual disease (MRD) in adult acute lymphoblastic leukemia (ALL). Blood 2009; 113(18): 4153–4162.

171. Giebel S, Stella-Holowiecka B, Krawczyk-Kulis M et al. Status of minimal residual disease determines outcome of autologous hematopoietic SCT in adult ALL. Bone Marrow Transplant 2009; 45: 1095–1101.

172. Pfeifer H, Wassmann B, Bethge W et al. Randomized comparison of prophylactic and minimal residual disease-triggered imatinib after allogeneic stem cell transplantation for BCR-ABL1 positive acute lymphoblastic leukemia. Leukemia 5 December 2012 [Epub ahead of print].

173. Topp MS, Kufer P, Gokbuget N, Goebeler M, Klinger M et al. Targeted therapy with the T-cell-engaging antibody blinatumomab of chemotherapy-refractory minimal residual disease in B-lineage acute lymphoblastic leukemia patients results in high response rate and prolonged leukemia-free survival. Journal of Clinical Oncology 2011; 29: 2493–2498.

174. Gawad C, Pepin F, Carlton VE et al. Massive evolution of the immunoglobulin heavy chain locus in children with B precursor acute lymphoblastic leukemia. Blood 2012; 120(22): 4407–4417.

175. Faham M, Zheng J, Moorhead M et al. Deep-sequencing approach for minimal residual disease detection in acute lymphoblastic leukemia. Blood 2012; 120(26): 5173–5180.

176. Pui CH, Robison LL, Look AT. Acute lymphoblastic leukaemia. Lancet 2008; 371(9617): 1030–1043.

177. Inaba H, Greaves M, Mulligan CG. Acute lymphoblastic leukaemia. Lancet 2013; 381(9881): 1943–1955.

178. Rowley JD. Letter: A new consistent chromosomal abnormality in chronic myelogenous leukaemia identified by quinacrine fluorescence and Giemsa staining. Nature 1973; 243(5405): 290–293.

179. Ben-Neriah Y, Daley GQ, Mes-Masson AM, Witte ON, Baltimore D. The chronic myelogenous leukemia-specific P210 protein is the product of the bcr/abl hybrid gene. Science 1986; 233(4760): 212–214.

180. Grosveld G, Verwoerd T, van Agthoven T, de Klein A, Ramachandran KL et al. The chronic myelocytic cell line K562 contains a breakpoint in bcr and produces a chimeric bcr/c-abl transcript. Molecular and Cellular Biology 1986; 6(2): 607–616.

181. Heisterkamp N, Stam K, Groffen J, de Klein A, Grosveld G. Structural organization of the bcr gene and its role in the Ph' translocation. Nature 1985; 315(6022): 758–761.

182. Mes-Masson AM, McLaughlin J, Daley GQ, Paskind M, Witte ON. Overlapping cDNA clones define the complete coding region for the P210c-abl gene product associated with chronic myelogenous leukemia cells containing the Philadelphia chromosome. Proceedings of the National Academy of Sciences USA 1986; 83(24): 9768–9772.

183. Shtivelman E, Lifshitz B, Gale RP, Canaani E. Fused transcript of abl and bcr genes in chronic myelogenous leukaemia. Nature 1985; 315(6020): 550–554.

184. Look AT. Oncogenic transcription factors in the human acute leukemias. Science 1997; 278(5340): 1059–1064.

185. Ford AM, Ridge SA, Cabrera ME, Mahmoud H, Steel CM et al. In utero rearrangements in the trithorax-related oncogene in infant leukaemias. Nature 1993; 363(6427): 358–360.

186. Gale KB, Ford AM, Repp R, Borkhardt A, Keller C et al. Backtracking leukemia to birth: identification of clonotypic gene fusion sequences in neonatal blood spots. Proceedings of the National Academy of Sciences USA 1997; 94(25): 13950–13954.

187. Mullighan CG. Genome sequencing of lymphoid malignancies. Blood 2013; 122(24): 3899–3907.

188. Mullighan CG, Goorha S, Radtke I, Miller CB, Coustan-Smith E et al. Genome-wide analysis of genetic alterations in acute lymphoblastic leukaemia. Nature 2007; 446(7137): 758–764.

189. Mullighan CG. Molecular genetics of B-precursor acute lymphoblastic leukemia. Journal of Clinical Investigation 2012; 122(10): 3407–3415.

190. Moorman AV, Richards SM, Martineau M, Cheung KL, Robinson HM et al. Outcome heterogeneity in childhood high-hyperdiploid acute lymphoblastic leukaemia. Blood 2003; 102(8): 2756–2762.

191. Tallen G, Ratei R, Mann G, Kaspers G, Niggli F et al. Long-term outcome in children with relapsed acute lymphoblastic leukaemia after time-point and site-of-relapse stratification and intensified short-course multidrug chemotherapy: results of trial ALL-REZ BFM 90. Journal of Clinical Oncology 2010; 28(14): 2339–2347.

192. Sutcliffe MJ, Shuster JJ, Sather HN, Camitta BM, Pullen J et al. High concordance from independent studies by the Children's Cancer Group (CCG) and Pediatric Oncology Group (POG) associating favorable prognosis with combined trisomies 4, 10, and 17 in children with NCI Standard-Risk B-precursor Acute Lymphoblastic Leukemia: a Children's Oncology Group (COG) initiative. Leukemia 2005; 19(5): 734–740.

193. Paulsson K, Johansson B. High hyperdiploid childhood acute lymphoblastic leukemia. Genes Chromosomes Cancer 2009; 48(8): 637–660.

194 Andersson A, Olofsson T, Lindgren D, Nilsson B, Ritz C et al. Molecular signatures in childhood acute leukemia and their correlations to expression patterns in normal hematopoietic subpopulations. Proceedings of the National Academy of Sciences USA 2005; 102(52): 19069–19074.

195. Ross ME, Zhou X, Song G, Shurtleff SA, Girtman K et al. Classification of pediatric acute lymphoblastic leukemia by gene expression profiling. Blood 2003; 102(8): 2951–2959.

196. Figueroa ME, Chen SC, Andersson AK, Phillips LA, Li Y et al. Integrated genetic and epigenetic analysis of childhood acute lymphoblastic leukemia. Journal of Clinical Investigation 2013; 123(7): 3099–3111.

197. Paulsson K, Horvat A, Strombeck B, Nilsson F, Heldrup J et al. Mutations of FLT3, NRAS, KRAS, and PTPN11 are frequent and possibly mutually exclusive in high hyperdiploid childhood acute lymphoblastic leukemia. Genes Chromosomes Cancer 2008; 47(1): 26–33.

198. Inthal A, Zeitlhofer P, Zeginigg M, Morak M, Grausenburger R et al. CREBBP HAT domain mutations prevail in relapse cases of high hyperdiploid childhood acute lymphoblastic leukemia. Leukemia: official journal of the Leukemia Society of America, Leukemia Research Fund, UK. 2012.

199. Mullighan CG, Zhang J, Kasper LH, Lerach S, Payne-Turner D et al. CREBBP mutations in relapsed acute lymphoblastic leukaemia. Nature 2011; 471(7337): 235–239.

200. Harrison CJ, Moorman AV, Broadfield ZJ, Cheung KL, Harris RL et al. Three distinct subgroups of hypodiploidy in acute lymphoblastic leukaemia. British Journal of Haematology 2004; 125(5): 552–559.

201. Heerema NA, Nachman JB, Sather HN, Sensel MG, Lee MK et al. Hypodiploidy with less than 45 chromosomes confers adverse risk in

childhood acute lymphoblastic leukemia: a report from the children's cancer group. Blood 1999; 94(12): 4036–4045.

202. Nachman JB, Heerema NA, Sather H, Camitta B, Forestier E et al. Outcome of treatment in children with hypodiploid acute lymphoblastic leukemia. Blood 2007; 110(4): 1112–1115.

203. Pui CH, Carroll AJ, Raimondi SC, Land VJ, Crist WM et al. Clinical presentation, karyotypic characterization, and treatment outcome of childhood acute lymphoblastic leukemia with a near-haploid or hypodiploid less than 45 line. Blood 1990; 75(5): 1170–1177.

204. Pui CH, Williams DL, Raimondi SC, Rivera GK, Look AT et al. Hypodiploidy is associated with a poor prognosis in childhood acute lymphoblastic leukemia. Blood 1987; 70(1): 247–253.

205. Raimondi SC, Zhou Y, Mathew S, Shurtleff SA, Sandlund JT et al. Reassessment of the prognostic significance of hypodiploidy in pediatric patients with acute lymphoblastic leukemia. Cancer 2003; 98(12): 2715–2722.

206. Carroll AJ, Heerema NA, Gastier-Foster JM, Astbury C, Pyatt R et al. Masked Hypodiploidy: Hypodiploid Acute Lymphoblastic Leukemia (ALL) in Children Mimicking Hyperdiploid ALL: A Report From the Children's Oncology Group (COG) AALL03B1 Study. ASH Annual Meeting Abstracts 2009; 114(22): 1580.

207. Holmfeldt L, Wei L, Diaz-Flores E, Walsh M, Zhang J et al. The genomic landscape of hypodiploid acute lymphoblastic leukemia. Nature Genetics 2013; 45(3): 242–252.

208. Powell BC, Jiang L, Muzny DM, Trevino LR, Dreyer ZE et al. Identification of TP53 as an acute lymphocytic leukemia susceptibility gene through exome sequencing. Pediatric Blood Cancer 2013; 60(6): E1–E3.

209. Golub T, McLean T, Stegmaier K, Ritz J, Sallan S et al. TEL-AML1: The most common gene rearrangement in childhood ALL. Blood 1995; 86(10): 2377.

210. Romana SP, Poirel H, Leconiat M, Flexor MA, Jonveaux MMP et al. High-frequency of T(12-21) in childhood B-lineage acute lymphoblastic-leukemia. Blood 1995; 86(11): 4263–4269.

211. Shurtleff SA, Buijs A, Behm FG, Rubnitz JE, Raimondi SC et al. TEL/AML1 fusion resulting from a cryptic t(12;21) is the most common genetic lesion in pediatric ALL and defines a subgroup of patients with an excellent prognosis. Leukemia 1995; 9(12): 1985–1989.

212. Burmeister T, Gokbuget N, Schwartz S, Fischer L, Hubert D et al. Clinical features and prognostic implications of TCF3-PBX1 and ETV6-RUNX1 in adult acute lymphoblastic leukemia. Hematology Hematology Journal 2010; 95(2): 241–246.

213. Aguiar RCT, Sohal J, vanRhee F, Carapeti M, Franklin IM et al. TEL-AML1 fusion in acute lymphoblastic leukaemia of adults. British Journal of Haematology 1996; 95(4): 673–677.

214. Al-Obaidi MSJ, Martineau M, Bennett CF, Franklin IM, Goldstone AH et al. ETV6/AML1 fusion by FISH in adult acute lymphoblastic leukemia. Leukemia 2002; 16(4): 669–674.

215. Raynaud S, Mauvieux L, Cayuela JM, Bastard C, BilhouNabera C et al. TEL/AML1 fusion gene is a rare event in adult acute lymphoblastic leukemia. Leukemia 1996; 10(9): 1529–1530.

216. Romana SP, Le Coniat M, Berger R. t(12;21): a new recurrent translocation in acute lymphoblastic leukemia. Genes Chromosomes Cancer 1994; 9(3): 186–191.

217. Golub TR, Barker GF, Bohlander SK, Hiebert SW, Ward DC et al. Fusion of the Tel Gene on 12p13 to the Aml1 Gene on 21q22 in Acute Lymphoblastic-Leukemia. Proceedings of the National Academy of Sciences USA 1995; 92(11): 4917–4921.

218. Romana SP, Mauchauffe M, Leconiat M, Chumakov I, Lepaslier D et al. The t(12-21) of acute lymphoblastic-leukemia results in a tel-aml1 gene fusion. Blood 1995; 85(12): 3662–3670.

219. Bohlander SK. ETV6: A versatile player in leukemogenesis. Seminars in Cancer Biology 2005; 15(3): 162–174.

220. Harewood L, Robinson H, Harris R, Al-Obaidi MJ, Jalali GR et al. Amplification of AML1 on a duplicated chromosome 21 in acute lymphoblastic leukemia: a study of 20 cases. Leukemia 2003; 17(3): 547–553.

221. Robinson HM, Broadfield ZJ, Barber KE, Cheung KL, Stewart ARM et al. Amplification of RUNX1 in acute lymphoblastic leukaemia is associated with intrachromosomal instability of the duplicated chromosome 21—a distinct mechanism? Journal of Medical Genetics 2005; 42: S20.

222. Robinson HM, Broadfield ZJ, Cheung KL, Harewood L, Harris RL et al. Amplification of AML1 in acute lymphoblastic leukemia is associated with a poor outcome. Leukemia 2003; 17(11): 2249–2250.

223. Strefford J, Van Delft F, Robinson HM, Worley H, Selzer R et al. Patients with RUNX1 (AML1) amplification exhibit consistent genomic amplification, chromosome instability and a distinct gene expression signature. Journal of Medical Genetics 2005; 42: S65–S.

224. Strefford JC, Van Delft F, Robinson HM, Worley H, Selzer R et al. Molecular characterization of AML1 (RUNX1) amplification: a poor risk chromosomal marker in acute lymphoblastic leukaemia (ALL). Chromosome Research 2005; 13: 151.

225. Stegmaier K, Pendse S, Barker GF, Brayward P, Ward DC et al. Frequent Loss of Heterozygosity at the Tel Gene Locus in Acute Lymphoblastic-Leukemia of Childhood. Blood 1995; 86(1): 38–44.

226. Bhojwani D, Pei D, Sandlund JT, Jeha S, Ribeiro RC et al. ETV6-RUNX1-positive childhood acute lymphoblastic leukemia: improved outcome with contemporary therapy. Leukemia 2012; 26(2): 265–270.

227. Ford AM, Bennett CA, Price CM, Bruin MCA, Van Wering ER et al. Fetal origins of the TEL-AML1 fusion gene in identical twins with leukemia. Proceedings of the National Academy of Sciences USA 1998; 95(8): 4584–4588.

228. Wiemels JL, Cazzaniga G, Daniotti M, Eden OB, Addison GM et al. Prenatal origin of acute lymphoblastic leukaemia in children. Lancet 1999; 354(9189): 1499–1503.

229. Wiemels JL, Ford AM, Van Wering ER, Postma A, Greaves M. Protracted and variable latency of acute lymphoblastic leukemia after TEL-AML1 gene fusion in utero. Blood 1999; 94(3): 1057–1062.

230. Mori H, Colman SM, Xiao ZJ, Ford AM, Healy LE et al. Chromosome translocations and covert leukemic clones are generated during normal fetal development. Proceedings of the National Academy of Sciences USA 2002; 99(12): 8242–8247.

231. Lausten-Thomsen U, Madsen HO, Vestergaard TR, Hjalgrim H, Nersting J et al. Prevalence of t(12;21)[ETV6-RUNX1]-positive cells in healthy neonates. Blood 2011; 117(1): 186–189.

232. Lilljebjorn H, Heidenblad M, Nilsson B, Lassen C, Horvat A et al. Combined high-resolution array-based comparative genomic hybridization and expression profiling of ETV6/RUNX1-positive acute lymphoblastic leukemias reveal a high incidence of cryptic Xq duplications and identify several putative target genes within the commonly gained region. Leukemia 2007; 21(10): 2137–2144.

233. Lilljebjorn H, Soneson C, Andersson A, Heldrup J, Behrendtz M et al. The correlation pattern of acquired copy number changes in 164 ETV6/RUNX1-positive childhood acute lymphoblastic leukemias. Human Molecular Genetics 2010; 19(16): 3150–3158.

234. Raynaud S, Cave H, Baens M, Bastard C, Cacheux V et al. The 12;21 translocation involving TEL and deletion of the other TEL allele: Two frequently associated alterations found in childhood acute lymphoblastic leukemia. Blood 1996; 87(7): 2891–2899.

235. SennanaSendi H, Dastugue N, Talmant P, Bastard C, Cacheux V et al. Deletions of the non-translocated allele of TEL (ETV6) seem to be constant in childhood B-lineage ALLs with a t(12;21). Results of a FISH study on 148 children included in the 58881 therapeutic trial from the CLCG (EORTC). Blood 1996; 88(10): 274.

236. Parker H, An Q, Barber K, Case M, Davies T et al. The complex genomic profile of ETV6-RUNX1 positive acute lymphoblastic leukemia highlights a recurrent deletion of TBL1XR1. Genes Chromosomes Cancer 2008; 47(12): 1118–1125.

237. Al-Shehhi H, Konn ZJ, Schwab CJ, Erhorn A, Barber KE et al. Abnormalities of the der(12)t(12;21) in ETV6-RUNX1 acute lymphoblastic leukemia. Genes Chromosomes Cancer 2013; 52(2): 202–213.

238. Imai Y, Kurokawa M, Tanaka K, Friedman AD, Ogawa S et al. TLE, the human homolog of Groucho, interacts with AML1 and acts as a repressor of AML1-induced transactivation. Biochemical and Biophysical Research Communication 1998; 252(3): 582–589.

239. Okuda T, vanDeursen J, Hiebert SW, Grosveld G, Downing JR. AML1, the target of multiple chromosomal translocations in human leukemia, is essential for normal fetal liver hematopoiesis. Cell 1996; 84(2): 321–330.

240. Wang Q, Stacy T, Miller JD, Lewis AF, Gu TL et al. The CBF beta subunit is essential for CBF alpha 2 (AML1) function in vivo. Cell 1996; 87(4): 697–708.

241. Fenrick R, Amann JM, Lutterbach B, Wang LL, Westendorf JJ et al. Both TEL and AML-1 contribute repression domains to the t(12;21) fusion protein. Molecular Cell Biology 1999; 19(10): 6566–6574.

242. Guidez F, Petrie K, Ford AM, Lu HF, Bennett CA et al. Recruitment of the nuclear receptor corepressor N-CoR by the TEL moiety of the childhood leukemia-associated TEL-AML1 oncoprotein. Blood 2000; 96(7): 2557–2561.

243. Andreasson P, Schwaller J, Anastasiadou E, Aster J, Gilliland DG. The expression of ETV6/CBFA2 (TEL/AML1) is not sufficient for the transformation of hematopoietic cell lines in vitro or the induction of hematologic disease in vivo. Cancer Genetics and Cytogenetics 2001; 130(2): 93–104.

244. Morrow M, Horton S, Kioussis D, Brady HJM, Williams O. TEL-AML1 promotes development of specific hematopoietic lineages consistent with preleukemic activity. Blood 2004; 103(10): 3890–3896.

245. Tsuzuki S, Seto M, Greaves M, Enver T. Modeling first-hit functions of the t(12;21) TEL-AML1 translocation in mice. Proceedings of the National Academy of Sciences USA 2004; 101(22): 8443–8448.

246. Bernardin F, Yang YD, Cleaves R, Zahurak M, Cheng LZ et al. TEL-AML1, expressed from t(12;21) in human acute lymphocytic leukemia, induces acute leukemia in mice. Cancer Research 2002; 62(14): 3904–3908.

247. Moorman AV, Chilton L, Wilkinson J, Ensor HM, Bown N et al. A population-based cytogenetic study of adults with acute lymphoblastic leukemia. Blood 2010; 115(2): 206–214.

248. Privitera E, Kamps MP, Hayashi Y, Inaba T, Shapiro LH et al. Different molecular consequences of the 1;19 chromosomal translocation in childhood B-cell precursor acute lymphoblastic leukemia. Blood 1992; 79(7): 1781–1788.

249. Raimondi SC, Behm FG, Roberson PK, Williams DL, Pui CH et al. Cytogenetics of pre-B-cell acute lymphoblastic leukemia with emphasis on prognostic implications of the t(1;19). Journal of Clinical Oncology 1990; 8(8): 1380–1388.

250. Crist WM, Carroll AJ, Shuster JJ, Behm FG, Whitehead M et al. Poor prognosis of children with pre-B acute lymphoblastic leukemia is associated with the t(1;19)(q23;p13): a Pediatric Oncology Group study. Blood 1990; 76(1): 117–122.

251. Hunger SP. Chromosomal translocations involving the E2A gene in acute lymphoblastic leukemia: clinical features and molecular pathogenesis. Blood 1996; 87(4): 1211–1224.

252. Kamps MP, Murre C, Sun XH, Baltimore D. A new homeobox gene contributes the DNA binding domain of the t(1;19) translocation protein in pre-B ALL. Cell 1990; 60(4): 547–555.

253. Mellentin JD, Nourse J, Hunger SP, Smith SD, Cleary ML. Molecular analysis of the t(1;19) breakpoint cluster region in pre-B cell acute lymphoblastic leukemias. Genes Chromosomes Cancer 1990; 2(3): 239–247.

254. Nourse J, Mellentin JD, Galili N, Wilkinson J, Stanbridge E et al. Chromosomal translocation t(1;19) results in synthesis of a homeobox fusion mRNA that codes for a potential chimeric transcription factor. Cell 1990; 60(4): 535–545.

255. Jeha S, Pei D, Raimondi SC, Onciu M, Campana D et al. Increased risk for CNS relapse in pre-B cell leukemia with the t(1;19)/TCF3-PBX1. Leukemia 2009; 23(8): 1406–1409.

256. Pui CH, Campana D, Pei D, Bowman WP, Sandlund JT et al. Treating childhood acute lymphoblastic leukemia without cranial irradiation. New England Journal of Medicine 2009; 360(26): 2730–2741.

257. Pui CH, Behm FG, Downing JR, Hancock ML, Shurtleff SA et al. 11q23/MLL rearrangement confers a poor prognosis in infants with

258. Rubnitz JE, Link MP, Shuster JJ, Carroll AJ, Hakami N et al. Frequency and Prognostic-Significance of Hrx Rearrangements in Infant Acute Lymphoblastic-Leukemia—a Pediatric-Oncology-Group Study. Blood 1994; 84(2): 570–573.

259. Pui CH, Kane JR, Crist WM. Biology and treatment of infant leukemias. Leukemia 1995; 9(5): 762–769.

260. Forestier E, Johansson B, Borgstrom G, Kerndrup G, Johannsson J et al. Cytogenetic findings in a population-based series of 787 childhood acute lymphoblastic leukemias from the Nordic countries. European Journal of Haematology 2000; 64(3): 194–200.

261. Forestier E, Johansson B, Gustafsson G, Borgstrom G, Kerndrup G et al. Prognostic impact of karyotypic findings in childhood acute lymphoblastic leukaemia: a Nordic series comparing two treatment periods. For the Nordic Society of Paediatric Haematology and Oncology (NOPHO) Leukaemia Cytogenetic Study Group. British Journal of Haematology 2000; 110(1): 147–153.

262. Harrison CJ. The detection and significance of chromosomal abnormalities in childhood acute lymphoblastic leukaemia. Blood Reviews 2001; 15(1): 49–59.

263. Harrison CJ, Hills RK, Moorman AV, Grimwade DJ, Hann I et al. Cytogenetics of childhood acute myeloid leukemia: United Kingdom Medical Research Council Treatment trials AML 10 and 12. Journal of Clinical Oncology 2010; 28(16): 2674–2681.

264. Balgobind BV, Zwaan CM, Pieters R, Van den Heuvel-Eibrink MM. The heterogeneity of pediatric MLL-rearranged acute myeloid leukemia. Leukemia 2011; 25(8): 1239–1248.

265. Forestier E, Heim S, Blennow E, Borgstrom G, Holmgren G et al. Cytogenetic abnormalities in childhood acute myeloid leukaemia: a Nordic series comprising all children enrolled in the NOPHO-93-AML trial between 1993 and 2001. British Journal of Haematology 2003; 121(4): 566–577.

266. Secker-Walker LM, Prentice HG, Durrant J, Richards S, Hall E, Harrison G. Cytogenetics adds independent prognostic information in adults with acute lymphoblastic leukaemia on MRC trial UKALL XA. MRC Adult Leukaemia Working Party. British Journal of Haematology 1997; 96(3): 601–610.

267. Cytogenetic abnormalities in adult acute lymphoblastic leukaemia: correlations with hematologic findings outcome. A Collaborative Study of the Group Francais de Cytogenetique Hematologique. Blood 1996; 87(8): 3135–3142.

268. Mancini M, Scappaticci D, Cimino G, Nanni M, Derme V et al. A comprehensive genetic classification of adult acute lymphoblastic leukemia (ALL): analysis of the GIMEMA 0496 protocol. Blood 2005; 105(9): 3434–3441.

269. Moorman AV, Harrison CJ, Buck GA, Richards SM, Secker-Walker LM et al. Karyotype is an independent prognostic factor in adult acute lymphoblastic leukemia (ALL): analysis of cytogenetic data from patients treated on the Medical Research Council (MRC) UKALLXII/Eastern Cooperative Oncology Group (ECOG) 2993 trial. Blood 2007; 109(8): 3189–3197.

270. Domer PH, Head DR, Renganathan N, Raimondi SC, Yang E, Atlas M. Molecular analysis of 13 cases of MLL/11q23 secondary acute leukemia and identification of topoisomerase II consensus-binding sequences near the chromosomal breakpoint of a secondary leukemia with the t(4;11). Leukemia 1995; 9(8): 1305–1312.

271. Felix CA, Hosler MR, Winick NJ, Masterson M, Wilson AE et al. ALL-1 gene rearrangements in DNA topoisomerase II inhibitor-related leukemia in children. Blood 1995; 85(11): 3250–3256.

272. Pui CH, Ribeiro RC, Hancock ML, Rivera GK, Evans WE et al. Acute myeloid leukemia in children treated with epipodophyllotoxins for acute lymphoblastic leukemia. New England Journal of Medicine 1991; 325(24): 1682–1687.

273. Moorman AV, Raimondi SC, Pui CH, Baruchel A, Biondi A et al. No prognostic effect of additional chromosomal abnormalities in

acute lymphoblastic leukemia. Journal of Clinical Oncology 1994; 12(5): 909–915.

children with acute lymphoblastic leukemia and 11q23 abnormalities. Leukemia 2005; 19(4): 557–563.

274. Pieters R, Schrappe M, De Lorenzo P, Hann I, De Rossi G et al. A treatment protocol for infants younger than 1 year with acute lymphoblastic leukaemia (Interfant-99): an observational study and a multicentre randomised trial. Lancet 2007; 370(9583): 240–250.

275. Dreyer ZE, Dinndorf PA, Camitta B, Sather H, La MK et al. Analysis of the role of hematopoietic stem-cell transplantation in infants with acute lymphoblastic leukemia in first remission and MLL gene rearrangements: a report from the Children's Oncology Group. Journal of Clinical Oncology 2011; 29(2): 214–222.

276. Mann G, Attarbaschi A, Schrappe M, De Lorenzo P, Peters C et al. Improved outcome with hematopoietic stem cell transplantation in a poor prognostic subgroup of infants with mixed-lineage-leukemia (MLL)-rearranged acute lymphoblastic leukemia: results from the Interfant-99 Study. Blood 2010; 116(15): 2644–2650.

277. Pui CH, Chessells JM, Camitta B, Baruchel A, Biondi A et al. Clinical heterogeneity in childhood acute lymphoblastic leukemia with 11q23 rearrangements. Leukemia 2003; 17(4): 700–706.

278. Mitchell C, Richards S, Harrison CJ, Eden T. Long-term follow-up of the United Kingdom medical research council protocols for childhood acute lymphoblastic leukaemia, 1980-2001. Leukemia 2010; 24(2): 406–418.

279. Pui CH, Pei D, Sandlund JT, Ribeiro RC, Rubnitz JE et al. Long-term results of St Jude Total Therapy Studies 11, 12, 13A, 13B, and 14 for childhood acute lymphoblastic leukemia. Leukemia 2010; 24(2): 371–382.

280. Schichman SA, Caligiuri MA, Gu Y, Strout MP, Canaani E et al. ALL-1 partial duplication in acute leukemia. Proceedings of the National Academy of Sciences USA 1994; 91(13): 6236–6239.

281. Bernard OA, Romana SP, Schichman SA, Mauchauffe M, Jonveaux P et al. Partial duplication of HRX in acute leukemia with trisomy 11. Leukemia 1995; 9(9): 1487–1490.

282. Caligiuri MA, Schichman SA, Strout MP, Mrozek K, Baer MR et al. Molecular rearrangement of the ALL-1 gene in acute myeloid leukemia without cytogenetic evidence of 11q23 chromosomal translocations. Cancer Research 1994; 54(2): 370–373.

283. Patel JP, Gonen M, Figueroa ME, Fernandez H, Sun Z et al. Prognostic relevance of integrated genetic profiling in acute myeloid leukemia. New England Journal of Medicine 2012; 366(12): 1079–1089.

284. Andersen MK, Christiansen DH, Kirchhoff M, Pedersen-Bjergaard J. Duplication or amplification of chromosome band 11q23, including the unrearranged MLL gene, is a recurrent abnormality in therapy-related MDS and AML, and is closely related to mutation of the TP53 gene and to previous therapy with alkylating agents. Genes Chromosomes Cancer 2001; 31(1): 33–41.

285. Meyer C, Schneider B, Jakob S, Strehl S, Attarbaschi A et al. The MLL recombinome of acute leukemias. Leukemia: Official Journal of the Leukemia Society of America, Leukemia Research Fund, UK 2006; 20(5): 777–784.

286. Bardini M, Spinelli R, Bungaro S, Mangano E, Corral L et al. DNA copy-number abnormalities do not occur in infant ALL with t(4;11)/MLL-AF4. Leukemia 2010; 24(1): 169–176.

287. Dobbins SE, Sherborne AL, Ma YP, Bardini M, Biondi A et al. The silent mutational landscape of infant MLL-AF4 pro-B acute lymphoblastic leukemia. Genes Chromosomes Cancer 2013; 52(10): 954–960.

288. Djabali M, Selleri L, Parry P, Bower M, Young BD et al. A trithorax-like gene is interrupted by chromosome 11q23 translocations in acute leukaemias. Nature Genetics 1992; 2(2): 113–118.

289. Simon J. Locking in stable states of gene expression: transcriptional control during Drosophila development. Current Opinion in Cell Biology 1995; 7(3): 376–385.

290. Nilson I, Lochner K, Siegler G, Greil J, Beck JD et al. Exon/intron structure of the human ALL-1 (MLL) gene involved in translocations to chromosomal region 11q23 and acute leukaemias. British Journal of Haematology 1996; 93(4): 966–972.

291. Zeleznik-Le NJ, Harden AM, Rowley JD. 11q23 translocations split the 'AT-hook' cruciform DNA-binding region and the transcriptional repression domain from the activation domain of the mixed-lineage leukemia (MLL) gene. Proceedings of the National Academy of Sciences USA 1994; 91(22): 10610–10614.

292. Xia ZB, Anderson M, Diaz MO, Zeleznik-Le NJ. MLL repression domain interacts with histone deacetylases, the polycomb group proteins HPC2 and BMI-1, and the corepressor C-terminal-binding protein. Proceedings of the National Academy of Sciences USA 2003; 100(14): 8342–8347.

293. Milne TA, Briggs SD, Brock HW, Martin ME, Gibbs D et al. MLL targets SET domain methyltransferase activity to Hox gene promoters. Molecular Cell 2002; 10(5): 1107–1117.

294. Nakamura T, Mori T, Tada S, Krajewski W, Rozovskaia T et al. ALL-1 is a histone methyltransferase that assembles a supercomplex of proteins involved in transcriptional regulation. Molecular Cell 2002; 10(5): 1119–1128.

295. Butler LH, Slany R, Cui X, Cleary ML, Mason DY. The HRX proto-oncogene product is widely expressed in human tissues and localizes to nuclear structures. Blood 1997; 89(9): 3361–3370.

296. Hsieh JJ, Ernst P, Erdjument-Bromage H, Tempst P, Korsmeyer SJ. Proteolytic cleavage of MLL generates a complex of N- and C-terminal fragments that confers protein stability and subnuclear localization. Molecular Cell Biology 2003; 23(1): 186–194.

297. Yokoyama A, Kitabayashi I, Ayton PM, Cleary ML, Ohki M. Leukemia proto-oncoprotein MLL is proteolytically processed into 2 fragments with opposite transcriptional properties. Blood 2002; 100(10): 3710–3718.

298. Yagi H, Deguchi K, Aono A, Tani Y, Kishimoto T, Komori T. Growth disturbance in fetal liver hematopoiesis of Mll-mutant mice. Blood 1998; 92(1): 108–117.

299. Yu BD, Hess JL, Horning SE, Brown GA, Korsmeyer SJ. Altered Hox expression and segmental identity in Mll-mutant mice. Nature 1995; 378(6556): 505–508.

300. Yu BD, Hanson RD, Hess JL, Horning SE, Korsmeyer SJ. MLL, a mammalian trithorax-group gene, functions as a transcriptional maintenance factor in morphogenesis. Proceedings of the National Academy of Sciences of the United States of America 1998; 95(18): 10632–10636.

301. Hess JL, Yu BD, Li B, Hanson R, Korsmeyer SJ. Defects in yolk sac hematopoiesis in Mll-null embryos. Blood 1997; 90(5): 1799–1806.

302. Corral J, Lavenir I, Impey H, Warren AJ, Forster A et al. An Mll-AF9 fusion gene made by homologous recombination causes acute leukemia in chimeric mice: a method to create fusion oncogenes. Cell 1996; 85(6): 853–861.

303. Krivtsov AV, Twomey D, Feng Z, Stubbs MC, Wang Y et al. Transformation from committed progenitor to leukaemia stem cell initiated by MLL-AF9. Nature 2006; 442(7104): 818–822.

304. Barabe F, Kennedy JA, Hope KJ, Dick JE. Modeling the initiation and progression of human acute leukemia in mice. Science 2007; 316(5824): 600–604.

305. Wei J, Wunderlich M, Fox C, Alvarez S, Cigudosa JC et al. Microenvironment determines lineage fate in a human model of MLL-AF9 leukemia. Cancer Cell 2008; 13(6): 483–495.

306. Zeisig BB, Garcia-Cuellar MP, Winkler TH, Slany RK. The oncoprotein MLL-ENL disturbs hematopoietic lineage determination and transforms a biphenotypic lymphoid/myeloid cell. Oncogene 2003; 22(11): 1629–1637.

307. Forster A, Pannell R, Drynan LF, McCormack M, Collins EC et al. Engineering de novo reciprocal chromosomal translocations associated with Mll to replicate primary events of human cancer. Cancer Cell 2003; 3(5): 449–458.

308. Metzler M, Forster A, Pannell R, Arends MJ, Daser A et al. A conditional model of MLL-AF4 B-cell tumourigenesis using invertor technology. Oncogene 2006; 25(22): 3093–3103.

309. Chen W, Li Q, Hudson WA, Kumar A, Kirchhof N, Kersey JH. A murine Mll-AF4 knock-in model results in lymphoid and

myeloid deregulation and hematologic malignancy. Blood 2006; 108(2): 669–677.

310. Krivtsov AV, Feng Z, Lemieux ME, Faber J, Vempati S et al. H3K79 methylation profiles define murine and human MLL-AF4 leukemias. Cancer Cell 2008; 14(5): 355–368.

311. Armstrong SA, Staunton JE, Silverman LB, Pieters R, den Boer ML, Minden MD, et al. MLL translocations specify a distinct gene expression profile that distinguishes a unique leukemia. Nature Genetics 2002; 30(1): 41–47.

312. Faber J, Krivtsov AV, Stubbs MC, Wright R, Davis TN et al. HOXA9 is required for survival in human MLL-rearranged acute leukemias. Blood 2009; 113(11): 2375–2385.

313. Li Z, Huang H, Chen P, He M, Li Y et al. miR-196b directly targets both HOXA9/MEIS1 oncogenes and FAS tumour suppressor in MLL-rearranged leukaemia. Nature communications 2012; 3: 688.

314. Mi S, Li Z, Chen P, He C, Cao D et al. Aberrant overexpression and function of the miR-17-92 cluster in MLL-rearranged acute leukemia. Proceedings of the National Academy of Sciences of the USA 2010; 107(8): 3710–3715.

315. Popovic R, Riesbeck LE, Velu CS, Chaubey A, Zhang J et al. Regulation of mir-196b by MLL and its overexpression by MLL fusions contributes to immortalization. Blood 2009; 113(14): 3314–3322.

316. Armstrong SA, Kung AL, Mabon ME, Silverman LB, Stam RW et al. Inhibition of FLT3 in MLL. Validation of a therapeutic target identified by gene expression based classification. Cancer Cell 2003; 3(2): 173–183.

317. Stubbs MC, Armstrong SA. FLT3 as a therapeutic target in childhood acute leukemia. Current Drug Targets 2007; 8(6): 703–714.

318. Stubbs MC, Kim YM, Krivtsov AV, Wright RD, Feng Z et al. MLL-AF9 and FLT3 cooperation in acute myelogenous leukemia: development of a model for rapid therapeutic assessment. Leukemia: Official Journal of the Leukemia Society of America, Leukemia Research Fund, UK 2008; 22(1): 66–77.

319. Jiang X, Huang H, Li Z, Li Y, Wang X et al. Blockade of miR-150 Maturation by MLL-Fusion/MYC/LIN-28 Is Required for MLL-Associated Leukemia. Cancer Cell 2012; 22(4): 524–535.

320. Mohan M, Herz HM, Takahashi YH, Lin C, Lai KC et al. Linking H3K79 trimethylation to Wnt signaling through a novel Dot1-containing complex (DotCom). Genes and Development 2010; 24(6): 574–589.

321. Okada Y, Feng Q, Lin Y, Jiang Q, Li Y et al. hDOT1L links histone methylation to leukemogenesis. Cell 2005; 121(2): 167–178.

322. Park G, Gong Z, Chen J, Kim JE. Characterization of the DOT1L network: implications of diverse roles for DOT1L. The Protein Journal 2010; 29(3): 213–223.

323. Yokoyama A, Lin M, Naresh A, Kitabayashi I, Cleary ML. A higher-order complex containing AF4 and ENL family proteins with P-TEFb facilitates oncogenic and physiologic MLL-dependent transcription. Cancer Cell 2010; 17(2): 198–212.

324. Zhang W, Xia X, Reisenauer MR, Hemenway CS, Kone BC. Dot1a-AF9 complex mediates histone H3 Lys-79 hypermethylation and repression of ENaCalpha in an aldosterone-sensitive manner. Journal of Biological Chemistry 2006; 281(26): 18059–18068.

325. Daigle SR, Olhava EJ, Therkelsen CA, Majer CR, Sneeringer CJ et al. Selective killing of mixed lineage leukemia cells by a potent small-molecule DOT1L inhibitor. Cancer Cell 2011; 20(1): 53–65.

326. Bernt KM, Zhu N, Sinha AU, Vempati S, Faber J et al. MLL-rearranged leukemia is dependent on aberrant H3K79 methylation by DOT1L. Cancer Cell 2011; 20(1): 66–78.

327. Grembecka J, He S, Shi A, Purohit T, Muntean AG et al. Menin-MLL inhibitors reverse oncogenic activity of MLL fusion proteins in leukemia. Nature Chemical Biology 2012; 8(3): 277–284.

328. Crist W, Carroll A, Shuster J, Jackson J, Head D et al. Philadelphia-Chromosome Positive Childhood Acute Lymphoblastic-Leukemia—Clinical and Cytogenetic Characteristics and Treatment Outcome—a Pediatric-Oncology-Group Study. Blood 1990; 76(3): 489–494.

329. Ribeiro RC, Abromowitch M, Raimondi SC, Murphy SB, Behm F et al. Clinical and Biologic Hallmarks of the Philadelphia-Chromosome in Childhood Acute Lymphoblastic-Leukemia. Blood 1987; 70(4): 948–953.

330. Suryanarayan K, Hunger SP, Kohler S, Carroll AJ, Crist W et al. Consistent Involvement of the Bcr Gene by 9-22 Breakpoints in Pediatric Acute Leukemias. Blood 1991; 77(2): 324–330.

331. Liu-Dumlao T, Kantarjian H, Thomas DA, O'Brien S, Ravandi F. Philadelphia-Positive Acute Lymphoblastic Leukemia: Current Treatment Options. Current Oncology Reports 2012.

332. Deklein A, Vankessel AG, Grosveld G, Bartram CR, Hagemeijer A et al. A Cellular Oncogene Is Translocated to the Philadelphia-Chromosome in Chronic Myelocytic-Leukemia. Nature 1982; 300(5894): 765–767.

333. Groffen J, Stephenson JR, Heisterkamp N, Deklein A, Bartram CR et al. Philadelphia Chromosomal Breakpoints Are Clustered within a Limited Region, Bcr, on Chromosome-22. Cell 1984; 36(1): 93–99.

334. Melo JV. The diversity of BCR-ABL fusion proteins and their relationship to leukemia phenotype. Blood 1996; 88(7): 2375–2384.

335. Sattler M, Griffin JD. Molecular mechanisms of transformation by the BCR-ABL oncogene. Seminars in Hematology 2003; 40(2 Suppl): 4–10.

336. Heerema NA, Harbott J, Galimberti S, Camitta BM, Gaynon PS et al. Secondary cytogenetic aberrations in childhood Philadelphia chromosome positive acute lymphoblastic leukemia are nonrandom and may be associated with outcome. Leukemia 2004; 18(4): 693–702.

337. Mullighan CG, Miller CB, Radtke I, Phillips LA, Dalton J et al. BCR-ABL1 lymphoblastic leukaemia is characterized by the deletion of Ikaros. Nature 2008; 453(7191): 110–114.

338. Iacobucci I, Storlazzi CT, Cilloni D, Lonetti A, Ottaviani E et al. Identification and molecular characterization of recurrent genomic deletions on 7p12 in the IKZF1 gene in a large cohort of BCR-ABL1-positive acute lymphoblastic leukemia patients: on behalf of Gruppo Italiano Malattie Ematologiche dell'Adulto Acute Leukemia Working Party (GIMEMA AL WP). Blood 2009; 114(10): 2159–2167.

339. Daley GQ, Van Etten RA, Baltimore D. Induction of chronic myelogenous leukemia in mice by the P210bcr/abl gene of the Philadelphia chromosome. Science. 1990; 247(4944): 824–830.

340. Williams RT, den Besten W, Sherr CJ. Cytokine-dependent imatinib resistance in mouse BCR-ABL+, Arf-null lymphoblastic leukemia. Genes and Development 2007; 21(18): 2283–2287.

341. Williams RT, Roussel MF, Sherr CJ. Arf gene loss enhances oncogenicity and limits imatinib response in mouse models of Bcr-Abl-induced acute lymphoblastic leukemia. Proceedings of the National Academy of Sciences USA 2006; 103(17): 6688–6693.

342. Arico M, Valsecchi MG, Camitta B, Schrappe M, Chessells J et al. Outcome of treatment in children with Philadelphia chromosome-positive acute lymphoblastic leukemia. New England Journal of Medicine 2000; 342(14): 998–1006.

343. Buchdunger E, Zimmermann J, Mett H, Meyer T, Muller M et al. Inhibition of the Abl protein-tyrosine kinase in vitro and in vivo by a 2-phenylaminopyrimidine derivative. Cancer Research 1996; 56(1): 100–104.

344. Schultz KR, Bowman WP, Aledo A, Slayton WB, Sather H et al. Improved Early Event-Free Survival With Imatinib in Philadelphia Chromosome-Positive Acute Lymphoblastic Leukemia: A Children's Oncology Group Study. Journal of Clinical Oncology 2009; 27(31): 5175–5181.

345. Kantarjian H, Giles F, Wunderle L, Bhalla K, O'Brien S et al. Nilotinib in imatinib-resistant CML and Philadelphia chromosome-positive ALL. New England Journal of Medicine 2006; 354(24): 2542–2551.

346. Ottmann O, Dombret H, Martinelli G, Simonsson B, Guilhot F et al. Dasatinib induces rapid hematologic and cytogenetic responses in adult patients with Philadelphia chromosome-positive

acute lymphoblastic leukemia with resistance or intolerance to imatinib: interim results of a phase 2 study. Blood 2007; 110(7): 2309–2315.

347. Seckerwalker LM, Craig JM, Hawkins JM, Hoffbrand AV. Philadelphia Positive Acute Lymphoblastic-Leukemia in Adults—Age Distribution, Bcr Breakpoint and Prognostic-Significance. Leukemia 1991; 5(3): 196–199.

348. Russell LJ, Capasso M, Vater I, Akasaka T, Bernard OA et al. Deregulated expression of cytokine receptor gene, CRLF2, is involved in lymphoid transformation in B-cell precursor acute lymphoblastic leukemia. Blood 2009; 114(13): 2688–2698.

349. Mullighan CG, Collins-Underwood JR, Phillips LA, Loudin MG, Liu W et al. Rearrangement of CRLF2 in B-progenitor- and Down syndrome-associated acute lymphoblastic leukemia. Nature Genetics 2009; 41(11): 1243–1246.

350. Chapiro E, Russell L, Lainey E, Kaltenbach S, Ragu C et al. Activating mutation in the TSLPR gene in B-cell precursor lymphoblastic leukemia. Leukemia 2010; 24(3): 642–645.

351. Hertzberg L, Vendramini E, Ganmore I, Cazzaniga G, Schmitz M et al. Down syndrome acute lymphoblastic leukemia: a highly heterogeneous disease in which aberrant expression of CRLF2 is associated with mutated JAK2: a report from the iBFM Study Group. Blood 2010; 115(5): 1006–1017.

352. Flex E, Petrangeli V, Stella L, Chiaretti S, Hornakova T et al. Somatically acquired JAK1 mutations in adult acute lymphoblastic leukemia. Journal of Experimental Medicine 2008; 205(4): 751–758.

353. Zhang J, Ding L, Holmfeldt L, Wu G, Heatley SL et al. The genetic basis of early T-cell precursor acute lymphoblastic leukaemia. Nature 2012; 481(7380): 157–163.

354. Levine RL, Gilliland DG. Myeloproliferative disorders. Blood 2008; 112(6): 2190–2198.

355. Toms AV, Deshpande A, McNally R, Jeong Y, Rogers JM et al. Structure of a pseudokinase-domain switch that controls oncogenic activation of Jak kinases. Nature Structural and Molecular Biology 2013; 20(10): 1221–1223.

356. Bercovich D, Ganmore I, Scott LM, Wainreb G, Birger Y et al. Mutations of JAK2 in acute lymphoblastic leukaemias associated with Down's syndrome. Lancet 2008; 372(9648): 1484–1492.

357. Mullighan CG, Zhang J, Harvey RC, Collins-Underwood JR, Schulman BA et al. JAK mutations in high-risk childhood acute lymphoblastic leukemia. Proceedings of the National Academy of Sciences USA 2009; 106: 9414–9418.

358. Kearney L, Gonzalez De Castro D, Yeung J, Procter J, Horsley SW et al. A specific JAK2 mutation (JAK2R683) and multiple gene deletions in Down syndrome acute lymphoblastic leukaemia. Blood 2008; 113: 646–648.

359. Tasian SK, Doral MY, Borowitz MJ, Wood BL, Chen IM et al. Aberrant STAT5 and PI3K/mTOR pathway signaling occurs in human CRLF2-rearranged B-precursor acute lymphoblastic leukemia. Blood 2012; 120(4): 833–842.

360. Maude SL, Tasian SK, Vincent T, Hall JW, Sheen C et al. Targeting JAK1/2 and mTOR in murine xenograft models of Ph-like acute lymphoblastic leukemia. Blood 2012; 120(17): 3510–3518.

361. Harvey RC, Mullighan CG, Chen IM, Wharton W, Mikhail FM et al. Rearrangement of CRLF2 is associated with mutation of JAK kinases, alteration of IKZF1, Hispanic/Latino ethnicity, and a poor outcome in pediatric B-progenitor acute lymphoblastic leukemia. Blood 2010; 115(26): 5312–5321.

362. Harvey RC, Mullighan CG, Wang X, Dobbin KK, Davidson GS et al. Identification of novel cluster groups in pediatric high-risk B-precursor acute lymphoblastic leukemia with gene expression profiling: correlation with genome-wide DNA copy number alterations, clinical characteristics, and outcome. Blood 2010; 116(23): 4874–4884.

363. Cario G, Zimmermann M, Romey R, Gesk S, Vater I et al. Presence of the P2RY8-CRLF2 rearrangement is associated with a poor prognosis in non-high-risk precursor B-cell acute lymphoblastic leukemia in

364. Ensor HM, Schwab C, Russell LJ, Richards SM, Morrison H et al. Demographic, clinical, and outcome features of children with acute lymphoblastic leukemia and CRLF2 deregulation: results from the MRC ALL97 clinical trial. Blood 2011; 117(7): 2129–2136.

365. Chen IM, Harvey RC, Mullighan CG, Gastier-Foster J, Wharton W, Kang H, et al. Outcome modeling with CRLF2, IKZF1, JAK, and minimal residual disease in pediatric acute lymphoblastic leukemia: a Children's Oncology Group study. Blood 2012; 119(15): 3512–3522.

366. Mullighan CG, Su X, Zhang J, Radtke I, Phillips LA et al. Deletion of IKZF1 and prognosis in acute lymphoblastic leukemia. New England Journal of Medicine 2009; 360(5): 470–480.

367. Den Boer ML, van Slegtenhorst M, De Menezes RX, Cheok MH, Buijs-Gladdines JG et al. A subtype of childhood acute lymphoblastic leukaemia with poor treatment outcome: a genome-wide classification study. Lancet Oncology 2009; 10(2): 125–134.

368. Loh ML, Zhang J, Harvey RC, Roberts K, Payne-Turner D et al. Tyrosine kinome sequencing of pediatric acute lymphoblastic leukemia: a report from the Children's Oncology Group TARGET Project. Blood 2013; 121(3): 485–488.

369. van der Veer A, Waanders E, Pieters R, Willemse ME, Van Reijmersdal SV et al. Independent prognostic value of BCR-ABL1-like signature and IKZF1 deletion, but not high CRLF2 expression, in children with B-cell precursor ALL. Blood 2013; 122(15): 2622–2629.

370. Roberts KG, Morin RD, Zhang J, Hirst M, Zhao Y et al. Genetic alterations activating kinase and cytokine receptor signaling in high-risk acute lymphoblastic leukemia. Cancer Cell 2012; 22(2): 153–166.

371. Bersenev A, Wu C, Balcerek J, Jing J, Kundu M et al. Lnk constrains myeloproliferative diseases in mice. Journal of Clinical Investigation 2010; 120(6): 2058–2069.

372. Weston BW, Hayden MA, Roberts KG, Bowyer S, Hsu J et al. Tyrosine Kinase Inhibitor Therapy Induces Remission in a Patient With Refractory EBF1-PDGFRB-Positive Acute Lymphoblastic Leukemia. Journal of Clinical Oncology 2013; 31(25): e413–e416.

373. Lengline E, Beldjord K, Dombret H, Soulier J, Boissel N et al. Successful tyrosine kinase inhibitor therapy in a refractory B-cell precursor acute lymphoblastic leukemia with EBF1-PDGFRB fusion. Haematologica 2013; 98(11): e146–e148.

374. Moorman AV, Richards SM, Robinson HM, Strefford JC, Gibson BE et al. Prognosis of children with acute lymphoblastic leukaemia (ALL) and intrachromosomal amplification of chromosome 21 (iAMP21). Blood 2007; 109(6): 2327–2330.

375. Robinson HM, Harrison CJ, Moorman AV, Chudoba I, Strefford JC. Intrachromosomal amplification of chromosome 21 (iAMP21) may arise from a breakage-fusion-bridge cycle. Genes, Chromosomes and Cancer 2007; 46(4): 318–326.

376. Strefford JC, van Delft FW, Robinson HM, Worley H, Yiannikouris O et al. Complex genomic alterations and gene expression in acute lymphoblastic leukemia with intrachromosomal amplification of chromosome 21. Proceedings of the National Academy of Sciences of the USA 2006; 103(21): 8167–8172.

377. Moorman AV, Robinson H, Schwab C, Richards SM, Hancock J et al. Risk-Directed Treatment Intensification Significantly Reduces the Risk of Relapse Among Children and Adolescents With Acute Lymphoblastic Leukemia and Intrachromosomal Amplification of Chromosome 21: A Comparison of the MRC ALL97/99 and UKALL2003 Trials. Journal of Clinical Oncology 2013; 31(27): 3389–3396.

378. Mullighan CG, Miller CB, Su X, Radtke I, Dalton J et al. ERG Deletions Define a Novel Subtype of B-Progenitor Acute Lymphoblastic Leukemia. Blood (ASH Annual Meeting Abstracts) 2007; 110(11): 691.

379. Zaliova M, Zimmermanova O, Dorge P, Eckert C, Moricke A, Zimmermann M, et al. ERG deletion is associated with CD2 and

attenuates the negative impact of IKZF1 deletion in childhood acute lymphoblastic leukemia. Leukemia 2015; 29(5): 1222.

380. Clappier E, Auclerc MF, Rapion J, Bakkus M, Caye A et al. An intragenic ERG deletion (ERG) is a marker of an oncogenic subtype of B-cell precursor acute lymphoblastic leukemia with a favorable outcome despite frequent IKZF1 deletions. Leukemia 2014; 28(1): 70–77.

381. Mullighan CG. Single nucleotide polymorphism microarray analysis of genetic alterations in cancer. Methods in Molecular Biology 2011; 730: 235–258.

382. Mullighan CG, Downing JR. Global genomic characterization of acute lymphoblastic leukemia. Seminars in Hematology 2009; 46(1): 3–15.

383. Kuiper RP, Schoenmakers EF, van Reijmersdal SV, Hehir-Kwa JY, van Kessel AG et al. High-resolution genomic profiling of childhood ALL reveals novel recurrent genetic lesions affecting pathways involved in lymphocyte differentiation and cell cycle progression. Leukemia 2007; 21(6): 1258–1266.

384. Kawamata N, Ogawa S, Zimmermann M, Kato M, Sanada M et al. Molecular allelokaryotyping of pediatric acute lymphoblastic leukemias by high-resolution single nucleotide polymorphism oligonucleotide genomic microarray. Blood 2008; 111(2): 776–784.

385. Fugmann SD, Lee AI, Shockett PE, Villey IJ, Schatz DG. The RAG proteins and V(D)J recombination: complexes, ends, and transposition. Annual Review of Immunology 2000; 18: 495–527.

386. Jung D, Giallourakis C, Mostoslavsky R, Alt FW. Mechanism and control of V(D)J recombination at the immunoglobulin heavy chain locus. Annual Review of Immunology 2006; 24: 541–570.

387. Waanders E, Scheijen B, van der Meer LT, van Reijmersdal SV, van Emst L et al. The origin and nature of tightly clustered BTG1 deletions in precursor B-cell acute lymphoblastic leukemia support a model of multiclonal evolution. PLoS Genetics 2012; 8(2): e1002533.

388. Meyer C, Zur Stadt U, Escherich G, Hofmann J, Binato R et al. Refinement of IKZF1 recombination hotspots in pediatric BCP-ALL patients. American Journal of Blood Research 2013; 3(2): 165–173.

389. Hauer J, Mullighan C, Morillon E, Wang G, Bruneau J et al. Loss of p19Arf in a Rag1(-/-) B-cell precursor population initiates acute B-lymphoblastic leukemia. Blood 2011; 118(3): 544–553.

390. Andersson AK, Ma J, Wang J, Chen X, Rusch M et al. Whole Genome Sequence Analysis of 22 MLL Rearranged Infant Acute Lymphoblastic Leukemias Reveals Remarkably Few Somatic Mutations: A Report From the St Jude Children's Research Hospital—Washington University Pediatric Cancer Genome Project. ASH Annual Meeting Abstracts 2011; 118(21): 69.

391. dChip website. Available from: <http://www.dchip.org>.

392. Radtke I, Mullighan CG, Ishii M, Su X, Cheng J et al. Genomic analysis reveals few genetic alterations in pediatric acute myeloid leukemia. Proceedings of the National Academy of Sciences USA 2009; 106(31): 12944–12949.

393. Zhang J, Mullighan CG, Harvey RC, Wu G, Chen X et al. Key pathways are frequently mutated in high-risk childhood acute lymphoblastic leukemia: a report from the Children's Oncology Group. Blood 2011; 118(11): 3080–3087.

394. Mullighan CG, Su X, Zhang J, Radtke I, Phillips LA et al. Deletion of IKZF1 and Prognosis in Acute Lymphoblastic Leukemia. New England Journal of Medicine 2009; 360: 470–480.

395. Iacobucci I, Lonetti A, Paoloni F, Papayannidis C, Ferrari A et al. The PAX5 gene is frequently rearranged in BCR-ABL1-positive acute lymphoblastic leukemia but is not associated with outcome. A report on behalf of the GIMEMA Acute Leukemia Working Party. Haematologica 2010; 95(10): 1683–1690.

396. Martinelli G, Iacobucci I, Storlazzi CT, Vignetti M, Paoloni F et al. IKZF1 (Ikaros) deletions in BCR-ABL1-positive acute lymphoblastic leukemia are associated with short disease-free survival and high rate of cumulative incidence of relapse: a GIMEMA AL WP report. Journal of Clinical Oncology 2009; 27(31): 5202–5207.

397. Georgopoulos K, Bigby M, Wang JH, Molnar A, Wu P et al. The Ikaros gene is required for the development of all lymphoid lineages. Cell 1994; 79(1): 143–156.

398. Ofverholm I, Tran AN, Heyman M, Zachariadis V, Nordenskjold M et al. Impact of IKZF1 deletions and PAX5 amplifications in pediatric B-cell precursor ALL treated according to NOPHO protocols. Leukemia 2013; 27(9): 1936–1939.

399. Kuiper RP, Waanders E, van der Velden VH, van Reijmersdal SV, Venkatachalam R et al. IKZF1 deletions predict relapse in uniformly treated pediatric precursor B-ALL. Leukemia 2010; 24(7): 1258–1264.

400. Yamashita Y, Shimada A, Yamada T, Yamaji K, Hori T et al. IKZF1 and CRLF2 gene alterations correlate with poor prognosis in Japanese BCR-ABL1-negative high-risk B-cell precursor acute lymphoblastic leukemia. Pediatric Blood Cancer 2013; 60(10): 1587–1592.

401. Buitenkamp TD, Pieters R, Gallimore NE, van der Veer A, Meijerink JP et al. Outcome in children with Down's syndrome and acute lymphoblastic leukemia: role of IKZF1 deletions and CRLF2 aberrations. Leukemia 2012; 26(10): 2204–2211.

402. Krentz S, Hof J, Mendioroz A, Vaggopoulou R, Dorge P et al. Prognostic value of genetic alterations in children with first bone marrow relapse of childhood B-cell precursor acute lymphoblastic leukemia. Leukemia 2013; 27(2): 295–304.

403. Asai D, Imamura T, Suenobu S, Saito A, Hasegawa D et al. IKZF1 deletion is associated with a poor outcome in pediatric B-cell precursor acute lymphoblastic leukemia in Japan. Cancer Medicine 2013; 2(3): 412–419.

404. Olsson L, Castor A, Behrendtz M, Biloglav A, Forestier E et al. Deletions of IKZF1 and SPRED1 are associated with poor prognosis in a population-based series of pediatric B-cell precursor acute lymphoblastic leukemia diagnosed between 1992 and 2011. Leukemia 2014; 28(2): 302–310.

405. Feng J, Tang Y. Prognostic significance of IKZF1 alteration status in pediatric B-lineage acute lymphoblastic leukemia: a meta-analysis. Leukemia Lymphoma 2013; 54(4): 889–891.

406. Yang YL, Hung CC, Chen JS, Lin KH, Jou ST et al. IKZF1 deletions predict a poor prognosis in children with B-cell progenitor acute lymphoblastic leukemia: A multicenter analysis in Taiwan. Cancer Science 2011; 102(10): 1874–1881.

407. Harvey RC, Mullighan CG, Wang X, Dobbin KK, Davidson GS et al. Identification of novel cluster groups in pediatric high-risk B-precursor acute lymphoblastic leukemia with gene expression profiling: correlation with genome-wide DNA copy number alterations, clinical characteristics, and outcome. Blood 2010; 116(23): 4874–4884.

408. Virely C, Moulin S, Cobaleda C, Lasgi C, Alberdi A et al. Haploinsufficiency of the IKZF1 (IKAROS) tumor suppressor gene cooperates with BCR-ABL in a transgenic model of acute lymphoblastic leukemia. Leukemia 2010; 24(6): 1200–1204.

409. Heltemes-Harris LM, Willette MJ, Ramsey LB, Qiu YH, Neeley ES et al. Ebf1 or Pax5 haploinsufficiency synergizes with STAT5 activation to initiate acute lymphoblastic leukemia. Journal of Experimental Medicine 2011; 208(6): 1135–1149.

410. Aifantis I, Raetz E, Buonamici S. Molecular pathogenesis of T-cell leukaemia and lymphoma. Nature Reviews Immunology 2008; 8(5): 380–390.

411. Nickoloff JA, De Haro LP, Wray J, Hromas R. Mechanisms of leukemia translocations. Current Opinion in Hematology 2008; 15(4): 338–345.

412. Cauwelier B, Dastugue N, Cools J, Poppe B, Herens C et al. Molecular cytogenetic study of 126 unselected T-ALL cases reveals high incidence of TCRbeta locus rearrangements and putative new T-cell oncogenes. Leukemia: official journal of the Leukemia Society of America, Leukemia Research Fund, UK 2006; 20(7): 1238–1244.

413. McKeithan TW, Shima EA, Le Beau MM, Minowada J, Rowley JD et al. Molecular cloning of the breakpoint junction of a human chromosomal 8;14 translocation involving the T-cell receptor alpha-chain gene and sequences on the 3' side of MYC. Proceedings of the National Academy of Sciences USA 1986; 83(17): 6636–6640.

414. Finger LR, Harvey RC, Moore RC, Showe LC, Croce CM. A common mechanism of chromosomal translocation in T- and B-cell neoplasia. Science 1986; 234(4779): 982–985.

415. Shima EA, Le Beau MM, McKeithan TW, Minowada J, Showe LC et al. Gene encoding the alpha chain of the T-cell receptor is moved immediately downstream of c-myc in a chromosomal 8;14 translocation in a cell line from a human T-cell leukemia. Proceedings of the National Academy of Sciences USA 1986; 83(10): 3439–3443.

416. Chen Q, Cheng JT, Tasi LH, Schneider N, Buchanan G et al. The tal gene undergoes chromosome translocation in T cell leukemia and potentially encodes a helix-loop-helix protein. EMBO 1990; 9(2): 415–424.

417. Xia Y, Brown L, Yang CY, Tsan JT, Siciliano MJ et al. TAL2, a helix-loop-helix gene activated by the (7;9)(q34;q32) translocation in human T-cell leukemia. Proceedings of the National Academy of Sciences USA 1991; 88(24): 11416–11420.

418. Mellentin JD, Smith SD, Cleary ML. lyl-1, a novel gene altered by chromosomal translocation in T cell leukemia, codes for a protein with a helix-loop-helix DNA binding motif. Cell 1989; 58(1): 77–83.

419. Wang J, Jani-Sait SN, Escalon EA, Carroll AJ, de Jong PJ et al. The t(14;21)(q11.2;q22) chromosomal translocation associated with T-cell acute lymphoblastic leukemia activates the BHLHB1 gene. Proceedings of the National Academy of Sciences USA 2000; 97(7): 3497–3502.

420. McGuire EA, Hockett RD, Pollock KM, Bartholdi MF, O'Brien SJ et al. The t(11;14)(p15;q11) in a T-cell acute lymphoblastic leukemia cell line activates multiple transcripts, including Ttg-1, a gene encoding a potential zinc finger protein. Molecular and Cellular Biology 1989; 9(5): 2124–2132.

421. Boehm T, Foroni L, Kaneko Y, Perutz MF, Rabbitts TH. The rhombotin family of cysteine-rich LIM-domain oncogenes: distinct members are involved in T-cell translocations to human chromosomes 11p15 and 11p13. Proceedings of the National Academy of Sciences USA 1991; 88(10): 4367–4371.

422. Royer-Pokora B, Loos U, Ludwig WD. TTG-2, a new gene encoding a cysteine-rich protein with the LIM motif, is overexpressed in acute T-cell leukaemia with the t(11;14)(p13;q11). Oncogene 1991; 6(10): 1887–1893.

423. Hatano M, Roberts CW, Minden M, Crist WM, Korsmeyer SJ. Deregulation of a homeobox gene, HOX11, by the t(10;14) in T cell leukemia. Science 1991; 253(5015): 79–82.

424. Kennedy MA, Gonzalez-Sarmiento R, Kees UR, Lampert F, Dear N et al. HOX11, a homeobox-containing T-cell oncogene on human chromosome 10q24. Proceedings of the National Academy of Sciences of the USA 1991; 88(20): 8900–8904.

425. Bernard OA, Busson-LeConiat M, Ballerini P, Mauchauffe M, Della Valle V et al. A new recurrent and specific cryptic translocation, t(5;14)(q35;q32), is associated with expression of the Hox11L2 gene in T acute lymphoblastic leukemia. Leukemia: official journal of the Leukemia Society of America, Leukemia Research Fund, UK 2001; 15(10): 1495–1504.

426. Weng AP, Ferrando AA, Lee W, Morris JPt, Silverman LB et al. Activating mutations of NOTCH1 in human T cell acute lymphoblastic leukemia. Science 2004; 306(5694): 269–271.

427. Gutierrez A, Sanda T, Grebliunaite R, Carracedo A, Salmena L et al. High frequency of PTEN, PI3K, and AKT abnormalities in T-cell acute lymphoblastic leukemia. Blood 2009; 114(3): 647–650.

428. Tosello V, Mansour MR, Barnes K, Paganin M, Sulis ML et al. WT1 mutations in T-ALL. Blood 2009; 114(5): 1038–1045.

429. O'Neil J, Grim J, Strack P, Rao S, Tibbitts D et al. FBW7 mutations in leukemic cells mediate NOTCH pathway activation and resistance to gamma-secretase inhibitors. Journal of Experimental Medicine 2007; 204(8): 1813–1824.

430. Clappier E, Cuccuini W, Kalota A, Crinquette A, Cayuela JM et al. The C-MYB locus is involved in chromosomal translocation and genomic duplications in human T-cell acute leukemia (T-ALL), the translocation defining a new T-ALL subtype in very young children. Blood 2007; 110(4): 1251–1261.

431. Lahortiga I, De Keersmaecker K, Van Vlierberghe P, Graux C, Cauwelier B et al. Duplication of the MYB oncogene in T cell acute lymphoblastic leukemia. Nature Genetics 2007; 39(5): 593–595.

432. Begley CG, Aplan PD, Davey MP, Nakahara K, Tchorz K et al. Chromosomal translocation in a human leukemic stem-cell line disrupts the T-cell antigen receptor delta-chain diversity region and results in a previously unreported fusion transcript. Proceedings of the National Academy of Sciences of the USA 1989; 86(6): 2031–2035.

433. Brown L, Cheng JT, Chen Q, Siciliano MJ, Crist W et al. Site-specific recombination of the tal-1 gene is a common occurrence in human T cell leukemia. EMBO 1990; 9(10): 3343–3351.

434. Aplan PD, Lombardi DP, Kirsch IR. Structural characterization of SIL, a gene frequently disrupted in T-cell acute lymphoblastic leukemia. Molecular and Cellular Biology 1991; 11(11): 5462–5469.

435. Aplan PD, Lombardi DP, Reaman GH, Sather HN, Hammond GD et al. Involvement of the putative hematopoietic transcription factor SCL in T-cell acute lymphoblastic leukemia. Blood 1992; 79(5): 1327–1333.

436. Bernard O, Lecointe N, Jonveaux P, Souyri M, Mauchauffe M et al. Two site-specific deletions and t(1;14) translocation restricted to human T-cell acute leukemias disrupt the 5' part of the tal-1 gene. Oncogene 1991; 6(8): 1477–1488.

437. Breit TM, Mol EJ, Wolvers-Tettero IL, Ludwig WD, van Wering ER et al. Site-specific deletions involving the tal-1 and sil genes are restricted to cells of the T cell receptor alpha/beta lineage: T cell receptor delta gene deletion mechanism affects multiple genes. Journal of Experimental Medicine 1993; 177(4): 965–977.

438. Baer R. TAL1, TAL2 and LYL1: a family of basic helix-loop-helix proteins implicated in T cell acute leukaemia. Seminars Cancer Biology 1993; 4(6): 341–347.

439. Bash RO, Hall S, Timmons CF, Crist WM, Amylon M et al. Does activation of the TAL1 gene occur in a majority of patients with T-cell acute lymphoblastic leukemia? A pediatric oncology group study. Blood 1995; 86(2): 666–676.

440. Aplan PD, Lombardi DP, Ginsberg AM, Cossman J, Bertness VL et al. Disruption of the human SCL locus by 'illegitimate' V-(D)-J recombinase activity. Science 1990; 250(4986): 1426–1429.

441. Ferrando AA, Neuberg DS, Staunton J, Loh ML, Huard C et al. Gene expression signatures define novel oncogenic pathways in T cell acute lymphoblastic leukemia. Cancer Cell 2002; 1(1): 75–87.

442. Hsu HL, Cheng JT, Chen Q, Baer R. Enhancer-binding activity of the tal-1 oncoprotein in association with the E47/E12 helix-loop-helix proteins. Molecular and Cellular Biology 1991; 11(6): 3037–3042.

443. Miyamoto A, Cui X, Naumovski L, Cleary ML. Helix-loop-helix proteins LYL1 and E2a form heterodimeric complexes with distinctive DNA-binding properties in hematolymphoid cells. Molecular and Cellular Biology 1996; 16(5): 2394–2401.

444. Shivdasani RA, Mayer EL, Orkin SH. Absence of blood formation in mice lacking the T-cell leukemia oncoprotein tal-1/SCL. Nature 1995; 373(6513): 432–434.

445. Robb L, Lyons I, Li R, Hartley L, Kontgen F et al. Absence of yolk sac hematopoiesis from mice with a targeted disruption of the scl gene. Proceedings of the National Academy of Sciences USA 1995; 92(15): 7075–7079.

446. Begley CG, Aplan PD, Denning SM, Haynes BF, Waldmann TA et al. The gene SCL is expressed during early hematopoiesis and encodes a differentiation-related DNA-binding motif. Proceedings of the National Academy of Sciences USA 1989; 86(24): 10128–10132.

447. Porcher C, Swat W, Rockwell K, Fujiwara Y, Alt FW et al. The T cell leukemia oncoprotein SCL/tal-1 is essential for development of all hematopoietic lineages. Cell 1996; 86(1): 47–57.

448. Hsu HL, Wadman I, Tsan JT, Baer R. Positive and negative transcriptional control by the TAL1 helix-loop-helix protein. Proceedings of the National Academy of Sciences USA 1994; 91(13): 5947–5951.

449. Park ST, Sun XH. The Tal1 oncoprotein inhibits E47-mediated transcription. Mechanism of inhibition. Journal of Biological Chemistry 1998; 273(12): 7030–7037.

450. Bain G, Engel I, Robanus Maandag EC, te Riele HP, Voland JR et al. E2A deficiency leads to abnormalities in alphabeta T-cell development and to rapid development of T-cell lymphomas. Molecular and Cellular Biology 1997; 17(8): 4782–4791.

451. Yan W, Young AZ, Soares VC, Kelley R, Benezra R et al. High incidence of T-cell tumors in E2A-null mice and E2A/Id1 double-knockout mice. Molecular and Cellular Biology 1997; 17(12): 7317–7327.

452. Begley CG, Green AR. The SCL gene: from case report to critical hematopoietic regulator. Blood 1999; 93(9): 2760–2770.

453. Van Vlierberghe P, van Grotel M, Beverloo HB, Lee C, Helgason T et al. The cryptic chromosomal deletion del(11)(p12p13) as a new activation mechanism of LMO2 in pediatric T-cell acute lymphoblastic leukemia. Blood 2006; 108(10): 3520–3529.

454. Valge-Archer VE, Osada H, Warren AJ, Forster A, Li J et al. The LIM protein RBTN2 and the basic helix-loop-helix protein TAL1 are present in a complex in erythroid cells. Proceedings of the National Academy of Sciences USA 1994; 91(18): 8617–8621.

455. Wadman I, Li J, Bash RO, Forster A, Osada H et al. Specific in vivo association between the bHLH and LIM proteins implicated in human T cell leukemia. EMBO 1994; 13(20): 4831–4839.

456. Larson RC, Osada H, Larson TA, Lavenir I, Rabbitts TH. The oncogenic LIM protein Rbtn2 causes thymic developmental aberrations that precede malignancy in transgenic mice. Oncogene 1995; 11(5): 853–862.

457. Neale GA, Rehg JE, Goorha RM. Ectopic expression of rhombotin-2 causes selective expansion of CD4-CD8- lymphocytes in the thymus and T-cell tumors in transgenic mice. Blood 1995; 86(8): 3060–3071.

458. Aplan PD, Jones CA, Chervinsky DS, Zhao X, Ellsworth M et al. An scl gene product lacking the transactivation domain induces bony abnormalities and cooperates with LMO1 to generate T-cell malignancies in transgenic mice. EMBO 1997; 16(9): 2408–2419.

459. Chervinsky DS, Zhao XF, Lam DH, Ellsworth M, Gross KW et al. Disordered T-cell development and T-cell malignancies in SCL LMO1 double-transgenic mice: parallels with E2A-deficient mice. Molecular and Cellular Biology 1999; 19(7): 5025–5035.

460. McCormack MP, Young LF, Vasudevan S, de Graaf CA, Codrington R et al. The Lmo2 oncogene initiates leukemia in mice by inducing thymocyte self-renewal. Science 2010; 327(5967): 879–883.

461. Argiropoulos B, Humphries RK. Hox genes in hematopoiesis and leukemogenesis. Oncogene 2007; 26(47): 6766–6776.

462. Dear TN, Sanchez-Garcia I, Rabbitts TH. The HOX11 gene encodes a DNA-binding nuclear transcription factor belonging to a distinct family of homeobox genes. Proceedings of the National Academy of Sciences USA 1993; 90(10): 4431–4435.

463. Allen JD, Lints T, Jenkins NA, Copeland NG, Strasser A et al. Novel murine homeo box gene on chromosome 1 expressed in specific hematopoietic lineages and during embryogenesis. Genes and Development 1991; 5(4): 509–520.

464. McGinnis W, Krumlauf R. Homeobox genes and axial patterning. Cell 1992; 68(2): 283–302.

465. Lu M, Gong ZY, Shen WF, Ho AD. The tcl-3 proto-oncogene altered by chromosomal translocation in T-cell leukemia codes for a homeobox protein. The EMBO 1991; 10(10): 2905–2910.

466. Dube ID, Kamel-Reid S, Yuan CC, Lu M, Wu X et al. A novel human homeobox gene lies at the chromosome 10 breakpoint in lymphoid neoplasias with chromosomal translocation t(10;14). Blood 1991; 78(11): 2996–3003.

467. Salvati PD, Ranford PR, Ford J, Kees UR. HOX11 expression in pediatric acute lymphoblastic leukemia is associated with T-cell phenotype. Oncogene 1995; 11(7): 1333–1338.

468. Ferrando AA, Herblot S, Palomero T, Hansen M, Hoang T et al. Biallelic transcriptional activation of oncogenic transcription factors in T-cell acute lymphoblastic leukemia. Blood 2004; 103(5): 1909–1911.

469. Watt PM, Kumar R, Kees UR. Promoter demethylation accompanies reactivation of the HOX11 proto-oncogene in leukemia. Genes, Chromosomes and Cancer 2000; 29(4): 371–377.

470. Roberts CW, Shutter JR, Korsmeyer SJ. Hox11 controls the genesis of the spleen. Nature 1994; 368(6473): 747–749.

471. Hawley RG, Hawley TS, Cantor AB. TLX1 (HOX11) immortalization of embryonic stem cell-derived and primary murine hematopoietic progenitors. Current Protocols in Stem Cell Biology 2008; Chapter 1: Unit 1F 7.

472. Keller G, Wall C, Fong AZ, Hawley TS, Hawley RG. Overexpression of HOX11 leads to the immortalization of embryonic precursors with both primitive and definitive hematopoietic potential. Blood 1998; 92(3): 877–887.

473. Hawley RG, Fong AZ, Reis MD, Zhang N, Lu M et al. Transforming function of the HOX11/TCL3 homeobox gene. Cancer Research 1997; 57(2): 337–345.

474. Cave H, Suciu S, Preudhomme C, Poppe B, Robert A et al. Clinical significance of HOX11L2 expression linked to t(5;14)(q35;q32), of HOX11 expression, and of SIL-TAL fusion in childhood T-cell malignancies: results of EORTC studies 58881 and 58951. Blood 2004; 103(2): 442–450.

475. Ballerini P, Blaise A, Busson-Le Coniat M, Su XY, Zucman-Rossi J et al. HOX11L2 expression defines a clinical subtype of pediatric T-ALL associated with poor prognosis. Blood 2002; 100(3): 991–997.

476. Berger R, Dastugue N, Busson M, Van Den Akker J, Perot C et al. t(5;14)/HOX11L2-positive T-cell acute lymphoblastic leukemia. A collaborative study of the Groupe Francais de Cytogenetique Hematologique (GFCH). Leukemia: official journal of the Leukemia Society of America, Leukemia Research Fund, UK 2003; 17(9): 1851–1857.

477. De Keersmaecker K, Real PJ, Gatta GD, Palomero T, Sulis ML et al. The TLX1 oncogene drives aneuploidy in T cell transformation. Nature Medicine 2010; 16(11): 1321–1327.

478. Nagel S, Scherr M, Kel A, Hornischer K, Crawford GE et al. Activation of TLX3 and NKX2-5 in t(5;14)(q35;q32) T-cell acute lymphoblastic leukemia by remote 3'-BCL11B enhancers and coregulation by PU.1 and HMGA1. Cancer Research 2007; 67(4): 1461–1471.

479. Nagel S, Kaufmann M, Drexler HG, MacLeod RA. The cardiac homeobox gene NKX2-5 is deregulated by juxtaposition with BCL11B in pediatric T-ALL cell lines via a novel t(5;14)(q35.1;q32.2). Cancer Research 2003; 63(17): 5329–5334.

480. Su XY, Busson M, Della Valle V, Ballerini P, Dastugue N et al. Various types of rearrangements target TLX3 locus in T-cell acute lymphoblastic leukemia. Genes, Chromosomes and Cancer 2004; 41(3): 243–249.

481. Van Vlierberghe P, Homminga I, Zuurbier L, Gladdines-Buijs J, van Wering ER et al. Cooperative genetic defects in TLX3 rearranged pediatric T-ALL. Leukemia: Official Journal of the Leukemia Society of America, Leukemia Research Fund, UK 2008; 22(4): 762–770.

482. Hayette S, Tigaud I, Maguer-Satta V, Bartholin L, Thomas X et al. Recurrent involvement of the MLL gene in adult T-lineage acute lymphoblastic leukemia. Blood 2002; 99(12): 4647–4649.

483. Rubnitz JE, Camitta BM, Mahmoud H, Raimondi SC, Carroll AJ et al. Childhood acute lymphoblastic leukemia with the MLL-ENL fusion and t(11;19)(q23;p13.3) translocation. Journal of Clinical Oncology: Official Journal of the American Society of Clinical Oncology 1999; 17(1): 191–196.

484. Ferrando AA, Armstrong SA, Neuberg DS, Sallan SE, Silverman LB et al. Gene expression signatures in MLL-rearranged T-lineage and B-precursor acute leukemias: dominance of HOX dysregulation. Blood 2003; 102(1): 262–268.

485. Dreyling MH, Martinez-Climent JA, Zheng M, Mao J, Rowley JD et al. The t(10;11)(p13;q14) in the U937 cell line results in the fusion of the AF10 gene and CALM, encoding a new member of the

AP-3 clathrin assembly protein family. Proceedings of the National Academy of Sciences of the USA 1996; 93(10): 4804–4809.

486. Asnafi V, Radford-Weiss I, Dastugue N, Bayle C, Leboeuf D et al. CALM-AF10 is a common fusion transcript in T-ALL and is specific to the TCRgammadelta lineage. Blood 2003; 102(3): 1000–1006.

487. Bohlander SK, Muschinsky V, Schrader K, Siebert R, Schlegelberger B et al. Molecular analysis of the CALM/AF10 fusion: identical rearrangements in acute myeloid leukemia, acute lymphoblastic leukemia and malignant lymphoma patients. Leukemia: Official Journal of the Leukemia Society of America, Leukemia Research Fund, UK 2000; 14(1): 93–99.

488. Dreyling MH, Schrader K, Fonatsch C, Schlegelberger B, Haase D et al. MLL and CALM are fused to AF10 in morphologically distinct subsets of acute leukemia with translocation t(10;11): both rearrangements are associated with a poor prognosis. Blood 1998; 91(12): 4662–4667.

489. Deshpande AJ, Cusan M, Rawat VP, Reuter H, Krause A et al. Acute myeloid leukemia is propagated by a leukemic stem cell with lymphoid characteristics in a mouse model of CALM/AF10-positive leukemia. Cancer Cell 2006; 10(5): 363–374.

490. Caudell D, Zhang Z, Chung YJ, Aplan PD. Expression of a CALM-AF10 fusion gene leads to Hoxa cluster overexpression and acute leukemia in transgenic mice. Cancer Research 2007; 67(17): 8022–8031.

491. Homminga I, Pieters R, Langerak AW, de Rooi JJ, Stubbs A et al. Integrated Transcript and Genome Analyses Reveal NKX2-1 and MEF2C as Potential Oncogenes in T Cell Acute Lymphoblastic Leukemia. Cancer Cell 2011; 19(4): 484–497.

492. Coustan-Smith E, Mullighan CG, Onciu M, Behm FG, Raimondi SC et al. Early T-cell precursor leukaemia: a subtype of very high-risk acute lymphoblastic leukaemia. Lancet Oncology 2009; 10(2): 147–156.

493. Inukai T, Kiyokawa N, Campana D, Coustan-Smith E, Kikuchi A et al. Clinical significance of early T-cell precursor acute lymphoblastic leukaemia: results of the Tokyo Children's Cancer Study Group Study L99-15. British Journal of Haematology 2012; 156(3): 358–365.

494. Wood B, Winter S, Dunsmore K, Raetz E, Borowitz MJ et al. Patients with Early T-Cell Precursor (ETP) Acute Lymphoblastic Leukemia (ALL) Have High Levels of Minimal Residual Disease (MRD) at the End of induction—A Children's Oncology Group (COG) Study. Blood (ASH Annual Meeting Abstracts) 2009; 114(22): 9.

495. Rothenberg EV, Moore JE, Yui MA. Launching the T-cell-lineage developmental programme. Nature Reviews Immunology 2008; 8(1): 9–21.

496. Korbel JO, Campbell PJ. Criteria for inference of chromothripsis in cancer genomes. Cell 2013; 152(6): 1226–1236.

497. Della Gatta G, Palomero T, Perez-Garcia A, Ambesi-Impiombato A, Bansal M et al. Reverse engineering of TLX oncogenic transcriptional networks identifies RUNX1 as tumor suppressor in T-ALL. Nature Medicine 2012; 18(3): 436–440.

498. Van Vlierberghe P, Ambesi-Impiombato A, Perez-Garcia A, Haydu JE, Rigo I et al. ETV6 mutations in early immature human T cell leukemias. Journal of Experimental Medicine 2011; 208(13): 2571–2579.

499. Shochat C, Tal N, Bandapalli OR, Palmi C, Ganmore I et al. Gain-of-function mutations in interleukin-7 receptor-alpha (IL7R) in childhood acute lymphoblastic leukemias. Journal of Experimental Medicine 2011; 208(5): 901–908.

500. Zenatti PP, Ribeiro D, Li W, Zuurbier L, Silva MC et al. Oncogenic IL7R gain-of-function mutations in childhood T-cell acute lymphoblastic leukemia. Nature Genetics 2011; 43(10): 932–939.

501. Ntziachristos P, Tsirigos A, Vlierberghe PV, Nedjic J, Trimarchi T et al. Genetic inactivation of the polycomb repressive complex 2 in T cell acute lymphoblastic leukemia. Nature Medicine 2012; 18(2): 298–303.

502. Neumann M, Coskun E, Fransecky L, Mochmann LH, Bartram I et al. FLT3 mutations in early T-cell precursor ALL characterize a stem cell like leukemia and imply the clinical use of tyrosine kinase inhibitors. PLoS One 2013; 8(1): e53190.

503. Neumann M, Heesch S, Gokbuget N, Schwartz S, Schlee C et al. Clinical and molecular characterization of early T-cell precursor leukemia: a high-risk subgroup in adult T-ALL with a high frequency of FLT3 mutations. Blood Cancer Journal 2012; 2(1): e55.

504. Morin RD, Johnson NA, Severson TM, Mungall AJ, An J et al. Somatic mutations altering EZH2 (Tyr641) in follicular and diffuse large B-cell lymphomas of germinal-center origin. Nature Genetics 2010; 42(2): 181–185.

505. Sneeringer CJ, Scott MP, Kuntz KW, Knutson SK, Pollock RM et al. Coordinated activities of wild-type plus mutant EZH2 drive tumor-associated hypertrimethylation of lysine 27 on histone H3 (H3K27) in human B-cell lymphomas. Proceedings of the National Academy of Sciences USA 2010; 107(49): 20980–20985.

506. Yap DB, Chu J, Berg T, Schapira M, Cheng SW et al. Somatic mutations at EZH2 Y641 act dominantly through a mechanism of selectively altered PRC2 catalytic activity, to increase H3K27 trimethylation. Blood 2011; 117(8): 2451–2459.

507. Simon C, Chagraoui J, Krosl J, Gendron P, Wilhelm B et al. A key role for EZH2 and associated genes in mouse and human adult T-cell acute leukemia. Genes and Development 2012; 26(7): 651–656.

508. Ley TJ, Ding L, Walter MJ, McLellan MD, Lamprecht T et al. DNMT3A mutations in acute myeloid leukemia. New England Journal of Medicine 2010; 363(25): 2424–2433.

509. Neumann M, Heesch S, Schlee C, Schwartz S, Gokbuget N et al. Whole-exome sequencing in adult ETP-ALL reveals a high rate of DNMT3A mutations. Blood 2013; 121(23): 4749–4752.

510. Shi J, Wang E, Zuber J, Rappaport A, Taylor M et al. The Polycomb complex PRC2 supports aberrant self-renewal in a mouse model of MLL-AF9;Nras(G12D) acute myeloid leukemia. Oncogene 2013; 32(7): 930–938.

511. Neff T, Sinha AU, Kluk MJ, Zhu N, Khattab MH et al. Polycomb repressive complex 2 is required for MLL-AF9 leukemia. Proceedings of the National Academy of Sciences USA 2012; 109(13): 5028–5033.

512. Kim W, Bird GH, Neff T, Guo G, Kerenyi MA et al. Targeted disruption of the EZH2-EED complex inhibits EZH2-dependent cancer. Nature Chemical Biology 2013; 9(10): 643–650.

513. De Keersmaecker K, Atak ZK, Li N, Vicente C, Patchett S et al. Exome sequencing identifies mutation in CNOT3 and ribosomal genes RPL5 and RPL10 in T-cell acute lymphoblastic leukemia. Nature Genetics 2013; 45(2): 186–190.

514. Van Vlierberghe P, Palomero T, Khiabanian H, Van der Meulen J, Castillo M et al. PHF6 mutations in T-cell acute lymphoblastic leukemia. Nature Genetics 2010; 42(4): 338–342.

515. Van Vlierberghe P, Patel J, Abdel-Wahab O, Lobry C, Hedvat CV et al. PHF6 mutations in adult acute myeloid leukemia. Leukemia 2011; 25(1): 130–134.

516. Todd MA, Picketts DJ. PHF6 interacts with the nucleosome remodeling and deacetylation (NuRD) complex. Journal of Proteome Research 2012; 11(8): 4326–4337.

517. Wang J, Leung JW, Gong Z, Feng L, Shi X, Chen J. PHF6 regulates cell cycle progression by suppressing ribosomal RNA synthesis. Journal of Biological Chemistry 2013; 288(5): 3174–3183.

518. Raimondi SC, Pui CH, Head DR, Rivera GK, Behm FG. Cytogenetically different leukemic clones at relapse of childhood acute lymphoblastic leukemia. Blood 1993; 82(2): 576–580.

519. Yang JJ, Bhojwani D, Yang W, Cai X, Stocco G et al. Genome-wide copy number profiling reveals molecular evolution from diagnosis to relapse in childhood acute lymphoblastic leukemia. Blood 2008; 112(10): 4178–4183.

520. Kawamata N, Ogawa S, Seeger K, Kirschner-Schwabe R, Huynh T et al. Molecular allelokaryotyping of relapsed pediatric acute lymphoblastic leukemia. International Journal of Oncology 2009; 34(6): 1603–1612.

521. Mullighan CG, Phillips LA, Su X, Ma J, Miller CB et al. Genomic analysis of the clonal origins of relapsed acute lymphoblastic leukemia. Science 2008; 322(5906): 1377–1380.

522. Blau O, Avigad S, Stark B, Kodman Y, Luria D et al. Exon 5 mutations in the p53 gene in relapsed childhood acute lymphoblastic leukemia. Leukemia Research 1997;21(8):721–729.

523. Diccianni MB, Yu J, Hsiao M, Mukherjee S, Shao LE, Yu AL. Clinical significance of p53 mutations in relapsed T-cell acute lymphoblastic leukemia. Blood 1994; 84(9): 3105–3112.

524. Gump J, McGavran L, Wei Q, Hunger SP. Analysis of TP53 mutations in relapsed childhood acute lymphoblastic leukemia. Journal of Pediatric Hematology and Oncology 2001; 23(7): 416–419.

525. Hof J, Krentz S, van Schewick C, Korner G, Shalapour S et al. Mutations and deletions of the TP53 gene predict nonresponse to treatment and poor outcome in first relapse of childhood acute lymphoblastic leukemia. Journal of Clinical Oncology 2011; 29(23): 3185–3193.

526. Hsiao MH, Yu AL, Yeargin J, Ku D, Haas M. Nonhereditary p53 mutations in T-cell acute lymphoblastic leukemia are associated with the relapse phase. Blood 1994; 83(10): 2922–2930.

527. Inthal A, Zeitlhofer P, Zeginigg M, Morak M, Grausenburger R et al. CREBBP HAT domain mutations prevail in relapse cases of high hyperdiploid childhood acute lymphoblastic leukemia. Leukemia 2012; doi:10.1038/leu.2012.60

528. Pasqualucci L, Dominguez-Sola D, Chiarenza A, Fabbri G, Grunn A et al. Inactivating mutations of acetyltransferase genes in B-cell lymphoma. Nature 2011; 471(7337): 189–195.

529. Kino T, Nordeen SK, Chrousos GP. Conditional modulation of glucocorticoid receptor activities by CREB-binding protein (CBP) and p300. Journal of Steroid Biochemistry and Molecular Biology 1999; 70(1–3): 15–25.

530. Lambert JR, Nordeen SK. CBP recruitment and histone acetylation in differential gene induction by glucocorticoids and progestins. Molecular Endocrinology 2003; 17(6): 1085–1094.

531. Meyer JA, Wang J, Hogan LE, Yang JJ, Dandekar S et al. Relapse-specific mutations in NT5C2 in childhood acute lymphoblastic leukemia. Nature Genetics 2013; 45(3): 290–294.

532. Tzoneva G, Perez-Garcia A, Carpenter Z, Khiabanian H, Tosello V et al. Activating mutations in the NT5C2 nucleotidase gene drive chemotherapy resistance in relapsed ALL. Nature Medicine 2013; 19(3): 368–371.

533. Taylor GM, Birch JM. The hereditary basis of human leukemia. In Henderson ES, Lister TA, Greaves MF, eds, Leukemia. Philadelphia: WB Saunders, 1996, 210–245.

534. Mullighan CG. Genetic variation and the risk of acute lymphoblastic leukemia. Leukemia Research 2010; 34(10): 1269–1270.

535. Shah S, Schrader KA, Waanders E, Timms AE, Vijai J et al. A recurrent germline PAX5 mutation confers susceptibility to pre-B cell acute lymphoblastic leukemia. Nature Genetics 2013; 45(10): 1226–1231.

536. Greaves MF, Maia AT, Wiemels JL, Ford AM. Leukemia in twins: lessons in natural history. Blood 2003; 102: 2321–2333.

537. Hasle H, Clemmensen IH, Mikkelsen M. Risks of leukaemia and solid tumours in individuals with Down's syndrome. Lancet 2000; 355: 165–169.

538. Vijayakrishnan J, Houlston RS. Candidate gene association studies and risk of childhood acute lymphoblastic leukemia: a systematic review and meta-analysis. Haematologica 2010; 95(8): 1405–1414.

539. Papaemmanuil E, Hosking FJ, Vijayakrishnan J, Price A, Olver B et al. Loci on 7p12.2, 10q21.2 and 14q11.2 are associated with risk of childhood acute lymphoblastic leukemia. Nature Genetics 2009; 41(9): 1006–1010.

540. Trevino LR, Yang W, French D, Hunger SP, Carroll WL et al. Germline genomic variants associated with childhood acute lymphoblastic leukemia. Nature Genetics 2009; 41(9): 1001–1005.

541. Sherborne AL, Hosking FJ, Prasad RB, Kumar R, Koehler R et al. Variation in CDKN2A at 9p21.3 influences childhood acute lymphoblastic leukemia risk. Nature Genetics 2010; 42(6): 492–494.

542. Yang W, Trevino LR, Yang JJ, Scheet P, Pui CH et al. ARID5B SNP rs10821936 is associated with risk of childhood acute lymphoblastic

543. leukemia in blacks and contributes to racial differences in leukemia incidence. Leukemia 2010; 24(4): 894–896.

543. Yang JJ, Cheng C, Devidas M, Cao X, Fan Y et al. Ancestry and pharmacogenomics of relapse in acute lymphoblastic leukemia. Nature Genetics 2011; 43(3): 237–241.

544. Migliorini G, Fiege B, Hosking FJ, Ma Y, Kumar R et al. Variation at 10p12.2 and 10p14 influences risk of childhood B-cell acute lymphoblastic leukemia and phenotype. Blood 2013; 122(19): 3298–3307.

545. Yang JJ, Cheng C, Yang W, Pei D, Cao X et al. Genome-wide interrogation of germline genetic variation associated with treatment response in childhood acute lymphoblastic leukemia. JAMA 2009; 301(4): 393–403.

546. Perez-Andreu V, Roberts KG, Harvey RC, Yang W, Cheng C et al. Inherited GATA3 variants are associated with Ph-like childhood acute lymphoblastic leukemia and risk of relapse. Nature Genetics 2013; 45(12): 1494–1498.

547. Auer F, Ruschendorf F, Gombert M, Husemann P, Ginzel S et al. Inherited susceptibility to pre B-ALL caused by germline transmission of PAX5 c.547G>A. Leukemia 2014; 28(5): 1136–1138.

548. Pui C-H, Evans W. Treatment of acute lymphoblastic leukemia. New England Journal of Medicine 2006; 354: 166–178.

549. Pui C, Sandlund J, Pei D et al. Improved outcome for children with acute lymphoblastic leukemia: results of Total Therapy Study XIIIB at St Jude Children's Research Hospital. Blood 2004; 104(9): 2690.

550. Gatta G, Capocaccia R, Stiller C et al. Childhood cancer survival trends in Europe: a EUROCARE Working Group study. Journal of Clinical Oncology 2005; 23(16): 3742.

551. Conter V, Aricò M, Basso G et al. Long-term results of the Italian Association of Pediatric Hematology and Oncology (AIEOP) Studies 82, 87, 88, 91 and 95 for childhood acute lymphoblastic leukemia. Leukemia 2010; 24(2): 255–264.

552. Möricke A, Zimmermann M, Reiter A et al. Long-term results of five consecutive trials in childhood acute lymphoblastic leukemia performed by the ALL-BFM study group from 1981 to 2000. Leukemia 2010; 24(2): 265–284.

553. Hunger S, Lu X, Devidas M et al. Improved survival for children and adolescents with acute lymphoblastic leukemia from 1990-2005: a report from the Children's Oncology Group. Journal of Clinical Oncology 2012; 30(14): 1663–1669.

554. Schmiegelow K, Forestier E, Hellebostad M et al. Long-term results of NOPHO ALL-92 and ALL-2000 studies of childhood acute lymphoblastic leukemia. Leukemia 2010; 24(2): 345–354.

555. Mitchell C, Richards S, Harrison C et al. Long-term follow-up of the United Kingdom medical research council protocols for childhood acute lymphoblastic leukaemia, 1980–2001. Leukemia 2010; 24(2): 406–418.

556. Pulte D, Gondos A, Brenner H. SEER Registry data on adult ALL. Improvement in survival in younger patients with acute lymphoblastic leukemia from the 1980s to the early 21st century. Blood 2009; 113: 1408–1411.

557. Veerman A, Kamps W, van den Berg H et al. Dexamethasone-based therapy for childhood acute lymphoblastic leukaemia: results of the prospective Dutch Childhood Oncology Group (DCOG) protocol ALL-9 (1997–2004). Lancet Oncology 2009; 10(10): 957–966.

558. Vrooman L, Neuberg D, Stevenson K et al. Dexamethasone and individualized asparaginase dosing are each associated with superior event-free survival in childhood acute lymphoblastic leukemia: results from DFCI-ALL Consortium Protocol 00–01 [Abstract]. Blood (ASH Annual Meeting Abstracts) 2009; 114(22):136. Abstract 321.

559. Hoelzer D, Thiel E, Loffler H et al. Prognostic factors in a multicentre study for treatment of acute lymphoblastic leukemia in adults. Blood 1988; 71: 123–131.

560. Boissel N, Auclerc M-F, Lhéritier V et al. Should adolescents with acute lymphoblastic leukemia be treated as old children or young adults? Comparison of the French FRALLE-93 and LALA-94 trials. Journal of Clinical Oncology 2003; 21: 774–780.

561. De Bont J, Holt B, Dekker A et al. Significant difference in outcome for adolescents with acute lymphoblastic leukemia treated on pediatric vs. adult protocols in the Netherlands. Leukemia 2004; 18: 2032–2035.

562. Huguet F, Leguay T, Raffoux E et al. Pediatric-inspired therapy in adults with Philadelphia chromosome-negative acute lymphoblastic leukemia: the GRAALL-2003 study. Journal of Clinical Oncology 2009; 27: 911–918.

563. Seibel N. Treatment of acute lymphoblastic leukemia in children and adolescents: peaks and pitfalls. Hematology American Society of Hematology Education Program 2008: 374–380.

564. Stock W, La M, Sanford B et al. What determines the outcomes for adolescents and young adults with acute lymphoblastic leukemia treated on cooperative group protocols? A comparison of Children's Cancer Group and Cancer and Leukemia Group B studies. Blood 2008; 112:1646–1654.

565. Testi A, Conter V, Vignetti M et al. Difference in outcome of adolescents (14–17 years) with acute lymphoblastic leukemia (ALL) enrolled in the Italian pediatric (AIEOP) and adult (GIMEMA) multicentre protocols [Abstract]. Journal of Clinical Oncology 2006; 24(18S): 9024.

566. Ramanujachar R, Richards S, Hann I et al. Adolescents with acute lymphoblastic leukemia: Outcome on UK national paediatric (ALL97) and adult (UKALLXII/E2993) trials. Pediatric Blood Cancer 2007; 48: 254–261.

567. Hallbook H, Gustafsson G, Smedmyr B et al. Treatment outcome in young adults and children >10 years of age with acute lymphoblastic leukemia in Sweden: a comparison between a pediatric protocol and an adult protocol. Cancer 2006; 107: 1551–1561.

568. Usvasalo A, Raty R, Knuutila S et al. Acute lymphoblastic leukemia in adolescents and young adults in Finland. Haematologica 2008; 93: 1161–1168.

569. Sive J, Buck G, Fielding A et al. Inability to tolerate standard therapy is a major reason for poor outcome in older adults with acute lymphoblastic leukemia (ALL): Results from the international MRC/ECOG trial. Blood (ASH Annual Meeting Abstracts) 2010; 116: 493.

570. Gökbuget N. Acute lymphoblastic leukemia in older patients. Haematology Education 2011; 5(1): 20–26.

571. Sive J, Buck G, Fielding A et al. Outcomes in older adults with acute lymphoblastic leukemia (ALL): results from the international MRC UKALL XII/ECOG2993 trial. British Journal of Haematology 2012; 157: 463–471.

572. Sancho M, Ribera J, Xicoy B et al. Results of the PETHEMA ALL-96 trial in elderly patients with Philadelphia chromosome-negative acute lymphoblastic leukemia. European Journal of Haematology 2007; 78(2): 102–110.

573. Gökbuget N, Hartog M, Dengler J et al. First analysis of prognostic factors in elderly Ph/BCR-ABL negative ALL including comorbidity scores: Different factors predict mortality and relapse. Onkologie 2008; 31: 14 (V29).

574. Goekbuget N, Leguay T, Hunault M et al. First European Chemotherapy Schedule for Elderly Patients with Acute Lymphoblastic Leukemia: Promising Remission Rate and Feasible Moderate Dose Intensity Consolidation [Abstract]. Blood 2008; 112: 304.

575. Hunault-Berger M, Leguay T, Thomas X et al. A randomized study of pegylated liposomal doxorubicin versus continuous-infusion doxorubicin in elderly patients with acute lymphoblastic leukemia: the GRAALL-SA1 study. Haematologica 2011; 96(2): 245–252.

576. Bassan R, Hoelzer D. Modern therapy of acute lymphoblastic leukemia. Journal of Clinical Oncology 2011; 29: 532–543.

577. Jabbour E, Faderl S, Kantarjian H. Adult acute lymphoblastic leukemia. Mayo Clinic Proceedings 2005; 80: 1517–1527.

578. Gokbuget N, Hoelzer D. Treatment of adult acute lymphoblastic leukemia. Hematology American Society of Hematology Education Program 2006; 133–141.

579. Stock W. Adolescents and young adults with acute lymphoblastic leukemia. Hematology American Society of Hematology Education Program 2010; 21–29.

580. Mitchell C, Richards S, Kinsey S et al. Benefit of dexamethasone compared with prednisolone for childhood acute lymphoblastic leukaemia: results of the UK Medical Research Council ALL97 randomized trial. British Journal of Haematology 2005; 129: 734–745.

581. Bostrom B, Sensel M, Sather H et al. Dexamethasone versus prednisone and daily oral versus weekly mercaptopurine for patients with standard-risk acute lymphoblastic leukemia: a report from the Children's Cancer Group. Blood 2003; 101: 3809–3817.

582. Inaba H, Pui CH. Glucocorticoid use in acute lymphoblastic leukemia. Lancet Oncology 2010; 11(11): 1096–1106.

583. Teuffel O, Kuster S, Hunger S et al. Dexamethasone versus prednisone for induction therapy in childhood acute lymphoblastic leukemia: a systemic review and meta-analysis. Leukemia 2011; 25(8) 1232–1238.

584. Schrappe M, Zimmermann M, Moricke A et al. Dexamethasone in induction can eliminate one third of all relapses in childhood acute lymphoblastic leukemia (ALL): results of an international randomized trial in 3655 patients (trial AIEOP-BFM ALL 2000). Blood (ASH Annual Meeting Abstracts) 2008; 112(11):9 (Abstr 7).

585. Pui C. Central nervous system disease in acute lymphoblastic leukemia: prophylaxis and treatment. Hematology American Society of Hematology Education Program 2006: 142–146.

586. Gottlieb A, Weinberg V, Ellison R et al. Efficacy of daunorubicin in the therapy of adult acute lymphocytic leukemia: a prospective randomized trial by cancer and leukemia group B. Blood 1984; 64: 267–274.

587. Bassan R, Lerede T, Rambaldi A et al. Role of anthracyclines in the treatment of adult acute lymphoblastic leukemia. Acta Haematologica 1996; 95: 188–192.

588. Cuttner J, Mick R, Budman D et al. Phase III trial of brief intensive treatment of adult acute lymphocytic leukemia comparing daunorubicin and mitoxantrone: a CALGB Study. Leukemia 1991; 5: 425–431.

589. Larson R, Dodge R, Burns C et al. A five-drug remission induction regimen with intensive consolidation for adults with acute lymphoblastic leukemia: cancer and leukemia group B study 8811. Blood 1995; 85: 2025–2037.

590. Thomas D, O'Brien S, Faderl S et al. Anthracycline dose intensification in adult acute lymphoblastic leukemia: lack of benefit in the context of the fractionated cyclophosphamide, vincristine, doxorubicin, and dexamethasone regimen. Cancer 2010; 116: 4580–4589.

591. Schrappe M, Reiter A, Ludwig W et al. Improved outcome in childhood acute lymphoblastic leukemia despite reduced use of anthracyclines and cranial radiotherapy: results of trial ALL-BFM 90. German-Austrian-Swiss ALL-BFM Study Group. Blood 2000; 95: 3310–3322.

592. Pieters R, Hunger S, Boos J et al. L-asparaginase treatment in acute lymphoblastic leukemia: a focus on Erwina asparaginase. Cancer 2011; 117(2): 238–249.

593. Amylon M, Shuster J, Pullen J et al. Intensive high-dose asparaginase consolidation improves survival for pediatric patients with T cell acute lymphoblastic leukemia and advanced stage lymphoblastic lymphoma: a Pediatric Oncology Group study. Leukemia 1999; 13:335–342.

594. Pession A, Valsecchi M, Masera G et al. Long-term results of a randomized trial on extended use of high dose L-asparaginase for standard risk childhood acute lymphoblastic leukemia. Journal of Clinical Oncology 2005; 23:7161–7167.

595. Wetzler M, Sanford B, Kurtzburg J et al. Effective aspargine depletion with pegylated asparaginase results in improved outcomes in adult acute lymphoblastic leukemia: Cancer and Leukemia Group B Study 9511. Blood 2007; 109: 4164–4167.

596. Goekbuget N, Baumann A, Beck J et al. PEG-asparaginase in adult acute lymphoblastic leukemia: efficacy and feasibility analysis with increasing dose levels. Blood 2008; 112(Suppl. 1): Abstract 302.

597. Avramis V, Sencer S, Periclou A et al. A randomized comparison of native Escherichia coli asparaginase and polyethylene glycol conjugated asparaginase for treatment of children with newly diagnosed standard-risk acute lymphoblastic leukemia: a Children's Cancer Group study. Blood 2002; 99: 1986–1994.

598. Liu C, Kawedia J, Cheng C et al. Clinical utility and implications of asparaginase antibodies in acute lymphoblastic leukemia. Leukemia 2012 (published online ahead of print April 9, 2012); doi:10.1038/leu.2012.102

599. Willer A, Gerss J, Konig T et al. Anti-Escherichia coli asparaginase antibody levels determine the activity of second-line treatment with pegylated E coli asparaginase: a retrospective analysis within the ALL-BFM trials. Blood 2011; 118: 5774–5782.

600. Kawedia J, Liu C, Pei D. Dexamethasone exposure and asparaginase antibodies affect relapse risk in acute lymphoblastic leukemia. Blood 2012; 119: 1658–1664.

601. Wang B, Relling M, Storm M et al. Evaluation of immunologic cross-reaction of antiasparaginase antibodies in acute lymphoblastic leukemia (ALL) and lymphoma patients. Leukemia 2003; 17: 1583–1588.

602. Vrooman L, Supko J, Neuberg D et al. Erwinia asparaginase after allergy to E. coli asparaginase in children with acute lymphoblastic leukemia. Pediatric Blood Cancer 2010; 54: 199–205.

603. Stock W, Douer D, DeAngelo D et al. Prevention and management of asparaginase/pegasparaginase-associated toxicities in adults and older adolescents: recommendations of an expert panel. Leukemia and Lymphoma 2011; 52(12): 2237–2257.

604. Grace R, Dahlberg S, Neuberg D et al. The frequency and management of asparaginase-related thrombosis in paediatric and adult patients with acute lymphoblastic leukemia treated on the Dana-Faber Cancer Institute consortium protocols. British Journal of Haematology 2011; 152(4): 452–459.

605. Kearney S, Dahlberg S, Levy D et al. Clinical course and outcome in children with acute lymphoblastic leukemia and asparaginase-associated pancreatitis. Pediatric Blood Cancer 2009; 53(2): 162–167.

606. Hunault-Berger M, Chevallier P, Delain M et al. Changes in antithrombin and fibrinogen levels during induction chemo therapy with L-asparaginase in adult patients with acute lymphoblastic leukemia or lymphoblastic lymphoma. Use of supportive coagulation therapy and clinical outcome: the CAPELAL study. Haematologica 2008; 93: 1488–1494.

607. Gaynon P, Angiolillo A, Carroll W et al. Long-term results of the children's cancer group studies for childhood acute lymphoblastic leukemia 1983–2002: a Children's Oncology Group Report. Leukemia 2010; 24(2): 285–297.

608. Sallan S, Gelber R, Kimball V et al. More is better! Update of Dana-Farber Cancer Institute/Children's Hospital childhood acute lymphoblastic leukemia trials. Haematology and Blood Transfusion 1990; 33: 459–466.

609. Asselin B, Devidas M, Wang C et al. Effectiveness of high-dose methotrexate in T-cell lymphoblastic leukemia and advanced-stage lymphoblastic lymphoma: a randomized study by the Children's Oncology Group (POG 9404). Blood 2011; 118: 874–883.

610. Kager L, Cheok M, Yang W et al. Folate pathway gene expression differs in subtypes of acute lymphoblastic leukemia and influence methotrexate pharmacodynamics. Journal of Clinical Investigation 2005; 1115: 110–117.

611. Marks D, Paietta E, Moorman A et al. T-cell acute lymphoblastic leukemia in adults: Clinical features, immunophenotype, cytogenetics, and outcome from the large randomized prospective trial (UKALL XII/ECOG 2993). Blood 2009; 114: 5136–5145.

612. Pui C, Relling M, Evans W. Role of pharmacogenomics and pharmacodynamics in the treatment of acute lymphoblastic leukemia. Best Practice and Research Clinical Haematology 2002; 15: 741–756.

613. Evans W, Relling M. Moving towards individualized medicine with pharmacogenomics. Nature 2004; 429: 464–468.

614. Schmiegelow K, Al-Modhwahi I, Anderson M et al. Methotrexate/6-mercaptopurine maintenance therapy influences the risk of a second malignant neoplasm after childhood acute lymphoblastic leukemia: results from the NOPHO ALL-92 study. Blood 2009; 113: 6077–6084.

615. Relling M, Gardner E, Sandborn W et al. Clinical Pharmacogenetics Implementation Consortium guidelines for thiopurine methyltransferase genotype and thiopurine dosing. Clinical Pharmacology and Therapeutics 2011; 89(3): 387–391.

616. Kamps W, Bokkerink J, Hakvoort-Cammel F et al. BFM-oriented treatment for children with acute lymphoblastic leukemia without cranial irradiation and treatment reduction for standard risk patients: results of DCLSG protocol ALL-8 (1991-1996). Leukemia 2002; 16: 1099–1111.

617. Pui C-H, Campana D, Pei, D et al. Treating childhood acute lymphoblastic leukemia without cranial irradiation. New England Journal of Medicine 2009; 360: 2730–2741.

618. Annino L, Vegna ML, Camera A et al. Treatment of adult acute lymphoblastic leukemia (ALL): long-term follow-up of the GIMEMA ALL 0288 randomized study. Blood 2002; 99(3): 863–871.

619. Kantarjian H, Thomas D, O'Brien S et al. Long-term follow-up results of hyperfractionated cyclophosphamide, vincristine, doxorubicin, and dexamethasone (Hyper-CVAD), a dose-intensive regimen, in adult acute lymphoblastic leukemia. Cancer 2004; 101: 2788–2801.

620. Kantarjian H, O'Brien S, Smith T et al. Results of treatment with hyper-CVAD, a dose-intensive regimen, in adult acute lymphoblastic leukemia. Journal of Clinical Oncology 2000; 18: 547–561.

621. Sancho J, Riberaa J, Oriol A et al. Central nervous system recurrence in adult patients with acute lymphoblastic leukemia: frequency and prognosis in 467 patients without cranial irradiation for prophylaxis. Cancer 2006; 106: 2540–2546.

622. Pui C, Cheng C, Leung W et al. Extended follow-up of long-term survivors of childhood acute lymphoblastic leukemia. New England Journal of Medicine 2003; 349(7): 640–649.

623. Goldsby R, Liu Q, Nathan P et al. Late-occurring neurologic sequelae in adult survivors of childhood acute lymphoblastic leukemia: a report from the Childhood Cancer Survivor Study. Journal of Clinical Oncology 2010; 28(2): 324–331.

624. Hill F, Richards S, Gibson B et al. Successful treatment without cranial radiotherapy of children receiving intensified chemotherapy for acute lymphoblastic leukaemia: results of the risk-stratified randomized central nervous system treatment trial MRC UKALL XI (ISRC TN 16757172). British Journal of Haematology 2004; 124(1): 33–46.

625. Tubergen D, Gilchrist G, O'Brien R et al. Prevention of CNS disease in intermediate-risk acute lymphoblastic leukemia: comparison of cranial radiation and intrathecal methotrexate and the importance of systemic therapy: a Children's Cancer Group report. Journal of Clinical Oncology 1993; 11(3): 520–526.

626. Matloub Y, Lindemulder S, Gaynon P et al. Intrathecal triple therapy decreases central nervous system relapse but fails to improve event-free survival when compared with intrathecal methotrexate: results of the Children's Cancer Group (CCG) 1952 study for standard-risk acute lymphoblastic leukemia, reported by the Children's Oncology Group. Blood 2006; 108: 1165–1173.

627. Richards S, Pui CH, Gayon P et al. Systematic review and meta-analysis of randomized trials of central nervous system directed therapy for childhood acute lymphoblastic leukaemia. Pediatric Blood Cancer 2012; doi: 10.1002/pbc.24228

628. Cave H, van der Werff ten Bosch J, Suciu S et al. Clinical significance of minimal residual disease in childhood acute lymphoblastic leukemia. European Organization for Research and Treatment of Cancer-Childhood Leukemia Cooperative Group. New England Journal of Medicine 1998; 339(9): 591–598.

629. Van Dongen J, Seriu T, Panzer-Grumayer E et al. Prognostic value of minimal residual disease in acute lymphoblastic leukemia in childhood. Lancet 1998; 352: 1731–1738.

630. Coustan-Smith E, Sancho J, Hancock M et al. Clinical importance of minimal residual disease in childhood acute lymphoblastic leukemia. Blood 2000; 96(8): 2691–2696.

631. Dworzak M, Froschi G, Printz D et al. Prognostic significance and modalities of flow cytometric minimal residual disease detection in childhood acute lymphoblastic leukemia. Blood 2002; 99(6): 1952–1958.

632. Zhou J, Goldwasser M, Li A et al. Quantitative analysis of minimal residual disease predicts relapse in children with B-lineage acute lymphoblastic leukemia in DFCI ALL Consortium Protocol 95-01. Blood 2007; 110(5): 1607–1611.

633. Borowitz M, Devidas M, Hunger S et al. Clinical significance of minimal residual disease in childhood acute lymphoblastic leukemia and the relationship to other prognostic factors. A Children's Oncology Group study. Blood 2008; 111(12): 5477–5485.

634. Basso G, Veltroni M, Valsecchi M et al. Risk of relapse of childhood acute lymphoblastic leukemia is predicted by flow cytometric measurement of residual disease on day 15 bone marrow. Journal of Clinical Oncology 2009; 27 (31): 5168–5174.

635. Conter V, Bartram C, Valsecchi M et al. Molecular response to treatment redefines all prognostic factors in children and adolescents with B-cell precursor acute lymphoblastic leukemia: results in 3184 patients of the AIEOP-BFM ALL 2000 study. Blood 2010; 115(16): 3206–3214.

636. Bassan R, Spinelli O, Oldani E et al. Improved risk classification of risk-specific therapy based on the molecular study of MRD in adult ALL. Blood 2009; 113(18): 4153–4162.

637. Stow P, Key L, Chen X et al. Clinical significance of low levels of minimal residual disease at the end of remission induction therapy in childhood acute lymphoblastic leukemia. Blood 2010; 115(23): 4657–4663.

638. Foroni L, Mortuza F, Papaioannou M et al. Minimal residual disease tests provide an independent predictor of clinical outcome in adult acute lymphoblastic leukemia. JCO 2002; 20: 1094–1104.

639. Krampera M, Vitale A, Vincenzi C et al. Outcome prediction by immunophenotypic minimal residual disease detection in adult T-cell acute lymphoblastic leukemia. British Journal of Haematology 2003; 120 (1): 74–79.

640. Vidriales M, Perez J, Lopez-Berges C et al. Minimal residual disease in adolescent (>14 years) and adult acute lymphoblastic leukemia (ALL): early immunophenotypical evaluation has high clinical value. Blood 2003; 101(12): 4695–4700.

641. Holowiecki J, Krawczyk-Kulis M, Giebel S et al. Status of minimal residual disease after induction predicts the outcome in both standard and high-risk Ph-negative adult acute lymphoblastic leukemia. The Polish Adult Leukemia Group ALL 4-2002 MRD study. British Journal of Haematology 2008; 142(2): 227–237.

642. Brüggemann M, Raff T, Thomas F et al. Clinical significance of minimal residual disease quantification in adult patients with standard-risk acute lymphoblastic leukemia. Blood 2006; 107: 1116–1123.

643. Raff T, Gokbuget N, Luschen S et al. Molecular relapse in adult standard-risk ALL patients detected by prospective MRD monitoring during and after maintenance treatment: data from the GMALL 06/99 and 07/03 trials. Blood 2007; 109(3): 910–915.

644. Goldstone A, Richards S, Lazarus H et al. In adults with standard-risk acute lymphoblastic leukemia, the greatest benefit is achieved from a matched sibling allogeneic transplantation in first complete remission, and an autologous transplantation is less effective than conventional consolidation/maintenance chemotherapy in all patients: final results of the International ALL Trial (MRC UKALL XII/ECOG E2993). Blood 2008; 111(4): 1827–1833.

645. Dhedin N, Dombret H, Thomas X et al. Autologous stem cell transplantation in adults with acute lymphoblastic leukemia in first complete remission: analysis of the LALA-85, -87 and -94 trials. Leukemia 2006; 20: 336–344.

646. Yanada M, Matsuo K, Suzuki T et al. Allogeneic hematopoietic stem cell transplantation as part of postremission therapy improves survival for adult patients with high-risk acute lymphoblastic leukemia: a meta-analysis. Cancer 2006; 106: 2657–2663.

647. Rowe J. Graft-versus-disease effect following allogeneic transplantation for acute leukaemia. Best Practice and Research Clinical Haematology 2008; 21: 485–502.

648. Thiebaut A, Vernant J, Degos L et al. Adult acute lymphocytic leukemia study testing chemotherapy and autologous and allogeneic transplantation. A follow-up report of the French protocol LALA 87. Hematology and Oncology Clinics of North America 2000; 14: 1353–1366.

649. Thomas X, Boiron J, Huguet F et al. Outcome of treatment in adults with acute lymphoblastic leukemia: analysis of the LALA-94 trial. Journal of Clinical Oncology 2004; 22: 4075–4086.

650. Hunault M, Harousseau J, Delain M et al. Better outcome of adult acute lymphoblastic leukemia after early genoidentical allogeneic bone marrow transplantation (BMT) than after late high-dose therapy and autologous BMT: a GOELAMS trial. Blood 2004; 104: 3028–3037.

651. Ribera J, Oriol A, Bethencourt C et al. Comparison of intensive chemotherapy, allogeneic or autologous stem cell transplantation as post-remission treatment for adult patients with high-risk acute lymphoblastic leukemia. Results of the PETHEMA ALL-93 trial. Haematologica 2005; 90: 1346–1356.

652. Cornelissen J, van der Holt B, Verhoef G et al. Myeloablative allogeneic versus autologous stem cell transplantation in adult patients with acute lymphoblastic leukemia in first remission: a prospective sibling donor versus no-donor comparison. Blood 2009; 113: 1375–1382.

653. Marks D, Perez W, He W et al. Unrelated donor transplants in adults with Philadelphia-negative acute lymphoblastic leukemia in first complete remission. Blood 2008; 112: 426–434.

654. Dahlke J, Kroger N, Zabelina T et al. Comparable results in patients with acute lymphoblastic leukemia after related and unrelated stem cell transplantation. Bone Marrow Transplant 2006; 37: 155–163.

655. Kiehl M, Kraut L, Schwerdtfeger R et al. Outcome of allogeneic hematopoietic stem-cell transplantation in adult patients with acute lymphoblastic leukemia: no difference in related compared with unrelated transplant in first complete remission. Journal of Clinical Oncology 2004; 22: 2816–2825.

656. Chim C, Lie A, Liang R et al. Long-term results of allogeneic bone marrow transplantation for 108 adult patients with acute lymphoblastic leukemia: favorable outcome with BMT at first remission and HLA-matched unrelated donor. Bone Marrow Transplant 2007; 40(4): 339–347.

657. Petersdorf E, Gooley T, Anasetti C et al. Optimizing outcome after unrelated marrow transplantation by comprehensive matching of HLA class I and II alleles in the donor and recipient. Blood 1998; 92(10): 3515–3520.

658. Gooley T, Chien J, Pergam S et al. Reduced mortality after allogeneic hematopoietic-cell transplantation. New England Journal of Medicine 2010; 363(22): 2091–2101.

659. Ottinger H, Ferencik S, Beelen D et al. Hematopoietic stem cell transplantation: contrasting the outcome of transplantations from HLA-identical siblings, partially HLA-mismatched related donors, and HLA-matched unrelated donors. Blood 2003; 102(3): 1131–1137.

660. Walter R, Pagel J, Gooley T et al. Comparison of matched unrelated and matched related donor myeloablative hematopoietic cell transplantation for adults with acute myeloid leukemia in first remission. Leukemia 2010; 24(7): 1276–1282.

661. Yakoub-Agha I, Mesnil F, Kuentz M et al. Allogeneic marrow stem-cell transplantation from human leukocyte antigen-identical siblings versus human leukocyte antigen-allelic-matched unrelated donors (10/10) in patients with standard-risk hematologic malignancy: a prospective study from the French Society of Bone Marrow Transplantation and Cell Therapy. Journal of Clinical Oncology 2006; 24(36): 5695–5702.

662. Laughlin M, Eapen M, Rubinstein P et al. Outcomes after transplantation of cord blood or bone marrow from unrelated donors in adults with leukemia. New England Journal of Medicine 2004; 351(22): 2265–2275.

663. Eapen M, Rocha V, Sanz G et al. Effect of graft source on unrelated donor haemopoietic stem-cell transplantation in adults with acute leukaemia: a retrospective analysis. Lancet Oncology 2010; 11(7): 653–660.

664. Ciceri F, Labopin M, Aversa F et al. A survey of fully haploidentical hematopoietic stem cell transplantation in adults with high-risk acute leukemia: a risk factor analysis of outcomes for patients in remission at transplantation. Blood 2008; 112(9): 3574–3581.

665. Huang X, Liu D, Liu K et al. Treatment of acute leukemia with unmanipulated HLA-mismatched/haploidentical blood and bone marrow transplantation. Biology of Blood and Marrow Transplantation 2009; 15(2): 257–265.

666. Martino R, Giralt S, Caballero M et al. Allogeneic hematopoietic stem cell transplantation with reduced-intensity conditioning in acute lymphoblastic leukemia: a feasibility study. Haematologica 2003; 88(5): 555–560.

667. Ram R, Storb R, Sandmaier B et al. Non-myeloablative conditioning with allogeneic hematopoietic cell transplantation for the treatment of high-risk acute lymphoblastic leukemia. Haematologica 2011; 96(8): 1113–1120.

668. Stein A, Palmer J, O'Donnell M et al. Reduced-intensity conditioning followed by peripheral blood stem cell transplantation for adult patients with high-risk acute lymphoblastic leukemia. Biology of Blood and Marrow Transplantation 2009; 15(11): 1407–1414.

669. Marks D, Wang T, Perez W et al. The outcome of full-intensity and reduced intensity conditioning matched sibling or unrelated donor transplantation in adults with Philadelphia chromosome-negative acute lymphoblastic leukemia in first and second complete remission. Blood 2010; 116(3): 366–374.

670. Mohty M, Labopin M, Tabrizzi R et al. Reduced intensity conditioning allogeneic stem cell transplantation for adult patients with acute lymphoblastic leukemia: a retrospective study from the European Group for Blood and Marrow Transplantation. Haematologica 2008; 93: 303–306.

671. Patel B, Kirkland K, Szydlo R et al. Favourable outcomes with alemtuzumab-conditioned unrelated donor stem cell transplantation in adults with high-risk Philadelphia chromosome-negative acute lymphoblastic leukaemia in first complete remission. Haematologica 2009; 94: 1399–1406.

672. Ram R, Gafter-Gvili A, Vidal L et al. Management of adult patients with acute lymphoblastic leukemia in first complete remission: systematic review and meta-analysis. Cancer 2010; 116(14): 3447–3457.

673. Gökbuget N, Kneba M, Raff T et al. Adult patients with acute lymphoblastic leukemia and molecular failure display a poor prognosis and are candidates for stem cell transplantation and targeted therapy. Blood 2012; 120: 1868–1876.

674. Hoelzer D, Thiel E, Loffler H et al. Prognostic factors in a multicentre study for treatment of acute lymphoblastic leukemia in adults. Blood 1988; 71(1): 123–131.

675. Moorman A, Harrison C, Buck G et al. Karyotype is an independent prognostic factor in adult acute lymphoblastic leukemia (ALL): analysis of cytogenetic data from patients treated on the Medical Research Council (MRC) UKALLXII/Eastern Cooperative Oncology Group (ECOG) 2993 trial. Blood 2007; 109: 3189–3197.

676. Pullarkat V, Slovak M, Kopecky K et al. Impact of cytogenetics on the outcome of adult acute lymphoblastic leukemia: results of Southwest Oncology Group 9400 study. Blood 2008; 111(5): 2563–2572.

677. Chen I, Harvey R, Mullighan C et al. Outcome modeling with CRLF2, IKZF1, JAK, and minimal residual disease in pediatric acute lymphoblastic leukemia: a Children's Oncology Group Study. Blood 2012; 119(15): 3512–3522.

678. Mullighan CG, Su X, Zhang J et al. Deletion of IKZF1 and prognosis in acute lymphoblastic leukemia. New England Journal of Medicine 2009; 360(5): 470–480.

679. Den Boer ML, van Slegtenhorst M, De Menezes RX et al. A subtype of childhood acute lymphoblastic leukaemia with poor treatment

680. Moorman AV, Schwab C, Ensor HM, Russell LJ, Morrison H et al. IGH@ translocations, CRLF2 deregulation and micro-deletions in adolescents and adults with acute lymphoblastic leukemia. Journal of Clinical Oncology July 30 2012. doi.10.1200/JCO.2011.40.3907

681. Beldjord K, Macintyre E, Lhéritier V, Boulland M-L, Leguay T et al. Minimal residual disease at 3 months, combined to the presence of IKZF1 deletion in B-lineage or absence of NOTCH1 pathway mutation in T-lineage, recapitulates the disease risk assessment in adults with Philadelphia chromosome-negative acute lymphoblastic leukemia—a GRAALL study [Abstract]. Blood 2011; 118: 572.

682. Hof J, Krentz S, van Schewick C et al. Mutations and deletions of the TP53 gene predict nonresponse to treatment and poor outcome in first relapse of childhood acute lymphoblastic leukemia. Journal of Clinical Oncology 2011; 29(23): 3185–3193.

683. Schrappe M, Aricò M, Harbott J et al. Philadelphia chromosome-positive (Ph+) childhood acute lymphoblastic leukemia: good initial steroid response allows early prediction of a favorable treatment outcome. Blood 1998; 92(8): 2730–2741.

684. Grosicki S, Holowiecki J, Giebel S et al. The early reduction of leukemic blasts in bone marrow on day 6 of induction treatment is predictive for complete remission rate and survival in adult acute myeloid leukemia; the results of multicentre, prospective Polish Adult Leukemia Group study. American Journal of Hematology 2011; 86(5): 437–439.

685. Patel B, Rai L, Buck G et al. Minimal residual disease is a significant predictor of treatment failure in non T-lineage adult acute lymphoblastic leukaemia: final results of the international trial UKALL XII/ECOG2993. British Journal of Haematology 2010; 148(1): 80–89.

686. Ribera J-M, Oriol A, Morgades M et al. Treatment of high-risk (HR) Philadelphia chromosome negative (Ph-) adult acute lymphoblastic leukemia (ALL) according to baseline risk factors and minimal residual disease (MRD): Results of the PETHEMA ALL-AR-03 trial including the use of propensity score (PS) method to reduce assignment bias. Blood 2009; 114(abstr 322): 136.

687. Secker-Walker L, Craig J, Hawkins J et al. Philadelphia positive acute lymphoblastic leukemia in adults: age distribution, BCR breakpoint and prognostic significance. Leukemia 1991; 5: 196–199.

688. Lee KH, Lee JH, Choi SJ et al. Clinical effect of imatinib added to intensive combination chemotherapy for newly diagnosed Philadelphia chromosome-positive acute lymphoblastic leukemia. Leukemia 2005; 19: 1509–1516.

689. Delannoy A, Delabesse E, Lheritier V et al. Imatinib and methylprednisolone alternated with chemotherapy improve the outcome of elderly patients with Philadelphia-positive acute lymphoblastic leukemia: results of the GRAALL AFR09 study. Leukemia 2006; 20: 1526–1532.

690. Tanguy-Schmidt A, de Labarthe A, Rousselot P et al. Long-term results of the imatinib GRAAPH-2003 study in newly diagnosed patients with de novo Philadelphia chromosome-positive acute lymphoblastic leukemia [Abstract]. Blood 2009; 114(abstr 3080).

691. Thomas DA, O'Brien SM, Faderl S et al. Long-term outcome after hyper-CVAD and imatinib (IM) for de novo or minimally treated Philadelphia chromosome-positive acute lymphoblastic leukemia (Ph-ALL) [Abstract]. Journal of Clinical Oncology 2010; 28(abstr 6506): 15S.

692. Druker BJ, Sawyers CL, Kantarjian H et al. Activity of a specific inhibitor of the BCR-ABL tyrosine kinase in the blast crisis of chronic myeloid leukemia and acute lymphoblastic leukemia with the Philadelphia chromosome. New England Journal of Medicine 2001; 344: 1038–1042.

693. Ottmann OG, Druker BJ, Sawyers CL et al. A phase 2 study of imatinib in patients with relapsed or refractory Philadelphia chromosome-positive acute lymphoid leukemias. Blood 2002; 100: 1965–1971.

outcome: a genome-wide classification study. Lancet Oncology 2009; 10(2): 125–134.

694. Schultz K, Bowman W, Aledo A et al. Improved early event-free survival with imatinib in Philadelphia chromosome-positive acute lymphoblastic leukemia: A Children's Oncology Group Study. Journal of Clinical Oncology 2009; 27(31): 5175–5181.

695. Rives S, Estella J, Gómez P et al. Intermediate dose of imatinib in combination with chemotherapy followed by allogeneic stem cell transplantation improves early outcome in paediatric Philadelphia chromosome-positive acute lymphoblastic leukemia (ALL): results of the Spanish Cooperative Group SHOP studies ALL-94, ALL-99 and ALL-2005. British Journal of Haematology 2011; 154: 600–611.

696. Thomas DA, O'Brien SM, Faderl S et al. Long-term outcome after hyper-CVAD and imatinib (IM) for de novo or minimally treated Philadelphia chromosome-positive acute lymphoblastic leukemia (Ph-ALL) [Abstract]. Journal of Clinical Oncology 2010; 28(abstr 6506): 15S.

697. Yanada M, Sugiura I, Takeuchi J et al. Prospective monitoring of BCR-ABL1 transcript levels in patients with Philadelphia chromosome-positive acute lymphoblastic leukaemia undergoing imatinib-combined chemotherapy. British Journal of Haematology 2008; 143(4): 503–510.

698. Wassmann B, Pfeifer H, Goekbuget N et al. Alternating versus concurrent schedules of imatinib and chemotherapy as front-line therapy for Philadelphia-positive acute lymphoblastic leukemia (Ph+ ALL) Blood 2006; 108: 1469–1477.

699. de Labarthe A, Rousselot P, Huguet-Rigal F et al. Imatinib combined with induction or consolidation chemotherapy in patients with de novo Philadelphia chromosome-positive acute lymphoblastic leukemia: results of the GRAAPH-2003 study. Blood 2007; 109: 1408–1413.

700. Ribera JM, Oriol A, Gonzalez M et al. Concurrent intensive chemotherapy and imatinib before and after stem cell transplantation in newly diagnosed Philadelphia chromosome-positive acute lymphoblastic leukemia. Final results of the CSTIBES02 trial. Haematologica 2010; 95(1): 87–95.

701. Stein A, O'Donnell M, Snyder D et al. Reduced-intensity stem cell transplantation for high-risk acute lymphoblastic leukaemia. Biology of Blood and Marrow Transplantation 2009; 15(11): 1407–1414.

702. Ravandi F, O'Brien S, Thomas D et al. First report of phase 2 study of dasatinib with hyper-CVAD for the frontline treatment of patients with Philadelphia chromosome-positive (Ph+) acute lymphoblastic leukemia. Blood 2010; 116(12): 2070–2077.

703. Vignetti M, Fazi P, Cimino G et al. Imatinib plus steroids induces complete remissions and prolonged survival in elderly Philadelphia chromosome-positive patients with acute lymphoblastic leukemia without additional chemotherapy: results of the Gruppo Italiano Malattie Ematologiche dell'Adulto (GIMEMA) LAL0201-B protocol. Blood 2007; 109: 3676–3678.

704. Ottmann OG, Wassmann B, Pfeifer H et al. Imatinib compared with chemotherapy as front-line treatment of elderly patients with Philadelphia chromosome-positive acute lymphoblastic leukemia (Ph+ALL) Cancer 2007; 109: 2068–2076.

705. Foà R, Vitale A, Vignetti M et al. Dasatinib as first-line treatment for adult patients with Philadelphia chromosome-positive acute lymphoblastic leukemia. Blood 2011; 118(25): 6521–6528.

706. Fielding AK, Buck G, Lazarus H et al. Imatinib significantly enhances long-term outcomes in Philadelphia positive acute lymphoblastic leukaemia; final results of the UKALLXII/ECOG2993 Trial [Abstract]. Blood 2010; 116: 493.

707. Chalandon Y, Thomas X, Hayette S et al. First results of the GRAAPH-2005 study in younger adult patients with de novo Philadelphia positive acute lymphoblastic leukemia [Abstract]. Blood 2008; 112: 12.

708. Rousselot P, Hayette S, Récher C et al. Dasatinib (Sprycel®) and low intensity chemotherapy for first-line treatment in elderly patients with de novo Philadelphia positive ALL (EWALL-PH-01): kinetics of response, resistance and prognostic significance [Abstract]. Blood 2010; 116: 172.

709. O'Hare T, Walters D, Stoffregen E et al. In vitro activity of Bcr-Abl inhibitors AMN107 and BMS-354825 against clinically relevant imatinib-resistant Abl kinase domain mutants. Cancer Research 2005; 65: 4500–4505.

710. Ottmann O, Dombret H, Martinelli G et al. Dasatinib induces rapid hematologic and cytogenetic responses in adult patients with Philadelphia chromosome positive acute lymphoblastic leukemia with resistance or intolerance to imatinib: interim results of a phase 2 study. Blood 2007; 110: 2309–2315.

711. Talpaz M, Shah N, Kartarjian H et al. Dasatinib in imatinib-resistant Philadelphia chromosome-positive leukemias. New England Journal of Medicine 2006; 354: 2531–2541.

712. Lilly M, Ottmann O, Shah N et al. Dasatinib 140mg once daily versus 70mg twice daily in patients with Ph-positive acute lymphoblastic leukemia who failed imatinib: Results from a phase 3 study. American Journal of Hematology 2010; 85: 164–170.

713. Takayama N, Sato N, O'Brien S et al. Imatinib mesylate has limited activity against the central nervous system involvement of Philadelphia chromosome-positive acute lymphoblastic leukemia due to poor penetration into cerebrospinal fluid. British Journal of Haematology 2002; 119: 106–108.

714. Porkka K, Koskenvesa P, Lundan T et al. Dasatinib crosses the blood-brain-barrier and is an efficient therapy for central nervous system Philadelphia chromosome-positive leukemia. Blood 2008; 112: 1005–1012.

715. Thomas D, Faderl S, Cortes J et al. Treatment of Philadelphia chromosome-positive acute lymphocytic leukemia with hyper-CVAD and imatinib mesylate. Blood 2004; 103: 4396–4407.

716. Pfeifer H, Goekbuget N, Volp C et al. Long-term outcome of 335 adult patients receiving Different schedules of imatinib and chemotherapy as front-line treatment for Philadelphia-positive acute lymphoblastic leukemia (Ph+ ALL). [Abstract]. Blood 2010; 116: 173.

717. Fielding A, Rowe J, Richards S et al. Prospective outcome data on 267 unselected adult patients with Philadelphia chromosome-positive acute lymphoblastic leukemia confirms superiority of allogeneic transplantation over chemotherapy in the pre-imatinib era: results from the International ALL trial MRC UKALLXII/ECOG2993. Blood 2009; 113(19): 4489–4496.

718. Mizuta S, Matsuo K, Yagasaki F et al. Pre-transplant imatinib-based therapy improves the outcome of allogeneic stem cell transplantation for BCR-ABL-positive acute lymphoblastic leukemia. Leukemia 2011; 25(1): 41–47.

719. Kebriaei P, Saliba R, Rondon G et al. Long-term follow of allogeneic hematopoietic stem cell transplantation for patients with Philadelphia chromosome-positive acute lymphoblastic leukemia: Impact of tyrosine kinase inhibitors on treatment outcome. Biology of Blood and Marrow Transplantation 2012; 18: 584–592.

720. Burke M, Cao Q, Trotz B et al. Allogeneic hematopoietic cell transplantation (allogeneic HCT) for treatment of pediatric Philadelphia chromosome-positive acute lymphoblastic leukemia (ALL). Pediatric Blood Cancer 2009; 53: 1289–1294.

721. Pane F, Cimino G, Izzo B et al. Significant reduction of the hybrid BCR/ABL transcripts after induction and consolidation therapy is a powerful predictor of treatment response in adult Philadelphia-positive acute lymphoblastic leukemia. Leukemia 2005; 19(4): 628–635.

722. Preudhomme C, Henic N, Cazin B et al. Good correlation between RT-PCR analysis and relapse in Philadelphia (Ph1)-positive acute lymphoblastic leukemia (ALL). Leukemia 1997; 11(2): 294–298.

723. Lee S, Kim D-W, Cho B-S et al. Impact of minimal residual disease kinetics during imatinib-based treatment on transplantation outcome in Philadelphia chromosome-positive acute lymphoblastic leukemia. Leukemia 2012; advance online publication, 6 July 2012. doi:10.1038/leu.2012.164

724. Soverini S, Vitale A, Poerio A et al. Philadelphia-positive acute lymphoblastic leukemia patients already harbor BCR-ABL kinase domain mutations at low levels at the time of diagnosis. Haematologica 2011; 96: 552–557.

725. Lee S, Kim D, Cho B et al. Risk factors for adults with Philadelphia-chromosome positive acute lymphoblastic leukaemia in remission treated with allogeneic bone marrow transplantation: the potential of real-time quantitative reverse transcription polymerase chain reaction. British Journal of Haematology 2003; 120(1): 145–153.

726. Hofmann W, Jones L, Lemp N et al. Ph(+) acute lymphoblastic leukemia resistant to the tyrosine kinase inhibitor STI571 has a unique BCR-ABL gene mutation. Blood 2002; 99: 1860–1862.

727. Hu Y, Liu Y, Pelletier S et al. Requirement of Src kinases Lyn, Hck and Fgr for BCR-ABL1-induced B-lymphoblastic leukemia but not chronic myeloid leukemia. Nat Genet 2004; 36: 453–461.

728. Pui C, Pei D, Sandlund J et al. Long-term results of St Jude total therapy studies 11, 12, 13A, 13B and 14 for childhood acute lymphoblastic leukemia. Leukemia 2010; 24: 371–382.

729. Nguyen K, Devidas M, Cheng S et al. Factors influencing survival after relapse from acute lymphoblastic leukemia: a Children's Oncology Group study. Leukemia 2008; 22: 2142–2150.

730. Rowe J, Buck G, Burnett A et al. Induction therapy for adults with acute lymphoblastic leukemia: results of more than 1500 patients from the international ALL trial. MRC UKALL XII/ECOG E2993. Blood 2005; 106: 3760–3767.

731. Gokbuget N, Hoelzer D, Arnold R, et al. Treatment of adult ALL according to protocols of the German Multicentre Study Group for Adult ALL (GMALL). Hematology and Oncology Clinics of North America 2000; 14: 1307–1325.

732. Linker C, Damon L, Ries C et al. Intensified and shortened cyclical chemotherapy for adult acute lymphoblastic leukemia. Journal of Clinical Oncology 2002; 20: 2464–2471.

733. Takeuchi J, Kyo T, Naito K et al. Induction therapy by frequent administration of doxorubicin with four other drugs, followed by intensive consolidation and maintenance therapy for adult acute lymphoblastic leukemia: the JALSG-ALL93 study. Leukemia 2002; 16: 1259–1266.

734. Giona F, Annino L, Rondelli R et al. Treatment of adults with acute lymphoblastic leukaemia in first bone marrow relapse: results of the ALL R-87 protocol. British Journal of Haematology 1997; 97(4): 896–903.

735. Montillo M, Tedeschi A, Centurioni R et al. Treatment of relapsed adult acute lymphoblastic leukemia with fludarabine and cytosine arabinoside followed by granulocyte colony-stimulating factor (FLAGGCSF). Leukemia and Lymphoma 1997; 25: 579–583.

736. Thomas D, Kantarjian H, Smith T et al. Primary refractory and relapsed adult acute lymphoblastic leukemia: characteristics, treatment results, and prognosis with salvage therapy. Cancer 1999; 86(7): 1216–1230.

737. Fielding A, Richards S, Chopra R et al. Outcome of 609 adults after relapse of acute lymphoblastic leukemia (ALL); an MRC UKALL12/ ECOG 2993 study. Blood 2007; 109(3): 944–950.

738. Einsiedel H, von Stackelberg A, Hartmann R et al. Long-term outcome in children with relapsed ALL by risk-stratified salvage therapy: results of trial acute lymphoblastic leukemia-relapse study of the Berlin-Frankfurt-Munster Group 87. Journal of Clinical Oncology 2005; 23: 7942–7950.

739. Tallen G, Ratei R, Mann G et al. Long-term outcome in children with relapsed acute lymphoblastic leukemia after time-point and site-of-relapse stratification and intensification short-course multidrug chemotherapy: results of trial ALL-REZ BFM 90. Journal of Clinical Oncology 2010; 28: 2339–2347.

740. Malempati S, Gaynon P, Sather H et al. Outcome after relapse among children with standard-risk acute lymphoblastic leukemia: Children's Oncology Group study CCG-1952. Journal of Clinical Oncology 2007; 25: 5800–5807.

741. Oriol A, Vives S, Hernandez-Rivas J et al. Outcome after relapse of acute lymphoblastic leukemia in adult patients included in four consecutive risk-adapted trials by the PETHEMA Study Group. Haematologica 2010; 95: 589–596.

742. Gökbuget N, Stanze D, Beck J et al. Outcome of relapsed adult lymphoblastic leukemia depends on response to salvage chemotherapy, prognostic factors, and performance of stem cell transplantation. Blood 2012; 120: 2032–2041.

743. Jeha S, Gaynon P, Razzouk B et al. Phase II study of clofarabine in pediatric patients with refractory or relapsed acute lymphoblastic leukemia. Journal of Clinical Oncology 2006; 24: 1917–1923.

744. Locatelli F, Testi A, Bernardo M et al. Clofarabine, cyclophosphamide and etoposide as single-course re-induction therapy for children with refractory/multiple relapsed acute lymphoblastic leukemia. British Journal of Haematology 2009; 147: 371–378.

745. Pigneux A, Sauvezie M, Vey N et al. Clofarabine combinations in adults with refractory/relapsed acute lymphoblastic leukemia (ALL): A GRAALL report [Abstract]. Blood 2011; 118(abstr 2586):

746. Gökbuget N, Basara N, Baurmann H et al. High single-drug activity of nelarabine in relapsed T-lymphoblastic leukemia/lymphoma offers curative option with subsequent stem cell transplantation. Blood 2011; 118: 3504–3511.

747. Berg S, Blaney S, Devidas M et al. Phase II study of nelarabine (compound 506U78) in children and young adults with refractory T-cell malignancies: a report from the Children's Oncology Group. Journal of Clinical Oncology 2005; 23: 3376–3382.

748. Topp M, Goekbuget N, Zugmaier G et al. Anti-CD19 BiTE blinatumomab induces high complete remission rate in adult patients with relapsed B-precursor ALL: Updated results of an ongoing phase II trial [Abstract]. Blood 2011; 118:(abstr 252).

749. Litzow M. Novel therapeutic approaches for acute lymphoblastic leukemia. Hematology and Oncology Clinics of North America 2011; 25(6): 1303–1317.

750. Lazarus H, Richards S, Chopra R et al. Central nervous system involvement in adult acute lymphoblastic leukemia at diagnosis: results from the international ALL trial MRC UKALL XII/ECOG E2993. Blood 2006; 108: 465–472.

751. Reman O, Pigneux A, Huguet F et al. Central nervous system involvement in adult acute lymphoblastic leukemia at diagnosis and/or at first relapse: results from the GET-LALA group. Leukemia Research 2008; 32: 1741–1750.

752. Clarke M, Gaynon P, Hann I et al. CNS-directed therapy for childhood acute lymphoblastic leukemia: Childhood ALL Collaborative Group overview of 43 randomized trials. Journal of Clinical Oncology 2003; 21: 1798–1809.

753. Buonamici S, Trimarchi T, Ruocco M et al. CCR7 signaling as an essential regulator of CNS infiltration in T-cell leukaemia. Nature 2009; 459: 1000–1004.

754. Robison L, Bhatia S. Late-effects among survivors of leukaemia and lymphoma during childhood and adolescence. British Journal of Haematology 2003; 122: 345–359.

755. Bowers D, Liu Y, Leisenring W et al. Late-occurring stroke among long-term survivors of childhood leukemia and brain tumors: a report from the Childhood Cancer Survivor Study. Journal of Clinical Oncology 2006; 24: 5277–5282.

756. Byrne J, Fears T, Mills J et al. Fertility in women treated with cranial radiotherapy for childhood acute lymphoblastic leukemia. Pediatric Blood Cancer 2004; 42: 589–597.

757. Mattano L, Sather H, Trigg M et al. Osteonecrosis as a complication of treating acute lymphoblastic leukemia in children: a report from the Children's Cancer Group. Journal of Clinical Oncology 2000; 18: 3262–3272.

758. Te Winkel M, Pieters R, Hop W et al. Prospective study on incidence, risk factors, and long-term outcome of osteonecrosis in pediatric acute lymphoblastic leukemia. Journal of Clinical Oncology 2011; 29: 4143–4150.

759. Patel B, Richards S, Rowe J et al. High incidence of avascular necrosis in adolescents with acute lymphoblastic leukaemia: a UKALL XII analysis. Leukemia 2008; 22(2): 308–312.

760. Kawedia J, Kaste S, Pei D et al. Pharmacokinetic, pharmacodynamic, and pharmacogenetic determinants of osteonecrosis in children with acute lymphoblastic leukemia. Blood 2011; 117: 2340–2347.

761. Singal P, Iliskovic N. Doxorubicin-induced cardiomyopathy. New England Journal of Medicine 1998; 339: 900–905.

762. Kimball V, Gelber R, Li F et al. Second malignancies in patients treated for childhood acute lymphoblastic leukemia. Journal of Clinical Oncology 1998; 16: 2848–2853.

763. Löning L, Zimmermann M, Reiter A et al. Secondary neoplasms subsequent to Berlin-Frankfurt-Münster therapy of acute lymphoblastic leukemia in childhood: significantly lower risk without cranial radiotherapy. Blood 2000; 95: 2770–2775.

764. Neglia JP, Meadows AT, Robison LL et al. Second neoplasms after acute lymphoblastic leukemia in childhood. New England Journal of Medicine 1991; 325(19): 1330–1336.

765. Tavernier E, Le Q, de Botton S et al. Secondary or concomitant neoplasms among adults diagnosed with acute lymphoblastic leukemia and treated according to the LALA-87 and LALA-94 trials. Cancer 2007; 110(12): 2747–2755.

CHAPTER 52

Chronic leukaemias

Hemant Malhotra, Lalit Kumar, Pankaj Malhotra, Devendra Hiwase, and Ravi Bhatia

Introduction to chronic leukaemia

The chronic leukaemias are a group of monoclonal haematological malignancies characterized by proliferation and accumulation of cells of one or more haematopoietic lineage. Even without treatment, survival is possible for several months, and sometimes several years. These are usually adult diseases with age of onset in the fifth or sixth decade in the majority of patients. Chronic lymphocytic leukaemia (CLL) is the most common haematological cancer seen in Africa and the Western hemisphere. However, in Asia chronic myeloid leukaemia (CML) is the most common adult leukaemia. Why CML is more common in Asia is not clear, but the aetio-pathogenesis is more likely to be due to genetic rather than environmental factors.

These two common chronic leukaemias (CML and CLL) and some other less common leukaemias will be discussed in this chapter.

Chronic myelogenous leukaemia

Epidemiology

CML is a clonal disorder of a leukaemic pluripotent stem cell that affects several lineages, primarily the myeloid lineage. The molecular hallmark of CML is the presence of the Philadelphia chromosome (reciprocal translocations of genetic material between chromosomes 9 and 22) which brings the BCR gene into proximity to the ABL gene, forming a new fusion chimeric gene—BCR–ABL—which has oncogenic potential and is responsible for the pathogenesis of the disease. The BCR–ABL gene is expressed in nearly all patients of CML and this fact has been utilized in the developments of specific tyrosine kinase inhibitor (TKI) therapies targeting the gene. Since the development and availability of these agents, there has been a paradigm shift in the treatment of CML with the majority of patients now experiencing multi-decade survival. These drugs have affected a change in the natural disease of the disease and form the model for targeted treatment of several other solid and haematological cancers.

The age-adjusted annual incidence of CML in the US from 2004–2008 was 1.6 cases/100 000 population, with an estimated 4 870 new cases expected in 2010 [1]. CML accounts for approximately 11% of all leukaemias. With the prolonged survival achieved with TKIs, CML prevalence in the US in the coming decades is expected to increase substantially. Mortality associated with CML decreased by 7.2% from 2003–2007. Overall five-year survival for US patients diagnosed with CML from 2001–2007 was 57.2%.

The exact incidence in Asian countries in not known, but CML is the most common adult leukaemia in this region and is much more common than CLL. The disease onset is reported to be about a decade earlier in Asian countries compared to the West, with more patients presenting in higher stages at diagnosis.

Staging and diagnostics

More than 80% of patients of CML are diagnosed in the chronic phase of the disease. The disease usually takes a triphasic clinical course—chronic phase (CP), accelerated phase (AP), and blastic phase (BP). Sometimes, the patient can progress directly from the CP to the BP without an intervening AP. In CP, the patient is usually asymptomatic or minimally symptomatic, and historically had a median survival of four to five years [2]. Approximately 10% of patients are diagnosed incidentally during workup for some other medical illness or on routine testing. Without adequate therapy, all patients will eventually go to an end-stage BP with a median survival of only three to six months. The BP is usually of myeloblastic type (50%) but could be of lymphoblastic type (20–30%) or of undifferentiated phenotype (25%) [3].

Different criteria have been used in the literature to define CP, AP, and BP; Table 52.1 presents some of the most frequently used criteria. The University of Texas MD Anderson Cancer Center (MDACC) classification [4] has been used in all studies with TKIs and most of the interferon studies and, therefore, is supported by the most data with modern therapy. Other criteria have been proposed, but some of these, such as the World Health Organization (WHO) proposal [5] have not been clinically validated. The expected survival in all stages has changed with the use of TKIs [6]. An analysis of 3 548 patients with CML referred to the MDACC from 1965–2010 indicated that the overall survival (OS) of patients has significantly improved in all CML phases [7].

For the patient in the CP of the disease, the prognosis can be further defined by the Sokal score [8], which uses clinical and laboratory parameters (age, spleen size, platelet count, and percentage of blasts in the peripheral blood) to define a risk score that is associated with long-term outcome. The three Sokal prognostic groups are identified with hazard ratios of <0.8, 0.8–1.2, and >1.2, with historical median survivals of 2.5, 3.5, and 4.5 years, respectively [8]. Although the score was designed long before the era of TKIs, it is still applicable today and the probability of response to these agents is greatly influenced by the Sokal risk score. Other prognostic scores such as the Hasford score, [9] and the EUTOS score [10] are less frequently used but may have similar prognostic implications.

Table 52.1 Criteria for diagnosis of accelerated and blast phase of common chronic leukaemia (CML)

Chronic phase: None of the criteria for accelerated phase or blast phase

Accelerated phase

	MDACC	IBMTR	WHO
Blasts, %	15–30	10–30	10–19
Blasts + promyelocytes, %	≥30	≥20	NA
Basophils, %	≥20	≥20*	≥20
Platelets	<100	Unresponsive increase or persistent decrease	$<100 \times 10^9$/L, or $>1000 \times 10^9$/L unresponsive to treatment
Cytogenetics	CE	CE	CE not at the time of diagnosis
WBC	NA	Difficult to control, or doubling in <5 days	NA
Anaemia	NA	Unresponsive	NA
Splenomegaly	NA	Increasing	NA
Other	NA	Chloromas, myelofibrosis	Megakaryocyte proliferation, fibrosis
Blast phase			
Blasts, %	≥30	≥30	≥20
Other	ED	ED	ED

*Basophils + eosinophils.

CE, clonal evolution; ED, extramedullary disease with localized immature blasts; MDACC, MD Anderson Cancer Center; IBMTR, International Bone Marrow Transplant Registry; WHO, World Health Organisation; NA, not applicable; WBC, white blood cell count.

Reproduced with permission from Swerdlow SH et al., *WHO Classification of Tumors of Hematopoietic and Lymphoid Tissues*, Fourth edition, Copyright, World Health Organization, Geneva, Switzerland, Copyright © 2008 World Health Organization.

Molecular biology

CML develops from transformation of a haematopoietic stem cell (HSC) by the BCR–ABL gene, which results from a chromosomal translocation that leads to juxtaposition of the 5' portion of the BCR gene on chromosome 22 and the 3' portion of the ABL gene on chromosome on chromosome 22 [11, 12]. The derivative shortened chromosome 22 is also referred to as the Philadelphia chromosome (Ph). The resulting messenger RNA usually contains an e13a2 (formerly b2a2) or e14a2 (or b3a2) BCR–ABL junction. Both BCR–ABL mRNA molecules translate into a 210-kd fusion protein (p210BCR–ABL) [13]. Other variant fusions can rarely give rise to oncogenic BCR–ABL proteins. The translocation is found in cells of multiple lineages, consistent with a HSC origin of the disease. CML patients may have a karyotype of normal appearance but have a cytogenetically occult BCR–ABL gene. It has been suggested that CML may have multistep pathogenesis, with clonal haematopoiesis preceding acquisition of the t(9;22) translocation [14]. However, expression of a BCR–ABL fusion gene in HSCs appears to be sufficient to initiate CML in various mouse models [15].

The mechanisms of BCR–ABL-mediated cellular transformation have been extensively studied [16]. The tyrosine kinase activity of the ABL protein is constitutively activated by addition of N-terminal BCR sequences, which promote protein dimerization, leading to phosphorylation of tyrosine residues in the kinase-activation loops and constitutive activation of kinase activity. The fusion of BCR sequences to ABL also adds new regulatory motifs to ABL. The uncontrolled kinase activity of BCR–ABL and enhanced interaction with a variety of effector proteins leads to deregulation of cell-signalling mechanisms that regulate proliferation. The BCR–ABL protein and associated biochemical pathways have been extensively studied. The ABL tyrosine kinase is crucial for oncogenic transformation, further substantiated by the success of kinase inhibitor therapy for CML. Other domains in BCR–ABL play important roles in regulating ABL kinase activity or connect to downstream signalling pathways. For example the amino-terminal coiled-coil oligomerization domain of BCR is an important activator of ABL kinase activity; phosphorylation of BCR at tyrosine 177 generates a GRB2-binding site, which is important for RAS activation; and mutations in the ABL SH2 domain reduces BCR–ABL induced myeloproliferation in mice. Many signalling proteins interact with BCR–ABL through various functional domains and are phosphorylated, leading to activation of signalling, through RAS, PI3K, AKT, JNK, and SRC family kinases, protein phosphatase, STATs, nuclear factor-B, and MYC. BCR–ABL also induces expression of cytokines such as interleukin-3, granulocyte colony-stimulating factor (G-CSF), and granulocyte–macrophage colony-stimulating factor (GM-CSF), potentially contributing to expansion of leukaemic cells.

Progression to AP and BC is associated with increase in immature blast cells. It is likely that a variety of molecular mechanisms contributes to maturation arrest, enhanced proliferation, survival, and increased tissue invasiveness in BC CML [17]. Increased BCR–ABL expression appears to be a key factor in the development of BC. Additional cytogenetic and molecular changes are frequently seen during progression. Genetic instability may be related to increased oxidative stress, reduced DNA repair, or reduced DNA damage response. Genetic changes observed in leukaemic cells from BP CML patients include non-random cytogenetic changes and point mutations in TP53, RB, and CDKN2A. The block in myeloid differentiation in BC may involve defects in haematopoietic transcriptional factors. The granulocyte/macrophage progenitor (GMP) pool is expanded in patients with BP CML, which may be related to increased WNT signalling and increased self-renewal capacity [18, 19].

Pathology

Patients usually present with leucocytosis, thrombocytosis, and anaemia. The total leukocyte count is usually over 25×10^9/L, and rises progressively without treatment. Granulocytes at all stages of differentiation are seen on differential counts. Granulocytes are usually normal in appearance. Circulating blasts between 0.5% and 10% are seen. Low or absent neutrophil alkaline phosphatase activity is seen in 90% of patients. The absolute basophil count is consistently increased. Basophils are usually less than 15% in CML CP. The absolute eosinophil count is usually increased, although the eosinophils percentage is usually not increased. The absolute lymphocyte count may be increased related to increased T cells. The platelet count is often elevated at diagnosis. Platelet function abnormalities with reduced second wave of aggregation to epinephrine may be seen. Most patients have reduced haematocrit at diagnosis. Small numbers of nucleated red blood cells and mild reticulocytosis may be seen. Clinical chemistry may reveal hyperuricaemia and hyperuricosuria, elevated serum LDH, increased serum vitamin B12-binding capacity related to release of transcobalamin I and II from mature neutrophils, and an average of tenfold increased serum B12 levels. Release of potassium from WBC during clotting may cause pseudohyperkalaemia. Consumption of glucose and oxygen by neutrophils after a sample is drawn may result in spurious hypoglycaemia or hypoxaemia.

Bone marrow (BM) examination usually shows marrow hypercellularity up to 75–90%. There is increased granulocytic/erythroid ratio. Eosinophils and basophils are often increased. Blasts usually represent less than 5% of cells in CP CML. Presence of more than 10% blasts indicate transformation to AP. Megakaryocytes are typically smaller and may be hypolobated. About 40–50% of patients show increased megakaryocyte proliferation. Collagen type III staining is typically increased. Increased reticulin fibrosis is seen in 50% of patients often associated with increased marrow megakaryocytes. The spleen shows infiltration of red pulp cords with granulocytes at various stages of maturation. Granulocytic cell infiltration may be seen in the portal areas and hepatic sinusoids of the liver.

On cytogenetic examination, the t(9;22)(q34;q11) is seen in more than 90% of patients. Additional chromosomal abnormalities, including -Y and +8, are seen in 20% of patients at diagnosis. 5% of patients show variant Ph chromosomes, with complex rearrangements. Cryptic or complex translocations can be detected by fluorescence in situ hybridization (FISH) or polymerase chain reaction (PCR) assays in a small proportion of patients where the t(9;22) may not be detected. Real-time quantitative polymerase chain reaction (RQ-PCR) provides an accurate measure of the total leukaemia cell mass. Circulating BCR–ABL transcript numbers and marrow cytogenetics should be studied in every new patient with CML before initiation of treatment.

Cytogenetics allows identification of unusual translocations or additional cytogenetic abnormalities. BCR–ABL RQ-PCR identifies whether the commonly observed transcripts, or a less common fusion transcript not amplified in the standard assay, are present. FISH on blood specimens using dual probes for the BCR and ABL genes is also useful for confirming the diagnosis, and may also detect deletions in the derivative 9q, which have prognostic significance [20].

Medical management

Chemotherapy

CML chemotherapy with busulfan (BU), introduced in the 1950s, is associated with serious adverse effects, including prolonged aplasia and pulmonary fibrosis. Treatment with hydroxyurea, started as an alternative to BU, is less toxic than BU, with the major adverse effect being reversible marrow suppression. Neither drug significantly suppresses the leukaemic clone. The main aim of treatment with these agents is to control disease and symptoms with initiation of treatment with imatinib (IM) or other disease-specific therapies.

Interferon

Interferon-α (IFN) was recognized to have efficacy in the treatment of CML in the 1980s. The activity of IFN in CML may be related to inhibition of proliferation, correction of altered microenvironmental interactions, or stimulation of immune response. Treatment of CP CML patients results in complete and partial cytogenetic remissions rates from 0% to 38% [21]. Remissions are more common in younger patients, less advanced stage disease, favourable prognostic stage, and those treated soon after diagnosis. Haematologic remissions usually occur within one to three months, and complete cytogenetic remissions 9 to 18 months, after starting IFN. Durable responses may be seen in patients who achieve a complete cytogenetic remission. Virtually all patients receiving IFN experience constitutional adverse effects. Acute adverse effects include flu-like symptoms such as fever, chills, and malaise. Additional more severe acute reactions and chronic complications can occur. These are usually dose- and duration-dependent, and may require discontinuation of treatment. Randomized studies show an improvement in survival rates with IFN treatment compared with BU or hydroxyurea [22–24]. Meta-analysis shows a five-year survival rate of 57% (50–59%) for IFN and 42% (29–44%) for chemotherapy [25]. IFN increases life expectancy by a median of approximately 20 months compared with chemotherapy. However, IFN may not enhance survival for patients in the late CP or with more than 10–30% blasts in peripheral blood. Adding cytosine arabinoside to IFN appears to enhance survival benefit but at the cost of increased toxicity [26]. Therefore, although IFN clearly is beneficial in patients with CML patients, benefit is limited by low levels of cytogenetic response and considerable toxicity. Its use in the modern treatment of CML patients has been replaced by use of IM and other TKIs, although there has been revived interest recently in combination treatment.

Tyrosine kinase inhibitors (TKIs)

The introduction of TKIs into clinical practice has dramatically changed CML treatment. TKI therapy induces remissions in most patients with CP CML, leading to excellent survival, and is now the mainstay of treatment. However in AP and BC CML, TKI resistance can occur, usually as a result of tyrosine kinase domain point mutations. Resistance to the first-generation TKI IM can often be treated by 'second generation' TKIs, such as dasatinib, nilotinib, bosutinib, or ponatinib. These drugs may be even more effective than IM for front line treatment of CML and the first two (dasatinib and nilotinib) have been approved in that indication.

IM mesylate (STI571; Gleevec®) is a small molecule kinase inhibitor of ABL-containing proteins, the platelet-derived growth factor receptor, and the c-KIT receptor [27]. IM competitively binds the ATP-binding site in the kinase domain of ABL, and blocks the ability of BCR–ABL to phosphorylate its substrates. Initial phase 1 and phase 2 trials established that IM induced haematologic and cytogenetic responses in most CP CML patients who had failed other treatments and was well tolerated [28]. The International Randomized Interferon and STI571 (IRIS) study compared IM (400 mg daily) with IFN-α plus cytosine arabinoside in 1106 newly-diagnosed CP CML patients. In the initial analysis, the estimated complete cytogenetic response (CCR) rate was 76.2% (95% CI, 72.5–79.9) in the IM group and was superior to 14.5% (95% CI, 10.5–18.5) in the IFN plus cytosine arabinoside group (p <0.001) at 18 months [29]. The estimated freedom from progression to AP or BC at 18 months was 96.7% in the IM group and 91.5% in the IFN group (p <0.001). IM was better tolerated than IFN therapy. A 60-month follow-up report for this study found an estimated cumulative incidence rate of complete haematological response (CHR), major cytogenetic response (MCR), and CCR of 98%, 92%, and 87% at 60 months for patients on first-line IM. The estimated event-free survival (EFS) at six years was 83%, and the estimated OS was 88% [30].

IM 400 mg daily is currently the standard dose for initiating therapy in newly-diagnosed CP CML patients. Higher dose IM (800 mg) provide faster responses CCR rates at six months (57% vs 45%, respectively), but there are no significant differences at 12 months (70% vs 66%, respectively) or 24 months (76% in both groups), with no difference in EFS, progression-free survival (PFS), or OS. However, a subset of patients that can tolerate higher doses of IM, may have a better response [31]. The results of IM therapy in the community setting may be somewhat less favourable. A report from the Hammersmith Hospital calculated that the five-year EFS on IM treatment was only 63% [32]. Pretreatment risk factors can predict the likelihood of achieving and maintaining response to IM. The risk of disease progression was higher for patients with a higher pretreatment Sokal score. The achievement of certain milestones of response can also predict prognosis as discussed in the next section. Lack of adherence to medication is a major underlying reason for failure of treatment [33, 34].

Results of IM therapy are poorer in AP patients, with haematologic response in 82% of patients, CHR in 34% of patients, MCR in 24% of patients, with 17% complete responses [35]. Estimated 12-month PFS rates were 59%. Myeloid BC patients treated with IM showed an overall response rate (ORR) of 52%, with 31% of patients having haematologic responses lasting at least four weeks [36]. The median survival was seven months. These results compare favourably with historical results showing three-month median survival for patients treated with chemotherapy. Although 60% of Ph-positive acute lymphoblastic leukemia, also known as acute lymphocytic leukaemia or acute lymphoid leukemia (ALL), patients responded to IM, the duration of response was relatively short, with a median estimated time-to-disease progression of only two months.

IM treatment may result in myelosuppression, which is more common in patients with advanced disease. Grade 3 and 4 neutropaenia is frequent, particularly in advanced phases. Central nervous system and gastrointestinal haemorrhages occur most frequently in patients in BC. For otherwise healthy patients in CP, the goal is to avoid potentially dangerous neutropaenia and platelet transfusion dependence. For patients with BC or AP disease, the approach is to balance risks and benefits, and support patients with critically low platelet count. For absolute neutrophil count <500/mm^3, IM is continued if the marrow is hypercellular or if there are >30% blasts. Where the marrow is hypocellular and the absolute neutrophil count (ANC) is <500/mm^3, IM may be held, the dose reduced or myeloid growth factors used [37]. Common IM-related non-haematologic adverse events include nausea, muscle cramps, fluid retention, diarrhoea, musculoskeletal pain, fatigue, and skin rashes. Grade 3 or 4 toxicity is uncommon, and the rate of discontinuance of therapy because of toxicity is 2–5%. Most adverse effects can be managed successfully with supportive measures.

Both de novo and acquired resistance may occur in IM-treated CML patients. The most common mechanism associated with resistance is point mutations in the BCR–ABL gene that prevent IM from inhibiting kinase activity, although BCR–ABL-independent mechanisms may also contribute to IM resistance in some patients. Over 90 different amino acid substitutions are reported to result in IM resistance, with varying frequency and degrees of IM resistance [38]. Cells with pre-existing BCR–ABL mutations that confer IM resistance may have a selective clonal growth advantage during IM treatment. A mutation resulting in substitution of isoleucine for threonine in the T315 position (T315I) affects residues that directly contact IM. ABL kinase P-loop mutations prevent conformational changes required for IM binding. Mutations in the activation loop result in the kinase being fixed in the active conformation and unable to acquire the inactive conformation required for IM binding. Resistance to the second-generation TKIs, dasatinib and nilotinib, is related to a much narrower spectrum of mutations. These mutations are non-overlapping, with the exception of the T315I mutation. Knowledge of BCR–ABL mutation status is being integrated into therapeutic decision-making algorithms for patients. Mutation analysis is recommended in IM-resistant patients planned to receive an alternative TKI [38].

BMS-354825 (dasatinib, Sprycel®) is a dual SRC–ABL kinase inhibitor exhibiting 300-fold higher potency against native BCR–ABL [39]. Dasatinib effectively inhibits most clinically-detected BCR–ABL kinase domain mutants at low nanomolar concentrations, except for T315I. Another compound, AMN107 (nilotinib, Tasigna®) was synthesized by modification of IM to enhance BCR–ABL kinase-binding activity [40]. Nilotinib binds ABL with increased avidity and can overcome resistance of most kinase domain mutants, with the exception of T315I. These agents have significant activity in IM-resistant CML, yielding CCR in approximately 50% of CP CML cases, and leading to stable responses [41, 42]. Both of these drugs have been evaluated as first-line therapy in newly diagnosed CP CML. The Dasatinib Versus Imatinib Study In Treatment-naive CML (DASISION) study tested 100 mg dasatinib daily versus 400 mg IM daily [43]. The Evaluating Nilotinib Efficacy and Safety in Clinical Trials Newly Diagnosed Patients (ENESTnd) study compared two nilotinib doses (400 mg twice daily and 300 mg twice daily) with IM 400 mg daily [44]. These studies found that dasatinib and nilotinib were superior to IM in achieving the primary endpoints (dasatinib: CCR by 12 months; nilotinib: major molecular response (MMR) at 12 months). Patients treated with nilotinib had a significantly reduced risk of progression. Based on these results, nilotinib and dasatinib have been approved for first-line therapy of newly-diagnosed CP CML patients. However, the choice of TKI in newly-diagnosed patients remains open to debate. Although dasatinib and nilotinib are associated with faster and deeper reduction in leukaemia burden, no differences in OS have yet been observed, and long-term data from the randomized clinical studies are needed to confirm the initial findings. IM is less expensive and there is longer experience with its use. A direct comparison between nilotinib and dasatinib has not been performed. Since their overall efficacy appears to be similar, the selection may be based primarily on side effect profile and convenience. Dasatinib treatment is associated with higher rates of myelosuppression and with pericardial and pleural effusion. In contrast, nilotinib can induce an increase in pancreatic enzymes, hyperglycaemia, and hyperbilirubinaemia. The fact that the T315I mutant is not responsive to either dasatinib or nilotinib underscores the need for drugs with T315I inhibitory activity [45]. The multi-target kinase inhibitor ponatinib (Iclusig®) is active against all BCR–ABL mutants, including T315I, and has shown promising activity in initial trials [45, 46].

An increasing proportion of TKI-treated patients appear to enter a molecular remission over time. However, even patients with negative PCR (so-called complete molecular response [CMR]) may retain significant numbers of residual malignant cells. Several groups have identified BCR–ABL-expressing leukaemia stem cells in patients with sustained undetectable molecular residual remission [47]. The STIM (Stop IMatinib) trial evaluated IM discontinuation in patients with sustained undetectable minimal residual disease (MRD) for >2 years. Approximately 40% of patients did not develop molecular recurrence after one year [48]. Patients with undetectable MRD after IM therapy continued to have BCR–ABL rearrangement detectable at the genomic level indicating persistence of residual leukaemic cells not detected by reverse transcription polymerase chain reaction (RT-PCR). These data suggest that IM may not eradicate the leukaemic clone and patients at present are recommended to continue medication indefinitely.

Allogeneic haematopoietic cell transplantation

HLA-matched sibling donor haematopoietic cell transplants (HCTs) were initially performed as therapy for CML patients in the 1980s and became the first curative treatments for CML. Data reported to the International Bone Marrow Transplant Registry (IBMTR) showed a probability of survival of 69% ± 2% for patients transplanted within the first year from diagnosis, and 57% ± 3% for patients transplanted more than one year from diagnosis. Several single institution studies demonstrate excellent outcomes with HCT, related to advances in preparative regimens, supportive care, and HLA typing for unrelated donors. For example, the Seattle group has reported a three-year post-transplant survival of 86% using a preparative regimen of targeted BU plus cyclophosphamide (CY) in consecutive CP CML patients [49]. The outcome of allogeneic HCT (alloHCT) in CML is influenced by the phase of disease, type of donor used (related or unrelated), the source of the stem cell product (marrow or peripheral blood), and the age of the patient. Outcomes are superior for HCT in CP compared to advanced phases of disease. Transplantation for patients in BC is associated with poor prognosis, related to a high rate of relapse and transplant-related mortality. Only a third of patients have HLA-matched family member donors. Advances in donor selection, graft-versus-host disease (GVHD) prophylaxis, and supportive care have resulted in continued improvements in outcome for matched unrelated donor transplants, which in many institutions are almost equivalent to those seen with matched sibling transplants. Registry data reports 65% survival at five years among younger patients transplanted within a year of diagnosis. Although marrow was initially used as the stem cell source, large randomized trials have shown that use of G-CSF mobilized peripheral blood haematopoietic cells leads to more rapid myeloid and platelet recovery when compared to marrow, without significant differences in GVHD and OS, although relapse rates may be lower in the peripheral blood group. For patients transplanted in CP, increased interval from diagnosis to transplant is associated with a worse outcome. The effect of delay could be related to the disease evolution over time and cumulative toxicity of prior therapy. Prevention of GHVD by removing T cells is associated with high rates of graft failure and relapse, leading to poorer DFS. These findings illustrated the critical role of the graft-vs-leukaemia (GVL) effect in eradicating CML following allogeneic transplantation. There has been interest in preventing GVHD without loss of GVL by combining T-cell depletion with delayed reinfusion of viable donor lymphocytes.

There is considerable evidence in support of GVL-effect in CML, including high rates of relapse following syngeneic and T-cell-depleted transplants, close association between acute and chronic GVHD and freedom from relapse, and the high response rate of post-transplant relapse to donor lymphocyte infusions. Reduced-intensity conditioning (RIC) approaches may potentially avoid the toxicities of conventional high-dose conditioning regimens while maintaining GVL effects. Reduced-intensity transplantation may be safe and effective for CP CML, but not be sufficient for advanced phase patients [50]. Donor lymphocyte (or leukocyte) infusion (DLI) can induce complete cytogenetic responses in 50–100% of patients with relapsed CP CML. The major complications of DLI are transient marrow failure and the development of GVHD. The overall incidence of GVHD following DLI can be reduced with fractionated administration of T cells and escalating dosage as required. Complications of recurrence of GVHD and granulocytopaenia were seen. More recently, IM has been shown to be active as post-transplant therapy.

Prior IM treatment does not appear to adversely affect transplant outcomes, with no difference in regimen-related mortality, survival, or relapse compared to historical controls, and similar cumulative incidence of acute and chronic GVHD. Conventional prognostic indicators continue to be the major predictors of transplant outcomes [51]. With the establishment of TKI as first-line therapy for CML, the number of patients undergoing allogeneic transplantation has dramatically declined. Currently, allogeneic transplantation is recommended for patients who have failed a second-generation TKI, with TKI-resistant mutations such as T315I, and in AP or blast phase. Allogeneic transplantation is an effective option for treatment for T315I-mutated leukaemias [52] and an effective salvage treatment for TKI-resistant patients [53]. Since patients with advanced disease have worse outcomes after transplantation, this procedure should be considered early for patients responding poorly to a second-generation TKI.

Disease monitoring

Monitoring response is critical even in the era of effective TKI therapies

TKIs are extremely effective in CML CP patients; however, 45% [54, 30] of IM-treated, 25–30% of dasatinib- [55, 56] and nilotinib- [44, 57, 58] treated patients discontinue first-line of therapy. The majority of these patients can be salvaged with second- and third-generation TKI therapy [59–61]. All current therapies are more effective in CP than advanced phase; hence, the aim of monitoring the response is to identify patients earlier who can benefit by switching to other effective therapies and preventing transformation to advanced phase disease. Multiple studies show that an early response can predict a long-term outcome. Clinicians have to be more vigilant during the initial two to three years of therapy, as the majority of events occurred within the first three years (5.2% per year, averaging out to 0.9% per year for the subsequent three years [30, 62]).

Tools for response monitoring and response definition

Integral parts of the initial assessment and monitoring include physical examination, complete blood count (CBC) examination, BM morphology, cytogenetic analysis, and molecular monitoring (Table 52.2). In a newly-diagnosed CML patient, TKI therapy progressively reduces the disease burden. Therefore, as the number of leukaemia cells decrease, the sensitivity of the techniques used to monitor the disease effectively must increase accordingly.

All patients treated with TKI therapy should have a CBC every two weeks until complete haematologic response (CHR) (see Table 52.2) is achieved, followed by further testing every three months, unless patients develop unexplained cytopaenias [63]. Cytopaenia in the first three to six months is not unexpected, but if it evolves at a later stage, the possibility of underlying marrow abnormalities should be considered.

Cytogenetic analysis

Bone marrow (BM) morphology and cytogenetic analysis are essential at diagnosis to confirm the diagnosis of CP CML and to establish a baseline regarding the presence of any additional cytogenetic abnormalities (ACA). European Leukemia Net (ELN) guidelines recommend cytogenetic analysis at three and six months after starting TKI therapy, and then every six months until complete cytogenetic response (CCR) is achieved and confirmed. Once CCR is achieved, BM cytogenetic analysis can be repeated once a year, if regular molecular monitoring cannot be assured [63]. BM cytogenetic testing is also recommended in patients with unexplained cytopaenia or loss of response. Typically, cytogenetic responses are divided into several categories (Table 52.2), which are usually determined by metaphase chromosome analysis (using at least 20 metaphases) of the BM.

Conventional cytogenetic testing can also detect additional chromosomal abnormalities in Ph+ chromosomes (ACA) and Ph- metaphase cells (other chromosomal abnormality, OCA). Approximately 5–12% of newly diagnosed CML CP patients and 30–80% of patients with AP and BC have ACA [64–67]. WHO recognizes ACA in Ph+ chromosomes evolving during therapy as a sign of disease progression to the AP; however, ACA at diagnosis is not recognized as a sign of advanced phase disease. ACA includes variant translocation, lack of Y chromosomes (-Y) and major and minor route ACA. Major route ACA includes trisomy 8, a second Ph+ chromosome, isochromosome (17)(q10), and trisomy 19. While minor route ACA includes t(3; 12), t(4;6), t(2;16), and t(1;21) (rarely observed in CML AP or BC) [65]. Five-year OS and PFS was significantly poorer in patients harbouring major route ACA (53% and 50%, respectively) compared with patients with minor route ACA (96% and 96%, respectively), -Y (87% and 88%, respectively), t(v;22) (87% and 81%, respectively), and t(9;22) (92% and 90%, respectively) [64]. Similarly the GIMEMA study also showed an inferior outcome in patients with ACA [68]. Variant Philadelphia chromosome translocations have been reported in 5–10% of patients and have no impact on cytogenetic or molecular responses or on outcome [69, 70]. Deletions of the derivative chromosome 9 [der(9)] are not associated with poor prognosis in patients treated

Table 52.2 Definition of response and frequency of monitoring newly diagnosed common chronic leukaemia chronic phase (CML CP) patients treated with first-line TKI therapy

Test	Frequency of monitoring	Definition of response
Complete blood count	◆ Baseline then ◆ Every 15 days until CHR, then ◆ Every three monthly unless otherwise required	◆ Complete haematological response: ◆ Platelets ≤ 450 × 10⁹/L ◆ WBC count ≤10 × 10⁹/L ◆ Differential without immature granulocytes and with ≤5% basophils and ◆ Non-palpable spleen
Cytogenetic (cytogenetic should be performed by chromosome banding analysis of bone marrow metaphase cells)	◆ Baseline then ◆ At 3 and 6 months then ◆ Every six months until confirmed CCyR, then ◆ Every 12 months if reliable molecular testing is not available	◆ Complete (CCgR): No Ph+ chromosome ◆ Partial (PCgR): 1% to 35% Ph+ metaphase ◆ Minor (mCgR): 36% to 65% Ph+ metaphase ◆ Minimal (minCgR): 66% to 95% Ph+ metaphase ◆ None (noCgR): >95% metaphase
BCR–ABL RQ-PCR BCR–ABL/control gene ratio on international scale	◆ Baseline ◆ Three monthly until stable MMR ◆ Then 3 to 6 monthly	◆ MMR: ≤0.1% BCR–ABL/housekeeping genes ratio on IS ◆ CMolR: Undetectable BCR–ABL1 mRNA transcripts by RQ-PCR and/or nested PCR in two consecutive blood samples of adequate quality (sensitivity >10⁴)
Mutation analysis	◆ Suboptimal response or failure ◆ Always required before changing to other TKI therapies	

with IM [71, 72]; hence, recent ELN guidelines do not consider it as a warning sign [63] unlike previous guidelines [73].

OCA has been reported in Ph⁻ cells of about 5% of patients who achieved CCR with IM [74–76]. The most common abnormality is trisomy 8 (50%), but deletion of chromosome 7 alone or with other abnormalities is observed in about 15% of cases [75]. In some cases, OCA has been associated with the development of a myelodysplastic syndrome or acute myeloid leukaemia, mainly in patients with a deletion of chromosome 7 and/or other complex abnormalities, but also in some patients with isolated trisomy 8 [76]. However, some patients remain in CCR and haematological remission after the detection of OCAs and, in some cases, OCAs may be transient. The presence of OCAs without dysplastic features in the blood is probably not an indication for a change in therapy based on our current understanding.

The limitations of BM conventional cytogenetic include a 10–25% failure rate or inadequate metaphase for analysis. FISH (see below) might be useful at this stage to determine if patients have achieved CCR. FISH is used in some countries for monitoring patient response.

Fluorescence in situ hybridization (FISH)

FISH studies use peripheral blood samples and analyse approximately 200 interphase cells. The sensitivity of dual-colour FISH ranges from 0.1–1%. FISH studies cannot be used interchangeably with metaphase cytogenetic analysis, as the long-term outcome data from prospective studies is based on conventional cytogenetic analysis but not on FISH. However, for 82% of patients there is correlation between CCR by FISH and conventional cytogenetic testing; 18% of patients in CCR by standard cytogenetic testing had 1% to >5% FISH-positive cells [77]. Whether patients in CCR (i.e., 0% Ph-positive by cytogenetic analysis) but FISH positive would have a similar or worse prognosis to FISH-negative patients is unknown. Clinicians should also be cautious in establishing response failure to treatment based on low levels of positivity by FISH. False-positive rates of 1–10% can also hinder interpretation of the findings. Another significant limitation of FISH technology is its inability to detect clonal chromosome abnormalities in Ph⁺ or Ph⁻ cells. With the availability of molecular monitoring, the value of FISH analysis in current clinical practice is limited.

Real-time quantitative polymerase chain reaction (RT-PCR)

Patients with leukaemia at presentation or relapse usually have a total burden of 10^{11} to 10^{12} malignant cells; cytogenetics and conventional FISH have a maximum sensitivity of 1%. Thus, a patient with negative results using these assays may harbour as many as 10^9 to 10^{10} residual leukaemic cells. Real-time quantitative PCR (RT-PCR) is a sensitive assay to detect minimal residual disease (MRD) and is commonly used for monitoring patients after achieving CCR. The level of BCR–ABL transcripts is calculated by normalizing the absolute value of BCR–ABL to that of a housekeeping gene. The three genes that have been studied extensively and appear most suitable for BCR–ABL quantitation are BCR, ABL, and b-glucuronidase (GUSB) [78]. Efforts are ongoing to standardize molecular responses derived in different laboratories using an International Scale. Expressing quantitative RT-PCR values on the International Scale using an individual conversion factor unique to each laboratory may facilitate comparisons of molecular response data [79].

We perform BCR–ABL1 PCR at baseline in all newly-diagnosed CML-CP patients to confirm the transcript type; uncommon rearrangements (e.g., e19a2, e14a3, and e13a3) may not be detectable by the standard PCR probes. Not having a baseline PCR on a patient with such abnormality could create confusion when subsequent evaluation comes with undetectable BCR–ABL transcripts, which could be interpreted wrongly as complete molecular response (CMR). Baseline absolute BCR–ABL1 transcript value does not influence the long-term outcome; however, transcript type may influence the outcome. Although CCR [80], MMR and MR⁴·⁵ were achieved earlier in patients with e14a2 transcript type, there was no difference in OS and PFS [81].

Correlation between cytogenetic response and molecular response

By assessing simultaneous blood real-time quantitative polymerase chain reaction (RQ-PCR) and BM cytogenetics, Ross et al. reported that 98% of patients who achieved 1–2 log (BCR–ABL1 1 to ≤10% IS) reduction from standardized baseline were in MCR, and 95% of patients who had achieved 2–3 log (1 to 0.1% IS) reductions were in CCR. The correlation between CCR and BCR–ABL1 transcript is better at 12 months of IM therapy, as compared with earlier time points [82].In the DASISION study, 96% and 83% of dasatinib and IM-treated patients achieving at least PCR had BCR–ABL1 transcript ≤10%, while only 68% and 26% of dasatinib and IM-treated patients achieving CCR had BCR–ABL1 ≤1% [83].

Target response during tyrosine kinase inhibitor therapy

There is substantial evidence that early molecular and cytogenetic responses predict long-term survival. Hence, the expert panel for the European Leukemia Net (ELN) provides guidelines for monitoring and milestone responses at different time points during TKI therapy [63] (see Baccarani et al. 2013 [73]). Optimal response means there is no indication that changing therapy may improve survival, while suboptimal response means that the patient may still have a substantial long-term benefit from continuing a specific treatment, but the chances of optimal outcome are reduced, so suboptimal responders may be eligible for alternative approaches. Failure means continuing the same therapy is unlikely to result in a favourable outcome and a change in therapy is recommended when possible [63]. These guidelines were developed and revised when only IM was available as first-line therapy; with the availability of second generation TKI as first-line therapy and the availability of more data, these guidelines are under revision. The current ELN recommendation and recent data demonstrating the impact of early molecular response on the long-term outcome are summarized below.

Target response at three months after starting tyrosine kinase inhibitor therapy

According to ELN criteria, achieving CHR at three months (96–100% of IM treated patients) and minor CR (80–82% of IM treated patients) is considered as an optimal response [63]. However, long-term OS and PFS are significantly lower in patients failing to achieve at least partial cytogenetic response (PCR) PCyR and/or BCR–ABL1 transcript ≤10% at three months (Table 52.3) [83–87]. Moreover, cumulative incidence of CCR and major molecular response (MMR, MR)⁴·⁵ at three years were significantly lower in patients failing to achieve BCR–ABL1 transcript ≤10% at three months [83, 86, 87]. 25–35% of IM [83, 86, 87], 9%

Table 52.3 Comparison of overall survival (OS) and progression-free survival (PFS) according to cytogenetic and molecular response at three months

Study	PCyR vs No PCyR		BCR–ABL1 ≤10% vs .>10%	
	OS	PFS	OS	PFS
German CML study (n = 460 patients) Five years follow-up	95% vs 87%; p = 0.03	94% vs 87%; p = 0.016	96% vs 87%; p <0.002	95.2% vs 87%; p <0.001
DASISION study (Three years follow-up)				
Dasatinib (n = 259)	96.4% vs 84.2%; p = 0.01	93.9% vs 71.3%; p = 0.21	95.9% vs 85.9%; p = 0.03	93.1% vs 68.2%; p = 0.0003
Imatinib (n = 260)	93.9% vs 93.1%; p = 0.36	93.7% vs 77.3%; p <0.002	96% vs 88%; p = 0.003	95.9% vs 75.3%; p< 0.0001
ENESTnd study (Three years follow-up)				
Nilotinib (n = 258)	NA	NA	95.6% vs 82.9%; p = 0.002	96.9% vs 86.7%; p = 0.003
Imatinib (n = 264)	NA	NA	95.3% vs 84.8%; p <0.0001	95.3% vs 83.8%; p <0.0001
Hammersmith study (n = 282)*< Eight year follow-up	NA	NA	93.3% vs 56.9%; p <0.01	92.8% vs 57%; p <0.01

*In Hammersmith study: Patients were divided into ≤9.84% and >9.84% BCR–ABL1 transcript at 3 months.

NA, data not available.

Source: data from de Lavallade H et al., Imatinib for newly diagnosed patients with chronic myeloid leukemia: incidence of sustained responses in an intention-to-treat analysis, *Journal of Clincal Oncology*, Volume 26, Issue 20, pp. 3358–3363, Copyright © 2008 by the American Society of Clinical Oncology; Marin D et al., Adherence is the critical factor for achieving molecular responses in patients with chronic myeloid leukemia who achieve complete cytogenetic responses on imatinib, *Journal of Clincal Oncology*, Volume 28, Issue 14, pp. 2381–2388 Copyright © 2010 by the American Society of Clinical Oncology; Talpaz M et al., A phase II study of STI571 in adult patients with Philadelphia chromosome positive chronic myelogenous leukemia in accelerated phase, *Blood*, Volume 96, Issue 11, 469A, Copyright © 2009 by American Society of Hematology; Kantarjian H et al., Nilotinib in imatinib-resistant CML and Philadelphia chromosome-positive ALL, *New England Journal of Medicine*, Volume 354, Number 24, pp. 2542–2551, Copyright © 2006 Massachussetts Medical Society.

of nilotinib-treated [86], and 16–19% [83, 85] of dasatinib-treated patients fail to achieve PCR and/or BCR–ABL1 transcript ≤10% at three months and are considered as a high-risk group. These patients would need a different approach. In the ongoing Australian TIDEL II study, IM (600 mg starting dose) treated patients failing to achieve ≤10%, 1%, and 0.1% BCR–ABL1 transcript at three, six, and 12 months, respectively, were changed to either high-dose IM (cohort I) or nilotinib (cohort II) therapy [88]. IM intolerant patients were switched to nilotinib in both cohorts. Although this strategy has achieved a higher rate of MMR at 12 months of 69% compared to 47% in TIDEL-I study (IM dose intensification), the improvement in molecular response is mostly attributable to improved responses in patients intolerant to IM. Deeper responses were uncommon (only 13% achieved MMR after changing over to nilotinib) in patients failed their early molecular targets response [88]. This suggests that patients failing to achieve early milestone response on IM therapy may not be effectively rescued with second generation TKI therapy. Patients treated with second generation TKI therapy and failing to achieve ≤10% and/or PCR at three months (10–15%) would also need an alternative approach. However, there is no good alternative therapy today that can match an expected survival greater than 98%. Further randomized clinical trials over the next few years should focus on addressing this issue.

Target response at six months after starting tyrosine kinase inhibitor therapy

According to ELN guidelines, achieving at least PCR (~89% of IM-treated patients) by six months of IM therapy is considered as an optimal response, while less than PCR (7% of IM-treated patients) and a lack of cytogenetic response (3% of IM-treated patients) is considered as a suboptimal response and failure, respectively [63]. Although ELN recommends changing therapy for IM failure patients, guidelines are vague for suboptimal responder patients. However, five-year OS (81.8% vs 91.7% vs 97.9%; p = 0.02) and PFS (73.4% vs 61.5% vs 92%; p = 0.002) was significantly lower in both IM failure and suboptimal responders compared to optimal responders [89]. Hence, patients failing to achieve at least PCyR at six months on IM therapy may benefit by changing to more potent second-generation TKI therapy. 67–73% of patients treated with dasatinib or nilotinib achieve CCR at six months [55, 44] and patients failing to achieve CCR at six months had poor EFS; these patients will also need alternative approach.

The landmark analysis of the IRIS study showed inferior EFS (56% at 84 months) in patients with BCR–ABL1 (IS) >10% at six months compared with patients with BCR–ABL1 0.1 to ≤1% and those with >1 to ≤10%, all of whom had EFS rates of 85% at 84 months (see Figure 52.1A and 52.1B) [90]. In the ENESTnd study, 97% and 84% of patients treated with nilotinib and IM achieved BCR–ABL1 ≤10% at six months [86]. In both treatment groups patients achieving BCR–ABL1 ≤10% at six months had significantly superior OS and PFS as compared to patients with >10% at six months. In both treatment arms, there was no significant survival difference in patients achieving BCR–ABL1 ≤1% and >1–10% [86]. While other groups reported inferior OS, PFS, and EFS in patients failing to achieve CCR or BCR–ABL1 transcript ≤1.67% by six months [84, 91, 92].

These data suggest that failing to achieve BCR–ABL1≤10% and/or PCR (suboptimal responders) at six months predict an inferior outcome and warrant changing therapy. Other groups have proposed more aggressive approaches and recommend changing therapy in patients failing to achieve CCR and/or ≤1% BCR–ABL1 transcript at six months [84, 91].

Target response at 12 months after starting tyrosine kinase inhibitor therapy

ELN guidelines consider less than PCR at 12 months as IM treatment failure while achieving CCR and PCR at 12 months as an optimal response and suboptimal response, respectively [63]. However, the five-year OS (85.4% vs 98.4%), PFS (73.4% vs 96.1%),

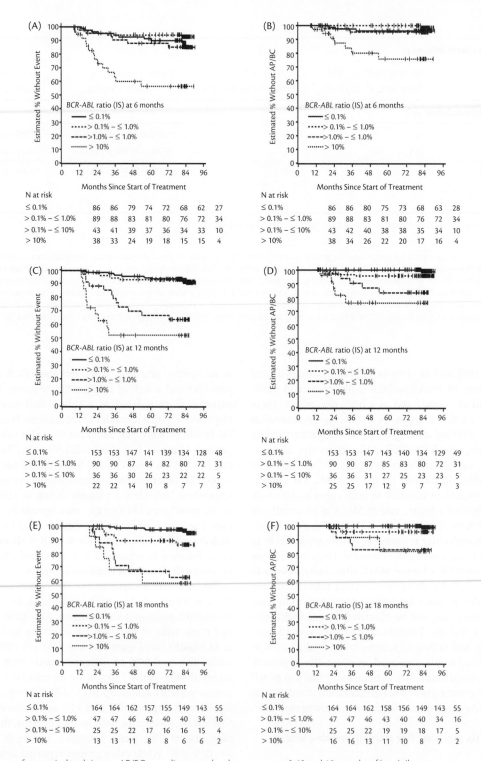

Fig. 52.1 Seven-year event-free survival and time to AP/BC according to molecular response at 6, 12 and 18 months of imatinib treatment.

Reproduced from Hughes TP et al., Long-term prognostic significance of early molecular response to imatinib in newly diagnosed chronic myeloid leukemia: an analysis from the International Randomized Study of Interferon and STI571 (IRIS), *Blood*, Volume 116, Issue 19, pp. 3758–3765, Copyright © 2010 American Society of Hematology.

and probability of achieving CCR (77.8% vs 100%) are significantly lower in suboptimal responders than patients achieving an optimal response at 12 months [89]. This is further substantiated by the three-year follow-up results of the DASISION study. Patients who had failed to achieve CCR at 12 months had significantly inferior PFS and OS in both IM- and dasatinib-treated patients [83].

Similarly, long-term follow-up of the IRIS study suggest that seven-year-EFS (91% vs 64%), OS (93% vs 85%), and PFS (96% vs 83%) was higher in IM-treated patients achieving BCR–ABL1 ≤1% compared with patients with >1% at 12 months (see Figure 52.1C and 52.1D) [90]. Patients with MMR (≤0.1%) and those with BCR–ABL1 (IS) level >0.1 to ≤1% had similar 84 months EFS rate [90]. In the DASISION study, in both dasatinib and IM-treated patients, there was also no difference in three-year PFS and OS in patients achieving CCR and MMR compared with patients with CCR but no MMR at 12 months [83].

These data suggests that failing to achieve CCR and/or ≤1% BCR–ABL1 on IM (28% of patients) [54, 89, 90], dasatinib (17% of patients), [83] or nilotinib (20% of patients) [93] warrants changing therapy; further clinical trial are required to address this issue.

Target response at 18 months after starting tyrosine kinase inhibitor therapy

The lack of CCR by 18 months of IM therapy is considered as IM failure and ELN guidelines suggest changing therapy [63]. However, the long-term outcome was superior in patients achieving MMR at 18 months compared with all other response categories with an EFS of 95% compared to 86%, 62%, and 58% for patients in the >0.1 to 1%, >1% to ≤10% and>10% categories, respectively (see Figure 52.1E and 52.1F) [90]. Moreover, 97% of patients with MMR at 18 months remained in CCR at 84 months compared with only 74% of the patients with molecular response >0.1 to ≤1.0% remaining in CCR (p <0.001) [90].

Target response beyond 18 months of first-line TKI therapy: the Holy Grail for most physicians treating CML is eradicating leukaemic stem cells, which is less likely in the majority of patients treated with TKI therapy. However 'operation cure' is possible which means patients can maintain CMR without TKI therapy. The term CMR does not always indicate eradication of leukaemia. Rather, it is used to describe the sustained undetectable BCR–ABL transcript with sensitive RQ-PCR assay (sensitivity with 4.5 to 5 logs). Up to 10^7 leukaemic cells could still be present in the absence of measurable BCR–ABL. Hence to avoid confusion, more recently MR^4 (≤0.01% IS), $MR^{4.5}$ (detectable transcript ≤0.0032% or undetectable BCR–ABL1 with sample sensitivity of ≥4.5) and MR^5 (≤0.001% IS) is commonly used to denote the log reduction below the standardized baseline [94].

Significantly more numbers of patients treated with dasatinib (22%), and nilotinib (32%) achieve $MR^{4.5}$ compared to IM-treated patients (12–15%) [83, 86, 87, 90]. Patients achieving CMR have the most favourable relapse-free survival rates: only one out of 28 patients in CMR lost CCR while 11 out of 48 patients in MMR lost CCR [95]. Another important benefit of achieving CMR is the possibility of maintaining a molecular response off TKI therapy. In the French Stop Imatinib (STIM) study, IM treatment was discontinued in patients with CML (n = 100) who were in CMR (>5-log reduction in BCR–ABL and ABL levels and undetectable transcripts on quantitative RT-PCR and who have received IM >2 years). Within six months of stopping IM therapy, 61% patients

developed molecular relapse while 39% patients remained in CMR off TKI therapy [48]. Similarly, in an Australian study, 40% patients remained in CMR off TKI therapy [96]. All patients developing molecular relapse re-responded to IM therapy. These studies suggest that about half of the patients who achieve and maintain CMR for two years on IM therapy remain in CMR after stopping IM. Many of these patients have remained in CMR off TKI therapy for three to four years. Currently, however, this approach should only be considered in the clinical trial setting; it cannot be recommended outside clinical trial scenarios.

Mutation screening

Mutations in the BCR–ABL kinase domain can cause or contribute to resistance to TKI therapy. This section will address the practical issues faced in clinical practice, such as when to screen for mutation? Which methods should be used? How to use mutation results for managing patients treated with TKI therapy?

Baseline BCR–ABL kinase domain mutations analysis is not recommended in newly-diagnosed CML CP. It can be performed in rare patients presenting in the AP or in BC. Due to the very low frequency of BCR–ABL kinase domain mutation in responding patients, screening at regular intervals is not recommended in all CML CP patients on therapy. Mutation analysis is recommended only in the case of failure, suboptimal response to IM therapy, and in patients with a rise in BCR–ABL transcript associated with a loss of MMR [63]. It has been estimated that, overall 29–43% of IM failure CML CP patients harbour BCR–ABL kinase domain mutations [97, 98]. Although differences exist in mutation incidence across different categories of 'failure', mutations are more frequent in patients with secondary resistance rather than patients who failed to achieve milestone response [63, 89, 99]. None of the patients who failed to achieve CHR or minor cytogenetic response by three and six months, respectively, had BCR–ABL1 kinase domain mutations [100]. On the other hand, the mutation detection rate was higher in patients who failed to achieve late ENL milestone responses: 24% and 22% patients who did not achieve MCR and CCR by 12 and 18 months, respectively, had BCR–ABL1 kinase domain mutations [89, 100]. Similarly, mutation rates were also higher in patients transforming to AP or BC (21%), and patients losing CHR (41%), CCR (13%), or MMR (13%) [98]. The mutation rate is lower in patients with a suboptimal response: 4%, 10%, and 0% of patients who did not achieve MCR, CCR, and MMR at 6, 12, and 18 months, respectively, had BCR–ABL1 kinase domain mutations [100].

Several groups reported that a rise in BCR–ABL1 transcript should be viewed as a trigger for BCR–ABL1 kinase domain mutation analysis; however, there is no agreement regarding the level of BCR–ABL1 transcript rise. Earlier studies suggested that patients with >2 to 2.6-fold rise BCR–ABL1 transcript have a high probability of detecting BCR–ABL1 kinase domain mutations [101, 102], while other groups reported a >5.5-fold rise [103] and NCCN guidelines suggest a >10 fold rise in BCR–ABL1 transcript is significant. Emerging consensus is that BCR–ABL kinase domain mutation should be checked in patients with a consistent rise in BCR–ABL1 transcript on two independent samples and associated with a loss of MMR. Patient compliance should be checked before requesting BCR–ABL1 kinase domain mutation studies [38].

BCR–ABL1 kinase domain mutations can be detected by direct sequencing with sensitivity to detect 10–20% of the mutant clone

[38]. Denaturing high-performance liquid chromatography followed by direct sequencing is another assay with increased sensitivity which can detect the mutant clone at levels down to 1–5%. Other methods used for mutation detection include sequencing after subcloning of PCR products, allele-specific oligonucleotide PCR, restriction-fragment-length polymorphism-based assays, and pyrosequencing. Although these are more sensitive methods for mutation detection, they may not be suitable for routine screening. Moreover, the clinical utility of very small mutant clones detected by these sensitive methods remains the source of conjecture. Hence, the ELN expert panel recommend direct sequencing for BCR–ABL kinase domain mutation screening [38].

In IM-treated patients, >90 BCR–ABL kinase domain mutations have been identified in association with resistance and they are located throughout the kinase domain. However, 15 common mutations account for >90% of all mutations detected during IM therapy. These common mutations include T315I, Y253F/H, E255D/K/R/V, M351T, G250A/E, F359C/L/V, and H396P/R [104, 105]. Although in the ENESTnd study mutation rate was lower in the nilotinib (3.9% vs 7%) group compared with IM-treated patients, most of the nilotinib-treated patients developed nilotinib-resistant (T315I, n = 3) or less sensitive mutations (E255K/V, F359C/V, Y253H; n = 6) [58, 93]. In the DASISION study, mutation rates were similar in dasatinib and IM-treated patients (3.8% vs 3.8%), but dasatinib-resistant mutations such as T315I (n = 7), F317L (n = 2), and V299L (n = 1) were commonly detected in the dasatinib group, while in IM-treated patients, there were ten different mutations and none of the patients developed the T315I mutation during three years of follow-up [55, 56].

Detection of some specific mutations can influence the choice of the second- or subsequent-line TKI. For patients with V299L, T315A, or F317L/V/I/C mutations, nilotinib is more effective, while for patients with Y253H, E255K/V, or E359V/C/I mutations dasatinib is probably more effective than nilotinib [38]. In the case of all other mutations except T315I, dasatinib and nilotinib are likely to be similarly effective. Moreover, patients with multiple mutations detected by multiplexed mass spectrometry assay is associated with lower rates of CCR (50% vs 21%; p = 0.003), MMR (31% vs 6%; p = 0.005), and higher rates of new resistant mutations (25% vs 56%; p = 0.009) [106].

A T315I mutation is refractory to dasatinib, bosutinib, and nilotinib. Phase II studies of ponatinib demonstrated efficacy in patients with T315I mutation. CCR and MMR were achieved in 66% and 50% of patients, respectively, in this scenario [107].

Management of the relapse/refractory patient

The role of high-dose imatinib in patients with imatinib resistance

Some patients who have suboptimal responses on standard-dose IM may benefit from higher dosing [108]. In one study, almost 50% of CP CML patients with disease resistance achieved MCR after having their dose escalated to 300–400 mg bid [109]. However, the response to high-dose IM appears to be transient and the therapy was poorly tolerated: 82% of patients discontinued high-dose IM (compared to 28% in the dasatinib arm, p < 0.0001). Most discontinuations (61%) in the high-dose IM group were due to a lack of response or disease progression [110, 111]. As the toxicity of high-dose IM is greater than standard-dose IM, it may not be a

viable option for many patients, particularly those who could not tolerate standard-dose IM.

The role of dasatinib in imatinib-resistant patients

Promising results of phase I and phase II studies were further substantiated by the phase III randomized study, demonstrating superior efficacy of dasatinib over high-dose IM in patients failing standard-dose IM therapy. Significantly higher CHR (93% vs 82%), CCR (40% vs 16%), and MMR (16% vs 4%) rates were achieved in the dasatinib arm as compared with high-dose IM [110, 111].

The six-year follow-up of another phase III, dasatinib dose optimization study in IM-resistant/intolerant CP CML patients (n = 670), demonstrated that dasatinib 100 mg/daily is as effective as 50 mg/bd, 140 mg/day and 70 mg/bd, with a significantly more favourable toxicity profile [112]. Comparable six-year OS (70–77%), PFS (40–51%), MMR (67–71%) rates were achieved in all four groups [112]. Although there was no difference in response rates between patients who had a baseline mutation and those who did not, a significant difference in response rates emerged when results were analysed according to the specific mutation developed. MCR (61% vs 46%), CCR (53% vs 32%), and MMR (38% vs 23%) were higher in patients harbouring mutations with low IC50 (≤3 nM; G250E, Y253F/H, M315T, E355G, F359V, V379I, L387M, H396P, H396R, M244V) compared with patients with intermediate sensitivity (IC50 >3 ≤60 nM; Q252H, E255K/V, V299L, and F317L/V) [113]. The responses were particularly poor in patients harbouring F317L (7%) and V299L (0%) and T315I (0%) mutations. Other studies also demonstrated lower response rates with dasatinib in patients with F317L [114, 115]. These data indicate that dasatinib is effective in the majority of patients with IM resistance except for patients with T315I, F317L, and V299L mutations.

Role of nilotinib in imatinib-resistant/intolerant patients

The phase II nilotinib registration study, demonstrated the efficacy of nilotinib in IM-resistant and -intolerant patients [104]. Of the 321 patients initially enrolled in the study, 98 (31%) were treated for at least four years; 224 (69.8%) patients discontinued therapy, primarily due to disease progression (30%) or adverse events (21%). The estimated OS and PFS at 48 months were 78% and 57%, respectively. MCR and CCR rates were 59% and 45%, respectively [59]. Baseline mutations (those detectable at the time of IM resistance) were present in 55% of IM-resistant patients [104]. After 12 months of therapy, MCR (49% vs 60%; p = 0.1), CCR (32% vs 40%; p = 0.2), and MMR (22% vs 29%; p = 0.3) were not significantly different in patients with or without baseline mutations [104]. However, when responses were analysed according to individual mutations, patients harbouring T315I, Y253H, E255V/K, and F359V/C had less favourable responses. None of the patients with resistant mutations achieved CCR by 12 months in contrast to 43% of patients with other mutations. Similarly, patients who failed nilotinib therapy displayed frequent mutations at 253, 255, 359, and 311 residues [104]. Thus for most IM-resistant patients, nilotinib is effective except for patients with T315I, Y253H, E255V/K, and F359V/C mutations [104].

Bosutinib in imatinib-resistant/intolerant CP CML patients

Bosutinib (SKI-606; Bosulif®) is an orally bioavailable dual Src/Abl inhibitor, 100- to 200-fold more potent (in vitro) than IM. In a phase I/II study of IM-resistant or -intolerant CP CML patients, 86%, 53%, and 41% of patients achieved CHR, MCR, and

CCR, respectively. At two-years OS and PFS were 92% and 79%, respectively [116].

Ponatinib in imatinib-resistant/intolerant CML CP patients

Ponatinib (AP24534; Iclusig®), an orally available TKI, is a potent pan-BCR–ABL inhibitor with activity against T315I. With median follow-up at 10 months, 66% and 50% patients with T315I mutation achieved CCR and MMR, respectively [107]. The response rate was dependent on the number of patients with prior TKI therapy; the CCR rate in patients who failed IM, two and three prior TKI therapies was 80%, 74%, and 48%, respectively. In the majority of patients the response rate was stable [107].

Allogeneic stem cell transplantation in imatinib-resistant patients

In the era of TKI therapy, alloSTC is restricted to patients with advanced phase disease (AP and BC) and CML CP patients failing at least two or three lines of TKI therapy and/or harbouring T315I mutations.

Monitoring of patients on second-generation tyrosine kinase inhibitor

Monitoring of IM-failure patients treated with second-line, second-generation TKI therapy (2GTKI) is guided by the phase of disease and the reason for starting 2GTKI (IM intolerance or resistance). IM-intolerant or slow-responding CP CML patients (patients who have demonstrated a progressive drop in Ph⁺ chromosomes and/or BCR–ABL1 transcript but failed to achieve target response) who are switched to 2GTKI can be monitored with CBE every two weeks; RQ-PCR for BCR–ABL1 every three months; and BM cytogenetic analysis at six months, 12 months, and then annually. Patients who lose a previously achieved response (but maintain CP) and/or have a rapidly rising BCR–ABL1 level or Ph⁺ metaphases should be monitored very closely with RQ-PCR for BCR–ABL1 monthly until a progressive fall in BCR–ABL1 is demonstrated and then be monitored three-monthly. These patients may need BM aspiration and cytogenetic analysis at three, six, and 12 months. The frequency of mutation analysis will depend on the baseline mutation status. Patients with baseline mutations probably need mutation analysis every three months as well as at the time of confirmed rise in BCR–ABL1 transcripts or Ph⁺ chromosomes. Patients without baseline mutations may not require regular mutation analysis unless the BCR–ABL1 value at three months is >10%.

The long-term response to second-line therapy depends on the disease phase at the time of starting therapy and response to prior IM therapy [59, 117]. Patients with haematologic resistance and ACA have poor outcome with second-line TKI therapy and are considered as a warning sign in ELN provisional guidelines [63]. Early response to 2GTKI can also predict the longer-term outcome. Current ELN guidelines do not provide definition of optimal response to second-line TKI therapy. However, suboptimal response to second-line therapy is defined as minor CR, PCR, and lack of MMR at three, six, and 12 month of second-line TKI therapy, respectively. Failure is defined as the development of new mutations and/or lack of cytogenetic response; minimal CR; and less than PCR at three, six, and 12 months, respectively [63]. Recent data suggest that PFS (63.5% vs 25.9%; p < 0.0001) and OS (85% vs 59.7%; p < 0.001) were significantly higher in dasatinib-treated patients achieving BCR–ABL1 transcript ≤10% at three months compared with patients with BCR–ABL1 transcript >10% [112].

Similarly, in IM-resistant/intolerant CML CP patients treated with nilotinib, BCR–ABL1 transcript levels at three and six months predicted four-year PFS and OS. The estimated PFS (85% vs 67% vs 42%; p <0.002) and OS (95% vs 81% and 71%; p = 0.03) at four years were significantly higher in patients achieving BCR–ABL1 transcript ≤1% at three months compared with patients with >1% to 10% and >10% at three months. At 24 months, MMR rates were significantly higher in patients with three-month BCR–ABL1 ≤1% compared with patients with 1–10% and >10% (86% vs 34% vs 9%; p <0.01) [59]. Similarly the BCR–ABL1 transcript level at six months also predicts long-term survival. The estimated PFS (86% vs 58% vs 39%; p <0.001) and OS (95% vs 82% vs 73%; p = 0.009) at 48 months were significantly higher in patients achieving BCR–ABL1 transcript ≤1% compared to patients > 1 to 10% and >10% at six months, respectively [59]. Patients with CCR at 12 months had a higher PFS compared with patients without CCR at 12 months (89% vs 56%; p <0.0001) [59].

Future directions in treatment for CML

With the remarkable progress in first-line treatment for CML, one of the major remaining problems related to CML treatment include the small subset of CML patients that do not achieve sustained adequate and sustained response to TKI treatment and continue to have a poor prognosis. Although BCR–ABL kinase domain mutations are a well-characterized mechanism of resistance, resistance is clearly a more complex phenomenon, and it is likely that additional mechanisms, including BCR–ABL-independent mechanisms, appear to contribute to resistance. Other than the T315I mutant, in vitro sensitivity does not correlate well with in vivo response. With the availability of pan-TKI inhibitors with anti-T315I activity, these BCR–ABL independent mechanisms may become the dominant resistance mechanisms. Patients with primary resistance to TKI usually do not have BCR–ABL kinase domain mutations. Patients showing poor initial PCR response to IM usually do not respond well to second-line inhibitors. These observations suggest that inter-patient biological heterogeneity may determine resistance. Improved understanding of such resistance mechanisms is critical for strategies to target the small population of CML patients that does not respond well to TKIs.

Another important issue in the future will be whether patients can actually be cured with TKI treatment. An increasing proportion of CML patients treated with TKI have undetectable BCR–ABL levels on RQ-PCR. These patients may still have significant numbers of residual malignant cells. Some patients can maintain a BCR–ABL-negative status for >1 year following discontinuation of IM treatment [118]. Although the long-term durability and frequency of such responses are not known, it may be argued that at least some of these patients are functionally 'cured'. The definition of a 'cure' for these patients remains unresolved. It has been argued that patients may be considered 'cured' if there is no clinical recurrence after stopping treatment. Such a situation may be similar to what is seen in some CML patients post allogeneic transplantation or in AML associated with the t(8;21). On the other hand, late relapses can be observed in some leukaemia patients in prolonged remission, suggesting that definition of cure is still uncertain. Additional factors related to the leukaemogenic potential of residual cells, and immune or microenvironmental factors may determine risk of relapse. In the future, a better understanding of these factors may allow improved prediction of patients in whom treatment can be stopped without recurrence, and support development of improved strategies to enhance the number of CML patients in whom TKI treatment can be stopped and who are effectively 'cured'. Several preclinical and clinical studies addressing these questions are already underway.

Chronic lymphocytic leukaemia

Epidemiology

CLL is a heterogeneous disease characterized by the progressive accumulation of functionally incompetent mature B lymphocytes. The clinical course is variable with an indolent, minimally symptomatic course in many patients for many years. CLL accounts for about 20–30% of leukaemia cases in the West and is the most common form of leukaemia among adults. The median age is 64 years and male to female ratio 1.2:1. The incidence of CLL is low in Japan, China, India, and other Asian countries. Based on hospital-based data, CLL accounts for <10% of leukaemia cases in these countries. CLL occurs at relatively younger age in Asia, at 55–58 years, and male to female ratio is 2.8:1; <20% of cases are diagnosed at an asymptomatic stage compared to 60–70% in the West [119–120].

Staging and diagnostics

Almost 20–60% of patients are diagnosed while asymptomatic on routine blood counts or during investigation for an unrelated illness. The remainder present with various symptoms including constitutional symptoms, such as fatigue, weight loss, and fever. Common signs include lymph node enlargement or lump in abdomen (splenomegaly). Sometimes, enlarged lymph nodes, with the development of an infection is the initial manifestation of disease. Bacterial infections, such as pneumonia, are more common in patients who present with advanced stage disease. Infections secondary to opportunistic organisms, particularly Herpes zoster, may occur. However, B symptoms (fever, night sweats, weight loss) are relatively uncommon in patients with CLL. In contrast to lymphoma, fever in the absence of infection is rare in CLL. An exaggerated skin reaction to bee stings or insect bites is frequent (Well's syndrome). Skin involvement occurs in fewer than 5% of cases. Leptomeningeal leukaemia is rare and, if present, is usually seen in patients with refractory disease. Physical findings include localized or generalized lymphadenopathy, splenomegaly (30–40% of cases), hepatomegaly (20% of cases), petechiae, and pallor.

Investigations

A list of investigations to be performed in a case of CLL is given below (Box 52.1). Haemogram (CBC) reveals lymphocytosis with an absolute lymphocyte count of 5000/μL or higher. CLL cells typically resemble small mature lymphocytes, have clumped chromatin, scanty cytoplasm, and lack nucleoli. Peripheral blood film usually shows the presence of 'smudge', 'smear', or basket cells, which are artefacts due to damaged lymphocytes during the slide preparation. For diagnosis of CLL, absolute lymphocyte count must be 5000/μL or above. The pathologic features of the lymph node are those of a small lymphocytic lymphoma. BM involvement could be interstitial, nodular or diffuse.

Immunophenotype

Flow cytometry of peripheral blood is the most common method for confirming the diagnosis of CLL. The monoclonal population of B cells in CLL expresses CD19, CD5, and CD23 and has reduced

---

Box 52.1 Investigation for the newly-diagnosed patient with CLL

1. Haemogram, peripheral smear, absolute lymphocyte count
2. Urine examination
3. Chest X-ray P/A view
4. Liver, renal function tests
5. Electrolytes, serum calcium/phosphate, uric acid
6. Electrocardiogram
7. Serum electrophoresis
8. Serum immunoglobulin (IgG, IgA) levels
9. CT scan of chests, abdomen, and pelvis
10. Bone marrow aspiration and biopsy
11. Immunophenotyping
12. β-2 microglobulin
13. Serum LDH

---

level of membrane IgM, IgD, and CD79b, a phenotype of mature, activated B lymphocytes. Other conditions which can mimic with are mantle cell lymphoma, indolent lymphoma, splenic villous lymphoma, hairy cell leukaemia (HCL), and pro-lymphocytic leukaemia. The latter has a typical phenotype that is positive for CD19, CD20, and surface membrane immunoglobulin and negative for CD5. Immuno-phenotyping is key in differentiating CLL from these disorders (Table 52.4).

CLL with >55% prolymphocytes is considered B-cell prolymphocytic leukaemia (PLL), whereas typical CLL is associated with 10–55% prolymphocytes and are traditionally classified as CLL/PLL. In such cases, on flow cytometry, transformed prolymphocytes (CLL/PLL) often retain CD5 expression. In contrast, de novo PLL are CD5 negative. Other laboratory abnormalities include elevated serum B2 microglobulin, but LDH is rarely elevated.

Diagnosis

Diagnostic criteria were proposed in 1989 by the International Workshop on CLL (IWCLL) and these have been revised by the National Cancer Institute-sponsored CLL Working Group (NCIWG) in 1996 [121]. For diagnosis, an absolute lymphocyte

Table 52.4 Immunophenotype of B-cell phenotype (B-CLL) and other related B-lympho-proliferative disorders

B-CLL Antigen	Mantle cell			Follicular
	Lymphoma	SLVL	NHL	
SIg	Weak	++	++	++
CD5	++	++	−	−
CD19	++	++	++	++
CD20	+	++	++	++
CD22	Weak or −	++	++	++
CD23	++	−	−	−
CD79b	Weak or −	++	++	++
FMC7	−	++	++	++
CD10	−	−	−	++

Abbreviations: sIg, surface immunoglobulin; SLVL, splenic lymphoma with villous lymphocytes.

Table 52.5 Binet staging of common chronic leukaemia (CLL)

Binet stage	Lymphocytosis	Lymph node areas	Hb (<11G %)	Platelets <100,000/cmm	Survival (years)
A	N/A	<3	No	No	12
B		3 or more	No	No	5
C		+/–	+/–	Yes or low Hb	2

Stage A includes Rai stage 0, 2/3rd of stage I and 1/3rd of stage II.

Reproduced with from Binet et al., A new prognostic classification of chronic lymphocytic leukemia derived from a multivariate survival analysis, Cancer, Volume 48, Issue 1, pp. 198–206, Copyright © 1981 American Cancer Society, with permission from John Wiley and Sons Ltd.

count of ≥5000/μL with lymphocytes co-expressing CD5 and a B-cell marker (CD19, CD20, and CD23) and BM lymphocytes of ≥30%. NCIWG criteria do not require a BM aspiration/biopsy for diagnosis. These criteria correlate well with modified Rai and Binet staging.

Staging

Two staging systems are popular: Rai staging in US [122] and Binet in Europe [123] (the Binet staging is given in Table 52.5). Based on the presence of lymph node, liver and spleen enlargement, Hb (G/dl), and platelet counts, CLL can be staged from stage 0 to IV (Rai Stage). There is good correlation between Rai staging and median OS. Binet staging divides CLL into stage A, B, and C, depending upon lymph node areas involved and haematological parameters. Almost 50–60% of patients have Rai stage 0 and I or Binet stage A at presentation.

Molecular biology and pathology

CLL is a clonal B-cell lymphoid leukaemia and is thought to originate from 'activated' B cells. Expression of the CD5 antigen is the hallmark of CLL cells; CD19, CD20, and CD23 are other B-cell markers expressed on CLL cells. Surface immunoglobulin, FMC7, CD22, CD11c, and CD79b are either weakly expressed or negative in CLL. Molecular changes leading to the pathogenesis of the disease are still poorly understood. Approximately 50–70% of CLL cases have somatic hypermutation of immunoglobulin variable gene (IgVH, a marker of B-cell maturation in the follicular germinal centre) and thus appear to arise from post-germinal B cells [124]. Remaining cases appear to arise from naive B cells; these have inferior outcome.

Cytogenetic abnormalities have been detected on conventional cytogenetics in 40–50% of patients. However, a low proliferative rate is a limitation for conventional cytogenetics. In the past decade, FISH using DNA probes has greatly enhanced the ability to detect molecular abnormalities in almost 80% of cases of CLL. 13q deletion is the most common genetic aberration present in CLL (55%) followed by 11q deletion (18%), 12q trisomy (16%), and 17p deletion (7%) [125, 126]. These abnormalities have been correlated with outcome. Patients with 17p or 11q deletion generally have more advanced disease with frequent splenomegaly, mediastinal, and abdominal lymphadenopathy and more extensive peripheral lymphadenopathy. Presence of 17p deletion correlates with low incidence of IgVH mutation and also resistance to fludarabine

therapy. In contrast, patients with leukaemic cells that have mutant IgVH genes usually present in an early clinical stage, frequently have 13q14 chromosomal deletions do not have alterations of p53, do not require therapy, and have a long survival [127, 128].

Zeta-associated protein (ZAP-70), a member of the Syk–ZAP-70 protein tyrosine kinase family, is normally expressed in T cells and natural killer cells, and has a critical role in the initiation of T-cell signalling. Expression of ZAP-70 has been shown to correlate inversely with IgVH gene mutation [126]. ZAP-70 is commonly measured by flow cytometry. A reliable flow cytometry strategy is needed to separate ZAP-70 expression on malignant CLL cells from that of back ground T- and NK-cell populations. More recently, a whole-genome sequencing study by a Spanish Group have identified four recurrent mutations in CLL; these are notch 1 (NOTCH1), exportin 1 (XPO1), myeloid differentiation primary response gene 88 (MYD88), and kelch-like 6 (KLHL6). Mutations in MYD88 and KLHL6 are predominant in cases of CLL with mutated immunoglobulin genes, whereas NOTCH1 and XPO1 mutations are mainly detected in patients with an unmutated IgVH gene. Based on the patterns of somatic mutation, supported by functional and clinical analyses, it appears that recurrent NOTCH1, MYD88, and XPO1 mutations are oncogenic changes that contribute to the clinical evolution of the disease [129].

Medical management of chronic lymphocytic leukaemia

All patients of CLL must initially be kept under observation before starting cytotoxic chemotherapy unless there is clear indication. The blood lymphocyte count must be charted at diagnosis and at each follow-up to determine the doubling time.

Indications for treatment

- Increasing BM failure (anaemia, thrombocytopaenia) [121]
- Auto-immune haemolytic anaemia
- Auto-immune thrombocytopaenia, poorly responsive to corticosteroid
- B symptoms (fever and night sweats without evidence of infection, weight loss >10% of normal body weight)
- Extreme fatigue. Rule out other causes of fatigue, e.g., cardiovascular disease, sleep apnoea, depression, hypothyroidism, or secondary malignancy
- Massive or progressive lymphadenopathy, massive splenomegaly
- Disease-related recurrent bacterial infections
- Short lymphocyte doubling time (>50% over two to three months); or if total number of lymphocytes is >150–300 × 10^9/L
- Leukostasis and hyperviscosity-related complications may requires leukapheresis

Many patients may have a slow course (smouldering CLL) and may not require treatment for a long period of time. Early treatment should not be considered for young patients with smouldering CLL until some evidence of progression occurs. Smouldering CLL is suggested by (i) Binet stage A disease, (ii) non-diffuse BM involvement, (iii) absolute lymphocyte count of <30 × 10^9/L, (iv) Hb >13g%, and (v) lymphocyte doubling time >12 months. Risk of progression for such patients is 14–17% at five years, with a clinical outcome similar to age-matched control population [128, 130].

General guidelines for stage-wise management

Early-stage disease (Binet stage A)

- Low-risk disease (smouldering CLL). Only follow-up initially; treatment only if progression.

- High-risk disease (includes one-third of stage IA). This is defined as (i) elevated β2 microglobulin or elevated thymidine kinase, (ii) lymphocyte doubling time <12 months, (iii) non-nodular BM infiltration. Treatment options are: (i) chlorambucil, (ii) fludarabine, (iii) fludarabine + cyclophosphamide, or (iv) observation.

Symptomatic Binet stage B and all patients of Binet stage C

In recent years, there are several options available for first-line therapy in CLL and also for patients who relapse. Selecting the best treatment for an individual patient is sometimes difficult and challenging. The various old and new drugs available and recommended for the treatment of CLL include fludarabine, chlorambucil, bendamustine, lenalidomide, and monoclonal antibodies (immunotherapy) such as rituximab and alemtuzumab, and multiple combinations of these agents.

Younger patients with unfavourable biological risk factors should be considered for high-dose chemotherapy and autologous or reduced-intensity alloSTC as part of a clinical trial. Patients either relapsing rapidly or not responding to first-line chlorambucil should be considered for fludarabine-containing regimens. Patients relapsing soon after or progressing while on fludarabine-based chemotherapy may be considered for treatment with alemtuzumab, possibly followed by autologous or alloSTC in the context of a clinical trial.

The majority of patients treated with these agents and combinations have a partial response. However, newer agents and combinations do produce more complete responses. Response criteria have been well defined (Table 52.6).

Commonly-used drugs and combinations

Alkylating agents, corticosteroids, and combinations

Before the availability of purine analogues, chlorambucil with/without prednisolone was the only available and commonly-used treatment of CLL, producing a response rate of between 35–75%

Table 52.6 Response criteria in common chronic leukaemia (CLL)

Complete response	• Resolution of constitutional symptoms
	• Resolution of lymphadenopathy and organomegaly
	• PB lymphocyte count <4000/cmm
	• ANC >1500/cmm, platelets >100,000/cmm
	• BM aspiration/biopsy—normal or nodular or focal infiltrate
Partial response	• Change from Binet stage C to A, B, or from stage B to A
	• More than 50% decrease in PB lymphocyte count
	• More than 50% decrease in size of Lymph nodes, spleen and liver size
	• Hb >11g%, ANC >1500/cmm, Platelets >100,000/cmm or an improvement of 50% in these values from baseline

but few complete remissions. The CHOP regimen (cyclophosphamide, doxorubicin, vincristine, and prednisolone) and other related regimens like CVP (cyclophosphamide, vincristine, and prednisolone) have not been shown to be more effective than chlorambucil [131–133]. Chlorambucil is still indicated for use in the low-risk patient and elderly patients who have a poor performance status. Alkylating agents like cyclophosphamide are still used in several regimens like FCR (fludarabine, cyclophosphamide, rituximab).

Bendamustine, another alkylating agent also having purine analogue properties, has been recently approved as front line therapy for CLL based on the results of a phase III trial [134]. This agent, although new to the US, has been in use in Eastern Europe for several years. Bendamustine in combination with rituximab is also recommended for previously untreated CLL based on data from another phase III study, as well as for patients relapsing after a purine analogue [135, 136].

Prednisolone or dexamethasone have activity in CLL and have been used in combination with chlorambucil. These agents are also a part of several effective CLL regimens, with or without rituximab. Infections remain a concern with prolonged corticosteroid use [137].

Purine analogues and combinations

Purine analogues (fludarabine, cladrabine, and pentostatin) form one of the most effective groups of drugs, which are part of most CLL regimens of treatment. When compared with chlorambucil and alkylating agent combinations (CHOP, CAP), fludarabine and fludarabine-containing combinations has been shown to produce more responses, more complete remissions, and a survival advantage in some studies [138–141].

Infections and myelosuppression are the major toxicities of purine analogues. The drug also suppresses both T and B lymphocytes with resultant increase in bacterial, viral and opportunistic infections [142, 143].

Combinations with purine analogues

Even though purine analogues have significant single-agent activity in CLL, they are most commonly used in combination with cyclophosphamide and/or rituximab.

- Fludarabine plus cyclophosphamide (FC). The combination of fludarabine and cyclophosphamide has shown a synergism which has been utilized in the treatment of patients of CLL [144]. Three randomized trials have shown the superiority of this combination over fludarabine alone. The FC regimen has been demonstrated to have higher overall response rates, higher complete response rates, and longer PFS over single-agent fludarabine [138, 145, 146]. Benefit with regards to OS is less clear. Even though the combination produces more myelosuppression, infection rates and mortality due infection have not been found to be increased. The FC regimen remains an important treatment option for the patient with good performance status who is unable to tolerate rituximab. The monoclonal antibody directed against CD20 (ofatumumab; Arzerra®) can be combined with the FC regimen to yield high complete response rates (30–50%) [147].

- Fludarabine plus rituximab. Fludarabine can be combined with the anti-CD20 monoclonal antibody, rituximab (Rituxan®), with preclinical and clinical synergy [148]. The FR combination regimen has been shown to be better than the two drugs used in a sequential fashion [149]. This regimen is a viable option for patients of CLL in the first-line setting [150]. When combined with the alkylating agent, cyclophosphamide, the FCR regimen can achieve a high complete remission rate.

♦ Fludarabine, cyclophosphamide, rituximab (FCR). The FCR regimen, combining the three most effective agents, is now one of the standard first-line treatments for CLL, with about 25–72% patients achieving a CR. However, grade 3 and 4 neutropaenia have been reported in 51% patients [151, 152]. There is presently no prospective head-to-head comparison between FCR vs FR, and therefore, neither can be labelled as superior. A trial designed to answer this question is presently ongoing. FCR has been compared with FC in two prospective, multicentre phase III clinical trials. Both have demonstrated the superiority of the former over the latter in terms to response rates, CR, PFS, and OS. Grade 3/4 neutropaenia was significantly more common in the three-drug regimen [153, 154]. Along with FR, FCR is currently the treatment of choice for first-line CLL and both regimens are acceptable for first-line treatment. The superiority of the three-drug regimen remains to be established.

Monoclonal antibodies and immunotherapy

♦ Rituximab. Rituximab, a chimeric monoclonal antibody which targets the CD20 receptor, is an effective drug in CLL and forms an integral part in most regiments. Single-agent responses are of short duration [155]. Combination of rituximab with purine analogues and/or alkylating agents significantly adds to activity and potency [152, 154, 156]. Several combination regimens are now standard of care first-line therapies. A combination of rituximab with an anti-CD52 monoclonal antibody (alemtuzumab) has also shown synergy and is a useful combination in patients, especially those who have bulky lymphadenopathy [157, 158]. Rituximab administration can be associated with significant infusion toxicities including rigors, anaphylactic reactions, and hypotension. As a rule, premedication with steroids and antihistaminics should be given to all patients and the infusion should be initiated slowly under careful monitoring of vital parameters.

♦ Alemtuzumab. Alemtuzumab (Lemtrada®) is a fully humanized monoclonal antibody targeting CD52, which is expressed in most patients with CLL. The initial approval of the drug was for patients who were refractory to fludarabine [159] but recently it has been approved for first-line use also. The drug is most effective on peripheral blood, BM, and spleen but has relatively less activity on bulky lymph nodes [160, 161]. There are some reports suggesting that alemtuzumab may have significantly more activity than standard treatment in high-risk patients who have 17p and 11q deletions [160, 162]. The drug has shown encouraging activity when combined with fludarabine [163, 164] and chlorambucil [162]. Anaphylactic and other infusion-related toxicities are troublesome. Subcutaneous administration of the drug is effective and is being tested in clinical trials [165, 166]. Because of activity on normal B and T lymphocytes, the major toxicities of alemtuzumab are cytopaenias and immune suppression with consequent increase in opportunistic infections especially *Pneumocystis jiroveci* pneumonias, and cytomegalovirus (CMV) (re)activation and infection. All patients receiving the drug should receive pneumocystis prophylaxis and be closely monitored for CMV infection [162, 167].

Prognostic factors

Clinical stage remains the most important prognostic factor in CLL. Other prognostic factors are listed below (Table 52.7) A number of biological markers, particularly serum markers, cytogenetic abnormalities, IgVH mutations, CD38, and ZAP-70 expression in leukaemic cells offer important, independent prognostic information.

Management of the relapse/refractory chronic lymphocytic leukaemia patient

The most important consideration in the choice of therapy for the patient who relapses is the initial treatment and the duration of response to the same. For example, for the patient who has been treated with the FCR regimen and has relapsed after more than 12 months, another trial of the same regimen is appropriate. For the patient with early relapse, a change of regimen is indicated. Bendamustine with rituximab (the BR regimen) is a useful combination in patients who relapse after a purine analogue-containing regimen (FR or FCR) with expected response rates of approximately 59% [168].

The anti-CD52 monoclonal antibody, alemtuzumab, is important as second-line treatment. The drug is indicated either alone or in combination with fludarabine or rituximab. In a phase II study of patients with relapsed CLL, the combination of fludarabine, alemtuzumab, and cyclophosphamide produced an overall RR of 67% with a CR rate of 30% [169].

Table 52.7 Prognostic factors in chronic lymphocytic leukaemia (CLL)

Factor	Outcome
Clinical stage	Rai stage 0 & 1: good, stage II intermediate, III–IV poor Binet stage A >B >C
Degree of BM infiltration	Nodular good, Diffuse poor
Absolute lymphocyte count	<30,000/cmm better than higher
Lymphocyte doubling time	>12 months better than <12 months
Serum levels of β- 2 microglobulin	Normal better than elevated
Serum levels of thymidine kinase	Normal better than elevated
CD38 expression	Negative good, high poor
Cytogenetic abnormality	13q del: good, 11q del: intermediate, del 17p: poor **Median OS:** 13q- =133m, 11q del (+) = 79 mon, 17 p del (+) = 72 mon
Mutation of IgVH gene	Unmutated poor (median OS 84 months, and PFS 68 months); mutated good (median OS not reached, 70% 12 year survival, PFS 141 months)*

Lumiliximab, an anti-CD23 monoclonal antibody, when used in combination with the FCR regimen can produce response rates of 65% (CR in 52%) in relapsed CLL patients and can be considered in this setting in clinical trials [170].

Ofatumumab (Arzerra®) is a new anti-CD20 humanized monoclonal antibody that binds to a distinct epitope from rituximab. Use of this agent in patients who are refractory to both fludarabine and alemtuzumab in early trials is impressive, with a reported RR of 58% [171]. Obinutuzumab, a glyco-engineered monoclonal antibody targeting the CD20 (also known as GA101), in combination with chlorambucil, has shown impressive activity, especially in patients with significant co-morbidities as compared to chlorambucil alone [172].

Another new concept in treating relapse/refractory CLL is the use of cyclin-dependent kinase pathway inhibitor alvocidib (also known as flavopiridol). In a phase II study, encouraging response rates of 48% have been reported in 117 relapsed CLL patients [173].

A recent major advance in the understanding and treatment of CLL has been the discovery and targeting of the Bruton's tyrosine kinase (BTK) pathway. BTK is an essential component of B-cell-receptor signalling, mediates interactions with the tumour microenvironment, and promotes the survival and proliferation of CLL cells. Ibrutinib (Imbruvica®), a first-in-class BTK inhibitor has shown very good results in a recent phase I/II multicentre study with overall RR of 71% and PFS rate of 75%; OS was 83% after more than two-years of follow-up [174].

There has been a reawakening of the use of immune-therapy in lymphoid malignancies, including CLL. In a recently published phase 1 clinical trial, autologous chimeric antigen receptor-modified T cells (CART) were infused in one heavily pretreated patient with relapsed refractory B-cell CLL. The patient achieved CR and continues to be in remission three months at the time of the report of the trial [175].

Future directions in chronic lymphocytic leukaemia

After a gap of several years, in recent times several new agents and strategies have emerged on the therapeutic front for the treatment of CLL. The most promising of these are the BTK inhibitors like ibrutinib, the immune-modulatory agent lenalidomide, and the use of modified autologous T-cells against the disease.

Lenalidomide (Revlimid®) is presently approved for use in multiple myeloma and in patients of myelodysplastic syndrome with 5q deletion. Several clinical trials have demonstrated significant activity of the drug in CLL in the relapse setting, either alone or in combination with rituximab. Lenalidomide has also been found useful in consolidation therapy after induction with FCR-like regimens [176–178].

Dasatinib (Sprycel®), used primarily in CML, has some activity as a single agent in relapsed or refractory CLL [179].

Other new agents include CAL-101, a phosphatidylinositol 3-kinase (PI3K) delta inhibitor [180]; TRU-016, a novel B-cell selective agent which targets CD 37 [181]; the new BTK inhibitor bafetinib; and the proteasome inhibitor carfilzomib [182].

Other less common chronic leukaemias

Hairy cell leukaemia

HCL is considered as one of the curable chronic B-cell lymphoproliferative neoplasms. The usual presentation is in a middle-aged man with splenomegaly and pancytopaenia. The diagnosis is made on finding hairy cells on peripheral blood film or on BM examination and immunophenotyping. Asymptomatic patients require observation and follow-up. Purine analogues are considered to be the first-line therapies of choice. Rituximab in combination with purine analogues is being tested in relapsed patients.

HCL has fascinated haematologists and oncologists ever since its first description more than fifty years ago [183]. Ewald first described it as leukaemic reticuloendotheliosis in 1923. But it was after Bouroncle's classic paper in 1958 and Schrek and Donnelly's observations of hair-like projections under phase contrast microscopy in 1966 that it came to be referred as HCL. Approximately 500–800 new patients are diagnosed every year [184]. Recent discovery of BRAF mutations in most patients with HCL and development of targeted therapy has renewed the interest of the researchers in this field [184–186].

Molecular biology and pathology of hairy cell leukaemia

HCL is a B-cell lymphoproliferative neoplasm. The cell of origin in HCL is the same as is proposed in CLL, i.e., antigen-experienced memory/marginal zone B cell. This was suggested with the demonstration of rearrangement of the B-cell receptor (BCR) Ig genes and heavy chains in hairy cells. Such is the similarity with CLL that HCL may also be differentiated into two types depending on mutation status of the immunoglobulin heavy chain (IGH) as mutated and unmutated HCL, with the same connotation as in CLL. However, the exact cell of origin remains debatable, as in CLL. HCL has a unique tumour mass distribution. Infiltration in the spleen occurs exclusively in the red pulp with sparing of the white pulp, liver involvement is restricted to sinusoids, and lymph node infiltration is rare [187]. This has been attributed to the interaction of the tumour necrosis factor alpha (TNFα) released by hairy cells and integrins $\alpha 4\beta 1$ and its ligand VCAM-1 expressed on endothelial cells [188]. The fibrosis seen in the involved tissues is thought to be due to the secretion of fibronectin by the hairy cells, which is an extracellular matrix ligand for a4b.

Staging and diagnostics of hairy cell leukaemia

The usual presentation of HCL is a middle-aged man with splenomegaly, pancytopaenia, and circulating hairy cells. The median age onset in HCL is 50 years and the male to female ratio is 4:1 [189]. About a quarter of patients present either with easy fatigability, infections, incidental splenomegaly, or abnormal blood counts. Splenomegaly is present in 90% and one-third have hepatomegaly. Though peripheral lymphadenopathy is uncommon (10%), abdominal lymphadenopathy at presentation is found in 17% and in 75% at autopsy.

Infection rates in HCL have varied from 32% in recent series to 68% in older series. Mortality due to infections has varied from 7% in older series [189] to 0.8% in recent series [190]. The commonest infections remain gram-positive and gram-negative bacteria. However, certain unusual organisms like atypical mycobacteria, Pneumocystis jirovecii, Legionella, Listeria, and fungi occur more frequently than in other lymphoproliferative disorders. The reason for higher infection rates in HCL is thought to be due to neutropaenia, monocytopaenia, T-cell, and NK-cell dysfunction [191].

Various autoimmune conditions like polyarteritis nodosa, scleroderma, and polymyositis have been shown to be associated with HCL. Presentation is often non-specific with symptoms of fever, malaise, weight loss, arthralgias, and palpable purpura. Skin biopsy

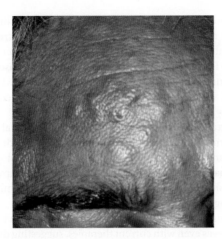

Fig. 52.2 Skin vasculitis in a patient with hairy cell leukaemia (HCL).

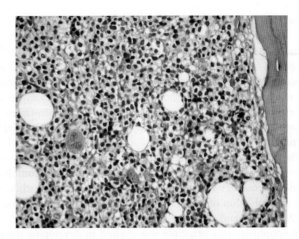

Fig. 52.4 HCL trephine: bone marrow trephine biopsy section showing interstitial excess of atypical lymphoid cells with conspicuous perinuclear halo giving the cells a 'fried egg' appearance (H&E stain, magnification 40×).

may reveal leucocytoclastic vasculitis (see Figure 52.2). The reason for this association is hypothesized to be antigenic cross reaction between hairy cell antigens and epitopes on endothelial cells as well as defective immune complex clearance by the functionally impaired immune mechanisms [192].

Laboratory investigations

A complete blood count with a peripheral blood film (PBF) examination offers the first clue to the diagnosis of HCL. Most patients have variable degree of cytopaenias and more than half have pancytopaenia [189]. Monocytopaenia is common in HCL. Romanovsky-stained PBF may reveal hairy cells in a few on light microscopy. These hairy cells are so-called because of their circumferential fine hairy-like cytoplasmic projections. These cells can be demonstrated to be TRAP (tartrate-resistant acid phosphatase) positive and is a useful test in centres without flow cytometry facilities. TRAP is not specific for HCL and can be seen in other conditions as well. BM aspiration may yield a dry tap due to the reticulin fibrosis. The cellularity of the aspirate may vary from hypercellular to hypocellular (see Figure 52.3). Trephine is therefore almost always informative (see Figure 52.4). BM infiltration is focal, diffuse, or interstitial. The mononuclear cells are

10–25μ in size, with a perinuclear zone of abundant pale region giving it a fried egg appearance, which is attributable to cytoplasmic retraction accentuated by reticulin fibrosis. Nuclei vary in size and shape and may be indented to bilobed. Other haematopoietic elements may or may not be adequately represented in the biopsy specimens. Reticulin fibrosis is increased. Immunohistochemistry on trephine is often not done in the era of immunophenotyping. Flow cytometry immunophenotyping is helpful in the classification of chronic lymphoproliferative disorders and often can differentiate HCL from others [193]. HCL is classified as a CD5 and CD23 negative CLPD. HCL is typically positive for B-cell markers CD19, CD20, CD22, CD79a, CD79b, and FMC7, and CD11c, CD25, CD71, CD103, CD123, which are specifically expressed in HCL [194]. One needs to be aware of the immunophenotypic variations that can be seen in up to 35% of the cases. It is vital to differentiate hairy cell variants on the basis of leucocytosis, lack of monocytopaenia and absent CD25 expression, as they respond poorly to standard treatment. Flow cytometry can be used to monitor residual disease after treatment [195].

Medical management of hairy cell leukaemia

The indication for treatment of HCL is similar to other chronic lymphoproliferative disorders. Only symptomatic disease needs intervention. Symptomatic cytopaenias, organomegaly, constitutional symptoms interfering in the activities of daily living of the patient are common indications for treatment. Even in the current era, there is a role for watchful-waiting. It is important to intervene if there is a rapid worsening of blood counts, as treatment itself entails a further risk of worsening the cytopaenias [196].

Splenectomy, which had been the treatment of choice for HCL for the last three decades, is no longer offered to patients due to its poor complete remission rates and durability. The mechanism of action of splenectomy has remained an enigma. It was thought to be due to sequestration. Response rates reported with splenectomy are in the range of 40–70%; however, durability is only 20 months [197]. An intriguing fact is that a minority of patients remain in complete remission for periods of 15–25 years. There have been studies showing a survival benefit as well as those refuting it. Despite this, the long-term results of splenectomy as a debulking procedure in HCL are not clear.

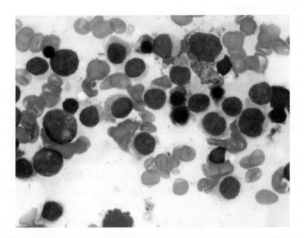

Fig. 52.3 HCL BM: bone marrow aspirate smear showing atypical lymphoid cells, slightly larger than mature lymphocytes, rounded nuclei, homogeneous chromatin, absent nucleoli, moderate amount of cytoplasm with fuzzy borders (May Grunwald Geimsa stain; magnification 100×).

Since its first use in 1984 for HCL, interferon-alpha (IFNα) has lost the battle to newer generation of drugs. IFN has an immunomodulatory effect by affecting other cytokines and promoting apoptosis. The dose of IFN used in HCL is two million IU/m2 subcutaneously three times a week for 12–18 months. Response rates range from 75–90%; though better than splenectomy, complete responses are only occasional. The median time-to-failure of response is 31.3 months. The toxicity profile of IFN has limited its current use.

The discovery of purine analogues came from the observation of adenosine deaminase (ADA) deficient severe combined immunodeficiency (SCID) in paediatric patients. These children had accumulation of deoxyadenosine triphosphates which led to DNA damage and defective repair, thereby leading to lymphocyte apoptosis. This principle was applied in developing purine analogues which irreversibly bind and inhibit ADA enzyme 2'-deoxycoformycin (pentostatin, [Nipent®]) or are resistant to the action of ADA 2-chlorodeoxyadenosine (cladribine; Leustatin®) [198,199]. The results with these two new agents were so remarkable that the response criteria were redefined. Complete response (CR) is defined as disappearance of hairy cells from the blood and BM, normalization of blood counts (haemoglobin>12 g/dL, platelet >100,000/μL, and absolute neutrophil count>1000/μL) and resolution of splenomegaly. Partial remission (PR) requires more than 50% reduction in hairy cells and splenomegaly with normalization of blood counts.

Following their discovery, many case series were published using pentostatin and cladribine. However, there is no clinical difference in outcomes when used as either first- or second-line therapy. The overall CR rate is 81% and DFS is 16 years. Achieving a CR is the only factor associated with relapse- free survival. Patients in CR at five years have a relapse risk of only 25% by 15 years [200]. Pentostatin is given as 4 mg/m2 intravenously every two-weekly until remission. Cladribine is traditionally given as a single cycle of 0.1 mg/kg/day continuous infusion for seven days. To overcome the inconvenience of seven-day continuous infusion, alternative dosing schedules were designed: daily intravenous pulse of 0.14 mg/kg for five days, weekly intravenous pulse of 0.15 mg/kg for six weeks, and daily subcutaneous injection of 3.4 mg/m2 for seven days. All these regimens were found to have equivalent efficacy, toxicity, and outcomes [201]. In the absence of randomized control trials, the choice between cladribine and pentostatin rests with the physician and the patient. Although some authors prefer to use pentostatin as it permits titration of dose and schedule with fewer episodes of febrile neutropaenia, cladribine is overall accepted as the first-line treatment of choice, with pentostatin reserved for relapses. The major concern with the use of these purine analogues is the immunosuppression that occurs after their use, increasing the predisposition to infections. CD4 lymphocyte count may take years to recover [202]. For patients presenting with severe cytopaenias and life-threatening infections, IFN or rituximab can be considered as a bridge to therapy with purine analogues. Currently, there are no established criteria or optimal methods for minimal residual disease (MRD) detection. In the absence of data supporting improved survival by MRD eradication, no recommendation can be made to treat MRD [203].

Late relapses (more than one year of purine nucleoside therapy) can be retreated with either the same or the other purine nucleoside with similar responses as those achieved after first line.

Early relapses (within one year) can be enrolled in clinical trials with novel agents, offered splenectomy, or may be treated with monoclonal antibodies like rituximab [204, 205]. Immunotoxin conjugates LMB-2 and BL22 have been used in relapsed patients with encouraging results. The most recent agent, HA22, has shown CR and PR of 34.6% and 38.5% in relapsed patients, respectively [206].

With current options, patients with HCL have survival approaching the normal population. The leading cause of death in HCL is infections and secondary malignancies [207]. The etiology for second malignancies has been variably attributed to therapy and HCL itself. This debate will continue, however, till more robust data are forthcoming.

Major long-term studies have not shown a plateau in relapse-free survival curves even with current therapies, suggesting disease control but not cure [208]. Recently, the association of BRAF V600E mutation with HCL was identified [185]. BRAF mutations have already been targets for treatment in melanoma and in pilot studies with HCL [186].

Prolymphocytic leukaemia

Prolymphocytic leukaemias (PLL) are rare lymphoproliferative disorders. Though they are labelled as chronic, their clinical behaviour is aggressive. They are of B and T cell type and both show poor response to chemotherapy or immunotherapy. Allogenic HSC transplantation is curative; however, because of old age of presentation, it is carried out only in a minority of patients.

Molecular biology and pathology

PLL are rare, constituting 2% of mature chronic lymphoproliferative disorders. The prolymphocyte cell is twice the size of a CLL lymphocyte (the term prolymphocyte is a misnomer) with prominent nucleus and nucleolus and faintly basophilic cytoplasm. First recognized in 1973 and 1974 as a variant of CLL, PLL is now considered a distinct clinical and pathologically entity with further subdivision into T- and B-cell type depending upon their cell of origin. 80% belong to the B-cell phenotype (B-PLL) and 20% belong to the T-cell phenotype (T-PLL) [209].These leukaemias are generally aggressive in their clinical behaviour and exhibit poor response to chemotherapy.

B-cell phenotype

B-cell phenotype (B-PLL) is diagnosed when the number of prolymphocytes in the peripheral blood is more than 55% (see Figure 52.5). Generally the patients are elderly and present with rapidly rising white cell count, progressive anaemia, thrombocytopaenia, and splenomegaly. Systemic B symptoms (fevers, weight loss, night sweats) are generally present. Significant lymphadenopathy is uncommon. Patients have hypergammaglobulinaemia and a small monoclonal band in their serum. The diagnosis is made on the morphology of the cells seen on the peripheral blood film (PBF) and on BM (see Figure 52.5). Immunophenotyping of these cells reveal B cells expressing surface IgM+/– IgD, CD19, CD20, CD22, CD79a, CD79b, FMC7, and bright kappa or lambda light-chain. CD5 and CD23 (hallmarks of CLL) are present in only 20% of cases. Cytogenetic profile shows del(17p) mutations in more than 50% of cases and presence of these mutations are generally responsible for chemoresistance. The differential diagnosis of B-PLL consists of leukaemic phase of mantle cell lymphoma (differentiated by cyclin D1 positivity and t(11;14)(q13;q32) translocations) and HCL

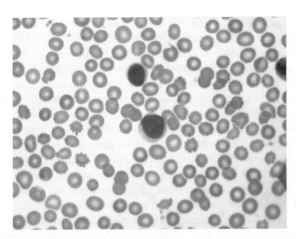

Fig. 52.5 Peripheral blood film showing a prolymphocyte, two times the size of mature lymphocyte, with opened up chromatin, prominent nucleoli, moderate amount of basophilic cytoplasm (May Grunwald Giemsa stain, magnification 100×).

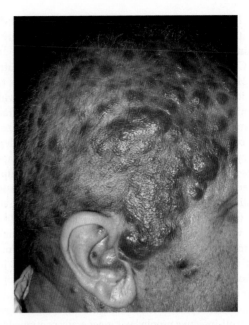

Fig. 52.6 Skin infiltration in a case of T-cell phenotype (T-PLL).

variants (differentiated by hairy cytoplasmic projections, CD11c, and CD103+).

Medical management of B-cell phenotype

Because of the rarity of this leukaemia, treatment guidelines are not available. The median age of the patients is 69 years and hence many of the patients are not candidates for aggressive therapies because of co-morbidities present at this age. Even with aggressive treatment approaches, the median survival rarely goes beyond three years. Before the availability of purine analogues, CHOP (cyclophosphamide, doxorubicin, vincristine [Oncovin®], prednisolone) was used to induce remission in symptomatic patients. Later, single-agent purine analogues were used in the treatment, with response rates approaching 50%. Combinations of purine analogues with cyclophosphamide increased the median survival of patients compared to that achieved by purine analogues alone. Because of strong CD20 expression, combinations of purine analogues with cyclophosphamide and antiCD20 antibody rituximab is an attractive treatment option [210]. Various chemotherapy drugs like mitoxantrone, bendamustine, and epirubicin have been used in combinations with each other to increase response rates. Presence of TP53 abnormalities confers primary resistance to purine analogues; in these patients alemtuzumab has been used successfully to treat this condition [211]. Eligible patients should undergo alloSTC to take the benefit of GVL effect in curing this disorder, though only a small percentage of patients undergo this procedure because of advanced age and co-morbidities. Most transplant physicians prefer reduced-intensity conditioning because of these reasons. Splenectomy has been used successfully as palliative therapy in very frail patients and in patients with poor performance status [212].

T-cell phenotype

The T-cell phenotype (T-PLL) is generally more aggressive in clinical behaviour and shows poorer response to chemotherapy than B-PLL [213]. The median age of presentation is between 65–70 years (similar to B-PLL). Patients with the genetic condition ataxia-telangiectasia have the ATM (ataxia-telangiectasia mutant) gene and tend to develop T-PLL at a younger age. The clinical features of T-PLL are similar to those seen in B-PLL with additional clinical findings in the skin (20% of cases) in the form of nodules, maculopapular rash, and erythroderma (see Figure 52.6); serous effusions in 12% of patients; and generalized lymphadenopathy in 46% of patients.

Molecular biology and pathology of the T-cell phenotype

Three morphological variants of T-PLL are described; typical (75%), small cell (20%), and cerebriform (5%). The immunophenotype of PLL cells is characteristically post-thymic phenotype (CD1a and TdT negative), pan T-cell positive (CD2, CD3, and CD7), and strongly positive CD52. In 60% of patients, the CD4+/CD8- phenotype is seen, while 15% of cells co-express CD4+/CD8+ and the same proportion co-express CD4-/CD8+. Clonal rearrangement of TCR is seen in almost all patients as well as genetic abnormalities involving chromosome 14 (most common), 11, and 8. Inversion and tandem translocation of chromosome 14 leads to activation and expression of proto-oncogene TCL1 that can also be used to detect residual disease post-chemotherapy either by immunohistochemistry or flow cytometry on BM samples. A host of other chromosomal abnormalities have been described, e.g., [t(X;14)(q28;q11)], idic(8p11), t(8;8), trisomy 8q, 11q23, loss at 22q, 13q, 6q, 9p, 12p, 17p and gains at 22q and 6p. T-PLL needs to be differentiated from other T-cell leukaemias mainly adult T-cell leukaemia lymphoma (ATLL), T-cell large granular lymphocytic leukaemia (T-LGL), and Sézary syndrome (SS). The differentiation from these disorders sometimes becomes difficult and morphology, immunophenotypic features, cytogenetics, and progression of the disease help in making this differentiation. A few investigations are very helpful, e.g., presence of human T-lymphotropic virus type 1 serology and hypercalcaemia in ATLL, granular lymphocyte with CD8, CD57, CD16+/- in T-LGL, and distinct morphology and skin findings in SS [214].

Medical management of T-cell phenotype

Similar to CLL, treatment is indicated only in symptomatic patients with progressive disease. Asymptomatic patients require closer clinical and laboratory monitoring than asymptomatic CLL patients. In the past, purine analogues were used to treat this condition with RR of 45% and CR of 9%. T-PLL cells strongly express CD52 antigen stimulating interest in the monoclonal antibody against CD52, alemtuzumab, which is the current treatment of choice [215]. Though the earliest use of this antibody was reported in 1989, it was only in 1997 that its effectiveness in achieving complete remission rates of 60% was reported in patients refractory to purine analogues. The mechanism of action of alemtuzumab in causing cell lysis is postulated to be due to antibody-dependent cellular cytotoxicity, complement activation, and direct apoptosis. When used as first-line agent, complete remission rates up to 81% have been achieved. However, most responses are transient and these patients require additional consolidative therapy in the form of HSC transplantation [216]. Eligible patients should undergo alloSCT, while other patients can be consolidated with autologous SCT to increase their DFS. Alemtuzumab is highly immunosuppressant agent and these patients should receive anti-infective prophylaxis with co-trimoxazole for *Pneumocystis jerovicii* and acyclovir or valcyclovir for herpes. CMV activation occurs in substantial number of patients, mandating weekly monitoring of CMV viremia. Anti-infective prophylaxis is generally continued for three months post-completion of treatment as CD4+ cells remain suppressed for a long period of time. Relapsed T-PLL cases have a poor prognosis and a combination of purine analogues with cytotoxic chemotherapy such as mitoxantrone and cyclophosphamide can be used. Eligible patients should be transplanted if possible [217]. Repeat treatment with alemtuzumab may work in a few patients in whom the CD52 expression is still present. As always, patients should be enrolled in well-designed clinical trials.

Large granular lymphocyte leukaemia and hairy cell leukaemia-variant

Large granular lymphocytic leukaemia (LGL) and HCL variant (HCL-v) are rare types of chronic lymphoproliferative disorders. LGL can be of T-cell and NK-cell origin, depending upon the phenotype. LGL is generally seen in patients with rheumatological or autoimmune disorders. HCL-v is now considered as separate disorder from classic HCL. HCL-v is generally more aggressive and shows poor response to chemotherapy or immunotherapy.

Large granular lymphocyte leukaemia

LGLs are distinct subset of lymphocytes 15–18 μm in size containing abundant azurophilic granules and constitute 10–15% of peripheral blood mononuclear cells. Loughran et al. in 1985 observed three patients who had increase in LGLs along with splenomegaly, chronic neutropaenia, and multiple auto-antibodies and named it as LGL leukaemia [218]. The WHO 2008 classification of tumours of haematopoietic and lymphoid tissues classify this leukaemia into T-cell large granular lymphocytic leukaemia and chronic lymphoproliferative disorders of NK cells, based on the immunophenotyping of the cells. These disorders are still controversial, as many believe that the T cell represents reactive proliferation and not malignant proliferation. Recently, the presence of STAT3 mutations has been documented in large number of patients, correlating with malignant potential of these disorders [219].

T-cell large granular lymphocytic leukaemia

T-cell large granular lymphocytic leukaemia (T-LGL) is diagnosed when the peripheral blood T lymphocytes (immunophenotypically CD3+, CD57+, CD56-) shows persistence of these cells numbering between 2–20 × 10^9/L for more than six months without any identifiable cause. This leukaemia represents 2–3% of mature lymphocytic leukaemia and 85% of LGL leukaemias. The majority of the cases occur between 45–75 years of age without any sex predilection. In 40–60% of cases, associated rheumatic (most common rheumatoid arthritis) or other autoimmune disorders are seen. Based on these associations, an immune aetiology has been proposed for this disorder [220]. Clinical presentation is mostly indolent with splenic enlargement. Haemogram shows either normal or low haemoglobin with severe neutropaenia and lymphocytosis and normal platelet count. Recurrent infections occur in 20–40% of cases because of neutropaenia. Asymptomatic patients require only observation and treatment of the underlying autoimmune or rheumatological disorder [221]. Symptomatic patients (fatigue, recurrent infections) are treated with low-dose methotrexate, corticosteroids, cyclophosphamide, or cyclosporine. Patients with severe neutropaenia but who are otherwise asymptomatic can be treated with intermittent granulocyte colony stimulating factors.

Chronic lymphoproliferative disorder of NK cells

These are rare disorders and constitute only 15% of LGL leukaemias [222]. These are diagnosed when NK cells numbering ≥2 × 10^9/L persist in the peripheral blood for more than six months without a clearly identifiable cause. The immunophenotype of the cells is CD3-, CD56+, and CD16+. The WHO 2008 classification has defined this as a provisional entity. The presentation is similar to T-LGL. The median age of onset is 60 years. There are a few differences with T-LGL in the form of slight male preponderance in the ratio of 3:2, absence of splenomegaly and lymphadenopathy, and less severe neutropaenia [223]. The treatment, however, is similar with asymptomatic patients require observation and symptomatic patients are treated with methotrexate, cyclophosphamide, corticosteroids, and cyclosporine [221].

Hairy cell leukaemia-variant (HCL-v)

Initially described as a variant of HCL, this disorder has now gained entry into the WHO classification of haematopoietic disorders as an independent provisional entity. The cells of HCL-v exhibit phenotypic features that overlap between classic HCL and B-PLL, hence the synonym prolymphocytic variant of HCL. It is a relatively uncommon condition and constitutes 10% of HCL cases and 0.4% of chronic lymphoproliferative disorders [224]. The median age of presentation is 71 years. Most patients have splenomegaly, high white blood cell count without monocytopaenia or neutropaenia, and thrombocytopaenia. The BM can easily be aspirated and is hypercellular. HCL-v cells are smaller than the HCL cells and show high nuclear cytoplasmic ratio and no ribosome-lamella complexes. The cells resemble prolymphocytes in the form of prominent nucleoli and basophilic cytoplasm. The immunephenotype consists of CD19, CD20, CD22+ve (B cell phenotype), CD11c+, CD10-, CD23-, CD25-, CD5-, and variable expression of CD103 and bright monotypic surface immunoglobulin [225]. The treatment consists of observation in asymptomatic patients. Symptomatic patients generally do not respond very well to purine analogues and IFN. Most patients are still treated with splenectomy. Weekly administration of monoclonal antibody against CD20 (rituximab) has shown promising results. Other therapies that have been used successfully are anti-CD22 and anti-CD25 immunotoxins, alemtuzumab, and HSC transplantation. The prognosis is less favourable than classic HCL patients [226].

References

1. National Cancer Institute. SEER stat fact sheets: chronic myeloid leukemia. Available at: <http://seer.cancer.gov/statfacts/html/cmyl.html>.

2. Cortes J. Natural history and staging of chronic myelogenous leukemia. Hematology and Oncology Clinics North America 2004; 18(3): 569–584.

3. Derderian PM, Kantarjian HM, Talpaz M, O'Brien S, Cork A et al. Chronic myelogenous leukemia in the lymphoid blastic phase: characteristics, treatment response, and prognosis. American Journal of Medicine 1993; 94(1): 69–74.

4. Kantarjian HM, Dixon D, Keating MJ, Talpaz M, Walters RS et al. Characteristics of accelerated disease in chronic myelogenous leukemia. Cancer 1988; 61(7): 1441–1446.

5. Vardiman JW, Harris NL, Brunning RD. The World Health Organization (WHO) classification of the myeloid neoplasms. Blood 2002; 100(7): 2292–2302.

6. Kantarjian HM, Talpaz M, O'Brien S, Jones D, Giles F et al. Survival benefit with imatinib mesylate versus interferon-alpha-based regimens in newly diagnosed chronic-phase chronic myelogenous leukemia. Blood 2006; 108(6): 1835–1840.

7. Quintas-Cardama A, Cortes JE, Jabbou E, et al. Improved survival in chronic myeloid leukemia (CML) since introduction of imatinib therapy: a single-institution experience in 1,570 patients referred within 1 month from diagnosis. Program and abstracts of the 2011 Annual Meeting of the American Society of Clinical Oncology, Chicago, Illinois, June 3–7, 2011, abstr 6557.

8. Sokal JE, Cox EB, Baccarani M, Tura S, Gomez GA et al. Prognostic discrimination in "good-risk" chronic granulocytic leukemia. Blood 1984; 63(4): 789–799.

9. Hasford J, Pfirrmann M, Hehlmann R, Allan NC, Baccarani M et al. A new prognostic score for survival of patients with chronic myeloid leukemia treated with interferon alfa. Writing Committee for the Collaborative CML Prognostic Factors Project Group. Journal of the National Cancer Institute 1998; 90(11): 850–858.

10. Hasford J, Baccarani M, Hoffmann V, Guilhot J, Saussele S et al. Predicting complete cytogenetic response and subsequent progression-free survival in 2060 patients with CML on imatinib treatment: the EUTOS score. Blood 2011; 118(3): 686–692.

11. DeKlein A, Van Kessel AG, Grosveld G, et al. A cellular oncogene is translocated to the Philadelphia chromosome in chronic myelocytic leukemia. Nature 1982; 300: 765–767.

12. Rowley JD. A new consistent chromosome abnormality in chronic myelogenous leukemia identified by quinacrine fluorescence and Giemsa staining. Nature 1973; 243: 209–213.

13. Bose S, Deininger M, Gora-Tybor J, Goldman JM, Melo JV. The presence of typical and atypical BCR-ABL fusion genes in leukocytes of normal individuals: biologic significance and implications for the assessment of minimal residual disease. Blood 1998; 92(9): 3362–3367.

14. Fialkow PJ, Jacobson RJ, Papayannopoulou T. Chronic myelocytic leukemia: clonal origin in a stem cell common to the granulocyte, erythrocyte, platelet and monocyte/macrophage. American Journal of Medicine 1977; 63(1): 125–130.

15. Daley GQ, Van Etten RA, Baltimore D. Induction of chronic myelogenous leukemia in mice by the P210bcr/abl gene of the Philadelphia chromosome. Science 1990; 247(4944): 824–830.

16. Ren R. Mechanisms of BCR-ABL in the pathogenesis of chronic myelogenous leukaemia. Nature Reviews Cancer 2005; 5(3): 172–183.

17. Perrotti D, Jamieson C, Goldman J, Skorski T. Chronic myeloid leukemia: mechanisms of blastic transformation. Journal of Clinical Investigation 2010; 120(7): 2254–2264.

18. Calabretta B, Perrotti D. The biology of CML blast crisis. Blood 2004; 103(11): 4010–4022.

19. Goldman JM, Melo JV. Chronic myeloid leukemia—advances in biology and new approaches to treatment. New England Journal of Medicine 2003; 349(15): 1451–1464.

20. Huntly BJ, Reid AG, Bench AJ, et al. Deletions of the derivative chromosome 9 occur at the time of the Philadelphia translocation and provide a powerful and independent prognostic indicator in chronic myeloid leukemia. Blood 2001; 98(6): 1732–1738.

21. Silver RT, Woolf SH, Hehlmann R, et al. An evidence-based analysis of the effect of busulfan, hydroxyurea, interferon, and allogeneic bone marrow transplantation in treating the chronic phase of chronic myeloid leukemia: developed for the American Society of Hematology. Blood 1999; 94(5): 1517–1536.

22. Interferon alfa-2a as compared with conventional chemotherapy for the treatment of chronic myeloid leukemia. The Italian Cooperative Study Group on Chronic Myeloid Leukemia. New England Journal of Medicine 1994; 330(12): 820–825.

23. Allan NC, Richards SM, Shepherd PC. UK Medical Research Council randomised, multicentre trial of interferon-alpha n1 for chronic myeloid leukaemia: improved survival irrespective of cytogenetic response. The UK Medical Research Council's Working Parties for Therapeutic Trials in Adult Leukaemia. Lancet 1995; 345(8962): 1392–1397.

24. Hehlmann R, Heimpel H, Kolb HJ, et al. The German CML study, comparison of busulfan vs. hydroxyurea vs. interferon alpha and establishment of prognostic score 1. Leukemia and Lymphoma 1993; 11(Suppl 1): 159–168.

25. Interferon alfa versus chemotherapy for chronic myeloid leukemia: a meta-analysis of seven randomized trials: Chronic Myeloid Leukemia Trialists' Collaborative Group. Journal of the National Cancer Institute 1997; 89(21): 1616–1620.

26. Guilhot F, Chastang C, Michallet M, et al. Interferon alfa-2b combined with cytarabine versus interferon alone in chronic myelogenous leukemia. French Chronic Myeloid Leukemia Study Group. New England Journal of Medicine 1997; 337(4): 223–229.

27. Druker B, Tamura S, Buchdunger E, et al. Effects of a selective inhibitor of the Abl tyrosine kinase on the growth of Bcr-Abl positive cells. Nature Medicine 1996; 2(5): 561–566.

28. Druker BJ, Talpaz M, Resta DJ, et al. Efficacy and safety of a specific inhibitor of the BCR-ABL tyrosine kinase in chronic myeloid leukemia. New England Journal of Medicine 2001; 344(14): 1031–1037.

29. O'Brien SG, Guilhot F, Larson RA, et al. Imatinib compared with interferon and low-dose cytarabine for newly diagnosed chronic-phase chronic myeloid leukemia. New England Journal of Medicine 2003; 348(11): 994–1004.

30. Hochhaus A, O'Brien SG, Guilhot F, et al. Six-year follow-up of patients receiving imatinib for the first-line treatment of chronic myeloid leukemia. Leukemia 2009; 23(6): 1054–1061.

31. Cortes J, Kantarjian H. How I treat newly diagnosed chronic phase CML. Blood 2012; 120(7): 1390–1397.

32. de Lavallade H, Apperley JF, Khorashad JS, et al. Imatinib for newly diagnosed patients with chronic myeloid leukemia: incidence of sustained responses in an intention-to-treat analysis. Journal of Clinical Oncology 2008; 26(20): 3358–3363.

33. Ibrahim AR, Eliasson L, Apperley JF, et al. Poor adherence is the main reason for loss of CCyR and imatinib failure for chronic myeloid leukemia patients on long-term therapy. Blood 2011; 117(14): 3733–3736.

34. Marin D, Bazeos A, Mahon FX, et al. Adherence is the critical factor for achieving molecular responses in patients with chronic myeloid leukemia who achieve complete cytogenetic responses on imatinib. Journal of Clinical Oncology 2010; 28(14): 2381–2388.

35. Talpaz M, Silver RT, Druker B, et al. A phase II study of STI571 in adult patients with Philadelphia chromosome positive chronic myelogenous leukemia in accelerated phase. Blood 2000; 96(11): 469A.

36. Sawyers CL, Hochhaus A, Feldman E, et al. Imatinib induces hematologic and cytogenetic responses in patients with chronic myelogenous leukemia in myeloid blast crisis: results of a phase II study. Blood 2002; 99(10): 3530–3539.

37. Deininger MW, O'Brien SG, Ford JM, Druker BJ. Practical management of patients with chronic myeloid leukemia receiving imatinib. Journal of Clinical Oncology 2003; 21(8): 1637–1647.

38. Soverini S, Hochhaus A, Nicolini FE, et al. BCR-ABL kinase domain mutation analysis in chronic myeloid leukemia patients treated with tyrosine kinase inhibitors: recommendations from an expert panel on behalf of European LeukemiaNet. Blood 2011; 118(5): 1208–1215.

39. Shah N, Nicoll J, Nagar B, et al. Multiple BCR-ABL kinase domain mutations confer polyclonal resistance to the tyrosine kinase inhibitor imatinib (STI571) in chronic phase and blast crisis chronic myeloid leukemia. Cancer Cell 2002; 2(2): 117.

40. Weisberg E, Manley PW, Breitenstein W, et al. Characterization of AMN107, a selective inhibitor of native and mutant Bcr-Abl. Cancer Cell 2005;7(2): 129–141.

41. Kantarjian H, Giles F, Wunderle L, et al. Nilotinib in imatinib-resistant CML and Philadelphia chromosome-positive ALL. New England Journal of Medicine 2006; 354(24): 2542–2551.

42. Talpaz M, Shah NP, Kantarjian H, et al. Dasatinib in imatinib-resistant Philadelphia chromosome-positive leukemias. New England Journal of Medicine 2006; 354(24): 2531–2541.

43. Cortes J, O'Brien S, Kantarjian H. Discontinuation of imatinib therapy after achieving a molecular response. Blood 2004; 104(7): 2204–2205.

44. Saglio G, Kim DW, Issaragrisil S, et al. Nilotinib versus imatinib for newly diagnosed chronic myeloid leukemia. New England Journal of Medicine 2010; 362(24): 2251–2259.

45. Santos FP, Quintas-Cardama A. New drugs for chronic myelogenous leukemia. Current Hematologic Malignancy Reports 201; 6(2): 96–103.

46. O'Hare T, Shakespeare WC, Zhu X, et al. AP24534, a pan-BCR-ABL inhibitor for chronic myeloid leukemia, potently inhibits the T315I mutant and overcomes mutation-based resistance. Cancer Cell 2009; 16(5): 401–412.

47. Chu S, McDonald T, Lin A, et al. Persistence of leukemia stem cells in chronic myelogenous leukemia patients in prolonged remission with imatinib treatment. Blood 2011; 118(20): 5565–5572.

48. Mahon FX, Rea D, Guilhot J, et al. Discontinuation of imatinib in patients with chronic myeloid leukaemia who have maintained complete molecular remission for at least 2 years: the prospective, multicentre Stop Imatinib (STIM) trial. Lancet Oncology 2010; 11(11): 1029–1035.

49. Radich JP, Gooley T, Bensinger W, et al. HLA-matched related hematopoietic cell transplantation for chronic-phase CML using a targeted busulfan and cyclophosphamide preparative regimen. Blood 2003; 102(1): 31–35.

50. Kebriaei P, Detry MA, Giralt S, et al. Long-term follow-up of allogeneic hematopoietic stem-cell transplantation with reduced-intensity conditioning for patients with chronic myeloid leukemia. Blood 2007; 110(9): 3456–3462.

51. Khoury HJ, Kukreja M, Goldman JM, et al. Prognostic factors for outcomes in allogeneic transplantation for CML in the imatinib era: a CIBMTR analysis. Bone Marrow Transplantation 2012; 47(6): 810–816.

52. Basak G, Torosian T, Snarski E, et al. Hematopoietic stem cell transplantation for T315I-mutated chronic myelogenous leukemia. Annals of Transplantation 2010; 15(2): 68–70.

53. Jabbour E, Cortes J, Kantarjian HM, et al. Allogeneic stem cell transplantation for patients with chronic myeloid leukemia and acute lymphocytic leukemia after Bcr-Abl kinase mutation-related imatinib failure. Blood 2006; 108(4): 1421–1423.

54. Druker BJ, Guilhot F, O'Brien SG, Gathmann I, Kantarjian H et al. Five-year follow-up of patients receiving imatinib for chronic myeloid leukemia. New England Journal of Medicine 2006; 355(23): 2408–2417.

55. Kantarjian H, Shah NP, Hochhaus A, Cortes J, Shah S et al. Dasatinib versus imatinib in newly diagnosed chronic-phase chronic myeloid leukemia. New England Journal of Medicine 2010; 362(24): 2260–2270.

56. Kantarjian HM, Shah NP, Cortes JE, Baccarani M, Agarwal MB et al. Dasatinib or imatinib in newly diagnosed chronic-phase chronic myeloid leukemia: 2-year follow-up from a randomized phase 3 trial (DASISION). Blood 2012; 119(5): 1123–1129.

57. Larson RA, Hochhaus A, Hughes TP, Clark RE, Etienne G et al. Nilotinib vs imatinib in patients with newly diagnosed Philadelphia chromosome-positive chronic myeloid leukemia in chronic phase: ENESTnd 3-year follow-up. Leukemia 2012; 26(10): 2197–2203.

58. Kantarjian HM, Hochhaus A, Saglio G, De Souza C, Flinn IW et al. Nilotinib versus imatinib for the treatment of patients with newly diagnosed chronic phase, Philadelphia chromosome-positive, chronic myeloid leukaemia: 24-month minimum follow-up of the phase 3 randomised ENESTnd trial. Lancet Oncology 2011; 12(9): 841–851.

59. GilesFJ, le Coutre PD, Pinilla-Ibarz J, Larson RA, Gattermann N et al. Nilotinib in imatinib-resistant or imatinib-intolerant patients with chronic myeloid leukemia in chronic phase: 48-month follow-up results of a phase II study. Leukemia 2012 .

60. Shah NP, Kantarjian HM, Kim DW, Rea D, Dorlhiac-Llacer PE et al. Intermittent target inhibition with dasatinib 100 mg once daily preserves efficacy and improves tolerability in imatinib-resistant and -intolerant chronic-phase chronic myeloid leukemia. Journal of Clinical Oncology 2008; 26(19): 3204–3212.

61. Shah NP, Kim DW, Kantarjian H, Rousselot P, Llacer PE et al. Potent, transient inhibition of BCR-ABL with dasatinib 100 mg daily achieves rapid and durable cytogenetic responses and high transformation-free survival rates in chronic phase chronic myeloid leukemia patients with resistance, suboptimal response or intolerance to imatinib. Haematologica 2010; 95(2): 232–240.

62. O'Brien SG, Guilhot F, Goldman JM, O'Brien SG, Guilhot F et al. International Randomized Study of Interferon versus STI571 (IRIS) 7-year follow-up: sustained survival, low rate of transformation and increased rate of major molecular response (MMR) in patients (pts) with newly diagnosed chronic myeloid leukemia in chronic phase (CML-CP) treated with imatinib (IM) [abstract]. Blood 2008; 112: 76.

63. Baccarani M, Cortes J, Pane F, Niederwieser D, Saglio G et al. Chronic myeloid leukemia: an update of concepts and management recommendations of European LeukemiaNet. Journal of Clinical Oncology 2009; 27(35): 6041–6051.

64. Fabarius A, Leitner A, Hochhaus A, Muller MC, Hanfstein B et al. Impact of additional cytogenetic aberrations at diagnosis on prognosis of CML: long-term observation of 1151 patients from the randomized CML Study IV. Blood 2011; 118(26): 6760–6768.

65. Mitelman F. The cytogenetic scenario of chronic myeloid leukemia. Leukemia and Lymphoma 1993; 11(Suppl 1): 11–15.

66. Mitelman F, Levan G, Nilsson PG, Brandt L. Non-random karyotypic evolution in chronic myeloid leukemia. International Journal of Cancer 1976; 18(1): 24–30.

67. Sokal JE, Gomez GA, Baccarani M, Tura S, Clarkson BD et al. Prognostic significance of additional cytogenetic abnormalities at diagnosis of Philadelphia chromosome-positive chronic granulocytic leukemia. Blood 1988; 72(1): 294–298.

68. Luatti S, Castagnetti F, Marzocchi G, Baldazzi C, Gugliotta G et al. Additional chromosomal abnormalities in Philadelphia-positive clone: adverse prognostic influence on frontline imatinib therapy: a GIMEMA Working Party on CML analysis. Blood 2012; 120(4): 761–767.

69. El-Zimaity MM, Kantarjian H, Talpaz M, O'Brien S, Giles F et al. Results of imatinib mesylate therapy in chronic myelogenous leukaemia with variant Philadelphia chromosome. British Journal of Haematology 2004; 125(2): 187–195.

70. Marzocchi G, Castagnetti F, Luatti S, Baldazzi C, Stacchini M et al. Variant Philadelphia translocations: molecular-cytogenetic characterization and prognostic influence on frontline imatinib therapy, a GIMEMA Working Party on CML analysis. Blood 2011; 117(25): 6793–6800.

71. Castagnetti F, Marzocchi G, Luatti S, Buontempo F, Baldazzi C et al. Deletions of the derivative chromosome 9 do not influence response to imatinib of early chronic phase chronic myeloid leukemia patients (a GIMEMA Working Party analysis). Blood 2006; 108(11): 2112.

72. Castagnetti F, Testoni N, Luatti S, Marzocchi G, Mancini M et al. Deletions of the derivative chromosome 9 do not influence the response and the outcome of chronic myeloid leukemia in early

chronic phase treated with imatinib mesylate: GIMEMA CML Working Party analysis. Journal of Clinical Oncology 2010; 28(16): 2748–2754.

73. Baccarani M, Deininger MW, Rosti G, Hochhaus A, Soverini S et al. European LeukemiaNet recommendations for the management of chronic myeloid leukemia 2013. Blood 2013; 122(6): 872–884. Available from: <http://dx.doi.org/10.1182/blood-2013-05-501569>.

74. Jabbour E, Kantarjian HM, Abruzzo LV, O'Brien S, Garcia-Manero G et al. Chromosomal abnormalities in Philadelphia chromosome negative metaphases appearing during imatinib mesylate therapy in patients with newly diagnosed chronic myeloid leukemia in chronic phase. Blood 2007; 110(8): 2991–2995.

75. O'Dwyer ME, Gatter KM, Loriaux M, Druker BJ, Olson SB et al. Demonstration of Philadelphia chromosome negative abnormal clones in patients with chronic myelogenous leukemia during major cytogenetic responses induced by imatinib mesylate. Leukemia 2003; 17(3): 481–487.

76. Medina J, Kantarjian H, Talpaz M, O'Brien S, Garcia-Manero G et al. Chromosomal abnormalities in Philadelphia chromosome-negative metaphases appearing during imatinib mesylate therapy in patients with Philadelphia chromosome-positive chronic myelogenous leukemia in chronic phase. Cancer 2003; 98(9): 1905–1911.

77. Testoni N, Marzocchi G, Luatti S, Amabile M, Baldazzi C et al. Chronic myeloid leukemia: a prospective comparison of interphase fluorescence in situ hybridization and chromosome banding analysis for the definition of complete cytogenetic response: a study of the GIMEMA CML WP. Blood 2009; 114(24): 4939–4943.

78. Hughes T, Deininger M, Hochhaus A, Branford S, Radich J et al. Monitoring CML patients responding to treatment with tyrosine kinase inhibitors: review and recommendations for harmonizing current methodology for detecting BCR-ABL transcripts and kinase domain mutations and for expressing results. Blood 2006; 108(1): 28–37.

79. Branford S, Fletcher L, Cross NC, Muller MC, Hochhaus A et al. Desirable performance characteristics for BCR-ABL measurement on an international reporting scale to allow consistent interpretation of individual patient response and comparison of response rates between clinical trials. Blood 2008; 112(8): 3330–3338.

80. Lucas CM, Harris RJ, Giannoudis A, Davies A, Knight K et al. Chronic myeloid leukemia patients with the e13a2 BCR-ABL fusion transcript have inferior responses to imatinib compared to patients with the e14a2 transcript. Haematologica 2009; 94(10): 1362–1367.

81. Hanfstein B, Erben P, Saussele S, Lauseker M, Proetel U et al. Distinct characteristics of e13a2 versus e14a2 BCR-ABL chronic myeloid leukemia under upfront treatment with imatinib—an analysis of the German CML Study IV. ASH Annual Meeting Abstracts 2011; 118(21): 3773.

82. Ross DM, Branford S, Moore S, Hughes TP. Limited clinical value of regular bone marrow cytogenetic analysis in imatinib-treated chronic phase CML patients monitored by RQ-PCR for BCR-ABL. Leukemia 2006; 20(4): 664–670.

83. Jabbour E, Shah N, Chuah C, Pavlovsky C, Mayer J et al. An exploratory analysis from 3 year DASISION follow-up examining the impact on patient outcomes of early complete cytogenetic responses at 3 months and major molecular responses at 12 months. Haematologica 2012; 97(abstr 1106): 454.

84. Marin D, Ibrahim AR, Lucas C, Gerrard G, Wang L et al. Assessment of BCR-ABL1 transcript levels at 3 months is the only requirement for predicting outcome for patients with chronic myeloid leukemia treated with tyrosine kinase inhibitors. Journal of Clinical Oncology 2011; 30(3): 232–238.

85. Marin D, Hedgley C, Clark RE, Apperley J, Foroni L et al. Predictive value of early molecular response in patients with chronic myeloid leukemia treated with first-line dasatinib. Blood 2012; 120(2): 291–294.

86. Hochhaus A, Guilhot F, Haifa Al-Ali K, Rosti G, Nakaseko C et al. Early BCR-ABL transcript levels predict future molecular response and long-term outcomes in newly daignosed patients with CML-CP: analysis of ENESTnd 3-year data (abstr 192). Haematologica 2012; 97(S1): 72.

87. Hochhaus A, Boqué C, Garelik MBB, Manos G, Steegmann JL. Molecular response kinetics and BCR-ABL reductions in patients with newly diagnosed chronic myeloid leukemia in chronic Phase (CML-CP) receiving dasatinib versus imatinib: DASISION 3-Year follow-up (abstr 584). Haematologica 2012; 97: 237.

88. Yeung DT, Osborn M, White DL, Branford S, Kornhauser M et al. upfront imatinib therapy in CML patients with rapid switching to nilotinib for failure to achieve molecular targets or intolerance achieves high overall rates of molecular response and a low risk of progression—an update of the TIDEL-II Trial. ASH Annual Meeting Abstracts 2011; 118(21): 451.

89. Marin D, Milojkovic D, Olavarria E, Khorashad JS, de Lavallade H et al. European LeukemiaNet criteria for failure or suboptimal response reliably identify patients with CML in early chronic phase treated with imatinib whose eventual outcome is poor. Blood 2008; 112(12): 4437–4444.

90. Hughes TP, Hochhaus A, Branford S, Muller MC, Kaeda JS et al. Long-term prognostic significance of early molecular response to imatinib in newly diagnosed chronic myeloid leukemia: an analysis from the International Randomized Study of Interferon and STI571 (IRIS). Blood 2010; 116(19): 3758–3765.

91. Jabbour E, Kantarjian HM, O'Brien S, Shan J, Quintas-Cardama A et al. Front-line therapy with second-generation tyrosine kinase inhibitors in patients with early chronic phase chronic myeloid leukemia: what is the optimal response? Journal of Clinical Oncology 2011; 29(32): 4260–4265.

92. Hanfstein B, Muller MC, Hehlmann R, Erben P, Lauseker M et al. Early molecular and cytogenetic response is predictive for long-term progression-free and overall survival in chronic myeloid leukemia (CML). Leukemia 2012; 26(9): 2096–2102.

93. Clark RE, Reiffers J, Kim D, Rosti G, Kurokawa M et al. Superior efficacy of nilotinib compared with imatinib in newly diagnosed patients with Ph+ chronic myeloid leukemia in chronic phase (CML-CP): ENESTnd 3-year follow-up (abstr 583). Haematologica 2012; 97: 237.

94. Cross NC, White HE, Muller MC, Saglio G, Hochhaus A. Standardized definitions of molecular response in chronic myeloid leukemia. Leukemia 2012; 26(10): 2172–2175.

95. Press RD, Galderisi C, Yang R, Rempfer C, Willis SG et al. A half-log increase in BCR-ABL RNA predicts a higher risk of relapse in patients with chronic myeloid leukemia with an imatinib-induced complete cytogenetic response. Clinical Cancer Research 2007; 13(20): 6136–6143.

96. Ross DM, Branford S, Seymour JF, Schwarer AP, Arthur C et al. Patients with chronic myeloid leukemia who maintain a complete molecular response after stopping imatinib treatment have evidence of persistent leukemia by DNA PCR. Leukemia 2010; 24(10): 1719–1724.

97. Soverini S, Colarossi S, Gnani A, Rosti G, Castagnetti F et al. Contribution of ABL kinase domain mutations to imatinib resistance in different subsets of Philadelphia-positive patients: by the GIMEMA Working Party on Chronic Myeloid Leukemia. Clinical Cancer Research 2006; 12(24): 7374–7379.

98. Branford S, Melo JV, Hughes TP. Selecting optimal second-line tyrosine kinase inhibitor therapy for chronic myeloid leukemia patients after imatinib failure—does the BCR-ABL mutation status really matter? Blood 2009; 114(27): 5426–5435.

99. Soverini S, Gnani A, Colarossi S. Abl kinase domain mutations are infrequent in early-chronic phase chronic myeloid leukemia patients resistant to imatinib Haematologica 2008; 93 (abstr 107).

100. Branford S, Goh H-G, Izzo B, Beppu L, Ortmann C-E et al. A review of mutation analysis in the TOPS trial of standard dose versus high dose IM in CML suggests that refinements to the ELN recommendations for mutation screening may be appropriate. Blood (ASH Annual Meeting Abstracts) 2010; 116 (abstr 889).

101. Branford S, Rudzki Z, Parkinson I, Grigg A, Taylor K et al. Real-time quantitative PCR analysis can be used as a primary screen to identify

patients with CML treated with imatinib who have BCR-ABL kinase domain mutations. Blood 2004; 104(9): 2926–2932.

102. Press RD, Willis SG, Laudadio J, Mauro MJ, Deininger MW. Determining the rise in BCR-ABL RNA that optimally predicts a kinase domain mutation in patients with chronic myeloid leukemia on imatinib. Blood [Evaluation Studies Research Support, N.I.H., Extramural Research Support, Non-U.S. Govt] 2009; 114(13): 2598–2605.

103. Saur G, Ivanova A, et al. Evaluation of BCR-ABL/ABL ratio increase that corresponds to BCR-ABL mutation in chronic myeloid leukemia patients treated by imatinib. Blood (ASH Annual Meeting Abstracts) 2010; 116(21): 3422.

104. Hughes T, Saglio G, Branford S, Soverini S, Kim DW et al. Impact of baseline BCR-ABL mutations on response to nilotinib in patients with chronic myeloid leukemia in chronic phase. Journal of Clinical Oncology 2009; 27(25): 4204–4210.

105. Apperley JF. Part I: mechanisms of resistance to imatinib in chronic myeloid leukaemia. Lancet Oncology 2007; 8(11): 1018–1029.

106. Parker WT, Ho M, Scott HS, Hughes TP, Branford S. Poor response to second-line kinase inhibitors in chronic myeloid leukemia patients with multiple low-level mutations, irrespective of their resistance profile. Blood 2012; 119(10): 2234–2238.

107. Cortes J, Kantarijain H, Shah N, Bixby D, Mauro M et al. Ponatinib in refractory Philadelphia chromosome-postive leukemias. New England Journal of Medicine 2012; 367(22): 2075–2088.

108. Bhamidipati PK, Kantarjian H, Cortes J, Cornelison AM, Jabbour E. Management of imatinib-resistant patients with chronic myeloid leukemia. Therapeutic Advances in Hematology 2013; 4(2): 103–117.

109. Kantarjian HM, Talpaz M, O'Brien S, Giles F, Garcia-Manero G et al. Dose escalation of imatinib mesylate can overcome resistance to standard-dose therapy in patients with chronic myelogenous leukemia. Blood 2003; 101(2): 473–475.

110. Kantarjian H, Pasquini R, Hamerschlak N, Rousselot P, Holowiecki J et al. Dasatinib or high-dose imatinib for chronic-phase chronic myeloid leukemia after failure of first-line imatinib: a randomized phase 2 trial. Blood 2007; 109(12): 5143–5150.

111. Kantarjian H, Pasquini R, Levy V, Jootar S, Holowiecki J et al. Dasatinib or high-dose imatinib for chronic-phase chronic myeloid leukemia resistant to imatinib at a dose of 400 to 600 milligrams daily: two-year follow-up of a randomized phase 2 study (START-R). Cancer 2009; 115(18): 4136–4147.

112. Rea D, Vellenga E, Junghanβ C, Baccarani M, Kantarjian K et al. Six-year follow-up of patients with imatinib-resistant or imatinib-intolerant chronic-phase chronic myeloid leukemia(CP-CML) receiving dasatinb. Haematologica 2012; 97 (abstr 0199): 80.

113. Muller MC, Cortes JE, Kim DW, Druker BJ, Erben P et al. Dasatinib treatment of chronic-phase chronic myeloid leukemia: analysis of responses according to preexisting BCR-ABL mutations. Blood 2009; 114(24): 4944–4953.

114. Jabbour E, Kantarjian HM, Jones D, Reddy N, O'Brien S et al. Characteristics and outcome of chronic myeloid leukemia patients with F317L BCR-ABL kinase domain mutation after therapy with tyrosine kinase inhibitors. Blood 2008; 112(13): 4839–4842.

115. Soverini S, Colarossi S, Gnani A, Castagnetti F, Rosti G et al. Resistance to dasatinib in Philadelphia-positive leukemia patients and the presence or the selection of mutations at residues 315 and 317 in the BCR-ABL kinase domain. Haematologica 2007; 92(3): 401–404.

116. Cortes JE, Kantarjian HM, Brummendorf TH, Kim DW, Turkina AG et al. Safety and efficacy of bosutinib (SKI-606) in chronic phase Philadelphia chromosome-positive chronic myeloid leukemia patients with resistance or intolerance to imatinib. Blood 2011; 118(17): 4567–4576.

117. Tam CS, Kantarjian H, Garcia-Manero G, Borthakur G, O'Brien S et al. Failure to achieve a major cytogenetic response by 12 months defines inadequate response in patients receiving nilotinib or dasatinib as second or subsequent line therapy for chronic myeloid leukemia. Blood 2008; 112(3): 516–518.

118. Ross DM, Branford S, Seymour JF, Schwarer AP, Arthur C et al. Safety and efficacy of imatinib cessation for CML patients with stable undetectable minimal residual disease: results from the TWISTER Study. Blood 2013; 122(4): 515–522.

119. Fleming AF. The epidemiology of lymphomas and leukemias in Africa: an overview. Leukemia Research 1985; 9: 735–740.

120. Yang C, Zhang X. Incidence survey of leukemia in China. Chinese Medical Sciences Journal 1991; 6: 65–70.

121. Hallek M, Cheson BD, Catovsky D, Caligaris-Cappio F, Dighiero G, et al. Guidelines for the diagnosis and treatment of chronic lymphocytic leukemia: a report from the International Workshop on Chronic Lymphocytic Leukemia updating the National Cancer Institute-Working Group 1996 guidelines. Blood 2008; 111: 5446–5456.

122. Rai KR, Sawitsky A, Cronkite EP, Chanana AD, Levy RN et al. Clinical staging of chronic lymphocytic leukemia. Blood 1975; 46: 219–234.

123. Binet JL, Auquier A, Dighiero G, Chastang C, Piguet H et al. A new prognostic classification of chronic lymphocytic leukemia derived from a multivariate survival analysis. Cancer 1981; 48: 198–206.

124. Chiorazzi N, Hatzki K, Albesiano E. B-cell chronic lymphocytic leukemia, a clonal disease with receptors that vary in specificity for (auto)antigens. Annals of the New York Academy of Sciences 2005; 1062: 1–12.

125. Cimmino A, Calin GA, Fabbri M, Iorio MV, Ferracin M et al. miR-15 and miR-16 induce apoptosis by targeting BCL2. Proceedings of the National Academy of Sciences USA 2005; 102: 13944–13949.

126. Calin GA, Ferracin M, Cimmino A, Di Leva G, Shimizu M et al. A MicroRNA signature associated with prognosis and progression in chronic lymphocytic leukemia. New England Journal of Medicine 2005; 353: 1793–1801.

127. Damle RN, Wasil T, Fais F, Ghiotto F, Valetto A et al. Ig V gene mutation status and CD38 expression as novel prognostic indicators in chronic lymphocytic leukemia. Blood 1999; 94: 1840–1847.

128. Hamblin TJ, Davis Z, Gardiner A, Oscier DG, Stevenson FK. Unmutated Ig V(H) genes are associated with a more aggressive form of chronic lymphocytic leukemia. Blood 1999; 94: 1848–1854.

129. Puente XS, Pinyol M, Quesada V, Conde L, Ordóñez GR et al. Whole-genome sequencing identifies recurrent mutations in chronic lymphocytic leukaemia. Nature 2011; 475(7354): 101–105.

130. Dighiero G, Maloum K, Desablens B, Cazin B, Navarro M et al. Chlorambucil in indolent chronic lymphocytic leukemia. French Cooperative Group on Chronic Lymphocytic Leukemia. New England Journal of Medicine 1998; 338: 1506–1514.

131. Raphael B, Andersen JW, Silber R, Oken M, Moore D et al. Comparison of chlorambucil and prednisone versus cyclophosphamide, vincristine, and prednisone as initial treatment for chronic lymphocytic leukemia: long-term follow-up of an Eastern Cooperative Oncology Group randomized clinical trial. Journal of Clinical Oncology 1991; 9: 770–776.

132. Jaksic B, Brugiatelli M, Krc I, Losonczi H, Holowiecki J et al. High dose chlorambucil versus Binet's modified cyclophosphamide, doxorubicin, vincristine, and prednisone regimen in the treatment of patients with advanced B-cell chronic lymphocytic leukemia. Results of an international multicenter randomized trial. Cancer 1997; 79: 2107–2114.

133. French Cooperative Group on Chronic Lymphocytic Leukemia. A randomized clinical trial of chlorambucil versus COP in stage B chronic lymphocytic leukemia. Blood 1990; 75: 1422–1425.

134. Knauf WU, Lissichkov T, Aldaoud A, Liberati A, Loscertales J et al. Phase III randomized study of bendamustine compared with chlorambucil in previously untreated patients with chronic lymphocytic leukemia. Journal of Clinical Oncology 2009; 27: 4378–4384.

135. Fischer K, Cramer P, Busch R, Böttcher S, Bahlo J et al. Bendamustine in combination with rituximab for previously untreated patients with chronic lymphocytic leukemia: a multicenter phase II trial of the

German Chronic Lymphocytic Leukemia Study Group. Journal of Clinical Oncology 2012; 30: 3209–3216.

136. Rummel MJ, Niederle N, Maschmeyer G, Banat GA, von Grünhagen U et al. Bendamustine plus rituximab versus CHOP plus rituximab as first-line treatment for patients with indolent and mantle-cell lymphomas: an open-label, multicentre, randomised, phase 3 non-inferiority trial. Lancet 2013; 381(9873): 1203–1210.

137. Castro JE, Sandoval-Sus JD, Bole J, Rassenti L, Kipps TJ. Rituximab in combination with high-dose methylprednisolone for the treatment of fludarabine refractory high-risk chronic lymphocytic leukemia. Leukemia 2008; 22: 2048–2053.

138. Eichhorst BF, Busch R, Hopfinger G, Pasold R, Hensel M et al. Fludarabine plus cyclophosphamide versus fludarabine alone in first-line therapy of younger patients with chronic lymphocytic leukemia. Blood 2006; 107: 885–891.

139. Rai KR, Peterson BL, Appelbaum FR, et al. Long-term survival analysis of the North American Intergroup Study C9011 comparing fludarabine (F) and chlorambucil (C) in previously untreated patients with chronic lymphocytic leukemia (CLL). Program and abstracts of the 51st American Society of Hematology Annual Meeting and Exposition, New Orleans, Louisiana, December 5–8, 2009; Abstract 536.

140. Johnson S, Smith AG, Löffler H, Osby E, Juliusson G et al. Multicentre prospective randomised trial of fludarabine versus cyclophosphamide, doxorubicin, and prednisone (CAP) for treatment of advanced-stage chronic lymphocytic leukaemia Lancet 1996; 347: 1432–1438.

141. Leporrier M, Chevret S, Cazin B, Boudjerra N, Feugier P et al. Randomized comparison of fludarabine, CAP, and ChOP in 938 previously untreated stage B and C chronic lymphocytic leukemia patients. Blood 2001; 98: 2319–2325.

142. Steurer M, Pall G, Richards S, Schwarzer G, Bohlius J et al. Purine antagonists for chronic lymphocytic leukaemia. Cochrane Database Systematic Reviews 2006; 3: CD004270.

143. Morrison VA, Rai KR, Peterson BL, Kolitz JE, Elias L et al. Impact of therapy with chlorambucil, fludarabine, or fludarabine plus chlorambucil on infections in patients with chronic lymphocytic leukemia: Intergroup Study Cancer and Leukemia Group B 9011. Journal of Clinical Oncology 2001; 19: 3611–3621.

144. Yanagihara ET, Blaisdell RK, Hayashi T, Lukes RJ. Malignant lymphoma in Hawaii-Japanese: a retrospective morphologic survey. Hematological Oncology 1989; 7: 219–232.

145. Flinn IW, Neuberg DS, Grever MR, Dewald GW, Bennett JM et al. Phase III trial of fludarabine plus cyclophosphamide compared with fludarabine for patients with previously untreated chronic lymphocytic leukemia: US Intergroup Trial E2997. Journal of Clinical Oncology 2007; 25: 793–798.

146. Catovsky D, Richards S, Matutes E, Oscier D, Dyer MJ et al. Assessment of fludarabine plus cyclophosphamide for patients with chronic lymphocytic leukaemia (the LRF CLL4 Trial): a randomised controlled trial. Lancet 2007; 370: 230–239.

147. Wierda WG, Kipps TJ, Dürig J, Griskevicius L, Stilgenbauer S et al. Chemoimmunotherapy with ofatumumab, fludarabine, and cyclophosphamide (O-FC) in previously untreated patients with chronic lymphocytic leukemia. Blood 2011; 117: 6450–6458.

148. Jazirehi AR, Huerta-Yepez S, Cheng G, Bonavida B. Rituximab (chimeric anti-CD20 monoclonal antibody) inhibits the constitutive nuclear factor-{kappa}B signaling pathway in non-Hodgkin's lymphoma B-cell lines: role in sensitization to chemotherapeutic drug-induced apoptosis. Cancer Research 2005; 65: 264–276.

149. Byrd JC, Peterson BL, Morrison VA, Park K, Jacobson R et al. Randomized phase 2 study of fludarabine with concurrent versus sequential treatment with rituximab in symptomatic, untreated patients with B-cell chronic lymphocytic leukemia: results from Cancer and Leukemia Group B 9712 (CALGB 9712). Blood 2003; 101: 6–14.

150. Woyach JA, Ruppert AS, Heerema NA, Peterson BL, Gribben JG et al. Chemoimmunotherapy with fludarabine and rituximab produces extended overall survival and progression-free survival in chronic lymphocytic leukemia: long-term follow-up of CALGB study 9712. Journal of Clinical Oncology 2011; 29: 1349–1355.

151. Wierda W, O'Brien S, Wen S, Faderl S, Garcia-Manero G et al. Chemoimmunotherapy with fludarabine, cyclophosphamide, and rituximab for relapsed and refractory chronic lymphocytic leukemia. Journal of Clinical Oncology 2005; 23: 4070–4078.

152. Tam CS, O'Brien S, Wierda W, Kantarjian H, Wen S et al. Long-term results of the fludarabine, cyclophosphamide, and rituximab regimen as initial therapy of chronic lymphocytic leukemia. Blood 2008; 112: 975–980.

153. Robak T, Dmoszynska A, Solal-Céligny P, Warzocha K, Loscertales J et al. Rituximab plus fludarabine and cyclophosphamide prolongs progression-free survival compared with fludarabine and cyclophosphamide alone in previously treated chronic lymphocytic leukemia. Journal of Clinical Oncology 2010; 28: 1756–1765.

154. Hallek M, Fischer K, Fingerle-Rowson G, Fink AM, Busch R et al. Addition of rituximab to fludarabine and cyclophosphamide in patients with chronic lymphocytic leukaemia: a randomised, open-label, phase 3 trial. Lancet 2010; 376: 1164–1174.

155. Hainsworth JD, Litchy S, Barton JH, Houston GA, Hermann RC et al. Single-agent rituximab as first-line and maintenance treatment for patients with chronic lymphocytic leukemia or small lymphocytic lymphoma: a phase II trial of the Minnie Pearl Cancer Research Network. Journal of Clinical Oncology 2003; 21: 1746–1751.

156. Robak T. Novel monoclonal antibodies for the treatment of chronic lymphocytic leukemia. Current Cancer Drug Targets 2008; 8(2): 156–171.

157. Frankfurt O, Hamilton E, Duffey S, et al. Alemtuzumab and rituximab combination therapy for patients with untreated CLL: a phase II trial. Program and abstracts of the 50th American Society of Hematology Annual Meeting and Exposition, San Francisco, California, December 6–9, 2008. Abstract 2098.

158. Zent CS, Ding W, Schwager SM, Reinalda MS, Hoyer JD et al. The prognostic significance of cytopenia in chronic lymphocytic leukemia/small lymphocytic lymphoma (CLL). British Journal of Haematology 2008; 141: 615–621.

159. Keating MJ, Flinn I, Jain V, Binet JL, Hillmen P et al. Therapeutic role of alemtuzumab (Campath-1H) in patients who have failed fludarabine: results of a large international study. Blood 2002; 99: 3554–3561.

160. Lozanski G, Heerema NA, Flinn IW, Smith L, Harbison J et al. Alemtuzumab is an effective therapy for chronic lymphocytic leukemia with p53 mutations and deletions. Blood 2004; 103: 3278–3281.

161. Moreton P, Kennedy B, Lucas G, Leach M, Rassam SM et al. Eradication of minimal residual disease in B-cell chronic lymphocytic leukemia after alemtuzumab therapy is associated with prolonged survival. Journal of Clinical Oncology 2005; 23: 2971–2979.

162. Hillmen P, Skotnicki AB, Robak T, Jaksic B, Dmoszynska A et al. Alemtuzumab compared with chlorambucil as first-line therapy for chronic lymphocytic leukemia. Journal of Clinical Oncology 2007; 25: 5616–5623.

163. Engert A, Gercheva L, Robak T, et al. Improved progression-free survival (PFS) of alemtuzumab (Campath, MabCampath) plus fludarabine (Fludara) versus fludarabine alone as second-line treatment of patients with B-cell chronic lymphocytic leukemia: preliminary results from a phase III randomized trial. Program and abstracts of the 51st American Society of Hematology Annual Meeting and Exposition, New Orleans, Louisiana, December 5–8, 2009. Abstract 537.

164. Engert A, Gercheva L, Pilipenko G, et al. Overall survival advantage and acceptable safety profile with fludarabine in combination with alemtuzumab (FluCam) in previously treated patients with advanced stage chronic lymphocytic leukemia. Program and abstracts of the 52nd American Society of Hematology Annual Meeting and Exposition, Orlando, Florida, December 4–7, 2010. Abstract 919.

165. Moreton P, Hillmen P. Alemtuzumab therapy in B-cell lymphoproliferative disorders. Seminars in Oncology 2003; 30: 493–501.

166. Stilgenbauer S, Cymbalista F, Leblond V, et al. Subcutaneous alemtuzumab combined with oral dexamethasone, followed by alemtuzumab maintenance or allo-SCT in CLL with 17p- or refractory to fludarabine: interim analysis of the CLL2O trial of the GCLLSG and FCGCLL/MW. Program and abstracts of the 52nd American Society of Hematology Annual Meeting and Exposition, Orlando, Florida, December 4–7, 2010. Abstract 920.

167. O'Brien SM, Keating MJ, Mocarski ES. Updated guidelines on the management of cytomegalovirus reactivation in patients with chronic lymphocytic leukemia treated with alemtuzumab. Clinical Lymphoma and Myeloma 2006; 7: 125–130.

168. Fischer K, Cramer P, Busch R, Stilgenbauer S, Bahlo J et al. Bendamustine combined with rituximab in patients with relapsed and/or refractory chronic lymphocytic leukemia: a multicenter phase II trial of the German Chronic Lymphocytic Leukemia Study Group. Journal of Clinical Oncology 2011; 29: 3559–3566.

169. Montillo M, Tedeschi A, Petrizzi VB, Ricci F, Crugnola M et al. An open-label, pilot study of fludarabine, cyclophosphamide, and alemtuzumab (FCC) in relapsed/refractory patients with B-cell chronic lymphocytic leukemia. Blood 2011; 118(15): 4079–4085 [Epub ahead of print].

170. Byrd JC, Kipps TJ, Flinn IW, Castro J, Lin TS et al. Phase 1/2 study of lumiliximab combined with fludarabine, cyclophosphamide, and rituximab in patients with relapsed or refractory chronic lymphocytic leukemia. Blood 2010; 115: 489–495.

171. Wierda WG, Kipps TJ, Mayer J, Stilgenbauer S, Williams CD et al. Ofatumumab as single-agent CD20 immunotherapy in fludarabine-refractory chronic lymphocytic leukemia. Journal of Clinical Oncology 2010; 28: 1749–1755.

172. Goede V, Fisher K, Bursch R, Engelke A, Eichhorst B et al. Obinutuzumab plus chlorambucil in patients with CLL and coexisting conditions. New England Journal of Medicine 2014; 370(12): 1101–1110. (Epub ahead of print).

173. Lin TS, Heerema NA, Lozanski G, et al. Flavopiridol (alvocidib) induces durable responses in relapse chronic lymphocytic leukemia (CLL) patients with high-risk cytogenetic abnormalities. Program and abstracts of the 50th American Society of Hematology Annual Meeting and Exposition, San Francisco, California, December 6–9, 2008. Abstract 46.

174. Byrd JC, Furman RR, Coutre SE, Flinn IW, Burger JA et al. Targeting BTK with ibrutinib in relapsed chronic lymphocytic leukemia. New England Journal of Medicine 2013; 369(1): 32–42.

175. Porter DL, Levine BL, Kalos M, Bagg A, June CH. Chimeric antigen receptor-modified T cells in chronic lymphoid leukemia. New England Journal of Medicine 2011; 365(8): 725–733.

176. Ferrajoli A, O'Brien S, Faderl SH, O'Brien SM, Gao H et al. Lenalidomide induces complete and partial remissions in patients with relapsed and refractory chronic lymphocytic leukemia. Blood 2008; 111: 5291–5297.

177. Chen CI, Bergsagel PL, Paul H, Xu W, Lau A et al. Single-agent lenalidomide in the treatment of previously untreated chronic lymphocytic leukemia. Journal of Clinical Oncology 2011; 29: 1175–1181.

178. Shanafelt T, Tun H, Hanson C, et al. Lenalidomide consolidation after first-line chemoimmunotherapy for patients with previously untreated CLL. Program and abstracts of the 52nd American Society of Hematology Annual Meeting and Exposition, Orlando, Florida, December 4–7, 2010. Abstract 1379.

179. Amrein PC, Attar EC, Takvorian T, Hochberg EP, Ballen KK et al. Phase II study of dasatinib in relapsed or refractory chronic lymphocytic leukemia. Clinical Cancer Research 2011; 17: 2977–2986.

180. Furman RR, Byrd JC, Brown JR, et al. CAL-101, an isoform-selective inhibitor of phosphatidylinositol 3-kinase (PI3K) delta, demonstrates clinical activity and pharmacodynamic effects in patients with relapsed or refractory chronic lymphocytic leukemia. Program and abstracts of the 52nd American Society of Hematology Annual Meeting and Exposition, Orlando, Florida, December 4–7, 2010. Abstract 55.

181. Furman RR, Andritsos L, Flinn IW, et al. Phase 1 dose escalation study of TRU-016, an anti-CD37 SMIP protein in relapsed and refractory CLL. Program and abstracts of the 52nd American Society of Hematology Annual Meeting and Exposition, Orlando, Florida, December 4–7, 2010. Abstract 56.

182. Burger JA, O'Brien S, Fowler N, et al. The Bruton's tyrosine kinase inhibitor, PCI-32765, is well tolerated and demonstrates promising clinical activity in chronic lymphocytic leukemia (CLL) and small lymphocytic lymphoma (SLL): an update on ongoing phase 1 studies. Program and abstracts of the 52nd American Society of Hematology Annual Meeting and Exposition, Orlando, Florida, December 4–7, 2010. Abstract 57.

183. Tallman MS, Polliack A. Historical aspects and milestones in the development of effective treatment for hairy cell leukemia. Leukemia and Lymphoma 2009; 50: 2–7.

184. Staines A, Cartwright RA. Hairy cell leukemia: descriptive epidemiology and a case control study. British Journal of Haematology 1993; 85: 714–717.

185. Tiacci E, Trifonov V, Schiavoni G, Holmes A, Kern W et al. BRAF mutations in hairy-cell leukemia. New England Journal of Medicine 2011; 364: 2305–2315.

186. Dietrich S, Glimm H, Andrulis M, von Kalle C, Ho AD et al. BRAF inhibition in refractory hairy-cell leukemia. New England Journal of Medicine 2012; 366: 2038–2040.

187. Swerdlow SH, Campo E, Harris NL, Pileri SA, Stein H et al. WHO Classification of Tumours of Haematopoietic and Lymphoid Tissues (4th ed.). Geneva: WHO press, IARC, 2008, 441.

188. Vincent AM, Burthem J, Brew R, Cawley JC. Endothelial interactions of hairy cells: the importance of a4b1 in the unusual tissue distribution of the disorder. Blood 1996; 88: 3945–3952.

189. Frassoldati A, Lamparelli T, Federico M, Annino L, Capnist G et al. Hairy cell leukemia: a clinical review based on 725 cases of the Italian co-operative group (ICGHCL). Leukemia and Lymphoma 1994; 13: 307–316.

190. Saven A, Burian C, Koziol JA, Piro LD. Long-term follow-up of patients with hairy cell leukemia after cladribine treatment. Blood 1998; 92: 1918–1926.

191. Forconi F. Hairy cell leukemia: biological and clinical overview from immunogenetic insights. Hematological Oncology 2011; 29: 55–66.

192. Hasler P, Kistler H, Gerber H. Vasculitides in hairy cell leukemia. Seminars in Arthritis and Rheumatism 1995; 25: 134–142.

193. Summers TA, Jaffe ES. Hairy cell leukemia diagnostic criteria and differential diagnosis. Leukemia Lymphoma 2011; 52: 6–10.

194. Dong HY, Weisberger J, Liu Z, Tugulea S. Immunophenotypic analysis of CD 103+ B-lymphoproliferative disorders: hairy cell leukemia and its mimics. American Journal of Clinical Pathology 2009; 131: 586–595.

195. Sausville JE, Salloum RG, Sorbara L, Kingma DW, Raffeld M et al. Minimal residual disease detection in hairy cell leukemia. Comparision of flow cytometric immunophenotyping with clonal analysis using consensus primer polymerase chain for the heavy chain gene. American Journal of Clinical Pathology 2003: 119: 213–217.

196. Grever MR. How I treat hairy cell leukemia. Blood 2010; 115: 21–28.

197. Habermann TM. Splenectomy, interferon, and treatments of historical interest in hairy cell leukemia. Hematology and Oncology Clinics North America 2006; 20: 1075–1086.

198. Tallman MS, Hakimian D. Purine nucleoside analogs: emerging roles in indolent lymphoproliferative disorders. Blood 1995; 86:2463–2474.

199. Johnston JB. Mechanism of action of pentostatin and cladribine in hairy cell leukemia. Leukemia and Lymphoma 2011; 52: 43–45.

200. Dearden CE, Else M, Catovsky D. Long term results for pentostatin and cladribine treatment of hairy cell leukemia. Leukemia and Lymphoma 2011; 52: 21–24.

201. Lauria F, Cencini E, Forconi F. Alternative methods of cladribine administration. Leukemia and Lymphoma 2011; 52: 34–37.

202. Seymour J, Talpaz M, Kurzrock R. Response duration and recovery of CD4+ lymphocytes following deoxycoformycin in

interferon-α- resistant hairy cell leukemia: 7-year follow-up. Leukemia 1997; 11: 42–47.

203. Ravandi F, Jorgensen JL, O'Brien SM, Verstovsek S, Koller CA et al. Eradication of minimal residual disease in hairy cell leukemia. Blood 2006; 107: 4658–4662.

204. Nieva J, Bethel K, Saven A. Phase II study of rituximab in the treatment of cladribine-failed patients with hairy cell leukemia. Blood 2003; 102: 810–813.

205. Kreitman RJ, Fitzgerald DJ, Pastan I. Approach to the patient after relapse of hairy cell leukemia. Leukemia and Lymphoma 2009; 50: 32–37.

206. Kreitman RJ, Arons E, Stetler-Stevenson M, Fitzgerald DJ, Wilson WH et al. Recombinant immunotoxins and other therapies for relapsed/refractory hairy cell leukemia. Leukemia and Lymphoma 2011; 52(Suppl 2): 82–86.

207. Hisada M, Chen BE, Jaffe ES, Travis LB. Second cancer incidence and cause specific mortality among 3104 patients with hairy cell leukemia: a population based study. Journal of the National Cancer Institute 2007; 99: 215–222.

208. Grever MR, Lozanski G. Modern strategies for hairy cell leukemia. Journal of Clinical Oncology 2011; 29: 583–590.

209. Dungarwalla M, Matutes E, Dearden CE. Prolymphocytic leukaemia of B- and T-cell subtype: a state-of-the-art paper. European Journal of Haematology 2008; 80: 469–476.

210. Tempescul A, Feuerbach J, Ianotto JC, Dalbies F, Marion V et al. A combination therapy with fludarabine, mitoxantrone and rituximab induces complete immunophenotypical remission in B-cell prolymphocytic leukaemia. Annals of Hematology 2009; 88: 85–88.

211. Dearden C. How I treat prolymphocytic leukemia. Blood 2012; 120: 538–551.

212. Kalaycio ME, Kukreja M, Woolfrey AE, Szer J, Cortes J et al. Allogeneic hematopoietic cell transplant for prolymphocytic leukemia. Biology of Blood and Marrow Transplantation 2010; 16: 543–547.

213. Khot A, Dearden C. T-cell prolymphocytic leukemia. Expert Reviews of Anticancer Therapy 2009; 9: 365–371.

214. Dearden CE. T-cell prolymphocytic leukemia. Clinical Lymphoma and Myeloma 2009; 9(Suppl 3): S239–S243.

215. Dearden CE, Khot A, Else M, Hamblin M, Grand E et al. Alemtuzumab therapy in T-cell prolymphocytic leukemia: comparing efficacy in a series treated intravenously and a study piloting the subcutaneous route. Blood 2011; 118: 5799–5802.

216. Krishnan B, Else M, Tjonnfjord GE, Cazin B, Carney D et al. Stem cell transplantation after alemtuzumab in T-cell prolymphocytic leukaemia results in longer survival than after alemtuzumab alone: a multicentre retrospective study. British Journal of Haematology 2010; 149: 907–910.

217. Wiktor-Jedrzejczak W, Dearden C, de Wreede L, van Biezen A, Brinch L et al. Hematopoietic stem cell transplantation in T-prolymphocytic leukemia: a retrospective study from the European Group for Blood and Marrow Transplantation and the Royal Marsden Consortium. Leukemia 2012; 26: 972–976.

218. Loughran TP Jr, Kadin ME, Starkebaum G, Abkowitz JL, Clark EA et al. Leukemia of large granular lymphocytes: association with clonal chromosomal abnormalities and autoimmune neutropenia, thrombocytopenia, and hemolytic anemia. Annals of Internal Medicine 1985; 102: 169–175.

219. Jerez A, Clemente MJ, Makishima H, Koskela H, Leblanc F et al. STAT3 mutations unify the pathogenesis of chronic lymphoproliferative disorders of NK cells and T cell large granular lymphocyte leukemia. Blood 2012; 120(15): 3048–3057.

220. Dearden C. Large granular lymphocytic leukaemia pathogenesis and management. British Journal of Haematology 2011; 152: 273–283.

221. Lamy T, Loughran TP Jr. How I treat LGL leukemia. Blood 2011; 117: 2764–2774.

222. Prochorec-Sobieszek M. Advances in diagnosis and treatment of large granular lymphocyte syndrome. Current Opinions in Hematology 2010 [Epub ahead of print].

223. Watters RJ, Liu X, Loughran TP Jr. T-cell and natural killer-cell large granular lymphocyte leukemia neoplasias. Leukemia and Lymphoma 2011; 52: 2217–2225.

224. Robak T. Hairy-cell leukemia variant: recent view on diagnosis, biology and treatment. Cancer Treatment Reviews 2011; 37: 3–10.

225. Robak T. Management of hairy cell leukemia variant. Leukemia and Lymphoma 2011; 52(Suppl 2): 53–56.

226. Jones G, Parry-Jones N, Wilkins B, Else M, Catovsky D. British Committee for Standards in Haematology. Revised guidelines for the diagnosis and management of hairy cell leukaemia and hairy cell leukaemia variant*. British Journal of Haematology 2012; 156: 186–195.

CHAPTER 53

Myeloma

Charlotte Pawlyn, Faith Davies, and Gareth Morgan

Introduction to myeloma

Multiple myeloma (myeloma or MM) is the second most common haematological malignancy in the UK and is characterized by the proliferation of clonal plasma cells in the bone marrow. It was first described in the mid-nineteenth century when a patient in London was noted to have a large amount of protein in his urine. His physicians, Dr William MacIntyre and Dr Thomas Watson, sent a sample of urine to Dr Henry Bence Jones, a well-recognized physician and chemical pathologist at St George's Hospital. Dr Jones described characteristic changes on heating and cooling the urine and quantified the protein and recognizing its diagnostic importance. After the patient's death, Dr John Dalrymple described cells—consistent with plasma cells—taken from the lumbar vertebrae and a rib, and in 1850 Dr McIntyre published a description of the case with characteristic clinical, urine protein, and bone marrow features [1, 2].

Myeloma is divided into a number of distinct clinical phases. The first, a premalignant stage termed MGUS (monoclonal gammopathy of undetermined significance) in asymptomatic patients, in which there is a population of clonal plasma cells that produce a monoclonal protein or 'paraprotein'. This syndrome is present in 3% of adults over the age of 60 [3] with a risk of progressing to myeloma of 1% per year [4]. The next stage, asymptomatic myeloma, has a higher percentage of plasma cells in the bone marrow but without end-organ damage. Myeloma requiring treatment is defined as disease causing detectable damage to the bones or kidneys and/or suppression of normal bone marrow function or disease defined by 'biomarkers of malignancy'. Plasma cell leukaemia is the most aggressive stage of disease and is characterized by the ability of plasma cells to survive outside of the protective bone marrow microenvironment.

Epidemiology

Myeloma is predominantly a disease of those aged over 60 and as such the incidence is increasing as the population ages. There are currently approximately 20 000 new cases diagnosed each year in the US and 4500 in the UK [5, 6]. Epidemiological studies have established increasing age, male gender, familial background, and a past history of MGUS as risk factors for MM [7, 8]. It has been suggested that myeloma is always preceded by MGUS as the abnormal plasma cells in both conditions share many of the same genetic abnormalities. Two long-term cohort studies support this view, which is now generally accepted [9–11], The risk of developing clinical myeloma is either related to the development of MGUS or to the transition from MGUS to MM, either of which can be contributed to by inherited genetic variation.

The male:female split observed is 60:40, both in clinical trial data and population statistics, with differences seen in the underlying cytogenetic abnormalities seen between sexes [8]. There is also a difference in incidence dependent on racial background, with a higher prevalence in African-Americans compared to those with a European background [10, 12, 13]. MGUS has a similar profile suggesting the higher prevalence in African-Americans is due to differences in the primary genetic event causing MGUS rather than the risk of progression from MGUS to MM. The rates in American Chinese, Japanese, and Mexican populations are lower than the general population [14, 15].

Myeloma risk has also been linked to a number of lifestyle and environmental factors including obesity [16], autoimmune disease [17], exposure to agricultural or chemical toxins [18], and radiation. The evidence for a familial basis for the development of multiple myeloma is not clear. Over 37 families with two or more affected members have been reported, but case control studies have not always yielded evidence as to whether or not family members of patients with multiple myeloma are at a significantly increased risk of developing the disease [19]. The first-degree relatives of patients with MGUS or MM have been shown to have a consistently increased risk of myeloma in epidemiological and case control studies [19–22]. The largest study to date, involving 11 752 MM patients diagnosed in Sweden between 1958 and 2002, showed that the risk of MM was increased fourfold in first-degree relatives (95% CI 1.81–8.41) [20]. Several other studies have also supported this data [23–28] and shown a possible increased risk of MM in family members of those with other cancers such as prostate cancer, melanoma, non-Hodgkin lymphoma, and chronic lymphocytic leukaemia [19, 20, 29, 30]. Collectively, these data are consistent with a two- to fourfold inherited genetic susceptibility to MM.

The possible cause for this inherited genetic risk has been identified in large genome-wide association studies [31–33]. These identified single nuclear polymorphisms (SNPs) at 2p23.3, 3p22.1, 3q26.2, 6p21.33, 7p15.3, 17p11.2, and 22q13.1, which were associated with increased risk of myeloma. These are associated with different genes (Table 53.1). These genes have not been previously investigated in the context of myeloma and further work is required to assess their functional role.

Molecular biology and pathology

Normal plasma cell development

The primary function of a plasma cell is to secrete antibody or immunoglobulin, molecules of which comprise two larger, heavy

Table 53.1 Single nuclear polymorphisms (SNP) identified in genome-wide association studies associated with an increased risk of myeloma and possible candidate genes associated with each SNP

SNP	Possible candidate genes	Function
2p23.3	DNMT3A	DNA methyltransferase
	DTNB	β-dystrobrevin, a component of the dystrophin-associated protein complex
3p22.1	CTNNB1	β catenin gene which activates transcription factors including MYC
	ULK4	Regulator of mTOR mediated autophagy
	TRAK1	Endocytic trafficking of the GABA(A) receptors
3q26.2	TERC	Involved in maintenance of telomere length
6p21.33	PSORS1C1	Psoriasis susceptibility gene
7p15.3	CDCA7L	Cell cycle regulation, directly interacts with MYC
	DNAH11	Dynein heavy-chain microtubule-dependent ATPase motor involved in respiratory cilia movement
22q13.1	CBX7	Encodes a polycomb group protein

chains and two smaller, light chains. In order to generate antibody diversity, a complex sequential system of rearrangements within the germline DNA of immunoglobulin genes has evolved. Heavy (H)-chain rearrangement precedes that of light (L)-chains and kappa (k)-light chain precedes lambda (l) during productive immunoglobulin gene rearrangement. One of a number of variable (V), diversity (D), and joining (J) sequences are brought together to form a functional IgH heavy-chain gene. Diversity results from the ability to use combinations of these different families and from the random insertion of nucleotides by the enzyme terminal deoxyribonucleotidyl transferase at the junctional regions. The same process is undertaken at the immunoglobulin light-chain locus. A functional immunoglobulin molecule is produced by fusion of a variable region with a constant region. The variable regions provide antibody specificity and the constant regions provide specific functions such as complement fixation and activation of other effector functions. The immunoglobulin gene product is present on the surface of a virgin B cell as a receptor. This is composed of the gene product, which provides the specificity, with CD79a and b, the B-cell receptor accessory molecule, and b2-microglobulin.

If virgin B cells encounter an antigen recognized by their surface receptor, they are stimulated to divide. A proportion of the cells produce low-affinity IgM antibodies and the remainder migrate to a germinal centre. Within the germinal centre, affinity maturation utilizes the process of somatic hypermutation (SHM) to introduce DNA mutation into the immunoglobulin (Ig) genes to produce highly specific and avid antibodies [34]. The functionality of these antibodies is potentiated by the ability to use different classes of heavy-chain, a process termed class switch recombination (CSR) as a result of which the class of immunoglobulin produced is changed from IgM or IgD to IgG, IgA, or IgE.

CSR and SHM are essential for the generation of effective antibodies and confer a major survival advantage. Both of these processes require the expression of activation-induced deaminase, which results in double strand breaks (DSBs) in the Ig loci. DSBs are necessary to carry out CSR and SHM and are usually successfully repaired. However, mis-joining of DSBs to others formed elsewhere in the genome is inevitable at a low rate and can result in mutations and chromosomal rearrangements, which can potentially lead to malignancy.

On leaving the germinal centre the plasma cell differentiates from a centroblast to a mature antibody-secreting cell. The main function of a plasma cell is to secrete immunoglobulin, so surface immunoglobulin is no longer expressed but is present in the cytoplasm. Similarly, the B-cell receptor accessory molecules, CD79a and b, are no longer expressed on the cell surface. There are a number of other changes in antigen expression, including downregulation of CD19 and upregulation of CD38 and CD138 (syndecan 1). This process of plasma cell development requires the coordination of several intracellular processes including cell cycle arrest, the compaction of chromatin, the downregulation of proteins not required to produce antibodies, and the upregulation of the protein-producing machinery of the cell. This series of events requires the coordinated expression of transcription factors. These molecules include IRF4, which results in the downregulation of BCL6, whilst BLIMP1 and XBP1 are upregulated. The final stages of plasma cell development depend critically on the expression of XBP1, which mediates the unfolded protein response (UPR). IRE1a senses intracellular stress and the accumulation of unfolded protein and results in the splicing of XBP1 to XBP1s which upregulates proteins providing key mechanisms to effectively manage the accumulation of proteins and promote cell growth and survival (Figure 53.1).

Once in the bone marrow, the normal plasma cell either dies as a result of resolution of the immune response or becomes a long-lived memory plasma cell and survives by interacting with the bone marrow microenvironment.

Myeloma initiation and progression

Myeloma development was previously thought to be the result of the sequential acquisition of aberrant lesions resulting in the transition from normal plasma cell to MGUS and then to MM. It is becoming increasingly clear that the molecular events acquired during this process are not acquired in a linear fashion and rather that branching non-linear pathways, as suggested by Darwin to explain the 'evolution of species', is a crucial feature of disease progression (Figure 53.2) [35]. The events that occur at the roots of the developing disease are either chromosomal translocations, thought to occur as a result of aberrant resolution of double strand breaks, or the acquisition of hyperdiploidy. These events are usually found in close to 100% of clonal cells and are therefore thought to be aetiologic events.

Aetiologic translocations result in oncogenes being placed under the control of strong immunoglobulin gene enhancers on chromosome 14 as shown in Table 53.2. These translocations have prognostic implications for cases in which they are detected, with t(4;14), t(14;16), and t(14;20) associated with poor-risk disease whilst t(11;14) is associated with standard risk. (Risk stratification of myeloma is discussed further below.) The deregulation of the G1/S transition in the cell cycle is recognized as a critical early event in myeloma pathogenesis. It is mediated via the upregulation

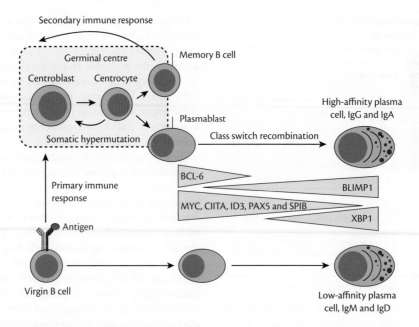

Fig. 53.1 The B-cell immune response. Encouraging antigen drives a virgin B cell to generate a low-affinity plasma cell or stimulates its migration to a germinal centre. In the germinal centre, affinity maturation occurs and is mediated through two processes: somatic hypermutation and antigen selection. Subsequently, class switch recombination (CSR) occurs, leading to the development of immunoglobulin (Ig) isotypes. Once this process is complete, the plasmablast leaves the germinal centre and migrates to the bone marrow where it becomes a long-lived plasma cell that produces antibody. The machinery that is necessary to generate these physiological DNA rearrangements can malfunction, leading to mutations in crucial oncogenes and tumour suppressor genes, and malignant change. Key challenges for a plasma cell include switching off cellular characteristics that are no longer required, such as cell cycling, activating programmes that are essential for antibody production, and undergoing apoptosis if they do not find a receptive niche in the bone marrow. Failure to complete these programmes correctly could potentially leave active cellular processes, which may result in the features of myeloma. The key transcription factors underlying this coordinated differentiation process are also showed.

BCL-6, B-cell lymphoma 6; BLIMP1, B-lymphocyte-induced maturation protein 1; CIIITA, MHC class II transactivator; ID3, DNA-binding protein inhibitor ID3; PAX5, paired-box gene 5; XBP1, X box-binding protein 1.

of cyclin-D as a result of the t(6;14) and t(11;14) translocations but also via non-translocation based upregulation of CCND2, including downstream of MAF and MMSET/FGFR3 activation. Loss of negative regulators of the cell cycle including RB1 and CDKN2C are also important in this transition and the mechanism causing their loss is discussed further below.

Secondary events

There are numerous further genetic events and intracellular pathways that are affected later in the disease process and collaborate with the aetiologic/initiating lesions previously described. These are summarized in the following sections:

Copy number abnormalities/chromosomal gains/losses

Loss or gain of whole or portions of chromosomes resulting in copy number alterations are common in myeloma. Interstitial losses of copy number cause deletion of tumour suppressor genes. Mostly, tumour suppressor genes need both allele copies to be deleted to produce an oncogenic phenotype and driver genes have been identified through analysing mutations along with copy number status. Genes known to be deleted with each chromosomal deletion are 1p: CDKN2C, FAF1, and FAM46C; 11q: BIRC2 and BIRC3; 13: RB1 and DIS3; 14q: TRAF3; 16q: CYLD and WWOX; and 17p: TP53. The latter (del17p) results in the deletion of a gene involved in mediating the apoptotic response to chemotherapy which may be the cause of the poor prognosis in these patients [36].

In contrast, copy number gains lead to the over-expression of oncogenes, for example 1q: CKS1B, ANP32E, BCL-9, and PDZK1.

Translocations

In addition to the translocations previously described, further translocations also occur later in the disease process and are not driven by CSR. These include t(8;14) which causes upregulation of *MYC*. In addition, less well-characterized translocations can occur not involving the immunoglobulin heavy-chain region.

Mutations

The incidence of non-synonymous mutations in myeloma is approximately 35 per case [37]. This number lies between the genetically simpler acute leukaemias and those present in highly complex epithelial tumours such as lung cancer. The few recurrently mutated genes are mostly known oncogenes but some novel genes have also been identified including FAM46C in 13% of cases and DIS3 in 11% of cases. There is a stark contrast to other haematological malignancies such as hairy cell leukaemia which is unified by mutations in the *BRAF* gene. The fact that this is not the case in myeloma supports the theory that it is deregulation of intracellular pathways that is critically important in the pathogenesis of myeloma. Particularly implicated are the RAS/MAPK pathway, constituents of which are mutated in approximately 50% of cases, implying that myeloma is a disease of aberrant RAS signalling.

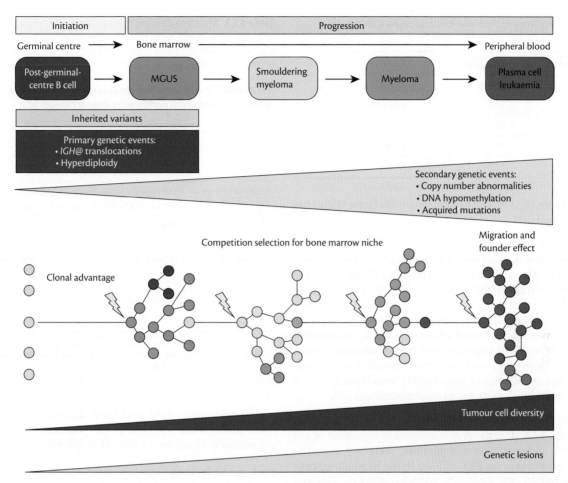

Fig. 53.2 Initiation and progression of myeloma. Monoclonal gammopathy of undetermined significance (MGUS) is an indolent, asymptomatic condition that transforms to myeloma at a rate of 1% per annum. Smouldering myeloma lacks clinical features; by contrast, symptomatic myeloma has various clinical features that are collectively referred to as calcium, renal, anaemia, and bone abnormalities (CRAB), which provide an indication that treatment is required. Later in the disease progression, the myeloma plasma cells are no longer restrained to growth within the bone marrow and can be found at extramedullary sites and as circulating leukaemic cells. It is thought that transition through these different states requires the acquisition of genetic abnormalities that lead to the development of the biological hallmarks of myeloma. The initial deregulated cell belongs to the MGUS clone; however, subsequent to the development of sufficient genetic abnormalities, it acquires a clonal advantage, expands and evolves. This clonal evolution is through the branching pathways that are typically associated with Darwin's explanation of the origin of species. During the evolution of MGUS to myeloma these processes lead to the development of numerous ecosystems, which correspond to the clinically recognized phases of disease. At the end of this evolutionary process, at the stage of plasma cell leukaemia (PCL), the clone is proliferative and no longer confined to the bone marrow; the clone expands rapidly and leads to patient death. Cells at this stage are substantially altered genetically, and the precursor subclones will be present at low levels because of competition for access to the stromal niches in the bone marrow: these clones may be eradicated by more aggressive clones. In evolutionary terms, this phase of disease could be considered to be initiated by a migration and founder effect whereby a cell that is able to survive and grow in the peripheral blood is faced with no competition, thus limiting its clonal expansion.

Abbreviation: IGH@, immunoglobulin heavy-chain locus.

Reprinted by permission from Macmillan Publishers Ltd: *Nature Reviews Cancer*, Morgan GJ et al., The genetic architecture of multiple myeloma, Volume 12, Issue 5, pp. 335–348, Copyright © 2012, Rights Managed by Nature Publishing Group.

Epigenetic aberrations

Epigenetic modifications regulate the process of normal B-cell development and plasma cell differentiation. Several specific epigenetic aberrations have been identified in myeloma pathogenesis. MMSET (WHSC1/NSD2) is a histone lysine methyltransferase of H3K36 that is over-expressed frequently in multiple myeloma as a result of the aetiologic translocation t(4;14) and is associated with a poor prognosis [38]. Other methyltransferases and histone demethylases are also implicated in myeloma pathogenesis including EZH2 (H3K27 methyltransferase) and UTX/KDM6A (H3K27 demethylase), which is mutated in 10% of cases [37].

DNA methylation changes have also been clearly demonstrated to be associated with disease progression [39]. At the transition from MGUS to myeloma, global hypomethylation with gene specific hypermethylation is seen, whilst at the transition from myeloma to plasma cell leukaemia there was re-methylation across the genome [39, 40]. There is also a distinct signature in different cytogenetic subgroups with the most distinct being the t(4;14) subgroup which over-expresses the histone methyltransferase MMSET.

Interaction with the bone marrow microenvironment

MM plasma cells rely on the protective bone marrow microenvironment in order to survive and this is particularly crucial for the myeloma progenitor cell. The interactions between the bone marrow niche and plasma cells have been well studied. The importance of several cytokine and adhesion molecule networks including interleukin 6 (IL-6), tumour necrosis factor α (TNFα), B-cell

Table 53.2 Frequency of translocations associated with the immunoglobulin heavy-chain gene enhancer

Translocation	Frequency	Gene
t(4;14)	11%	MMSET/FGFR3
t(6;14)	<1%	CCND3
t(11;14)	14%	CCND1
t(14;16)	3%	MAF
t(14;20)	1.5%	MAFB

activating factor (BAFF), and hepatocyte growth factor (HGF) has been established [41].

MYC dysregulation

MYC dysregulation is associated with poor prognosis and aggressive disease features. It is present in 15–20% of patients at diagnosis [42, 43]. It can be the result of the (8;14) translocation described previously but *MYC* translocations do not always involve the *IGH* gene, with 40% of translocations involving different partner genes. Moreover, when the *IGH* locus is involved, the breakpoint does not usually occur within switch regions or V(D)J sequences, and the translocation is often complex with more than two chromosomes involved or with associated segmental amplification or inversion [44]. In addition, *MYC* may be upregulated through mutations or other mechanisms [45].

Dysregulation of intracellular pathways

Ras/Raf/MEK/ERK. This pathway is involved in regulation of cell proliferation, differentiation and survival. There is a high frequency of mutations in the ERK pathway shown by whole-genome sequencing (*NRAS* 24%, *KRAS* 27%, and *BRAF* 4%) [37]. This suggests that the ERK pathway is crucial to myeloma cell development.

PI3K/Akt/mTOR. Upregulation of PI3K enhances cell survival by reducing apoptosis. Whilst there are no mutations seen in the PI3K pathway it is known to be deregulated with phosphorylated AKT, indicative of PI3K activity, in 50% of cases. IL-6, IGF-1, and HGF all induce Akt phosphorylation, which in turn activates several downstream targets including mammalian target of rapamycin (mTOR), GSK-3B, and forkhead transcription factor (FKHR). Akt activation has been linked to resistance to dexamethasone-induced apoptosis, mediated through inactivation of capsase-9 [46]. In addition, DEP domain-containing mTOR-interacting protein (DEPTOR) is upregulated, often as a result of MAF translocations [47, 48].

NF-kB. The NF-kB pathway is upregulated in myeloma cells and causes disruption of cell cycle and apoptotic pathways. It also has a role in bone marrow stromal cells where it triggers cytokines such as Il-6 and BAFF [49–54]. 11q, 16q, and 14q deletions, some interstitial copy number gains, and some mutations affect genes involved in the Nf-kB pathway further indicating that upregulation of this pathway is important in myeloma.

JAK/STAT. This pathway has been shown to be upregulated in 50% of myeloma samples [55].

Clinical presentation

Myeloma causes clinical disease though the accumulation of malignant plasma cells in the bone marrow which secrete a monoclonal immunoglobulin called a 'paraprotein'. Presenting symptoms include anaemia in 50–75% of patients, hypercalcaemia (15%),

Table 53.3 Myeloma defining events. Clonal bone marrow plasma cells >=10% or biopsy proven bony or extramedullary plasmacytoma and either evidence of end organ damage (1) or a biomarker of malignancy (2)

(1) Evidence of end organ damage that can be attributed to the underlying plasma cell proliferative disorder specifically:	
Hypercalcaemia	Serum calcium >0.25mmol/L (>1mg/dL) higher than the upper limit of normal or >2.75 mmol/L (>11 mg/dL)
Renal insufficiency	Creatinine clearance <40ml /min or serum creatinine >177umol/L (>2 mg/dL)
Anaemia	Haemoglobin value of >20 g/L below the lower limit of normal , or a haemoglobin value <100g/L
Bone lesions	One or more osteolytic lesions on skeletal radiography, CT or PET-CT.

(2) Any one or more of the following biomarkers of malignancy:
Clonal bone marrow plasma cell percentage >= 60%
Involved:uninvolved serum free light chain ratio >=100
>1 focal lesions on MRI studies

Reproduced from Criteria for the classification of monoclonal gammopathis, Multiple myeloma and related disorders: A report of the International Myeloma Working Group, *British Journal of Haematology*, Volume 121, Issue 5, pp. 749–757, Copyright © 2003 John Wiley and Sons Ltd, with permission from John Wiley and Sons Ltd.

renal impairment (20%), and bone disease (70–80%) [56–58]. These clinical features are part of the diagnostic criteria for initiating treatment in myeloma (Table 53.3) [58, 59].

Lytic bone lesions

The cellular proliferation of myeloma cells in the axial skeleton produces the bone pain and destruction that dominates the clinical picture of myeloma. Malignant plasma cells uncouple the process of normal bone formation by osteoblasts and bone resorption by osteoclasts. The result is osteolytic lesions, which are present in 60–70% of patients at diagnosis [60]. Lytic lesions increase the risk of skeletal-related events defined as pathological fractures, spinal cord compression, the requirement for radiotherapy or surgery, and hypercalcaemia. Although bone pain may be gradual in onset, pathological fractures are frequent and are usually indicated by the sudden onset of local tenderness and pain. Fracture may be caused by minor trauma. Loss of height due to collapse of vertebrae and kyphosis are common.

Hypercalcaemia

Bone destruction releases calcium into the blood resulting in hypercalcaemia. Approximately one-fifth of patients will be hypercalcaemic at presentation and about half of these will have symptoms on close questioning. Many more patients will become hypercalcaemic during the course of their illness. Symptoms include nausea, vomiting, polyuria, polydipsia, constipation, or confusion. Characteristically, despite hypercalcaemia and radiological bone destruction, the serum alkaline phosphatase is not greatly raised because of the lack of osteoblastic bone regeneration.

Immunoparesis

Myeloma patients are immunosuppressed and susceptible to bacterial infections, particularly with gram positive bacteria. The causes of this immunodeficiency are complex but mainly involve abnormalities of immunoglobulin production. Patients may be hypogammaglobulinaemic and demonstrate an impairment of the primary immune response, while the secondary immune response and cellular immunity remain relatively preserved in untreated patients. The risk of infection is particularly important in early phases of anti-myeloma therapy. In cases of hypogammaglobulinaemia and recurrent infection intravenous immunoglobulin supplementation may be helpful. Patients with MGUS may also be immunosuppressed with an increased risk of developing bacterial and viral infections at twice the rate of controls [61, 62].

Renal failure

20–30% of patients have renal impairment at diagnosis and up to 10% may require dialysis [63]. The most direct mechanism of renal failure is a result of the precipitation of immunoglobulin free light-chains in the lumen of the distal tubule causing intratubular obstruction resulting in interstitial inflammation and fibrosis and classical cast nephropathy. Light-chains may also cause damage in the glomerulus, such as that seen in amyloid light-chain amyloidosis (AL) and light-chain deposition disease, or in the proximal tubule which characteristically presents with acquired Fanconi syndrome or progressive renal fibrosis [64]. Renal failure can also be caused by hypercalcaemia leading to dehydration, infection, contrast media, non-steroidal anti-inflammatory drugs, and (rarely) as a result of renal vein thrombosis. These factors may also precipitate cast nephropathy. The presence of a high urine albumin should raise the suspicion of amyloid deposition or light-chain deposition disease [65]. The advent of tests to monitor light-chains in the blood has enabled early intervention prior to renal failure to reduce serum free light-chains.

Cytopenias

Bone marrow occupancy by plasma cells reduces the ability of normal bone marrow precursors from developing, leading to anaemia, thrombocytopenia, and neutropenia. Anaemia is often compounded by low erythropoietin levels due to renal failure.

Hyperviscosity

Symptoms of hyperviscosity may be seen with very high concentrations of monoclonal protein (typically IgA >40g/L or IgG >60g/L) which may lead to hypervolaemia. The clinical hyperviscosity/hypervolaemia syndrome includes a predisposition to bleeding, particularly from mucosal surfaces, and dilatation and segmentation of retinal and conjunctival veins. A range of central nervous system disturbances are seen, characterized by headache, drowsiness, weakness, and confusion that may progress to epileptic fits, paralysis, and coma. Symptomatic hyperviscosity should be treated as a medical emergency.

Soft tissue plasmacytomas

Extramedullary plasmacytomas may be present at diagnosis and involvement of almost every organ has been described. Extradural deposits may occur with resultant cord compression.

Cryoglobulins

Some 5% of myeloma paraproteins can precipitate in the cold [66] but this usually does not result in clinical problems. Occasionally, cryoglobulinaemia in myeloma can produce vascular problems, leg ulcers, and Raynaud's phenomenon as well as renal, central nervous system, and gastrointestinal disorders. Biopsies will usually show a vasculitis. In severe cases, peripheral gangrene, renal failure, severe purpura, or gastrointestinal perforation can result, so that vigorous treatment of the underlying myeloma and avoidance of cold exposure is indicated.

Other biochemical findings

Hyponatraemia and a low anion gap

Cationic proteins can lead to an artefactual hyponatraemia associated with retention of chloride and bicarbonate, leading to a low anion gap, usually not requiring treatment.

Hyperlipidaemia

The finding of high- and low-density lipoproteins to paraprotein has been described, which can lead to the clinical syndrome of xanthomatosis and marked serum lipidaemia.

Hyperuricaemia

Hyperuricaemia results from an increased cell turnover and decreased renal excretion of urate; theoretically, this could be a factor in the development of renal failure in myeloma. Prophylactic allopurinol is widely recommended at the time of initiating treatment.

Diagnostic investigations

Patients with a detected paraprotein or clinically suspected myeloma should be investigated as outlined in Figure 53.3. Specific clinical scenarios prompting investigation include:

- Unexplained anaemia, hypercalcaemia, or hyperviscosity
- Identified serum or urine paraprotein/abnormal serum free light-chain ratio
- Lytic lesions detected on radiological imaging
- Cast nephropathy, amyloid or light-chain deposition on biopsy (renal or other)
- Immunoparesis
- Plasma cells seen on blood film

Tables 53.3 and 53.4 summarize the International Myeloma Working Group (IMWG) diagnostic criteria for myeloma, asymptomatic myeloma, and MGUS updated in 2014.

The investigations essential to make the diagnosis of myeloma and stage the disease are described in the following section.

Detection and quantification of the monoclonal protein

This is done by serum and urine electrophoresis (SPEP/UPEP) where the abnormal accumulation of a large amount of protein of exactly the same size causes a 'spike' that can be quantified. This detects the whole immunoglobulin molecule that is overproduced. The presence of a spike of any level is always abnormal though may be due to a number of different underlying causes and is not always indicative of a neoplastic process. The type of paraprotein present is identified by immunofixation, which uses antisera specific to the different potential immunoglobulin types to identify them.

More recently, assays have been developed to identify the production of light-chains, which are usually produced in excess of heavy-chains during the antibody development process and so are likely to be detectable at high levels when immunoglobulin

(A)

Blood tests	Bone marrow	Imaging studies	Protein studies
Full blood count and Erythrocyte Sedimentation Rate (ESR) Serum Urea and electrolytes (U+Es) and live function (LFTs) Serum albumin, calcium and uric acid B_2 microglobulin C-reactive protein (CRP) Lactate dehydrogenase (LDH) Vitamin B12 and folate Coagulation screen Blood film	Aspirate for morphology, flow cytometry iFISH and cytogenetics Trephine See part (B), (C) and (D)	As per local protocols to look for evidence of myeloma related bone disease. MRI in case of suspected cord compression See part (E), (F), (G), (H)	Serum protein electrophoresis, immunofixation and M-protein quantification Serum immunoglobulins Serum Free light chain levels and ratio Urine electrophoresis and immunofixation 24 hour urine for creatinine clearance and urinary protein or urinary protein: creatinine ratio

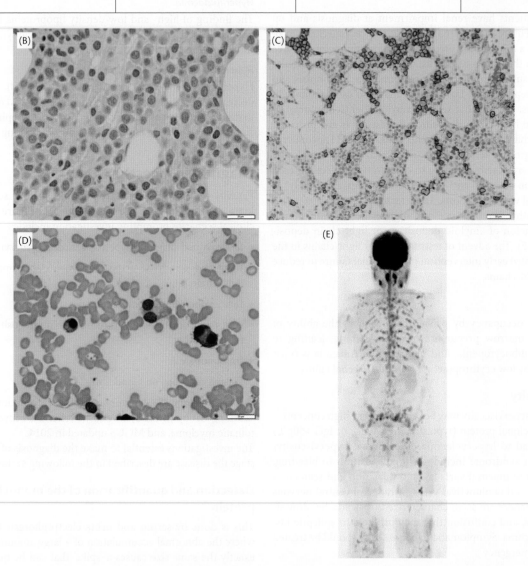

Fig. 53.3 (A) Basic diagnostic work up for myeloma/suspected plasma cell dyscrasia. In patients with MGUS, bone marrow and imaging studies are not considered essential provided there is no evidence of end-organ damage and the disease is classified as low risk for progression, i.e., IgG paraprotein <15g/L with normal SFLC ratio and no symptoms or other clinical features of concern. (B) Haematoxylin and eosin stain (× 60) of bone marrow trephine demonstrating asynchronous plasma cells in a patient with relapsing myeloma. (C) CD138 immunohistochemical staining (× 10) of bone marrow trephine highlights plasma cell infiltrate and enables quantification. (D) Bone marrow aspirate (× 60) demonstrating abnormal plasma cells including binucleate forms in a newly-diagnosed patient. (E) Whole-body diffusion weighted MRI demonstrating multi-focal bone disease throughout the axial skeleton. (F) 18F-FDG PET-CT of a 67-year-old myeloma patient with widespread FDG avid sites of disease infiltration seen in the skeletal system. (G) Sagittal T1 weighted MRI, and (H) axial T2 weighted MRI. Images show classical malignant collapse: bulging posterior cortex, involvement of pedicles, and soft tissue component causing compromise to the spinal canal.

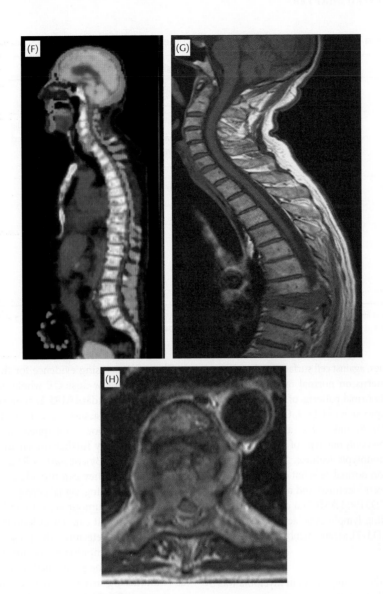

Fig. 53.3 Continued

production is in overdrive. They may be overproduced along with a detectable paraprotein and are called serum free light-chains (SFLC). The use of free light-chain assays, however, has also enabled the detection of measurable protein in patients who would have been previously classified as non-secretory (i.e., without a detectable paraprotein or urine protein by SPEP or UPEP but with an infiltrate of plasma cells on bone marrow) [34]. Rare true non-secretory disease is, therefore, now classified as the absence of paraprotein by SPEP, immunofixation and UPEP, and normal SFLC analysis. In a cohort of 2709 MRC myeloma trial patients in the UK, 85% secreted a whole paraprotein (56% IgG, 27% IgA and 2% IgD). In those who produced a whole paraprotein there were sufficient FLC secreted to exceed the renal threshold and become detectable in urine in 70%; in over 90% the SFLC ratio was abnormal. In 13% of the total cohort only SFLC were secreted and just 2% were oligo/non-secretory [67].

Assessment of plasma cell infiltration by bone marrow aspirate and trephine

The proportion of plasma cells in normal bone marrow is usually less than 4% of nucleated cells, although a working level of 5% is often taken as normal. In reactive plasmacytoses, the proportion of plasma cells may exceed 30%, emphasizing how difficult it is to define a normal level for plasma cells. The morphology and distribution of plasma cells can help in distinguishing reactive from malignant proliferations. The morphological features that differentiate malignant plasma cells from their normal counterparts include a considerable variation in size, shape, basophilia, nuclear maturity, and the number of nuclei present within the plasma cells [68, 69]. The trephine biopsy is most useful in distinguishing reactive plasmacytoses from myelomatous infiltration. Normal plasma cells usually occur singly and in close proximity to the bone marrow microvasculature. In myeloma, this distribution is altered and plasma cells are situated between fat cells away from the vasculature. Within the bone marrow the plasma-cell infiltration is uneven, so that the percentage infiltration in a single trephine biopsy might not be representative of the level of infiltration in the marrow as a whole. When infiltration is heavier, in addition to focal deposits it can become diffuse.

A sample of the bone marrow aspirate should also be sent for flow cytometry assessment. Flow cytometry allows the determination of neoplastic vs normal plasma cells. This is done by using antibodies,

Table 53.4 International Myeloma Working Group criteria for diagnosis of other plasma cell dyscrasias

	MGUS	Light-chain MGUS	Smouldering myeloma
Clonal plasma cells present in bone marrow	<10%	<10%	≥10% but <60%
Monoclonal protein	Serum: <30 g/L Urine: <500mg/24hrs	Serum: None but abnormal serum free light chain ratio (<0.26 or >1.65) with elevated level of involved light chain. Urine: <500mg/24hrs	Serum: ≥30 g/L Urine: >=500mg/24 hr
End organ damage attributable to underlying plasma cell proliferation	No	No	No
Other features	Non-IgM in most cases precedes progression to myeloma or solitary plasmacytoma. IgM – more likely to progress to Waldenström's macroglobulinaemia		

Source: data from *The Lancet Oncology*, Volume 15, Issue 11, S Vincent Rajkumar et al., International Myeloma Working Group updated criteria for the diagnosis of multiple myeloma, pp. e538–e548, Copyright © 2014 Elsevier Ltd, http://www.sciencedirect.com/science/journal/14702045.

labelled with fluorescent moieties, against cell surface markers known to be present in different patterns on normal or malignant cells. Myeloma plasma cells show abnormal patterns of expression of cell surface proteins with under-expression of CD19, CD 27, and CD45, over-expression of CD38, CD138, and CD56, and asynchronous expression of CD20. They express only one type of light-chain, kappa or lambda, consistent with monotypic features. Several other cell surface glycoproteins, present on normal cells but over-expressed on myeloma plasma cells, have been identified and are also targets for therapy. These include CS1 (CD319/SLAMF7) a cell surface receptor that belongs to the signalling lymphocytic activation molecule (SLAM) family and HM1.24 (CD317), a transmembrane glycoprotein.

Cytogenetics

Previously the only way to analyse cytogenetics in myeloma was by G-banded chromosome profiling of chromosomes in metaphase. The problems with this technology are the time and cost involved, and that metaphases are often not achievable and reciprocal translocations can be missed. Interphase fluorescence in situ hybridization (FISH) is now commonly used, with fluorescently-labelled probes which hybridize to the regions of DNA of interest. This remains an expensive technique, however, and for this diagnostic information to be more widely available and at a lower cost, new modalities—particularly to look for translocations associated with adverse outcomes—are being developed, such as polymerase chain reaction (PCR) techniques [70].

Bone imaging

Skeletal survey has been the gold standard for the detection of myeloma-associated lytic lesions, which appear as radiolucent areas on plain film skeletal survey of at least the skull, ribs, pelvis, entire spine, and both humeri and femora. The procedure is time-consuming, interpreter-dependent, and not very sensitive; in addition, it is necessary to lose >30% of trabecular bone to detect a lytic lesion on a plain film. There is also difficulty in detecting bone healing and a new vertebral collapse, for example, may not necessarily represent new disease.

There is increasing evidence for the use other imaging modalities, including low-dose CT, whole-body diffusion-weighted MRI, PET-CT, and standard MRI. Low-dose CT can image all bones and more accurately assess the extent of bone destruction, identifying lesions that would not appear on a skeletal survey. It does not, however, give any further information about activity or viability of tumour cells. By contrast, MRI and PET-CT give a more functional image as they can provide a surrogate for tumour activity. Using MRI scanning, signal changes can indicate when the marrow is infiltrated by tumour cells. In addition, MRI is the best way to image the spine. It can detect lesions in areas difficult to interpret on plain films, determine the presence and extent of spinal cord or nerve root compression and identify soft tissue masses. A spinal MRI should be performed in all patients otherwise classified as smouldering myeloma to rule out lesions that would prompt treatment. PET-CT is able to identify metabolically active lesions by the uptake of fluorodeoxyglucose (FDG) in cells with high glucose demand but is not as sensitive as MRI at detecting lesions in the spine.

Each modality, therefore, has advantages and disadvantages and should be considered based on the clinical history and availability until clinical trial data is available to further inform choice. The radiation dose of each approach should also be considered in an era where patients are surviving beyond ten years. These more sensitive imaging techniques can upgrade disease in a number of cases, which may have an impact on response and progression data from clinical trials. It is important to note that isotope bone scans are not useful in myeloma because the lesions are lytic and do not take up the scan isotope which recognizes sclerotic lesions only.

Disease risk assessments

Monoclonal gammopathy of undetermined significance (MGUS) risk stratification

The risk of progression from MGUS to myeloma has been linked to the size of the paraprotein (>15g/L), type of paraprotein (non-IgG), and the concurrent presence of an abnormal free light-chain (SFLC) ratio [71]. The absolute risk is 5% at 20 years for patients with no risk factors with this increasing to 21% with one risk factor, 37% with two and 58% with three. Flow cytometry can also provide useful information regarding risk of progression with the percentage of clonal plasma cells correlating with risk along with the trajectory of increase in the paraprotein. These risk factors should be considered when approaching the workup of a patient with apparent MGUS. However, the consensus opinion is that a bone marrow aspirate and imaging investigations may not be indicated in cases where the paraprotein is an IgG <15g/L and the SFLC ratio is normal, provided there are no other clinical features of MM.

Smouldering risk stratification

The risk of progression from smouldering myeloma (SMM) to multiple myeloma has been shown to be increased with the coexistence of paraprotein level >30g/L and >10% plasma cells in the bone marrow [71]. In another study, the presence of aberrant plasma cells by immunophenotyping and the presence of immunoparesis predicted for shorter time to progression [72]. It is becoming increasingly clear that there are two populations of SMM: one with a poor prognosis and rapid transition to myeloma and the other behaving more like MGUS. Separating these subtypes of disease accurately is difficult using flow cytometry alone, although gene expression profiling may help.

Myeloma risk stratification

Diagnostic investigations can be used to assess disease risk. The international staging system (ISS) scoring system has now replaced the previously used Durie-Salmon criteria. The ISS risk stratification combines β_2 microglobulin (β_2M) and albumin at diagnosis and correlates with disease outcome, even in the era of novel therapies. For stage I, serum β2 microglobulin is <3.5 mg/L and albumin ≥35 g/L; stage II does not meet the criteria for stage I or III, and stage III serum β2 microglobulin is ≥5.5 mg/L [73]. This essentially combines an assessment of the burden of disease and renal function (β_2M) with an assessment of overall patient condition (albumin). Using this model, patients are classified in three groups with very different median overall survival: 62 months for stage I, 44 months for stage II, and 29 months for stage III. However, MM is a heterogeneous disease at the cellular level and an increased knowledge of the impact of genetic events combined with the ISS can give improved prognostic accuracy. The most important genetic predictors of an adverse outcome are the t(4;14), del17p, and 1q+ abnormalities. The IMWG has therefore divided patients into iFISH-ISS groups with group I comprising those patients with ISS stage I or II with no adverse cytogenetic lesions, group 2 ISS 3 with no adverse lesions or ISS stage I with an adverse lesion, and group 3 ISS stage II or III with an adverse cytogenetic lesion. The four-year progression-free survival (PFS) and overall survival (OS) estimates are 44%, 23%, and 12% for PFS and 76%, 52%, and 33% for OS, respectively (p <0.0001 in each case), showing that the criteria were clearly prognostic. Accuracy was confirmed on subgroup analysis according to age, treatment strategy, etc. [74]. In addition, it has been shown that accumulating more than one adverse genetic lesion predicts for a worse survival [75].

A number of different gene expression signatures using microarrays technology have been reported. Although the technology used is now well understood and validated there is very little overlap in signatures defined by different groups [76, 77]. This lack of concordance may signify different aspects of myeloma biology and attempts are being made to unify gene expression profiling prognostic signatures using prognostic modelling [78].

Other predictors for a poor response to therapy and shorter OS include the presence of blastic morphology and renal failure at diagnosis. The purpose of using these risk stratification approaches should be to move away from treating all myelomas alike to tailoring treatment towards a particular risk group. Several groups have developed models for this but none has yet been universally adopted [79].

Response assessment

Disease response can be monitored by repeat measurement of the serum paraprotein and serum free light-chains. It is important to remember, however, that the half-lives of these vary from two to four hours for SFLC to 25 days for IgG, which should be considered when interpreting results. Repeat bone marrow aspirates are performed to look for evidence of plasma cells by morphology both on the aspirate and trephine. More recently, multiparameter flow cytometry, clonal specific PCR techniques and next-generation sequencing approaches have become available to look for a low level of plasma cells remaining that would not be visible using other techniques and in the absence of an abnormal paraprotein or SFLC analysis. This is termed minimal residual disease (MRD). PCR techniques are time-consuming, whilst flow cytometry is more widely available. Using standardized, eight-colour flow panels, the presence of one malignant cell in 1×10^6 cells can be detected.

The response of disease to treatment has been standardized and the IMWG criteria are shown in Table 53.5 [80]. The inclusion of the stringent complete response (sCR) criteria, including the absence of MRD by flow cytometry and a normal SFLC ratio, reflects the correlation between MRD negativity and improved survival [81, 82]. The clinical benefit rate (CBR) for a drug is defined as the proportion of patients achieving at least a minimal response (MR) to a treatment. This is used for responses to agents given in the relapsed disease setting when the depth of response is less critical but disease control is a more central focus.

Management at diagnosis

Patients with myeloma-defining events (criteria in Table 53.3) require immediate treatment as without treatment OS is only ten months. Increasingly, agents have become available that modify the natural history of disease and can prevent end-organ damage. These have improved outcomes with significant numbers of survivors at ten years, leading some investigators to talk of a cure for myeloma [83]. In addition, these agents are being increasingly evaluated earlier in the natural history of the disease such as in high-risk smouldering myeloma, especially for younger patients.

Monoclonal gammopathy of undetermined significance/smouldering myeloma

There is no evidence that any intervention currently available is able to delay the progression of MGUS to myeloma. Therefore, at this stage there is no indication that population screening would be of benefit. Once identified, MGUS patients should be followed depending on their risk of transformation to multiple myeloma. The risk of progression remains fairly constant throughout the lifetime of an individual and so follow-up should be lifelong. Several conditions have been linked to MGUS indirectly associated with

Table 53.5 International Myeloma Working Group response criteria

sCR (stringent complete response)	As CR (below) plus normal SFLC ratio and absence of clonal plasma cells by immunohistochemistry or flow cytometry
CR (complete response)	Negative immunofixation of serum and urine
	Disappearance of any soft tissue plasmacytomas and <5% plasma cells in bone marrow
	(In the case of SFLC only myeloma CR also requires normalization of SFLC ratio)
VGPR (very good partial response)	Serum and urine M-protein detectable by immunofixation but not on electrophoresis or >= 90% reduction in serum M-protein plus urine M-protein level <100 mg/24hrs
	(In the case of SFLC only myeloma then reduction in the difference between involved and uninvolved SFLC by >= 90%)
PR (partial response)	>= 50% reduction of serum M-protein and reduction in 24 hours urinary M-protein by >= 90% or to <200 mg/24 hrs
	If the serum and urine M-protein are unmeasurable, a >= 50% decrease in the difference between involved and uninvolved SFLC is required
	In non-secretory myeloma a >= 50% reduction in bone marrow plasma cells (provided baseline was >= 30%)
	If soft tissue plasmacytoma present the >= 50% reduction in size
SD (stable disease)	Not meeting criteria for sCR, CR, VGPR, PR, or PD
PD (progressive disease)	Increase of >= 25% from lowest response value in one or more of:
	Serum M-protein (absolute increased must be >= 5g/L)
	Urine M-protein (absolute increased must be >= 200 mg/24hrs)
	If serum and urine M-protein are unmeasurable, the difference between involved and uninvolved SFLC (absolute increase must be >100 mg/L)
	Bone marrow plasma cell percentage (absolute percentage must be >10%)
	Bone lesion or soft tissue plasmacytoma (or the development of new lesions)
	Or
	Development of hypercalcaemia that can be attributed solely to the plasma cell proliferative disorder
Only used in the setting of response assessment for novel agents used in relapsed refractory patients:	
MR (minimal response)	>= 25% (but <= 49%) reduction of serum M-protein and reduction in 24 hr urine M-protein by 50–90% plus 25–50% reduction in size of plasmacytomas if present and no increase in number of bone lesions
CBR (clinically beneficial response)	MR, PR, VGPR, CR, and sCR combined

Adapted by permission from Macmillan Publishers Ltd: *Leukemia*, Durie BG et al., International uniform response criteria for multiple myeloma, Volume 20, Issue 9, pp. 1467–1473, Copyright © 2009 Nature Publishing Group. All rights reserved.

the paraprotein and these should be monitored during follow-up. These include an increased risk of infections as a result of immunodeficiency from a reduced level of uninvolved immunoglobulins [14], osteoporosis [84, 85], venous thromboembolism [86] and malignancy [87]. Patients with osteoporosis should be managed with bisphosphonates and calcium/vitamin D supplements. Related to their paraprotein, patients may develop cryoglobulinaemia, neuropathy, and renal impairment. If patients develop severe symptoms directly attributed to the MGUS clone, then treatment to eradicate the clone should be initiated.

Patients with high-risk MGUS (defined as paraprotein >15g/L, non IgG paraprotein, or the presence of an abnormal SFLC ratio) and those meeting the criteria for asymptomatic myeloma should be followed-up in a specialist haematology clinic. Trials of treatment of high-risk smouldering myeloma show that early intervention may be beneficial, with some studies already reporting an increased OS for early treatment [88]. It is recommended that patients with high-risk smouldering myeloma should receive bisphosphonate therapy [89].

Serious conditions, discussed in the following section, manifested by a small paraprotein that should be actively managed include POEMS syndrome and amyloid (discussed below).

Myeloma treatment

Strategy

The ultimate aim of myeloma treatment is to completely eradicate the clonal plasma cells to achieve a cure. In many cases this is not achieved and the goal shifts to maintaining a low level of disease for as long as possible, postponing relapse and the point at which patients require further treatment. The depth of response to treatment predicts for time-to-progression, so that achieving maximal response, where no clonal cells are detectable by any currently available technologies, is the target of initial therapy (Figure 53.4).

Current strategies of treatment utilize blocks of therapy, termed induction and consolidation, to exert as much pressure as possible on the clonal cells, using different modalities of treatment in each, so that subclones resistant to the first type of chemotherapy given may also succumb. Consolidation therapy can be in the form of

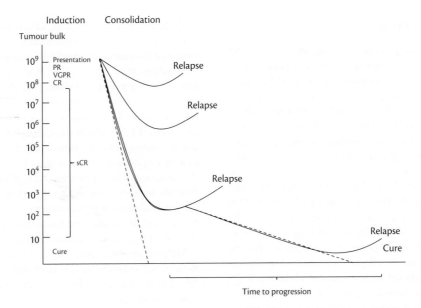

Fig. 53.4 The graph shows the hypothesized tumour bulk on the y axis with the number of clonal cells present. At present our diagnostic criteria (CR, VGPR, etc.) define a small range of reduction in tumour cells. Trial data suggests that the greater the reduction in tumour bulk for example achieving an sCR rather than PR following ASCT is associated with a longer overall survival. Reducing the tumour burden still further by the use of consolidation chemotherapy may improve outcomes further. Improved methods of detection of residual clonal cells to lower levels may help us make more informed decisions about further treatment requirements enabling the reduction of tumour bulk still further and ultimately curing patients of disease.

an autologous transplant and/or further blocks of chemotherapy, given after or without autologous transplant. Maintenance chemotherapy involves continuing treatment to kill remaining myeloma stem cells as they come into cell cycle and to control any residual cells. The aim of maintenance is to modify the disease biology and prolong survival; it is of crucial importance for a maintenance regimen to maintain quality of life.

The mainstay of induction treatment over the past ten years has been the so-called 'novel' drugs bortezomib, a proteasome inhibitor, and thalidomide and lenalidomide, immunomodulatory agents. In the UK, five-year survival rates increased from 26% between 1996–2000 to 37% between 2005–2009. Median OS for younger, fitter patients eligible for autologous stem cell transplant is now greater than six years, with a recent study in the US showing median OS not reached at 5.9 years of follow-up for those <65 years and 5.0 years for those aged >65 years. These improvements in OS were particularly notable in the older population [83]. The majority (62%) of patients included in this analysis received a lenalidomide-containing regimen with >90% receiving at least one novel agent. PFS also continues to improve; in patients treated with bortezomib-containing regimens PFS was 35.9 months for those eligible for autologous stem cell transplant (ASCT) in a recent meta-analysis [90]. This compares to 20.3 months for those receiving a thalidomide-containing regimen in a meta-analysis of transplant-ineligible patient trials [91]. As treatment continues to improve, it takes longer for survival data to mature so that surrogate markers of benefit, e.g., response rates, are increasingly important.

The improvements seen in survival rates have mainly been for patients with low-risk disease as defined by cytogenetics. Patients at higher risk are generally either poorly responsive or resistant to first-line treatment or have a good response but relapse quickly. It is thought that their outcomes could be improved by using more intensive chemotherapy regimens followed by continuous therapy in order to achieve and maintain remission.

Novel agents are commonly given in combination with steroids (dexamethasone or prednisolone) and with the oral alkylating agents melphalan or cyclophosphamide. The use of anthracyclines, such as doxorubicin, has declined since the arrival of novel agents but are still used in certain situations. Benefit from combining two novel agents has also been demonstrated. The modes of action and side effects of commonly used drugs are summarized in Box 53.1.

When deciding on a treatment schedule for myeloma patients it is important to consider both the age and comorbidities of the patient. Younger, fitter patients generally have their response to induction chemotherapy consolidated with an autologous stem cell transplant whilst older or less fit patients likely will not tolerate the intensive chemotherapy given during this procedure.

Younger/fitter patients
Induction
The novel agents thalidomide, bortezomib, and lenalidomide have significantly improved patient outcomes. They are used as induction therapy for myeloma in two, three, or four drug combinations, which are capable of inducing rapid disease response and lasting remissions. Which drugs are combined in the first-line setting should be determined by patient factors such as pre-existing neuropathy (for lenalidomide and thalidomide) or the presence of renal failure, which may require the avoidance of certain therapies, and tumour factors. For example, there is evidence that bortezomib can overcome the poor prognosis associated with the t(4;14) cytogenetic lesion and also is the most effective agent for patients presenting with renal failure. The availability of certain drugs in specific clinical settings or limitations by funding bodies or regulatory approvals in different countries also need to be taken into account.

Benefit has been demonstrated from the combination of novel agents with dexamethasone and a third agent (often the alkylating agent cyclophosphamide). Clinical trials have demonstrated benefit from the use of three drugs over two [104, 105]. Four drug

---

Box 53.1 Drugs used in myeloma

Bortezomib (Velcade®) is a proteasome inhibitor, which works by multiple mechanisms including targeting the unfolded protein response (UPR), inducing endoplasmic reticulum (ER) stress, inhibiting NFkB and suppressing several anti-apoptotic proteins [92]. It is usually given as a 21-day cycle of treatment with subcutaneous injections twice weekly for two weeks followed by a week off. Common side effects include thrombocytopenia, peripheral neuropathy, autonomic neuropathy, gastrointestinal toxicity, and fatigue. The use of the subcutaneous administration route and weekly dosing has reduced the incidence of neuropathy compared to intravenous use [93]. There are standard dose reduction protocols shown in the summary of product characteristics to be followed in the event of these side effects occurring during treatment. Bortezomib is commonly given in combination with the steroid dexamethasone and the alkylating agent cyclophosphamide. It may also be combined with immunomodulatory drugs with evidence that this improves response rates. Bortezomib is safe to give even at low GFR and due to this and its rapid reduction in tumour bulk is considered standard first-line treatment in patients presenting with renal function. There is some evidence that it can overcome the adverse risk associated with t(4;14) myeloma.

Thalidomide was the first in the family of immunomodulatory drugs (IMiD) to be used in the treatment of myeloma. It has been shown to block several pathways important for disease progression in myeloma. It was initially investigated due to its known anti-angiogenic properties but also inhibits IL-6, activates apoptosis and augments natural killer cell function and number thereby enhancing the anti-myeloma immune response [94–96]. More recently, it has been shown that many of these effects occur as a result of IMiDs binding to the intracellular protein cereblon and it is reported that low cereblon expression is correlated with drug resistance and poor survival but measuring cereblon levels is difficult and we need antibodies that can measure the protein and studies to address the impact of reduction in its expression level [97, 98].

Thalidomide is usually given continuously as a 21-day cycle. Common side effects include peripheral neuropathy, constipation, fatigue, bradycardia, skin rashes, thyroid dysfunction and, rarely, cytopenias. When given in combination regimens it is associated with an increased risk of thromboembolism and so thromboprophylaxis is given whilst patients are on therapy. The teratogenic effects of thalidomide should be carefully considered and patients counselled to avoid pregnancy; both in females of childbearing potential and in the partner of male patients. Schemes for pregnancy counselling and regimens for testing are followed strictly prior to prescribing. It is commonly given with dexamethasone and cyclophosphamide. It may also be combined with proteasome inhibitors or older agents such as bendamustine.

Lenalidomide (Revlimid®) is a newer, more efficacious, oral IMiD with a similar mechanism of action to thalidomide but with a slightly different side effect profile with a higher incidence of cytopenias but lower risk of peripheral neuropathy. It is usually given as a 28-day cycle with three weeks of daily treatment followed by a week break due to the higher incidence of cytopenias. The risk of teratogenicity persists. Combination treatment

with dexamethasone is usual. Lenalidomide is renally excreted and so needs to be dose reduced in renal failure with close monitoring of haematologic toxicities in case it accumulates.

Bendamustine is an anti-tumour agent with mechanisms of action similar to both alkylating agents and purine analogues. It can induce both single and double strand breaks in DNA, which are more durable than those seen with other agents, and result in impaired DNA synthesis and repair [99, 100]. It is administered intravenously and commonly given on days one and eight of a 28-day cycle or one and two of a 28-day cycle. Studies have demonstrated efficacy in relapsed myeloma in combination with steroids and novel chemotherapy agents. Due to its similarity to purine analogues it is recommended that patients who receive bendamustine should have irradiated blood products to prevent the risk of transfusion associated graft-vs-host disease [101].

Melphalan is an alkylating agent and can be given intravenously, for example as the high dose chemotherapy prior to ASCT or as oral tablets for older, less fit patients often in combination regimens.

Cyclophosphamide is an alkylating agent, which has substantially less mutagenic toxicity than melphalan [102]. It is administered orally in combination with either IMiDs or proteasome inhibitors as part of induction or relapse regimens. It is also used as a mobilization agent for stem cell harvesting.

Doxorubicin (Adriamycin®) is an anthracycline which was previously commonly used as induction treatment for myeloma. Its use has been superseded following the introduction of novel agents, however, it is still used in certain contexts, for example in the treatment of highly aggressive or proliferative disease. It has well-recognized side effects of cardiotoxicity with cumulative dosing and can also cause hair loss, cytopenias, and will discolour urine for 24–48 hours after administration.

Corticosteroids usually dexamethasone or prednisolone, have activity against myeloma as single agents but also show additive and synergistic activity with other chemotherapeutic agents and are included in almost all combination regimens.

Pomalidomide is a new generation IMiD which has a high potency in vitro and a similar side effect profile to lenaliomide. It has anti-angiogenic, anti-proliferative (NFkB inhibition), pro-apoptotic, and immunomodulatory properties including downregulation of inflammatory cytokines and stimulation of cytotoxic T-cells. It is structurally similar to lenalidomide and thalidomide but differs functionally and in its side effect profile, the most common side effects being myelosuppression and venous thromboembolism. It is an oral drug, recently licenced, and is administered on day 21 of a 28-day cycle in combination with low-dose dexamethasone. Pomalidomide plus low-dose dexamethasone prolonged PFS to 4 months vs 1.9 months for patients treated with high-dose dexamethasone alone in a recent phase III clinical trial [103].

Carfilzomib is a new generation epoxyketone proteasome inhibitor which irreversibly binds and inhibits the 20S subunit of the proteasome. This leads to more sustained inhibition. It is more potent that bortezomib in vitro and demonstrates less cross reactivity with off-target enzymes with lower rates of peripheral neuropathy in early stage clinical trials. A phase III trial directly comparing bortezomib and dexamethasone to carfilzomib and dexamethasone in the relapse setting is ongoing. Its use earlier in the disease course is also being investigated in three or four drug combinations both in young patients and the elderly. Other proteasome inhibitors in development include NPI-0052 (marizomib) which inhibits all three catalytic subunits of the 20S proteasome and MLN9708 (ixazomib) which is administered orally.

combinations published to date show no further benefit over three, largely due to increased toxicity [106], however the availability of new agents with better side effect profiles are enabling this to be studied further in current trials. Regimens commonly used with good response rates include:

- Bortezomib (Velcade®) and dexamethasone—VD [107]

- Cyclophosphamide, bortezomib, and dexamethasone—CVD [108, 109]

- Cyclophosphamide, thalidomide (Thalomid®), and dexamethasone—CTD [104]

- Lenalidomide (Revlimid®) and dexamethasone—RD [110]

- Bortezomib, thalidomide, and dexamethasone—VTD [111]

- Bortezomib, lenalidomide, and dexamethasone—VRD

These regimens have not been evaluated in head-to-head clinical trials, but examples of their response rates following induction chemotherapy from different trials are shown in Figure 53.5.

Two approaches to induction treatment are either to give a fixed number of cycles or to continue treatment to maximum response prior to stem cell transplant. There are no data comparing these approaches directly; however, trial data suggests that reaching a complete response to induction treatment is associated with prolonged PFS and OS [104, 112, 113].

Autologous stem cell transplant

Consolidation of response to induction therapy with an autologous stem cell transplant (auto-ASCT) following high-dose melphalan is the current standard of care in fit patients, supported by several large phase III studies [114, 115]. Induction treatment aims to maximize response whilst preserving bone marrow stem cell function and enabling stem cell harvesting. Patient stem cells are mobilized using growth factor granulocyte colony stimulating factor (GCSF) and/or cyclophosphamide chemotherapy and collected from peripheral blood by apheresis. There is little evidence generated from comparison of mobilization regimens; pragmatically, harvesting is better at maximum response with only low levels of residual disease and seems to be associated with less myeloma cell contamination of the stem cell product. In patients who fail to mobilize with these regimens, it may be due to continued infiltration of the bone marrow in which case further treatment may be appropriate. The aim at the time of harvesting is to collect enough stem cells for more than one possible autologous stem cell transplant and to store cells for patients in case they are needed for a repeat transplant in the future.

The standard dose of melphalan administered prior to stem cell return is 200 mg/m^2, with a lower dose used in renal failure. Carefully selected patients can increasingly be maintained at home after this procedure until they become neutropenic, at which point they should be reverse-barrier nursed in hospital. Studies have evaluated the use of tandem autografts, a second autograft shortly

after the first, with results suggesting late benefit in patients who do not respond to the first [116, 117] and trials are ongoing to address the value of this approach. While the necessity of auto-ASCT in the era of novel therapies is being questioned, currently available evidence suggests that it remains the standard of care for younger, fitter patients.

Allogeneic transplant

Allogeneic transplant (allo-ASCT) has previously been described as the only way of achieving a 'cure' in myeloma. This is mediated via a graft-vs-myeloma effect, whereby the donor lymphocytes recognize the myeloma cells as 'foreign' and destroy them. This effect is demonstrated by achieving a complete response of disease with repeat donor lymphocyte infusions [118]. However, the graft-vs-myeloma effect is not very strong and so it is essential that patients are in very good and stable remissions prior to allograft and it cannot be relied upon to eradicate aggressive end-stage disease. This had led to the use of an allo-ASCT prior to mini-allograft as an effective strategy.

Allografting has significant transplant-related mortality and risk of graft-vs-host disease with associated morbidity, especially in the elderly. Trials to assess allografts in the context of molecularly defined high-risk disease at presentation are currently underway to further inform the place of allografting in myeloma.

Consolidation

Achieving a complete response following induction and ASCT predicts for longer survival [119]. However, improving the response to the level of the relatively recently defined sCR—where minimal residual disease is no longer detectable—is even better [81, 120]. Strategies to achieve sCR include the use of consolidation chemotherapy after ASCT. This can improve response rates, a benefit that has been demonstrated with the use of single-agent bortezomib [121] and bortezomib combined with thalidomide/dexamethasone [122] showing benefit over thalidomide/dexamethasone alone. The triplet combination also improved PFS. Lenalidomide has also been used in this setting with improved response rates when given after a single ASCT [123]. Further trials are ongoing with lenalidomide in combination with bortezomib and also comparisons of consolidation with a second ASCT or bortezomib, lenalidomide, and dexamethasone, or no consolidation.

Maintenance

Maintenance therapy has been used historically in myeloma with alkylating agents, steroids, interferon and, most recently, thalidomide. Steroids and interferon have shown improved PFS, and interferon was associated with a statistically significantly improved OS in a large meta-analysis [124], but use was often accompanied by side effects limiting prolonged treatment [125–127]. Thalidomide as a maintenance treatment is associated with improved PFS but with less clear impact on OS [128–130]. The MRC Myeloma IX study showed a prolonged PFS, though not OS, for thalidomide in patients with favourable cytogenetics, and no prolonged PFS and a worse OS for patients with unfavourable cytogenetics [131]. This result is supported by one previous study [128] though the results are different in other studies [132]. Meta-analyses showed an OS benefit [133–135] but there are limitations to the use of thalidomide maintenance; for example, early cessation of treatment is evident with the median duration of therapy on the MRC Myeloma IX study only nine months for younger, fitter patients.

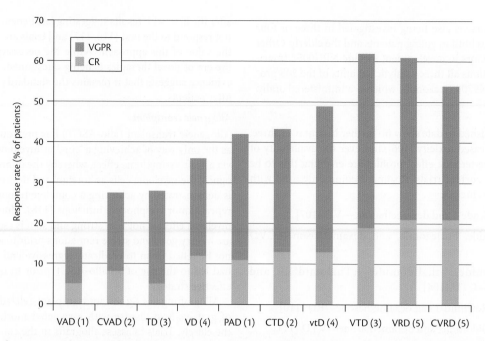

Fig. 53.5 An example of response rates (VGPR or CR) with different regimens for transplant eligible (younger, fitter) patients. It should be noted that these data are taken from different trials with varying populations and some are based on small single-centre experiences that have yet to mature with survival data. It demonstrates, however, an overview of the differences between older agents such as VAD or CVAD, the use of doublets such at TD or VD and the improved responses seen with triplet or quadruplet regimens.

VGPR, very good partial response; CR, complete response; VAD, vincristine, adriamycin, dexamethasone; CVAD, cyclophosphamide, vincristine, adriamycin, dexamethasone; TD, thalidomide, dexamethasone; VD, bortezomib, dexamethasone; PAD, bortezomib, adriamycin, dexamethasone; CTD, cyclophosphamide, thalidomide, dexamethasone; vtD, bortezomib, thalidomide, dexamethasone (reduced doses of bortezomib and thalidomide); VTD, bortezomib, thalidomide, dexamethasone (standard doses); VRD, bortezomib, lenalidomide, dexamethasone; CVRD, cyclophosphamide, bortezomib, lenalidomide, dexamethasone.

The newer and more tolerable IMiD (structural and functional analogues of thalidomide) lenalidomide has more recently been used in trials of maintenance therapy with promising results and demonstration of prolonged OS in one of three studies [123, 136, 137]. There have been some reports of an increase in second primary malignancies with the use of lenalidomide [138] but the absolute risk is very low, likely to be outweighed by the benefit of maintenance treatment. Taken together with data post-ASCT and at relapse long-term exposure to this agent is beneficial.

The impact of maintenance with bortezomib is difficult to determine as it has been used following different induction regimens in clinical trials. It has been shown to be safe and tolerable, however, either as a single agent or in combination with thalidomide [130, 139] and its use is being further investigated.

Older, fit patients

There is no consensus of the age at which ASCT is contraindicated. Decisions regarding whether to use this treatment should be based on individual patients' biological status and an informed decision following discussion between doctor and patient. Pragmatically, in our experience, it is rarely appropriate to use full-dose ASCT in those much over 70 years. Until recently, for those not thought to be fit for ASCT, melphalan and prednisolone (MP) had been the standard of care. The addition of novel agents to this regimen has improved outcomes, although with slightly higher rates of side effects for the combinations of melphalan, thalidomide, and prednisolone (MPT); cyclophosphamide, thalidomide, and dexamethasone (CTDa); and melphalan, bortezomib, and prednisolone (VMP) [91, 113, 140, 141]. The use of lenalidomide and low-dose dexamethasone for this group of patients is also becoming increasingly attractive due to its excellent tolerability with good safety and efficacy data for this group of patients in the relapsed setting [142]. A first line phase 3 study comparing MPT to lenalidomide plus low-dose dexamethasone for 18 cycles or lenalidomide plus low-dose dexamethasone to disease progression shows an OS and PFS benefit for the latter treatment [143].

Frail, older patients

Human aging is associated with deterioration in physiological reserve including organ function and haematopoietic reserve. As 37% of myeloma patients are over the age of 75 at the time of diagnosis, a significant number will fall into the category of frail and elderly and will not be able to tolerate full drug doses [144]. They are more likely to have co-morbid conditions and so will be more susceptible to side effects and drug interactions. Their OS is shorter than younger or fitter patients. For example, in a recent trial comparing MPR to MP, despite younger patients having good responses and improved PFS, those age >75 years did not have any benefit with 20% of patients discontinuing treatment due to toxicities [145].

It is important to screen for frailty and vulnerability in order to identify this group by using validated indices and also to carefully evaluate cardiac, respiratory, renal, hepatic, and neurological function. Comorbidities, disability, and frailty should be taken into account. Alkylating agents may be inappropriate in the presence of impaired haematopoietic reserve and dose reductions of other agents, especially steroids, should be considered. Specific clinical trials are needed in this group to better define optimum treatments.

Bisphosphonates

Myeloma bone disease is a central feature of MM and is actively managed by bisphosphonates. There is evidence for many bisphosphonates, including clodronate, zolendronic acid, and pamidronate, in reducing skeletal-related events (SREs) and pain [146]. Zolendronic acid has also been shown to reduce SREs following diagnosis, even in patients with no bone disease at baseline and with improved overall survival in a large phase III study [60, 147, 148], suggesting that it may exert a direct anti-myeloma effect. There was continued benefit from the use of bisphosphonates beyond two years in patients who were not in a CR; for these patients administration continues indefinitely [89]. The IMWG consensus recommendations include the use of bisphosphonates for all MM patients receiving first-line therapy, regardless of the presence of osteolytic bones lesions on conventional radiography. This recommendation was made even though as yet it is unknown whether bisphosphonates offer any advantage to patients with no bone disease as determined by MRI or PET-CT.

The side effects of bisphosphonates include renal impairment and osteonecrosis of the jaw. The latter is slightly higher with the use of zoledronic acid compared with other bisphosphonates and a dental assessment is indicated prior to commencing treatment. Renal function should be monitored and dose adjustments made as necessary. Calcium and vitamin D deficiency can be prevented by using supplements.

Myeloma emergencies and complications

Discussion of the management of patients with myeloma tends to focus upon specific measures to reduce the tumour bulk. However, it is also of immediate clinical concern to first treat medical emergencies arising as a result of myeloma.

Spinal cord compression

Cord compression in myeloma can be caused by a spinal plasmacytoma invading into the spinal canal causing compression of the cord in association with a paraspinal mass or as a result of vertebral collapse. Extramedullary deposits of myeloma near the dura may also impact on the spinal canal, but myeloma within the substance of the spinal cord is rare. Patients present with pain in the spine as well as neurological symptoms including numbness, limb weakness, difficulty walking, and loss of bowel or bladder function. Patients should be educated to be aware of the emergence of these signs and symptoms.

As myeloma is a chemo- and radio-sensitive malignancy, optimal management may differ from other cancers. Pain relief should be commenced and urgent MRI imaging of the whole spine is performed to elucidate the exact location, cause, and extent of cord compromise. If the compression is related to bone, surgical intervention may be required. More commonly, it is the result of soft tissue or plasmacytoma encroachment into the spinal canal in a patient with a known diagnosis of myeloma, immediate high-dose steroids and definitive treatment with anti-myeloma therapy is initiated as soon as possible. Radiotherapy to affected spine may also be appropriate. If the diagnosis is unknown and patients present for the first time with spinal cord compression, a neurosurgical procedure to obtain tissue may be required. Patients with spinal cord compression are at high risk of venous thromboembolism due to their immobility and underlying disease.

Vertebral collapse

In patients presenting with acute back pain, vertebral compression fractures should be considered. Balloon kyphoplasty or vertebroplasty may relieve symptoms and improve function and quality of life [89, 149]. This may alter the forces exerted on adjacent vertebrae with risk of further compression, so the whole spine should be carefully imaged prior to intervention. These procedures should not delay the commencement of systemic therapy at diagnosis; sometimes, it may be more appropriate to wait until induction chemotherapy has been completed.

Hypercalcaemia

Treatment of hypercalcaemia must begin with correction of salt and water depletion and high fluid throughput of three to four litres of normal saline per day with careful monitoring of fluid balance and serum electrolytes. The use of loop diuretics will help to maintain fluid output in the rehydrated patient and increase calcium loss in the urine by depressing renal calcium reabsorption.

Amino-bisphosphonates are the drugs of choice for the treatment of hypercalcaemia. When given intravenously, they will rapidly inhibit bone resorption and lower serum calcium levels. Zoledronic acid is more potent at controlling hypercalcaemia than pamidronate and is the bisphosphonate of choice in this setting. Bisphosphonates are remarkably free from acute side effects and normocalcaemia may be sustained for three to four weeks after a single treatment. Doses need to be adjusted in the presence of renal failure.

Hyperviscosity

Symptoms of hyperviscosity include blurred vision, headaches, mucosal bleeding, and heart failure. Symptoms rarely occur until an IgM level of at least 30 g/L, an IgA level of 40 g/L, or an IgG level of 60 g/L are reached [150]. It is possible to measure plasma viscosity; however, the results are often not immediately available. Therapy with plasmapheresis and saline and albumin replacement is, therefore, commenced based upon the presence of symptoms alone. This should also be combined with a strategy to reduce the level of paraprotein directly with systemic therapy.

Renal failure

As previously described, the causes of renal failure in myeloma are multifactorial. Even in patients with apparently normal renal function, the maintenance of a fluid intake of at least three litres per day is important [151]. Precipitating factors of renal failure (such as hypercalcaemia, dehydration, infection, and hyperuricaemia) should be treated, as should the underlying myeloma. Other precipitating factors, such as the use of non-steroidal anti-inflammatory drugs and aminoglycoside antibiotics should be avoided. If the underlying myeloma responds to chemotherapy, renal function should improve and may normalize in many patients. The best responses in renal recovery are associated with a rapid normalization of serum free light-chain levels; the speed of reduction is more important than the agent used. Some agents, such as lenalidomide and cyclophosphamide, need to be dose adjusted whereas bortezomib can be used safely at the usual dose. The use of plasmapheresis to remove light-chains directly from the blood has not been successful [152] but the use of high-cut-off haemodialysis membranes is now being investigated in clinical trials. Patients requiring long-term dialysis for renal failure may still be safely given high-dose therapy and ASCT with a reduced melphalan dose [153].

Pain control

Bone pain is challenging because of its severity and the relationship of pain to movement. Patients may be pain-free at rest but severely limited on any movement ('incident pain') and their analgesic requirements are therefore closely related to mobility. A clinical assessment will often reveal clinical evidence of nerve entrapment or pathological fractures which can be amenable to local measures. However, opiate analgesics remain the mainstay of pain control and specialist pain management teams are often valuable. Non-steroidal anti-inflammatory drugs should be avoided due to the additive risk of renal impairment. Although a sudden exacerbation of pain may indicate a pathological fracture, this can occur in myeloma without radiological evidence of fracture or progression of the underlying disease. In this circumstance, these episodes may be self-limiting, presumably resulting from fractures not visible on radiographs or from subperiosteal haemorrhages. Low-dose radiotherapy (up to 30 Gy) can be beneficial for bone pain and to prevent impending fracture.

Neuropathic pain is a well-recognized side effect of both the proteasome inhibitor bortezomib and the immunomodulatory drugs. It is best managed with dose reductions but calcium channel blockers (such as gabapentin) or serotonin noradrenaline reuptake inhibitors (such as amitriptyline) may also be beneficial.

Fractures

Fractures can occur in any weight-bearing bone or in ribs. Internal fixation of long bones is desirable to minimize pain, speed mobilization, and avoid non-union. Bones at risk of pathological fracture identified on imaging should have pre-emptive internal fixation. Rib fractures are usually managed with analgesia and maintenance of mobility.

Anaemia

The aetiology of anaemia in myeloma is multifactorial, resulting from the combined effects of bone marrow infiltration, renal failure, the blunting of the erythropoietin response by cytokines and the effects of chemotherapy. Adequate specific therapy will usually correct the anaemia in patients responding to treatment and transfusions will maintain adequate control in others. Anaemia may be an indication of active myeloma requiring specific treatment. Recombinant human erythropoietin can be considered [154] although its benefit-risk ratio should be carefully considered, particularly in the context of IMiD treatment which can increase the risk of venous thromboembolism [155].

Prevention of infection

Recurrent bacterial infections are a major cause of morbidity and mortality in patients with myeloma. The risk of infection is highest in the first few months after diagnosis and decreases with response to therapy [156] but still remains the major contributor to early deaths [57]. The most commonly identified pathogens are *Streptococcus pneumonia*, *Haemophilus influenza*, and *Escherichia coli* [148–159]. Febrile patients with neutropenia or severe systemic infections are hospitalized and given broad-spectrum antibiotics and G-CSF (granulocyte-colony stimulating factor) where appropriate. Aminoglycosides are avoided because of the likely additive impact on renal function. Routine prophylactic antibiotics are not currently recommended. Patients are offered vaccination against seasonal influenza, *Streptococcus pneumonia*, and *Haemophilus influenza*, but the vaccination may not produce an effective

response due to defective immune systems. Patients with proven hypogammaglobulinaemia may benefit from prophylactic intravenous immunoglobulin replacement.

Antiviral, antifungal, and *Pneumocystis jirovecci* prophylaxis should be given during and following an ASCT and with other immunosuppressive agents.

Prevention of venous thromboembolism

Myeloma increases the risk of venous thromboembolism (VTE), which occurs in up to 10% of patients, usually within four months of diagnosis. This risk is increased by the use of IMiD drugs; this is negligible when they are used as a single agent but higher when combined with steroids [160] or anthracyclines [161, 162]. When patients are prescribed immunomodulatory drugs in combination regimens they should begin thromboprophylaxis. The type of prophylaxis is determined by individual patient risk, with those at low risk receiving aspirin and those at higher risk either prophylactic low molecular weight heparin or warfarin [163]. Factors in the high-risk category include patient-related factors (e.g., previous VTE, co-morbidities), disease-related factors (e.g., new diagnosis of myeloma, high disease burden, hyperviscosity), and treatment-related factors (e.g., combination with high-dose steroids).

Patient information and psychological support

Patients should be given information about their disease and advised of the steps to take in the event of disease- or treatment-related adverse events, such as neutropenic sepsis, drug reactions, or new symptoms of disease. A multidisciplinary approach to the whole patient and appropriate referrals to psychological and palliative care support are important.

Relapse

Despite improvements in myeloma therapy with the advent of novel agents, disease relapse inevitably occurs in most patients. With progressive relapses, the disease becomes more difficult to treat and progression-free periods between treatments shorten [164].

Monitoring during treatment

Myeloma patients are generally monitored regularly in a specialist haematology clinic, at two- to three-monthly intervals after disease remission. This enables the close monitoring of patient symptoms, blood parameters, and paraprotein/SFLC quantification to enable early detection of relapsing disease. Traditionally, treatment is initiated when there are disease-related symptoms, organ, or tissue impairment (rising calcium, renal failure, cytopenias, new bone lesions) or if there is a steep rise in the paraprotein or SFLC. In the latter case, treatment should be started in the absence of symptoms to prevent rapid clinical deterioration. More recently, with the advent of new drugs which modify the disease natural history, there has been a tendency to start treatment earlier as soon as clinical relapse can be predicted. The IMWG have defined relapse criteria [165].

Investigations at relapse

Relapse should be confirmed by repeating the bone marrow biopsy and imaging. Assessment of risk status should also be repeated. A short PFS, often defined as <one year, following first-line therapy predicts for poor OS Cytogenetic risk factors at relapse are

comparable to those at diagnosis, although there is no clear indication of whether relapsed patients with different risk status should be treated differently. As treatments become available to target specific genetic lesions this will be of even greater importance.

The molecular events acquired as myeloma progresses are not acquired in a linear fashion but in branching non-linear pathways resulting in different clonal populations with different molecular characteristics, a concept termed intraclonal heterogeneity. These clones compete for dominance and at each relapse the dominant clone may have different features. This suggests that the sequence in which treatments with different mechanisms of action are used may affect clonal selection and, therefore, clinical outcomes. It also has an impact on the development of targeted treatments, as a treatment targeting a lesion found in only a minor subclone will not successfully eradicate the whole population. Instead, combination treatments or targeted therapies targeting a 'founder' lesion (i.e., present in a high percentage of clonal cells) should be used.

Assessment of relapse

The age and performance status of the patient at the time of relapse will help determine what type of agents may be tolerable. Side effects often accumulate with therapy and should be carefully assessed, including the presence of neuropathy, risk factors for venous thromboembolism, and the remaining bone marrow reserve. The stage of disease and number of relapses should also be considered; these have been defined by the IMWG to improve consistency in reporting of clinical trials at every stage of disease [165].

Primary refractory disease

Patients are defined as primary refractory if they have never achieved at least a minimal response (MR) to any therapy. This includes patients who have stable disease on all therapies and those who have progressive disease having never responded.

Relapse

Relapse is defined as patients who have had a period of time (at least 60 days) off therapy and have disease progression requiring treatment.

Relapsed and refractory

Patients are described as 'relapsed and refractory' if they have achieved at least MR to prior therapy but have not achieved MR on salvage therapy or relapse within 60 of salvage therapy.

The assessment of disease response to relapse treatment should also be considered differently from induction treatment. Especially in later stages of disease, it becomes more important to maintain a stable disease state rather than aim for complete response. In this setting, the clinical benefit rate (defined as response ≥MR) of an agent should be considered.

Relapsed disease management

Generally, patients who have been treated first-line with a proteasome inhibitor will be commenced on an IMiD-containing regimen or vice versa. If a thalidomide-based treatment has been used first-line then bortezomib is generally preferred at relapse, with lenalidomide reserved for subsequent relapse. If the patient had a good response to previous bortezomib treatment (usually considered as a response of ≥PR lasting >six months) then retreatment with the same agent might be considered [166]. If not, then a new

agent should be initiated. Treatment with bortezomib is unaffected by prior lenalidomide [167, 168] and vice versa [169].

For patients who have previously had an ASCT with a disease-free period of 18–24 months, a repeat ASCT is feasible with good response rates with a median PFS of 17 months [170]. Importantly, even if response duration has been short in a relapsed patient with no other therapeutic options, high dose melphalan supported by stem cells may be acceptable.

For patients on maintenance treatment, for example with the IMiD lenalidomide, in addition to increasing the dose to its full therapeutic level it is possible to add another agent to their regimen (e.g., steroids +/− cyclophosphamide) at the first sign of relapse to control their disease without the need to change the chemotherapy regimen completely [171].

Relapsed and refractory disease management

Patients relapsing after prior exposure to both IMiDs and bortezomib have a poor prognosis with a median OS of six months [172]. This is a setting in which novel drugs have been evaluated with accelerated approval in the US. For example, the new generation IMiD pomalidomide has recently been licensed in the US and Europe for patients with MM relapsed and refractory to both bortezomib and lenalidomide [103]. Other options include combinations of novel agents, such as lenalidomide and bortezomib [173], the new proteasome inhibitor carfilzomib (which has efficacy even in patients with bortezomib-refractory disease) [174], or older agents such as bendamustine (see Box 53.1). There have been particularly promising results for antibody-targeted therapies (e.g., anti-CD38, anti-CD138 and anti-CS1). In addition, trials are ongoing for oral proteasome inhibitors, epigenetic therapies including histone deacetylase inhibitors, and molecularly-targeted treatment strategies.

Other plasma cell dyscrasias

Plasma cell leukaemia

Plasma cell leukaemia (PCL) is termed primary if it presents *de novo* or secondary if it presents as the end-stage of multiply-relapsed myeloma. Primary PCL is the most aggressive form of plasma cell dyscrasia and is traditionally characterized by the presence of more than 20% plasma cells in the peripheral blood and an absolute plasma cell count greater than $2 \times 10^9/l$ [175] although this may underestimate the true incidence [176]. Prospective studies are required to investigate whether a lower cut-off would be more valid as even a few circulating plasma cells may indicate a highly proliferative and aggressive process.

PCL represents a stage of disease where plasma cells are no longer dependent on the bone marrow microenvironment. Patients often present with a high tumour burden and aggressive, rapidly developing clinical symptoms including anaemia, bleeding due to thrombocytopenia, and hypercalcaemia. Markers of disease activity including B_2microglobulin and LDH may be elevated and morphology often reveals anaplastic or plasmablastic plasma cells with a high proliferative index. Loss of interaction with the bone marrow microenvironment is demonstrated by the loss of CD56 on immunophenotyping. Extramedullary disease is common and should be investigated with whole-body imaging techniques. Bone lytic lesions are, however, less common than in myeloma [177]. Prognosis is poor with median OS less than one year in most studies [177–179] and the improvement in survival for myeloma patients over the last decade has not been seen in PCL.

The goals of treatment are to rapidly control disease to minimize the risk of early death and to achieve complete responses if possible. The high tumour burden places patients with PCL at higher risk of tumour lysis syndrome when chemotherapy is commenced so that strategies to prevent this should be considered. Intensive chemotherapy regimens combining novel drugs, including bortezomib with different classes of chemotherapy and steroids, are often used. Examples include VDT-PACE (bortezomib, dexamethasone, thalidomide, doxorubicin, cisplatin, cyclophosphamide, and etoposide) given prior to ASCT [176]. Bortezomib is thought to improve disease outcome and is used in varying combinations if high-dose regimens would not be tolerated [180–182]. In younger patients, myeloablative or reduced intensity allografts and tandem autografts have also been used if they are in deep stable responses.

POEMS

POEMS is a paraneoplastic syndrome associated with plasma cell dyscrasias. It is characterized by the presence of Polyneuropathy, Organomegaly, Endocrinopathy, Monoclonal plasma cell disorder, and Skin changes. It may also include other features including papilloedema, fluid overload, sclerotic bone lesions, and elevated red blood cells or platelets [183, 184]. In contrast to other plasma cells dyscrasias, the levels of the cytokine vascular endothelial growth factor (VEGF) correlate with disease activity and it is more commonly associated with a lambda light-chain producing plasma cell clones. It should be considered in cases of myeloma where the symptoms are not typical, for example when neuropathy, endocrine abnormalities and volume overload predominate over bone pain.

Certain features of POEMS are associated with a worse overall survival including extravascular fluid overload, respiratory symptoms [185], reduced lung diffusing capacity [186], and fingernail clubbing [187]. There is also a relationship between VEGF levels and response to treatment, with lower levels predicting for better response [188].

POEMS is isolated to a solitary site, like solitary plasmacytoma of bone (SPB) as described, extramedullary plasmacytoma, or isolated to a few lesions of bone with no evidence of bone marrow involvement, then treatment should be with localized radiotherapy with an improvement in symptoms in half of patients [186], although this may take months to occur. The largest retrospective analysis of these patients showed a four-year PFS of 52% and OS of 97%. If there is evidence of a clonal plasma cell population on bone marrow biopsy or other evidence of disseminated disease then radiotherapy is not expected to be curative and treatment with systemic chemotherapy should be initiated even if the plasma cell percentage is very small. The treatment approach follows the same principles as for myeloma, although the low tumour burden often enables the avoidance of induction chemotherapy with its associated side effects, instead proceeding directly to ASCT. ASCT in POEMS is associated with relatively high peri-transplant complications but good long-term outcomes. Patients may have a poor pulmonary reserve as a result of neuromuscular impairment and a reduction in lung diffusion capacity. There is also a relatively high incidence of engraftment syndrome [189]; treatment-related morbidity and mortality can be reduced by actively monitoring and treatment with corticosteroids.

Post-transplant, the observed OS is 94% and PFS 75% at five years [190], with a median survival of 13 years [187].

Symptomatic improvement is often slow but continues over time and has been seen up to three years following treatment. VEGF levels and lesions on PET scanning can be monitored and specific organ response criteria have been suggested. VEGF levels correlate better with disease activity than paraprotein quantification or PET-CT lesions.

Amyloidosis

Amyloidosis is a condition characterized by the deposition of insoluble, fibrillar protein in the extracellular space leading to organ dysfunction. AL amyloid is the term used to describe this protein resulting from the deposition of light-chains produced by clonal plasma cells. These can cause systemic proteotoxicity. AL amyloid can result from myeloma or from a small clone of plasma cells in MGUS. Protein deposition can occur in virtually all organs but predominantly symptoms result from cardiac (70%), renal (70%), liver (17%), neurological (15%), or gastrointestinal (10%) involvement [191]. Amyloidosis may also be associated with coagulopathy due to factor X deficiency, as a result of vitamin K-dependent clotting factors binding to amyloid deposits [192]. Demonstration of amyloid deposition in the tissue is performed by Congo red staining, but further characterization of the amyloid type is also necessary to guide the correct treatment and requires the use of mass spectrometry proteomics. Typing of the amyloid protein is particularly important in MGUS as it is possible for patients with MGUS to have co-incidental AA (a complication of a number of inflammatory diseases and infections) or other types of amyloid protein, the management of which would be very different to that of AL amyloid. Following diagnosis, each organ system should be fully evaluated and investigations to look for clonal plasma cells, if their presence is not already known, should be undertaken. A SAP (serum amyloid P) scan is performed to look for the distribution and amount of amyloid. Cardiac function should also be carefully assessed, which is best done with cardiac MRI scanning.

Prognosis in amyloid is most closely associated with cardiac status. The Mayo clinic staging system divides patients into three groups based on cardiac troponin and NT-BNP (N-terminal pro-brain natriuretic peptide) results with prognosis 3.5 months (stage III, both levels high), 10.5 months (stage II, one level high), and 26.4 months (stage I, both levels normal) [193]. It has been suggested that patients with MGUS and an abnormal SFLC ratio should be screened with regular NT-BNP measurement to prompt investigations to detect amyloid early and to start chemotherapy before cardiac symptoms become apparent [191].

Treatment for amyloid is aimed at rapidly reducing the abnormal light-chain production by targeting the plasma cell clone. In addition to their prognostic role, cardiac biomarkers are also important in determining appropriate therapy. Patients with cardiac disease (high NT-BNP or clinical symptoms) are in a high-risk group for treatment in which aggressive chemotherapies or ASCT would not be tolerated without a high incidence of complications. The presence of cardiac disease should, therefore, be thoroughly investigated and assessed prior to transplant to determine an individual's risk. Patients at high risk need gentler, but rapidly acting regimens; bortezomib is often used. For patients at lower risk, more aggressive chemotherapy and/or ASCT regimens are preferred [191]. If patients do not have overt myeloma, have a low burden of disease, and have low cardiac risk they can proceed directly to ASCT but may also benefit from consolidation chemotherapy with bortezomib or thalidomide after the ASCT, which has been shown to increase CR rates [194, 195]. Intermediate-risk patients are commonly given melphalan and dexamethasone, which induces good responses [196] although newer agents are being investigated. Where stem cell preservation is important and where improvement in organ function may enable ASCT, melphalan should be avoided and regimens of cyclophosphamide, thalidomide, and dexamethasone or cyclophosphamide, bortezomib, and dexamethasone are used [197]. The aim of treatment is a CR or at least a very good partial remission (VGPR). Haematologic and cardiac response is assessed frequently to enable therapy to be switched to a different agent and prevent progression of target organ damage if there is not a good response.

Solitary plasmacytoma of bone (SPB)

Less than 5% of patients with plasma cell malignancies present with a single bone lesion, a condition known as solitary plasmacytoma of bone (SPB). SPB occurs mainly in the axial skeleton. To meet diagnostic criteria there must be <10% plasma cells on bone marrow biopsy, a single area of disease, and no related organ or tissue impairment. There may be a small paraprotein or abnormal free light-chain ratio. The key to successful treatment is to accurately rule out the presence of disease elsewhere as truly isolated lesions can be treated with radiotherapy alone with the expectation of cure.

Extramedullary plasmacytoma (EMP)

EMP is defined as localized plasma cell neoplasms that arise in tissues other than bone. They occur most commonly in the upper air passages and oral cavity. As with SPB, there must be <10% plasma cells on bone marrow biopsy, a single area of disease, and no related organ or tissue impairment. These cases are often marginal zone lymphomas with plasma-cell differentiation and can be cured with surgical resection (although this is often technically impossible due to the location of disease) or radiotherapy. For patients with EMP that do not respond or relapse, treatment with lymphoma chemotherapy regimens should be considered, as it is more closely related to marginal zone lymphoma than myeloma.

Acknowledgment

We would like to thank Dr Attygalle and Dr Messiou for their help with the images in Figure 53.3.

References

1. Clamp JR. Some aspects of the first recorded case of multiple myeloma. Lancet 1967; 2(7530): 1354–1356. PubMed PMID: 4170040.
2. Kyle RA. Multiple myeloma: an odyssey of discovery. British Journal of Haematology. 2000; 111(4): 1035–1044. PubMed PMID: 11167737.
3. Kyle RA, Therneau TM, Rajku mar SV, Larson DR, Plevak MF et al. Prevalence of monoclonal gammopathy of undetermined significance. New England Journal of Medicine. 2006; 354(13): 1362–1369. PubMed PMID: 16571879.
4. Kyle RA, Remstein ED, Therneau TM, Dispenzieri A, Kurtin PJ et al. Clinical course and prognosis of smoldering (asymptomatic) multiple myeloma. New England Journal of Medicine. 2007; 356(25): 2582–2590. PubMed PMID: 17582068.
5. Jemal A, Siegel R, Xu J, Ward E. Cancer statistics, 2010. CA A Cancer Journal for Clinicians 2010; 60(5): 277–300. PubMed PMID: 20610543. Epub 2010/07/09.
6. Cancer Research UK, UK Cancer Incidence (2010) by Country Summary, April 2013.
7. Morgan GJ, Davies FE, Linet M. Myeloma aetiology and epidemiology. Biomedicine and Pharmacotherapy 2002; 56(5): 223–234. PubMed PMID: 12199621. Epub 2002/08/30.
8. Boyd KD, Ross FM, Chiecchio L, Dagrada G, Konn ZJ et al. Gender disparities in the tumor genetics and clinical outcome of multiple myeloma. Cancer epidemiology, biomarkers & prevention : a publication of the American Association for Cancer Research, cosponsored by the American Society of Preventive Oncology. 2011; 20(8): 1703–1707. PubMed PMID: 21680536.
9. Landgren O, Kyle RA, Pfeiffer RM, Katzmann JA, Caporaso NE et al. Monoclonal gammopathy of undetermined significance (MGUS) consistently precedes multiple myeloma: a prospective study. Blood 2009; 113(22): 5412–5417. PubMed PMID: 19179464. Pubmed Central PMCID: 2689042. Epub 2009/01/31.
10. Landgren O, Weiss BM. Patterns of monoclonal gammopathy of undetermined significance and multiple myeloma in various ethnic/racial groups: support for genetic factors in pathogenesis. Leukemia 2009; 23(10): 1691–1697. PubMed PMID: 19587704. Epub 2009/07/10.
11. Weiss BM, Abadie J, Verma P, Howard RS, Kuehl WM. A monoclonal gammopathy precedes multiple myeloma in most patients. Blood 2009; 113(22): 5418–5422. PubMed PMID: 19234139. Pubmed Central PMCID: 2689043. Epub 2009/02/24.
12. Landgren O, Rajkumar SV, Pfeiffer RM, Kyle RA, Katzmann JA et al. Obesity is associated with an increased risk of monoclonal gammopathy of undetermined significance among black and white women. Blood 2010; 116(7): 1056–1059. PubMed PMID: 20421448. Pubmed Central PMCID: 2938127. Epub 2010/04/28.
13. Greenberg AJ, Vachon CM, Rajkumar SV. Disparities in the prevalence, pathogenesis and progression of monoclonal gammopathy of undetermined significance and multiple myeloma between blacks and whites. Leukemia 2012; 26(4): 609–614.
14. Kyle RA, Therneau TM, Rajkumar SV, Offord JR, Larson DR et al. A long-term study of prognosis in monoclonal gammopathy of undetermined significance. New England Journal of Medicine 2002; 346(8): 564–5649. PubMed PMID: 11856795.
15. Landgren O, Gridley G, Turesson I, Caporaso NE, Goldin LR et al. Risk of monoclonal gammopathy of undetermined significance (MGUS) and subsequent multiple myeloma among African American and white veterans in the United States. Blood 2006; 107(3): 904–906. PubMed PMID: 16210333.
16. Soderberg KC, Kaprio J, Verkasalo PK, Pukkala E, Koskenvuo M et al. Overweight, obesity and risk of haematological malignancies: a cohort study of Swedish and Finnish twins. European Journal of Cancer 2009; 45(7): 1232–1238. PubMed PMID: 19091543.
17. Lindqvist EK, Goldin LR, Landgren O, Blimark C, Mellqvist UH et al. Personal and family history of immune-related conditions increase the risk of plasma cell disorders: a population-based study. Blood 2011; 118(24): 6284–6291. PubMed PMID: 21998210. Epub 2011/10/15.
18. Ruder AM, Hein MJ, Hopf NB, Waters MA. Mortality among 24,865 workers exposed to polychlorinated biphenyls (PCBs) in three electrical capacitor manufacturing plants: a ten-year update. International Journal of Hygiene and Environmental Health 2014; 217(2–3): 176–187. PubMed PMID: 23707056. Epub 2013/05/28.
19. Bourguet CC, Grufferman S, Delzell E, DeLong ER, Cohen HJ. Multiple myeloma and family history of cancer. A case-control study. Cancer 1985; 56(8): 2133–2139. PubMed PMID: 4027940.
20. Altieri A, Chen B, Bermejo JL, Castro F, Hemminki K. Familial risks and temporal incidence trends of multiple myeloma. European Journal of Cancer 2006; 42(11): 1661–1670. PubMed PMID: 16753294. Epub 2006/06/07.
21. Ogmundsdottir HM, Einarsdottir HK, Steingrimsdottir H, Haraldsdottir V. Familial predisposition to monoclonal gammopathy of unknown significance, Waldenstrom's macroglobulinemia, and multiple myeloma. Clinical Lymphoma Myeloma and Leukemia 2009; 9(1): 27–29. PubMed PMID: 19362965.

22. Ogmundsdottir HM, Haraldsdottirm V, Johannesson GM, Olafsdottir G, Bjarnadottir K et al. Familiality of benign and malignant para-proteinemias. A population-based cancer-registry study of multiple myeloma families. Haematologica 2005; 90(1): 66–71. PubMed PMID: 15642671. Epub 2005/01/12.

23. Camp NJ, Werner TL, Cannon-Albright LA. Familial myeloma. New England Journal of Medicine 2008; 359(16): 1734–1735. PubMed PMID: 18923179. Epub 2008/10/17.

24. Dilworth D, Liu L, Stewart AK, Berenson JR, Lassam N, Hogg D. Germline CDKN2A mutation implicated in predisposition to multiple myeloma. Blood 2000; 95(5): 1869–1871. PubMed PMID: 10688850. Epub 2000/02/26.

25. Eriksson M, Karlsson M. Occupational and other environmental factors and multiple myeloma: a population based case-control study. British Journal of Industrial Medicine 1992; 49(2): 95–103. PubMed PMID: 1536825. Pubmed Central PMCID: 1012073. Epub 1992/02/01.

26. Eriksson M, Hallberg B. Familial occurrence of hematologic malignancies and other diseases in multiple myeloma: a case-control study. Cancer Causes Control 1992; 3(1): 63–67. PubMed PMID: 1536915. Epub 1992/01/01.

27. Landgren O, Kristinsson SY, Goldin LR, Caporaso NE, Blimark C et al. Risk of plasma cell and lymphoproliferative disorders among 14621 first-degree relatives of 4458 patients with monoclonal gammopathy of undetermined significance in Sweden. Blood 2009; 114(4): 791–795. PubMed PMID: 19182202. Pubmed Central PMCID: 2716021.

28. Vachon CM, Kyle RA, Therneau TM, Foreman BJ, Larson DR et al. Increased risk of monoclonal gammopathy in first-degree relatives of patients with multiple myeloma or monoclonal gammopathy of undetermined significance. Blood 2009; 114(4): 785–790. PubMed PMID: 19179466. Pubmed Central PMCID: 2716020.

29. Brown LM, Linet MS, Greenberg RS, Silverman DT, Hayes RB et al. Multiple myeloma and family history of cancer among blacks and whites in the U.S. Cancer 1999; 85(11): 2385–2390. PubMed PMID: 10357409. Epub 1999/06/05.

30. Linet MS, McLaughlin JK, Harlow SD, Fraumeni JF. Family history of autoimmune disorders and cancer in multiple myeloma. International Journal of Epidemiology 1988; 17(3): 512–513. PubMed PMID: 3209328. Epub 1988/09/01.

31. Broderick P, Chubb D, Johnson DC, Weinhold N, Forsti A et al. Common variation at 3p22.1 and 7p15.3 influences multiple myeloma risk. Nature Genetics 2012; 44(1): 58–61. PubMed PMID: 22120009.

32. Chubb D, Weinhold N, Broderick P, Chen B, Johnson DC et al. Common variation at 3q26.2, 6p21.33, 17p11.2 and 22q13.1 influences multiple myeloma risk. Nature Genetics 2013; 45(10): 1221–1225. PubMed PMID: 23955597.

33. Martino A, Campa D, Jamroziak K, Reis RM, Sainz J et al. Impact of polymorphic variation at 7p15.3, 3p22.1 and 2p23.3 loci on risk of multiple myeloma. British Journal of Haematology 2012; 158(6): 805–809. PubMed PMID: 22823248.

34. Gonzalez D, van der Burg M, Garcia-Sanz R, Fenton JA, Langerak AW et al. Immunoglobulin gene rearrangements and the pathogenesis of multiple myeloma. Blood 2007; 110(9): 3112–3121. PubMed PMID: 17634408.

35. Morgan GJ, Walker BA, Davies FE. The genetic architecture of multiple myeloma. Nature Reviews Cancer 2012; 12(5): 335–348. PubMed PMID: 22495321.

36. Bourdon JC. p53 and its isoforms in cancer. British Journal of Cancer 2007; 97(3): 277–282. PubMed PMID: 17637683. Pubmed Central PMCID: 2360320. Epub 2007/07/20.

37. Chapman MA, Lawrence MS, Keats JJ, Cibulskis K, Sougnez C et al. Initial genome sequencing and analysis of multiple myeloma. Nature 2011; 471(7339): 467–472. PubMed PMID: 21430775. Pubmed Central PMCID: 3560292.

38. Kuo AJ, Cheung P, Chen K, Zee BM, Kioi M et al. NSD2 links dimethylation of histone H3 at lysine 36 to oncogenic programming. Molecular Cell 2011; 44(4): 609–620. PubMed PMID: 22099308. Pubmed Central PMCID: 3222870.

39. Walker BA, Wardell CP, Chiecchio L, Smith EM, Boyd KD et al. Aberrant global methylation patterns affect the molecular pathogenesis and prognosis of multiple myeloma. Blood 2011; 117(2): 553–562. PubMed PMID: 20944071.

40. Salhia B, Baker A, Ahmann G, Auclair D, Fonseca R, Carpten J. DNA methylation analysis determines the high frequency of genic hypomethylation and low frequency of hypermethylation events in plasma cell tumors. Cancer Research 2010; 70(17): 6934–6944. PubMed PMID: 20736376. Epub 2010/08/26.

41. Mitsiades CS, Mitsiades NS, Munshi NC, Richardson PG, Anderson KC. The role of the bone microenvironment in the pathophysiology and therapeutic management of multiple myeloma: interplay of growth factors, their receptors and stromal interactions. European Journal of Cancer 2006; 42(11): 1564–1573. PubMed PMID: 16765041.

42. Avet-Loiseau H, Gerson F, Magrangeas F, Minvielle S, Harousseau JL et al. Rearrangements of the c-myc oncogene are present in 15% of primary human multiple myeloma tumors. Blood 2001; 98(10): 3082–3086. PubMed PMID: 11698294. Epub 2001/11/08.

43. Walker BA, Wardell C, Brioli A, Kaiser MF, Begum DB et al. Translocations at 8q24 juxtapose MYC with genes that harbor super-enhancers resulting in overexpression and poor prognosis in myeloma patients 2014; 4: e1914.

44. Dib A, Gabrea A, Glebov OK, Bergsagel PL, Kuehl WM. Characterization of MYC translocations in multiple myeloma cell lines. Journal of the National Cancer Institute Monographs 2008; 39: 25–31. PubMed PMID: 18647998. Pubmed Central PMCID: 2737184. Epub 2008/07/24.

45. Cobbold LC, Wilson LA, Sawicka K, King HA, Kondrashov AV et al. Upregulated c-myc expression in multiple myeloma by internal ribosome entry results from increased interactions with and expression of PTB-1 and YB-1. Oncogene 2010; 29(19): 2884–2891. PubMed PMID: 20190818. Epub 2010/03/02.

46. Hideshima T, Nakamura N, Chauhan D, Anderson KC. Biologic sequelae of interleukin-6 induced PI3-K/Akt signaling in multiple myeloma. Oncogene 2001; 20(42): 5991–6000. PubMed PMID: 11593406. Epub 2001/10/11.

47. Boyd KD, Walker BA, Wardell CP, Ross FM, Gregory WM et al. High expression levels of the mammalian target of rapamycin inhibitor DEPTOR are predictive of response to thalidomide in myeloma. Leukemia and Lymphoma 2010; 51(11): 2126–2129. PubMed PMID: 20858096.

48. Peterson TR, Laplante M, Thoreen CC, Sancak Y, Kang SA et al. DEPTOR is an mTOR inhibitor frequently overexpressed in multiple myeloma cells and required for their survival. Cell 2009; 137(5): 873–886. PubMed PMID: 19446321. Pubmed Central PMCID: 2758791.

49. Chauhan D, Uchiyama H, Akbarali Y, Urashima M, Yamamoto K et al. Multiple myeloma cell adhesion-induced interleukin-6 expression in bone marrow stromal cells involves activation of NF-kappa B. Blood 1996; 87(3): 1104–1112. PubMed PMID: 8562936. Epub 1996/02/01.

50. Tai YT, Li XF, Breitkreutz I, Song W, Neri P et al. Role of B-cell-activating factor in adhesion and growth of human multiple myeloma cells in the bone marrow microenvironment. Cancer Research 2006; 66(13): 6675–6682. PubMed PMID: 16818641.

51. Annunziata CM, Davis RE, Demchenko Y, Bellamy W, Gabrea A et al. Frequent engagement of the classical and alternative NF-kappaB pathways by diverse genetic abnormalities in multiple myeloma. Cancer Cell 2007; 12(2): 115–130. PubMed PMID: 17692804. Pubmed Central PMCID: 2730509.

52. Keats JJ, Fonseca R, Chesi M, Schop R, Baker A et al. Promiscuous mutations activate the noncanonical NF-kappaB pathway in multiple myeloma. Cancer Cell 2007; 12(2): 131–144. PubMed PMID: 17692805. Pubmed Central PMCID: 2083698. Epub 2007/08/19.

53. Demchenko YN, Glebov OK, Zingone A, Keats JJ, Bergsagel PL et al. Classical and/or alternative NF-kappaB pathway activation in multiple

myeloma. Blood 2010; 115(17): 3541–3552. PubMed PMID: 20053756. Pubmed Central PMCID: 2867265. Epub 2010/01/08.

54. Demchenko YN, Kuehl WM. A critical role for the NFkB pathway in multiple myeloma. Oncotarget 2010; 1(1): 59–68. PubMed PMID: 20890394. Pubmed Central PMCID: 2947827. Epub 2010/10/05.

55. Bharti AC, Donato N, Aggarwal BB. Curcumin (diferuloylmethane) inhibits constitutive and IL-6-inducible STAT3 phosphorylation in human multiple myeloma cells. Journal of Immunology 2003; 171(7): 3863–3871. PubMed PMID: 14500688. Epub 2003/09/23.

56. Palumbo A, Anderson K. Multiple myeloma. New England Journal of Medicine 2011; 364(11): 1046–1060. PubMed PMID: 21410373.

57. Augustson BM, Begum G, Dunn JA, Barth NJ, Davies F et al. Early mortality after diagnosis of multiple myeloma: Analysis of patients entered onto the United Kingdom Medical Research Council trials between 1980 and 2002—Medical Research Council Adult Leukaemia Working Party. Journal of Clinical Oncology 2005; 23(36): 9219–9226. PubMed PMID: 16275935.

58. Kyle RA, Rajkumar SV. Criteria for diagnosis, staging, risk stratification and response assessment of multiple myeloma. Leukemia 2009; 23(1): 3–9. PubMed PMID: 18971951. Pubmed Central PMCID: 2627786.

59. Rajkumar SV et al. International Myeloma Working Group updated criteria for the diagnosis of multiple myeloma. Lancet Oncology 2014; 15(12): e538–548.

60. Morgan GJ, Davies FE, Gregory WM, Szubert AJ, Bell SE et al. Effects of induction and maintenance plus long-term bisphosphonates on bone disease in patients with multiple myeloma: the Medical Research Council Myeloma IX Trial. Blood 2012; 119(23): 5374–5383. PubMed PMID: 22498739.

61. Kristinsson SY, Bjorkholm M, Andersson TM, Eloranta S, Dickman PW et al. Patterns of survival and causes of death following a diagnosis of monoclonal gammopathy of undetermined significance: a population-based study. Haematologica 2009; 94(12): 1714–1720. PubMed PMID: 19608666. Pubmed Central PMCID: 2791946.

62. Gregersen H, Madsen KM, Sorensen HT, Schonheyder HC, Ibsen JS et al. The risk of bacteremia in patients with monoclonal gammopathy of undetermined significance. European Journal of Haematology 1998; 61(2): 140–144. PubMed PMID: 9714528.

63. Dimopoulos MA, Terpos E, Chanan-Khan A, Leung N, Ludwig H et al. Renal impairment in patients with multiple myeloma: a consensus statement on behalf of the International Myeloma Working Group. Journal of Clinical Oncology 2010; 28(33): 4976–4984. PubMed PMID: 20956629.

64. Davenport A, Merlini G. Myeloma kidney: advances in molecular mechanisms of acute kidney injury open novel therapeutic opportunities. Nephrology, Dialysis, Transplantation: Official Publication of the European Dialysis and Transplant Association 2012; 27(10): 3713–3718. PubMed PMID: 23114897.

65. Hutchison CA, Batuman V, Behrens J, Bridoux F, Sirac C et al. The pathogenesis and diagnosis of acute kidney injury in multiple myeloma. Nature Reviews Nephrology 2012; 8(1): 43–51. PubMed PMID: 22045243. Pubmed Central PMCID: 3375610.

66. Kyle RA. Multiple myeloma: review of 869 cases. Mayo Clinic Proceedings Mayo Clinic 1975; 50(1): 29–40. PubMed PMID: 1110582.

67. Drayson M, Begum G, Basu S, Makkuni S, Dunn J, Barth N et al. Effects of paraprotein heavy and light chain types and free light chain load on survival in myeloma: An analysis of patients receiving conventional-dose chemotherapy in Medical Research Council UK multiple myeloma trials. Blood 2006; 108(6): 2013–2019. PubMed PMID: 16728700. Epub 2006/05/27.

68. Hayhoe FGJ, Swirsky DM, Bevan PC. Morphological aspects. In Delamore IW, ed, Multiple Myeloma and Other Paraproteinaemias. Edinburgh: Churchill Livingstone, 1986, 75–102.

69. Bartl R, Frisch B. Bone marrow biopsy and aspiration for diagnosis of multiple myeloma In Malpas JS, Bergsagel DE, Kyle R, Anderson K, eds, Myeloma: Biology and Management. Oxford: Oxford University Press, 1998, 89–131.

70. Kaiser MF, Walker BA, Hockley SL, Begum DB, Wardell CP et al. A TC classification-based predictor for multiple myeloma using multiplexed real-time quantitative PCR. Leukemia 2013; 27(8): 1754–1757. PubMed PMID: 23318961.

71. Kyle RA, Rajkumar SV. Monoclonal gammopathy of undetermined significance and smouldering multiple myeloma: emphasis on risk factors for progression. British Journal of Haematology 2007; 139(5): 730–743. PubMed PMID: 18021088.

72. Perez-Persona E, Vidriales MB, Mateo G, Garcia-Sanz R, Mateos MV et al. New criteria to identify risk of progression in monoclonal gammopathy of uncertain significance and smoldering multiple myeloma based on multiparameter flow cytometry analysis of bone marrow plasma cells. Blood 2007; 110(7): 2586–2592. PubMed PMID: 17576818.

73. Greipp PR, San Miguel J, Durie BG, Crowley JJ, Barlogie B et al. International staging system for multiple myeloma. Journal of Clinical Oncology 2005; 23(15): 3412–3420. PubMed PMID: 15809451.

74. Avet-Loiseau H, Durie BG, Cavo M, Attal M, Gutierrez N et al. Combining fluorescent in situ hybridization data with ISS staging improves risk assessment in myeloma: an International Myeloma Working Group collaborative project. Leukemia 2013; 27(3): 711–717. PubMed PMID: 23032723.

75. Boyd KD, Ross FM, Chiecchio L, Dagrada GP, Konn ZJ et al. A novel prognostic model in myeloma based on co-segregating adverse FISH lesions and the ISS: analysis of patients treated in the MRC Myeloma IX trial. Leukemia 2012; 26(2): 349–355. PubMed PMID: 21836613.

76. Decaux O, Lode L, Magrangeas F, Charbonnel C, Gouraud W et al. Prediction of survival in multiple myeloma based on gene expression profiles reveals cell cycle and chromosomal instability signatures in high-risk patients and hyperdiploid signatures in low-risk patients: a study of the Intergroupe Francophone du Myelome. Journal of Clinical Oncology 2008; 26(29): 4798–4805. PubMed PMID: 18591550.

77. Shaughnessy JD, Jr., Zhan F, Burington BE, Huang Y, Colla S et al. A validated gene expression model of high-risk multiple myeloma is defined by deregulated expression of genes mapping to chromosome 1. Blood 2007; 109(6): 2276–2284. PubMed PMID: 17105813.

78. Chng WJ, Dispenzieri A, Chim CS, Fonseca R, Goldschmidt H et al. IMWG consensus on risk stratification in multiple myeloma. Leukemia 2014; 28(2): 269–277. PubMed PMID: 23974982.

79. Kumar SK, Mikhael JR, Buadi FK, Dingli D, Dispenzieri A et al. Management of newly diagnosed symptomatic multiple myeloma: updated Mayo Stratification of Myeloma and Risk-Adapted Therapy (mSMART) consensus guidelines. Mayo Clinic Proceedings Mayo Clinic 2009; 84(12): 1095–1110. PubMed PMID: 19955246. Pubmed Central PMCID: 2787395.

80. Durie BG, Harousseau JL, Miguel JS, Blade J, Barlogie B, Anderson K, et al. International uniform response criteria for multiple myeloma. Leukemia 2006; 20(9):1467–1473. PubMed PMID: 16855634.

81. Rawstron AC, Child JA, de Tute RM, Davies FE, Gregory WM et al. Minimal Residual Disease Assessed by Multiparameter Flow Cytometry in Multiple Myeloma: Impact on Outcome in the Medical Research Council Myeloma IX Study. Journal of Clinical Oncology 2013; 31(20): 2540–2547. PubMed PMID: 23733781.

82. Paiva B, Vidriales MB, Cervero J, Mateo G, Perez JJ et al. Multiparameter flow cytometric remission is the most relevant prognostic factor for multiple myeloma patients who undergo autologous stem cell transplantation. Blood 2008; 112(10): 4017–4023. PubMed PMID: 18669875. Pubmed Central PMCID: 2581991.

83. Kumar SK, Dispenzieri A, Lacy MQ, Gertz MA, Buadi FK et al. Continued improvement in survival in multiple myeloma: changes in early mortality and outcomes in older patients. Leukemia 2014; 28(5): 1122–1128. PubMed PMID: 24157580.

84. Bida JP, Kyle RA, Therneau TM, Melton LJ, 3rd, Plevak MF et al. Disease associations with monoclonal gammopathy of undetermined significance: a population-based study of 17,398 patients. Mayo Clinic Proceedings Mayo Clinic 2009; 84(8): 685–693. PubMed PMID: 19648385. Pubmed Central PMCID: 2719521.

85. Gregersen H, Jensen P, Gislum M, Jorgensen B, Sorensen HT et al. Fracture risk in patients with monoclonal gammopathy of undetermined significance. British Journal of Haematology 2006; 135(1): 62–67. PubMed PMID: 16925792.

86. Gregersen H, Norgaard M, Severinsen MT, Engebjerg MC, Jensen P et al. Monoclonal gammopathy of undetermined significance and risk of venous thromboembolism. European Journal of Haematology 2011; 86(2): 129–134. PubMed PMID: 20942842.

87. Roeker LE, Larson DR, Kyle RA, Kumar S, Dispenzieri A et al. Risk of acute leukemia and myelodysplastic syndromes in patients with monoclonal gammopathy of undetermined significance (MGUS): a population-based study of 17 315 patients. Leukemia 2013; 27(6): 1391–1393. PubMed PMID: 23380709. Pubmed Central PMCID: 3676476.

88. Mateos MV, Hernandez MT, Giraldo P, de la Rubia J, de Arriba F et al. Lenalidomide plus dexamethasone for high-risk smoldering multiple myeloma. New England Journal of Medicine 2013; 369(5): 438–447. PubMed PMID: 23902483.

89. Terpos E, Morgan G, Dimopoulos MA, Drake MT, Lentzsch S et al. International Myeloma Working Group recommendations for the treatment of multiple myeloma-related bone disease. Journal of Clinical Oncology 2013; 31(18): 2347–2357. PubMed PMID: 23690408.

90. Sonneveld P, Goldschmidt H, Rosinol L, Blade J, Lahuerta JJ et al. Bortezomib-based versus nonbortezomib-based induction treatment before autologous stem-cell transplantation in patients with previously untreated multiple myeloma: a meta-analysis of phase III randomized, controlled trials. Journal of Clinical Oncology 2013; 31(26): 3279–3287. PubMed PMID: 23897961.

91. Fayers PM, Palumbo A, Hulin C, Waage A, Wijermans P et al. Thalidomide for previously untreated elderly patients with multiple myeloma: meta-analysis of 1685 individual patient data from 6 randomized clinical trials. Blood 2011; 118(5): 1239–1247. PubMed PMID: 21670471.

92. Hideshima T, Mitsiades C, Akiyama M, Hayashi T, Chauhan D et al. Molecular mechanisms mediating antimyeloma activity of proteasome inhibitor PS-341. Blood 2003; 101(4): 1530–1534. PubMed PMID: 12393500.

93. Moreau P, Pylypenko H, Grosicki S, Karamanesht I, Leleu X et al. Subcutaneous versus intravenous administration of bortezomib in patients with relapsed multiple myeloma: a randomised, phase 3, non-inferiority study. Lancet Oncology 2011; 12(5): 431–440. PubMed PMID: 21507715.

94. Davies FE, Raje N, Hideshima T, Lentzsch S, Young G et al. Thalidomide and immunomodulatory derivatives augment natural killer cell cytotoxicity in multiple myeloma. Blood 2001; 98(1): 210–216. PubMed PMID: 11418482.

95. Mitsiades N, Mitsiades CS, Poulaki V, Chauhan D, Richardson PG et al. Apoptotic signaling induced by immunomodulatory thalidomide analogs in human multiple myeloma cells: therapeutic implications. Blood 2002; 99(12): 4525–4530. PubMed PMID: 12036884.

96. Hideshima T, Chauhan D, Shima Y, Raje N, Davies FE et al. Thalidomide and its analogs overcome drug resistance of human multiple myeloma cells to conventional therapy. Blood 2000; 96(9): 2943–2950. PubMed PMID: 11049970.

97. Zhu YX, Braggio E, Shi CX, Bruins LA, Schmidt JE et al. Cereblon expression is required for the antimyeloma activity of lenalidomide and pomalidomide. Blood 2011; 118(18): 4771–4779. PubMed PMID: 21860026. Pubmed Central PMCID: 3208291.

98. Schuster SR, Kortuem KM, Zhu YX, Braggio E, Shi CX et al. The clinical significance of cereblon expression in multiple myeloma. Leukemia Research 2014; 38(1): 23–28. PubMed PMID: 24129344.

99. Leoni LM, Bailey B, Reifert J, Bendall HH, Zeller RW et al. Bendamustine (Treanda) displays a distinct pattern of cytotoxicity and unique mechanistic features compared with other alkylating agents. Clinical Cancer research 2008; 14(1): 309–317. PubMed PMID: 18172283.

100. Hartmann M, Zimmer C. Investigation of cross-link formation in DNA by the alkylating cytostatic IMET 3106, 3393 and 3943. Biochimica et Biophysica Acta. 1972; 287(3): 386–389. PubMed PMID: 4629776.

101. Pratt G, Bowcock S, Lai M, Bell S, Bird J et al. United Kingdom Myeloma Forum (UKMF) position statement on the use of bendamustine in myeloma. International Journal of Laboratory Hematology 2014; 36(1): 20–28. PubMed PMID: 23615178.

102. Cuzick J, Erskine S, Edelman D, Galton DA. A comparison of the incidence of the myelodysplastic syndrome and acute myeloid leukaemia following melphalan and cyclophosphamide treatment for myelomatosis. A report to the Medical Research Council's working party on leukaemia in adults. British Journal of Cancer 1987; 55(5): 523–529. PubMed PMID: 3300761. Pubmed Central PMCID: 2001731.

103. Miguel JS, Weisel K, Moreau P, Lacy M, Song K et al. Pomalidomide plus low-dose dexamethasone versus high-dose dexamethasone alone for patients with relapsed and refractory multiple myeloma (MM-003): a randomised, open-label, phase 3 trial. Lancet Oncology 2013; 14(11): 1055–1066. PubMed PMID: 24007748.

104. Morgan GJ, Davies FE, Gregory WM, Bell SE, Szubert AJ et al. Cyclophosphamide, thalidomide, and dexamethasone as induction therapy for newly diagnosed multiple myeloma patients destined for autologous stem-cell transplantation: MRC Myeloma IX randomized trial results. Haematologica 2012; 97(3): 442–450. PubMed PMID: 22058209. Pubmed Central PMCID: 3291601.

105. Lokhorst HM, van der Holt B, Zweegman S, Vellenga E, Croockewit S et al. A randomized phase 3 study on the effect of thalidomide combined with adriamycin, dexamethasone, and high-dose melphalan, followed by thalidomide maintenance in patients with multiple myeloma. Blood 2010; 115(6): 1113–1120. PubMed PMID: 19880501.

106. Kumar S, Flinn I, Richardson PG, Hari P, Callander N et al. Randomized, multicenter, phase 2 study (EVOLUTION) of combinations of bortezomib, dexamethasone, cyclophosphamide, and lenalidomide in previously untreated multiple myeloma. Blood 2012; 119(19): 4375–4382. PubMed PMID: 22422823.

107. Moreau P, Avet-Loiseau H, Facon T, Attal M, Tiab M et al. Bortezomib plus dexamethasone versus reduced-dose bortezomib, thalidomide plus dexamethasone as induction treatment before autologous stem cell transplantation in newly diagnosed multiple myeloma. Blood 2011; 118(22): 5752–5758. PubMed PMID: 21849487.

108. Harousseau JL, Attal M, Avet-Loiseau H, Marit G, Caillot D et al. Bortezomib plus dexamethasone is superior to vincristine plus doxorubicin plus dexamethasone as induction treatment prior to autologous stem-cell transplantation in newly diagnosed multiple myeloma: results of the IFM 2005-01 phase III trial. Journal of Clinical Oncology 2010; 28(30): 4621–4629. PubMed PMID: 20823406.

109. Reeder CB, Reece DE, Kukreti V, Chen C, Trudel S et al. Cyclophosphamide, bortezomib and dexamethasone induction for newly diagnosed multiple myeloma: high response rates in a phase II clinical trial. Leukemia 2009; 23(7): 1337–1341. PubMed PMID: 19225538. Pubmed Central PMCID: 2711213.

110. Rajkumar SV, Jacobus S, Callander NS, Fonseca R, Vesole DH et al. Lenalidomide plus high-dose dexamethasone versus lenalidomide plus low-dose dexamethasone as initial therapy for newly diagnosed multiple myeloma: an open-label randomised controlled trial. Lancet Oncology; 11(1): 29–37. PubMed PMID: 19853510. Pubmed Central PMCID: 3042271.

111. Cavo M, Tacchetti P, Patriarca F, Petrucci MT, Pantani L et al. Bortezomib with thalidomide plus dexamethasone compared with thalidomide plus dexamethasone as induction therapy before, and consolidation therapy after, double autologous stem-cell transplantation in newly diagnosed multiple myeloma: a randomised phase 3 study. Lancet 2010; 376(9758): 2075–2085. PubMed PMID: 21146205.

112. O'Shea D, Giles C, Terpos E, Perz J, Politou M et al. Predictive factors for survival in myeloma patients who undergo autologous stem cell transplantation: a single-centre experience in 211 patients.

Bone Marrow Transplantation 2006; 37(8): 731–737. PubMed PMID: 16501593.

113. Morgan GJ, Davies FE, Gregory WM, Russell NH, Bell SE et al. Cyclophosphamide, thalidomide, and dexamethasone (CTD) as initial therapy for patients with multiple myeloma unsuitable for autologous transplantation. Blood 2011; 118(5): 1231–1238. PubMed PMID: 21652683. Pubmed Central PMCID: 3152492.

114. Child JA, Morgan GJ, Davies FE, Owen RG, Bell SE et al. High-dose chemotherapy with hematopoietic stem-cell rescue for multiple myeloma. New England Journal of Medicine 2003; 348(19): 1875–1883. PubMed PMID: 12736280.

115. Attal M, Harousseau JL, Stoppa AM, Sotto JJ, Fuzibet JG et al. A prospective, randomized trial of autologous bone marrow transplantation and chemotherapy in multiple myeloma. Intergroupe Francais du Myelome. New England Journal of Medicine. 1996; 335(2): 91–97. PubMed PMID: 8649495.

116. Cavo M, Tosi P, Zamagni E, Cellini C, Tacchetti P et al. Prospective, randomized study of single compared with double autologous stem-cell transplantation for multiple myeloma: Bologna 96 clinical study. Journal of Clinical Oncology: Official Journal of the American Society of Clinical Oncology 2007; 25(17): 2434–2441. PubMed PMID: 17485707.

117. Kumar A, Kharfan-Dabaja MA, Glasmacher A, Djulbegovic B. Tandem versus single autologous hematopoietic cell transplantation for the treatment of multiple myeloma: a systematic review and meta-analysis. Journal of the National Cancer Institute 2009; 101(2): 100–106. PubMed PMID: 19141779.

118. Lokhorst HM, Schattenberg A, Cornelissen JJ, van Oers MH, Fibbe W et al. Donor lymphocyte infusions for relapsed multiple myeloma after allogeneic stem-cell transplantation: predictive factors for response and long-term outcome. Journal of Clinical Oncology 2000; 18(16): 3031–3037. PubMed PMID: 10944138.

119. Chanan-Khan AA, Giralt S. Importance of achieving a complete response in multiple myeloma, and the impact of novel agents. Journal of Clinical Oncology 2010; 28(15): 2612–2624. PubMed PMID: 20385994.

120. Barlogie B, Anaissie E, Haessler J, van Rhee F, Pineda-Roman M et al. Complete remission sustained 3 years from treatment initiation is a powerful surrogate for extended survival in multiple myeloma. Cancer 2008; 113(2): 355–359. PubMed PMID: 18470907.

121. Mellqvist UH, Gimsing P, Hjertner O, Lenhoff S, Laane E et al. Bortezomib consolidation after autologous stem cell transplantation in multiple myeloma: a Nordic Myeloma Study Group randomized phase 3 trial. Blood 2013; 121(23): 4647–4654. PubMed PMID: 23616624. Pubmed Central PMCID: 3674665.

122. Cavo M, Pantani L, Petrucci MT, Patriarca F, Zamagni E et al. Bortezomib-thalidomide-dexamethasone is superior to thalidomide-dexamethasone as consolidation therapy after autologous hematopoietic stem cell transplantation in patients with newly diagnosed multiple myeloma. Blood 2012; 120(1): 9–19. PubMed PMID: 22498745.

123. Attal M, Lauwers-Cances V, Marit G, Caillot D, Moreau P et al. Lenalidomide maintenance after stem-cell transplantation for multiple myeloma. New England Journal of Medicine 2012; 366(19): 1782–1791. PubMed PMID: 22571202.

124. Fritz E, Ludwig H. Interferon-alpha treatment in multiple myeloma: meta-analysis of 30 randomised trials among 3948 patients. Annals of Oncology: Official Journal of the European Society for Medical Oncology/ESMO 2000; 11(11): 1427–1436. PubMed PMID: 11142483.

125. Cunningham D, Powles R, Malpas J, Raje N, Milan S et al. A randomized trial of maintenance interferon following high-dose chemotherapy in multiple myeloma: long-term follow-up results. British Journal of Haematology 1998; 102(2): 495–502. PubMed PMID: 9695964.

126. Shustik C, Belch A, Robinson S, Rubin SH, Dolan SP et al. A randomised comparison of melphalan with prednisone or dexamethasone as induction therapy and dexamethasone or observation as maintenance therapy in multiple myeloma: NCIC CTG MY.7. British Journal of Haematology 2007; 136(2): 203–211. PubMed PMID: 17233817.

127. Myeloma Trialists' Collaborative G. Interferon as therapy for multiple myeloma: an individual patient data overview of 24 randomized trials and 4012 patients. British Journal of Haematology 2001;113(4): 1020–1034. PubMed PMID: 11442498.

128. Attal M, Harousseau JL, Leyvraz S, Doyen C, Hulin C et al. Maintenance therapy with thalidomide improves survival in patients with multiple myeloma. Blood 2006; 108(10): 3289–3294. PubMed PMID: 16873668.

129. Spencer A, Prince HM, Roberts AW, Prosser IW, Bradstock KF et al. Consolidation therapy with low-dose thalidomide and prednisolone prolongs the survival of multiple myeloma patients undergoing a single autologous stem-cell transplantation procedure. Journal of Clinical Oncology 2009; 27(11): 1788–1793.

130. Sonneveld P, Schmidt-Wolf IG, van der Holt B, El Jarari L, Bertsch U et al. Bortezomib induction and maintenance treatment in patients with newly diagnosed multiple myeloma: results of the randomized phase III HOVON-65/ GMMG-HD4 trial. Journal of Clinical Oncology 2012; 30(24): 2946–2955. PubMed PMID: 22802322.

131. Morgan GJ, Gregory WM, Davies FE, Bell SE, Szubert AJ et al. The role of maintenance thalidomide therapy in multiple myeloma: MRC Myeloma IX results and meta-analysis. Blood 2012; 119(1): 7–15. PubMed PMID: 22021371.

132. Barlogie B, Anaissie E, van Rhee F, Shaughnessy JD, Szymonifka J et al. Reiterative survival analyses of total therapy 2 for multiple myeloma elucidate follow-up time dependency of prognostic variables and treatment arms. Journal of Clinical Oncology 2010; 28(18): 3023–3027.

133. Ludwig H, Durie BG, McCarthy P, Palumbo A, San Miguel J et al. IMWG consensus on maintenance therapy in multiple myeloma. Blood 2012; 119(13): 3003–3015. PubMed PMID: 22271445. Pubmed Central PMCID: 3321864.

134. Morgan GJ, Gregory WM, Davies FE, Bell SE, Szubert AJ et al. The role of maintenance thalidomide therapy in multiple myeloma: MRC Myeloma IX results and meta-analysis. Blood 2012; 119(1): 7–15. PubMed PMID: 22021371. Epub 2011/10/25.

135. Hahn-Ast C vL-TM, van Heteren P, Mückter S, Brossart P, Glasmacher A. Improved progression-free and overall survival with thalidomide maintenance therapy after autologous stem cell transplantation in multiple myeloma: a meta-analysis of five randomized trials. Haematologica 2011 June 1, 2011; 96(supplement 2):16th Congress of the European Hematology Association, London, United Kingdom, June 2–9, 2011: Abstr 884.

136. McCarthy PL, Owzar K, Hofmeister CC, Hurd DD, Hassoun H et al. Lenalidomide after stem-cell transplantation for multiple myeloma. New England Journal of Medicine 2012; 366(19): 1770–1781. PubMed PMID: 22571201. Pubmed Central PMCID: 3744390.

137. Palumbo A, Hajek R, Delforge M, Kropff M, Petrucci MT et al. Continuous lenalidomide treatment for newly diagnosed multiple myeloma. New England Journal of Medicine 2012; 366(19): 1759–1769. PubMed PMID: 22571200.

138. Dimopoulos MA, Richardson PG, Brandenburg N, Yu Z, Weber DM et al. A review of second primary malignancy in patients with relapsed or refractory multiple myeloma treated with lenalidomide. Blood 2012; 119(12): 2764–2767. PubMed PMID: 22323483.

139. Mateos MV, Oriol A, Martinez-Lopez J, Gutierrez N, Teruel AI et al. Maintenance therapy with bortezomib plus thalidomide or bortezomib plus prednisone in elderly multiple myeloma patients included in the GEM2005MAS65 trial. Blood 2012; 120(13): 2581–2588. PubMed PMID: 22889759.

140. Kapoor P, Rajkumar SV, Dispenzieri A, Gertz MA, Lacy MQ et al. Melphalan and prednisone versus melphalan, prednisone and thalidomide for elderly and/or transplant ineligible patients with multiple myeloma: a meta-analysis. Leukemia 2011; 25(4): 689–696. PubMed PMID: 21233832.

141. San Miguel JF, Schlag R, Khuageva NK, Dimopoulos MA, Shpilberg O et al. Bortezomib plus melphalan and prednisone for initial treatment of multiple myeloma. New England Journal of Medicine 2008; 359(9): 906–917. PubMed PMID: 18753647.

142. Chanan-Khan AA, Lonial S, Weber D, Borrello I, Foa R et al. Lenalidomide in combination with dexamethasone improves survival and time-to-progression in patients >/=65 years old with relapsed or refractory multiple myeloma. International Journal of Hematology 2012; 96(2): 254–262. PubMed PMID: 22752567. Pubmed Central PMCID: 3670754.

143. Benboubker et al. Lenalidomide and dexamethasone in transplant-ineligible patients with myeloma. New England Journal of Medicine 2014; 371: 906–917.

144. Palumbo A, Bringhen S, Ludwig H, Dimopoulos MA, Blade J et al. Personalized therapy in multiple myeloma according to patient age and vulnerability: a report of the European Myeloma Network (EMN). Blood 2011; 118(17): 4519–4529. PubMed PMID: 21841166.

145. Palumbo A, Falco P, Falcone A, Benevolo G, Canepa L et al. Melphalan, prednisone, and lenalidomide for newly diagnosed myeloma: kinetics of neutropenia and thrombocytopenia and time-to-event results. Clinical Lymphoma and Myeloma 2009; 9(2): 145–150. PubMed PMID: 19406725.

146. Mhaskar R, Redzepovic J, Wheatley K, Clark OA, Miladinovic B et al. Bisphosphonates in multiple myeloma: a network meta-analysis. The Cochrane Database of Systematic Reviews 2012; 5: CD003188. PubMed PMID: 22592688.

147. Morgan GJ, Child JA, Gregory WM, Szubert AJ, Cocks K et al. Effects of zoledronic acid versus clodronic acid on skeletal morbidity in patients with newly diagnosed multiple myeloma (MRC Myeloma IX): secondary outcomes from a randomised controlled trial. Lancet Oncology 2011; 12(8): 743–752. PubMed PMID: 21771568. Pubmed Central PMCID: 3148431.

148. Morgan GJ, Davies FE, Gregory WM, Cocks K, Bell SE et al. First-line treatment with zoledronic acid as compared with clodronic acid in multiple myeloma (MRC Myeloma IX): a randomised controlled trial. Lancet 2010; 376(9757): 1989–1999. PubMed PMID: 21131037. Pubmed Central PMCID: 3639680.

149. Bouza C, Lopez-Cuadrado T, Cediel P, Saz-Parkinson Z, Amate JM. Balloon kyphoplasty in malignant spinal fractures: a systematic review and meta-analysis. BMC Palliative Care 2009; 8: 12. PubMed PMID: 19740423. Pubmed Central PMCID: 2746801.

150. Mehta J, Singhal S. Hyperviscosity syndrome in plasma cell dyscrasias. Seminars in Thrombosis and Hemostasis 2003; 29(5): 467–471. PubMed PMID: 14631546.

151. Cooper EH, Forbes MA, Crockson RA, MacLennan IC. Proximal renal tubular function in myelomatosis: observations in the fourth Medical Research Council trial. Journal of Clinical Pathology 1984; 37(8): 852–858. PubMed PMID: 6206095. Pubmed Central PMCID: 498880.

152. Clark WF, Stewart AK, Rock GA, Sternbach M, Sutton DM et al. Plasma exchange when myeloma presents as acute renal failure: a randomized, controlled trial. Annals of Internal Medicine 2005; 143(11): 777–784. PubMed PMID: 16330788.

153. Raab MS, Breitkreutz I, Hundemer M, Benner A, Klaus J et al. The outcome of autologous stem cell transplantation in patients with plasma cell disorders and dialysis-dependent renal failure. Haematologica 2006; 91(11): 1555–1558. PubMed PMID: 17082013.

154. Rizzo JD, Brouwers M, Hurley P, Seidenfeld J, Arcasoy MO et al. American Society of Clinical Oncology/American Society of Hematology clinical practice guideline update on the use of epoetin and darbepoetin in adult patients with cancer. Journal of Clinical Oncology 2010; 28(33): 4996–5010. PubMed PMID: 20975064.

155. Anaissie EJ, Coleman EA, Goodwin JA, Kennedy RL, Lockhart KD et al. Prophylactic recombinant erythropoietin therapy and thalidomide are predictors of venous thromboembolism in patients with multiple myeloma: limited effectiveness of thromboprophylaxis. Cancer 2012; 118(2): 549–557. PubMed PMID: 21720994.

156. Lenhoff S, Hjorth M, Holmberg E, Turesson I, Westin J et al. Impact on survival of high-dose therapy with autologous stem cell support in patients younger than 60 years with newly diagnosed multiple myeloma: a population-based study. Nordic Myeloma Study Group. Blood 2000; 95(1): 7–11. PubMed PMID: 10607678.

157. Savage DG, Lindenbaum J, Garrett TJ. Biphasic pattern of bacterial infection in multiple myeloma. Annals of Internal Medicine 1982; 96(1): 47–50. PubMed PMID: 6976144.

158. Jacobson DR, Zolla-Pazner S. Immunosuppression and infection in multiple myeloma. Seminars in oncology. 1986; 13(3): 282–290. PubMed PMID: 3532328.

159. Rayner HC, Haynes AP, Thompson JR, Russell N, Fletcher J. Perspectives in multiple myeloma: survival, prognostic factors and disease complications in a single centre between 1975 and 1988. Quarterly Journal of Medicine 1991;79(290):517–525. PubMed PMID: 1946932.

160. Cavo M, Zamagni E, Cellini C, Tosi P, Cangini D et al. Deep-vein thrombosis in patients with multiple myeloma receiving first-line thalidomide-dexamethasone therapy. Blood 2002; 100(6): 2272–2273. PubMed PMID: 12229885.

161. Schutt P, Ebeling P, Buttkereit U, Brandhorst D, Opalka B et al. Thalidomide in combination with vincristine, epirubicin and dexamethasone (VED) for previously untreated patients with multiple myeloma. European Journal of Haematology 2005; 74(1): 40–46. PubMed PMID: 15613105.

162. Schutt P, Ebeling P, Buttkereit U, Brandhorst D, Opalka B et al. Thalidomide in combination with dexamethasone for pretreated patients with multiple myeloma: serum level of soluble interleukin-2 receptor as a predictive factor for response rate and for survival. Annals of Hematology 2005; 84(9): 594–600. PubMed PMID: 15744524.

163. Palumbo A, Rajkumar SV, Dimopoulos MA, Richardson PG, San Miguel J et al. Prevention of thalidomide- and lenalidomide-associated thrombosis in myeloma. Leukemia 2008; 22(2): 414–423. PubMed PMID: 18094721.

164. Kumar SK, Therneau TM, Gertz MA, Lacy MQ, Dispenzieri A et al. Clinical course of patients with relapsed multiple myeloma. Mayo Clinic Proceedings Mayo Clinic 2004; 79(7): 867–874. PubMed PMID: 15244382.

165. Rajkumar SV, Harousseau JL, Durie B, Anderson KC, Dimopoulos M et al. Consensus recommendations for the uniform reporting of clinical trials: report of the International Myeloma Workshop Consensus Panel 1. Blood 2011; 117(18): 4691–4695. PubMed PMID: 21292775. Pubmed Central PMCID: 3710442.

166. Sood R, Carloss H, Kerr R, Lopez J, Lee M et al. Retreatment with bortezomib alone or in combination for patients with multiple myeloma following an initial response to bortezomib. American Journal of Hematology 2009; 84(10): 657–660. PubMed PMID: 19731393.

167. Dimopoulos MA, Christoulas D, Roussou M, Kastritis E, Migkou M et al. Lenalidomide and dexamethasone for the treatment of refractory/relapsed multiple myeloma: dosing of lenalidomide according to renal function and effect on renal impairment. European Journal of Haematology 2010; 85(1): 1–5. PubMed PMID: 20192988.

168. Sonneveld P, Hajek R, Nagler A, Spencer A, Blade J et al. Combined pegylated liposomal doxorubicin and bortezomib is highly effective in patients with recurrent or refractory multiple myeloma who received prior thalidomide/lenalidomide therapy. Cancer 2008; 112(7): 1529–1537. PubMed PMID: 18300257.

169. Richardson P, Jagannath S, Hussein M, Berenson J, Singhal S et al. Safety and efficacy of single-agent lenalidomide in patients with relapsed and refractory multiple myeloma. Blood 2009; 114(4): 772–778. PubMed PMID: 19471019.

170. Mansi JL, Cunningham D, Viner C, Ellis E, Meldrum M et al. Repeat administration of high dose melphalan in relapsed myeloma. British Journal of Cancer 1993; 68(5): 983–987. PubMed PMID: 8217614. Pubmed Central PMCID: 1968739.

171. van de Donk NW, Wittebol S, Minnema MC, Lokhorst HM. Lenalidomide (Revlimid) combined with continuous oral

cyclophosphamide (endoxan) and prednisone (REP) is effective in lenalidomide/dexamethasone-refractory myeloma. British Journal of Haematology 2010; 148(2): 335–337. PubMed PMID: 20085583.

172. Kumar SK, Lee JH, Lahuerta JJ, Morgan G, Richardson PG et al. Risk of progression and survival in multiple myeloma relapsing after therapy with IMiDs and bortezomib: a multicenter international myeloma working group study. Leukemia 2012; 26(1): 149–157. PubMed PMID: 21799510.

173. Richardson PG, Weller E, Jagannath S, Avigan DE, Alsina M et al. Multicenter, phase I, dose-escalation trial of lenalidomide plus bortezomib for relapsed and relapsed/refractory multiple myeloma. Journal of Clinical Oncology 2009; 27(34): 5713–5719. PubMed PMID: 19786667. Pubmed Central PMCID: 2799050.

174. Vij R, Wang M, Kaufman JL, Lonial S, Jakubowiak AJ et al. An open-label, single-arm, phase 2 (PX-171-004) study of single-agent carfilzomib in bortezomib-naive patients with relapsed and/or refractory multiple myeloma. Blood 2012; 119(24): 5661–5670. PubMed PMID: 22555973.

175. Kyle RA, Maldonado JE, Bayrd ED. Plasma cell leukemia. Report on 17 cases. Archives of Internal Medicine 1974; 133(5): 813–818. PubMed PMID: 4821776.

176. Fernandez de Larrea C, Kyle RA, Durie BG, Ludwig H, Usmani S et al. Plasma cell leukemia: consensus statement on diagnostic requirements, response criteria and treatment recommendations by the International Myeloma Working Group. Leukemia 2013; 27(4): 780–791. PubMed PMID: 23288300.

177. Tiedemann RE, Gonzalez-Paz N, Kyle RA, Santana-Davila R, Price-Troska T et al. Genetic aberrations and survival in plasma cell leukemia. Leukemia 2008; 22(5): 1044–1052. PubMed PMID: 18216867.

178. Dimopoulos MA, Palumbo A, Delasalle KB, Alexanian R. Primary plasma cell leukaemia. British Journal of Haematology 1994; 88(4): 754–759. PubMed PMID: 7819100.

179. Ramsingh G, Mehan P, Luo J, Vij R, Morgenszturn D. Primary plasma cell leukemia: a Surveillance, Epidemiology, and End Results database analysis between 1973 and 2004. Cancer 2009; 115(24): 5734–5739. PubMed PMID: 19877113.

180. Esparis-Ogando A, Alegre A, Aguado B, Mateo G, Gutierrez N et al. Bortezomib is an efficient agent in plasma cell leukemias. International Journal of Cancer Journal International du Cancer 2005; 114(4): 665–667. PubMed PMID: 15609327.

181. Musto P, Rossini F, Gay F, Pitini V, Guglielmelli T et al. Efficacy and safety of bortezomib in patients with plasma cell leukemia. Cancer 2007; 109(11): 2285–2290. PubMed PMID: 17469169.

182. D'Arena G, Valentini CG, Pietrantuono G, Guariglia R, Martorelli MC et al. Frontline chemotherapy with bortezomib-containing combinations improves response rate and survival in primary plasma cell leukemia: a retrospective study from GIMEMA Multiple Myeloma Working Party. Annals of Oncology: Official Journal of the European Society for Medical Oncology/ESMO 2012; 23(6): 1499–1502. PubMed PMID: 22039089.

183. Dispenzieri A. How I treat POEMS syndrome. Blood 2012;119(24): 5650–5658. PubMed PMID: 22547581. Pubmed Central PMCID: 3425020.

184. Dispenzieri A. POEMS syndrome: update on diagnosis, risk-stratification, and management. American Journal of Hematology 2012; 87(8): 804–814. PubMed PMID: 22806697.

185. Allam JS, Kennedy CC, Aksamit TR, Dispenzieri A. Pulmonary manifestations in patients with POEMS syndrome: a retrospective review of 137 patients. Chest 2008; 133(4): 969–974. PubMed PMID: 18198255.

186. Humeniuk MS, Gertz MA, Lacy MQ, Kyle RA, Witzig TE et al. Outcomes of patients with POEMS syndrome treated initially with radiation. Blood 2013; 122(1): 68–73. PubMed PMID: 23699599.

187. Dispenzieri A, Kyle RA, Lacy MQ, Rajkumar SV, Therneau TM et al. POEMS syndrome: definitions and long-term outcome. Blood 2003; 101(7): 2496–2506. PubMed PMID: 12456500.

188. Scarlato M, Previtali SC, Carpo M, Pareyson D, Briani C et al. Polyneuropathy in POEMS syndrome: role of angiogenic factors in the pathogenesis. Brain: A Journal of Neurology 2005; 128(Pt 8): 1911–1920. PubMed PMID: 15975949.

189. Dispenzieri A, Lacy MQ, Hayman SR, Kumar SK, Buadi F et al. Peripheral blood stem cell transplant for POEMS syndrome is associated with high rates of engraftment syndrome. European Journal of Haematology 2008; 80(5): 397–406. PubMed PMID: 18221391. Pubmed Central PMCID: 2327207.

190. D'Souza A, Lacy M, Gertz M, Kumar S, Buadi F et al. Long-term outcomes after autologous stem cell transplantation for patients with POEMS syndrome (osteosclerotic myeloma): a single-center experience. Blood 2012; 120(1): 56–62. PubMed PMID: 22611150.

191. Merlini G, Wechalekar AD, Palladini G. Systemic light chain amyloidosis: an update for treating physicians. Blood 2013; 121(26): 5124–5130. PubMed PMID: 23670179.

192. Thompson CA, Kyle R, Gertz M, Heit J, Pruthi R et al. Systemic AL amyloidosis with acquired factor X deficiency: A study of perioperative bleeding risk and treatment outcomes in 60 patients. American Journal of Hematology 2010; 85(3): 171–173. PubMed PMID: 20052750. Pubmed Central PMCID: 2896569.

193. Dispenzieri A, Gertz MA, Kyle RA, Lacy MQ, Burritt MF et al. Prognostication of survival using cardiac troponins and N-terminal pro-brain natriuretic peptide in patients with primary systemic amyloidosis undergoing peripheral blood stem cell transplantation. Blood 2004; 104(6): 1881–1887. PubMed PMID: 15044258.

194. Cohen AD, Zhou P, Chou J, Teruya-Feldstein J, Reich L et al. Risk-adapted autologous stem cell transplantation with adjuvant dexamethasone +/- thalidomide for systemic light-chain amyloidosis: results of a phase II trial. British Journal of Haematology 2007; 139(2): 224–233. PubMed PMID: 17897298.

195. Landau H, Hassoun H, Rosenzweig MA, Maurer M, Liu J et al. Bortezomib and dexamethasone consolidation following risk-adapted melphalan and stem cell transplantation for patients with newly diagnosed light-chain amyloidosis. Leukemia 2013; 27(4): 823–828. PubMed PMID: 23014566.

196. Palladini G, Russo P, Nuvolone M, Lavatelli F, Perfetti V et al. Treatment with oral melphalan plus dexamethasone produces long-term remissions in AL amyloidosis. Blood 2007; 110(2): 787–788. PubMed PMID: 17606766.

197. Wechalekar AD, Goodman HJ, Lachmann HJ, Offer M, Hawkins PN et al. Safety and efficacy of risk-adapted cyclophosphamide, thalidomide, and dexamethasone in systemic AL amyloidosis. Blood 2007; 109(2): 457–464. PubMed PMID: 16990593.

CHAPTER 54

Malignant lymphomas

Frank Kroschinsky, Friedrich Stölzel, Stefano A. Pileri,
Björn Chapuy, Rainer Ordemann, Christian Gisselbrecht,
Tim Illidge, David C. Hodgson, Mary K. Gospodarowicz,
Christina Schütze, and Gerald G. Wulf

Epidemiology

The incidence of lymphomas in the Western world until recently was quoted to be 10–15/100 000 inhabitants per year with rising incidence with age. However, a Surveillance, Epidemiology, and End Results (SEER) study reporting registry data of lymphoma patients by WHO subtype between 1975 and 2001 in the US showed a rising incidence of lymphomas, with a plateau since the mid-1990s with an age-standardized incidence rate of 33.4/100 000 per year [1]. The European HAEMACARE project showed an age-standardized incidence rate of lymphomas according to the WHO subtypes in Europe of 24.5/100 000, which is considerably lower as compared to the earlier reported US data [2]. The distribution of different lymphoma subtypes (excluding plasma cell neoplasms) of the HAEMACARE project are depicted as crude incidence rates per 100 000 in Figure 54.1.

Both of these studies suggest increasing lymphoma incidences with age and lower incidence rates for lymphoma in women than in men. Improved diagnostic practice and the emergence of infections with the human immunodeficiency virus (HIV) and subsequent acquired immunodeficiency syndrome (AIDS) may partly explain this increase. Interestingly, the US SEER data demonstrated varying incidence patterns for Asian Americans, whites, and blacks with, for example, lower rates of chronic lymphatic leukaemia (CLL) and small lymphocytic lymphoma (SLL) in Asian Americans, which has also been reported in general for Asians. Both hairy cell leukaemia and follicular lymphoma (FL) were found to have higher incidences in white Americans, while plasma cell neoplasias and T/NK-cell lymphomas were found to be more frequent in black Americans. With FL being one of the most frequent non-Hodgkin lymphomas (NHLs) in the US and in Europe, it is rarely observed in developing countries—interestingly, an association of smoking and FL seems to exist [3]. Regardless of race, the SEER data demonstrated a male predominance for Burkitt lymphoma and hairy cell leukaemia. Interestingly, diffuse large B-cell lymphoma (DLBCL) was the most frequent lymphoma in whites and Asian Americans, whereas in African Americans DLBCL was second. These varying incidence rates amongst different ethnic groups, genders, and age groups (with increasing incidence for almost all lymphomas with age) may reflect a major role for host susceptibility in lymphoid malignancies. Hence, national registry data from Germany demonstrate

an increased proportion of NHL and a decreased proportion of Hodgkin lymphoma (HL), consistent with an ageing society, which might be applicable also for other developed countries and societies [4]. Geographical differences were reported in the HAEMACARE project in Europe but speculated to be confounders, due to differences in diagnostic procedures and under-reporting. However, besides diagnostic and regulatory issues, incidence and diagnosis across the world are highly variable since there exist infectious predispositions which are known initiators and mediators of NHL (and HL) such as viral infections with, for example, Epstein–Barr virus (EBV) in endemic Burkitt lymphoma (together with malaria) in the lymphoma belt of Africa [5], HIV-associated EBV-positive Burkitt lymphoma [6], and *HTLV1/2* in T-NHL in southern Japan [7]. Other infection-associated predispositions which are not specifically geographically associated but result in higher incidence of NHL include *Helicobacter pylori* and *Helicobacter heilmani* in mucosa-associated lymphatic tissue-lymphoma (MALT lymphoma), *Chlamydophilia* (formerly Chlamydia) *psittaci* in ocular adnexal marginal zone lymphoma (MZL), *Borrelia afzelii* in cutaneous B-cell lymphoma (also known as borrelial lymphocytoma), and *Hepatitis C virus* (HCV) in MZLs. Furthermore, increased incidence occur in patients who are immunocompromised due to previous cytotoxic therapies such as chemotherapy and/or ionizing radiation therapy, immunosuppressive agents for autoimmune diseases, constitutional immunosuppression in inherited immunodeficiency syndromes, or acquired immunosuppression due to HIV infection. Individuals with AIDS have a 1000-fold increased risk of suffering from NHL, and NHL constitutes one of the AIDS-defined malignancies [8]. Although antiviral therapies effectively prolong the lives of patients with HIV, the risk of developing NHL for HIV-positive patients is higher in those receiving highly active antiretroviral therapy (HAART), whereas NHL is less frequently observed in patients without adequate HIV treatment (which is likely explained by their shorter overall survival). Typically, HIV-positive patients most often present with aggressive B-NHL, advanced stage disease, and often extranodal disease [9]. Another aspect affecting treatment results and survival, which has been demonstrated for other malignancies and which was studied in DLBCL, was that patients with a low socio-economic status (SES) have greater than a one-third higher mortality rate from lymphoma

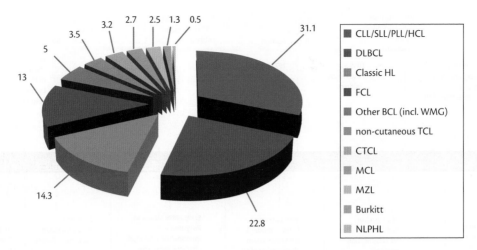

Fig. 54.1 Crude incidence rates (IR) of lymphoid malignancies per 100 000 in Europe according to the Data of the HAEMACARE project.
CLL, chronic lymphocytic leukaemia; SLL, small lymphocytic lymphoma; PLL, prolymphocytic leukaemia; HCL, hairy cell leukaemia; DLBCL, diffuse large B-cell lymphoma; HL, Hodgkin lymphoma; FCL, follicular cell lymphoma; other BCL (including WMG), other B-cell lymphomas (including Waldenström's macroglobulinaemia); TCL, T-cell lymphoma; CTCL, cutaneous T-cell lymphoma; MCL, mantle cell lymphoma; MZL, marginal zone lymphoma; NLPHL, nodular lymphocyte predominant Hodgkin lymphoma.
Source: data from HAEMACARE.

and from all other non-lymphoma related causes as compared to patients with a higher SES. Additionally, this increased mortality rate was even higher in those patients who were under the age of 65 years or unmarried [10].

Genome-wide association studies (GWAS) using next-generation sequencing (NGS) technologies will help to unravel the geographical differences, differing ethnic incidence ratios, and uneven gender distributions of lymphoma. The roles of certain single-nucleotide polymorphisms (SNPs) as factors for increasing or reducing individual risk for certain NHL subtypes are currently being discovered and interpreted [11–14]. Whether, or how, individual genetic variability needs to be considered in future treatment plans has not yet been properly addressed. International collaborative efforts such as the InterLymph Consortium are currently running advanced molecular epidemiological studies, which will hopefully shed more light on the genetic backgrounds, predispositions, susceptibilities, and their clinical implications for lymphomas.

History

A comprehensive overview of the description, hypotheses, and classifications of lymphomas which have influenced the medical community over the decades is depicted in Figure 54.2. However, as outlined at the end of the previous section, there are currently a multitude of collaborative efforts combining epidemiologic, genetic, and medical data to not only illuminate the mechanistic backgrounds which occur in the heterogeneous group of lymphomas but also to demonstrate how these findings might be translated from bench to bedside to improved patient outcomes. A comprehensive 4th WHO classification of lymphomas was published in 2008 by the International Agency for Research on Cancer (IARC) [15]. The WHO Classification on Lymphoid tumours (see pp. 812–813) depicts the mature B-cell, T-cell, and NK-cell neoplasms as well as HL and post-transplant lymphoproliferative disorders (PTLD). Although many genetic alterations were acknowledged in the 2008 WHO classification, data from microarray studies, GWAS, or mutational profiling were not been taken into account since they were regarded to be premature for inclusion. However, future classifications will most likely include more genetic characteristics to improve diagnosis, classification, risk-prognostication, and treatment modalities for malignant lymphomas.

Clinical entities

In the daily clinical setting, NHLs are dichotomized as either low-grade or high-grade NHL, with a comparable separation into indolent and aggressive NHL. However, although these distinctions are commonly used, they are poorly defined. In general, aggressive NHL such as DLBCL or Burkitt lymphoma will result in short- or very short-term progressive disease and lead to death when not treated immediately. This depends on the NHL-bulk burden, stage, and accompanying complications. But, when treated appropriately, aggressive NHL now has a high rate of complete remission and long-term survival. On the other hand, low-grade or indolent NHL, such as FL or CLL, might be clinically either asymptomatic or oligosymptomatic, not progressive, and not necessitate the early initiation of therapy. Depending on symptoms, age, and patient preferences, as well as predicted treatment success, patients might be monitored to determine the time when therapy should be initiated. Some patients will never require treatment. However, separating NHL into these two clinical entities also means that some NHLs, such as mantle cell lymphoma (MCL), which are traditionally thought to be indolent may also have courses which are more like aggressive NHL, with fast-progressing and highly-symptomatic disease such that a delay of treatment cannot be advised.

HL is a B-cell-derived malignancy of the lymphatic system. Two groups of histological types are defined: nodular lymphocyte predominant (LP) and the classic HL (CHL), the latter accounting for 95% of all HL cases. This includes four subtypes: nodular sclerosis, mixed cellularity, lymphocyte-rich, and lymphocyte-depleted HL. The annual incidence is about three cases per 100 000. Patients with HL present with indolent lymphadenopathy, most commonly located in the neck, in supraclavicular areas, and mediastinal nodes. About 40% of patients show B-symptoms such as fever, weight loss, and night sweats.

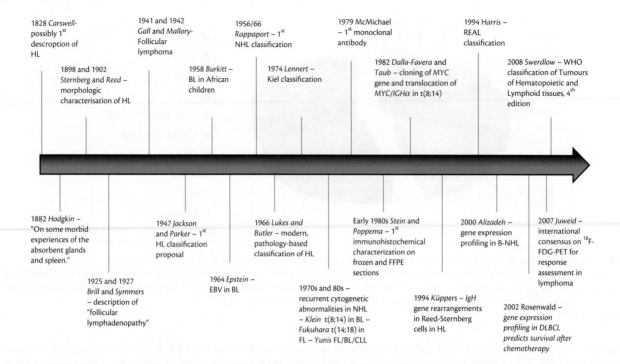

Fig. 54.2 Historical overview of lymphoma from discovery and first description to recent classification systems and genetic studies which might be incorporated in future considerations regarding classifications, aetiology, and pathogenesis.

Other clinically-used terms include the distinction of nodal versus extranodal disease, which are usually included in the Ann Arbor classification or International Prognostic Index (IPI) but do not have any prognostic or therapeutic implications alone, except when affecting adjacent organ function such as pericardial effusion or infiltration into the cerebrospinal fluid (discussed in the next section).

Medical management

Since the type of lymphoma and the areas of involvement vary, clinical symptoms and complications are very heterogeneous. Clinically, aggressive and indolent lymphomas differ with patients suffering from aggressive lymphomas presenting with a short history of lymphadenopathy, organomegaly (especially splenomegaly and hepatomegaly), and B-symptoms (defined by weight loss >10% within six months, night sweats defined by the need to change pyjamas, and fever defined as increased temperatures above 38 °C). Elevated serum markers, reflecting a high cell-cycle turnover of malignant cells, such as serum lactate dehydrogenase (LDH), uric acid, β_2-microglobulin (β_2M), or soluble interleukin-2 receptor (sIL-2R) may be measured. These are most prominent in patients diagnosed with DLBCL, Burkitt lymphoma, T-cell lymphomas, MCL, or B- and T-lymphoblastic lymphoma/leukaemia. In contrast, indolent lymphomas have usually slow-progressing lymphadenopathy or organomegaly and only modest serum marker elevations. The most frequent lymphomas in this category are FL, CLL/SLL, and MZL.

Possible oncologic emergencies amongst malignant lymphomas which might be present at initial diagnosis but can also occur or progress during treatment or relapse include:

- tumour lysis syndrome (TLS)—typically in lymphomas with high tumour burden

- hyperleukocytosis (or even leukostasis)—typically in B- and T-lymphoblastic lymphoma/leukaemia

- hyperviscosity syndrome—typically in lymphoplasmacytic lymphoma due to high IgM serum levels

- pericardial or pleural effusion due to extranodal infiltration leading to cardiopulmonary insufficiency

- spinal cord/intracerebral CNS compression or neoplastic meningitis

- superior or inferior vena cava obstruction

- acute airway obstruction due to mediastinal lymphoma leading to tracheal or bronchial obstruction

- bowel or ureteral obstruction

- venous thromboembolism

The approach to a patient with suspected lymphoma includes a meticulous patient history and physical examination, focusing on lymph node sites, extranodal sites such as skin, testis, salivary glands amongst others, pleural or pericardial effusion, vena cava syndrome, and neurologic abnormalities indicative of CNS involvement. Furthermore, it must be emphasized that, whenever possible and desired, fertility preservation by obtaining a germline specimen and subsequent cryopreservation in women and men in their reproductive life time should be planned after definite diagnosis. Laboratory workup should include a complete blood count to assess cytopaenias or hyperleukocytosis, serum-calcium level (albumin-bound calcium and ionized calcium) to assess hypercalcaemia, serum-uric acid level to assess hyperuricaemia, serum-LDH level to assess the tumour burden, prognosis (in aggressive lymphomas), and lymphoma growth and shrinkage during treatment. The latter clinical setting can also be ascertained by measuring serum-β_2M or sIL-2R. Other routine laboratory studies should include immunoglobulin analysis, HIV and Hepatitis B and C serology, and other standard laboratory analyses for kidney, liver, endocrine function tests as well as coagulation analysis. In B- or T-lymphoblastic lymphoma/leukaemia or MCL, leukaemic dissemination allows for fluorescence-activated cell sorting (FACS) analysis or cytogenetic analysis by conventional G-banding or fluorescent in situ hybridization (FISH) from peripheral blood samples. In case of suspected CNS disease lumbar puncture needs to be performed; CSF should be examined for absolute cell count, cytomorphologic assessment, FACS, and histologic workup including histochemical staining procedures. Gene-expression profiling using microarray technologies is able to distinguish GCB-type from ABC-type DLCBL (GCB refers to germinal centre B-like DLBCL and ABC refers to activated B-like DLBCL). This aids in diagnostic workup and prognostication since GCB-type DLCBL has a better prognosis compared to ABC-type DLBCL [16]. A biopsy of an enlarged lymph node is mandatory for definite diagnosis and classification. Although fine needle aspiration (FNA) is widely used in clinical practice, it should be performed only by trained clinicians and analysed only by specialty-trained cytomorphologists and flow cytometrists [17]. However, FNA might only serve as a screening procedure and might have—especially in the non-well trained setting—a high false-negative rate of diagnosis leading to unnecessary delay and misguided treatment [18]. Therefore, a tissue biopsy of an intact lymph node for complete and accurate histopathology (including histologic, immunologic, molecular, and cytogenetic analysis) is recommended in all cases where a lymph node is accessible for excision. Generally, lymph nodes with a diameter of 1.5 to 2 cm have the highest diagnostic yield [19, 20]. In case lymph nodes are not accessible for excision, computed tomography (CT)-guided biopsies might be performed to obtain tissue for a diagnostic workup. Since approximately one-third of lymphomas present at initial diagnosis with bone marrow (BM) involvement, BM examination by trephine biopsy with at least 2 cm length should be performed in all lymphoma patients at least once at initial diagnosis. Low-grade lymphomas have a higher tendency to be present in the BM while the more aggressive lymphoma subtypes occur more often in the lymph nodes [21].

Routine imaging studies which need to be performed at initial diagnosis include contrast-enhanced CT of the neck, chest, abdomen, and pelvis to accurately stage a patient according to the Ann Arbor staging classification [22]. Positron emission tomography (PET) scanning using ^{18}F-Fluoro-deoxyglucose (^{18}F-FDG), either alone or in combination with CT (^{18}F-FDG-PET-CT), is not only feasible in detecting neoplastic infiltrated/transformed lymph nodes and extranodal sites in high-grade and aggressive lymphomas but is also superior to CT-based staging alone [23, 24]. Although there exist concerns about the reproducibility of ^{18}F-FDG-PET scan interpretation, its definite role for evaluating treatment response in various settings and its unknown prognostic role on the IPI (see Risk prognostication, below), an international consensus set the following recommendations in 2007 [25]:

- visual assessment alone is adequate when interpreting ^{18}F-FDG-PET findings as positive or negative, when evaluating response to treatment after completion of therapy
- ^{18}F-FDG-PET scanning after chemotherapy or chemoimmunotherapy should be performed at least three weeks—but preferably

six to eight weeks after—completion of therapy and eight to twelve weeks after radiation or radiochemotherapy

- mediastinal blood pool activity is recommended as the reference background activity to define ^{18}F-FDG-PET positivity of a residual mass ≥2 cm in greatest transverse diameter, regardless of its location
- a smaller residual mass or lymph node should be considered positive if its activity is above that of the surrounding background
- attenuation-corrected ^{18}F-FDG-PET is recommended
- outside of clinical trials or prospective registries, there is currently no routine role for ^{18}F-FDG-PET during the course of therapy

As a result of the 12th international conference on malignant lymphoma in Lugano in June 2013, recommendations were made for initial evaluation, staging, and response assessment of Hodgkin and non-Hodgkin lymphoma [26]. The Lugano workshop led to the following revised criteria (in addition to the above mentioned) for staging and response assessment in patients with lymphoma:

- FDG-PET was formally incorporated into standard staging for FDG-avid lymphomas
- a modified Ann Arbor staging system is recommended for primary nodal lymphomas
- if a PET-CT is performed, a bone marrow biopsy is no longer indicated in patients with HL
- a bone marrow biopsy is only recommended in patients with DLBCL if the PET is negative and identifying a discordant histology is important for patient management
- FDG-PET should be performed for response assessment in FDG-avid lymphoma , using the 5-point scale, while CT is preferred for low or variable FDG-avid lymphoma

Furthermore, the International Conference on Malignant Lymphomas Imaging Working Group has published a recent summary of recommendations for interpretation of PET-CT scans and the roles of PET-CT for staging, interim PET, and at the end of treatment [27]. These imaging procedures, which partly determine the stage of the underlying lymphoma according to the Ann Arbor classification, however, do not solely prognosticate a patient's individual risk. Over the course of time, individual prognostic scoring systems have been developed for several NHL entities which might be applied for individual risk-prognostication, decision for treatment strategies, and trial designs, discussed in the following section.

Risk prognostication

In 1993, an international consortium published collaborative data on a prognostic model for aggressive NHL [28]. Based on previously reported factors, which might influence patient outcome, the consortium used retrospective patient data to report what has been widely applied since, the International Prognostic Index and the age-adjusted IPI (aaIPI). In the meantime, prognostic indices for other NHL entities have been established for survival prognostication. Interestingly, the IPI and the aaIPI also keep their prognostic value in the rituximab era, with improved outcome within each IPI group but maintaining the order of IPI groups [29]. Nowadays, not only the original publications but also internet-based calculators or mobile applications based on the original literature can easily be used to calculate these indices.

Pathology of malignant lymphomas

The 4th edition of the WHO Classification

In 2008, the WHO released a new edition of the Classification of Tumours of Haematopoietic and Lymphoid Tissues [30], as the 2001 version had become outdated very soon after its publication (Box 54.1). In line with the concepts of the Revised European-American (REAL) Classification [31], it consisted of a

---

Box 54.1 2008 WHO Classification: Lymphoid tumours

Precursor B- and T-cell neoplasms

Precursor B lymphoblastic leukaemia/lymphoma

  B lymphoblastic leukaemia/lymphoma, NOS
  B lymphoblastic leukaemia/lymphoma with recurrent genetic abnormalities
  B lymphoblastic leukaemia/lymphoma with t(9;22)(q34;q11.2; BCR-ABL1
  B lymphoblastic leukaemia/lymphoma with t(v;11Q23); MLL rearranged
  B lymphoblastic leukaemia/lymphoma with t(12;21)(p13;22); TEL_AML1,(ETV 6-RUNX1)
  B lymphoblastic leukaemia/lymphoma with hyperdiploidy
  B lymphoblastic leukaemia/lymphoma with hypodiploidy (hypodiploid ALL)
  B lymphoblastic leukaemia/lymphoma with t(5;14)(q31;q32); IL3-IGH
  B lymphoblastic leukaemia/lymphoma with t(1;19)q23;p13.3); E2A-PBX1 (TCF3-PBX1)

Precursor T lymphoblastic leukaemia/lymphoma

Mature B-cell neoplasms

Chronic lymphocytic leukaemia/ small lymphocytic lymphoma

B-prolymphocytic leukaemia

Splenic marginal zone lymphoma

Hairy cell leukaemia

Splenic B-cell lymphoma/leukaemia, unclassifiable

  Splenic diffuse red pulp small B-cell lymphoma
  Hairy cell leukaemia

Lymphoplasmacytic lymphoma/ Waldenström macroglobulinaemia

Heavy-chain disease

  Alpha heavy-chain disease
  Gamma heavy-chain disease
  Mu heavy-chain disease

Plasma cell myeloma

Solitary plasmacytoma of bone

Extraosseous plasmacytoma

Extranodal marginal zone lymphoma (MALT lymphoma)

Nodal marginal zone lymphoma

  Paediatric nodal marginal zone lymphoma

Follicular lymphoma

  Paediatric follicular lymphoma

Mantle cell lymphoma

Diffuse large B-cell lymphoma (DLBCL), NOS

  T-cell/histiocyte rich large B-cell lymphoma
  Primary DLBCL of CNS
  Primary cutaneous DLBCL, leg type

DLBCL associated with chronic inflammation

Lymphomatoid granulomatosis

Mediastinal (thymic) large B-cell lymphoma

Intravascular large B-cell lymphoma

ALK positive large B-cell lymphoma

Plasmablastic lymphoma

Large B-cell lymphoma arising in HHV8-associated multicentric Castleman disease

Primary effusion lymphoma

Burkitt lymphoma

B-cell lymphoma, unclassifiable, with features intermediate between diffuse and

  Large B-cell lymphoma and Burkitt lymphoma

B-cell lymphoma, unclassifiable, with features intermediate between diffuse and

  Large B-cell lymphoma and classical Hodgkin lymphoma

Mature T-cell and NK-cell neoplasms

T-cell prolymphocytic leukaemia

T-cell large granular lymphocytic leukaemia

Chronic lymphoproliferative disorder of NK-cells

  Aggressive NK-cell leukaemia
  Systemic EBV positive T-cell lymphoproliferative disease of childhood
  Hydroa vacciniforme-like lymphoma
  Adult T-cell leukaemia/lymphoma
  Extranodal NK/T-cell lymphoma nasal-type
  Enteropathy-type T-cell lymphoma
  Hepatosplenic T–cell lymphoma
  Subcutaneous panniculitis-like T-cell lymphoma

Mycosis fungoides

Sézary syndrome

Primary cutaneous CD30-positive T-cell lymphoproliferative disorders

  Primary cutaneous anaplastic T-cell lymphoma (ALCL) Lymphomatoid papulosis

Primary cutaneous gamma-delta T-cell lymphoma

Primary cutaneous CD8 positive aggressive epidermotropic cytotoxic T-cell Lymphoma

Primary cutaneous CD4 positive aggressive small-medium T-cell lymphoma

Peripheral T-cell lymphoma, NOS

Angioimmunoblastic T-cell lymphoma

Anaplastic large-cell lymphoma, ALK positive

Anaplastic large-cell lymphoma, ALK negative

Hodgkin lymphoma

Nodular Lymphocyte predominant Hodgkin lymphoma

Classical Hodgkin lymphoma

   Nodular sclerosis classical Hodgkin lymphoma

   Mixed cellularity classical Hodgkin lymphoma

   Lymphocyte-rich classical Hodgkin lymphoma

   Lymphocyte-depleted classical Hodgkin lymphoma

Post-transplant lymphoproliferative disorders (PTLD)

Early lesions

   Plasmacytic hyperplasia

   Infectious mononucleosis-like PTLD

Polymorphic PTLD

Monomorphic PTLD (B- and T/NK-cell types)

Classical Hodgkin lymphoma type PTLD.

Reproduced with permission from Swerdlow SH et al., *WHO Classification of Tumours of Haematopoietic and Lymphoid Tissues, Fourth Edition*, World Health Organization, Geneva, Switzerland, Copyright © 2008.

list of clinicopathologic entities, each defined by the amalgamation of morphology, phenotype, cytogenetics, molecular features, and clinical data along with the recognition of a normal counterpart. The entities were subdivided into accepted and provisional, depending on their unanimous acknowledgment or the need for further validation before definitive acceptance. In particular, by comparison with the previous edition, several well-known lymphoma entities were revised and new entities were included. Thus, among peripheral B-cell lymphomas (BCL), international consensus guidelines were adopted for CLL, lymphoplasmacytic lymphoma (LPL), Waldenström macroglobulinaemia (WM), and plasma cell myeloma (PCM). In the field of CLL, the concept of monoclonal B-cell lymphocytosis (MBL) was incorporated, representing an important practical issue [32]. In addition, the EORTC consensus classification of cutaneous lymphomas was included [33]. The grading of FL was simplified by combining grades 1 and 2 and maintaining grades 3A and 3B. The latter was a matter of debate, since it might be related to DLBCL of the GCB type more than to the remaining FLs. Finally, it was decided to maintain the term FL only for cases with a pure follicular growth pattern. Furthermore, the borders of FL were broadened by

quoting the paediatric, intestinal, other extranodal, and in situ variants. In the section on MCL, in situ and indolent variants were reported as the possible result of multi-step lymphomagenesis. The spectrum of DLBCL was significantly enlarged by establishing the basic distinction between a not otherwise specified form on the one hand and subtypes and special types on the other. Notably, some provisional entities were set up: splenic B-cell lymphoma/leukaemia, unclassifiable (including diffuse red pulp small B-cell lymphoma and hairy cell leukaemia variants), paediatric nodal MZL (to be distinguished from atypical MZ hyperplasia with monotypic Ig expression), EBV-positive DLBCL of the elderly, and borderline lesions between DLBCL and BL or CHL. In particular, the term BCL was considered unclassifiable, with features intermediate between DLBCL and BL. This was applied to cases resembling BL but presented with evident pleomorphism or to typical BL carrying aberrant phenotype and/or genetic features. These cases have a *MYC*-complex karyotype and require treatment as BL [34]. BCL-unclassifiable, with features intermediate between DLBCL and CHL, more often presents in males aged between 30–40 years with a bulky mediastinal mass [35]. Morphologically and phenotypically, it shows features between CHL and DLBCL, especially primary mediastinal large B-cell lymphoma (PMBL) [35]. The behaviour is more aggressive than the one of CHL or PMBL [35]. At the time being, the optimal treatment remains matter of debate.

Peripheral T-cell lymphomas (PTCL) were also extensively revised. The chapters on PTCL-not otherwise specified (NOS) and angioimmunoblastic T-cell lymphoma (AITL) were expanded. The former included the follicular variant; similar to AITL, it is related to follicular T-helper (FTH) lymphocytes [36]. There is increasing evidence that the FTH signature is not restricted to AITL—as originally thought [37]—but does also occur in a group of PTCLs that do not fulfil the diagnostic criteria for AITL [38]. In the 4th edition of the WHO Classification, anaplastic large-cell lymphoma (ALCL) was subdivided into two categories: ALK⁺ and ALK⁻, characterized by the occurrence or absence of genetic alterations involving *ALK*. In particular, the former carries the t(2;5) translocation and variants, causing ALK gene and protein over-expression. On immunohistochemistry, the latter is aberrantly detected in the nucleus and/or cytoplasm based on the translocation at work [30]. At the present time, ALK⁺ ALCL is regarded as a distinct entity, most frequently occurring in children/adolescents and with a good response to therapy if the IPI is below 3 [30]. The genetic aberration that leads to ALK over-expression drives lymphomagenesis and can represent the target for tailored therapies and vaccination. ALK⁻ ALCL is morphologically and phenotypically indistinguishable from the ALK⁺ form, showing the same 'hallmark' cells, cohesive growth pattern, diffusion through sinuses, CD30 expression (that represents the target of brentuximab vedotin [38]), positivity for cytotoxic markers, possible lack of CD45, frequent EMA expression, variable staining for T-cell markers, general negativity for CD15, PAX5/BSAP, and EBV, and frequent clonal *TCR@* rearrangement [30]. The ALK⁻ ALCL category was debated at the time of the classification writing, since it was argued that it should be combined with PTCL-NOS. Finally, the decision was taken to maintain it distinct from both ALK⁺ ALCL and PTCL-NOS. This decision has later found validation in studies, which showed that, although more aggressive than the ALK⁺ form, ALK⁻ ALCL has a response to therapy superior to PTCL-NOS [39]. Also, the gene signature of ALK$^-$ ALCL is distinct from that of PTCL-NOS, revealing instead deregulation of several pathways in common with ALK$^+$ ALCL [40]. More recently, massive parallel genome sequencing has allowed the identification of a t(6;7)(p25.3;q32.3) translocation in about 30% of ALK$^-$ ALCLs, causing down-regulation of *DUSP22* and up-regulation of *MIR29* micro-RNAs [41]. In the 2008 WHO Classification, the category of enteropathy-associated T-cell lymphoma (EATL) was introduced, which is much more restrictive than the enteropathy-type of the 3rd edition by indicating evidence of coeliac disease (CD). However, a variant of EATL (termed type II) was described that can also occur in the absence of risk factors or clinical signs of CD. This is characterized by monomorphic small-to-medium sized elements, expressing CD8 and CD56, and carrying *MYC* amplifications; it likely represents an entity distinct from EATL. The term 'subcutaneous panniculitis-like T-cell lymphoma' was restricted to neoplasms of peripheral α/β T-lymphocytes, characterized by a five-year OS of about 80% with conservative therapies [42]. Tumours with similar morphology, but γ/δ phenotype, were assigned to a new category termed primary cutaneous γ/δ T-cell lymphoma, with a 15-month OS [42]. Novel entities were the EBV$^+$ lymphoproliferative disorders of childhood, related to a cytotoxic defect of the host response to the virus and commonly affecting children in Mexico, Taiwan and Japan [43]. Two variants of the condition are known: systemic EBV$^+$ lymphoproliferative disease of children [43] and Hydroa vacciniforme-like lymphoma [44]. The former usually develops within the context of chronic active EBV infection and is rapidly fatal due to the onset of a haemophagocytic syndrome and/or multi-organ failure [43]. The latter, which is associated with insect bites and sun exposure, is limited to the skin and lasts 10–15 years before systemic progression [44]. Finally, the 4th edition of the WHO Classification ruled out the so-called NK/T-cell lymphoma, blastic type that originates from plasmacytoid dendritic cells, and listed some further provisional NK/T-cell entities. These include chronic lymphoproliferative disorders of NK-cells, clinically similar to LGL but lacking both clonality and malignancy [45], primary cutaneous CD8$^+$ aggressive epidermotropic cytotoxic T-cell lymphoma, and primary cutaneous CD4$^+$ small/medium T-cell lymphoma that is a very indolent condition, simply requiring complete excision when presenting in a solitary form [46].

Present challenges and pathobiology

The frequency of monoclonal B-cell lymphocytosis (MBL) tends to increase with age [31]. The elements sustaining it are clonal and carry the same phenotype as CLL [31]. However, only about 1% of cases progress to overt CLL [31]. Elements carrying the t(14;18) can be frequently detected in the peripheral blood of healthy individuals [41], their incidence becoming even higher in HCV$^+$ subjects [47]. Epidemiological studies, however, indicate that this finding does not predict FL development [41]. The same holds true for t(11;14), although its detection is much rarer than that of t(14;18) [48]. Notably, both of these conditions have potential counterparts at the tissue level commonly denoted as FL and MCL in situ [49, 50], although the term 'intrafollicular' would be more appropriate. The former corresponds to the presence of some germinal centres (GCs) consisting of BCL2$^+$/t(14;18)$^+$ monotonous elements, within the context of an otherwise normal lymph node [49]. The latter is characterized by the accumulation of cyclin D1$^+$/t(11;14)$^+$ cells in the inner layer of the mantle zone of some

follicles in a preserved lymph node structure [50]. Notably, both conditions undergo progression to an overt lymphoma in only a few patients [49, 50].

Another challenging issue is the occurrence of indolent variants of usually progressive or aggressive diseases. This is the case of 'indolent MCL', clinically characterized by splenomegaly, BM involvement, leukaemic spread, and lack of lymphadenopathy. Immunohistochemistry is negative for SOX11, a finding recently questioned by some authors [51]. Molecular biology indicates a post-GC derivation with a high load of somatic mutations. Notably, SNP arrays reveal one or two genetic lesions instead of the complex karyotype of usual MCL. Examples of FL are analogously encountered in children and adults that turn BCL2$^-$/t(14;18)$^-$. These are monoclonal at PCR, graded 3A or 3B, and display a very high proliferation rate. Interestingly, they lack *TP53* and/or *MYC* abnormalities in contrast to aggressive FLs that are also BCL2$^-$/t(14;18)$^-$ [52]. Thus, the distinction of such cases from follicular hyperplasia on the one hand and highly aggressive FL on the other is of pivotal importance. In fact, stage I patients are cured by the excision of the affected node. Similar findings have been reported in the setting of the so-called paediatric-type MZL that—when observed in adults—is cured by surgery [53].

In the 2008 WHO Classification, the diagnosis of some lymphomas still represents an exclusion process. Thus, nodal and extranodal MZLs are reported to be CD5, CD10, BCL6, CD23, and cyclin D1-negative, findings which excludes CLL/SLL, FL and MCL [30]. Very recently, however, a monoclonal antibody against a formalin-resistant epitope, the IRTA1 molecule, has been developed [54]. This reacts with most nodal and extranodal MZLs, but not the splenic variant. Interestingly, its application to more than 2100 cases showed that no other lymphoid tumours are stained with the exception of some DLBCLs with para-sinusoidal distribution (which might also have MZ origin) or of FLs with MZ differentiation. In addition, in conjunction with FISH studies, it showed that the colonization of pre-existing follicles by neoplastic cells is associated with loss of IRTA1 and re-exposure of BCL6 in the absence of CD10, an observation questioning the criteria previously used for the 'exclusion' diagnosis.

As previously mentioned, the opportunity to maintain type II EATL within the same box as type I is matter of debate. In fact, it has recently been reported that most if not all 'type II' EATLs stem from γδ T-lymphocytes, type I being an αβ T-cell tumour [55]. Thus, 'type II' might represent a different entity and thus deserve a different name.

Recently developed high-throughput technologies have allowed in-depth exploration of the mechanisms sustaining the development, progression, and chemoresistance of malignant lymphomas. Relevant information is coming from next generation sequencing (NGS) that can lead to the discovery of mutations driving their pathogenesis. Besides the t(6;7) detected in about one third of ALK$^-$ ALCLs, many recurrent genetic aberrations have been discovered in the setting of malignant lymphomas. Thus, all hairy cell leukaemia cases carry a heterozygous mutation in *BRAF* resulting in the BRAF V600E variant protein provided with oncogenic properties [56]. Importantly, this mutation does not occur in other B-cell lymphomas and can represent the rationale for the usage of specific inhibitors of active BRAF [56]. In CLL, NGS has shown that the recurrent *NOTCH1*, *MYD88*, and *XPO1* mutations are oncogenic and contribute to disease evolution [57]. In particular, Fabbri et al.

[58] reported *NOTCH1* mutations in 8.3% of patients at diagnosis, with prevalence rising up to 31% and 20.8% in patients with Richter transformation and chemorefractory disease, respectively. In conjunction with the fact that they are detected in only 3.2% of MBLs, these findings suggest that *NOTCH1* mutations represent an acquired lesion strictly related to disease progression. The application of NGS to FL and DLBCL has shown that they harbour frequent structural alterations inactivating *CREBBP* and, more rarely, *EP300*, two highly-related histone and non-histone acetyl-transferases (HATs) acting as transcriptional co-activators in multiple signalling pathways [59]. Overall, about 39% of DLBCLs and 41% of FLs display genomic deletions and/or somatic mutations that remove or inactivate the HAT coding domain of these genes. Such lesions are usually mutually exclusive and affect one allele, suggesting that reduction in HAT dosage is important for lymphomagenesis by mediating inactivation of *BCL6* and activation of *TP53*, and drugs targeting acetylation/de-acetylation mechanisms might be effective in this setting. The mutation of *MYD88* has been reported in different lymphoma categories [60]. MYD88 transduces signals from Toll-like, IL1, and IL18 receptors to the NF-κB transcription factors that, in turn, regulate the production of cytokines and anti-apoptotic molecules. It can be the target of specific inhibitors. Whole-transcriptome paired-end sequencing has revealed that *CIITA* (*MHC2TA*) breaks are highly recurrent in PMBL (38%) and CHL (15%) [61]. Functional consequences of *CIITA* fusions are down-regulation of surface HLA class II expression and over-expression of CD274/PD-L1 and PDCD1LG2/PD-L2, respectively, causing reduced tumour cell immunogenicity and antitumour immune responses. Last, but not least, *IDH2* and *TET2* mutations have been reported in PTCLs, the former being associated with AITL [62].

The goal of these technologies is to identify novel targets for tailored therapies. Interesting data have been obtained in PTCL-NOS, which has a poor response to conventional drugs including anthracyclines, with a five-year OS of 20% [63]. Recent gene expression profiling (GEP) studies have provided hints for the usage of tyrosine kinase (TKI), histone deacetylase and proteasome inhibitors [64]. In particular, aberrant activation of tyrosine kinases seems to commonly occur in PTCLs and TKIs have been found effective in ex vivo models [64].

Molecular genetics

Over the last decade, advances in technology and decreasing costs for NSG experiments have greatly increased our molecular understanding of lymphomas to the extent that not only have new categories of lymphomas been defined, but these technologies are becoming increasingly instrumental for the prediction of outcome and for identifying rationally-designed targeted treatments. While the initial landscape of frequent genetic alterations in almost all lymphoma subtypes has been reported, current efforts will shed light on the less frequent genetic alterations and the clonality of genetic events within a tumour sample. Emerging data suggest that single tumour samples harbour multiple genetic drivers and current and future efforts need to fully unveil their complex functional interplay. Therefore, we will now show in certain aggressive B-cell lymphomas how technology has been used to deepen our understanding of the molecular genetics, to predict outcome, and to identify rationally-defined targeted treatments.

Diffuse large B-cell lymphoma
Germinal centre origin
DLBCLs largely originate from germinal centres (GC), where high-affinity antibodies during humoral immune responses are formed by somatic hypermutation (SHM) and where the heavy-chain of the antibody changes from IgM and IgD to IgG, IgA, or IgE by class switch recombination (CSR) [65]. Both processes, SHM and CSR, are associated with DNA strand breaks, single nucleotide changes, small deletions, and duplications in somatic cells [65]. Consequently, these processes and the high proliferation rate in the GC predispose normal GC B-cells to malignant transformation. As a result, DLBCLs exhibit multiple low-frequency genetic alterations including chromosomal translocations, somatic mutations, and copy number alterations (CNAs) [65].

Transcriptional heterogeneity
Given the intrinsic clinical heterogeneity and numbers and types of genetic alterations in DLBCL, investigators have sought additional comprehensive classification systems to identify groups of tumours with similar molecular traits in various settings. By profiling samples at diagnosis and samples from patients who relapse after cyclophosphamide, doxorubicin, vincristine, and prednisone (CHOP), gene expression profiling has been used to identify signatures of resistance in patients [66]. This led to the identification of the protein kinase PKCß as a rational therapeutic target, prompting subsequent preclinical work and resulting in clinical testing of enzostaurin, a PKCß inhibitor, in DLBCL [67].

Transcriptional profiling has also been used to define DLBCL subsets that share certain features with normal B-cell subtypes, leading to the widely used cell-of-origin (COO) classification [68]. COO-defined DLBCLs distinguish tumours that share transcriptional signatures with GC-derived B-cells (GCB-type) and other tumours that share signatures with in vitro activated GC-B-cells (ABC-type), suggesting that each subtype originates from different stages of B-cell differentiation by acquisition of distinct oncogenic events during lymphomagenesis [68]. Therefore, each subtype is characterized by certain biological features, most notably increased NF-κB activity and less favourable outcome in ABC-type DLBCLs (see [68] for details).

An alternative transcriptional-profiling classification, termed comprehensive consensus clustering (CCC classification), identifies DLBCL subtypes solely on the basis of distinctions within primary tumours and includes three groups: B-cell receptor (BCR-type), oxidative phosphorylation (OxPhos-type), and host-response (HR-type) [69]. Within this classification, OxPhos DLBCLs have increased expression of genes regulating oxidative phosphorylation, mitochondrial function, and electron transport, resulting in different fuel utilization and metabolism of the DLBCL cell, a putatively targetable feature [69, 70]. The HR-type DLBCLs have certain genetic features with the pathological defined subtype 'T-cell histiocyte rich B-cell lymphoma'. The BCR DLBCLs rely on tonic B-cell receptor signalling owing to increased expression and activation of members of the BCR-signalling cascade [69, 71]. Hence, these tumours are susceptible to various inhibitors of the BCR-signalling cascade in vitro and in vivo [71, 72]. This led to the clinical development of various BCR-signalling inhibitors, from which SYK and BTK inhibitors are the most clinically advanced and tested in clinical trials [73]. Recently, ABC DLBCLs have been reported to be sensitive to upstream modulation of BCR signalling, underscoring the importance of targeting this critical survival pathway in DLBCLs [74, 75].

Structural basis of underlying biological heterogeneity

Somatic mutations

The initial landscape of somatic mutations in primary DLBCL was reported by several independent groups which were limited by sample size [76–79]. As a consequence, only ten reported mutations show a high concordance between the four different cohorts using different deep-sequencing approaches (RNA Seq and whole-exome sequencing) suggesting the potential relevance of these identified recurrent mutations. However, this also underscores that to capture the full spectrum of genetic driver events (so-called 'long tail') larger, more comprehensive studies need to be performed.

One of the most frequent events reported in these studies were inactivating somatic mutations in *TP53,* found in only about 20% of patients. This is remarkable, since inactivating mutations of *TP53* in certain solid neoplasms occur in up to 100% of patients [77–80] and suggests that in DLBCL additional means of inactivating *TP53* exists (see Copy number alterations, below). In addition, infrequent mutations in cyclin D3 (*CCND3*) have been reported [78, 81]. While for some of the identified mutations the associated biology has been addressed, for the majority of mutations a functional evaluation is pending. Of note, several gain of function mutations have been linked to be the structural basis of ABC-type DLBCLs, such as activating mutations in *CD79B, MYD88,* and *CARD11* [68, 82, 83]. In addition, mutations in *FBXO11*, which encodes an F-box protein, are important to diminish the post-transcriptional degradation and thereby stabilizing BCL6, a master regulator of DLBCL biology [84–86]. Furthermore, epigenetic modifiers are frequently altered in DLBCL, such as *EZH2, MLL2,* and *MEF2B*, as well as *CREBBP* [74, 76–78, 84] (see also above).

Copy number alterations

Initial work focused on the identification of individual CNAs in smaller cohorts, which resulted in the discovery of deletions in the tumour suppressor genes *CDKN2A, RB1,* and *TP53* [78, 88–90]. With the advent of whole-genome approaches, larger cohorts were analyzed more comprehensively and several CNAs were captured concordantly, especially with respect to their differential distribution across the COO-defined subtypes of DLBCLs [91, 92]. These studies used array Comparative Genomic Hybridization (aCGH) to identify CNAs and tried to link certain CNAs to putative target genes. They reported deletion of 9p24/*CDKN2A*, trisomy 3, and amplification of chromosome 19 to be enriched in ABC-type DLBCLs. Additionally, *REL* amplification on chromosome 2 and deletion of the *PTEN* tumour suppressor are enriched in GCB-type DLBCLs [91, 92].

Recently, higher resolution technologies, such as HD-SNP arrays, allowed a more fine-grained analysis of the precise boundaries of CNAs, the associated candidate 'driver genes', and implicated pathways [93]. By integrating high-density copy number data with transcriptional profiles and performing pathway analysis in 180 primary DLBCLs, a recent study identified a comprehensive set of CNAs within the *CDKN2A-TP53-RB-E2F* axis that decreased p53 activity, perturbed cell-cycle regulation, and provided a structural basis for increased proliferation in DLBCL [93]. Since DLBCLs have infrequent inactivating somatic mutations of *TP53* and *RB1*, these data define an alternative copy number-dependent mechanism of deregulating p53 and *E2F1*-mediated cell cycle progression [93]. Of note, two-thirds of primary DLBCLs had multiple complementary CNA of p53 and cell-cycle components and were named 'complex DLBCLs', while the remaining third largely lacked these lesions ('clean DLBCLs'). Patients treated with rituximab-CHOP (R-CHOP) and with complex CNA patterns had a five-year OS of only 62%, whereas those with clean CNA signatures were all cured [93]. The association between CN complexity and outcome added prognostic value to the IPI and/or transcriptional COO categories [93]. Most interestingly, this genetic signature not only predicts outcome, but is amenable to targeted treatment with pan cyclin-dependent kinase inhibition or BET-bromodomain inhibition in vitro and in vivo [93, 94].

Translocations

Several groups reported independently on the unfavourable prognostic value of aggressive lymphomas that contain chromosomal translocations of both *MYC* and *BCL2*, commonly referred to as 'double hit DLBCL'. Initial reports used this term for DLBCLs with a chromosomal rearrangement, but as the prognosis of patients with positive immunohistochemistry for both oncogenes is also poor, this definition now also includes these cases. These 'double hit lymphomas' occur in both GCB-type and ABC-type DLBCL and their clinical management is a major challenge to active clinical investigation [95–97].

Primary mediastinal large B-cell lymphoma

Gene expression profiling (GEP) has also been used to distinguish a large B-cell lymphoma with evident different clinical features and defined a new entity of lymphoma, primary mediastinal large B-cell lymphomas (PMBL) [98, 99]. In the new WHO classification, PMBL has been fully recognized as its own entity [100]. Patients presenting with PMBL are predominantly women, with a median age of ~35 years old and an inferior outcome with standard treatment [101]. GEP revealed that PMBLs share features of CHL, such as constitutive activation of the NF-κB survival pathway [98–101]. Interestingly, an additional similarity between CHL and PMBL is the amplification of 9p24, resulting in the increased expression of several oncogenes, including *JAK2, JMJD2C,* and the two PD-1 ligands, PD-L1 (*CD274*) and PD-L2 (*PDCD1LG2*) [102, 103]. Thereby, *JAK2* co-operates with the demethylase *JMJD2C* in promoting an open chromatin structure allowing the expression of several survival genes, including *MYC* [102]. Besides promoting proliferation itself, *JAK2* also amplifies the expression of the PD-1 ligands [103, 104]. Both the PD-1 ligands, PD-L1 and PD-L2, are also targets of chromosomal translocation from transcription factor *CIITA* in cHL and PMBL [105]. The multiple genetic bases of deregulated PD-1 expression reflect an effective immune evasion strategy of the CHL tumour cells against infiltrating T-cells [103, 104]. Neutralizing antibodies against PD-1 and PD-L1 were tested in phase III trials with great success, even in diseases without a genetic basis of PD-L1/L2 deregulation [106, 107]. Most notably, this genetic basis of deregulated PD-1 ligand expression prompted the clinical evaluation of PD-1 blockade in CHL. The clinical trial evaluating the PD-1 antibody nivolumumab in multiple pretreated CHL has recently been published, reporting an overall response rate of 87% [108]. This data resulted in breakthrough status assignment by the FDA and is an example of a rationally-defined target by whole genome technologies.

Burkitt lymphoma

Transcriptional profiling was further used to define boundaries between DLBCLs and Burkitt lymphoma (BL) [109, 110]. This distinction is clinically relevant, since BL, also a GCB-derived disease with lower prevalence, resembles DLBCL in some cases morphologically and cytogenetically [100]. However, BL benefits from a more aggressive treatment than DLBCLs upfront. To that end, two independent groups demonstrated that transcriptional profiles derived from classical DLBCL and BL define both entities, but also highlighted an additional molecular BL (mBL). mBL is not morphologically distinguishable from DLBCL, but shares molecular features of BL and has inferior outcome when treated with DLBCL protocols [109, 110].

Multi-step-model-pathogenesis of Burkitt lymphoma

A hallmark event of BL is the translocation of the MYC proto-oncogene into the Ig locus, resulting in deregulated expression of *MYC* in virtual all cases of BL [100]. Transgenic expression of *MYC* leads to increased proliferation, metabolic reprogramming, and increased genomic instability of the transformed cell, and also to increased apoptosis. To overcome apoptosis, additional alterations have been postulated, but besides inactivation of *TP53* no other co-operating transforming event has been implicated in the lymphomagenesis of BL [111]. Recently, two studies have implicated additional activating events, augmenting the BCR signalling through the PI3K pathway as a major second event in the pathogenesis of BL in humans and mice [81, 112]. Human RNA-Seq data were combined with functional and structural data to implicate activating mutations in the transcription factor, *TCF3*, and inactivating mutation in its negative regulator, *ID3*, resulting in augmentation of tonic BCR signalling, and thereby providing the survival signal to overcome the pro-apoptotic part of the transgenic expression of *MYC* [81]. Consistently, mice engineered to express *MYC* and a constitutive active form of PI3K ectopically in GCB cells, resulted in the development of lymphomas after a longer latency, representing a faithful BL mice model [81, 112]. Both studies revealed mutations in cyclin D3 (*CCND3*) as tertiary events in human and mice, resulting in prolonged stability of *CCND3* [81, 112]. Thus, BL requires a multi-step lymphomagenesis, potentially targetable with compounds inhibiting the PI3K pathway and cyclin D-dependent kinases [81, 112].

Chemotherapy

Chemotherapy is the backbone of lymphoma treatment. In 1976 McKelvey et al. [113] established the combination of CHOP (cyclophosphamide, doxorubicin, vincristine, and prednisone) which became the gold standard of treatment in many malignant lymphomas. Depending on the stage of the disease and risk factors, about 30–50% of patients with aggressive lymphomas were cured with CHOP or CHOP-like regimens in the pre-rituximab era. Due to lower proliferative activity, chemotherapy has only palliative effects in indolent lymphomas. Chemotherapy is used in combination with CD20-antibody rituximab in all BCLs today. The majority of chemotherapy trials in the 1980s and 1990s included patients with BCLs as well as those with diseases of T-cell phenotype. However, in patients with (non-cutaneous and non-leukaemic) peripheral T-cell lymphomas, both response and survival after chemotherapy are worse compared to the diseases of B-cell origin [114].

Aggressive B-cell lymphomas

Aggressive B-cell lymphomas represent a clinically-defined group of entities with similar biology and prognosis. In terms of treatment, the category includes the numerous variants and subtypes of DLBCL and grade 3 FLs. MCL is also regarded as an aggressive B-cell lymphoma for which different treatment algorithms are increasingly being identified. The treatment of lymphoblastic, Burkitt and Burkitt-like lymphomas follow the complex chemotherapy concepts of acute leukaemia due to their even more aggressive behaviour.

In the 1980s, several modifications of the CHOP protocol (MACOP-B, m-BACOD, ProMACE-CytaBOM) showed superior response rates (RR) and survival in advanced NHL in phase 2 trials (overview in [115]). However, the results of these complex regimens with up to eight cytotoxic drugs could not be reproduced in a large multicentre trial in the US [116]. In patients with limited disease, combinations of a reduced number of chemotherapy cycles followed by radiotherapy of involved sites has been regarded an effective approach. Longer follow-up of a Southwest Oncology Group (SWOG) trial comparing three cycles of CHOP followed by involved-field radiation (IFRT) vs eight cycles of chemotherapy did not confirm initial promising results in terms of survival advantage for combined modality [117, 118]. Therefore, full-course CHOP-based chemotherapy remains the standard of care for patients with aggressive B-cell lymphomas.

In the 1990s, the German High-Grade Non-Hodgkin Lymphoma Study Group (DSHNHL) evaluated the effects of adding etoposide, which had been shown high single-agent activity in lymphomas, to standard CHOP protocol (CHOEP). Etoposide was given at a dose of 100 mg/m^2 on three consecutive days. In an initial phase 2 study [119], 60 previously untreated patients with aggressive lymphomas (67% with stage III/IV) received six cycles of CHOEP and IFRT. Forty-nine patients (82%) achieved a complete remission, most of them (n = 45, 75%) after the fourth chemotherapy cycle and before radiotherapy was started. Toxicity was manageable. The rate of overall response was 93%; OS depended on stage and lymphoma subtype and was about 50%. The results were reproduced in a phase 3 trial comparing CHOEP with an approach of alternating dose-intensified CHOP and IVEP (ifosfamide, vindesine, etoposide, prednisone), showing no superior benefit for alternating regimens, concluding that both are effective treatment protocols for aggressive histologic-type malignant lymphomas [120].

The second approach of the DSHNHL to improve outcome in aggressive lymphomas was to increase dose intensity by shortening the intervals between treatment cycles. A faster sequence of cytotoxic effects should cause more intense cell death and impairment of tumour regrowth. This concept is based not only on the known strong dose-response relationship in chemosensitive diseases, but also on kinetic models of tumour cell growth and development of chemoresistance [121]. In addition, interval reduction was facilitated by the availability of haematopoietic growth factors, which made the haematological toxicity manageable.

Both methods of intensification (addition of etoposide, interval reduction) were investigated in the large German multicentre NHL-B trial. Between 1993 and 2000 almost 1700 patients with aggressive NHL (B- as well as T-cell lymphomas) were randomized to receive standard CHOP or CHOEP every three weeks (CHOP-21, CHOEP-21) or every two weeks (CHOP-14, CHOEP-14). The feasibility of the presumably most effective, but also most toxic treatment, with two-weekly CHOEP had been tested in a phase 2 trial [122]. In this pilot study, 30 patients with aggressive lymphomas received a total of 159 cycles of CHOEP-14 chemotherapy. G-CSF was given between day four and 13, and blood counts recovered completely in all cycles. Non-haematological toxicity was tolerable.

The NHL-B trial included ≤60-year-old patients with low-risk (LDH within normal range) aggressive lymphoma (NHL-B1) and all patients aged between 61 and 75 years (NHL-B2). Data of an interim analysis in 959 patients demonstrated that administration of standard-dosed and intensified chemotherapy cycles was safe and practicable in all age and risk groups [123]. For young patients with normal LDH level, CHOEP-21 was identified as the optimal regimen based on outcome and toxicity results. Complete remission (87.6% vs 79.4%, p = 0.003) and five-year-event-free survival (EFS) (69.2% vs 57.6%, p = 0.004) rates were superior to standard CHOP [124]. In contrast, two-weekly CHOP was defined to be the new standard in older patients (CR rate 76.1% vs 60.1% and five-year EFS 43.8% vs 32.5% compared to CHOP-21) [125]. The different results were interpreted to be attributable to the inclusion of patients with highly proliferative tumours in the NHL-B2 trial, whereas in the NHL-B1 study (for the younger population) elevation of LDH was an exclusion criterion. In patients >60, CHOEP-14 was associated with increased toxicities and treatment delay.

The substitution of doxorubicin by idarubicin within the CHOEP-protocol (CIVEP) was investigated in a phase 2 trial. Idarubicin had demonstrated greater cytotoxicity than daunorubicin or doxorubicin in various cell line models and showed reduced cardiac toxicity in clinical studies. However, the use within the CIVEP protocol was accompanied with increased haematotoxicity without improvement in efficacy [126, 127].

The further investigations regarding chemotherapy of lymphoma focused on three items. First, are there six or eight cycles of chemotherapy necessary to cure patients? Second, what are the best chemotherapy concepts for patients with different risk profiles? Third, are there results for treatment intensification reproducible if chemotherapy is combined with rituximab?

Eight vs six cycles of chemotherapy

Treatment of aggressive lymphomas with eight cycles of chemotherapy was established empirically based on the concept of remission 'induction' and 'consolidation' and became the standard of care, which was also used in large multicentre trials [116, 117]. Patients treated in the French GELA LNH98-5 trial, which established R-CHOP combination in first-line treatment of DLBCL, also received eight cycles of immunochemotherapy [128]. The addition of rituximab significantly improved CR-rates (76% vs 63%, p = 0.005) and survival (two-year-EFS, 57% vs 38%, p <0.001; two-year-OS, 70% vs 57%, p = 0.007). Furthermore, risk of early progression and death also were reduced significantly. The results were confirmed with longer follow-up [129].

A randomized comparison of six vs eight cycles of chemotherapy, with or without rituximab, was performed in the RICOVER-60 trial of the DSHNHL [130]. More than 1200 patients between 61 and 80 years with DLBCL were included. The study confirmed the superiority of R-CHOP over CHOP alone. In addition, no further improvement was observed with more than six cycles of CHOP or

R-CHOP. Therefore, six cycles of R-CHOP-14 were recommended as the preferred regimen in elderly patients with DLBCL.

Chemotherapy in the rituximab era

The implementation of rituximab in the treatment of aggressive B-cell lymphoma improves patient outcome markedly. Furthermore, the question arose as to whether there are benefits from different strategies of dose intensification.

The role of etoposide-supplemented CHOP was redefined by the MInT-Trial [131]. This international study primarily compared CHOP-like chemotherapy with and without CD20-antibody in young patients (18–60 years) with good-prognosis DLBCL. Different chemotherapy protocols could have been used (CHOP-21, CHOEP-21, MACOP-B, PMitCEBO). While there was a significant improvement of EFS at three years with CHOEP-21 alone compared to CHOP-21 alone, no benefit with CHOEP was demonstrated if chemotherapy was combined with rituximab. Therefore, six cycles of CHOP-21 plus rituximab was defined as a standard of care in the young good-risk DLBCL population.

The optimal number and interval of chemotherapy cycles was addressed again by two large European multicentre studies. First, the French trial (LNH03-6B) included patients between 60–80 years with newly-diagnosed DLBCL and at least one risk factor according to aaIPI [132]. Compared to the German RICOVER-60 study, the LNH03-6B population was slightly older and the risk profile was higher. Patients were randomized to receive eight cycles of R-CHOP-14 or eight cycles of R-CHOP-21. The two-weekly regimen did not improve outcome, but, apart from a higher number of red cell transfusions, did also not increase toxicity. A major finding was that relative dose intensities for cyclophosphamide and doxorubicin were significantly lower in the dose-dense R-CHOP-14 arm after two, four, and eight cycles. This might be attributed also to an inconsistent use of granulocyte colony stimulating factor (GCSF), which was administered in (only) about 90% of cycles in the two-weekly regimen arm.

The second trial was undertaken by the UK Clinical Research Network and compared six cycles of R-CHOP-14 and eight cycles of R-CHOP-21 in adult DLBCL patients [133]. GCSF was given in all patients with R-CHOP-14. The median relative dose intensities of the individual cytotoxic drugs achieved almost 100% of planned doses in both arms. However, superiority of two-weekly chemotherapy could not be demonstrated in any subgroups (e.g., age, risk profile, ABC/GCB phenotype). Therefore, the conclusion was that R-CHOP-21 remains the standard of care in first-line treatment of DLBCL.

Chemotherapy of younger patients in different risk groups

Ongoing efforts target on the identification of different risk groups among lymphoma patients and on the identification of treatment strategies with the best efficacy at minimal toxicity.

Previous trials mainly addressed age or risk-adapted concepts. Algorithms for first-line treatment commonly assign young patients <60 years into a good-risk and a poor-risk group based on the IPI criteria. For poor-risk patients (IPI category high-intermediate and high-risk) more intensive chemotherapy regimen, with or without autologous transplantation, was evaluated in numerous studies. None of them could conclusively demonstrate an improvement in long-term outcome. Treatment with eight cycles of biweekly R-CHOEP showed encouraging efficacy in a randomized comparison with repetitive autografting within the German MegaCHOEP trial (3-year EFS, 69.5% vs 61.4%; PFS, 73.7% vs 69.8%; OS, 84.6% vs 77.0 %) [134].

A major finding of the MInT trial was that young good-risk patients can be divided in two different prognostic subgroups: favourable (IPI = 0, no bulk) or less favourable (IPI = 1 and/ or bulk) [131]. This study also evaluated the question of which size of bulky disease has an impact on outcome. Although the cut-off point remains arbitrary, a diameter of 10 cm was recommended as a suitable margin [135] to define populations with significantly different survival after R-CHOP. Ongoing German multicentre studies are investigating, for the young good-risk patients with less favourable profile, outcomes after six cycles of R-CHOP-14 (vs six cycles of R-CHOP-21) and the effect of a reduced number of chemotherapy cycles (from six to four) in those with favourable prognosis.

The French GELA group studied a more complex approach consisting of induction treatment and consolidation in young good-risk patients (LNH03-2B) [136]. Four cycles of ACVBP chemotherapy (see Table 54.1) combined with rituximab and intrathecal MTX administration once per cycle were administered, followed by sequential consolidation courses including methotrexate,

Table 54.1 Commonly-used chemotherapy regimen in aggressive non-Hodgkin lymphoma

(R)-CHO(E)P [113, 124, 128]	Dose		Route	Schedule
Rituximab	375	mg/m²	iv infusion	day 0 (or 1)
Cyclophosphamide	750	mg/m²	iv infusion	day 1
Doxorubicin	50	mg/m²	iv infusion	day 1
Vincristine	1.4*	mg/m²	iv bolus	day 1
Etoposide	100	mg/m²	iv infusion	days 1 to 3
Prednisone	100	mg	iv bolus or po	days 1 to 5
repeat on day 22				
or day 15 → G-CSF	5	µg/kg	*sc injection*	*days 4 to 13*
R-ACVBP [136]				
Rituximab	375	mg/m²	iv infusion	day 0 (or 1)
Doxorubicin	75	mg/m²	iv bolus	day 1
Cyclophosphamide	1200	mg/m²	iv infusion	day 1
Vindesine	2	mg/m²	iv bolus	days 1 and 5
Bleomycin	10	mg/m²	iv bolus	days 1 and 5
Prednisone	60	mg/m²	iv bolus or po	days 1 to 5
Methotrexate	15	mg	intrathecal bolus	day 1
repeat on day 15				
→ G-CSF	5	µg/kg	*sc injection*	*days 6 to 13*
R-DHAP [185, 188]				
Rituximab	375	mg/m²	iv infusion	day 0 (or 1)
Dexamethasone	40	mg	iv infusion	day 1

(continued)

Table 54.1 Continued

(R)-CHO(E)P [113, 124, 128]	Dose		Route	Schedule
Cytarabine	2 × 2000	mg/m²	iv infusion	day 2
Cisplatin	100	mg/m²	iv continuous infusion	day 1
repeat on day 22				
R-ICE [186, 187]				
Rituximab	375	mg/m²	iv infusion	day 0 (or 1)
Ifosfamide	5000	mg/m²	iv continuous infusion	day 2
Carboplatin	AUC	5	iv infusion	day 2
Etoposide	100	mg/m²	iv infusion	days 1 to 3
repeat on day 22				
(R)-DexaBEAM [191, 192]				
Rituximab	375	mg/m²	iv infusion	day 0 (or 1)
Dexamethasone	3×8	mg	p.o.	days 1 to 10
Carmustine	60	mg/m²	iv infusion	day 2
Etoposide	75 (to 100)	mg/m²	iv infusion	days 4 to 7
Cytarabine	2x 100	mg/m²	iv infusion	days 4 to 7
Melphalan	20	mg/m²	iv infusion	day 3
repeat on day 22				
R-DA-EPOCH***	Dose		Route	Schedule
Rituximab	375	mg/m²	iv infusion	day 0 (or 1)
Etoposide	50	mg/m²	iv continuous infusion	days 1 to 4
Vincristine	0.4	mg/m²	iv continuous infusion	days 1 to 4
Doxorubicin	10	mg/m²	iv continuous infusion	days 1 to 4
Prednisone	2 × 60	mg/m²	iv bolus or p.o.	days 1 to 5
→ G-CSF	5	µg/kg	*s.c. injection*	*day 6 to ANC recovery*

* max. 2.0 mg.

** Treatment concept includes four induction courses of R-ACVBP followed by sequential consolidation with two cycles of high-dose methotrexate (3 g/m²), four cycles of rituximab (375 mg/m²), ifosfamide (1500 mg/m²), and etoposide (300 mg/m²), and finally two cycles of subcutaneous cytarabine (100 mg/m² days 1 to 4), all courses given every two weeks.

*** DA—dose adjustment: presented doses are administered in cycle 1; subsequent doses are adjusted on the haematotoxicity after previous cycle (for details see reference [193]).

ifosfamide, and cytarabine. This concept was randomly compared to eight cycles of R-CHOP-21; radiotherapy was not permitted. Overall response was not different between the arms. In contrast, OS was significantly better in the R-ACVBP patients (92% vs 84% at three years, p = 0.0071). Toxicity was higher with the intensive regimen but was judged to be manageable. Five deaths unrelated to lymphoma occurred after R-ACVBP, but only three deaths in the CHOP group.

At present, new diagnostic tools and therapeutic approaches are under investigation. Tumour response by interim-PET after two, three, or four treatment cycles has been shown to be predictive for relapse rates and survival in small studies. Whether decision on therapy intensification (or de-escalation) can be made on this information is controversial. Furthermore, the use of new antibodies or signal inhibitors as adjuncts to chemotherapy could be an option in poor-prognosis patients.

Mantle cell lymphoma

Treatment of MCL has been changed over the last decade. The addition of rituximab to chemotherapy, the use of cytarabine, and the implementation of autologous transplant have improved patient outcome markedly [137].

The Houston group demonstrated promising results in patients with aggressive mantle cell lymphomas using a regimen of HyperCVAD alternating with high-dose methotrexate/cytarabine, both in combination with rituximab [138]. After ten years of follow-up, median OS was not reached and the median time-to-treatment failure (TTF) was 4.6 years for the entire study population and 5.9 years for patients ≤65 years. Similar concepts were evaluated by two European trials. Alternating courses of dose-intensified (Maxi-)CHOP and high-dose cytarabine (patients ≤60 years, 4 × 3 g/m²; patients >60 years, 4x2 g/m²) followed by BCNU, etoposide, cytarabine, and melphalan or cyclophosphamide (BEAM or BEAC) and stem cell rescue were given to 160 untreated patients in the Nordic MCL2 trial. In long-term follow-up, median OS and response duration were more than ten years [139].

The European MCL Network compared, in a randomized study, six courses of standard R-CHOP with alternating cycles of R-CHOP (× 3) and R-DHAP (× 3) in <65-year-old patients with stage II–IV disease [140]. Responding patients received autologous stem cell transplantation (ASCT) after TBI-containing conditioning. Response rates were high after autografting in both arms (97% vs 98%). TTF was significantly improved after CHOP/dexamethasone/high-dose ara-C/cisplatin (DHAP)/ASCT in all risk groups and there was a better OS for intermediate and high-risk patients. Furthermore, molecular remission was found to be a prognostic factor independent of the mantle cell lymphoma international prognostic index (MIPI), and the number of patients without minimal residual disease (MRD) was significantly higher in the DHAP arm [141].

For elderly patients or patients who are not suitable for intensive chemotherapy, immunochemotherapy remains the standard of care. Rituximab in combination with six to eight cycles of CHOP or six courses of bendamustine (90 mg/m² day 1 and 2, q4w) have been shown to be safe and effective regimens [142, 143]. Maintenance therapy with rituximab (375 mg/m² q2m) compared to interferon-alpha significantly reduced the risk of progression or death in a randomized trial [142]. Therefore, rituximab maintenance should be given to elderly patients responding to induction

treatment. While rituximab maintenance has also been shown to prolong response duration in relapsed or refractory patients responding to salvage chemotherapy [144], the role is not yet clear in patients after first-line ASCT.

During the last years, treatment options in mantle cell lymphomas were expanded by the development and introduction of new drugs. Temsirolimus, an inhibitor of the mammalian target of rapamycin (mTOR), has demonstrated to be effective in relapsed or refractory MCL. Twenty-two per cent of patients who received temsirolimus 175 mg intravenously weekly followed by 75 mg weekly showed a complete (2%) or partial (20%) response. Median progression-free survival (PFS) was significantly improved (4.8 vs 1.9 months, p = 0.0009) compared to other cytotoxic or antibody regimens [145]. Grade 3 or 4 adverse events were observed in about 90% of patients with temsirolimus, mainly cytopaenias and asthaenia.

A more promising approach is represented by the inhibition of Bruton's tyrosine kinase (BTK). The BTK-inhibitor ibrutinib was investigated in a phase 2 trial for patients with advanced, extensively pretreated, relapsed, or refractory disease. Ibrutinib was given at doses of 560 mg orally per day until progression or toxicity. Sixty-eight percent of patients responded completely (21%) or partially (47%). Median duration of response was 17.5 months. Side effects were mild or moderate, primarily with gastrointestinal symptoms. Grade 3 or 4 haematotoxicity occurred only in about 15% of cases [146].

Nowadays, proteasome inhibitors represent an established treatment option in multiple myeloma. This approach was also tested in patients with MCL. The use of bortezomib as a salvage regimen showed RRs in non-randomized trials in about 30–50% and promising PFS of up to 12 months [147].

Indolent B-cell lymphomas

In contrast to aggressive NHL, in which in almost all cases treatment is indicated after definitive diagnosis, disease management and treatment decisions are more complex in the indolent lymphomas. Although modern immunochemotherapy is able to reduce tumour burden substantially and complete remission can be documented in conventional and PET imaging, these treatment options have no curative potential due to the different biology of these entities.

An algorithm for decision-making in indolent nodal B-cell lymphomas is presented in Figure 54.3. Histological diagnosis should be followed by common staging procedures including CT (or MRI) scans and BM examination. Radiotherapy should be offered to patients in early-stage (Ann Arbor stage I or II, i.e., follicular) lymphoma, because there is a chance for long-lasting disease control, or even cure (dose, technique and results are discussed in chapter 'Role of radiotherapy').

This approach is supported by results from a recent retrospective SEER database study on effectiveness of first-line strategies in stage I FL [148]. Patients who underwent complete ('rigorous') staging had significantly better PFS than those who did not. Patients after systemic treatment (rituximab ± chemotherapy ± radiation) showed significantly improved PFS than patients after radiotherapy alone, but differences in OS were not observed.

A change of strategy has also been observed in patients with advanced, but asymptomatic, indolent lymphomas, with consensus for watchful waiting due to the lack of curative treatment options.

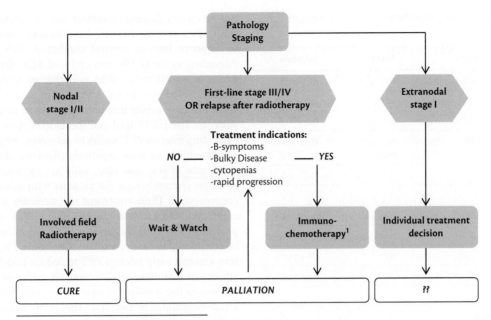

Fig. 54.3 Algorithm for treatment of decision making in indolent lymphomas (follicular, marginal zone, and lymphoplasmacytic).

A large British trial demonstrated a clinical benefit for patients with advanced stage, but non-bulky and asymptomatic FL, by treatment with rituximab monotherapy [148]. There was a significant longer PFS and time-to-next-therapy in patients who had received rituximab induction (375 mg/m² weekly, × 4) or rituximab induction followed by maintenance treatment (375 mg/m² q2mo × 12) compared to patients with observation only. Toxicity of antibody therapy was limited and also quality of life was not impaired; therefore, rituximab monotherapy should be considered for these patients.

The initiation of systemic treatment is clearly indicated in patients with symptomatic disease. Standard of care is a combination of chemotherapy and rituximab. Induction treatment includes six (to eight) cycles of immunochemotherapy followed by maintenance therapy with rituximab alone. Results with different commonly-used chemotherapy regimen are summarized in Table 54.2. Rituximab significantly improves treatment results, but there are different contributions with several chemotherapy regimens. The Italian FOLL05 [149] trial showed superiority of anthracycline-containing combinations CHOP and fludarabine/mitoxantrone (FM) over cyclophosphamide, vincristine, and prednisone (CVP) in RR and TTF. Data for OS in the different arms are not available because the study was not powered for this analysis. The German GLSG demonstrated in a randomized study higher RRs and reduced haematotoxicity after CHOP compared to MCP (mitoxantrone, chlorambucil, prednisolone) in patients with FL and MCLs [150]. However, there was no impact on survival.

The use of monochemotherapy with bendamustine instead of a combination regimen was investigated by the German STiL group. Bendamustine is an alkylating agent which was synthesized in the 1960s in Germany. The chemical structure is similar to classic alkylating drugs but also to purine analogues. This is hypothesized to be the background for high activity also in alkylator-resistant lymphomas [151]. Superior clinical efficacy was demonstrated

in a randomized trial comparing bendamustine to CHOP, both in combination with rituximab, in patients with indolent and MCLs [143]. More than 50% of patients in both arms had FLs, and less than 20% had MCL. Median PFS was significantly longer after R-bendamustine than after R-CHOP (69.5 vs 31.2 months, p <0.0001) for the entire group. The improvement was also found in MCL (35.4 vs 22.1 months, p = 0.0044) and Waldenström macroglubulinaemia (69.5 vs 28.1 months, p = 0.0033), but not in patients with mantle zone lymphoma (57.2 vs 47.2 months, p = 0.3249). Furthermore, the safety profile of bendamustine was much better: less haematotoxicity and infections, less peripheral neuropathy and stomatitis, and no alopecia. Therefore, R-bendamustine has been established as one of the preferred regimen in these entities.

Hodgkin lymphomas

Staging in HL is based on the Ann Arbor classification [152]. Regarding this classification and depending on precisely-defined risk factors, patients are classified into three risk groups (limited, intermediate, or advanced stages) defined by co-operative research groups (EORTC, GELA, GHSG, NCCN). The intensity of treatment depends on this stratification [153–155].

Treating patients with multi-agent chemotherapy and radiotherapy has led to significantly improved prognosis over the last decades, with five-year survival rates over 90%. The first modern combination chemotherapy, MOPP (mechlorethamine, vincristine, procarbazine, prednisone), was established by DeVita and colleagues [156]. A number of modifications were made to the original MOPP regimen by others intending to reduce toxicity. Bonadonna and colleagues established an alternative protocol, ABVD (doxorubicin, bleomycin, vinblastine, and dacarbazine), which was effective in the treatment of patients who had failed MOPP [157]. In advanced HL, the regimen was as effective as MOPP and in combination superior to MOPP alone [158, 159]. Other alternative

Table 54.2 Commonly-used chemotherapy regimen in indolent non-Hodgkin lymphoma

R-CVP [203]	Dose	Route	Schedule
Rituximab	375 mg/m²	iv infusion	d 0 (or 1)
Cyclophosphamide	750 mg/m²	iv infusion	day 1
Vincristine	1.4* mg/m²	iv bolus	day 1
Prednisone	40 mg/m²	iv bolus or orally	days 1 to 5
repeat on day22			
R-MCP [205]			
Rituximab	375 mg/m²	iv infusion	day 0 (or 1)
Mitoxantrone	8 mg/m²	iv infusion	days 1 and 2
Chlorambucil	3 x 3 mg/m²	po	days 1 to 5
Prednisolone	25 mg/m²	po	days 1 to 5
repeat on day 29			
R-Bendamustine [143]			
Rituximab	375 mg/m²	iv infusion	day 0 (or 1)
Bendamustine	90 mg/m²	iv infusion	days 1 and 2
repeat on day 29			
R-CHVP [206]			
Rituximab	375 mg/m²	iv infusion	day 0 (or 1)
Cyclophosphamide	600 mg/m²	iv infusion	day 1
Doxorubicin	25 mg/m²	iv bolus	day 1
Etoposide	100 mg/m²	iv infusion	day 1
Prednisolone	40 Mg	po	days 1 to 5
repeat on day 29			
R-FM [149]			
Rituximab	375 mg/m²	iv infusion	day 0 (or 1)
Fludarabine	25 mg/m²	iv infusion	days 1 to 3
Mitoxantrone	10 mg/m²	iv infusion	day 1
repeat on day 22			

* max. 2.0 mg.

chemotherapy regimens have been developed for the treatment of HL [160, 161].

For patients in the favourable risk group, combined modality treatment of two to three cycles chemotherapy and radiotherapy is the standard treatment of care demonstrated by the GHSG HD7 trial and the EORTC-GELA H8-F trial [162, 163]. The randomized HD10 trial of the German Hodgkin Study Group (GHSG) showed that two cycles of ABVD followed by 20 Gy of radiotherapy is sufficient and less toxic. Therefore, this approach is now the standard of care within the GHSG and an increasing number of centres worldwide [164].

For intermediate stage patients, four cycles of chemotherapy (ABVD) followed by 30 Gy IFRT is the standard of care [165]. However, the ideal chemotherapy and radiation regimens are

not yet clearly defined. Therefore, several randomized trials from the GHSG and the EORTC have investigated different regimes to improve tumour control combined with reduced toxicity. According to the GHSG two cycles of BEACOPP$_{escalated}$ plus two cycles of ABVD followed by radiotherapy with 30 Gy is recommended based on the final evaluation of the HD14 trial [166]. It is still a matter of debate if radiotherapy can be suspended in selected patients. The HD17 trial and the EORTC/GELA H10U trial are evaluating interim PET results to determine whether radiotherapy can possibly be omitted in patients after chemotherapy.

Because of response rates and toxicity, the intensity of combination chemotherapy for patients with advanced-stage HL is controversial. Three treatment regimens are widely used: six to eight cycles of escalated BEACOPP, ABVD, or the Stanford V protocol [167–169]. Additional localized radiotherapy needs to be considered in case of residual lymphoma. Ongoing studies take into account early interim PET to reduce toxicity without losing efficacy of treatment. In Germany six cycles of BEACOPP$_{escalated}$ represents the standard of care for patients with advanced-stage HL demonstrated by the HD15 trial [170]. In case of PET-positive residual mass ≥2.5 cm after chemotherapy consolidation radiotherapy should be performed. Because of toxicity, patients older than 60 years should be treated with six to eight cycles of ABVD [171].

In relapsed disease, conventional salvage chemotherapy and high-dose chemotherapy with autologous haematopoietic cell transplantation (HCT) is considered the treatment of choice. For reducing tumour burden and mobilization of stem cells, several salvage regimens are used such as DHAP or ICE (ifosfamide/carboplatin/etoposide) [172, 173]. Allogeneic stem cell transplantation (alloSCT) can be considered in case of repeated relapse. However, this approach is not standard and should be conducted only within clinical trials [174–176].

Patients with progressive, resistant disease in a palliative situation can benefit by gemcitabine-based chemotherapy and/or regional radiotherapy. Brentuximab vedotin (Adcetris®) is approved by the US and European authorities for the treatment of relapsed or refractory HL in patients with progressive disease after ASCT, or after two chemotherapy regimens in patients ineligible for transplantation [177].

In recent years, new less toxic, targeted drugs are emerging such as the monoclonal antibody brentuximab targeting CD30, bi-specific antibodies, immunomodulatory drugs, HDAC, and mTOR inhibitors [178]. Recent data of PD-1 immune checkpoint blockade in HL are very promising [179]. All of these are being evaluated in clinical trials.

Concerning nodular lymphocyte pre-dominant HL, stage IA patients are usually treated with radiotherapy alone. All other LP patients are treated as cHL patients [180]. LP HL express CD20, so that anti-CD20 monoclonal antibodies have been shown to be effective [181].

Chemotherapy for relapsed or refractory disease

Treatment decisions in relapsed or refractory disease must address lymphoma histology as well as patient age and comorbidities.

In elderly and frail patients, palliative conventional chemotherapy can reduce symptom burden and improve survival. The choice of regimen depends on previous therapies and individual reserves of haematopoietic and organ functions. The majority of patients with relapsed aggressive lymphomas are pretreated with CHOP-like regimens; salvage treatment with an anthracycline-based combination has to respect the previous cumulative dose of these drugs because of their potential cardiotoxic effects. The aza-anthracenedione derivate pixantrone should have less cardiotoxicity and was investigated in heavily pretreated patients with relapsed and refractory aggressive NHL. Pixantrone given at a dose of 85 mg/m^2 (intravenously, days 1, 8, 15, repeated day 28, up to six infusions) showed superior complete response (CR) or unconfirmed CR (CRu) rate (20% vs 7%, p = 0.021) in a randomized multicentre study compared to other single-agent chemotherapy including vinorelbine, oxaliplatin, ifosfamide, etoposide, mitoxantrone, or gemcitabine [182].

ASCT offers a chance for cure to younger and eligible patients. The sensitivity of relapsed disease to chemotherapy is one of the major prognostic factors for outcome after transplantation. There are two groups of chemotherapy regimen which are used to treat relapsed (or refractory) patients who have a transplant option; in B-cell lymphomas all combinations are given together with rituximab today.

First, platinum-based regimens, including DHAP, was established as an effective treatment in the late 1980 [183]. Later, the ICE protocol was developed [184, 185]. RRs range from 50–70% with CRs in 25–40% of patients. A recent randomized study comparing R-DHAP and R-ICE in salvage treatment of DLBCL patients showed no significant differences in response and event-free survival between the two regimens [186]. There were more grade 3 to 4 haematological toxicities and a higher number of severe renal adverse events after R-DHAP.

Second, modifications of the BEAM-conditioning regimen, such as miniBEAM [187, 188] or DexaBEAM [189–191], were evaluated in several studies in HL as well as NHL, where limited efficacy was seen. A retrospective study in patients with peripheral T-cell lymphomas showed superior RRs after DexaBEAM than after ICE (overall response 69% vs 20%, p = 0.01) prior to autologous transplantation [192]. However, there is no randomized prospective trial comparing DexaBEAM or platin-regimens in salvage treatment of lymphoma.

Role of immunotherapy

Tumour immunotherapy consists of both and 'active' and 'passive' approaches. The principle of active immunotherapy is to generate a host immune response, as in tumour vaccination strategies. In contrast, passive immunotherapy most commonly involves administering monoclonal antibodies (mAb) leading to antibody effector mechanisms including the recruitment of host immune cells to generate antibody-dependent cellular cytotoxicity (ADCC). Although considerable progress has been made in developing active immunotherapy with vaccinations, cellular therapy, and immunoregulatory mAb, all of which are now emerging as potentially important therapeutic approaches, it is the delivery of passive immunotherapy with mAb that has led to improvements in outcome for patients in a wide range of lymphomas.

More than 20 years elapsed after the advent of mAb technology in 1976 [194], before mAb began to fulfil their early promise as effective anticancer therapeutics in the routine care of lymphomas.

Numerous B- and T-cell antigens have been assessed as potential targets for mAb therapy, including the B-cell antigens CD19, CD22, CD37, HLA DR and the B-cell receptor (BCR) in B-cell malignancies as well as CD4, CD8, CD52 and, more recently, CD30 in T-cell and HL [195, 196]. CD20 was found to have favourable characteristics being expressed specifically within the B-cell lineage from pre-B-cells to mature B-cells in normal and malignant B-cells, resulting in lymphoid progenitors not being depleted after anti-CD20 mAb therapy due to the absence of CD20 on their surface, allowing them to replenish the B-cell population after anti-CD20 mAb therapy [197]. Anti-CD20 mAbs have subsequently dominated clinical development in B-cell malignancies, as unconjugated mAb and in radioimmunotherapy (RIT).

Rituximab is a chimeric mAb that targets the B-cell specific antigen CD20 and was the first mAb approved for the treatment of cancer by the US Food and Drug Administration (FDA) in 1997. The overall response rates (ORR) in patients with relapsed FL was around 50%, although single-agent complete RRs were modest at around 6% [198]. However, when rituximab was combined with chemotherapy, greatly enhanced RRs and improvements in PFS and OS in a wide range of B-cell malignancies were observed, with no or modest increases in toxicity compared to chemotherapy alone [199–207]. The initial data emerged from older patients (60–80 years) with untreated DLBCL [199]. This important finding was subsequently confirmed in young patients with good-prognosis DLBCL in the MINT (MAbthera International Study) trial. Here the addition of rituximab increased the three-year EFS compared with those assigned chemotherapy alone by 20% (79% vs 59%) and increased three-year OS by 9% (93% vs 84%) [200].

There have been numerous large international studies confirming the improved RRs, PFS, and OS for the addition of rituximab to combination chemotherapy in the initial treatment of advanced stage FL and other indolent lymphomas for patients requiring treatment (see Table 54.3) and confirmed in a meta-analysis [207]. However, the optimal combination of chemotherapy to deliver with rituximab as induction or initial treatment for patients that require therapy remains controversial. Whilst the use of anthracyclines as used in R-CHOP regimens led to higher ORR and CR rates, it is at the price of increased acute and late toxicity. The use of maintenance rituximab in patients who have achieved at least a partial response after induction chemotherapy was explored by the European Organisation for Research and Treatment of Cancer phase III trial EORTC 20981 in relapsed/resistant FL [209]. Rituximab maintenance significantly improved PFS compared with observation (median of 3.7 years vs 1.3 years). With longer-term follow-up, the superior PFS has been maintained but improvement of OS did not reach statistical significance, possibly because of the unbalanced use of rituximab in post-protocol salvage treatment. Rituximab maintenance was associated with a significant increase in grades 3 to 4 infections (9.7% vs 2.4%) [209]. More recently, in a large international randomized study the potential benefits of the addition of maintenance rituximab given two-monthly over two years was investigated. The PFS was 74.9% in the rituximab maintenance group and 57.6% in the observation group but OS did not differ significantly between the groups [208].

Over the last decade, many new insights have been discovered regarding the mechanism of action of anti-CD20 mAbs, which eliminate their targets by engaging in a range of antibody effector

Table 54.3 Immunochemotherapy trials in advanced indolent lymphoma

Study	Treatment	N	Median FU months	ORR %	CR %	Median TTP/TTF/ EFS months	OS %
Marcus et al. 2006 [203]	CVP	159	53	57	10	15	77
	R-CVP	162		81	41	34	83
						p < .0001	p = .0290
Hiddemann et al. 2005 [204]	CHOP-IFN	205	18	90	17	29	90
	R-CHOP-IFN	223	96		20	NR	95
						p < .001	p = .016
Herold et al. 2007 [205]	MCP-IFN	96	47	75	25	26	74
	R-MCP-IFN	105		92	50	NR	87
						p < .0001	p = .0096
Salles et al. 2008 [206]	CHVP-IFN	183	42	73	63	46	84
	R-CHVP-IFN	175		84	79	67	91
						p < .0001	p = .029
				3-yrs TTF%			
Federico et al. 2013 [149]	R-CVP	168	46	88	67	46	n.d.
	R-CHOP	165	62	93	73	62 p = .003	n.d.
	R-FM	171	59	91	72	59 p = .006	n.d.

pathways. These include mAb Fc-FcγR interactions [210,211] including ADCC and phagocytosis, complement-dependent cytotoxicity (CDC), and the direct induction of programmed cell death (PCD) (reviewed in [199]). Several mechanisms of resistance to rituximab have been postulated including increased mAb metabolism, reduced tumour penetration, impaired mAb binding, 'shaving' loss/ or modulation of CD20, resistance of tumour cells to mAb-effector mechanisms, and impaired immune effector cell recruitment or function [212]. The contribution of these mechanisms to resistance to rituximab seen in the clinic currently remains unclear.

Currently, there are several new-generation anti-CD20 mAbs undergoing clinical investigation, engineered to provide theoretical advantages over rituximab. These anti-CD20 mAb include obinutuzumab [GA101], ofatumumab, PRO13192, AME133V, and multiple biosimilars [212–216]. Newer generation anti-CD20 mAb have been designed to deliver improved effector functions including enhanced FcγR binding, CDC, or PCD. Ofatumumab is at the most advanced stage of clinical development and binds a unique epitope on CD20, resulting in an unusually high ability to activate CDC. Ofatumumab has received FDA approval for use in fludarabine and alemtuzumab-refractory CLL, yet its clinical superiority over rituximab has yet to be determined [213]. Obinutuzumab (GA101) is another anti-CD20 which is at an advanced stage of clinical development. GA101 has a glyco-engineered Fc fragment with non-fucosylated oligosaccharides to enhance the interaction with FcγR, particularly FcγRIIIa, therefore enhancing ADCC and inducing direct cell death [216]. The efficacy of these next-generation mAbs compared to rituximab as initial therapy in combination with chemotherapy are being determined in large ongoing randomized clinical trials as well as efficacy in rituximab-refractory disease. Many of these ongoing clinical trials are using increased dose of anti-CD20 mAb used in comparison to the standard 375 mg/m² rituximab dose, making comparison of therapeutic efficacy more difficult.

Radioimmunotherapy

The radiosensitivity of malignant lymphomas makes the systemic delivery of targeted radiation in the form of radioimmunotherapy (RIT) a logical approach. RIT involves the administration of mAb or mAb-derived constructs which are chemically conjugated to therapeutic radioisotopes targeted to tumour. A wide variety of different mAb, delivery schedules, radioisotopes, and doses of radioactivity have been tested in RIT, resulting in impressive responses in the treatment of follicular NHL [217]. Various isotopes have been studied, but the commonest isotopes used in routine clinical practice are iodine-131 (^{131}I) and yttrium-90 (^{90}Y), due to their favourable emission characteristics which are shown in Table 54.4.

The ^{131}I-tositumomab regimen (Bexxar®) is completed within one to two weeks and consists of a tracer dose of the radioimmunoconjugate followed by the therapeutic dose 7 to 14 days later. Whole-body gamma camera imaging is performed three times over the week following the trace-labelled infusion to calculate

Table 54.4 Comparing the characteristics of Iodine-131 and Yttrium-90

	Iodine-131 (^{131}I)	Yttrium-90 (^{90}Y)
Emission	Β and γ	β only
B-particle energy	0.6 MeV	2.3 MeV
B-particle path length	0.8 mm	5.3 mm
Physical half-life	8.1 days	2.6 days
Conjugation to mAb	Direct	Via chelator, tiuxetan
Radiation protection measures	4 to 6 day inpatient stay in shielded room	Outpatient

the whole-body half-time and the dose required for the therapeutic infusion to deliver a 65 to 75 cGy whole body dose (WBD) depending on the baseline platelet count. ^{90}Y-ibritumomab tiuxetan consists of an IgG1 anti-CD20 mAb, the murine parent immunoglobulin of rituximab, covalently attached to a metal chelator molecule tiuxetan [217].

In a pivotal study of 60 extensively pretreated patients, a single administration of ^{131}I-tositumomab was administered and disease responses compared to their previous responses to chemotherapy for follicular or transformed FL. ^{131}I-tositumomab therapy was shown to provide greatly superior relapse-free survival compared to the last qualifying chemotherapy [218]. A RR of 68%, CR rate of 30%, and a median duration of response of 14.7 months were reported in a heavily-pretreated 'rituximab refractory' patient population to rituximab treated with ^{131}I-tositumomab in [219]. For ^{90}Y-ibritumomab tiuxetan, the phase II trial in heavily pretreated rituximab-refractory disease also showed an ORR of 74% and a CR rate of 15%, with a time-to-progression of 6.8 months in all patients and 8.7 months in responders [220].

Over the last ten years, both licensed RIT reagents, namely ^{131}I tositumomab and ^{90}Y-ibritumomab tiuxetan, have demonstrated high clinical efficacy in follicular and transformed disease leading to durable remissions. RIT delivers durable remissions for some patients and an analysis of the long-term follow-up of patients treated with ^{131}I-tositumomab demonstrated an RR of 47% to 68%, with CR rates between 20% and 38% [221]. At a median follow-up of 5.3 years, five-year PFS was 17%, and 32% of the 250 patients studied had a time-to-progression of $\geq$ 1 year. For these patients, the median duration of response of 45.8 months and had not been reached for those who achieved a CR [221]. Higher RRs and durable responses were also observed with ^{90}Y-ibritumomab tiuxetan with the observed median duration of remission approaching two years [222, 223].

RIT consolidation therapy after first-line cytoreduction with chemotherapy or immunochemotherapy has also been extensively investigated, initially with several phase II trials involving ^{90}Y ibritumomab and ^{131}I tositumomab. The largest phase II trial in 90 patients used ^{131}I tositumomab as consolidation therapy after six cycles of CHOP without rituximab. The ORR was 91%, including a 69% CR rate. After a median follow-up of 5.1 years, the estimated five-year OS rate was 87%, and the PFS rate was encouraging at 67% [224]. This regimen was subsequently compared in a randomized study to six cycles of R-CHOP and no statistically significant differences in PFS, OS, or serious toxicities are yet demonstrable with either regimen. However, the median times to progression not yet reached for either treatment [225].

A phase III study investigated ^{90}Y ibritumomab tiuxetan given as consolidation therapy versus observation in previously untreated stage III/IV FL, following induction with a wide range of different chemotherapy regimens. Although the median PFS in the ^{90}Y-ibritumomab group was highly significantly improved from 14 months in the control group to 49 months in those that received RIT, no OS advantage has yet been seen [226]. The marked improvement in CR rates and PFS in this study along with excellent PR to CR/CRu conversion rates and a favourable tolerability profile led to the approval of ^{90}Y ibritumomab tiuxetan in April 2008 by the European Medicines Agency (EMEA) as consolidation therapy after remission induction in previously untreated patients with FL. However, around 86% of the patients in this study were not treated with the current established standard of care with rituximab-containing chemotherapy. This lack of a current standard of care in the initial treatment has led to a poor uptake of this consolidation approach in modern management of FL, as uncertainty remains as to whether the similar benefits would be seen after rituximab-chemotherapy combinations.

RIT has been tested as a single-treatment approach in untreated FL. Seventy-six patients with stage III or IV FL received, as an initial therapy, a single-course of treatment with 131I-tositumomab therapy. The ORR was 95% and 75% achieved a CR. After a median follow-up of 5.1 years, the five-year PFS was 59%, with a median PFS of 6.1 years [227]. The mature results of phase II studies with ^{90}Y ibritumomab tiuxetan in newly diagnosed patients with FL are yet to be published.

Both licensed RIT approaches are well-tolerated during treatment and non-haematologic toxicities following treatment are relatively uncommon and generally minor. The most common, clinically significant, non-haematologic toxicities are similar to ^{90}Y ibritumomab and include fever, chills, asthaenia, and nausea. Myelosuppression is the primary toxicity with neutropaenia and thrombocytopaenia occurring several weeks after treatment and recovering to pretreatment levels after two to three months. The risk of myelodysplastic syndrome (MDS) occurring after lower BM doses of radioactivity delivered by RIT, however, appears to be modest at around (1–4%) [221, 222]. The introduction of RIT into clinical practice has been slow, given the activity of the RIT drugs, and uncertainty remains as to when and how best to integrate RIT into the treatment of FL. The treatment is well-tolerated by older patients and is an effective approach for relapsed FL, but further randomized studies demonstrating efficacy compared with current standards of care with rituximab/chemotherapy combination regimens will be required before these drugs are used more frequently.

Antibody drug conjugates

Antibody drug conjugates (ADCs) offer the potential to target the tumour specifically with mAb and deliver potent drug therapies with minimal or less systemic toxicity. Although initial early phase clinical trial results were disappointing, much was learnt about the chelate chemistry and the nature of conjugated cytotoxic agents. Recently highly-promising results have been achieved with this class of drugs using brentuximab vedotin (SGN-35) which combines an anti-CD30 monoclonal antibody and the antitubulin agent monomethyl auristatin E. The CD30 antigen was first identified in the Reed Sternberg malignant cell of HL and emerged as a promising potential target for antibody treatment. Although the first-generation monoclonal anti-CD30 antibodies proved disappointing with little clinical efficacy, the delivery of ADC against CD30 proved the validity of targeting CD30 with high RRs in the phase I study [228]. In the pivotal phase II study, performed in a treatment-refractory population who had relapsed post-ASCT, an RR of 75% and a CR of 34% was observed. The median duration of response was 6.7 months, and 20.5 months in those who achieved CR [229].

Brentuximab vedotin has also demonstrated high efficacy in patients with systemic ALCL recurrent disease with 86% achieving an objective response, 57% a CR, and 29% a partial remission. The median duration of overall response and CR was 12.6 and 13.2 months, respectively. Treatment-emergent adverse events included peripheral sensory neuropathy, fatigue, nausea, and neutropaenia; however, the majority of these were mild to moderate [230]. Grade 3/4 toxicity was primarily haematologic, with just over 5% of subjects experiencing at least one episode of neutropaenia, peripheral neuropathy, thrombocytopaenia, or anaemia. These results led to the accelerated approval of brentuximab vedotin (Adcetris®) by the US FDA in 2011 for the treatment of the treatment of relapsed or refractory HL in patients with progressive disease after ASCT, or after two chemotherapy regimens in patients ineligible for transplantation. Brentuximab vedotin was also approved for patients with ALCL who failed at least one prior treatment. Brentuximab vedotin is the first new therapy approved for the treatment of HL in over 30 years.

There are numerous ongoing studies in combination with chemotherapy in CD30-positive malignancies that will help define the role of this antibody–drug conjugate (ADC) in lymphoma management. The high durable RR of brentuximab vedotin has increased the interest in the use of ADC in treatment of lymphoma and there many drugs in this class in development. One such drug, inotuzumab ozogamicin (CMC-544), is in advanced clinical development having completed promising early phase clinical trials; phase III clinical trials are underway [231].

Role of stem cell transplantation

The introduction of high-dose therapy (HDT) followed by ASCT or alloSCT has led to substantial progress in the treatment of patients with NHLs. Haematopoietic reconstitution with peripheral blood progenitor cells (PBPC), improvement in supportive care, as well as the availability of matched unrelated donors has led to the widespread use of transplantation in the treatment of patients with lymphomas. However, the integration of the anti CD20 antibody, rituximab, has dramatically improved the prognosis of patients with B-cell lymphoma. The role of SCT for patients with B-cell lymphoma needs to be re-evaluated and will be discussed along with other lymphoma entities.

Because HDT and SCT are procedures with high acute and long-term toxicities, most studies have limited the use of this procedure to patients under the age of 65 who have good performance status and organ function. The clinical indications for HDT include several categories of patients, such as those who are refractory to initial treatment or with a poor prognosis, resistant relapse, or sensitive relapse. However, only patients sensitive to chemotherapy are eligible for this procedure. While the vast majority of patients who undergo ASCT have DLBCL, ASCT has also been used to treat patients with other types of low-grade lymphomas who have failed conventional treatment or with T-cell lymphomas. Until recently, the use of alloSCT was limited, but its application is expanding with the progress in donor selection and the use of reduced-intensity conditioning regimens (RIC) prior to alloSCT [232].

Principles of conditioning regimens

The principle underlying the use of SCT in haematological malignancies is that a more intensive cytoreductive therapy may result in an increase in the rate of CR. However, 'dose-response' is a concept that can be interpreted in many ways, including an increase in the peak dose level with a single very high dose of chemotherapy, the area under the curve or the dose intensity expressed by mg/m2/week [233]. In the setting of ASCT, pulsed multidrug high-dose regimens are generally given together after a period of standard- or high-dose induction chemotherapy. Nevertheless, drug sensitivity is required so that the procedure can participate in disease eradication. Until the last decade, it was thought that the mechanism of curing a malignancy was entirely due to conditioning therapy and that the transplant was a supportive measure that allowed for supralethal treatment.

However, this mechanism does not apply to all antineoplastic agents; in particular, myelosuppression is not the dose-limiting toxicity for agents such as cisplatin, and is not fully limiting for etoposide or cyclophosphamide. However, most other agents used in preparative regimens are highly toxic to stem cells and require obligate stem-cell support to rescue the patient from potentially lethal aplasia. In practice, there are two main advantages for using stem-cell support during treatment. First, the duration of acute myelosuppression is dramatically reduced, and second, a broader array of non–cross-resistant agents is available.

Because ASCT relies on the principle of dose escalation (usually less than tenfold) before toxicity in non-haematopoietic organs occurs, only a few drugs can be used. Alkylating agents are particularly suitable for ASCT because their doses can be easily intensified as their main toxicity is haematologic. In addition, they possess significant antitumour activity against lymphomas and their drug-resistance mechanism is not attributable to the multidrug resistance gene. Furthermore, a five-fold increased dose can be safely administered, thereby attaining a concentration that should be able to overcome drug resistance [234].

Preparative regimens

Combination of drugs without total-body irradiation

This type of conditioning regimen is preferred for several major reasons: several centres lack access to adequate radiation facilities, long-term side effects have been more frequently described with total-body irradiation (TBI) than with combination chemotherapy [235], and some lymphoma patients have already received the maximum tolerated dose (MTD) of radiation to critical organs.

The choice of drugs was initially classified into regimens that combined BEAM or cyclophosphamide, BCNU, etoposide (CBV), which are the most popular regimens used for lymphoma patients [236–238]. More intensive therapy adds high-dose mitoxantrone to CBV or escalates the dose of cytarabine or etoposide in the BEAM regimen [239, 240].

Some conditioning regimens have been developed for treating cerebral lymphoma. These use drugs that cross the blood-brain barrier, such as thiotepa, carmustine, etoposide, thiotepa, busulfan, and cyclophosphamide [241, 242].

Dose escalation studies conducted with the major regimens used to treat lymphoma patients have demonstrated non-haematologic toxicities, mainly pulmonary or hepatic, for agents such as carmustine or busulfan.

Tandem transplant

Promising results have been reported for treating multiple myeloma with a total therapy that consists of two ASCTs performed at three-month intervals. Recent trials have suggested that ASCT may offer a measurable advantage and that a second transplant is feasible [243].

Sequential high-dose chemotherapy with peripheral blood progenitor cells support

New schedules for the escalation of chemotherapy can take advantage of the use of both growth factors and stem-cell support to modify the established MTD and to maximize the dose intensity. The use of such a strategy as a first-line therapy rather than as consolidation therapy may offer the potential benefits of the most active drugs to more lymphoma patients with poor prognoses [244]. In this setting, the pulsed multidrug doses are generally lower per cycle than those used in myeloablative conditioning regimens. However, after four to six cycles with repeated PBPC support, the total dose may remain the same. A German study group performed a randomized study to compare standard chemotherapy to repetitive HDT supported by the reinfusion of progenitor cells [245], but they did not observe a benefit for this approach in DLBCL patients with poor prognoses. Nevertheless, despite the generally reversible haematotoxicity of a chosen drug, the blood concentrations of the drugs did not reach the same peaks levels that were necessary to overcome drug-resistance mechanisms.

Combination of drugs with total-body irradiation

Early preparative regimens utilized cyclophosphamide with TBI [246], and subsequent studies evaluated the use of alternative cytotoxic drugs, such as cytarabine, etoposide, and melphalan [247]. TBI dose-escalation studies have shown that the MTD was 10 Gy when given in a single dose and 16 Gy when given in 2 Gy fractions twice a day [248]. The dose-limiting toxicities were stomatitis, veno-occlusive disease, and skin lesions. Additionally, preparative regimens combining more than one cytotoxic drug with TBI have been studied. The rationale was that combinations of drugs have been shown to be superior to single agents and that dose escalation should be possible without the marked overlapping of toxicities. The results of phase II studies have led to the establishment of the ranges of doses that can be given safely to the majority of patients. An alternative could be to replace TBI with radioimmunoconjugates as part of the preparative regimen to selectively irradiate residual tumour cells [249]. Unfortunately, a randomized study comparing rituximab-BEAM to ^{131}I tositumomab-BEAM in patients with a relapsed DLBCL did not demonstrate any benefit for this new conditioning regimen [250].

Over the last decade, a new concept involving RIC prior to alloSCT was developed [251]. This technique emphasized the importance of immune cells that were transferred along with the graft for eradicating the tumour. As such, a myeloablative conditioning regimen was no longer a crucial prerequisite for successful alloSCT. This concept was also adopted because it decreased transplant-related mortality (TRM) to the point that this procedure can now be offered to virtually any elderly patient without serious co-morbidity. Encouraging results for this regimen have also been observed in patients with a DLBCL [252].

Stem cell source

The best source of progenitor cells for reconstitution following HDT in lymphoma is still a matter of debate. The use of a sibling or a matched unrelated donor as a source of stem cells that are not contaminated with lymphoma cells, that have not been exposed to cytotoxic agents, and that may induce a graft-vs-lymphoma effect is attractive. However, complications resulting from graft-vs-host disease and increased immunosuppression are associated with an increase in mortality compared to the use of stem cells from an autologous source. Until now, in most of the patients with lymphoma long-term survival is similar or inferior to that resulting from autoSCT, despite a decrease in the relapse rate post-alloSCT [253].

The use of PBPCs has become increasingly common, and it is the main source of stem cells for ASCT and, increasingly, for alloSCT. In addition, the current use of PBPC has shortened the duration of severe hypoplasia to a median time of 12 days [254]. The procedure is also easier to perform than BM collection in an operating room. The collection of stem cells can be performed as an outpatient procedure and involves apheresis to reach a minimal of $>2 \times 10^6$ CD34 + cells/kg cells. The mobilization of stem cells is performed with chemotherapy and haematopoietic growth factors or with growth factors alone and has a success rate of 90% in relapsed lymphoma patients [255]. In cases of collection failure, the use of plerixafor in combination with growth factors can rescue half of the cases [256].

The use of purging for ASCT is also a controversial issue. However, the debate has been partially resolved through the use of rituximab for therapy, which also reduces the stem cell contamination in B-cell lymphoma. In fact, in a randomized study in FL, the PFS and OS curves of patients receiving rituximab and those who did not receive rituximab prior to the collection of stem cells and transplantation were similar [257].

Evaluation of the toxicity of the conditioning regimens

Overall toxicity

TRM and mortality following transplantation have often been considered as a necessary compromise for achieving long-term survival. Earlier studies in ASCT reported that the percentage of TRM was above 10%, and this rate remains at 7% in the European Bone Marrow Transplantation (EBMT) registry [258]. However, several major advances over the past ten years have dramatically changed the toxicities associated with treatment. The observed mortality rate has been lowered to 3.5% [258].

More generally, the choice of the conditioning regimen depends on the severity of the disease.

Conventional alloSCT showed disappointing results in the treatment of patients with relapsed DLBCL and was associated with a devastatingly high TRM of up to 50%. RIC alloSCT is also associated with a variable TRM, but this averaged 20% in most reports [252, 259] thus accounting for the increased use of alloSCT in the treatment of lymphoma.

Role of radiotherapy

Radiation therapy (RT) has been used in the management of malignant lymphoid malignancies for over 80 years. Most lymphoid malignancies are very radiosensitive and moderate doses of radiotherapy result in a durable local control. However, most lymphomas even when localized at presentation are associated with occult systemic disease and recurrence after local radiotherapy is common. Therefore, with the development of effective chemotherapy a systemic treatment approach is now the mainstay of the management for most lymphomas.

In general, radiotherapy is used as primary curative therapy in stage I and II FL and MZL and as part of combined modality approach in DLBCL, primary mediastinal lymphomas, and NK-T cell lymphomas. The technical aspects of treatment planning for lymphomas are highly dependent on the location and extent of the target volume. In general, RT planning involves the use of immobilization devices, CT-assisted tumour localization and planning, and computerized calculation of dose distributions. The goal of these steps is to achieve dose uniformity in the target volume while minimizing RT dose to normal tissues.

Radiation volumes are defined using the information on planning CT that allows accurate delineation of target and normal tissue in a 3D perspective. The planning of radiation includes a determination of gross tumour volume (GTV), clinical target volume (CTV), and planning target volume (PTV). GTV is important in patients treated with RT alone and those with residual disease after chemotherapy. CTV includes the pretreatment tumour and what is considered to be the relevant tissues that contain microscopic disease. PTV includes an appropriate margin to the CTV to account for movement and set up variation during treatment delivery.

The toxicity of RT depends on three main factors: radiation dose, volume of tissue irradiated, and the area of the body exposed to radiation. While the acute toxicity of radiotherapy is mild to moderate, the main concern is that of late radiation toxicity that may become clinically significant decades later. In the last decade, there have been significant technologic advances that facilitate the delivery of therapeutic radiation dose to tumour while effectively protecting normal tissues.

Early-stage follicular lymphoma

Several studies have described ten-year PFS rates of approximately 50% and OS rates of 60–70% following RT alone for early-stage FL [260–263]. The large majority of relapses are in untreated sites, with long-term local relapse rates typically <10%. With follow-up longer than 15 years, there appears to be plateau in the risk of relapse, suggesting that some patients with localized disease can be cured with RT [263]. Further, a majority of patients treated with initial RT will not require chemotherapy 15 years after initial diagnosis. The contrast between the high local control rate and the suboptimal disease-free survival (DFS) illustrates in part the limitation of conventional staging investigations in identifying which patients have truly localized disease.

Radiotherapy dose

A phase III randomized study compared 24 Gy versus 40–45Gy among patients receiving RT for indolent lymphomas [264]. With 289 patients (361 sites) randomized, there was no significant difference between the dose levels in terms of in-field progression, PFS, or OS. Among 248 patients receiving RT as first-line therapy, there was no difference in PFS, with 64% in the 24 Gy arm and 54% in the high-dose arm without recurrence at last follow-up. These findings are consistent with single-arm studies demonstrating excellent local control with doses ≈30 Gy, indicating that higher doses are rarely warranted. RT target volumes should encompass enlarged nodes seen on CT-imaging and other sites consistent with lymphomatous involvement on MRI or FDG-PET, as needed. It is acceptable also to cover adjacent uninvolved nodal regions, but extended-field RT is not useful, as it does not appear to enhance disease control compared to smaller fields, though it does substantially increase the normal tissue dose [265].

Palliative radiation therapy for indolent lymphoma

Indolent lymphoma is a highly radiosensitive disease, and the use of low-dose short fractionation RT (i.e., two fractions of 2 Gy each)

can provide excellent palliation of local symptoms among patients with recurrent disease. The largest study of low-dose RT included 109 patients (304 sites) with recurrent indolent lymphoma treated with 4 Gy in one or two fractions. The ORR was 92% with a median duration time until local relapse of 25 months [266]. Other single-institution studies have also demonstrated similar results, with median local control duration typically of one to two years. This is a highly effective treatment option for patients with relapsed disease with symptoms caused by local bulk [266–268].

Mucosa-associated lymphatic tissue lymphoma

Moderate dose (i.e., 25–30Gy) RT can produce long-term cure for localized extranodal MALT lymphomas. A study of 144 patients treated with RT alone reported ten-year OS and relapse-free rates (RFR) of 89% and 74%, respectively. The ten-year RFRs for thyroid and gastric lymphoma were 95% and 92%. However, for salivary gland and orbital lymphoma, RFRs were 68% and 67%, respectively, due to recurrence in paired organs for lymphomas arising in these sites [269, 270].

A full description of the principles of RT-planning for low-grade MALT lymphomas is beyond the scope of this chapter. In general, the CTV should encompass the entire organ, not only the area where abnormalities are seen on imaging or direct visualization. For example, for gastric MALT the entire stomach is generally treated, and the entire orbit is encompassed in retro-orbital cases. Prophylactic coverage of the regional lymph nodes is not necessary for indolent histologies, although for high-grade extranodal lymphomas it is often done [271]. The expected target organ motion, the spatial variation in daily set-up, and the radiosensitivity of adjacent normal tissues requires individualization of treatment with respect to the design of an appropriate RT pan.

Diffuse large B-cell lymphoma

The role of RT in the treatment of DLBCL has been the subject of randomized trials, but applying the results of these trials in the context of modern practice is challenging. This is due to several factors: the systemic therapy regimens employed have become outdated (for example, due to the absence of rituximab), studies were underpowered to detect clinically important differences in outcome, FDG-PET imaging was not available, and also results among seemingly similar trials differed with respect to the benefit of RT. A SWOG study compared eight cycles of CHOP chemotherapy with three cycles of CHOP plus IFRT (40–55 Gy) [272]. The study included 442 patients with stage I (bulky) or II non-bulky disease. Patients receiving combined modality therapy had superior PFS (77% vs 64% with chemotherapy alone) and OS (82% vs 72%, respectively (p = 0.02). In a follow-up analysis nine years following randomization, the advantage of combined modality therapy was no long statistically significant [273]. An Eastern Cooperative Oncology Group (ECOG) study, randomized 215 patients with stage I–II diffuse aggressive NHL, including bulky stage II disease who had achieved a complete response to eight cycles of CHOP chemotherapy to 30 Gy IFRT or no further therapy. Six-year FFS was 70% with the addition of RT, compared to 53% among patients receiving chemotherapy alone (p = 0.05) and six-year OS was also 12% better, though this difference was not statistically significant [274]. Although these results indicated a significant benefit with the use of combined modality therapy, other randomized trials have found no benefit when more intensive chemotherapy regimens are used, or when only elderly patients are enrolled [275, 276].

An obvious limitation of these trials is the absence of rituximab as part of the therapy. The landmark trials demonstrating the benefit of rituximab in addition to CHOP chemotherapy employed RT to sites of bulk (variably defined between >5cm to >10cm) and extranodal involvement. Approximately 50% of patients on these trials received RT based on these criteria. A prospective non-randomized study compared patients treated on the RICOVER-60 trial with six cycles of R-CHOP-14 + two cycles of R with 36Gy to bulky sites >7.5cm with 164 patients treated with the same systemic therapy without RT. After adjusting for other prognostic factors, the omission of RT was associated with a significantly inferior results (HR = 2.7 for EFS, p = 0.011; HR = 4.3 for OS, p = 0.02) [277]. Similarly, a study of 292 patients with skeletal involvement treated on German High-grade Non-Hodgkin Lymphoma Study Group trials, including those treated with rituximab, reported that the use of RT among patients with skeletal involvement was associated with significantly superior EFS (p = 0.001) and better OS (p = 0.11) than treatment with systemic therapy alone [278]. The subsequent German High Grade Lymphoma Group study, UNFOLDER, includes patients aged <60 years with aaIPI of 0–1, and initially included a 2 × 2 randomization of R-CHOP on a 14-day vs 21-day schedule, and a randomization of RT vs no RT for patients with initial disease bulk >7.5 cm who were in CR after chemotherapy. In July 2012, the RT randomization was discontinued after an interim analysis revealed poorer outcome among patients treated with systemic therapy only, indicating that combined modality therapy remains the standard of care among patients with bulk disease.

Single-arm studies also support the use of abbreviated chemotherapy (i.e., three cycles of R-CHOP) with 30–36 Gy IFRT for patients with 0–1 IPI factor. This treatment can yield 3–8 year PFS of >80% with minimal acute toxicity and limited exposure to anthracyclines [279].

For patients with a complete response to RT, 30–36 Gy are typically considered adequate. For patients with a PR, there are very limited dose-response data, but in these cases 36–45 Gy may be warranted, particularly in circumstances in which both anatomic and functional imaging are abnormal [280, 281].

Primary mediastinal B-cell lymphoma

Primary mediastinal DLBCL is a distinct clinicopathologic entity typically presenting as a large mediastinal mass in a young patients. Because of the young age of affected patients and the recognized delayed toxicity of mediastinal RT, its role has been controversial [282]. Non-randomized retrospective studies have demonstrated superior PFS and OS among patients receiving combined modality therapy compared to chemotherapy alone. Todeschini et al., for example, reported that among 138 patients with PMBL five-year OS was 90% among those receiving RT compared to 78% without (p = 0.04) [283]. More recently, Xu et al. evaluated 79 patients with PMBL who received CHOP chemotherapy with (n = 39) or without rituximab (n = 40), and 60 patients received additional radiotherapy, and found OS and PFS rates for early-stage patients were 73.6% and 69.9% for chemotherapy and radiotherapy, and 50.8% (p = 0.076) and 36.9% (p = 0.008) for chemotherapy alone, respectively [284]. There is great interest in the use of dose-intensive regimens as a means of reducing the need for RT. Recognizing the need to evaluate RT in a randomized setting, the International Extranodal Lymphoma Study Group (IELSG) has initiated a randomized trial comparing systemic therapy alone (including rituximab) with or without RT. Very promising results were reported from a prospective phase 2 study in 51 PMBL patients using an intensive, toxicity-adjusted, infusional regimen (DA-EPOCH plus rituximab). None of the patients received radiotherapy. After a median follow-up of five years EFS and OS were 93% and 97%, respectively; late morbidities or cardiac toxicities were not observed.

Sinonasal NK/T lymphoma

Due to the relatively chemotherapy-resistant nature of NK lymphoma, initial therapy with combined chemoradiation remains the standard of care for stage I/II disease. Several retrospective studies have demonstrated superior PFS with the use of combined-modality therapy compared to systemic therapy alone [285, 286]. Aviles et al. randomized 427 patients with stage I/II NK/T lymphoma to RT alone, chemotherapy alone, or combined modality therapy, and reported superior PFS with combined modality therapy (9% vs 78% with chemotherapy alone and 40% with RT alone, and better five-year survival (86% vs 95% CI 81–90%) for CT; 64% (95% CI 59–70%) for RT; and 45% (95% CI 39–51%) for C (p < 0.001) [287]. Initial treatment with CHOP-21 is associated with progression prior to completion of six cycles in a substantial proportion of patients and, more recently, the early introduction of RT with dose-intensive chemotherapy regimens has been advocated [288].

The RT dose required to control localized NK/T lymphoma is 45–50 Gy. Intensity-modulated RT can be used to reduce the dose to the anterior chamber of the eye and the parotid glands, thereby reducing the late toxicity of RT compared to conventional lateral parallel-opposed beams that would have been used historically (Figure 54.4).

Hodgkin lymphomas

In the modern era of HL management, RT is still an important component of treatment for many patients. Since modern therapy options have significantly improved cure rates, the vast majority of patients will survive HL and thus will face potential late effects of therapy such as secondary cancers or late cardiovascular effects. Consequently, for favourable and intermediate-risk patients, efforts have been focused on retaining high cure rates while reducing the risk of adverse late effects. Currently, the intensity of chemotherapy and the selection of patients to receive RT depend on the disease stage, the presence of risk factors, and potentially early response to treatment. Reduction of therapy-related toxicity has been achieved by the replacement of alkylator-intensive chemotherapy regimens for early-stage disease with less toxic and more effective regimens, through the judicious selection of appropriate patients to receive RT and the minimization of normal tissue dose among those receiving it. The goal of modern smaller field RT (i.e., IFRT or involved-node RT (INRT)) is to reduce both treatment volume and treatment dose while maintaining efficacy and minimizing acute and late sequelae [289–291].

The principal objective of RT in HL is to treat involved lymph nodes (as INRT or involved-site RT) with or without contiguous adjacent nodes (in the case of IFRT) to a dose associated with a high likelihood of tumour eradication [292].

It is strongly recommended that all HL patients should be treated within a multidisciplinary clinical setting to facilitate the thoughtful balance of treatment intensity and toxicity.

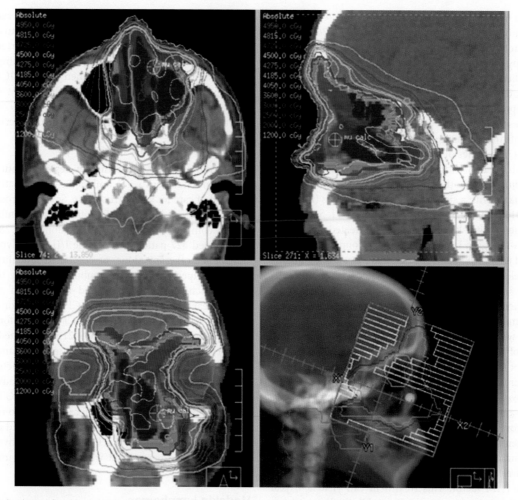

Fig. 54.4 RT dose distribution for sinonasal NK-T cell lymphoma. The use of intensity-modulated RT (IMRT) allows reduction of dose to optic structures and salivary glands, minimizing the risk of visual complications or xerostomia.

3D simulation and treatment planning

Recent recommendations for radiotherapy field and dose guidelines of the International Lymphoma Radiation Oncology Group (ILROG) can be found by Specht et al. [293] or the German evidence-based guidelines for HL by Eich et al. [294] or by Participants of the Lymphoma Radiotherapy Group by Hoskin et al. [295].

Planning requires modern 3D-CT-based simulation and planning capabilities. The capacity to fuse other additional imaging such as [18F] FDG-PET and MRI to planning CT datasets often enhances treatment planning.

The optimal irradiation technique includes pretreatment simulation and requires the use of 3D (i.e., CT-based) treatment planning, well-collimated megavoltage photon beams (dual-energy linear accelerator), nodal volumes, and normal tissues individually contoured to the patient´s anatomy and tumour configuration, an adequate dose, fractionated treatment, and accurate verification of patient positioning during therapy. As normal tissue dose is now well recognized as an important clinical consideration, contouring of normal tissues (i.e., 'organs at risk' such as breast, heart, and thyroid) should be viewed as an important part of treatment planning for HL. Newer treatment techniques, including intensity-modulated radiation therapy (IMRT), breath-hold, image-guided RT, and 4D

imaging, should be implemented when their use is expected to decrease significantly the risk for normal tissue damage while still achieving the primary goal of local tumour control.

Radiotherapy target definition

The International Commission on Radiation Units and Measurements (ICRU) Report 83 [296] concepts of volume determination are used for RT planning. A GTV may be defined as all individual nodes or extranodal sites of disease that are enlarged on CT, or avid on [18F] FDG-PET. The post-chemotherapy residual GTV should be outlined on the simulation study. The CTV would be defined as the original (before any intervention) GTV and includes the initial (pre-chemotherapy) location and extent of nodal disease (GTV plus the entire involved lymph node region(s)), excluding uninvolved organs.

When the target is moving, most commonly in the chest and upper abdomen with respiratory movements, an internal target volume (ITV) is defined [297] as the CTV plus a margin taking into account uncertainties in size, shape, and position of the CTV within the patient. The optimal way is to use 4D CT simulation to obtain the ITV margins. In sites (e.g., the neck) that are unlikely to change shape or position during or between treatments, outlining the ITV is not required. The PTV would include the CTV (or ITV if created) plus a margin for set-up uncertainties in patient positioning, typically 0.5–1.5 cm. In the setting, if there is a large mediastinal mass, the post-chemotherapy treatment fields can usually conform to the width of the residual disease (unless there was pulmonary parenchymal extension), although the superior and inferior field margins should encompass the initial extent of disease.

Irradiation dose recommendations for combined modality therapy

The determinants of dose prescription for HL include the histologic subtype, clinical risk factors, and patient age.

Classical Hodgkin lymphoma

Early stage (favourable prognosis) CS IA–IIB (no risk factors)
Combined-modality treatment is the standard treatment for patients with clinical stage I/II HL. In early-stage CHL, RT is often part of the treatment program after adequate systemic chemotherapy in all age groups. Although chemotherapy alone can produce excellent disease control for selected early-stage patients, RT improves freedom from treatment failure even in patients with negative PET scans [298, 299] and allows treatment with fewer chemotherapy cycles [289]. In a recent systematic review, combined-modality treatment was found to improve tumour control and OS in patients with early-stage HL [300].

For patients with early-stage CHL in CR after chemotherapy, the dose to the CTV is determined on the basis of the results of the German Hodgkin Studies HD 10 and 11 [289, 301]. For patients with favourable characteristics according to the German criteria, the dose is 20 Gy, whereas for patients with unfavourable characteristics it is 30 Gy.

In most circumstances, the current standard treatment for these patients is combined-modality therapy consisting of ABVD × 2 (–4) cycles followed by IFRT or involved-site radiation with 20 Gy [302–307].

An alternative treatment regimen consists of Stanford V × 8 weeks followed by IFRT.

Intermediate stage (unfavourable prognosis) CS IA/B to IIA/B (risk factors, bulky/non-bulky disease)
In most circumstances, the current standard treatment for these patients is combined-modality therapy consisting of poly-chemotherapy such as escalated BEACOPP × 2 plus ABVD × 2 followed by an IFRT with 30 Gy [290, 301, 307, 308]. In North America the standard poly-chemotherapy regimen for unfavourable bulky disease would be ABVD × 4–6 or Stanford V × 12 weeks. PET/CT is applied for restaging. Based on the DEAUVILLE PET criteria [309], further treatment decisions (ABVD × 4 +/- IFRT 30 Gy) are made. The results of the preplanned interim analysis of the randomized EORTC/LYSA/FIL Intergroup H10 trial [310] evaluated whether INRT could be omitted without compromising PFS in patients attaining a negative early PET scan after ABVD × 2 as compared with standard combined-modality treatment. The combined-modality treatment resulted in fewer early progressions in clinical stage I/II HL, although early outcome was excellent in both arms.

Advanced stage (unfavourable prognosis) CS IIB, III, IV
The role of additive RT is controversial and the appropriate use of RT in advanced-stage disease is certainly challenging to define. In advanced disease, many centres treat patients with intensive poly-chemotherapy alone (especially in the absence of bulky

disease). Only if a CR is not achieved will localized additive RT be used for residual lymphoma after full chemotherapy [311, 312]. The target in this situation is the residual mass after chemotherapy [313].

In advanced-stage HL two PET-based ABVD escalation or BEACOPP de-escalation trials aimed at determining the feasibility of omitting radiotherapy in interim PET-negative patients. Patients with a [18F] FDG-PET positive residual tumour after the end of chemotherapy (escalated BEACOPP or ABVD × 6 or Stanford V) should receive local radiotherapy with 30 Gy [314–316].

Nodular lymphocyte-predominant Hodgkin lymphoma early-stage IA

Nodular lymphocyte-predominant Hodgkin lymphoma (NLPHL) (stage IA) is treated with IFRT alone. The guidelines of the German Hodgkin Study Group (GHSG) for NLPHL recommend a dose of 30 Gy as sufficient [317, 318]. All fields are treated with fractions of 1.8 to 2.0 Gy, depending on the field size and patient tolerance. No advantage has been shown for doses over 30 to 35 Gy, which is the recommended dose to the CTV [319].

Nodular lymphocyte-predominant Hodgkin lymphoma >stage IA

NLPHL (>stage IA) is treated according to (the same stage) CHL with combined-modality therapy (chemotherapy followed by IFRT) [320, 321].

Ongoing clinical trials will help to clarify the role of systemic chemotherapy or antibody-based approaches in the treatment of these patients.

Paediatric Hodgkin lymphoma

A full review of RT for paediatric HL is beyond the scope of this chapter. However, paediatric protocols in both North America and Europe have typically prescribed ≈20 Gy to most patients, with only few selected patients with partial response receiving and a RT dose of 30 Gy. The marginal benefit of an additional boost dose is unclear. In contrast, adult protocols typically prescribe 30 Gy, with very favourable-risk patients receiving 20 Gy.

Peripheral T-cell lymphomas

According to the WHO classification 2008 mature T-cell and NK-cell neoplasms can be divided into cutaneous, extranodal, nodal, and leukaemic subtypes, all occurring at incidences below 1 in 100 000 people per year [322, 323]. The clinically aggressive extranodal and nodal types of T-cell lymphoma are considered as PTCL based on their descendency from peripheral (mature) T cells. Within PTCL, further histologic subtypes can be distinguished at variable prevalence depending on patient age and geography (see above). In Western countries the most common entities encompass PTCL-NOS (30%), ALCL (20%), AITL (15%), and the NK/T-cell lymphomas (15%) [323, 324]. Further subtypes of PTCL are the EATLs, of which the classical EATL mostly incurs in the small bowel and is associated with coeliac disease in patients from Northern Europe, while the monomorphic variant (type II EATL) appears to have a broader geographic distribution. The hepatosplenic T-cell lymphoma, mostly of γδ T-cell receptor type, occurs in male adolescents and young adults, 20% of which are associated with chronic immunosuppression [325, 326]. As for extranodal PTCL involving the skin, the cutaneous γδ T-cell lymphomas represent a rapidly progressive disease demanding intensive systemic treatment, compared to the mostly indolent course of the αβ T-cell receptor-positive subcutaneous panniculitis-like T-cell lymphoma, in part occurring in association with systemic lupus erythematosus in some patients [327, 328].

Detailed immunohistopathological evaluation and molecular studies, in many cases involving reference pathology, are essential for diagnostic accuracy [323]. In cases of ALCL the expression of CD30 on the tumour cells as well as the mutational status for the ALK, constitutively activated mostly by fusion to the nucleophosmin gene (NPM) through t(2;5) or alternative partners is important for therapeutic stratification. In paediatric patients, elevated levels of antibody titers against the NPM/ALK fusion protein were found to be prognostic for favourable outcome [329]. Besides the serological screen for antiviral titres applicable to any lymphoma patient, initial workup of PTCL patients should also include T-lymphotropic virus-1 (HTLV-1) serology in order to identify HTLV-1 positive adult T-cell lymphoma/leukaemia. EBV serology is necessary to identify patients at risk for EBV-reactivation associated with lymphoma-mediated or treatment-associated immunosuppression [330]. PCR for plasma levels of EBV genome copy numbers allows monitoring of EBV-reactivation, and may serve to follow disease in some entities, particularly NK/T cell lymphoma, nasal type [331]. Further immunological and molecular markers for outcome prediction are currently under investigation, yet without current impact on the treatment stratification [332].

Staging of patients with PTCL follows standard studies, with 18-fluoro-2-deoxyglucose FDG-PET as a helpful measure to detect and follow extranodal manifestations [333]. The IPI is well suited for outcome prognosis with current treatment regimens [334], though a revised international index integrating BM involvement (PIT) has been proposed [335].

So far, evidence for treatment recommendation in PTCL patients has been derived from retrospectives analyses and phase II clinical trials only; results of current phase III protocols specifically designed to optimize the treatment of patients with PTCL are expected.

Extranodal NK/T-cell lymphoma, nasal type

Due to its prevalence in Asian and Native Americans of Mexico, Central America, and South America, knowledge about treatment strategies of extranodal NK/T-cell lymphoma, nasal type mainly stems from Asian register analyses and studies. In limited stages I and II, IFRT should be applied with curative intent. Sequential or concurrent chemotherapy further improves treatment results, leading to OS rates of 78–86% by combinations of radiotherapy with platinum-based chemotherapy [336]. The optimal protocol of either concurrent, e.g., the 2/3 DeVIC-protocol, or sequential regimens is currently accruing [336–338]. In advanced stages, systemic chemotherapy is mandatory. Results with CHOP-based regimens had been unsatisfactory with one-year OS rates of only 20%, due to the low susceptibility of the NK/T-lymphoma cells towards anthracyclines. Treatment protocols integrating ifosfamide, asparaginase, methotrexate and etoposide, e.g., the SMILE protocol, or platinum-based combinations have demonstrated improved efficacy in the salvage setting [337, 339], and should therefore be offered as first-line treatment. Consolidation of remission by high-dose chemotherapy followed by either ASCT or alloSCT is an option in first-line treatment, and should clearly be evaluated in the salvage setting.

Anaplastic large-cell lymphoma

ALCL predominantly occurs in paediatric patients and young adults, and usually responds well to current paediatric or adult chemotherapy protocols [340]. For adult patients with ALK-positive ALCL, six courses of CHOEP in trials of the German High Grade Lymphoma Group (DSHNHL) or ACVBP-been based protocols in studies of the GELA (Groupe d'etudes lymphomes adultes) lead to five-year OS rates of 90% [334, 341]. For adult patients with ALK-negative ALCL, the outcome under CHOP or CHOEP as a primary therapy is worse, so that consolidation of remission by high-dose therapy and ASCT represents an option to achieve a five-year OS rate of 70% [342]. Due to the high expression of CD30 on the ALCL lymphoma cell surface, brentuximab vedotin, a conjugate of a monoclonal anti-CD30 antibody and the microtubulin inhibitor monomethyl-Auristatin E, has significant cytostatic activity against ALCL lymphoma cells and has been available for patients since 2012. The RR as a single agent is as high as 86% in the situation of relapsed disease [343], opening a window towards definitive therapy with high-dose therapy for some patients. Whether brentuximab vedotin has a role as part of first-line treatment regimens for patients with ALCL is currently under investigation in a prospective phase III trial.

Peripheral T-cell lymphomas (angioimmunoblastic T-cell lymphoma, peripheral T-cell lymphomas not otherwise specified)

The majority of patients with PTCL, i.e., those with NOS and AITL and those with rare subtypes, are treated with six to eight courses of CHOP-based regimens, resulting in five-year OS rates of 20–50%, depending on clinical risk factors summoned in the IPI [344, 323]. The addition of etoposide to the CHOP-backbone (CHOEP) increases the RR, particularly in the ALK-negative ALCL patients [334, 342], albeit at cost of increased toxicity in elder patients; thus, CHOEP may be offered to select patients age <60 years. Novel agents to be added to, or to substitute parts of, the CHOP or CHOEP-backbone of are currently under investigation. Eligible patients are candidates for consolidating high-dose therapy with ASCT, which in several phase II studies showed five-year OS rates of 50% [342, 345, 346]. However, despite early-dose intensification, approximately 25% of patients experience primary progression or early relapse of lymphoma.

In the relapse situation, intensified multiagent platinum-based cytostatic drug combinations like ICE, DHAP, or gemcitabine-based combinations have shown significant efficacy against PTCL and thus offer a bridge for eligible patients towards definitive high-dose therapy followed by ASCT or alloSCT [335, 345, 347, 349]. For patients not eligible for multiagent chemotherapy, several agents have shown single-agent cytostatic activity and acceptable toxicity, namely the methotrexate analogue pralatrexate, the HDAC inhibitor romidepsin, as well as gemcitabine, bendamustine and the IMID lenalidomide [349–352]. Based on the results of phase II trials, both romidepsin and pralatrexate have gained FDA approval as single agents for patients with relapsed PTCL. Despite transient antitumour efficacy, both intensified cytostatic drug combinations and novel agents are not sufficient to secure long-term disease control [353]. In cohorts of patients eligible for high-dose therapy and HLA-compatible donors, alloSCT have provided DFS at rates of 40–50% [354–357], offering alloSCT as a therapeutic option with curative intent.

References

1. Morton LM, Wang SS, Devesa SS, Hartge P, Weisenburger DD et al. Lymphoma incidence patterns by WHO subtype in the United States, 1992–2001. Blood 2006; 107(1): 265–276.

2. Sant M, Allemani C, Tereanu C, De Angelis R, Capocaccia R et al. Incidence of hematologic malignancies in Europe by morphologic subtype: results of the HAEMACARE project. Blood 2010; 116(19): 3724–3734.

3. Gibson TM, Smedby KE, Skibola CF, Hein DW, Slager SL et al. Smoking, variation in N-acetyltransferase 1 (NAT1) and 2 (NAT2), and risk of non-Hodgkin lymphoma: a pooled analysis within the InterLymph consortium. Cancer Causes Control 2013; 24(1): 125–134.

4. Haberland J WU, Barnes B, Bertz J, Dahm S, Laudi A et al. Kurzfristige Prognosen der Krebsmortalität in Deutschland bis 2015. UMID 2012; 3: 17–23.

5. van den Bosch CA. Is endemic Burkitt's lymphoma an alliance between three infections and a tumour promoter? Lancet Oncology 2004; 5(12): 738–746.

6. Carbone A. Emerging pathways in the development of AIDS-related lymphomas. Lancet Oncology 2003; 4(1): 22–29.

7. Arisawa K, Soda M, Endo S, Kurokawa K, Katamine S et al. Evaluation of adult T-cell leukemia/lymphoma incidence and its impact on non-Hodgkin lymphoma incidence in southwestern Japan. International Journal of Cancer 2000; 85(3): 319–324.

8. Clarke CA. Changing incidence of Kaposi's sarcoma and non-Hodgkin's lymphoma among young men in San Francisco. AIDS 2001; 15(14): 1913–1925.

9. Levine AM, Shibata D, Sullivan-Halley J, Nathwani B, Brynes R et al. Epidemiological and biological study of acquired immunodeficiency syndrome-related lymphoma in the County of Los Angeles: preliminary results. Cancer Research 1992; 52(19 Suppl): 5482s–5484s.

10. Tao L, Foran JM, Clarke CA, Gomez SL, Keegan TH. Socioeconomic disparities in mortality after diffuse large B-cell lymphoma in the modern treatment era. Blood 2014; 123(23): 3553–3562.

11. Conde L, Halperin E, Akers NK, Brown KM, Smedby KE et al. Genome-wide association study of follicular lymphoma identifies a risk locus at 6p21.32. Nature Genetics 2010; 42(8): 661–664.

12. Nieters A, Conde L, Slager SL, Brooks-Wilson A, Morton L et al. PRRC2A and BCL2L11 gene variants influence risk of non-Hodgkin lymphoma: results from the InterLymph consortium. Blood 2012; 120(23): 4645–4648.

13. Skibola CF, Bracci PM, Halperin E, Conde L, Craig DW et al. Genetic variants at 6p21.33 are associated with susceptibility to follicular lymphoma. Nature Genetics 2009; 41(8): 873–875.

14. Smedby KE, Foo JN, Skibola CF, Darabi H, Conde L et al. GWAS of follicular lymphoma reveals allelic heterogeneity at 6p21.32 and suggests shared genetic susceptibility with diffuse large B-cell lymphoma. PLoS Genetics 2011; 7(4): e1001378.

15. Swerdlow SH CE, Harris NL, Jaffe ES, Pileri SA, Stein H et al. WHO Classification of Tumours of Haematopoietic and Lymphoid Tissues. 2008: 140–141.

16. Alizadeh AA, Eisen MB, Davis RE, Ma C, Lossos IS et al. Distinct types of diffuse large B-cell lymphoma identified by gene expression profiling. Nature 2000; 403(6769): 503–511.

17. Florentine BD, Staymates B, Rabadi M, Barstis J, Black A. The reliability of fine-needle aspiration biopsy as the initial diagnostic procedure for palpable masses: a 4-year experience of 730 patients from a community hospital-based outpatient aspiration biopsy clinic. Cancer 2006; 107(2): 406–416.

18. Hehn ST, Grogan TM, Miller TP. Utility of fine-needle aspiration as a diagnostic technique in lymphoma. Journal of Clinical Oncology 2004; 22(15): 3046–3052.

19. Pangalis GA, Vassilakopoulos TP, Boussiotis VA, Fessas P. Clinical approach to lymphadenopathy. Seminars in Oncology 1993; 20(6): 570–582.

20. Slap GB, Connor JL, Wigton RS, Schwartz JS. Validation of a model to identify young patients for lymph node biopsy. JAMA 1986; 255(20): 2768–2773.

21. Conlan MG, Bast M, Armitage JO, Weisenburger DD. Bone marrow involvement by non-Hodgkin's lymphoma: the clinical significance of morphologic discordance between the lymph node and bone marrow. Nebraska Lymphoma Study Group. Journal of Clinical Oncology 1990; 8(7): 1163–1172.

22. Lister TA, Crowther D, Sutcliffe SB, Glatstein E, Canellos GP et al. Report of a committee convened to discuss the evaluation and staging of patients with Hodgkin's disease: Cotswolds meeting. Journal of Clinical Oncology 1989; 7(11): 1630–1636.

23. Freudenberg LS, Antoch G, Schutt P, Beyer T, Jentzen W et al. FDG-PET/CT in re-staging of patients with lymphoma. European Journal of Nuclear Medicine and Molecular Imaging 2004; 31(3): 325–329.

24. Kwee TC, Kwee RM, Nievelstein RA. Imaging in staging of malignant lymphoma: a systematic review. Blood 2008; 111(2): 504–516.

25. Juweid ME, Stroobants S, Hoekstra OS, Mottaghy FM, Dietlein M et al. Use of positron emission tomography for response assessment of lymphoma: consensus of the Imaging Subcommittee of International Harmonization Project in Lymphoma. Journal of Clinical Oncology 2007; 25(5): 571–578.

26. Cheson BD, Fisher RI, Barrington SF et al. Recommendations for initial evaluation, staging, and response assessment of Hodgkin and non-Hodgkin lymphoma: the Lugano classification. Journal of Clinical Oncology 2014; 32(27): 3059–3068. 10.1200/JCO.2013.54.8800.

27. Barrington SF, Mikhaeel NG, Kostakoglu L et al. Role of imaging in the staging and response assessment of lymphoma: consensus of the International Conference on Malignant Lymphomas Imaging Working Group. Journal of Clinical Oncology 2014; 32(27): 3048–3058. 10.1200/JCO.2013.53.5229.

28. A predictive model for aggressive non-Hodgkin's lymphoma. The International Non-Hodgkin's Lymphoma Prognostic Factors Project. New England Journal of Medicine 1993; 329(14): 987–994.

29. Ziepert M, Hasenclever D, Kuhnt E, Glass B, Schmitz N et al. Standard International prognostic index remains a valid predictor of outcome for patients with aggressive CD20+ B-cell lymphoma in the rituximab era. Journal of Clinical Oncology 2010; 28(14): 2373–2380.

30. Swerdlow S, Campo E, Harris NL et al. WHO Classification of tumors of hematopoietic and lymphoid tissues. Lyon: IARC, 2008, 429.

31. Harris N, Jaffe E, Stein H et al. A Revised European-American Classification of lymphoid neoplasms: a proposal from the International Lymphoma Study Group. Blood 1994; 84(5): 1361–1392.

32. Marti GE, Rawstron AC, Ghia P et al. Diagnostic criteria for monoclonal B-cell lymphocytosis. British Journal of Haematology 2005; 130(3), 325–332.

33. Burg G, Kempf W, Cozzio A et al. WHO/EORTC classification of cutaneous lymphomas 2005: histological and molecular aspects. Journal of Cutaneous Pathology 2005; 32(10), 647–674.

34. Cong P, Raffeld M, Teruya-Feldstein J et al. In situ localization of follicular lymphoma: description and analysis by laser capture microdissection. Blood 2002; 99(9), 3376–3382.

35. Hummel M, Bentink S, Berger H et al. A biologic definition of Burkitt's lymphoma from transcriptional and genomic profiling. New England Journal of Medicine 2006; 354(23): 2419–2430.

36. Traverse-Glehen A, Pittaluga S, Gaulard P et al. Mediastinal gray zone lymphoma: the missing link between classic Hodgkin's lymphoma and mediastinal large B-cell lymphoma. American Journal of Surgical Pathology 29(11): 1411–1421.

37. Piccaluga PP, Agostinelli C, Califano A et al. Gene expression analysis of angioimmunoblastic lymphoma indicates derivation from T follicular helper cells and vascular endothelial growth factor deregulation. Cancer Research 2007; 67(22): 10703–10710.

38. Agostinelli C, Hartmann S, Klapper W et al. Peripheral T cell lymphomas with follicular T helper phenotype: a new basket or a distinct

entity? Revising Karl Lennert's personal archive. Histopathology 2011; 59(4): 679–691.

39. Younes A, Bartlett NL, Leonard JP et al. Brentuximab vedotin (SGN-35) for relapsed CD30-positive lymphomas. New England Journal of Medicine 2010; 363(19): 1812–1821.

40. Savage KJ, Harris NL, Vose JM et al. ALK- anaplastic large-cell lymphoma is clinically and immunophenotypically different from both ALK+ ALCL and peripheral T-cell lymphoma, not otherwise specified: report from the International Peripheral T-Cell Lymphoma Project. Blood 2008; 111(12): 5496–5504.

41. Bekkenk MW, Vermeer MH, Jansen PM et al. Peripheral T-cell lymphomas unspecified presenting in the skin: analysis of prognostic factors in a group of 82 patients. Blood 2003; 102(6): 2213–2219.

42. Feldman AL, Dogan A, Smith DI et al. Discovery of recurrent t(6;7) (p25.3;q32.3) translocations in ALK-negative anaplastic large cell lymphomas by massively parallel genomic sequencing. Blood 2011; 117(3): 915–919.

43. Willemze R, Jansen PM, Cerroni L et al. Subcutaneous panniculitis-like T-cell lymphoma: definition, classification, and prognostic factors: an EORTC Cutaneous Lymphoma Group Study of 83 cases. Blood 2008; 111(2): 838–845.

44. Quintanilla-Martinez L, Kumar S, Fend F et al. Fulminant EBV(+) T-cell lymphoproliferative disorder following acute/chronic EBV infection: a distinct clinicopathologic syndrome. Blood 2000; 96(2): 443–451.

45. Barrionuevo C, Anderson VM, Zevallos-Giampietri E et al. Hydroa-like cutaneous T-cell lymphoma: a clinicopathologic and molecular genetic study of 16 pediatric cases from Peru. Applied Immunohistochemistry and Molecular Morphology 2002; 10(1): 7–14.

46. Rabbani GR, Phyliky RL, Tefferi A. A long-term study of patients with chronic natural killer cell lymphocytosis. British Journal of Haematology 1999; 106(4): 960–966.

47. Summers KE, Goff LK, Wilson AG et al. Frequency of the Bcl-2/IgH rearrangement in normal individuals: implications for the monitoring of disease in patients with follicular lymphoma. Journal of Clinical Oncology 2001; 19(2): 420–424.

48. Zignego AL, Ferri C, Giannelli F et al. Prevalence of bcl-2 rearrangement in patients with hepatitis C virus-related mixed cryoglobulinemia with or without B-cell lymphomas. Annals of Internal Medicine 2002; 137(7): 571–580.

49. Lecluse Y, Lebailly P, Roulland S et al. t(11;14)-positive clones can persist over a long period of time in the peripheral blood of healthy individuals. Leukemia 2009; 23(6): 1190–1193.

50. Richard P, Vassallo J, Valmary S et al. 'In situ-like' mantle cell lymphoma: a report of two cases. Journal of Clinical Oncology 2006; 59(9): 995–996.

51. Fernandez V, Salamero O, Espinet B et al. Genomic and gene expression profiling defines indolent forms of mantle cell lymphoma. Cancer Research 2010; 70(4): 1408–1418.

52. Gagyi E, Balogh Z, Bodor C et al. Somatic hypermutation of IGVH genes and aberrant somatic hypermutation in follicular lymphoma without BCL-2 gene rearrangement and expression. Haematologica 2008; 93(12): 1822–1828.

53. Gitelson E, Al-Saleem T, Robu V, Millenson MM, Smith MR. Pediatric nodal marginal zone lymphoma may develop in the adult population. Leukemia Lymphoma 2010; 51(1): 89–94.

54. Falini B, Agostinelli C, Pucciarini A et al. The IRTA1 molecule is selectively expressed in nodal and extranodal marginal zone lymphomas. Histopathology 2012; 61(5): 930–941 [Epub ahead of print].

55. Chan JK, Chan AC, Cheuk W et al. Type II enteropathy-associated T-cell lymphoma: a distinct aggressive lymphoma with frequent gammadelta T-cell receptor expression. American Journal of Surgical Pathology 2011; 35(10): 1557–1569.

56. Tiacci E, Trifonov V, Schiavoni G et al. BRAF mutations in hairy-cell leukemia. New England Journal of Medicine 2011; 364(24): 2305–2315.

57. Puente XS, Pinyol M, Quesada V et al. Whole-genome sequencing identifies recurrent mutations in chronic lymphocytic leukaemia. Nature 2011; 475(7354): 101–105.

58. Fabbri G, Rasi S, Rossi D et al. Analysis of the chronic lymphocytic leukemia coding genome: role of NOTCH1 mutational activation. Journal of Experimental Medicine 2011; 208(7): 1389–1401.

59. Pasqualucci L, Dominguez-Sola D, Chiarenza A et al. Inactivating mutations of acetyltransferase genes in B-cell lymphoma. Nature 2011; 471(7337): 189–195.

60. Ngo VN, Young RM, Schmitz R et al. Oncogenically active MYD88 mutations in human lymphoma. Nature 2011; 470(7332): 115–119.

61. Steidl C, Shah SP, Woolcock BW et al. MHC class II transactivator CIITA is a recurrent gene fusion partner in lymphoid cancers. Nature 2011; 471(7338): 377–381.

62. Cairns RA, Iqbal J, Lemonnier F et al. IDH2 mutations are frequent in angioimmunoblastic T-cell lymphoma. Blood 2012; 119(8): 1901–1903.

63. Vose J, Armitage J and Weisenburger D. International peripheral T-cell and natural killer/T-cell lymphoma study: pathology findings and clinical outcomes. Journal of Clinical Oncology 2008; 26(25): 4124–4130.

64. Piccaluga PP, Agostinelli C, Califano A et al. Gene expression analysis of peripheral T cell lymphoma, unspecified, reveals distinct profiles and new potential therapeutic targets. Journal of Clinical Investigation 2007; 117(3): 823–834.

65. Klein U, Dalla-Favera R. Germinal centres: role in B-cell physiology and malignancy. Nature Reviews Immunology 2008; 8(1): 22–33.

66. Shipp MA et al. Diffuse large B-cell lymphoma outcome prediction by gene-expression profiling and supervised machine learning. Nature Medicine 2002; 8(1): 68–74.

67. Robertson MJ et al. Phase II study of enzastaurin, a protein kinase C beta inhibitor, in patients with relapsed or refractory diffuse large B-cell lymphoma. Journal of Clinical Oncology 2007; 25(13): 1741–1746.

68. Lenz G, Staudt LM. Aggressive lymphomas. New England Journal of Medicine 2010; 362(15): 1417–1429.

69. Monti S et al., Molecular profiling of diffuse large B-cell lymphoma identifies robust subtypes including one characterized by host inflammatory response. Blood 2005; 105(5): 1851–1861.

70. Caro P, Kishan AU, Norberg E, Stanley IA, Chapuy B. Metabolic Signatures Uncover Novel Targets in Molecular Subsets of Diffuse Large B-Cell Lymphoma. Cancer Cell 2012; 22(4): 547–560.

71. Chen L et al. SYK-dependent tonic B-cell receptor signaling is a rational treatment target in diffuse large B-cell lymphoma. Blood 2008; 111(4): 2230–2237.

72. Cheng S et al. SYK inhibition and response prediction in diffuse large B-cell lymphoma. Blood 2011; 118(24): 6342–6352.

73. Friedberg JW et al. Inhibition of Syk with fostamatinib disodium has significant clinical activity in non-Hodgkin lymphoma and chronic lymphocytic leukemia. Blood 2010; 115(13): 2578–2585.

74. Davis RE et al. Chronic active B-cell-receptor signalling in diffuse large B-cell lymphoma. Nature 2010; 463(7277): 88–92.

75. Yang Y et al. Exploiting synthetic lethality for the therapy of ABC diffuse large B cell lymphoma. Cancer Cell 2012; 21(6): 723–737.

76. Lohr JG et al. Discovery and prioritization of somatic mutations in diffuse large B-cell lymphoma (DLBCL) by whole-exome sequencing. Proceedings of the National Academy of Sciences USA 2012; 109(10): 3879–3884.

77. Morin RD et al. Frequent mutation of histone-modifying genes in non-Hodgkin lymphoma. Nature 2011; 476(7360): 298–303.

78. Pasqualucci L et al. Analysis of the coding genome of diffuse large B-cell lymphoma. Nature Genetics 2011; 43(9): 830–837.

79. Zhang J, Grubor V, Love CL, Banerjee A, Richards KL, et al. Genetic heterogeneity of diffuse large B-cell lymphoma. Proceedings of the National Academy of Sciences 2013; 110(4): 1398–1403. doi: 10.1073/pnas.1205299110. Epub 2013 Jan 4.

80. Young KH et al. Structural profiles of TP53 gene mutations predict clinical outcome in diffuse large B-cell lymphoma: an international collaborative study. Blood 2008; 112(8): 3088–3098.

81. Schmitz R, Young RM, Ceribelli M, Jhavar S, Xiao W, et al. Burkitt lymphoma pathogenesis and therapeutic targets from structural and functional genomics. Nature 2012; 490(7418): 116–120. doi: 10.1038/nature11378. Epub 2012 Aug 12.

82. Lenz G et al. Oncogenic CARD11 mutations in human diffuse large B cell lymphoma. Science 2008; 319(5870): 1676–1679.

83. Ngo VN et al. Oncogenically active MYD88 mutations in human lymphoma. Nature 2011; 470(7332): 115–119.

84 Duan S et al. FBXO11 targets BCL6 for degradation and is inactivated in diffuse large B-cell lymphomas. Nature 2012; 481(7379): 90–93.

85. Pasqualucci L et al. Molecular pathogenesis of non-Hodgkin's lymphoma: the role of Bcl-6. Leukemia Lymphoma 2003; 44(Suppl 3): S5–S12.

86. Staudt LM, Dave S. The biology of human lymphoid malignancies revealed by gene expression profiling. Advances in Immunology 2005; 87: 163–208.

87. Morin RD et al. Somatic mutations altering EZH2 (Tyr641) in follicular and diffuse large B-cell lymphomas of germinal-center origin. Nature Genetics 2010; 42(2): 181–185.

88. Jardin F et al. Diffuse large B-cell lymphomas with CDKN2A deletion have a distinct gene expression signature and a poor prognosis under R-CHOP treatment: a GELA study. Blood 2010; 116(7): 1092–1104.

89. Sanchez-Beato M, Sanchez-Aguilera M, Piris MA. Cell cycle deregulation in B-cell lymphomas. Blood 2003; 101(4): 1220–1235.

90. Winter JN et al. Expression of p21 protein predicts clinical outcome in DLBCL patients older than 60 years treated with R-CHOP but not CHOP: a prospective ECOG and Southwest Oncology Group correlative study on E4494. Clinical Cancer Research 2010; 16(8): 2435–2442.

91. Bea S et al. Diffuse large B-cell lymphoma subgroups have distinct genetic profiles that influence tumor biology and improve gene-expression-based survival prediction. Blood 2005; 106(9): 3183–3190.

92. Lenz G et al. Molecular subtypes of diffuse large B-cell lymphoma arise by distinct genetic pathways. Proceedings of the National Academy of Sciences USA 2008; 105(36): 13520–13525.

93. Monti S et al. Integrative Analysis Reveals an Outcome-Associated and Targetable Pattern of p53 and Cell Cycle Deregulation in Diffuse Large B Cell Lymphoma. Cancer Cell 2012; 22(3): 359–372.

94. Chapuy B, McKeown MR, Lin CY, Monti S, Roemer MG, et al. Discovery and characterization of super-enhancer-associated dependencies in diffuse large B cell lymphoma. Cancer Cell 2013; 24(6): 777–790.

95. Horn H, Ziepert M, Becher C, Barth TF, Bernd HW et al. MYC status in concert with BCL2 and BCL6 expression predicts outcome in diffuse large B-cell lymphoma. Blood 2013; 121: 2253–2263.

96. Hu S, Xu-Monette ZY, Tzankov A, Green T, Wu L et al. MYC/BCL2 protein co-expression contributes to the inferior survival of activated B-cell subtype of diffuse large B-cell lymphoma and demonstrates high-risk gene expression signatures: a report from The International DLBCL Rituximab-CHOP Consortium Program Study. Blood 2013; 121(20): 4021–4031.

97. Johnson NA, Slack GW, Savage KJ, Connors JM, Ben-Neriah S et al. Concurrent expression of MYC and BCL2 in diffuse large B-cell lymphoma treated with rituximab plus cyclophosphamide, doxorubicin, vincristine, and prednisone. Journal of Clinical Oncology 2012; 30(28): 3452–3459.

98. Savage KJ et al. The molecular signature of mediastinal large B-cell lymphoma differs from that of other diffuse large B-cell lymphomas and shares features with classical Hodgkin lymphoma. Blood 2003; 102(12): 3871–3879.

99. Rosenwald A et al. Molecular diagnosis of primary mediastinal B cell lymphoma identifies a clinically favorable subgroup of diffuse large B cell lymphoma related to Hodgkin lymphoma. Journal of Experimental Medicine 2003; 198(6): 851–862.

100. Swerdlow S, Campo E, Harris NL et al. WHO Classification of tumors of hematopoietic and lymphoid tissues, 4th ed. Lyon: IARC, 2008, 429.

101. Steidl C, Gascoyne RD. The molecular pathogenesis of primary mediastinal large B-cell lymphoma. Blood 2011; 118(10): 2659–2669.

102. Rui L et al. Cooperative epigenetic modulation by cancer amplicon genes. Cancer Cell 2010; 18(6): 590–605.

103. Green MR et al. Integrative analysis reveals selective 9p24.1 amplification, increased PD-1 ligand expression, and further induction via JAK2 in nodular sclerosing Hodgkin lymphoma and primary mediastinal large B-cell lymphoma. Blood 2010; 116(17): 3268–3277.

104. Pardoll DM. The blockade of immune checkpoints in cancer immunotherapy. Nat Rev Cancer 2012; 12(4): 252–264.

105. Steidl C et al. MHC class II transactivator CIITA is a recurrent gene fusion partner in lymphoid cancers. Nature 2011; 471(7338): 377–381.

106. Brahmer JR et al. Safety and activity of anti-PD-L1 antibody in patients with advanced cancer. New England Journal of Medicine 2012; 366(26): 2455–2465.

107. Topalian SL et al. Safety, activity, and immune correlates of anti-PD-1 antibody in cancer. New England Journal of Medicine 2012; 366(26): 2443–2454.

108. Ansell SM, Lesokhin AM, Borrello I, Halwani A, Scott EC, et al. PD-1 blockade with nivolumab in relapsed or refractory Hodgkin's lymphoma. The New England Journal of Medicine 2015; 372(4): 311–319.

109. Dave SS et al. Molecular diagnosis of Burkitt's lymphoma. New England Journal of Medicine 2006; 354(23): 2431–2442.

110. Hummel M et al. A biologic definition of Burkitt's lymphoma from transcriptional and genomic profiling. New England Journal of Medicine 2006; 354(23): 2419–2430.

111. Gaidano G et al. p53 mutations in human lymphoid malignancies: association with Burkitt lymphoma and chronic lymphocytic leukemia. Proceedings of the National Academy of Sciences USA 1991; 88(12): 5413–5417.

112. Sander S et al. Synergy between PI3K Signaling and MYC in Burkitt Lymphomagenesis. Cancer Cell 2012; 22(2): 167–179.

113. McKelvey EM, Gottlieb JA, Wilson HE, Haut A, Talley RW et al. Hydroxyldaunomycin (Adriamycin)combination chemotherapy in malignant lymphoma. Cancer 1976; 38(4): 1484–1493.

114. Gisselbrecht C, Gaulard P, Lepage E, Coiffier B, Brière J et al. Prognostic significance of T-cell phenotype in aggressive non-Hodgkin's lymphomas. Groupe d'Etudes des Lymphomes de l'Adulte (GELA). Blood 1998; 92(1): 76–82.

115. Kimby E, Brandt L, Nygren P, Glimelius B for the SBU-Group. A systematic overview of chemotherapy effects in aggressive non-Hodgkin's lymphoma. Acta Oncology 2001; 40(2/3): 198–212.

116. Fisher RI, Gaynor ER, Dahlberg S, Oken MM, Grogan TM et al. Comparison of a standard regimen (CHOP) with three intensive chemotherapy regimens for advanced non-Hodgkin's lymphoma. New England Journal of Medicine 1993; 328(14): 1002–1006.

117. Miller T, Dahlberg S, Cassady J, et al. Chemotherapy alone compared with chemotherapy plus radiotherapy for localized intermediate- and high-grade non-Hodgkin's lymphoma. New England Journal of Medicine 1998; 339: 21–26.

118. Miller T, Leblanc M, Spier C, et al. CHOP alone compared to CHOP plus radiotherapy for early stage aggressive non-Hodgkin's lymphomas: Update of the Southwest Oncology Group (SWOG) randomized trial. Blood 2001; 98 (abstr 3024).

119. Köppler H, Pflüger KH, Eschenbach I, Pfab R, Lennert K et al. CHOP-VP16 chemotherapy and involved field irradiation for high grade non-Hodgkin's lymphomas: a phase II multicentre study. British Journal of Cancer 1989; 60: 79–82.

120. Köppler H, Pflüger KH, Eschenbach I, Pfab R, Birkmann J et al. Randomised comparison of CHOEP versus alternating hCHOP/IVEP for high-grade non-Hodgkin's lymphomas: Treatment results and prognostic factor analysis in a multi-centre trial. Annals of Oncology 1994; 5: 49–55.

121. Gregory SA, Trümper L. Chemotherapy dose intensity in non-Hodgkin's lymphoma: is dose intensity an emerging paradigm for better outcomes? Annals of Oncology 2005; 16: 1413–1424.

122. Trümper L, Renner Ch, Nahler M, Engert A, Koch P et al. Intensification of the CHOEP regimen for high-grade non-Hodgkin's lymphoma by G-CSF: feasibility of a 14-day regimen. Onkologie 1994; 17: 69–71.

123. Wunderlich A, Kloess M, Reiser M, Rudolph C, Truemper L et al. on behalf of the German High-Grade Non-Hodgkin's Lymphoma Study Group (DSHNHL). Practicability and acute haematological toxicity of 2- and 3-weekly CHOP and CHOEP chemotherapy for aggressive non-Hodgkin's lymphoma: results from the NHL-B trial of the German High-Grade Non-Hodgkin's Lymphoma Study Group (DSHNHL). Annals of Oncology 2003; 14: 881–893.

124. Pfreundschuh M, Trümper L, Kloess M, Schmits R, Feller AC et al. for the German High-Grade Non-Hodgkin's Lymphoma Study Group. Two-weekly or 3-weekly CHOP chemotherapy with or without etoposide for the treatment of young patients with good-prognosis (normal LDH) aggressive lymphomas: results of the NHL-B1 trial of the DSHNHL. Blood 2004; 104(3): 626–633.

125. Pfreundschuh M, Trümper L, Kloess M, Schmits R, Feller AC et al. for the German High-Grade Non-Hodgkin's Lymphoma Study Group. Two-weekly or 3-weekly CHOP chemotherapy with or without etoposide for the treatment of elderly patients with aggressive lymphomas: results of the NHL-B2 trial of the DSHNHL. Blood 2004; 104(3): 634–641.

126. Hohloch K, Zwick C, Ziepert M, Hasenclever D, Kaiser U et al. for the German High-Grade Non-Hodgkin´s Lymphoma Study Group (DSHNHL). Significant dose escalation of idarubicin in the treatment of aggressive non-Hodgkin lymphoma leads to increased hemato-toxicity without improvement in efficacy in comparison to stand-ard CHOEP-14: 9-year follow up results of the CIVEP trial of the DSHNHL. SpringerPlus 2014; 3: 5.

127. Kroschinsky F, Schleyer E, Renner U, Schimming C, Schimmelpfennig C et al. Increased myelotoxicity of idarubicin: is there a pharmacological basis? Results of a pharmacokinetic and an in vitro cytotoxicity study. Cancer Chemotherapy and Pharmacology 2004; 53(1): 61–67.

128. Coiffier B, Lepage E, Briere J, Herbrecht R, Tilly H et al. CHOP chemotherapy plus rituximab compared with CHOP alone in elderly patients with diffuse large-B-cell lymphoma. New England Journal of Medicine 2002; 346(4): 235–242.

129. Feugier P, Van Hoof A, Sebban C, Solal-Celigny P, Bouabdallah R et al. Long-term results of the R-CHOP study in the treatment of elderly patients with diffuse large B-cell lymphoma: a study by the Groupe d'Etude des Lymphomes de l'Adulte. Journal of Clinical Oncology 2005; 23(18): 4117–4126.

130. Pfreundschuh M, Schubert J, Ziepert M, Schmits R, Mohren M et al. German High-Grade Non-Hodgkin Lymphoma Study Group (DSHNHL). Six versus eight cycles of bi-weekly CHOP-14 with or without rituximab in elderly patients with aggressive CD20+ B-cell lymphomas: a randomised controlled trial (RICOVER-60). Lancet Oncology 2008; 9(2): 105–116.

131. Pfreundschuh M, Kuhnt E, Trümper L, Osterborg A, Trneny M et al. MabThera International Trial (MInT) Group. CHOP-like chemother-apy with or without rituximab in young patients with good-prognosis diffuse large-B-cell lymphoma: 6-year results of an open-label randomised study of the MabThera International Trial (MInT) Group. Lancet Oncology 2011; 12(11): 1013–1022.

132. Delarue R, Tilly H, Mounier N, Petrella T, Salles G et al. Dose-dense rituximab-CHOP compared with standard rituximab-CHOP in elderly patients with diffuse large B-cell lymphoma (the LNH03-6B study): a randomised phase 3 trial. Lancet Oncology 2013; 14(6): 525–533.

133. Cunningham D, Hawkes EA, Jack A, Qian W, Smith P et al. Rituximab plus cyclophosphamide, doxorubicin, vincristine, and prednisolone in patients with newly diagnosed diffuse large B-cell non-Hodgkin lymphoma: a phase 3 comparison of dose intensification with 14-day versus 21-day cycles. Lancet 2013; 381(9880): 1817–1826.

134. Schmitz N, Nickelsen M, Ziepert M, Haenel M, Borchmann P et al. Conventional chemotherapy (CHOEP-14) with rituximab or high-dose chemotherapy (Mega-CHOEP) with rituximab for young, high-risk patients with aggressive B-cell lymphoma: an open-label, randomized, phase 3 trial (DSHNHL 2001-1). Lancet Oncology 2012; 13: 1250–1259.

135. Pfreundschuh M, Ho AD, Cavallin-Stahl E, Wolf M, Pettengell R et al. MabThera International Trial (MInT)Group. Prognostic significance of maximum tumour (bulk) diameter in young patients with good-prognosis diffuse large-B-cell lymphoma treated with CHOP-like chemotherapy with or without rituximab: an exploratory analysis of the MabThera International Trial Group (MInT) study. Lancet Oncology 2008; 9(5): 435–444.

136. Récher C, Coiffier B, Haioun C, Molina TJ, Fermé C et al. Groupe d'Etude des Lymphomes de l'Adulte. Intensified chemotherapy with ACVBP plus rituximab versus standard CHOP plus rituximab for the treatment of diffuse large B-cell lymphoma (LNH03-2B): an open-label randomised phase 3 trial. Lancet 2011; 378: 1858–1867.

137. Abrahamsson A, Dahle N, Jerkeman M. Marked improvement of overall survival in mantle cell lymphoma: a population based study from the Swedish Lymphoma Registry. Leukemia Lymphoma 2011; 52(10): 1929–1935.

138. Romaguera JE, Fayad LE, Feng L, Hartig K, Weaver P et al. Ten-year follow-up after intense chemoimmunotherapy with Rituximab-HyperCVAD alternating with Rituximab-high dose methotrexate/cytarabine (R-MA) and without stem cell transplanta-tion in patients with untreated aggressive mantle cell lymphoma. British Journal of Haematology 2010; 150(2): 200–208.

139. Geisler CH, Kolstad A, Laurell A, Jerkeman M, Räty R et al. Nordic Lymphoma Group. Nordic MCL2 trial update: six-year follow-up after intensive immunochemotherapy for untreated mantle cell lymphoma followed by BEAM or BEAC + autologous stem-cell support: still very long survival but late relapses do occur. British Journal of Haematology 2012; 158(3): 355–362.

140. Hermine O, Hoster E, Szymczyk M, Walewski J, Ribrag V et al. Alternating courses of 3x CHOP and 3x DHAP plus rituximab fol-lowed by a high-dose ARA-C containing myeloablative regimen and autologous stem cell transplantation (ASCT) is superior to 6 courses CHOP plus rituximab followed by myeloablative radiochemotherapy and ASCT in mantle cell lymphoma: Final results of the MCL Younger Trial of the European Mantle Cell Lymphoma Network (MCL net). Blood 2012; 120(21): abstr 150.

141. Pott C, Hoster E, Delfau-Larue MH, Beldjord K, Böttcher S et al. Molecular remission is an independent predictor of clinical outcome in patients with mantle cell lymphoma after combined immuno-chemotherapy: a European MCL intergroup study. Blood 2010; 115(16): 3215–3223.

142. Kluin-Nelemans HC, Hoster E, Hermine O, Walewski J, Trneny M et al. Treatment of older patients with mantle-cell lymphoma. New England Journal of Medicine 2012; 367(6): 520–531.

143. Rummel MJ, Niederle N, Maschmeyer G, Banat GA, von Grünhagen U et al. Study group indolent Lymphomas (StiL). Bendamustine plus rituximab versus CHOP plus rituximab as first-line treatment for patients with indolent and mantle-cell lymphomas: an open-label, multicentre, randomised, phase 3 non-inferiority trial. Lancet 2013; 381(9873): 1203–1210.

144. Forstpointner R, Unterhalt M, Dreyling M, Böck HP, Repp R et al. German Low Grade Lymphoma Study Group (GLSG). Maintenance therapy with rituximab leads to a significant prolongation of response duration after salvage therapy with a combination of rituximab, fludarabine, cyclophosphamide, and mitoxantrone (R-FCM) in patients with recurring and refractory follicular and mantle cell lymphomas: Results of a prospective randomized study of the German Low Grade Lymphoma Study Group (GLSG). Blood 2006; 108(13): 4003–4008.

145. Wang ML, Rule S, Martin P, Goy A, Auer R et al. Targeting BTK with ibrutinib in relapsed or refractory mantle-cell lymphoma. New England Journal of Medicine 2013; 369(6): 507–516.

146. Holkova B, Grant S. Proteasome inhibitors in mantle cell lymphoma. Best Practice and Research Clinical Haematology 2012; 25: 133–141.

147. Friedberg JW, Byrtek M, Link BK, Flowers C, Taylor M et al. Effectiveness of first-line management strategies for stage I follicular lymphoma: analysis of the National LymphoCare Study. Journal of Clinical Oncology 2012; 30(27): 3368–3375.

148. Ardeshna KM, Qian W, Smith P, Braganca N, Lowry L et al. Rituximab versus a watch-and-wait approach in patients with advanced-stage, asymptomatic, non-bulky follicular lymphoma: an open-label randomised phase 3 trial. Lancet Oncology 2014; 15(4): 424–435.

149. Federico M, Luminari S, Dondi A, Tucci A, Vitolo U et al. R-CVP versus R-CHOP versus R-FM for the initial treatment of patients with advanced-stage follicular lymphoma: results of the FOLL05 trial conducted by the Fondazione Italiana Linfomi. Journal of Clinical Oncology 2013; 31(12): 1506–1513.

150. Nickenig C, Dreyling M, Hoster E, Pfreundschuh M, Trumper L et al. German Low-Grade Lymphoma Study Group. Combined cyclophosphamide, vincristine, doxorubicin, and prednisone (CHOP) improves response rates but not survival and has lower hematologic toxicity compared with combined mitoxantrone, chlorambucil, and prednisone (MCP) in follicular and mantle cell lymphomas: results of a prospective randomized trial of the German Low-Grade Lymphoma Study Group. Cancer 2006; 107(5): 1014–1022.

151. Jacobson CA, Freedman AS. First-line treatment of indolent lymphoma: axing CHOP? Lancet 2013; 381(9873): 1163–1165.

152. Carbone PP, Kaplan HS, Musshoff K et al. Report of the Committee on Hodgkin Lymphoma Staging Classification. Cancer Research 1971; 31: 1860–1861.

153. Lister TA, Crowther D, Sutcliffe SB et al. Report of a committee convened to discuss the evaluation and staging of patients with Hodgkin's disease: Cotswolds meeting. Journal of Clinical Oncology 1989; 7: 1630–1636.

154. Eichenauer DA, Engert A, Dreyling M. Hodgkin's lymphoma: ESMO clinical practice guidelines for diagnosis, treatment and follow-up. Annals Oncology 2011; 22(Suppl 6): vi55–vi58

155. Klimm B, Goergen H, Fuchs M et al. Impact of risk factors on outcomes in early-stage Hodgkin's lymphoma: an analysis of international staging definitions. Annals of Oncology 2013; 24(12): 3070–3076

156. DeVita V, Serpick A, Carbone P. Combination chemotherapy in the treatment of advanced Hodgkin's disease. Annals of Internal Medicine 1970; 73: 881.

157. Bonadonna G, Zucali R, Monfardini S et al. Combination chemotherapy of Hodgkin´s disease with adriamycin, bleomycin, vinblastine, and imidazole carboximide versus MOPP. Cancer 1975; 36: 252–259.

158. Santoro A, Bonadonna G, Bonfante V, Valagussa P. Alternating drug combinations in the treatment of advanced Hodgkin's disease. New England Journal of Medicine 1982; 306: 770–775.

159. Bonadonna G, Valagussa P, Santoro A: Alternating non-cross-resistant combination chemotherapy or MOPP in stage IV Hodgkin's disease. A report of 8-year results. Annals of Internal Medicine 1986; 104: 739.

160. Diehl V, Franklin J, Hasenclever D et al. BEACOPP, a new dose-escalated and accelerated regimen, is at least as effective as COPP/ABVD in patients with advanced-stage Hodgkin's lymphoma: interim report from a trial of the German Hodgkin's Lymphoma Study Group. Journal of Clinical Oncology 1998; 16: 3810.

161. Bartlett NL, Rosenberg SA, Hoppe RT et al. Brief chemotherapy, Stanford V, and adjuvant radiotherapy for bulky or advanced-stage Hodgkin's disease: a preliminary report. Journal of Clinical Oncology 1995; 13: 1080.

162. Engert A, Franklin J, Eich HT et al. Two cycles of doxorubicin, bleomycin, vinblastine, and dacarbazine plus extended-field radiotherapy is superior to radiotherapy alone in early favorable Hodgkin's lymphoma: final results of the GHSG HD7 trial. Journal of Clinical Oncology 2007; 25: 3495–3502.

163. Ferme C, Eghbali H, Meerwaldt JH et al. Chemotherapy plus involved-field radiation in early-stage Hodgkin's disease. New England Journal of Medicine 2007; 357: 1916–1927.

164. Engert A, Plütschow A, Eich HT et al. Reduced treatment intensity in patients with early-stage Hodgkin's lymphoma. New England Journal of Medicine 2010; 363(7): 640–652.

165. Eich HT, Diehl V, Görgen H et al. Intensified chemotherapy and dose-reduced involved-field radiotherapy in patients with early unfavorable Hodgkin's lymphoma: final analysis of the German Hodgkin Study Group HD11 trial. Journal of Clinical Oncology 2010; 28: 4199–4206.

166. Von Tresckow B, Plütschow A, Fuchs M et al. Dose-intensification in early unfavorable Hodgkin Lymphoma: Final analysis of the GHSG HD14 trial. Journal of Clinical Oncology 2012; 30: 907–913.

167. Canellos GP, Niedzwiecki D, Johnson JL. Long-term follow-up of survival in Hodgkin's lymphoma. New England Journal of Medicine 2009; 361(24): 2390–2391.

168. Gordon LI, Hong F, Fisher RI, et al. Randomized phase III trial of ABVD versus Stanford V with or without radiation therapy in locally extensive and advanced-stage Hodgkin lymphoma: An intergroup study coordinated by the Eastern Cooperative Oncology Group (E2496). Journal of Clinical Oncology 2013; 31: 684–691.

169. Engert A, Diehl V, Franklin J et al. Escalated-dose BEACOPP in the treatment of patients with advanced-stage Hodgkin's lymphoma: 10 years of follow-up of the GHSG HD9 study. Journal of Clinical Oncology 2009; 27(27): 4548–4554.

170. Engert A, Haverkamp H, Kobe C et al.: Reduced intensity of chemotherapy and PET-guided radiotherapy in patients with advanced stage Hodgkin lymphoma: an open-label, randomized phase 3 trial. Lancet 2012; 379: 1791–1799.

171. Ballova V, Rüffer JU, Haverkamp H et al. A prospectively randomized trial carried out by the Germany Hodgkin Study Group (GHSG) for elderly patients with advanced Hodgkin's disease comparing BEACOPP baseline and COPP-ABVD (study HD9elderly). Annals of Oncology 2005; 16(1): 124–131.

172. Josting A, Müller H, Borchmann P et al. Dose intensity of chemotherapy in patients with relapsed Hodgkin's lymphoma. Journal of Clinical Oncology 2010; 28(34): 5074–5080.

173. Rancea M, Monsef I, von Tresckow B et al. high-dose chemotherapy followed by autologous stem cell transplantation for patients with relapsed/refractory Hodgkin lymphoma. Cochrane database Systematic Reviews 2013; 6: CD009411.

174. Thomson KJ, Peggs KS, Smith P et al. Superiority of reduced-intensity allogeneic transplantation over conventional treatment for relapse of Hodgkin's lymphoma following autologous stem cell transplantation. Bone Marrow Transplantation 2008; 41(9): 765.

175. Peggs KS, Hunter A, Chopra R et al. Clinical evidence of a graft-versus-Hodgkin's-lymphoma effect after reduced-intensity allogeneic transplantation. Lancet 2005; 365(9475): 1934.

176. Sarina B, Castagna L, Farina L et al. Allogeneic transplantation improves the overall and progression-free survival of Hodgkin lymphoma patients relapsing after autologous transplantation: a retrospective study based on the time of HLA typing and donor availability. Blood 2010; 115(18): 3671.

177. Younes A, Bartlett NL, Leonard JP et al. Brentuximab vedotin (SGN-35) for relapsed CD30-positive lymphomas. New England Journal of Medicine 2010; 363: 1812–1821.

178. Diefenbach C, Steidl C. New strategies in Hodgkin lymphoma: better risk profiling and novel treatments. Clinical Cancer Research 2013; 19(11): 2797–2803.

179. Ansell SM, Lesokhin AM, Borrello I, Halwani A, Scott EC, et al. PD-1 blockade with nivolumab in relapsed or refractory Hodgkin's lymphoma. New England Journal of Medicine 2015; 372(4): 311–319.

180. Nogova L, Reineke T, Brillant C et al. Extended field radiotherapy, combined modality treatment or involved field radiotherapy for

patients with stage IA lymphocyte-predominant Hodgkin's lymphoma: a retrospective analysis from the German Hodgkin Study Group (GHSG). Annals of Oncology 2005; 16(10): 1683–1687.

181. Ekstrand BC, Lucas JB, Horwitz SM et al. Rituximab in lymphocyte-predominant Hodgkin disease: results of a phase 2 trial. Blood 2003; 101(11): 4285–4289.

182. Pettengell R, Coiffier B, Narayanan G, de Mendoza FH, Digumarti R et al. Pixantrone dimaleate versus other chemotherapeutic agents as a single-agent salvage treatment in patients with relapsed or refractory aggressive non-Hodgkin lymphoma: a phase 3, multicentre, open-label, randomised trial. Lancet Oncology 2012; 13(7): 696–706.

183. Velasquez WS, Cabanillas F, Salvador P, McLaughlin P, Fridrik M et al. Effective salvage therapy for lymphoma with cisplatin in combination with high-dose Ara-C and dexamethasone (DHAP). Blood 1988; 71: 117–122.

184. Moskowitz CH, Bertino JR, Glassman JR, Hedrick EE, Hunte S et al. Ifosfamide, carboplatin, and etoposide: a highly effective cytoreduction and peripheral-blood progenitor-cell mobilization regimen for transplant-eligible patients with non-Hodgkin's lymphoma. Journal of Clinical Oncology 1999; 17(12): 3776–3785.

185. Kewalramani T, Zelenetz AD, Nimer SD, et al. Rituximab and ICE as second-line therapy before autologous stem cell transplantation for relapsed or primary refractory diffuse large B-cell lymphoma. Blood 2004 103: 3684–3688.

186. Gisselbrecht C, Glass B, Mounier N, Singh Gill D, Linch DC et al. Salvage regimens with autologous transplantation for relapsed large B-cell lymphoma in the rituximab era. Journal of Clinical Oncology 2010; 28(27): 4184–4190.

187. Girouard C, Dufresne J, Imrie K, Stewart AK, Brandwein J et al. Salvage chemotherapy with mini-BEAM for relapsed or refractory non-Hodgkin's lymphoma prior to autologous bone marrow transplantation. Annals of Oncology 1997; 8(7): 675–680.

188. Martín A, Fernández-Jiménez MC, Caballero MD, Canales MA, Pérez-Simón JA et al. Long-term follow-up in patients treated with Mini-BEAM as salvage therapy for relapsed or refractory Hodgkin's disease. British Journal of Haematology 2001; 113(1): 161–171.

189. Pfreundschuh MG, Rueffer U, Lathan B, Schmitz N, Brosteanu O et al. Dexa-BEAM in patients with Hodgkin's disease refractory to multidrug chemotherapy regimens: a trial of the German Hodgkin's Disease Study Group. Journal of Clinical Oncology 1994; 12(3): 580–586.

190. Reiser M, Josting A, Dias Wickramanayake P, Draube A, Scheid C et al. Dexa-BEAM is not effective in patients with relapsed or resistant aggressive high-grade non-Hodgkin's lymphoma. Leukemia Lymphoma 1999; 33(3–4): 305–312.

191. Atta J, Chow KU, Weidmann E, Mitrou PS, Hoelzer D et al. Dexa-BEAM as salvage therapy in patients with primary refractory aggressive non-Hodgkin lymphoma. Leukemia Lymphoma 2007; 48(2): 349–356.

192. Mikesch JH, Kuhlmann M, Demant A, Krug U, Thoennissen GB et al. DexaBEAM versus ICE salvage regimen prior to autologous transplantation for relapsed or refractory aggressive peripheral T cell lymphoma: a retrospective evaluation of parallel patient cohorts of one center. Annals of Hematology 2013; 92(8): 1041–1048.

193. Dunleavy K, Pittaluga S, Maeda LS, Advani R, Chen CC et al. Dose-adjusted EPOCH-rituximab therapy in primary mediastinal B-cell lymphoma. New England Journal of Medicine 2013; 368(15): 1408–1416.

194. Kohler G, Milstein C. Continuous cultures of fused cells secreting antibody of predefined specificity. Nature 1975; 256(5517): 495–497.

195. Grossbard ML, Press OW, Appelbaum FR, Bernstein ID, Nadler LM. Monoclonal antibody-based therapies of leukemia and lymphoma. Blood 1992; 80: 863–878.

196. Cheson BD, John P. Leonard Monoclonal Antibody Therapy for B-Cell Non-Hodgkin's Lymphoma New England Journal of Medicine 2008; 359: 613–626.

197. Reff ME, Carner K, Chambers KS, Chinn PC, Leonard JE et al. Depletion of B cells in vivo by a chimeric mouse human monoclonal antibody to CD20. Blood 1994; 83(2): 435–445.

198. McLaughlin P, Grillo-Lopez AJ, Link BK et al. Rituximab chimeric anti-CD20 monoclonal antibody therapy for relapsed indolent lymphoma: half of patients respond to a four-dose treatment program. Journal of Clinical Oncology 1998; 16(8): 2825–2833.

199. Coiffier B, Lepage E, Briere J et al. CHOP Chemotherapy plus Rituximab Compared with CHOP Alone in Elderly Patients with Diffuse Large-B-Cell Lymphoma. New England Journal of Medicine 2002; 346(4): 235–242.

200. Pfreundschuh M, Trümper L, Osterborg A, Pettengell R, Trneny M et al. CHOP-like chemotherapy plus rituximab versus CHOP-like chemotherapy alone in young patients with good-prognosis diffuse large-B-cell lymphoma: a randomised controlled trial by the MabThera International Trial (MInT) Group. Lancet Oncology 2006; 7(5): 379–391.

201. Pfreundschuh M, Kuhnt E, Trümper L, Osterborg A, Trneny M et al. MabThera International Trial (MInT) Group. CHOP-like chemotherapy with or without rituximab in young patients with good-prognosis diffuse large-B-cell lymphoma: 6-year results of an open-label randomised study of the MabThera International Trial (MInT) Group. Lancet Oncology 2011; 12(11): 1013–1022.

202. Cunningham D, Smith P, Mouncey P, Qian W, Jack AS et al. R-CHOP14 versus R-CHOP21: Result of a randomized phase III trial for the treatment of patients with newly diagnosed diffuse large B-cell non-Hodgkin lymphoma Journal of Clinical Oncology 2011; 29(suppl, abstr 8000).

203. Marcus R, Imrie K, Belch A et al. CVP chemotherapy plus rituximab compared with CVP as first-line treatment for advanced follicular lymphoma. Blood 2005; 105(4): 1417–1423.

204. Hiddemann W, Kneba M, Dreyling M et al. Frontline therapy with rituximab added to the combination of cyclophosphamide, doxorubicin, vincristine, and prednisone (CHOP) significantly improves the outcome for patients with advanced-stage follicular lymphoma compared with therapy with CHOP alone: results of a prospective randomized study of the German Low-Grade Lymphoma Study Group. Blood 2005; 106(12): 3725–3732.

205. Herold M, Haas A, Srock S, Neser S, Al-Ali KH et al. East German Study Group Hematology and Oncology Study. Rituximab added to first-line mitoxantrone, chlorambucil, and prednisolone chemotherapy followed by interferon maintenance prolongs survival in patients with advanced follicular lymphoma: an East German Study Group Hematology and Oncology Study. Journal of Clinical Oncology 2007; 25(15): 1986–1992.

206. Salles G, Mounier N, de Guibert S, Morschhauser F, Doyen C et al. Rituximab combined with chemotherapy and interferon in follicular lymphoma patients: results of the GELA-GOELAMS FL2000 study. Blood 2008; 112(13): 4824–4831.

207. Schulz H, Bohlius JF, Trelle S et al. Immunochemotherapy With Rituximab and Overall Survival in Patients With Indolent or Mantle Cell Lymphoma: A Systematic Review and Meta-analysis. Journal of the National Cancer Institute 2007; 99(9): 706–714.

208. Salles G, Seymour JF, Offner F, López-Guillermo A, Belada D et al. Rituximab maintenance for 2 years in patients with high tumour burden follicular lymphoma responding to rituximab plus chemotherapy (PRIMA): a phase 3, randomised controlled trial. Lancet 2011; 377(9759): 42–51.

209. van Oers MH, Van Glabbeke M, Giurgea L, Klasa R, Marcus RE et al. Rituximab maintenance treatment of relapsed/resistant follicular non-Hodgkin's lymphoma: long-term outcome of the EORTC 20981 phase III randomized intergroup study. Journal of Clinical Oncology 2010; 28(17): 2853–2858.

210. Clynes RA, Towers TL, Presta LG, Ravetch JV. Inhibitory Fc receptors modulate in vivo cytotoxicity against tumor targets. Nature Medicine 2000; 6(4): 443–446.

211. Cartron G, Dacheux L, Salles G et al. Therapeutic activity of humanized anti-CD20 monoclonal antibody and polymorphism in IgG Fc receptor Fcgamma RIIIa gene. Blood 2002; 99(3): 754–758.

212. Alduaij W, Illidge TM. The future of anti-CD20 monoclonal antibodies: are we making progress? Blood 2011; 117(11): 2993–3001.

213. Wierda WG, Kipps TJ, Mayer J et al. Ofatumumab as single-agent CD20 immunotherapy in fludarabine-refractory chronic lymphocytic leukemia. Journal of Clinical Oncology 2010; 28(10): 1749–1755.

214. Morschhauser F, Marlton P, Vitolo U et al. Results of a phase I/II study of ocrelizumab, a fully humanized anti-CD20 mAb, in patients with relapsed/refractory follicular lymphoma. Annals of Oncology 2010; 21(9): 1870–1876.

215. Morschhauser F, Leonard JP, Fayad L et al. Humanized anti-CD20 antibody, veltuzumab, in refractory/recurrent non-Hodgkin's lymphoma: phase I/II results. Journal of Clinical Oncology 2009; 27(20): 3346–3353.

216. Mossner E, Brunker P, Moser S et al. Increasing the efficacy of CD20 antibody therapy through the engineering of a new type II anti-CD20 antibody with enhanced direct and immune effector cell-mediated B-cell cytotoxicity. Blood 2010; 115(22): 4393–4402.

217. Illidge TM, Johnson PW. The emerging role of radioimmunotherapy in haematological malignancies. British Journal of Haematology 2000; 108: 679–688.

218. Kaminski MS, Zelenetz AD, Press OW Saleh M Leonard J et al. Pivotal study of iodine I 131 tositumomab for chemotherapy-refractory low-grade or transformed low-grade B-cell non-Hodgkin's lymphomas. Journal of Clinical Oncology 2001; 19: 3918–3928.

219. Horning SJ, Younes A, Jain V, Kroll S, Lucas J et al. (2005) Efficacy and safety of tositumomab and iodine-131 tositumomab (Bexxar) in B-cell lymphoma, progressive after rituximab. Journal of Clinical Oncology 23: 712–719.

220. Witzig TE, Flinn IW, Gordon LI, Emmanouilides C, Czuczman MS et al. Treatment With Ibritumomab Tiuxetan Radioimmunotherapy in Patients With Rituximab-Refractory Follicular Non-Hodgkin's Lymphoma. Journal of Clinical Oncology 2002; 20: 3262–3269.

221. Fisher RI, Kaminski MS, Wahl RL, Knox SJ et al. Tositumomab and iodine-131 tositumomab produces durable complete remissions in a subset of heavily pretreated patients with low-grade and transformed non-Hodgkin's lymphomas. Journal of Clinical Oncology 2005; 23: 7565–7573.

222. Witzig TE, White CA, Gordon LI, Wiseman GA, Emmanouilides C et al. Safety of yttrium-90 ibritumomab tiuxetan radioimmunotherapy for relapsed low-grade, follicular, or transformed non-Hodgkin's lymphoma. Journal of Clinical Oncology 2003; 21: 1263–1270.

223. Gordon LI, Molina A, Witzig T, Emmanouilides C, Raubitschek A et al. Durable responses after ibritumomab tiuxetan radioimmunotherapy for CD20+ B-cell lymphoma: long-term follow-up of a phase 1/2 study. Blood 2004; 103: 4429–4431.

224. Press OW, Unger JM, Braziel RM, Maloney DG, Miller TP et al. Phase II trial of CHOP chemotherapy followed by tositumomab/iodine I-131 tositumomab for previously untreated follicular non-Hodgkin's lymphoma: five-year follow-up of Southwest Oncology Group Protocol S9911. Journal of Clinical Oncology 2006; 24(25): 4143–4149.

225. Press OW, Unger JM, Rimsza LM, Friedberg JW, LeBlanc M, et al. Phase III randomized intergroup trial of CHOP plus rituximab compared with CHOP chemotherapy plus (131)iodine-tositumomab for previously untreated follicular non-Hodgkin lymphoma: SWOG S0016. Journal of Clinical Oncology 2013; 31(3): 314–320. doi: 10.1200/JCO.2012.42.4101. Epub 2012 Dec 10.

226. Morschhauser F, Radford J, Van Hoof A, Vitolo U, Soubeyran P et al. Phase III trial of consolidation therapy with yttrium-90-ibritumomab tiuxetan compared with no additional therapy after first remission in advanced follicular lymphoma. Journal of Clinical Oncology 2008; 26(32): 5156–5164.

227. Kaminski MS, Tuck M, Estes J, Kolstad A, Ross CW et al. 131I-tositumomab therapy as initial treatment for follicular lymphoma. New England Journal of Medicine 2005; 352: 441–449.

228. Younes A, Bartlett NL, Leonard JP, Kennedy DA, Lynch CM et al. Brentuximab vedotin (SGN-35) for relapsed CD30-positive lymphomas. New England Journal of Medicine 2010; 363(19): 1812–1821.

229. Younes A, Gopal AK, Smith SE, Ansell SM, Rosenblatt JD et al. Results of a pivotal phase II study of brentuximab vedotin for patients with relapsed or refractory Hodgkin's lymphoma. Journal of Clinical Oncology 2012; 30(18): 2183–2189.

230. Pro B, Advani R, Brice P, Bartlett NL, Rosenblatt JD et al. Brentuximab vedotin (SGN-35) in patients with relapsed or refractory systemic anaplastic large-cell lymphoma: results of a phase II study. Journal of Clinical Oncology 2012; 30(18): 2190–2196.

231. Advani A, Coiffier B, Czuczman MS, Dreyling M, Foran J et al. Safety, pharmacokinetics, and preliminary clinical activity of inotuzumab ozogamicin, a novel immunoconjugate for the treatment of B-cell non-Hodgkin's lymphoma: results of a phase I study. Journal of Clinical Oncology 2010; 28(12): 2085–2093.

232. Schmitz N, Nickelsen M, Glass B. Autologous or allogeneic transplantation in B- and T-cell lymphomas. Best Practice and Research in Clinical Haematology 2012; 25: 61–73.

233. Dembo AJ. Time-dose factors in chemotherapy: expanding the concept of dose-intensity. Journal of Clinical Oncology 1987; 5: 694–696.

234. Vose JM:. Dose-intensive ifosfamide for the treatment of non-Hodgkin's lymphoma. Seminars in Oncology 1996; 23: 33–37.

235. Michel G, Socie G, Gebhard F et al. Late effects of allogeneic bone marrow transplantation for children with acute myeloblastic leukemia in first complete remission: the impact of conditioning regimen without total-body irradiation—a report from the Societe Francaise de Greffe de Moelle. Journal of Clinical Oncology 1997; 15: 2238–2246.

236. Mills W, Chopra R, McMillan A et al. BEAM chemotherapy and autologous bone marrow transplantation for patients with relapsed or refractory non-Hodgkin's lymphoma. Journal of Clinical Oncology 1995; 13: 588–595.

237. Wheeler C, Antin JH, Churchill WH et al. Cyclophosphamide, carmustine, and etoposide with autologous bone marrow transplantation in refractory Hodgkin's disease and non-Hodgkin's lymphoma: a dose-finding study. Journal of Clinical Oncology 1990; 8: 648–656.

238. Haioun C, Lepage E, Gisselbrecht C et al. Comparison of autologous bone marrow transplantation with sequential chemotherapy for intermediate-grade and high-grade non-Hodgkin's lymphoma in first complete remission: a study of 464 patients. Groupe d'Etude des Lymphomes de l'Adulte. Journal of Clinical Oncology 1994; 12: 2543–2551.

239. Attal M, Canal P, Schlaifer D et al. Escalating dose of mitoxantrone with high-dose cyclophosphamide, carmustine, and etoposide in patients with refractory lymphoma undergoing autologous bone marrow transplantation. Journal of Clinical Oncology 1994; 12: 141–148.

240. Mills W, Strang J, Goldstone AH et al. Dose intensification of etoposide in the BEAM ABMT protocol for malignant lymphoma. Leukemia Lymphoma 1995; 17: 263–270.

241. Soussain C, Hoang-Xuan K, Taillandier L et al. Intensive chemotherapy followed by hematopoietic stem-cell rescue for refractory and recurrent primary CNS and intraocular lymphoma: Societe Francaise de Greffe de Moelle Osseuse-Therapie Cellulaire. Journal of Clinical Oncology 2008; 26: 2512–2518.

242. Korfel A, Elter T, Thiel E et al. Phase II study of central nervous system (CNS)-directed chemotherapy including high-dose chemotherapy with autologous stem cell transplantation for CNS relapse of aggressive lymphomas. Haematologica 2012; 98: 364–370.

243. Morschhauser F, Brice P, Ferme C et al. Risk-adapted salvage treatment with single or tandem autologous stem-cell transplantation for first relapse/refractory Hodgkin's lymphoma: results of the prospective

multicenter H96 trial by the GELA/SFGM study group. Journal of Clinical Oncology 2008; 26: 5980–5987.

244. Stoppa AM, Bouabdallah R, Chabannon C et al. Intensive sequential chemotherapy with repeated blood stem-cell support for untreated poor-prognosis non-Hodgkin's lymphoma. Journal of Clinical Oncology 1997; 15: 1722–1729.

245. Schmitz N, Nickelsen M, Ziepert M et al. Conventional chemotherapy (CHOEP-14) with rituximab or high-dose chemotherapy (MegaCHOEP) with rituximab for young, high-risk patients with aggressive B-cell lymphoma: an open-label, randomised, phase 3 trial (DSHNHL 2002-1). Lancet Oncology 2012; 13: 1250–1259.

246. Petersen FB, Appelbaum FR, Hill R et al. Autologous marrow transplantation for malignant lymphoma: a report of 101 cases from Seattle. Journal of Clinical Oncology 1990; 8: 638–647.

247. Blume KG, Forman SJ, O'Donnell MR et al. Total body irradiation and high-dose etoposide: a new preparatory regimen for bone marrow transplantation in patients with advanced hematologic malignancies. Blood 1987; 69: 1015–1020.

248. Petersen FB, Buckner CD, Appelbaum FR et al. Etoposide, cyclophosphamide and fractionated total body irradiation as a preparative regimen for marrow transplantation in patients with advanced hematological malignancies: a phase I study. Bone Marrow Transplantation 1992; 10: 83–88.

249. Gisselbrecht C, Vose J, Nademanee A et al. Radioimmunotherapy for stem cell transplantation in non-Hodgkin's lymphoma: in pursuit of a complete response. Oncologist 2009; 14(Suppl 2): 41–51.

250. Vose JM, Carter S, Burns LJ et al. Phase III randomized study of rituximab/carmustine, etoposide, cytarabine, and melphalan (BEAM) compared with iodine-131 tositumomab/BEAM with autologous hematopoietic cell transplantation for relapsed diffuse large B-cell lymphoma: results from the BMT CTN 0401 trial. Journal of Clinical Oncology 2013; 31: 1662–1668.

251. Storb R, Yu C, Barnett T et al. Stable mixed hematopoietic chimerism in dog leukocyte antigen-identical littermate dogs given lymph node irradiation before and pharmacologic immunosuppression after marrow transplantation. Blood 1999; 94: 1131–1136.

252. van Kampen RJ, Canals C, Schouten HC et al. Allogeneic stem-cell transplantation as salvage therapy for patients with diffuse large B-cell non-Hodgkin's lymphoma relapsing after an autologous stem-cell transplantation: an analysis of the European Group for Blood and Marrow Transplantation Registry. Journal of Clinical Oncology 2011; 29: 1342–1348.

253. van Besien K, Loberiza FR, Jr., Bajorunaite R et al. Comparison of autologous and allogeneic hematopoietic stem cell transplantation for follicular lymphoma. Blood 2003; 102: 3521–3529.

254. Schmitz N, Linch DC, Dreger P et al. Randomised trial of filgrastim-mobilised peripheral blood progenitor cell transplantation versus autologous bone-marrow transplantation in lymphoma patients. Lancet 1996; 347: 353–357.

255. Gisselbrecht C, Glass B, Mounier N et al. Salvage regimens with autologous transplantation for relapsed large B-cell lymphoma in the rituximab era. Journal of Clinical Oncology 2010; 28: 4184–4190.

256. Lanza F, Lemoli RM, Olivieri A et al. Factors affecting successful mobilization with plerixafor: an Italian prospective survey in 215 patients with multiple myeloma and lymphoma. Transfusion 2014; 54(2): 331–339.

257. Pettengell R, Schmitz N, Gisselbrecht C et al. Rituximab purging and/or maintenance in patients undergoing autologous transplantation for relapsed follicular lymphoma: a prospective randomized trial from the lymphoma working party of the European group for blood and marrow transplantation. Journal of Clinical Oncology 2013; 31: 1624–1630.

258. Majolino I, Pearce R, Taghipour G et al. Peripheral-blood stem-cell transplantation versus autologous bone marrow transplantation in Hodgkin's and non-Hodgkin's lymphomas: a new matched-pair analysis of the European Group for Blood and Marrow Transplantation Registry Data. Lymphoma Working Party of the European Group for Blood and Marrow Transplantation. Journal of Clinical Oncology 1997; 15: 509–517.

259. Passweg JR, Baldomero H, Bregni M et al. Hematopoietic SCT in Europe: data and trends in 2011. Bone Marrow Transplant 2013; 48(9): 1161–1167.

260. Wilder RB, Jones D, Tucker SL et al. Long-term results with radiotherapy for Stage I-II follicular lymphomas. International Journal of Radiation Oncology Biology Physics 2001; 51: 1219–1227.

261. Petersen PM, Gospodarowicz M, Tsang R et al. Long-term outcome in stage I and II follicular lymphoma following treatment with involved field radiation therapy alone. Journal of Clinical Oncology 2004; 22(14S): 563.

262. Guadagnolo BA, Li S, Neuberg D et al. Long-term outcome and mortality trends in early-stage, Grade 1-2 follicular lymphoma treated with radiation therapy. International Journal of Radiation Oncology Biology Physics 2006; 64: 928–934.

263. Charpentier A-M, Tsang R, Pintilie M et al. Managing Stage I-II Follicular Lymphoma with Upfront Definitive Radiation Therapy: the Forty Year Experience of the Princess Margaret Cancer Centre. Haematological Oncology 2013; 31: 166, abstr 062.

264. Lowry L, Smith P, Qian W et al. Reduced dose radiotherapy for local control in non-Hodgkin lymphoma: a randomised phase III trial. Radiotherapy and Oncology 2011; 100: 86–92.

265. Campbell BA, Voss N, Woods R et al. Long-term outcomes for patients with limited stage follicular lymphoma: involved regional radiotherapy versus involved node radiotherapy. Cancer 2010; 116: 3797–3806.

266. Haas RL, Poortmans P, de Jong D et al. High response rates and lasting remissions after low-dose involved field radiotherapy in indolent lymphomas. Journal of Clinical Oncology 2003; 21: 2474–2480.

267. Haas RL, Poortmans P, de Jong D et al. Effective palliation by low dose local radiotherapy for recurrent and/or chemotherapy refractory non-follicular lymphoma patients. European Journal of Cancer 2005; 41: 1724–1730.

268. Chan EK, Fung S, Gospodarowicz M et al. Palliation by low-dose local radiation therapy for indolent non-Hodgkin lymphoma. International Journal of Radiation Oncology Biology Physics 2011; 81: e781–e786.

269. Zucca E, Conconi A, Pedrinis E et al. Nongastric marginal zone B-cell lymphoma of mucosa-associated lymphoid tissue. Blood 2003; 101: 2489–2495.

270. Goda JS, Gospodarowicz M, Pintilie M et al. Long-term outcome in localized extranodal mucosa-associated lymphoid tissue lymphomas treated with radiotherapy. Cancer 2010; 116: 3815–3824.

271. Tsang RW, Gospodarowicz MK. Radiation therapy for localized low-grade non-Hodgkin's lymphomas. Hematology and Oncology 2005; 23: 10–17.

272. Miller, TP, Dahlberg, S, Cassady, JR, Adelstein, DJ, Spier, CM, et al. Chemotherapy alone compared with chemotherapy plus radiotherapy for localized intermediate- and high-grade non-Hodgkin's lymphoma. New England Journal of Medicine 1998; 339: 21–26.

273. Miller T, Leblanc M, Spier C et al. CHOP alone compared to CHOP plus radiotherapy for early stage aggressive non-Hodgkin's lymphomas: Update of the Southwest Oncology Group (SWOG) randomized trial. Blood 2001; 98.

274. Horning SJ, Weller E, Kim K et al. Chemotherapy with or without radiotherapy in limited-stage diffuse aggressive non-Hodgkin's lymphoma: Eastern Cooperative Oncology Group Study 1484. Journal of Clinical Oncology 2004; 22(15): 3032–3038.

275. Bonnet C, Fillet G, Mounier N et al. CHOP alone compared with CHOP plus radiotherapy for localized aggressive lymphoma in elderly patients: a study by the Groupe d'Etude des Lymphomes de l'Adulte. Journal of Clinical Oncology 2007; 25: 787–792.

276. Reyes F, Lepage E, Ganem G et al. ACVBP versus CHOP plus radiotherapy for localized aggressive lymphoma. New England Journal of Medicine 352: 1197–1205.

277. Held G, Murawski N, Ziepert M, Fleckenstein J, Pöschel V, et al. Role of radiotherapy to bulky disease in elderly patients with aggressive

B-cell lymphoma. Journal of Clinical Oncology 2014; 32(11): 1112–1118.

278. Held G, Zeynalova S, Murawski N et al. The impact of rituximab and radiotherapy on outcome of patients with aggressive B-cell lymphoma and skeletal involvement. Haematological Oncology 2013; 31: 129, abstr 098.

279. Shenkier TN, Voss N, Fairey R et al. Brief chemotherapy and involved-region irradiation for limited-stage diffuse large-cell lymphoma: an 18-year experience from the British Columbia Cancer Agency. Journal of Clinical Oncology 2002; 20: 197–204.

280. Ng AK. Diffuse large B-cell lymphoma. Seminars in Radiation Oncology 2007; 17: 169–175.

281. Wirth A. The rationale and role of radiation therapy in the treatment of patients with diffuse large B-cell lymphoma in the rituximab era. Leukemia Lymphoma 2007; 48: 2121–2136.

282. Martelli M, Ferreri AJ, Johnson P. Primary mediastinal large B-cell lymphoma. Critical Reviews Oncology/Hematology 2008; 68: 256–263.

283. Todeschini G, Secchi S, Morra E et al. Primary mediastinal large B-cell lymphoma (PMLBCL): long-term results from a retrospective multicentre Italian experience in 138 patients treated with CHOP or MACOP-B/VACOP-B. British Journal of Cancer 2004; 90: 372–376.

284. Xua L-M, Fanga H, Wanga W-H, Jina J, Wanga S-L. Prognostic significance of rituximab and radiotherapy for patients with primary mediastinal large B-cell lymphoma receiving doxorubicin-containing chemotherapy. Leukemia Lymphoma 2013; 54(8): 1684–1690.

285. Wang B, Lu JJ, Ma X et al. Combined chemotherapy and external beam radiation for stage IE and IIE natural killer T-cell lymphoma of nasal cavity. Leukemia Lymphoma 2007; 48: 396–402.

286. Guo Y, Lu JJ, Ma X et al. Combined chemoradiation for the management of nasal natural killer (NK)/T-cell lymphoma: elucidating the significance of systemic chemotherapy. Oral Oncology 2008; 44: 23–30.

287. Aviles A, Neri N, Fernandez R et al. Combined therapy in untreated patients improves outcome in Nasal NK/T lymphoma: results of a clinical trial. Medical Oncology 2013; 30: 637.

288. Kim WS, Song SY, Ahn YC et al. CHOP followed by involved field radiation: is it optimal for localized nasal natural killer/T-cell lymphoma? Annals of Oncology 2001; 12: 349–352.

289. Engert A, Plutschow A, Eich HT et al. Reduced treatment intensity in patients with early-stage Hodgkin's lymphoma. New England Journal of Medicine 2010; 363: 640–652.

290. von Tresckow B, Plutschow A, Fuchs M et al. Dose-intensification in early unfavorable Hodgkin's lymphoma: final analysis of the German Hodgkin Study Group HD14 trial. Journal of Clinical Oncology 2012; 30: 907–913.

291. Straus DJ. Chemotherapy alone for early-stage Hodgkin's lymphoma. New England Journal of Medicine 2012; 366: 470–471.

292. Yahalom J, Ryu J, Straus DJ et al. Impact of adjuvant radiation on the patterns and rate of relapse in advanced-stage Hodgkin's disease treated with alternating chemotherapy combinations. Journal of Clinical Oncology 1991; 9: 2193–2201.

293. Specht L, Yahalom J, Illidge T et al. Modern radiation therapy for Hodgkin lymphoma: field and dose guidelines from the International Lymphoma Radiation Oncology Group (ILROG). International Journal of Radiation Oncology Biology Physics 2015; 92(1): 11–31.

294. Eich HT, Kriz J, Schmidberger H et al. The German evidence-based guidelines for Hodgkin's lymphoma. Aspects for radiation oncologists. Strahlenther Onkologie 2013; 189: 445–457.

295. Hoskin PJ, Diez P, Williams M et al. Recommendations for the use of radiotherapy in nodal lymphoma. Clinical Oncology (Royal College of Radiologists) 2013; 25: 49–58.

296. DeLuca P, Jones D, Gahbauer R et al. Prescribing, recording, and reporting photon-beam intensity-modulated radiation therapy (IMRT). Journal of the ICRU 2010; 10: 1–106.

297. ICRU: (International Commission on Radiation Units and Measurements). Prescribing, recording, and reporting photon therapy. (Supplement to ICRU Report 50). ICRU Report 62, 1999.

298. Radford J, Illidge T, Counsell N, Hancock B, Pettengell R, et al. Results of a trial of PET-directed therapy for early-stage Hodgkin's lymphoma. The New England Journal of Medicine 2015; 372(17): 1598–1607. doi: 10.1056/NEJMoa1408648.

299. Radford J, Illidge T, Counsell N, Hancock B, Pettengell R, et al. Results of a trial of PET-directed therapy for early-stage Hodgkin's lymphoma. The New England Journal of Medicine 2015; 372(17): 1598–1607. doi: 10.1056/NEJMoa1408648.

300. Herbst C, Rehan FA, Brillant C et al. Combined modality treatment improves tumor control and overall survival in patients with early stage Hodgkin's lymphoma: a systematic review. Haematologica 2010; 95: 494–500.

301. Eich HT, Diehl V, Gorgen H et al. Intensified chemotherapy and dose-reduced involved-field radiotherapy in patients with early unfavorable Hodgkin's lymphoma: final analysis of the German Hodgkin Study Group HD11 trial. Journal of Clinical Oncology 2010; 28: 4199–4206.

302. Specht L, Gray RG, Clarke MJ et al. Influence of more extensive radiotherapy and adjuvant chemotherapy on long-term outcome of early-stage Hodgkin's disease: a meta-analysis of 23 randomized trials involving 3,888 patients. International Hodgkin's Disease Collaborative Group. Journal of Clinical Oncology 1998; 16: 830–843.

303. Noordijk EM, Carde P, Dupouy N et al. Combined-modality therapy for clinical stage I or II Hodgkin's lymphoma: long-term results of the European Organisation for Research and Treatment of Cancer H7 randomized controlled trials. Journal of Clinical Oncology 2006; 24: 3128–3135.

304. Ferme C, Eghbali H, Meerwaldt JH, et al. Chemotherapy plus involved-field radiation in early-stage Hodgkin's disease. New England Journal of Medicine 2007; 357: 1916–1927.

305. Herbst C, Rehan FA, Skoetz N, et al. Chemotherapy alone versus chemotherapy plus radiotherapy for early stage Hodgkin lymphoma. Cochrane Database Systematic Reviews: CD007110, 2011.

306. Hoskin PJ, Smith P, Maughan TS, et al. Long-term results of a randomised trial of involved field radiotherapy vs extended field radiotherapy in stage I and II Hodgkin lymphoma. Clinical Oncology (Royal College Radiologists) 2005; 17: 47–53.

307. Engert A, Schiller P, Josting A, et al. Involved-field radiotherapy is equally effective and less toxic compared with extended-field radiotherapy after four cycles of chemotherapy in patients with early-stage unfavorable Hodgkin's lymphoma: results of the HD8 trial of the German Hodgkin's Lymphoma Study Group. Journal of Clinical Oncology 2003; 21: 3601–3608.

308. Engert A, Haverkamp H, Kobe C, et al. Reduced-intensity chemotherapy and PET-guided radiotherapy in patients with advanced stage Hodgkin's lymphoma (HD15 trial): a randomised, open-label, phase 3 non-inferiority trial. Lancet 2012; 379: 1791–1799.

309. Meignan M, Gallamini A, Haioun C, et al. Report on the Second International Workshop on interim positron emission tomography in lymphoma held in Menton, France, 8–9 April 2010. Leukemia Lymphoma 2010; 51: 2171–2180.

310. Raemaekers JM, Andre MP, Federico M, et al. Omitting radiotherapy in early positron emission tomography-negative stage I/II Hodgkin lymphoma is associated with an increased risk of early relapse: Clinical results of the preplanned interim analysis of the randomized EORTC/LYSA/FIL H10 trial. Journal of Clinical Oncology 2014; 32: 1188–1194.

311. Borchmann P, Haverkamp H, Diehl V, et al. Eight cycles of escalated-dose BEACOPP compared with four cycles of escalated-dose BEACOPP followed by four cycles of baseline-dose BEACOPP with or without radiotherapy in patients with advanced-stage Hodgkin's lymphoma: final analysis of the HD12 trial of the German Hodgkin Study Group. Journal of Clinical Oncology 2011; 29: 4234–4242.

312. Aleman BM, Raemaekers JM, Tirelli U, et al. Involved-field radiotherapy for advanced Hodgkin's lymphoma. New England Journal of Medicine 2003; 348: 2396–2406.

313. Bartlett NL, Rosenberg SA, Hoppe RT, et al. Brief chemotherapy, Stanford V, and adjuvant radiotherapy for bulky or advanced-stage Hodgkin's disease: a preliminary report. Journal of Clinical Oncology 1995; 13: 1080–1088.

314. Brincker H, Bentzen SM. A re-analysis of available dose-response and time-dose data in Hodgkin's disease. Radiotherapy and Oncology 1994; 30: 227–230.

315. Vijayakumar S, Myrianthopoulos LC. An updated dose-response analysis in Hodgkin's disease. Radiotherapy and Oncology 1992; 24: 1–13.

316. Hutchings M, Barrington SF. PET/CT for therapy response assessment in lymphoma. Journal of Nuclear Medicine 2009; 50(Suppl 1): 21S–30S.

317. Duhmke E, Franklin J, Pfreundschuh M, et al. Low-dose radiation is sufficient for the noninvolved extended-field treatment in favorable early-stage Hodgkin's disease: long-term results of a randomized trial of radiotherapy alone. Journal of Clinical Oncology 2001; 19: 2905–2914.

318. Nogova L, Reineke T, Brillant C, et al. Lymphocyte-predominant and classical Hodgkin's lymphoma: a comprehensive analysis from the German Hodgkin Study Group. Journal of Clinical Oncology 2008; 26: 434–439.

319. Wirth A, Yuen K, Barton M, et al. Long-term outcome after radiotherapy alone for lymphocyte-predominant Hodgkin lymphoma: a retrospective multicenter study of the Australasian Radiation Oncology Lymphoma Group. Cancer 2005; 104: 1221–1229.

320. Savage KJ, Skinnider B, Al-Mansour M, et al. Treating limited-stage nodular lymphocyte predominant Hodgkin lymphoma similarly to classical Hodgkin lymphoma with ABVD may improve outcome. Blood 2011; 118: 4585–4590.

321. Canellos GP, Mauch P. What is the appropriate systemic chemotherapy for lymphocyte-predominant Hodgkin's lymphoma? Journal of Clinical Oncology 2010; 28: e8.

322. Campo E, Swerdlow SH, Harris NL et al. The 2008 WHO classification of lymphoid neoplasms and beyond: evolving concepts and practical applications. Blood 2011; 117: 5019–5032.

323. Vose J, Armitage J, Weisenburger D. International peripheral T-cell and natural killer/T-cell lymphoma study: pathology findings and clinical outcomes. Journal of Clinical Oncology 2008; 26: 4124–4130.

324. Rudiger T, Weisenburger DD, Anderson JR et al. Peripheral T-cell lymphoma (excluding anaplastic large-cell lymphoma): results from the Non-Hodgkin's Lymphoma Classification Project. Annals of Oncology 2002; 13: 140–149.

325. Belhadj K, Reyes F, Farcet JP et al. Hepatosplenic gammadelta T-cell lymphoma is a rare clinicopathologic entity with poor outcome: report on a series of 21 patients. Blood 2003; 102: 4261–4269.

326. Malamut G, Chandesris O, Verkarre V et al. Enteropathy associated T cell lymphoma in celiac disease: a large retrospective study. Digestive and Liver Disease 2013; 45: 377–384.

327. Hoque SR, Child FJ, Whittaker SJ et al. Subcutaneous panniculitis-like T-cell lymphoma: a clinicopathological, immunophenotypic and molecular analysis of six patients. British Journal of Dermatology 2003; 148: 516–525.

328. Toro JR, Liewehr DJ, Pabby N et al. Gamma-delta T-cell phenotype is associated with significantly decreased survival in cutaneous T-cell lymphoma. Blood 2003; 101: 3407–3412.

329. Mussolin L, Damm-Welk C, Pillon M et al. Use of minimal disseminated disease and immunity to NPM-ALK antigen to stratify ALK-positive ALCL patients with different prognosis. Leukemia 2013; 27: 416–422.

330. Kluin-Nelemans HC, Coenen JL, Boers JE, van Imhoff GW, Rosati S. EBV-positive immunodeficiency lymphoma after alemtuzumab-CHOP therapy for peripheral T-cell lymphoma. Blood 2008; 112: 1039–1041.

331. Suzuki R, Yamaguchi M, Izutsu K et al. Prospective measurement of Epstein-Barr virus-DNA in plasma and peripheral blood mononuclear cells of extranodal NK/T-cell lymphoma, nasal type. Blood 2011; 118: 6018–6022.

332. Gaulard P, de LL. Pathology of peripheral T-cell lymphomas: where do we stand? Seminars in Hematology 2014; 51: 5–16.

333. Casulo C, Schoder H, Feeney J et al. 18F-fluorodeoxyglucose positron emission tomography in the staging and prognosis of T cell lymphoma. Leukemia Lymphoma 2013; 54: 2163–2167.

334. Schmitz N, Trumper L, Ziepert M et al. Treatment and prognosis of mature T-cell and NK-cell lymphoma: an analysis of patients with T-cell lymphoma treated in studies of the German High-Grade Non-Hodgkin Lymphoma Study Group. Blood 2010; 116: 3418–3425.

335. Went P, Agostinelli C, Gallamini A et al. Marker expression in peripheral T-cell lymphoma: a proposed clinical-pathologic prognostic score. Journal of Clinical Oncology 2006; 24: 2472–2479.

336. Suzuki R. Pathogenesis and treatment of extranodal natural killer/T-cell lymphoma. Seminars in Hematology 2014; 51: 42–51.

337. Yamaguchi M. Current and future management of NK/T-cell lymphoma based on clinical trials. International Journal of Hematology 2012; 96: 562–571.

338. Lee J, Kim CY, Park YJ, Lee NK. Sequential chemotherapy followed by radiotherapy versus concurrent chemoradiotherapy in patients with stage I/II extranodal natural killer/T-cell lymphoma, nasal type. Blood Research 2013; 48: 274–281.

339. Jaccard A, Gachard N, Marin B et al. Efficacy of L-asparaginase with methotrexate and dexamethasone (AspaMetDex regimen) in patients with refractory or relapsing extranodal NK/T-cell lymphoma, a phase 2 study. Blood 2011; 117: 1834–1839.

340. Le Deley MC, Rosolen A, Williams DM et al. Vinblastine in children and adolescents with high-risk anaplastic large-cell lymphoma: results of the randomized ALCL99-vinblastine trial. Journal of Clinical Oncology 2010; 28: 3987–3993.

341. Sibon D, Fournier M, Briere J et al. Long-term outcome of adults with systemic anaplastic large-cell lymphoma treated within the Groupe d'Etude des Lymphomes de l'Adulte trials. Journal of Clinical Oncology 2012; 30: 3939–3946.

342. D'Amore F, Relander T, Lauritzsen GF et al. Up-front autologous stem-cell transplantation in peripheral T-cell lymphoma: NLG-T-01. Journal of Clinical Oncology 2012; 30: 3093–3099.

343. Pro B, Advani R, Brice P et al. Brentuximab vedotin (SGN-35) in patients with relapsed or refractory systemic anaplastic large-cell lymphoma: results of a phase II study. Journal of Clinical Oncology 2012; 30: 2190–2196.

344. Savage KJ, Chhanabhai M, Gascoyne RD, Connors JM. Characterization of peripheral T-cell lymphomas in a single North American institution by the WHO classification. Annals of Oncology 2004; 15: 1467–1475.

345. Rodriguez J, Conde E, Gutierrez A et al. Prolonged survival of patients with angioimmunoblastic T-cell lymphoma after high-dose chemotherapy and autologous stem cell transplantation: the GELTAMO experience. European Journal of Haematology 2007; 78: 290–296.

346. Reimer P, Schertlin T, Rudiger T et al. Myeloablative radiochemotherapy followed by autologous peripheral blood stem cell transplantation as first-line therapy in peripheral T-cell lymphomas: first results of a prospective multicenter study. Journal of Hematology 2004; 5: 304–311.

347. Wulf GG, Hasenkamp J, Jung W et al. Reduced intensity conditioning and allogeneic stem cell transplantation after salvage therapy integrating alemtuzumab for patients with relapsed peripheral T-cell non-Hodgkin's lymphoma. Bone Marrow Transplantation 2005; 36: 271–273.

348. Kim MK, Kim S, Lee SS et al. High-dose chemotherapy and autologous stem cell transplantation for peripheral T-cell lymphoma: complete response at transplant predicts survival. Annals of Hematology 2007; 86: 435–442.

349. Arkenau HT, Chong G, Cunningham D et al. Gemcitabine, cisplatin and methylprednisolone for the treatment of patients with peripheral T-cell lymphoma: the Royal Marsden Hospital experience. Haematologica 2007; 92: 271–272.

350. O'Connor OA, Pro B, Pinter-Brown L et al. Pralatrexate in patients with relapsed or refractory peripheral T-cell lymphoma: results from the pivotal PROPEL study. Journal of Clinical Oncology 2011; 29: 1182–1189.

351. Damaj G, Gressin R, Bouabdallah K et al. Results from a prospective, open-label, phase II trial of bendamustine in refractory or relapsed T-cell lymphomas: the BENTLY trial. Journal of Clinical Oncology 2013; 31: 104–110.

352. Morschhauser F, Fitoussi O, Haioun C et al. A phase 2, multicentre, single-arm, open-label study to evaluate the safety and efficacy of single-agent lenalidomide (Revlimid) in subjects with relapsed or refractory peripheral T-cell non-Hodgkin lymphoma: the EXPECT trial. European Journal of Cancer 2013; 49: 2869–2876.

353. Mak V, Hamm J, Chhanabhai M et al. Survival of patients with peripheral T-cell lymphoma after first relapse or progression: spectrum of disease and rare long-term survivors. Journal of Clinical Oncology 2013; 31: 1970–1976.

354. Corradini P, Dodero A, Zallio F et al. Graft-versus-lymphoma effect in relapsed peripheral T-cell non-Hodgkin's lymphomas after reduced-intensity conditioning followed by allogeneic transplantation of hematopoietic cells. Journal of Clinical Oncology 2004; 22: 2172–2176.

355. Le GS, Milpied N, Buzyn A et al. Graft-versus-lymphoma effect for aggressive T-cell lymphomas in adults: a study by the Societe Francaise de Greffe de Moelle et de Therapie Cellulaire. Journal of Clinical Oncology 2008; 26: 2264–2271.

356. Jacobsen ED, Kim HT, Ho VT et al. A large single-center experience with allogeneic stem-cell transplantation for peripheral T-cell non-Hodgkin lymphoma and advanced mycosis fungoides/Sezary syndrome. Annals of Oncology 2011; 22: 1608–1613.

357. Dodero A, Spina F, Narni F et al. Allogeneic transplantation following a reduced-intensity conditioning regimen in relapsed/refractory peripheral T-cell lymphomas: long-term remissions and response to donor lymphocyte infusions support the role of a graft-versus-lymphoma effect. Leukemia 2012; 26: 520–526.

CHAPTER 55

Sarcomas of soft tissues and bone

Alessandro Gronchi, Angelo P. Dei Tos, and Paolo G. Casali

Introduction to soft tissue sarcomas

Soft tissue sarcomas (STSs) represent a heterogeneous group of rare mesenchymal malignancies, with an annual incidence of approximately 5/100 000 [1]. Bone sarcomas are even rarer, with an incidence of around 0.3/100 000/year [1].

The median age of incidence of soft tissue sarcomas (STSs) is about 60 years, but varies according to histology (e.g., rhabdomyosarcoma and Ewing sarcoma occur in children and young adults, whereas pleomorphic sarcomas affect adults and the elderly). The main sites of occurrence also depend on histology, but generally the most frequently affected sites are the lower limbs, followed by upper limbs, trunk, and head and neck region. Some sites are related to specific histologies, such as the retroperitoneum for well-differentiated/dedifferentiated liposarcoma and leiomyosarcoma. Visceral primary locations are quite rare, with the exception of uterine leiomyosarcomas, with an incidence of 0.5/100,000/year, but STSs are possible in any visceral site [2, 3].

The age incidence of bone sarcomas is bimodal, with osteosarcoma and Ewing sarcoma prevailing in the second decade and chondrosarcoma in the sixth. The most frequent site of occurrence is the lower limbs, followed by the pelvis.

Surgery is the mainstay of local treatment of all sarcomas. Adjuvant radiation therapy (RT) is often used in high-grade STSs and Ewing sarcoma, while adjuvant/neoadjuvant chemotherapy can be offered in selected STSs and is part of the standard treatment of osteosarcoma and Ewing sarcoma. Of course, histology, not age, determines clinical decisions, so that osteosarcoma, Ewing sarcoma, or rhabdomyosarcoma in an adult are treated in the same way as in children. The role of medical therapy is limited in chondrosarcoma, while molecularly-targeted therapies are expected to find a role in chordoma.

Sarcomas show some peculiarities in their natural history, which have therapeutic implications. A considerable number of sarcomas typically metastasize to the lungs before spreading to other organs, and typically they lack lymph node regional extension, although exceptions exist with regard to selected histological types. Thus, surgery of isolated lung metastases is performed, especially when prognostic factors are favourable, that is, when the number of lesions is limited and the disease-free interval is reasonably long. If and how to combine surgery of isolated lung metastases with chemotherapy is uncertain, although unfavourable prognostic factors encourage the inclusion of medical therapy in the treatment program. Likewise, in most histologies, lymph nodes are generally not routinely a target of surgical exploration, unless they are clinically involved.

Staging and diagnosis

To better define the extent of extremity and truncal STSs, including depth of invasion and relationship with neurovascular structures, a contrast-enhanced MRI of the affected site is the preferred imaging study. To establish the diagnosis, a percutaneous core needle biopsy is the preferred method. Fine needle aspiration biopsy can be an alternative only in centres with a specific expertise in cytological diagnosis of sarcoma. If percutaneous core needle biopsy fails, an open biopsy is indicated. Histological diagnosis should always be obtained before making any treatment decision. Further staging studies for patients with extremity STS should include abdominal and chest contrast-enhanced CT. A bone scan is not routinely recommended if the chest and the abdomen are clear, unless clinical signs of bone involvement are apparent. Patients with abdominal visceral, pelvic, and retroperitoneal sarcomas should undergo contrast-enhanced CT imaging of the abdomen, pelvis, and chest. Patients with breast STS should undergo contrast-enhanced MRI imaging to define depth of extension; mammography is not routinely useful. Positron emission tomography (PET) is rarely indicated in routine sarcoma care. PET scans should only be ordered selectively, when attempting to resolve an ambiguous finding on other imaging or gauging treatment responses under specific circumstances.

In bone sarcomas, a plain radiograph of the affected site is the primary study. Subsequent imaging should include contrast-enhanced CT to study bone involvement and MRI to study soft tissue extension. To establish the diagnosis, a percutaneous trocar biopsy is the preferred method. If percutaneous trocar biopsy fails, an open biopsy is indicated. Histological diagnosis should always be obtained before making any treatment decision. Further staging studies include contrast-enhanced abdominal and chest CT, bone scan and/or PET scan to identify possible skip lesions in the affected bone. In Ewing sarcoma (also named primitive Peripheral Neuro-Ectodermic Tumor [pPNET]) a bone marrow aspiration biopsy is part of the staging workup, although some concerns about its value have been recently raised.

Pathology

Sarcomas are pathologically classified on the basis of a combination of clinical, morphologic, and genetic features. The radiological appearance may be relevant for the pathologic diagnosis of bone sarcomas. In general, bone and STSs are regarded as major diagnostic challenges. This is certainly due their rarity, but also to their inherent morphologic features. For example, some of the common diagnostic criteria of malignancy used in common cancers (i.e., increased mitotic activity, cytologic atypia, and hypercellularity) do not always apply to sarcomas, requiring highly specific diagnostic expertise.

An accurate recognition of the many histologic subtypes currently represents a major requirement for proper therapeutic planning. In the past, diagnostic accuracy was less crucial when treatment options were limited. By contrast, recent therapeutic advances have made proper sarcoma classification mandatory, especially in regard to proper subtyping. This makes case referral to specialized centres strongly advised with regard to pathologic diagnosis.

During the last decade, the classification of soft tissue and bone sarcomas has significantly evolved. A major step forward was the publication of the 2002 WHO classification of bone and soft tissue tumours [2], which for the first time established a strong integration between morphology and genetics. The main conceptual advances can be summarized as follows:

1. Integration of morphologic, immunophenotypic, and genetic findings, whereas classification was previously based on pure morphology.

2. Clear definition of the category of borderline (intermediate grade) mesenchymal neoplasms:

   a. Identification of locally aggressive, non-metastasizing tumours (i.e., desmoid fibromatosis).

   b. Identification of neoplasms which rarely metastasize (<2% of cases) (i.e., plexiform fibrohistiocytic tumour).

3. Definition of atypical lipomatous tumour as a synonym (based on morphology and genetics) for well-differentiated liposarcoma (WDLPS) occurring at surgically amenable anatomic sites. This important terminological shift acknowledged the fact that WDPLSs never metastasize and, when superficially located, are cured by complete surgery.

4. Reappraisal of obsolete diagnostic labels such as malignant fibrous histiocytoma (MFH), haemangiopericytoma (HPC), and fibrosarcoma.

5. Recognition of newly-described tumour entities.

The 2002 WHO classification was updated very recently and the current classification scheme for bone and STSs is reported in Boxes 55.1 and 55.2 [3]. Labels such as MFH and HPC do not exist anymore. The main practical advantage of the current classification is to identify morphologically/genetically/clinically homogenous subgroups, setting the stage for the development of more effective therapeutic strategies. The use of the WHO classification is strongly endorsed by several clinical practice guidelines to promote the adoption of a homogeneous nomenclature [4]

Morphologic characterization of sarcomas

As highlighted by Box 55.1 and 55.2, the classification of sarcomas is pragmatically conceived according to histogenetic criteria, that is, it refers to the morphologic similarity to a hypothetic normal tissue of 'origin'. This approach is practical, but does not reflect biologic reality. Any tumour, in fact, does not originate from normal tissue, but most likely from immature mesenchymal progenitor cells, which can undergo variable differentiation steps and thus generate distinct morphologies [5].

Box 55.1 Updated WHO classification of malignant and intermediate malignancy soft tissue neoplasms

Adipocytic tumours

- Atypical lipomatous tumours/well-differentiated liposarcoma (lipoma-like, sclerosing, and inflammatory variants)
- Spindle cell liposarcoma
- Myxoid/round cell liposarcoma
- Pleomorphic liposarcoma

Fibroblastic/myofibroblastic tumours

- Desmoid fibromatosis
- Dermatofibrosarcoma protuberans (DFSP)
- Fibrosarcomatous DFSP
- Atypical fibroxanthoma
- Solitary fibrous tumour
- Inflammatory myofibroblastic tumour
- Low-grade myofibroblastic sarcoma
- Infantile fibrosarcoma
- Myxofibrosarcoma
- Myxoinflammatory fibroblastic sarcoma
- Low-grade fibromyxoid sarcoma
- Sclerosing epithelioid fibrosarcoma

So-called fibrohistiocytic tumours

- Plexiform fibrohistiocytic tumour
- Giant cell tumour of soft tissue

Smooth muscle tumours

- Leiomyosarcoma

Pericytic (perivascular) tumours muscle tumours

- Malignant glomus tumour

Skeletal muscle tumours

- Embryonal rhabdomyosarcoma
- Alveolar rhabdomyosarcoma
- Pleomorphic rhabdomyosarcoma
- Spindle cell/sclerosing rhabdomyosarcoma

Vascular tumours

- Kaposiform haemangioendothelioma
- Retiform haemangioendothelioma
- Papillary intralymphatic angioendothelioma
- Composite haemangioendothelioma
- Kaposi sarcoma
- Pseudomyogenic 'epithelioid sarcoma-like' haemangioendothelioma

- Epithelioid haemangioendothelioma
- Angiosarcoma of soft tissue

Chondro-osseous tumours

- Extraskeletal osteosarcoma

Gastrointestinal stromal tumour

Nerve sheath tumours

- Malignant peripheral nerve sheath tumours
- Malignant granular cell tumour

Tumours of uncertain differentiation

- Angiomatous fibrous histiocytoma
- Hyalinizing angiectatic tumour of soft parts
- Ossifying fibromyxoid tumour
- Myoepithelioma
- Phosphaturic mesenchymal tumour
- Synovial sarcoma
- Epithelioid sarcoma
- Alveolar soft part sarcoma
- Clear cell sarcoma
- Extraskeletal myxoid chondrosarcoma
- Mesenchymal chondrosarcoma
- Desmoplastic small round cell tumour
- Extrarenal rhabdoid tumour
- PEComa
- Intimal sarcoma
- Undifferentiated sarcomas (pleomorphic, epithelioid, spindle cell, and round cell)

Reproduced with permission from Fletcher C et al., *WHO Classification of Tumours of Soft Tissue and Bone, Fourth Edition*, World Health Organization, Geneva, Switzerland, Copyright © 2013 World Health Organization.

Box 55.2 Updated WHO classification of malignant and intermediate malignancy bone neoplasms.

Cartilage tumours

- Chondrosarcoma
- Dedifferentiated chondrosarcoma
- Mesenchymal chondrosarcoma
- Clear cell chondrosarcoma

Osteogenic tumours

- Low-grade central osteosarcoma
- Conventional osteosarcoma
- Teleangiectatic osteosarcoma
- Small cell osteosarcoma
- Paraosteal osteosarcoma
- Periosteal osteosarcoma
- High-grade surface osteosarcoma

Fibrogenic tumours

- Desmoplastic fibroma of bone
- Undifferentiated high-grade pleomorphic sarcoma

Ewing sarcoma

Notochordal tumours

- Chordoma

Vascular tumours

- Epithelioid haemangioendothelioma
- Angiosarcoma

Smooth muscle tumours

- Leiomyosarcoma

Adipocytic tumours

- Liposarcoma

Epithelial tumours

- Adamantinoma

Reproduced with permission from Fletcher C et al., WHO *Classification of Tumours of Soft Tissue and Bone, Fourth Edition*, World Health Organization, Geneva, Switzerland, Copyright © 2013 World Health Organization.

The diagnostic process toward a correct diagnosis of a sarcoma can be summarized as follows:

1. Recognition of the key morphologic features (i.e., cell shape, pattern of growth, and background).

2. Integration of a panel of immunophenotypic markers.

3. Integration of genetic features when deemed necessary.

Of course, the precise knowledge of the clinical picture (age, sex, anatomic site, clinical presentation, imaging) is mandatory, underlining the crucial importance of a multidisciplinary management of sarcomas, even in the diagnostic workup. Radiological imaging plays a role in the diagnosis of bone sarcomas, wherein it can undoubtedly guide the evaluation of surgical biopsies.

Morphologic evaluation of soft tissue tumours takes into consideration the following microscopic features:

1. cell shape: spindled, rounded, epithelioid, or pleomorphic (Figure 55.1).

2. pattern of growth: fascicular, storiform, alveolar, or solid (Figure 55.2).

3. background: fibrillary, myxoid, or desmoplastic.

4. vascularization.

The combination of these morphologic features allows the identification of a restricted number of diagnostic options. A conclusive assignment to a specific diagnostic label is then generally achieved by the integration of immunophenotypic data and, when necessary, molecular assessments. It should be always

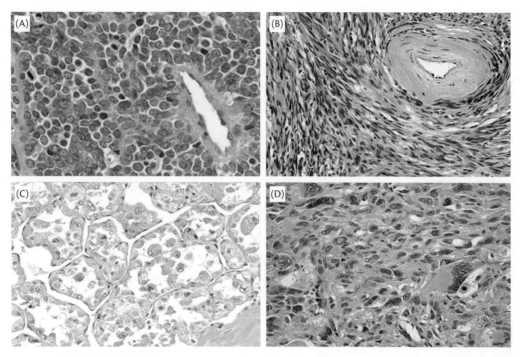

Fig. 55.1 Cell shape represents an important clue to sarcoma classification. (A) Round cell morphology, (B) spindle cell morphology, (C) epithelioid cell morphology, (D) pleomorphic cell morphology.

emphasized that sarcoma diagnosis is extremely complex and that, even in expert hands, approximately 10% of lesions cannot be classified by using current classification criteria. Instead of arbitrarily forcing the inclusion of these cases into a specific label, it is preferable to adopt a descriptive approach highlighting the morphologic characteristics that may help predict their clinical behaviour.

As already noted, the diagnostic approach to bone sarcomas includes a broad use of both clinical findings and radiological imaging. Morphologically, the identification of malignant cartilaginous and osteoid matrix is an important clue to the diagnosis of chondrosarcoma and osteosarcoma, respectively. Among primary bone tumours, immunohistochemistry (IHC) plays its greatest role in the differential diagnosis of Ewing sarcoma and chordoma,

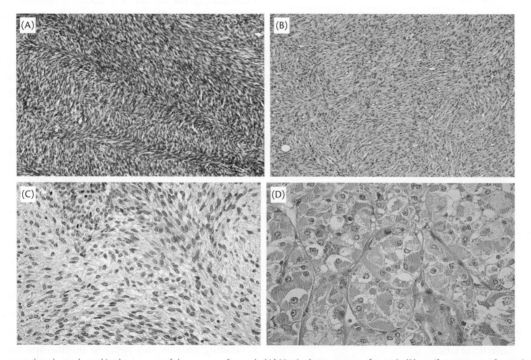

Fig. 55.2 Cell shape needs to be evaluated in the context of the pattern of growth. (A) Herringbone pattern of growth, (B) storiform pattern of growth, (C) fascicular pattern of growth, (D) alveolar pattern of growth.

whereas molecular genetics is a key tool in the differential diagnosis of Ewing sarcoma.

Immunophenotypic characterization of sarcomas

Immunohistochemistry is extremely useful in allowing an accurate classification of sarcomas [3]. As already mentioned, IHC appears to be more useful in the diagnosis of soft tissue than bone sarcomas, wherein the number of differentiation markers is much fewer. Table 55.1 summarizes the most commonly used

Table 55.1 Selected immunophenotypic markers utilized in bone and soft sarcoma diagnosis

Antibody	Histotype	Specificity
ALK	Inflammatory myofibroblastic tumour	++--
Beta-catenin	Desmoid fibromatosis	++++
CD31	Vascular tumours	+++-
	Histiocytes	
CD34	DFSP	-----
	Solitary fibrous tumour	
	Vascular tumours	
CD99	Ewing sarcoma	+++-
	Synovial sarcoma	
CD117 (KIT)	Gastrointestinal stromal tumour	++--
	Melanocytic tumours	
	Seminoma	
	Mast cell diseases	
Cytokeratin AE1/AE3	Synovial sarcoma	+----
	Epithelioid sarcoma	
	Desmoplastic small round cell tumour	
	Myoepithelioma	
h-Caldesmon	Leiomyosarcoma	+++-
Desmin	Rhabdomyosarcoma	++--
	Leiomyosarcoma	
	Desmoplastic small round cell tumour	
	Ossifying fibromyxoid tumour	
DOG1	Gastrointestinal stromal tumour	++++
EMA	Synovial sarcoma	+----
	Myoepithelial tumours	
ERG	Vascular tumours	++++
FVIII-RA	Vascular tumours	++++
FLI-1	Ewing sarcoma	++--
	Vascular tumours	
GFAP	Glial tumours	++--
	Neural tumours	
	Myoepithelial tumours	
HHSV8	Kaposi sarcoma	++++
HMB45	PEComa	
	Clear cell sarcoma	
	Melanocytic tumours	

(continued)

Table 55.1 Continued

Antibody	Histotype	Specificity
INI1 (loss of expression)	Epithelioid sarcoma	+++-
	Myoepithelioma	
MDM2	Well-differentiated/dedifferentiated liposarcoma	+++-
	Low-grade central osteosarcoma	
Myogenin	Rhabdomyosarcoma	++++
MUC4	Low-grade fibromyxoid sarcoma	++++
Smooth muscle actin	Leiomyosarcoma	++--
	Myofibroblastic tumours	
S100 protein	Neural tumours	-----
	Myoepithelial tumours	
	Melanocytic tumours	
	Clear cell sarcoma	
	Synovial sarcoma	
SOX9	Chondrogenic tumours	+++-
TFE3	Alveolar soft part sarcoma	
	PEComa	
TLE1	Synovial sarcoma	+++-
WT1 (n-terminal)	Desmoplastic small round cell tumour	+++-

immunohistochemical markers as well as their potential diagnostic value. It should be stressed that, with extremely rare exceptions, no immunophenotypic marker possesses absolute specificity. The immediate consequence is that the evaluation of any panel of immunoreagents should be conducted rigorously and integrated with morphology. The use of single markers should be avoided.

Histologic grading of sarcomas

The histological type does not represent the unique feature on which therapeutic decision-making is based. Analogous to other fields of oncologic pathology, several morphologic grading systems have been developed to predict prognosis. It is a broadly shared opinion that the grading system generated by the Federation Nationale des Centres de Lutte Contre le Cancer (FNCLCC) in France represents a suitable option. This grading system is based on the integration of three microscopic parameters [6–8] (Box 55.3):

1. Differentiation.

2. Mitotic index, expressed as the number of mitoses in ten high power fields (HPF).

3. Necrosis.

To avoid misunderstandings, a few important caveats should be underscored.

1. Grading systems only complement, and do not replace, histologic diagnosis. In fact, grading is performed once the histologic label is properly assigned.

2. Grading systems only apply to surgical specimens. As the use of core biopsies is rapidly expanding, one should integrate

Box 55.3 Grading system for sarcoma developed by FNCLCC

Differentiation

Score 1: Sarcomas exhibiting morphology clearly related to a normal adult mesenchymal tissue (i.e., well-differentiated liposarcoma)

Score 2: Sarcomas of certain histotype (i.e., myxoid liposarcoma)

Score 3: Undifferentiated or embryonal sarcomas, sarcoma with uncertain differentiation

Mitotic index

Score 1: 0–9 mitoses/10HPF*

Score 2: 10–19 mitoses/10HPF

Score 3: > 19 mitoses/10HPF

*HPF (high power field) = 0.1734 mm^2

Amount of necrosis

Score 0: no necrosis

Score 1: tumour necrosis <50%

Score 2: tumour necrosis >50%

Grade

Grade 1: score from 1 to 3

Grade 2: score from 4 to 5

Grade 3 score from 6 to 8

Reproduced from Trojani M et al., Soft tissue sarcomas of adults; study of pathological prognostic variables and definitely of histopathological grading system, *International Journal of Cancer*, Volume 33, Issue 1, pp. 37–421, Copyright © 1984 Wiley-Liss Inc., a Wiley Company, with permission from John Wiley and Sons Ltd.

morphology with radiological imaging. Obviously, clinicians need to be aware of the limitation of this approach.

3. Histologic grading does not apply to all histological types, since some of them are related to a selective biologic potential, whatever the grading morphological assignment.

Grading systems are far from being prognostically optimal. In particular, they often fail to discriminate prognosis within the Grade 2 ('intermediate') category. It is possible that in the future a molecularly-based approach such as The Complexity Index in Sarcoma (CINSARC, see below) may replace microscopic grading systems, provided that current technical limitations are standardized [9].

Molecular characterization of sarcomas

Sarcomas, like tumours of the haemato-lymphoid organs, are frequently associated with relatively specific genetic alterations, such as chromosome translocations, amplification of proto-oncogenes, and loss of tumour suppressor genes. A significant number of sarcomas—in particular, pleomorphic sarcomas and leiomyosarcoma—actually exhibit more complex genetic aberrations that still need to be further elucidated. Table 55.2

Table 55.2 Chromosome translocation occurring in mesenchymal tumours of bone and soft tissue

Tumour	Genetic mutation	Gene involved
Alveolar rhabdomyosarcoma	t(2;13)(q35;q14)	PAX3-FOXO1A
	t(1;13)(p36;q14)	PAX7-FOXO1A
Alveolar soft part sarcoma	t(X;17)(p11.2;q25)	ASPL-TFE3
Angiomatoid fibrous histiocytoma	t(12;22)(q13;q12)	ATF1-EWSR1
	t(2;22)(q34;q12)	CREB1-EWSR1
Aneurysmal bone cyst	t16;17)(q22;p13)	CDH11-USP6
Atypical lipomatous tumour/ dedifferentiated liposarcoma	Amplification	MDM2
Central/periosteal osteosarcoma	Point mutation	IDH1/IDH2
Clear cell sarcoma	t(12;22)(q13;q12)	ATF1-EWSR1
	t(2;22)(q34;q12)	CREB1-EWSR1
Dermatofibrosarcoma protuberans	t(17;22)(q22;q13)	COL1A1-PDGFB
Desmoid type fibromatosis	Activating mutation	BCTN1
Desmoplastic round cell tumour	t(11;22)(p13;q12)	WT1-EWSR1
Endometrial stromal sarcoma	t(7;17)(p15;q21)	JAZF1-JJAZ1
	t(6;7)(p21;p15)	PHF1-JAZF1
	t(6;10)(p21;p11)	PHF1-EPC1
Ewing sarcoma/PNET	t(11;22)(q24;q12)	EWSR1-FLI1
	t(21;22)(q22;q12)	EWSR1-ERG
	t(7;22)(p22;q12)	EWSR-ETV1
	t(17;22)(q12;q12)	EWSR1-EIAF
	t(16;21)(q13;q22)	FUS-ERG
	t(2;22)(q33;q12)	EWSR1-FEV
	t(20;22)(q13;q12)	EWSR1-NFATC2
	t(6;22)(p21;q12)	EWSR1-POU5F1
	t(4;19)(q35;q13)	CIC-DUX4
Extraskeletal myxoid chondrosarcoma	t(9;22)(q22;q12)	EWSR1–NR4A3
	t(9;15)(q22;q21)	TCF12–NR4A3
		TFG–NR4A3
Fibrous dysplasia/ intramuscular myxoma	Activating mutation	GNAS1
Infantile fibrosarcoma	t(12; 15)(p13;q25)	ETV6-NTRK3
Inflammatory myofibroblastic tumour	t(2;19)(p23;p13.1)	ALK-TPM4
	t(1;2)(q22-23;p23)	TPM3-ALK
Low-grade fibromyxoid sarcoma	t(7;16)(q33;p11)	FUS-BBF2H7
	t(11;16)(p11;p11)	CREB3L1-FUS
Myxoid-round cell liposarcoma	t(12;16)(q13;p11)	FUS-DDIT3
	t(12;22)(q13;q12)	EWSR1-DDIT3
Neuroblastoma	Amplification	N-MYC

(continued)

Table 55.2 Continued

Tumour	Genetic mutation	Gene involved
Pericytoma with t(7;12)	t(7;12)(p22;q13)	*ACTB-GLI*
Pigmented villonodular synovitis	t(1;2)(p13;q37)	*COL6A-CSF1*
Soft tissue and bone myoepithelioma	t(1;22)(q23;q12)	*EWSR1-PBX1*
	t(19;22)(q13;q12)	*EWSR1-ZNF444*
Synovial sarcoma	t(X;18)(p11;q11)	*SS18-SSX1*
		SS18-SSX2
		SS18-SSX4

Table 55.3 Genetic abnormalities shared by different tumour types

ETV6-NTRK3 / t(12;15)	Infantile fibrosarcoma
	Acute myeloid leukaemia
	Secretory carcinoma of the breast
ALK gene fusions	Inflammatory myofibroblastic tumour
	Large cell anaplastic lymphoma
	Lung carcinoma
FUS-ERG / t(16;21)	Ewing sarcoma
	Acute myeloid leukaemia
ASPL-TFE3 / t(X;17)	Alveolar soft part sarcoma
	Subset of paediatric renal cell carcinoma
EWS-ATF1/t(12;22) and EWS-CREB1/ t(2;22)	Clear cell sarcoma
	Angiomatoid fibrous histiocytoma

summarizes the most common genetic aberrations observed in soft tissue and bone sarcomas. This represents an incomplete list, as new aberrations are continuously reported as a consequence of broader applications of genetic analysis [10]. It is also possible that in the future some histological types will be defined on the basis of their molecular characteristics rather than on morphology, as anticipated in small subsets of undifferentiated round cell sarcomas of bone [11].

Chromosome translocations not only shed light on the mechanism of sarcomagenesis, but also represent a powerful diagnostic tool (Figure 55.3). As with IHC, molecular genetic findings need to be interpreted in the context of morphology. In fact, contrary to general belief, they lack absolute specificity (Table 55.3). An example is the rearrangement of the ALK gene that can occur in subsets of non-Hodgkin lymphoma, lung cancer, and inflammatory myofibroblastic tumour [12].

The most common diagnostic applications of genetic testing in sarcoma are the following:

1. Challenging differential diagnoses (i.e., poorly differentiated round cell synovial sarcoma vs Ewing sarcoma; dedifferentiated liposarcoma vs retroperitoneal leiomyosarcoma).

2. Atypical anatomical sites (i.e., visceral locations).

3. Discrepancies between morphological and immunophenotypic findings.

Chromosome translocations do not represent the only diagnostically relevant genetic alterations. Detection of MDM2 amplification (or over-expression of the protein thereof) represents a key tool in

the recognition of well-differentiated as well as of dedifferentiated liposarcoma [13, 14]. An important example of diagnostic application of molecular genetics is the detection of mutations of the β-catenin gene in desmoid fibromatosis [15].

During the last decade, several attempts have been made to determine the prognostic value of molecular genetic findings. Most analyses have focused on Ewing sarcoma, alveolar rhabdomyosarcoma, and synovial sarcoma. Results have been conflicting; as of today no meaningful molecular prognostic stratification can be foreseen [16–20]. A notable exception is the recently published molecular signature called CINSARC (The Complexity Index in Sarcoma) that may allow better separation of intermediate-grade sarcomas [9]. Nonetheless, this attempt is based on the use of a relatively complex technique (CGH-array) and requires availability of fresh material. Both factors may unfortunately hamper the application of CINSARC on a large-scale basis.

The indisputable efficacy of KIT/PDGFRA inhibition in GIST has certainly boosted interest in targeted therapy in solid cancers, including rare ones. There exists a need for biomarkers capable of predicting response to novel treatments and identifying a preclinical rationale for their potential use. The opportunity to target ALK in inflammatory myofibroblastic tumour, PDGFβ in DFSP, mTOR in malignant PEComas and lymphangioleiomyomatosis, MDM2 in dedifferentiated liposarcoma, and KDR in angiosarcoma, are all examples of potential clinical applications [21–25] New molecular techniques such as next-generation sequencing associated with functional genomics approaches will clarify which of the many detected genetic aberrations actually represent true drivers of oncogenesis [26].

The challenge of achieving diagnostic accuracy in sarcomas

Diagnostic accuracy, both in morphology and molecular biology, is a key factor for optimal therapeutic planning. However, as sarcomas are rare diseases, it is a challenging goal [27]. As mentioned, inherent diagnostic difficulties and the low number of cases entail the risk of erroneous disease recognition. For these reasons, pathologic second opinions at reference centres or within health networks are strongly advised. In addition, as molecular testing is increasingly utilized in the diagnostic workup of sarcomas, and the quality of molecular diagnostics also tends to be extremely variable

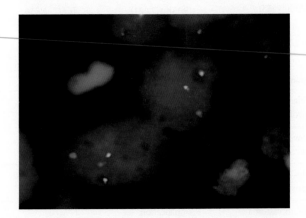

Fig. 55.3 EWSR1 rearrangement detected by fluorescence in situ hybridization (FISH).

and dependent on local expertise, it seems important that ad hoc external quality assurance programs are implemented [28].

Surgical management of soft tissue and bone sarcomas

Basic principles

Sarcomas usually present as solid masses. The periphery of the lesion is the most vital part of the mass. It is generally surrounded by a pseudocapsule of variable thickness consisting of compressed tumour cells embedded in a fibrovascular tissue, rarely associated with an inflammatory component, and in continuity with the surrounding normal tissues. This is the reason why a simple excision, i.e., enucleation, cannot be curative, even if most sarcomas do not seem to infiltrate surrounding structures.

Indeed, sarcomas respect anatomical borders. Thus, the local anatomy influences tumour growth by setting natural barriers to their extension. In general, sarcomas take the path allowed by least resistance anatomical planes and initially grow within the anatomical compartment in which they arose. Only at a later stage are the walls of that compartment violated (i.e., the cortex of a bone or the aponeurosis of a muscle) and the tumour breaks into another compartment. Most bone sarcomas are bicompartmental at the time of presentation: they destroy the overlying cortex and extend directly into the adjacent soft tissues. STSs may arise between compartments (thus being extracompartmental) or in anatomical sites that are not walled off by anatomical barriers, such as the intermuscular or subcutaneous planes. In the latter case, they remain extracompartmental and only at a later stage break into the adjacent compartment.

There are four basic types of excisions [29], depending on the relationship of the dissection plane to the surface of the tumour. An 'intralesional' excision is performed within the tumour mass and results in removal of only a portion, so that macroscopic tumour is left behind. In a 'marginal' excision, the dissection plane crosses the pseudocapsule of the tumour. Such an excision may leave microscopic disease, and microscopic margins may be either positive or negative, depending on the type of tumour and surrounding tissues. 'Wide' excision entails removing the tumour with a cuff of

circumferential healthy tissue. However, the adequate thickness of this cuff varies broadly according to the type of tissue. It should be of some centimetres along the longitudinal plane of the muscle. It can be one centimetre along the axial plane of the muscle. It can be few millimetres, or even less, in proximity of tissues particularly resistant to tumour, such as peritoneum or pleura. If not infiltrated, the underlying structures can be safely preserved. If infiltrated, their removal should always be considered. 'Radical' resection implies removal of the tumour and the whole anatomical compartment in which it is located. Of course, a compartmental resection does not define per se the quality of surgical margins, since it can achieve a wide or a borderline margin, depending on how close the tumour is to the border of the compartment.

The quality of surgical margins is critical and ideally should be always evaluated by both the operating surgeon and the pathologist [30]. The closest margin should be identified and extensively sampled. Microscopically, margins are defined as negative, when the tumour edge is covered by at least one mm of healthy tissue, or positive when the tumour edge is covered by less than one mm of healthy tissue or is found at the inked surface [31–35].

In principle, the aim of surgery is to resect the tumour surrounded by healthy tissue and to avoid positive surgical margins. In fact, the risk of local failure doubles in case of positive margins, despite the use of post-operative RT, with a subsequent impact on distant outcome and survival (Table 55.4). While the initial prognosis mainly depends on the biology of the tumour, once a patient has 'survived' the first period and the systemic risk dependent on tumour biology becomes weaker, the quality of surgery appears as the strongest prognosticator for outcome [31–35]. Two factors can explain the impact of positive surgical margins on survival: a relatively slight increase in the risk of subsequent systemic spread in case of recurrence and a direct impact of local recurrence that may lead to death in some sites [35–36]. In the case of pathological positive margins, re-excision should always be considered whenever feasible [30, 37–39]. This does not apply when a positive margin is planned in advance in order to preserve an important structure for function-sparing (i.e., a motor nerve), provided adequate RT is delivered (especially in the preoperative setting) [40–43].

Table 55.4 Incidence of local recurrence, distant metastases and death in major published series of extremities soft tissue sarcoma, according to microscopic surgical margins

| | 5-yrs LR | | 5-yrs DM | | 5-yrs CSD | | 10-yrs LR | | 10-yrs DM | | 10-yrs CSD | |
	M+	M–	M+	M–	M+	M–	M+	M–	M+	M–	M+	M–
Trovik et al. (2000) [32]	36%	18%	28%	28%	NR	NR	NR	NR	NR	NR	NR	NR
Zagars et al. (2003) [33]	36%	12%	25%	28%	31%	25%	44%	14%	33%	33%	39%	34%
Stojadinovic et al. (2002) [34]	35%	18%	32%	24%	30%	20%	NR	NR	NR	NR	NR	NR
Gronchi et al. (2010) [35]	26%	10%	20%	21%	29%	16%	30%	12%	24%	24%	38%	19%

LR, incidence of local recurrence; DM, incidence of distant metastases; CSD, incidence of disease specific death; M+, positive microscopic surgical margins; M–, negative microscopic surgical margins.

The same principles should be applied to tumours located outside the limbs and trunk wall, although wide margins may be more difficult to obtain and a careful balance between morbidity and chances of cure should always be made on a case-by-case basis [44].

The ability to reconstruct large defects by pedicled or free flaps, to restore function by replacing bone, vessels, nerves, and to perform major visceral resections, whenever needed to improve quality of surgery, should be part of proper planning before the surgical procedure is undertaken. Therefore, a careful multidisciplinary approach is needed in all cases for proper treatment delivery [30].

Soft tissue sarcoma

Surgery of STSs primarily consists of the resection of the tumour surrounded by a cuff of healthy tissue [45]. In extremities and trunk walls, this basically implies the resection of surrounding soft tissues, mainly muscles, subcutaneous fat, and skin (Figure 55.4). The necessity to cover the soft tissue loss by a flap transposition depends on several factors, such as the site and size of the defect, exposed structures (bone, vessels, nerves), and functional restoration. Vessels, nerves, and bone are always resected when directly invaded/encased, while their resection has to be discussed on a case-by-case basis when their periosteum, adventitia, or epineurium are infiltrated without invasion of the underlying structure.

Similar principles apply to surgery of retroperitoneal sarcomas [46]. In fact, unlike primary epithelial solid tumours, which are usually confined to a single organ and can generally be removed with resection of that organ, retroperitoneal STS commonly abuts multiple surrounding organs. Paralleling surgery in extremities, tumours should be systematically resected en bloc with surrounding tissues, which at this site are mainly the adjacent viscera even when not overtly involved, to minimize the risk of microscopically positive margins (Figure 55.5). Indeed, not all uninvolved adjacent viscera/structures are routinely resected en bloc with the tumour [47–53]. The objective is to achieve a wide microscopic margin along most surfaces, even by removing additional dispensable organs, while performing what is essentially a marginal excision along critical structures. In general, the ipsilateral kidney,

colon, and mesocolon and at least a portion of the psoas can be safely and relatively easily resected without serious consequences. Resection of the pancreatic body and tail and spleen can usually be performed with a relatively low short-term morbidity. Resection of other structures, including—but not limiting to—the aorta, inferior vena cava, iliac vessels, femoral nerve, diaphragm, duodenum, head of the pancreas, uncinate process, liver, and bone (specifically vertebral bodies) entails significant resections with ensuing greater morbidity, so that it is not performed unless macroscopic invasion is documented. This extended approach has been systematically adopted only in the recent years, with a significant improvement in local control in all patients and of survival in patients affected by low/intermediate grade sarcomas, whose outcome had been dominated by inoperable local recurrences [47–61] (Table 55.5).

Similar principles do apply, as long as it is feasible, also to tumours at other sites (mediastinum, head and neck) [30], a systematic description of which goes beyond the scope of the present text.

Since the STS family is made up of at least 50 histological subtypes, these general principles can be applied differently in selected subtypes, as follows.

Atypical lipomatous tumour/well-differentiated liposarcoma

This low-grade tumour, when arising in the extremity, has a relatively low rate of recurrence, may not recur for a relatively long interval, and has minimal or no risk of distant metastatic spread and death, unless dedifferentiation occurs [62]. In fact, dedifferentiation in general entails a risk of metastatic spread as high as 20%, but in extremities dedifferentiation develops only rarely (less than 5% of cases) [62, 63]. In other words, a well-differentiated liposarcoma in extremities only occasionally poses a life threat. Furthermore, low-grade recurrent atypical lipomatous tumours (ALTs) may grow slowly for years. Therefore, such tumours can be resected with a modest positive margin, especially when preserving limb function is an issue. The same low-grade tumour, however, becomes a life-threatening disease when located to the retroperitoneum, even if lacking areas of dedifferentiation [64]. In fact, as discussed above, local control is an issue for retroperitoneal sarcomas, and patients often die of local regional failures without developing distant

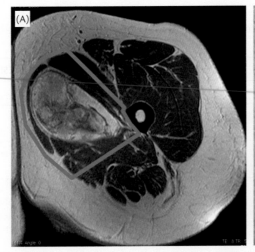
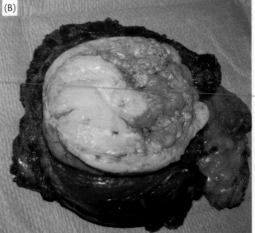

Fig. 55.4 (A) Contrast-enhanced T1 weighted MRI of myxoid liposarcoma of the left thigh, originating in the abductor compartment. The planned resection line is shown in blue. (B) Surgical specimen cut through the longest diameter. The tumour is surrounded by a cuff of healthy tissue.

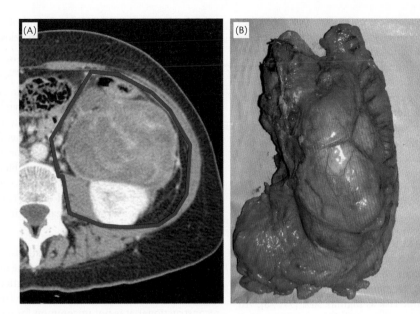

Fig. 55.5 (A) Contrast-enhanced CT scan of left retroperitoneal liposarcoma. The planned resection line is shown in blue. (B) The surgical specimen. The tumour is covered by the left kidney and colon (and psoas muscle in the back, not shown here).

metastases. An extended surgical approach for well-differentiated liposarcoma located at this site is therefore recommended [44].

Myxoid/round cell liposarcoma

This tumour predominantly occurs in the extremities [65]. It can be found even in the trunk, but almost always as a metastasis from a primary tumour located in extremities. Pure myxoid liposarcoma rarely metastasizes, while the risk increases when a round cell component is present in more than 5% of the tumour [65–68]. At variance with most other sarcomas, metastases can occur in the soft tissues, abdomen, mediastinum, and bone before affecting the lung [65–68]. Chemotherapy and RT may be particularly active [69–71]. Therefore, preoperative therapies, either by single or combined modalities, are often offered to reduce surgical morbidity and increase chances of cure [72, 73].

Dermatofibrosarcoma protuberans

Dermatofibrosarcoma protuberans (DFSP) is a superficial tumour, which infiltrates soft tissues for centimetres beyond the obvious margins of the lesion and can recur locally following inadequate

Table 55.5 Local recurrence-free survival and overall survival in major published series of retroperitoneal soft tissue sarcoma

	Study period	Median FU	No patients	Complete resection (%)	5-years LRFS	5-years OS
Lewis et al. 1998 [54]	1982–1997	28	231	80	59	54
Stoeckle et al. 2001 [55]	1980–1994	47	165	65	42	49
Ferrario et al. 2003 [56]	1977–2001	41	79	99	43	65
Hassan et al. 2004 [58]	1983–1995	36	97	78	56	51
Lehnert et al. 2009 [60]	1998–2002	89	71	70	59	65
Bonvalot et al. 2010 [51]	2000–2008	37	249	93	78	65
Gronchi et al. 2012 [53]	2002–2008	48	136	94	79	68

FU: follow-up; N.: number; LRFS: local recurrence free survival; OS: overall survival; in bold: series of patients systematically resected by an extended approach.

resection [74]. However, the more common variety of DFSP has no metastatic potential. The goal of surgery should be to achieve negative margins, often necessitating reconstruction by plastic surgery [74–76]. When cosmetic/function preservation is an issue, limited positive margins may be accepted, and a wider resection postponed when a recurrence occurs. Since DFSP is usually a relatively superficial tumour, resection of muscles deep to the tumour is often unnecessary. Approximately 5–10% of patients with DFSP present as a more aggressive fibrosarcomatous variant, which may more often recur locally and potentially spread [74]. These patients should be treated as those having a 'conventional' sarcoma, with limited positive margins being only occasionally acceptable.

Leiomyosarcoma

This sarcoma may arise from skin, soft tissues, visceral organs, or vessels and it is one of the commonest histological subtypes [77]. The approach to skin leiomyosarcoma is easy, since the invasion of surrounding tissues is limited and the metastatic potential almost nil. On the contrary, soft tissues leiomyosarcoma often presents as large masses and has a systemic risk as high as 50% [77, 78]. An extended soft tissue en bloc resection with the mass is required. Adjuvant treatments are often discussed with the patient, although their impact on local and distant outcome is limited. Gastrointestinal (GI) leiomyosarcomas are rare [79]. They are treated by the resection of the affected GI tract. Adjacent organs are resected only if directly infiltrated. They typically have a high metastatic risk and spread to liver before other organs. Vascular leiomyosarcomas predominantly arise from veins and often abut outside the vessel extending in the soft tissues [80, 81]. The affected vascular tract should be resected en bloc with adjacent soft tissues. Intravascular tumour thrombi may be present and should be removed en bloc with the disease. Frozen margin specimens over the vessel should be taken to ensure free margins. The metastatic risk is significant, although a fraction of them may have a long natural history.

Pleomorphic liposarcoma, unclassified pleomorphic sarcoma, synovial sarcoma

These tumours, although different from a histological and biological standpoint, are usually approached the same way [82–86]. They predominantly affect the extremities and present as large and deeply located masses. They have a significant metastatic risk and are often treated by combined modalities. The surgical approach consists of the standard procedures described above.

Myxofibrosarcoma

This malignant tumour, when located superficially, infiltrates through soft tissue (subcutaneous fat and investing fascia) some centimetres beyond the ostensible margins of the visible or palpable mass. When located intramuscularly, the extension of the infiltration is usually limited by anatomical barriers, although it has a higher propensity to invade them as compared to other histological subtypes. Myxofibrosarcoma most commonly arises in the extremities of elderly individuals. It demonstrates a 30% rate of local recurrence and a 16% rate of distant recurrence [87–90]. Eventually, multiple local recurrences may lead to amputation. Therefore, it is critical to pursue aggressive local therapy. Wide surgical margins (≥2 cm beyond the clinical boundaries of the palpable mass in general and up to 4 cm for the superficial ones) should be the goal of surgery, which often requires complex wound closure or flap reconstruction by a plastic and reconstructive surgeon, as well as

resection/reconstruction of vessels and nerves. RT, either preoperatively or post-operatively (described below), may be considered.

Malignant peripheral nerve sheath tumours

These tumours often arise from a major peripheral nerve, which can be identified macroscopically. They can occur sporadically or in the context of neurofibromatosis type 1 syndrome. The high-grade variant is marked by an early propensity for distant metastases [91–93]. When originating from a peripheral nerve, they also may spread along the nerve fibres proximally or distally. Wider margins at this level should be obtained (if possible at least 4 cm of macroscopic healthy nerve) to limit this loco-regional failure, which eventually may reach the spinal cord. Frozen sections may help ensure the accomplishment of clear margins.

Angiosarcoma

Management of primary and radiation-associated (secondary) angiosarcoma is challenging because of the multifocality of this disease [94–97]. Scalp angiosarcoma is a particularly insidious malignancy. While radical surgery is possible (requiring complex flap reconstructions), it is not uncommon for patients to develop local recurrences immediately outside the margins of resection even if the margins of the initial resection were widely negative, with or without RT. Angiosarcoma is sensitive to systemic chemotherapy and to RT. Since surgery is rarely curative, it should not be considered as the only treatment choice, especially for scalp angiosarcoma. Surgery may be reserved for patients who are experiencing problems with local control (bleeding from a fungating tumour) or who only appear to have a solitary site of disease by both clinical examination and imaging while undergoing systemic therapy.

Epithelioid and clear cell sarcomas

Both of these tumours tend to affect young adults and to occur in distal extremities. At variance with all other histological subtypes, they may give rise to in-transit metastasis along the affected limb and to loco-regional lymph node metastases [98–100]. Accurate staging of the whole limb is mandatory and sentinel lymph node biopsy should be considered as part of the routine approach to primary disease. Their sensitivity to conventional chemotherapy is at best limited. A more aggressive variant of epithelioid sarcoma tends to occur to the limb roots and the trunk and is called proximal-type epithelioid sarcoma [101]. This variant behaves as a very aggressive unclassified sarcoma, having a high risk of hematogenous distant spread. Loco-regional lymph nodes are only rarely involved [102]. Its sensitivity to conventional chemotherapy is higher, but fast progression after response is often observed. If a preoperative treatment is planned, the status of the disease has to be carefully monitored.

Radiation-induced sarcomas

Radiation-induced sarcomas are rare and include a variety of histological subtypes, the most common of which are pleomorphic undifferentiated sarcoma, angiosarcoma, malignant peripheral nerve sheath tumours, and leiomyosarcoma [103, 104]. Beside the inherent characteristics of each histological subtype, they are all marked by a high propensity to locally recur, given the difficulty in obtaining clear margins. In fact, it is very difficult to distinguish tumour infiltration of healthy tissues from radiation-induced changes around the tumour site. The tumour should be excised with as much surrounding tissue as possible. Often, if not always, this requires plastic surgery and liberal vascular and nerve resection and reconstruction. Systemic chemotherapy and re-irradiation are often considered, given the overall dismal prognosis.

Bone sarcomas

Surgery of bone sarcomas primarily consists of resection of the affected bone, surrounded by healthy tissue whenever needed and feasible [105, 106]. Adequate staging by bone scan and cross-sectional imaging should be performed to understand the extent of the disease in the affected bone and the presence of satellite or skip lesions. Resected peripheral bones are usually replaced by prostheses of variable lengths and complexity [107, 108]. Bone pure allografts can also be used, especially when tendon and joints need to be replaced. In the last years, composed allografts (bone grafts + prostheses) have been successfully used in several conditions [109, 110]. Thus, the rate of primary amputation today does not exceed 10% [107, 110]. The replacement of axial bones (pelvis and spine) is more difficult, while they are frequently affected in adult bone sarcomas. In fact, osteosarcoma and Ewing sarcoma predominantly affect the limbs, while many chondrosarcomas and all chordomas affect central bones.

For tumours located in the pelvis, hindquarter amputations can still be an option, although followed by significant disability. Rehabilitation is difficult and patients often require prosthetics or remain in a wheel chair for the rest of their life. Nevertheless, this is still an option in several presentations. In fact, reconstruction is a challenge for most pelvic tumours. The pelvic anatomy (presence of sciatic and femoral nerves, iliac vessels, sacral plexus, and pelvic viscera) adds to the complexity of the osteo-muscular resection and may sometimes render an amputation more suitable than a conservative procedure.

There are three types of conservative resections [111]. Type I is the easiest and is used for tumours confined in the iliac wing. It consists of resections of the iliac bone without interrupting the continuity between the sacrum and the rest of the pelvic bones of the affected site. Type II is the most complex, since it involves the acetabulum. Different types of reconstruction have been attempted over the years with prosthesis or bone allografts. None of them has proved to be really successful. The failure rate is as high as 30–50% [112, 113]. This should be factored in the decision before surgery is undertaken. Type III involves the pubis and is used for tumours confined to the pubic bone and ileo-pubic and/or ischiopubic branches. No reconstruction is needed as for type I. Tumours may obviously extend beyond one segment of the pelvic bone and the resection include more than one type.

For tumours located to the sacrum, the complexity of the intervention increases with the level of resection, although reconstructions are almost never needed, even for total sacrectomy [114]. For tumours located below S3, the resection is straightforward and followed by a complete recovery of the pelvic functions, if at least both S3 roots are preserved. For tumours located above S3, morbidity depends on the number of roots resected. In fact, if both S2 are preserved, there is still a 40% chance of complete recovery of the pelvic functions. If both S2 roots are transected, the pelvic functions are lost and rehabilitation is needed to live with fecal incontinence and neurologic bladder. From S1 on the resection determines also impairment of the motor/sensitive function of the limbs [115]. For tumours located to the mobile spine, a reconstruction is always needed and usually consists of a segmental arthrodesis obtained through osteosynthesis and bone grafts. Morbidity is mainly related to the extent of resection in soft tissues, the number of roots and the number of vertebral bones resected [116]. Dorsal vertebral bones resection is followed by more limited morbidity, if compared to lumbar and cervical bones, since the latter always affect the function of at least one of the lower or upper limbs.

Surgery of bone tumours in general and all the more of pelvic/spine tumours should be performed only by a dedicated team with specific expertise in this difficult field.

Osteosarcoma

Osteosarcoma is the most common primary bone sarcoma and is usually marked by a high grade of aggressiveness [117]. It typically occurs during childhood and adolescence. More rarely it can occur in young adults. Histologic variants include low-grade central, conventional, teleangiectatic, small cell, paraosteal, periosteal, and high-grade surface osteosarcoma. In patients over the age of 40, it is usually associated with a pre-existent condition such as Paget's disease or irradiated bone [118, 119]. Paraosteal, periosteal, and low-grade central osteosarcomas tend to occur in the third decade of life. Between 80–90% of the tumours occur in the metaphysis of long bone with the most common sites being the distal femur, proximal tibia, and proximal humerus. Surgery and chemotherapy are the mainstays of therapy. Given the sensitivity of osteosarcoma to chemotherapy, surgery is commonly performed after three to four courses of chemotherapy, which is continued post-operatively [120, 121]. Pathologic evaluation of tumour response to chemotherapy has a significant prognostic value. Parosteal osteosarcoma is a distinct variant of osteosarcoma. Its incidence is estimated to be 4% of all osteosarcomas. It arises from the cortical bone and generally occurs in an older age group and has a better overall prognosis than osteosarcoma, since it may also have a low histological grade of aggressiveness. 50% of cases exhibit overt cartilaginous differentiation. The treatment program may vary according to the grade and be surgery alone for the low-grade variant. Periosteal osteosarcoma is a rare cortical variant of osteosarcoma that arises superficially on the cortex, most often on the tibial shaft, and can also occur in patients over 50 years of age. It may also have a more limited aggressiveness as compared to the more common osteosarcoma [122, 123]. Surgery for all osteosarcomas always consists in the resection of the affected bone. Reconstruction is performed as described above.

Ewing sarcoma/pPNET

Ewing sarcoma represents the prototype of round cell sarcomas. Typically it strongly expresses CD99, and harbours a typical chromosomal translocation that fuses in most cases the *EWSR1* gene on chromosome 22 with a variety of partner genes (*FLI1* in approximately 85% of cases), belonging to the ETS family of transcription factors (Table 55.2). Ewing sarcoma is marked by high aggressiveness and early distant spread. They may occur either in bones or soft tissues. Ewing sarcoma of bone occurs predominantly in the diaphysis or metaphyseal-dyaphyseal portion of long bones of skeletally immature patients. The peak incidence is the second decade of life. It is exceedingly rare in very young patients and in those over the age of 30. Extraskeletal Ewing sarcoma represents approximately 20% of all Ewing sarcomas, tends to occur at an older age, and exhibits the same morphological and molecular features of the skeletal counterpart. Treatment is made up of surgery, chemotherapy and RT [124, 125]. Given the high sensitivity of these tumours to chemotherapy, the local treatment is almost always preceded by induction chemotherapy. Histopathologic evaluation of tumour necrosis after induction chemotherapy has prognostic value. In general, there is retrospective evidence that adding surgery to chemotherapy and RT improves the final outcome. However, for proximally located or trunk lesions, where surgery may result in excessive morbidity, RT may be delivered as definitive treatment. Surgical resection in selected presentations may also be placed at the end of the chemotherapy program.

Chondrosarcoma

The most useful prognostic tools in chondrosarcoma, both in terms of surgical planning and prognosis, is histological grading [126, 127]. There are a few distinct, relatively rare, histological variants of chondrosarcoma, in addition to the conventional type. These include clear cell, mesenchymal, and dedifferentiated chondrosarcoma. Primary chondrosarcomas are not associated with a pre-existing lesion (90% of the cases). Secondary chondrosarcomas are associated with pre-existing chondroid lesions such as enchondroma, osteochondroma, chondroblastoma, chondromyxofibroma, periosteal chondroma, and synovial chondromatosis (10% of the cases). The majority of conventional chondrosarcomas occur between the ages of 40 and 60. The most common sites are the pelvis, femur, and shoulder girdle. Low-grade chondrosarcomas originating from the limbs can be treated by intralesional curettage and application of local adjuvants, such as phenol, ethanol, and liquid nitrogen. As an alternative for small lesions, radiofrequency ablation and, more recently, cryoablation are occasionally used. Intermediate- and high-grade chondrosarcomas as well as low-grade chondrosarcomas located in the pelvis or shoulder girdle have to be treated by conventional resections and reconstructions. Adjuvant RT is not routinely administered, since chondrosarcoma has long been considered radioresistant. Nonetheless, recent data on the administration of radiotherapy with heavy particles have raised potential benefit for problematic sites. Confirmatory studies are needed to include these new modalities as part of a standard approach. Chemotherapy is not routinely recommended, save for specific subtypes. Dedifferentiated chondrosarcoma may be treated by employing chemotherapy regimens similar to those used for high-grade sarcomas [128, 129]. This is most true of mesenchymal chondrosarcoma, for which chemotherapy regimens similar to those used in Ewing sarcoma may be selected.

Chordoma

Chordomas are definitely rare, affecting 0.1 individuals in 100 000 per year. They occur predominantly between the age of 50 and 70, although the ones located at the base of the skull may occur in young adults. The most common site of origin is the sacrum (it is the most common primary bone tumour of the sacrum), followed by the clivus and base of the skull in general. More rarely it affects the mobile spine. It is never found outside the vertebral bodies. Resection of the affected bone can be challenging because of extension into surrounding soft tissues, spinal cord or central nervous system, viscera, and major vessels. Surgery has always been considered the mainstay of therapy, although often followed by significant long-term morbidity [130, 131]. Only recently, with the introduction of heavy particles, i.e., protons and carbon ions (RT

that allows the delivery of higher doses by sparing normal tissues), combined approaches or radiotherapy alone have been proposed as an alternative to conventional surgery with the goal of reducing surgical sequelae [132, 133]. Confirmatory studies are needed, though the rarity of these tumours, along with their variability in clinical presentation, make studies all the more difficult, especially when the goal is to compare long-term complications from different treatment modalities.

Radiation therapy

Soft tissue sarcoma

In general, limb-sparing surgery relies on complementary RT, to minimize risk of local recurrence, as demonstrated in two pivotal trials--one with brachytherapy (BRT) and one with post-operative external beam radiotherapy (EBRT) [134, 135]. RT reduces the risk of local recurrence from greater than 30% to less than 10% in most series, but does not impact distant failure or overall survival.

EBRT may be delivered preoperatively or postoperatively [136]. When given preoperatively, the goal of radiation is to treat the margins to minimize the risk of recurrence, not necessarily to reduce the size of the tumour per se. A randomized comparison between pre- and post-operative EBRT has been performed. There was no difference in local recurrence rates [137]. Preoperative EBRT was associated with a doubling in the rate of wound complications (35% vs 17%) but with a lower rate of late complications and tissue fibrosis and better functional outcomes. Postoperative EBRT generally covers a larger field (including drain sites) and used a higher dose than preoperative EBRT. This is particularly important in young adults of childbearing age with proximal thigh STS: preoperative EBRT may spare the gonads whereas postoperative radiation may not [136].

Moreover, data from retrospective series suggest that the administration of preoperative RT minimizes the risk of limited close or positive margins [40–43]. Therefore, whenever preservation of function is a goal and the tumour abuts critical structures, preoperative EBRT should be considered.

Brachytherapy (BRT) may be delivered through after-loading catheters placed across the tumour bed at the end of surgery [138]. The goal of BRT is to deliver additional radiation to a close margin (including neurovascular structures) with minimal treatment to surrounding tissue, particularly when further EBRT is no longer feasible. When the final pathologic margins are confirmed, the appropriate catheters may be loaded with radioactive seeds once or twice a day for a defined treatment period concentrated over the close margins. To minimize wound complications, catheters should not be loaded until at least postoperative day five. To minimize the risk of dislodging the catheters, any drains placed at the time of surgery should remain in place until the catheters have been removed.

Intraoperative RT (IORT) has also been studied in extremity STS, but it has failed to improve results of conventional EBRT. It is therefore not routinely used in clinical practice [138].

Patients with small (<5 cm), superficial, well-circumscribed STS resected with a wide margin (>1 cm) of non-neoplastic tissue or a biologic barrier (fascia) may not require RT, provided that they can be reliably followed for local recurrence [139]. The same may apply to low-grade tumours, independent of tumour location and size. Of note, myxoid/round cell liposarcoma and angiosarcoma are more sensitive to EBRT than all other histological subtypes [71]. Therefore, EBRT is more liberally used in patients affected by these tumours, especially in the preoperative setting.

In retroperitoneal sarcomas (RPS), the role of RT is controversial, in the absence of phase III randomized controlled trial data. While RT unequivocally reduces the risk of local recurrence in patients with extremity STS, this has not been proven in RPS [140]. Furthermore, the proximity of radiosensitive tissues and organs, such as the liver and small intestine, together with the large size of the radiation field, limit its utility. Those who utilize RT generally deliver it preoperatively, when the bulk of the tumour itself displaces uninvolved organs out of the radiation field [141]. There is one ongoing randomized trial assessing the efficacy of preoperative RT in patients with RPS.

IORT has also been studied in RPS, with results similar to those achieved in the extremities [142].

Bone sarcoma

In general, osteosarcoma and adult bone sarcoma (chondrosarcoma and chordoma) are considered radioresistant tumours [143–146]. No randomized trials have been performed to formally address radiation in these tumours. On the contrary, Ewing sarcoma is highly radiosensitive [147]. RT is therefore part of Ewing sarcoma treatment program, while other bone tumours have only been rarely treated by EBRT, and then predominantly in a palliative setting. The introduction of heavy-particle RT has allowed the possibility to increase dose delivery, sparing normal tissues [4]. Both chordomas and chondrosarcoma located to difficult sites (base of the skull and spine) have then been treated with these new methodologies in recent years with promising results [143–146]. Confirmatory studies are needed to understand whether this modality could complement or even substitute for surgery.

Medical therapy

The efficacy of chemotherapy in adult STS has long been confined to the low/intermediate spectrum, with doxorubicin and ifosfamide as the only active drugs, whether used alone or in combination. More recently, some cytotoxics were proven to have significant antitumour activity in selected STS subtypes, while new molecular targeted agents are progressively entering the medical armamentarium. Therefore, medical therapy of adult STS is much broader today. While this evolution is in progress, single-agent doxorubicin might still be regarded as a standard medical therapy by some, while a set of old and new agents are increasingly used at many institutions for 'precision' therapeutic choices. The quality of evidence backing this shift is a limiting factor and a reason for discrepancies across institutions. In fact, STS are a family of rare tumours, so that clinical studies regarding selected histologies are all the more difficult to carry out.

With regard to strategy, medical therapy always needs to be combined with other treatment modalities in localized STS and is considered an essentially palliative modality in advanced STS. This differentiates adult STS from small round blue cell sarcomas of childhood, in which chemotherapy has a comparatively much higher efficacy and an eradicating potential in some presentations. Actually, adjuvant chemotherapy is not standard treatment in adult STS, although, in the high-risk setting, many institutions share the decision with the patient to undertake it. In addition, chemotherapy may be employed to down-stage localized, surgically problematic STS, possibly in combination with RT. Metastatic STS are treated with chemotherapy, unless surgery of isolated lung metastases is used alone, as is the case when prognostic factors are good. As long as the number of available agents, and regimens, increases, clinical decision-making may be problematic in regard to how many lines of medical therapy should be resorted to in the palliative setting.

Active drugs and regimens in soft tissue sarcoma

Doxorubicin is still regarded as the most active agent in adult STS. It is reasonable to place its response rate at around 20%. In the metastatic setting, median duration of tumour response is slightly less than one year. Ifosfamide was later shown to exert an antitumour activity which can be viewed as essentially similar to doxorubicin. Therefore, the potential for cytoreduction of single-agent chemotherapy, whether doxorubicin or ifosfamide, is low and its prognostic impact is limited in the advanced disease.

Doxorubicin and ifosfamide can be combined, to potentially increase their efficacy. Currently available randomized clinical trials have failed, however, to show any major improvement in the average adult STS patient [148]. However, data from randomized trials point to an increased progression-free survival and response frequency with multiagent chemotherapy. Uncontrolled studies report better results, which suggest a selection bias, by which larger studies might have been less selective, thus diluting what the effect of multiagent chemotherapy may be in some clinical presentations. The toxicity of the combination of doxorubicin and ifosfamide, administered over three to five days with mesna (Uromitexan®) and hydration, and recycled every three weeks, is definitely higher than single-agent chemotherapy with either doxorubicin or ifosfamide. With a full-dose doxorubicin plus ifosfamide regimen, most patients experience profound neutropenia, though lasting a few days, while platelets are relatively spared, with a few patients requiring platelet transfusions. Neutropenic fever is experienced by a substantial number of patients in some cycles, so that granulocyte colony stimulating factors are generally used. Thus, while doxorubicin is a safe standard choice for palliating an advanced disease, a full-dose doxorubicin + ifosfamide regimen may be used when tumour response, or major antitumour activity, is a clinical goal, after considering age, performance status, and co-morbidities. Thus, the combination of doxorubicin plus ifosfamide will be preferred when chemotherapy is used as an adjuvant, or when the goal is to down-stage an advanced, or surgically problematic, localized STS. It may also be an option when any major symptom needs prompt palliation. In general, the good performance status of many adult STS patients—advanced though their disease may be—is an additional factor which tends to favour multiagent chemotherapy to maximize the treatment effect. It goes without saying that there is a high variability across institutions in these treatment choices, depending on whether a conservative or a more aggressive approach is preferred.

Both doxorubicin and ifosfamide can be regarded as wide-spectrum agents across all adult STS histological subtypes. Indeed, while this is true of doxorubicin, ifosfamide seems to have limited activity in leiomyosarcomas [149]. On the contrary, it has major activity in synovial sarcoma. Ifosfamide is generally used in the 6–9 g/sqm dose range every three weeks. When used at doses in the 12–15 g/sqm range, it is termed 'high-dose' [150].

If administered over four to five days, its toxicity profile includes high-grade neutropaenia, though of limited duration. CNS symptoms are uncommon in adults, though minor drowsiness may be a sign. While urothelial toxicity is prevented by the standard administration of mesna, renal damage is generally avoided by appropriate hydration, although signs of tubular toxicity may be encountered. A better toxicity profile is associated with high-dose ifosfamide administered as a prolonged 14-day infusion through a portable external pump, every four weeks [151]. High-dose ifosfamide may be active in a proportion of patients already exposed to standard-dose ifosfamide. This makes it a second-line option in patients previously treated with doxorubicin and ifosfamide. Otherwise, in patients treated with doxorubicin alone, it can be used also at standard doses with the same aim. In patients who responded to doxorubicin, other anthracyclines can be employed in the second-line setting as well, although the top cumulative dose is a limiting factor for treatment duration, so that high-dose ifosfamide may again be an alternate choice. Liposomal doxorubicin may be an option.

Dacarbazine (DTIC) is an agent which was included in the multiagent regimens CYVADIC and its ifosfamide-containing 'upgrade', MAID. Currently, its added value is felt to be limited, so that multiagent first-line chemotherapy is most often doxorubicin plus ifosfamide without dacarbazine. However, an exception may be the use of dacarbazine in leiomyosarcomas, an entity which may be less sensitive to ifosfamide. Thus it may be added to doxorubicin in the first-line therapy of leiomyosarcomas, or it can be used as a further-line single-agent choice in leiomyosarcoma. Its toxicity profile is good with currently available antiemetic coverage. Its oral counterpart, temozolomide, which is converted into its active metabolite in plasma, has been shown to have some activity in leiomyosarcoma as well [152].

In fact, there is currently a trend towards tailoring medical therapy to the histological sarcoma subtype [153]. Amongst cytotoxics, for example, gemcitabine (Gemzar®) has distinct activity in leiomyosarcoma and angiosarcomas [154, 155]. Angiosarcomas are also the only histological subtype in which taxanes have some antitumour activity in sarcomas; low-dose paclitaxel, given every 7 to10 days, is effective in angiosarcoma [156]. In this histology, the onset of tumour resistance may be relatively fast, but the substantial cytoreduction which can be achieved may be exceedingly useful in combination with surgery and/or RT, especially in the loco-regional advanced setting.

Docetaxel (Taxotere®) was combined with gemcitabine to give rise to the GEMTAX regimen [157]. Given the lack of activity of taxanes in all STS histologies with the exception of angiosarcoma, the assumption is that this combination may exploit a synergy between the two agents. Data are conflicting, however, about the clinical added value of the combination in comparison to gemcitabine alone. GEMTAX seems mainly active in leiomyosarcoma, and possibly pleomorphic sarcoma and angiosarcoma. Of course, tolerability of single-agent gemcitabine is much higher than the combination, so that its use may be all the more interesting for palliation of recurrent, metastatic leiomyosarcoma.

A marine-derived agent which was shown to be active in advanced STS is trabectedin [158]. The two histologies where trabectedin is most active are leiomyosarcomas and liposarcomas, although other subtypes may be sensitive, in particular synovial sarcoma. Indeed, when liposarcomas are split into their two main subtypes, i.e.,

well- and dedifferentiated and myxoid/round cell liposarcomas, the activity profile of trabectedin looks markedly different. In fact, trabectedin shows a definitely higher response frequency in myxoid/round cell liposarcomas [70, 72], a longer duration of response, and a higher chance of a new response after treatment interruption following best response [159]. This has been shown retrospectively, while proof of a peculiar mechanism of action was provided as well. In fact, myxoid/round cell liposarcomas are a translocation-related STS, and trabectedin apparently displaces the fusion protein from target genes, thus displaying a kind of 'targeted' mechanism of action. Myxoid/round cell liposarcomas are a chemosensitive histology, marked by a relatively 'slow' natural history, which adds to the value of therapy per se. Trabectedin is generally well-tolerated, provided patients do not have liver function abnormalities at baseline, in particular cholestasis. Proper dose reductions and delays are suggested for liver alterations during therapy. Steroid premedication and a maximum dose per cycle may be useful to minimize toxicity. This may be limited to fatigue following administration, nausea in some patients, and laboratory evidence of increased transaminases. Major myelosuppression is unlikely, though it may occur and be prolonged, while rhabdomyolysis is exceedingly rare.

A well-known molecularly-targeted agent, imatinib (Gleevec®), has a specific role in STS, namely in DFSP [21]. This is a surgically-curable disease in most cases [74], but there are instances in which medical therapy can be useful because the tumour is locally advanced and cytoreduction can make surgery feasible or, rarely, metastases have developed. Imatinib has a high response frequency, possibly related to the fact that DFSP is a translocation-related STS, with increased stimulation of platelet derived growth factor receptor beta (PDGFRβ) as a result of the fusion protein activity. It is worth distinguishing typical DFSP from its 'fibrosarcomatous' variant. Imatinib is active also in these cases, but the duration of response is shorter [160].

Other highly specific subgroups which may be sensitive to molecularly-targeted therapies include ALK-rearranged inflammatory myofibroblastic tumours, which may be responsive to crizotinib (Xalkori®) [161]. Likewise, malignant PEComas are marked by a degree of disruption of the mTOR pathway and a proportion of these tumours are responsive to mTOR inhibitors [22]. Formal clinical studies are lacking at the moment, and the therapeutic value of these target therapies in these histologies is yet to be defined.

In a randomized clinical trial with broad eligibility criteria, mTOR inhibitors have been shown to slightly prolong progression-free survival in advanced sarcomas when given as a maintenance therapy following best response to standard chemotherapy [162].

The antiangiogenic agent pazopanib (Votrient®) was shown to significantly prolong progression-free survival when given for advanced, previously treated, non-adipogenic STS [163]. It is possible that pazopanib exerts a more specific antitumour activity in selected histologies, namely synovial sarcomas and leiomyosarcomas. Some antitumour activity has also been shown also for other antiangiogenic agents, including sorafenib, sunitinib, cediranib, and bevacizumab. Sunitinib (Sutent®) has been shown to result in tumour shrinkage in alveolar soft part sarcoma and solitary fibrous tumours, possibly through its activity on PDGFR [164, 165]. Cediranib (Recentin®) was also shown to be active in alveolar soft part sarcoma. The combination of temozolomide and bevacizumab (Avastin®) was shown to be active in solitary fibrous tumour [166]. A variety of molecularly-targeted agents are under investigation today in STSs. Likely, they will provide their best benefit in selected histologies expressing specific biomarkers. The development of new agents in this way, i.e., looking for biomarkers within selected STS subtypes, is challenging due to the small numbers of patients.

Medical therapy in the multidisciplinary treatment strategy of soft tissue sarcomas

Positioning of medical therapy in the treatment strategy of adult STS is problematic and reflects uncertainties in the potential of available agents and regimens.

Chemotherapy was tested as an adjuvant as from the 1970s, with a series of randomized clinical trials employing doxorubicin or doxorubicin-based regimens. These studies varied widely in sample size as well as eligibility criteria. Second-generation trials employed anthracyclines and ifosfamide. An Italian randomized trial tested a full-dose epirubicin plus ifosfamide regimen for five courses vs no medical therapy after surgery. It enrolled around one hundred patients with an advantage in overall survival which led to its early interruption [167]. On longer follow-up, the magnitude of the benefit and its statistical significance decreased. A large randomized trial from the EORTC, of five courses of doxorubicin plus ifosfamide vs no medical therapy after surgery, has been recently reported to be negative [168]. Prognostically, the patient population of this trial was slightly more favourable than the Italian trial. In brief, the largest trials, both of first- and second-generation, have been negative, while some smaller trials provided positive results. The former may have been less selective, as opposed to the latter, which might have highlighted benefits confined to the highest-risk patient subgroups. When published randomized trials of adjuvant chemotherapy were pooled together in a meta-analyses, a statistically significant benefit was shown in terms of overall survival, distant relapse-free survival, and local relapse-free survival. In the last published meta-analysis, the absolute risk reduction was in the range of 5–10% for all these end-points [169]. The main weakness is the presence of large negative trials, as opposed to some positive small studies, with marginal statistical significance [167]. In brief, the absolute benefit is likely limited, in the 10% range, and the uncertainty is high. This is widely felt to justify a policy of shared decision-making with patients in conditions of uncertainty, obviously selecting high-risk presentations. In practice, these are marked by a high malignancy grade, tumour size in excess of 5 cm, and deep location for limb STS. Clinical decisions by analogy may be allowed in rare tumours, so that adjuvant chemotherapy may be proposed also in non-limb sarcomas, including visceral, when the risk is high as well. An anthracycline plus ifosfamide regimen is generally selected, although leiomyosarcomas might benefit more from the combination of doxorubicin with dacarbazine or gemcitabine with docetaxel. Less chemo-responsive histologies are usually excluded, while waiting for more mature data about the activity in the advanced setting of selected molecularly targeted agents for some of them.

When the decision is made to use chemotherapy in the localized disease setting, one may well choose to administer medical therapy before surgery. This may provide benefit in quality of surgical margins or function-sparing surgical options. A randomized trial compared three courses of preoperative full-dose epirubicin plus ifosfamide chemotherapy with the same preoperative treatment followed by two further cycles of the same regimen [170]. No difference was found. Though lacking a no-adjuvant therapy control arm, the results of the treatment arm of the previous Italian randomized trial were reproduced in this study. An option may thus be to administer three cycles of full-dose multiagent chemotherapy, possibly before surgery, to exploit both the systemic potential of adjuvant treatment in high-risk adult STS and the local benefit for subsequent surgery. A currently ongoing trial randomizes patients between three pre-operative cycles of full-dose epirubicin plus ifosfamide and three cycles of a histology-driven chemotherapy. A trial is ongoing in uterine leiomyosarcomas comparing no further treatment after surgery versus four courses of GEMTAX followed by four courses of doxorubicin.

The natural history of a distinct proportion of adult STS is marked by the presence of 'isolated' lung metastases, i.e., in the absence of extrapulmonary disease. Complete surgery of all visible lesions, if feasible, is then standard treatment. The treatment goal is to pursue eradication in a small proportion of these patients and achieve a meaningful disease-free interval in a number of them. It is unknown whether adding chemotherapy might increase the cure rate, although it probably increases relapse-free interval. In these patients, however, medical therapy at relapse might bring the same prognostic benefit in the context of a palliative approach. Prognostic factors for complete surgery of isolated lung metastases are tumour aggressiveness, reflected by the previous relapse-free interval (or the doubling time on serial assessments, if available) and the number of metastases [171]. The value of thresholds is questionable, but a number of metastases of around four or five and a previous relapse-free interval in the range of one to two years may be used to separate patients with a bad or a good prognosis. In the lack of available clinical trials, therefore, many clinicians do not use chemotherapy when prognostic factors are favourable and share the decision with the patient whether to use it or not when prognostic factors are poor. If selected, chemotherapy may be administered preoperatively, with the opportunity to monitor tumour response and thus tailor treatment accordingly.

Chemotherapy is an obvious choice in the advanced metastatic setting, although its benefit may be limited, with median overall survival intervals of less than one year. Median duration of tumour response is in the same range. It cannot be ruled out, however, that an aggressive use of all medical options available, depending on tumour histology, may translate into an effect on survival and quality of life, although obviously within the context of palliative intent. The availability of new agents and their potential in selected histologies definitely encourages the clinician to embark in several 'further-line' medical therapies. The prognostic impact of an aggressive medical approach to the advanced disease is unknown, while its impact on costs and toxicity is obvious. The natural history of metastatic adult STS is marked by a relatively limited extent of disease for long periods of time, as may be the case when metastases are confined to the lungs. Thus, performance status is often preserved along the natural history of an advanced disease. A few symptoms may be dominating, with dyspnoea prevailing, carrying all the palliative problems therefrom. Merging symptomatic measures with reasonable attempts through a specific medical therapy may be the best choice in several cases. However, clinical decision-making is especially challenging when disease is advanced, performance status is good, and convincing histology-driven medical options are potentially available.

Isolated limb perfusion

This treatment is reserved for limb-threatening STS. This procedure involves placing vascular access catheters into the main artery and vein of the affected extremity and perfusing with high-dose chemotherapy (usually melphalan) and tumour necrosis factor alpha (TNFα) under hyperthermic conditions. Isolated limb perfusion (ILP) is generally performed as an open procedure with cutdown directly onto the vessel and is delivered in the neoadjuvant setting.

ILP with chemotherapy alone has uniformly failed in the treatment of unresectable extremity STSs. The addition of TNF-α to this treatment approach has proved to be critical in improving the outcome of locally advanced extremity STS [172].

TNF-α has an early and a late effect; it enhances tumour-selective drug uptake during the perfusion and also plays an essential role in the subsequent selective destruction of the tumour vasculature. These effects result in a high response rate, which translates into limb salvage in most cases. Several single-institution reports have confirmed the safety and efficacy of this procedure.

Medical therapy of adult Ewing sarcomas

Ewing sarcoma may occasionally occur in adults. In adults, extraskeletal presentations are more common than in children. Indeed, extraskeletal Ewing sarcoma may occur to any site, from soft tissues (e.g., of limbs or superficial trunk) to viscera (e.g., kidney, etc.). The overall treatment strategy, including medical therapy, should follow the same principles applied in younger patients and the prognostic impact of treatment should thus parallel in principle what is achievable today in younger ages, though in all series there is an unfavourable prognostic trend as age increases. Likewise, treatment does not change in principle whether the patient has skeletal or extraskeletal disease. Of course, tolerability of treatments may decrease as long as age increases, especially with regard

to the duration of chemotherapy foreseen by standard protocols for skeletal Ewing sarcoma of children and adolescents. In several institutions, a duration of chemotherapy approaching nine courses is often applied. It is not known to which extent the approach to the exceedingly rare subcutaneous Ewing sarcomas might be less aggressive, given their good prognosis.

Active agents are doxorubicin, cyclophosphamide, ifosfamide, vincristine, etoposide, and actinomycin D, so that many of these drugs are usually incorporated in protocols employed both in adults and in children and adolescents [173, 174]. Upfront chemotherapy is often used, followed by surgery of residual localized disease and consolidation chemotherapy. RT is often used in adults, lacking of some constraints in sites which may apply to children.

An open question has to do with the value of high-dose intensification therapy for patients who do not respond optimally to preoperative chemotherapy and for high-risk and metastatic patients. Indeed, there is retrospective evidence that high-dose consolidation therapy may be effective for patients with isolated lung metastases, while disease diffusely metastatic to bone and/or bone marrow is not [175]. However, lacking positive controlled evidence, high-dose therapy is not standard treatment today in any presentation. With regard to extraskeletal Ewing sarcomas, pathologic criteria to assess tumour response to preoperative chemotherapy in bone Ewing sarcoma do not apply [176], and there is uncertainty as to how to stratify prognosis on the basis of the clinical presentation.

Salvage medical therapy may include high-dose ifosfamide, cyclophosphamide + topotecan, temozolomide + irinotecan, or gemcitabine + docetaxel [177–180].

Medical therapy of adult bone sarcomas

Osteosarcoma may occasionally occur in adults. The overall treatment strategy, including medical therapy, should follow the same

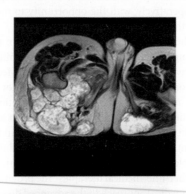
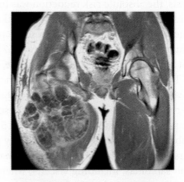

baseline

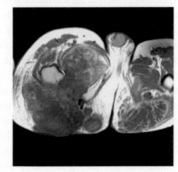
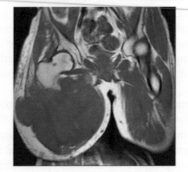

+4 months

Fig. 55.6 Non dimensional tumour response in a chordoma patient to imatinib mesylate.

principles applied in younger patients. Thus, it will include chemotherapy in all cases, with the exception of low-grade osteosarcomas, i.e., paraosteal and periosteal osteosarcoma, and low-grade chondroblastic osteosarcoma of the skull. Clearly, there may be a problem of treatment tolerability depending on age, e.g., ≥ 40. This mainly affects the use of high-dose methotrexate. In fact, in most institutions standard chemotherapy for osteosarcoma includes doxorubicin, cisplatin, and high-dose methotrexate [181]. Randomized evidence in favour of the addition of the latter is lacking, but retrospective studies are available and randomized comparisons have not replicated expected results for standard treatment. High-dose methotrexate may be less tolerated in older patients, so that there are protocols in >40-year-old patients, including high-dose methotrexate only for suboptimally-responding patients. Ifosfamide and etoposide may be added as well in those patients with suboptimal tumour response to preoperative chemotherapy. Aside from high-dose methotrexate, principles of treatment should be the same as in children or adolescents. This means that preoperative chemotherapy is generally used, although with a lack of any randomized evidence supporting the added value of placing medical therapy preoperatively instead of postoperatively. Preoperative chemotherapy is followed by surgery, then by consolidation chemotherapy, which may be tailored to the degree of pathologic response. A macrophage activator, muramil tripeptide, has been associated to some benefit when given upfront in a single randomized trial, with reference to the subgroup receiving ifosfamide (which, however, was shown to be devoid of any added value in the same study), so that its incorporation in standard protocols is still controversial [182]. In metastatic osteosarcoma, treatment is often the same as for localized disease with the addition of surgery of lung metastases, if isolated (i.e., in the absence of extrapulmonary lesions). The prognosis of osteosarcoma patients with isolated lung metastases occurring d'emblée may even parallel prognosis of localized disease when the tumour burden is very low, and in any case benefit from the same approach as for localized disease, plus surgery of lung nodules. When the relapse occurs to the lungs exclusively, the number of lesions and the disease-free interval dictate to which extent further chemotherapy is combined with surgery of metastases, if complete excision of all nodules is feasible [183]. Even the choice of second-line chemotherapy is based on previous treatments and tumour response. High-dose ifosfamide may be an option, while alternate agents are lacking for an effective salvage medical therapy in relapsing osteosarcoma patients, who generally receive virtually all active drugs first-line.

The medical therapy of chondrosarcoma has been poorly investigated [184]. However, it is logical to assume that low-grade chondrosarcomas are poorly responsive to cytotoxic chemotherapy. High-grade chondrosarcomas may have a higher sensitivity to agents used for high-grade sarcomas in general, while it is not yet understood to what extent drugs specifically active in osteosarcoma may be used as well. Mesenchymal chondrosarcomas are aggressive tumours which may display a sensitivity profile such that regimens used in Ewing sarcomas are often used.

Chordomas are poorly sensitive to cytotoxic chemotherapy, with the possible exception of the rare dedifferentiated chordomas. In the last years, molecularly-targeted therapies have been shown to be active in this disease, though their efficacy within the overall treatment strategy is yet to be elucidated. Imatinib has antitumour activity, which is likely related to its anti-PDGFRβ effect [185]. Responses are often unidimensional (Figure 55.6) and

progression-free survival may be in the one-year range. The combination of imatinib with mTOR inhibitors is currently investigated, with evidence of more pronounced dimensional responses. The dual histogenetic profile of chordomas may justify the evidence of activity which was provided for anti-EGFR agents, though it seems to be less remarkable. Strategically, medical therapy may currently find a place in metastatic chordomas as well as locally advanced tumours for which surgery and RT cannot be foreseen, or possibly can be envisaged in case of tumour response.

References

1. Gatta G, van der Zwan JM, Casali PG, Siesling S, Dei Tos AP et al. Rare cancers are not so rare: the rare cancer burden in Europe. European Journal of Cancer 2011; 47: 2493–2511.
2. Fletcher CDM, Unni KK, Mertens F. WHO Classification of Tumours. Pathology and Genetics of Tumours of Soft Tissue and Bone. Lyon: IARC Press, 2002.
3. Fletcher CDM, Bridge JA, Hogendoorn PCW, Mertens F eds. WHO Classification of Tumours of Soft Tissue and Bone. Lyon: IARC, 2013.
4. Bone Sarcomas: ESMO Clinical Practice Guidelines for diagnosis, treatment and follow-up. The ESMO/European Sarcoma Network Working Group. Annals of Oncology 2012; 23(Suppl 7): v100–v109.
5. Mohseny AB, Hogendoorn PC. Concise review: mesenchymal tumors: when stem cells go mad. Stem Cells 2011; 29: 397–403.
6. Trojani M, Contesso G, Coindre JM, Rouesse J, Bui NB et al. Soft-tissue sarcomas of adults; study of pathological prognostic variables and definition of a histopathological grading system. International Journal of Cancer 1984; 33: 37–42.
7. Coindre JM, Terrier P, Bui NB, Bonichon F, Collin F et al. Prognostic factors in adult patients with locally controlled soft tissue sarcoma. A study of 546 patients from the French Federation of Cancer Centers Sarcoma Group. Journal of Clinical Oncology 1996; 14: 869–877.
8. Guillou L, Coindre JM, Bonichon F, Nguyen BB, Terrier P et al. Comparative study of the National Cancer Institute and French Federation of Cancer Centers Sarcoma Group grading systems in a population of 410 adult patients with soft tissue sarcoma. Journal of Clinical Oncology 1997; 15: 350–362.
9. Chibon F, Lagarde P, Salas S, Pérot G, Brouste V et al. Validated prediction of clinical outcome in sarcomas and multiple types of cancer on the basis of a gene expression signature related to genome complexity. Nature Medicine 2010; 16: 781–787.
10. Romeo S, Dei Tos AP. Clinical application of molecular pathology in sarcomas. Current Opinions in Oncology 2011; 23: 379–384.
11. Pierron G, Tirode F, Lucchesi C, Reynaud S, Ballet S, et al. A new subtype of bone sarcoma defined by BCOR-CCNB3 gene fusion. Nature Genetics 2012; 44: 461–466.
12. Mano H. ALKoma: A cancer subtype with a shared target. Cancer Discovery 2012; 2(6): 495–502.
13. Dei Tos AP, Doglioni C, Piccinin S, Sciot R, Furlanetto A et al. Coordinated expression and amplification of the MDM2, CDK4, and HMGI-C genes in atypical lipomatous tumours. Journal of Pathology 2000; 190: 531–536.
14. Binh MB, Sastre-Garau X, Guillou L, de Pinieux G, Terrier P et al. MDM2 and CDK4 immunostainings are useful adjuncts in diagnosing well-differentiated and dedifferentiated liposarcoma subtypes: a comparative analysis of 559 soft tissue neoplasms with genetic data. American Journal of Surgical Pathology 2005; 29: 1340–1347.
15. Lazar AJ, Tuvin D, Hajibashi S, Habeeb S, Bolshakov S et al. Specific mutations in the beta-catenin gene (CTNNB1) correlate with local recurrence in sporadic desmoid tumors. American Journal of Pathology 2008; 173: 1518–1527.
16. Kawai A, Woodruff J, Healy JH, Brennan MF, Antonescu CR et al. SYT-SSX gene fusion as a determinant of morphology and prognosis in synovial sarcoma. New England Journal of Medicine 1998, 338: 153–160.

17. Ladanyi M, Antonescu CR, Leung DH, Woodruff JM, Kawai A et al. Impact of SYT-SSX fusion type on the clinical behavior of synovial sarcoma: a multi-institutional retrospective study of 243 patients. Cancer Research 2002; 62: 135–140.

18. Guillou L, Benhattar J, Bonichon F, Gallagher G, Terrier P et al. Histologic grade, but not SYT-SSX fusion type, is an important prognostic factor in patients with synovial sarcoma: a multicenter, retrospective analysis. Journal of Clinical Oncology 2004; 22: 4040–4050.

19. Stegmaier S, Poremba C, Schaefer KL, Leuschner I, Kazanowska B et al. Prognostic value of PAX-FKHR fusion status in alveolar rhabdomyosarcoma: a report from the cooperative soft tissue sarcoma study group (CWS). Pediatric Blood Cancer 2011; 57: 406–414.

20. Le Deley MC, Delattre O, Schaefer KL, Burchill SA, Koehler G et al. Impact of EWS-ETS fusion type on disease progression in Ewing Sarcoma/Peripheral Primitive Neuroectodermal Tumor: prospective results from the cooperative Euro-E.W.I.N.G. 99 trial. Journal of Clinical Oncology 2010; 28: 1982–1988.

21. Rutkowski P, Van Glabbeke M, Rankin CJ, Ruka W, Rubin BP et al. Imatinib mesylate in advanced dermatofibrosarcoma protuberans: pooled analysis of two phase II clinical trials. Journal of Clinical Oncology 2010; 28: 1772–1779.

22. Wagner AJ, Malinowska-Kolodziej I, Morgan JA, Qin W, Fletcher CD et al. Clinical activity of mTOR inhibition with sirolimus in malignant perivascular epithelioid cell tumors: targeting the pathogenic activation of mTORC1 in tumors. Journal of Clinical Oncology 2010; 28: 835–840.

23. McCormack FX, Inoue Y, Moss J, Singer LG, Strange C et al. Efficacy and safety of sirolimus in lymphangioleiomyomatosis. New England Journal of Medicine 2011; 364: 1595–1606.

24. Singer S, Socci ND, Ambrosini G, Sambol E, Decarolis P et al. Gene expression profiling of liposarcoma identifies distinct biological types/subtypes and potential therapeutic targets in well-differentiated and dedifferentiated liposarcoma. Cancer Research 2007; 67: 6626–6636.

25. Antonescu CR, Yoshida A, Guo T, Chang NE, Zhang L et al. KDR activating mutations in human angiosarcomas are sensitive to specific kinase inhibitors. Cancer Research 2009, 69: 7175–7179.

26. Barretina J, Taylor BS, Banerji S, Ramos AH, Lagos-Quintana M et al. Subtype-specific genomic alterations define new targets for soft-tissue sarcoma therapy. Nature Genetics 2010; 42: 715–721.

27. Ray-Coquard I, Montesco MC, Coindre JM, Dei Tos AP, Lurkin A et al. Sarcoma: concordance between initial diagnosis and centralized expert review in a population-based study within three European regions. Annals of Oncology 2012; 23(9): 2442–2449.

28. Hostein I, Debiec-Rychter M, Olschwang S, Bringuier PP, Toffolati L et al. A quality control program for mutation detection in KIT and PDGFRA in gastrointestinal stromal tumours. Journal of Gastroenterology 2011; 46: 586–594.

29. Enneking WF, Spanier SS, Malawer MM. The effect of the anatomic setting on the results of surgical procedures for soft parts sarcoma of the thigh. Cancer 1981; 47(5): 1005–1022.

30. ESMO/European Sarcoma Network Working Group. Soft tissue and visceral sarcomas: ESMO Clinical Practice Guidelines for diagnosis, treatment and follow-up. Annals of Oncology 2012; 23(Suppl 7): vii92–vii99.

31. Gronchi A, Casali PG, Mariani L, Miceli R, Fiore M et al. Status of surgical margins and prognosis in adult soft tissue sarcomas of the extremities: a series of patients treated at a single institution. Journal of Clinical Oncology 2005; 23: 96–104.

32. Trovik CS, Bauer HC, Alvegard TA, Anderson H, Blomqvist C et al. Surgical margins, local recurrence and metastasis in soft tissue sarcomas: 599 surgically-treated patients from the Scandinavian Sarcoma Group register. European Journal of Cancer 2000; 36: 710–716.

33. Zagars GK, Ballo MT, Pisters PW, Pollock RE, Patel SR et al. Surgical margins and re-excision in the management of patients with soft tissue sarcoma using conservative surgery and radiation therapy. Cancer 2003; 97: 2530–2543.

34. Stojadinovic A, Leung DHY, Hoos A, Jaques DP, Lewis JJ et al. Analysis of the prognostic significance of microscopic margins in 2084 localized primary adult soft tissue sarcomas. Annals of Surgery 2002; 235: 424–434.

35. Gronchi A, Lo Vullo S, Colombo C, Collini P, Stacchiotti S et al. Extremity soft tissue sarcoma in a series of patients treated at a single institution: the local control directly impacts survival. Annals of Surgery 2010; 251: 512–517.

36. Gronchi A, Miceli R, Colombo C, Collini P, Stacchiotti S et al. Primary Extremity Soft Tissue Sarcoma: outcome improvement over time at a single institution. Annals of Oncology 2011; 22(7): 1675–1681.

37. Giuliano AE, Eilber FR. The rationale for planned reoperation after unplanned total excision of soft tissue sarcomas. Journal of Clinical Oncology 1985; 3: 1344–1348.

38. Lewis JJ, Leung D, Espat J, Woodruff JM, Brennan MF. Effect of re-excision in extremity soft tissue sarcoma. Annals of Surgery 2000; 231: 655–663.

39. Fiore M, Casali PG, Miceli R, Mariani L, Bertulli R et al. Prognostic effect of re-excision in adult soft tissue sarcoma of the extremities. Annals of Surgical Oncology 2006; 13(1): 110–117.

40. Gerrand CH, Wunder JS, Kandel RA, O'Sullivan B, Catton CN et al. Classification of positive margins after resection of soft-tissue sarcoma of the limb predicts the risk of local recurrence. Journal of Bone and Joint Surgery (British Ed.) 2001; 83(8): 1149–1155.

41. Dagan R, Indelicato DJ, McGee L, Morris CG, Kirwan et al. The significance of a marginal excision after preoperative radiation therapy for soft tissue sarcoma of the extremity. Cancer 2012; 118(12): 3199–3207.

42. Al Yami A, Griffin AM, Ferguson PC, Catton CN, Chung PW et al. Positive surgical margins in soft tissue sarcoma treated with preoperative radiation: is a postoperative boost necessary? International Journal of Radiation Oncology Biology Physics 2010; 77(4): 1191–1197.

43. Gronchi A, Verderio P, De Paoli A, Ferraro A, Tendero O et al. Quality of surgery and neoadjuvant combined therapy in the ISG-GEIS trial on soft tissue sarcomas of limbs and trunk wall. Annals of Oncology 2013; 24(3): 817–823.

44. Colombo C, R Randall L, Andtbacka RH, Gronchi A. A new surgical perspective in soft tissue sarcoma (STS) management: more conservative in ESTS (Extremity Soft Tissue Sarcoma), more extended in RSTS (Retroperitoneal Soft Tissue Sarcoma). Expert Reviews of Anticancer Therapy 2012; 12(8): 1079–1087.

45. Kawaguchi N, Ahmed AR, Matsumoto S, Manabe J, Matsushita Y. The concept of curative margin in surgery for bone and soft tissue sarcoma. Clinical Orthopaedics and Related Research 2004; 419: 165–172.

46. Bonvalot S, Raut CP, Pollock RE, Rutkowski P, Strauss DC et al. Technical considerations in surgery for retroperitoneal sarcomas: position paper from E-Surge, a master class in sarcoma surgery, and EORTC–STBSG. Annals of Surgical Oncology 2012; 19: 2981–2991.

47. Gronchi A, Lo Vullo S, Fiore M, Mussi C, Stacchiotti S et al. Aggressive surgical policies in a retrospectively reviewed single-institution case series of retroperitoneal soft tissue sarcoma patients. Journal of Clinical Oncology 2009; 27: 24–30.

48. Bonvalot S, Rivoire M, Castaing M, Stoeckle E, Le Cesne A et al. Primary retroperitoneal sarcomas: a multivariate analysis of surgical factors associated with local control. Journal of Clinical Oncology 2009; 27: 31–37.

49. Pisters PW. Resection of some—but not all—clinically uninvolved adjacent viscera as part of surgery for retroperitoneal soft tissue sarcomas. Journal of Clinical Oncology 2009; 27: 6–8.

50. Gronchi A, Bonvalot S, Le Cesne A, Casali PG. Resection of uninvolved adjacent organs can be part of surgery for retroperitoneal soft tissue sarcoma. Journal of Clinical Oncology 2009; 27: 2106–2107.

51. Bonvalot S, Miceli R, Berselli M, Causeret S, Colombo C et al. Aggressive surgery in retroperitoneal soft tissue sarcoma carried out at high-volume centers is safe and is associated with improved local control. Annals of Surgical Oncology 2010; 17: 1507–1514.

52. Raut CP, Swallow CJ. Are radical compartmental resections for retroperitoneal sarcomas justified? Annals Surgical Oncology 2010; 17: 1481–1484.

53. Gronchi A, Miceli R, Colombo C, Stacchiotti S, Collini P et al. Frontline extended surgery is associated with improved survival in

retroperitoneal low-intermediate grade soft tissue sarcomas. Annals of Oncology 2012; 23(4): 1067–1073.

54. Lewis JJ, Leung D, Woodruff JM, Brennan MF. Retroperitoneal soft-tissue sarcoma: analysis of 500 patients treated and followed at a single institution. Annals of Surgery 1998; 228: 355–365.

55. Stoeckle E, Coindre JM, Bonvalot S, Kantor G, Terrier P et al. Prognostic factors in retroperitoneal sarcoma: a multivariate analysis of a series of 165 patients of the French Cancer Center Federation Sarcoma Group. Cancer 2001; 92: 359–368.

56. Ferrario T, Karakousis CP. Retroperitoneal sarcomas: grade and survival. Archives of Surgery 2003; 138: 248–251.

57. Kilkenny JW, Bland KI, Copel EM. Retroperitoneal sarcoma: The University of Florida experience. Journal of the American College of Surgeons 1996; 182: 329–339.

58. Hassan I, Park SZ, Donohue JH, Nagorney DM, Kay PA et al. Operative management of primary retroperitoneal sarcomas: a reappraisal of an institutional experience. Annals of Surgery 2004; 239: 244–250.

59. van Dalen T, Plooij JM, van Coevorden F, van Geel AN, Hoekstra HJ et al. Long-term prognosis of primary retroperitoneal soft tissue sarcoma. European Journal of Surgical Oncology 2007; 33: 234–238.

60. Lehnert T, Cardona S, Hinz U, Willeke F, Mechtersheimer G et al. Primary and locally recurrent retroperitoneal soft-tissue sarcoma: local control and survival. European Journal of Surgical Oncology 2009; 35: 986–993.

61. Strauss DC, Hayes AJ, Thway K, Moskovic EC, Fisher C et al. Surgical management of primary retroperitoneal sarcoma. British Journal of Surgery 2010; 101: 520–523.

62. Sommerville SM, Patton JT, Luscombe JC, Mangham DC, Grimer RJ. Clinical outcomes of deep atypical lipomas (well-differentiated lipoma-like liposarcomas) of the extremities. ANZ Journal of Surgery 2005; 75(9): 803–806.

63. Hogg ME, Wayne JD. Atypical lipomatous tumor/well-differentiated liposarcoma: what is it? Surgical Oncology Clinics of North America 2012; 21(2): 333–340.

64. Mussi C, Collini P, Miceli R, Barisella M, Mariani L et al. Prognostic impact of dedifferentiation in retroperitoneal liposarcoma: a series of patients surgically treated at a single institution. Cancer 2008; 113: 1657–1665.

65. Fiore M, Grosso F, Lo Vullo S, Pennacchioli E, Stacchiotti S et al. Myxoid/round cell and pleomorphic liposarcoma: prognostic factors and survival in a series of patients treated at a single institution. Cancer 2007; 109: 2522–2531.

66. Antonescu CR, Tschernyavsky SJ, Decuseara R, Leung DH, Woodruff JM et al. Prognostic impact of P53 status, TLS-CHOP fusion transcript structure, and histological grade in myxoid liposarcoma: a molecular and clinicopathologic study of 82 cases. Clinical Cancer Research 2001; 7(12): 3977–3987.

67. Hoffman A, Ghadimi MP, Demicco EG, Creighton CJ, Torres K et al. Localized and metastatic myxoid/round cell liposarcoma: clinical and molecular observations. Cancer 2013; 119(10): 1868–1877.

68. Moreau LC, Turcotte R, Ferguson P, Wunder J, Clarkson P et al. Myxoid\round cell liposarcoma (MRCLS) revisited: an analysis of 418 primarily managed cases. Annals of Surgical Oncology 2012; 19(4): 1081–1088.

69. Jones RL, Fisher C, Al-Muderis O, Judson IR. Differential sensitivity of liposarcoma subtypes to chemotherapy. European Journal of Cancer 2005; 41(18): 2853–2860.

70. Grosso F, Jones RL, Demetri GD, Judson IR, Blay JY et al. Efficacy of trabectedin (ET-743) in advanced pre- treated myxoid liposarcomas. Lancet Oncology 2007; 8(7): 595–602.

71. Chung PW, Deheshi BM, Ferguson PC, Wunder JS, Griffin AM et al. Radiosensitivity translates into excellent local control in extremity myxoid liposarcoma: a comparison with other soft tissue sarcomas. Cancer 2009; 115(14): 3254–3261.

72. Gronchi A, Bui BN, Bonvalot S, Pilotti S, Ferrari S et al. Phase II clinical trial of neoadjuvant trabectedine in patients with advanced localized myxoid liposarcoma. Annals of Oncology 2012; 23(3): 771–776.

73. Wang WL, Katz D, Araujo DM, Ravi V, Ludwig JA et al. Extensive adipocytic maturation can be seen in myxoid liposarcomas treated with neoadjuvant doxorubicin and ifosfamide and pre-operative radiation therapy. Clinical Sarcoma Research 2012; 2(1): 25.

74. Fiore M, Miceli R, Mussi C, Lo Vullo S, Mariani L et al. Dermatofibrosarcoma protuberans treated at a single institution: a surgical disease with a high cure rate. Journal of Clinical Oncology 2005; 23: 7669–7675.

75. Miller SJ, Alam M, Andersen JS, Berg D, Bichakjian CK et al. Dermatofibrosarcoma protuberans. Journal of the National Comprehensive Cancer Network 2012; 10(3): 312–328.

76. Cai H, Wang Y, Wu J, Shi Y. Dermatofibrosarcoma protuberans: clinical diagnoses and treatment results of 260 cases in China. Journal of Surgical Oncology 2012; 105(2): 142–148.

77. Colombo C, Miceli R, Collini P, Radaelli S, Palassini E et al. Leiomyosarcoma and sarcoma with myogenic differentiation: two different entities or two faces of the same disease? Cancer 2012; 118(21): 5349–5357.

78. Gladdy RA, Qin LX, Moraco N, Agaram NP, Brennan MF et al. Predictors of survival and recurrence in primary leiomyosarcoma. Annals of Surgical Oncology 2013; 20(6): 1851–1857.

79. Aggarwal G, Sharma S, Zheng M, Reid MD, Crosby JH et al. Primary leiomyosarcomas of the gastrointestinal tract in the post-gastrointestinal stromal tumor era. Annals of Diagnostic Pathology 2012; 16(6): 532–540.

80. Fiore M, Colombo C, Locati P, Berselli M, Radaelli S et al. Surgical technique, morbidity, and outcome of primary retroperitoneal sarcoma involving inferior vena cava. Annals of Surgical Oncology 2012; 19(2): 511–518.

81. Abraham JA, Weaver MJ, Hornick JL, Zurakowski D, Ready JE. Outcomes and prognostic factors for a consecutive case series of 115 patients with somatic leiomyosarcoma. Journal of Bone and Joint Surgery America 2012; 94(8): 736–744.

82. Fletcher CD, Gustafson P, Rydholm A, Willén H, Akerman M. Clinicopathologic re-evaluation of 100 malignant fibrous histiocytomas: prognostic relevance of subclassification. Journal of Clinical Oncology 2001; 19: 3045–3050.

83. Carneiro A, Francis P, Bendahl PO, Fernebro J, Akerman M et al. Indistinguishable genomic profiles and shared prognostic markers in undifferentiated pleomorphic sarcoma and leiomyosarcoma: different sides of a single coin? Laboratory Investigation 2009; 89(6): 668–675.

84. Canter RJ, Qin LX, Maki RG, Brennan MF, Ladanyi M et al. A synovial sarcoma-specific preoperative nomogram supports a survival benefit to ifosfamide-based chemotherapy and improves risk stratification for patients. Clinical Cancer Research 2008; 14(24): 8191–8197.

85. Ferrari A, Gronchi A, Casanova M, Meazza C, Gandola L et al. Synovial sarcoma: a retrospective analysis of 271 patients of all ages treated at a single institution. Cancer 2004; 101(3): 627–634.

86. Ghadimi MP, Liu P, Peng T, Bolshakov S, Young ED et al. Pleomorphic liposarcoma: clinical observations and molecular variables. Cancer 2011; 117(23): 5359–5369.

87. Sanfilippo R, Miceli R, Grosso F, Fiore M, Puma E et al. Myxofibrosarcoma: prognostic factors and survival in a series of patients treated at a single institution. Annals of Surgical Oncology 2011; 18(3): 720–725.

88. Haglund KE, Raut CP, Nascimento AF, Wang Q, George S et al. Recurrence patterns and survival for patients with intermediate- and high-grade myxofibrosarcoma. International Journal of Radiation Oncology Biology Physics 2012; 82(1): 361–367.

89. Mutter RW, Singer S, Zhang Z, Brennan MF, Alektiar KM. The enigma of myxofibrosarcoma of the extremity. Cancer 2012; 118(2): 518–527.

90. Look Hong NJ, Hornicek FJ, Raskin KA, Yoon SS, Szymonifka J et al. Prognostic factors and outcomes of patients with myxofibrosarcoma. Annals of Surgical Oncology 2013; 20(1): 80–86.

91. Anghileri M, Miceli R, Fiore M, Mariani L, Ferrari A et al. Malignant peripheral nerve sheath tumors: prognostic factors and survival in a series of patients treated at a single institution. Cancer 2006; 107(5): 1065–1074.

92. Kolberg M, Høland M, Agesen TH, Brekke HR, Liestøl K et al. Survival meta-analyses for >1800 malignant peripheral nerve sheath tumor patients with and without neurofibromatosis type 1. Neurological Oncology 2013; 15(2): 135–147.

93. Kamran SC, Howard SA, Shinagare AB, Krajewski KM, Jagannathan JP et al. Malignant peripheral nerve sheath tumors: prognostic impact of rhabdomyoblastic differentiation (malignant triton tumors), neurofibromatosis 1 status and location. European Journal of Surgical Oncology 2013; 39(1): 46–52.

94. Lindet C, Neuville A, Penel N, Lae M, Michels JJ et al. Localised angiosarcomas: the identification of prognostic factors and analysis of treatment impact. A retrospective analysis from the French Sarcoma Group (GSF/GETO). European Journal of Cancer 2013; 49(2): 369–376.

95. Fayette J, Martin E., Piperno-Neumann S, Le Cesne A, Robert C et al. Angiosarcomas, a heterogeneous group of sarcomas with specific behavior depending on primary site: a retrospective study of 161 cases. Annals of Oncology 2007; 18: 2030–2036.

96. Fury MG, Antonescu CR, Van Zee KJ, Brennan MF, Maki RG. A 14-year retrospective review of angiosarcoma: clinical characteristics, prognostic factors, and treatment outcomes with surgery and chemotherapy. Cancer Journal 2005; 11: 241–247.

97. Lahat G, Dhuka AR, Hallevi H, Xiao L, Zou C et al. Angiosarcoma: clinical and molecular insights. Annals of Surgery 2010; 251: 1098–1106.

98. Sakharpe A, Lahat G, Gulamhusein T, Liu P, Bolshakov S et al. Epithelioid sarcoma and unclassified sarcoma with epithelioid features: clinicopathological variables, molecular markers, and a new experimental model. Oncologist 2011; 16(4): 512–522.

99. Baratti D, Pennacchioli E, Casali PG, Bertulli R, Lozza L et al. Epithelioid sarcoma: prognostic factors and survival in a series of patients treated at a single institution. Annals of Surgical Oncology 2007; 14(12): 3542–3551.

100. Hocar O, Le Cesne A, Berissi S, Terrier P, Bonvalot S et al. Clear cell sarcoma (malignant melanoma) of soft parts: a clinicopathologic study of 52 cases. Dermatology Research and Practice 2012; 2012:984096. doi: 10.1155/2012/984096. Epub 2012 May 30.

101. Andreou D, Boldt H, Werner M, Hamann C, Pink D et al. Sentinel node biopsy in soft tissue sarcoma subtypes with a high propensity for regional lymphatic spread—results of a large prospective trial. Annals of Oncology 2013 24(5): 1400–1405.

102. Hornick JL, Dal Cin P, Fletcher CD. Loss of INI1 expression is characteristic of both conventional and proximal-type epithelioid sarcoma. American Journal of Surgical Pathology 2009; 33(4): 542–550.

103. Sheth GR, Cranmer LD, Smith BD, Grasso-Lebeau L, Lang JE. Radiation-induced sarcoma of the breast: a systematic review. Oncologist 2012; 17(3): 405–418.

104. Gladdy RA, Qin LX, Moraco N, Edgar MA, Antonescu CR et al. Do radiation-associated soft tissue sarcomas have the same prognosis as sporadic soft tissue sarcomas? Journal of Clinical Oncology 2010; 28(12): 2064–2069.

105. Enneking WF. A system for staging musculoskeletal neoplasms. Clinical Orthopaedic and Related Research 1986; 204: 9–24.

106. Enneking WF. An abbreviated history of orthopaedic oncology in North America. Clinical Orthopaedic and Related Research 2000; 374: 115–124.

107. Gherlinzoni F, Picci P, Bacci G, Campanacci D. Limb sparing versus amputation in osteosarcoma. Correlation between local control, surgical margins and tumor necrosis. Instituto Rizzoli experience. Annals of Oncology 1992; 3(Suppl 2): S23–S27.

108. Mankin HJ, Doppelt SH, Sullivan TR, Tomford WW. Osteoarticular and intercalary allograft transplantation in the management of malignant tumors of bone. Cancer 1982: 50: 613–630.

109. Mankin HJ, Fogelson JF, Thrasher AZ, Jaffer F. Massive resection and allograft transplantation in the treatment of malignant bone tumors. New England Journal of Medicine 1976: 294: 1247–1255.

110. White J, Toy P, Gibbs P, Enneking W, Scarborough M. The current practice of orthopaedic oncology in North America. Clinical Orthopaedic and Related Research 2010; 468(11): 2840–2853.

111. Enneking WF, Durnham WK. Resection and reconstruction for primary neoplasms involving the innominate bone. Journal of Bone and Joint Surgery American 1996; 6: 266–267.

112. Schwartz A, Eckardt MD, Beauchamp CP. Internal hemipelvectomy of musculoskeletal tumors—indications and options for reconstruction. US Journal of Oncology and Hematology 2011; 7: 123–125.

113. Sherman CE, O'Connor MI, Sim FH. Survival, local recurrence, and function after pelvic limb salvage at 23 to 38 years of followup. Clinical Orthopaedic and Related Research 2012; 470(3): 712–727.

114. Gennari L, Azzarelli A, Quagliuolo V. A posterior approach for the excision of sacral chordoma. Journal of Bone and Joint Surgery (British Ed.) 1987; 69(4): 565–568.

115. Todd LT Jr, Yaszemski MJ, Currier BL, Fuchs B, Kim CW et al. Bowel and bladder function after major sacral resection. Clinical Orthopaedic and Related Research 2002; 397: 36–39.

116. Mukherjee D, Chaichana KL, Parker SL, Gokaslan ZL, McGirt MJ. Association of surgical resection and survival in patients with malignant primary osseous spinal neoplasms from the Surveillance, Epidemiology, and End Results (SEER) database. European Spine Journal 2013; 22(6): 1375–1382.

117. Malhas AM, Grimer RJ, Abudu A, Carter SR, Tillman RM et al. The final diagnosis in patients with a suspected primary malignancy of bone. Journal of Bone and Joint Surgery (British Ed.) 2011; 93-B: 980–983.

118. Hansen MF, Seton M, Merchant A. Osteosarcoma in Paget's disease of bone. Journal of Bone and Mineral Research 2006; 21(Suppl 2): 58–63.

119. Grimer RJ, Cannon SR, Taminiau AHM, Bielack S, Kempf-Bielack B et al. Osteosarcoma over the age of forty. European Journal of Cancer 2003; 39: 157–163.

120. Bielack SS, Machatschek JN, Flege S, Jürgens H. Delaying surgery with chemotherapy for osteosarcoma of the extremities. Expert Opinion on Pharmacotherapy 2004; 5: 1243–1256.

121. Goorin AM, Schwartzentruber DJ, Devidas M, Gebhardt MC, Ayala AG et al. Presurgical chemotherapy compared with immediate surgery and adjuvant chemotherapy for nonmetastatic osteosarcoma: Pediatric Oncology Group Study POG-8651. Journal of Clinical Oncology 2003; 21: 1574–1580.

122. Grimer RJ, Bielack S, Flege S, Cannon SR, Foleras G et al. Periosteal osteosarcoma—a European review of outcome. European Journal of Cancer 2005; 41: 2806–2811.

123. Cesari M, Alberghini M, Vanel D, Palmerini E, Staals EL et al. Periosteal osteosarcoma: a single institution experience. Cancer 2011; 117(8): 1731–1735.

124. Schuck A, Ahrens S, Paulussen M, Kuhlen M, Könemann S et al. Local therapy in localized Ewing tumors: results of 1058 patients treated in the CESS 81, CESS 86, and EICESS 92 trials. International Journal of Radiation Oncology Biology Physics 2003; 55: 168–177.

125. Bernstein M, Kovar H, Paulussen M Randall RL, Schuck A et al. Ewing's sarcoma family of tumors: current management. Oncologist 2006; 11: 503–519.

126. Gelderblom H, Hogendoorn PCW, Dijkstra SD, van Rijswijk CS, Krol AD et al. The clinical approach towards chondrosarcoma. Oncologist 2008; 13: 320–329.

127. Riedel RF, Larrier N, Dodd L, Kirsch D, Martinez S et al. The clinical management of chondrosarcoma. Current Treatment Options in Oncology 2009; 10: 94–106.

128. Dickey ID, Rose PS, Fuchs B, Wold LE, Okuno SH et al. Dedifferentiated chondrosarcoma: the role of chemotherapy with updated outcomes. Journal of Bone and Joint Surgery American 2004; 86-A: 2412–2418.

129. Grimer RJ, Gosheger G, Taminiau A, Biau D, Matejovsky Z et al. Dedifferentiated chondrosarcoma: prognostic factors and outcome from a European group. European Journal of Cancer 2007; 43: 2060–2065.

130. Stacchiotti S, Casali PG, Lo Vullo S, Mariani L, Palassini E et al. Chordoma of the Mobile Spine and Sacrum: A Retrospective Analysis of a Series of Patients Surgically Treated at Two Referral Centers. Annals of Surgical Oncology 2010; 17: 211–219.

131. Boriani S, Bandiera S, Biagini R, Bacchini P, Boriani L et al. Chordoma of the mobile spine: fifty years of experience. Spine 2006; 31: 493–503.

132. Noel G, Feuvret L, Ferrand R, Boisserie G, Mazeron JJ et al. Radiotherapeutic factors in the management of cervical-basal chordomas and chondrosarcomas. Neurosurgery 2004; 55: 1252–1260.

133. Schulz-Ertner D, Nikoghosyan A, Thilmann C, Haberer T, Jäkel O et al. Results of carbon ion radiotherapy in 152 patients. International Journal of Radiation Oncology Biology Physics 2004; 58: 631–640.

134. Pisters PWT, Harrison LB, Leung DHY, Woodruff JM, Casper ES et al. Long-term results of a prospective randomized trial of adjuvant brachytherapy in soft tissue sarcoma. Journal of Clinical Oncology 1996; 14: 859–868.

135. Yang JC, Chang AE, Sindelar WF, Danforth DN, Topalian SL et al. Randomized prospective study of the benefit of adjuvant radiation therapy in the treatment of soft tissue sarcomas of the extremity. Journal of Clinical Oncology 1998; 16: 197–203.

136. Pisters PW, O'Sullivan B, Maki RG. Evidence-based recommendations for local therapy for soft tissue sarcomas. Journal of Clinical Oncology 2007; 25(8): 1003–1038.

137. O'Sullivan B, Davis AM, Turcotte R, Bell R, Catton C et al. Preoperative versus postoperative radiotherapy in soft-tissue sarcoma of the limbs: a randomised trial. Lancet 2002; 359: 2235–2241.

138. Delaney TF. Radiation therapy: neoadjuvant, adjuvant, or not at all. Surgical Oncology Clinics of North America 2012; 21(2): 215–241.

139. ESMO/European Sarcoma Network Working Group. Soft tissue and visceral sarcomas: ESMO Clinical Practice Guidelines for diagnosis, treatment and follow-up. Annals of Oncology 2012; 23(Suppl 7): vii92–vii99.

140. Le Péchoux C, Musat E, Baey C, Al Mokhles H, Terrier P et al. Should adjuvant radiotherapy be administered in addition to front-line aggressive surgery (FAS) in patients with primary retroperitoneal sarcoma? Annals of Oncology 2013; 24(3): 832–837.

141. Pawlik TM, Pisters PW, Mikula L, Feig BW, Hunt KK et al. Long-term results of two prospective trials of preoperative external beam radiotherapy for localized intermediate- or high-grade retroperitoneal soft tissue sarcoma. Annals of Surgical Oncology 2006; 13(4): 508–517.

142. McBride SM, Raut CP, Lapidus M, Devlin PM, Marcus KJ et al. Locoregional recurrence after preoperative radiation therapy for retroperitoneal sarcoma: adverse impact of multifocal disease and potential implications of dose escalation. Annals of Surgical Oncology 2013; 20(7): 2140–2147.

143. Engelsman M, DeLaney TF, Hong TS. Proton radiotherapy: the biological effect of treating alternating subsets of fields for different treatment fractions. International Journal of Radiation Oncology Biology Physics 2011; 79(2): 616–622.

144. DeLaney TF, Liebsch NJ, Pedlow FX, Adams J, Dean S et al. Phase II study of high-dose photon/proton radiotherapy in the management of spine sarcomas. International Journal of Radiation Oncology Biology Physics 2009; 74(3): 732–739.

145. Nishida Y, Kamada T, Imai R, Tsukushi S, Yamada Y et al. Clinical outcome of sacral chordoma with carbon ion radiotherapy compared with surgery. International Journal of Radiation Oncology Biology Physics 2011; 79(1): 110–116.

146. Nikoghosyan AV, Rauch G, Münter MW, Jensen AD, Combs SE et al. Randomised trial of proton vs. carbon ion radiation therapy in patients with low and intermediate grade chondrosarcoma of the skull base, clinical phase III study. BMC Cancer 2010; 10: 606.

147. Potratz J, Dirksen U, Jürgens H Craft A. Ewing sarcoma: clinical state-of-the-art. Pediatric Hematology and Oncology 2012; 29(1): 1–11.

148. Judson I, Verweij J, Gelderblom H, Hartmann JT, Schöffski P et al. Doxorubicin alone versus intensified doxorubicin plus ifosfamide for first-line treatment of advanced or metastatic soft-tissue sarcoma: a randomised controlled phase 3 trial. Lancet Oncology 2014; 15(4): 415–423.

149. Lorigan P, Verweij J, Papai Z, Rodenhuis S, Le Cesne A et al. Phase III trial of two investigational schedules of ifosfamide compared with standard-dose doxorubicin in advanced or metastatic soft tissue sarcoma: a European Organisation for Research and Treatment of Cancer Soft Tissue and Bone Sarcoma Group Study. Journal of Clinical Oncology 2007; 25: 3144–3150.

150. Le Cesne A, Antoine E, Spielmann M, Le Chevalier T, Brain E et al. High-dose ifosfamide: circumvention of resistance to standard-dose ifosfamide in advanced soft tissue sarcomas. Journal of Clinical Oncology 1995; 13: 1600–1608.

151. Meazza C, Casanova M, Luksch R, Podda M, Favini F et al. Prolonged 14-day continuous infusion of high-dose ifosfamide with an external portable pump: feasibility and efficacy in refractory pediatric sarcoma. Pediatric Blood Cancer 2010; 55: 617–620.

152. Garcia del Muro X, Lopez-Pousa A, Martin J, Buesa JM, Martinez-Trufero J et al. Spanish Group for Research on Sarcomas. A phase II trial of temozolomide as a 6-week, continuous, oral schedule in patients with advanced soft tissue sarcoma: a study by the Spanish Group for Research on Sarcomas. Cancer 2005; 104: 1706–1712.

153. Casali PG. Histology- and non-histology-driven therapy for treatment of soft tissue sarcomas. Annals of Oncology 2012; 23(Suppl 10): 167–169.

154. Duffaud F, Pautier P, Bui Nguyen B, Hensley ML, Rey A et al. A pooled analysis of the final results of the two randomized Phase II studies comparing gemcitabine (G) vs gemcitabine + docetaxel (G+D) in patients (pts) with metastatic/relapsed leiomyosarcoma (LMS). Annals of Oncology 2010; 21(Suppl 8): viii408.

155. Stacchiotti S, Palassini E, Sanfilippo R, Vincenzi B, Arena MG et al. Gemcitabine in advanced angiosarcoma: a retrospective case series analysis from the Italian Rare Cancer Network. Annals of Oncology 2012; 23: 501–518.

156. Penel N, Bui BN, Bay JO, Cupissol D, Ray-Coquard I, et al. Phase II trial of weekly paclitaxel for unresectable angiosarcoma: the ANGIOTAX Study. Journal of Clinical Oncology 2008; 26: 5269–5274.

157. Maki RG, Wathen JK, Patel SR, Priebat DA, Okuno SH et al. Randomized phase II study of gemcitabine and docetaxel compared with gemcitabine alone in patients with metastatic soft tissue sarcomas: results of sarcoma alliance for research through collaboration study 002. Journal of Clinical Oncology 2007; 25: 2755–2763.

158. Demetri GD, Chawla SP, von Mehren M, Ritch P, Baker LH et al. Efficacy and safety of trabectedin in patients with advanced or metastatic liposarcoma or leiomyosarcoma after failure of prior anthracyclines and ifosfamide: results of a randomized phase II study of two different schedules. Journal of Clinical Oncology 2009; 27: 4188–4196.

159. Grosso F, Sanfilippo R, Virdis E, Piovesan C, Collini P et al. Trabectedin in myxoid liposarcomas (MLS): a long-term analysis of a single-institution series. Annals of Oncology 2009; 20: 1439–1444.

160. Stacchiotti S, Pedeutour F, Negri T, Conca E, Marrari A et al. Dermatofibrosarcoma protuberans-derived fibrosarcoma: clinical history, biological profile and sensitivity to imatinib. International Journal of Cancer 2011; 129: 1761–1772.

161. Butrynski JE, D'Adamo DR, Hornick JL, Dal Cin P, Antonescu CR et al. Crizotinib in ALK-rearranged inflammatory myofibroblastic tumor. New England Journal of Medicine 2010; 363: 1727–1733.

162. Demetri GD, Chawla SP, Ray-Coquard IL, Le Cesne A, Staddon AP et al. Results of an international randomized phase III trial of the mammalian target of rapamycin inhibitor ridaforolimus versus placebo to control metastatic sarcomas in patients after benefit from prior chemotherapy. Journal of Clinical Oncology 2013; 31(19): 2485–2492.

163. van der Graaf WT, Blay JY, Chawla SP, Kim DW, Bui-Nguyen B et al. EORTC Soft Tissue and Bone Sarcoma Group; PALETTE study group. Pazopanib for metastatic soft-tissue sarcoma (PALETTE): a randomised, double-blind, placebo-controlled phase 3 trial. Lancet 2012; 379: 1879–1886.

164. Stacchiotti S, Negri T, Zaffaroni N, Palassini E, Morosi C et al. Sunitinib in advanced alveolar soft part sarcoma: evidence of a direct antitumor effect. Annals of Oncology 2011; 22: 1682–1690.

165. Stacchiotti S, Negri T, Palassini E, Conca E, Gronchi A et al. Sunitinib malate and figitumumab in solitary fibrous tumor: patterns and molecular bases of tumor response. Molecular Cancer Therapy 2010; 9: 1286–1297.

166. Park MS, Patel SR, Ludwig JA, Trent JC, Conrad CA et al. Activity of temozolomide and bevacizumab in the treatment of locally advanced, recurrent, and metastatic hemangiopericytoma and malignant solitary fibrous tumor. Cancer 2011; 117(21): 4939–4947.

167. Frustaci S, Gherlinzoni F, De Paoli A, Bonetti M, Azzarelli A et al. Adjuvant chemotherapy for adult soft tissue sarcomas of the extremities and girdles: results of the Italian randomized cooperative trial. Journal of Clinical Oncology 2001; 19: 1238–1247.

168. Woll PJ, Reichardt P, Le Cesne A, Bonvalot S, Azzarelli A et al. EORTC Soft Tissue and Bone Sarcoma Group and the NCIC Clinical Trials Group Sarcoma Disease Site Committee. Adjuvant chemotherapy with doxorubicin, ifosfamide, and lenograstim for resected soft-tissue sarcoma (EORTC 62931): a multicentre randomised controlled trial. Lancet Oncology 2012; 13: 1045–1054.

169. Pervaiz N, Colterjohn N, Farrokhyar F, Tozer R, Figueredo A et al. A systematic meta-analysis of randomized controlled trials of adjuvant chemotherapy for localized resectable soft-tissue sarcoma. Cancer 2008; 113: 573–581.

170. Gronchi A, Frustaci S, Mercuri M, Martin J, Lopez-Pousa A et al. Short, full-dose adjuvant chemotherapy in high-risk adult soft tissue sarcomas: a randomized clinical trial from the Italian Sarcoma Group and the Spanish Sarcoma Group. Journal of Clinical Oncology 2012; 30: 850–856.

171. Roth JA, Putnam JB Jr, Wesley MN, Rosenberg SA. Differing determinants of prognosis following resection of pulmonary metastases from osteogenic and soft tissue sarcoma patients. Cancer 1985; 55: 1361–1366.

172. Deroose JP, Eggermont AM, van Geel AN, Burger JW, den Bakker MA et al. Long-term results of tumor necrosis factor alpha- and melphalan-based isolated limb perfusion in locally advanced extremity soft tissue sarcomas. Journal of Clinical Oncology 2011; 29: 4036–4044.

173. Nesbit ME Jr, Gehan EA, Burgert EO Jr, Vietti TJ, Cangir A et al. Multimodal therapy for the management of primary, nonmetastatic Ewing's sarcoma of bone: a long-term follow-up of the First Intergroup study. Journal of Clinical Oncology 1990; 8: 1664–1674.

174. Grier HE, Krailo MD, Tarbell NJ, Link MP, Fryer CJ et al. Addition of ifosfamide and etoposide to standard chemotherapy for Ewing's sarcoma and primitive neuroectodermal tumor of bone. New England Journal of Medicine 2003; 348: 694–701.

175. Luksch R, Tienghi A, Hall KS, Fagioli F, Picci P et al. Primary metastatic Ewing's family tumors: results of the Italian Sarcoma Group and Scandinavian Sarcoma Group ISG/SSG IV Study including myeloablative chemotherapy and total-lung irradiation. Annals of Oncology 2012; 23: 2970–2976.

176. Picci P, Rougraff BT, Bacci G, Neff JR, Sangiorgi L et al. Prognostic significance of histopathologic response to chemotherapy in non-metastatic Ewing's sarcoma of the extremities. Journal of Clinical Oncology 1993; 11: 1763–1769.

177. Ferrari S, del Prever AB, Palmerini E, Staals E, Berta M et al. Response to high-dose ifosfamide in patients with advanced/recurrent Ewing sarcoma. Pediatric Blood Cancer 2009; 52: 581–584.

178. Farhat R, Raad R, Khoury NJ, Feghaly J, Eid T et al. Cyclophosphamide and topotecan as first-line salvage therapy in patients with relapsed Ewing sarcoma at a single institution. Journal of Pediatric Hematology and Oncology 2013; 35(5): 356–360.

179. Casey DA, Wexler LH, Merchant MS, Chou AJ, Merola PR et al. Irinotecan and temozolomide for Ewing sarcoma: the Memorial Sloan-Kettering experience. Pediatric Blood Cancer 2009; 53: 1029–1034.

180. Rapkin L, Qayed M, Brill P, Martin M, Clark D et al. Gemcitabine and docetaxel (GEMDOX) for the treatment of relapsed and refractory pediatric sarcomas. Pediatric Blood Cancer 2012; 59: 854–858.

181. Ferrari S, Ruggieri P, Cefalo G, Tamburini A, Capanna R et al. Neoadjuvant chemotherapy with methotrexate, cisplatin, and doxorubicin with or without ifosfamide in nonmetastatic osteosarcoma of the extremity: an Italian sarcoma group trial ISG/OS-1. Journal of Clinical Oncology 2012; 30: 2112–2118.

182. Meyers PA, Schwartz CL, Krailo MD, Healey JH, Bernstein ML et al. Children's Oncology Group. Osteosarcoma: the addition of muramyl tripeptide to chemotherapy improves overall survival—a report from the Children's Oncology Group. Journal of Clinical Oncology 2008; 26: 633–638.

183. Putnam JB Jr, Roth JA, Wesley MN, Johnston MR, Rosenberg SA. Survival following aggressive resection of pulmonary metastases from osteogenic sarcoma: analysis of prognostic factors. Annals of Thoracic Surgery 1983; 36: 516–523.

184. Riedel RF, Larrier N, Dodd L, Kirsch D, Martinez S et al. The clinical management of chondrosarcoma. Current Treatment Options in Oncology 2009; 10: 94–106.

185. Stacchiotti S, Longhi A, Ferraresi V, Grignani G, Comandone A et al. Phase II study of imatinib in advanced chordoma. Journal of Clinical Oncology 2012; 30: 914–920.

CHAPTER 56

Craniospinal malignancies

Puneet Plaha, Allyson Parry, Pieter Pretorius,
Michael Brada, Olaf Ansorge, and Claire Blesing

Tumours of the central nervous system

Epidemiology and aetiology

Compared with other cancers, primary neoplasms of the brain and spinal cord in adults are relatively rare. They comprise approximately 1.5% of all cancers. There are an estimated 6.4 new cases per 100 000 people per year and the lifetime risk is 0.6% [1].

The aetiology of most primary brain tumours is unknown; random somatic mutations in glial progenitor cells are thought to be the initiating event in gliomagenesis. Iatrogenic or environmental exposure to radiation is an established cause. For example, radiotherapy (RT) involving the cranium for childhood malignancies results in a 500-fold increased risk for meningioma after 40 years of follow-up compared to the normal population [2]. Genetic tumour predisposition syndromes or phakomatoses often have a nervous system component (Table 56.1). Lifestyle factors are not thought to contribute significantly to brain tumour development.

Classification, pathology, and molecular genetics

The WHO classification of brain tumours

Classification schemes are constantly evolving and aim to integrate historically-determined concepts with insights from molecular biology. Since its inception in 1979, the World Health Organization (WHO) classification of tumours of the central nervous system (CNS) has included a malignancy grading system (WHO grade I, II, III, and IV) that is applied across the diverse range of primary brain tumours. The purpose of the WHO grading system is to provide clinicians with guidance about prognosis. For example, a WHO grade I tumour (pilocytic astrocytoma, meningioma) has generally low proliferative potential and may be cured by surgery alone, whereas a WHO grade IV tumour (glioblastoma) has a high proliferation rate and is usually treated with surgery and adjuvant radio/chemotherapy. Although tumour grade is a strong independent predictor of outcome, it is important to remember that the site of a tumour in relationship to functional domains of the brain is equally important. For example, a benign (WHO grade I) convexity meningioma can be removed completely with resulting cure whilst the same grade I tumour located at the edge of the foramen magnum is relatively inaccessible and may result in fatal brainstem compression. Further, it should be remembered that the WHO grade reflects natural history following surgery, not adjuvant radio/chemotherapy.

The 2007 WHO scheme (Table 56.2) is a histological classification system; brain tumours are classified according to their presumed cell lineage (e.g., astrocyte or oligodendrocyte progenitor cell). This morphological approach is increasingly supplemented by molecular genetic data, and it is becoming clear that the molecular characteristics of histologically identical tumours are more powerful predictors of outcome or treatment response than histology alone. This will be reflected in the forthcoming amendment of the WHO classification scheme [3].

The role of neuropathology in the diagnosis of brain tumours

Modern CT and MRI techniques have revolutionized the initial diagnostic approach to a patient with a suspected brain tumour. However, in the vast majority of cases a biopsy is required to establish the nature of the neoplasm. Often only a small needle biopsy is obtained. In these circumstances the neurosurgeon works with a neuropathologist during the operation to establish whether diagnostic tissue has been obtained. These intraoperative consultations provide instant feedback and, due to the soft texture of most CNS neoplasms, are carried out via touch or squash preparations. The final diagnosis is obtained from tissue sections and molecular genetic data. This is synthesized in a report that may also take into account MRI appearances and possible sampling bias.

Cell of origin and recurrence after therapy

Both morphology and expression of lineage specific markers is used to infer the likely cell of origin of a brain tumour. This underpins the current classification system. A small number of proteins, detectable by immunohistochemistry, allow the distinction of glial, neuronal, and other lineages. Whether tumours arise from dedifferentiated mature cells or lineage-restricted precursors remains uncertain; however, there is increasing evidence supporting the idea that a small number of stem-like cells within an otherwise heterogeneous tumour are responsible for tumour progression, therapeutic resistance, and subsequent recurrence of malignant gliomas. Such 'tumour-initiating cells' are the focus of extensive research. Figure 56.1 shows a model of presumed histogenesis of common brain cancers.

Molecular pathogenesis of brain tumours

Most primary brain tumours occur sporadically; fewer than 5% occur in the context of hereditary tumour predisposition syndromes (Table 56.1). These often manifest with multiple stigmata reflecting the diverse tissues derived from the neuroectoderm. It is noteworthy that sporadic counterparts of familial brain tumours

Table 56.1 Inherited tumour syndromes and their nervous system lesions

Syndrome	Gene	Chr	Nervous system	Skin	Other
NF-1	NF1	17q11	Neurofibromas, MPNST, optic nerve glioma (pilocytic astrocytomas), astrocytomas	Café au lait spots, axillary freckling, cutaneous neurofibromas	Iris hamartomas (Lisch nodules), phaeochromocytoma, osseous lesions, leukaemia
NF-2	NF2	22q12	Schwannomas (bilateral, vestibular, and peripheral), meningiomas, ependymomas (spinal), astrocytomas, glial hamartias, calcifications	—	Posterior lens opacities, retinal hamartomas
vHL	VHL	3p25	Haemangioblastoma	—	Retinal haemangioblastoma, renal cell carcinoma, phaeochromocytoma, visceral cysts
TSC	TSC1 TSC2	9p34 16p13	Subependymal giant cell astrocytoma, cortical tubers	Angiofibroma, subungual fibroma, *peau chagrin*	Cardiac rhabdomyoma, duodenal polyps, lung and kidney cysts, renal angiomyolipoma, lymphangioleiomyomatosis
LFS-1	TP53	17p13	Astrocytomas (GBM), PNETs	—	Breast ca, sarcomas
Cowden	PTEN	10q23	Dysplastic gangliocytoma of the cerebellum (Lhermitte-Duclos), megalencephaly	Trichilemmoma, fibromas	Hamartomatous polyps of the colon, thyroid neoplasms, breast carcinoma
Turcot	APC hMLH1 hPSM2	5q21 3p21 7p22	Medulloblastoma, Glioblastoma	Café-au-lait spots (hMLH1)	Colorectal polyps
Gorlin	PTCH	9q31	Medulloblastoma	Basal cell carcinomas, palmar and plantar pits	Jaw cysts, ovarian fibroma, skeletal abnormalities
MRT	INI1	22q11.2	AT/RT	—	Renal rhabdoid tumours

Abbreviations: NF, neurofibromatosis; vHL, von Hippel-Lindau; TSC, tuberous sclerosis; LFS, Li-Fraumeni syndrome; MRT, malignant rhabdoid tumour predisposition syndrome. MPNST, malignant peripheral nerve sheath tumour; GBM, glioblastoma; AT/RT, atypical teratoid rhabdoid tumour; PNET, primitive neuroectodermal tumour.

Adapted with permission from Louis DN, Ohgaki H, Wiestler OD, Cavenee WK. (Eds.), *World Health Organization Classification of Tumours of the Central Nervous System*, International Agency for Research on Cancer (IARC), Lyon, France, Copyright © 2007.

(e.g., meningiomas, a hallmark of neurofibromatosis type 2) often carry mutations at the same locus (tumour suppressor gene), but manifest at an older age, as predicted by Knudson's two-hit hypothesis.

Insights from high-throughput tissue analyses

Brain cancers (gliomas) were amongst the first neoplasms subjected to systematic genomic and transcriptomic analysis. This has resulted in the identification of molecular subtypes of histologically identical tumours that may guide individualized treatments. However, translation into the clinic remains challenging. A few common themes have emerged from these studies. For example, the evolutionary history of a presumed cell of origin of a primary brain tumour is reflected in the number (and type) of mutations and epigenetic marks. For example, age and site-specific molecular signatures may be observed in glioblastoma, the most common malignant glioma. Mutations in the histone gene *H3F3A* (K27) occur in ~80% of midline glioblastoma in children but are rare in adults. Mutations in IDH1 or IDH2 are seen in young adults, particularly in hemispheric tumours, but are absent in older adults. IDH1/2 glioblastomas often arise from lower grade precursor tumours, whereas EGFR-mutated tumours often present de novo (Figure 56.2).

High-throughput analyses are rapidly evolving and the reader is advised to refer to online resources for up-to-date information [4, 5].

Tumour heterogeneity and evolution of resistance to treatment

The high-throughput datasets described above have two main limitations: they are generally static (reflecting one time-point of a highly dynamic process) and the use of bulk tissue as source material do not (yet) provide information about specific subpopulations of cells that may be most relevant for tumour progression. Tumour cell heterogeneity likely underpins also the emergence of therapy-resistant subclones. Analysis of sequential biopsies allows the construction of temporo-spatial evolutionary trees of genomic changes associated with tumour progression and treatment-induced changes [6]. These studies suggest that, in diffuse gliomas, recurrences not occurring under the selective pressure of temozolomide are seeded by cells derived from the initial tumour at early stages of their evolution, whereas those recurring after chemotherapy show distinct pathways to tumour progression. These observations suggest that it will be difficult to design effective therapies based on the molecular signature of a single (pretreatment) biopsy.

Clinical manifestations of brain tumours

Brain tumours can present with a wide range of clinical symptoms and signs, which are largely dependent on both the location in the brain and the rate of tumour growth. Patients with rapidly growing tumours are more likely to present with headaches due to raised intracranial pressure, seizures, and focal symptoms and signs. In

Table 56.2 WHO (2007) classification of nervous system tumours

Astrocytic tumours	I	II	III	IV		I	II	III	IV
Subependymal giant cell astrocytoma	•				Central neurocytoma		•		
Pilocytic astrocytoma	•				Extraventricular neurocytoma		•		
Pilomyxoid astrocytoma		•			Cerebellar liponeurocytoma		•		
Diffuse astrocytoma		•			Paraganglioma of the spinal cord	•			
Pleomorphic xanthoastrocytoma		•			Papillary glioneuronal tumour	•			
Anaplastic astrocytoma			•		Rosette-forming glioneuronal tumour of the fourth ventricle	•			
Glioblastoma				•					
Giant cell glioblastoma				•	**Pineal tumours**				
Gliosarcoma				•	Pineocytoma	•			
Oligodendroglial tumours					Pineal parenchymal tumour of intermediate differentiation		•	•	
Oligodendroglioma		•							
Anaplastic oligodendroglioma			•		Pineoblastoma				•
Oligoastrocytic tumours					Papillary tumour of the pineal region		•	•	
Oligoastrocytoma		•			**Embryonal tumours**				
Anaplastic oligoastrocytoma			•		Medulloblastoma				•
Ependymal tumours					CNS primitive neuroectodermal tumour (PNET)				•
Subependymoma	•				Atypical teratoid / rhabdoid tumour				•
Myxopapillary ependymoma	•				**Tumours of the cranial and paraspinal nerves**				
Ependymoma		•			Schwannoma	•			
Anaplastic ependymoma			•		Neurofibroma	•			
Choroid plexus tumours					perineuroma	•	•	•	
Choroid plexus papilloma	•				Malignant peripheral nerve sheath tumour (MPNST)		•	•	•
Atypical choroid plexus papilloma		•			**Meningeal tumours**				
Choroid plexus carcinoma			•		Meningioma	•			
Other neuroepithelial tumours					Atypical meningioma		•		
Angiocentric glioma	•				Anaplastic / malignant meningioma			•	
Choroid glioma of the third ventricle		•			Haemangiopericytoma		•		
Neuronal and mixed neuronal-glial tumours					Anaplastic haemangiopericytoma			•	
Gangliocytoma	•				Haemangioblastoma	•			
Ganglioglioma	•				**Tumours of the sellar region**				
Anaplastic ganglioglioma			•		Craniopharyngioma	•		•	
Desmoplastic infantile astrocytoma and ganglioglioma	•				Granular cell tumour of the neurohypophysis	•			
Dysembryoplastic neuroepithelial tumour	•				Pituicytoma	•			
					Spindle cell oncocytoma of the adenohypophysis	•			

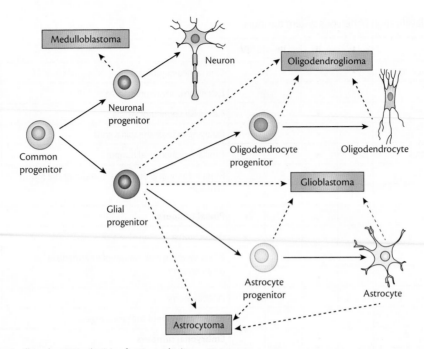

Fig. 56.1 Glioneuronal precursor cells and presumed origin of common brain tumours.

Reprinted by permission from Macmillan Publishers Ltd: *Nature Reviews Cancer*, Jason T. Huse and Eric C. Holland, Targeting brain cancer: Advances in the molecular pathology of malignant glioma and medulloblastoma, Volume 10, Issue 5, pp. 319–331, Copyright © 2010, Rights Managed by Nature Publishing Group.

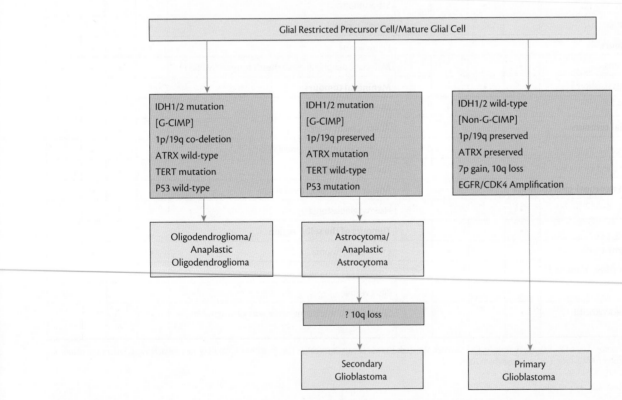

Fig. 56.2 Common molecular signatures of diffuse gliomas in adults. The constellation of a relatively small set of genetic alterations can be used to refine the classification of the main morphological categories of diffuse glioma (oligodendroglioma, astrocytoma, glioblastoma). Primary and secondary glioblastoma are morphologically indistinguishable but genetically distinct. Some of the markers are of prognostic (IDH1/2) or predictive (1p/19q) value (or both). Stratification by tumour genotype will be essential for future trial design.

Abbreviation: G-CIMP, Glioma CpG Island Methylator Phenotype.

contrast, many patients with low-grade gliomas present after a seizure but are otherwise completely well. With the increase in the availability of MRI scanning, asymptomatic tumours are also detected.

Headache, often an early symptom in the patient's history, is rarely the only symptom in a patient without abnormal neurological signs. Headache may be caused by raised intracranial pressure from peritumoural vasogenic oedema or from obstructive hydrocephalus (which occurs more commonly with posterior fossa tumours). Whilst headaches due to raised intracranial pressure have typical features (e.g., more severe when recumbent, associated with vomiting, and possibly visual obscuration), many patients have headaches (especially initially) which do not have any concerning 'red flag' features.

Seizures are a common presenting symptom, but these may be unrecognized focal or partial seizures. Patients can present with less focal signs such as personality or cognitive change. These symptoms are often detected after obtaining a corroborative history from a relative. Rapidly growing gliomas which involve the corpus callosum often present with striking cognitive change and sometimes incontinence, whereas slower growing tumours may present with more insidious cognitive and behavioural change (e.g., with a low-grade orbito-frontal meningioma).

Focal symptoms at presentation depend on the location of the tumour. Dysphasia may occur with lesions in the dominant frontal or temporal lobe and focal weakness or sensory symptoms may occur with lesions located in the frontal or parietal lobes, respectively. Patients may not always be aware of a visual field defect and instead present as a consequence of this (e.g., after repeated driving accidents) or an asymptomatic field defect may be detected on examination.

Compression of the quadrigeminal plate, due to intrinsic tumours in the posterior part of the third ventricle and in the pineal region, leads to palsy of upward gaze, ptosis, and pupillary dilation (Parinaud's syndrome) in addition to hydrocephalus. Tumours affecting the thalamus and basal ganglia tend to cause contralateral motor and sensory deficit and occasional impairment of consciousness.

Neuroradiology

CT and MRI allow non-invasive visualization of the CNS parenchyma as well as the cerebrospinal fluid (CSF) spaces, blood vessels, the adjacent skull, scalp, skull-base, and orbits. In addition to the macroscopic structural and anatomical information provided by standard CT and MRI imaging techniques, functional, ultrastructural, and pathophysiological information can also be obtained with contrast-enhanced techniques, diffusion-weighted imaging, diffusion tractography, perfusion imaging, MR-spectroscopy, and functional MRI. The structural imaging capabilities and, to a lesser extent, these more advanced techniques have made CT and MRI indispensable to the modern practice of neurology, neurosurgery, and neuro-oncology. Nuclear medicine techniques, including PET-CT, have a limited role in neuro-oncology.

The differential diagnosis of ring-enhancing intracranial mass lesions include metastases, glioblastoma multiforme (GBM), acute inflammatory demyelination, bacterial abscess, and a number of other infectious conditions such as toxoplasmosis, tuberculoma, and cysticercosis (Box 56.1). Diffusion-weighted imaging (DWI) can be used to distinguish between a bacterial brain abscess and a tumour by evaluating the diffusion characteristics of the fluid component

---

Box 56.1 Information to consider when generating a differential diagnosis of CNS mass lesions.

1. Age of the patient
2. Clinical presentation

   seizure

   neurological deficit

   headache

   length of history
3. History of a disease or syndrome, e.g., a phacomatosis, AIDS or a known systemic malignancy
4. Location of the lesions

   intra-axial vs extra-axial

   supratentorial vs infratentorial

   gray matter vs white matter vs both

   specific sites: brainstem, spinal cord, pituitary, suprasellar, pineal, intraventricular

   internal auditory meatus/cerebellopontine angle
5. Number of lesions
6. Imaging characteristics on unenhanced CT/MRI

   signal characteristics on MRI, density characteristics on CT

   diffusion characteristics on DWI

   size

   border characteristics

   surrounding vasogenic oedema
7. Contrast enhancement characteristics

   solid

   ring

   smooth ring

   irregular ring

   incomplete ring

---

of the lesion. Pus in bacterial abscesses demonstrates markedly restricted diffusion while necrotic tumour material demonstrates facilitated diffusion, except in rare instances where haemorrhage has occurred into the necrotic tumour centre. The absence of restricted diffusion in the fluid component of a ring-enhancing lesion has a high negative predictive value for excluding a bacterial abscess [7].

MR-spectroscopy is a well-established technique that allows the relative abundance of various metabolites within brain parenchyma to be determined. Standard brain MR-spectroscopy techniques target compounds such as choline, creatine, N-acetyl aspartate, lipids, lactate, various amino acids, and myo-inositol. Certain inferences can be drawn from the relative abundance of these metabolites and it offers information that is complimentary to the information obtained from standard MR imaging and perfusion imaging. MR spectroscopy techniques can be adapted to detect new target metabolites; for example, much research is currently aimed at MR-spectroscopic detection of 2-hydroxyglutarate (2-HG), an oncometabolite resulting from enzymatic activity of the mutated IDH gene product [8].

Medical management of central nervous system tumours

Patients with brain tumours often develop a number of general medical issues requiring management [9]. Many patients have seizures and need treatment with anti-convulsant medication. Consideration should be given to the potential interaction between enzyme-inducing anti-epileptic drugs, steroids, and some chemotherapy agents. It appears that the use of non-enzyme-inducing agents is increasing. The prophylactic use of anti-epileptic drugs in patients with gliomas who have never had seizures is not currently recommended [10].

Corticosteroids (usually dexamethasone up to 24 mg/daily in divided doses) are commonly used in patients who present with features of raised intracranial pressure and significant neurological deficits. Following debulking surgery, the dose should be reduced rapidly and titrated against symptoms; it should be discontinued where possible to avoid long-term effects, of which proximal myopathy is particularly disabling. Where possible, steroids should not be used prior to biopsy if the differential diagnosis includes primary cerebral lymphoma.

The risk of venous thromboembolism is increased in patients with malignant gliomas [9, 11]. However, the risk of intratumoural haemorrhage whilst on anticoagulation therapy is relatively low [9, 12] and, therefore, unless there are other specific contraindications to anticoagulation therapy or an existing intratumoural haemorrhage, it is reasonable to anticoagulate patients with malignant glioma and venous thromboembolism using low molecular weight heparin.

Many patients with brain tumours suffer with depression associated with the knowledge of the diagnosis of such serious consequence [13]. Patients and their family and friends require intensive psychological support, both in hospital and in the community. In addition, patients should be offered intensive rehabilitation to overcome or to learn to cope with disability caused by the tumour and its treatment.

Surgery for intracranial tumours

Biopsy is used to obtain adequate and representative tissue for histopathology and molecular/genetic diagnosis. This can be performed using stereotactic frame-based or frameless neuronavigation techniques to localize small lesions with precision. Craniotomy and complete resection, debulking, or subtotal resection of the tumour is carried out to reduce mass effect on adjacent structures and prevent or improve neurological deficit. Cytoreduction also helps reduce surrounding brain oedema and steroid intake, thus improving the patient's quality of life and possibly prolonging survival.

Preoperative planning is important and resection can be maximized using functional MRI (fMRI) and diffusion tensor tractography (DTI) [14, 15]. While fMRI is able to highlight localization of function within the cortex, DTI represents the only technique able to elucidate white matter structures in vivo. During tumour resection, these systems become less accurate because of brain shift which occurs as a result of the craniotomy and CSF release. Intraoperative

MR imaging can provide scans of adequate resolution to visualize any residual tumour during surgery [16]. Intraoperative ultrasound provides a less expensive option by providing real-time images of the tumour; however, it is limited by spatial resolution and difficulty in outlining tumour margins [16, 17].

Tumour visualization using high-definition microscopic images and intraoperative fluorescence modules, especially tumour fluorescence derived from 5-aminolevulinic acid (ultraviolet light 440 nm), enables more complete resection of contrast-enhancing malignant glioma. High-definition endoscopes with wide viewing angles complement the microscope by providing excellent illumination and panoramic view, especially for skull-base approaches to look beyond the surgeon's direct field of view. They have revolutionized trans-sphenoidal and extended endonasal approaches [18]; more recently, they have been used to resect intraparenchymal tumours [19].

Radiotherapy for central nervous system tumours

Radiotherapy (RT) plays an integral part in the management of many patients with benign and malignant brain and spine tumours. RT is delivered in multiple daily fractions to minimize side effects to normal tissues. A radical course of treatment may deliver up to 33 fractions with a maximum dose of 60–70 Gy and a palliative course only 2 to 15 fractions. Stereotactic radiosurgery (SRS) is delivered in one to five high-dose fractions as an ablative treatment. This may be used to treat many benign conditions such as vestibular schwannoma, meningioma, arteriovenous malformation, trigeminal neuralgia, pituitary adenoma, as well as limited volume (<20 cm^3) brain metastases.

Chemotherapy is delivered concurrently with RT for indications such as glioblastoma, where temozolomide improves prognosis significantly, leading to 27% of patients living beyond two years and 9.8% beyond five years [20, 21]. For patients with anaplastic oligodendroglioma and 1p19q co-deletion who are treated with RT and procarbazine, lomustine, and vincristine (PCV) chemotherapy, the median overall survival (OS) exceeds 12 years [22]. Thus, attention to reducing the risks of late radiation toxicity in this patient group as well as those with intrinsically good prognosis has become more pertinent [23, 24].

Radiotherapy technique

Planning and delivery of RT include reproducible patient immobilization and a planning CT with the patient in the treatment position. The CT is fused to diagnostic pre- and post-operative MRI or CT [25]. Amino acid-labelled PET-CT is an investigational tool which has shown promise in helping to define recurrent high-grade glioma treated with stereotactic re-irradiation [26]. Gross tumour volume (GTV) and clinical target volume (CTV) are delineated and an appropriate departmental margin to planning target volume (PTV) is calculated using the Van Herk formula [27]. Van Herk formula: CTV-PTV margin = $2.5\Sigma + 0.7\sigma$ (Σ = SD systematic error; σ = SD random error). The critical normal tissue organs-at-risk (OAR) are delineated and a planning organ-at-risk volume (PRV) margin added using the modified van Herk formula, which takes into account the fact that OAR will not be irradiated from all directions. OAR-PRV margin = $1.3\Sigma + 0.5\sigma$ [28].

SRS may be delivered using a modified linear accelerator, multi-headed cobalt (e.g., Gamma Knife®), or a focused robotic arm on a linear accelerator (e.g. CyberKnife®) system. All three systems achieve largely similar dose distributions [29, 30].

Heavy-particle accelerators, such as proton beam, can deliver treatment to large volumes (such as craniospinal axis [CSA]) or localized stereotactic treatment). The dose distribution of the proton beam consists of an entrance region where there is a slowly increasing dose, followed by a rapid rise to a maximum dose (the Bragg peak) and a fall off to near zero. Proton beam therapy is delivered using two to six beams. Proton beam therapy (PBT) is now considered to be superior to photon RT for paediatric CNS tumours due to the lower normal tissue dose; ocular melanomas and chordoma are indications for this approach [31].

Adverse effects of central nervous system irradiation

The acute reactions to CNS irradiation occur during or immediately after a treatment course. These include tiredness, skin reaction (erythema, desquamation), and hair loss, which usually commence three weeks after the start of RT. Neurological deterioration, headache, and nausea, due usually to cerebral oedema, can be controlled with steroids (dexamethasone in doses of 2–16 mg per day). However, these symptoms could also signify ongoing tumour growth.

Delayed radiation reactions may be either 'early delayed' appearing a few weeks to a few months after RT or 'late delayed' starting months to years later [32]. The early delayed reaction is usually one of transient demyelination due to temporary depletion of oligodendroglia [33]. Late delayed damage results from the combination of oligodendroglial loss and endothelial damage, leading to demyelination and necrosis.

The somnolence syndrome represents an early delayed radiation reaction in the brain and in adults is characterized by a transient period of exhaustion at two weeks and drowsiness, lethargy, and anorexia at 4–6 weeks after irradiation.

The incidence and severity of late radiation damage are dose- and volume-dependent and can also be increased by chemotherapy, age, diabetes, and spatial factors. Necrosis appears a median of one to two years following RT, whilst cognitive decline develops over many years [34]. For radiosurgery, the volume of the brain receiving >12 Gy correlates with both the incidence of radiation necrosis and asymptomatic radiologic changes. For fractionated RT without chemotherapy, if the dose per fraction is <2.5 Gy there is a 5% necrosis risk at 72 Gy and 10% risk at 90 Gy [34]. Twice-daily fractionation and fraction sizes of >2.5 Gy have higher and less predictable necrosis risks. Adult survivors of radical brain irradiation at or below the standard tolerance limits may develop neuropsychological sequelae; these have also been described for lower doses of radiation when combined with chemotherapy. Ongoing deterioration at 12 years post-RT can be seen in over 50% of patients with low-grade glioma. White matter hyperintensities and global cortical atrophy were associated with worse cognitive functioning in several domains [35]. Irradiation of the pituitary and hypothalamus may lead to pituitary failure [36]. Cerebrovascular accidents (CVA) occur at increased frequency following brain irradiation.

Radiation carries a risk of the development of new primary tumours within the radiation treatment field. The latency is 7–30 years and the risk is in the order of 0.5–3% at 30 years after RT for benign CNS disease [37]. Patients with tumour-prone conditions such as neurofibromatosis NF1 and NF2, von Hippel-Lindau, and Gorlin's syndromes who receive RT or radiosurgery for benign CNS conditions such as acoustic neuroma have a much higher risk of developing either malignant transformation (e.g., ten-fold risk in acoustic neuroma for NF2 patients) or second malignancy (9.5-fold risk of meningioma for NF2 patients) than those without tumour-prone conditions [37]. RT or radiosurgery should be used with great caution in these patients. Tolerance doses for normal tissues within the CNS have been estimated by the Quantitative Analysis of Normal Tissue Effects in the Clinic (QUANTEC) [38, 39].

Re-irradiation of central nervous system tumours

A meta-analysis of brain re-irradiation (interval between courses, 3–55 months) found no cases of necrosis when the total radiation dose was <100 Gy (normalized to 2 Gy/fraction; a/b ratio, 2) [40]. Data on re-irradiation of the spinal cord in animals and humans suggest partial repair of RT-induced subclinical damage becoming evident about six months post-RT and increasing over the next two years. For re-irradiation of the full cord cross-section at 2 Gy per day after prior conventionally fractionated treatment, cord tolerance appears to increase at least 25% at six months after the initial course of RT based on animal and human studies [41]. For the brain, 50% of repair of damaged tissues after one year can be assumed in order to calculate potential retreatment doses [34, 38, 39, 42].

Chemotherapy

The response of intracranial tumours to chemotherapy depends on drug delivery and the individual sensitivity of tumour cells. Factors influencing drug delivery to CNS tumours include blood flow, permeability across capillaries and cell membranes, and the half-life of the drug. Cerebral capillary endothelial cells differ from endothelium at other sites by the presence of tight intercellular junctions on a basement membrane which lacks fenestrations and which restrict the passage of material across the capillary wall. This is defined as the blood brain barrier (BBB). The ability of a drug to cross the BBB is determined by its molecular weight and lipophilicity, so water-soluble drugs of molecular weight more than 200 kDa penetrate poorly. However, it is the transfer of drugs across the tumour endothelial membrane which is of most relevance to drug delivery. The capillary permeability of brain tumour vasculature varies in different regions of the tumour as well as between tumours, even of the same histological type, and the precise role of the blood-tumour barrier in determining chemoresponsiveness is not known. This blood-tumour permeability results in the enhancement seen on contrast imaging studies; however, the infiltration of tumour cells extends well beyond the enhancing edge on imaging.

The intrinsic cellular chemosensitivity of intracranial tumours relates to tumour histology. Germinomas, primitive neuroectodermal tumours, and primary cerebral lymphomas are chemoresponsive. The management of glial tumours has been transformed over the past 15 years due to the positive additive effect of the alkylating agent temozolomide on survival following surgery and RT for glioblastoma [20, 21]. Temozolomide also has a role to play in monotherapy for some elderly patients with glioblastoma and also patients with recurrent high-grade glioma [43]. Patients with anaplastic oligodendroglioma have a high response rate to a combination of procarbazine, lomustine, and vincristine (PCV), which has now been shown to improve OS following RT for those patients with 1p19q co-deletion. [22]. Monoclonal antibodies target agents and small molecules such as VEGF inhibitors (bevacizumab and cediranib), and integrin inhibitors which inhibit angiogenesis (cilengitide) are being extensively studied in CNS tumours due to the high vascularity of high-grade gliomas. However, to date these have not impacted on survival for these patients in the adjuvant or recurrent setting [44, 45].

Clinical management of brain tumours
Glioma

High-grade glioma—glioblastoma multiforme
Radiology. The cardinal imaging features of a glioblastoma are irregular peripheral enhancement around an area or areas of necrosis and variable amounts of vasogenic oedema in the surrounding white matter (see Figure 56.3). 99% of glioblastomas are supratentorial. The amount of oedema has a great influence

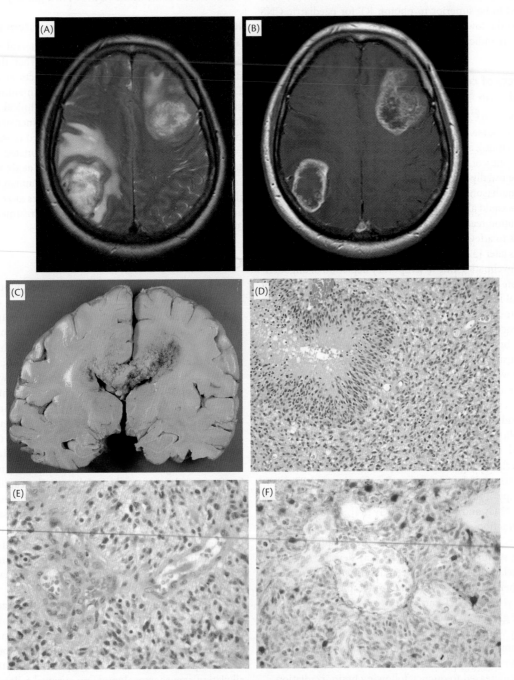

Fig. 56.3 Multifocal GBM: axial T2-weighted (A) and gadolinium enhanced T1-weighted (B) MR images demonstrate large intra-axial tumours in the left frontal and right parietal lobes. Note the typical imaging features of irregular peripheral enhancement, central necrosis, and surrounding oedema. (C) Macroscopic specimen showing necrotic tumour crossing the corpus callosum. (D) Pseudopalisading microscopic necrosis and (E) microvascular proliferation are characteristic. (F) Tumour cells express GFAP (brown stain), which leaves the proliferating vessels unstained.

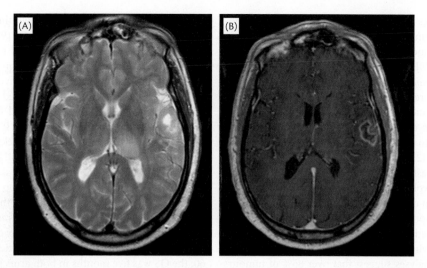

Fig. 56.4 Incompletely enhancing GBM: in addition to the peripherally-enhancing tumour seen in the left temporal lobe on the T1-weighted gadolinium enhanced image (B), there is an area of high signal in the left thalamus on the T2-weighted image (A). This area does not show contrast enhancement on the T1-weighted image.

on the amount of mass effect and, when a sizable rim-enhancing lesion has little or no oedema, it is more likely to be a GBM than a metastases or abscess. Other frequent findings are smaller enhancing satellite nodules, spread along white matter tracts such as the corpus callosum and areas of contiguous or non-contiguous non-enhancing solid tumours that correspond histologically to the WHO grade II or III tumour. These areas are better appreciated on MRI (see Figure 56.4) than CT, often involve cortical or deep grey matter structures and their presence indicates a slightly better prognosis [46]. The uncommon glioblastomas with the IDH1 mutation commonly have areas of non-enhancing tumour and most IDH1-mutated tumours involve the frontal lobes [47].

MR spectroscopy of the solid-enhancing portions of the tumour demonstrates a markedly raised choline:NAA ratio and perfusion imaging demonstrates a markedly increased cerebral blood volume (rCBV).

Surgery. High-grade gliomas are diffusely invasive tumours and patients undergo either a biopsy or tumour resection. A biopsy of the enhancing part of the tumour on a T1-weighted post-contrast MRI scan is offered to patients with poor WHO performance status despite being on steroids, and for those with diffuse or multifocal tumours and tumours in deep locations (e.g., thalamus, brainstem). The risk associated with biopsy is relatively low with a negative biopsy rate and mortality of approximately 5% and 1%, respectively [48, 49].

The infiltrating nature of gliomas means they cannot be completely excised and the majority will recur within 2 cm of their original location [50]. The goal of tumour resection is to obtain tissue for histological diagnosis, decompress tumour-mass effect, and extend tumour-free and patient survival. Extent of resection and residual tumour volume correlate with survival and recurrence, with thresholds of 70% and 5 cm³, respectively [51]. Resection >90% is associated with significantly greater one-year survival (76.5%) than resection <90% [52].

Safe extensive resection has been possible with the aid of intra-operative MR guidance (iMR), intraoperative tumour fluorescence techniques, cortical mapping, and intraoperative high-frequency ultrasound [53]. iMR (either low or high field) achieves greater extent of resection compared to conventional neuronavigational techniques with a trend towards improved survival [54–59]. 5-aminolevulinic acid (5-ALA)-induced fluorescence has been recently used for better in situ visualization of high-grade gliomas. The patient drinks an oral preparation of the drug three to four hours prior to surgery. ALA is a natural precursor in the haem-biosynthetic pathway and accumulates protoporphyrin IX in malignant cells to allow visualization with a modified microscope emitting blue light (440 nm) compared to surrounding normal brain. A randomized, controlled multicentre trial showed that gross total resection was achieved in 65% patients assigned to 5-ALA arm in comparison to 36% assigned to white light (p <0.0001) with a longer 6-month progression-free survival (41% vs 21.1%) [60]. Since then, studies have shown the superiority of 5-ALA resections compared to conventional white light resection [61, 62] and combined 5-ALA with iMR [63] and 5-ALA with cortical mapping [64] in improving survival. Sodium fluorescein is another fluorescent dye that accumulates in malignant glioma cells and is visualized under 560 nm wavelength fluorescent light source [65]. Recent studies have demonstrated its safety [66] and role in improving gross total resection and quality of life [67].

The median survival for glioblastoma patients is 14 months after maximal resective surgery and adjuvant radiochemotherapy [20]. Further maximal resective surgery following recurrence is offered to patients with a good performance status and who can have further chemotherapy. Surgery in this group of patients is beneficial [68] and improves median overall survival from six months following one resection to 26 months after three or four resections [69]. Because local recurrence is the failure pattern of the current therapeutic strategy for glioblastoma, local drug delivery has emerged as an alternative/adjunct to systemic drug delivery. This is primarily in two forms: implantation of biodegradable BCNU (Gliadel®) wafers along the wall of the resection cavity, and convection-enhanced delivery (CED) of various chemo- and immunotherapy agents.

Gliadel® wafers have been implanted both after primary resective surgery [70] and following tumour recurrence [71] with mixed outcome [72–74]. A recent meta-analysis showing improved survival compared to placebo with no increased incidence of adverse events

[75]. A number of studies using different combination of chemo- and immuno-therapy using CED for recurrent glioma have thus far shown mixed results and failed to show any clinically significant survival advantage [76–78].

Radiotherapy and chemotherapy. Adjuvant RT has an established role following biopsy or resection in the management of patients with malignant glioma due to the high local recurrence rate following surgery alone. In early randomized studies, whole-brain RT (WBRT) was shown to prolong median survival from 18 weeks with no treatment up to 42 weeks after 60 Gy WBRT [79, 80].

With improved contrast-enhanced imaging, current standard practice is to treat the involved field using conformal RT. The optimal total dose is 60 Gy in doses of 1.8–2 Gy per fraction, reducing to 55 Gy for specific tumour locations such as brainstem and optic chiasm. The margin added to the GTV (defined as the enhancing tumour and resection cavity) is based on patterns of failure following RT. Retrospective analyses suggest that over 85% of tumours recur within 2 cm of the GTV [81]. This holds true for patients treated with 60 Gy RT and temozolomide chemotherapy [82, 83]. Serial stereotactic biopsy specimens showed infiltrating tumour cells extending up to 2 cm beyond the enhancing tumour edge [84]. Thus, the recommended CTV is 2 cm beyond the GTV, unless limited by anatomical barriers to tumour growth (skull, ventricles, falx, etc.) [85, 86].

The addition of alkylating agent temozolomide to radical RT (60 Gy) followed by six subsequent cycles has resulted in a significant survival advantage over RT alone, leading to 27% of patients living beyond two years and 9.8% beyond five years vs 11% and 2%, respectively, for RT alone in the EORTC trial [20, 21]. This is now standard of care for patients up to 70 years of age with WHO performance status ≤2. Cytotoxicity of temozolomide is mediated mainly through methylation of the O^6 position of guanine. This DNA damage is rapidly repaired by MGMT. Epigenetic silencing of MGMT has been proposed as a predictive factor for benefit from treatment with alkylating agents. The EORTC study group carried out a post hoc analysis of outcome dependent on methylation of the MGMT gene for 206 out of the 573 patients included in the randomized study. Patients with this genetic alteration had a better two- and five-year survival with temozolomide (48.9%, 13.8%) than for the patients with unmethylated MGMT gene (14.8% and 8.3%) [87]. Methylation of the MGMT gene is a prognostic factor, but its predictive role is still to be quantified in prospective studies.

Two large studies (AVAGlio and RTOG 0825) investigated the addition of the VEGF inhibitor bevacizumab (Avastin®) to RT and temozolomide for glioblastoma. The agent adds to toxicity but failed to demonstrate an OS benefit [44, 45].

Glioblastoma in the elderly. Glioblastoma is a disease that primarily affects the elderly population (>65 years) and the incidence in this group continues to rise [88, 89]. There is class I evidence in the literature that maximal resection of high-grade glioma in the elderly is warranted and yields improved survival without an increase in surgical morbidity [90]. Although the number of patients in the trial was small, resection had an average survival of 24.5 weeks, compared with 12 weeks following stereotactic biopsy [90]. A number of other single-centre studies have shown the same [91–96].

Along with tumour grade and performance status, age is an important prognostic factor for patients with brain tumours. This may be related to age-adapted patterns of care as well as treatment independent intrinsic factors, such as the virtual absence of the good prognostic IDH-1 mutation within tumours in the malignant glioma population aged over 60 [97]. The tolerance of the brain to radiation may also be affected by age. From the Central Brain Tumour Registry of the US, the median age at diagnosis for glioblastoma is 64 and the two- and five-year survival for those over this age is 5.5% and 1.4% compared with 34.3% and 16% for 19–44 year olds [98]. Median survival for elderly patients with high-grade glioma unfit for or declining RT is poor, and in an unselected retrospective group it was ten weeks.

A series of clinical trials have investigated the best treatment for elderly patients. The French study showed that patients over 70 years of age randomized to best supportive care survived 16.9 weeks which was significantly shorter than 29.1 weeks for those treated with focal RT (50 Gy in 1.8 Gy fractions) [99]. A Canadian study looked at a shorter course of 40 Gy delivered in 2.66 Gy fractions compared with 60 Gy in 2 Gy fractions for patients aged over 60; the OS was five months in both arms [100]. Methylation of the MGMT gene occurs in just under half of patients with GBM, and this is also seen in the population over 65 years [101]. Two large phase 3 trials have looked at temozolomide in older patients. The Nordic trial randomized 291 patients over 60 years to four-weekly temozolomide versus hypofractionated RT (34 Gy in 3.4 Gy fractions) or conventional RT (60 Gy in 2 Gy fractions). Survival with temozolomide (8.4 months) or hypofractionated RT (7.5 months) was longer than conventional RT (six months), particularly in those over 70 (p = 0.02) [102]. The German NOA-08 trial included 373 patients aged over 65 with KPS (Karnofsky Performance Status Scale) 60% or higher. Dose-dense temozolomide (100 mg/m², 1 week on, 1 week off) was compared with conventional RT (60 Gy in 2 Gy fractions); survival was similar (8.6 vs 9.6 months HR 1.09) [103]. 60% of the patients in the studies had undergone partial or complete resection. Both studies found that patients with methylation of the MGMT gene treated with temozolomide lived longer (9.7 months) compared with those without the genetic change (6.8 months, HR 0.56).

For patients aged over 70, treatment stratification by methylation status is evidence-based. Those who are methylation MGMT positive can be offered first-line temozolomide, and those without should be offered RT alone using shorter regimens such as 34 Gy in 10 fractions [104]. Patients aged 60–70 and PS 0–1 benefit from combined temozolomide and RT (60 Gy) [21].

High-grade glioma (HGG)—anaplastic gliomas
Anaplastic astrocytoma, anaplastic oligodendroglioma, and anaplastic oligoastrocytoma

Imaging. Like grade II astrocytomas, these tumours generally show relatively uniform high signal on T2-weighted images and relatively low density on CT. The majority (>80%) of anaplastic astrocytomas (AA) (WHO grade III) show at least some contrast enhancement, either a focal nodule of enhancement or patchy areas of enhancement within part of the tumour (see Figure 56.5). This enhancement may be relatively subtle and MRI has a greater sensitivity than CT in this regard. The contrast-enhancing components of the tumours often demonstrate lower signal on T2 than the surrounding non-enhancing areas as seen in Figure 56.5. This corresponds to higher density on CT and a degree of restricted diffusion on DWI—all imaging features of increased cellularity.

While necrosis with peripheral enhancement is not a feature of these tumours, focal areas or well-circumscribed cystic change is

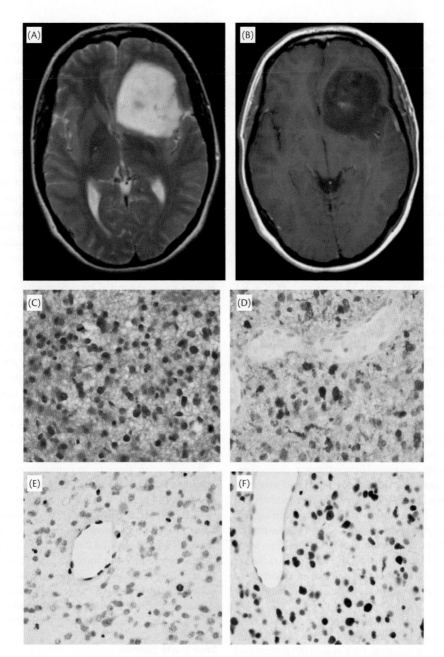

Fig. 56.5 Grade III astrocytoma: axial T2-weighted (A) and gadolinium enhanced T1-weighted (B) MR images demonstrate a large intra-axial tumour in the left frontal lobe. The tumour is of predominantly high signal on T2 and intermediate signal on T1 with a focal area of contrast enhancement indicating the high grade component of the lesion. (C) Atypical glial cells with mitoses set in a fibrillar matrix. (D) Tumour cells express the protein product of the IDH1R132H mutation and have (E) lost nuclear ATRX expression (note preserved staining in endothelial and other non-neoplastic cells). (F) Strong nuclear p53 over-expression suggests the presence of a TP53 mutation. The constellation of these changes is highly characteristic of diffuse astrocytoma (see schematic in Figure 56.2).

occasionally seen. Most AAs are supratentorial; the pons is the most common infratentorial location. MR spectroscopy demonstrate raised choline:NAA ratio and perfusion imaging demonstrate an increased relative cerebral blood volume (rCBV).

Radiotherapy and chemotherapy. Anaplastic gliomas are distinct from glioblastoma in tumour cell genetics. The treatment strategy for anaplastic tumours should therefore be tailored by the presence or absence of these genetic changes. 1p19q co-deletion is seen in 75% of anaplastic oligodendroglioma (AO), 60% of anaplastic oligoastrocytoma (AOA), and 15% of AA, conferring both a better prognosis, as well as higher response likelihood to chemotherapy

when the deletion is present. Methylation of the MGMT gene is present in 70% of AO and AOA and 50% of AA. IDH1 mutation occurs in a similar percentage of cases. Both methylation MGMT and IDH1 mutation are independent predictors of a better prognosis [105].

Given the very long survival of some patients with anaplastic glioma, trials to reduce treatment have been conducted. RT (60 Gy in 1.8–2 Gy fractions treating GTV + 2 cm) was compared with a six-month course of chemotherapy (PCV or temozolomide) for 318 patients in the NOA-04 trial [105]. The progression-free survival (PFS) (30.6 months for RT and 31.9 months for chemotherapy

HR = 1) and OS at 48 months (72% for RT and 65% for chemotherapy) were not statistically different. More patients receiving RT showed a response or stable disease compared with chemotherapy (p = 0.08). Overall, 24% of patients had a partial or complete response and 66% stable disease. Only 50% of patients have so far required second-line treatment. The AA subgroup had the worst prognosis; PFS was 10.8 months with RT and 18.2 months with chemotherapy compared with 52 months for either treatment for AO and AOA. For this poorer prognosis group, the ongoing CATNON/BR14 study is evaluating the role of temozolomide in addition to RT for anaplastic glioma patients without 1p19q loss.

The EORTC 26951 and RTOG 9402 studies of patients with anaplastic oligodendroglioma treated with RT, with or without PCV chemotherapy, did not initially show a survival difference. However, the 12-year follow-up of the EORTC study has shown that the median survival is significantly longer for RT and PCV (42.3 vs 30.6 months; HR 0.75). For the subgroup of patients with 1p19q co-deletion the OS exceeds 12 years with PCV + RT against 9.3 years for RT alone (HR 0.56) [22]. The RTOG 9402 study did not show an OS benefit by adding PCV (median survival 54 months; HR 0.79, p = 0.1), but for those patients with 1p19q co-deletion median survival with PCV + RT was 14.7 vs 7.3 years without chemotherapy (HR 0.59, p = 0.03). No survival benefit was seen for the addition of chemotherapy for patients without 1p19q co-deletion [106].

Management of recurrent high-grade glioma. Most patients with high-grade malignant glioma ultimately fail locally or loco-regionally. In parallel with improvements outlined above in the initial treatments of these tumours, salvage strategies including re-operation, re-irradiation, interstitial brachytherapy, chemotherapy, and use of targeted agents have been developed and may have a role in selected patients [107]. There have been no randomized trials comparing these options. It is important to distinguish recurrence from pseudo-progression which occurs in one-fifth of patients treated with RT and temozolomide [108]. Therefore, adjuvant temozolomide should be continued if the early post-radiation scan suggests pseudo-progression, unless there is evidence of clinical deterioration or further disease progression on subsequent imaging.

Stratifying patients with recurrent disease into prognostic groups is helpful in planning treatment. A minority of patients will be suitable for second surgery or re-irradiation. Park et al. [109] determined prognostic factors for 34 patients who underwent re-operation for recurrent GBM. A validation cohort (109 patients) were scored one point for each of KPS ≤80, tumour volume ≥50 cm³, or tumour in an eloquent area (motor, speech, or middle cerebral artery [MCA] region). Good (zero points), intermediate (one to two points), and poor (three points) prognostic groups had median survivals of 9.2, 6.3, and 1.9 months (p <0.001). Other factors that help in decision making are the histologic grade, relapse-free interval, and local vs diffuse recurrence. At the time of re-resection for high-grade glioma, insertion of carmustine wafers prolongs survival modestly (31 vs 23 weeks with placebo, p = 0.006) [110].

Focal re-irradiation using single-fraction (SRS) or fractionated (fSRT) stereotactic radiation can be used for small volume recurrence. As with surgery, prognostic factors to guide re-irradiation include small tumour volume, young age, good performance status, and treatment-free interval (a radiation repair factor of 50% can be used 12 months after RT). SRS delivering a marginal dose of 15–18 Gy in a single fraction to a tumour size 10–20cm³, results in medial survival of 8–11 months and 22% necrosis rate at re-operation [111]. Tumour volumes up to 50cm³ treated with hypofractionated schedules (e.g., 25–35Gy in 3–7 Gy fractions) result in median survivals of 8–11 months with low necrosis rates [111]. Alternatively, fSRT using 1.5–2 Gy fractions can be used to deliver a total retreatment dose of 36 Gy along with systemic therapy such as bevacizumab giving a median survival of ten months [112] or RT alone up to 45–54 Gy depending on fraction size, previous dose, and time since treatment [42].

Brachytherapy can be used to deliver high localized radiation doses to the resection cavity following re-operation. This treatment is delivered using ^{125}I implanted seeds or afterloaded ^{192}I seeds or solution (GliaSite). Median survival is in the order of 8–10 months [111]. However, radionecrosis is seen in about 40% of cases.

Systemic therapy has a role to play in recurrent high-grade glioma. A randomized study of 447 patients with recurrent high-grade glioma following initial treatment with RT alone, showed no difference in survival between procarbazine, vincristine, and CCNU (lomustine) (PCV) vs temozolomide (6.7 vs 7.2 months) [113]. For patients who have completed six months of adjuvant temozolomide, re-exposure to that drug following a treatment-free interval of over two months results in a 30% six-month PFS [114]. Dose-dense temozolomide is less effective than conventional dosing in temozolomide-naïve patients [113]. Alternative options include lomustine (CCNU) or carmustine (BCNU) single-agent therapy with a 19% PFS at six months and response rate of 4% [115], or the PCV combination with a median survival 6.7 months and PFS 3.6 months [113].

Bevacizumab alone or in combination with chemotherapy has not been shown to prolong survival in recurrent HGG. Evidence from the phase 2 BRAIN study comparing bevacizumab alone or with irinotecan for 167 patients with recurrent GBM following adjuvant RT and temozolomide showed no difference between the arms with a PFS of 4.2 months and OS of 8–9 months. Steroid doses were reduced in most patients [116]. Bevacizumab appears to reduce permeability with normalization of vessels, reduced oedema, and improved oxygenation, hence the reduced steroid dependence; however, there is a rebound increase in vascular permeability and oedema when this treatment is ceased.

Low-grade gliomas

Imaging. Grade 2 astrocytomas show relatively uniform high signal on T2-weighted MRI images, low density on CT and do not show contrast enhancement (Figure 56.6). They may be well-circumscribed and can resemble an infarct on both imaging modalities. DWI demonstrates facilitated diffusion which provides a reliable distinction from an acute infarct. MR spectroscopy demonstrates an increase in myoinositol and a slightly raised choline: NAA ratio. Perfusion imaging shows a low rCBV. An increase in rCBV is an indication of high-grade transformation and can precede the onset of contrast enhancement by up to 12 months [117]. Larger tumour size at presentation and the growth rate in the first six months predict earlier high grade transformation [118].

Oligodendrogliomas usually involve the cortex and subcortical white matter of the cerebral hemispheres and are often indistinguishable on imaging from grade II or III astrocytomas unless they contain calcification, seen in more than two-thirds of oligodendroglioma but rarely in astrocytoma. MR spectroscopy and

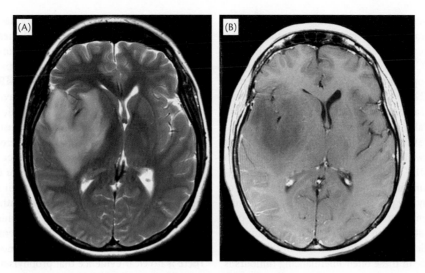

Fig. 56.6 Grade II astrocytoma: axial T2-weighted (A) and gadolinium enhanced T1-weighted (B) MR images demonstrate a large intra-axial tumour in the right frontotemporal region. The tumour is of high signal on T2 and intermediate signal on T1 with no contrast enhancement.

perfusion findings also overlap with those of grade II and grade III astrocytomas. A small minority of oligodendrogliomas present as intraventricular or extra-axial masses. Compared to astrocytomas, imaging is relatively poor at distinguishing between WHO grade II and III oligodendrogliomas since the presence or absence of contrast enhancement is a less reliable indicator of grade.

Pilocytic astrocytomas are rare in adults compared to children and the anatomical distribution differs with supratentorial lesions outnumbering the cerebellar and brainstem lesions more commonly encountered in children. In the cerebral hemispheres, these tumours usually have a heterogeneous appearance with mixed solid and cystic areas, with avid contrast enhancement of some or all of the solid areas often with focal areas of calcification on CT. Surrounding vasogenic oedema is uncommon. Pilocytic astrocytoma in the cerebrum can resemble various other tumours including oligodendroglioma, glioblastoma, ganglioglioma, and pleomorphic xanthroastrocytoma.

Optic nerve gliomas are usually pilocytic astrocytomas but are usually infiltrative, leading to fusiform enlargement of the optic nerve, often extending to the chiasm and beyond. Contrast enhancement is also more variable in optic pathways pilocytic astrocytomas and is occasionally absent.

Surgery. These low-grade tumours grow continuously [119–121] and may transform into higher grade gliomas, leading to neurological disability and ultimately death. Therefore, surgical management paradigms have changed in the last decade. The shift has been from regular imaging surveillance (with or without a biopsy) to aggressive surgical resection including awake craniotomy with intraoperative neurophysiology mapping as the first treatment option to prolong PFS and OS [122].

To maximize the extent of resection, a craniotomy is performed with the patient awake under local anaesthesia or asleep for the initial craniotomy and then awake after the dura is opened. With the patient awake, intraoperative electrostimulation is now considered the gold standard. Eloquent cortical and subcortical white fibre tracts (motor, somatosensory, optic radiation, language, and spatial cognition) are stimulated to define their relationship to the tumour and preserve them during tumour resection [123]. This has resulted

in reduction in neurological deficit from up to 28% (without awake mapping) to less than 2% with more evidence pointing towards functional mapping-guided resection rather than image-guided resection. Duffau et al. recently introduced the concept of 'supratotal resection' where a tumour is resected with an additional margin beyond the signal abnormality visible on the FLAIR-weighted MRI scan, as it has been shown that isolated tumour cells exist beyond the signal abnormality. This has resulted in a significantly lower rate of anaplastic transformation when compared to a control group who underwent a 'complete' resection [124]. An aggressive surgical approach also results in improvement in quality of life, especially with reduction in seizures.

Pilocytic astrocytomas are grade 1 benign tumours and carry an excellent prognosis. Therefore, the aim of surgery is a complete resection without producing a deficit. In children and young adults the cerebellum is a common site and the tumour presents as a cyst with enhancing mural nodule. A suboccipital craniotomy is commonly performed and the mural nodule excised. The cyst wall is non-neoplastic and need not be removed unless it enhances as well. Invasion of brainstem or involvement of cranial nerves or blood vessels may limit resection. Prognosis is good and the residual tumour may show arrested growth or even spontaneous regression and if there is a recurrence on serial MR imaging, patients can be re-operated upon [125, 126].

Intrinsic low-grade glioma of the brainstem can undergo stereotactic biopsy. Surgical resection is usually not possible given its eloquent location. Some patients require a CSF diversion procedure (endoscopic third ventriculostomy or ventriculoperitoneal shunt) for obstructive hydrocephalus. Resection is indicated for tumours with a dorsal exophytic component in the fourth ventricle or the cerebellopontine angle as these are generally benign and amenable to radical subtotal resection [127].

Subependymomas of the fourth ventricle are approached through a suboccipital craniotomy and telovelar approach and should be resected as fully and safely as possible. Damage to the floor of the fourth ventricle can lead to neurological deficit. Surgery reduces the tumour burden and re-establishes the flow of cerebrospinal fluid [128].

Radiotherapy and chemotherapy. The role of RT in the treatment of low-grade gliomas (grade 2 astrocytoma, oligodendroglioma, mixed oligoastrocytoma) was investigated in two large EORTC randomized trials. EORTC 22844 showed no difference in survival between immediate post-operative RT of 45 Gy with 59.4 Gy in 1.8 Gy fractions [129]. Trial 22845 compared immediate RT (54 Gy in 1.8 Gy fractions) with the same given on tumour progression. Again, the overall median survival (7.2 years) and five-year survival (60%) were the same [130]. There was no difference in the rate of malignant progression between the two arms, but early RT improved PFS from 3.4 to 5.3 years (p <0.0001). RT stabilizes or improves neurological deficit caused by the tumour and often reduces the frequency of seizures which accompany the presentation of low-grade tumours. RT is currently recommended following evidence of tumour progression following surgical excision or biopsy or for symptomatic tumours. The recommended radiation dose is 54 Gy in 1.8 Gy fractions. The extent of disease in these often-unenhancing tumours is usually defined as the region of T2 hyper-intensity on MRI [131], with a 1 cm surrounding margin to give CTV.

From the EORTC studies, five independent poor prognostic factors have been determined: age >40, astrocytoma subtype, tumours >6 cm, those crossing midline, and presence of neurologic deficit before surgery. The presence of three or more risk factors determines a higher risk group with a median survival of three years. The low-risk group (0–2 risk factors) has a median survival of over seven years [132].

Chemotherapy in low-grade glioma has a potential role following RT. The US RTOG 9802 trial treated 251 patients with unfavourable low-grade glioma (age >40 or subtotal resection or biopsy irrespective of age) with RT, 54 Gy in 1.8 Gy fractions. Patients were then randomized to receive six cycles of PCV or no further treatment [133]. Median OS was not statistically different between the arms (>8.5 years vs 7.5 years) as was five-year survival (72% vs 63%). PFS at five years was, however, improved by the addition of chemotherapy (63% vs 46%, p = 0.005). Molecular markers IDH1, methylation MGMT, and 1p19q co-deletion are good prognostic features in low-grade gliomas [134]. Phase 2 studies indicate a potential role for temozolomide in low-grade gliomas, and several intergroup studies comparing RT with temozolomide in low-grade gliomas stratifying by molecular characteristics are in progress.

Brainstem gliomas. Glial tumours may involve any of the structures from the thalamus and hypothalamus through the midbrain to the pons and medulla. In adults, half are diffusely infiltrating non-enhancing low-grade gliomas. When treated with RT, 62% of patients improve and the median survival exceeds seven years. 30% are malignant glioma with poor response to chemo/RT and have a median survival of 11 months. Just under 10% of cases are focal tectal glioma, often presenting with hydrocephalus, and prognosis exceeds ten years without irradiation [135].

Ependymoma

Ependymomas occur more commonly in children than adults, and account for less than 10% of CNS tumours, and typically arise within or adjacent to the ependymal lining of the ventricular system. Tumours may be low grade (1 or 2) or anaplastic (grade 3). In adults, 75% of ependymomas arise within the spinal canal, and up to 10% of patients have spinal metastases. Neuroaxis MRI should be carried out on all patients and CSF cytology should be examined for posterior fossa lesions and all anaplastic tumours.

Imaging. The majority of intracranial ependymomas arise in the wall of the fourth ventricle and these tumours often fill the ventricle and extend through one or more of its outflow foramina into the cisterna magna leading to obstructive hydrocephalus. Signal heterogeneity is common on MRI due to cystic change. Focal haemorrhage, calcification, and avid contrast enhancement is often seen.

Supratentorial ependymomas are usually much larger than fourth ventricular tumours at the time of presentation and most are within the brain parenchyma rather than intraventricular. It is rarely possible to make a prospective radiological diagnosis of a supratentorial ependymoma since their imaging features overlap significantly with those of a number of other lesions including glioblastoma, ganglioglioma, and pleomorphic xanthroastrocytoma.

Radiotherapy. Retrospective studies demonstrate good long-term control following partial or complete tumour excision and RT [136]. There is no clear evidence that prophylactic spinal irradiation prevents isolated spinal metastases, particularly if the primary tumour remains uncontrolled. The consensus view is that ependymomas should be treated with local irradiation to the site of the tumour and the appropriate margin, regardless of tumour grade and site. The technique and doses used are the same as those employed for other low-grade gliomas (54 Gy in 1.8 Gy fractions) increasing to 59.4 Gy in 1.8 Gy fractions for anaplastic tumours outside of the brainstem [137].

The overall five-year survival of adult patients with cranial ependymomas is 67–85% and PFS is 63%. The prognosis is related to the histological grade, the extent of surgical resection, patient age, and performance status [136].

Patients with sub-ependymoma have a good prognosis following resection alone, and adjuvant RT is not routinely given.

Medulloblastoma/primitive neuro-ectodermal tumours (PNET)

Clinical presentation and diagnosis. Patients with medulloblastoma may present with raised intracranial pressure (usually due to hydrocephalus), cerebellar signs, and occasionally brainstem cranial nerve palsies.

Imaging. Medulloblastomas are usually solid, well-circumscribed intra-axial lesions of the cerebellum. The high cellularity of these lesions is reflected in their slightly hyperdense (compared to normal brain parenchyma) appearance on unenhanced CT scan and this corresponds to a slightly hypodense appearance on T2-weighted images and moderate diffusion restriction on DWI. Contrast enhancement is variable with some tumours enhancing avidly and relatively uniformly while some show only patchy enhancement and a small minority show no enhancement at all. Subarachnoid dissemination in the intracranial and spinal canal is a frequent finding.

Surgery. A medulloblastoma is approached by posterior fossa craniotomy and usually removal of the posterior arch of C1. The approach depends on the anatomical location of the tumour but the telovelar approach is the best choice for tumours in the fourth ventricle and avoids post-operative mutism [138]. The goal of surgery is gross total resection and the extent of resection correlates with five-year survival [139–143]. >1.5cm^3 of residual tumour on the post-operative MRI scan in children >3 years with no tumour dissemination correlates with good prognosis [144]. Some patients who present with obstructive hydrocephalus require preoperative CSF diversion (endoscopic third ventriculostomy or ventriculo-peritoneal shunt) [145, 146].

Radiotherapy. Patients are classified according to extent of disease using the Modified Chang criteria [147]. Those with localized primary disease and negative spinal MRI and CSF cytology are M0. Positive CSF cytology alone is M1, intracranial metastatic disease M2, and macroscopic disease within the spinal area is M3, and outside the CNS is M4. Low-risk patients are those with <1.5 cm^3 post-op residual, >3 years old and M0. All other patients are high risk. Post-operative CSA RT is indicated in all patients regardless of the extent of tumour resection. For M0 disease, the CSA being treated to 35 Gy in 1.66 Gy fractions. The posterior fossa or site of supratentorial primitive neuro-ectodermal tumours (PNET) plus margin is boosted to a further dose of 20 Gy in 1.66 Gy fractions. For patients with M1–M3 disease, the CSA should be treated to a higher dose of 40 Gy in 1.66 Gy fractions and a further boost of 15 Gy in 1.66 Gy fractions to the primary site, and spinal seedlings should be treated with a RT boost to a small volume to the level of spinal cord tolerance (5–10 Gy in 1.66 Gy fractions). UK national guidelines are available from the British Neuro-Oncology Society [148].

Chemotherapy. The use of adjuvant chemotherapy in paediatric medulloblastoma has been extensively tested in sequential intergroup studies; however, there have been no trials in adults. As the natural history of adult medulloblastoma is similar to that in children, similar indications for chemotherapy could be accepted. The regimens used are those tested in randomized trials in children [149].

Prognosis. The extent of disease defined by the Modified Chang criteria, age, completeness of resection, histological subtype, and genetic markers are prognostic indicators [150]. For adults, with low-risk disease treated with the paediatric HIT 2000 protocol (CSA RT 35.2 Gy and boost total 55.2 Gy then lomustine, vincristine, cisplatin chemotherapy), a prospective study of 70 adults showed the four-year survival of 89% [151]. Most patients who relapse do so at the primary site.

The prognosis of patients with metastatic medulloblastoma is poor 23–30% of patients relapse. Up to 10% of patients disease recurs outside the CNS, particularly in the bone marrow and systemic spread may be seen in the absence of a ventricular shunt. Recurrent tumours may be chemoresponsive, although they are rarely curable. Stem cell transplant results in a disease-free survival in 24% of patients at ten years [152].

Pineal tumours

Clinical presentation. Tumours arising from the pineal gland can be germ cell tumours, pineal cell tumours, and gliomas (see Table 56.3). Due to their location, obstruction of the cerebral aqueduct with obstructive hydrocephalus is a common complication. Other features reflect the involvement of adjacent structures, such as the midbrain, hypothalamus, and the brainstem. Compression of the quadrigeminal plate causes paresis of upward gaze and the pupils become unresponsive to light or accommodation (Parinaud's syndrome). Downward gaze paresis usually indicates further inferior tumour extension. The duration of symptoms relates to tumour growth rate, and for slow-growing germinoma could be as long as 20–30 months.

Germinomas make up the majority of germ cell tumours. On CT, germinomas are slightly hyperdense and engulf the normal pineal

Table 56.3 Histology and characteristics of pineal region tumours

Germ cell tumours (GCTs)	Germinoma (equivalent of testicular seminoma) may have ß-HCG up to 50
	Malignant non-germinomatous germ cell tumour (MNGGCT) 80% have αFP>25+/- ß-HCG >50 (yolk sac and choriocarcimoma subtypes)
	Embryonal carcinoma—immature germ cells
	Teratoma—differentiated germ cells
Pineal parenchymal tumours	Pineocytoma (grade I)
	Pineal tumour of intermediate differentiation (grade II or III)
	Papillary pineal tumour (grade II or III)
	Pineoblastoma (grade IV managed with CSA RT as per PNET)
Astrocytic tumours (see section on Glioma)	High-grade astrocytic tumour
	Low-grade astrocytic tumour
	Tectal plate tumour

calcification. Avid uniform contrast enhancement is the rule with germinomas. Metastases to the anterior recesses of the third ventricle are often seen. Pineal germ cell tumours, like their systemic testicular counterparts, may secrete alpha-fetoprotein and human chorionic gonadotrophin into the cerebrospinal fluid and systemic circulation. The presence of αFP is specific for teratoma, while ß-HCG levels may be elevated by either teratoma or germinoma.

Pineal cell tumours, pineocytomas and pineoblastomas, also show enhancement on CT and MRI but in contrast to germinomas, they expand the normal pineal calcification leading to the 'exploded pineal' appearance on CT. Pineoblastomas can grow large and invade surrounding structures.

Diagnosis and staging. Patients with pineal region tumours should have preoperative craniospinal MRI, CSF cytology, as well as serum and CSF αFP and ß-HCG. Key distinctions are made between secreting (αFP>25 and/or ß-HCG >50) and non-secreting germinoma, and between localized and metastatic disease (multifocal cranial disease, positive spine MRI or CSF cytology). Immediate post-operative imaging to define resection extent is recommended. The presence of positive tumour markers along with clinical and neuroradiological picture of germ cell tumour (GCT) is sufficient to start therapy without histological confirmation. All other tumours should have a biopsy at the minimum. UK national guidelines for pineal region tumours are available [148].

Surgery. Surgical management of pineal tumours includes an endoscopic third ventriculostomy and endoscopic tumour biopsy with CSF sampling for tumour markers which is usually the first-line treatment, although occasionally a ventriculoperitoneal shunt may need to be performed [153–156].

Patients who need a surgical resection can undergo four possible surgical approaches: (a) transcallosal interforniceal, (b) transventricular, (c) occipital transtentorial, and (d) infratentorial supracerebellar. For benign or low-grade tumours a complete surgical resection results in excellent long-term recurrence-free survival [157, 158]. The benefit of maximal surgical resection for malignant tumours is less clearly defined and is weighed against the potential morbidity of an aggressive approach [159, 160] although, a recent meta-analysis showed a graded increase in five-year survival with increasing degrees of resection (84% for gross total, 53% subtotal, and 29% debulking for pineoblastoma) [161].

Chemotherapy and radiotherapy

Germinoma. For patients with non-secreting germinoma, 97% long-term survival has been achieved following CSA RT (24 Gy in 1.6 Gy fractions) followed by a boost of 16 Gy in 1.6 Gy fractions to the primary tumour (in the SIOP CNS GCT 96 study). Long-term outcomes with CSA RT are excellent for patients with metastatic germinoma, (98%) [162]. Attempts to reduce the radiation volume with the addition of chemotherapy and using involved-field RT, resulted in an unacceptably high risk of leptomeningeal relapse [162]. The ongoing European SIOP CNS CGT II study investigates chemotherapy followed by whole ventricular irradiation and a boost for any residual tumour for localized non-metastatic non-secreting germinoma. In the USA, whole ventricular irradiation with tumour boost to a total dose 40–45 Gy is standard of care for localized germinoma.

Malignant non-germinoma germ cell tumour (secreting CGTs) MNGGCT. The prognosis for patients with MNGGCT is poorer than for germinoma. The tumour is less radiosensitive and RT alone is ineffective (20–40% long-term survival). Patients treated following the SIOP 96 protocol with initial chemotherapy (cisplatin or carboplatin, ifosfamide, and etoposide) for 4–6 cycles followed by surgical resection of any residual, and then focal irradiation (54 Gy in 1.8 Gy fractions) for non-metastatic disease had a PFS of 67%. Those with metastatic disease treated with chemotherapy and CSA RT (30 Gy in 1.5 Gy fractions) with a boost to tumour (24 Gy in 1.6 Gy fractions) and spinal metastatic boost (16 Gy in1.6 Gy fractions) have a PFS of 72% [163]. The ongoing SIOP CNS GCT II study is evaluating high-dose chemotherapy for those with high-risk MNGGCT.

Pineal parenchymal tumours (PPT). These compose 30% of pineal region tumours. Surgery for pineocytoma, followed by local RT for residual disease (50–55 Gy), yields a five-year survival of 86%. SRS gave ten-year survival rates of 67% in a small study of eight patients with PPT and should be considered experimental [164]. If surgical resection is complete, an expectant policy can be adopted.

PPT of intermediate differentiation and papillary tumours are rare, and some reports include cases with CSF dissemination. Management should include maximal surgical excision, and local or CSA irradiation depending on disease extent.

Pineoblastoma has a higher risk of leptomeningeal dissemination and should be treated as per PNET above with CSA RT.

Primary cerebral lymphoma

Clinical presentation and diagnosis. Lymphoma infiltrates the white matter tracts to produce an array of symptoms including focal weakness or language deficits, cognitive, and behavioural changes. Lymphoma can also invade the meninges producing cranial nerve deficits and cognitive change. Infiltration of the spinal nerve roots can also cause specific sensory motor deficits or migratory pain syndromes. Systemic involvement (suggested by concurrent 'B' symptoms such as weight loss and fever) is rare in primary cerebral lymphoma.

Uveitis may precede or accompany other neurological features in 5–10% of patients. Patients may present with 'floaters' and blurred vision and infiltrates may be seen on slit lamp examination [165].

Patients with intravascular lymphoma may present to a neurologist with lacunar strokes due to obstruction of the brain arterioles by malignant lymphocytes. Intravascular lymphoma is a systemic non-Hodgkin lymphoma which causes systemic symptoms such as night sweats, hepatosplenomegaly, or pancytopaenia [166].

Diagnosis. UK national guidelines for the diagnosis and management of CNS lymphoma are available [148]. Up to 12.5% of patients with disease apparently confined to the CNS are found to have extraneural involvement. Staging investigations should include an MRI scan of the brain and spine; CT scan of the chest, abdomen, and pelvis; serum LDH and HIV serology; CSF protein, glucose, cytology; flow cytometry; and IG gene rearrangement. Cytological examination of either vitreous or CSF can provide a diagnosis of primary cerebral lymphoma, although the sensitivity of this test is variable [167]. As well as ophthalmic examination and bone marrow histology for all patients, elderly males should undergo testicular ultrasound.

In immunosuppressed patients, examination of the CSF with Epstein–Barr virus (EBV) specific polymerase chain reaction (PCR) primers can be used to aid the diagnosis, although this has a low positive predictive value [168]. In view of the morbidity of treatment, neuropsychological baseline testing should be considered.

Imaging. The most common forms of PCNSL (diffuse large B-cell lymphoma) cause multifocal, relatively well-circumscribed intra-axial mass lesions, mostly in the supratentorial compartment. The disease involves regions that abut the CSF spaces, particularly the periventricular white matter including the corpus callosum. On CT, these tumours are of noticeably higher density than the surrounding brain parenchyma (Figure 56.7) and demonstrate a degree of restricted diffusion on DWI reflecting the high cellularity of these tumours. Avid uniform contrast enhancement and prominent surrounding vasogenic oedema are characteristic. The solid pattern of enhancement indicates the absence of macroscopic necrosis and this is a useful distinguishing feature between PCNSL and GBM. Necrosis has been described in PCNSL in immunosuppressed patients but even in that clinical context it is a rare finding.

A dramatic response to steroid treatment can occur with potentially complete resolution of all the imaging findings—a response that may last for weeks or even months before recurrence in the same or different anatomical locations in the CNS. Treatment with corticosteroids should therefore be avoided before attempting a tissue diagnosis.

Prognosis. The International Extra-nodal Lymphoma Study Group (IELSG) scoring system is based on age (>60 years), performance status (>1), raised LDH, raised CSF protein, and deep brain-matter involvement. High (score 4–5), medium (score 2–3), and low risk (score 0–1) categories gave two-year survival rates of 15%, 48%, and 80% [169].

Surgery. The mainstay of treatment is chemotherapy; therefore, a craniotomy and tumour resection is not warranted [170]. Tissue diagnosis is required prior to starting treatment and a stereotactic biopsy (framebased or frameless) is an excellent means of obtaining tissue.

Chemotherapy and radiotherapy. Chemotherapy is the first-line treatment for patients who are fit. High-dose methotrexate (≥3 g/m^2) has good CNS penetration and has the best outcome, particularly if combined with cytarabine and WBRT. Such treatment

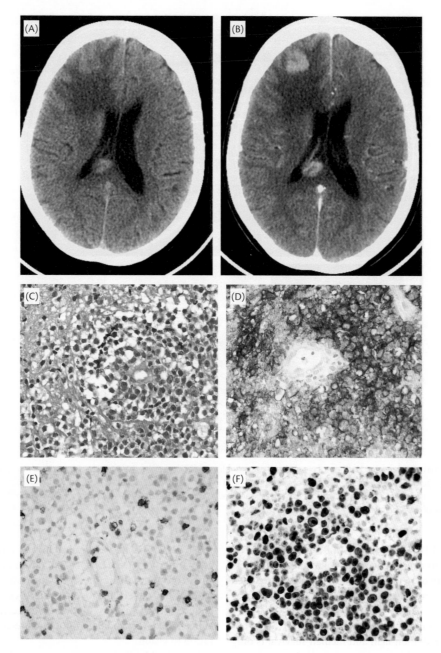

Fig. 56.7 PCNSL pre- (A) and post-contrast (B) CT images demonstrate the typical appearance of PCNSL. The lesions in the right frontal lobe and corpus callosum are both in contact with the CSF spaces, are slightly hyperdense on the unenhanced image and show avid, solid enhancement after contrast administration. The florid oedema seen around the right frontal lesion is also a typical feature. (C) Angiocentric growth of large atypical lymphoid cells that (D) strongly express the B-cell marker CD20. (E) T-cell marker CD3 is restricted to small non-neoplastic lymphocytes. (F) The proliferation fraction is very high (MIB-1/KI-67). Most primary CNS lymphomas are of diffuse large B-cell type.

resulted in a 47% three-year survival vs 34% for HD-MTX and WBRT alone in one study [171].

A more recent study of 44 patients given HD-MTX, rituximab, and temozolomide-induction therapy followed by etoposide and cytarabine consolidation therapy without WBRT resulted in a CR rate of 66%, and four-year survival estimate of 65% [172]. This regimen is now being tested in a larger intergroup study.

The ongoing role of WBRT in PCNSL is uncertain. Omission of WBRT (45 Gy) following HD-MTX + ifosfamide resulted in an inferior outcome in terms of PFS (18.3 vs 11.9 months); however, neurotoxicity was seen in 49% of those receiving WBRT against 26%

who did not and OS was unchanged [173]. Unlike other settings, in PCNSL RT at doses of 40 Gy has been associated with late cognitive decline, dementia, ataxia, and urinary incontinence, especially in those >60 years old. The heightened sensitivity to irradiation might be explained by the tumour's highly diffuse, angiocentric growth pattern, as well as that most patients receive high-dose methotrexate, a potent neurotoxin [34].

Consolidation WBRT (45 Gy in 25 Gy fractions) may be considered in patients under the age of 60 following HD-MTX as this reduces the relapse risk from 83% to 25% and improved three-year survival (92% vs 60%) compared with lower-dose WBRT (30.6 Gy)

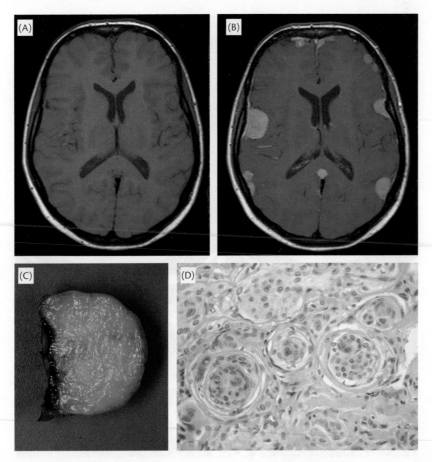

Fig. 56.8 Multiple meningiomas in a patient with NF2: axial pre- (A) and post-gadolinium (B) T1-weighted MR images demonstrate multiple avidly enhancing durally-based mass lesions. The tumours are isointense to cortex on the unenhanced images and therefore difficult to identify on that image. (C) Macroscopic meningioma specimen, cross section. Note dural base to the left of the image and well-circumscribed nature of the tumour. (D) Whorls and lobules of meningothelial cells are a characteristic feature of these neoplasms.

following CHOD-BVAM [174]. However, WBRT may not have an overall benefit for patients over the age of 60 following chemotherapy, due to the high rate of neurotoxicity; if it is used, a reduced dose of 30.6 Gy in 17 fractions results in the same relapse risk as 45 Gy [174].

WBRT alone has a complete response rate of over 50%, but 61% relapse within the radiation field and median survival is only 11 months. RT has a role to play in patients progressing on, or not tolerating, chemotherapy, where three-year survival rates of 33% and 60% have been seen [175]. A dose of 36 Gy in 1.8 Gy fractions WBRT followed by a 9 Gy boost is often used.

Meningioma

Presenting features. Slow-growing meningiomas may remain clinically silent despite reaching a relatively large size. With more frequent use of MRI, small incidental asymptomatic meningiomas are found. Meningiomas impinging on local brain structures may present with focal neurological deficit and epilepsy; features of increased intracranial pressure occur relatively late. In older patients, an enlarging mass may cause global deterioration of intellectual function and personality changes. Meningiomas of the olfactory groove may cause anosmia; parasellar and suprasellar meningiomas may compress the optic chiasm and result in visual deficit. Clivus and foramen magnum region tumours impinge on

the lower cranial nerves, brainstem, and midbrain, presenting with cranial nerve deficit. Lesions extending into the orbit, cavernous sinus, or compressing the optic apparatus may lead to proptosis with visual deficit and occasionally oculomotor, trochlear, and abducent nerve palsies. Optic nerve sheath meningiomas, which are generally very indolent tumours, present with gradual deterioration in vision.

Imaging. Meningiomas are extra-axial, durally-based tumours with the rare exception of intraventricular meningiomas. Approximately 90% are supratentorial with the convexities and parafalcine regions the most common locations. The commonest growth pattern is the so-called 'globose' meningioma—a sessile or less commonly pedunculated mass attached to the dura (Figure 56.8). Less common are the so called 'en plaque' tumours that have a more carpet-like growth pattern and often an intraosseous component characterized by hyperostosis of the involved bone. The greater wing of the sphenoid bone is the most common location of this type of meningioma.

The majority of meningiomas enhance uniformly and avidly. A 'dural tail' of congested enhancing dura can be seen on MRI in up to 60% of meningiomas. Approximately 20% demonstrate some degree of calcification on CT. Most are relatively isointense to cortex on T1 and T2-weighted images and can therefore be relatively inconspicuous unless contrast-enhanced images are performed.

Heavily-calcified meningiomas are hypointense on all pulse sequences and some histological types of meningiomas such as the microcystic and secretory types can be markedly hyperintense on T2-weighted images. Oedema is commonly seen, especially around larger meningiomas.

Surgery is the mainstay of treatment and the goal of surgery is complete macroscopic resection of the tumour with its dural attachment and also the bone if it is involved. This is dependent on tumour location, consistency, size, relationship and involvement of adjacent neurovascular structures and, in recurrent cases, previous RT or surgery.

The general principles of meningioma surgery are:

1. Early interruption of blood supply to the tumour (consider preoperative embolization in some cases).

2. Internal tumour decompression (suction, ultrasonic aspirator, coagulation).

3. Arachnoid plane dissection with minimal retraction on adjacent brain (separate the tumour capsule from the surrounding brain, neurovascular structures).

The Simpson classification of meningioma resection is: grade I, complete removal, including resection of dura and bone; grade II, complete tumour removal with coagulation of dural attachment; grade III, complete tumour removal without resection or coagulation of dural attachments; grade IV, subtotal removal; and grade V, decompression. This classification remains useful for evaluating recurrences and in Simpson's series, grade I through to grade IV tumours had recurrence rates of 9%, 19%, 29%, and 40%, respectively, at ten years follow-up [176]. However, a recent study has shown no statistical difference in recurrence rate between grade I to IV resections at five years, so the benefit of more aggressive attempts to resect tumour with dura and bone was negligible compared with simply removing the entire tumour or even leaving small amounts of tumour attached to critical structures [177].

Tumours arising from the convexity can be completely resected with a rim of surrounding normal dura (usually 2 cm) and also any infiltrated bone. The dural defect after resection can be reconstructed using either autologous pericranial flap (vascularized or non-vascularized) or a synthetic dural substitute. The craniectomy defect after bone resection can be replaced either with acrylic or titanium mesh.

Parasagittal and falx meningiomas can be removed in their entirety, although a key factor in this is the anatomical location of the tumour in relation to the superior sagittal sinus (SSS) and the extent of sinus invasion [178]. As part of the preoperative workup it is important to perform a venogram (MR or CT) to assess the patency of the SSS.

A meningioma which only involves the falx can be resected with its base and the defect in the falx replaced either with autologous tissue (pericranium or temporalis fascia) or a synthetic dural substitute. The management of meningioma which involves the SSS is more controversial. Sindou et al. have described a grading system for meningioma based on extent of invasion of the SSS [178]. Depending on the extent of tumour invasion into the SSS they advocate either coagulating the invading tumour or resecting the sinus wall and repairing it directly or with autologous patch or a vein bypass. The final option is sinus resection with no venous bypass. It may be best to leave the residual tumour and follow up with

MR imaging; if the residual grows, RT may be used. It is generally agreed that a partially occluded sinus in its anterior one-third can be resected as the risk of a venous infarction is very low. Resection of the posterior two-thirds of a partially occluded sinus carries a high risk of venous infarction.

Tumours of the anterior skull base can be approached by a craniotomy (bifrontal/anterior interhemispheric/pterional/subfrontal) or an extended endoscopic transplanum/transtuberculum approach [179, 180]. A recent meta-analysis showed that an open transcranial approach results in higher resection rate with lower postoperative CSF leak [181].

Lateral sphenoid wing meningioma are similar to convexity tumours and a Simpson grade I resection can be achieved. Medial sphenoid wing meningiomas tend to encase the internal carotid and middle cerebral artery; therefore, a total removal is not possible [182].

Meningiomas at other sites, such as the cerebellopontine angle, the clivus, or the anterior part of the foramen magnum, are accessible through a retrosigmoid /translabyrinthine or far lateral approach. Their removal carries a higher morbidity, especially involving the lower cranial nerves [183]. Some centres perform an endoscopic endonasal transclival approach to resect clival tumours [184, 185].

Radiotherapy is very effective in controlling the growth of surgically inaccessible meningiomas. It is used principally for the treatment of progressive benign (grade I) skull-base meningiomas and recurrent benign meningiomas at other sites not amenable to surgical excision, such as tumours involving but not occluding the venous sinuses.

Many meningiomas remain slow growing without threat to function and there is no evidence to suggest that earlier treatment is associated with better tumour control or survival outcome, although there are no randomized studies to assess this. The decision to proceed with treatment depends on the rate of growth, the presence and progression of neurological deficit caused by the tumour, and the perceived risk from uncontrolled growth.

The optimum treatment approach is the use of fractionated conformal or high precision stereotactic RT, which achieves disease control in most tumours with little or no radiation-induced toxicity [186]. As in other benign intracranial tumours, the GTV is defined on contrast-enhanced MRI (in three orthogonal planes) co-registered with planning CT scan. The PTV incorporates margin around the tumour of 3–5mm. There is no reliable dose response data and most series reporting outcome have used doses between 50 and 56 Gy at 1.8–1.6 Gy per fraction. Intensity-modulated radiation therapy (IMRT), while theoretically allowing for reduced dose to adjacent structures, has not been convincingly demonstrated to improve outcome either in terms of tumour control or toxicity [187]. Similarly, the reported results of proton RT for benign meningiomas are not superior, either in terms of disease control or toxicity, with a suggestion of higher incidence of side effects [188, 189].

The reported actuarial local tumour control following RT of benign meningioma is in the region of 90% at five years and 80–90% at ten years [186, 190, 191] and this is similar following high-precision treatment [186, 187]. The control rate of progressive optic nerve sheath meningiomas can be up to 100% at five and ten years. Similarly, the local control rate of progressive grade I parasellar/cavernous sinus meningiomas can reach 100% at five and ten years [186, 187].

Small meningiomas away from critical structures such as the optic apparatus, brainstem, and cranial nerves have been treated with single fraction radiosurgery with reported five- and ten-year control rates of cavernous meningiomas in the region of 90% at ten years [192]. Hypofractionated RT regimens should only be used with caution within prospective trials.

The evidence for benefit of RT for grade II tumours in terms of achieving long-term disease control is limited to small, largely retrospective, series [186]. While historically the reported recurrence rate is in the region of 90% for subtotally and 50% for completely excised tumours, with the use of MRI a proportion of completely excised grade II meningiomas do not recur and the current policy is to consider fractionated RT to patients with incompletely excised and offer to those with recurrent grade II tumours.

Pituitary adenoma

Clinical presentation. Non-functioning pituitary adenomas become symptomatic due to the involvement of the visual pathways (typically bitemporal hemianopia) or due to hypopituitarism. Rarely, the tumour mass may involve cranial nerves in the cavernous sinus. Spontaneous haemorrhage into such tumours (pituitary apoplexy) results in abrupt loss of vision with severe headache and impaired consciousness. Functioning pituitary adenomas present with features of a pituitary mass and endocrine syndromes such as acromegaly with elevated growth hormone (GH), Cushing syndrome with excess ACTH secretion, and features of excess prolactin secretion in prolactinoma.

Imaging. Pituitary adenomas are usually solid tumours and depending on their size, they can cause expansion of the pituitary fossa and extension into the suprasellar cistern and/or the cavernous sinuses. Macroadenomas can cause chiasmal compression. The tumours are slightly hypointense to normal pituitary tissue on T1-weighted images and slightly hyperintense on T2. They enhance less avidly and somewhat slower than normal pituitary tissue. Gadolinium-enhanced T1-weighted images therefore increase the sensitivity for detecting microadenomas and the sensitivity is further increased if dynamic (rapid sequence) imaging is performed during contrast administration; microadenomas are most conspicuous as relatively non-enhancing nodule surrounded by enhancing pituitary tissue on the early images.

Surgery is the first-line treatment for non-functioning pituitary adenomas. The aim of surgery is to maximally resect the tumour, obtain tissue for histopathology diagnosis, and, importantly, relieve compression on the pituitary and optic chiasm to possibly preserve and restore function.

Surgical access is through the sphenoid sinus either using an endonasal or sublabial approach and takes advantage of the close proximity of the sphenoid sinus to the sella and pituitary tumour. Tumour resection can be performed with the microscope or endoscope. More recently, an endoscopic endonasal approach is preferred by surgeons as it has the added advantage of extended approaches where bone of the rostral, anterior skull-base can be removed (transplanum/transtuberculum) for better access to large suprasellar pituitary tumours [193–196]. This also provides a wide panoramic view without brain and optic chiasm retraction and has a rapid recovery time and lower surgical morbidity and mortality (<1%) [193, 194, 197–200]. A trans-sphenoidal approach improves vision in the majority of patients with complete recovery seen in 35–39% and partial improvement in 50–60% of patients

[200–203]. The most common complication after surgery is diabetes insipidus, seen in 15% of patients (up to 2% being permanent) [204, 205].

A trans-sphenoidal approach is now also the treatment of choice for elderly patients compared to a transcranial approach with a significantly lower mortality [202, 206].

Transcranial approaches (pterional craniotomy or subfrontal approach) are usually advocated for tumours with eccentric extensions into the frontal, temporal, or posterior fossa [207, 208]. They are now typically performed as part of a staged procedure after an endonasal trans-sphenoidal approach first.

Radiotherapy. Fractionated RT for progressive unresectable or recurrent pituitary tumours achieves excellent tumour control and, in functioning tumours, normalization of hormone levels albeit with delay of some years [209]. However, pituitary adenomas have an indolent natural history with little threat from a non-functioning adenoma mass to the optic apparatus unless in close proximity to it, and in the absence of local invasion minimal risk to other surrounding neural structures. The current policy is therefore to manage residual non-functioning pituitary adenomas following surgery with a policy of surveillance, which generally consists of annual MRI imaging and, in tumours close to the optic apparatus, regular ophthalmological assessment. RT is recommended at progression, especially if considered as a threat to functions or if enlarging tumour may require further surgery in the future and RT would be aimed at avoiding it.

In patients with residual secreting tumours, the aim is to achieve normalization of hormone levels and this generally means the use of irradiation in the presence of an elevated hormone following surgery regardless of the size of the residual tumour mass. Nevertheless, a debate exists on the relative value of somatostatin analogues and radiation in achieving the normalization of growth hormone. The current cost of life-long use of somatostatin analogues tends to favour RT in patients with apparently normalized GH levels on medical treatment, to allow for its subsequent withdrawal.

The principal RT option for the treatment of pituitary adenomas is fractionated 3D conformal RT using various forms of immobilization (mask or a relocatable frame) combined with image guidance to achieve high precision of treatment. The GTV/CTV-PTV margin is generally in the region of 3–5mm. The majority of functioning and non-functioning adenomas are effectively treated with a dose of 45 Gy in 1.8 Gy fractions [210]. There is no data to suggest dose-response relationship in terms of disease control or the rate of normalization of hormonal levels.

Following fractionated conventional and high-precision stereotactic RT of non-functioning pituitary adenomas, the ten-year control rate is in the region of 90–95% [209–211]. Fractionated RT to pituitary adenomas is associated with 1–2% risk of radiation optic neuropathy and 20–30% risk of developing pituitary hormone deficiency requiring replacement therapy [211, 212]. Although there is an increased risk of stroke associated with stroke mortality [213, 214] and increased risk of second brain tumours presumed at least in part to be radiation-induced [215], the increased risk may also be associated with the pituitary disorder itself.

Small functioning and non-functioning pituitary adenomas have been treated with single-fraction radiosurgery. The overall inferior results compared to conventionally fractionated treatment in terms of tumour control would argue against the routine use of radiosurgery. The current evidence also does not support the hypothesis that high single radiation doses alter the rate of decline of elevated hormone levels [209].

Craniopharyngioma

Clinical presentation. The presenting features of craniopharyngioma similarly to non-functioning adenomas include symptoms of compression of visual pathways, hypothalamus, and the pituitary. The cystic component of craniopharyngioma can involve frontal and temporal lobes and can extend to the posterior fossa. Craniopharyngiomas can cause raised intracranial pressure due to third ventricular compression and obstructive hydrocephalus; in older patients, this may present with non-specific dementia-like features. Endocrine disturbances in addition to frequent hypopituitarism also include diabetes insipidus, which is unusual in pituitary adenomas.

Imaging. Craniopharyngiomas are predominantly suprasellar multicystic lesions with solid enhancing components. Calcification is seen in most paediatric tumours and up to 50% of adult tumours. The MRI signal characteristics of the fluid contents vary according to the protein content of the cyst fluid and the presence of haemorrhage and can be strikingly hyper- or hypointense on either T1 or T2-weighted images. Larger tumours can cause compression of the optic chiasm and even obstructive hydrocephalus.

Surgery. Surgery has an important role in the management of craniopharyngioma. Two main surgical strategies have been adopted. The first is aggressive surgical resection to achieve a gross total resection. This has been advocated as a curative measure. The second option is subtotal or partial resection, but tumour recurrence is higher with subtotal resection with recurrence rate of 25–100% compared to 0–62% with gross total resection [216–222]. Therefore, RT as an adjuvant to subtotal resection is now recommended. Recent studies have found no significant difference in PFS or OS between gross total resection and subtotal resection with adjuvant RT [223–227]. However, the incidence of surgical complications (panhypopituitarism, diabetes insipidus, and hypothalamic injury) which have long-term sequelae and affect quality of life are less with a conservative approach [225, 228, 229].

The two main surgical access routes for craniopharyngioma are trans-sphenoidal (microscopic or endoscopic) or transcranial (pterional, subfrontal). The trans-sphenoidal approach was traditionally used only for small intrasellar and infradiaphragmatic tumours [217] but over the past few years the advent of extended endoscopic approaches (EEA) has resulted in achieving resection of supradiaphragmatic/suprasellar lesions [230–233]. The initial concern with this approach was the high CSF leak rate, but advancement in closure techniques using a multilayered closure or a vascularized nasoseptal flap has reduced the CSF leak rates to less than 5% [234–236].

The wide panoramic view of the EEA has certain advantages such as lack of brain and optic apparatus retraction/manipulation, excellent visualization of the floor of the third ventricle and anatomy of the suprasellar space. The main limitation of this approach is significant tumour lateral to the carotid arteries. The transcranial approach is preferred by some surgeons with suprasellar tumour extension and is particularly helpful with tumours with significant lateral extension and vascular encasement. A recent meta-analysis and review has shown better gross total resection, less neurological morbidity, better visual outcome, and lesser incidence of diabetes insipidus with an EEA compared to transcranial surgery [237, 238].

A craniopharyngioma with an intraventricular component or completely intraventricular can be accessed through an endoscopic intraventricular approach [155, 239, 240].

Patients who present with acute hydrocephalus secondary to a suprasellar tumour obstructing the third ventricle require urgent surgical intervention by either direct tumour decompression or insertion of an external ventriculostomy. Tumours with a large suprasellar cystic component can undergo endoscopic intraventricular cyst fenestration with insertion of a ventricular access device to facilitate reaspiration if the cyst recurs [239].

Radiotherapy is part of the management of patients with incompletely resected and recurrent craniopharyngioma. While the relatively high recurrence rate of apparently completely excised craniopharyngiomas also suggested the use of irradiation in this group of patients, with improved imaging surveillance is a reasonable alternative with early institution of RT with evidence of tumour progression to avoid the need for additional surgery.

Fractionated high-precision conformal RT is the gold standard (see above). The techniques include multiple non-coplanar fixed-field treatment, IMRT, or arcing techniques. Fractionated radiation is delivered in daily fractions of 1.6–1.8 Gy per fraction to a total dose of 50 Gy in 28–30 fractions [240].

Following conventional RT, the ten-year PFS and OS rates are 75–90% [240, 241]. The results following high-precision fractionated treatment are similar, albeit less mature, with five-year PFS rates over 90% and up to 100% five-year survival [240, 242].

The results of single-fraction radiosurgery are disappointing, with five-year local PFS rates in the region of 60–70% even though smaller tumours tend to be treated with this technique [240]. Hypofractionated regimens should be used with caution as long-term results are not available. There is limited data on the use of protons to assess the comparative efficacy and toxicity.

Before, during, and after RT, 10–20% patients may develop cystic enlargement of the craniopharyngioma, which does not signify treatment failure [243]. If this occurs, and causes visual impairment and/or hydrocephalus, early recognition and treatment in the form of cyst aspiration is essential [243].

Spinal tumours

Clinical presentation

Spinal tumours cause local pain at the site of the lesion and impaired neurological function at and below the spinal level. Pain due to bone or spinal-root involvement is localized to the level of the lesion and may significantly predate other symptoms. It is usually worse at night and coughing or straining may exacerbate it and provoke paraesthesiae or temporary impairment of neurological function. Pain from intramedullary tumours is less severe.

Spinal compression by tumours causes segmental loss of power and tendon reflexes. Below this level it causes impairment of long-tract function, with loss of sensation and motor deficit (paraparesis or paraplegia) with hyper-reflexia and dysfunction in bladder and bowel sphincter control (usually urinary retention and constipation or incontinence). Laterally placed tumours may cause a Brown-Séquard syndrome with loss of motor function ipsilaterally and of sensation contralaterally.

Clinical features may indicate the level of spinal compression due to a tumour but confirmatory radiological investigations are essential. In adults, the spinal cord segmental level differs from that of the bony vertebral level. Thus, below the level of the axis (C2) in the cervical and thoracic region the approximate segmental level of the cord can be obtained by adding two to the corresponding vertebral level. The spinal cord terminates at the conus medullaris at the level of L1–L2 lumbar vertebrae, so that the lumbar segments of the spinal cord lie at the T11–T12 vertebral levels, with the sacral spinal segments at the L1–L2 level. Below the conus the lumbar and sacral nerve roots form the cauda equina.

Specific syndromes. Spinal tumours may arise within the spinal theca (intradural), in the substance of the cord (intramedullary) or in the subarachnoid space (extramedullary), or they may lie outside the theca (extradural).

Intradural intramedullary tumours (e.g., ependymomas) result in diffuse spinal cord swelling over several spinal segments, often in the cervical or upper thoracic region and can be associated with cyst formation centrally in the spinal medulla. They initially result in loss of local function over several spinal segments, particularly involving crossing spinothalamic tract fibres, as well as pain and subsequent loss of neurological function below the level of the tumour. The cyst may give rise to a syringomyelic clinical picture, with a predominant loss of spinothalamic sensation and impaired tendon reflexes at the level of the tumour. A late, but diagnostic, feature of intrinsic spinal cord tumour is sacral sparing. Tumours in the conus or in the filum terminale cause cauda equina and conus involvement. The cauda equina syndrome typically presents with local pain (rectal or genital), backache, loss of sphincter tone and function, and lower limb flaccid paralysis. Perianal sensory loss (saddle anaesthesia) is a frequent early sign.

Intradural extramedullary tumours (schwannomas or meningiomas) may present with spinal root involvement, pain, and impaired neurological function due to spinal compression. In the cervical region, combined intradural and extradural components are often found, while in the thoracic region tumours are sometimes wholly extradural. Large extraspinal components may present with a mass in the neck or mediastinum.

Extradural tumours, which are most frequently metastatic, present with pain and features of spinal cord compression which are dominated by motor impairment, initially as mild spastic paraparesis. This is accompanied by sphincter disturbance and ascending sensory loss, often starting as paraesthesiae.

Imaging

* *Pilocytic astrocytomas:* These are more common in children and vary from relatively well-circumscribed enhancing lesions with or without juxtatumoural cysts or syrinx formation, most commonly in the cervical cord, to more diffuse lesions that can involve the whole cord with marked expansion of the cord. Widening of the spinal canal is occasionally seen and reflects the slow-growing nature of these lesions.

* *Grade II—IV astrocytomas:* These tumours are characterized by cord expansion and T2 hyperintensity usually involving several adjacent segments. The cervical cord is more commonly involved than the thoracic cord. Contrast enhancement is almost always evident in grade III and IV tumours and subarachnoid spread as well as intratumoural haemorrhage are features that suggest grade IV tumours.

* *Spinal cord ependymomas:* Ependymomas that occur within the spinal cord are usually WHO grade II or III, as opposed to the

grade I myxopapillary ependymomas that usually affect the filum terminale. Cord ependymomas also occur more commonly in the cervical cord (Figure 56.9) but are usually better circumscribed than diffuse astrocytomas with avid contrast enhancement. Polar cysts are commonly seen in the superior and/or inferior aspect of the tumour and haemosiderin staining in the cyst walls is responsible for low signal seen in the fundus of the cyst walls on T2-weighted images in up to half of tumours—the so called 'cap sign'. Syrinx formation is also a common feature as in other cord tumours.

* *Spinal cord metastases:* Cord metastases are very rare compared to brain metastases. Unlike cord ependymomas and astrocytomas, metastases are usually quite small (typically less than 1.5 cm in maximum extent) and do not have a predilection for any particular segment of the cord. Avid contrast enhancement and extensive cord oedema extending several segments above and below the tumour are typical features (Figure 56.10).

Surgery. The surgical approach to most spinal tumours is by a non-destabilizing standard posterior laminectomy or laminoplasty performed at the level of the lesion and extended rostral and caudal to it determined by the pre-operative MRI scan. This gives good access to all posteriorly-located and some postero-laterally-located tumours. Tumours located anterior to the spinal cord require more direct open approaches through the mouth, neck, chest, or abdomen [244–247] or endoscopic-assisted to minimize retraction and injury to the spinal cord [248]. Occasionally, even these tumours can be resected through a standard posterior approach with varying degrees of lateral bone resection, dentate ligament division, and gentle cord rotation [245].

In meningioma, the aim of surgery is complete tumour removal, which is usually possible through an exposure by posterior laminectomy and with opening of the spinal theca. The rostral and caudal pole of the tumour is exposed. Depending on the size and consistency of the tumour, it is internally debulked with an ultrasonic aspirator or laser, which facilitates visualization and development of the tumour margins. There is usually a good arachnoid plane which separates the tumour capsule from the spinal cord, nerve roots, or cauda equine rootlets. This plane is developed and the tumour separated off the normal tissue. The dural attachment can either be resected and autologous tissue or synthetic graft sewn, or the base cauterized.

The above basic principles apply to neurofibromas as well. Typically, these tumours arise from the dorsal nerve root and tumour removal requires identification and division of the proximal and distal nerve root tumour attachments. It is possible to preserve the ventral root, which is tightly applied to the ventral tumour surface. Large tumours with dumb-bell–shaped extension through the root sleeve, however, usually necessitate resection of the entire spinal nerve. Patients rarely have a significant nerve deficit due to compensation by adjacent roots.

Intramedullary tumours are generally approached by posterior laminectomy and dural opening. Most centres perform spinal cord monitoring (somatosensory-evoked potentials [SSEP]) and motor-evoked potentials (MEP) to predict potential postoperative neurological deficit, although there is no good correlation between change in amplitude and outcome [249].

Usually a midline myelotomy is performed although with eccentric tumours a myelotomy over its most superficial part causes least

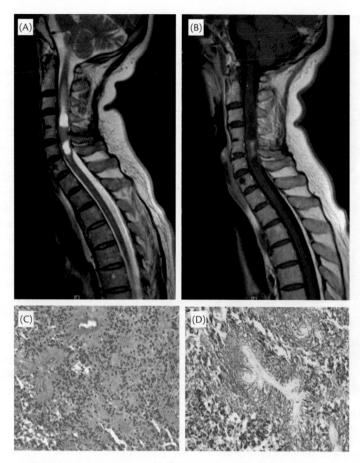

Fig. 56.9 Spinal cord ependymoma: sagittal T2-weighted (A) and gadolinium enhanced T1-weighted (B) MR images demonstrate an avidly enhancing intramedullary tumour in the cervical cord with 'polar' cysts at the superior and inferior aspects of the solid, enhancing component of the tumour. Note the modest amount of cord oedema above and below the cystic components. (C) Perivascular pseudorosettes with (D) strongly GFAP positive processes radiating towards a vessel are characteristic of ependymomas.

neurological damage. The tumour is resected 'inside to outside' using an ultrasonic aspirator. The most important factor governing surgical outcome and extent of resection is the plane between the tumour and the spinal cord. Where a plane can be developed between the tumour and the cord (cavernoma, ependymoma, some low-grade astrocytomas and haemangioblastoma) an attempt at gross total resection is an option. Where the plane is poorly defined (high-grade astrocytoma or some low-grade astrocytoma) a biopsy or subtotal resection is recommended [250]. Cystic component within the tumour can be aspirated or drained.

Recently, 5-ALA fluorescence-guided resection has been performed in ependymoma to visualize the tumour margin and safely achieve maximum tumour resection [251].

Radiotherapy. Primary intramedullary tumours are treated by radical spinal irradiation to spinal cord tolerance doses. The clinical target volume based on MRI should include the whole circumference of the spinal canal and tumour extension with a 1–2 cm margin. The beam may traverse sensitive structures such as the kidneys, small bowel, and lungs, and the chosen technique has to take into account their limits of radiation tolerance. In whole-spine irradiation as part of craniospinal axis radiotherapy, the superior margin is matched to the cervical extension of the whole-brain field. In-field segments and intensity modulation can be used to ensure dose homogeneity throughout the target volume.

Spinal cord tolerance to irradiation. The spinal cord is a 'serial' rather than 'parallel' organ, which means that a small area of damage to the organ can be catastrophic to function. Using conventional fraction sizes of 1.8–2 Gy to the full-thickness cord, the estimated risk of myelopathy is <1% and <10% at 54 Gy and 61 Gy, respectively, with a calculated strong dependence on dose/fraction ($a/b = 0.87$ Gy). Reports of myelopathy from stereotactic radiosurgery to spinal lesions appear rare (<1%) when the maximum spinal cord dose is limited to the equivalent of 13 Gy in a single fraction or 20 Gy in three fractions [41].

Re-irradiation of spinal cord tumours. Data on re-irradiation of the spinal cord in animals and humans suggest partial repair of RT-induced subclinical damage becoming evident about 6 months post-RT and increasing over the next two years. For re-irradiation of the full cord cross-section at 2 Gy per day after prior conventionally fractionated treatment, cord tolerance appears to increase at least 25% six months after the initial course of RT based on animal and human studies [41].

Spinal ependymomas

Surgery. Gross total resection is the aim of filum terminale and conus medullaris tumours and has a lower risk of a recurrence than subtotal resection [252]. Filum tumours are resected by first dividing the filum above the lesion to prevent retraction and then below

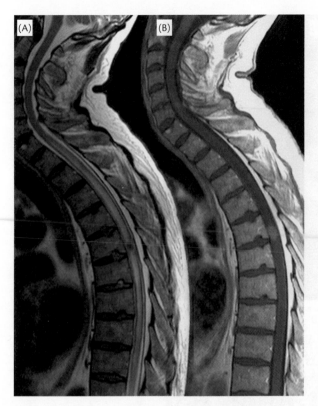

Fig. 56.10 Spinal cord metastases from breast cancer: sagittal T2-weighted (A) and gadolinium enhanced T1-weighted (B) MR images demonstrate an avidly enhancing intramedullary tumour at the T5 level with extensive oedema in the thoracic cord above and below the lesion. The tumour itself is visible on the T2-weighted image as a focus of intermediate signal outlined by the high signal oedema in the swollen cord. Note: no histology.

the lesion. The filum is differentiated from nerve roots by its whiter appearance, vessels on its surface, and, more definitely, by intraoperative stimulation and anal sphincter EMG recording. Tumour of the conus medullaris does not usually invade the conus and can be separated from it. Sometimes a subtotal resection is accepted to prevent damage to the conus.

Intramedullary ependymoma usually have a clear cleavage plane and a complete surgical removal reduces the likelihood of a recurrence [253] but aggressive resection is associated with high complication rate [254].

Radiotherapy. Spinal ependymoma account for 60–80% of spinal gliomas. There are no randomized trials on the role of adjuvant RT following surgical excision; however, total excision has a very good survival (86% at 10 years) and adjuvant RT is not generally used [255]. However, following less radical surgical procedures (partial excision or biopsy alone) if RT (50 Gy in 1.5–2 Gy fractions) is used, 50–60% of patients remain alive and free of tumour progression at five and ten years [256]. Irradiation is confined to the region of the tumour and the margin of potential spread. The use of more extensive irradiation, including brain and whole spinal cord, is not advocated; however, all patients should have imaging of the whole neuroaxis to exclude the possibility of primary intracranial disease with drop spinal metastases.

Anaplastic ependymoma of the spinal cord is rare (5% of spinal ependymoma) and surgical biopsy or excision should be followed by local RT (50–55 Gy in 1.6–1.8 Gy fractions).

Spinal astrocytoma

Surgery. The optimal management of malignant intramedullary spinal cord astrocytomas remains controversial. The principles of surgical approach to these tumours however are the same as other intramedullary tumours. Most AA patients undergo a subtotal resection given the lack of a clear tumour-spinal cord plane and have a decreased OS (38% vs 78%) at four years compared to those who have a complete resection [257]. However, complete resection of a glioblastoma is usually not possible [257, 258]. Surgery carries a high risk of neurological deterioration [258].

Radiotherapy. Since the biological nature of spinal cord high-grade glioma is identical to that of the brain, RT remains a key adjuvant treatment [259]. Radical surgery and RT of spinal GBM is associated with poor survival, similar to historical controls of diagnostic biopsy and RT [257]. The rationale for post-operative RT is equivalent to that for the treatment of intracranial gliomas, treating all high-grade tumours and incompletely resected low-grade tumours due to the high risk of neurological compromise if left untreated. Doses of 50–55 Gy in 1.6–1.8 Gy fractions are administered. For patients with glioblastoma, temozolomide should be given concurrently with the RT as for cranial GBM, and if there is already very poor neurological function due to cord disruption, radiation doses up to 60 Gy could be justified. Neurological deficit due to tumour or surgery is rarely relieved by RT and patients with high-grade tumours have very poor prognosis [260, 261].

Brain metastases

Clinical presentation

Brain metastases are the most common intracranial tumours in adults, accounting for over half of brain tumours. Up to 20% of patients with systemic malignancy will develop brain metastases, but the frequency appears to be increasing with the increased control of extra-cerebral disease from improved systemic therapy that may lack CNS penetration. Most malignant tumours are associated with the development of brain metastases through haematogenous spread. The risk of brain metastases is highest in patients with lung cancer (20% of cases), melanoma (7%), renal cell cancer (7%), breast cancer (5%), and colorectal cancer (1%) [262]. The most frequent presentation is of multiple lesions within the brain parenchyma; less frequent are single metastases or meningeal disease.

Patients with brain metastases present with typical features of a gradually expanding tumour mass and associated oedema with headache, focal neurological dysfunction, cognitive dysfunction, and seizures. Confusional states and multiple neurological deficits are common. Less commonly, intratumoural haemorrhage, obstructive hydrocephalus, or embolization by tumour cells is seen.

Approximately two-thirds of patients presenting with brain metastases have a known underlying primary tumour, usually with metastatic disease at other sites. In the absence of known malignant disease, if imaging suggests brain metastases and the patient is fit enough to undergo treatment, it is necessary to search for a primary cancer (CT chest and abdomen or PET CT). 60% of cases will have an underlying lung cancer. However, in the 25% of cases where no primary is detected, biopsy of the brain metastasis must be undertaken to obtain histological diagnosis.

In some cancer types, genetic modification may be seen in the metastasis not present in the primary cancer. For example, Her-2 overexpression in breast cancer or BRAF mutation in melanoma may occur in the brain lesions, which may determine treatment options which can cross the blood brain barrier (lapatinib and vemurafenib, respectively). Therefore, a biopsy of brain metastases in a patient with known metastatic cancer may be required to direct subsequent treatment.

Imaging

Parenchymal brain metastases are much more common than leptomeningeal metastases. Metastases can occur anywhere in the brain parenchyma but favour the junction of the cortex with the white matter. The vast majority of metastases show contrast enhancement. Necrosis and surrounding oedema are commonly seen, particularly with larger lesions.

Leptomeningeal metastases are more difficult to detect and can be very subtle, even on gadolinium-enhanced MRI. The cerebellar folia, cranial nerves, and internal auditory meatus are common locations for leptomeningeal metastases.

Treatment

The aim of therapy is palliation. Corticosteroids improve symptoms in up to 60 per cent of patients. A randomized trial compared 16 mg with 4 mg of dexamethasone for patients with brain metastases, KPS ≤80, and no impending risk of herniation. There was no difference in degree of KPS improvement between the doses, and toxic effects were worse with the higher dose [263]. Tapering of dose from 4 mg should be carried out over four weeks following palliative treatment. This may be sufficient palliation in patients with extensive systemic metastatic disease when prognosis is 1–2 months. Further treatment should be determined by the patient's overall prognosis. Patients with brain metastases can be divided into three prognostic groups from the RTOG recursive partitioning analysis (RPA) [264]. The RPA has recently been validated for updated treatment modalities stereotactic radiosurgery (SRS) and fractionated stereotactic radiation therapy (fSRT) [265].

Using this analysis, RPA class I tumours (KPS ≥70, <65 years, controlled primary, no extracranial metastases) have a median survival of 7.1 months. Class III tumours, in patients with KPS <70 have a median survival of 2.3 months. For class II, who are neither class I nor III, the median survival is intermediate at 4.2 months. Patients with class I and some class II have a favourable prognosis. Those with limited brain metastases (1–3) and controlled systemic disease have the best overall prognosis with a median survival of over a year; treatment should be focused on eradication or control of the brain metastases, including surgery or radiosurgery.

Patients with an unfavourable prognosis (most in class II and all in class III) should have treatment focused on control of symptoms caused by the brain metastases.

Surgery

Surgery is usually reserved for patients with a single symptomatic accessible metastatic deposit. Following gross total resection alone, local disease control at one year is around 50% [266, 267]. Surgery also has a role in patients with multiple metastases if one is symptomatic or life-threatening (as in the posterior fossa) [268].

Occasionally, patients with two or three lesions that can all be removed by one or more craniotomies are still considered surgical candidates. The aim of surgery is to reduce the mass effect from the lesion and possibly improve neurological deficits. Resecting the metastases reduces the surrounding oedema and, as a consequence, reduces the need for steroid medications and, consequently, their long-term side effects.

However, the decision to proceed with surgery is multifactorial and depends on the patient's age, Karnofsky score, extracranial disease (controlled or progressing), number, size, location, and histological type of metastasis (if known primary) as shown below. Surgery is generally indicated for tumours of ~3 cm, but not for small tumours (<1 cm), and ≤3 lesions (although it is possible to resect the large one if symptomatic and >3 cm). Surgery is generally reserved for superficial or supratentorial lesions, rather than for those in the thalamus, deep basal ganglia, or brainstem. For surgery, patients should generally have KPS ≤ 70, with controlled extracranial disease. Optimal primary tumour types include solid tumours such as those of the breast, colon, or lung, melanoma, and renal cancers rather than lymphoma, small cell lung cancer, or germ cell tumours.

The aim of surgery is en bloc resection, but sometimes this might not be possible depending on tumour location and size. The lesion is localized using a neuronavigation system. Patients undergoing a piecemeal resection have an increased risk of leptomeningeal dissemination compared to en bloc resection [269–271]. Some authors advocate a wider resection incorporating up to 5mm of adjacent brain to reduce local recurrence [272].

Radiotherapy

Favourable prognostic group

Stereotactic radiosurgery, used either alone or in combination with whole-brain irradiation, achieves local tumour control and survival of approximately 11 months, similar to neurosurgical excision [266]. It can be considered a non-invasive alternative to surgery in patients with low-volume brain metastases, particularly where risks of morbidity are high with surgery. The decision to use SRS/fSRT must, however, balance the likely benefits against the risk of complications, including radio-necrosis. Evidence suggests that radio-necrosis becomes more likely as the total brain volume treated increases; if the brain volume receiving >12Gy is >8.5 cm^3, the necrosis rate is 10% [273]. An upper limit of 20 cm^3 has been identified as a reasonable cut-off point for metastatic disease burden to receive SRS [274]. A total volume of 20 cm^3 could accommodate a single tumour of approximately 3.2 cm diameter or a number of smaller tumours.

The addition of whole brain radiotherapy (WBRT) to radiosurgery or surgery for patients with 1–3 brain metastases improves local and distant brain control but there is no difference in median survival (10.7 months) or quality of life from the EORTC 22952 study. Patients treated with radiosurgery alone were found to have better neurocognitive outcomes as compared to patients treated with WBRT and radiosurgery [266]. Radiosurgery to the tumour bed with a 2 mm margin following surgical excision of isolated metastases is an alternative approach to avoid WBRT and reduce local relapse. This technique is currently being tested in intergroup studies [275].

Radiosurgery boost with WBRT may improve local disease control in selected participants compared to WBRT alone, although the median survival of six months remains unchanged for participants with multiple (>3) brain metastases [276].

Unfavourable prognostic group

Whole brain radiation (WBRT) provides effective palliation and can produce neurological improvement in 64–85% of patients. A Cochrane review of 39 randomized trials involving over 10,000 patients concluded that none of the RCTs with altered WBRT dose-fractionation schemes as compared to the standard (30 Gy in ten daily fractions or 20 Gy in four or five daily fractions) found a benefit in terms of overall survival, neurologic function, or symptom control [277]. Case series indicate that the median survival increases by 3–6 months with the use of palliative WBRT; however, the benefit of WBRT as compared to supportive care alone has only been studied in one RCT. The MRC QUARTZ trial group has recently published interim results of a study of patients with non-small cell lung cancer and inoperable brain metastases. The first 151 patients given optimal supportive care, with or without WBRT (20 Gy in five fractions), had a median survival of 50 days and no difference in quality of life scores. 50% of patients were RPA class III [278]. It may be that supportive care alone, without WBRT, is appropriate for some patients, particularly those with advanced disease and poor performance status [279]. In a cohort study of 3459 patients with brain metastases, 17% lived for less than six weeks after their WBRT [280].

Chemotherapy

Systemic chemotherapy administered to patients with brain metastases of chemosensitive tumours, such as lymphoma, teratoma, small cell lung cancer, and breast cancer, can induce clinical responses, particularly in previously untreated patients. More recent evidence has become available on the use of targeted agents crossing the blood brain barrier for brain metastases. The BRAF inhibitor, vemurafenib, has shown activity for melanoma patients who exhibit V600 BRAF mutations with brain metastases. A 50% response rate was seen in non-pretreated patients [281] lasting 8–32 weeks, and a 75% response rate following cranial radiotherapy [282]. Lapatinib is an oral small molecule tyrosine kinase inhibitor also crossing the blood brain barrier that interrupts Her-2 receptor pathways. Its use resulted in prolonged median survival for Her-2 positive breast cancer patients with brain metastases (19 months) compared with trastuzumab (12 months), a monoclonal antibody inhibitor of Her-2 receptor [283].

Metastatic spinal tumours

Although uncommon, spinal tumours may present with symptoms mimicking many benign disorders, frequently delaying diagnosis. These include back pain, sometimes radiating to other parts of the body; loss of sensation, especially in the arms or legs; difficulty in walking; decreased sensitivity; loss of bowel or bladder function; and muscle weakness depending on which nerve or part of the spinal cord is compressed. Spinal tumours progress at different rates. In general, cancerous spinal tumours grow more quickly, and noncancerous spinal tumours tend to develop very slowly. Metastatic tumours to the spine are usually extradural, arising from bony or surrounding soft tissue metastatic masses. Rarely, deposits may be intramedullary. The neurological deficit is the result of the combination of local cord oedema, ischaemia, and direct pressure.

The aim of therapy is functional improvement and pain control. Survival depends usually on the extent of metastatic disease and the tumour type, as well as treatment. The functional outcome after therapy is largely dependent on pretreatment neurologic status. Education for patients and health care staff about symptoms that warrant immediate evaluation to detect malignant spinal cord compression (MSCC) is key to early diagnosis and therapy. A recent study indicates that 62% of patients are ambulatory at the time of diagnosis [284]. Rapid diagnosis and treatment are also key to maintaining or regaining ambulation. MRI of the whole spine should be conducted for suspected cases of MSCC.

Treatment guidelines

Patients are frequently in severe pain. Corticosteroids are the initial treatment in patients with suspected spinal cord compression and usually relieve pain within a few hours; however, opioids are also usually required. Treatment with higher doses than those given conventionally (dexamethasone 4 mg, 6 hourly) results in higher adverse events, but no improved pain control or neurological outcome [285].

Spinal stability should be assessed using the SINS score (spinal instability neoplastic score) which considers disease location at junctions in the spine, mechanical pain, bone lesion type, spinal alignment, vertebral body collapse, and involvement of posterolateral spinal elements [286]. If the spine is unstable (score 13–18) patients should be nursed horizontally in bed, and a surgical approach considered. An indeterminate score 7–12 should involve surgical consultation. An unstable spine will not respond to radiotherapy and should be treated surgically with fixation, or—if there is no epidural disease— with percutaneous vertebroplasty followed by radiotherapy.

The choices of treatment for patients with stable spinal disease include decompressive surgery, radiotherapy, or both. In patients with chemosensitive tumours, chemotherapy may be the initial treatment. Patients with spinal metastasis who do not have acute neurological deterioration may require workup to identify the primary tumour and to obtain histological confirmation of malignancy. The role of surgery is dependent on a number of factors including patient age, histopathology of the primary tumour, number of spinal metastases, and systemic disease (controlled vs uncontrolled). Solitary metastasis with indolent tumours (renal cell cancer, melanoma, some adenocarcinomas, thyroid, and sarcoma) may be candidates for attempted cure with en bloc resection (total spondylectomy) [287–290].

Patients with stable spines, who are able to walk, could be considered for chemotherapy for very chemosensitive tumours (teratoma or lymphoma); radiotherapy alone if the tumour is very radiosensitive (small cell carcinoma, germ cell tumour, lymphoma, leukaemia, and multiple myeloma); or, for the majority of patients, surgical decompression followed by radiotherapy (30Gy in ten fractions). This latter approach results in maintained ambulation in 94% treated with surgery and RT versus 74% for RT alone [291].

Surgical decompression is done through either an anterior approach or a posterior laminectomy. Most cases require a metallic instrumented fixation and fusion to maintain spinal stability. When an anterior approach is employed, an anterior plate spanning one level above and one level below the vertebrectomy defect is generally used to support the cage or cement reconstruction in the vertebral body. In posterior decompression, posterolateral lateral mass or pedicle instrumentation is usually employed, spanning at least two levels above and below the tumour.

In non-ambulant patients with a single area of compression, paraplegia of <48 hours, prognosis of > 3 months, controlled metastatic disease elsewhere, and non-radioresponsive tumours, surgical decompression followed by radiotherapy (20–30Gy) should also be considered. This strategy results in regained ambulation in 62% compared to 19% for RT alone. Survival is similar between both treatment groups [291]. Spinal cord compression by a tumour of unknown primary site or progression of signs despite radiotherapy are also indications for surgery. Laminectomy alone has been shown to be no better than radiotherapy and should not be used.

Patients without the good prognostic features outlined above should be considered for treatment with palliative radiotherapy. Thirty percent of those who are non-ambulatory will regain the ability to walk, but only 2–6% of fully paraplegic patients will do so following radiotherapy alone. This is more likely for patients whose symptoms develop slowly (>2 weeks), treatment is started <12 hours after loss of ambulation, and bladder and bowel function are retained [292].

An optimal radiotherapy regimen has not been defined; in patients with a limited prognosis a dose of 20 Gy in five fractions by direct field is usually adequate. A single fraction of 8 Gy should be considered for patients with MSCC who have progressive neoplastic disease, poor performance status, and survival <6 months. In these patients, there is no benefit in a more protracted course of RT [293]. Prognosis for patients with MSCC who are ambulatory prior to RT is 8–10 months, compared with 2–4 months for non-ambulatory patients.

More radical RT is reserved for solitary lesions such as plasmacytoma (40 Gy in 20 fractions).

Skull base tumours

Clinical features

The most frequent site of primary bone tumours of the skull is the base of the cranium, with rare involvement of other regions. The most common tumours are chordomas and chondrosarcomas, with occasional osteomas, giant cell tumours of the bone, and osteosarcomas. Base of skull (clivus) tumours present with symptoms of local bone destruction (usually pain) and gradually progressive features of cranial nerve, brainstem, or mid-brain compression. Tumours may also invade other surrounding structures, such as the sphenoid sinus, pituitary fossa, orbits, and nasopharynx, with attendant focal clinical features.

Surgery

Surgery is the primary treatment but the tumour site and extensive invasion of surrounding structures make complete excision difficult.

Radiotherapy

The five-year progression-free survival of patients with chordoma treated with photon radiotherapy (50 Gy) after incomplete resection or biopsy alone is 20–30% and the median survival is five years [294].

High-energy charged-particle radiation (protons and helium ions) has been employed in the treatment of skull-base chordomas and low-grade chondrosarcomas. Due to the sharp dose gradient fall off, a higher dose (70 Cobalt-Gy equivalent) can be delivered to the skull-base tumour with reduced risk of normal tissue complications to the brainstem, optic chiasm, and spinal cord compared with photon RT. In addition, the low-dose radiation to normal tissues beyond the target volume is significantly lower with protons, and the rate of second malignancy following proton therapy appears to be half that of conventional radiotherapy (6.45% vs 12%). Published case series of 416 patients with chordoma treated with proton therapy has shown five-year local control and overall survival rates of 69% and 80%, respectively [295]. The results for chondrosarcoma are higher with ten-year local control and survival rates over 98% following 72 Cobalt Gy-equivalent proton therapy [296].

There are concerns about proton therapy, however. The radiobiological effectiveness (RBE) value for proton therapy has been calculated to be 1.1 compared with photon therapy. However, it is possible that the value varies between tumour and normal tissues, so better estimates of RBE for normal tissues are required to be certain of likely long-term risks to normal tissues. The recent developments in photon radiotherapy (IMRT, volumetric modulated arc therapy, relocatable frameless stereotactic immobilization, improved dose optimization and calculation) permit delivery of photon radiotherapy to higher doses. Randomized trials comparing photon therapy and proton treatment for indications such as skull base chordoma and chondrosarcoma should be conducted [297].

Vestibular schwannoma

Clinical presentation

Vestibular schwannomas are benign encapsulated tumours of the eighth cranial nerve, representing 8% of intracranial tumours in surgical series, either as sporadic tumours or as part of neurofibromatosis (NF2). They arise from the vestibular nerve within the internal auditory meatus and commonly present with unilateral progressive deafness. However, symptoms may not occur until the tumour has expanded into the cerebello-pontine angle, causing ataxia and involvement of the trigeminal and facial nerves. The mid-brain and pons may be compressed and hydrocephalus may develop. Large tumours may also involve the adjacent seventh or fifth (trigeminal) nerves with associated clinical signs. Schwannomas may rarely involve the trigeminal, glossopharyngeal, vagus, or hypoglossal nerves and these may also affect the cerebello-pontine angle. They are well-circumscribed, avidly-enhancing solid tumours, but larger lesions can have areas of non-enhancing cystic degeneration.

Vestibular schwannomas are graded according to local tumour extension and size. Histologically, they are highly cellular with interlacing bundles of spindle cells whose nuclei are often in parallel arrays, alternating with lesser-textured, often partially cystic areas.

Surgery

Tumours may be resected by retrosigmoid, subtemporal, or translabyrinthine routes. Given the success with stereotactic radiosurgery in controlling tumours <3 cm with improved facial nerve function (98%) and hearing preservation compared to surgery [298–302], surgery is usually reserved as first-line treatment for tumours >3cm.

Gross total resection with facial nerve preservation remains the ideal goal to lower the rate of recurrence [303–305]; however, this is also associated with a higher rate of facial nerve palsy with increasing tumour size. A recent large meta-analysis (>11,000 patients) showed 90% facial nerve preservation with tumour <2 cm vs 67% with >2 cm [306]; therefore, most surgeons now accept a subtotal resection with preservation of facial nerve function [307, 308] or follow it with planned radiosurgery [309].

Radiotherapy

Radiotherapy has been employed in the treatment of inaccessible or incompletely excised schwannomas of the eighth and other cranial nerves. Treatment is delivered with stereotactic immobilization and delivered as a single fraction (SRS) or fractionated (fSRT) [310]. The outcomes are similar, with long-term tumour control rates of 93% at ten years and hearing preservation 70% at ten years for SRT (up to 54 Gy in 1.8 Gy fractions) and SRS (<13 Gy to 80% isodose). However, when SRS delivered >13Gy to 80% isodose, this resulted in higher rates of hearing loss (25% preservation at ten years) [311]. The choice of treatment modality is governed by a number of factors. If a vestibular schwannoma is <3.5 cm, watch and wait, SRS, or surgery are options. If it is larger than 3.5 cm or presents with local compressive symptoms, then SRS should not be used, and surgical excision and/or fractionated SRT should be used. The likelihood of hearing preservation following treatment should also be considered in the choice of treatment.

Vestibular schwannoma in neurofibromatosis type II (NF2)

Patients with NF2 are a particular challenge because they usually have bilateral vestibular schwannomas and a higher risk of radiation-induced malignancy. Treatment is indicated when there is brainstem compression, deterioration in hearing, and/or facial nerve dysfunction. Surgery is usually carried out; however, hearing preservation is problematic with bilateral disease. VEGF is highly expressed in vestibular schwannoma in NF2 [312]. Bevacizumab, the monoclonal antibody targeting VEGF, has been used in patients with progressive vestibular schwannoma with NF2. In one study, 55% of 31 patients showed a response in terms of initial tumour reduction and hearing improvement. This improvement was durable; 61% had stable or improved hearing and 54% had stable or reduced tumour size at three years [312, 313].

Choroid plexus tumours

Imaging. Choroid plexus papillomas (CPP) are more common than choroid plexus carcinomas and occur predominantly in the trigone of the lateral ventricles in children. When they occur in adults, the fourth ventricle is the most common location. The tumours have an irregular frond-like outline and usually enhance avidly but heterogeneously. Calcification is seen in approximately 25% of CPP on CT.

Drop metastases are occasionally seen in patients with CPP. Choroid plexus carcinomas typically occur in the lateral ventricles of children under the age of five; although they resemble CPP on imaging, they tend to be larger and show infiltration of surrounding brain. Hydrocephalus is a common complication.

Surgery. Surgery is the treatment of choice in benign CPP and gross total resection is associated with excellent outcome and low recurrence rate. Patients with recurrence are offered further surgery rather than radiation therapy [314, 315].

Radiotherapy. Following incomplete excision, radiotherapy has been employed with variable results [316]. It is recommended as routine treatment only in patients with gross macroscopic residual disease and in those with recurrent tumour and should be delivered by localized irradiation in doses of 50–55 Gy as for low-grade gliomas.

CPP is a rare malignant variety, to be distinguished histologically from metastatic adenocarcinoma and ependymoma. Despite aggressive treatment with surgery, radiotherapy, or chemotherapy, the prognosis is poor with high risk of CSF dissemination. Review of published case series suggests that five-year overall survival is 59.5% and progression-free survival is 37.2%. Treatment with craniospinal axis irradiation resulted in better outcomes than focal irradiation [317].

Further reading

Bartlett F, Kortmann R, Saran F. Medulloblastoma: overview. Clinical Oncology 2013; 25: 36–45.

Hart MG, Garside R, Rogers G, Stein K, Grant R. Temozolomide for high grade glioma (Cochrane Review). The Cochrane Library 2013; 4:1–58.

Huse JT, Holland EC. Targeting brain cancer: advances in the molecular pathology of malignant glioma and medulloblastoma. Nature Reviews Cancer 2010; 10: 319–331. doi:10.1038/nrc2818.

Jefferies SJ, Harris FP, Price SJ, Collins VP, Watts C. High Grade Glioma—the arrival of the molecular diagnostic era for patients over the age of 65 years in the UK. Clinical Oncology 2013; 25: 391–393.

Louis DN, Perry A, Burger P, Ellison DW, Reifenberger G et al. International Society of Neuropathology—Haarlem Consensus Guidelines for Nervous System Tumor Classification and Grading. Brain Pathology 2014; 24: 429–435. doi: 10.1111/bpa.12171.

Louis D et al. (Eds.), World Health Organization Classification of Tumours of the Central Nervous System, International Agency for Research on Cancer (IARC), Lyon, France, 2007.

Pignatti F, van den Bent M, Curran D et al. Prognostic factors for survival in adult patients with cerebral low-grade glioma. Journal of Clinical Oncology 2002; 20(8): 2076–2084.

Weller M, Cloughesy T, Perry JR, Wick W. Standards of care for treatment of recurrent glioblastoma—are we there yet? Neuro-oncology 2013; 15: 4–27.

References

1. http://seer.cancer.gov/statfacts/html/brain.html [accessed February 2015].

2. JRSM Open. 2014; 5(4): 2054270414524567. doi: 10.1177/2054270414524567

3. Louis DN, Perry A, Burger P, Ellison DW, Reifenberger G, et al. International Society of Neuropathology—Haarlem consensus guidelines for nervous system tumor classification and grading. Brain Pathology 2014; 24(5): 429–435. doi: 10.1111/bpa.12171. Epub 2014 Sep 10.

4. http://cancergenome.nih.gov/.

5. http://cancer.sanger.ac.uk/cancergenome/projects/cosmic/.

6. Johnson BE, Mazor T, Hong C, Barnes M, Aihara K, et al. Mutational analysis reveals the origin and therapy-driven evolution of recurrent glioma. Science 2014; 343(6167): 189–193. doi: 10.1126/science.1239947. Epub 2013 Dec 12.

7. Reddy JS, Mishra AM, Behari S et al. The role of diffusion-weighted imaging in the differential diagnosis of intracranial cystic

mass lesions: a report of 147 lesions. Surgical Neurology 2006; 66(3): 246–250.

8. Andronesi OC, Kim G, Gerstner E et al. Detection of 2-hydroxyglutarate in IDH-mutated glioma patients by in vivo spectral-editing and 2D correlation magnetic resonance spectroscopy. Science Translational Medicine 2012; 4(116): 116ra4.

9. Wen PY, Schiff D, Kesari S, Drappatz J, Gigas D, Doherty L. Medical management of patients with brain tumours. Journal of Neuro-Oncology 2006; 80: 313–332.

10. Glantz MJ, Cole BF, Forsyth PA et al. Practice parameter: anti-convulsant prophylaxisin patients with newly diagnosed brain tumours: report of the Quality Standards Subcommittee of the American Academy of Neurology. Neurology 2000; 54: 1886–1893.

11. Gerber DE, Grossman SA, Streiff MB. Management of venous throm-boembolism in patients with primary and metastatic brain tumors. Journal of Clinical Oncology 2006; 24: 1310–1318.

12. Ruff RL, Posner JB. Incidence and treatment of peripheral venous thrombosis in patients with glioma. Annals of Neurology 1983; 13: 334–346.

13. Litofsky NS, Farace E, Anderson F Jr, Meyers CA, Huang W, Laws ER Jr. Depression in patients with high-grade glioma: results of the Glioma Outcomes Project. Neurosurgery 2004; 54: 358–366.

14. Dimou S, Battisti RA, Hermens DF, Lagopoulos J. A systematic review of functional magnetic resonance imaging and diffusion tensor imag-ing modalities used in presurgical planning of brain tumour resection. Neurosurgical Review 2013; 36(2): 205–214; discussion 14.

15. Alexander AL, Lee JE, Lazar M, Field AS. Diffusion tensor imaging of the brain. Neurotherapeutics 2007; 4(3): 316–329.

16. Gerganov VM, Samii A, Akbarian A, Stieglitz L, Samii M, Fahlbusch R. Reliability of intraoperative high-resolution 2D ultrasound as an alternative to high-field strength MR imaging for tumor resection con-trol: a prospective comparative study. Journal of Neurosurgery 2009; 111(3): 512–519.

17. Selbekk T, Jakola AS, Solheim O, Johansen TF, Lindseth F et al. Ultrasound imaging in neurosurgery: approaches to minimize surgi-cally induced image artefacts for improved resection control. Acta Neurochirurgica (Wien) 2013; 155(6): 973–980.

18. Kassam AB, Prevedello DM, Carrau RL, Snyderman CH, Thomas A et al. Endoscopic endonasal skull base surgery: analysis of complica-tions in the authors' initial 800 patients. Journal of Neurosurgery 2011; 114(6): 1544–1568.

19. Kassam AB, Engh JA, Mintz AH, Prevedello DM. Completely endoscopic resection of intraparenchymal brain tumors. Journal of Neurosurgery 2009; 110(1): 116–123.

20. Stupp R, Mason W, Van der Bent M et al Radiotherapy plus con-comitant and adjuvant temozolamide for glioblastoma. New England Journal of Medicine 2005; 352: 987–996.

21. Stupp R, Hegi M, Mason W et al. Effects of radiotherapy with concomi-tant and adjuvant temozolamide versus radiotherapy alone on survival in glioblastoma in a randomised phase III study: 5-year analysis of the EORTC-NCIC trial. Lancet Oncology 2009; 10: 459–466.

22. Van den Bent, Brandes AA, Taphoorn MJ, Kros JM, Kouwenhoven MC et al. Adjuvant procarbazine, lomustine and vincristine chemotherapy in newly diagnosed anaplastic oligodendroglioma; long term follow up of EORTC brain tumour group study 26951. Journal of Clinical Oncology 2013; 31(3): 344–350.

23. Morris DE, Kimple RJ. Normal tissue tolerance for high grade gliomas: is it an issue? Seminars in Radiation Oncology 2009; 19: 187–192.

24. Creak AL, Tree A, Saran F. Radiotherapy planning n high-grade gliomas: a survey of current UK practice. Clinical Oncology 2011; 23: 189–198.

25. Farace P, Giri MG, Meliado G, Amelio D, Widesott L et al. Clinical target volume delineation in glioblastomas: pre-operative versus post-operative/pre-radiotherapy MRI. British Journal of Radiology 2011; 84(999): 271–278.

26. Grosu A, Weber WA. PET for radiation treatment planning of brain tumours. Radiotherapy and Oncology 2010; 96: 325–327.

27. van Herk M, Remeijer P, Rasch C, Lebesque JV. The probability of cor-rect target dosage: dose-population histograms for deriving treatment margins in radiotherapy. International Journal of Radiation Oncology Biology Physics 2000; 47(4): 1121–1235.

28. McKenzie A, van Herk M, Mijnheer B. Margins for geometric uncertainty around organs at risk in radiotherapy. Radiotherapy and Oncology 2002; 62: 299–307.

29. Gevaert T, Verellen D, Tournel K et al. Setup accuracy of the Novalis ExacTrac 6DOF system for frameless radiosurgery. International Journal of Radiation Oncology Biology Physics 2012; 82: 1627–1635.

30. Gevaert T, Levivier M, Lacournerie T et al. Dosimetric comparison of different treatment modalities for stereotactic radiosurgery of arteriovenous malformations and acoustic neuroma. Radiotherapy and Oncology 2013; 106: 192–197.

31. Allen AM, Pawlicki T, Dong L et al. An evidence based review of proton beam therapy: the report of ASTRO's emerging technology committee. Radiotherapy and Oncology 2012; 103: 8–12.

32. Sheline GE. Normal tissue tolerance and radiation therapy of glio-mas of the adult brain. In Bleehen NM ed., Tumours of the Brain. Berlin: Springer-Verlag, 1986, 141–160.

33. Mastaglia FL, McDonald WI, Watson JV, Yogendran K. Effects of X-radiation of the spinal cord: an experimental study of the morpho-logical changes in central nerve fibres. Brain 1976; 99: 101–122.

34. Lawrence YR, Allen Li X, Naqa IE et al. Radiation dose-volume effects in the brain. International Journal of Radiation Oncology Biology Physics 2010; 76(3): S20–S27.

35. Duow L, Klein M, Fagal S et al. Cognitive and radiological effects of radiotherapy in patients with low-grade glioma: long-term follow up. Lancet Neurology 2009; 8: 810–818.

36. Taphoorn MJB, Heimans JJ, van der Veen EA, Karim ABMF. Endocrine function in long-term survivors of low-grade supratentorial glioma treated with radiation therapy. Journal of Neuro-Oncology 1995; 25: 97–102.

37. Evans DRG, Birch JM, Ramsden RT, Sharif S, Baser ME. Malignant transformation and new primary tumours after therapeutic radiation for benign disease: substantial risks in certain tumour prone syn-dromes. Journal of Medical Genetics 2006; 43: 289–294.

38. Mayo C, Martel M, Marks LB. Radiation dose volume effects of optic nerves and chiasm. International Journal of Radiation Oncology Biology Physics 2010; 76(3): S28–S35.

39. Mayo C, Yorke E, Merchant TE. Radiation associated brainstem injury. International Journal of Radiation Oncology Biology Physics 2010: 76(3): S36–S41.

40. Mayer R, Sminia P. Re-irradiation tolerance of the human brain. International Journal of Radiation Oncology Biology Physics 2008; 70: 1350–1360.

41. Kirkpatrick JP, Van der Kogel AJ, Schultheiss TE. Radiation dose-volume effects in the spinal cord. International Journal of Radiation Oncology Biology Physics 2010; 76(3): S42–S49.

42. Jones B, Grant W. Retreatment of central nervous system tumours. Clinical Oncology 2014; 26: 407–418.

43. Hart MG, Garside R, Rogers G, Stein K, Grant R. Temozolomide for high grade glioma (Cochrane Review). The Cochrane Library 2013; 4: 1–58.

44. Gilbert MR, Dignam J, Won M et al. RTOG 0825: Phase III double-blind placebo-controlled trials evaluating bevacizumab (Bev) in patients with newly diagnosed glioblastoma (GBM). Journal of Clinical Oncology 2013; 31 suppl (abstr 1).

45. Wick W, Cloughsey TF, Nishikawa R et al. Tumour response based on adapted Macdonald criteria and assessment of pseudoprogres-sion (PsPD) in the phase III AVAglio trial of bevacizumab (Bv) plus temozolamide (T) and radiotherapy (RT) in newly diagnosed glioblastoma (GBM) Journal of Clinical Oncology 2013; 31 suppl (abstr 2002).

46.   Pope WB, Sayre J, Perlina A, Pablo Villablanca J, Mischel PS et al. MR imaging correlates of survival in patients with high-grade gliomas. AJNR American Journal of Neuroradiology 2005; 26: 2466–2474.

47.   Carrillo JA, Lai A, Nghiemphu PL, Kim HJ, Phillips HS et al. Relationship between tumor enhancement, edema, IDH1 mutational status, MGMT promoter methylation, and survival in glioblastoma. AJNR American Journal of Neuroradiology 2012; 33: 1349–1355.

48.   Hall WA. The safety and efficacy of stereotactic biopsy for intracranial lesions. Cancer 1998; 82(9): 1749–1755.

49.   Kingkham PN, Knifed E, Tamber MS, Bernstein M. Complications in 622 cases of frame-based stereotactic biopsy, a decreasing procedure. Canadian Journal of Neurological Sciences 2008; 35(1): 79–84.

50.   Petrecca K, Guiot MC, Panet-Raymond V, Souhami L. Failure pattern following complete resection plus radiotherapy and temozolomide is at the resection margin in patients with glioblastoma. Journal of Neurooncology 2013; 111(1): 19–23.

51.   Chaichana KL, Jusue-Torres I, Navarro-Ramirez R, Raza SM, Pascual-Gallego M et al. Establishing percent resection and residual volume thresholds affecting survival and recurrence for patients with newly diagnosed intracranial glioblastoma. Neuro- Oncology 2014; 16(1): 113–122. doi: 10.1093 [Epub 2013].

52.   Orringer D, Lau D, Khatri S, Zamora-Berridi GJ, Zhang K et al. Extent of resection in patients with glioblastoma: limiting factors, perception of resectability, and effect on survival. Journal of Neurosurgery 2012; 117(5): 851–859.

53.   Serra C, Stauffer A, Actor B, Burkhardt JK, Ulrich NH et al. Intraoperative high frequency ultrasound in intracerebral high-grade tumors. Ultraschall in der Medizin 2012; 33(7): E306–E312.

54.   Kubben PL, ter Meulen KJ, Schijns OE, ter Laak-Poort MP, van Overbeeke JJ, van Santbrink H. Intraoperative MRI-guided resection of glioblastoma multiforme: a systematic review. Lancet Oncology 2011; 12(11): 1062–1070.

55.   Lenaburg HJ, Inkabi KE, Vitaz TW. The use of intraoperative MRI for the treatment of glioblastoma multiforme. Technology in Cancer Research & Treatment 2009; 8(2): 159–162.

56.   Hatiboglu MA, Weinberg JS, Suki D, Rao G, Prabhu SS et al. Impact of intraoperative high-field magnetic resonance imaging guidance on glioma surgery: a prospective volumetric analysis. Neurosurgery 2009; 64(6): 1073–1081; discussion 81.

57.   Muragaki Y, Iseki H, Maruyama T, Kawamata T, Yamane F et al. Usefulness of intraoperative magnetic resonance imaging for glioma surgery. Acta Neurochirurgica 2006 (Suppl.); 98: 67–75.

58.   Nimsky C, Ganslandt O, Buchfelder M, Fahlbusch R. Intraoperative visualization for resection of gliomas: the role of functional neuro-navigation and intraoperative 1.5 T MRI. Neurological Research 2006; 28(5): 482–487.

59.   Bohinski RJ, Kokkino AK, Warnick RE, Gaskill-Shipley MF, Kormos DW et al. Glioma resection in a shared-resource magnetic resonance operating room after optimal image-guided frameless stereotactic resection. Neurosurgery 2001; 48(4): 731–742; discussion 42-4.

60.   Stummer W, Pichlmeier U, Meinel T, Wiestler OD, Zanella F, Reulen HJ. Fluorescence-guided surgery with 5-aminolevulinic acid for resection of malignant glioma: a randomised controlled multicentre phase III trial. Lancet Oncology 2006; 7(5): 392–401.

61.   Panciani PP, Fontanella M, Schatlo B, Garbossa D, Agnoletti A et al. Fluorescence and image guided resection in high grade glioma. Clinical Neurology and Neurosurgery 2012; 114(1): 37–41.

62.   Stummer W, Tonn JC, Mehdorn HM, Nestler U, Franz K et al. Counterbalancing risks and gains from extended resections in malignant glioma surgery: a supplemental analysis from the randomized 5-aminolevulinic acid glioma resection study. Clinical article. Journal of Neurosurgery 2011; 114(3): 613–623.

63.   Tsugu A, Ishizaka H, Mizokami Y, Osada T, Baba T et al. Impact of the combination of 5-aminolevulinic acid-induced fluorescence with intraoperative magnetic resonance imaging-guided surgery for glioma. World Neurosurgery 2011; 76(1–2): 120–127.

64.   Feigl GC, Ritz R, Moraes M, Klein J, Ramina K et al. Resection of malignant brain tumors in eloquent cortical areas: a new multimodal approach combining 5-aminolevulinic acid and intraoperative monitoring. Journal of Neurosurgery 2010; 113(2): 352–357.

65.   Li Y, Rey-Dios R, Roberts DW, Valdes PA, Cohen-Gadol AA. Intraoperative fluorescence-guided resection of high-grade gliomas: a comparison of the present techniques and evolution of future strategies. World Neurosurgery 2014; 82(1–2): 175–185 [Epub 9 July 2013].

66.   Schebesch KM, Proescholdt M, Hohne J, Hohenberger C, Hansen E et al. Sodium fluorescein-guided resection under the YELLOW 560 nm surgical microscope filter in malignant brain tumor surgery—a feasibility study. Acta Neurochirurgica (Wien). 2013; 155(4): 693–699.

67.   Liu JG, Yang SF, Liu YH, Wang X, Mao Q. Magnetic resonance diffusion tensor imaging with fluorescein sodium dyeing for surgery of gliomas in brain motor functional areas. Chinese Medical Journal (English edition) 2013; 126(13): 2418–2423.

68.   Bloch O, Han SJ, Cha S, Sun MZ, Aghi MK et al. Impact of extent of resection for recurrent glioblastoma on overall survival: clinical article. Journal of Neurosurgery 2012; 117(6):1032–1038.

69.   Chaichana KL, Zadnik P, Weingart JD, Olivi A, Gallia GL et al. Multiple resections for patients with glioblastoma: prolonging survival. Journal of Neurosurgery 2013; 118(4): 812–820.

70.   Westphal M, Ram Z, Riddle V, Hilt D, Bortey E. Gliadel wafer in initial surgery for malignant glioma: long-term follow-up of a multicenter controlled trial. Acta Neurochirurgica (Wien) 2006; 148(3): 269–275; discussion 75.

71.   Brem H, Piantadosi S, Burger PC, Walker M, Selker R et al. Placebo-controlled trial of safety and efficacy of intraoperative controlled delivery by biodegradable polymers of chemotherapy for recurrent gliomas. The Polymer-brain Tumor Treatment Group. Lancet 1995; 345(8956): 1008–1012.

72.   Noel G, Schott R, Froelich S, Gaub MP, Boyer P et al. Retrospective comparison of chemoradiotherapy followed by adjuvant chemotherapy, with or without prior gliadel implantation (carmustine) after initial surgery in patients with newly diagnosed high-grade gliomas. International Journal of Radiation Oncology Biology Physics 2012; 82(2): 749–755.

73.   Salvati M, D'Elia A, Frati A, Brogna C, Santoro A, Delfini R. Safety and feasibility of the adjunct of local chemotherapy with biodegradable carmustine (BCNU) wafers to the standard multimodal approach to high grade gliomas at first diagnosis. Journal of Neurosurgical Sciences 2011; 55(1): 1–6.

74.   Attenello FJ, Mukherjee D, Datoo G, McGirt MJ, Bohan E et al. Use of gliadel (BCNU) wafer in the surgical treatment of malignant glioma: a 10-year institutional experience. Annals of Surgical Oncology 2008; 15(10): 2887–2893.

75.   Hart MG, Grant R, Garside R, Rogers G, Somerville M, Stein K. Chemotherapy wafers for high grade glioma. Cochrane Database of Systematic Reviews 2011(3): CD007294.

76.   Lidar Z, Mardor Y, Jonas T, Pfeffer R, Faibel M et al. Convection-enhanced delivery of paclitaxel for the treatment of recurrent malignant glioma: a phase I/II clinical study. Journal of Neurosurgery 2004; 100(3): 472–479.

77.   Bogdahn U, Hau P, Stockhammer G, Venkataramana NK, Mahapatra AK et al. Targeted therapy for high-grade glioma with the TGF-beta2 inhibitor trabedersen: results of a randomized and controlled phase IIb study. Neuro-Oncology 2011; 13(1): 132–142.

78.   Carpentier A, Metellus P, Ursu R, Zohar S, Lafitte F et al. Intracerebral administration of CpG oligonucleotide for patients with recurrent glioblastoma: a phase II study. Neuro-Oncology 2010; 12(4): 401–408.

79.   Walker MD, Strike TA, Sheline GE. An analysis of dose-effect relationship in the radiotherapy of malignant gliomas. International Journal of Radiation Oncology Biology Physics 1979; 5: 1725–1731.

80.   Kristiansen K, Hagen S, Kollevold T et al. Combined modality therapy of operated astrocytomas grade III and IV. Confirmation of the value of postoperative irradiation and lack of potentiation of bleomycin on survival time. Cancer 1981; 47: 649–652.

81. Hess CF, Scaaf JC, Kortmann RD, Schabet M, Bamberg M. Malignant glioma: patterns of failure following individually tailored limited volume irradiation. Radiotherapy and Oncology 1994; 30: 146–149.

82. Minniti G, Amelio D, Amichetti M, Salvati M, Muni R et al. Patterns of failure and comparison of different target volume delineations in patients with glioblastoma treated with conformal radiotherapy plus concomitant and adjuvant temozolomide. Radiotherapy and Oncology 2010; 97(3): 377–381.

83. McDonald MW, Shu HKG, Curran WJ, Crocker IR. Pattern of failure after limited margin radiotherapy and temozolamide for glioblastoma. International Journal of Radiation Oncology Biology Physics 2011; 79(1): 130–136.

84. Kelly PJ, Daumas-Duport C, Scheithauer BW et al. Stereotactic histologic correlations of computed tomography and magnetic resonance imaging defined abnormalities in patients with glial neoplasms. Mayo Clinic Proceedings 1987; 62(6): 450–459.

85. Jansen EP, Dewit LG, van Herk M, Bartelink H. Target volumes in radiotherapy for high-grade malignant glioma of the brain. Radiotherapy and Oncology 2000; 56(2): 151–156.

86. Stall B, Zach L, Ning H, Ondos J, Arora B et al. Comparison of T2 and FLAIR imaging for target delineation in high grade gliomas. Radiation Oncology 2010; 5: 5.

87. Hegi M, Diserens AC, Gorlia T, Hamou MF, de Tribolet N et al. MGMT gene silencing and benefit from temozolomide in glioblastoma. New England Journal of Medicine 2005; 352: 997–1003.

88. Brandes A, Fiorentino MV. Treatment of high-grade gliomas in the elderly. Oncology 1998; 55(1): 1–6.

89. Davis FG, Freels S, Grutsch J, Barlas S, Brem S. Survival rates in patients with primary malignant brain tumors stratified by patient age and tumor histological type: an analysis based on Surveillance, Epidemiology, and End Results (SEER) data, 1973–1991. Journal of Neurosurgery 1998; 88(1): 1–10.

90. Vuorinen V, Hinkka S, Farkkila M, Jaaskelainen J. Debulking or biopsy of malignant glioma in elderly people—a randomised study. Acta Neurochirurgica (Wien) 2003; 145(1): 5–10.

91. Whittle IR, Denholm SW, Gregor A. Management of patients aged over 60 years with supratentorial glioma: lessons from an audit. Surgical Neurology 1991; 36(2): 106–111.

92. Whittle IR, Basu N, Grant R, Walker M, Gregor A. Management of patients aged >60 years with malignant glioma: good clinical status and radiotherapy determine outcome. British Journal of Neurosurgery 2002; 16(4): 343–347.

93. Piccirilli M, Bistazzoni S, Gagliardi FM, Landi A, Santoro A et al. Treatment of glioblastoma multiforme in elderly patients. Clinico-therapeutic remarks in 22 patients older than 80 years. Tumori 2006; 92(2): 98–103.

94. Combs SE, Wagner J, Bischof M, Welzel T, Wagner F et al. Postoperative treatment of primary glioblastoma multiforme with radiation and concomitant temozolomide in elderly patients. International Journal of Radiation Oncology Biology Physics 2008; 70(4): 987–992.

95. Mukerji N, Rodrigues D, Hendry G, Dunlop PR, Warburton F, Kane PJ. Treating high grade gliomas in the elderly: the end of ageism? Journal of Neuro-Oncology 2008; 86(3): 329–336.

96. Scott JG, Suh JH, Elson P, Barnett GH, Vogelbaum MA et al. Aggressive treatment is appropriate for glioblastoma multiforme patients 70 years old or older: a retrospective review of 206 cases. Neuro-Oncology 2011; 13(4): 428–436.

97. Weller M, Platten M, Roth P, Wick W. Geriatric neuro-oncology: from mythology to biology. Current Opinion in Neurobiology 2011; 24: 599–604.

98. www.cbtrus.org.

99. Keime-Guibert F, Chinot O, Taillandier L et al. Radiotherapy for glioblastoma in the elderly. New England Journal of Medicine 2007; 356: 1527–1535.

100. Roa W, Brasher PM, Bauman G et al. Abbreviated course of radiation therapy in older patients with glioblastoma multiforme: a prospective randomised clinical trial. Journal of Clinical Oncology 2004; 22: 1583–1588.

101. Brandes A, Franceschi E, Tosani A et al. Temozolamide concomitant and adjuvant to radiotherapy in elderly patients with glioblastoma: correlation with MGMT promoter methylation status. Cancer 2009; 115(15): 3512–3518.

102. Malmstrom A, Gronberg BH, Marosi C et al. Temozolamide versus standard 6 week radiotherapy versus hypofractionated radiotherapy in patients older than 60 years with glioblastoma: the Nordic randomised phase 3 trial. Lancet Oncology 2012; 13(9): 916–926.

103. Wick W, Platten M, Meisner C et al. Temozolamide chemotherapy alone versus radiotherapy alone for malignant astrocytoma in the elderly: the NOA-08 randomised phase 3 trial. Lancet Oncology 2012; 13(7): 707–715.

104. Jefferies SJ, Harris FP, Price SJ, Collins VP, Watts C. High grade glioma—the arrival of the molecular diagnostic era for patients over the age of 65 years in the UK. Clinical Oncology 2013; 25: 391–393.

105. Wick W, Hartmann C, Engel C et al. NOA-04 randomized phase iii trial of sequential radiochemotherapy of anaplastic glioma with procarbazine, lomustine, and vincristine or temozolomide. Journal of Clinical Oncology 2009; 27: 5874–5880.

106. Cairncross G, Wang M, Shaw E et al. Phase III trial of chemoradiotherapy for anaplastic oligodendroglioma: long-term results of RTOG 9402. Journal of Clinical Oncology 2013; 31(3): 337–343.

107. Weller M, Cloughesy T, Perry JR, Wick W. Standards of care for treatment of recurrent glioblastoma—are we there yet? Neuro-oncology 2013; 15: 4–27.

108. Chamberlain MC, Glantz MJ, Chalmers L et al. Early necrosis following concurrent Temodar and radiotherapy in patients with glioblastoma. Journal of Neuro-Oncology 2007; 82(1): 81.

109. Park JK, Hodges T, Arko L et al. Scale to predict survival after surgery for recurrent glioblastoma multiforme. Journal of Clinical Oncology 2010; 28(24): 3838–3843.

110. Brem H, Piantodosi S, Burger P et al. Placebo-controlled trial of safety and efficacy of intraoperative controlled delivery by biodegradable polymers of chemotherapy for recurrent gliomas. Lancet 1995; 345: 1008–1012.

111. Niyazi M, Siefart A, Schwarz SB et al. Therapeutic options for recurrent malignant glioma. Radiotherapy and Oncology 2011; 98: 1–14.

112. Niyazi M, Ganswindt U, Schwarz SB et al. Irradiation and bevacizumab in high-grade glioma retreatment settings. International Journal of Radiation Oncology Biology Physics 2012; 82(1): 67–76.

113. Brada M, Stenning S, Gabe R et al Temozolamide versus procarbazine, lomustine and vincristine in recurrent high-grade glioma. Journal of Clinical Oncology 2010; 28(30): 4601.

114. Perry JR, Belanger K, Mason WP et al. Phase II trial of continuous dose-intense temozolamide in recurrent malignant glioma: RESCUE study. Journal of Clinical Oncology 2010; 28(12): 2051–2057.

115. Brandes AA, Torsoni A, Amista P et al. Howe effective is BCNU in recurrent glioblastoma in the modern era? A phase II trial. Neurology 2004; 63(7): 1281.

116. Cloughesy T, Vredenburgh JJ, Day B et al. Updated safety and survival of patients with relapsed glioblastoma treated with bevacizumab in the BRAIN study. Journal of Clinical Oncology 2010; 28(15s): 2008.

117. Nasuda Danchaivijitr, Waldman AD, Tozer DJ et al. Low-grade gliomas: do changes in rCBV measurements at longitudinal perfusion-weighted MR imaging predict malignant transformation? Radiology 2008; 247: 170–178.

118. Caseiras GB, Ciccarelli O, Altmann DR, Benton CE, Tozer DF et al. Low-grade gliomas: six-month tumor growth predicts patient outcome better than admission tumor volume, relative cerebral blood volume, and apparent diffusion coefficientt. Radiology 2009; 253: 505–512.

119. Mandonnet E, Delattre JY, Tanguy ML, Swanson KR, Carpentier AF et al. Continuous growth of mean tumor diameter in a subset of grade II gliomas. Annals of Neurology 2003; 53(4): 524–528.

120. Pallud J, Fontaine D, Duffau H, Mandonnet E, Sanai N et al. Natural history of incidental World Health Organization grade II gliomas. Annals of Neurology 2010; 68(5): 727–733.

121. Pallud J, Mandonnet E, Duffau H, Kujas M, Guillevin R et al. Prognostic value of initial magnetic resonance imaging growth rates for World Health Organization grade II gliomas. Annals of Neurology 2006; 60(3): 380–383.

122. Smith JS, Chang EF, Lamborn KR, Chang SM, Prados MD et al. Role of extent of resection in the long-term outcome of low-grade hemispheric gliomas. Journal of Clinical Oncology 2008; 26(8): 1338–1345.

123. Sanai N, Berger MS. Intraoperative stimulation techniques for functional pathway preservation and glioma resection. Neurosurgical Focus 2010; 28(2): E1.

124. Yordanova YN, Moritz-Gasser S, Duffau H. Awake surgery for WHO Grade II gliomas within 'noneloquent' areas in the left dominant hemisphere: toward a 'supratotal' resection. Clinical article. Journal of Neurosurgery 2011; 115(2): 232–239.

125. Ogiwara H, Bowman RM, Tomita T. Long-term follow-up of pediatric benign cerebellar astrocytomas. Neurosurgery 2012; 70(1): 40–147; discussion 7–8.

126. Palma L, Celli P, Mariottini A. Long-term follow-up of childhood cerebellar astrocytomas after incomplete resection with particular reference to arrested growth or spontaneous tumour regression. Acta Neurochirurgica (Wien) 2004; 146(6): 581–588; discussion 8.

127. Klimo P Jr, Pai Panandiker AS, Thompson CJ, Boop FA, Qaddoumi I et al. Management and outcome of focal low-grade brainstem tumors in pediatric patients: the St. Jude experience. Journal of Neurosurgery Pediatrics 2013; 11(3): 274–281.

128. Jain A, Amin AG, Jain P, Burger P, Jallo GI et al. Subependymoma: clinical features and surgical outcomes. Neurological Research 2012; 34(7): 677–684.

129. Karim ABMF, Maat B, Hatlevoll R et al. Randomized trial on dose-response in radiation therapy of low-grade cerebral glioma: European Organization for Research and Treatment of Cancer (EORTC) study 22844. International Journal of Radiation Oncology Biology Physics 1996; 36(3): 549–556.

130. Karim ABMF, Afra D, Cornu P et al. Randomized trial of the efficacy of radiotherapy for low-grade glioma in the adult: European Organization for Research and Treatment of Cancer Study 22845 with the Medical Research Council study BR04: An interim analysis. International Journal of Radiation Oncology Biology Physics 2002; 52: 316–324.

131. Musat E, Roelofs E, Bar-Deroma R, Fenton P, Gulyban A et al. Dummy run and conformity indices in the ongoing EORTC low-grade glioma trial 22033–26033: first evaluation of quality of radiotherapy planning. Radiotherapy and Oncology 2010; 95(2): 218–224.

132. Pignatti F, van den Bent M, Curran D et al. Prognostic factors for survival in adult patients with cerebral low-grade glioma. Journal of Clinical Oncology 2002; 20(8): 2076–2084.

133. Shaw ED, Wang M, Coons SW et al. Randomized trial of radiation therapy plus procarbazine, lomustine, and vincristine chemotherapy for supratentorial adult low-grade glioma: initial results of RTOG 9802. Journal of Clinical Oncology 2012; 30(25): 3065–3070.

134. Leu S, von Felten S, Frank S, et al. IDH/MGMT-driven molecular classification of low-grade glioma is a strong predictor for long-term survival. Neuro-Oncology 2013; 15(4): 469–479.

135. Guillamo JS, Monjour A, Taillandier L et al. Brainstem gliomas in adults: prognostic factors and classification. Brain 2001; 124(12): 2528–2539.

136. Metellus P, Barrie M, Figarella-Branger D et al. Multicentric French study on adult intracranial ependymomas: prognostic factors analysis and therapeutic considerations from a cohort of 152 patients. Brain 2007; 130(5): 1338–1349.

137. Iqbal MS, Lewis J. An overview of the management of adult ependymomas with emphasis on relapsed disease. Clinical Oncology 2013; 25: 726–733.

138. Sutton LN, Phillips PC, Molloy PT. Surgical management of medulloblastoma. Journal of Neuro-Oncology 1996; 29(1): 9–21.

139. Park TS, Hoffman HJ, Hendrick EB, Humphreys RP, Becker LE. Medulloblastoma: clinical presentation and management. Experience at the hospital for sick children, Toronto, 1950–1980. Journal of Neurosurgery 1983; 58(4): 543–552.

140. Jaing TH, Wu CT, Chen SH, Hung PC, Lin KL et al. Intracranial tumors in infants: a single institution experience of 22 patients. Child's Nervous System 2011; 27(3): 415–419.

141. Lang SS, Beslow LA, Gabel B, Judkins AR, Fisher MJ et al. Surgical treatment of brain tumors in infants younger than six months of age and review of the literature. World Neurosurgery 2012; 78(1–2): 137–144.

142. Khafaga Y, Kandil AE, Jamshed A, Hassounah M, DeVol E, Gray AJ. Treatment results for 149 medulloblastoma patients from one institution. International Journal of Radiation Oncology Biology Physics 1996; 35(3): 501–516.

143. Muzumdar D, Deshpande A, Kumar R, Sharma A, Goel N et al. Medulloblastoma in childhood—King Edward Memorial hospital surgical experience and review: comparative analysis of the case series of 365 patients. Journal of Pediatric Neurosciences 2011; 6(Suppl 1): S78–S85.

144. Albright AL, Wisoff JH, Zeltzer PM, Boyett JM, Rorke LB, Stanley P. Effects of medulloblastoma resections on outcome in children: a report from the Children's Cancer Group. Neurosurgery 1996; 38(2): 265–271.

145. Bhatia R, Tahir M, Chandler CL. The management of hydrocephalus in children with posterior fossa tumours: the role of pre-resectional endoscopic third ventriculostomy. Pediatric Neurosurgery 2009; 45(3): 186–191.

146. Di Rocco F, Juca CE, Zerah M, Sainte-Rose C. Endoscopic third ventriculostomy and posterior fossa tumors. World Neurosurgery 2013; 79(2 Suppl): S18 e5–e9.

147. Chang CH, Housepian EM, Herbert C. An operative staging system and a megavoltage radiotherapeutic technique for cerebellar medulloblastomas. Radiology 1969; 93(6): 1351–1359.

148. <www.bnos.org.uk/rare_tumours.html>.

149. Packer RJ, Gajjar A, Vezina G et al. Phase III study of craniospinal radiation therapy followed by adjuvant chemotherapy for newly diagnosed average-risk medulloblastoma. Journal of Clinical Oncology 2006; 24(25): 4202–4208.

150. Bartlett F, Kortmann R, Saran F. Medulloblastoma: overview. Clinical Oncology 2013; 25: 36–45.

151. Friedrich C, von Bueren AO, von Hoff K et al. Treatment of adult nonmetastatic medulloblastoma patients according to the paediatric HIT 2000 protocol: a prospective multicentre study. European Journal of Cancer 2013; 49(4): 893–903.

152. Dunkel IJ, Gardner SL, Garvin JH et al. High dose carboplatin, thitepa and etoposide with autologous stem cell rescue for patients with previously irradiated recurrent medulloblastoma. Neuro-Oncology 2010; 12(3): 297–303.

153. Parker JJ, Waziri A. Preoperative evaluation of pineal tumors. Neurosurgery Clinics of North America 2011; 22(3): 353–358, vii–viii.

154. Constantini S, Mohanty A, Zymberg S, Cavalheiro S, Mallucci C et al. Safety and diagnostic accuracy of neuroendoscopic biopsies: an international multicenter study. Journal of Neurosurgery Pediatrics 2013; 11(6): 704–709.

155. Oppido PA, Fiorindi A, Benvenuti L, Cattani F, Cipri S et al. Neuroendoscopic biopsy of ventricular tumors: a multicentric experience. Neurosurgery Focus 2011; 30(4): E2.

156. Morgenstern PF, Souweidane MM. Pineal region tumors: simultaneous endoscopic third ventriculostomy and tumor biopsy. World Neurosurgery 2013; 79(2 Suppl): S18 e9–e13.

157. Clark AJ, Sughrue ME, Ivan ME, Aranda D, Rutkowski MJ et al. Factors influencing overall survival rates for patients with pineocytoma. Journal of Neuro-Oncology 2010; 100(2): 255–260.

158. Clark AJ, Ivan ME, Sughrue ME, Yang I, Aranda D et al. Tumor control after surgery and radiotherapy for pineocytoma. Journal of Neurosurgery 2010; 113(2): 319–324.

159. Lutterbach J, Fauchon F, Schild SE, Chang SM, Pagenstecher A et al. Malignant pineal parenchymal tumors in adult patients: patterns of care and prognostic factors. Neurosurgery 2002; 51(1): 44–55; discussion 55-6.

160. Fauchon F, Jouvet A, Paquis P, Saint-Pierre G, Mottolese C et al. Parenchymal pineal tumors: a clinicopathological study of 76 cases. International Journal of Radiation Oncology Biology Physics 2000; 46(4): 959–968.

161. Tate M, Sughrue ME, Rutkowski MJ, Kane AJ, Aranda D et al. The long-term postsurgical prognosis of patients with pineoblastoma. Cancer 2012; 118(1): 173–179.

162. Calaminus G, Kortmann R, Worch J et al. SIOP CNS GCT 96: final report of outcome of a prospective, multinational nonrandomized trial for children and adults with intracranial germinoma, comparing craniospinal irradiation alone with chemotherapy followed by focal primary site irradiation for patients with localized disease. Neuro-Oncology 2013; 15(6): 788–796.

163. Calaminus G, Frappaz D, Kortmann R et al. Localized and metastatic nongerminoma treated according to the SIOP CNS GCT 96 protocol: update on risk profiles and outcome. Neuro-Oncology 2008; 10(3): 418.

164. Mori Y, Kobayashi T, Hasegawa T et al. Stereotactic radiosurgery for pineal and related tumours. Progress in Neurological Surgery 2009; 23: 106.

165. Akpek EK, Ahmed I, Hochberg FH et al. Intraocular-CNS lymphoma: clinical features, diagnosis, and outcomes. Ophthalmology 1999; 106: 1805–1810.

166. Glass J, Hochberg FH, Miller DC. Intravascular lymphomatosis: a systemic disease with neurologic manifestations. Cancer 1993; 71: 3156–3164.

167. Hochberg FH, Baehring JM, Hochberg EP et al. Primary CNS lymphoma. Nature Clinical Practice Neurology 2007; 3(1): 24–35.

168. Ivers LC, Kim AY, Sax PE et al. Predictive value of polymerase chain reaction of cerebrospinal fluid for detection of Epstein–Barr virus to establish the diagnosis of HIV related primary central nervous system lymphoma. Clinical Infectious Diseases 2004; 38: 1629–1632.

169. Ferreri AJ, Blay JY, Reni M et al. Prognostic scoring system for primary CNS lymphoma: The International Extranodal Lymphoma Study Group Experience. Journal of Clinical Oncology 2003; 21: 266–272.

170. Murray K, Kun L, Cox J. Primary malignant lymphoma of the central nervous system. Results of treatment of 11 cases and review of the literature. Journal of Neurosurgery 1986; 65(5): 600–607.

171. Ferreri AJ, Reni M, Foppoli M et al. High-dose cytarabine plus high-dose methotrexate versus high-dose methotrexate alone in patients with primary CNS lymphoma: a randomised phase 2 trial. Lancet 2009; 374: 1512.

172. Rubenstien JL, His ED, Johnson JL et al. Intensive chemotherapy and immunotherapy in patients with newly diagnosed primary CNS lymphoma: CALGB 50202 (Alliance 50202). Journal of Clinical Oncology 2013; 31(25): 3061–3068.

173. Thiel E, Korfel A, Martus P et al. High-dose methotrexate with or without whole brain radiotherapy for primary CNS lymphoma (G-PCNSL-SG-1): a phase 3, randomised, non-inferiority trial. Lancet Oncology 2010; 11(11): 1036–1047.

174. Bessell EM, Lopez-Guillermo A, Villa S et al. Importance of radiotherapy in the outcome of patients with primary CNS lymphoma: an analysis of the CHOD/BVAM regimen followed by two different radiotherapy treatments. Journal of Clinical Oncology 2002; 20: 231–236.

175. Muirhead R, Murray EC, Bell SL et al. Is there a role for radiotherapy in the primary management of Central Nervous System lymphoma? A single-centre case series. Clinical Oncology 2013; 25: 400–405.

176. Simpson D. The recurrence of intracranial meningiomas after surgical treatment. Journal of Neurology, Neurosurgery and Psychiatry 1957; 20(1): 22–39.

177. Sughrue ME, Kane AJ, Shangari G, Rutkowski MJ, McDermott MW et al. The relevance of Simpson Grade I and II resection in modern neurosurgical treatment of World Health Organization Grade I meningiomas. Journal of Neurosurgery 2010; 113(5): 1029–1035.

178. Sindou MP, Alvernia JE. Results of attempted radical tumor removal and venous repair in 100 consecutive meningiomas involving the major dural sinuses. Journal of Neurosurgery 2006; 105(4): 514–525.

179. Gardner PA, Kassam AB, Thomas A, Snyderman CH, Carrau RL et al. Endoscopic endonasal resection of anterior cranial base meningiomas. Neurosurgery 2008; 63(1): 36–52; discussion 52-4.

180. de Divitiis E, Cavallo LM, Esposito F, Stella L, Messina A. Extended endoscopic transsphenoidal approach for tuberculum sellae meningiomas. Neurosurgery 2008; 62(6 Suppl 3): 1192–1201.

181. Komotar RJ, Starke RM, Raper DM, Anand VK, Schwartz TH. Endoscopic endonasal versus open transcranial resection of anterior midline skull base meningiomas. World Neurosurgery 2012; 77(5–6): 713–724.

182. Sughrue ME, Rutkowski MJ, Chen CJ, Shangari G, Kane AJ et al. Modern surgical outcomes following surgery for sphenoid wing meningiomas. Journal of Neurosurgery 2013; 119(1): 86–93.

183. Talacchi A, Biroli A, Soda C, Masotto B, Bricolo A. Surgical management of ventral and ventrolateral foramen magnum meningiomas: report on a 64-case series and review of the literature. Neurosurgical Review 2012; 35(3): 359–367; discussion 367–8.

184. Fraser JF, Nyquist GG, Moore N, Anand VK, Schwartz TH. Endoscopic endonasal minimal access approach to the clivus: case series and technical nuances. Neurosurgery 2010; 67(3 Suppl Operative): ons 150–8; discussion ons 158.

185. Fraser JF, Nyquist GG, Moore N, Anand VK, Schwartz TH. Endoscopic endonasal transclival resection of chordomas: operative technique, clinical outcome, and review of the literature. Journal of Neurosurgery 2010; 112(5): 1061–1069.

186. Brada M, Minniti G, Weber DC. Fractionated radiation for meningiomas. In Black P, Necmettin Pamir M, Fahlbusch R, Meningiomas: A Comprehensive Text. Elsevier, 2010.

187. Combs SE, Adeberg S, Dittmar JO, Welzel T, Rieken S et al. Skull base meningiomas: long-term results and patient self-reported outcome in 507 patients treated with fractionated stereotactic radiotherapy (FSRT) or intensity modulated radiotherapy (IMRT). Radiotherapy and Oncology 2013; 106(2): 186–191.

188. Wenkel E, Thornton AF, Finkelstein D, Adams J, Lyons S et al. Benign meningioma: partially resected, biopsied, and recurrent intracranial tumors treated with combined proton and photon radiotherapy. International Journal of Radiation Oncology Biology Physics 2000; 48(5): 1363–1370.

189. Weber DC, Lomax AJ, Rutz HP, Stadelmann O, Egger E et al. Spot-scanning proton radiation therapy for recurrent, residual or untreated intracranial meningiomas. Radiotherapy and Oncology 2004; 71(3): 251–258.

190. Goldsmith BJ, Wara WM, Wilson CB, Larson DA (1994). Postoperative irradiation for subtotally resected meningiomas. A retrospective analysis of 140 patients treated from 1967 to 1990. Journal of Neurosurgery 1994; 80(2): 195–201.

191. Nutting C, Brada M, Brazil L, Sibtain A, Saran F et al. Radiotherapy in the treatment of benign meningioma of the skull base. Journal of Neurosurgery 1999; 90(5): 823–827.

192. Kondziolka D, Mathieu D, Lunsford LD, Martin JJ, Madhok R et al. Radiosurgery as definitive management of intracranial meningiomas. Neurosurgery 2008; 62(1): 53–58; discussion 58–60.

193. Di Maio S, Cavallo LM, Esposito F, Stagno V, Corriero OV, Cappabianca P. Extended endoscopic endonasal approach for selected pituitary adenomas: early experience. Journal of Neurosurgery 2011; 114(2): 345–353.

194. Kassam A, Snyderman CH, Mintz A, Gardner P, Carrau RL. Expanded endonasal approach: the rostrocaudal axis. Part I. Crista galli to the sella turcica. Neurosurgical Focus 2005; 19(1): E3.

195. Koutourousiou M, Gardner PA, Fernandez-Miranda JC, Paluzzi A, Wang EW, Snyderman CH. Endoscopic endonasal surgery for giant pituitary adenomas: advantages and limitations. Journal of Neurosurgery 2013; 118(3): 621–631.

196. McLaughlin N, Eisenberg AA, Cohan P, Chaloner CB, Kelly DF. Value of endoscopy for maximizing tumor removal in endonasal transsphenoidal pituitary adenoma surgery. Journal of Neurosurgery 2013; 118(3): 613–620.

197. Nakao N, Itakura T. Surgical outcome of the endoscopic endonasal approach for non-functioning giant pituitary adenoma. Journal of Clinical Neuroscience 2011; 18(1): 71–75.

198. Cavallo LM, Solari D, Esposito F, Cappabianca P. Endoscopic endonasal approach for pituitary adenomas. Acta Neurochirurgica (Wien) 2012; 154(12): 2251–2256.

199. Sanai N, Quinones-Hinojosa A, Narvid J, Kunwar S. Safety and efficacy of the direct endonasal transsphenoidal approach for challenging sellar tumors. Journal of Neuro-Oncology 2008; 87(3): 317–325.

200. Losa M, Mortini P, Barzaghi R, Ribotto P, Terreni MR et al. Early results of surgery in patients with nonfunctioning pituitary adenoma and analysis of the risk of tumor recurrence. Journal of Neurosurgery 2008; 108(3): 525–532.

201. Gnanalingham KK, Bhattacharjee S, Pennington R, Ng J, Mendoza N. The time course of visual field recovery following transphenoidal surgery for pituitary adenomas: predictive factors for a good outcome. Journal of Neurology, Neurosurgery, and Psychiatry 2005; 76(3): 415–419.

202. Grossman R, Mukherjee D, Chaichana KL, Salvatori R, Wand G et al. Complications and death among elderly patients undergoing pituitary tumour surgery. Clinical Endocrinology (Oxford) 2010; 73(3): 361–368.

203. Fraser CL, Biousse V, Newman NJ. Visual outcomes after treatment of pituitary adenomas. Neurosurgery Clinics of North America 2012; 23(4): 607–619.

204. Nemergut EC, Zuo Z, Jane JA Jr, Laws ER Jr. Predictors of diabetes insipidus after transsphenoidal surgery: a review of 881 patients. Journal of Neurosurgery 2005; 103(3): 448–454.

205. Greenman Y, Stern N. How should a nonfunctioning pituitary macroadenoma be monitored after debulking surgery? Clinical Endocrinology (Oxford) 2009; 70(6): 829–832.

206. Sheehan JM, Douds GL, Hill K, Farace E. Transsphenoidal surgery for pituitary adenoma in elderly patients. Acta Neurochirurgica (Wien) 2008; 150(6): 571–574; discussion 4.

207. Raza SM, Boahene KD, Quinones-Hinojosa A. The transpalpebral incision: its use in keyhole approaches to cranial base brain tumors. Expert Review of Neurotherapeutics 2010; 10(11): 1629–1632.

208. Raza SM, Quinones-Hinojosa A, Lim M, Boahene KD. The transconjunctival transorbital approach: a keyhole approach to the midline anterior skull base. World Neurosurgery 2013; 80(6): 864–871 [Epub 2012 Jun 19].

209. Brada M, Jankowska P. Radiotherapy for pituitary adenomas. Endocrinology and Metabolism Clinics of North America 2008; 37(1): 263–275, xi.

210. Minniti G, Gilbert DC, Brada M. Modern techniques for pituitary radiotherapy. Reviews in Endocrine and Metabolic Disorders 2009; 10: 135–144.

211. Brada M, Rajan B, Traish D, Ashley S, Holmes-Sellors PJ. The long-term efficacy of conservative surgery and radiotherapy in the control of pituitary adenomas. Clinical Endocrinology (Oxford) 1993; 38(6): 571–578.

212. Fernandez A, Brada M, Zabuliene L, Karavitaki N, Wass JA. Radiation-induced hypopituitarism. Endocrine Related Cancer 2009; 16(3): 733–772.

213. Brada M, Ashley S, Ford D, Traish D, Burchell L, Rajan B. Cerebrovascular mortality in patients with pituitary adenoma. Clinical Endocrinology (Oxford) 2002; 57(6): 713–717.

214. Brada M, Ford D, Ashley S, Bliss JM, Crowley S et al. Risk of second brain tumour after conservative surgery and radiotherapy for pituitary adenoma. British Medical Journal 1992; 304(6838): 1343–1346.

215. Minniti G, Traish D, Ashley S, Gonsalves A, Brada M. Risk of second brain tumor after conservative surgery and radiotherapy for pituitary adenoma: update after an additional 10 years. Journal of Clinical Endocrinology and Metabolism 2005; 90(2): 800–804.

216. Karavitaki N, Cudlip S, Adams CB, Wass JA. Craniopharyngiomas. Endocrine Reviews 2006; 27(4): 371–397.

217. Yasargil MG, Curcic M, Kis M, Siegenthaler G, Teddy PJ, Roth P. Total removal of craniopharyngiomas. Approaches and long-term results in 144 patients. Journal of Neurosurgery 1990; 73(1): 3–11.

218. Zuccaro G. Radical resection of craniopharyngioma. Child's Nervous System 2005; 21(8–9): 679–690.

219. Di Rocco C, Caldarelli M, Tamburrini G, Massimi L. Surgical management of craniopharyngiomas—experience with a pediatric series. Journal of Pediatric Endocrinology and Metabolism 2006; 19(Suppl 1): 355–366.

220. Mortini P, Losa M, Pozzobon G, Barzaghi R, Riva M et al. Neurosurgical treatment of craniopharyngioma in adults and children: early and long-term results in a large case series. Journal of Neurosurgery 2011; 114(5): 1350–1359.

221. Elliott RE, Wisoff JH. Surgical management of giant pediatric craniopharyngiomas. Journal of Neurosurgery Pediatrics 2010; 6(5): 403–416.

222. Muller HL, Gebhardt U, Schroder S, Pohl F, Kortmann RD et al. Analyses of treatment variables for patients with childhood craniopharyngioma—results of the multicenter prospective trial KRANIOPHARYNGEOM 2000 after three years of follow-up. Hormone Research in Paediatrics 2010; 73(3): 175–180.

223. Karavitaki N, Brufani C, Warner JT, Adams CB, Richards P et al. Craniopharyngiomas in children and adults: systematic analysis of 121 cases with long-term follow-up. Clinical Endocrinology (Oxford) 2005; 62(4): 397–409.

224. Clark AJ, Cage TA, Aranda D, Parsa AT, Sun PP et al. A systematic review of the results of surgery and radiotherapy on tumor control for pediatric craniopharyngioma. Child's Nervous System 2013; 29(2): 231–238.

225. Schoenfeld A, Pekmezci M, Barnes MJ, Tihan T, Gupta N et al. The superiority of conservative resection and adjuvant radiation for craniopharyngiomas. Journal of Neuro-Oncology 2012; 108(1): 133–139.

226. Yang I, Sughrue ME, Rutkowski MJ, Kaur R, Ivan ME et al. Craniopharyngioma: a comparison of tumor control with various treatment strategies. Neurosurgical Focus 2010; 28(4): E5.

227. Moon SH, Kim IH, Park SW, Kim I, Hong S et al. Early adjuvant radiotherapy toward long-term survival and better quality of life for craniopharyngiomas—a study in single institute. Child's Nervous System 2005; 21(8–9): 799–807.

228. Schubert T, Trippel M, Tacke U, van Velthoven V, Gumpp V et al. Neurosurgical treatment strategies in childhood craniopharyngiomas: is less more? Child's Nervous System 2009; 25(11): 1419–1427.

229. Muller HL. Childhood craniopharyngioma—current concepts in diagnosis, therapy and follow-up. Nature Reviews Endocrinology 2010; 6(11): 609–618.

230. Kassam AB, Gardner PA, Snyderman CH, Carrau RL, Mintz AH, Prevedello DM. Expanded endonasal approach, a fully endoscopic transnasal approach for the resection of midline suprasellar craniopharyngiomas: a new classification based on the infundibulum. Journal of Neurosurgery 2008; 108(4): 715–728.

231. Schwartz TH, Fraser JF, Brown S, Tabaee A, Kacker A, Anand VK. Endoscopic cranial base surgery: classification of operative approaches. Neurosurgery 2008; 62(5): 991–1002; discussion 1002-5.

232. Frank G, Pasquini E, Doglietto F, Mazzatenta D, Sciarretta V et al. The endoscopic extended transsphenoidal approach for craniopharyngiomas. Neurosurgery 2006; 59(1 Suppl 1): ONS75–83; discussion ONS75-83.

233. Gardner PA, Prevedello DM, Kassam AB, Snyderman CH, Carrau RL, Mintz AH. The evolution of the endonasal approach for craniopharyngiomas. Journal of Neurosurgery 2008; 108(5): 1043–1047.

234. Hadad G, Bassagasteguy L, Carrau RL, Mataza JC, Kassam A et al. A novel reconstructive technique after endoscopic expanded endonasal approaches: vascular pedicle nasoseptal flap. Laryngoscope 2006; 116(10): 1882–1886.

235. Leng LZ, Greenfield JP, Souweidane MM, Anand VK, Schwartz TH. Endoscopic, endonasal resection of craniopharyngiomas: analysis of outcome including extent of resection, cerebrospinal fluid leak, return to preoperative productivity, and body mass index. Neurosurgery 2012; 70(1): 110–123; discussion 23-4.

236. Snyderman CH, Pant H, Carrau RL, Prevedello D, Gardner P, Kassam AB. What are the limits of endoscopic sinus surgery?: the expanded endonasal approach to the skull base. Keio Journal of Medicine 2009; 58(3): 152–160.

237. Elliott RE, Jane JA Jr, Wisoff JH. Surgical management of craniopharyngiomas in children: meta-analysis and comparison of transcranial and transsphenoidal approaches. Neurosurgery 2011; 69(3): 630–643; discussion 43.

238. Komotar RJ, Starke RM, Raper DM, Anand VK, Schwartz TH. Endoscopic endonasal compared with microscopic transsphenoidal and open transcranial resection of craniopharyngiomas. World Neurosurgery 2012; 77(2): 329–341.

239. Cinalli G, Spennato P, Cianciulli E, Fiorillo A, Di Maio S, Maggi G. The role of transventricular neuroendoscopy in the management of craniopharyngiomas: three patient reports and review of the literature. Journal of Pediatric Endocrinology and Metabolism 2006; 19(Suppl 1): 341–354.

240. Aggarwal A, Fersht N, Brada M. Radiotherapy for craniopharyngioma. Pituitary 2013; 16(1): 26–33.

241. Rajan B, Ashley S, Gorman C, Jose CC, Horwich A et al. Craniopharyngioma—long-term results following limited surgery and radiotherapy. Radiotherapy and Oncology 1993; 26(1): 1–10.

242. Minniti G, Saran F, Traish D, Soomal R, Sardell S et al. Fractionated stereotactic conformal radiotherapy following conservative surgery in the control of craniopharyngiomas. Radiotherapy and Oncology 2007; 82(1): 90–95.

243. Rajan B, Ashley S, Thomas DG, Marsh H, Britton J, Brada M. Craniopharyngioma: improving outcome by early recognition and treatment of acute complications. International Journal of Radiation Oncology Biology Physics 1997; 37(3): 517–521.

244. O'Toole JE, McCormick PC. Midline ventral intradural schwannoma of the cervical spinal cord resected via anterior corpectomy with reconstruction: technical case report and review of the literature. Neurosurgery 2003; 52(6): 1482–1485; discussion 5-6.

245. Angevine PD, Kellner C, Haque RM, McCormick PC. Surgical management of ventral intradural spinal lesions. Journal of Neurosurgery: Spine 2011; 15(1): 28–37.

246. McCormick PC. Retropleural approach to the thoracic and thoracolumbar spine. Neurosurgery 1995; 37(5): 908–914.

247. Lubelski D, Abdullah KG, Steinmetz MP, Masters F, Benzel EC et al. Lateral extracavitary, costotransversectomy, and transthoracic thoracotomy approaches to the thoracic spine: review of techniques and complications. Journal of Spinal Disorders & Techniques 2013; 26(4): 222–232.

248. Ponce FA, Killory BD, Wait SD, Theodore N, Dickman CA. Endoscopic resection of intrathoracic tumors: experience with and long-term results for 26 patients. Journal of Neurosurgery: Spine 2011; 14(3): 377–381.

249. Kothbauer K, Deletis V, Epstein FJ. Intraoperative spinal cord monitoring for intramedullary surgery: an essential adjunct. Pediatric Neurosurgery 1997; 26(5): 247–254.

250. Nadkarni TD, Rekate HL. Pediatric intramedullary spinal cord tumors. Critical review of the literature. Child's Nervous System 1999; 15(1): 17–28.

251. Inoue T, Endo T, Nagamatsu K, Watanabe M, Tominaga T. 5-aminolevulinic acid fluorescence-guided resection of intramedullary ependymoma: report of 9 cases. Neurosurgery 2013; 72(2 Suppl Operative): ons159–168; discussion ons68.

252. Feldman WB, Clark AJ, Safaee M, Ames CP, Parsa AT. Tumor control after surgery for spinal myxopapillary ependymomas: distinct outcomes in adults versus children: a systematic review. Journal of Neurosurgery: Spine 2013; 19(4): 471–476.

253. Hoshimaru M, Koyama T, Hashimoto N, Kikuchi H. Results of microsurgical treatment for intramedullary spinal cord ependymomas: analysis of 36 cases. Neurosurgery 1999; 44(2): 264–269.

254. Kucia EJ, Bambakidis NC, Chang SW, Spetzler RF. Surgical technique and outcomes in the treatment of spinal cord ependymomas, part 1: intramedullary ependymomas. Neurosurgery 2011; 68(1 Suppl Operative): 57–63; discussion 63.

255. Sgouros S, Malluci CL, Jackowski A. Spinal ependymomas—the value of postoperative radiotherapy for residual disease control. British Journal of Neurosurgery 1996; 10(6): 559–566.

256. Whitaker SJ, Bessell ED, Ashley S, Bloom HJG, Bell BA, Brada M. Postoperative radiotherapy in the management of spinal cord ependymomas. Journal of Neurosurgery 1991; 74: 720–728.

257. McGirt MJ, Goldstein IM, Chaichana KL, Tobias ME, Kothbauer KF, Jallo GI. Extent of surgical resection of malignant astrocytomas of the spinal cord: outcome analysis of 35 patients. Neurosurgery 2008; 63(1): 55–60; discussion 60-1.

258. Raco A, Piccirilli M, Landi A, Lenzi J, Delfini R, Cantore G. High-grade intramedullary astrocytomas: 30 years' experience at the Neurosurgery Department of the University of Rome 'Sapienza'. Journal of Neurosurgery: Spine 2010; 12(2): 144–153.

259. Benes V 3rd, Barsa P, Benes V Jr, Suchomel P. Prognostic factors in intramedullary astrocytomas: a literature review. European Spine Journal 2009; 18(10): 1397–1422.

260. Linstadt DE, Wara WM, Leibel SA, Gutin PH, Wilson CB, Sheline GE. Postoperative radiotherapy of primary spinal cord tumors. International Journal of Radiation Oncology Biology Physics 1989; 16: 1397–1403.

261. Huddart R, Traish D, Ashley S, Moore A, Brada M. Management of spinal astrocytoma with conservative surgery and radiotherapy. British Journal of Neurosurgery 1993; 7: 473–481.

262. Barnholz-Sloan JS, Sloan AE, Davis FG et al. Incidence proportions of brain metastases in patients diagnosed (1973 to 2001) in the Metropolitan Detroit Cancer Surveillance System. Journal of Clinical Oncology 2004; 22(14): 2865.

263. Vecht CJ, Hovestadt A, Verbiest HBC et al. Dose-effect relationship of dexamethasone on Karnofsky performance in metastatic brain tumours: a randomized study of doses of 4, 8 and 16 mg per day. Neurology 1994; 44: 675–680.

264. Gaspar L, Scott C, Rotman M et al. Recursive partitioning analysis (RPA) of prognostic factors in three Radiation Therapy Oncology Group (RTOG) brain metastases trials. International Journal of Radiation Oncology Biology Physics 1997; 37(4): 745.

265. Rodriges G, Gonzalez-Maldonado, Bauman G et al. A statistical comparison of prognostic index systems for brain metastases after stereotactic radiosurgery or fractionated stereotactic radiation therapy. Clinical Oncology 2013; 25: 227–235.

266. Kocher M, Soffietti R, Abacioglu U, Villa S, Fauchon F et al. Adjuvant whole-brain radiotherapy versus observation after radiosurgery or surgical resection of one to three cerebral metastases: results of the EORTC 22952-26001 study. Journal of Clinical Oncology 2011; 29(2): 134–141.

267. Patchell RA, Tibbs PA, Regine WF, Dempsey RJ, Mohiuddin M et al. Postoperative radiotherapy in the treatment of single metastases to the brain: a randomized trial. Journal of the American Medical Association 1998; 280(17): 1485–1489.

268. Ampil FL, Nanda A, Willis BK, Nandy I, Meehan R. Metastatic disease in the cerebellum. The LSU experience in 1981–1993. American Journal of Clinical Oncology 1996; 19(5): 509–511.

269. Suki D, Abouassi H, Patel AJ, Sawaya R, Weinberg JS, Groves MD. Comparative risk of leptomeningeal disease after resection or stereotactic radiosurgery for solid tumor metastasis to the posterior fossa. Journal of Neurosurgery 2008; 108(2): 248–257.

270. Suki D, Hatiboglu MA, Patel AJ, Weinberg JS, Groves MD et al. Comparative risk of leptomeningeal dissemination of cancer after surgery or stereotactic radiosurgery for a single supratentorial solid tumor metastasis. Neurosurgery 2009; 64(4): 664–674; discussion 74–6.

271. Ahn JH, Lee SH, Kim S, Joo J, Yoo H et al. Risk for leptomeningeal seeding after resection for brain metastases: implication of tumor location with mode of resection. Journal of Neurosurgery 2012; 116(5): 984–993.

272. Yoo H, Kim YZ, Nam BH, Shin SH, Yang HS et al. Reduced local recurrence of a single brain metastasis through microscopic total resection. Journal of Neurosurgery 2009; 110(4): 730–736.

273. Minniti G, Clarke E, Lanzetta G et al. Stereotactic radiosurgery for brain metastases: analysis of outcome and risk of brain radionecrosis. Radiation Oncology 2011; 6: 48.

274. Ernst-Stecken, Ganslandt O, Lambrecht U et al. Phase II trial of hypofractionated stereotactic radiotherapy for brain metastases: results and toxicity Radiotherapy and Oncology 2006; 81: 18–24.

275. Choi CY, Chang SD, Gibbs IC et al. Stereotactic radiosurgery of the postoperative resection cavity for brain metastases: prospective evaluation of target margin on tumor control. International Journal of Radiation Oncology Biology Physics 2012; 84(2): 336–342.

276. Andrews DW, Scott CB, Sperduto PW, Flanders AE, Gaspar LE et al. Whole brain radiation therapy with or without stereotactic radiosurgery boost for patients with one to three brain metastases: phase III results of the RTOG 9508 randomised trial. Lancet 2004; 363(9422): 1665–1672.

277. Cochrane Database of Systematic Reviews 2012, Issue 4. Art. No.: CD003869.

278. Langley RE, Stephens RJ, Nankivell M et al. Interim data from the Medical Research Council QUARTZ Trial: does whole brain radiotherapy affect the survival and quality of life of patients with brain metastases from non-small cell lung cancer. Clinical Oncology 2013; 25(3): e23–30.

279. Tsao MN, Lloyd N, Wong RKS, Chow E, Rakovitch E et al. Whole brain radiotherapy for the treatment of newly diagnosed multiple brain metastases. Cochrane Database of Systematic Reviews 2012; 4: CD003869.

280. Windsor AA, Koh ES, Allen S et al. Poor outcome after whole brain radiotherapy in patients with brain metastases: results from an International Multicentre Cohort Study. Clinical Oncology 2013; 2013: 674–680.

281. Dzienis MR, Atkinson V. Response rate to vemurafenib in BRAF-positive melanoma brain metastases. Journal of Clinical Oncology 2013; 31(15 Suppl): 9081.

282. Narayana A, Matthew M, Tarn M et al. Vemurafenib and radiation therapy in melanoma brain metastases. Journal of Neuro-Oncology 2013; 113(3): 411–416.

283. Kaplan MA, Isikdogan A, Koca D et al. Lapatinib or trastuzumab? Which anti-Her2 treatment is more effective in the treatment of patients with HER2-positive breast cancer with brain metastases? An Anatolian Society of Medical Oncology Study. Journal of Clinical Oncology 2012; 30(15 Suppl): 638.

284. Rades D, Huttenlocher S, Dunst J et al. Matched pair analysis comparing surgery followed by radiotherapy and radiotherapy alone for metastatic spinal cord compression. Journal of Clinical Oncology 2010; 28(22): 3597.

285. George R, Jeba J, Ramkumar G et al. Interventions for the treatment of metastatic extradural spinal cord compression in adults. Cochrane Database Systemic Reviews 2008; 4: CD006716.

286. Fourney DR, Frangou EM, Ryken TC et al. Spinal Instability Neoplastic Score: an analysis of reliability and validity from the spine oncology study group. Journal of Clinical Oncology 2011; 29(22): 3072.

287. Kato S, Murakami H, Demura S, Yoshioka K, Kawahara N et al. More than 10-year follow-up after total en bloc spondylectomy for spinal tumors. Annals of Surgical Oncology 2013 Oct 23.

288. Demura S, Kawahara N, Murakami H, Abdel-Wanis ME, Kato S et al. Total en bloc spondylectomy for spinal metastases in thyroid carcinoma. Journal of Neurosurgery: Spine 2011; 14(2): 172–176.

289. Sakaura H, Hosono N, Mukai Y, Ishii T, Yonenobu K, Yoshikawa H. Outcome of total en bloc spondylectomy for solitary metastasis of the thoracolumbar spine. Journal of Spinal Disorders & Techniques 2004; 17(4): 297–300.

290. Fourney DR, Abi-Said D, Rhines LD, Walsh GL, Lang FF et al. Simultaneous anterior-posterior approach to the thoracic and lumbar spine for the radical resection of tumors followed by reconstruction and stabilization. Journal of Neurosurgery 2001; 94(2 Suppl): 232–244.

291. Patchell RA, Tibbs PA, Regine F et al. Direct decompressive surgical resection in the treatment of spinal cord compression caused by metastatic cancer: a randomised trial. Lancet 2005; 366(9486): 643–648.

292. Zaidat OO, Ruff RL. Treatment of spinal epidural metastasis improves patient survival and functional state. Neurology 2002; 58(9): 1360.

293. Maranzano E, Trippa F, Casale M et al. 8 Gy single-dose radiotherapy is effective in metastatic spinal cord compression: results of a phase III randomized multicentre Italian trial. Radiotherapy and Oncology 2009; 93: 174–179.

294. Catton C, O'Sullivan B, Bell R, Laperriere N, Cummings B et al. Chordoma: a long-term follow up after radical photon irradiation. Radiology and Oncology 1996; 41(1): 67–72.

295. Amichetti M, Cianchetti M, Amelio D et al. Proton therapy in chordoma of the base of skull: a systematic review. Neurosurgical Review 2009; 32: 403–416.

296. Rosenberg AE, Nielson GP, Keel SB et al. Chondrosarcoma of the base of the skull, a clinicopathologic study of 200 cases with emphasis on its distinction from chordoma. American Journal of Surgical Pathology 1999; 23(11): 1370.

297. de Ruysscher D, Chang JY. Clinical controversies: proton therapy for thoracic tumours. Seminars in Radiation and Oncology 2013; 23(2): 115–119.

298. Regis J, Pellet W, Delsanti C, Dufour H, Roche PH et al. Functional outcome after gamma knife surgery or microsurgery for vestibular schwannomas. Journal of Neurosurgery 2002; 97(5): 1091–1100.

299. Pollock BE, Lunsford LD, Kondziolka D, Flickinger JC, Bissonette DJ et al. Outcome analysis of acoustic neuroma management: a comparison of microsurgery and stereotactic radiosurgery. Neurosurgery 1995; 36(1): 215–224; discussion 24-29.

300. Maniakas A, Saliba I. Microsurgery versus stereotactic radiation for small vestibular schwannomas: a meta-analysis of patients with more than 5 years' follow-up. Otology & Neurotology 2012; 33(9): 1611–1620.

301. Myrseth E, Moller P, Pedersen PH, Vassbotn FS, Wentzel-Larsen T, Lund-Johansen M. Vestibular schwannomas: clinical results and quality of life after microsurgery or gamma knife radiosurgery. Neurosurgery 2005; 56(5): 927–935; discussion 927-35.

302. Lobato-Polo J, Kondziolka D, Zorro O, Kano H, Flickinger JC, Lunsford LD. Gamma knife radiosurgery in younger patients with vestibular schwannomas. Neurosurgery 2009; 65(2): 294–300; discussion 300-1.

303. Ahmad RA, Sivalingam S, Topsakal V, Russo A, Taibah A, Sanna M. Rate of recurrent vestibular schwannoma after total removal via different surgical approaches. Annals of Otology, Rhinology & Laryngology 2012; 121(3): 156–161.

304. Arlt F, Trantakis C, Seifert V, Bootz F, Strauss G, Meixensberger J. Recurrence rate, time to progression and facial nerve function in microsurgery of vestibular schwannoma. Neurological Research 2011; 33(10): 1032–1037.

305. Sughrue ME, Kaur R, Rutkowski MJ, Kane AJ, Kaur G et al. Extent of resection and the long-term durability of vestibular schwannoma surgery. Journal of Neurosurgery 2011; 114(5): 1218–1223.

306. Sughrue ME, Yang I, Aranda D, Rutkowski MJ, Fang S et al. Beyond audiofacial morbidity after vestibular schwannoma surgery. Journal of Neurosurgery 2011; 114(2): 367–374.

307. Seol HJ, Kim CH, Park CK, Kim DG, Chung YS, Jung HW. Optimal extent of resection in vestibular schwannoma surgery: relationship to recurrence and facial nerve preservation. Neurologia Medico-Chirurgica (Tokyo) 2006; 46(4): 176–180; discussion 80-1.

308. Bloch O, Sughrue ME, Kaur R, Kane AJ, Rutkowski MJ et al. Factors associated with preservation of facial nerve function after surgical resection of vestibular schwannoma. Journal of Neuro-Oncology 2011; 102(2): 281–286.

309. van de Langenberg R, Hanssens PE, van Overbeeke JJ, Verheul JB, Nelemans PJ et al. Management of large vestibular schwannoma. Part I. Planned subtotal resection followed by gamma knife surgery: radiological and clinical aspects. Journal of Neurosurgery 2011; 115(5): 875–884.

310. Murphy ES, Suh JH. Radiotherapy for vestibular schwannomas: a critical review. International Journal of Radiation Oncology Biology Physics 2011; 79(4): 985–997.

311. Combs SE, Welzel T, Kessel K. Hearing preservation after radiotherapy for vestibular schwannomas is comparable to hearing deterioration in healthy adults and is accompanied by local tumor control and a highly preserved quality of life (QOL) as patients' self-reported outcome. Radiotherapy and Oncology 2013; 106: 175–180.

312. Plotkin SR, Stemmer-Rachamimov AO, Barker FG et al. Hearing improvement after bevacizumab in patients with neurofibromatosis type 2. New England Journal of Medicine 2009; 361(4): 358–367.

313. Plotkin SR, Merker VL, Halpin C. Bevacizumab for progressive vestibular schwannoma in neurofibromatosis type 2: a retrospective review of 31 patients. Otology & Neurotology 2012; 33(6): 1046–1052.

314. Krishnan S, Brown PD, Scheithauer BW, Ebersold MJ, Hammack JE, Buckner JC. Choroid plexus papillomas: a single institutional experience. Journal of Neuro-Oncology 2004; 68(1): 49–55.

315. Safaee M, Clark AJ, Bloch O, Oh MC, Singh A et al. Surgical outcomes in choroid plexus papillomas: an institutional experience. Journal of Neuro-Oncology 2013; 113(1): 117–125.

316. McGirr SJ, Ebersold MJ, Scheithauer BW, Quast LM, Shaw EG. Choroid plexus papillomas: long-term follow-up results in a surgically treated series. Journal of Neurosurgery 1988; 69: 843–849.

317. Mazloom A, Wolff JE, Paulino AC. The impact of radiotherapy fields in the treatment of patients with choroid plexus carcinoma. International Journal of Radiation Oncology Biology Physics 2010; 78(1): 79–84.

CHAPTER 57

Tumours of the eye and orbit

Daniel G. Ezra, Geoffrey E. Rose, Jacob Pe'er, Sarah E. Coupland, Stefan Seregard, G.P.M. Luyten, and Annette C. Moll

Introduction to adult tumours of the eye and orbit

Eyelid tumours

Tumours of the eyelid are the most frequent seen in ophthalmic practice and the periocular skin is one of the commonest sites for non-melanoma skin cancers. Numerous tumour types arise from the eyelid, as it is contains many different tissues that are capable of undergoing benign or malignant transformation. The eyelid skin is extremely thin (less than 1 mm), but contains all of the normal skin elements, as well as the adnexal elements, such as fine hairs, and rudimentary sebaceous and sweat glands. Beneath the skin is the orbicularis oculi muscle, under which lies the tarsal plate that provides support for the meibomian glands. The bulbar surface of the tarsal plate is lined with conjunctiva that is tightly adherent to the substantia propria [1].

Eyelid tumours are thought to account for 5% of all non-melanoma skin cancers [2], and, whilst prevalence data is limited, about 60 000 malignant eyelid tumours are diagnosed annually in the US [3].

Symptoms and signs

As the face is the most examined area of the body, patients will often present early having noticed a lump in the eyelid region, although some such tumours may be neglected, particularly in the elderly. Periocular tumours are usually slow growing, with local invasion and disruption of normal anatomical structures a feature of malignancy. This disruption is particularly evident at the lid margin, where the complex and close arrangement of structures is disrupted even by very small tumours. In contrast, benign lesions may distort, but do not destroy, normal structures. Although patients will only very rarely present with pain, this important symptom might suggest bony invasion as a result of late presentation, or perineural invasion by malignant tumours, particularly squamous cell carcinoma (SCC).

Conjunctival invasion or pagetoid spread is a particular feature of sebaceous carcinoma and can commonly present with symptoms of a red or sore eye suggestive of blepharitis; as such, the clinician should consider conjunctival biopsy in all patients having persistent unilateral ocular surface 'inflammation'. Areas of diffuse induration are a feature of eyelid tumours and scirrhous cutaneous lesions can commonly cause eyelid retraction and cicatricial ectropion.

Clinical history, examination, and imaging

The central objective in the evaluation of any eyelid lesion is to differentiate between benign and malignant lesions. The most important feature of the history is that of progressive growth: benign lesions and the more common malignant tumours, such as basal cell carcinoma (BCC), are usually indolent in nature and typically grow slowly. In contrast, more aggressive tumours such as melanoma can proliferate more rapidly. Other features suggestive of malignancy include irritation, crusting, bleeding with minor trauma, and failure of any such lesion to heal within 3–4 weeks.

A full examination should include the skin, conjunctiva, eyelid margin, and eyelashes. Although examination can be done with magnifiers or other aides, it is usually performed using slit-lamp biomicroscopy by specialists. Other systems, such as dermatoscopy, also have a particular role for pigmented lesions. The nature of the lesion should be examined, including the tarsal conjunctiva and ocular surface, and a full orbital examination performed where orbital invasion is suspected. Rolled 'pearly' borders and indurated or hardened areas are suggestive of malignancy (e.g., BCC), as is a loss of mobility over the underlying structures.

The lymphatic drainage from the medial end of the eyelids is to the submandibular nodes and that of the lateral ends to the preauricular nodes; all assessments of eyelid tumours should include examination of these lymph node groups. This is particularly important where more aggressive malignancies (such as melanoma, SCC, or sebaceous carcinoma) are suspected. Examination of periocular cutaneous sensation is particularly important with SCC that has a predilection for perineural invasion that can cause periocular pain or numbness.

Imaging is imperative where larger tumours appear to be involving the orbit: CT has advantages over MRI, providing thinner cuts with less motion artefact, better details of bone involvement, and greater inherent contrast within the orbital structures. In some cases, however, MRI may be of value in imaging anterior orbital structures, as it offers better differentiation of soft tissues.

Malignant tumours

BCC is the most common malignant eyelid tumour in Caucasians [4]. The age-adjusted incidence of BCC in men and women is equal and about 14 per 100 000 per year [5]. BCCs typically appear on sun-exposed areas, being most common on the lower eyelid (50%), followed by the medial canthal area (36%), and are rarer on the upper lid (8%) or lateral canthus (6%); this periocular distribution is explained by the shielding of upper lid skin by the eyebrow and plication of the upper eyelid skin when the eye is open [6]. In addition to sun exposure, patients on long-term immunosuppression are at a higher risk of developing skin cancers (with BCC being the most common). Xeroderma pigmentosum is an autosomal recessive condition, with an inability to repair cellular damage due to UV exposure, and affected patients develop pigmented lesions early in life followed by the appearance of BCCs. Gorlin's, or basal cell naevus, syndrome is an autosomal dominant condition characterized by the development of numerous BCCs, especially on the sun-exposed areas such as face and hands [6].

Several different histological subtypes of BCC are described, which underlie differences in clinical presentation, and include nodular, ulcerative, cystic, morphoeic, and pigmented BCCs. The most common BCC (60%) is nodular, that presents as a raised nodule with well demarcated, pearly, and telangiectatic borders; with growth, the centre may become ulcerated and umbilicated. Morphoeic BCCs are the second most common lesion and can look innocuous, with borders that are difficult to identify and a surface that may be sore or crusted. BCCs can often present as pigmented lesions and hence should enter the differential diagnosis for a periocular pigmented lesion. Occasionally BCCs can present as a cystic lesions containing mucinous material and, without biopsy, these can be difficult to distinguish from other benign periocular cysts.

BCCs very rarely metastasize and their morbidity arises from local invasion into adjacent tissues, with neglected tumours invading the orbit or mid-face.

Sebaceous carcinoma is a malignancy arising from the meibomian glands, sebaceous glands aligned vertically in the tarsus and being unconnected with hairs [1]. The incidence of this tumour varies widely with geographical location, forming ~9% of periocular malignancies in the West but 30–40% in Southern and Eastern Asia, and described as 'more common than BCCs' in some reports [8]. Unlike sebaceous adenomas, sebaceous carcinoma is only rarely related to Muir-Torre syndrome [9]. This tumour usually presents in older patients, most commonly in their seventies, and three-quarters occur in women. It can masquerade as other conditions, such as recurrent chalazion, chronic unilateral conjunctivitis or blepharitis. The correct histological diagnosis can also be difficult to determine, with up to a half of biopsies being misinterpreted as SCC. Metastasis is estimated at 8% and can develop up to five years after initial treatment of the eyelid lesion [10].

Sebaceous carcinoma has a propensity for intraepithelial, pagetoid spread which is believed to increase the risk of invasion and metastasis. All cases of sebaceous carcinoma require mapping biopsies of the bulbar and tarsal conjunctiva to exclude pagetoid spread and, if epithelial involvement is identified, surgical clearance might require orbital exenteration [11].

SCCs are related to chronic sun exposure, commonly presenting as ulcerated or hyperkeratotic lesions. A well-described feature is the development of a cutaneous horn or scaly surface. The differential diagnosis for these lesions includes fast-growing keratoacanthomas or actinic keratoses. SCC arising primarily on the exposed bulbar conjunctiva is commonly associated with immunosuppression due to HIV infection. Periocular skin SCC behaves similarly to SCC occurring elsewhere, with low metastatic potential and low mortality. Local spread to regional lymph nodes may occur in a quarter of patients and a lymph node assessment is essential if SCC is suspected. Death is usually a result of perineural invasion, often through the frontal nerve, into the CNS (8%) or due to distant metastasis (6%) [12].

Cutaneous melanoma of the eyelid is rare, comprising 1% of all melanomas [13]. Risk factors for melanoma are similar to those of other malignant tumours—including sun exposure, a family history, fair skin, and older age. Periocular radiotherapy is also a risk factor, particularly for patients previously treated for retinoblastoma who may have required high dose external beam radiotherapy. Lentigo maligna melanoma is the most common head and neck form of cutaneous melanoma, and is also the most common form of eyelid melanoma. Whilst these lesions often occur *de novo*, up to a half of melanomas arise from a predisposing lesion such as lentigo maligna (i.e., in situ melanoma), congenital naevus, and rarely, a naevus of Ota [14]. Eyelid melanomas can also arise from an extension of a conjunctival melanoma crossing the muco-cutaneous junction and invading the adjacent skin. Some evidence suggests that eyelid melanoma might have a more favourable prognosis than other melanomas of the head and neck [15].

Merkel cell tumours, which typically occur in elderly females, progress at an extraordinarily rapid rate of growth, often doubling in size within two or three weeks. They require aggressive therapy by wide surgical clearance, but still carry a relatively poor prognosis.

Principles of management

Periocular skin tumours present unique difficulties in management due to the proximity of the globe and orbital contents, and the high density of regional innervation also makes perineural spread a significant problem for some tumour types. Although only 15–20% of lid lesions are malignant [4], an accurate clinical diagnosis and determination of malignant potential can be challenging. If there is any doubt, an incisional biopsy should be taken as an initial step, unless a sentinel lymph node biopsy is planned, when this should be performed prior to tumour manipulation.

Whilst there is significant variation in the practical management of these tumours, the universal principle is to eradicate the tumour with maximal preservation of function and physical appearance. After correct diagnosis, it is essential to ensure adequate clearance of the tumour. To this end, excision is usually performed with histological clearance either as a two-stage procedure (using frozen section and fast paraffin techniques) or by using Mohs' micrographic surgery. Mohs' surgery, both by limiting loss of normal tissues and by increasing the proportion of tumour-free survivors, is becoming increasingly popular as the treatment of choice for periocular BCCs—particularly in high-risk areas, such as the inner canthus, or with morphoeic tumours. Additional difficulties are presented with sebaceous carcinoma, where multiple conjunctival mapping biopsies are required to evaluate the presence or extent of any pagetoid tumour spread.

Defects are generally reconstructed using combinations of direct closure techniques, flaps or free grafts, although small defects can often be left to heal spontaneously over a few weeks. Orbital invasion is a devastating complication of eyelid tumours and the patient will generally require orbital exenteration. Whilst exenteration improves survival outcomes for most tumours, there is evidence that it has no impact on survival in melanoma [14].

The proximity of the eye globe makes 5-fluorouracil and imiquimod less tolerated as treatment options for periocular BCCs, as they can cause significant ocular surface inflammation. Other modalities, such as radiotherapy and cryotherapy, also have a role in more conservative treatment.

Orbital tumours

Malignant tumours of the orbit arise as primary disease, by secondary direct spread from the paranasal sinuses or lacrimal sac, or as metastases from remote primary tumours. The US National

Cancer Institute reports an annual incidence of periocular malignancy—albeit of the eye *and* orbit—to be up to 1 in 100 000, with 13% arising under the age of 20 years and a fifth arising in each of the decades from 55 and 65 years of age [16]. Orbital malignancy equally affects men and women, with an estimated cumulative lifetime risk of 0.08% [16].

Symptoms and signs

The presentation of orbital tumours varies with the predominant location of the mass: for example, anterior masses generally causing a visible and palpable localized eyelid swelling and displacement of the globe. In contrast, tumours in the posterior half of the orbit cause progressive proptosis and are often associated with ill-defined periocular swelling. This swelling, often worse on wakening, is both due to displacement of normal orbital fat and due to vascular congestion at the orbital apex. True binocular diplopia is a common feature of orbital malignancy and can arise from restriction of globe movements by sheer tumour bulk, or by malignant infiltration of the three nerves supplying the extraocular muscles. Ptosis is usually due to eyelid swelling, but more rarely arises from tumour invasion of the upper branch of the oculomotor nerve within the orbit. Optic neuropathy—with reduced visual acuity, reduced colour perception, or visual field impairment—is rare with orbital malignancy, but can arise from compression of the optic nerve. Malignancies of the lacrimal drainage system and the maxilla, that may secondarily invade the orbit, are often associated with a watering eye and, more rarely, with ipsilateral epistaxis.

Orbital malignancies are typically painless unless associated with bone erosion, the exception being lacrimal gland carcinoma—commonly accompanied by chronic ache that is thought to arise from perineural infiltration [17]. Cancers arising in the paranasal sinuses will commonly cause pain that may be referred to the head or the teeth. Periocular sensory loss, whilst a good guide to the location of an orbital lesion, is most commonly due to non-malignant processes [18].

Clinical history, examination, and imaging

A thorough medical history should be taken, as the progression of symptoms provides a good idea of the likely diagnosis. This is well illustrated with orbital apex syndromes, where loss of multiple functions (e.g., ocular motility, periocular sensation, and visual impairment) occur within hours, the apex lesion is probably inflammatory or vascular. In contrast, a step-wise progression over months is probably a malignant infiltration sequentially impairing the many nerves at the apex. Clearly a history of systemic malignancy is important, even if many years before, and the enquiry should also address epiphora, nasal symptoms or surgery, and dental or pharyngeal pain.

Ophthalmic examination should include an assessment of orbital signs and also a check for intraocular malignancy that can spread outside the globe. Likewise, it is imperative to check the nasal space and search for regional lymphadenopathy. Where the length of history is uncertain, reference to past photographs can be valuable; a sole photograph is best for such comparison, as downward displacement of the resting lower lid—with an apparent 'rising sun' corneal configuration—is one of the earliest signs of proptosis.

Whilst most tumours in the orbit will cause proptosis or eyelid fullness, certain malignant tumours—such as metastatic breast or lung carcinoma—can generate a desmoplastic scirrhous response with secondary enophthalmos, or eyelid 'hangup' on downgaze due to fibrosis of the levator muscle [19]. Facial weakness is another—easily-overlooked—periocular clinical sign that is of particular importance with periocular malignancy, as it can occur as a result of malignant infiltration of the preauricular lymph nodes.

Thin-slice CT is the primary investigation of choice for orbital disease as it demonstrates in fine detail the micro-invasion of cortical bone, tumour calcification, and defines the macroscopic extent of disease. MRI can be a useful secondary imaging for soft-tissue detail within the skull-base, details of meningeal involvement, and the assessment of water content within abnormal tissues. Ultrasonography has a minor role in orbital disease: it is invaluable for imaging intraocular disease and measuring tumour dimensions, at assessing the scleral thickness for tumour invasion, and—using the Doppler colour imaging mode—for the assessment of blood-flow within the orbital tissues.

Immunohistochemical studies of the biopsy tissue may help identify the site of the primary tumour. Likewise, specific blood tests may be indicated for various systemic malignancies.

Orbital tumours in adults

Lymphoma is the main orbital malignancy, and will be discussed separately below. Lacrimal gland carcinoma is very rare, but sadly involves younger people and carries a poor prognosis [2]. Adenoid cystic carcinoma is the commonest epithelial malignancy, but others include primary adenocarcinoma, mucoepidermoid carcinoma, or SCC. Malignant mixed tumours arise within previously benign pleomorphic adenomas and may present with recent change in a longstanding known orbital asymmetry. These tumours often cause some inflammatory signs with pain and, because of this risk, any 'dacryoadenitis' lasting for more than three months should be considered for biopsy. Incisional biopsy is performed through the upper lid skin crease and, if proven to be carcinoma, consideration given to the macroscopic removal of tumour with later high-dose (about 5500 cGy) fractionated radiotherapy to both the orbit, superior orbital fissure, and anterior cavernous sinus—treatment for the latter two sites reducing recurrence due to perineural spread of the tumour. Implantation brachytherapy has been used to treat the tumour 'bed' but it does not treat the critical areas of the superior orbital fissure or cavernous sinus. Orbital exenteration and deliberate breach of the lateral wall should probably be avoided, as it does not improve survival [20], and tends to seed tumour into the cranial diploe with relentless recurrence of disease. Exenteration might, however, have a role in treating these patients where combined with preoperative intra-arterial chemoreductive therapy—the current suggested regimen is cisplatin and doxorubicin—and later radiotherapy [21].

The orbit is not infrequently invaded by malignancy arising in the globe such as choroidal melanoma, eyelids (commonly BCC), or the paranasal sinuses. Invasive malignancies of sinus origin include squamous carcinomas, lymphomas, adenocarcinomas, esthesioneuroblastomas, and melanomas. Orbital invasion by these tumours tends to be manifest as restriction of ocular motility and displacement of the globe. Such cases usually require partial or complete orbital exenteration during resection of the primary site of disease, together with adjunctive radiotherapy in many cases.

Metastases, whilst common within the choroid, comprise a minority of orbital malignant diseases. Some of the commonest

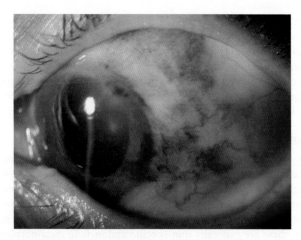

Fig. 57.1 Primary acquired melanosis presented as diffuse superficial conjunctival pigmentation with corneal involvement.

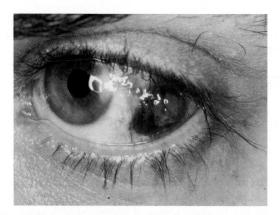

Fig. 57.2 Large conjunctival melanoma on the temporal bulbar conjunctiva.

primary sites are the breast, cutaneous melanoma, prostate, and lung. Whilst most metastases will generally present with rapidly progressive and painful proptosis that looks rather 'inflammatory', scirrhous carcinoma of breast or lung can cause enophthalmos. With secondary melanomas, the growth may be so rapid that the lesion looks like a well-defined benign lesion such as cavernous haemangioma—but the history should clinch the correct diagnosis. Clearly, these patients must be managed in a multidisciplinary team.

Conjunctival melanoma

Conjunctival melanoma is a rare tumour of middle-aged and older persons, mostly in Caucasians and more commonly in males, with an annual incidence of 0.2–0.8 per million in Caucasian populations [22, 23]. Conjunctival melanoma is unilateral and arises most commonly in the perilimbal, interpalpebral, and bulbar conjunctiva, plica semilunaris, and caruncle (Figures 57.1 and 57.2). Conjunctival melanoma arising from primary acquired melanosis or conjunctival melanocytic intraepithelial neoplasia (PAM/C-MIN) with atypia is most common (70%). However, it may be multifocal and may appear simultaneously or sequentially in different parts of the conjunctiva. Conjunctival melanoma that arises from a naevus or *de novo* appears clinically as a solitary pigmented or non-pigmented vascularized nodule, commonly in the limbal area.

The definitive diagnosis of conjunctival melanoma is made by histopathological examination. Most cases can be diagnosed with confidence by light microscopic features. Four types of atypical melanocytes have been described in conjunctival melanoma: small polyhedral, spindle, balloon, and round epithelioid cells with eosinophilic cytoplasm. The invasive melanoma is often accompanied by conjunctival melanoma in situ in the adjacent epithelium. Any breeching of the basement membrane by atypical melanocytes in conjunctival melanoma in situ should be considered as microinvasive melanoma. Atypical melanocytes within the epithelium of subepithelial cysts can give rise to multiple foci of invasive melanoma [24].

If in doubt, immunohistochemical stains such as HMB-45 or Melan-A can be used to highlight the neoplastic melanocytes, and Ki-67 proliferation index may help to differentiate melanoma from

naevi. BRAF mutations are found in about half of conjunctival melanomas while BRAF mutations are seldom encountered in uveal melanomas [25].

There are several histopathological features that predict adverse prognosis in conjunctival melanoma, including depth of invasion measured with an ocular micrometer from the basement membrane to the deepest point of invasion. Other histological prognostic factors are pagetoid spread, mixed cell tumours versus spindle cell tumours, lymphatic invasion, high mitotic count, and high cell proliferation indices. The presence of previous primary acquired melanosis (PAM) does not appear to be a prognostic indicator [26].

The primary treatment of conjunctival melanoma is surgical excision of the entire tumour when possible. When limbal and scleral involvement are suspected, scleroconjunctivectomy can be considered [27]. Most surgeons will add adjuvant treatment, including cryotherapy, ruthenium brachytherapy, and proton beam radiotherapy. Topical mitomycin C and topical interferon alpha-2b have also been used successfully as adjuvant treatment, especially in melanoma originating from PAM with atypia [28]. Exenteration of the orbit is reserved only as a palliative treatment for advanced stages.

Local recurrence of conjunctival melanoma, when treated by surgical excision alone, has been reported in 56–65% of patients, and nearly half develop more than one recurrence. Risk factors for local recurrences are melanoma originating in PAM with atypia, located other than at the limbus and bulbar conjunctiva, involvement of surgical margins, and failure to perform adjuvant therapy. Local recurrences are managed as primary melanoma.

Conjunctival melanoma may spread locally via 'in-transit' metastases to local lymphatics within the conjunctiva. Spread of conjunctival melanoma to the nasolacrimal duct, the nasal cavity and paranasal sinuses, has been attributed to shedding of exfoliated melanoma cells in the tear film. Rarely, conjunctival melanoma invades the eyeball or the orbit. Conjunctival melanoma can metastasize to any organ in the body; in half of them regional lymph nodes (preauricular and submandibular) will be involved before systemic spread. The rate of conjunctival melanoma-related mortality ranges, according to several studies, between 12–19% in five years and 23–30% in ten years. The most important clinical risk factors are tumour location and tumour thickness. Tumour locations with high risk of metastases are non-bulbar conjunctival melanomas, i.e., those in the palpebral conjunctiva, fornices, plica, and caruncle. The critical thickness is 0.8 mm, above which there is continuous worsening in prognosis with increasing tumour thickness [29, 30].

Uveal melanoma

Uveal melanoma is distinctly different from cutaneous melanoma. The incidence is stable rather than increasing. Most data argue against ultraviolet radiation as a significant cause of uveal melanoma, and the molecular mechanisms operating in uveal melanoma are not akin to those identified in cutaneous melanoma. Significant advances have been made in treatment of the primary disease with a number of eye-preserving options now available. Mortality has, however, remained unchanged with nearly half of patients ultimately developing metastatic disease. To date, no treatment for disseminated uveal melanoma has proven efficacious in a randomized clinical trial.

Aetiology

Uveal melanoma arises from the melanocytes of the uveal tract, i.e. from the neural crest-derived, non-epithelial, pigment-containing cells of the choroid, ciliary body, and iris stroma. Melanoma of the eye and ocular adnexa, so-called ocular melanoma, comprises about 5% of all melanoma and more than 85% of ocular melanoma is of uveal origin [31]. Only 5% of uveal melanoma arises from the iris; the vast majority of uveal melanoma originates from the choroid posterior to the equator. It is widely assumed that most lesions arise from uveal naevi that have transformed into melanoma. Because the prevalence of uveal naevi is 4–6.5% in the general population, the risk for a naevus without atypical features to develop into a melanoma is markedly low. Individuals with syndromes like oculo(dermal) melanocytosis are at an increased risk to develop uveal melanoma [32], but the majority occur in patients with no apparent predisposing condition. Most cases present in a sporadic setting and familial uveal melanoma is distinctly uncommon, although an increasing number of families with germline BAP-1 mutations and familial uveal melanoma are now being reported [33, 34]. There are a few case reports of families with the familial atypical multiple mole melanoma syndrome (FAMMM) with some family members featuring an associated uveal melanoma [31]. A possible link, albeit probably not strong, between uveal and cutaneous melanoma is supported by data indicating a 75% increased risk for patients with uveal melanoma to develop skin melanoma [35]. Also, case-control studies suggesting that atypical (dysplastic) naevi are more prevalent in patients with uveal melanoma. Nevertheless, the incidence of uveal melanoma is largely stable in many countries and does not parallel the rapid increase seen in cutaneous melanoma [36, 37]. Although there are a few reports of uveal melanoma being more frequent in welders, occupational exposure to ultraviolet radiation has not been associated with uveal melanoma [38]. A few case-control studies on sunlight, and hence ultraviolet radiation, exposure have generated conflicting results [39]. Moreover, unlike cutaneous or conjunctival melanoma, mutations in the BRAF and NRAS genes are uncommon events in uveal melanoma [27, 40, 41]. Uveal melanoma is much more prevalent in Caucasians than in African Americans, perhaps by as much as a 20-fold difference in the age-adjusted incidence rate. In largely Caucasian populations, the annual incidence ranges approximately

from 5–10 cases per million [31, 38]. Notably, uveal melanoma is a disease of the middle-aged and elderly and is rare in children and young adolescents [42]. There are some data suggesting that predisposing conditions like oculo(dermal) melanocytosis are more frequent in young patients with uveal melanoma [42]. Bilateral disease is an extremely uncomment event, without a clear association to any known genetic predisposition [43].

Signs and symptoms

Approximately 70–87% of patients with uveal melanoma experience symptoms at the time of referral to an ocular oncologist [44]. A substantial proportion of patients are diagnosed with uveal melanoma following a routine ophthalmological examination or fundus photography for an unrelated condition. When symptoms are present, these are generally non-specific and include metamorphopsia (distorted vision in which straight lines appear wavy), blurred vision, a visual field defect and, rarely, ocular pain. Generally, a uveal melanoma grows slowly and symptoms accumulate over a considerable period of time. Nevertheless, an associated serous retinal detachment may sometimes progress rapidly and cause a sudden onset of symptoms. An iris melanoma is located on the anterior iris surface and as such recognizable to the patient or relatives as a brown spot on iris. Diffuse iris melanoma with raised intraocular pressure may sometimes cause iris atrophy and a change in iris colour (typically to a greenish hue) that sets the eye apart from the fellow eye; i.e., iris heterochromia.

Diagnosis

Although initial misdiagnosis of a uveal melanoma by an ophthalmologist reportedly occurs in one of four patients [45], an ophthalmologist specialized in ocular oncology can make the diagnosis by clinical appearance assisted by non-invasive techniques in 95% of cases. The most frequently used non-invasive technique is ultrasonography. This is available in frequencies ranging from 10–50 MHz featuring different resolution and depth penetration. Other techniques like fluorescein angiography, optical coherence tomography, indocyaninine green angiography, and MRI may provide additional information. The typical choroidal melanoma is a 10–15 mm dome-shaped or mushroom-shaped (this signifies a rupture of Bruch's membrane) solid tumour with a colour ranging from greyish to dark brown, but rarely black (Figure 57.3). Many lesions are clinically non-pigmented (whitish) and larger lesions may feature an associated serous retinal detachment. The diffuse choroidal melanoma is a rare subtype (1–3% of choroidal melanoma), typically a flat pigmented lesion extending to more than one quadrant of the ocular fundus. This subtype is notoriously difficult to diagnose for the inexperienced physician, but carries a significant mortality and a tendency to grow extrasclerally. Other rare subtypes include the annular (ring-like) ciliary body melanoma and the retroinvasive melanoma which may invade the optic nerve. Sometimes, lesions like peripheral choroidal haemorrhagic retinopathy, choroidal metastases, uveal effusion syndrome, hamartoma of the retinal pigment epithelium, posterior scleritis, choroidal haemangioma and subretinal haemorrhage may simulate a posterior uveal melanoma.

Uveal melanoma is almost unique among cancers in that the clinical diagnosis often is not verified by cytological or histopathological examination. For tumours large enough to warrant

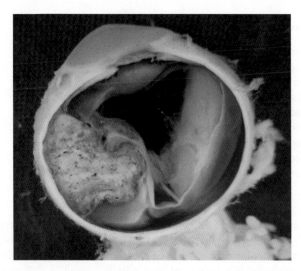

Fig. 57.3 Enucleated eye with large (15 × 15 × 12 mm) choroidal melanoma. The tumour is mushroom-shaped and the retina is partially detached.

enucleation, the clinical diagnosis is highly accurate at 99.7% [46]. For smaller uveal melanoma or clinically atypical tumours, any diagnostic uncertainty can be resolved by any of a range of biopsy techniques. Although symptoms like progressive visual field loss and blurred vision are not specific for uveal melanoma, they usually lead to a prompt ophthalmological examination. Nevertheless, significant delays in referral to a dedicated ocular oncology centre remain a concern [45]. Small indeterminate melanocytic lesions are sometimes observed for growth before treatment is initiated, in particular when treatment is likely to be associated with significant visual loss. Features of indeterminate melanocytic lesions of the choroid, such as thickness greater than 2 mm, subretinal fluid, orange pigment within the tumour, clinical symptoms, location within 3 mm of the optic disc, acoustic hollowness by ultrasonography, and absence of a halo are associated with increased risk for growth [27] (Figure 57.4). The risk

for growth is more than 50% at five-years follow-up when two or more risk factors are present [27]. Although not always appropriate, growth of indeterminate melanocytic lesion of the choroid is then often used as a surrogate measure for malignant transformation. Because uveal melanoma is distinctly rare, but choroidal naevi occur in approximately 4–6.5% of a Caucasian population, the features predictive for growth help to identify the very few lesions at significant risk for malignant transformation. It is widely assumed that uveal melanoma may metastasize when quite small and given the impact early treatment may have on visual function, this has generated significant controversy of when to treat small melanocytic lesions [47].

Management of primary disease

In the US, there has been a dramatic shift towards the use of eye-preserving options for uveal melanoma. During 1973–74, nearly all patients with uveal melanoma had surgery, almost always enucleation of the eye, but in 2004–2006 only ~25% of patients with uveal melanoma had surgery as the first option. Radiotherapy, largely episcleral brachytherapy, has become much more common as the first line of treatment in up to 62.5% of patients [48]. This change has been stimulated by evidence that survival is not compromised for patients with medium-sized tumours who have primary radiotherapy rather than enucleation and by the introduction of standardized plaques for episcleral brachytherapy as a result of the Collaborative Ocular Melanoma Study (COMS) [49]. Another of the COMS trials showed that pre-enucleation radiotherapy for uveal melanoma provided no survival benefit [50]. Treatment is not standardized among centres and patients with similarly-sized tumours may receive different treatment. Enucleation is a reasonable option for many large tumours and tumours adjacent to the optic disc where poor visual outcome is expected. Episcleral brachytherapy using a radioactive plaque (Figure 57.5) may be performed under local anaesthesia or general anaesthesia. A range of radionucleotides with different characteristics are available (Table 57.1), but ruthenium-106 is more widely used in Europe and iodine-125 in North America. Tissue penetration is greater for iodine and centres with access to both radionuclides often use ruthenium for small and medium-sized tumours and iodine for larger tumours. Typically, tumour regression is slow and may take 6–9 months to become apparent. Local recurrence may occur after many years and periodic monitoring of the irradiated tumour, typically for life, is therefore important. A number of side effects occur following

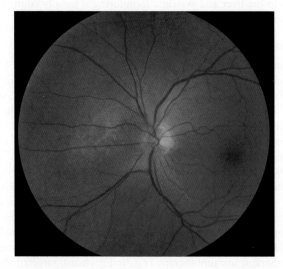

Fig. 57.4 Juxtapapillary choroidal naevus with significant characteristics predicting growth.

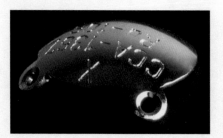

Fig. 57.5 Ruthenium-106 applicator for episcleral brachytherapy. The outer surface includes a silver lining to minimize radiation to normal tissue. The inner surface contains the radioactive source and is molded to fit the curvature of the eye. Two eyelets allow for suturing the radioactive plaque to the scleral surface.

Table 57.1 Radionuclides in current use for episcleral brachytherapy of uveal melanoma

Element	Nuclide	Energy (MeV)	Half-life
Iodine	I-125	2.40	59 days
Ruthenium	Ru-106	6.55	374 days
Iridium	Ir-192	1.46	74 days
Palladium	Pd-103	2.67	17 days
Gold	Au-198	1.37	2.7 days
Strontium	Sr-90	6.70	29 years

Adapted from Seregard S et al., Uveal malignant melanoma: management options—brachytherapy, Chapter 41 in Singh A et al., (Eds.), *Clinical Ophthalmic Oncology*, Copyright © 2007 Elsevier Inc. All rights reserved, with permission from Elsevier.

plaque radiotherapy (Figure 57.6) and radiation retinopathy is seen in up to half of eyes treated (Box 57.1), but this complication is also frequent after any form of teletherapy.

A juxtapapillary choroidal melanoma is difficult to treat with episcleral brachytherapy and may alternatively be managed with proton beam radiotherapy. Some centres use this technique as the first option for most uveal melanoma [51]. To avoid significant side effects from radiation, large tumours may be fragmented and removed by a vitreous cutter (endoresection) after radiotherapy [52]. Primary endoresection not preceded by radiotherapy is highly controversial, although a histopathological study of eyes enucleated after primary endoresection suggest that tumour seeding is a rare event [53, 54]. Some tumours may also be managed by trans-scleral local resection (exoresection), often combined with plaque radiotherapy, which reduces the rate of local tumour recurrence [55]. Alternative radiation techniques to treat uveal melanoma include fractionated stereotactic radiotherapy and single-fraction radiosurgery. Primary transpupillary thermotherapy is now rarely used as the sole therapy

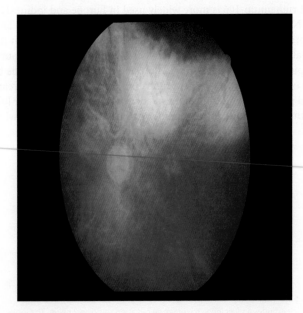

Fig. 57.6 Choroidal melanoma 6.5 years after iodine brachytherapy. There is significant tumour regression, but also side effects, such as choroidal atrophy and radiation optic neuropathy.

Box 57.1 Complications following episcleral brachytherapy

Ocular perforation
Uveal effusion
Diplopia
Choroidal atrophy
Radiation-induced cataract
Radiation optic neuropathy
Radiation retinopathy
Neovascular glaucoma
Scleral melting

because of an increased risk for local recurrence and is now typically combined with brachytherapy [56]. A circumscribed iris melanoma has traditionally either been observed (because of the excellent prognosis for this subgroup) or surgically excised. A diffuse iris melanoma is often monitored until any raised intraocular pressure cannot be controlled by topical or oral medication, or diode laser cyclo-photocoagulation. For this subtype, surgical intervention typically entails enucleation of the eye. Recently, proton beam irradiation for both subtypes of iris melanoma has been advocated as an alternative to enucleation or local excision. Irradiation may subsequently be combined with a shunt to control intraocular pressure [57].

Follow-up

Patients with uveal melanoma treated with an eye-preserving option are usually monitored for life at regular intervals. This includes comparison with standardized pre-treatment fundus photographs and often ultrasonography. Patients with extrascleral growth found at or after enucleation may need periodic imaging of the orbit to exclude an orbital recurrence. Fine stippled episcleral pigment deposits, which may appear a few years after brachytherapy for uveal melanoma, may be pigment lodged in macrophages rather than extrascleral tumour growth [58]. Although an effective treatment for metastatic uveal melanoma is still lacking, an increasing number of ocular oncologists advise periodic extraocular monitoring for metastatic disease. Uveal melanoma preferentially disseminates to the liver and systemic monitoring is usually confined to this site.

Management of systemic disease

Metastases are detected at the time of diagnosis in less than 1% of patients with uveal melanoma. Nevertheless, prolonged follow-up reveals disseminated disease in more than half of patients at 35 years after diagnosis. Although most patients with metastatic disease are identified during the first five years after diagnosis, 20–33% of deaths even after 15 to 35 years following the diagnosis of uveal melanoma are attributable to melanoma [59]. The liver is involved in 90% of metastatic uveal melanoma and frequently the presenting site of widespread disease. Traditionally, patients with systemic uveal melanoma often received treatment similar to patients with systemic cutaneous melanoma, but therapy is now more specific. Current strategies to manage systemic uveal melanoma include partial hepatectomy, radiofrequency ablation, selective internal radiotherapy, immunotherapy (e.g., ipilimumab), targeted therapies, liver chemoembolization, intrahepatic arterial chemotherapy, systemic chemotherapy, or combinations of the above [60].

Quality of life

The diagnosis of ocular cancer generates significant anxiety and depression in patients. Symptoms like fatigue and insomnia are prevalent [61]. There are some data to suggest that anxiety diminishes faster after diagnosis in patients with enucleation than in patients managed by brachytherapy [62]. Visual function is initially better in patients with brachytherapy, but this difference is reduced over time as radiation-related side effects emerge [62]. Differences between individuals may be significant and there is scope for personalized treatment [63] in particular, as a consistent survival benefit for radical treatment such as enucleation has not been shown.

Histopathology

For many decades, the cell type of uveal melanoma has been known to correlate with prognosis. Traditionally, tumour cells are characterized as spindle or epithelioid depending on their morphology and prognosis is poorer for tumours with epithelioid cells. Tumours may be described as containing a mixed cell type when both spindle cells and epthelioid cells are present, but there is no consensus as to how many epithelioid tumour cells make a melanoma an epithelioid melanoma. Uveal melanoma may occasionally be largely necrotic, but the original cell type is usually discernible. When a choroidal melanoma grows it will eventually rupture Bruch's membrane causing a mushroom or collar-stud appearance. The retina is typically eroded rather than frankly invaded by a choroidal melanoma. Likewise, the sclera is often only minimally invaded by a choroidal melanoma, but tumour cells may gain access to one or more of the routes taken by nerves and vessels which traverse the sclera and then reach the surface of the eye. By histopathological examination, the tumour cells of medium-sized and larger tumours invade trans-scleral emissary canals in more than half of cases and extrascleral growth is evident in 8% of cases [46]. Similarly, intravascular tumour growth is found in nearly 40% of eyes following enucleation for uveal melanoma. In most cases this occurs within the tumour proper or away from the tumour, but within the eye [64]. All intraocular vascular channels are presumed to be part of the blood vasculature as lymphatics have not been detected within the eye. This is consistent with tumour seeding from uveal melanoma believed to be almost exclusively haematogenous. A number of histopathologic parameters have been found to correlate with prognosis including nucleolar size, the number of cycling tumour cells, tumour cell mitotic count, extravascular matrix patterns (particularly the presence of closed connective tissue loops), microvascular density, and tumour-infiltrating macrophages [65–70]. Eyes with irradiated tumours may be secondarily enucleated for local recurrence or ocular complications or both. Typically, these irradiated tumours feature secondary changes like obliterated blood vessels and tumour cells with intracytoplasmatic vacuolization [71]. Although the number of cycling tumour cells is much reduced after radiotherapy there may be still be proliferating tumour cells present in eyes enucleated for ocular complications but with clinically- regressed tumours [72, 73]. Intriguingly, data suggest that in 40% of eyes enucleated for presumed failed brachytherapy, the clinically increased tumour size cannot be histopathologically confirmed [71].

Prognosis

Although significant progress has been made in the management of the primary uveal melanoma, prognosis for life has largely remained unchanged [74]. Notably, the mortality rate is higher than for patients with cutaneous melanoma and nearly half of patients with uveal melanoma will die with metastatic disease [31]. Most of these will die during the first five years after diagnosis [75], but some patients develop systemic disease several decades after diagnosis [76]. It is widely assumed that tumours spread when quite small, usually several years before diagnosis, and that metastases then remain unnoticed in the liver for many years [47, 77]. When metastatic disease becomes clinically evident, the median survival is 6–12 months, but 22% of patients survive more than four years after diagnosis of metastases [59, 78]. Most patients have hepatic metastases as the first site of presentation of disseminated uveal melanoma [78]. Large tumours, anteriorly- located tumours (except iris melanoma which have an excellent prognosis), tumours with specific extracellular matrix patterns and tumours containing epithelioid cells, cells with large nucleoli or a large proportion of cycling tumour cells carry a worse prognosis [66, 67, 77]. Moreover, tumours with chromosomal aberrations like monosomy 3 and gain of chromosome 8q are associated with poor survival [79, 80]. These latter findings have prompted a surge in using prognostic tumour biopsies to make tissue or cells available for molecular testing. Fluorescence in-situ hybridization FISH has been used extensively to study chromosomal abnormalities, but the technique lacks standardization and results have not always been consistent [81]. Increasingly sophisticated methods, like multiplex ligation probe dependent amplification, now more reliably predicts survival [82, 83]. Nevertheless, tumour significant heterogeneity for chromosomal aberrations across the tumour necessitates multifocal tumour sampling [84, 85]. Gene expression profiling has also been able to identify a subgroup of uveal melanoma associated with a very high mortality rate [86]. This method has recently evolved into a commercially available platform for molecular prognostic testing in patients with uveal melanoma validated by a large set of patents [87, 88]. To date, there is no independent study comparing the prognostic accuracy of gene expression profiling with that of DNA-based techniques. It could be argued that there is no use in genetic testing for uveal melanomas if there is no successful treatment for metastatic disease. Speaking against this line of thought is the increasing pressure from patients to know whether they have a 'good' or 'bad' uveal melanoma. Further, the frequency of screening can be adjusted according to whether the patient is at high or low risk of developing disseminated tumour. Those patients at high risk can be screened more intensively (possibly with techniques of greater resolution, e.g., MRI) with the aim of detecting the metastases earlier and allowing possibly for surgical removal. Finally, those patients at high risk of metastatic uveal melanoma will be those to consider for clinical trial enrolment, including those trials in adjuvant therapy [89].

Lymphoproliferative tumours

Conjunctival lymphomas

Conjunctival lymphoid tumours may be subdivided into reactive lymphoid hyperplasia, atypical lymphoid hyperplasia, and the more common conjunctival lymphoma. These tumours belong to the group of ocular adnexal lymphomas that may affect also the orbit and eyelids.

Conjunctival lymphomas usually occur in adults and can present as an isolated primary lesion of the conjunctiva; however, in up to one-third of patients it is a manifestation of systemic lymphoma that can be present simultaneously with the conjunctival disease or during follow-up. Lymphomas may involve additional ocular sites, mainly the orbit. Most patients are symptomatic, presenting with a conjunctival mass or irritation and, less commonly, ptosis, epiphora, proptosis, and diplopia. Lymphomas of the conjunctiva appear as an elevated pink mass, commonly termed a 'salmon patch' (Figure 57.7). These lesions are commonly located at the bulbar conjunctiva and fornix, usually hidden by the eyelids. Biopsy is needed to establish the histopathological diagnosis, i.e., to differentiate lymphomas from reactive lymphoid hyperplasia and to subtype the lymphoma [90]. The vast majority of the conjunctival lymphomas are low-grade non-Hodgkin B-cell lymphoma, usually extranodal marginal zone B-cell lymphoma. Other subtypes are diffuse large B-cell lymphoma, follicular lymphoma, mantle cell lymphoma, plasmacytoma, and lymphoplasmocytic lymphoma [90].

In all cases of conjunctival lymphoma, systemic evaluation should be performed to determine the extent (or stage) of the disease. Conjunctival lymphomas are treated using surgical excision, cryotherapy, low-dose external beam radiation, and brachytherapy. Recently, intravenous or intralesional rituximab has been used [91]. Since many low-grade conjunctival lymphomas are indolent or progress very slowly, observation and periodic follow-up has been advocated. The mortality rate of conjunctival lymphoma is usually low; however, this is dependent on the lymphoma subtype and the stage of the disease at presentation.

Lymphoma of the retina

Vitreoretinal lymphoma

Vitreoretinal lymphoma (VRL) is a lymphoma of high-grade malignancy, usually of B-cell type, which is often associated with cerebral disease. CNS lymphoma (CNSL) may occur prior to, concurrently, or subsequent to the ocular disease.

Clinical features

VRL most often affects elderly patients (i.e., over the age of 60 years) and the incidence is dramatically increasing. Infrequently, however, they are seen in younger, possibly immunocompromised,

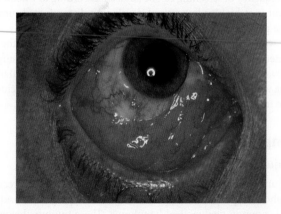

Fig. 57.7 Diffuse conjunctival lymphoma presented as elevated pink mass occupying most of the bulbar conjunctiva and lower fornix.

individuals (Table 57.2). VRL are bilateral in about 60–90% of patients but are often asymmetrical at presentation. The eye is involved in about 20% of primary CNSL, but the brain ultimately becomes involved in about 80% of VRL arising initially in the eye.

Usually VRL can be distinguished from uveitis clinically, although there are overlaps, which may be pronounced in eyes with a large component of reactive inflammation. Lymphomatous deposits initially accumulate around the retinal blood vessels and can be visible ophthalmoscopically as perivascular sheathing, mimicking vasculitis. Multiple, tiny, cream-coloured deposits can develop, resembling peripheral drusen or a white-dot syndrome. These may result in punched-out, atrophic retinal pigment epithelium (RPE) lesions. The lymphomatous infiltrations become more extensive, eventually involving the full thickness of the retina, which, on ophthalmoscopy, becomes opaque. The tumour cells seem to permeate the RPE, accumulating as clumps in the subretinal space on Bruch's membrane. The overlying RPE atrophies, leaving a fine pigment dusting over the amelanotic tumour surface. Fluorescein angiography (FA) shows a variety of features, such as staining of subretinal deposits, RPE window defects, diffuse RPE mottling or stippling, and rarely, vascular leakage and macular oedema [92]. The so-called leopard skin appearance on FA is considered to be pathognomic for VRL.

Histology, immunohistology, and genetics of vitreoretinal lymphoma

In most centres, diagnostic pars plana vitrectomies are performed to establish the diagnosis of VRL. The laboratory techniques applied to achieve diagnosis consist of cytology, immunohistochemistry, flow cytometry, polymerase chain reaction (PCR) for clonality analysis, and cytokine profiling.

Histologically, VRL can be subtyped in most cases as a diffuse large B-cell lymphoma (DLBCL) [90]. VRL is characterized by a subretinal or perivascular retinal infiltration of pleomorphic medium-to-large sized cells with minimal basophilic cytoplasm, indented or folded nuclei, and prominent, often multiple, nucleoli. Atypical mitotic figures can be seen.

Immunohistochemically, VRL are characterized by the following expression profile: positivity for B-cell antigens (CD79a, CD20, PAX-5), as well as for BCL-2, MUM1/IRF4, OCT2, BOB.1, BCL-6+/-, CD10-/+, Pu.1-/+. They are usually monotypical for IgM on immunohistochemistry [93]. Staining with Ki-67 shows that the tumour cell growth fraction is very high (i.e., about 80–90%). Clonality assessment can also be performed on DNA extracted from VRL using PCR directed against the immunoglobulin heavy and light chains in B-cell lymphomas, and against the T-cell receptor in the case of rare T-cell lymphomas.

Treatment of vitreoretinal lymphoma

The treatment of VRL remains controversial and varies considerably between centres, including external beam radiotherapy, intravitreal therapies (with or without CNS radiotherapy), and autologous bone marrow transplantation with chemotherapy. Low-dose external beam radiotherapy induces clearance of the vitreous opacities and regression of the subretinal tumour deposits, leaving behind areas of atrophy. In time, there can be radiation-induced complications such as retinopathy and cataract. Intraocular methotrexate is effective [94]. Rituximab has recently been shown to induce regression of VRL, whether given intravitreally or systemically, although recurrence is common [91]. Intraocular rituximab seems to be

Table 57.2 Summary of the clinical, morphological, immunophenotypical, and genotypic features of the various types of intraocular lymphoma

Lymphoma	Clinical features	Most common subtype	Morphology	Immunoprofile of neoplastic cells	Genotype	Putative cell of origin
Vitreoretinal	60–70 years 'Floaters' Painless decrease in VA Subretinal infiltrates Often bilateral RPE changes on FA CNS involvement (70–80% of patients)	DLBCL	Medium large cells with minimal cytoplasm and prominent nuclei. Often admixed macrophages	CD79a+ CD20+ PAX5+ BCL2+ MUM1/IRF4+ BCL6+/– CD10–/+ OCT2+ BOB1+ Pu1– High Ki–67 rate: >80%	Very high somatic IgH mutation load Few ongoing somatic mutations Chromosomal translocations in 50%: t(14;18) (q31;q21)	Two different types: (a) Early post–germinal centre B cell = DLBCL of ABC type (b) Germinal centre cell = DLBCL of GCB type
Choroidal	50–60 years Blurring of vision Metamorphopsia Clear vitreous Diffuse thickening of choroid Usually unilateral Extraocular extension No CNS involvement	*Primary:* EMZL	Small centrocyte–like cells with varying plasmacellular differentiation Few admixed reactive T–cells Necrosis rare	CD79a+ CD20+ BCL2+ CD43+/– IgM+ CD5– CD23– CyclinD1– CD10– Low Ki–67 rate: 5–15%	Moderate somatic IgH mutation load Few ongoing somatic mutations Chromosomal abnormalities: t(11;18)(q21;q21)	Post–germinal centre (memory) B cell
Choroidal	Previous history of systemic NHL Decrease in VA Possibly bilateral	*Secondary:* Dependent on systemic NHL	Dependent on systemic NHL	Dependent on systemic NHL	Dependent on systemic NHL	Dependent on systemic NHL
Iridal	Pain Redness Photophobia Pseudohypopyon Usually unilateral Often ultimate systemic dissemination	DLBCL TCL NOS		CD79a+ CD20+ CD3– High Ki–67 rate: >80% CD3+ CD4+ CD20– High Ki–67 rate: >80%	Not known	Not known Neoplastic peripheral T–cell
Ciliary Body#	Raised IOP Ciliary body mass	EMZL	Small centrocyte–like cells with varying plasmacellular differentiation Few admixed reactive cells Necrosis rare	CD79a+ CD20+ CD43+/– IgM+ CD5– CD23– CyclinD1– Low Ki–67 rate: 5–15%	Not known	Not known

Abbreviations: VA, Visual acuity; FA, fluorescein angiography; IOP, intraocular pressure; CNS, central nervous system; DLBCL, diffuse large B-cell lymphoma; EMZL, extranodal marginal zone B-cell lymphoma; NHL, Non Hodgkin lymphoma; CD, cluster of differentiation; ABC, activated B-cell type; GCB, germinal centre B-cell type; t(N1;N2), chromosomal translocation between chromosome N1 and N2. #, represents features of only one case.

well-tolerated by the eye and the risks of this treatment are the same as any invasive procedure (i.e., endophthalmitis, haemorrhage, and cataract).

Prognosis

As mentioned above, approximately 80% of patients with primary VRL subsequently develop lymphoma of the brain, spinal cord, or meninges. Whether this is the result of metastatic spread or multifocal tumour development is not known at present. Whether ocular treatment influences the prognosis for survival is also not clear. There is some evidence that early systemic treatment for VRL delays the onset of CNS disease, prolonging survival [90, 95]. The onset of cerebral disease in VRL portends a poor prognosis.

Uveal lymphoma

Lymphoid proliferations of the uvea can be divided into two main groups: primary uveal tumours and secondary intraocular manifestations of systemic lymphoma. Primary uveal lymphoma is rare and can be further divided according to location: primary choroidal lymphoma, primary ciliary body lymphoma, and primary iridal lymphoma, with the first being the most common.

Primary choroidal lymphoma

Primary choroidal lymphoma was first described in 1920, and occurs as a unilateral tumour in the absence of systemic disease at diagnosis. Due to the usual low-grade nature of these tumours, they were previously erroneously termed reactive lymphoid hyperplasia or uveal pseudotumours. Subsequent investigations including clonality analysis using PCR have provided evidence that the majority of these tumours are low-grade B-cell lymphomas. Most primary choroidal lymphomas can be sub-typed as extranodal marginal zone B-cell lymphomas (EMZL), with clinical, morphological, immunophenotypical, and genetic features similar to EMZL in other locations [reviewed in 96].

Secondary choroidal lymphomas

Intraocular lymphoma secondary to disseminated, systemic NHL is usually confined to the choroid [97]. Rarely, systemic lymphoma can present with anterior segment disease such as pseudohypopyon or iris infiltration.

The most common systemic lymphoma subtype involving the choroid is DLBCL. This is followed by multiple myeloma, extramedullary plasmacytoma, lymphoplasmacytic lymphoma/immunocytoma, marginal zone B-cell lymphoma of either the gastric mucosa or lung, and B-cell chronic lymphocytic leukaemia.

The treatment of patients with secondary intraocular lymphoma is dependent on the underlying systemic NHL and the extent of its dissemination. Similarly, the prognosis of the patients is associated with this and the response to therapy.

Metastatic tumours to the eye

Haematogenous dissemination of tumour cells from primary carcinomas in other parts of the body can form secondary tumours most frequently in the choroid (Table 57.3). Less frequent tumours can develop in the iris and ciliary body. Increased incidence of these primary carcinomas and prolonged survival had led to an increased incidence of metastatic tumours to the eye. The metastatic lesions involve both eyes in 25% of the cases and often multiple lesions can

Table 57.3 Primary sites of choroidal metastases

Males (n= 137)	Females (n = 287)
Lung 40%	Breast 70%
Unknown (30%)	Lung (10%)
Gastrointestinal (10%)	Unknown (10%)
Kidney (5%)	Others (<5%)
Prostate (5%)	Gastrointestinal (<5%)
Skin (<5%)	Skin (<1%)
Others (<5%)	Kidney (<1%)
Breast (1%)	

Source: data from Shields CL et al., Survey of 520 eyes with uveal metastases, *Ophthalmology*, Volume 104, Issue 8, pp. 1265–1676, Copyright © 1997 American Academy of Ophthalmology. Published by Elsevier Inc. All rights reserved.

be observed. The frequent primary sites are breast cancer in females and lung cancer in males [98].

Clinical signs

The clinical signs and symptoms depend on the location of the tumour. Tumours located in the iris are often without signs or symptoms and appear as a small gray or gelatinous lump. Patients with posteriorly-located choroidal lesions often complain of vision loss, blurring, or visual disturbances. Indirect ophthalmoscopy will show an irregular and ill-defined, commonly pale yellow, slightly elevated lesion with exudative retinal detachment. Ultrasonography will usually show a relative flat lesion, sometimes lobulated with high internal reflectivity on the A-scan. In difficult cases, fine-needle aspirate biopsy can be of help when the diagnosis cannot be made with non-invasive techniques. In those cases with suspected choroidal metastases and with an unknown primary tumour, a CT-scan of the thorax and abdomen is indicated to rule out the most common primary tumours.

Treatment and prognosis

Survival of the patient strongly depends on the primary tumour. Since the primary tumours are widely disseminated the prognosis of these patients are poor, particularly with primary lung carcinoma and gastrointestinal carcinomas. The primary goal for the treatment is to preserve vision and palliate pain. Most patients will be treated locally with external beam irradiation, while others are treated with systemic chemotherapy or hormone therapy [99, 100].

References

1. Ezra DG, Beaconsfield M, Collin R. Surgical anatomy of the upper eyelid: old controversies, new concepts. Expert Review of Ophthalmology 2009; 4: 47–57.
2. Cook BE Jr, Bartley GB. Treatment options and future prospects for the management of eyelid malignancies: an evidence-based update. Ophthalmology 2001;108: 2088–2098.
3. Piest KL. Malignant lesions of the eyelids. Journal of Dermatologic Surgical Oncology 1992; 18: 1056–1059.
4. Deprez M, Uffer S. Clinicopathological features of eyelid skin tumors. A retrospective study of 5504 cases and review of literature. American Journal of Dermatopathology 2009; 31: 256–262.
5. Cook BE Jr, Bartley GB. Epidemiologic characteristics and clinical course of patients with malignant eyelid tumors in an incidence cohort in Olmsted County, Minnesota. Ophthalmology 1999; 106: 746–750.

6. Gayre S. Outcomes of excision of 1750 eyelid and periocular skin basal cell and squamous cell carcinomas by modified en face frozen section margin-controlled technique. International Ophthalmology Clinics 2009; 49: 97–110.

7. Abdi U, Tiyagi N, Maheshwari V, Gogi R, Tyagi SP. Tumours of the eyelid: a clinic-pathologic study. Journal of the Indian Medical Association 1996; 94: 405–409.

8. Ni C, Searl SS, Kuo PK et al. Sebaceous cell carcinomas of the ocular adnexa. International Ophthalmology Clinics 1982; 22: 23–61.

9. Rishi K, Font RL. Sebaceous gland tumors of the eyelids and conjunctiva in the Muir-Torre syndrome: a clinicopathologic study of five cases and literature review. Ophthalmic Plastic and Reconstructive Surgery 2004; 20: 31–36.

10. Shields JA, Demirci H, Marr BP, Eagle RC Jr, Shields CL. Sebaceous carcinoma of the eyelids. Ophthalmology 2004; 111: 2151–2157.

11. Putterman AM. Conjunctival map biopsy to determine pagetoid spread. American Journal of Ophthalmology 1986; 102: 87–90.

12. Faustina M, Diba R, Ahmadi MA, Esmaeli B. Patterns of regional and distant metastasis in patients with squamous cell carcinoma. Ophthalmology 2004; 111: 1930–1932.

13. Vaziri M, Buffam FV, Martinka M, Oryschak A, Dhaliwal H et al. Clinicopathologic features and behavior of cutaneous eyelid melanoma. Ophthalmology 2002; 109: 901–918.

14. Boulos PR, Rubin AD. Cutaneous melanomas of the eyelid. Seminars in Ophthalmology 2006; 21: 195–206.

15. Polito E, Leccisotti A. Primary and secondary orbital melanomas: a clinical and prognostic study. Ophthalmic Plastic and Reconstructive Surgery 1995; 11: 169–181.

16. Surveillance Epidemiology and End Results Stat Fact Sheets: Eye and Orbit; <http://seer.cancer.gov/faststats/selections>.

17. Wright JE, Rose GE, Garner A. Primary malignant neoplasms of the lacrimal gland. British Journal of Ophthalmology 1992; 76: 401–417.

18. Rose GE, Wright JE. Trigeminal sensory loss and orbital disease. British Journal of Ophthalmology 1994; 78: 427–429.

19. Uddin JM, Rose GE. Downgaze 'hang-up' of the upper eyelid in patients with adult-onset ptosis: an important sign of possible orbital malignancy. Ophthalmology 2003; 110: 1433–1436.

20. Binning MJ, Liu JK, Kestle JR, Brockmeyer DL, Walker ML. Optic pathway gliomas: a review. Neurosurgery Focus 2007; 23: E2.

21. Tse DT, Benedetto P, Dubovy S, Schiffman JC, Feuer WJ. Clinical analysis of the effect of intraarterial cytoreductive chemotherapy in the treatment of lacrimal gland adenoid cystic carcinoma. American Journal of Ophthalmology 2006; 141: 44–53.

22. Shields CL, Shields JA. Tumors of the conjunctiva and cornea. Survey of Ophthalmology 2004; 49: 3–24. Review.

23. Folberg R. Melanocytic lesions of the conjunctiva. In Spencer WH. Ophthalmic Pathology, 4th ed. Philadelphia: WB Saunders, 1996, 125–155.

24. Jakobiec FA, Folberg R, Iwamoto T. Clinicopathologic characteristics of premalignant and malignant melanocytic lesions of the conjunctiva. Ophthalmology 1989; 96: 147–166. Review.

25. Cruz F 3rd, Rubin BP, Wilson D et al. Absence of BRAF and NRAS mutations in uveal melanoma. Cancer Research 2003; 63(18): 5761–5766.

26. Folberg R, McLean IW, Zimmerman LE. Primary acquired melanosis of the conjunctiva. Human Pathology 1985; 16: 129–135.

27. Shields CL, Shields JA, Gunduz K, Cater J, Mercado GV et al. Conjunctival melanoma: risk factors for recurrence, exenteration, metastasis, and death in 150 consecutive patients. Archives in Ophthalmology 2000; 118(11): 1497–1507.

28. Pe'er J, Frucht-Pery J. The treatment of primary acquired melanosis (PAM) with atypia by topical mitomycin C. American Journal of Ophthalmology 2005; 139: 229–234.

29. Damato B, Coupland SE. Conjunctival melanoma and melanosis: a reappraisal of terminology, classification and staging. Clinical and Experimental Ophthalmology 2008; 36: 786–795.

30. Yousef YA, Finger PT. Predictive value of the seventh edition American Joint Committee on Cancer staging system for conjunctival melanoma. Archives of Ophthalmology 2012; 130: 599–606.

31. Singh AD, Bergman L, Seregard S. Uveal melanoma: epidemiologic aspects. Ophthalmology Clinics of North America 2005; 18(1): 75–84, viii.

32. Singh AD, De Potter P, Fijal BA et al. Lifetime prevalence of uveal melanoma in white patients with oculo(dermal) melanocytosis. Ophthalmology 1998; 105(1): 195–198.

33. Abdel-Rahman MH, Pilarski R, Cebulla CM et al. Germline BAP1 mutation predisposes to uveal melanoma, lung adenocarcinoma, meningioma, and other cancers. Journal of Medical Genetics 2011; 48(12): 856–859.

34. Carbone M, Ferris LK, Baumann F et al. BAP1 cancer syndrome: malignant mesothelioma, uveal and cutaneous melanoma, and MBAITs. Journal of Translational Medicine 2012; 10: 179.

35. van Hees CL, Jager MJ, Bleeker JC et al. Occurrence of cutaneous and uveal melanoma in patients with uveal melanoma and their first degree relatives. Melanoma Research 1998; 8(2): 175–180.

36. Hu DN, Yu GP, McCormick SA et al. Population-based incidence of uveal melanoma in various races and ethnic groups. American Journal of Ophthalmology 2005; 140(4): 612–617.

37. Stang A, Schmidt-Pokrzywniak A, Lehnert M et al. Population-based incidence estimates of uveal melanoma in Germany. Supplementing cancer registry data by case-control data. European Journal of Cancer Preview 2006; 15(2): 165–170.

38. Lutz JM, Cree I, Sabroe S et al. Occupational risks for uveal melanoma results from a case-control study in nine European countries. Cancer Causes Control 2005; 16(4): 437–447.

39. Singh AD, Rennie IG, Seregard S et al. Sunlight exposure and pathogenesis of uveal melanoma. Survey of Ophthalmology 2004; 49(4): 419–428.

40. Cohen Y, Goldenberg-Cohen N, Parrella P et al. Lack of BRAF mutation in primary uveal melanoma. Investigative Ophthalmology and Visual Science 2003; 44(7): 2876–2878.

41. Kilic E, Bruggenwirth HT, Verbiest MM et al. The RAS-BRAF kinase pathway is not involved in uveal melanoma. Melanoma Research 2004; 14(3): 203–205.

42. Singh AD, Shields CL, Shields JA, Sato T. Uveal melanoma in young patients. Archives of Ophthalmology 2000; 118(7): 918–923.

43. Singh AD, Shields CL, Shields JA, De Potter P. Bilateral primary uveal melanoma. Bad luck or bad genes? Ophthalmology 1996; 103(2): 256–262.

44. Eskelin S, Kivela T. Mode of presentation and time to treatment of uveal melanoma in Finland. British Journal of Ophthalmology 2002; 86(3): 333–338.

45. Damato EM, Damato BE. Detection and time to treatment of uveal melanoma in the United Kingdom: an evaluation of 2,384 patients. Ophthalmology 2012; 119(8): 1582–1589.

46. Histopathologic characteristics of uveal melanomas in eyes enucleated from the Collaborative Ocular Melanoma Study. COMS report 6. American Journal of Ophthalmology 1998; 125(6): 745–766.

47. Singh AD. Uveal melanoma: implications of tumor doubling time. Ophthalmology 2001; 108(5): 829–831.

48. Collaborative Ocular Melanoma Study G. Trends in size and treatment of recently diagnosed choroidal melanoma, 1987–1997: findings from patients examined at collaborative ocular melanoma study (COMS) centers: COMS report 20. Archives of Ophthalmology 2003; 121(8): 1156–1162.

49. Jampol LM, Moy CS, Murray TG, Reynolds SM, Albert DM, Schachat AP. The COMS randomized trial of iodine 125 brachytherapy for choroidal melanoma: IV. Local treatment failure and enucleation in the first 5 years after brachytherapy. COMS report no. 19. Ophthalmology 2002;109(12): 2197–2206.

50. Hawkins BS, Collaborative Ocular Melanoma Study G. The Collaborative Ocular Melanoma Study (COMS) randomized trial of pre-enucleation radiation of large choroidal melanoma: IV. Ten-year mortality findings and prognostic factors. COMS report no. 24. American Journal of Ophthalmology 2004; 138(6): 936–951.

51. Gragoudas ES, Marie Lane A. Uveal melanoma: proton beam irradiation. Ophthalmology Clinics of North America 2005; 18(1): 111–118, ix.

52. Damato BE. Local resection of uveal melanoma. Developmental Ophthalmology 2012; 49: 66–80.

53. Damato B, Groenewald C, McGalliard J, Wong D. Endoresection of choroidal melanoma. British Journal of Ophthalmology 1998; 82(3): 213–218.

54. Hadden PW, Hiscott PS, Damato BE. Histopathology of eyes enucleated after endoresection of choroidal melanoma. Ophthalmology 2004; 111(1): 154–160.

55. Damato B. Adjunctive plaque radiotherapy after local resection of uveal melanoma. Frontiers of Radiation Therapy and Oncology 1997; 30: 123–132.

56. Singh AD, Kivela T, Seregard S et al. Primary transpupillary thermotherapy of 'small' choroidal melanoma: is it safe? British Journal of Ophthalmology 2008; 92(6): 727–728.

57. Sharkawi E, Oleszczuk JD, Bergin C, Zografos L. Baerveldt shunts in the treatment of glaucoma secondary to anterior uveal melanoma and proton beam radiotherapy. British Journal of Ophthalmology 2012; 96(8): 1104–1107.

58. Toivonen P, Kivela T. Pigmented episcleral deposits after brachytherapy of uveal melanoma. Ophthalmology 2006; 113(5): 865–873.

59. Singh AD, Borden EC. Metastatic uveal melanoma. Ophthalmology Clinics of North America 2005; 18(1): 143–150, ix.

60. Giuliari GP, Sadaka A. Uveal metastatic disease: current and new treatment options (review). Oncology Reports 2012; 27: 603–617.

61. Brandberg Y, Kock E, Oskar K et al. Psychological reactions and quality of life in patients with posterior uveal melanoma treated with ruthenium plaque therapy or enucleation: a one year follow-up study. Eye (London) 2000; 14(Pt 6): 839–846.

62. Melia M, Moy CS, Reynolds SM et al. Quality of life after iodine 125 brachytherapy vs enucleation for choroidal melanoma: 5-year results from the Collaborative Ocular Melanoma Study: COMS QOLS Report 3. Archives in Ophthalmology 2006; 124(2): 226–238.

63. Damato B, Heimann H. Personalized treatment of uveal melanoma. Eye (London) 2013; 27: 172–179 [published online 23 November 2012].

64. Ly LV, Odish OF, Wolff-Rouendaal D et al. Intravascular presence of tumor cells as prognostic parameter in uveal melanoma: a 35-year survey. Investigative Ophthalmology & Visual Science 2010; 51(2): 658–665.

65. McLean IW, Keefe KS, Burnier MN. Uveal melanoma. Comparison of the prognostic value of fibrovascular loops, mean of the ten largest nucleoli, cell type, and tumor size. Ophthalmology 1997; 104(5): 777–780.

66. Seregard S, Oskarsson M, Spangberg B. PC-10 as a predictor of prognosis after antigen retrieval in posterior uveal melanoma. Investigative Ophthalmology & Visual Science 1996; 37(7): 1451–1458.

67. Seregard S, Spangberg B, Juul C, Oskarsson M. Prognostic accuracy of the mean of the largest nucleoli, vascular patterns, and PC-10 in posterior uveal melanoma. Ophthalmology 1998; 105(3): 485–491.

68. Folberg R, Rummelt V, Parys-Van Ginderdeuren R et al. The prognostic value of tumor blood vessel morphology in primary uveal melanoma. Ophthalmology 1993; 100(9): 1389–1398.

69. Foss AJ, Alexander RA, Jefferies LW et al. Microvessel count predicts survival in uveal melanoma. Cancer Research 1996; 56(13): 2900–2903.

70. Makitie T, Summanen P, Tarkkanen A, Kivela T. Tumor-infiltrating macrophages (CD68(+) cells) and prognosis in malignant uveal melanoma. Investigative Ophthalmology & Visual Science 2001; 42(7): 1414–1421.

71. Avery RB, Diener-West M, Reynolds SM et al. Histopathologic characteristics of choroidal melanoma in eyes enucleated after iodine 125 brachytherapy in the collaborative ocular melanoma study. Archives of Ophthalmology 2008; 126(2): 207–212.

72. Seregard S, Lundell G, Lax I et al. Tumour cell proliferation after failed ruthenium plaque radiotherapy for posterior uveal melanoma. Acta Ophthalmologica Scandinavica 1997; 75(2): 148–154.

73. Pe'er J, Gnessin H, Shargal Y, Livni N. PC-10 immunostaining of proliferating cell nuclear antigen in posterior uveal melanoma. Enucleation

74. Singh AD, Topham A. Survival rates with uveal melanoma in the United States: 1973–1997. Ophthalmology 2003; 110(5): 962–965.

75. Bergman L, Seregard S, Nilsson B et al. Uveal melanoma survival in Sweden from 1960 to 1998. Investigative Ophthalmology & Visual Science 2003; 44(8): 3282–3287.

76. Kujala E, Makitie T, Kivela T. Very long-term prognosis of patients with malignant uveal melanoma. Investigative Ophthalmology & Visual Science 2003; 44(11): 4651–4659.

77. Seregard S, Kock E. Prognostic indicators following enucleation for posterior uveal melanoma. A multivariate analysis of long-term survival with minimized loss to follow-up. Acta Ophthalmologica Scandinavica 1995; 73(4): 340–344.

78. Rietschel P, Panageas KS, Hanlon C et al. Variates of survival in metastatic uveal melanoma. Journal of Clinical Oncology 2005; 23(31): 8076–8080.

79. Prescher G, Bornfeld N, Becher R. Nonrandom chromosomal abnormalities in primary uveal melanoma. Journal of the National Cancer Institute 1990; 82(22): 1765–1769.

80. Aalto Y, Eriksson L, Seregard S et al. Concomitant loss of chromosome 3 and whole arm losses and gains of chromosome 1, 6, or 8 in metastasizing primary uveal melanoma. Investigative Ophthalmology & Visual Science 2001; 42(2): 313–317.

81. Singh AD, Aronow ME, Sun Y et al. Chromosome 3 status in uveal melanoma: a comparison of fluorescence in situ hybridization and single-nucleotide polymorphism array. Investigative Ophthalmology & Visual Science 2012; 53(7): 3331–3339.

82. Damato B, Dopierala J, Klaasen A et al. Multiplex ligation-dependent probe amplification of uveal melanoma: correlation with metastatic death Investigative Ophthalmology & Visual Science 2009; 50(7): 3048–3055.

83. Lake SL, Kalirai H, Dopierala J et al. Comparison of formalin-fixed and snap-frozen samples analyzed by multiplex ligation-dependent probe amplification for prognostic testing in uveal melanoma. Investigative Ophthalmology & Visual Science 2012; 53(6): 2647–2652.

84. Dopierala J, Damato BE, Lake SL et al. Genetic heterogeneity in uveal melanoma assessed by multiplex ligation-dependent probe amplification. Investigative Ophthalmology & Visual Science 2010; 51(10): 4898–4905.

85. Schoenfield L, Pettay J, Tubbs RR, Singh AD. Variation of monosomy 3 status within uveal melanoma. Archives of Pathology & Laboratory Medicine 2009; 133(8): 1219–1222.

86. Onken MD, Worley LA, Ehlers JP, Harbour JW. Gene expression profiling in uveal melanoma reveals two molecular classes and predicts metastatic death. Cancer Research 2004; 64(20): 7205–7209.

87. Onken MD, Worley LA, Tuscan MD, Harbour JW. An accurate, clinically feasible multi-gene expression assay for predicting metastasis in uveal melanoma. Journal of Molecular Diagnostics 2010; 12(4): 461–468.

88. Onken MD, Worley LA, Char DH. Collaborative Ocular Oncology Group report number 1: prospective validation of a multi-gene prognostic assay in uveal melanoma. Ophthalmology 2012; 119(8): 1596–1603.

89. Damato B. Progress in the management of patients with uveal melanoma. The 2012 Ashton Lecture. Eye 2012; 26(9): 1157–1172.

90. Chan CC. Primary intraocular lymphoma: clinical features, diagnosis, and treatment. Clinical Lymphoma 2003; 4(1): 30–31.

91. Ferreri AJ, Govi S, Colucci A, Crocchiolo R, Modorati G. Intralesional rituximab: a new therapeutic approach for patients with conjunctival lymphomas. Ophthalmology 2011; 118: 24–28.

92. Turaka K, Bryan JS, De Souza S et al. Vitreoretinal lymphoma: changing trends in diagnosis and local treatment modalities at a single institution. Clinical Lymphoma Myeloma and Leukemia 2012; 12(6): 412–417.

93. Coupland SE. Molecular pathology of lymphoma. Eye (London) 2013; 27(2): 180–189.

94. Fishburne BC, Wilson DJ, Rosenbaum JT, Neuwelt EA. Intravitreal methotrexate as an adjunctive treatment of intraocular lymphoma. Archives of Ophthalmology 1997; 115(9): 1152–1156.

95. Pe'er J, Hochberg FH, Foster CS. Clinical review: treatment of vitreoretinal lymphoma. Ocular Immunology and Inflammation 2009; 17(5): 299–306.

96. Baryla J, Allen LH, Kwan K, Ong M, Sheidow T. Choroidal lymphoma with orbital and optic nerve extension: case and review of literature. Canadian Journal of Ophthalmology 2012; 47(1): 79–81.

97. Shields CL, Shields JA, Carvalho C, Rundle P, Smith AF. Conjunctival lymphoid tumors: clinical analysis of 117 cases and relationship to systemic lymphoma. Ophthalmology 2001; 108(5): 979–984.

98. Shields CL, Shields JA, Gross NE, Schwartz GP, Lally SE. Survey of 520 eyes with uveal metastases. Ophthalmology 1997; 104: 1265–1676.

99. Giuliari GP, Sadaka A. Uveal metastatic disease: current and new treatment options (review). Oncology Reports 2012; 27: 603–617.

100. Chen CJ, McCoy AN, Brahmer J, Handa JT. Emerging treatments for choroidal metastases. Survey of Ophthalmology 2011; 56: 511–521.

CHAPTER 58

Endocrine cancers

Andrew Weaver, Anthony P. Weetman, Oliver Gimm, Ashley Grossman, Petra Sulentic, Bertram Wiedenmann, Ursula Plöckinger, Ulrich-Frank Pape, John Wass, Angela Rogers, and Wouter de Herder

Thyroid cancers

Thyroid cancers account for less than 1% of all malignancies but are the most frequent cancers of the endocrine organs. The commonest type of thyroid cancer is papillary carcinoma, accounting for 60% of cases, followed by follicular carcinoma (15% of cases). Papillary thyroid cancer may be induced by exposure to radiation. Thyroid cancer typically presents as an asymptomatic thyroid nodule, usually diagnosed by fine needle aspiration biopsy. Treatment is typically by total or near total thyroidectomy, followed by the administration of radio-iodine to destroy any remaining thyroid tissue (followed by long-term thyroid replacement therapy).

Medullary thyroid carcinoma (MTC) arises from parafollicular C cells and comprises 5–10% of all thyroid cancers. Hereditary autosomal dominant forms are associated with germline point mutations in the *RET* proto-oncogene and occur as part of multiple endocrine neoplasia (MEN) type 2A or 2B, or as isolated familial medullary carcinoma. MTCs typically present with a solitary thyroid nodule, accompanied in 50% of cases by cervical lymphadenopathy, and can be associated with unusual hormonal effects, including secretory diarrhoea. The diagnosis is often made by fine needle aspiration biopsy and elevated serum calcitonin. Treatment is by total thyroidectomy, followed by monitoring of serum calcitonin levels (and long-term thyroid replacement therapy). Testing for the presence of *RET* mutations (see Chapter 13.10) allows family testing, with prophylactic thyroidectomy recommended for affected individuals. Rare thyroid tumours include: anaplastic carcinomas, which present as a rapidly enlarging and fixed thyroid mass, sometimes with local pain and are typically rapidly fatal; sarcomas; and primary lymphomas which usually also present as a rapidly enlarging thyroid mass in a patient with Hashimoto's thyroiditis. Squamous cell carcinomas may also present as an enlarging thyroid mass. Much information on the evidence base for the optimum diagnosis and management of thyroid cancers can be found in published guidelines [1–4].

Primary thyroid follicular epithelial tumours

See Table 58.1.

Aetiology

Excessive stimulation of the thyroid by thyroid-stimulating hormone (TSH) accounts for the higher proportion of follicular carcinomas compared with papillary carcinomas in iodine-deficient areas. The thyroid-stimulating antibodies of Graves' disease do not increase the risk of developing thyroid cancer, but incidental thyroid tumours that arise in this disorder may behave more aggressively because of activation of TSH receptors. Low-dose external beam radiation (10–1500 cGy) to the head and neck increases the risk of papillary thyroid cancer 10 to 30 years after exposure. Higher thyroid

Table 58.1 Classification of thyroid malignancies

Primary thyroid follicular epithelial tumours	Differentiated (papillary, follicular)
	Poorly differentiated (insular, other)
	Undifferentiated (anaplastic)
C-cell epithelial tumours	
Primary non-epithelial tumours	Lymphoid origin (lymphoma, plasmacytoma)
	Mesenchymal cell origin (sarcoma)
	Other (teratoma)
Secondary nonthyroidal tumours	Metastases
	Extension of tumour from adjacent structures

---

radiation doses, including those arising from radio-iodine given for treatment of hyperthyroidism, are not associated with an increased risk of malignancy because thyroid cells are destroyed rather than transformed. However, death from thyroid cancer, which is an unusual outcome, may be slightly increased by radio-iodine treatment, suggesting an effect of radiation on tumour dedifferentiation. In Belarus, the incidence of papillary carcinomas in children and young adults has increased 60-fold after the disastrous release of radio-iodine and other radionuclides from the Chernobyl nuclear reactor. The increase has been greatest in those aged less than four years at the time of exposure and is due to the potent mutagenic effects of radio-iodine on the growing thyroid gland.

Familial forms of papillary and follicular carcinomas exist but are unusual (less than 5% of cases). There are also associations with familial adenomatosis polyposis, including the Gardner syndrome variant (OMIM [Online Medelian Inheritance in Man] 175100), Cowden's disease (multiple hamartoma syndrome, OMIM 158350), Peutz-Jeghers syndrome (OMIM 175200), the Carney complex (OMIM 160980), and ataxia-telangiectasia (OMIM 208900). Papillary carcinomas do not arise from hyperplastic nodules or adenomas. In about one-third of these tumours one of several distinct rearrangements of the *RET* proto-oncogene, a member of the receptor tyrosine kinase family, occurs. The resulting chimeric oncogenes are termed *RET/PTC* (for papillary thyroid carcinoma). *RET/PTC3* is particularly linked to radiation. Around 40% of papillary carcinomas have mutations in the *BRAF* gene which encodes a serine-threonine kinase, and these tumours tend to be more aggressive and present more often with extrathyroidal invasion. Less than 10% of papillary carcinomas have mutations in the *NTRK1* oncogene.

Activation of the *RAS* oncogene occurs in around 20% of follicular and papillary thyroid cancers. Combinations of *RET, BRAF,* and *RAS* mutations do not occur in the same tumour, implying activation of the MAPK cascade as a critical step in carcinogenesis. Follicular carcinomas probably arise, at least in some cases, from follicular adenomas. Rarely, follicular carcinomas are associated with activating mutations of the genes encoding the TSH receptor or G α-protein, similar to those found in toxic adenoma. Anaplastic carcinoma may arise in a papillary or follicular carcinoma and is associated with mutations of several genes including *CTNNB1* and the p53 tumour suppressor gene.

Epidemiology

Papillary microcarcinomas are tumours less than 1 cm in diameter that occur in up to 36% of autopsy specimens and up to 24% of surgical thyroidectomies. Clearly, most of these do not become malignant. Excluding tumours that are found coincidentally, the annual incidence of thyroid follicular epithelial cancer is around 4 per 100 000. In iodine-sufficient countries, more than 80% of these are papillary carcinoma, about 10% are follicular carcinoma, and 5–10% are anaplastic carcinoma. Women are two to four times more likely to develop thyroid cancer than men, and the peak incidence is between 30 and 50 years of age.

Clinical features

Most patients present with an asymptomatic thyroid nodule; this may be noticed by themselves or their relatives, or sometimes the nodule is detected during physical examination for another complaint. The difficulty in making a diagnosis arises because thyroid nodules are frequent, and only about 5% of palpable thyroid nodules are malignant. Diffuse or multinodular thyroid enlargement occurs in around 10% of the population and is four times more common in women than in men. Solitary thyroid nodules occur in up to 5% of the population and are usually hyperplastic or colloid nodules; 5–20% of them are neoplastic, but this figure includes follicular adenomas as well as malignant tumours.

It can be seen that determining which thyroid nodules are malignant poses a dilemma that has been exacerbated by the widespread use of ultrasound examination of the neck. Up to 60% of adult thyroids have nodules detectable by high-resolution ultrasound scanning. Another problem is determining which nodules warrant investigation in a multinodular goitre. It seems reasonable to perform fine needle aspiration biopsy of so-called dominant nodules, as well as those nodules in which there are any suspicious ultrasonographic features (microcalcification, hypoechogenicity, and nodular hypervascularity) and any nodules that have demonstrated recent change in size.

There are usually no symptoms or signs to indicate that a solitary thyroid nodule is malignant because most tumours progress slowly and present before disease is advanced. Age and sex are important considerations, since a malignancy is more likely in a solitary nodule when the patient is a child or an adolescent, is over 60 years old, or is a man between the ages of 20 and 60 years. Previous exposure to radiation and a family history of thyroid cancer should also arouse suspicion. A carcinoma is more likely if the nodule has grown recently or is hard, irregular, or fixed on palpation. Clinical assessment should include careful examination of the cervical, submental, and supraclavicular lymph nodes. Late-presenting features include hoarseness, dysphagia, or dyspnoea which may indicate local invasion, but these symptoms can occasionally occur with an enlarging benign goitre. Rarely, the diagnosis only becomes apparent when metastatic disease is detected in bone or lung. The relatively indolent presentation of papillary and follicular thyroid carcinoma contrasts with that of anaplastic carcinoma in which a rapidly enlarging and fixed thyroid mass occurs, sometimes with local pain. Extension to the oesophagus, trachea, and/or recurrent laryngeal nerves is frequent, and the overlying skin may also be infiltrated.

Pathology

There are several variants of papillary thyroid carcinoma united by their characteristic cytological features (Figure 58.1). The nuclei are large, clear ('Orphan Annie', after the eyes of the cartoon character), and have longitudinal grooves and invaginations of cytoplasm (Figure 58.1A). Two-thirds of tumours are unencapsulated and display papillary and follicular structures; the remainder are the encapsulated, follicular, tall cell, sclerosing, and clear cell variants.

The encapsulated variant has a better-than-average prognosis and the tall cell variant a worse prognosis. Half of papillary carcinomas contain degenerate calcified papillae, termed psammoma bodies. The tumour is multicentric in up to 80% of cases if the resected thyroid is examined carefully.

Metastasis is via the lymphatics, and local lymph nodes are infiltrated in 40–50% of cases (more in young patients). Distant metastases are found in less than 5% of patients at presentation, with the lung being the most common site. Follicular carcinoma is characterized by follicular differentiation with a solid growth pattern and without the nuclear features of papillary carcinoma. The tumour is encapsulated, but there is invasion of the capsule and vessels (Figure 58.1B). This invasion is the crucial feature which distinguishes follicular carcinoma from follicular adenoma, self-evidently a distinction only possible by histological examination. Minimally and widely invasive subtypes are recognized, the

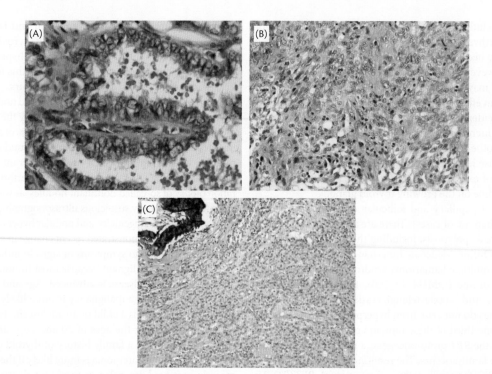

Fig. 58.1 Histopathological features of thyroid follicular epithelial carcinoma. (A) Papillary carcinoma with a central papilla, which has many overlapping and pleomorphic nuclei. Nuclear pallor and grooves are seen. (B) Anaplastic thyroid carcinoma is seen with poorly defined, pleomorphic cells. No overt papillary or follicular features are present. (C) Follicular carcinoma, showing microfollicles, is seen within the bone (calcified tissue at top).
Images reproduced courtesy of Dr K. Suvarna.

latter having a worse prognosis. When 75% or more of the tumour cells exhibit oxyphilic staining due to mitochondrial accumulation, it is called a Hürthle (or oncocytic) cell carcinoma, which probably also has a worse prognosis. Lymph node metastases with oncocytic tumours are unusual, as is multicentricity in the thyroid. Metastasis occurs via the bloodstream, typically to bone and lungs.

When follicular differentiation is poor or absent, the tumour is classified as an insular carcinoma with a poor prognosis. In anaplastic carcinoma there is no capsule, the cells are atypical, including spindle, multinuclear, and squamoid forms, and mitoses are frequent (Figure 58.1C).

Diagnosis

Thyroid epithelial cancers generally fail to affect thyroid function. However, this should be evaluated in all patients presenting with a thyroid nodule; a low circulating level of TSH strongly suggests an autonomous benign nodule. Anaplastic carcinoma may occasionally cause hypothyroidism, but the most frequent cause of an elevated level of TSH with a hard, nodular thyroid is Hashimoto's thyroiditis (OMIM 140300). Some of the glands in these cases are so irregular that a malignancy may be suspected. There is no increased or decreased risk of thyroid epithelial carcinoma in Hashimoto's thyroiditis, but thyroid lymphoma almost always occurs in association with autoimmune thyroiditis. Therefore, any dominant or atypical area in a Hashimoto's goitre requires careful evaluation. Thyroid peroxidase and/or thyroglobulin antibodies occur in about a quarter of patients with thyroid follicular epithelial carcinoma, coincident with the presence of a lymphocytic infiltrate which, in turn, is associated with a slightly more favourable prognosis. Although the serum thyroglobulin concentration is extremely useful in follow-up, as discussed below, this investigation is useless in

diagnosis; levels may not be elevated with some cancers and, even when elevated, cannot be causally distinguished from those that occur in benign adenoma, multinodular goitre, Graves' disease (OMIM 275000), or destructive thyroiditis.

Neither radionuclide nor ultrasound imaging are able to diagnose malignancy accurately. Radionuclide scanning can be performed with Tc pertechnetate or radio-iodine (^{131}I or ^{123}I), with similar information being obtained from either nuclide. Most thyroid cancers fail to take up radionuclide ('cold' nodules), but the more frequent benign lesions such as colloid nodules, cysts, adenomas, and thyroiditis behave similarly. About 20% of nodules have normal or increased radionuclide uptake. Malignancy cannot be excluded with these appearances, however. The only exception is when the nodule is 'hot' and the surrounding thyroid tissue fails to take up radionuclide, indicating the presence of a toxic adenoma which is almost invariably benign. This type of nodule will cause suppression of TSH and will be suspected from routine testing of thyroid function. In summary, radionuclide scanning usually adds little to the diagnosis.

The role of ultrasonography is more controversial but it is increasingly being used in the initial evaluation. Predicting the presence of malignancy based on the echo pattern of the tumour, and more recently using colour-flow Doppler imaging, may be successful in up to 80% of cases, but this depends on the operator having considerable experience. As well as the poor specificity of ultrasonography, the technique is so sensitive that many small unsuspected nodules will be uncovered, complicating the evaluation. Ultrasonography is useful for accurate measurement of thyroid and nodule size, which can be helpful in monitoring patients, for detecting lymphadenopathy, and for guiding biopsy, although this procedure is usually performed without imaging. Fine needle aspiration biopsy is undoubtedly the current technique of choice for investigation of a thyroid nodule. Local anaesthetic is not needed because the procedure causes little discomfort. It is usual to take two to six biopsies to increase the sample yield. Essentially three diagnoses are possible: benign (65–75% of specimens), malignant (5%), and indeterminate (20–30%), but an experienced cytopathologist is needed to obtain reliable results. Papillary carcinoma is readily diagnosed by fine needle aspiration biopsy, and medullary carcinoma and lymphoma can also be detected by the use of immunohistochemical staining, although lymphoma frequently requires core or open biopsy for confirmation.

Follicular carcinomas cannot be distinguished cytologically from follicular adenomas, and these tumours account for the bulk of needle aspiration specimens labelled indeterminate (or suspicious). Open biopsy is the only secure diagnostic method in this setting. About 15% of biopsies reported in experienced centres are considered unsuitable for diagnosis. It is relatively simple to repeat the biopsy, but a persistently equivocal biopsy should be grounds for considering surgery since malignant tumours will be found in about a half of these cases. A cyst may be aspirated during biopsy. If this fails to reaccumulate and no lesion remains palpable, a malignancy is highly unlikely, but recurrence of a cyst may indicate malignant disease and require surgery for definitive diagnosis. Overall, the sensitivity and specificity of fine needle aspiration biopsy is greater than 90%.

Molecular diagnosis

The most common molecular alterations in thyroid cancer include *BRAF* and *RAS* point mutations and *RET/PTC* and *PAX8/PPARγ* rearrangements. These genetic alterations are found in more than 70% of all papillary and follicular thyroid cancers. The diagnostic role of *BRAF* mutations has been studied most extensively. The *BRAF V600E* mutation can also be used for tumour prognostication as this mutation may be associated with a higher rate of tumour recurrence and tumour-related mortality. The use of these and other emerging molecular markers are expected to improve accuracy of diagnosis, allowing for more individualized surgical and post-surgical management. However, we are a little time away before these investigations become routine in the majority of thyroid clinics.

Treatment

Surgical excision

A total or near total thyroidectomy should usually be performed since thyroid carcinomas are often bilateral and removal of thyroid tissue facilitates subsequent ablation by radio-iodine. Unilateral total lobectomy is indicated for microcarcinoma. In papillary carcinoma, the central lymph nodes should be dissected, as should all palpable nodes. Central lymph node removal is also indicated in follicular carcinoma with histological evidence of extrathyroidal spread.

Radio-iodine therapy

After surgery, radio-iodine can be administered to remove any remaining thyroid tissue, which then allows thyroglobulin or iodine whole body scanning to be used in follow-up to detect metastases. This treatment also destroys occult carcinoma and, by scanning after ablation, metastatic disease is revealed. Local policies vary, but in most centres an ablation dose of 1100 MBq to 3700 MBq I is given one to three months after surgery. Recent studies have shown an equivalent outcome after either 1100 or 3700 MBq, with the higher dose having more adverse effects, so the lower dose is preferable for low-moderate risk tumours [5].

A pretreatment scan is not required because virtually all patients have persistent thyroid remnants no matter how apparently complete the surgery was. Radio-iodine ablation is indicated in all patients with a tumour >4 cm diameter, or any tumour size with gross extra-thyroidal extension, or with distant metastases present, whereas it is not indicated for a tumour ≤1 cm diameter and on histological examination the diagnosis is a classical papillary or follicular variant carcinoma, or a follicular minimally invasive carcinoma with no angioinvasion or invasion of thyroid capsule [2]. Disease presentations between these descriptors require careful consideration and discussion with the patient. There are persuasive arguments that low-risk patients with papillary carcinoma may not benefit from radio-iodine ablation and clinical staging scores (see below) may help to identify such patients.

In approximately 15% of patients, a second treatment dose of iodine is necessary to achieve ablation. Iodine exposure, including iodine-containing contrast media, may prevent accumulation of iodine during treatment. High levels of stimulation by TSH are required to produce maximum uptake of iodine; this has been achieved traditionally by a period of three to four weeks without thyroxine replacement and can thus lead to the development of severe hypothyroid symptoms. The short action of liothyronine, 20 μg three times daily, as a replacement is therefore preferable in the weeks before scanning and iodine treatment, because only two weeks are needed when this is stopped to increase endogenous TSH (which should be >30 mU/L). Even this short period without thyroid hormone may be troublesome for the patient. Recombinant TSH suitable for intramuscular administration is now available and can be given without cessation of thyroid hormone replacement. This is now the preparation method of choice in patients without high-risk disease or a recurrence, or in those who cannot tolerate hypothyroidism clinically, and it offers a better quality of life during treatment.

Systemic therapy for radio-iodine resistant thyroid cancer

Until recently, doxorubicin has been considered a systemic treatment by default, albeit with limited systematic evaluation of clinical benefit. The introduction of biologics, specifically tyrosine kinase inhibitors (TKIs), has radically altered this landscape. The pathways that are most likely targeted include the *BRAF V600E* mutation, which is present in approximately 45% of papillary thyroid cancer but is less common in follicular thyroid cancer [6]. *RAS* mutations are more common in follicular thyroid cancer, with mutations in *HRAS, NRAS,* or *KRAS* detectable in approximately 40% of FTC [7]. A number of TKIs and other biologics have been tested in thyroid cancer, including cediranib, lenalidomide, cabozantinib, dabrafenib, trametinib, everolimus, lenvatinib, pazopanib, selumetinib, sunitinib, vandetinib, and vemurafenib, although sorafenib is the only FDA-approved drug available for standard therapy in differentiated thyroid cancer (see section below on MTC concerning approval of vandetanib).

Most drugs have been primarily been evaluated in phase II trials in radio-iodine-resistant differentiated (not MTC or undifferentiated) thyroid cancer. However, sorafenib was approved based on data from the DECISION study in 417 patients treated with either sorafenib or placebo [8]. The primary endpoint of improved progression-free survival (PFS) was met with sorafenib at 10.8 months vs placebo at 5.8 months. Responses were seen in 12% with sorafenib and 0.5% with placebo, and stable disease in 42%

and 33%, respectively. Toxicities, including hand-foot syndrome, fatigue, and diarrhoea, were common, as when sorafenib is used in hepatocellular carcinoma, although these were considered manageable. To date, there are results from phase II studies suggesting that second-line TKI therapy may be helpful, although there are no studies demonstrating an optimal sequence, nor any prospective data validating predictive biomarkers. The likeliest target that may prove useful is the *BRAF V-600E* mutation, in which case one of the BRAF inhibitors might be considered.

Long-term thyroid replacement therapy

The last aspect of treatment is to maintain the patient for life on levothyroxine. This is given to high-risk patients at doses sufficient to suppress levels of TSH to below 0.1 mU/L, because TSH is a growth factor for thyroid carcinoma. In almost all patients, satisfactory suppression of TSH can be achieved without inducing thyrotoxic symptoms. The effective levothyroxine dosage is 2.2–2.8 µg/kg body weight, i.e., doses average between 150µg–200µg per day. The optimum level of TSH is unknown, but higher levels of TSH (0.1–0.5 mU/L) can be accepted in low-risk patients, and some form of risk stratification within the first year after initial treatment is helpful in determining the degree of TSH suppression to be aimed for [2].

Anaplastic carcinoma

Anaplastic carcinoma is usually rapidly fatal. The tumour rarely takes up radio-iodine. Surgery has a very limited role in relieving obstructive symptoms, and external beam radiotherapy is useful for short-term palliation. The place of chemotherapy remains to be fully established, although individual patients may achieve a partial remission with treatment, usually given as some combination of paclitaxel or docetaxel, doxorubicin and cisplatin, with or without radiotherapy [4].

Follow-up

Lifelong follow-up is recommended for papillary and follicular cancer because they may recur many years after apparent cure. Serum thyroglobulin measurement and ultrasound of the neck should be performed 9–12 months after initial resection and radio-iodine ablation to provide a baseline measurement for follow-up [2]. Detectable levels of thyroglobulin after thyroid ablation indicate persistent or recurrent disease. Measuring thyroglobulin levels is especially valuable after recombinant TSH stimulation, as the rise in TSH will promote thyroglobulin production and exaggerate any increase. This is particularly useful in initial follow-up and in following high-risk patients; in those at low risk who have a negative neck ultrasound thyroglobulin may be measured routinely without TSH stimulation. If thyroglobulin is detectable, the patient should have a whole body iodine scan and any recurrent disease can then be treated with a therapeutic dose of 5500 MBq I. It is usual to perform a diagnostic total body scan after initial radio-iodine ablation. If there is residual radio-iodine uptake, SPECT-CT scanning may provide useful localization information in some cases [2].

Repeated scans thereafter have now been superseded by measurement of thyroglobulin and low-risk cases may be assessed adequately by thyroglobulin measurement alone. The only exception is in the patient with thyroglobulin antibodies that interfere with many assays for thyroglobulin. If this is the case, repeated scans are the only way to ensure that the patient remains free of disease, although some argue monitoring the thyroglobulin antibody

level fall is a surrogate marker for the thyroglobulin level itself. Ultrasonography is useful to confirm the presence of loco-regional recurrence without distant metastases, and these tumour deposits are best dealt with surgically. For metastatic disease, usually in the lung, treatment with radio-iodine can be repeated every four to six months, but there is little benefit above a cumulative dose of 18 500 MBq. Bone metastases may respond to iodine or external beam radiotherapy. The best survival in metastatic thyroid cancer occurs in young patients with small metastases, indicating the overall value of early treatment for this disease.

Prognosis

At least nine scoring systems have been advocated to assess prognosis in papillary and follicular carcinoma, of which the TNM classification system is now the most popular. These systems generally take into account the age and sex of the patient, tumour characteristics (especially size, extension, and metastases), and completeness of excision.

With appropriate treatment the rate of recurrence of papillary carcinoma is about 15%, and the cause-specific death rate is approximately 5% at 20 years. In other words, 85% of these patients present with features of the group with the best prognosis, i.e., achieving a score of less than six in the system described in Table 58.2. In follicular carcinoma, the cause-specific survival rate is 80% at 20 years after treatment and 70% at 30 years. However, in the subgroup with metastases at presentation the ten-year survival is only 20%. The median survival time for anaplastic carcinoma is four to 12 months and those with distant metastases at presentation have a median survival time of only three months.

Special problems in pregnancy

A solitary nodule in a pregnant woman should be evaluated by fine needle aspiration biopsy. If the biopsy suggests malignancy and the nodule is growing significantly, surgery can be undertaken in the second or third trimester, but otherwise this is best deferred until after delivery. Women receiving radio-iodine ablation should avoid pregnancy for at least six months after all radioactive treatment has been administered.

Table 58.2 The predictive value of a scoring system in determining outcome in papillary carcinoma. The scoring system is used to divide patients into four prognostic groups. The overall score is the sum of the following: 3.1 (if ≤39 years old) or 0.08 × patient age (if ≥40 years old); 0.3 × size of tumour in centimetres; 1, if resection is incomplete; 1, if there is extrathyroidal extension; 3, if there are metastases

Score	20-year survival (%)
<6	99
6–6.99	89
7–7.99	56
≥8	24

A patient with a past history of thyroid cancer on suppressive doses of levothyroxine who becomes pregnant is likely to require an increased dose of levothyroxine during their pregnancy in order to keep the TSH level suppressed. After delivery of the baby their levothyroxine dose can be reduced to pre-pregnancy levels.

Primary thyroid lymphoma

Less than 5% of thyroid malignancies are non-Hodgkin's B-cell lymphoma (OMIM 605027). The peak incidence is between 50 and 80 years of age, and women are affected three times more frequently than men. The typical presentation is a rapidly enlarging thyroid mass in a patient with Hashimoto's thyroiditis. The clinical features may suggest anaplastic carcinoma. The diagnosis can be made by fine needle aspiration biopsy and confirmed by large needle or open biopsy. Accurate staging is then necessary to plan treatment, which may include external beam radiotherapy and anthracycline-based lymphoma chemotherapy. Intensive treatment has produced eight-year survival rates of over 90%. Recent results with rituximab, a monoclonal antibody directed against B cells, have shown some evidence of therapeutic benefit.

Medullary carcinoma of the thyroid

MTC was first described in 1959 by Hazard and colleagues as a distinct entity [9]. It can occur in a sporadic (about 75%) and a hereditary (about 25%) form. As of today, surgery is the only curative treatment. Current research is therefore concentrating on alternative treatment modalities.

Epidemiology

MTC is a rare malignancy. Reliable data regarding the incidence of MTC do not exist but it is believed that MTC accounts roughly for about 5% to 10% of all thyroid malignancies (<http://www.baets.org.uk/guidelines/>).

Hereditary medullary thyroid carcinoma

The aetiology of hereditary MTC is well known although our understanding of the pathogenesis is still incomplete. Clinically, three different forms of hereditary MTC are distinguished, namely familial MTC (FMTC), multiple endocrine neoplasia 2A (MEN 2A), and MEN 2B (Table 58.3), often also summarized as MEN 2 [10].

Molecular biology and pathology

Germline *RET* mutations in MEN 2

Germline mutations of the *RET* proto-oncogene have been shown to be associated with all three types of hereditary MTC. They can roughly be divided into extracellular and intracellular mutations. With regard to the extracellular mutations, one of five particular cysteine codons in exon 10 (C609, C611, C618, and C620) or exon 11 (C634) is affected in the majority of cases. In rare instances, mutations in exon 5 or exon 8 may be found. In contrast, intracellular mutations in exons 13–16 associated with MEN 2 always affect non-cysteine amino acids.

Association of *RET* genotype with disease features

While about 85% of MEN 2A have a codon 634 mutation, only 30% of FMTC families have a codon 634 mutation [11]. Actually, it would appear that the distribution of mutations among the cysteine codons is more even in FMTC families. Even though some mutations have only been found in patients with FMTC and not in MEN 2A patients, it is not recommended that these patients should forego phaeochromocytoma and pHPT surveillance.

The most common mutations associated with MEN 2B are located in the intracellular tyrosine kinase domain and affect non-cysteine amino acids. The most common of these mutations (>95%) is found in exon 16 (M918T) [14]; the next common, in exon 15 (A883F), probably accounts for approximately 2–3% of MEN 2B cases [15]. These two mutations have not yet been reported in patients with MEN 2A or FMTC. There does not appear to be any clinical difference between M918T cases and A883F ones. There are some rare

Table 58.3 Phenotypes in familial medullary thyroid carcinoma (FMTC), MEN 2A, and MEN 2B

Clinical Findings			FMTC	MEN 2A	MEN 2B
Medullary thyroid carcinoma	70–100%	90–100%	100%		
Phaeochromocytoma		–		40–60%	40–60%
Primary hyperparathyroidism	–		15–25%	–	
Ganglioneuromatosis		–		–	+
Intraoral neuromas		–		–	>90%
Neuromas of the lips		–		–	>60%
'Bumpy lips'			–	–	>95%
Medullated corneal fibres	–		–	+	

MEN 2A, multiple endocrine neoplasia type 2A.

MEN 2B, multiple endocrine neoplasia type 2B.

– Phenotype is not part of the syndrome.

+ Phenotype is not part of the syndrome; the frequency, however, is not well documented.

Source: data from Brauckhoff M et al., Premonitory symptoms preceding metastatic medullary thyroid cancer in MEN 2B: An exploratory analysis, *Surgery*, Volume 144, Issue 6, pp. 1044–1050, Copyright © 2008 Elsevier; and Gimm O., Familial Endocrine Conditions, in Hubbard JG et al. (Eds.), *Endocrine Surgery: Principles and Practice*, Springer Science and Business Media, New York, USA, Copyright © 2009.

reports of patients with *RET* double-mutations and a MEN 2B-like phenotype [12, 13].

Despite great advances in the study of genetics and genotype-phenotype association in MEN 2, unanswered questions remain. For instance, the onset of carcinogenesis can differ in family members harbouring the same mutations. In addition, it is unknown why some family members develop phaeochromocytomas and/or pHPT while others do not. GFR alpha 4 has been reported to be a modifying factor [16].

Sporadic medullary thyroid carcinoma

From the clinical point of view, the term sporadic indicates the absence of any family history of MTC or MEN 2 component tumours. However, the term sporadic MTC should only be used if no MEN 2-specific germline *RET* mutation was found [12].

Most recently, mutually exclusive somatic mutations in *RET* and *RAS* have been reported recently in about 90% of sporadic MTCs, suggesting that these oncogenes are predominant drivers [17].

Medullary thyroid carcinoma

MTC derives from the parafollicular C-cells. It is therefore sometimes even named C-cell carcinoma. C cells produce calcitonin and staining with calcitonin is the best diagnostic criterion. Less well-differentiated tumours, especially metastases, may show weak or absent calcitonin staining. CEA is the second most important hormone produced by C cells. Both calcitonin and CEA are used as blood tumour markers. Beside calcitonin and CEA, MTC may synthesize various other hormonal or non-hormonal substances, for example polypeptide hormones (adrenocorticotrophin [ACTH], somatostatin, vasoactive intestinal peptide), bioactive amines and enzymes (dopamine, histaminase, serotonin), amyloid, melanin, or nerve growth factor.

MTC is typically a circumscribed, rounded tumour that occurs in the middle or upper third of the thyroid lobe, where the concentration of C cells is greatest. Macroscopically, MTC is solid, firm, and usually not encapsulated. Calcification is often present. Microscopically, partial encapsulation of the tumour may be seen, but usually there is clear microscopic evidence of infiltration into the surrounding tissue. Amyloid deposition is a typical, but not invariable, feature. Structurally, MTC is a great imitator. Hereditary MTC is often multicentric whereas sporadic MTC is usually unicentric.

C-cell hyperplasia

In hereditary MTC, C-cell carcinoma seems to occur after development of C-cell hyperplasia (increased number of C cells). According to the WHO, the most accepted definition of C-cell hyperplasia is defined as more than 50 C-cells per low-power field [18]. This morphological (neoplastic) change is rarely seen in sporadic MTC. However, exceptions are reported in either instance and C-cell hyperplasia has also been reported in healthy individuals (reactive). Thus, C-cell hyperplasia is not a reliable finding in distinguishing hereditary from sporadic MTC.

TNM classification and staging

TNM classification and staging for MTC can be found on the website of the American Cancer Society: <http://www.cancer.org/cancer/thyroidcancer/detailedguide/thyroid-cancer-staging>.

Molecular diagnosis

Apparently sporadic medullary thyroid carcinoma

Today, it is standard practice that every new patient with apparently sporadic MTC should undergo germline mutation analysis of *RET* (Figure 58.2). Following genetic counselling that should be offered to any patient with MTC, patients can be easily screened by analysing DNA extracted from peripheral blood leucocytes (Figure 58.2A).

The reasons for advocating a consequent screening procedure are diverse. After exclusion of a germline *RET* mutation, these individuals, and subsequently their family members, can be excluded from further screening procedures for MTC or accompanying disorders (e.g., phaeochromocytoma). Therefore, it may very well be justified to screen a 70-year-old female with MTC for *RET* mutation, not for her own risk but to exclude the possibility that her descendants are at risk (Figure 58.2B).

RET mutation analysis should begin with exons 11 and 10 where mutations are found most often. If no mutations are found, exons 13, 14, and 15 followed by exons 5 and 8 need to be analysed. Analysis of exons 16 and 15 seems to be indicated if MEN 2B is suspected.

A hereditary background is highly unlikely, although possible, if analysis of all exons mentioned above is negative for specific *RET* mutations. To exclude administrative errors, a confirmation of the test would be desirable but is not established in all countries.

Known MEN 2 family

Given the current state of knowledge, any patient with MEN 2-specific *RET* mutation must be assumed to be at high risk of developing MTC.

Diagnosis and staging

The female to male ratio of both sporadic and hereditary MTC is approximately 1:1. Both sporadic and hereditary MTC can present clinically with a morphological change of the thyroid, possibly palpable during physical examination but almost never causing any functional disorder of the thyroid. The majority of patients (50–80%) with sporadic MTC and also those with hereditary MTC who are not diagnosed by screening procedures (= index patients) usually have lymph node metastases at the time of diagnosis. Thus, cervical lymph node metastases may be the initial symptom of MTC. In advanced stages, symptoms may arise from effects caused by extensive production of calcitonin, especially diarrhoea.

MTC is not just one type of thyroid cancer; it is a special form with its own biological behaviour and, therefore, needs to be treated differently from other thyroid cancers. Therefore, the diagnosis of MTC should be made preoperatively if possible. Reoperation due to avoidable incorrect initial treatment is not only accompanied by a higher morbidity rate but the chance of biochemical cure is certainly lower [19].

Fine needle aspiration cytology

In the case of suspected cancer based on clinical evaluation or ultrasound, a fine needle aspiration cytology (FNAC) either of the thyroid or regional lymph nodes should be performed [20].

Calcitonin and carcinoembryonic antigen

Before *RET* was identified as the MEN 2 disease-causing gene, all at-risk patients had to be screened via calcitonin. This is best

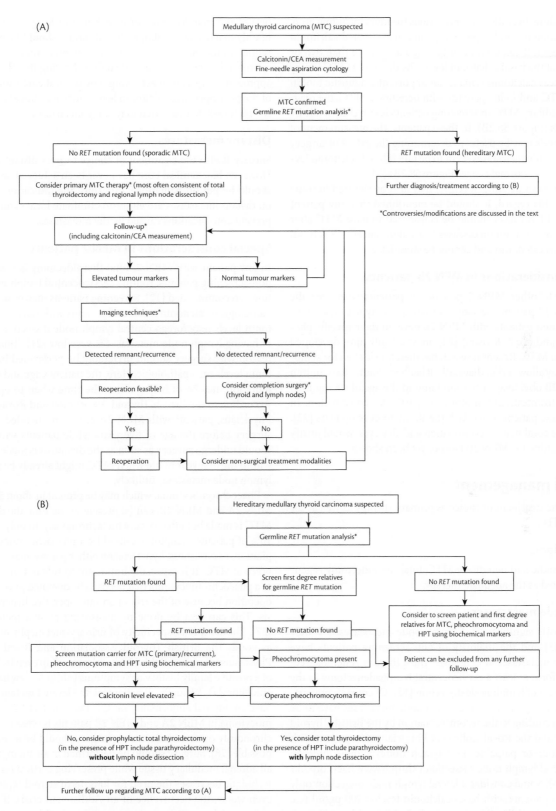

(A)

Medullary thyroid carcinoma (MTC) suspected

↓

Calcitonin/CEA measurement
Fine-needle aspiration cytology

↓

MTC confirmed
Germline *RET* mutation analysis*

No *RET* mutation found (sporadic MTC)　　　　　　*RET* mutation found (hereditary MTC)

Consider primary MTC therapy* (most often consistent of total thyroidectomy and regional lymph node dissection)　　　　Further diagnosis/treatment according to (B)

*Controversies/modifications are discussed in the text

Follow-up*
(including calcitonin/CEA measurement)

Elevated tumour markers　　　　Normal tumour markers

Imaging techniques*

Detected remnant/recurrence　　　　No detected remnant/recurrence

Reoperation feasible?　　　　Consider completion surgery* (thyroid and lymph nodes)

Yes　　　　No

Reoperation　→　Consider non-surgical treatment modalities

(B)

Hereditary medullary thyroid carcinoma suspected

↓

Germline *RET* mutation analysis*

RET mutation found　　　　Screen first degree relatives for germline *RET* mutation　　　　No *RET* mutation found

RET mutation found　　No *RET* mutation found　　　Consider to screen patient and first degree relatives for MTC, pheochromocytoma and HPT using biochemical markers

Screen mutation carrier for MTC (primary/recurrent), pheochromocytoma and HPT using biochemical markers　→　Pheochromocytoma present　　Patient can be excluded from any further follow-up

Calcitonin level elevated?　←　Operate pheochromocytoma first

No, consider prophylactic total thyroidectomy (in the presence of HPT include parathyroidectomy) **without** lymph node dissection　　　Yes, consider total thyroidectomy (in the presence of HPT include parathyroidectomy) **with** lymph node dissection

Further follow up regarding MTC according to (A)

Fig. 58.2 (A) Diagnostic and therapeutic strategy in apparently sporadic MTC. (B) Diagnostic and therapeutic strategy in suspected hereditary MTC.

done by measuring basal calcitonin. Calcitonin can even be stimulated with either calcium (2 mg/kg body weight of 10% Ca^{2+} injected intravenously in 1 min) or pentagastrin (0.5 μg/kg body weight, diluted in 5–10 ml sterile saline, injected intravenously in 5–15 s) or a combination of both. Calcitonin levels are determined

immediately before and 2 and 5 minutes after injection of the provocative reagent. Stimulation of calcitonin seems to be of most value in patients when the diagnosis MTC is questioned (e.g., if no thyroid nodule is found or if basal calcitonin is only slightly elevated). A variety of other conditions (e.g., pregnancy, contraceptive pill, renal failure, liver disease, and various tumours including lung, breast cell tumours, and hepatomas) can cause elevated calcitonin levels. However, if calcitonin can be stimulated more than two or three times of the basal calcitonin levels, the diagnosis MTC is very likely. Whereas calcitonin remains an important diagnostic tool in sporadic MTC and index patients with hereditary MTC, the diagnosis of hereditary MTC in screening patients is currently made by *RET* analysis (Figure 58.2B). In these patients, the measurement of calcitonin levels may be useful in determining the extent of surgery since lymph node metastases seem to be rare if basal calcitonin levels are within the normal range (Figure 58.2B) [21].

Carcinoembryonic antigen (CEA) may also be elevated in some patients. In this regard, it should be mentioned that any patient with elevated CEA level should be considered to have MTC after exclusion of more common diseases (e.g. colon cancer). CEA is not as sensitive as calcitonin and cannot be stimulated.

Special considerations in MEN 2B patients

In contrast to other MEN 2 patients or patients with sporadic MTC, MEN 2B patients develop a specific phenotype (Table 58.3). However, when patients with MEN 2B develop their specific phenotype (around age 3–8 years) [22], most already have developed metastasized MTC. Recent research has therefore looked for symptoms that may allow earlier diagnosis. It has been found that children with MEN 2B obviously very soon (around the age of six months) develop gastrointestinal symptoms, in particular constipation. In addition, these patients often lack the ability to develop tears [22]. Whether the combination constipation and 'dry eyes' would justify genetic screening for MEN 2B has not yet been shown.

Surgical management

Surgery is the treatment of choice as primary therapy as well as for recurrent MTC.

Thyroid gland

In both sporadic and hereditary MTC, total thyroidectomy is generally accepted as the adequate therapy.

Lymph node metastases

The prognostic significance of lymph node metastases is widely accepted [23] and the majority of non-screening patients have lymph node metastases at diagnosis. Thus, there is general agreement to perform at least a cervicocentral lymphadenectomy as the minimal extent of lymph node dissection [12]. Of course, compartments involved by macroscopic lymph node metastases have to be dissected. According to the recommendation by the British Thyroid Association and the Royal College of Physicians, any patient with pT2–4 tumour or palpable neck lymph nodes should undergo bilateral lateral lymph node dissection (<http://www.baets.org.uk/guidelines/>). Some consider a lateral lymph node dissection only necessary in patients with basal calcitonin levels >400 pg/ml (ca. 177 pmol/l) [12] while others recommend a bilateral lateral lymph node dissection if basal calcitonin levels are higher than 200 pg/ml (ca. 58 pmol/l) [24].

In any case, the surgical technique of the lymph node dissection should be performed in a systematic manner, i.e., that the removal of all lymph nodes in one region should be performed en bloc with the surrounding adipose tissue while preserving vital vessels, nerves and muscles. Any form of 'berry-picking', i.e., the removal of only macroscopic enlarged lymph nodes should be restricted to reoperations once a region has been cleared systematically. This approach is justified by several studies showing that the systematic approach is superior in achieving biochemical cure (normalization of the post-operative calcitonin level) since it removes even normal lymph nodes that very well may carry metastases.

Distant metastases

Surgery is also the treatment of choice to treat distant metastases. However, biochemical cure has never been achieved and the focus should be put on palliation [25]. Thus, the indications to operate on distant metastases are either to eliminate local symptoms or to prevent complications caused by the metastases.

Special considerations in MEN 2 patients

In any patient with MEN 2, total thyroidectomy is mandatory. In non-screening patients, routine cervicocentral lymph node dissection is recommended [12]. Screening patients may or may not have pathological calcitonin levels and patients with normal basal calcitonin levels may forego central lymph node dissection as the risk of having lymph node metastases is very low [21]. This is also the reason why surgery should preferably be performed before calcitonin levels turn pathologic. Here, the patient's age and the specific mutation may be of help guiding the time when to operate [26]. According to the British Thyroid Association and Royal College of Physicians, patients with MEN 2A are recommended to undergo surgery before the age of five years while patients with MEN 2B should undergo surgery as soon as the diagnosis is made, preferably within the first year of life when MTC might already be present but lymph node metastases unlikely.

Phaeochromocytoma, which may be present in about 50% in both MEN 2A and MEN 2B, can be present at the time the diagnosis of MTC is made but often occurs metachronously. In only up to about 10% of patients, symptoms caused by a phaeochromocytoma (palpitation, nervousness, hypertension either paroxysmal or sustained) precede MTC. It is especially important to rule out the coexistence of a phaeochromocytoma that needs to be operated prior to an MTC operation because of the risk of an intraoperative hypertensive crisis. This can best be done by measuring plasma-metanephrines [27]. The sensitivity/specificity of urinary-metanephrines is almost as good. The British Thyroid Association and Royal College of Physicians recommend this biochemical workup even in the absence of a positive family history or symptoms (<http://www.baets.org.uk/guidelines/>). Virtually all patients with elevated metanephrines do have an adrenal abnormality on CT. Due the fact that phaeochromocytoma in MEN 2A and MEN 2B patients is often bilateral (synchronously or metachronously), surgery should be as restrictive as possible [28]. Surgery should be performed in an attempt to remove all adrenal medullary tissue while preserving cortical function. This technique decreases the need for long-term steroid replacement or, even worse, the occurrence of an Addisonian crisis. If performed appropriately, the risk of recurrence is low. In this regard, it needs to be emphasized that phaeochromocytomas in MEN 2A and MEN 2B are malignant in less than 5%.

Up to 20–30% patients with MEN 2A will develop primary hyperparathyroidism (pHPT). The association of parathyroid disease with MEN 2A is regarded as being genetically determined and not a response to elevated calcitonin levels. pHPT is rarely present when MTC is diagnosed. Thus, pHPT is most often diagnosed during follow-up of patients operated on for MTC. As in sporadic cases, calcium and parathormone should be measured to diagnose pHPT. There is no need for prophylactic parathyroidectomy. Once pHPT is diagnosed or when operating on the thyroid gland, all four parathyroids should be identified and all enlarged parathyroids (rarely more than one) should be removed. In the rare event of enlargement of all four parathyroids, the least single pathological gland needs to be identified. The least pathological part should either remain in situ or should be autotransplanted into the sternomastoid muscle. Similar results could be achieved with either technique. In MEN 2B, pHPT is not more often present than in the general population.

Residual/recurrent medullary thyroid carcinoma

Even if primary therapy in a patient with sporadic MTC consists of total thyroidectomy and bilateral lymph node dissection, normal calcitonin levels can only be achieved in up to 40–50% (Figure 58.2A). There is general agreement that post-operative elevated calcitonin levels indicate residual tumour. However, despite elevated calcitonin levels, imaging techniques often fail to detect residual C cells. This situation probably reflects the limitations of imaging techniques available today since they fail to detect micrometastases. Common sites for distant metastases are lung, liver, and bone.

Localization and confirmation

Imaging studies are recommended in patients with a basal calcitonin levels of ≥150 pg/ml (= 44 pmol/L) [12]. For the detection of loco-regional and mediastinal metastases, CT is recommended. Concerning liver metastases, multidetector-CT or MRI is advised. In patients having basal calcitonin levels <150 pg/ml (~ 44 pmol/L), the indication to perform imaging studies should be made on an individual basis.

Larger metastases might very well be detectable using CT or MRI. Occult metastases, however, are rarely detectable using either technique. Due to the nature of C-cell metastasis (multiple, micronodular, involving the whole organ), laparoscopy has been successfully used to identify liver metastases [29]. Less invasive techniques used successfully include ^{99m}Tc-dimercaptosuccinic acid (DMSA), ^{131}I-MIBG, ^{111}In- or ^{99m}Tc-octreotide, and ^{18}FDG-PET (<http://www.baets.org.uk/guidelines/>) [30]. However, no single diagnostic technique is able to reliably demonstrate the full extent of disease in patients with recurrent or metastatic MTC.

If in doubt, a localized remnant/recurrent tumour should be subject to FNAC if accessible.

Reoperation

The indication for reoperation may be given: (1) if primary therapy did not consist of total thyroidectomy and either if the post-operative calcitonin level is elevated in patients with sporadic MTC or in any patients with hereditary MTC regardless of the post-operative calcitonin level; and (2) in cases of proven or suspected residual lymph node metastases. If a patient with sporadic MTC underwent less than total thyroidectomy, indication for reoperation is not necessarily given if the thyroid remnant is small and calcitonin levels after stimulation are within normal levels [31]. However, in the case of elevated calcitonin levels, completion

thyroidectomy and/or loco-regional lymph node dissection is recommended. In contrast, in hereditary MTC a completion of the thyroidectomy is always advised since every single C cell has the potential of developing MTC.

If either lymph node metastasis or recurrent disease is proven by imaging techniques/FNAC, the indication for reoperation is given in most cases.

In the presence of distant metastases, the extent of reoperation should be evaluated individually. In addition to the patient's age and general condition, the tumour dynamic should be taken into account. The latter can be assessed by looking at the doubling-time of both calcitonin and CEA (see prognosis).

Radiation

MTC is generally not very sensitive to radiation. Although there are some studies reporting a reduced risk of local recurrence after radiation, surgery should be performed if feasible. The reasons are the disadvantages of radiation:

1. Many patients experience distressing long-term side effects of cough and dryness due to the high doses needed.
2. Scarring of the neck makes assessment of future local recurrence (clinically and using imaging techniques) and reoperation difficult.

A plausible consensus is as follows:

1. If surgical treatment appears successful (defined as normal calcitonin level after stimulation), there is no need for radiation.
2. In cases of biochemical or clinical evidence of persistent/recurrent disease, reoperation would be the preferred treatment.
3. Radiation should be avoided until local disease is either symptomatic or rapidly progressing, and not amenable to reoperation.
4. In some rare instances, a combination of 'debulking' surgery and radiotherapy may be appropriate.
5. Radiation may be useful in treating symptomatic distant metastases, such as bone metastases.

Radio-iodine treatment

Because MTC does not derive from follicular cells, there is no uptake of radio-iodine and therefore no indication to treat these patients with radio-iodine.

Chemotherapy and other treatment modalities

Some experimental studies with chemotherapy are promising. Currently, one of the best results has been achieved by combining dacarbazine, fluorouracil, and doxorubicin [12].

New therapeutic approaches such as TKIs have been studied in recent years. For vandetanib, an inhibitor of vascular endothelial growth factor receptor (VEGFR), the epidermal growth factor receptor (EGFR), and the RET-tyrosine kinase, a significantly prolonged PFS has recently been shown in a phase III study [32]. However, the rate of adverse side effects (such as diarrhoea, rash, nausea, hypertension, headache) requiring intervention was quite high (26–56%). In animal studies, an improved efficacy was shown combining radioimmunotherapy and antiangiogenic therapy [33]. Concerning irinotecan, a reduced toxicity was shown when using octreotide-marked liposomes in comparison to 'free' irinotecan in in vitro studies [34]; clinical results have not yet been published.

Molecular-targeted therapy is most promising and we should expect new treatment options in the near future.

Prognosis

Most long-term studies report a five-year survival rate of 80–90% and a ten-year survival rate of 60–70%. Probably more than 50% of all patients with sporadic MTC will die of their disease.

Like most cancers, prognosis has been shown to depend on tumour stage [35]. Besides tumour stage, post-operative calcitonin level is the most powerful prognostic factor. In this regard, the term 'biochemical cure' needs to be explained. 'Biochemical cure' simply demonstrates the absence of pathological calcitonin levels after treatment. It does not necessarily mean that the patient is really cured (without tumour). Indeed, rising levels of calcitonin after apparent 'biochemical cure' have been reported although reoperation rarely had to be performed in these cases. In contrast, falling calcitonin levels have been observed without treatment. In these instances, falling calcitonin levels may indicate a dedifferentiation of the MTC with consequent decreased calcitonin expression rather than spontaneous regression. CEA levels seem to correlate inversely with calcitonin and correlate most likely better with the overall tumour mass in patients with less-differentiated MTC [36].

It has repeatedly been shown that the prognosis can be well assessed by looking at the doubling-time of both calcitonin and CEA [37, 38]. A doubling-time of less than six months correlates with a poor prognosis while one more than two years correlates with a good prognosis.

Follow-up

Following surgery, all patients need lifelong replacement of levothyroxine (L-T4). The dose of L-T4 should be adjusted according to periodic measurements of serum thyrotropin (TSH) that should be within the normal range. Patients who undergo treatment for MTC have to be followed-up lifelong in intervals usually between 6–12 months. Shorter follow-up might be justified if tumour progression is suspected. In this respect, there is generally no difference between sporadic and hereditary cases. However, it is unknown whether screening patients who underwent prophylactic thyroidectomy and histologically only showed C-cell hyperplasia need to undergo follow-up at all. In the case of follow-up, the basal calcitonin should be measured yearly. There is controversy about whether basal calcitonin or CEA levels correlate with the amount of disease (see prognosis), but agreement that elevated post-operative levels almost generally indicate persistent disease. If either basal or stimulated calcitonin level is abnormal, further investigations may be indicated to localize the residual disease. If medical management is not altered as a response to calcitonin levels in individual cases, there is no need to subject the patient to repeated tests.

Adrenal tumours

Adrenocortical tumours

The adrenal cortex comprises 90% of the normal adult adrenal gland and weighs up to 4 g. It consists of three zones: the outer zona glomerulosa (15% of the cortex), which expresses the enzyme 18-oxidase and can thus secrete aldosterone; the middle zona fasciculata (75% of the cortex); and inner zona reticularis which express the enzyme 17α-hydroxylase and can secrete cortisol, androgens, oestrogens, and weak mineralocorticoids. Tumours arising from the adrenal cortex are divided into benign and malignant; either can be functioning or non-functioning, the latter being a not uncommon incidental finding during abdominal imaging with either CT or MRI scanning. The great majority of adrenocortical tumours are benign and hormonally silent (non-functioning). Functioning tumours of the zona glomerulosa and fasciculata give rise to Conn's and Cushing's syndrome, respectively. Virilizing and feminizing tumours, probably arising from the zona reticularis, are more rare; however, tumours secreting combinations of adrenocortical steroids have also been described [39, 40].

Cushing's syndrome

Epidemiology

Cushing's syndrome is due to an adrenal adenoma in 10–30% of cases and shows a marked female preponderance of 4–5:1. Adrenal adenomas may occur at any age; bilateral adenomas are rare, but occur as part of familial adenomas [39].

Aetiology and pathogenesis

The cause of these tumours is essentially unknown, but adenomas have developed in a setting of chronic ACTH excess and micronodular adrenal hyperplasia [39, 40]. Loss of function of a tumour suppresser gene, the *MEN1* gene, and steroidogenic acute regulatory (STAR) protein mRNA are under investigation [41].

Pathology and biology

Adenomas are usually small (average diameter of 4 cm), encapsulated, and consist of mixtures of compact zona reticularis and clear zona fasciculata-type cells (see Figure 58.3). In Cushing's syndrome associated with primary adrenocortical disease, increased cortisol secretion suppresses ACTH synthesis and secretion, therefore inducing contralateral adrenal cortex atrophy [42].

Diagnosis and staging

Patients with adrenal adenomas usually present with the gradual onset of symptoms and signs of hypercortisolism. The presence of proximal myopathy, vascular fragility, and thin skin can be used to clinically differentiate them from other pseudo-Cushingoid states [43]. Benign adenomas are usually pure cortisol secretors, and hirsutism and other androgenic effects are usually absent. However, components of the syndrome due to mineralocorticoid excess (hypertension, hypokalaemia) and virilization have been described.

The mainstay of diagnosis of Cushing's syndrome is the demonstration of inappropriate and excessive secretion of cortisol [42, 43]. Measuring the 24-hour excretion of urinary free cortisol (UFC) was previously used, but is of low sensitivity. However, the 2 mg/day low-dose dexamethasone suppression test (LDDST), measuring the 9 am serum cortisol before and after the administration of dexamethasone 0.5 mg strictly six-hourly for 48 h, has a 98% sensitivity in demonstrating autonomy in cortisol secretion using a cut-off cortisol value for suppression of 50 nmol/l. All patients with adrenal adenomas fail to show suppression [43] (Figure 58.5). As a screening test, measurement of the 9 am serum cortisol after dexamethasone 1 mg at midnight has very high sensitivity but rather low specificity.

The differential diagnosis is made from the other causes of Cushing's syndrome, pituitary adenoma (Cushing's disease) and ectopic ACTH-secretion, by measurement of ACTH levels which are persistently very low or undetectable [42, 43].

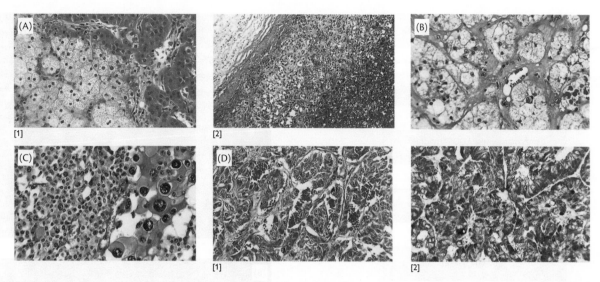

Fig. 58.3 High power photomicrographs of four adrenal tumours. Each is stained with haematoxylin and eosin and magnified ×400. (A) Adrenal adenoma causing Cushing's syndrome. [1] Note uniform, large clear cells resembling those from the zona fasciculata. [2] Atrophic adrenal cortex adjacent to the adenoma. (B) Adrenal aldosteronoma with typical spironolactone bodies. (C) Adrenal carcinoma with nuclear pleomorphism (D) Adrenal phaeochromocytoma. [1] Typical pleomorphic cells with cytoplasmic basophilia and background vascularity. [2] Finely granular cytoplasm indicative of plentiful chromaffin granules (characteristic chromogranin staining).

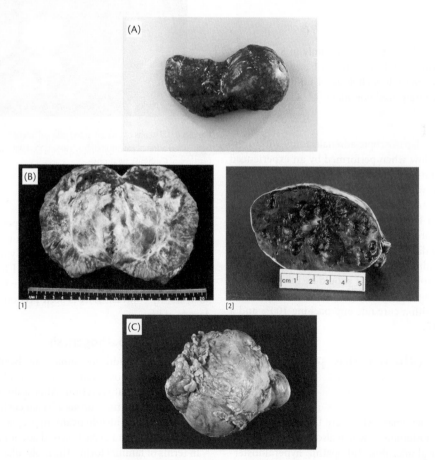

Fig. 58.4 Typical macroscopic appearance of three adrenal tumours (A) Adrenal cortical adenoma causing Cushing's syndrome: the adrenal gland weighing 14 g (normal 4–6 g for a surgically excised gland) in the medial aspect (left) of which is a well-circumscribed adrenal cortical adenoma measuring 2 × 1.5 cm. (B) Adrenal cortical carcinoma causing Cushing's syndrome. [1] A very large cortical carcinoma (9 cm) removed at postmortem examination. The specimen is attached to the inferior vena cava, which has been opened as far as the right atrium and ventricle. [2] An adrenal cortical carcinoma weighing 240 g. The tumour is encapsulated and composed of brown tissue with extensive areas of haemorrhage in the centre of the tumour. (C) Adrenal phaeochromocytoma: a well-defined adrenal tumour composed of slightly variegated pink tissue with extensive central necrosis.

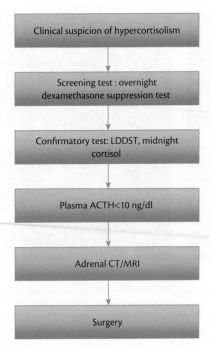

Clinical suspicion of hypercortisolism

↓

Screening test : overnight
dexamethasone suppression test

↓

Confirmatory test: LDDST, midnight
cortisol

↓

Plasma ACTH<10 ng/dl

↓

Adrenal CT/MRI

↓

Surgery

Fig. 58.5 Algorithm for suspected hypercortisolism.

By means of CT and MRI it is possible not only to localize the tumour, but to distinguish possible malignancy based on imaging characteristics (see Figure 58.6). Iodocholesterol and NP-59 radionuclide isotope scans are rarely used nowadays [44, 45].

Management

The treatment of choice is laparoscopic adrenalectomy with overall morbidity being very low when performed by an experienced surgeon [46]. Post-operatively, the contralateral atrophic adrenal gland may take from weeks to years to recover; it is therefore important to cover the surgical procedure with hydrocortisone 50–100 mg six-hourly for two to three days, and thereafter maintain the patient on standard steroid replacement with hydrocortisone (10 mg, 5 mg, 5 mg daily), until gradual normalization of the hypothalamo-pituitary-adrenal axis is obtained. Patients should be followed up and cortisol replacement should be increased during stress. Appropriate diagnosis and surgical treatment of adrenal adenomas is associated with a cure rate approaching 100% and a normal survival curve [47].

Conn's syndrome (aldosterone-producing adenomas)

Classification

Aldosterone-producing adenomas (APAs) are the most common form of primary hyperaldosteronism, which also includes bilateral hyperplasia of the zona glomerulosa (idiopathic hyperaldosteronism, IHA), primary adrenal hyperplasia (PAH, where the zona glomerulosa of one adrenal becomes hyperplastic and histopathologically resembles unilateral IHA, but biochemically behaves as APA), adrenal carcinoma, and two genetic familial varieties (type 1 which is called glucocorticoid-remediable aldosteronism [GRA] and type 2 variant which is not glucocorticoid sensitive).

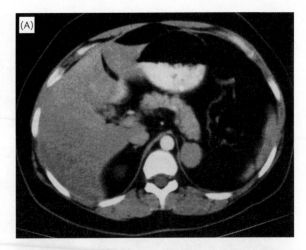

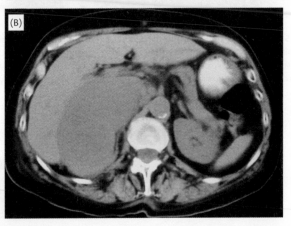

Fig. 58.6 CT scans of (A) left-sided adrenal adenoma and (B) a massive right-sided adrenal carcinoma, both associated with the clinical and biochemical features of Cushing's syndrome.

Epidemiology

Approximately 0.5–2% of unselected hypertensive individuals have primary hyperaldosteronism due to an adrenal adenoma. IHA is much more common, but may be simply one end of the spectrum of low-renin hypertension. There is a 2:1 female to male incidence in adenomas, which seem to congregate in the age range of 30 to 50 years. By contrast, IHA is seen predominantly in men in sixth decade of life.

Aetiology and pathogenesis

Increasingly, sporadic adenomas have been associated with mutations of sodium/potassium channels leading to constitutive activation of hormonal secretion. After a discrete adenoma has been removed, the non-tumourous adrenal cortical zona glomerulosa is often found to be histologically hyperplastic, with multiple small cortical nodules and even a second adenoma [48].

In terms of familial forms, the molecular basis of GRA is known. It is a rare, autosomal dominant disorder resulting from a heritable mutation that causes the fusion of genes encoding the promoter for 11β-hydroxylase and aldosterone secretion, and is under ACTH control [48, 68]. Studies in type 2 variant of familial hyperaldosteronism show loss of heterozygosity of the *MEN1* gene, but further studies are needed [68].

Pathology

The typical Conn's tumour is less than 2 cm and microscopically composed of mixture of zona glomerulosa, zona fasciculata cells, and hybrid cells with characteristics of both layers (see Figure 58.3B)

Diagnosis and staging

Patients with Conn's adenomas classically present with the triad of hypertension, hypokalaemic alkalosis, and muscle weakness. Spontaneous hypokalaemia occurs in 80%; but patients can be normokalaemic at the start, and develop hypokalaemia within three to five days of initiation of a liberal sodium intake (150 mEq/day). Hypokalaemia in a setting of a low to moderate dose of potassium-wasting diuretics can also be indicative. Symptoms induced by hypokalaemia are weakness, muscle cramping, paraesthesia, tetany, polyuria, and polydipsia due to hypokalaemia-induced nephrogenic diabetes insipidus. In IHA there may be less severe hypokalaemia or even normokalaemia.

The diagnosis of primary hyperaldosteronism (PA) is based on the demonstration of high-normal or frankly elevated levels of aldosterone with concomitantly suppressed plasma renin activity (Figure 58.7). There is no single specific and sensitive screening test. Random plasma aldosterone/renin activity can be used for screening, with high accuracy, also leading to a marked increase in a detection rate in PA [69, 70] (see Figure 58.7). Some authorities specify renin/aldosterone ratios suggestive of Conn's syndrome, but is should be recognized that these are very assay- and unit-dependent.

In the next step it is important to differentiate Conn's syndrome from hyperplasia, as the former is amenable to surgical treatment while the latter is usually treated medically. Basal levels of potassium, renin, and/or aldosterone are poor discriminators. Differentiating can be made by examining the response of serum aldosterone to 4-h ambulation between 8 am and 12 pm. As with adenomas, the tumour is ACTH-sensitive and aldosterone falls over the morning, while IHA is angiotensin-dependent and therefore aldosterone rises. However, the test has a low accuracy [48]. Adenomas also produce an excess of 18-hydroxycorticosterone, an intermediate precursor of aldosterone that facilitates the biochemical diagnosis. 18-hydroxycorticosterone levels are also elevated in glucocorticoid-sensitive hyperaldosteronism (GSA) [49].

Adrenal imaging with CT or MRI scan also plays a role in distinguishing these two entities, but even in expert hands the small size of many of these tumours, plus the presence of adrenal incidentalomas, suggest that it is only diagnostic in young patients with a nodule >1cm on one side and a normal contralateral adrenal. A more accurate technique is venous catheterization with sampling of both adrenals for aldosterone and the inferior vena cava to demonstrate a gradient, with a simultaneous cortisol sample to ensure correct placement within the adrenal veins (an aldosterone/cortisol ratio of >4:1 between the affected and unaffected site is indicative of an adenoma). This method has a near 100% sensitivity and a positive predictive value of 90%, but requires expert interventional radiology [44].

NP-59 I-iodomethyl-19-norcholesterol scintigraphy under dexamethasone suppression has also been used to distinguish adenoma from hyperplasia. Unilateral NP-59 uptake is regarded as sufficient evidence of an adenoma, while in IHA neither gland is visualized, but the test is now rarely used [45].

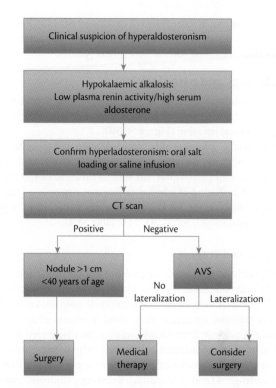

Fig. 58.7 Algorithm for suspected hyperaldosteronism.

Management

Having distinguished between an adenoma and IHA, a four- to six-week course of treatment with spironolactone should be given (100–400 mg daily) to assess reversibility of blood pressure, replete potassium levels, and desuppress the contralateral adrenal in patients with adenomas. Laparoscopic adrenalectomy is the treatment of choice as these tumours are relatively small [46]. One year post-operatively, 70% of patients are normotensive, falling to 50% after five years; however, normal potassium balance is permanent. Patients with GSA are treated with dexamethasone, while patients with carcinomas have an overall poor prognosis but may initially respond to mitotane.

Adrenal carcinoma

Epidemiology

Malignant neoplasms of the adrenal cortex account for 0.05–0.2% of all cancers and occur in two peaks; the first peak before the age of five and the second in the fourth to fifth decade. There is a female predominance, accounting for 65–90%, while bilateral tumours have been reported in 2–10% of the cases. These tumours account, in general, for one-third of adrenal tumours presenting with Cushing's syndrome [40, 50, 51].

Aetiology and pathogenesis

Adrenal carcinomas (AC), apart from sporadic variants whose pathogenesis remain unclear, have been described in siblings and can be associated with several syndromes. This implies a high probability that there may be an inherited component, seen in the Li–Fraumeni syndrome (germline mutations of p53 tumour suppressor gene). There is also evidence to suggest that environmental pollutants may play a causative role in some forms of childhood AC [52]. Rarely, AC can arise from ectopic adrenocortical tissue and from patients with uncontrolled congenital adrenal hyperplasia [44, 51].

Microbiology and pathology

Adrenal carcinomas are large (90–95% larger than 6 cm), encapsulated tumours with areas of haemorrhage, necrosis, calcification, and signs of local invasion (Figure 58.3B).

Histologically, pleomorphic, lipid-deplete cells, with varying mitotic activity, nuclear atypia and hyperchromasia, aneuploidy (83% of all carcinomas), as well as invasion of the capsule (Figure 58.3C). Staging of adrenal carcinomas depends on tumour size, nodal involvement, invasion of adjacent tissue, and the presence of metastases [40, 50, 51, 53, 54] (Table 58.4).

Diagnosis and staging

Approximately 50% of adult carcinomas are non-functional, and most of these patients first present with advanced metastatic disease to lungs, liver, or bone, before primary diagnosis is established. In 50% of patients a palpable abdominal mass and abdominal or flank pain is present. Sometimes tumours are discovered as 'incidentalomas'. Unlike adrenal adenomas, which predominantly secrete cortisol, carcinomas often secrete a variety of other steroids, mainly androgens (androstenedione, dehydroepiandrosterone sulphate [DHEAS]). This is especially the case in children, where isolated Cushing's syndrome is seen only in 3%. The majority present with virilization (40%) or the combination of Cushing's syndrome and virilization (50%). Virilization can cause isosexual precocious puberty in young girls [40, 50, 51]. An elevated blood pressure is seen in >50% of childhood adrenal carcinomas, mostly associated with cortisol hypersecretion. The median age at diagnosis in children is 4.3 years, with girls predominating over boys (5.3/1) below the age of four years [52].

Cushing's syndrome presents in 30% of adults (20–30% of cases of adrenal Cushing's are due to a carcinoma), virilization in 20%, and the combination of the two in 10 to 20%. Feminization and hyperaldosteronism are relatively rare manifestations; even rarer are hypoglycaemia and polycythaemia [40].

Diagnosis

The diagnostic tools are those used for Cushing's syndrome due to an adenoma, while measurement of adrenal androgens facilitates the diagnosis. Imaging with either CT (the presence of a large unilateral adrenal mass with irregular borders) or MRI scanning is often virtually diagnostic of an adrenal carcinoma (Figure 58.6B). On imaging, such tumours exceed 6 cm, although 16% may be less than 6 cm and resemble adenomas.

Management

Untreated, the median survival in adrenocortical carcinomas is less than three months. Patients with functional adrenal carcinomas present at earlier phase, and therefore have better prognosis. More than 50% of adrenal carcinomas are metastatic at the time of diagnosis. Radical excision with en bloc resection of any local invasion or distant metastasis if possible prolongs survival [71, 72].

The mainstay of pharmacotherapy is mitotane, which acts by blocking adrenal steroid 11β-hydroxylation and altering extra-adrenal metabolism of cortisol and androgens, but also exerts a direct tumouricidal effect. At high doses, if not limited by side-effects, it controls hypercortisolism in 50–60% of patients, although objective tumour responses (>50% reduction in tumour bulk) occur in less than 20% of such patients [55]. However, the extent to which mitotane can increase the length of time between recurrences remains to be assessed [56, 73, 74]. The dose should be rapidly increased, dependent on side effects and a therapeutic range of 14–20 mg/L is optimal; this should be monitored as levels below this are less effective, while above this toxic side effects are limiting. Hydrocortisone replacement may need to be added, with high doses often being required. Mitotane increases cortisol-binding globulin (CBG) so monitoring must be with salivary cortisol or UFC.

Metyrapone and the antifungal agent ketoconazole can be used to control cortisol secretion [56]. Chemotherapy is of limited efficacy, but the combination of etoposide, platinum, and doxorubicin is marginally more effective than streptozocin. Other regimens may be attempted, but none is in widespread use. Targeted therapy with IGF1 receptor antagonism has been tried but appears to

Table 58.4 Staging of adrenocortical carcinoma

Stage	T, N, Mα	Macfarlane (1958) [53]	Lee et al. (1995) [54]
I	T1, N0, M0	Tumour <5cm, confined to the adrenal gland	T1 (<5cm), N0, M0
II	T2, N0, M0	Tumour >5cm, confined to the adrenal gland	T2 (>5cm), N0, M0
III	T1 or T2, N1, M0 T3, N0, M0	Tumour confined to the adrenal gland with involvement of local lymph nodes, or, tumour extending beyond the adrenal gland but not invading adjacent organs	T3/T4 (local invasion as shown by histological evidence of adjacent organ invasion, direct tumour extension to IVC, or tumour thrombus within the IVC or renal vein) and/or N1 (positive renal lymph nodes), M0
IV	T3 or T4, N1, M0 any T, M1	Tumour extending beyond the adrenal gland, invading adjacent organs, and involving local lymph nodes, or any tumour with metastases	T1-4, N0-1, M1 (distance metastases)

Abbreviations: T, Tumour; N, lymph node; M, Metastases; 0, negative.

Adapted from Macfarlane DA, *Cancer of the adrenal cortex: the natural history, prognosis, and treatment in a study of 55 cases*, Hunterian Lecture delivered at the Royal College of Surgeons of England, March 1958, Copyright © 1958, the Royal College of Surgeons. Reproduced with permission; and adapted from *Surgery*, Volume 118, Issue 6, Lee JE et al., Surgical management, DNA content, and patient survival in adrenal cortical carcinoma, pp. 1090–1098, Copyright © 1995 Published by Mosby, Inc., with permission from Elsevier, <http://www.sciencedirect.com/science/journal/00396060>. Based on radiology, intraoperative evaluation, and permanent-section histopathological evaluation of the resected specimen.

be ineffective. Combining mitotane with cytotoxic chemotherapy shows no prolongation of survival, but requires further study [75].

Radiotherapy to the tumour bed can be used, in case of a high risk for local recurrence [40, 55, 56, 76].

In general, the great majority of patients show local invasion, with or without metastases, and despite aggressive surgical therapy the five-year survival is currently only 15–25% [40, 50, 55, 56]. A five-year survival rate of 46% has been described in patients with adrenal carcinoma in whom complete margin-negative tumour resection was achieved irrespective of adjuvant mitotane treatment [54], while others have advocated that immediate adjuvant long-term therapy with mitotane may also be beneficial [57, 73].

Virilizing tumours

Epidemiology

Virilizing adrenal tumours are rare, more common in childhood, but may present at any age and predominantly in women (75%). When present, they are usually carcinomas.

Microbiology and pathology

Virilizing adrenal tumours are well-encapsulated. Tumours secrete a variety of adrenal androgens proportionally with tumour size (mainly DHEAS, as well as testosterone and androstenedione), but a combined pattern with glucocorticoid and mineralocorticoid excess is seen in older patients with more malignant tumours. Small lesions are more often benign than larger ones, but the distinction is often less clear cut than for cortisol-producing adenomas and even large tumours may well be benign [58].

Diagnosis and staging

Signs and symptoms are mainly due to the excess androgen production. Young prepubertal women present with virilization and accelerated growth, while adult women experience menstrual irregularities, male-type alopecia, hoarseness of the voice, increased libido, and/or increased muscle mass. In men, symptoms may be minimal, except in childhood when they can induce isosexual precocious puberty [58].

The differential diagnosis is between congenital adrenal hyperplasia (CAH) in young girls and the polycystic ovary syndrome (PCO) in adult females.

Baseline testosterone levels >6 nmol/l are suggestive of the presence of a tumour, but there is significant overlap with values obtained from patients without tumours; however, a tumour is unlikely if androgens suppress following dexamethasone administration [59].

In women with PCO the onset of symptoms usually dates from puberty and is progressive, in contrast to women with tumours whose presentation is more acute. In CAH patients 82% have some sort of unilateral mass, while only 11% have bilateral adrenal enlargement, thus limiting the diagnostic specificity of adrenal imaging [59].

In cases of tumours, adrenal imaging with CT or MRI scanning will identify most of these tumours, which are usually greater than 2 cm; simultaneous adrenal and ovarian venous catheterization and sampling is rarely necessary.

Management

These tumours grow slowly and metastasize late. Surgical excision is the treatment of choice while the role of radiotherapy has not been clearly defined. Mitotane has also been used as adjunctive treatment, although at present there is no effective tumouricidal agent. Symptoms and signs of virilization may regress with cyproterone acetate or flutamide.

Feminizing tumours

Epidemiology

Feminizing adrenal tumours are rare, constituting less than 10% of adrenal tumours, 90% being seen in males, aged 25–45 years. Clearly, this figure may be an underestimate, as signs of hyperoestrogenism are clearly more subtle in women [60].

Microbiology and pathology

Feminizing adrenal tumours are always malignant although cases of benign tumours have been described in childhood suggesting adenoma-to-carcinoma transformation. There are no microscopic criteria to distinguish malignant from benign tumours. The majority of these tumours are large, often weighing more than 1 kg. Functionally, they produce oestrogenic steroids such as oestradiol, oestrone, and oestriol, and most of them have elevated levels of urinary oestrogens [60, 61].

Diagnosis and staging

In males, tumours present with gynaecomastia and evidence of hypogonadism. Half of patients may have a palpable abdominal mass. In females, isosexual precocious puberty may be seen in childhood, although normal menstruation is not achieved due to the unopposed oestrogen action on the uterus; elderly women can present with the acute onset of postmenopausal bleeding [60]. The elevated oestrogen levels are unresponsive to dynamic endocrine tests, ACTH-stimulation, GnRH-analogue, and dexamethasone suppression, although tumours with positive 'chorionic' and 'pituitary-gonadotrophin' tests have been described. Adrenal imaging with CT or MRI scanning will almost always identify such tumours.

Management

Surgical excision is the only available treatment; although there are a few studies describing partial responses of such tumours to non-specific cytotoxic chemotherapy or mitotane, experience is limited. The overall prognosis is poor [61].

Incidentally-discovered adrenal masses

Epidemiology

Adrenal masses are found in around 4% of patients imaged with CT scanning for reasons other than suspected adrenal pathology; such lesions are referred to as adrenal 'incidentalomas'. The majority are not diagnosed in life, considering their prevalence is four-fold greater at autopsy, but incidence has been increasing proportionally to the increased use of imaging interventions [62, 77]. They occur equally in both sexes, and are rare under the age of 30 years; their prevalence increasing with age. They are more common in the obese, diabetics, hypertensives, and patients with MEN 1 [50, 62]. The majority are benign adenomas, with the majority of the rest comprising adrenal carcinomas, phaeochromocytomas, and secondary metastases.

Management

See Figure 58.8. Lesions can be unilateral- or bilateral-differential diagnoses in Tables 58.5 and 58.6. The diagnostic approach in

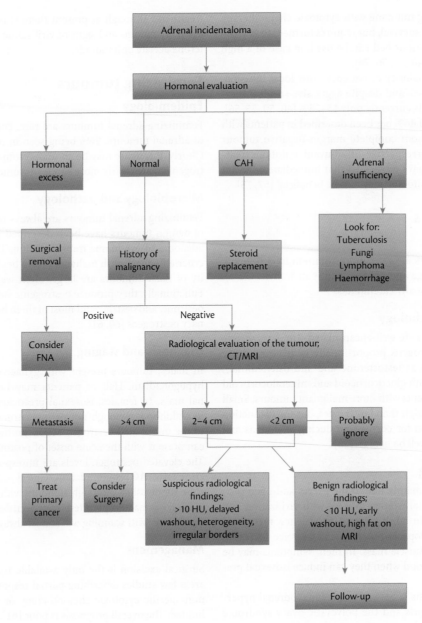

Fig. 58.8 Algorithm for an incidentally-discovered adrenal mass.

Table 58.5 Differential diagnosis of unilateral adrenal mass.

(A) Functional lesions	(1) Adrenal adenoma
	(2) Adrenal carcinoma
	(3) Phaeochromocytoma
	(4) Hyperplasia mimicking unilateral enlargement
(B) Non-functional lesions	(1) Adrenal adenoma
	(2) Adrenal carcinoma
	(3) Ganglioneuroma
	(4) Myelolipoma
	(5) Haemorrhage
	(6) Metastasis

Table 58.6 Differential diagnosis of bilateral adrenal mass.

(A) Functional lesions	(1) ACTH-dependent Cushing's syndrome
	(2) Congenital adrenal hyperplasia
	(3) Phaeochromocytoma
	(4) Micronodular adrenal disease
	(5) Idiopathic bilateral adrenal hypertrophy
(B) Non-functional lesions	(1) Infections (tuberculosis, fungi)
	(2) Infiltration (leukaemia, lymphoma)
	(3) Replacement (amyloidosis)
	(4) Haemorrhage
	(5) Bilateral metastases

patients with adrenal incidentalomas should focus on two main questions: whether the lesion is malignant, and whether it is hormonally active, in order to decide on the treatment if needed.

In case of bilateral 'incidentalomas' which represent 11–16% of lesions, the differential diagnosis is very broad, and clinical and biochemical evaluation is important given the potential for the presence of congenital adrenal hyperplasia (11% of all cases). However, there is also the rare occurrence of primary adrenal insufficiency due to bilateral destruction by solid tumour metastases, haematological malignancy, haemorrhage, or infectious (CMV, mycobacterium, fungal) or granulomatous disease [59, 62].

All patients should undergo biochemical assessment regardless of history and clinical findings [59, 78–80]. The majority of 'incidentalomas' are benign cortical adenomas, either non-secretory or of low secretory capacity [62]. Increasing data suggest that many apparent non-secretory adrenal adenomas do in fact show low-grade cortisol secretion, which may have metabolic effects, but whether all should then be removed is controversial. In the case of an adrenal mass which has been deemed hormonally non-secretory, the possibility of primary or metastatic malignancy must be excluded. Attempts to separate benign from malignant lesions on the basis of size (greatest diameter) criteria have been shown to be of limited value [62]. Therefore, the initial radiological investigation recommended to differentiate between adenomas and non-adenomas is unenhanced CT with the use of an attenuation value of ≤10 Hounsfield units (HU) highly indicative of a benign adenoma. In case of a higher baseline attenuation value, delayed contrast-enhanced CT studies should be performed with rapid washout indicative of a benign tumour [44, 78, 80]. MR should be considered when CT is inconclusive, as in-phase/out-of-phase imaging can be used to indicate a high fat content and hence benign behaviour [44, 62].

Fine needle aspiration under CT guidance may be used only in selected cases suspicious of metastases (after biochemical exclusion of phaeochromocytoma), because it is not useful in separating benign from malignant primary adrenal tumours [59, 62, 78]. Furthermore, suspected malignant adrenal tumours should *not* undergo biopsy because of the risk of dissemination.

Adrenocortical scintigraphy ^{131}I-6β-iodomethylnorcholesterol has been used but now is mainly of historical interest [63, 81].

All adrenal tumours with suspicious radiological findings, most functional tumours, and all tumours more than 4 cm in size that lack characteristic benign imaging features should be surgically excised [78–80]. Adrenal tumours may increase in size, develop overt or subclinical hormone secretion or feature malignant transformation. Therefore, radiological and hormonal follow-up should be recommended to the patients. More investigations are needed for the establishment of long-term follow-up protocols [77, 79]. For masses that appear to be benign (<10 HU; washout, >50% by MRI), small (<3 cm), and completely nonfunctioning, probably all that is required is one further imaging at 3–6 months [79].

Adrenomedullary tumours

Phaeochromocytomas and paragangliomas

Neuroendocrine tumours originated from chromaffin adrenal cells are called phaechromocytomas, while those arising in extra-adrenal sympathetic and parasympathetic paraganglia are called paragangliomas. The majority (80%) of tumours are located intra-adrenally, while sympathetic paragangliomas are in the abdominal preaortic sympathetic plexuses, paravertebral sympathetic chain, organ of Zuckerkandl, and, rarely, urinary bladder. Parasympathetic paragangliomas are most commonly found in the head and neck (HNPGLs) [64, 82].

Such tumours usually store and secrete catecholamines. They present a heterogeneous group of chromaffin cell neoplasms with different ages of onset, secretory profiles, locations, and potential for malignancy according to underlying genetic mutations [83].

Epidemiology

Phaeochromocytomas are rare tumours, showing no sexual predominance, occurring at any age, although most commonly in the third and fourth decades. A significant number of phaeochromocytomas (>50%) are found at autopsy having escaped diagnosis in life [87]. Tumours account for less than 1% of cases of hypertension, but importance of diagnostics is in potential lethal consequences if unrecognized and untreated [64, 65, 83]. Their prevalence is much higher in incidentalomas (4.2–6.5%), and therefore all adrenal incidentalomas should be screened for phaeochromocytoma irrespective of the presence of catecholamine excess [83].

Aetiology and pathogenesis

Phaeochromocytomas and sympathetic paragangliomas usually produce catecholamines or their metabolites. HNPGLs rarely produce significant amount of catecholamines (less than 5%) Catecholamines are metabolized within tumour cells: noradrenaline to normetanephrine and adrenaline to metanephrine [82]. Significant intra-tumour metabolism of catecholamines occurs in large tumours; conversely, small lesions can be disproportionally symptomatic because of high concentrations of catecholamines [64].

Relative catecholamine levels differ in different tumours; most phaeochromocytomas secrete noradrenaline predominantly, while in MEN 2 the secretory product is adrenaline. Dopamine, metabolized to 3-methoxytyramine, is seen in some succinate dehydrogenase (SDH)-B-related paragangliomas [82, 83]. Phaeochromocytomas may produce vasoactive peptides that reduce vascular responsiveness; thus, some patients with high catecholamine levels can be completely asymptomatic, while in others adrenoceptor blockade is ineffective in controlling hypertension [64].

Most phaeochromocytomas are sporadic, but 30% are hereditary. Three classical syndromes, connected to a loss of function in tumour suppressor genes and inherited in an autosomal dominant pattern, are associated with adrenal phaeochromocytoma: Von Hippel-Lindau (VHL) syndrome, multiple endocrine neoplasia type 2 (MEN 2), and neurofibromatosis type 1 (NF1). The MEN 2 syndrome, NF1, and VHL show prevalence of phaeochromocytomas in 40–50%, 1 % and 15% of patients, respectively. Phaeochromocytomas may be the only manifestation in about 25% of carriers of a MEN 2A mutation and in about 40% of carriers of the VHL syndrome. Mutations of all four SDH complex subunits (A, B, C, and D), and of the succinate dehydrogenase assembly factor 2 (SDHAF2) predispose to paragangliomas, while mutations of the transmembrane protein 127 (TMEM127) and the MAX-gene are associated with susceptibility to phaeochromocytomas and paragangliomas. In general, these traits are inherited in an autosomal dominant pattern, with SDH-D being inherited from the father due to imprinting [82, 83].

Microbiology and pathology

Lesions vary in size, are well encapsulated, and highly vascular (Figure 58.3C). Microscopically, all phaeochromocytomas and paragangliomas display similar histopathological characteristics (Figure 58.3D).

Approximately 10–20% of tumours are malignant. Signs of capsular invasion and vascular penetration are not proof of malignancy, which is clear if metastatic lesions to the bone, liver, lungs, and within the tumour bed are present. Paragangliomas are more likely to show malignant behaviour, as are tumours in the context of SDH-B mutations [64, 82].

Diagnosis and staging

Patients with phaeochromocytomas present with a diversity of symptoms, due to secreted catecholamines and other active substances.

The classic triad of severe headache, diaphoresis, and palpitations carries a high degree of specificity (94%) and sensitivity (91%) for phaeochromocytoma in the hypertensive population. Symptoms may vary in frequency and duration. Other symptoms in acute attack include tremor, pallor, weakness, nausea, and panic attacks. The hypertension is sustained in 50% of patients, paroxysmal in about 35% but absent in approximately 10–20%. Orthostatic hypotension can occur because of hypovolaemia and impaired arterial and venous constriction responses. Hypertensive crises with induction of anaesthesia, hypertensive encephalopathy, or spells suggestive of seizure disorder should all evoke suspicion of an underlying phaeochromocytoma. Cardiovascular and cerebrovascular complications can occur, including sudden left ventricular failure, pulmonary oedema, dysrhythmias, circulatory shock, myocardial infarction, dilated cardiomyopathy, cerebral infarction, and intracranial haemorrhage. Less specific signs and symptoms such as heat intolerance, weight loss, carbohydrate intolerance, pyrexia of unknown origin, and constipation mimicking pseudo-obstruction and paralytic ileus, have been described.

Other active secreted substances have been described: ACTH, vasoactive intestinal peptide, parathyroid hormone or parathyroid-hormone-related protein secretion [61].

Certain drugs can precipitate a hypertensive crisis in the presence of a phaeochromocytoma, which include tricyclic antidepressants, anti-dopaminergic agents (such as sulpiride and metoclopramide), and naloxone. β-adrenoreceptor blockers can also precipitate a hypertensive crisis if not preceded by adequate α-adrenoreceptor blockade.

Diagnosis is made by the demonstration of inappropriately high circulating plasma free or urinary fractionated metanephrines, followed by anatomical localization with imaging techniques due to the variable location of these tumours (Figure 58.9).

Biochemical testing should be performed in symptomatic patients, in patients with adrenal incidentalomas, or those in an increased hereditary risk [82]. Initial testing should include measurement of urinary or plasma metanephrines, or both if available. Measurement of plasma-free and urinary metanephrines show similarly high specificity, but overall plasma levels offer higher sensitivity [83].

If plasma metanephrines are more than four-fold above the upper reference limit there is a close to 100% probability of a tumour. Levels above the normal range but less than this can be seen in patients with acute, debilitating, non-endocrine illness [66]

and can be discriminated from true phaeochromocytomas by the clonidine suppression test. Raised urinary dopamine and high levels of 3-methoxytyramine may indicate malignancy, the latter being typically raised in paragangliomas [82, 83].

After biochemical diagnosis confirmation, anatomical localization is necessary due to the variable location of these tumours. CT scanning is very accurate in the detection of adrenal phaeochromocytomas with sensitivities ranging from 93–100%, although it lacks in specificity as it fails to distinguish between phaeochromocytomas, adrenal adenomas, and myelolipomas (Figure 58.10). MRI is a superior method in detecting adrenal and extra-adrenal tumours, demonstrates a bright hyperintense signal on T2 settings [44, 84]. Whole-body MRI may be included in initial anatomical imaging, especially in case of a strong clinical suspicion of extra-adrenal or extra-abdominal lesions [83].

To functionally confirm an adrenal mass as a phaeochromocytoma, prior to surgery, ^{123}I-meta-iodobenzylguanidine (^{123}I-MIBG) scintigraphy is helpful, and will identify some 80–90% of phaeochromocytomas. Considering the method shows reduced sensitivity in detecting paragangliomas, familial paraganglioma syndromes, and metastases, additional PET scanning with a range of labelled ligands (^{18}F-FDG, FDOPA, ^{11}C-HED) provides an alternative functional imaging approach with improved resolution over scintigraphy [82, 83]. In general, FDG-PET is most readily available, and is particularly useful for identifying tumours in patients with SDH mutations. However, ^{123}I-MIBG has the advantage that in patients with malignant tumours it can assess suitability for ^{131}I-MIBG therapy.

Management

Laparoscopic surgery is first choice technique for resection of adrenal and extra-adrenal tumours. The possibility of cortical-sparing surgery in hereditary syndromes with frequent bilateral disease, in order to avoid medical adrenal replacement therapy, remains controversial because of possible disease recurrence. Preoperatively, all patients should be given adequate alpha-blockade to achieve expansion of the intravascular volume and a reduction the frequency and severity of intraoperative pressor episodes. At least two weeks prior to surgery patients are started with oral phenoxybenzamine, usually at a dose of 1 mg/kg. Alternatives include calcium channel blockers and selective α1-adrenoreceptor blocking agents such as doxazocin or terazosin. However, significant elevations of blood pressure can still be seen during surgical manipulation of the tumour and thus nitroprusside should be available during operation. Beta-adrenoreceptor blockade may be used for control of tachyarrhythmias and angina, but always after prior α-adrenoceptor blockade, otherwise unopposed catecholamine induced vasoconstriction can result in dangerous blood pressure elevations. Patients with phaeochromocytomas have a high volume requirement both during and after surgery and plasma expanders may be necessary. Perioperatively, the use of morphine or phenothiazines should be avoided as these agents can precipitate hypertensive crises or hypotension. Enflurane and isoflurane are the anaesthetics preferentially used as they do not sensitize the myocardium to catecholamines and minimize the risk of arrhythmias. Post-operatively, the blood pressure may remain elevated for a few weeks and around 75% of patients become normotensive. Surgical mortality is now extremely low with adequate preparation and thus complete cure is the rule in patients undergoing elective procedures.

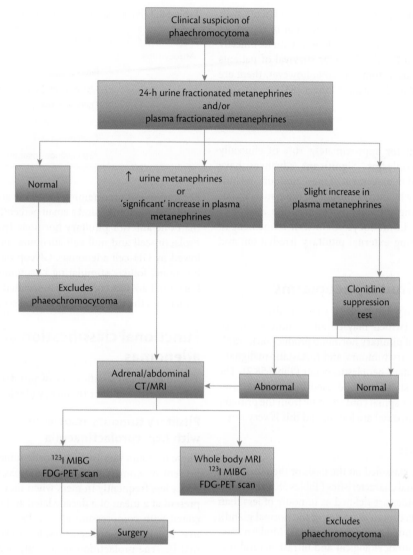

Fig. 58.9 Algorithm for suspected phaeochromocytoma.

Post-operative follow-up is necessary, not only for patients with identified mutations of disease causing genes, but for all patients because there is currently no reliable pathological technique which can rule out the potential for malignancy or recurrence.

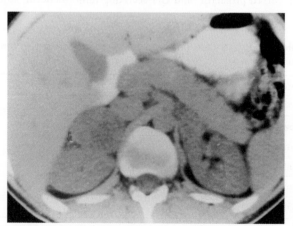

Fig. 58.10 CT scan of a large right-sided and smaller left-sided adrenal phaeochromocytoma.

Malignant phaeochromocytomas

Malignancy is diagnosed in terms of metastatic spread, which may occur years (median 5.6 years) after surgical excision. As mentioned, there are no histopathologic features to predict malignancy. There is a greater tendency to malignancy with paragangliomas, tumours in young people, female sex, large, familial lesions, and those associated with other endocrine or neoplastic disorders. These tumours are usually associated with increased dopamine and methoxytyramine secretion. There is no definitive consensus on therapy aimed at the tumour; ^{131}I-MIBG is used for patients with positive scintigraphy [82, 85]. Chemotherapy with a combination of cyclophosphamide, vincristine, and dacarbazine (CVD) is preferred in patients with negative [123I]-MIBG scintigraphy and in those with rapidly progressing tumours, regardless of MIBG uptake. The CVD combination can provide tumour regression and symptom relief in up to 50% of patients, but the responses are usually short and are seen in only 30% of patients [64, 82, 86]. Only a third of patients will respond to either of treatments; CVD and ^{131}I-MIBG [82], and it is unclear as to whether survival is increased. Temozolomide can be used as a second-line chemotherapeutic agent, while targeted therapy with sunitinib has shown some responses, albeit short-lived

[83]. Radiation therapy may provide palliation in patients with skeletal lesions [82]. There have also been a number of reports of treating inoperable primary and metastatic lesions with technically challenging embolization [67]. The five-year survival of patients with malignant phaeochromocytomas is 20%; however, there are patients who have survived for 20 years or longer [83].

Pituitary tumours

Pituitary tumours account for approximately 10% of clinically apparent intracranial neoplasms. Significant advances have improved the diagnosis and management of these tumours, including imaging of the pituitary by nuclear magnetic resonance, radio-immunoassay of circulating pituitary hormones, the advent of microsurgical techniques, immunocytochemistry, refinement of techniques for administering external pituitary irradiation, and new drug therapies.

Classification of pituitary neoplasms

Neoplasms of the pituitary (Box 58.1) may be divided into adenomas or carcinomas (which may be either functioning or non-functioning in terms of pituitary hormone production), craniopharyngiomas, other primary tumours, and metastatic malignancies. A number of parapituitary neoplasms occur (Table 58.7). The term pituitary carcinoma should not be used unless metastases within the nervous system or spinal cord separate from the primary tumour (or outside the neuroaxis) are found, and this is very rare.

Pituitary adenomas

Pituitary adenomas can be classified on the basis of their anatomical, histological, or functional characteristics (Tables 58.8 and 58.9). Anatomically, microadenomas are defined as tumours of less than 10 mm in diameter (the maximum diameter of the normal gland), and larger tumours are defined as macroadenomas. Modern classification based upon immunocytological and ultrastructural features of the tumour cell identifies the five major cell types of the anterior pituitary:

1. the lactotroph, producing prolactin;

2. the somatotroph, producing growth hormone (GH);

3. the corticotroph, producing adrenocorticotrophic hormone (ACTH);

4. the thyrotroph, producing thyroid stimulating hormone (TSH); and

5. the gonadotroph, producing luteinizing hormone (LH) and follicle-stimulating hormone (FSH).

Similarly, adenomas which immunostain for these hormones but do not secrete them can be identified. Some adenomas are

Box 58.1 Classification of pituitary neoplasms

Adenomas: functioning or apparently non-functioning
Carcinomas: functioning or apparently non-functioning
Craniopharyngiomas
Other pituitary tumours
Metastatic malignancies

Table 58.7 Hypothalamic and parapituitary neoplasms

Ganglioneuroma	Meningioma	Reticulosis
Astrocytoma	Chordoma	
	Pinealoma	
	Optic-nerve glioma	
	Ependymoma	
	Dermoid cyst	
	Epidermoid cyst	
	Arteriovenous malformation	

negative to immunostaining for all the anterior pituitary hormones (null-cell adenomas) and a small percentage immunostain for more than one anterior pituitary hormone (plurihormonal adenomas). Prolactin-cell and null-cell adenomas occur most commonly, followed by GH-cell adenomas. Glycoprotein hormones (luteinizing hormone, follicle-stimulating hormone, and thyroid-stimulating hormone) are less commonly associated with adenoma formation; sometimes the tumours stain for and secrete the α-subunit.

Functional classification of pituitary adenomas

The functional classification of pituitary adenomas is discussed below in order of their frequency (Table 58.8).

Pituitary tumours associated with hyperprolactinaemia

These tumours vary from microadenomas, which more commonly present in women, to macroadenomas. Although prolactinomas occur less frequently in men, when they do, they tend to be larger, present at a mean of a decade later, and are more likely to be associated with compression effects. Patients with macroprolactinomas usually have prolactin levels >3000 mU/l (normal up to 360 mU/l). True prolactinomas are only occasionally associated with lower circulating prolactin levels between 2000 and 3000 mU/l. Some large non-secreting pituitary tumours may also cause mild hyperprolactinaemia (<2000 mU/l) [88]. Intrasellar and suprasellar craniopharyngiomas, meningiomas, or any other parapituitary lesion may also cause a mild hyperprolactinaemia (<2000 mU/l) [89]. Mixed prolactin- and GH-secreting tumours occur, so that

Table 58.8 Pituitary adenomas and their relative incidence (per cent) in surgical material

Prolactin-cell (lactrotroph) adenomas	28
Null-cell (non-functioning) adenomas	26
Growth hormone-cell (somatotroph) adenomas	15
Corticotroph-cell adenomas	14 (45% silent)
Plurihormonal adenomas	12
Gonadotroph-cell adenomas	4
Thyrotroph-cell adenomas	1

Reprinted from *Endocrinology and Metabolism Clinics of North America*, Volume 16, Kovacs K, and Horvath E, Pathology of pituitary tumours, pp. 529–551, Copyright © 1987 Elsevier, with permission from Elsevier, <http://www.sciencedirect.com/science/journal/08898529>

Table 58.9 Anterior pituitary cell types, staining reaction, and mean secretory-granule diameter

Cell type	Hormone produced	Staining reactions of cytoplasmic granules		Mean granule diameter (nm)	Main distributor
		Mallory	PAS-OG		
Acidophil	Prolactin	Red	Yellow	550	Random
Acidophil	Growth hormone	Red	Yellow	450	Posterolateral
Basophil	ACTH	Blue	Red	360	Anterior median and anterolateral border
Basophil	LH, FSH	Blue	Red	200	Posterior median
Basophil	TSH	Blue	Red	135	Anterior median and anterolateral border

Abbreviations: ACTH, adrenocorticotrophic hormone; LH, luteinizing hormone; FSH, follicle-stimulating hormone; TSH, thyroid-stimulating hormone; PAS-OG, periodic acid-Schiff-Orange G.

some patients with hyperprolactinaemia may have the features of acromegaly.

Pituitary tumours associated with no elevation of circulating anterior pituitary hormones

These tumours tend to be macroadenomas and present with local pressure effects. They also may present with features of hypopituitarism.

Pituitary tumours associated with high levels of circulating growth hormone

These tumours cause acromegaly and/or gigantism and are commonly macroadenomas. They tend to be more aggressive and rapidly enlarging in younger patients. Approximately 35% of patients with acromegaly also have hyperprolactinaemia, which is due either to a plurihormonal tumour or a large somatotroph adenoma compressing the pituitary stalk. Less than 1% of patients with acromegaly have a large pituitary full of hyperplastic somatroph cells rather than a tumour, associated with elevated levels of GH-releasing hormone, usually from a carcinoid tumour of the pancreas or lung.

Pituitary tumours associated with Cushing's syndrome

Cushing's disease may be associated with normal or elevated ACTH levels, but in Nelson's syndrome (enlargement of the pituitary and skin pigmentation following bilateral adrenalectomy) the level of ACTH is invariably greatly elevated. Corticotroph adenomas are frequently microadenomas. Only rarely are they large, and in these circumstances they may be highly invasive.

Pituitary tumours associated with high gonadotrophin(s)

Pituitary tumours may secrete FSH alone, which is more common than LH secretion alone or both LH and FSH. They usually present as macroadenomas with space-occupying symptoms.

Pituitary tumours associated with thyrotoxicosis and high levels of thyroid-stimulating hormone

The tumours are usually macroadenomas and may also secrete prolactin.

Pituitary carcinomas

Primary carcinomas of the anterior lobe are very rare indeed and originate in adenohypophyseal cells. Most frequently they are non-secreting, but may secrete ACTH, prolactin, or GH.

Craniopharyngiomas

These tumours account for 2–5% of all intracranial neoplasms and arise in the remnants of Rathke's pouch, which is the dorsally directed outgrowth of the foetal stomatodeum [90]. They are more frequently suprasellar than intrasellar. They may be solid or cystic and are usually benign. These tumours present with hypopituitarism due to compression of the hypothalamus or, in the case of intrasellar tumours, the anterior pituitary. They most frequently present in children, but can occur throughout life. Suprasellar tumours may present with diabetes insipidus, and some patients have mild hyperprolactinaemia (see above).

Other primary tumours of the pituitary

Sarcomas of the pituitary occur. These are very rare and may occasionally be seen after irradiation of the pituitary.

Metastatic malignancies

Secondary tumours of the pituitary and parapituitary region are infrequent and rarely recognized clinically. They occur most frequently in patients with primary tumours of the breast, but bronchial, prostatic, and colonic neoplasms may also metastasize here.

Hypothalamic and parapituitary neoplasms

These are shown in Table 58.7.

Epidemiology of anterior pituitary tumours

Most pituitary tumours have an equal sex incidence, exceptions being tumours that secrete prolactin and ACTH, which are more common in women. They may occur at any age, although the greater frequency is between 30 and 50 years. A UK population-based study found the prevalence of pituitary adenomas to be 77.6/100 000 population, with a preponderance of prolactinoma (57%), and lower rates of the other subtypes (non-functioning adenoma [28%], acromegaly [11%], and Cushing's disease [2%]) [91].

Aetiology of anterior pituitary tumours

The aetiology of pituitary tumours is largely unknown and it is probable that there are various causes for their development. All cell types in the pituitary can become neoplastic.

Genetic factors play a role in some tumours, such as those associated with MEN type 1 or type 4 or Carney complex caused by mutations in the *PRKAR1A* gene. More recently, familial isolated pituitary adenoma (FIPA) has been shown to be associated with mutations in the tumour suppressor *AIP* gene in 20% of cases [92].

Clinical aspects of non-functioning pituitary tumours

These tumours most frequently present as large masses associated with local pressure effects. Microadenomas may be diagnosed incidentally on brain imaging performed for another disease. Rarely, because of bleeding into the pituitary tumour, they may present with the acute onset of headache associated with visual disturbance and meningism due to blood in the cerebrospinal fluid—pituitary apoplexy, which can be rarely fatal due to sudden hypopituitarism.

Clinical features

Local pressure

Headache is the most frequent symptom. It may be due to stretching of the dura above the pituitary. If there is upward extension of the pituitary tumour, pressure on the optic chiasm results in a bitemporal field defect. A decrease in visual acuity may occur due to optic atrophy, which may be irreversible if the pressure on the chiasm is long-standing [93].

Lateral extension of the tumour may cause interference of the function of the third, fourth, or sixth cranial nerves.

Hormonal changes

These occur with great frequency in patients with pituitary tumours. The most common cause of hypopituitarism is a pituitary tumour in adults and a craniopharyngioma in children. In progressive hypopituitarism, there is usually a characteristic order in the development of trophic-hormone deficiency. Usually, GH and LH secretions fail first, followed later by that of FSH, ACTH, and TSH. Prolactin deficiency is rare.

GH deficiency causes short stature in children and sometimes, but not always, retarded skeletal development. There are a number of important features of GH deficiency in adults, including impaired psychological well-being, increased abdominal adiposity, and reduced muscle strength (Box 58.2), and we now recognize that these are frequently reversible when GH is administered to adults.

In men with gonadotrophin deficiency, there is decreased libido, impotence, and a decrease in sperm count. Testicular size decreases and the testes may become soft. In addition, there is loss of pubic, axillary, and facial hair in both sexes. In women, a decrease in libido may occur and dyspareunia or amenorrhoea due to decreased oestrogen secretion is also seen. Infertility is common in both sexes. Prolactin deficiency is rare, and most commonly pressure by a functionless tumour on the pituitary stalk results in elevation of circulating prolactin levels. Hyposecretion of TSH in children causes growth retardation. In adults, when hypothyroidism develops, the swelling of the subcutaneous tissue is less prominent in pituitary

---

Box 58.2 Characteristic clinical features of growth hormone deficiency in adults

Increased fat mass
Reduced lean body mass
Decreased extracellular water
Low bone density
Impaired cardiac function
Poor physical performance
Impaired psychological well-being

---

hypothyroidism than in the primary form of the disease. Secretion of ACTH is associated with the features of corticosteroid deficiency, but in pituitary ACTH deficiency there is pallor of the skin, unlike most causes of primary adrenal failure. Deficiency of antidiuretic hormone causes diabetes insipidus. Cranial diabetes insipidus most commonly occurs after pituitary surgery. Patients with hypopituitarism may have anaemia associated with hypogonadism.

Investigation of patients with pituitary disease

Assessment of pituitary function

Anterior pituitary function

It is essential to assess and correct anterior pituitary function before testing that of the posterior pituitary. This is because cortisol and thyroxine deficiency may decrease the symptoms of diabetes insipidus by decreasing the glomerular filtration rate.

Basal serum hormone levels of thyroxine, cortisol, prolactin, LH, FSH, TSH, testosterone, or oestradiol should be assessed.

The insulin hypoglycaemia test is the standard way of assessing ACTH and GH reserves and is safe if adequate precautions are taken.

Posterior pituitary function

Posterior pituitary function is tested with a water-deprivation test, prior to which other causes of polyuria (including diabetes mellitus, chronic renal failure, hypercalcaemia, and hypokalaemia) must be excluded, as these impair the efficiency of antidiuretic-hormone action.

Neuro-ophthalmological investigation

Neuro-ophthalmological examination, particularly formal perimetry, aids diagnosis, determines type and timing of treatment, and serially helps to follow the progress of the disorder.

Radiological investigation

Magnetic resonance imaging

MRI with dedicated pituitary sequences (thin slices, small field of view, and dynamic contrast acquisition) is recommended as the routine examination for evaluating pituitary and parapituitary tumours. Post contrast and thin section dynamic contrast enhanced pituitary MRI imaging has significantly improved diagnostic accuracy. A pituitary microadenoma and macroadenoma are shown in Figures 58.11 and 58.12.

Surgical management of anterior pituitary tumours

Trans-sphenoidal pituitary surgery, using either the fully endoscopic endonasal or trans-septal approach, by an experienced pituitary neurosurgeon has revolutionized the management of pituitary tumours. Successful surgery is more likely to be achieved for microadenomas than for macroadenomas (in the treatment of acromegaly, for example, 80–85% of microadenomas have safe GH levels after surgery, but this figure falls to 50–60% for macroadenomas). Mortality is very low (<1%) and complications—haemorrhage, cerebrospinal fluid leak, and meningitis—are rare (1% each). Hypopituitarism is seen after trans-sphenoidal surgery and the frequency with which this complication is seen depends on the size of the pituitary tumour.

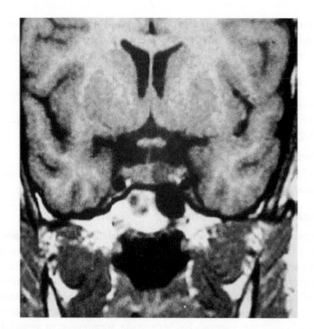

Fig. 58.11 A left-sided pituitary microadenoma is shown on MRI.

Transfrontal surgery, involving the lifting of a bone flap and frontal lobe retraction, has a greater morbidity and mortality than trans-sphenoidal surgery. The main indication for it is the decompression of the optic chiasm in patients with a large and inaccessible suprasellar extension (greater than 2 or 3 cm). Surgery using this route virtually never results in complete removal of the tumour and subsequent radiotherapy is necessary as 80% of tumours will recur.

Radiotherapy management of anterior pituitary tumours

External beam radiotherapy has been used for many years in the treatment of pituitary tumours to good effect [94]. Many studies have demonstrated the effectiveness of gamma knife radiosurgery in non-functional pituitary tumours with significant decreases in tumour dimensions occurring one year following treatment.

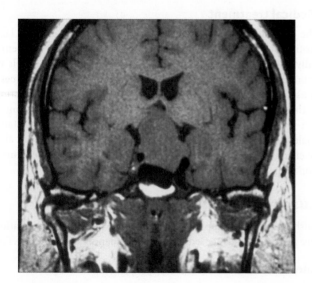

Fig. 58.12 A large extrasellar pituitary tumour (non-functioning) with suprasellar extension is shown on MRI.

Hypopituitarism following radiotherapy develops rarely and late, but this means that after radiotherapy patients need a yearly assessment of pituitary function. Less than 5% of pituitary adenomas recur if external pituitary irradiation is given. Late malignancy in the field of irradiation is reported to occur at 1.9% at 20 years, but these data are based on small numbers [95].

Functioning pituitary tumours

Prolactinoma

In women, prolactinomas tend to present earlier than in men. Furthermore, in women they tend to be smaller at presentation. Therefore, local effects of a pituitary tumour secreting prolactin occur commonly in men. In these patients pituitary function may also be affected as described above.

Symptoms of hyperprolactinaemia

High prolactin levels cause amenorrhoea or oligomenorrhoea, galactorrhoea, and infertility in women in the reproductive phase of life and relative or absolute impotence in men. Patients also have acne, a greasy skin, and hirsutism because prolactin enhances adrenal androgen secretion. In men, galactorrhoea is less frequent and gynaecomastia is a rare feature. Soft testes may eventually occur and testosterone levels, particularly in those patients who have long-standing hyperprolactinaemia, tend to fall, due to hypopituitarism.

Diagnosis of prolactinoma

The diagnosis is made by taking one or two basal, unstressed, blood samples for prolactin estimation. Once drugs and hypothyroidism have been excluded, hypothalamo-pituitary disease is by far the commonest cause of hyperprolactinaemia.

Management of prolactinoma

The aims of treatment are to reduce prolactin levels to normal, remove the tumour mass with the preservation of anterior pituitary function, and not cause significant side effects, particularly hypopituitarism. The choice of therapy depends on the size of the tumour, the presence of local complicating factors, the degree of elevation of serum prolactin, and the expertise that is locally available. In all but the largest tumours compressing local structures, medical treatment with dopamine agonists should be attempted as first-line therapy. In a large proportion of patients (85–90%) this will suppress prolactin levels to normal without side effects and will cause a resumption of normal gonadal function without the risk of hypopituitarism.

Medical therapy

Dopamine agonists are first-line therapy for prolactinomas. These drugs suppress prolactin by stimulating dopamine receptors present on the prolactin-secreting cells of the pituitary tumour. They can be used either on its own as primary therapy or as an adjunct in the treatment of patients with macroprolactinomas whose levels of prolactin are not adequately normalized by surgery or pituitary irradiation. Most experience has been gained with bromocriptine (an ergot alkaloid that works as a long-acting dopamine agonist) and cabergoline—a longer acting dopamine agonist administrable once or twice per week.

Surgery

Pituitary surgery is only indicated when medical therapy has either failed to reduce the prolactin level to normal or is not tolerated by the patient. Prolactinomas may re-develop after surgery.

Radiotherapy

External pituitary irradiation is also used in the treatment of prolactinoma [96]. It is clear that it arrests tumour growth, prevents further enlargement subsequently during pregnancies, and gradually decreases the circulating levels of prolactin. It may take between five and ten years to reduce prolactin levels to normal when off medical therapy.

Acromegaly

If GH hypersecretion occurs before fusion of the epiphyses, gigantism results. If secretion occurs after fusion, the acromegaly syndrome develops often over many years and this is much more common than gigantism as most tumours occur during adulthood.

Clinical features

Symptoms directly related to excessive GH secretion are numerous (Table 58.10).

Additionally, type 2 diabetes mellitus may occur in 30% of patients with acromegaly because GH hypersecretion results in hyperinsulinism and insulin resistance. Patients with persistent hypercalcaemia usually have multiple endocrine adenomas involving the pituitary and parathyroid glands and parathyroid hyperplasia may be seen.

Diagnosis of acromegaly

The chemical diagnosis of acromegaly is made by an oral glucose tolerance test (75 g), during which GH levels fail to suppress to <0.33 mcg/l. GH stimulates the production of insulin-like growth

Table 58.10 Presentation of acromegaly based on 310 patients

Presenting chief complaint	Frequency (%)
Menstrual disturbance	13
Change in appearance	11
Headaches	8
Paraesthesias/carpal tunnel syndrome	6
Diabetes mellitus/impaired glucose tolerance	5
Heart disease	3
Visual impairment	3
Decreased libido/impotence	3
Arthropathy	3
Thyroid disorder	2
Hypertension	1
Gigantism	1
Fatigue	0.3
Hyperhidrosis	0.3
Somnolence	0.3
Other	5
Chance (detected by unrelated physical or dental examination or radiograph)	40

Source: data from Molitch ME, Clinical manifestations of acromegaly, *Clinical Endocrinology and Metabolism*, Volume 21, Issue 3, pp. 597–614, Copyright © Endocrine Society.

factor 1 (IGF-1) and levels of this peptide are almost invariably raised at diagnosis. This peptide, in contrast to GH, does not show wide variations during the day.

Investigations

Radiology

99% of patients have a pituitary tumour detectable on MRI scanning. Formal visual field testing should also be carried out.

Biochemical investigations

GH levels should be assessed in samples obtained five or six times throughout the day.

Management of acromegaly

Acromegaly is a disease which approximately halves life expectancy [97]. Increased mortality is due to cardiovascular and cerebrovascular causes related to hypertension and diabetes mellitus [97] and to respiratory causes. Mortality is also increased for malignant causes and, in particular, the incidence of colonic cancer is significantly increased [98]. Therefore, it is important to treat patients with acromegaly once the diagnosis has been made. Suppression of mean GH levels to <1mcg/l are not associated with increased mortality [97].

Surgery

Definitive treatment usually involves trans-sphenoidal surgery. The best results follow surgery for microadenomas where there has been an early diagnosis and prompt definitive therapy. In experienced hands, up to 85% of patients with microadenomas can expect to be cured by trans-sphenoidal surgery. Larger tumours, and most particularly tumours which extend out of the sella turcica, are cured by trans-sphenoidal surgery in less than 40% of patients.

External beam pituitary irradiation

If surgery is unsuccessful at reducing GH to safe levels, external beam pituitary irradiation is considered afterwards. Several studies suggest that the response of GH to pituitary irradiation is dependent on the pre-irradiation GH concentration and the length of time after treatment. GH levels continue to fall up to at least 15 years after external pituitary irradiation.

Medical treatment

The long-acting somatostatin analogues, octreotide and lanreotide, may be used post-operatively for patients not biochemically cured by surgery. They normalize GH and IGF-1 levels in approximately 40% of post-operative patients. Medical treatment is used whilst awaiting the effects of external pituitary irradiation in those patients not completely cured by surgery. Pegvisomant, a GH-receptor antagonist, is used in those resistant to somatostatin analogues. Cabergoline, usually at a dose of 3 mg weekly, may also be effective (in 20–30% of cases) in reducing GH levels in conjunction with somatostatin analogues.

Cushing's disease

Cushing's disease is applies to inappropriate elevation of circulating free glucocorticoids caused by a pituitary adenoma secreting ACTH.

Clinical features

The clinical features include a rounded, plethoric face, and central obesity. Myopathy induces wasting of the arms and legs. Loss of libido, amenorrhoea, and galactorrhoea may occur, particularly if there is associated prolactin production by a pituitary tumour. Hirsutism and acne also occur. In patients with long-standing Cushing's syndrome, vertebral collapse occurs as a result of osteoporosis. Psychiatric manifestations, particularly depression, are seen in 50–60% of patients with this syndrome.

Differential diagnosis and investigation

There is no single, reliable test for the diagnosis of Cushing's syndrome, which may be difficult because intermittent, mild, and atypical forms of the disease occur [99]. Firstly, Cushing's syndrome must be diagnosed and secondly, the differential diagnosis must be established. Diagnosis is achieved with a low-dose dexamethasone test (0.5 mg six-hourly for 48 h) where there is failure of suppression of serum cortisol to <50 nmol/l after dexamethasone. In the differential diagnosis of Cushing's syndrome, the level of ACTH is important. It is undetectable in patients with adrenal adenoma or carcinoma. The major diagnostic problem involves differentiating Cushing's syndrome due to ectopic ACTH production by occult neoplasms from Cushing's disease (Table 58.11). Cushing's disease is suggested, if, when giving the patient dexamethasone 8 mg daily for 48 h (2 mg six-hourly), there is a >50% suppression of plasma cortisol. Unfortunately, some patients with ectopic ACTH production may show such suppression, while 10% of patients with Cushing's disease fail to suppress. Ectopic ACTH secretion is suggested by the presence of hypokalaemia, provided the patient is not taking diuretics.

Management of Cushing's disease

Surgery

Trans-sphenoidal pituitary surgery is the first-line treatment option for patients with Cushing's disease. Cure rates vary according to the criteria used but the immediate post-operative cure rate is 70 to 80% with an experienced neurosurgeon level when biochemical cure is defined as a circulating cortisol level <50 mU/l post-operatively.

Pituitary irradiation

Pituitary irradiation using the standard technique described above is most frequently indicated after unsuccessful surgery. Pituitary irradiation is particularly effective in the treatment of children with Cushing's disease.

Table 58.11 Response to tests used to differentiate ectopic ACTH secretion from Cushing's disease

	Ectopic ACTH (% of cases)	Cushing's disease (% of cases)
Hypokalaemia <3.2 mmol/l	100	10
Diabetes mellitus	78	38
Dexamethasone 8 mg/day (no suppression)	89	22
No response to metyrapone	50	36
CRH test excessive response	0	>90

Abbreviation: CRH, corticotrophin-releasing hormone.

Source: data from Trainer PJ and Grossman A, The diagnosis and differential diagnosis of Cushing's syndrome, *Clinical Endocrinology*, Volume 34, Issue 4, pp. 317–320, Copyright © 1991 John Wiley and Sons Ltd.

Medical treatment

Medical treatment may be used as an adjunct to surgery and radiotherapy while the effects of radiotherapy are awaited or, alternatively, for the preoperative treatment of patients. Metyrapone, an 11β-hydroxylase inhibitor, inhibits the synthesis of cortisol. Mitotane is an adrenolytic agent which may be used together with metyrapone in patients who are not responding adequately to this drug alone. It has a slow onset of action. Side effects include hypercholesterolaemia, and cerebellar ataxia because of its incorporation into cerebellar neurones. Both metyrapone and mitotane may result in adrenal insufficiency and so require careful monitoring of cortisol levels. Patients may require hydrocortisone replacement. Most recently, the somatostatin analogue, pasireotide, which stimulates somatostatin receptor subtypes 2 and 5 has been licensed for use in patients with Cushing's disease who fail to be biochemically cured. It is effective in ~30% of cases but may cause deterioration in glucose tolerance.

Gastroenteropancreatic neuroendocrine neoplasms

Introduction

Neuroendocrine neoplasias (NEN) of the gastroenteropancreatic (GEP) system are rare (incidence 1–4/100 000 worldwide) and affect both sexes equally. Although derived from endocrine precursor cells, less than half of all patients present with a classical functional hormone hypersecretion syndrome caused by the excessive and unregulated secretion of peptide hormones, neuropeptides, or neurotransmitters. In contrast to other epithelial tumours of the GEP-system, symptoms related to tumour burden usually develop late and are associated with advanced tumour stages, whether or not the symptoms are related to hormone hypersecretion (functioning NEN) or to tumour mass effects (e.g., small bowel obstruction, bile duct occlusion). Insulinomas are an exception to this rule because they manifest themselves at an early tumour stage in most cases with a specific and rather easily recognized clinical syndrome. Less than 10% of all patients present with a specific family history, whereby the GEP primary is almost exclusively located in the foregut (especially in the pancreas, duodenum, stomach, and bronchus). This hereditary tumour syndrome is termed 'multiple endocrine neoplasia, type 1' (MEN 1).

Tumour classification

Gastroenteropancreatic neuroendocrine neoplasias (GEP-NEN) are classified according to:

♦ primary tumour localization within the GEP-system

♦ tumour stage according to UICC (Union for International Cancer Control)/ AJCC (American Joint Committee on Cancer)/ENETS (European Neuroendocrine Tumor Society)

♦ tumour grading according to the Ki67-proliferative index

♦ functionality (i.e. a clinically manifest hormone hypersecretion syndrome)

♦ association with the MEN 1-syndrome.

30–40% of all tumours cause specific symptoms and syndromes (see Table 58.12) related directly to the excessive release of their functional secretory products (e.g., gastrin or serotonin) [100]. As a general rule, hindgut tumours (i.e., NEN originating from the colorectum)

are almost always non-functional. By contrast, midgut tumours present with carcinoid syndrome in many cases and then are usually metastatic, while foregut tumours—if hormonally active—present with either the Whipple's triad (symptoms known or likely to be caused by hypoglycaemia, low plasma glucose measured at the time of the symptoms, and relief of symptoms when the glucose is raised to normal), a Zollinger–Ellison syndrome or, more rarely, with glucagonoma syndrome or Verner–Morrison syndrome (see Table 58.12).

In the recent years, the WHO has published a new classification of NEN specifically addressing GEP-NEN (Table 58.13). This classification largely relies on the classification proposals made by ENETS and has been confirmed by several studies [101, 102]. It is important to realize that the proliferative capacity as indicated by either mitotic count or Ki67-labelling index by immunohistochemistry is now considered a most important prognostic factor of GEP-NEN. Thus, GEP-NEN with a proliferative capacity of no more than one mitosis per high power field (HPF) or no more than 2% Ki67-positive tumour cells are considered grade 1 (G1) neuroendocrine tumours (NET-G1) and may still be labelled with the traditional term 'carcinoid tumour'. GEP-NEN with an intermediate proliferative capacity of 2 to 20 mitoses per HPF or 3–20% Ki67-positive tumour cells are classified as grade 2 (G2) neuroendocrine tumours (NET-G2); the term 'carcinoid' is, however, no longer considered appropriate for these NET-G2. Finally, NEN with more than 20 mitoses or more than 20% Ki67-positive tumour cells are now termed grade 3 (G3) neuroendocrine carcinomas (NEC-G3) according to WHO, ENETS, AJCC, and UICC. WHO-grading according to Ki67-index or mitotic count as well as TNM (tumour node metastasis)-classification have proven to provide significant prognostic stratification (Table 58.14).

The efforts towards a clinically and prognostically relevant classification for NEN have also lead to a NEN-specific TNM-classification by ENETS which was largely adopted by the AJCC and the UICC; the latter varies from the ENETS proposal only for early stage appendiceal and pancreatic NEN [103–105].

Almost 90% of all GEP-NEN are well differentiated, as reflected by their slow rate of growth. In cases where there is a family history, tumours of the parathyroid and the pituitary can also occur (MEN 1). However, the subgroup of highly proliferative, poorly differentiated, and rapidly progressing neuroendocrine carcinomas (NEC-G3; see Tables 58.13 and 58.14) exists and requires an appropriately modified diagnostic and therapeutic approach.

Aetiology and frequency

Since cells of the diffuse endocrine system can be found anywhere within the GEP-system, primary NEN can also be found in essentially any GEP localization. However, in approximately 6–10% of all cases an advanced, metastatic NEN is found and no explicit primary tumour organ can be identified in spite of extensive and sensitive clinical investigation (CUP, cancer of unknown primary). Depending on the primary tumour localization the frequency of NEN varies considerably; however, NEN of the stomach, the appendix, and the rectum represent the most frequent NEN and by far the majority of them are early stage, non-metastatic tumours (10–15% of all NEN each) [106]. In contrast, small intestinal and pancreatic NEN, while also representing approximately 15% of all GEP-NEN each, are mostly advanced metastatic tumours. Other localizations such as duodenum (~ 4%), colon (~ 5%), and oesophagus (<1%) are much rarer [107].

NEN metastasize by lymphatic and hematogenous spread to numerous localizations; almost any location in the body has been described as a metastatic site (e.g., orbits, heart, breast, skin, adrenal glands, etc.) in addition to the most frequent sites as listed in Table 58.15.

The majority of neuroendocrine GEP tumours are sporadic without a family history of a hereditary syndrome. With the exception of a small subgroup of patients, until now no clear genetic cause has been found for the sporadic form [108, 109]. In contrast, most patients with multiple neuroendocrine neoplasia-type 1 possess a genetic defect of the so-called *MEN 1* or *menin* gene (90%). Studies have shown that *menin* acts as a tumour-suppressor gene. Therefore, *menin* modifications may affect the cellular replication of neuroendocrine cells [109–113].

Histology, routine laboratory testing, and neuroendocrine cell biology

Independent of the functional state, conventional histology of GEP-NEN typically shows a homogeneous array of small round cells, each with a uniform nucleus and cytoplasm, but mitoses are rare. The low proliferation index can be determined immunohistochemically using antibodies against the proliferation marker Ki67 (usually less than 5% of cells are proliferating) (Figure 58.13). Higher proliferation rates correspond to less differentiated NET-G2 and, in some cases, even to poorly-differentiated neuroendocrine carcinomas of the small- or large-cell type. In the common form of well-differentiated neuroendocrine tumours (NET-G1/2), malignancy can only be diagnosed by the detection of distant metastases or tumour invasion into neighbouring structures (e.g., nerve sheaths, blood and lymph vessels, or lymph nodes) [114]. Most NETs produce multiple gastrointestinal hormones, neurotransmitters, and neuropeptides. However, only some of the hormone-active components are released into the bloodstream. Thus, if immunoreactivity for various peptide hormones is demonstrated in the tissue section, this neither necessarily implies their release into the bloodstream nor a clinical manifestation of a functional hypersecretion syndrome. By contrast, chromogranin A (a packaging protein of secretory granules), is synthesized and released in almost all tumour cells. Hence, both immunohistologic as well as laboratory blood tests should be restricted to the use of chromogranin A as a broad-spectrum marker for the presence of neuroendocrine tumours. Only in selected cases, defined by a specific history suggesting the excessive release of a given hormone, are specific hormone determinations of use [100]. NEN cells are characterized by a cell type-specific synthesis of secretory vesicles. These vesicles are characterized by a specific vesicular envelope (membrane) and content (core). To release the vesicular content into the bloodstream, second messenger systems (for example, calcium, cGMP, or cAMP) are required. These second messengers permit the release of hormones, neuropeptides, and neurotransmitters in an 'on demand' or regulated fashion. While peptide hormones and neuropeptides, together with the so-called packaging proteins of the granin family (e.g., chromogranin A), are contained in secretory granules, neurotransmitters are mainly contained within neuroendocrine small synaptic-like vesicles [100].

Adequate histopathological diagnosis requires the use of immunohistochemical techniques based on molecular markers for these two types of vesicles. Chromogranin A is used both immunohistochemically and serologically to identify secretory granules (Figure 58.13). For neuroendocrine small synaptic-like vesicles, synaptophysin is now established as a routine immunohistochemical

Table 58.12 Hormone hypersecretion syndromes in NEN: syndrome characteristics, mediators, and diagnostic testing

Syndrome/tumour	Secreted hormone(s)	Primary tumour	Diagnostic test	Symptoms
Carcinoid syndrome (classical)	Serotonin (substance P, neuropeptide K, tachykinines)	Small intestine (mostly ileum), bronchial system, pancreas (rarely), rectum (extremely rarely)	5-HIAA in 24-hour- urine (acidified), serum chromogranin A (CgA)	Facial flushing (85%), secretory diarrhoea (75%), carcinoid heart disease (Hedinger's syndrome; 25%), wheezing (<10%)
Carcinoid syndrome (atypical)	Histamine (bradykinines)	Stomach (rarely)	Methylimidazole acetic acid in 24-hour- urine	Facial flushing, wheezing
Zollinger–Ellison syndrome (ZES) or gastrinoma	Gastrin	Duodenum (30%), pancreas (70%)	Serum gastrin, secretin-test, gastric 24-hour-pH-metry	Recurrent peptic ulcer disease (atypically localized, multiple), secretory diarrhoea, steatorrhoea, maldigestion
Insulinoma	Insulin (rarely proinsulin)	Pancreas	Serum glucose, serum insulin, serum proinsulin (rarely), C-peptide, 72-hour-fasting-test	Whipple's triad: fasting (hyperinsulinaemic) hypoglycaemia, neuroglycopaenia, reversibility after glucose application
Glucagonoma	Glucagon	Pancreas	Serum glucose, serum glucagon	Diabetes mellitus, necrolytic migratory erythema, anaemia, malnutrition (weight loss)
Verner–Morrison syndrome or VIPoma	VIP	Pancreas (90%)	Serum VIP, venous blood gas analysis	WDHA-syndrome: watery diarrhoea, hypokalaemia, achlorhydria, metabolic acidosis, occasionally facial flushing
Somatostatinoma	Somatostatin	Pancreas (50%), duodenum (periampullary region, 50%)	Serum somatostatin	Steatorrhoea, diarrhoea, cholelithiasis, diabetes mellitus
Ectopic ACTHoma	ACTH	Bronchial system	Serum ACTH, cortisol in 24-hour- urine dexamethasone suppression test	Cushing's syndrome
Non-functioning NET (G1/2)	None, causing clinical symptoms	Whole GEP-system	Serum chromogranin A (CgA)	None
Non-functioning NEC (G3)	None, causing clinical symptoms	Whole GEP-system	Neuron-specific enolase (NSE), serum chromogranin A (CgA)	None

Abbreviations: 5-HIAA, 5-hydroxy-indole acetic acid; ACTH, adrenocorticotrophic hormone; VIP, vasoactive intestinal peptide.

marker molecule with the highest sensitivity for the diagnosis of a neuroendocrine neoplasm (Figure 58.13). Due to their poor specificity regarding neuroendocrine neoplasms, neuron-specific enolase (NSE) and CD56 (NCAM) should be abandoned as immunohistologic markers for NEN.

Clinical syndromes

Neuroendocrine specific symptoms and syndromes are caused by the excessive release of hormones, neuropeptides, and neurotransmitters. As already pointed out, hormone hypersecretion is mainly

observed from a primary tumour located in the pancreas and duodenum, whereas neurotransmitters and neuropeptides are mainly released by tumours located in the distal small intestine. Specific hormone hypersecretion (i.e. functional) syndromes, the respective hormones or amines thought to mediate the symptoms, and the laboratory tests are summarized in Table 58.12.

Non-specific symptoms are frequently observed in GEP-NEN with abdominal pain (50–60% of all patients), unexplained weight loss (20%), fatigue (15%), small bowel obstruction (~12%), gastrointestinal bleeding (~10%), night sweats (~8%), jaundice (~4%),

Table 58.13 Classification of neuroendocrine neoplasms according to WHO 2010 [214–216]

WHO 2010	Histological differentiation grade	Grading Ki67-index mitotic rate	WHO 2000 (old)
NET-G1	Well differentiated	≤ 2% <2/10HPF	WDET/C
NET-G2	Well differentiated	3–20% 2–20/10HPF	WDET/C
NEC-G3 - Large cell phenotype - Small cell phenotype	Poorly differentiated	>20% >20/10HPF	PDEC
Exception: NET-G3	Well differentiated	>20% >20/10HPF	Increasingly described novel subgroup

Abbreviations: G1/2/3, grade; HPF, high power field (40-fold magnification); NET, neuroendocrine tumour; NEC, neuroendocrine carcinoma; PDEC, poorly differentiated endocrine carcinoma; WDET, well differentiated (neuro-)endocrine tumour; WDEC, well differentiated (neuro-)endocrine carcinoma.

and fever of unknown cause (~2%) as the most frequent symptoms ultimately leading to the diagnosis of a NEN.

Specific aspects of diagnosis and therapy of GEP-NEN

Functional tumours

Neuroendocrine neoplasms of the pancreas, duodenum, and stomach

NEN of the pancreas have also been called islet-cell tumours or endocrine pancreatic tumours (EPT). Since many of these tumours produce hormones (e.g., gastrin and vasoactive intestinal polypeptide [VIP]) that are not found in the normal untransformed endocrine pancreas, it is assumed that these tumours derive directly from transformed pancreatic stem cells. The

Table 58.14 Prognosis of GEP-NEN according to WHO-classification and TNM-staging groups

	GEP-NEN	Small intestine	Pancreas
Prognostic factor	5-YSR	5-YSR	5-YSR
G1	80–90%	90–95%	85–90%
G2	65–80%	70–85%	60–80%
G3	10–33%	20–50%	15–35%
Stage I–IIIa 'limited disease'	80–90%	85–95%	75–90%
Stage IIIb–IV 'extensive disease'	50–70%	60–75%	50–60%

Abbreviation: 5-YSR, 5-year survival rate.

Table 58.15 Sites and frequency of metastases of NEN

Localization	Frequency
Lymphonodular	~80%
Hepatic	~70%
Peritoneal	~20%
Osseous	~10%
Pulmonary	up to 10%
Other intra-abdominal organs	up to 7%
CNS	up to 3%

tumorigenesis of duodenal and gastric neuroendocrine tumours is even less clear [115].

Insulinoma/hypoglycaemia syndrome

The incidence of insulin-secreting neuroendocrine tumours, or insulinomas, is approximately 0.1–0.4 per 100 000 of the population worldwide, affecting both sexes equally [116]. Insulinomas can occur at any age. Most insulinomas (approximately 90%) are small (less than 2 cm), non-metastatic, and occur as solitary tumours. They are almost exclusively confined to the pancreas. Multiple, synchronously- or metachronously-occurring insulinomas are observed in only a few cases (less than 7%). In all of these, MEN 1 has to be excluded [110, 116–120]. In cases of malignant insulinoma, the 10-year survival rate is less than 30% [116]. Moreover, in these cases, the release of insulin into the bloodstream may lead to less functionality due to the secretion of incompletely-processed 'immature' insulin.

Diagnosis

To diagnose an insulin-secreting neuroendocrine tumour, the first step is to take the patient's history (reports of psychiatric and neurological symptoms, alterations or even loss of consciousness, e.g. related to hypoglycaemia), and the second is to perform a 72-hour fasting test combined with repeated determinations of glucose and insulin levels. In this context, C-peptide determinations to exclude exogenous insulin administration may be unnecessary. The test is diagnostic if the fasting glucose level is less than 2.5 mmol (45 mg/dl) with inappropriately high levels of insulin more than 70 pM (486 μIU/mL) and C-peptide (more than 500 pM) [121]. Alternatively, diagnostic challenge tests using a euglycaemic hyperinsulinaemic-clamp method [122] or diazoxide or calcium stimulation may be used in doubtful situations [121, 123, 124]. The localization of insulinomas is often difficult due to their small size (1–2 cm in diameter). For preoperative localization, endoscopic ultrasound (EUS) has the highest sensitivity (85%) [125]. A similar sensitivity is observed for the more invasive and rarely required procedure of intra-arterial calcium stimulation and selective portal venous sampling [121]. Other procedures such as transabdominal ultrasound (US), computed tomography (CT), and magnetic resonance imaging (MRI) detect less than half of all cases [126]. Similarly, somatostatin-receptor scintigraphy (SRS) has a low sensitivity in benign cases. This is best explained by the low expression of somatostatin-receptor subtypes-2 and -5 bound by somatostatin analogues such as octreotide [127]. However, in malignant insulinomas, sensitivities for SRS of up to 90% have been reported [128]. Positron emission tomography (PET)-scanning

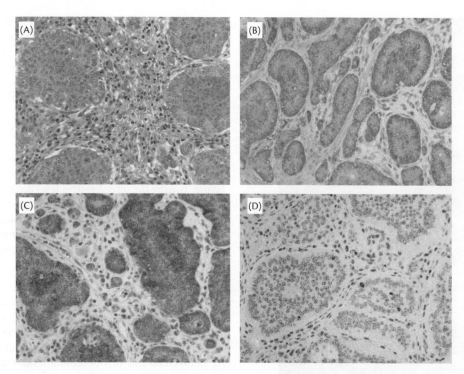

Fig. 58.13 Histological diagnosis of neuroendocrine tumours. (A) Conventional haematoxylin and eosin (H&E) staining of an ileal NET. (B) Immunohistochemical detection with antibodies against chromogranin A. (C) Synaptophysin. (D) Ki67; note that chromogranin A and synaptophysin antibodies react exclusively with tumour cells. Ki67 positivity is observed in a few tumour cells.

using either Gallium-68-DOTATOC/TATE (Ga-DOTATOC/TATE) or even the glucagon-like peptide-1(GLP-1)-analogue exendin-1 may provide more sensitive and specific means for insulinoma detection currently under development [128]. So far, no convincing data exist to include metaiodobenzylguanidine (MIBG)-scintigraphy into tumour staging. Intraoperatively, palpation as well as intraoperative ultrasound (IOUS) both detect insulinomas with a high degree of sensitivity (approximately 90%) (see Figure 58.14 which shows diagnostic images of a pancreatic neuroendocrine tumour with metastases to the liver).

Therapy

Curative tumour resection represents the therapy of choice: experienced centres report a cure rate of 90%; the procedures may involve open or laparoscopic resection of tumour, the latter for pancreatic tail insulinomas in particular. In patients with unresectable and metastatic disease (approximately 10%), symptomatic antisecretory therapy with diazoxide (a membrane, hyperpolarizing, potassium-channel opener) and one of the somatostatin analogues (SSA), octreotide or lanreotide, can improve hypoglycaemia (see Table 58.17) [129]. However, somatostatin analogues have to be used cautiously as reduced glucagon release may interfere with counter-regulatory mechanisms [130]. The somatostatin receptor-non-specific SSA pasireotide as well as the mTOR inhibitor everolimus may provide additional, off-label treatment for symptom control in otherwise uncontrolled patients [130]. To further control symptoms and with antiproliferative intent, the nitrosourea streptozocin in combination with 5-fluorouracil (5-FU) or doxorubicin can be effectively used (see Table 58.18) [131–133]. Tumour-volume reduction by embolizing liver metastases can be

employed in patients with extensive liver metastases [134–136]. Prognosis relates to tumour stage, differentiation, and proliferation. The 10-year survival rate for patients with metastatic disease is under 30% [116].

Gastrinoma/Zollinger–Ellison syndrome

Gastrin-secreting neuroendocrine tumours, or gastrinomas, are epithelial tumours characterized by the excessive release of gastrin into the bloodstream, which gives rise to the Zollinger–Ellison syndrome [137]. This syndrome, initially described by Zollinger and Ellison, consists of a triad of extensive peptic ulcerations in the upper gastrointestinal tract, excessive acid secretion in the stomach (combined in some cases with secretory diarrhoea), as well as solitary or multiple islet-cell tumours of the pancreas or duodenum (see Figure 58.15A and 58.15B). Gastrinomas usually become manifest between the third and fifth decades of life, although they are also occasionally observed during childhood. Up to 25% of all gastrinomas occur in association with MEN 1 [110, 117–120, 138–140]. At the time of presentation, about two-thirds of all patients already have metastatic disease [126, 141, 142]. Approximately 30–50% of all gastrinoma primaries occur extrapancreatically, with the primary (or primaries) located in the duodenal wall. Due to their small size, they are often missed endoscopically as well as surgically [125]. The prognosis for patients with extrapancreatic primaries appears to be better than that for patients with intrapancreatic tumours.

Clinical features

Multiple, small (less than 1 cm) peptic ulcerations are found in the oesophagus, stomach, post-bulbar duodenum, and even proximal jejunum. Approximately one-third of all patients complain of secretory diarrhoea in the presence, or even absence, of peptic

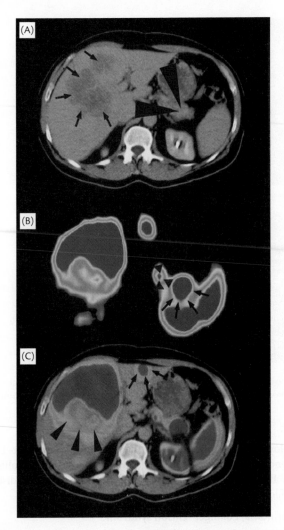

Fig. 58.14 Imaging diagnosis of a pancreatic neuroendocrine tumour metastatic to the liver. (A) Abdominal CT showing the larger of the two pancreatic primaries (arrowheads, right) and liver metastases (arrows, left). (B) Somatostatin receptor scintigraphy with two pancreatic tumours (small arrowheads) and liver metastases (small arrows). (C) Image fusion of CT and SRS indicating that part of the liver metastasis (arrowheads) is devoid of somatostatin receptors, probably representing necrotic tissue. The metastasis in the right liver lobe (arrows) was not detected by the abdominal CT. Note that the spleen on the right shows unspecific uptake.

ulcerations. Secretory diarrhoea is caused by the excessive release of hydrochloric acid which leads to protein denaturation in the intestinal lumen and wall. This in turn leads to a partial villous atrophy as well as malabsorption and steatorrhoea.

Diagnosis

Based on the clinical features given above, the final diagnosis is made by both laboratory testing and imaging procedures. The biochemical diagnosis is traditionally established if: unstimulated gastric acid secretion (BAO, basal acid output) exceeds 15 mval/h (more than 5 mval/h after partial gastric resection) together with an increased gastrin level of more than 150 pg/ml; high serum gastrin levels (more than 1000 pmol/ml) exist, and achlorhydria or hypochlorhydria is excluded [123, 143]. In patients with moderately high gastrin levels (150 to 1000 pg/ml) the diagnosis is made using a secretin-challenge provocation test (2 U/kg body weight). An increased gastrin level of

more than 200 pg/ml is pathognomonic. In rare cases, a gastrinoma can be only diagnosed by a pathological secretin test in the absence of a raised basal gastrin concentration [144]. However, positive secretin tests together with hypochlorhydria have been reported in only a few cases. The use of 24-hour transnasal pH-metry presenting unregulated pH-decrease below 4, particularly at night, may replace gastric acid secretion measurement.

Hypergastrinaemia is most often observed in patients treated with proton-pump inhibitors and H 2-receptor antagonists, and, less commonly, in patients with chronic atrophic gastritis, pernicious anaemia, hypercalcaemia, short-bowel syndrome, and renal failure. Usually the serum gastrin level does not exceed 500 pg/ml. However, in these cases, the secretin test will be negative. Due to the high frequency of MEN 1 associated with gastrinomas, serum prolactin, calcium, and phosphate concentrations should be analysed in parallel for the diagnosis of a prolactinoma and/or primary hyperparathyroidism [120, 140].

Imaging procedures

After the biochemical diagnosis has been established, the location and size of the primary, its local spread, as well as lymph node and liver metastases have all to be considered. Intrapancreatic gastrinomas are usually less than 2 cm in diameter at initial diagnosis. Between 80 and 90% of tumour lesions can be detected in the so-called gastrinoma triangle (cranial axis: cystic and common bile duct; caudal axis: distal two-thirds of the duodenum and medial axis: border of the pancreatic head and body). Most are located at the right side of the superior mesenteric artery. In those patients with a primary tumour located outside the pancreas (especially duodenum), the diagnosis is even more difficult. Only the EUS and SRS (see Figure 58.13) imaging modalities possess sensitivities between 85 and 90% [125, 128]. When these two procedures are combined, almost all tumours are detectable. For IOUS and intraoperative palpation, sensitivities range from 70 to 90%. In cases of suspected duodenal gastrinomas, intraoperative transduodenal illumination has the highest sensitivity, even allowing the detection of lesions in the few millimetre range. US and CT usually suffice for the detection of liver metastases (Figure 58.16). However, SRS and MRI represent the most sensitive methods for detecting the bony metastasis most frequently observed in neuroendocrine foregut tumours.

Therapy

The therapy of choice is surgery with a curative intent. Postoperative cure has been reported in more than 50% of cases (40–90%) [145]. In contrast to sporadic gastrinomas, patients with MEN 1 should be submitted to surgery only in selected cases [121, 145]. This stems from the finding that patients with MEN 1 develop multiple tumours at different times. In addition, different clinical courses are observed between families. Thus, symptomatic therapy with antisecretory agents represents the first treatment of choice (see Table 58.17) [141, 146, 147]. About 50% of all patients are not amenable to curative surgery. Provided tumour progression is evident, these patients should be treated with systemic chemotherapy using streptozocin in combination with 5-FU or doxorubicin. Objective response rates of approximately 50% have been reported, together with a survival benefit of 12 years in two phase-III studies [131, 133]. An alternative or sequential treatment option—particularly for pancreatic NET—is targeted treatment by either everolimus or sunitinib which have both proven a substantial prolongation of progression-free survival of pancreatic NET in phase III trials (see Table 58.18) [131, 133].

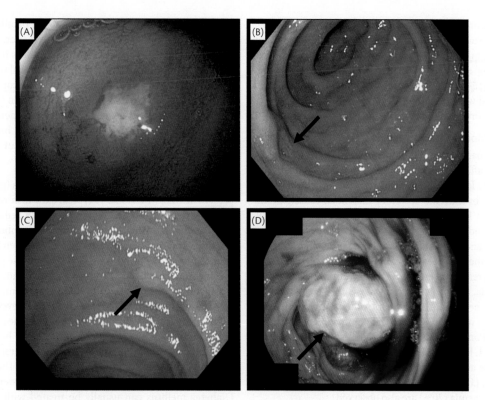

Fig. 58.15 Endoscopic appearance of NET-manifestations. (A) Small bulbar duodenal ulcer in Zollinger–Ellison syndrome (ZES). (B) Atypical, postbulbar duodenal ulcer in ZES (arrow), recognize small intestinal Kercking's folds. (C) Small ileal NET (arrow). (D) Large ileal NET protruding into the caecum (arrow).

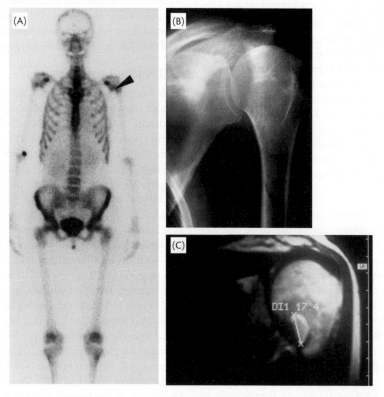

Fig. 58.16 Imaging diagnosis of a pancreatic NET metastatic to the bone. (a) Scintigraphic bone scan (SRS) showing a faint uptake in a bony metastasis located in the left shoulder (arrow). Note that the primary tumour and the liver metastasis had been resected. (b) No bony lesion was visualized in the left proximal humerus on conventional radiography. (c) However, magnetic resonance imaging of the left shoulder demonstrated a bony metastasis in the left humerus. Note that a bony metastasis can be missed by conventional radiography.

Patients who are unresponsive to chemotherapy and who have a functional tumour state unresponsive to extensive acid suppression with proton-pump inhibitors (PPIs) may be subjected to embolization of liver metastases, provided the major tumour burden is confined to the liver [134–136]. It is debatable whether embolization has to be performed with or without a chemotherapeutic agent (e.g., streptozocin or doxorubicin) coupled to an embolizate [146].

VIPoma/Verner–Morrison syndrome

NETs secreting vasoactive intestinal polypeptides (VIP) (VIPomas) occur in later life, affecting women slightly more often than men. Tumours are usually localized in the pancreatic head. They are clinically characterized by extreme secretory diarrhoea caused by the excessive release of VIP, which results in dehydration, hypochlorhydria/achlorhydria, and hypokalaemia [121]. This syndrome was first described by Priest and Alexander followed by Verner and Morrison one year later. Since the diarrhoea clinically resembles cholera, VIPoma is also termed 'pancreatic cholera' or WDHA syndrome (watery diarrhoea, hypokalaemia, and achlorhydria/acidosis). Whereas secretory diarrhoea presents the diagnostic hallmark, other symptoms include dehydration (100%), weight loss (100%), abdominal pain (60%), and flushing (20%). VIPomas are also observed in a small percentage of patients with MEN 1. Diagnosis is made on the basis of a stool volume of more than 1 litre as well as an increased VIP plasma concentration. Hypokalaemia (100%), hypochlorhydria (70%), hypercalcaemia (40%), and hypoglycaemia (20%) are also observed.

Imaging procedures

Tumours are usually large (more than 3 cm) at presentation, often located in the pancreatic tail, and are metastatic in two-thirds of all cases. Conventional imaging procedures such as US, CT, and MRI usually suffice to determine the tumour extent [121].

Antisecretory treatment using somatostatin analogues, such as octreotide or lanreotide, represent the therapy of choice (see Table 58.17). A reduction of the stool volume is usually observed within hours. In advanced cases, unresponsive to somatostatin analogues, (chemo)embolization for liver metastases, cytoreductive therapy using streptozocin together with 5-FU or doxorubicin, or debulking surgery may be considered (see Table 58.18) [148, 149]. For proliferation control, targeted treatments may also be considered (see 'Medical therapy' section below). For resectable tumours, surgery with a curative intent represents the therapy of choice [141, 147].

Somatostatinoma

Due to its many and varied functions, somatostatin secreted by neuroendocrine tumours (somatostatinomas) may cause diabetes mellitus, diarrhoea/steatorrhoea, gallstones, and hyperchlorhydria. In addition, weight loss might also be found as a characteristic clinical feature [121]. However, a large series of somatostatin-producing NET has not been able to identify any patient presenting with the postulated specific clinical syndrome, thus challenging the latter [121]. Somatostatin-producing NEN are considered slow growing in comparison to other functional neuroendocrine tumours. Diagnosis is made by the detection of increased serum somatostatin levels. Primary tumours are often found at a pancreatic or duodenal, mostly periampullary, location. At first presentation, pancreatic somatostatin-producing NEN are frequently already large in size and metastatic (90%). Thus, conventional imaging procedures allow complete staging of the tumour extent. Extrapancreatic tumours are usually smaller in size and metastatic in only 50% of cases. Extrahepatic somatostatinomas are often found in the

duodenum, especially in the region of the papilla. In the latter case, an association with von Recklinghausen's (neurofibromatosis type 1, NF1) disease has been described. Tumours in the duodenal wall are difficult to localize; therefore, conventional imaging procedures, with the exception of endoscopy and endoscopic ultrasound, may miss the lesion. Due to its common location in the foregut, surgical exploration may be considered in well-documented patients whose diagnosis is based solely on the results of biochemical testing. Treatment strategies adhere to the principles of pancreatic NEN.

Glucagonoma

Glucagon-secreting neuroendocrine tumours (glucagonomas) may present with skin lesions. A typical skin rash of necrolytic migratory erythema is observed, together with reduced glucose tolerance or diabetes mellitus. Moreover, thrombotic complications, anaemia, and psychiatric disturbances are often found. Serum concentrations of all amino acids, especially those generated by gluconeogenesis, are reduced and thus rather pronounced weight loss is frequently observed due to protein catabolism. Diagnosis is made on the basis of an increased serum glucagon level of more than 1000 pg/ml. Most primary tumours are found in the pancreas (especially body and tail). An association with MEN 1 has to be considered [121]. At presentation, tumours are usually already large (5–10 cm) and can be localized as mentioned above. Therapy includes the standard regimens used to treat other neuroendocrine tumours. Diabetes mellitus can usually be treated with oral antidiabetics; only 25% of patients require insulin treatment. Peri- and postoperative antithrombotic therapy is necessary to prevent thrombotic complications in patients undergoing surgery. Somatostatin analogues can improve skin lesions, but do not affect diabetes mellitus. Chemotherapy and targeted therapies as employed for the treatment of other pancreatic neuroendocrine tumours may be considered (see Tables 58.17 and 58.18) [147, 148, 150].

ACTH-producing tumours

Both well-differentiated and dedifferentiated neuroendocrine tumours may secrete ACTH, leading to a paraneoplastic Cushing's syndrome. In some rare cases, a Zollinger–Ellison, or even a carcinoid syndrome, may coexist. The prognoses for patients varies. These tumours are often large at presentation, proliferate variably, and may therefore not be amenable to curative or even debulking surgery. However, some small undifferentiated neuroendocrine carcinomas in the lung may present at early stage with a paraneoplastic Cushing's syndrome. Therapy with somatostatin analogues or chemotherapy using streptozocin and either 5-fluorouracil or doxorubicin may be of use in the case of NET (G1/2) [147, 148, 150]. In dedifferentiated NEC (G3), treatment with cisplatin and etoposide (VP-16) appears to be palliative in only a few cases. Non-suppressibility of cortisol by dexamethasone is diagnostic. ACTH may be either normal (but elevated with respect to the cortisol concentration) or elevated. Since tumours are large, conventional imaging procedures suffice for tumour staging in most cases. Therapy should be palliative, treating Cushing's syndrome with ketoconazole or metyrapone (see Tables 58.17 and 58.18) [151]. In the case of bronchial NEN, however, tumour localization may be difficult as the tumour is small and manifests clinically with a Cushing's syndrome. In these cases, SRS or either Ga-DOTATOC/TATE- (for NET) or fluoro-18-D-glucose-FDG PET/CT (for NEC) may be of help [152]. Differentiation of Cushing's syndrome and pituitary-derived Cushing's disease may be difficult.

Growth hormone-releasing hormone-secreting neuroendocrine tumours

Growth hormone-releasing hormone (GHRH)-secreting neuroendocrine tumours (GHRHomas) are extremely rare. They occur primarily in the pancreas (30%), lung (50%), and small intestine (10%), with most pancreatic GHRHomas located in the pancreatic tail. Some 30% of all GHRHomas occur together with MEN 1. At presentation, tumours are usually larger than 5 cm and, relatively commonly, occur together with gastrinomas. Based on the hypersecretion of GHRH, acromegaly is the leading clinical sign. Diagnosis is usually made by detecting the presence of both a pancreatic tumour and acromegaly. Cushing's syndrome together with Zollinger–Ellison syndrome can be observed in approximately 40% of all patients. However, most cases are diagnosed retrospectively after pituitary surgery for a supposed growth hormone (GH)-secreting pituitary tumour, since histology identifies somatotrophic hyperplasia rather than adenoma tissue. Biochemical testing should demonstrate non-suppressibility of GH by an oral glucose load in addition to a low GHRH concentration. Tumour localization and treatment are the same as for glucagonomas, with somatostatin analogues as the preoperative first-line treatment [121].

Other functional tumours

Due to the extremely low incidence of other functional neuroendocrine tumours (e.g., neurotensinomas), the reader is directed to Öberg [141] and Kulke and Mayer [153].

Neuroendocrine tumours of the intestine

Carcinoid syndrome/'serotoninomas'

Neuroendocrine tumours of the distal small intestine are characterized by the synthesis and release of low molecular-weight neurotransmitters (e.g., serotonin) as well as neuropeptides (e.g., tachykinins). When released in an unregulated mode and in excessive amounts into the bloodstream, these secretory compounds as well as many other (so far unidentified) factors lead to the so-called carcinoid syndrome. Approximately 80% of all neuroendocrine tumours of the distal small intestine (midgut origin) become functional when metastases are formed (see Figure 58.15C and 58.15D). Typically, these tumours grow slowly, reflecting WHO-grade 1 or 2. Usually, this slow tumour progress leads—even in metastatic disease—to a median overall survival (especially in the elderly) of up to 10 or even 20 years [154–156]. Therefore, patients with midgut tumours have a better prognosis compared to those with foregut tumours (see Table 58.14). The incidence of NET of the small intestine (formerly termed carcinoids of the midgut) is approximately 1.0 per 100 000 of the population worldwide, affecting middle or older ages and both sexes equally [154]. Primary tumours are usually small (less than 1 cm), solitary to multiple, and thus often escape imaging procedures (see 'Diagnosis' section below). Ileal and jejunal carcinoids are common and metastasize earlier than the most common appendiceal and rectal neuroendocrine tumours.

Diagnosis

Diagnosis is first accomplished by a clinical history of at least one of the symptoms observed in the carcinoid syndrome [157]. Symptoms of the carcinoid syndrome vary, with diarrhoea and flushing observed in approximately 80% of all patients at initial presentation [154, 157]. Bronchial wheezing as in asthma is observed in only less than 10% of all cases [154, 157]. Flushing is characterized by a reddening of the upper part of the body, particularly affecting the face, neck, and the upper part of the sternum; teleangiectasias may remain permanently in some patients. In advanced cases, functional NET of the small intestine can manifest with severe flushing, leading to a loss of consciousness combined with low or high blood pressure, all contributing to the clinical picture of the so-called malignant flush. Together with an endocardial fibrosis (30–40% of all cases), cardiac arrhythmias and severe right heart insufficiency are observed [154, 157]. In patients with local disease, the 10-year survival rate is more than 80% while it decreases to 50–60% in metastatic patients [155, 158]. With the advent of effective antisecretory treatment, endocardial fibrosis is often the life-limiting factor, progressing independently of symptom control.

Biochemical diagnosis is made by the determination of 5-hydroxyindoleacetic acid (5-HIAA) levels in urine (sampled for 24 h) and chromogranin A levels in serum (see Table 58.12). To avoid false-positive 5-HIAA results, certain precautions concerning food intake, prior and during urine sampling, have to be observed. This includes the avoidance of foods containing serotonin, such as pineapples, bananas, cheese, etc. [142, 159]. Imaging diagnosis is made by transabdominal ultrasound and computed tomography. For identification of the primary tumour, classic enteroclysis according to Sellink can be used. Somatostatin receptor scintigraphic scan (SRS) and the even more sensitive Ga-DOTATOC/TATE-PET/CT will be useful for identifying metastases and also the primary. MRI is useful for detecting small volume and diffuse metastatic disease to the liver or the bones; the use of liver-specific imaging techniques (contrast-media enhanced or diffusion weighted imaging) can significantly improve imaging results and thereby influence therapeutic management decisions (Figure 58.17) [121].

Therapy

Locally or locoregionally confined NEN of the small intestine should in general be surgically (but not endoscopically) resected [160]. Appendiceal carcinoids—a special subgroup—are observed during 0.3% of all appendectomies [155]. These tumours are practically always non-metastatic and are cured by surgery. Tumours tend to calcify with increasing age, especially when located in the tip of the appendix. Neuroendocrine tumours located in the appendiceal base (10%) have a worse prognosis. Despite a tumorous infiltration of the serosa and surrounding fatty tissue, only tumours larger than 1–2 cm in diameter appear to become metastatic and therefore these should be resected using surgical oncological techniques [121, 156]. In practical terms, appendiceal carcinoids incidentally found by appendectomy should only be considered for reoperation when they are larger than 1 cm, located at the appendiceal base, and infiltrating neighbouring structures. Tumour infiltration by the mesoappendix and vessels, however, is a clear indication for (extended) ileocaecal resection. An extended right hemicolectomy should be performed in cases of extensive lymph node metastasis [121]. In the elderly patient, even metastatic tumours tend to grow extremely slowly. Thus, surgery should only be considered in this subgroup of patients when obstructive tumour growth is either imminent or apparent. If somatostatin analogue therapy is planned, surgery combined with a prophylactic cholecystectomy should be performed to prevent the development of cholecystolithiasis (gall-stone formation is one of the possible side effects of somatostatin and its analogues).

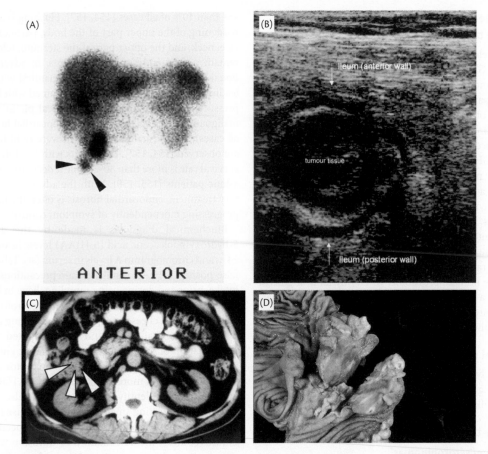

Fig. 58.17 Imaging of a neuroendocrine ileal primary. (A) Positive somatostatin receptor scintigraphic scan (SRS) in a neuroendocrine tumour of the ileum (arrowheads). (B) Abdominal CT of the abdomen demonstrating the neuroendocrine tumour in the ileum. Note that SRS was used for guided diagnostics in (A), i.e., CT was performed after localization of the tumour by SRS. (C) Transabdominal ultrasound also demonstrating the ileal primary. (D) Resected specimen demonstrating the ileal primary.

The value of debulking surgery, particularly in patients with multiple liver metastases, is questionable [121, 158, 161–163]. Perioperative treatment with somatostatin analogues is highly recommended for patients with a carcinoid syndrome, as a carcinoid crisis may be provoked during intraoperative tumour manipulation. Patients who are not candidates for surgery should be treated primarily with biotherapy (namely, somatostatin analogues and interferon-a), provided tumour progression has been verified during a treatment-free observation period (usually for longer than 3–6 months) (see Tables 58.17 and 58.18) [147, 164–166]. Only in patients unresponsive to biotherapy may chemoembolization or even chemotherapy be tried (Figure 58.18). However, only low response rates (less than 30%) are observed using the latter therapeutic regimen (see also 'Medical therapy' section for further details) [132, 141, 147, 167].

Non-functional neuroendocrine tumours of the pancreas and intestine

Introduction

Symptoms and signs

Non-functional neuroendocrine tumours are characterized by the hypersecretion of polypeptides or peptides (e.g., chromogranin A or pancreatic polypeptide (PP)) not causing a specific clinically manifest symptomatology [123, 141, 142, 168]. Approximately 50–65% of all neuroendocrine tumours are non-functional.

Primaries are most commonly located in the rectum and pancreas; however, they can also be found in other locations such as the small and large intestine and even in the ovary, prostate, and liver. Non-functional NEN manifest clinically only when a luminal obstruction of the intestine, the bile duct, or even of the urinary tract is observed, or when larger tumor masses are observed. In some cases, abdominal pain can be the presenting symptom due to metastatic mesenteric root infiltration. In this case, intestinal absorption is often impaired. Rectal NEN are usually small (more than 1 cm), yellow-greyish in colour, and located in the submucosa. Almost all rectal NEN occur 4–13 cm proximal of the dentate line as solitary tumours [121]. Often, they are removed endoscopically.

Diagnosis

Due to the lack of functionality/hormonal activity, specific symptoms and syndromes are missing. Therefore, patients present at the first visit with unspecific symptoms related to:

1. liver metastases (protrusion of the right upper abdomen and/or abdominal pain due to an extended liver capsule);

2. gastrointestinal obstruction, an acute abdomen, complete or incomplete mechanical obstruction;

3. obstruction of the biliary and/or pancreatic tract (jaundice, acute pancreatitis); and

4. fatigue and weight loss.

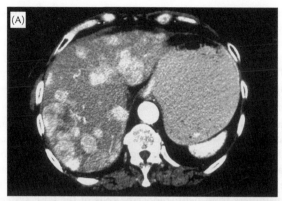

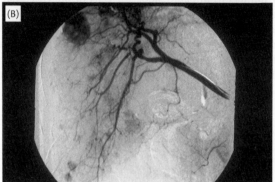

Fig. 58.18 Imaging diagnosis of liver metastases. (A) Computed tomogram of multiple liver metastases visualized using an intravenous contrast agent. (B) Angiographic detection also demonstrates multiple hypervascularized metastases of variable size. Note the large lesion in the upper left of the image. Hypervascularized lesions can be treated by (chemo)embolization.

The initial diagnosis of a non-functioning NET is frequently made by the ultrasonic detection of liver metastases in patients presenting with non-specific abdominal symptoms. After histological diagnosis staging with standard imaging modalities (US, CT, or MRI) provides information on the extent of tumour spread and tumour volume [121, 153, 169]. Recently, SRS and PET/CT have been increasingly used as the first imaging procedure since most non-functional tumours are positive by this functional imaging procedure [154, 157, 142, 169]. A whole-body scan allows 'guided diagnostics' for consecutive, selective imaging procedures

or even allows somatostatin receptor imaging and cross-sectional imaging at the same time ('one-stop imaging') (see Figure 58.14). Non-functional NET of the stomach, duodenum, and pancreas are best visualized using EUS, since this has the highest sensitivity for detecting primary tumours and local infiltration, particularly when larger vessels and lymph nodes are involved. US, CT, and MRI are utilized for determining the extent of distant metastases [110, 144].

Therapy
Since the natural clinical course of non-functional tumours is similar to that of functional tumours, therapy follows the same guidelines as for the latter [144].

NEN of the stomach
Gastric NEN are an increasingly diagnosed entity due to frequent endoscopic procedures of the upper gastrointestinal (GI)-tract (Table 58.16). However, they provide a rather heterogeneous group of organ-specific neoplasms according to their pathophysiologic association to hypergastrinaemia (types 1 and 2), their association with chronic atrophic gastritis and hypochlorhydria (type1, ECLoma) or with a Zollinger–Ellison syndrome of a MEN-1-associated gastrinoma (type 2), their sporadic occurrence (types 3 and 4), and their proliferative capacity according to a Ki67-index below 20% (G1 or 2, type 3) or higher than 20% (G3, type 4, see Table 58.16). The diagnosis is usually endoscopic, followed by EUS, US, CT, MRI, and somatostatin receptor imaging for staging in cases of suspected advanced stages. The therapy is usually oncologic resection (which may include endoscopic resection in early stage cases of type 1 and 2 gastric NET if larger than 1 cm but smaller than 2 cm). The palliative treatment options adhere to the general principles of treatment of advanced NEN although data are almost unavailable [110, 144].

Principles of the therapy of GEP-NEN
Surgery
For all GEP-NEN, surgery represents the therapy of first choice bearing the only potential for long-term cure. In patients with a known primary tumour and only local spread, radical surgery has to be performed to remove the primary as well as lymph nodes following the same standard oncological procedures used for resecting adenocarcinomas within the GI tract [158, 161–163, 170]. Liver transplantation may only be considered in very few and highly

Table 58.16 Subclassification of gastric NEN

	Type 1	Type 2	Type 3	Type 4
Prevalence of all gastric NEN [%]	70–80	5–6	10–20	<5
Tumour characteristics	Small (<1–2 cm), in 65% multiple, 78% polypoid	Mostly small (<1–2 cm) and multiple, polypoid	Solitary, large (>2cm), polypoid and ulcerated	Solitary, large (>2cm), polypoid, mostly ulcerated
Associated disease	Chronic atrophic gastritis (CAG)	Gastrinoma and ZES MEN 1	None	None
WHO classification	G1/2-NET	G1/2-NET	Mostly G2-NET	G3-NEC
Serum gastrin levels	↑	↑↑	Normal	Normal
Gastric pH	↑↑	↓↓	Normal	Normal
Metastases [%]	2–5	5–15	30–80	50–100
Estimated tumour-related deaths [%]	0	<10	25–30	60–95

selected instances of unresectable hepatic metastases arising from intestinal or pancreatic GEP-NET (G1/2) with lasting evidence of absent extrahepatic disease (possible only after successful and complete primary tumour resection) [160, 171–179].

Medical Therapy

Medical treatment of GEP-NEN generally covers two biological aspects of the disease: control of hormone hypersecretion symptoms (i.e. functionality, Table 58.16) and control of proliferation.

While specific symptom management (i.e. anti-hormonal) needs to be considered according to the respective functional syndrome (Table 58.17), medical antiproliferative treatment (Table 58.18) is considered according to NEN-grading and primary tumour localization. In any case, surgical resectability needs to be ruled out prior to treatment initiation.

Biotherapy

The use of pharmacologically modified biological peptides (such as the somatostatin analogues (SSA) octreotide, lanreotide, or pasireotide) and recombinant human interferon-α (IFN-α) or its PEGylated form (PEG-IFN-α) is usually termed biotherapy in contrast to chemotherapy. Although biologically, biotherapy also represents a targeted approach against specific NET-cell targets, SSA and IFN-α are usually not included in the term 'molecular targeted therapy' (see 'Molecular targeted therapy' section).

Somatostatin analogues

Somatostatin analogues (SSA) are synthetic derivatives of human somatostatin-14, with half-lives ($t\frac{1}{2}$, 180–210 min) greatly exceeding that of the naturally occurring somatostatin ($t/\frac{1}{2}$, 2–3 min). Somatostatin and its analogues (octreotide, lanreotide, and pasireotide) inhibit the release of hormones, neuropeptides, and neurotransmitters from neuroendocrine cells of the GEP system by activating somatostatin receptors on the surface of NET cells. While octreotide and lanreotide act primarily through somatostatin receptors subtype 2 and 5, pasireotide is less selective and also binds to subtypes 1 and 3; by this pasireotide may mediate additional effects for symptom and proliferation control currently

Table 58.17 Symptom management for functioning NEN

Carcinoid syndrome CS	Somatostatin analogues (SSA) effectively control hypersecretion of serotonin and other mediators of CS
	Somatostatin receptor subtype-specific SSA:
	◆ Octreotide: 50–500 µg s.c. bid or tid
	◆ Octreotide long-acting release LAR: 10–30 mg i.m., monthly
	◆ Lanreotide autogel: 60–120 mg deep s.c., monthly
	◆ Peri-interventional continuous i.v. infusion: initial 100 µg bolus, then 50 µg per hour; not approved but common practice
	Somatostatin receptor-non-specific SSA:
	◆ Pasireotide: 600–1200 µg s.c. bid; not approved
	Interferon-alpha (IFN-α) effectively controls hypersecretion of serotonin and other mediators of CS:
	◆ IFN-α2b: 3–5 Mio Units s.c., three times weekly
	◆ PEG- IFN-α2b: 90–180 µg s.c., once weekly
	Tryptophane hydroxylase inhibitor telotristate etiprate specifically inhibits synthesis of serotonin: not approved, under development
Insulinoma syndrome (Whipple's triad)	Diazoxide controls insulin hypersecretion by inhibiting K_{ATP}-channels:
	◆ 25–150 mg bid or tid
	SSA may control insulin hypersecretion:
	Somatostatin receptor subtype-specific SSA:
	◆ Octreotide and lanreotide: for dosing see CS
	Somatostatin receptor-non-specific SSA may very effectively control insulin hypersecretion:
	◆ Pasireotide: 600–1200 µg s.c. bid; not approved, under development
	Everolimus may provide additional control of insulin hypersecretion in refractory cases not amenable to surgical treatment:
	◆ 5–10 mg p.o. daily; not approved, individual approach
Zollinger–Ellison syndrome ZES (gastrinoma)	Proton-pump inhibitors (PPI) very effectively control gastric acid hypersecretion of ZES:
	◆ Pantoprazole: 40 mg p.o. tid, up to six times daily
	◆ Omeprazole: 40 mg p.o. tid, up to six times daily
	◆ Esomeprazole: 40 mg p.o. tid, up to six times daily
	Sufficient gastric acid suppression may be monitored by use of 24-hour pH-metry
	SSA may control hypersecretion of gastrin in cases of insufficient control by PPIs
	Somatostatin receptor subtype-specific SSA:
	◆ Octreotide and lanreotide: for dosing see CS
Glucagonoma syndrome	Standard antidiabetic treatment
	SSA effectively control hypersecretion of glucagon
	Somatostatin receptor subtype-specific SSA:
	◆ Octreotide and lanreotide: for dosing see CS

(continued)

Table 58.17 Continued

Verner–Morrison syndrome (VIPoma)	SSA effectively control hypersecretion of VIP
	Somatostatin receptor subtype-specific SSA:
	◆ Octreotide and lanreotide: for dosing see CS
	Additional standard antidiarrhoeal treatment may be necessary:
	◆ Loperamide: 2–4 mg p.o. tid
	◆ Tinctura opii 1%: titrate according to effect
	Monitoring of blood bicarbonate/base excess by blood gas analysis and subsequent substitution of bicarbonate may be required in individual cases
Atypical carcinoid syndrome	SSA may effectively control hypersecretion of histamine
	Somatostatin receptor subtype-specific SSA:
	◆ Octreotide and lanreotide: for dosing see CS
	Anti-histaminic drugs may provide some additional anti-histaminergic symptom control
Ectopic Cushing's syndrome (ACTHoma)	Ketoconazole can provide control of steroid hormone synthesis until definitive treatment:
	◆ 50–300 mg p.o. tid according to effect
	SSA may provide some additional control of ACTH hypersecretion
	Somatostatin receptor subtype-specific SSA:
	◆ Octreotide and lanreotide: for dosing see CS
	Somatostatin receptor-non-specific SSA effectively control ACTH hypersecretion in Cushing's disease and may be tried in refractory cases of peripheral, autonomous ACTH secretion:
	◆ Pasireotide: 600–1200 μg s.c. bid; not approved, under development
Somatostatinoma	No specific antisecretory treatment available
	Standard antidiabetic treatment in case of diabetes mellitus
	Standard endoscopic (ERCP) or surgical treatment for gall stone disease

under investigation. Hence, specific symptoms caused by the excessive release of secretory products can be inhibited. SSAs represent the therapy of choice for the carcinoid syndrome. A subcutaneous injection of 0.05 or 1.0 mg of octreotide three times per day will usually control diarrhoea and flushing within a few hours in 50–90% of patients [147, 148, 164, 166, 180, 181]. SSA has also proved effective in control of peptide hormone secretion in glucagonomas or VIPomas (Table 58.16). Depot formulations given either intramuscularly (octreotide) or subcutaneously (lanreotide) every four weeks have been shown to control symptoms (see Table 58.16) [148]. The development of gallstones during long-term SSA therapy is observed in 10–60% of all patients [148]; however, only a small percentage of these patients become symptomatic. Further side effects include a temporary exocrine pancreatic insufficiency and initial abdominal pain, which subsides after several days of treatment [141, 147, 148]. In some cases (especially with high dosages), substitution of pancreatic enzymes due to long-term exocrine pancreatic insufficiency may have to be initiated. Pasireotide, due to its less selective mode of action may cause additional side effects, such as disturbances of glucose homeostasis including diabetes mellitus. Occasionally, a complete or partial response with SSA therapy has been observed in well differentiated G1/2-NET [148]. In general, however, SSA treatment has been demonstrated to significantly increase progression-free survival in NET from the midgut (PROMID-trial with octreotide) [182] or of gastrointestinal and pancreatic origin (CLARINET-trial with lanreotide) [147, 148, 164, 165, 183, 184]. The median time to progression varies between 14 months in the PROMID trial and 32.8 months during treatment in the CLARINET trial; However, these trial designs are not directly comparable and thus the results cannot directly be compared.

Therefore—beyond antisymptomatic treatment—SSA may also be considered for long-term antiproliferative control in patients who do not need a cytoreductive strategy although not all countries have approved these drugs for that indication. In late 2014, the US FDA approved lanreotide for the treatment of patients with unresectable, well- or moderately- differentiated, locally-advanced or metastatic GEP-NETs to improve progression-free survival.

Interferon-α

Interferon-α (IFN-α) represents an alternative treatment to the use of SSA as monotherapy for metastatic neuroendocrine tumours of the GEP system [150, 185, 186]. Apart from its known antiviral action, an antiproliferative effect for IFN-α has also been demonstrated [186, 187]. Studies show that IFN-α has a direct action on the cell cycle as well as on chromogranin A expression. In contrast to SSA, control of symptoms takes several days to develop [141]. Similar to SSA, stable disease can be observed in about half of all patients in whom tumour progression had been documented prior to treatment; an objective response (mostly partial remission) may, however, be observed in up to 20% of treated NET patients. A clinical response can be achieved using 5 million units of IFN-α three times per week. In contrast to SSA, side effects are more significant, including influenza-like symptoms (fatigue, myalgia, arthralgia, and headache) [141, 148, 165]. Furthermore, latent autoimmune diseases can become manifest during IFN-α treatment. Myelotoxicity, neuropsychiatric abnormalities, and fatigue syndromes may also have to be considered as side effects. In relation to the location of the primary tumour, patients with NET of the small intestine tend to respond better to IFN-α treatment than those with pancreatic or other gastrointestinal NET [141].

Table 58.18 Antiproliferative medical treatment for NEN

Systemic therapy for NET (G1/2)	
Biotherapy SSA	Somatostatin analogues (SSA) prolong regression-free survival in both small intestinal and pancreatic NET Somatostatin receptor subtype-specific SSA: ♦ Octreotide long-acting release LAR: 10–30 mg i.m. monthly ♦ Lanreotide autogel: 60–120 mg deep s.c. monthly treat until PD Side effects: nausea, vomiting, mild diarrhoea or steatorrhoea, elevated liver enzymes, gall stones, hair loss, disturbed glucose tolerance, bradycardia (rarely)
Biotherapy Interferon-alpha	Interferon-alpha (IFN-α) may induce a tumour-control in 30-40% of pNET ♦ IFN-α2b: 3–5 Mio Units s.c. three times weekly ♦ PEG- IFN-α2b: 90–180 μg s.c. once weekly treat until PD (not approved by authorities) Side effects: flu-like syndrome, fever, chills, myalgia, cephalgia, fatigue, weight loss, anaemia, leukopaenia, thrombocytopaenia, symptoms of depression, activation of autoimmune diseases
Molecular targeted therapy: Everolimus	Everolimus induces SD/PR in app. 70% and prolongs PFS against placebo from 4.6 to 11.0 months ♦ Everolimus: 10 mg daily treat until PD Side effects: stomatitis, rash, pruritus, fatigue, cephalgia, infections, oedema, loss of appetite, diarrhoea, nausea, dysgeusia, epistaxis, anaemia, thrombocytopaenia, hyperglycaemia, pneumonitis, weight loss
Molecular targeted therapy: Sunitinib	Sunitinib induces SD/PR in app. 70% and prolongs PFS against placebo from 5.5 to 14.0 months ♦ Sunitinib: 37.5 mg daily treat until PD Side effects: diarrhoea, nausea, vomiting, anorexia, stomatitis, rash, dysgeusia, hand-foot-syndrome, hair-colour-changes, fatigue, epistaxis, neutropaenia, thrombocytopaenia, hypertension, insomnia, weight loss
Molecular targeted therapy: Bevacizumab	Bevacizumab may induce prolonged PFS as a reserve medication alone or in combination with SSA or TMZ: ♦ Bevacizumab (in combination with SSA) 15 mg/kg BW, i.v. over 1–2 hours, on day 1 repeat on day 21, treat until PD (not approved by authorities) ♦ Bevacizumab (in combination with TMZ) 5 mg/kg BW, i.v. over 1–2 hours, day 1 repeat on day 15, treat until PD (not approved by authorities) Side effects: allergic reactions, nausea, vomiting, fatigue, cephalgia, thrombosis, arterial hypertension, proteinuria, wound healing defects, spontaneous GI-perforations, tumour-associated bleeding episodes
Chemotherapy: Streptozocin-based	Combination chemotherapy of streptozocin (STZ) with either 5-fluorouracil (5FU) or doxorubicin (DOX) induces PR in 30–40% and SD in additional 20–30% ♦ STZ/5FU: STZ 500 mg/m² BSA, i.v. over 1 hour, days 1–5 5FU 400 mg/m² BSA, i.v. as bolus, days 1–5 repeat both on day 43, treat until best response or for 9 cycles ♦ STZ/DOX: STZ 500 mg/m² BSA, i.v. over 1 hour, days 1–5 DOX 50 mg/m² BSA, i.v. over 1 hour, days 1 and 22 repeat both on day 43, treat until best response or for 9 cycles CAVE: cumulative DOX-dose: 500 mg/m² Side effects: nausea, vomiting, diarrhoea, constipation, mucositis, hand-foot-syndrome, renal insufficiency, leukopaenia, neutropaenia, thrombocytopaenia, anaemia, cardiotoxicity (DOX)
Chemotherapy: Temozolomide-based	Combination chemotherapy of temozolomide (TEM) with capecitabine (CAP) induces PR in 40–70% and SD in additional 20% ♦ TEM 200 mg/m² BSA, dialy p.o., days 10–14 CAP 750 mg/m² BSA, bid p.o., days 1–14 repeat both on day 29, treat until PD (not approved by authorities) Side effects: nausea, vomiting, diarrhoea, mucositis, hand-foot-syndrome, fatigue, anaemia, leukopaenia, neutropaenia, thrombocytopaenia, herpes viridae infections, elevated liver enzymes This may also be applied to NET-G3 or NEC with a Ki67-index below 55%

(continued)

Table 58.18 Continued

Systemic therapy for NEC (G3)	
Chemotherapy: Cisplatin-based	Combination chemotherapy of cisplatin with etoposide (VP16) induces CR/PR in 60–70% NEC with TTP of app. 9–11 months
	◆ Cisplatin 45 mg/m^2 BSA, i.v. over 1–2 hours, days 2 and 3
	Etoposide 130 mg/m^2 BSA, i.v. over 1–2 hours, days 1–3
	repeat both on day 29, treat until PD (not approved by authorities)
	Side effects: nausea, vomiting, diarrhoea, mucositis, hand-foot-syndrome, distal polyneuropathy, hearing loss, renal insufficiency, leukopaenia, neutropaenia, thrombocytopaenia, anaemia
Chemotherapy: Oxaliplatin-based	Combination chemotherapy of oxaliplatin (OX) with either 5-fluorouracil (5FU) and folinic acid (FOL) or capecitabine (CAP) may induce tumour control in 30–40% of rapidly progressing pNET or such with high tumour load
	◆ FOLFOX: OX 85 mg/m^2 BSA, i.v. over 2 hours, day 1
	FOL 200 mg/m^2 BSA, i.v. over 2 hours, days 1 and 2
	5FU 400 mg/m^2 BSA, i.v. as bolus, days 1 and 2
	5FU 600 mg/m^2 BSA, 22-hour-infusion, days 1 and 2
	repeat both on day 15, treat until PD (not approved by authorities)
	◆ CAPOX: OX 130 mg/m^2 BSA, i.v. over 2 hours, day 1
	CAP 1000 mg/m^2 BSA, bid p.o., days 2–15
	repeat both on day 21, treat until PD (not approved by authorities)
	Side effects: nausea, vomiting, diarrhoea, constipation, mucositis, hand-foot-syndrome, distal polyneuropathy, leukopaenia, neutropaenia, thrombocytopaenia, anaemia, mild renal insufficiency
Chemotherapy: Irinotecan-based	Combination chemotherapy of irinotecan (IRI) with 5-fluorouracil (5FU) and folinic acid (FOL) may induce tumour-control in 30–40% of NEC as a second-line therapy
	◆ FOLFIRI: IRI 180 mg/m^2 BSA, i.v. over 2 hours, day 1
	FOL 400 mg/m^2 BSA, i.v. over 2 hours, day 1
	5FU 400 mg/m^2 BSA, i.v. as bolus, day 1
	5FU 1200 mg/m^2 BSA, 46-hour-infusion, days 1 and 2
	repeat both on day 15, treat until PD (not approved by authorities)
	Side effects: nausea, vomiting, diarrhoea, mucositis, hand-foot-syndrome, distal polyneuropathy, oropharyngel dyskinesia, leukopaenia, neutropaenia, thrombocytopaenia, anaemia

SSA and IFN-α combination therapy

A combination of IFN-α with SSA has been used to control symptoms as well as tumour-cell proliferation. So far, a synergistic effect has been demonstrated only in a relatively small number of cases. However, patients with progressive disease treated with monotherapy can be prescribed combination therapy, albeit for a limited time [188–190, 191].

Molecular targeted therapy

Molecular targeted therapy addressing signal transduction pathways within the NET cell have recently become a treatment option for well-differentiated G1/2-NET. Their mode of actions include inhibition of growth factor signalling (sunitinib, everolimus), inhibition of metabolic signalling (everolimus), inhibition of proliferation and induction of apoptosis (sunitinib, everolimus), and inhibition of angiogenesis (sunitinib, everolimus).

Everolimus

Recently, the mTOR-inhibitor everolimus has been extensively studied in G1/2-NETs that were not amenable to curative surgical treatment. The RADIANT-3 trial in advanced pancreatic NET demonstrated a significantly prolonged duration of progression-free survival in everolimus-treated EPT patients in comparison to placebo-treated patients of 11 versus 5 months when actively progressing patients were treated; this led to authority approval of

everolimus in progressive pancreatic NET [192]. In non-pancreatic NET everolimus has also been extensively studied and showed some effect in combination with octreotide in patients with progressive non-pancreatic NET; predefined statistical significance was, however, not met in this placebo-controlled phase III trial although longer follow-up is underway. Everolimus is therefore under further investigation in the treatment of non-pancreatic NET as is the mTOR-inhibitor temsirolimus [193].

Sunitinib

In a study design similar to that used with everolimus, the multiple tyrosine kinase inhibitor sunitinib was studied in progressive non-functioning pancreatic NET (G1/2) in a phase III trial and demonstrated good efficacy with a prolongation of progression-free survival from 5 months in the placebo arm to approximately 11 months in the treatment group [190]. Although—as with the mTOR-inhibitors—some toxicities have to be considered, this has led to authority approval of the substance for proliferation control of progressive pancreatic NET (G1/2) [194].

Bevacizumab

The anti-vascular endothelial growth factor (VEGF)-antibody bevacizumab has also been applied to NET in several phase-II trials and is currently under investigation for this indication [195]. The mostly hypervascularized NET treatment with this antibody has led to the proof of concept of antiangiogenic treatment in NET in a study combining pancreatic and intestinal NET [196].

Chemotherapy

In the early 1980s, chemotherapy represented the only systemic therapeutic option for the treatment of GEP-NET (G1/2). Based on the relatively high response rates (approximately 50%) achieved in the treatment of non-metastatic and metastatic insulinomas, the initial monotherapy with streptozocin has been extended to the treatment of patients with other neuroendocrine tumours, and in various drug combinations [131–133, 197]. Published data on a variety of combination therapies have demonstrated objective response rates for pancreatic NET ranging from 30 to 60%. By contrast, NET of the midgut have lower response rates (10–30%) [167]. The duration of remission is considerably shorter for patients with midgut tumours compared to those with pancreatic NET (less than 2 years). So far, the most comprehensive study of NET of the foregut showed that a combination of streptozocin together with doxorubicin is slightly superior to a combination of streptozocin plus 5-fluorouracil [133]. These findings are in contrast to those of an earlier study by the same group, which demonstrated similar response rates for both treatment regimens [131]. Thus, based on the lower side effects associated with 5-fluorouracil, streptozocin together with 5-fluorouracil is favoured by most centres [198].

In recent years, an oral combination regimen of temozolomide and capecitabine has been suggested to have efficacy in pancreatic and non-pancreatic NET. Objective radiological response rates of up to 70% and disease stabilization in the majority of the remaining patients have been observed, thus leading to a new treatment option in progressive NET. However, authority approval is not available; a prospective controlled trial is currently accruing patients in the US cooperative groups [199].

In metastatic poorly differentiated NEC (G3), a combination treatment using etoposide (VP-16) and cisplatin led to response rates in approximately 50% of patients [197]. However, objective response (in some cases even complete remissions) lasted only a few months (about 3 months) and was complicated by considerable side effects including nausea, leukopaenia, thrombocytopaenia, anaemia, and neuropathy. Other platinum-based regimens such as FOLFOX or CAPOX may be considered due to less toxicity and probably equal efficacy although no controlled comparative trial data are available [200]. As second-line treatment temozolomide- or irinotecan-based treatments have been suggested but not tested in prospective phase III trials [201].

Loco-regional and locally ablative therapies
(Chemo) embolization

Because of the frequent hypervascularization of neuroendocrine hepatic metastases, superselective occlusion of the hepatic artery represents a therapeutic option for both the control of symptoms and control of proliferation of liver metastases. During the last decade, superselective embolization, with or without chemotherapeutic agents coupled to microspheres, has shown response rates ranging from 30 to 80%. However, in inexperienced hands this technique can lead to a mortality rate of more than 5%. Studies have suggested that a combination of chemoembolization together with systemic chemotherapy can lead to response rates of up to 80% [134–136]. These promising data have still to be evaluated in prospective studies. Additional locally ablative treatment options such as radiofrequency ablation (RFA), catheter-guided [192]-Ir-irradiation (after-loading), or SIRT (selective intra-arterial radionuclide therapy with ^{90}Y) may be performed in experienced centres [190].

Peptide receptor-mediated radionuclide therapy (PRRT)

Overexpression of somatostatin receptors on the surface of tumour cells of NEN (most of them being NET-G1/2) has opened the option of peptide receptor-mediated radionuclide therapy as a highly tumour-specific treatment modality. Using either ^{90}Yttrium or ^{177}Lutetium as cytotoxic radioemitters, a tumour tissue-specific systemic treatment has become available for NET from any origin as long as there is sufficient somatostatin receptor expression on the tumour tissues evident on somatostatin receptor imaging. Retrospective and prospective cohort studies as well as one phase II trial have provided evidence for good efficacy for symptom and tumour growth control of NET in response to this treatment modality. Progression-free survival ranges from 12 months in progressive NET to over 4 years in pretreatment stable NET. Side effects like nephro-, myelo-, and gastrointestinal toxicity need to be considered but are usually well manageable. Since hitherto there are no comparative data of PRRT versus medical treatment options available, a clear-cut recommendation of when to apply PRRT within the sequelae of systemic treatments in NET is, as of now, still not possible [202–205].

Selective internal radionuclide therapy (SIRT)

A combination of a trans-arterial hepatic loco-regional treatment and locally applied radiotherapy can be achieved by combining a trans-arterial catheter approach to otherwise uncontrollable liver disease caused by NET with the advantage of radionuclide-covered microbeads or resin. The latter lead to arterial tumour vessel occlusion and the radionuclide (^{90}Yttrium) additional tumour irradiation. This approach may achieve additional control of liver disease in some advanced NET patients in experienced centres [182].

Carcinoid heart disease (CHD, Hedinger's syndrome)

Up to 30% of patients with mostly small intestinal NET suffering from the carcinoid syndrome experience an endocardial fibrosis mediated by serotonin and other mediators released by (mostly hepatic) tumour manifestations into the systemic circulation. This endocardial fibrosis can lead to thickening and retraction of the leaflets of the right ventricular valvular system and, by this mechanism, to severe life-limiting right heart failure [206]. To date, right heart valvular surgery is available for interdisciplinary treatment of this severe condition in experienced cardiothoracic surgical centres; however, a catheter-based approach to right heart valvular replacement has been reported recently [143, 207–209].

Experimental and future approaches

Novel substances like telotristat etiprate [210], pasireotide [211], temsirolimus [196], and pazopanib [212] are currently under investigation for a potential role in medical NEN treatment as well as several combination treatments with the aim to improve efficacy while not increasing toxicity. Also some comparative trials comparing either chemotherapy to targeted therapy or somatostatin analogue treatment to PRRT are currently recruiting and will provide important information in the future on the role of specific treatments within the therapy sequelae in individual patients—a hitherto unclear issue [121, 159, 213].

Summary

For appropriate prognostic and therapeutic stratification of GEP-NEN, adequate histopathological grading according to WHO criteria (Ki67-index) and clinicopathological staging according to either ENETS or UICC criteria is essential. Early and metastatic GEP-NEN can be treated by various modalities. Resection (mostly surgical but also—if accessible and feasible—endoscopic) represents the main treatment of choice, allowing the only cure of NEN disease. In patients with functional unresectable tumour disease, the control of hypersecretion (i.e. the control of symptoms) is best achieved using biotherapy with secretory inhibitors such as somatostatin analogues and interferon-α. However, in patients with documented tumour progression or where there is a lack of symptom control provided by the current biotherapy, an increase in the dose of the somatostatin analogues may be employed. Alternatively, a combination of somatostatin analogues with interferon-α can be successful in some cases. Patients with metastatic disease confined primarily to the liver and displaying significant functionality can be additionally treated by loco-regional or locally ablative techniques. Patients with pancreatic NET (G1/2) should be treated antiproliferatively when there is documented tumour progression. In such cases, streptozocin-based combination chemotherapy or molecular targeted treatments are available. There is increasing evidence that small intestinal NET (G1/2) may benefit from the antiproliferative treatment with somatostatin analogues independently from control of functionality. However, in this group fewer options are available as compared to pancreatic NET in case of progression. PRRT provides an effective antiproliferative (and in some cases symptomatic control) treatment option for all somatostatin receptor-positive NET. Novel treatments and combination as well as sequential treatments are currently under investigation. In patients with NEC-G3, platinum-based combination remains the cornerstone of treatment except for the few early resectable cases. Regular, long-term follow-up visits are essential in patients with GEP-NEN.

Further reading

Fernandez A, Karavitaki N, Wass JA. Prevalence of pituitary adenomas: a community-based, cross-sectional study in Banbury (Oxfordshire, UK). Clinical Endocrinology 2010; 72(3): 377–382.

Rajasekaran S, Vanderpump M, Baldeweg S, Drake W, Reddy N et al. UK guidelines for the management of pituitary apoplexy. Clinical Endocrinology 2011; 74(1): 9–20.

References

1. Cooper DS, Doherty GM, Haugen BR, Kloos RT, Lee SL et al. Revised American Thyroid Association management guidelines for patients with thyroid nodules and differentiated thyroid cancer. Thyroid 2009; 19: 1167–1214.

2. Perros P, Boelaert K, Colley S, Evans C, Evans RM et al. Guidelines for the management of thyroid cancer. Clinical Endocrinology (Oxford) 2014; 81 (Suppl 1): 1–122.

3. Wells SA Jr, Asa SL, Dralle H, Elisei R, Evans DB et al. Revised American Thyroid Association guidelines for the management of medullary thyroid carcinoma. Thyroid 2015 (March 26). [Epub ahead of print].

4. Smallridge RC, Ain KB, Asa SL, Bible KC, Brierley JD et al. American Thyroid Association guidelines for management of patients with anaplastic thyroid cancer. Thyroid 2012; 22: 1104–1139.

5. Cheng W, Ma C, Fu H, Li J, Chen S et al. Low- or high-dose radioiodine remnant ablation for differentiated thyroid carcinoma: a meta-analysis. Journal of Clinical Endocrinology and Metabolism 2013; 98: 1353–1360.

6. Fukushima T, Suzuki S, Mashiko M et al. BRAF mutations in papillary carcinomas of the thyroid. Oncogene 2003; 22: 6455–6457.

7. Garcia-Rostan G, Zhao H, Camp RL et al. ras mutations are associated with aggressive tumor phenotypes and poor prognosis in thyroid cancer. Journal of Clinical Oncology 2003; 21: 3226–3235.

8. Brose MS, Nutting CM, Jarzab B et al. Sorafenib in radioactive iodine-refractory, locally advanced or metastatic differentiated thyroid cancer: a randomised, double-blind, phase 3 trial. Lancet 2014; 384: 319–328.

9. Hazard JB, Hawk WA, Crile G. Medullary (solid) carcinoma of the thyroid—a clinicopathologic entity. Journal of Clinical Endocrinology and Metabolism 1959; 19: 152–161.

10. Wells SA Jr, Pacini F, Robinson BG, Santoro M. Multiple endocrine neoplasia type 2 and familial medullary thyroid carcinoma: an update. Journal of Clinical Endocrinology and Metabolism 2013; 98(8): 3149–3164.

11. Eng C, Clayton D, Schuffenecker I, Lenoir G, Cote G et al. The relationship between specific RET proto-oncogene mutations and disease phenotype in multiple endocrine neoplasia type 2: International RET Mutation Consortium. Journal of the American Medical Association 1996; 276: 1575–1579.

12. Kloos RT, Eng C, Evans DB, Francis GL, Gagel RF et al. Medullary thyroid cancer: management guidelines of the American Thyroid Association. Thyroid 2009; 19(6): 565–612.

13. Wohllk N, Schweizer H, Erlic Z, Schmid KW, Walz MK et al. Multiple endocrine neoplasia type 2. Best Practice and Research in Clinical Endocrinology and Metabolism 2010; 24(3): 371–387.

14. Hofstra RM, Landsvater RM, Ceccherini I, Stulp RP, Stelwagen T et al. A mutation in the RET proto-oncogene associated with multiple endocrine neoplasia type 2B and sporadic medullary thyroid carcinoma [see comments]. Nature 1994; 367(6461): 375–376.

15. Gimm O, Marsh DJ, Andrew SD, Frilling A, Dahia PL et al. Germline dinucleotide mutation in codon 883 of the RET proto-oncogene in multiple endocrine neoplasia type 2B without codon 918 mutation. Journal of Clinical Endocrinology and Metabolism 1997; 82(11): 3902–3904.

16. Vanhorne JB, Andrew SD, Harrison KJ, Taylor SA, Thomas B et al. A model for GFR alpha 4 function and a potential modifying role in multiple endocrine neoplasia 2. Oncogene 2005; 24(6): 1091–1097.

17. Agrawal N, Jiao Y, Sausen M, Leary R, Bettegowda C et al. Exomic sequencing of medullary thyroid cancer reveals dominant and mutually exclusive oncogenic mutations in RET and RAS. Journal of Clinical Endocrinology and Metabolism 2013; 98(2): E364–E369.

18. Gimm O, Morriso CD, Suster S, Komminoth P, Mulligan LM et al. Multiple endocrine neoplasia type 2. In DeLellis RA, Lloyd RV, Heitz PU, Eng C, eds. World Health Organization Classification of Tumours Pathology and Genetics Tumours of Endocrine Organs. Lyon: IARC Press, 2004, 211–217.

19. Machens A, Dralle H. Benefit-risk balance of reoperation for persistent medullary thyroid cancer. Annals of Surgery 2013; 257(4): 751–757.

20. Collins BT, Cramer HM, Tabatowski K, Hearn S, Raminhos A et al. Fine needle aspiration of medullary carcinoma of the thyroid. Cytomorphology, immunocytochemistry and electron microscopy. Acta Cytology 1995; 39(5): 920–930.

21. Machens A, Lorenz K, Dralle H. Individualization of lymph node dissection in RET (rearranged during transfection) carriers at risk for medullary thyroid cancer: value of pretherapeutic calcitonin levels. Annals of Surgery 2009; 250(2): 305–310.

22. Brauckhoff M, Machens A, Hess S, Lorenz K, Gimm O et al. Premonitory symptoms preceding metastatic medullary thyroid cancer in MEN 2B: an exploratory analysis. Surgery 2008; 144(6): 1044–1050; discussion 1050–1053.

23. Machens A, Dralle H. Prognostic impact of N staging in 715 medullary thyroid cancer patients: proposal for a revised staging system. Annals of Surgery 2013; 257(2): 323–329.

24. Machens A, Dralle H. Biomarker-based risk stratification for previously untreated medullary thyroid cancer. Journal of Clinical Endocrinology and Metabolism 2010; 95(6): 2655–2663.

25. Martinez SR, Beal SH, Chen A, Chen SL, Schneider PD. Adjuvant external beam radiation for medullary thyroid carcinoma. Journal of Surgery and Oncology 2010; 102(2): 175–188.

26. Machens A, Niccoli-Sire P, Hoegel J, Frank-Raue K, van Vroonhoven TJ et al. Early malignant progression of hereditary medullary thyroid cancer. New England Journal of Medicine 2003; 349(16): 1517–1525.

27. Lenders JW, Pacak K, Walther MM, Linehan WM, Mannelli M et al. Biochemical diagnosis of phaeochromocytoma: which test is best? Journal of the American Medical Association 2002; 287(11): 1427–1434.

28. Thosani S, Ayala-Ramirez M, Palmer L, Hu MI, Rich T et al. The characterization of phaeochromocytoma and its impact on overall survival in multiple endocrine neoplasia type 2. Journal of Clinical Endocrinology and Metabolism 2013; 98(11): E1813–E1819.

29. Tung WS, Vesely TM, Moley JF. Laparoscopic detection of hepatic metastases in patients with residual or recurrent medullary thyroid cancer. Surgery 1995; 118(6): 1024–1029, discussion 1029–1030.

30. Sager S, Kabasakal L, Ocak M, Maecke H, Uslu L et al. Clinical value of technetium-99m-labeled octreotide scintigraphy in local recurrent or metastatic medullary thyroid cancers: a comparison of lesions with 18F-FDG-PET and MIBI images. Nuclear Medicine Communications 2013; 34(12): 1190–1195.

31. Miyauchi A, Matsuzuka F, Hirai K, Yokozawa T, Kobayashi K et al. Prospective trial of unilateral surgery for nonhereditary medullary thyroid carcinoma in patients without germline RET mutations. World Journal of Surgery 2002; 26(8): 1023–1028.

32. Wells SA Jr, Robinson BG, Gagel RF, Dralle H, Fagin JA et al. Vandetanib in patients with locally advanced or metastatic medullary thyroid cancer: a randomized, double-blind phase III trial. Journal of Clinical Oncology 2012; 30(2): 134–141.

33. Kraeber-Bodere F, Bodet-Milin C, Niaudet C, Sai-Maurel C, Moreau A et al. Comparative toxicity and efficacy of combined radioimmunotherapy and antiangiogenic therapy in carcinoembryonic antigen-expressing medullary thyroid cancer xenograft. Journal of Nuclear Medicine 2010; 51(4): 624–631.

34. Iwase Y, Maitani Y. Octreotide-targeted liposomes loaded with CPT-11 enhanced cytotoxicity for the treatment of medullary thyroid carcinoma. Molecular Pharmacology 2011; 8(2): 330–337.

35. Yip DT, Hassan M, Pazaitou-Panayiotou K, Ruan DT, Gawande AA et al. Preoperative basal calcitonin and tumor stage correlate with postoperative calcitonin normalization in patients undergoing initial surgical management of medullary thyroid carcinoma. Surgery 2011; 150(6): 1168–1177.

36. Machens A, Ukkat J, Hauptmann S, Dralle H. Abnormal carcinoembryonic antigen levels and medullary thyroid cancer progression: a multivariate analysis. Archives of Surgery 2007; 142(3): 289–293, discussion 294.

37. Barbet J, Campion L, Kraeber-Bodere F, Chatal JF. Prognostic impact of serum calcitonin and carcinoembryonic antigen doubling-times in patients with medullary thyroid carcinoma. Journal of Clinical Endocrinology and Metabolism 2005; 90(11): 6077–6084.

38. Laure Giraudet A, Al Ghulzan A, Auperin A, Leboulleux S, Chehboun A et al. Progression of medullary thyroid carcinoma: assessment with calcitonin and carcinoembryonic antigen doubling times. European Journal of Endocrinology 2008; 158(2): 239–246.

39. Ross NS, Aron DC. Hormonal evaluation of the patient with an incidentally discovered adrenal mass. New England Journal of Medicine 1990; 323: 1401–1405.

40. Latronico AC, Choruses GP. Adrenocortical tumors. Journal of Clinical Endocrinology and Metabolism 1997; 82: 1317–1325.

41. Liu J, Heikkila P, Kahri AI, Voutilainen R. Expression of the steroidogenic acute regulatory protein mRNA in adrenal tumours and cultured adrenal cells. Journal of Endocrinology 1996; 150: 43–50.

42. Trainer PJ, Grossman A. The diagnosis and differential diagnosis of Cushing's syndrome. Clinical Endocrinology 1991; 34: 317–330.

43. Newell-Price J, Trainer P, Besser M, Grossman A. The diagnosis and differential diagnosis of Cushing's syndrome and pseudo-Cushing's states. Endocrine Reviews 1998; 19: 647–672.

44. Reznek RH, Armstrong P. The adrenal gland. Clinical Endocrinology 1994; 40: 561–576.

45. Britton KE. Editorial. Imaging of the adrenal cortex: Why and wherefore. Nuclear Medicine Communications 1992; 13: 485–487.

46. Cuesta MA, Bonjer HJ, Mourik JC. Endoscopic adrenalectomy: the adrenals under the scope. Clinical Endocrinology 1996; 44: 349–351.

47. Bertanga C, Orth DN. Clinical and laboratory findings and results of therapy in 58 patients with adrenocortical tumours admitted to a single medical center (1951–1978). American Journal of Medicine 1981; 71: 855–875.

48. Gordon RD, Klemm SA, Tunny TJ, Stowasser M. Primary hyperaldosteronism: hypertension with a genetic basis. Lancet 1990; 340: 159–161.

49. Stowasser M, Bachmann AW, Tunny TJ, Gordon RD. Production of 18-oxo-cortisol in subtypes of primary hyperaldosteronism. Clinical and Experimental Pharmacology and Physiology 1996; 23: 591–593.

50. Pommier RF, Brennan MF. An eleven year experience with adrenocortical carcinoma. Surgery 1992; 112: 963–971.

51. Barzilay JI, Pazianos A. Adrenocortical carcinoma. Urological Clinics of North America 1989; 16: 457–469.

52. Sandrini R, Ribeiro PC, DeLacerda L. Childhood adrenocortical tumors. Journal of Clinical Endocrinology and Metabolism 1997; 82: 2027–2031.

53. Macfarlane DA. Cancer of the adrenal cortex: the natural history, prognosis and treatment in a study of fifty-five cases. Annals of Royal College of Surgeons of England 1958; 23: 115–165.

54. Lee EJ, Berger HD, El-Naggar AK et al. Surgical management, DNA content, and patient survival in adrenal cortical carcinoma. Surgery 1995; 118: 1090–1098.

55. Luton JP, Cerdas S, Billaud L et al. Clinical features of adrenocortical carcinoma, prognostic factors, and the effect of mitotane therapy. New England Journal of Medicine 1990; 322: 1195–1201.

56. Schteingart DE. Treating adrenal cancer. Endocrinologist, 1992; 2: 149–157.

57. Kasperlik-Zahuska AA, Migdalska MB, Zglczynski S, Makowska MA. Adrenocortical carcinoma. A clinical study and treatment results of 52 patients. Cancer 1995; 75: 2587–2591.

58. Kirk JMW, Perry LA, Kirby RS, Besser GM, Savage MO. Female pseudohermaphroditism due to a maternal adrenocortical tumour. Journal of Clinical Endocrinology and Metabolism 1990; 70: 1280–1284.

59. Cook DM, Loriaux L. The incidental adrenal mass. American Journal of Medicine 1996; 101: 88–96.

60. Mc Kenna TJ, O'Connell Y, Cunningham S, McCave M, Culliton M. Steroidgenesis in an estrogen producing adrenal tumor in a young woman: Comparison with steroid profiles associated with cortisol and androgen producing tumors. Journal of Clinical Endocrinology and Metabolism 1990; 70: 28–34.

61. Goto T, Murakami O, Sato F, Haraguchi M, Yokoyama K et al. Oestrogen producing adrenocortical adenoma: clinical, biochemical and immunohistochemical studier. Clinical Endocrinology 1996; 45: 643–648.

62. Kloos RT, Gross MD, Francis IR, Korobkin M, Shapiro B. Incidentally discovered adrenal masses. Endocrine Reviews 1995; 16: 460–484.

63. Gross MD, Shapiro B, Francis IR et al. Scintigraphic evaluation of clinically silent adrenal masses. Journal of Nuclear Medicine 1994; 35: 1145–1152.

64. Bravo EL. Evolving concepts in the pathophysiology, diagnosis and treatment of phaeochromocytoma. Endocrine Reviews 1994; 15: 356–368.

65. Bouloux P-M G, Fakeeh M. Investigation of phaeochromocytoma. Clinical Endocrinology 1995; 43: 657–664.

66. Ross GA, Newbould E, Thomas J et al. Plasma and urinary catecholamine concentrations in normal and patient populations. Annals of Clinical Biochemistry 1993; 30: 38–44.

67. Pattarino F, Bouloux PM. The diagnosis of malignancy in phaeochromocytoma. Clinical Endocrinology 1996; 44: 239–241.

68. Funder JW. The genetic basis of primary aldosteronism. Current Hypertension Reports 2012; 14(2): 120–124.

69. Mulatero P, Stowasser M, Loh KC, Fardella CE, Gordon RD et al. Increased diagnosis of primary aldosteronism, including surgically correctable forms, in centers from five continents. Journal of Clinical Endocrinology and Metabolism 2004; 89(3): 1045–1050.

70. Funder JW, Carey RM, Fardella C, Gomez-Sanchez CE, Mantero F et al. Case detection, diagnosis, and treatment of patients with primary aldosteronism: an endocrine society clinical practice guideline. Journal of Clinical Endocrinology and Metabolism 2008; 93(9): 3266–3281.

71. Datrice NM, Langan RC, Ripley RT, Kemp CD, Steinberg SM et al. Operative management for recurrent and metastatic adrenocortical carcinoma. Journal of Surgical Oncology 2011;

72. Kemp CD, Ripley RT, Mathur A et al. Pulmonary resection for metastatic adrenocortical carcinoma: the National Cancer Institute experience. Annals of Thoracic Surgery 2011; 92(4): 1195–1200.

73. Terzolo M, Angeli A, Fassnacht M, Daffara F, Tauchmanova L et al. Adjuvant mitotane treatment for adrenocortical carcinoma. New England Journal of Medicine 2007; 356(23): 2372–2380.

74. Grubbs EG, Callender GG, Xing Y, Perrier ND, Evans DB et al. Recurrence of adrenal cortical carcinoma following resection: surgery alone can achieve results equal to surgery plus mitotane. Annals of Surgical Oncology 2009;

75. Fassnacht M, Terzolo M, Allolio B, Baudin E, Haak H et al. Combination chemotherapy in advanced adrenocortical carcinoma. New England Journal of Medicine 2012; 366(23): 2189–2197.

76. Polat B, Fassnacht M, Pfreundner L, Guckenberger M, Bratengeier K et al. Radiotherapy in adrenocortical carcinoma. Cancer 2009; 115(13): 2816–2823

77. Yener S, Ertilav S, Secil M et al. Prospective evaluation of tumor size and hormonal status in adrenal incidentalomas. Journal of Endocrinological Investigation 2010; 33(1): 32–36.

78. Terzolo M, Stigliano A, Chiodini I, Loli P, Furlani L et al. AME position statement on adrenal incidentaloma. European Journal of Endocrinology 2011; 164(6): 851–870.

79. Nieman LK. Approach to the patient with an adrenal incidentaloma. Journal of Clinical Endocrinology and Metabolism 2010; 95(9): 4106–4113.

80. Zeiger MA, Siegelman SS, Hamrahian AH. Medical and surgical evaluation and treatment of adrenal incidentalomas. Journal of Clinical Endocrinology and Metabolism 2011; 96(7): 2004–2015.

81. Yoh T, Hosono M, Komeya Y et al. Quantitative evaluation of norcholesterol scintigraphy, CT attenuation value, and chemical-shift MR imaging for characterizing adrenal adenomas. Annals of Nuclear Medicine 2008; 22(6): 513–519.

82. Chen H, Sippel RS, O'Dorisio MS, Vinik AI, Lloyd RV et al. The North American Neuroendocrine Tumor Society consensus guideline for the diagnosis and management of neuroendocrine tumors: phaeochromocytoma, paraganglioma, and medullary thyroid cancer. Pancreas 2010; 39(6): 775–783.

83. Därr R, Lenders JWM, Hofbauer LC, Naumann B, Bornstein SR et al. Phaeochromocytoma: update on disease management. Therapeutic Advances in Endocrinology and Metabolism 2012; 3(1): 11–26.

84. Blake MA, Kalra MK, Maher MM, Sahani DV, Sweeney AT et al. Phaeochromocytoma: an imaging chameleon. Radiographics 2004; 24(Suppl 1): S87–S99.

85. Gedik GK, Hoefnagel CA, Bais E, Olmos RA. 131I-MIBG therapy in metastatic phaeochromocytoma and paraganglioma. European Journal of Nuclear Medicine and Molecular Imaging 2008; 35(4): 725–733.

86. Averbuch SD, Steakley CS, Young RC et al. Malignant phaeochromocytoma: effective treatment with a combination of cyclophosphamide, vincristine, and dacarbazine. Annals of Internal Medicine 1988; 109(4): 267–273.

87. Beard CM, Sheps SG, Kurland LT, Carney JA, Lie JT. Occurrence of phaeochromocytoma in Rochester, Minnesota, 1950 through 1979. Mayo Clinic Proceedings 1983; 58(12): 802–804.

88. Karavitaki N, Thanabalasingham G, Shore HC, Trifanescu R, Ansorge O et al. Do the limits of serum prolactin in disconnection hyperprolactinaemia need re-definition? A study of 226 patients with histologically verified non-functioning pituitary macroadenoma. Clinical Endocrinology 2006; 65(4): 524–549.

89. Korevaar T, Wass JA, Grossman AB, Karavitaki N. Disconnection hyperprolactinaemia in nonadenomatous sellar/parasellar lesions practically never exceeds 2000 mU/l. Clinical Endocrinology 2012; 76(4): 602–603.

90. Karavitaki N, Wass JA. Non-adenomatous pituitary tumours. Best Practice and Research Clinical Endocrinology and Metabolism 2009; 23(5): 651–665.

91. Fernandez A, Karavitaki N, Wass JA. Prevalence of pituitary adenomas: a community-based, cross-sectional study in Banbury (Oxfordshire, UK). Clinical Endocrinology 2010; 72(3): 377–382.

92. Igreja S, Chahal HS, King P, Bolger GB, Srirangalingam U et al. Characterization of aryl hydrocarbon receptor interacting protein (AIP) mutations in familial isolated pituitary adenoma families. Human Mutation 2010; 31(8): 950–960.

93. Moore KP, Wass JA, Besser GM. Late diagnosis of pituitary and parapituitary lesions causing visual failure. British Medical Journal 1986; 293(6547): 609–610.

94. Jones A. Radiation oncogenesis in relation to the treatment of pituitary tumours. Clinical Endocrinology 1991; 35(5): 379–397.

95. Brada M, Ford D, Ashley S, Bliss JM, Crowley S et al. Risk of second brain tumour after conservative surgery and radiotherapy for pituitary adenoma. British Medical Journal 1992; 304(6838): 1343–1346.

96. Tsagarakis S, Grossman A, Plowman PN, Jones AE, Touzel R et al. Megavoltage pituitary irradiation in the management of prolactinomas: long-term follow-up. Clinical Endocrinology 1991; 34(5): 399–406.

97. Holdaway IM, Rajasoorya RC, Gamble GD. Factors influencing mortality in acromegaly. Journal of Clinical Endocrinology and Metabolism 2004; 89(2): 667–674.

98. Jenkins PJ, Fairclough PD, Richards T, Lowe DG, Monson J et al. Acromegaly, colonic polyps and carcinoma. Clinical Endocrinology 1997; 47(1): 17–22.

99. Trainer PJ, Grossman A. The diagnosis and differential diagnosis of Cushing's syndrome. Clinical Endocrinology 1991; 34(4): 317–330.

100. Wiedenmann B, John M, Ahnert-Hilger G, Riecken EO. Molecular and cell biological aspects of neuroendocrine tumors of gastroenteropancreatic system. Journal of Molecular Medicine 1998; 76: 637–647.

101. Pape UF, Jann H, Müller-Nordhorn J, Bockelbrink A, Berndt U et al. Prognostic relevance of a novel TNM classification system for upper gastroenteropancreatic neuroendocrine tumors. Cancer 2008; 113: 256–265.

102. Jann H, Roll S, Couvelard A, Hentic O, Pavel M et al. Neuroendocrine tumors of midgut and hindgut origin: tumor-node-metastasis classification determines clinical outcome. Cancer 2011; 117: 3332–3341.

103. Rindi G, Klöppel G, Ahlmann H et al. TNM staging of foregut (neuro)endocrine tumors: a consensus proposal including a grading system. Virchows Arch 2006; 449: 395–401.

104. Rindi G, Klöppel G, Couvelard A et al. TNM staging of midgut and hindgut (neuro)endocrine tumors: a consensus proposal including a grading system. Virchows Archiv 2007; 451: 757–762.

105. Sobin LH, Gospodarowicz MK, Wittekind C (eds). TNM Classification of Malignant Tumours. West Sussex, Oxford, Hoboken: Wiley & Blackwell, 2009.

106. Yao JC, Hassan M, Phan A et al. One hundred years after 'carcinoid': epidemiology of and prognostic factors for neuroendocrine tumors in 35,825 cases in the United States. Journal of Clinical Oncology 2008; 26: 3063–3072.

107. Pape UF, Berndt U, Muller-Nordhorn J, Bohmig M, Roll S et al. Prognostic factors of long-term outcome in gastroenteropancreatic neuroendocrine tumours. Endocrine Related Cancer 2008; 15: 1083–1097.

108. Heppner C, Kester MB, Agarwal SK et al. Somatic mutation of the MEN1 gene in parathyroid tumors. Nature Genetics 1997; 16: 375–378.

109. Toliat MR, Berger W, Ropers HH, Neuhaus P, Wiedenmann B. Mutations in the MEN 1 gene in sporadic neuroendocrine tumours of the gastroenteropancreatic system. Lancet 1997; 350: 1223.

110. Carney JA. Familial multiple endocrine neoplasia syndromes: components, classification, and nomenclature. Journal of Internal Medicine 1998; 243: 425–432.

111. Chandrasekharappa SC, Manickam P, Guru SC, Marx SJ, Skarulis MC et al. Positional cloning of the gene for multiple endocrine neoplasia-type 1. Science 1997; 276: 404–407.

112. The European Consortium on MEN 1. Identification of the multiple endocrine neoplasia type 1 (MEN 1) gene. Human Molecular Genetics 1976; 6: 1177–1183.

113. Zhuang Z et al. Mutations of the MEN1 tumor suppressor gene in pituitary tumors. Cancer Research 1997; 57: 5446–5451.

114. Capella C, Heitz PU, Höfler H, Solcia E, Klöppel G. Revised classification of neuroendocrine tumors of the lung, pancreas and gut. Digestion 1994; 55: 11–23.

115. Bieligk S, Jaffe BM. Islet cell tumors of the pancreas. Surgical Clinics of North America 1995; 75: 1025–1040.

116. Service FJ, McMahon MM, O'Brien PC, Ballard DJ. Functioning insulinoma—incidence, recurrence and long-term survival of patients: a 60-year study. Mayo Clinical Proceedings 1991; 66: 711–719.

117. Brandi ML. Multiple endocrine neoplasia type I. General features and new insights into etiology. Journal of Endocrinological Investigation 1991; 14: 61–62.

118. Pearce SHS. Multiple endocrine neoplasia type 1 (MEN1): recent advances. Clinical Endocrinology 1997; 47: 513–514.

119. Skogseid B, Eriksson B, Lundqvist G, Lörelius LE, Rastad J et al. Multiple endocrine neoplasia type 1: a 10-year prospective screening study in four kindreds . Journal of Clinical Endocrinology and Metabolism 1991; 73: 281–287.

120. Trump D, Farren B, Wooding C, Pang JT, Besser GM et al. Clinical studies of multiple endocrine neoplasia type 1 (MEN 1). Quarterly Journal of Medicine 1996; 89: 653–669.

121. Wiedenmann B, Jensen RT, Mignon M et al. Preoperative diagnosis and surgical management of neuroendocrine gastroenteropancreatic tumors: general recommendations by a consensus workshop. World Journal of Surgery 1998; 22: 309–318.

122. Gin H, Catargi B, Rigalleau V, Rullier E, Roger P, Tabarin A. Experience with the Biostator for diagnosis and assisted surgery of 21 insulinomas. European Journal of Endocrinology 1998; 139: 371–377.

123. Öberg K. The ultimate biochemical diagnosis of gastroenteropancreatic tumours. Digestion 1996; 1: 45–47.

124. Perry RR, Vinik AI. Clinical review: diagnosis and management of functioning islet cell tumors. Journal of Clinical Endocrinology and Metabolism 1995; 80: 2273–2278.

125. Zimmer T, Ziegler K, Bader M et al. Localisation of neuroendocrine tumours of the upper gastrointestinal tract. Gut 1994; 35: 471–475.

126. Modlin IM, Tang LH. Approaches to the diagnosis of gut neuroendocrine tumors: the last word (today). Gastroenterology 1997; 112: 583–590.

127. John M, Meyerhof W, Richter D, Waser B, Schaer J-C et al. Positive somatostatin receptor scintigraphy correlates with the presence of somatostatin receptor subtype 2 and 5. Gut 1996; 38: 33–39.

128. Krenning EP, Kwekkeboom DJ, Oei HY, de Jong RJ, Dop FJ et al. Somatostatin receptor scintigraphy in carcinoids, gastrinomas and Cushing's syndrome. Digestion 1994; 55: 54–59.

129. Von Eyben FE, Grodum E, Gjessing HJ, Hagen C, Bech Nielsen H. Metabolic remission with octreotide in patients with insulinoma. Journal of Internal Medicine 1994; 235: 245–248.

130. Stehouwer CDA, Lems WF, Fischer HRA, Hackeng WHL, Naafs MAB. Aggravation of hypoglycemia in insulinoma patients by the long-acting somatostatin analogue octreotide (Sandostatin®). Acta Endocrinologica 1989; 121: 34–40.

131. Moertel CG, Hanley JA, Johnson LA. Streptozotocin alone compared with streptozotocin plus fluorouracil in the treatment of advanced islet-cell carcinoma. New England Journal of Medicine 1980; 303: 1189–1194.

132. Moertel CG, Johnson CM, McKusick MA et al. The management of patients with advanced carcinoid tumors and islet cell carcinomas. Annals of Internal Medicine 1994; 120: 302–309.

133. Moertel CG, Lefkopoulo M, Lipsitz S, Hahn RG, Klaassen D. Streptozotocin–doxorubicin, streptozotocin–fluorouracil, or chlorozotocin in the treatment of advanced islet-cell carcinoma. New England Journal of Medicine 1992; 326: 519–523.

134. Marlink RG, Lokich JJ, Robins JR, Clouse ME. Hepatic arterial embolization for metastatic hormone-secreting tumors: technique, effectiveness, and complications. Cancer 1990; 65: 2227–2232.

135. Perry LJ, Stuart K, Stokes KR, Clouse ME. Hepatic arterial chemoembolization for metastatic neuroendocrine tumors. Surgery 1994; 116: 1111–1117.

136. Ruszniewski P, Rougier P, Roche A, Legmann P, Sibert A et al. Hepatic arterial chemoembolisation in patients with liver metastases of endocrine tumors. Cancer 1993; 71: 2624–2630.

137. Chiba T, Yamatani T, Yamaguchi A, Morishita T, Nakamura A et al. Mechanism for increase of gastrin release by secretin in Zollinger–Ellison syndrome. Gastroenterology 1989; 96: 1439–1444.

138. Lamers CBHW. Gastrinoma in multiple endocrine neoplasia type 1. Acta Oncologica 1991; 30: 489–492.

139. Lehy T, Cadiot G, Mignon M, Ruszniewski P, Bonfils S. Influence of multiple endocrine neoplasia type 1 on gastric endocrine cells in patients with the Zollinger–Ellison syndrome. Gut 1992; 33: 1275–1279.

140. Shepherd JJ, Challis DR, Davies PF, McArdle JP, Teh BT, Wilkinson S. Multiple endocrine neoplasm, type 1: gastrinomas, pancreatic neoplasms, microcarcinoids, the Zollinger–Ellison syndrome, lymph nodes, and hepatic metastases. Archives of Surgery 1993; 128: 1133–1142.

141. Öberg K. Neuroendocrine gastrointestinal tumours. Annals of Oncology 1996; 7: 453–463.

142. Scherübl H, Faiss S, Zimmer T, Riecken EO, Wiedenmann B. Neuroendocrine tumors of the gastroenteropancreatic system: diagnostic advances. Onkologie 1996; 19: 119–124.

143. Otte A, Mueller-Brand J, Dellas S, Nitzsche EU, Herrmann R, Maecke HR. Yttrium-90-labelled somatostatin analogue for cancer treatment. Lancet 1998; 351: 417–418.

144. Zimmer T, Stölzel U, Bäder M et al. Brief report: a duodenal gastrinoma in a patient with diarrhea and normal serum gastrin concentrations. New England Journal of Medicine 1995; 333: 634–636.

145. Skogseid B, Oberg K, Eriksson B, Juhlin C, Grandberg D et al. Surgery for asymptomatic pancreatic lesion in multiple endocrine neoplasia type I. World Journal of Surgery 1996; 20: 872–877.

146. Ahlman H, Westberg G, Wangberg B et al. Treatment of liver metastases of carcinoid tumors. World Journal of Surgery 1996; 20: 196–202.

147. Faiss S, Scherübl H, Riecken EO, Wiedenmann B. Drug therapy in metastatic neuroendocrine tumors of the gastroenteropancreatic system. Recent Results in Cancer Research 1996; 142: 193–207.

148. Arnold R, Frank M. Gastrointestinal endocrine tumours: medical management. Baillieres Clinical Gastroenterology 1996; 10: 737–759.

149. O'Dorisio TM, Mekhjian HS. Medical therapy of VIPomas. Endocrinology and Metabolism Clinics of North America 1989; 18: 545–556.

150. Öberg K, Eriksson B. The role of interferons in the management of carcinoid tumors. British Journal of Haematology 1991; 79: 74–77.

151. Tabarin A, Navarranne A, Guérin J, Corcuff JB, Parneix M, Roger P. Use of ketoconazole in the treatment of Cushing's disease and ectopic ACTH syndrome. Clinical Endocrinology 1991; 34: 63–69.

152. Tabarin A, Valli N, Chanson P et al. Usefulness of somatostatin receptor scintigraphy in patients with occult ectopic adrenocorticotropin syndrome. Journal of Clinical Endocrinology and Metabolism 1999; 84: 1193–1202.

153. Kulke MH, Mayer RJ. Carcinoid tumors. New England Journal of Medicine 1999; 340: 858–868.

154. Creutzfeldt W. Carcinoid tumors: development of our knowledge. World Journal of Surgery 1996; 20: 126–131.

155. Modlin IM, Sandor A. An analysis of 8305 cases of carcinoid tumors. Cancer 1997; 79: 813–829.

156. Moertel CG. An Odyssey in the land of small tumors. Journal of Clinical Oncology 1987; 5: 1503–1522.

157. Bax NDS, Woods HF, Batchelor A, Jennings M. Clinical manifestations of carcinoid disease. World Journal of Surgery 1996; 20: 142–146.

158. Wängberg B, Westberg G, Tylen U et al. Survival of patients with disseminated midgut carcinoid tumors after aggressive tumor reduction. World Journal of Surgery 1996; 20: 892–899.

159. Pape UF, Höcker M, Seuß U, Wiedenmann B. New molecular aspects in diagnosis and therapy of neuroendocrine tumors of the gastro-enteropancreatic system. Recent Results in Cancer Research 1999; 153: 45–60.

160. Pape UF, Perren A, Niederle B et al. Management of patients with neuroendocrine neoplasms from the jejuno-ileum and the appendix including goblet cell carcinomas. Neuroendocrinology 2012; 95: 135–156.

161. McEntee GP, Nagorney DM, Kvols LK, Moertel CG, Grant CS. Cytoreductive hepatic surgery for neuroendocrine tumors. Surgery 1990: 108: 1091–1096.

162. Que FG, Nagorney DM, Batts KP, Linz LJ, Kvols LK. Hepatic resection for metastatic neuroendocrine carcinomas. American Journal of Surgery 1995; 169: 36–43.

163. Soreide O, Berstad T, Bakka A et al. Surgical treatment as a principle in patients with advanced abdominal carcinoid tumors. Surgery 1992; 111: 48–54.

164. Arnold R, Trautmann ME, Creutzfeldt W, Benning R, Benning M et al. Somatostatin analogue octreotide and inhibition of tumour growth in metastatic endocrine gastroenteropancreatic tumours. Gut 1996; 38: 430–438.

165. Faiss S, Rath U, Mansmann U et al. Ultra-high-dose lanreotide treatment in patients with metastatic neuroendocrine gastroenteropancreatic tumors. Digestion 1999; 60: 469–476.

166. Kvols LK, Moertel CG, O'Connell MJ, Schutt AK, Rubin J, Hahn RG. Treatment of the malignant carcinoid syndrome. Evaluation of a long-acting somatostatin analogue. New England Journal of Medicine 1986; 315: 663–666.

167. Engström PF, Lavin PT, Moertel CG, Folsch E, Douglass HO. Streptozotocin plus fluorouracil versus doxorubicin therapy for metastatic carcinoid tumors. Journal of Clinical Oncology 1984; 2: 1255–1259.

168. Stridsberg M, Öberg K, Li Q, Engström U, Lundquist G. Measurements of chromogranin A, chromogranin B (secretogranin I), chromogranin C (secretogranin II) and pancreastatin in plasma and urine from patients with carcinoid tumors and endocrine pancreatic tumors. Journal of Endocrinology 1995; 144: 45–59.

169. Kwekkeboom DJ, Krenning EP. Somatostatin receptor scintigraphy in patients with carcinoid tumors. World Journal of Surgery 1996; 20: 157–161.

170. Norton JA, Sugarbaker PH, Doppman JL et al. Aggressive resection of metastatic disease in selected patients with malignant gastrinoma. Annals of Surgery 1986; 203: 352–359.

171. Bechstein WO, Neuhaus P. Liver transplantation for hepatic metastases of neuroendocrine tumors. Annals of the New York Academy of Sciences 1994; 733: 507–514.

172. Dousset B, Saint-Marc O, Pitre J, Soubrane O, Houssin D, Chapuis Y. Metastatic endocrine tumors: medical treatment, surgical resection, or liver transplantation. World Journal of Surgery 1996; 20: 908–915.

173. Makowka L, Tzakis AG, Mazzaferro V et al. Transplantation of the liver for metastatic endocrine tumors of the intestine and pancreas. Surgery, Gynecology and Obstetrics 1989; 168: 107–110.

174. O'Toole D, Grossman A, Gross D et al. ENETS Consensus Guidelines for the standards of care in neuroendocrine tumors: biochemical markers. Neuroendocrinology 2009; 90: 194–202.

175. Delle Fave G, Kwekkeboom DJ, Van Cutsem E et al. ENETS Consensus Guidelines for the management of patients with gastroduodenal neoplasms. Neuroendocrinology 2012; 95: 74–87.

176. Caplin M, Sundin A, Nillson O et al. ENETS Consensus Guidelines for the management of patients with digestive neuroendocrine neoplasms: colorectal neuroendocrine neoplasms. Neuroendocrinology 2012; 95: 88–97.

177. Jensen RT, Cadiot G, Brandi ML, de Herder WW, Kaltsas G et al. ENETS Consensus Guidelines for the management of patients with digestive neuroendocrine neoplasms: functional pancreatic endocrine tumor syndromes. Neuroendocrinology 2012; 95: 98–119.

178. Falconi M, Bartsch DK, Eriksson B, Klöppel G, Lopes JM et al. Neuroendocrine neoplasms of the digestive system. Pancreatic non-functioning neoplasms. Neuroendocrinology 2012; 95: 120–134.

179. Pavel M, Baudin E, Couvelard A et al. ENETS Consensus Guidelines for the management of patients with liver and other distant metastases from neuroendocrine neoplasms of foregut, midgut, hindgut, and unknown primary. Neuroendocrinology 2012; 95: 157–176.

180. Kvols LK, Reubi JC. Metastatic carcinoid tumors and the malignant carcinoid syndrome. Acta Oncologica 1993; 32: 197–201.

181. Schally AV. Oncological applications of somatostatin analogs. Cancer Research 1998; 48: 6977–6985.

182. King J, Quinn R, Glenn D et al. Radioembolization with selective internal radiation microspheres for neuroendocrine liver metastases. Cancer 2008; 113: 921–929.

183. Caplin ME, Pavel M, Ćwikła JB et al. Lanreotide in metastatic enteropancreatic neuroendocrine tumors. New England Journal of Medicine 2014; 371: 224–233.

184. Caplin ME, Rusziewski PB, Pavel ME et al. Progression-free survival (PFS) with lanreotide autogel/depot (LAN) in enteropancreatic NETs patients: the CLARINET extension study. Journal of Clinical Oncology 2014; 32: 5s (suppl; abstr 4107).

185. Öberg K, Eriksson B, Janson ET. The clinical use of interferons in the management of neuroendocrine gastroenteropancreatic tumors. Annals of the New York Academy of Sciences 1994; 733: 471–478.

186. Öberg K, Funa K, Alm G. Effects of leucocyte interferon on clinical symptoms and hormone levels in patients with mid-gut carcinoid tumors and carcinoid syndrome. New England Journal of Medicine 1983; 309: 129–133.

187. Joensuu H, Kumpulainen E, Gröhn P. Treatment of metastatic carcinoid tumour with recombinant interferon alfa. European Journal of Cancer 1992; 28A: 1650–1653.

188. Janson ET, Ahlström H, Andersson T, Öberg KE. Octreotide and interferon alfa: a new combination for the treatment of malignant carcinoid tumours. European Journal of Cancer 1992; 28A: 1647–1650.

189. Janson ET et al. Treatment with alpha-interferon versus alpha-interferon in combination with streptozotocin and doxorubicin in patients with malignant carcinoid tumors: a randomized trial. Annals of Oncology 1992; 3: 635–638.

190. Joensuu H, Kätkä K, Kujari H. Dramatic response of a metastatic carcinoid tumour to a combination of interferon and octreotide. Acta Endocrinologica 1992; 126: 184–185.

191. Faiss S, Pape UF, Böhmig M, Dörffel Y, Mansmann U et al. Prospective, randomized, multicenter trial on the antiproliferative effect of lanreotide, interferon-alfa, and their combination for therapy of metastatic neuroendocrine gastroenteropancreatic tumors—the International Lanreotide and Interferon Alfa Study Group. Journal of Clinical Oncology 2003; 21: 2689–2696.

192. Yao J, Shah MH, Ito T et al. Everolimus for advanced pancreatic neuroendocrine tumors. New England Journal of Medicine 2011; 364: 514–523.

193. Pavel ME, Hainsworth JD, Baudin E et al. Everolimus plus octreotide long-acting repeatable for the treatment of advanced neuroendocrine tumours associated with carcinoid syndrome (RADIANT-2): a randomised, placebo-controlled, phase 3 study. Lancet 2011; 378: 2005–2012.

194. Raymond E, Dahan L, Raoul JL, Bang YJ, Borbath I et al. Sunitinib malate for the treatment of pancreatic neuroendocrine tumors. New England Journal of Medicine 2011; 364: 501–513.

195. Yao J, Phan A, Hoff PM et al. Targeting vascular endothelial growth factor in advanced carcinoid tumor: a random assignment phase II study of depot octreotide with bevacizumab and pegylated interferon alfa-2b. Journal of Clinical Oncology 2008; 26: 1316–1323.

196. Hobday TJ, Qin R, Reidy-Lagunes D et al. Multicenter phase II trial of temsirolimus and bevacizumab in pancreatic neuroendocrine tumors. Journal of Clinical Oncology 2015; 33: 1551–1556.

197. Moertel CG, Kvols LK, O'Connell MJ, Rubin J. Treatment of neuroendocrine carcinomas with combined etoposide and cisplatin. Cancer 1991; 68: 227–232.

198. Dilz LM, Denecke T, Steffen IG et al. Streptozocin/5-fluorouracil chemotherapy is associated with durable response in patients with advanced pancreatic neuroendocrine tumours. European Journal of Cancer 2015; 51: 1253–1262.

199. Strosberg JR, Fine RL, Choi J, Nasir A, Coppola D et al. First-line chemotherapy with capecitabine and temozolomide in patients with metastatic pancreatic endocrine carcinomas. Cancer 2011; 117: 268–275.

200. Bajetta E, Catena L, Procopio G et al. Are capecitabine and oxaliplatin (XELOX) suitable treatments for progressing low-grade and high-grade neuroendocrine tumours? Cancer Chemotherapy and Pharmacology 2007; 59: 637–642.

201. Welin S, Sorbye H, Sebjornsen S et al. Clinical effect of temozolomide-based chemotherapy in poorly differentiated endocrine carcinoma after progression on first-line chemotherapy. Cancer 2011; 117: 4617–4622.

202. Kwekkeboom DJ, de Herder WW, Kam BL et al. Treatment with the radiolabeled somatostatin analog [177Lu-DOTA0,Tyr3] octreotate: toxicity, efficacy, and survival. Journal of Clinical Oncology 2008; 26: 2124–2130.

203. Ezziddin S, Opitz M, Attassi M et al. Impact of the Ki-67 proliferation index on response to peptide receptor radionuclide therapy. European Journal of Nuclear Medicine and Molecular Imaging 2011; 38: 459–466.

204. Bushnell DL Jr, O'Dorisio TM, O'Dorisio MS et al. 90Y-Edotreotide for metastatic carcinoid refractory to octreotide. Journal of Clinical Oncology 2010; 28: 1652–1659.

205. Imhof A, Brunner P, Marincek N et al. Response, survival, and long-term toxicity after therapy with the radiolabeled somatostatin analogue [90Y-DOTA]-TOC in metastasized neuroendocrine cancers. Journal of Clinical Oncology 2011; 29: 2416–2423.

206. Møller JE, Pellikka PA, Bernheim AM et al. Prognosis of carcinoid heart disease: analysis of 200 cases over two decades. Circulation 2005; 112: 3320–3327.

207. Krenning EP, Kooij PP, Bakker WH et al. Radiotherapy with a radiolabeled somatostatin analogue, [111In-DTPA-D-Phe1]-octreotide: a case history. Annals of the New York Academy of Sciences 1994; 733: 496–506.

208. Krenning EP, de Jong M, Kooij PP, Breeman WA, Bakker WH et al. Somatostatin receptor: scintigraphy and radionuclide therapy. Digestion 1996; 57: 57–61.

209. Laule M, Pschowski R, Pape UF, Pavel M, Stangl V, Baumann G, Wiedenmann B, Stangl K. Staged catheter-based valve treatment of severe carcinoid heart disease. Neuroendocrinology. doi:10.1159/000437167 [Epub ahead of print].

210. Pavel M, Hörsch D, Caplin M et al. Telotristat etiprate for carcinoid syndrome: a single-arm, multicenter trial. Journal of Clinical Endocrinology and Metabolism 2015; 100: 1511–1519.

211. Kvols LK, Oberg KE, O'Dorisio TM et al. Pasireotide (SOM230) shows efficacy and tolerability in the treatment of patients with advanced neuroendocrine tumors refractory or resistant to octreotide LAR: results from a phase II study. Endocrine-Related Cancer 2012; 19: 657–666.

212. Grande E, Capdevila J, Castellano D et al. Pazopanib in pretreated advanced neuroendocrine tumors: a phase II, open-label trial of the Spanish Task Force Group for Neuroendocrine Tumors (GETNE). Annals of Oncology 2015 (10 June); pii: mdv252 [Epub ahead of print]. PMID: 26063633. doi: 10.1093/annonc/mdv252.

213. Bilchik AJ, Saranton T, Foshag LJ, Giuliano AE, Ramming KP. Cryosurgical palliation of metastatic neuroendocrine tumors resistant to conventional therapy. Surgery 1997; 122: 1040–1048.

214. Klimstra DS, Arnold R, Capella C et al. Neuroendocrine neoplasms of the pancreas. In Bosman FT, Carneiro F, Hruban RH, Theise ND eds, WHO Classification of Tumours of the Digestive System. Lyon: IARC, 2010, 322–326.

215. Klimstra DS, Arnold R, Capella C et al. Neuroendocrine neoplasms of the colon and the rectum. In Bosman FT, Carneiro F, Hruban RH, Theise ND eds, WHO Classification of Tumours of the Digestive System. Lyon: IARC, 2010, 174–177.

216. Capella C, Arnold R, Klimstra DS et al. Neuroendocrine neoplasms of the small intestine. In Bosman FT, Carneiro F, Hruban RH, Theise ND eds, WHO Classification of Tumours of the Digestive System. Lyon: IARC, 2010, 102–107.

CHAPTER 59

Cancer of unknown primary site

Nicholas Pavlidis and George Pentheroudakis

Introduction to cancer of unknown primary

Cancer of unknown primary (CUP) is considered to be a neglected and orphan disease, refractory to standard chemotherapy and of a short survival in the majority of cases. In general, both diagnostic and therapeutic approaches for these patients remain a real dilemma for practising oncologists and a continuum issue for the health care system. Clinical, translational, and basic research is still a challenge for several specialized centres worldwide. For optimal diagnosis and treatment, CUP multidisciplinary teams should be established in major referral hospitals. Today, evidence-based guidelines are of paramount importance for the optimal management of these patients and for health economic policies.

CUP represents a heterogeneous group of histologically-confirmed metastatic malignancies for which a thorough medical history and a careful physical examination along with an extensive diagnostic workup fail to detect the primary site. These tests consist of full blood count, biochemistry tests, urinalysis, stool occult blood testing, specific immunohistochemistry, imaging technology (chest X-ray, computed tomography (CT) of the thorax, abdomen and pelvis, mammography and positron emission tomography (PET) in some cases) [1, 2]. Although molecular technology with multigene profiling platforms offers high sensitivity in detecting the primary site, their use in daily practice has not yet been introduced [3].

According to NICE (National Institute for Health and Clinical Experience) the definition of CUP is divided into: (a) malignancy of undefined primary origin (before comprehensive investigation); (b) provisional carcinoma of unknown primary (before specialist review and further specialized investigations); and (c) confirmed carcinoma of CUP (no detection of primary despite (a) and (b) investigations) [4].

Epidemiology

The median age at presentation is 65 years and males are affected more commonly than females. In general, CUP accounts for 2.3–4.2% of all human malignancies and it represents the seventh to eighth most common cancer and the fourth most frequent cause of death [1, 2]. The annual age-adjusted incidence per 100 000 population in the US is 7–12 cases, in Australia 18–19 cases, and in The Netherlands 5.3–6.7 cases (Table 59.1). CUP represents approximately 40 000 new cases per year in the US and 2500 in The Netherlands [5–7].

CUP is not very well-defined as a discrete classification within the International Classification of Disease (ICD) nomenclature. The ICD codes used for CUP registrations are ICD C77–C80 [8].

Recent data from the Sweden Family Cancer Database suggest that the cause of death in CUP patients frequently matched the cancer diagnosed in a family member, implying that the metastasis had probably undergone a phenotypic change of the primary cancer. The strongest data were correlated with lung, kidney, liver, and ovarian cancers, although independent significant association was also found with other malignancies such as colorectal, pancreatic, breast, and prostate cancer [9].

An increased risk of subsequent cancers in CUP patients has been reported in both Swedish and Swiss cancer databases, ranging from 1.4–1.69 (standardized incidence ratio). Significant excess risks were observed for cancer of prostate, oral cavity, pharynx, and skin [10–12].

Biologically, CUP follows a process of type 2 progression (a malignant clone to begin with) and not of a type 1 (from a premalignant lesion to malignant lesion) [13].

CUP patients carry a unique natural history which is not similar to patients diagnosed with known primary cancers. It is characterized by an early dissemination (50% of CUP patients present with multiple sites of metastases), a short history of symptoms and signs related to metastatic lesions, an aggressive behaviour, and an unpredictable metastatic pattern. The unpredictable metastatic pattern refers to the differences in the incidence of metastatic sites at diagnosis, between known and unknown primary tumours. Pancreatic cancer presenting as CUP has a four- to five-fold higher

Table 59.1 Incidence of CUP worldwide

Country	Incidence %
Switzerland	2.3
USA	2.3
Finland	2.5
UK	2.6
Japan	3.0
Russia	3.6
Netherlands	4.0
Australia	4.2

Source: data from Muir C, Cancer of unknown primary site, *Cancer*, Volume 75, Supplement 1, pp. 353–356, Copyright © 1995 American Cancer Society; van de Wonw AJ et al., Epidemiology of unknown primary tumors: Incidence and population—based survival of 1285 patients in Southeast Netherlands, 1984–1992, *European Journal of Cancer*, Volume 38, Issue 3, pp. 409–413, Copyright © 2002 Elsevier Science Ltd; and Coates M, and Armstrong B, New South Wales Central Cancer Registry, *Cancer in New South Wales, Incidence and Mortality*, Cancer Council, NSW, Australia, Copyright © 1995.

incidence of presenting with bone and lung involvement as compared to known primary pancreatic tumours [1, 2].

Molecular biology

Chromosomal instability, oncogenes, and oncoproteins

Aneuploidy is seen in 70–90% of solid tumours and probably reflects derangements of chromosomal replication during cell division. Hedley et al. established aneuploidy in 70% of 152 CUP, without any relationship to patterns of metastatic involvement or survival [14]. Abnormalities of the short arm of chromosome 1 (1p) were reported in 12 of 13 CUP, a finding consistent with the common occurrence of 1p structural alterations in advanced solid tumours [15].

Oncogenes are overexpressed or amplified in many solid tumours. The encoded proteins favour malignant transformation and survival by activating cellular proliferation, inducing cell migration, inhibiting apoptosis, and promoting neoangiogenesis. C-Myc, Ras, and human epidermal growth factor receptor (EGFR) (HER)-2 proteins were studied by immunohistochemistry (IHC) in 26 cases of CUP and were over-expressed in less than a third of cases for any of the studied proteins [16]. Hainsworth et al. examined 100 CUP and similarly observed HER-2 overexpression in 11% of specimens, with no differences in overall survival (OS) between patients with overexpressing and non-overexpressing HER-2 tumours [17]. Fizazi et al. found HER-2 IHC overexpression in only two of 56 CUP cases (4%); with no association of HER-2 status with histological differentiation, treatment activity, or clinical outcome [18]. Rashid et al. reported HER-2 IHC expression in 68% and overexpression in 24% of 76 cases of CUP [19]. Van de Wouw et al. also observed IHC HER2 overexpression in 16 of 45 CUP cases (35%) [20].

EGFR is a transmembrane protein that recently came under scrutiny after accumulating knowledge of its role in malignant transformation. Fizazi et al. reported IHC EGFR protein overexpression in two of 56 CUP specimens (4%), whereas Rashid et al. reported it in 46 of 76 CUP samples (61%) [18, 19]. These discrepant results serve to emphasize the heterogeneity of this group of tumours. Both studies, however, failed to establish any correlation between EGFR protein staining and clinicopathological parameters or prognosis. Dova et al. studied 50 patients with CUP and found EGFR protein expression in 74% of tumours (12% with overexpression) with no prognostic utility and with absence of activating mutations in exons 18, 19, 21 [21].

In IHC studies, Fizazi et al. reported c-Kit protein overexpression in six of 56 CUP samples (11%), while Rashid et al. reported it in three of 76 cases (4%) [18, 19]. Dova et al. screened 50 CUP specimens and found c-Kit protein overexpression in 13%. Moreover, we observed no activating mutations in exon 11 of the c-kit and exons 12 and 18 of the PDGFR genes by means of PCR-single strand conformational polymorphism (SSCP) [21, 22]. In all studies, c-Kit protein expression failed to demonstrate prognostic utility for response to therapy or survival.

MET is a transmembrane receptor that is activated upon binding of hepatocyte growth factor and has been incriminated in relaying survival signals to the interior of cancer cell upon therapeutic blockade of other receptors such as EGFR and HER2. Recently, Stella et al. screened 23 patients with CUP and reported presence of activating mutations in eight tumours (30%) [23]. The CUP mutation rate of MET (30%) is strikingly higher than that reported for other known primary tumours (4%).

Tumour- and metastasis-suppressor genes and proteins

Tumour-suppressor genes encode proteins that suppress malignant transformation, survival, and metastatic dissemination by maintaining the integrity of cellular DNA and by controlling vital cell cycle processes, with the 'guardian of the genome', p53, being the most investigated. Briasoulis et al. studied IHC p53 expression in 47 patients with CUP and found strong immunoreactivity in 24 (53%) suggesting accumulation of a mutated, abnormally stable protein [24]. The expression of p53 protein by itself had no prognostic value for treatment benefit or survival. Van de Wouw et al. found no prognostic value of IHC p53 detection, present in 23 of 48 tumours [48%] in a relatively large series of CUP patients from the Netherlands, whereas Bar-Eli et al. reported p53 exon 5–9 gene mutations in 6/15 CUP (26%) [20, 25].

Metastasis-suppressor genes have been recently recognized as genes that modulate the capability of the malignant clone for systemic dissemination without affecting the primary tumour malignant transformation process. Loss of function of the metastasis-suppressor KiSS-1 was seen in several human malignancies and was correlated with advanced stage and poor prognosis. Dova et al. screened 50 cases of CUP for KiSS-1 gene mutations by PCR-SSCP and direct sequencing and found only one mutated sample (242C>G resulting in P81R) [26].

Angiogenesis and hypoxic phenotype

Hillen et al. reported that tumour microvessel density was an adverse prognostic factor for outcome in 39 patients with liver metastases of unknown primary [27]. In a more recent study, van de Wouw et al. found no prognostic value of IHC CD34 (a microvessel density marker) and VEGF-A IHC detection (26%) for the outcome of 46 patients with CUP [20]. Karavasilis et al. studied the expression of VEGF-A, the main protein mediating angiogenesis, and thrombospondin-1 (TSP-1), an inhibitor of vessel formation, in 81 patients with CUP [28, 29]. Strong expression of VEGF and its inhibitor, TSP-1, was seen 83% and 20% of tumours, respectively. Rashid et al. recently observed VEGF expression by IHC in half of 75 CUP [19]. Despite reliance on neoplastic vessels, tumours are relatively hypoxic compared to normal tissues. Recently, Koo et al. reported a hypoxic phenotype, defined by IHC expression of Hypoxia-Inducible Factor 1a (HIF1a), Glucose Transporter 1 (GLUT1), and COX2, in 25% of 69 patients with CUP tumours [30]. In those patients, the tumoural hypoxic phenotype was significantly associated with worse survival.

Collectively, these data draw the picture of a highly-active angiogenic profile of CUP metastases. Although these features are not different from those seen in several advanced malignancies of known primary site, they provide a sound basis for implementation of therapies modulating angiogenesis.

Pharmacogenomics and circulating tumour cells

Pentheroudakis et al. studied the presence of circulating tumour cells (CTC) in 24 patients with CUP by immunofluorescent detection of cytokeratins CK 8, 18, 19, leukocyte antigen CD45, and nuclear antigen DAPI [31]. CTC were observed in 15 out of 24 (62.5%) evaluable patients (median 1 CTC/million peripheral blood mononuclear cell (PBMNC), range 0–20), while nine had no detectable CTC. The presence and number of CTCs at various cut-offs had no prognostic utility for OS or progression-free survival (log rank p > 0.05).

Souglakos et al. extracted mRNA from 62 paraffin-embedded CUP tumours and applied qRTPCR in order to study the transcription of DNA-repair, hypoxia, and cell-cycle control genes [32]. Among ten studied genes, the DNA repair gene ERCC1, the angiogenesis regulator TXR1, and the hypoxic factor HIF1a were significantly associated with patient outcome, though not with response to chemotherapeutic agents.

The cancer of unknown primary site genetic signature hypothesis

What does one mean by the term 'genuine' CUP? This refers to the possibility that a CUP tumour may possess not only a genetic signature specific for the primary site (since it unavoidably did originate somewhere in the body) but also a second genetic signature that is primary-independent, pro-metastatic, and possibly CUP-specific. This CUP multigene expression signature may be responsible for the early spread of the malignant clone to metastatic sites, regression of the primary, and distinct natural history from other common tumours and fulminant course of the disease. Whether there is a 'core' CUP signature common in all CUP tumours remains to be seen.

Overall, the search for a molecular CUP signature relied on rather random studies of single genes or proteins and did not disclose presence of a molecular trait that is a consistent CUP characteristic (Table 59.2). It is very likely that the CUP signature is complex and multigene, in which case multiplex or genome-wide expression profiling platforms should be utilized in order to identify it. In addition to genes being transcribed to messenger RNA, the complex mosaic of microRNAs, 20-nucleotide short RNA segments which regulate the translation of mRNA, is an additional layer of complexity worth investigating [33].

Pathology

Histologically, CUP is categorized into four major types. The most common type is adenocarcinoma of well- to moderate-differentiation (50%), followed by poorly or undifferentiated adenocarcinomas (30%), squamous cell carcinoma (15%), and undifferentiated neoplasms (5%). With modern immunohistochemistry undifferentiated neoplasms can be better characterized as non-specified carcinomas, neuroendocrine tumours, lymphomas, germ-cell tumours, melanomas, and sarcomas, or embryonal malignancies (Table 59.3) [1, 2].

The main diagnostic goal in CUP patients is to identify the primary site. The tools for this investigation include diagnostic pathology with specific immunohistochemistry, molecular technology, imaging technology, endoscopic workup, and occasional serum tumour markers. Molecular technology with gene profiling assays is not in routine use due to high cost and doubtful contribution to patients' outcome.

Light microscopy

Light microscopic examination, using routine staining with haematoxylin and eosin or other staining, i.e., mucicarmine, Alcian Blue, or periodic acid-Schiff, is only able to characterize cell morphology

Table 59.2 Selected publications of molecular aberrations reported in CUP

Investigator	Method	No of CUP	Molecular aberration
Hedley	Karyotypic analysis	152	Aneuploidy in 70%
Hainsworth	IHC	100	HER2 overexpression in 11%
Rashid	IHC	76	HER2 overexpression in 24%
Dova	IHC	50	EGFR overexpression in 12%
	PCR		No EGFR gene amplification nor activating mutations
Dova	IHC	50	cKIT overexpression in 13%
	PCR		No cKIT or PDGFR activating mutations
Stella	PCR	23	MET activating mutations in 30%
Van de Wou	IHC	48	p53 overexpression in 48%
Karavasilis	IHC	75	VEGF-A overexpression in 83%
			TSP1 overexpression in 20%
			MMP2 overexpression in 49%
			MMP9 overexpression in 36%
Koo	IHC	69	Hypoxic phenotype (HIF1a/GLUT1/COX2 +) in 25%
Pentheroudakis	IF	24	CTC present in 62%
Souglakos	PCR	62	Prognostic significance for ERCC1, TXR1, HIF1a mRNA

and tumour differentiation, but it is unsuccessful in identifying the primary site.

Immunohistochemistry

Immunohistochemical investigations by using a series of monoclonal or polyclonal antibodies against several structural tissue components are very useful in identifying the tumour origin in

Table 59.3 Histological classification of CUP with the ICD-0 morphology code

Adenocarcinoma (M8140/3)	
◆ Well to moderately differentiated	50%
◆ Poorly differentiated or undifferentiated	30%
Squamous cell carcinoma (M8070/3)	15%
Undifferentiated neoplasms	5%
◆ Non-specified carcinoma	
◆ Neuroendocrine tumours (M8246/3)	
◆ Lymphomas (M9590/3)	
◆ Germ cell tumours (M 9064/3O)	
◆ Melanomas (M 8720/3)	
◆ Sarcomas (M 8800/3)	
◆ Embryonal malignancies (M 9070/3)	

Table 59.4 An immunohistochemistry algorithm for CUP diagnosis

Step 1 (detects broad types of cancer)

Tumour type	Immunoperoxidase stains
Carcinoma	Pan-Cytokeratin, EMA
Lymphoma	CLA, (CD45RB), EMA (±)
Sarcoma	Vimentin, desmin, S100, alpha-smooth muscle actin, myoD1, CD34, c-kit, CD99
Melanoma	S100, HMB45, Melan-A

Step 2 (detects broad types of carcinoma)

Carcinoma type	
Adenocarcinoma	Light microscopy, PAS, CK7, CK20
Squamous cell carcinoma	CK5/6, p63
Neuroendocrine carcinoma	Chromogranin, synaptophysin, PG9.5, CD56
Germ-cell carcinoma	PLAP, OCT4, AFP, HCG

Step 3 (detects origin of adenocarcinoma)

Adenocarcinoma type	
Breast cancer	ER, GCDFP-15, mamaglobulin, CK7+/CK20-
Ovarian cancer	CA125, mesothelin, WT1, ER, CK7+/CK20-
Endometrial cancer	CK7+/CK20-, CA125, ER
Prostate Cancer	PSA, PAP, CK7-/CK20-
Colon cancer	CDX2, CEA, CK7-/CK20+
Pancreatic cancer	CK7+/CK20±, CA 125, mesothelin
Liver cancer	Hepar-1, AFP, polyclonal CEA, CD10, CD13
Lung cancer	TTF1, CK7+/CK20-
Kidney cancer	CD10, CK7-/CK20-
Thyroid cancer	TTF1, thyroglobulin

Reprinted from *Seminars in Oncology*, Volume 36, Issue 1, Oien KA, Pathologic evaluation of unknown primary cancer, pp. 8–37, Copyright © 2009 Elsevier Inc., with permission from Elsevier, <http://www.sciencedirect.com/science/journal/00937754>.

metastatic adenocarcinomas or poorly differentiated carcinomas. Antibodies against cytokeratins, and especially against CK7 and CK 20, have opened up a helpful diagnostic avenue (Table 59.4) [34, 35].

Chromosomal diagnosis

The detection of chromosomal abnormalities could be helpful in specific cases as in germ cell CUP (detection of an isochromosome of the short arm of chromosome 12i (12p) or a deletion in 12p), peripheral neuroectodermal tumours, or in Ewing's sarcomas (translocation t [11, 22] [q 24; q 12] [36, 37].

Diagnostic investigations

Imaging

Computed tomography

The sensitivity of whole-body CT-scans to detect a primary site is around 30–35%, recognizing that small lesions can be missed by CTs. CT scans are also used for CUP staging [38].

Magnetic resonance imaging

MRI is very useful in identifying mainly occult breast primary tumours. Its sensitivity could be as high as 60% [39].

[111]In Octreoscan

This is useful in detecting neuroendocrine CUP tumours expressing enhanced somatostatin receptors [40].

Mammography

Mammography is used to detect breast primary sites in women with isolated axillary lymph node involvement by an adenocarcinoma. However, its sensitivity is not as high as MRI of the breast [41].

FDG-PET/CT-scan

FDG-PET/CT scans have proven to be useful in CUP patients for the detection of primary site [42, 43]. In a recent meta-analysis, in a total sample size of 433 patients, the overall primary tumour detection rate, pooled sensitivity, and specificity of FDG-PET/CT scans were 37%, 84%, and 84%, respectively. The most common primaries discovered are those of head, neck, and lung [44]. NICE UK recommendations offer 'FDG-PET/CT scan for CUP patients presenting with cervical lymphadenopathy with no primary tumour identified on ear, nose and throat panendoscopy, if radical treatment is considered to be an option' [4].

Endoscopy

Endoscopic investigations should be limited to CUP patients with particular symptoms or signs, i.e., bronchoscopy in patients with haemoptysis or cough and negative imaging studies, or colonoscopy in patients with constipation, diarrhoea or overt blood loss. Extensive endoscopic evaluation in the absence of clinical or laboratory findings should be avoided, since sensitivity is extremely low [1, 2].

Serum tumour markers

Measurement of serum tumour markers has no diagnostic, prognostic, or predictive value in CUP patients.

Routine evaluation of epithelial serum tumour markers (CEA, CA 15-3, CA 19-9, and CA 125) might show non-specific overexpression, since almost 70% of patients express more than two markers in their serum.

However, some serum markers could be helpful in certain clinicopathological subsets, i.e., AFP or β-HCG in poorly-differentiated carcinomas with midline distribution, PSA in men with unique osteoblastic metastases, CA 125 in primary peritoneal adenocarcinoma, or CA 15-3 in women with isolated axillary nodal adenocarcinoma [45].

Multidisciplinary management of clinicopathological subsets

CUP is a heterogeneous group of diseases that is classified as favourable, specific, or good prognosis subsets and unfavourable, non-specific, or poor prognosis subsets. This classification is based on age, sex, histopathology, clinical presentation, and organ or tissue involvement. This classification offers great help to the practising oncologist for both diagnostic and therapeutic management and provides at the same time prognostic and predictive value (Table 59.5) [1, 2].

Prognostic and predictive factors

Several prognostic factors have been reported for patients diagnosed with CUP. From various multivariate analyses, significant

Table 59.5 Clinicopathological subsets and patients

Favourable or specific CUP subsets	Unfavourable or non-specific CUP subsets
Women with serous-papillary adenocarcinoma of peritoneal cavity	Adenocarcinoma metastatic to the liver or other organ
Women with adenocarcinoma involving only axillary lymph nodes	Malignant ascites from a non-papillary adenocarcinoma
Poorly-differentiated carcinoma with midline distribution	Multiple cerebral metastases from adenocarcinoma or squamous cell carcinoma
Squamous cell carcinoma involving cervical lymph nodes	Multiple lung or pleural metastases from adenocarcinoma
Neuroendocrine carcinoma of unknown primary	Multiple metastatic bone disease from an adenocarcinoma without a serum PSA elevation.
Adenocarcinoma with a colon-cancer profile	Squamous-cell carcinoma of the abdominal cavity
Men with blastic bone metastases and elevated serum PSA levels	
Patients with limited disease	
Melanoma of unknown primary with localized nodal disease	

Reprinted from *Critical Reviews in Oncology/Hematology*, Volume 69, Issue 3, Pavlidis N and Fizazi K, Carcinoma of unknown primary (CUP), pp. 271–279, Copyright © 2009 Published by Elsevier Ireland Ltd., with permission from Elsevier, <http://www.sciencedirect.com/science/journal/10408428>.

adverse prognostic indicators related to histology, clinical picture or serum markers have been identified. Among them, these factors are male sex, age >64, PS >1, number of metastatic sites, liver metastases, poorly-differentiated histology, weight loss, lymphopaenia, leukocytosis, elevated serum LDH, elevated alkaline phosphatase levels, and low albumin levels [46, 47].

Classification of clinicopathological subsets

Women with serous papillary adenocarcinoma of the peritoneal cavity

This subset is also called primary peritoneal adenocarcinoma and accounts for 7–20% of all pelvic or peritoneal serous papillary cancers. It seems to affect women three to seven years older than ovarian carcinoma patients, with a median age of 55–65 years.

The clinical manifestation of this disease is similar to stage III or IV ovarian cancer patients. The main symptoms and signs are abdominal pain and distention, ascites, and palpable masses. Signs of constipation with intestinal obstruction are more commonly seen in late stages. The disease is predominantly located in the peritoneal, mesenteric, omental, and ovarian surfaces as well as in pelvic and retroperitoneal nodes. Visceral organs are involved in less than 15% of the cases.

Serum CA 125 is a useful tumour marker since it is elevated in up to 90% of patients. Histopathologically, these are serous papillary adenocarcinomas, with or without psammoma bodies. Almost half of these patients are diagnosed with poorly-differentiated tumours. Immunohistochemistry is positive for pancytokeratins, CK7, epithelial membrane antigen, CA 125, B 72.3, ER, mesothelin, and WT 1 [48].

Women with isolated axillary nodal metastases from adenocarcinoma

This CUP subset affects women with a mean age of 52 years, most commonly postmenopausal. A quarter of these patients have a positive family history for malignancy. They present with axillary lymphadenopathy of either N1 (48%) or N2-3 disease (52%).

The detection of an occult primary tumour in the breast can be achieved by MRI or mastectomy in 60% and 70% of cases, respectively. Ductal carcinomas are the most common histology (83%) with a good to moderate differentiation in the majority of the patients. Oestrogen and progesterone receptors are expressed in around 40%, while HER 2 is overexpressed in 30% [49].

Poorly-differentiated carcinoma with midline distribution

This is a predominantly male disease occurring at a median age of 56 years. It presents with nodal involvement of midline distribution affecting mainly mediastinal, retroperitoneal, or supraclavicular lymph nodes. In some cases, peripheral nodes, lung, or pleural metastatic lesions can also be observed. These tumours are relatively aggressive with rapid growth. Elevated alpha-fetoprotein and β-chorionic gonadotropin levels are found in less than 20% of the patients.

Histologically, these tumours are characterized as poorly differentiated or undifferentiated carcinomas without the expression of any specific immunoperoxidase staining, apart from the presence of an i(12p) chromosomal abnormality-favouring germ cell tumour in some patients [50].

Squamous cell carcinoma involving cervical lymph nodes

This subset represents 5% of patients and affects middle-aged or elderly mainly male patients with a strong history of tobacco and alcohol abuse. Clinical presentation is characterized by unilateral enlargement of upper or middle cervical lymph nodes.

Histopathology is compatible with squamous cell carcinoma. Occasionally, the detection of Epstein–Barr or human papilloma virus, with the support of molecular techniques, could be helpful in distinguishing nasopharyngeal from oropharyngeal primary tumours [51, 52].

Neuroendocrine carcinomas of unknown primary

CUP neuroendocrine tumours account for 13% of all neuroendocrine tumours and are diagnosed as low-grade or high-grade malignancies. High-grade neuroendocrine tumours are the most common, representing almost 80% of all cases. These are poorly-differentiated tumours with disseminated disease and a rapidly-growing behaviour. Low-grade tumours are mainly located in the liver and manifest with symptoms associated with secretion of vasoactive peptides.

Histologically, they are diagnosed with small cells with little cytoplasm and dark nuclei, positive for neuroendocrine immunohistochemical stains (chromogranin, synaptophysin, PGP 9.5, CD56) [53].

Adenocarcinoma with a colon cancer profile

This CUP subset has recently been described and refers to patients with a mean age of 58 years who present with predominantly liver and peritoneal metastases and less commonly with lungs, pleura bones, or ovarian secondary lesions. Laboratory investigations show a normal colonoscopy and histology compatible with adenocarcinoma or poorly-differentiated adenocarcinoma stained with CK20, CDX2, and CEA [54, 55].

Men with blastic metastases and elevated serum PSA

This is a very rare CUP subset consisting of male patients with osteoblastic metastases, localized or diffuse bone pains, elevated serum PSA levels, and a histology revealing metastatic adenocarcinoma with a positive staining for PSA marker [1, 2].

Patients with limited disease

Patients with this subset are presented with: (a) a single lesion in several sites, i.e., lymph nodes, skin, liver, bone, lung, brain, or adrenal gland; or (b) with isolated inguinal lymphadenopathy, mainly of squamous cell histology [1, 2].

Melanoma of unknown primary with isolated nodal disease

This subset accounts for 3.2% of all melanoma patients. Clinically, it presents either as local nodal or as visceral metastatic disease. Cases with local nodal disease present with localized symptomatology, in contrast to the visceral type where more systemic symptoms and signs are present. Histopathology with light microscopy and immunohistochemistry reveal features of a melanoma [56].

Unfavourable or non-specific subsets

The incidence of the unfavourable group accounts for 80% of all CUP patients. The most common subset in this group is that of metastatic liver disease. Other organs involved by metastatic lesions are lymph nodes (35%), lungs (31%), bones (28%), and brain (15%). The most frequent histologic malignancy is adenocarcinoma (64%) followed by undifferentiated carcinoma (20%), neuroendocrine (9%), and squamous cell carcinoma (3%). These patients present with miscellaneous symptoms and signs related to the underlying metastatic organ [1, 2, 57, 58].

Treatment of clinicopathological subsets

Women with serum papillary adenocarcinoma of the peritoneal cavity

These women should be treated as FIGO stage III ovarian carcinoma with optimal surgical cytoreduction followed by platinum/taxane systemic chemotherapy. Data derived from a systemic review of 25 clinical series of a total of 579 patients with primary serous peritoneal adenocarcinoma showed response rates and survival similar to serous ovarian cancer. Median response rate was around 80% (53–100%) with clinical and pathological complete responders of 50–70% and 10–15%, respectively. The feasibility of optimal surgical debulking ranged between 13–79% of patients. Mean overall survival is 30 months (15 to 42 months) with longer survival seen more often in patients who underwent optimal debulking [48].

Women with isolated axillary nodal metastases from adenocarcinoma

The management of these patients includes locoregional and systemic treatment. Locoregional therapy is identical to stage II or III breast cancer. For patients with N1 disease (mobile nodes), axillary clearance followed by either simple mastectomy or breast irradiation should be offered. Adjuvant chemotherapy followed by endocrine treatment should be provided for premenopausal women, while postmenopausal women should receive only endocrine therapy with tamoxifen or aromatase inhibitors.

For patients with N2 disease (fixed nodes), neoadjuvant chemotherapy should be considered. In non-responding or elderly patients, radical radiotherapy is recommended. For patients with positive hormone receptors, adjuvant endocrine treatment should be provided. In addition, trastuzumab should be added to HER-2 positive patients according to the guidelines for stage III breast cancer.

Prognostic data from a recent systematic review including 24 clinical studies with 689 patients in this subset, demonstrated that prognosis is similar to stage II–III breast cancer. Two important prognostic factors were: (a) the number of involved axillary nodes and (b) the absence of residual gross disease.

Loco-regional failure in locally irradiated patients is around 15–25% and mean five-year overall survival is 72% with a median follow-up of 62 months. The impact of adjuvant systemic treatment at three-year overall survival is estimated to be approximately 22%. One should keep in mind that all therapeutic data in these patients are based on type 3 level of evidence [49].

Poorly differentiated carcinoma with midline distribution

Although these patients have a relatively poorer outcome comparing to germ cell tumours, they should still be treated with platinum-based combination chemotherapy. A systematic review of ten published studies and 703 patients reports response rates of 50% (42–64%) with 20–25% complete responses. Median survival is 12 months (8–15 months) and almost 10–15% of patients can enjoy long-term DFS. Favourable prognostic factors are: (a) low tumour burden, (b) absence of visceral disease, (c) good performance status, (d) female gender, and (e) platinum-based regimens [50].

Squamous cell carcinoma involving cervical lymph nodes

This subset of CUP patients should be managed according to locally advanced squamous carcinoma of the head and neck. Loco-regional treatment with radiotherapy to the pharyngeal axis and bilateral neck with or without radical neck dissection is recommended. Concurrent chemotherapy is also used in most cases.

The most prominent prognostic factors are lymph node stage and extracapsular spread followed by other less important factors such as good performance status, young age, absence of weight loss, and low-grade histology. Five-year survival or long-term disease control is around 50–60%, while the majority of these patients are considered cured [51].

Neuroendocrine carcinoma of unknown primary

Treatment provided to high-grade and low-grade neuroendocrine CUP tumours differs between patients. Patients with high grade neuroendocrine tumours are managed with platinum-based chemotherapy regimens containing mainly etoposide. Overall response rates are around 50–70% with 15–20% complete responders, a median survival of 15.5 months (range 12–40 months) and a two–year survival rate of 33–50%. On the contrary, patients with low-grade tumours are treated with somatostatin analogues or chemoembolization and can exhibit a median survival of 40 months and a five-year survival rate of 35–45%.

The above data are retrieved from a recent systematic review of 39 studies including 500 patients diagnosed with neuroendocrine carcinoma of unknown primary [53].

Adenocarcinoma with a colon-cancer profile

This favourable subset of patients is treated with colorectal chemotherapy regimens. Overall response rate is up to 70% with some complete responders. Median survival is around 20–24 months [54, 55].

Table 59.6 Treatment recommendations and prognosis in favourable CUP subsets

CUP subsets	Therapeutic recommendations	Prognosis
Women with serous papillary adenocarcinoma of the peritoneal cavity	Optimal surgical debulking followed by platinum-based combinations	Mean overall survival is 30 months and is 2–6 months less compared to primary ovarian cancer. Optimal debulking offers long-term survival of 15–42 months
Women with adenocarcinoma involving only axillary lymph nodes	Axillary nodal dissection, mastectomy or breast irradiation followed by adjuvant chemotherapy and/or endocrine treatment according to the biological characteristics	Mean 5-year overall survival is 72%. The impact of adjuvant systemic treatment is 22% at 3-year survival
Poorly differentiated carcinoma with midline distribution	Chemotherapy with platinum-containing regimens	Median survival is 12 months (8–15 months) and 10–15% are long-term disease-free survivors
Squamous cell carcinoma involving cervical lymph nodes	Neck dissection and/or irradiation of bilateral neck and head-neck axis. Concurrent chemotherapy seems to be beneficial for N_2 or N_3 disease	5-year survival or disease control is 50–60%. Most of these patients are considered cured
Neuroendocrine carcinomas of unknown primary	Platinum—etoposide combination chemotherapy for poorly differentiated tumours and somatostatin analogues for low-grade tumours	High-grade tumours: median survival is 15.5 months, 2-year survival: 33–50%. Low-grade tumours: median survival 40 months 5-year survival: 35–45%
Men with blastic bone metastases and elevated PSA	Endocrine treatment with LHRH agonists and/or antiandrogens	
Adenocarcinoma with a colon cancer profile	Colorectal chemotherapy regimens	Median overall survival is 20–24 months
Patients with limited disease	Surgical excision ± radiotherapy	Long-term survivors
Melanoma of unknown primary with isolated disease	Surgical treatment with local radiotherapy and adjuvant chemo-immunotherapy	Median survival: 24–165 months 5-year survival: 29–76% 10-year survival: 19–63%

Men with blastic bone metastases and elevated serum PSA levels

These patients should be treated empirically with androgen suppression treatment similar to metastatic prostate cancer [1, 2].

Patients with single operable metastatic deposit

This rare entity should be treated with local excision, with or without radiotherapy [1, 2].

Melanoma of unknown primary with localized nodal disease

Patients with localized disease should be treated surgically. Local radiotherapy as well as adjuvant chemoimmunotherapy are recommended post-operatively. Prognostically, two groups of patients have been described: localized nodal disease group and the metastatic visceral group. Survival rates differ substantially between these two groups. Localized nodal disease has a median survival between 24 and 165 months and a five-year and ten-year survival between 29–76% and 19–63%, respectively. The metastatic visceral group exhibits a median survival between three and 13 months and a five-year survival of 6–18%. Lymph node number, female gender, age, and surgical management are considered as favourable prognostic factors [56].

Table 59.6 summarizes the therapeutic recommendations and prognosis of favourable CUP subsets.

Unfavourable or non-specific subsets

Unfavourable subsets constitute a majority (75–80%) of CUP patients. Unfortunately, most of these subsets remain relatively unresponsive to systemic chemotherapy. Despite the availability of several cytostatic drugs active in various solid tumours, there is no evidence that chemotherapy benefits this particular group of patients. Although responses can be seen, survival benefit is lacking [57].

The most common agents in current use are platinum compounds, mainly cisplatin or carboplatin, and taxanes, either paclitaxel or docetaxel. Other drugs used in combination are gemcitabine, oxaliplatin, capecitabine, vinorelbine, etoposide, or anthracyclines. The most frequent combinations used as first-line treatment include carboplatin, cisplatin, paclitaxel, docetaxel, gemcitabine, or etoposide. In general, response rates vary between 20–40% with very few complete responders. OS is 9–11 months and 1-year survival is around 30% [59].

Table 59.7 Palliative regimens for unfavourable CUP patients

Drugs	Dosage
Carboplatin	AUC 5 Q 3 weeks
Paclitaxel	175 mg/m², Q 3 weeks
Carboplatin	AUC 5 Q 3 weeks
Docetaxel	75 mg/m², Q 3 weeks
Cisplatin	60–75 mg/m², Q 3 weeks
Gemcitabine	1000 mg/m², Q 3 weeks
Cisplatin	75 mg/m², Q 3 weeks
Etoposide	100 mg/m² days 1–3, Q 3 weeks
Irinotecan	160 mg/m², Q 3 weeks
Oxaliplatin	80 mg/m², Q 3 weeks
Irinotecan	100 mg/m², Q 3 weeks
Gemcitabine	1000 mg/m², Q 3 weeks
Oxaliplatin	85–130 mg/m², Q 3 weeks
Capecitabine (oral)	2000 mg/m², days 1–14, Q 3 weeks

The subset of patients with mainly liver metastases is one of the most common unfavourable subsets. The results from five studies published with more than 700 patients showed that the response rate was less than 20% and the median survival was 5.5 months [57]. Some authors claim that since 2000, with the availability of newer drugs, response rates and OS have been improved. Here, one should be cautious since CUP patients enrolled in clinical trials are selected patients with younger age and better performance status [60].

Nevertheless, according to the available guidelines, unfavourable CUP patients of relatively young age and good performance status should be considered for platinum-based chemotherapy. Alternatively, best supportive care should be recommended [61]. Table 59.7 demonstrates commonly used low-toxicity palliative chemotherapy regimens for poor-risk CUP patients.

Conclusion

The description and management of CUP is a constantly evolving story, encompassing, as it does, evolution in novel imaging and genomic classifiers of disease. As stated in the early chapters of this book, the ultimate key to this heterogeneous set of diseases may come from massive DNA sequencing efforts and the discovery of druggable, actionable, driver mutations.

Further reading

Dennis JL, Hvidsten TR, Wit EC, et al. Markers of adenocarcinoma characteristics of the site of origin: development of a diagnostic algorithm. Clinical Cancer Research 2005; 11: 3766–3772.

Golfinopoulos V, Pentheroudakis G, Salanti G, Nearchou AD, Ioannidis JP et al. Comparative survival with diverse chemotherapy regimens for cancer of unknown primary site: multiple-treatments meta-analysis. Cancer Treatment Reviews 2009; 35: 570–573.

Greco FA, Pavlidis N. Treatment for patients with unknown primary carcinoma and unfavourable prognostic factors. Seminars in Oncology 2009; 36(1): 65–74.

Horlings HM, van Laar RK, Kerst JM, et al. Gene expression profiling to identify the histogenetic origin of metastatic adenocarcinomas of unknown primary. Journal of Clinical Oncology 2008; 26(27): 4435–4441.

Monzon F, Koen TJ. Diagnosis of metastatic neoplasms: molecular approaches for identification of tissue of origin. Archives of Pathology and Laboratory Medicine 2010; 134: 216–224.

Oien KA. Pathologic evaluation of unknown primary cancer. Seminars in Oncology 2009; 36: 8–37.

Pentheroudakis G, Briasoulis E, Pavlidis N. Cancer of Unknown Primary: Missing primary or missing biology? The Oncologist 2007; 12: 418–425.

Pentheroudakis G, Golfinopoulos V, Pavlidis N. Switching benchmarks in cancer of unknown primary: from autopsy to microarray. European Journal of Cancer 2007; 43 (14): 2026–2036.

Stella GM, Benvenuti S, Gramaglia D, Scarpa A, Tomezzoli A et al. MET mutations in cancers of unknown primary origin (CUPs). Human Mutation 2011; 32(1): 44–50.

References

1. Pavlidis N, Briasoulis E, Haisworth J, Greco FA. Diagnostic and therapeutic management of cancer of an unknown primary. European Journal of Cancer 2003; 39: 1990–2005.
2. Pavlidis N, Fizazi K. Carcinoma of unknown primary. Critical Reviews in Oncology and Hematology 2009; 69: 271–278.
3. Pentheroudakis G, Golfinopoulos V, Pavlidis N. Switching benchmarks in cancer of unknown primary: from autopsy to microarray. European Journal of Cancer 2007; 43 (14): 2026–2036.
4. <www.nice.org.uk/guidance/index>.
5. Muir C. Cancer of unknown primary site. Cancer 1995; 75: 353–356.
6. van de Wonw AJ, Janssen-Heijnen MLG, Coebergh JWW, Hillen HF. Epidemiology of unknown primary tumors: incidence and population—based survival of 1285 patients in Southeast Netherlands, 1984–1992. European Journal of Cancer 2002; 38: 409–413.
7. Coates M, Armostrong B. NSW Central Cancer Registry. Cancer in New South Wales. Incidence and mortality. NSW, Cancer Council, 1995.
8. Fritz A, Percy C, Jack A et al., eds. International Classification of Diseases for Oncology (ICD-0), 3rd edition. Geneva World Health Organization, 2000.
9. Hemminki K, Ji J, Sundquist j, Shu X. Familial risks in cancer of unknown primary: tracking the primary sites. Journal of Clinical Oncology 2011; 29(4): 435–440.
10. Shu X, Sundquist K, Sundquist J, Hemminki K. Time trends in incidence, causes of death, and survival of cancer of unknown primary in Sweden. European Journal of Cancer Preview 2012; 21(3): 281–288.
11. Shu X, Lik HY, Ji J et al. Subsequent cancers in patients diagnosed with cancer of unknown primary (CUP: etiological insights). Annals of Oncology 2012; 23(1): 269–275.
12. Levi F, Blanc-Moya R, Maspoli-Conconi M, et al. Second neoplasms after cancers of unknown primary. Annals of Oncology 2011; 22(6): 1464–1465.
13. Frost P, Raber Mn, Abbruzzese JL. Unknown primary tumors as a unique clinical and biologic entity: a hypothesis. Cancer Bulletin 1989; 41: 139–141.
14. Hedley DW, Leary JA, Kirsten F. Metastatic adenocarcinoma of unknown primary site: abnormalities of cellular DNA content and survival. European Journal of Cancer Clinical Oncology 1985; 21: 185–189.
15. Abbruzzese JL, Lenzi R, Raber MN et al. The biology of unknown primary tumours. Seminars in Oncology 1993; 20: 238–243.
16. Pavlidis N, Briasoulis E, Bai M et al. Overexpression of C-myc, Ras and C-erbB-2 oncoproteins in carcinoma of unknown primary origin. Anticancer Research 1995; 15: 2563–2567.
17. Hainsworth JD, Lennington WJ, Greco FA. Overexpression of Her-2 in patients with poorly differentiated carcinoma or poorly differentiated adenocarcinoma of unknown primary site. Journal of Clinical Oncology 2000; 18: 632–635.
18. Fizazi K, Voigt JJ, Lesimple T et al. Carcinoma of unknown primary (CUP): Are the tyrosine kinase receptors HER-2, EGF-R, and c-Kit suitable targets for therapy? Proceedings of the American Society of Clinical Oncology 2003; 22: 3549.
19. Rashid A, Hess KR, Lenzi R et al. Overexpression and prevalence of molecular markers in patients with cancer of unknown primary (CUP). Proceedings of the American Society of Clinical Oncology 2005; 24: 9683.
20. Van de Wouw AJ, Jansen RL, Griffioen AW et al. Clinical and immunohistochemical analysis of patients with unknown primary tumour. A search for prognostic factors in UPT. Anticancer Research 2004; 24: 297–301.
21. Dova L, Georgiou I, Vartholomatos G et al. EGFR and C-KIT/CD117 gene mutational screening and oncoprotein expression in patients with cancer of unknown primary: Implications for molecular pathophysiology and therapy. European Journal of Cancer 2005; 3: 424.
22. Dova L, Pentheroudakis G, Golfinopoulos V, Malamou-Mitsi V, Georgiou I et al. Targeting c-KIT, PDGFR in cancer of unknown primary: a screening study for molecular markers of benefit. Journal of Cancer Research Clinical Oncology 2008; 134(6): 697–704.
23. Stella GM, Benvenuti S, Gramaglia D, Scarpa A, Tomezzoli A et al. MET mutations in cancers of unknown primary origin (CUPs). Human Mutation 2011; 32(1): 44–50.
24. Briasoulis E, Tsokos M, Fountzilas G et al. Bcl2 and p53 protein expression in metastatic carcinoma of unknown primary origin: Biological and clinical implications. A Hellenic Cooperative Oncology Group study. Anticancer Research 1998; 18: 907–1914.
25. Bar-Eli M, Abbruzzese JL, Lee-Jackson D et al. p53 gene mutation spectrum in human unknown primary tumors. Anticancer Research 1993; 13: 1619–1623.

26. Dova L, Golfinopoulos V, Pentheroudakis G, Georgiou I, Pavlidis N. Systemic dissemination in cancer of unknown primary is independent of mutational inactivation of the KiSS-1 metastasis-suppressor gene. Pathology and Oncology Research 2008; 14(3): 239–241.

27. Hillen HF, Hak LE, Joosten-Achjanie SR et al. Microvessel density in unknown primary tumors. International Journal of Cancer 1997; 74: 81–85.

28. Karavasilis V, Malamou-Mitsi V, Briasoulis E et al. Angiogenesis in cancer of unknown primary: clinicopathological study of CD34, VEGF and TSP-1. BMC Cancer 2005; 5: 25–32.

29. Karavasilis V, Malamou-Mitsi V, Briasoulis E et al. Matrix metalloproteinases in carcinoma of unknown primary. Cancer 2005; 104: 2282–2287.

30. Koo JS and Kim H. Hypoxia-related protein expression and its clinicopathologic implication in carcinoma of unknown primary. Tumour Biology 2011; 32(5): 893–904.

31. Pentheroudakis G, Apostolaki S, Stoyianni A, Karaxalios D, Patramani S et al. Circulating tumour cells in cancer of unknown primary site: correlation with clinico pathologic characteristics and prognosis. Annals in Oncology 2010; 21(Suppl 8): abstr 865.

32. Souglakos J, Pentheroudakis G, Papadaki C, Cervantes A, Petrakis D et al. Prognostic significance of gene expression profile in patients with carcinomas of unknown primary. Annals in Oncology 2010; 21(Suppl 8): abstr 128P.

33. Fabbri M, Calin GA. Epigenetics and miRNAs in human cancer. Advances in Genetics 2010; 70: 87–99.

34. Dennis JL, Hvidsten TR, Wit EC, et al. Markers of adenocarcinoma characteristics of the site of origin: development of a diagnostic algorithm. Clinical Cancer Research 2005; 11: 3766–3772.

35. Oien KA. Pathologic evaluation of unknown primary cancer. Seminars in Oncology 2009; 36: 8–37.

36. Motzer RJ, Rodriguer E, Reuter VE, et al. Molecular and cytogenetic studies in the diagnosis of patients with poorly differentiated carcinomas of unknown primary site. Journal of Clinical Oncology 1995; 13: 274–282.

37. Ilson DH, Motzer RJ, Rodriguez E, et al. Genetic analysis in the diagnosis of neoplasm of unknown primary tumor site. Seminars in Oncology 1993; 20: 229–237.

38. Karsell PR, Sheedy PF, O'Connell MJ. Computed tomography in search of cancer of unknown origin. Journal of the American Medical Association 1982; 248: 340–343.

39. Orel SG, Weinstein SP, Schmoll MD et al. Breast MR imaging in patients with axillary node metastases and unknown primary malignancy. Radiology 1999; 212: 543–549.

40. Hillel PG, van Beek EJ, Taylor C et al. The clinical impact of a combined gamma camera/CT imaging system on somatostatin receptor imaging of neuroendocrine tumours. Clinical Radiology 2006; 61: 579–587.

41. Baron PL, Moore MP, Kinne DW et al. Occult breast cancer presenting with axillary metastases. Updated management. Archives of Surgery 1990; 125: 210–214.

42. Rusthoven KE, Koshy M, Paulino AC. The role of fluorodeoxyglucose position emission tomography in cervical lymph node metastases from an unknown primary tumor. Cancer 2004; 101: 2641–2646.

43. Fencil P, Belohvaleu Ö, Skopalova M et al. Prognostic and diagnostic accuracy of [18 F] FDG-PET/CT in 190 patients with carcinoma of unknown primary. European Journal of Nuclear Medicine and Molecular Imaging 2007; 34: 1783–1792.

44. Delgado-Bolton RC, Fernander-Peper A, Gonraler-Mate A et al. Meta-analysis of the performance of 18F-FDG PET in primary tumor detection in unknown primary tumors. Journal of Nuclear Medicine 2003; 44: 1301–1314.

45. Pentheroudakis G, Pavlidis N. Serum Tumor Markers. In Wick MR ed. Metastatic Carcinomas of Unknown Origin, 1st Edition. New York: Demos Medical Publishing, 2008, 165–175.

46. Culine S. P rognostic factors in unknown primary cancer. Seminars of Oncology 2009; 36: 60–64.

47. Pavlidis N, Petrakis D, Golfinopoulos V, Penthertoudakis G. Long-term survivors among patients with cancer of unknown primary. Critical Reviews in Oncology and Hematology 2012; 84(1): 85–92.

48. Pentheroudakis G, Pavlidis N. Serous papillary peritoneal carcinoma: Unknown primary tumour, ovarian cancer counterpart or a distinct entity? A systematic review. Critical Reviews in Oncology and Hematology 2010; 75: 27–42.

49. Pentheroudakis G, Lazaridis G, Pavlidis N. Axillary nodal metastases from carcinoma of unknown primary (CUPAX): a systematic review of published evidence. Breast Cancer Research and Treatment 2010; 119: 1–11.

50. Pentheroudakis G, Stoyianni A, Pavlidis N. Cancer of unknown primary patient's with midline nodal distribution: Midway between poor and favourable prognosis? Cancer Treatment Reviews 2011; 37(2): 120–126.

51. Pavlidis N, Pentheroudakis G, Plataniotis G. Cervical lymph node metastases of squamous cell carcinoma from an unknown primary site: a favourable prognosis subset of patients with CUP. Clinical and Translational Oncology 2009; 11: 340–348.

52. Jereczek-Fossa BA, Jassem J, Orecchia R. Cervical lymph node metastases of squamous cell carcinoma from an unknown primary. Cancer Treatment Reviews 2004; 30(2): 153–164.

53. Stoyianni A, Pentheroudakis G, Pavlidis N. Neuroendocrine carcinoma of unknown primary. A systematic review of the literature and a comparative study with other neuroendocrine tumors. Cancer Treatment Reviews 2011; 37(5): 358–365.

54. Varadhachary GR, Raber MN, Matauroros A et al. Carcinoma of unknown primary with a colon-cancer profile—changing paradigm and emerging definitions. Lancet Oncology 2008; 9: 596–599.

55. Hainsworth JD, Schnabel CA, Erlander MG, Haines DW 3rd, Greco FA, et al. A retrospective study of treatment outcomes in patients with carcinoma of unknown primary site and a colorectal cancer molecular profile. Clinical Colorectal Cancer 2012; 11(2): 112–118. doi: 10.1016/j.clcc.2011.08.001. Epub 2011 Oct 14.

56. Kamposioras K, Pentheroudakis G, Pectasides D, Pavlidis N. Malignant melanoma of unknown primary site. To make the long story short. A systematic review of the literature. Critical Reviews in Oncology and Hematology 2011; 78(2): 112–126.

57. Lazaridis G, Pentheroudakis G, Fountzilas G, Pavlidis N. Liver metastases from cancer of unknown primary (CUPL): a retrospective analysis of presentation, management and prognosis in 49 patients and systematic review of the literature. Cancer Treatment Reviews 2008; 34(8): 693–700.

58. Golfinopoulos V, Pentheroudakis G, Salanti G, Nearchou AD, Ioannidis JP et al. Comparative survival with diverse chemotherapy regimens for cancer of unknown primary site: multiple-treatments meta-analysis. Cancer Treatment Reviews 2009; 35: 570–573.

59. Pavlidis N. Forty years experience of treating cancer of unknown primary. Acta Oncologica 2007; 46: 592–601.

60. Greco FA, Pavlidis N. Treatment for patients with unknown primary carcinoma and unfavourable prognostic factors. Seminars of Oncology 2009; 36(1): 65–74.

61. Fizazi K, Greco FA, Pavlidis N, Pentheroudakis G. Cancers of unknown primary site: ESMO Clinical Practice Guidelines for diagnosis, treatment and follow—up. Annals in Oncology 2011; 22(Suppl 6): vi64–vi68.

INDEX

Page numbers followed by *b, f* or *t* refer to boxes, figures or tables respectively. Alphabetical order is letter-by-letter.

A

ABC-02 trial 526
aberrant crypt foci (ACF) 451–2
abiraterone 612
ABL1 gene 720
  see also BCR-ABL1 fusion gene
absorption
  of carcinogens 145
  of drugs 189, 210, 211
accelerated radiotherapy (AF) 178
accountability for reasonableness rationing
    system 234*b*
accuracy of biomarker tests 105
achalasia 365
acidophils of the anterior pituitary 939*t*
acinar cell carcinoma (pancreatic) 483*f*, 484
acinar pattern lung carcinoma 631*f*
acne treatment 690
acromegaly 939, 942, 951
ACTH (adrenocorticotrophic hormone)
  in Cushing syndrome due to adrenal
    adenoma 928
  ectopic ACTHoma 945*t*, 950, 955*t*
  pituitary tumours
    non-functioning 940
    secreting ACTH 939, 942–3
actinic keratoses 693, 694
  appearance 694*f*, 695*f*
  treatment 694–5
active surveillance
  prostate cancer 610–11
  renal cancer 617
ACTS-GC trial 401, 401*t*
acute abdomen 537
acute leukaemia of ambiguous lineage 705
acute lymphoblastic leukaemia (ALL) 712–30
  chemotherapy 724–6
    for CNS disease 726, 730
    late adverse effects 730
    in Ph+ ALL (with imatinib) 727
  CNS disease 718, 726, 730
  CSCs 87*t*
  early T-cell precursor 722
  genetic profiles 713, 715–16
    B-cell lineages 716–21
    diagnosis-relapse changes 723
    and risk of ALL 723
    T-cell lineages 717*t*, 721–2
  incidence 715
  minimal residual disease 713–15, 726, 728–9

  Philadelphia chromosome-positive
    B-ALL 713, 715, 719, 727–9
  prognosis 712–15
  relapsed
    genetic changes compared with
      diagnosis 723
    treatment 729–30
  risk stratification 713
  stem cell transplantation
    allogeneic 713–14, 726–7, 727–8
    autologous 714
    Ph+ ALL 727–8
  survival rates 723–4
  targeted therapies 713, 714, 719
    Ph+ ALL 727–9
    relapsed disease 730
acute myeloid leukaemia (AML) 699–712
  causes and risk factors 131, 706
  chemotherapy
    induction 702, 704, 706–9
    maintenance 711–12
    older patients 704, 708–9
    post-remission 709–10
    relapsed disease 712
  classification 705
  clinical presentation 704–5
  CSCs 87*t*, 88, 90, 705
  diagnosis 705
  general management 706
  genetic profiles 699–702, 705, 711, 718
  incidence 702
  minimal residual disease 712
  in older patients 702–4, 708–9, 710, 711
  prognosis 700*f*, 730
    mutational profiling 699, 701–2, 711
  relapsed disease 712
  stem cell transplantation
    allogeneic 699, 710–11, 712
    autologous 710
  survival rates 702–4, 707*f*
  targeted therapies 89, 90, 707, 712
acute phase proteins 113
acute promyelocytic leukaemia (APL) 704–5,
    705
adenocarcinoma
  cervical 577
  gastric *see* gastric cancer
  lung 130, 629–30, 630–1, 644
  oesophageal 365, 367–9
    Siewert classification 369–70

    treatment 376, 377–8, 381, 382
  ovarian *see* ovarian cancer
  pancreatic *see* pancreatic cancer
  salivary gland 336
  sinonasal 334, 336*t*, 340, 342
adenoid cystic carcinoma 337
adenoma
  adrenal
    aldosterone-producing (Conn's
      syndrome) 929*f*, 930–1
    cortisol-producing (Cushing
      syndrome) 928–30, 929*f*
    incidentaloma 933–5
  colorectal 408, 411, 452, 456
  gallbladder 509
  gastric 393
  pituitary 886–7, 938–9
  pleomorphic 336, 906
adenomatoid tumour (peritoneal) 535
adenosine deaminase (ADA) 772
adenosquamous carcinoma
  lung 633
  pancreatic 483*f*
Adjuvant! Online 560
administration routes for drugs 190–1, 210, 683
adnexal transposition 582–3
adnexectomy 583
adolescents
  acute lymphoblastic leukaemia 724, 730
  hereditary syndromes 288
  HPV vaccination 258
  UV exposure 676
adoption by cancer survivors 317
adoptive immunotherapy 687, 712, 770
adrenaline 930
adrenal tumours 928–38
  adenoma
    aldosterone-producing (Conn's
      syndrome) 929*f*, 930–1
    cortisol-producing (Cushing
      syndrome) 928–30, 929*f*
  carcinoma 931–3
  causes and risk factors 928, 930, 931–2
  diagnosis 928, 931, 932, 933, 934*t*, 935, 936
  epidemiology 928, 930, 931, 933, 935
  feminizing 933
  histopathology 929*f*, 932
  imaging 930*f*, 931, 932, 935, 936, 937*f*
  incidentalomas 933–5
  macroscopic appearance 929*f*

adrenal tumours (*Cont.*)
  metastatic from lung 646
  phaeochromocytoma and
      paraganglioma 926, 929*f*, 935–7
    malignant 937–8
  staging 932*t*
  treatment 930, 931, 932–3, 933, 935, 936–8
  virilizing 932, 933
adrenocorticotrophic hormone *see* ACTH
adult T-cell leukaemia/lymphoma (ATL) 139, 832
  see also T-ALL (T-lineage ALL)
Advanced Market Commitment
    (AMC) 259–60
aesthesioneuroblastoma 335, 342
aetiology
  acute lymphoblastic leukaemia 723
  acute myeloid leukaemia 706
  adrenal tumours
    aldosterone-producing adenoma 930
    carcinoma 931–2
    cortisol-producing adenoma 928
    phaeochromocytoma/paraganglioma 935
  alcohol consumption 157, 320*t*, 366*t*, 446, 546
    plus smoking 130, 329
  bacterial infections 388, 389, 509, 510, 808
  bladder cancer 613
  body weight 155–6, 237, 320*t*, 367, 445, 546
  brain tumours 867
  breast cancer 156*t*, 546–7
    negative risk factors 158, 319, 546
    radiotherapy 151, 152
    smoking 131, 132
  cervical cancer 131, 139, 576
  chemicals *see* carcinogens, chemical
  cholangiocarcinoma 509–10, 511
  colorectal cancer 156, 157, 444–6
  diabetes mellitus 445–6
  diet 156–8, 365, 388, 445, 465, 546
  endometrial cancer 156*t*, 576, 578
  gallbladder cancer 508–9, 510
  gastric cancer 156*t*, 388, 389
  head and neck cancer 130, 157, 329, 340
  liver cancer 131, 140, 157, 508, 510–11
  liver flukes 509–10, 511
  lung cancer
    occupational carcinogens 151, 628
    radon 151, 628
    smoking 127–8, 130, 132, 628
  lymphoma 808
  melanoma 674–5, 676, 905, 908
  mesothelioma 533–4, 659
  myeloma 782, 783–4
  oesophageal cancer 156*t*, 157, 365, 367
  ovarian cancer 576
  pancreatic cancer 156*t*, 478
  phaeochromocytoma 935
  physical activity 156
  pituitary tumours 939
  prostate cancer 157, 609
  radiation 150–1, 444–5, 706, 919
    radiotherapy 151–3, 419, 560, 873, 905, 918–19
    radon 151, 628
  renal cancer 616–17
  skin cancer
    eyelid 904–5
    melanoma 674–5, 676
    non-melanoma 690–1, 693, 696
  smoking 127–32, 134, 366*t*, 446, 478, 628

passive 132
  plus alcohol 130, 329
  thyroid cancer 151, 918–19
  urothelial cell cancer 615
  uveal melanoma 908
  vaginal cancer 576
  viruses 136–40, 329, 510–11, 576, 808, 832
  vulvar cancer 576
afatinib 644, 645
aflatoxin 145*t*, 157
aflibercept 54, 428–9
AFP (alpha-fetoprotein)
  liver cancer 514
  pineal germ cell tumours 881
  testicular cancer 607, 608
age
  acute lymphoblastic leukaemia 712, 724–5
  acute myeloid leukaemia 702–4, 708–9, 710, 711
  breast cancer screening 268–9
  HPV vaccination 258
  melanoma 676, 678
  multidisciplinary care 205, 464–5
  of survivors of cancer 312
  see also elderly patients
AIDS-associated tumours 137–9, 808
AIO-04 trial 418
AIP gene 939
AKT signalling pathway (protein kinase B) 11, 26, 27*f*
  cell cycle/CDK activation 28
  mesothelioma 534
  metabolic reprogramming 120
  myeloma 786
  see also PI3K signalling pathway
5-ALA (5-aminolevulinic acid) 693, 872, 875, 889
AL amyloid 800–1
ALCL (anaplastic large-cell lymphoma) 813–14, 825–6, 832
alcohol consumption 157
  breast cancer 546
  colorectal cancer 446
  oesophageal cancer 157, 366*t*
  plus smoking 130, 329
  survivors of cancer 320*t*
aldehyde dehydrogenase-1 (ALDH-1) 89
aldosterone-producing adenoma 929*f*, 930–1
alectinib 646
alemtuzumab 769, 773, 774
ALK1-7 (activin-receptor-like kinases) 29
ALK/ALK (anaplastic lymphoma kinase)
  lung cancer 629–30, 646
  lymphoma 813–14, 832
  sarcoma 850, 858
alkylating agents
  carcinogenic 128, 144*t*, 157, 706
  chemotherapeutic 187, 212*t*
    see also bendamustine;
      cyclophosphamide; dacarbazine;
      ifosfamide; melphalan; streptozocin;
      temozolomide
ALL *see* acute lymphoblastic leukaemia
all-trans retinoic acid (ATRA) 699, 704
alpha blockers 936
alpha-fetoprotein (AFP)
  liver cancer 514
  pineal germ cell tumours 881
  testicular cancer 607, 608
alternative hypothesis 222*f*
alvocidib (flavopiridol) 770

amelanotic melanoma 676
American College of Surgeons Oncology Group
    Z001 trial 68, 555
American Society of Clinical Oncology
    (ASCO), on patient care 230, 232, 233, 240
Ames test 147
aminoazo dyes 144*t*
5-aminolevulinic acid (5-ALA) 693, 872, 875, 889
AML *see* acute myeloid leukaemia
AML15 trial 707
AML17 trial 706
AMPK (AMP-activated protein kinase) 27, 47, 120–1
amputation 683, 855
amrubicin 648
amyloidosis 800–1
anaemia
  melanoma 685
  myeloma 787, 798
analgesia 296
  bone pain 612, 688, 798
  chronic pain 315
  in pancreatic cancer 497
  spinal tumours 892
anal sphincter preservation in rectal
    surgery 411, 417, 418
anaphase promoting complex (APC) 29, 33, 36
anaplastic carcinoma
  pancreatic 483*f*, 484
  thyroid 918, 919, 920*f*, 922
anaplastic glioma 876–8
  oligodendroglioma 872, 874, 878
anaplastic large-cell lymphoma (ALCL) 813–14, 825–6, 832
anastomosis
  colonic/rectal 412, 454
  oesophageal 374, 375
  pancreatic 486
  ureterocolic 446
androgens
  deprivation therapy 187, 264–5, 612
  virilizing tumours 932, 933
aneuploidy 77
  acute lymphoblastic leukaemia 716–17
  chronic myeloid leukaemia 760
  unknown primary 966
angiogenesis 49–57
  growth factors 11, 16, 17, 50–1
  as a hallmark of cancer 5, 119
  and metastasis 66
  molecular biology 49–51
  non-angiogenic growth 119
  unknown primary 966
  see also anti-angiogenesis agents
angiogenic vascular cells (AVC) 8, 51
angioimmunoblastic T-cell lymphoma
    (AITL) 813
angiosarcoma 854, 857, 858
animal testing 147, 214–15
anomalous pancreatic biliary duct (APBD)
    junction 508–9
anthracyclines
  acute lymphoblastic leukaemia 725
  acute myeloid leukaemia 702, 706, 708*f*
  breast cancer 549–51, 561
  cardiotoxicity 315, 730
  as a cause of AML 706
  liver cancer 518, 519, 521
  lymphoma (CHOP) 817–18

mechanism of action 186
mesothelioma 539
myeloma 793, 794*b*
oesophageal cancer 378, 382
pharmacokinetics 212*t*
sarcoma 857, 859
anti-androgens 187, 264–5, 612
anti-angiogenesis agents 49, 51–7
adverse effects 53
brain tumours 876, 878
breast cancer 54, 563
colorectal cancer 52, 427–8, 429–31, 432,
459–60
gastro-oesophageal cancers 382, 404
liver cancer 51, 54, 519–21
lung cancer 644
mechanism of action 52–3, 187–8
neuroendocrine tumours 51, 956*t*, 957
ovarian cancer 51–2, 53–4, 593, 618–19
pancreatic cancer 496
preventing tumour rebound after
chemotherapy 66
renal cancer 51–2, 618–19
sarcoma 858
thyroid cancer 921–2
vestibular schwannoma 894
anti-apoptosis proteins 16, 42–3, 389
inhibitors 44, 542
antibiotics
anti-bacterial 392, 798
anti-tumour 187, 212*t*
see also bleomycin; doxorubicin; epirubicin
antibodies
deficiency in myeloma 786–7, 798
detection in myeloma 787–9
production 782–3, 815
see also monoclonal antibody therapies
anti-convulsant agents 872
antidepressants 297
antidiuretic hormone 940
anti-folate analogues 187, 212*t*
see also methotrexate; pemetrexed
antimetabolites 187, 212*t*
see also 5-fluorouracil; capecitabine;
cytarabine; gemcitabine; methotrexate;
pemetrexed
anti-oestrogens 187, 262–3
see also tamoxifen
antisense oligonucleotides 17, 44
anxiety 318
APC (adenomatous polyposis coli) 29
attenuated form 288, 450
colorectal cancer 29, 77, 450
gastric cancer 288, 390, 393
APC (anaphase promoting complex) 33, 36
APL (acute promyelocytic leukaemia) 704–5,
705
apoptosis 4, 42
and CRP 113
extrinsic pathway 43–4
gastric cancer 389
and genetic instability 79
intrinsic pathway 42–3
and p53 5, 28, 61
radiation-induced 174
and TGFβ 16
as a therapeutic target 44, 542
apparent diffusion coefficient (ADC) 338
appendiceal carcinoids 951
appetite promoters 308
area under the curve (AUC) 210

ARF (alternative reading frame) 28
ARID5B gene 723
aristolochic acid 615
aromatase inhibitors 187
breast cancer 262–3, 562
aromatic amines 128, 144*t*, 157
arsenic 690
arsenic trioxide 690, 704
ARTIST trial 400, 401*t*
asbestos 533–4, 628, 659
imaging 661
ascites 64, 537
Asia
chronic lymphocytic leukaemia 766
chronic myeloid leukaemia 754
gastric cancer 388, 397–8, 399, 400
liver flukes 511
nasopharyngeal carcinoma 342
L-asparaginase 725
aspirin (ASA) 114
colorectal cancer prevention 264, 446
astrocytoma 869*t*
high-grade 876–8, 877*f*
low-grade 878, 879, 879*f*
pilocytic 879, 888
spinal 888, 890
ASXL1 gene 701, 702
Atg genes (autophagy-related) 27, 46–7
ATM/ATM (ataxia telangiectasia mutated) 28,
36, 76, 277*t*, 773
atom bomb survivors 150, 706
ATP 44
see also energy metabolism of cancer cells
ATRA (all-trans retinoic acid) 699, 704
atrophic gastritis 388, 392–3
ATR protein kinase (ATR-related) 28, 36, 76
atypical carcinoid 632, 648, 945*t*, 955*t*
atypical fibroxanthoma 697
atypical lipomatous tumour (well-differentiated
liposarcoma) 845, 849*t*, 852–3
audits, in surgery 169–70, 423
Auer rods 705*f*
Aurora kinases 35
Australia
cost of cancer care 239–40
skin cancers 675–6, 690
autophagy 4–5, 45–7
regulation by mTOR pathway 27, 47, 120
AVANT trial 52, 459
Avastin® *see* bevacizumab
axillary management in breast cancer 555, 558
axillary nodal metastases of unknown
primary 969, 970
axitinib 52, 53, 619
azacitidine 709

B
Bak (Bcl-2 protein) 42–3
Balkan endemic nephropathy 615
B-ALL (B-lineage ALL) 713, 716–21
see also acute lymphoblastic leukaemia
Bannayan–Riley–Ruvalcaba syndrome 451
BAP1 gene (BRCA1 associated protein-1) 660,
675, 908
barium studies 371
Barrett metaplasia 375
Barrett oesophagus 367, 368, 369
treatment 372
basal cell carcinoma (BCC) 690, 691–3
eyelid 904–5
basal cell hyperplasia, oesophageal 365–6

basaloid squamous carcinoma 332
base excision repair (BER) pathway 75–6
MUTYH 75, 450
PARP/PARP-1 77, 84, 548
basement membrane 51, 65
basophil granulocytes 756
basophils of the anterior pituitary 939*t*
Bax (Bcl-2 protein) 42–3
BCC (basal cell carcinoma) 690, 691–3
eyelid 904–5
B cells
B-ALL 713, 716–21
B-cell lymphoma *see* lymphoma
B-CLL 766–70, 813
genetic profiles 767, 814–15
and skin cancer 690
B-PLL 766, 772–3
EBV infection 136
hairy cell leukaemia 770–2, 814
role in the immune system 111, 782–3, 784*f*
BCG (Bacillus Calmette-Guérin) intravesical
immunotherapy 615
Bcl-2 protein family 42–3
BCL2 in DLCBL 816
as therapeutic targets 44
BCL (B-cell lymphoma) *see* lymphoma
BCLC (Barcelona Clinic for Liver Cancer)
staging 515, 516*f*
B-CLL (B-lineage CLL) 766–70, 813
genetic profiles 767, 814–15
and skin cancer 690
BCOR/ BCORL1 complex 701
BCR-ABL1 fusion gene
acute lymphoblastic leukaemia 715, 719
chronic myeloid leukaemia 754, 755, 756,
757–8, 760
mutations conferring resistance to TKIs 757,
763–4
PCR 760
targeted therapy *see* bosutinib; dasatinib;
imatinib
BCR-ABL1-like acute lymphoblastic
leukaemia 719–20
BCR-type DLBCL 815
Beclin 1 (Atg6) 46, 47
Bence Jones protein 782
see also paraprotein
bendamustine
chronic lymphocytic leukaemia 768, 769
lymphoma 821
myeloma 794*b*
benzene 128, 706
benzo(a)pyrene 128
BER pathway *see* base excision repair (BER)
pathway
β$_2$-microglobulin 783, 791
bevacizumab (Avastin®) 49, 52*t*, 54
adverse effects 53
brain tumours 876, 878
breast cancer 54, 563
colorectal cancer 52, 427–8, 429–30, 432,
459
liver cancer 519, 520
lung cancer 643
micrometastatic disease 52–3, 459
neuroendocrine tumours 956*t*, 957–8
oesophageal cancer 382
ovarian cancer 53–4, 593
pancreatic cancer 496
vestibular schwannoma 894
bevatuzumab 90

bHLH gene family 721, 722
bias
    in biomarker tests 102
    in clinical trials 222–3, 223–4
    in screening outcomes 267
bidi smoking 131–2
BIG1.98 trial 562
bilateral salpingo-oophorectomy 280, 586
bile acids 445
biliary cancers *see* cholangiocarcinoma;
        gallbladder cancer
biliary cysts 509
biliary excretion of drugs 214
biliary obstruction
    biliary cancers 513–14, 522, 524–5, 526*f*
    pancreatic cancer 497, 498
Binet staging of CLL 767*t*
bioavailability of drugs 189, 210, 211
biobanks 101–2, 106
biochemistry
    acute myeloid leukaemia 706
    chronic myeloid leukaemia 756
    myeloma 787, 788*f*
bioinformatics 9–10, 660, 702
biologically optimal dose (BOD) 224
biological therapies *see* targeted therapies
biomarkers 98–107
    CSCs/CTCs 87–8*t*, 90, 93–4
    discovery of new markers 101–4
    of DNA repair capacity 84, 448, 639
    ethics of research biopsies 232
    pharmacodynamic 100–1, 209–10, 215–16
    pharmacogenomic 98, 99–100
    physiological 101
    predictive 53, 84, 99, 101*t*, 106
        in breast cancer 549–51, 561
    prognostic 99, 100*b*, 106
    quality control 106
    of radiosensitivity 84, 176, 184
    risk markers 98
    surrogate endpoints in clinical trials 223,
        494, 497
    tumour markers 98–9
        AFP 514, 607, 608, 881
        CA19-9 497
        CA-125 538, 969
        calcitonin 924–6, 927, 928
        CEA 466, 926, 928
        hCG 607, 608, 881
        in lymphoma 810
        in mesothelioma 538
        PSA 273, 610, 611, 612, 970
        unknown primary cancer 968, 969
    validation of new markers 105–6, 216
    see also immunohistochemistry;
        immunophenotype
biopsy 102
    bone marrow
        acute myeloid leukaemia 705
        chronic myeloid leukaemia 759–60
        hairy cell leukaemia 771
        myeloma 788*f*, 789–90
    brain tumours 867, 875, 882, 890
    ethics in clinical trials 231–2
    head and neck cancer 334, 353
    liver cancer 514
    lung cancer 633, 634
    lymphoma 811, 882
    melanoma 677
    mesothelioma 661

pancreatic cancer 484–5
prostate cancer 610
sarcoma 844
thyroid cancer 921, 924
bisphosphonates
    breast cancer 563
    in hypercalcaemia 797
    myeloma 792, 797
bladder cancer 613–15
bladder dysfunction 316, 611
BL (Burkitt lymphoma) 39, 136, 808, 817
bleomycin 187, 212*t*, 316, 609
blinatumomab 730
blinding in RCT design 222–3
blood product transfusions 706
blood tests 104*t*
    acute myeloid leukaemia 706
    chronic lymphocytic leukaemia 766
    chronic myeloid leukaemia 756, 759*t*
    hairy cell leukaemia 771
    myeloma 787, 788*f*
    plasma cell leukaemia 799
    prolymphocytic leukaemia 773*f*
    see also tumour markers
blood–brain barrier (BBB), drugs crossing 211,
        826, 873, 892
Bloom's syndrome 277*t*
B lymphocytes *see* B cells
BM *see* bone marrow
BMPR1A gene 451
body image 303
    breast-conserving surgery 163, 307
    stomas 316, 465
body weight
    liver imaging 512
    as a risk factor 155–6, 237, 320*t*, 367, 445,
        546
    weight gain in survivors of cancer 316
    weight loss in cancer 63–4, 497
BOND-1/BOND-2 trials 429, 430
bone
    metastasis to 62–3, 64
        from breast cancer 560, 563–4
        from melanoma 685, 688
        from neuroendocrine tumours 949*f*
        from prostate cancer 64, 612
        PSA-elevated unknown primary 970, 971
        treatment of bone pain 612, 688
    myeloma
        complications of the disease 786, 797, 798
        imaging 788*f*, 789*f*, 790
    osteonecrosis, steroid-induced 730
    osteoporosis (post-treatment) 316, 317
    pain 612, 688, 786, 798
    sarcoma
        chemotherapy 856, 860–1
        classification 846*b*
        diagnosis 844–5, 847–8, 850
        genetic profiles 849–50
        grading 848–9
        histopathology 847–8
        imaging 844
        incidence 844
        radiotherapy 857, 893
        surgery 855–6
    scintigraphy
        metastatic disease 610, 949*f*
        myeloma 790
    skull base tumours 335*t*, 336*t*, 893–4
    sinonasal 334, 340–2

solitary plasmacytoma 801
bone marrow (BM)
    biopsy
        acute myeloid leukaemia 705
        chronic myeloid leukaemia 759–60
        hairy cell leukaemia 771
        myeloma 788*f*, 789–90
    suppression by chemotherapy agents 191,
        192
    transplantation *see* haematopoietic stem cell
        transplantation
bone-modifying agents 563–4
Bonferroni adjustment 226
bortezomib
    mantle cell lymphoma 820
    myeloma 793, 794*b*, 795, 796, 798, 799
    plasma cell leukaemia 800
bosutinib 764–5
bowel cancer
    colorectal *see* colorectal cancer
    neuroendocrine 951–3
    small bowel metastases 685
bowel dysfunction 316, 419
bowel preparation for colorectal surgery 411
Bowen's disease 694, 694*f*, 695, 695*f*, 696
    penile 603
B-PLL (B-cell prolymphocytic leukaemia) 766,
        772–3
brachytherapy 180, 181*f*
    brain tumours 878
    cervical cancer 588, 594–5
    colorectal cancer 463
    endometrial cancer 589–90, 596
    image-guided adaptive ('3D') 588, 595
    oesophageal cancer 377, 382
    orbital tumours 906
    ovarian cancer 588
    prostate cancer 611
    sarcoma 856
    uveal melanoma (episcleral) 909–10, 911
    vaginal cancer 590
BRAF oncogene 25
    colorectal cancer 429, 449, 460
    gastric cancer 389
    hairy cell leukaemia 772, 814
    melanoma 674, 678, 680, 907
        BRAF inhibitor treatment 682, 685–6, 892
    thyroid cancer 919, 921
        BRAF inhibitor treatment 921–2
Bragg peak 179
brain abscesses 871
brain irradiation, adverse effects 730, 873, 883,
        891
brainstem tumours 879
brain tumours
    causes and risk factors 867
    cell of origin 867, 870*f*
    chemoradiotherapy 872, 876
        high-grade (anaplastic) glioma 878
    chemotherapy 873–4
        high-grade (anaplastic) glioma 878
        local delivery 875–6
        low-grade glioma 880
        lymphoma 882–3
        medulloblastoma 881
        non-germinoma germ cell tumour
            (pineal) 882
    classification 867, 869*t*
    clinical presentation 868–71, 880, 882, 886,
        887, 890–1

complications 872
diagnosis 867, 871b
  lymphoma 811, 882
  pineal tumours 881
  site of origin of metastatic disease 890
elderly patients 876
genetic profiles 122, 868, 870f, 877
genetic syndromes 868t
histopathology 874f, 877f, 883f
imaging 871–2
  choroid plexus 894
  craniopharyngioma 887
  ependymoma 880
  glioblastoma 874–5, 874f, 875f
  high-grade (anaplastic) glioma 876–7,
    877f
  intraoperative 872, 875
  low-grade glioma 878–9, 879f
  lymphoma 882, 883f
  medulloblastoma 880
  meningioma 884–5, 884f
  metastatic disease 891
  pineal tumours 881
  pituitary adenoma 886
incidence 867
lymphoma 811, 826, 882–4, 914
macroscopic appearance 874f, 884f
metastatic from other sites 62–3, 64, 890
  from ALL 718, 726, 730
  from breast 565, 892
  from lung 646, 647, 648
  from melanoma 685, 688, 689, 892
  pharmacodynamic resistance 646
  prophylactic irradiation 647, 648
  treatment 565, 891–2
molecular biology 87t, 867–8
multidisciplinary care 872
palliative care 565, 891
parapituitary 938t
  see also pituitary tumours
prognosis 867, 876, 878, 881, 882, 891
radiotherapy 872–3
  choroid plexus 894
  craniopharyngioma 887
  in the elderly 876
  ependymoma 880
  glioblastoma 876
  high-grade (anaplastic) glioma 877–8
  low-grade glioma 880
  lymphoma 883–4
  medulloblastoma 881
  meningioma 885–6
  metastatic disease 565, 646, 647, 648, 685,
    688, 891–2
  pineal tumours 882
  pituitary adenoma 886–7
recurrence 868, 875, 878
resistance to treatment 868
surgery 872
  choroid plexus 894
  craniopharyngioma 887
  glioblastoma 875, 876
  low-grade glioma 879
  medulloblastoma 880–1
  meningioma 885
  metastatic disease 891
  pineal tumours 881–2
targeted therapies 874, 876, 878
  metastatic disease 892
see also skull base tumours

BRCA1/BRCA2 genes
  DNA repair function 76, 77, 548
  hereditary cancer syndromes 165–6, 280,
    546–7
  testing for presence in breast cancer 282
breast calcifications 268f, 269f
breast cancer 546–65
  axillary management 555, 558
    occult primaries 969, 970
  basal-like subtype (triple-negative) 547, 548,
    552, 560–1
  carcinoma in situ 552
    detected at screening 269
    radiotherapy 559
    surgery 554
  case study 564–5
  causes and risk factors 156t, 546–7
    negative risk factors 158, 319, 546
    radiotherapy 151, 152
    smoking 131, 132
  chemotherapy
    adjuvant 559, 560–1
    metastatic disease 561–2
    neoadjuvant 549, 555–6, 559, 561
    occult primaries 970
    prediction of response 549–51, 561
    and radiotherapy 559
    and trastuzumab 563
  classification
    histopathological 551–2
    molecular 547–8, 552
  cost of care 237, 238
  diagnosis 553
  diet 319, 546
  endocrine therapy 187, 562, 970
    in combination with RT 559
    prediction of response 551
    prevention 262–3
  ER-positive 547, 548, 552–3
    chemotherapy 561
    endocrine therapy 562
    targeted therapies 563
  genetic profiles 99, 547–51, 561
  genetic syndromes 165–6, 280, 546–7
  genetic testing for BRCA mutations 282
  HER2-positive subtype 547–8
    chemotherapy 560
    radiotherapy + trastuzumab 559
    targeted therapies 67, 238, 553, 562–3,
      564–5, 892
  histopathology 551–3, 560–1
  incidence 262, 546
  luminal subtypes 547, 561
  lymph node involvement
    chemo/radiotherapy 68, 558–9
    sentinel node surgery 168, 555
  lymphoedema 316, 560
  in men 166, 559
  metastatic
    bone-modifying agents 563–4
    chemotherapy 561–2
    endocrine therapy 562
    miRNA 67
    radiotherapy 559–60, 565
    targeted therapies 54, 67, 564–5, 892
  molecular biology 547–51, 552
    CSCs 87t
    metastasis 67, 549, 564
    subtypes 547–8, 552, 560–1
  multidisciplinary care 199, 200t, 564–5

occult primaries 968, 969, 970
palliative care 559–60
prevention
  anti-hormones 262–3
  protective factors 158, 319, 546
  surgery 280, 554
prognosis
  genetic profiles 99, 548–51, 561
  histopathological profiles 552–3, 560–1
  screening-detected disease 269
QoL issues 307
radiotherapy (adjuvant) 556–60
  risk of second cancer 152, 153
recurrence
  re-irradiation 559
  risk 549–51, 552, 556, 561
  salvage surgery 168
screening 166, 267–70
staging 553, 553–4
surgery 168, 307, 553–6
  audits 170
  breast conservation 163, 554, 555–6
  carcinoma in situ 554
  lymph node resection 168, 555
  margins of resection 165, 554
  prophylactic 280, 554
  shared decision-making 170–1
survivors 152–3, 319
targeted therapies 54, 67, 562–3,
  564–5, 892
  in combination with RT 559
  costs 238
  resistance 548
treatment planning 168, 552–3
triple-negative (basal-like) 547, 548, 552,
  560–1
breastfeeding 158, 546
Breast Health Global Initiative 252
Brenner tumours 580
brentuximab vedotin 822, 825–6, 832
Breslow thickness 678
brivanib 54, 520
bromocriptine 941
bronchogenic lung cancer 631, 632
bronchoscopy 634
Bruton's tyrosine kinase (BTK) pathway 770
  inhibitors 770, 820
Burkitt lymphoma (BL) 39, 136, 808, 817
busulfan 756

C
C80405 trial 429
CA19-9 497
CA-125 538, 969
cabergoline 941, 942
cabizataxel 612
cachexia 63–4, 497
E-cadherin (CDH1) 29, 391, 396
CAIRO 3 trial 432
calcitonin 924–6, 927, 928
calcium
  and cancer risk 157
  hypercalcaemia in myeloma 786, 797
Canada 239
cancer-associated fibroblasts (CAF) 8, 67, 549
cancer control planning 245–52
  challenges 251–2
  international initiatives 246, 252
  key elements 246
  the process 246–51

cancer stem cells (CSCs) 86–95
　acute myeloid leukaemia 87t, 88, 90, 705
　biomarkers 87–8t, 90
　brain tumours 867
　cellular origin 89–90
　dynamic model 91–3
　functional traits 86–9
　gastric cancer 392
　melanoma 87–8t, 91–2, 674
　and metastasis 93–4
　pancreatic 481
　radiotherapy 89, 173–4, 175, 176
　resistance to therapy 9, 89, 91
　as therapeutic targets 90–1, 93
　tumour microenvironment 8–9, 89
cancer of unknown primary (CUP) 966–72
　brain metastases 890
　clinical types 969–70
　epidemiology 966–7
　head and neck cancer 349–51, 968, 969, 970
　histopathology 967–8
　imaging 349, 968
　melanoma 688, 970, 971
　molecular biology 966–7, 968
　neuroendocrine tumours 944, 968, 969, 970
　prognosis 968–9, 971t
　treatment 349–50, 970–2
capecitabine 212t
　breast cancer 562
　colorectal cancer 425, 458–9
　gastric cancer 382, 403
　pancreatic cancer 495
　squamous cell carcinoma 696
carbonic anhydrase IX (CAIX/CA9) 122, 619
carboplatin 187, 212t
　lung cancer
　　NSCLC 639t, 641, 643
　　SCLC 648
　mesothelioma 540
　ovarian cancer 592–3
　testicular cancer 608
carcinoembryonic antigen (CEA) 466, 926, 928
carcinogenesis 7–8
　BCR-ABL1 fusion gene 755
　chemicals 143–5
　　asbestos 533–4, 659
　　tobacco smoke 127–9
　dietary causes 157, 388
　genetic events 38–9, 72–9
　H. pylori infection 388, 389
　ionizing radiation 150
　oesophageal irritation 365, 367
　two-hit model 279, 705
　UV light 674
　viruses 136–40, 329, 330f, 577
carcinogens, chemical 142–7
　arsenic 690
　asbestos 533–4, 628, 659
　benzene 128, 706
　in biliary cancers 509, 510
　genotoxic 143, 144
　initiators 143
　in meat 157
　metabolism 145–7
　non-genotoxic 143–4
　progressors 143
　promoters 143
　in sinonasal cancer 340
　tests for 147
　tobacco smoke 127–8

in urinary tract cancers 613, 615
carcinoids 944, 945t, 951–2, 954t
　atypical 632, 648, 945t, 955t
　heart disease 951, 958
　lung 632, 648–9
cardiac disease
　amyloidosis 800
　carcinoid syndrome 951, 958
cardiopulmonary invasion of lung cancer 635
cardiotoxicity of cancer treatment 315, 377,
　　559, 560, 730, 823
care plans
　palliative care 297
　for survivors of cancer 246, 320–1
carfilzomib 794b
carotid body tumours 355, 356
caspases 42, 43, 44
catecholamine-producing tumours see
　　phaeochromocytoma
β-catenin (and Wnt pathway) 29
　gastric cancer 390, 393
　pancreatic cancer 481
catumaxomab 91, 115
cauda equina syndrome 888
C cells (parafollicular cells) 924
CCND1 gene 331, 366
CCND3 gene 816, 817
CD3 112
　anti-CD3 (blinatumomab) 730
　anti-CD3/EPCAM (catumaxomab) 91, 115
CD4+ T cells (helper T-cells) 111, 112, 114
CD5 766
CD8+ T-cells (cytotoxic T-cells) 6, 111, 112,
　　114
CD19 766
CD20 713, 766, 823
　anti-CD20 823–4
　　conjugated to radioisotopes 824–5
　　see also ofatumumab; rituximab
CD23 766
　anti-CD23 (lumiliximab) 770
CD30 825
　anti-CD30 (brentuximab) 822, 825–6, 832
CD33 707
CD34 705
CD44/CD44v 90, 392
　anti-CD44v6 (bevatuzumab) 90
CD52, anti-CD52 (alemtuzumab) 769, 773, 774
CD56 799, 945
CD79a/CD79b 783
CD123 90
CD antigens
　on cancer stem cells 87t
　chronic lymphocytic leukaemia 767
　HCL 771
　HCL-v 774
　LGL 774
　myeloma 790
　prolymphocytic leukaemia 772, 773
Cdh1 (APC activator subunit) 36
CDH1 gene (E-cadherin) 29, 391, 396
CDK see cyclin-dependent kinases
CDKN1B gene 390
CDKN2A gene/p16 protein
　acute lymphoblastic leukaemia 723
　DLBCL 816
　FAMMM syndrome 166
　head and neck cancer 329–31
　melanoma 675, 686
　mesothelioma 534, 660

oesophageal cancer 367
p14ARF 480
p16INK4A 480
　pancreatic cancer 479, 480
CEA (carcinoembryonic antigen) 466, 926, 928
CEBPA gene 699, 702
CEBPE gene 723
cediranib 54, 858
celiac nerve blocks 497
cell cycle 31–9
　checkpoints 31, 36, 84
　deregulation in cancer 38–9, 84
　　myeloma 783–4
　phases 28, 31
　regulation 3–4, 28–9, 31–3
　　DNA repair 28, 36–7, 84
　　DNA replication 31, 34
　　G1 to S phase 33–4, 84
　　mitosis 34–6
cell death 4–5, 42–7
　and inflammation 112
　radiation-induced 174
　see also apoptosis; autophagy
cell growth/proliferation
　and chemotherapy efficacy 188–9, 193–4
　as a hallmark of cancer 3–5
　non-angiogenic 119
　signalling pathways 11–18, 23–30
cerebellar tumours 879
cereblon 794b
cerebrospinal fluid (CSF) 811, 881, 882
ceritinib 646
Cervarix® (HPV vaccine) 258
cervical cancer
　case study 593–5
　causes and risk factors 131, 139, 576
　chemoradiotherapy 587–8, 593–5
　chemotherapy 591–2
　genetic profiles 577
　histopathology 577
　HPV infection 139, 258, 577
　imaging 581, 594f
　incidence 258, 576, 577
　lymph node involvement 577, 581–2, 595
　metastatic 592
　molecular biology 577
　multidisciplinary care 593–5
　premalignant lesions 272, 577
　radiotherapy 587–8, 593–5
　　surgery to reduce morbidity from 582–3
　screening 258, 272–3
　surgery 581–3, 593
cervical glandular intraepithelial neoplasia
　　(CGIN) 272
cervical intraepithelial neoplasia (CIN) 272,
　　577
cetuximab 83, 213t
　basal cell carcinoma 693
　colorectal cancer 418, 429, 429–30, 432,
　　459–60
　head and neck cancer 346, 348, 352–3
　lung cancer 643
　pancreatic cancer 496
CEUS (contrast-enhanced ultrasound) 512
CHARTWEL trial 641
checklists, surgical 167
chemokines 8, 110
chemoprevention 262
　breast cancer 262–3
　colorectal cancer 114, 115, 263–4, 446–7

lung cancer 265
prostate cancer 264–5
skin cancer 697–8
chemoradiotherapy (CRT) 83, 176
  brain tumours 872, 876
    high-grade (anaplastic) glioma 878
  cervical cancer 587–8, 593–5
  colorectal cancer
    adjuvant 415, 418
    neoadjuvant 168, 416–19, 453
    restaging 410, 418
  gastric cancer 400
  head and neck cancer
    laryngeal/hypopharyngeal 348–9
    nasopharyngeal 343
    oropharyngeal 346
    sinonasal lymphoma 829, 832
    unknown primary site 350
  lung cancer
    NSCLC (locally advanced) 640–1
    SCLC 646–7
  lymphoma 822, 828–9, 831
  mesothelioma 669
  oesophageal cancer 372, 377, 378–9
    adjuvant 381
    neoadjuvant 379, 380–1
  pancreatic cancer 489–94
    adjuvant 491, 493–4
    neoadjuvant 492–3, 494, 498
    unresectable locally advanced 490–1
  vulvar cancer 591
chemotherapy 186–94
  acute lymphoblastic leukaemia 724–6
    for CNS disease 726, 730
    late adverse effects 730
    in Ph+ ALL (with imatinib) 727
  acute myeloid leukaemia
    induction 702, 704, 706–9
    maintenance 711–12
    older patients 704, 708–9
    post-remission 709–10
    relapsed disease 712
  acute promyelocytic leukaemia 704
  adjuvant, principles of use 193
  administration routes 190–1, 210, 683
  adverse effects 193, 315–16, 464–5, 730
    carcinogenesis 706
    in combination therapy 192
  amyloidosis 801
  bladder cancer 615
  brain tumours 873–4
    high-grade (anaplastic) glioma 878
    local delivery 875–6
    low-grade glioma 880
    lymphoma 882–3
    medulloblastoma 881
    non-germinoma germ cell tumour
      (pineal) 882
  breast cancer
    adjuvant 559, 560–1
    metastatic disease 561–2
    neoadjuvant 549, 555–6, 561
    occult primaries 970
    prediction of response 549–51, 561
    and radiotherapy 559
    and trastuzumab 563
  and cell growth kinetics 188–9, 193–4
  cervical cancer 591–2
  cholangiocarcinoma 525–6
  chronic lymphocytic leukaemia 768

chronic myeloid leukaemia 756
clinical trials see clinical trials
colorectal cancer
  adjuvant 419–22, 458–62
  effect on fertility 464–5
  metastatic disease 52, 67–8, 423–7,
    431–3
combination therapy 191–3
dose 190, 191
  metronomic dosing vs MTD 66
  optimization 220–1
drug shortages 232, 233t, 238
endometrial cancer 592
gallbladder cancer 524, 525
gastric cancer 402–3
  adjuvant 400–1
  palliative 402–3
  perioperative 400
head and neck cancer
  laryngeal/hypopharyngeal 348–9
  nasopharyngeal 343–4
  oral cavity 345
  oropharyngeal 346
  palliative 352, 354
  salivary gland 354
  sinonasal 342
isolated limb perfusion/infusion (ILP/
  ILI) 683, 696, 860
liver cancer 518–19
  chemosaturation technique 517
  in combination with targeted
    therapies 521
  HBV reactivation 521–2
  TACE 516, 517, 521
lung cancer
  carcinoid tumours 648–9
  elderly patients 643
  LCNEC 649
  NSCLC (early stage) 638–9
  NSCLC (first-line therapy) 641–3
  NSCLC (locally advanced) 640–1
  NSCLC (maintenance therapy) 643
  NSCLC (metastatic) 641, 642t
  NSCLC (second-line therapy) 644
  NSCLC (with targeted therapies) 629,
    643–4, 645
  SCLC 68, 647–8
lymphoma 817
  aggressive B-cell 817–20
  CNS disease 882–3
  Hodgkin 821–2
  indolent B-cell 821, 822t, 824t
  mantle cell 820
  NK/T-cell 832
  pre-transplant conditioning 826–7
  relapsed disease 822–3
  T-cell lymphomas 832
mechanisms of action 186–8, 191
melanoma 683, 687
mesothelioma
  adjuvant 665–7
  intraoperative 540–2, 667
  neoadjuvant 667–9
  systemic 538–40, 664–5
myeloma 792–3
  at relapse 799
  consolidation 795
  induction 793–5
  maintenance 793, 795–6
  older patients 796

neoadjuvant, principles of use 193–4
neuroendocrine tumours 648–9, 948,
  956–7t, 958
oesophageal cancer 377–8
  adjuvant 381
  neoadjuvant 379–80
  palliative 381–2
ovarian cancer 68, 587, 592–3, 596, 597
pancreatic cancer 494–6, 496–7
  before chemoradiotherapy 490–1
penile cancer 603, 606
phaeochromocytoma 937
pharmacogenetics 99–100, 190, 215
pharmacokinetics 189–90, 209, 210–15
plasma cell leukaemia 800
POEMS syndrome 800
prolymphocytic leukaemia 773
prostate cancer 612
rationing 232, 233t, 238
resistance
  in CSCs 9, 89
  increases with subsequent cycles
    189, 191
  multidrug 89, 191–2
  in SCLC/ovarian cancer 68
sarcoma
  bone 856, 860–1
  soft tissue 857–60
skin cancer
  BCC 693
  melanoma 683, 687
  Merkel cell carcinoma 697
  SCC 694, 696
testicular cancer 608, 609
thymic tumours 656, 657
thyroid cancer 922, 927
topical 603, 683, 693, 694–5
treatment intervals 191
unknown primary site 970, 971–2
vaginal cancer 592
vulvar cancer 592
Chernobyl accident 150–1, 706, 919
childbearing, breast cancer risk 546
Child-Pugh score 514
children
  cancer in see paediatric cancer
  of survivors of cancer 319
China
  HBV vaccination 257
  lifestyle effects 156t
  nasopharyngeal carcinoma 342
  smoking 132
CHK1/CHK2 proteins (checkpoint) 76, 84
CHL see Hodgkin lymphoma
chlorambucil 768
cholangiocarcinoma
  causes and risk factors 509–10, 511
  chemotherapy 525–6
  clinical presentation 525
  ERCP 513–14
  histopathology 511, 526f
  imaging 512, 513–14, 525f
  incidence 509
  surgery 525
cholangioscopy 514
cholecystectomy 445, 522–3
choledochal cysts 509
cholelithiasis 508–9
chondrosarcoma 846b, 849t, 856, 857, 861
  head and neck 336, 893–4

CHOP chemotherapy 817–18
  R-CHOP 823
    aggressive B-cell lymphoma 818–20
    indolent B-cell lymphoma 821
    mantle cell lymphoma 820
  T-cell lymphomas 832
chordoma 856, 857, 861
  skull base 893–4
choriocarcinoma 67
choroidal lymphoma 913t, 914
choroidal melanoma 908–11
choroid plexus tumours 869t, 894
chromogranin A 944
chromosome behaviour during mitosis 35–6
chromosome instability (CIN) 72, 77
  acute lymphoblastic leukaemia 715–23
  acute myeloid leukaemia 699
  carcinogens promoting 144
  chronic lymphocytic leukaemia 767
  chronic myeloid leukaemia 754, 755, 756,
    759–60
  colorectal cancer 447, 460–1
  DLBCL 816
  melanoma 677–8
  mesothelioma 660
  myeloma 783–4
  sarcoma 849–50t, 850
  telomere shortening 7, 78
  unknown primary 966, 968
chronic lymphocytic leukaemia (CLL) 766–70,
  813
  genetic profiles 767, 814–15
  and skin cancer 690
chronic myeloid leukaemia (CML) 754–66
  chemotherapy 756
  clinical presentation 756
  CSCs 89, 90
  epidemiology 754
  genetic profiles 755, 756
    monitoring changes 759–60, 763–4
  histopathology 756
  interferon 756
  molecular biology 755–6
  prognosis 754
  staging 754, 755t
  stem cell transplantation 758, 765
  targeted therapies 754, 756–8
    may be stopped without recurrence 765–6
    monitoring response 758–63, 765
    refractory/recurrent disease 764–5
    resistance 89, 757, 763–4, 765
chylothorax 374
cigarettes see smoking
cigars 131, 628
CIITA gene 815
ciliary body lymphoma 913t
CIN (cervical intraepithelial neoplasia) 272,
  577
CIN (chromosome instability) see chromosome
  instability
circulating tumour cells (CTCs) 67, 93–4
  unknown primary 966–7
circumcision 603
cirrhosis 508, 510, 514, 515
cisplatin 187, 212t
  basal cell carcinoma 693
  bladder cancer 615
  breast cancer 562
  cervical cancer 591–2
  in combination therapies 192
  gastric cancer 400, 402, 403

head and neck cancer 342, 344, 345, 348,
  352, 354
  lung cancer
    neuroendocrine tumours 649
    NSCLC 639, 640, 641–3
    SCLC 646–7, 647–8
  mesothelioma 539, 540, 541, 664–5
  neuroendocrine tumours 649, 957t
  oesophageal cancer 377, 378, 382
  penile cancer 606
CKI (cyclin-dependent kinase inhibitors) 28,
  33, 34
  CDKN1B 390
  p16 see p16 protein/CDKN2A gene
cladribine 772
CLASSIC trial 401, 401t
class switch recombination 783
clathrin-coated vesicles 24
clearance of drugs 214
clear cell carcinoma
  endometrial 579
  ovarian 580
  renal 616, 617, 618–19
  vaginal 581
clear cell sarcoma 849t, 854
CLEOPATRA trial 564–5
clinical benefit rate 497
clinical nurse specialists 196, 198
clinical trials 220–6
  adaptive design 225
  analysis 220, 225–6
    interim 221, 224
    ITT principle 226
    multiple comparisons 226
    surrogate endpoints 223
  biomarker discovery 102, 103f
  design 220–5
  endpoints 223
    secondary 226
    surrogate 223, 494, 497
  ethics 221, 229–32
  for individualized treatments 184
  Phase I 220–1, 223, 224
    ethics 229–31
  Phase II 221
  Phase II/III combined 224–5
  Phase III 221–3
    endpoints 223, 225–6
    placebo use 231
    QoL assessment 307–9
    research biopsies 231–2
  QoL assessment 303, 307–9
  randomization
    Phase II studies 221
    Phase III studies 222
  sample size/power 223–4
  for screening tests 267
CLL see chronic lymphocytic leukaemia
clofarabine 709, 730
Clonorchis spp. 509–10, 511
Cmax (peak concentration) of a drug 210
CML see chronic myeloid leukaemia
CNOT3 gene 722
CNS tumours see brain tumours; spinal
  tumours
cognitive changes
  brain tumours 871
  iatrogenic 315, 730, 873
cohesin 35, 701
cohort-of-three design 220–1, 224
COLOFOL trial 422

colonization 5
colonography 271, 453
colonoscopy
  diagnostic 453
  screening 271, 465
  see also sigmoidoscopy
ColoPrint® 461
colorectal cancer (CRC) 444–67
  adenoma 408, 411, 452, 456
  anti-inflammatory agents 114, 115, 264,
    446–7
  case study 433
  causes and risk factors 156, 157, 444–6
  chemoradiotherapy
    adjuvant 415, 418
    neoadjuvant 168, 416–19, 453
    restaging after 410, 418
  chemotherapy
    adjuvant 419–22, 458–62
    effect on fertility 464–5
    metastatic disease 52, 67–8, 423–7, 431–3
  clinical presentation 408
  diagnosis 408, 453
  diet 157, 445, 465
  in the elderly 418, 424, 459, 464
  exercise 156, 465
  genetic profiles 99, 444, 447–50, 460–2
    BRAF and KRAS 429, 449, 460
  hereditary syndromes 277t, 278f, 280–2,
    449–51
    FAP see familial adenomatous polyposis
    HNPCC see Lynch syndrome
  histopathology 452–3
  imaging 408–11, 453, 466
  incidence 263, 278t, 444
  lymph node involvement
    imaging 409–10
    management 415, 419
    prognosis 452
    risk of metastasis in early cancer 457t
  macroscopic appearance 411f, 452
  metastatic 423–33
    chemotherapy 52, 67–8, 423–7, 431–3
    follow-up scans 422
    HIPEC 167, 457
    to the liver 67–8, 204, 431–2, 457, 463, 513
    multidisciplinary care 204, 433
    to the ovary 580
    peritoneal 167, 457, 534
    radiotherapy 415, 419, 463
    resection of distant metastases 68, 431–2,
      457
    survival rates 423t
    targeted therapies 52, 427–31, 432, 433,
      459–60
    treatment holidays 432–3
    treatment intention 431–2
  molecular biology 447–50
    CSCs 87t
    inflammation 444
    risk stratification for adjuvant
      therapy 460–2
  mortality 263
  multidisciplinary care 201t, 204, 433, 454,
    463–6
  neuroendocrine tumours 944, 952
  palliative care 424, 432, 456
  premalignant lesions 408, 411, 451–2, 456
  prevention
    lifestyle changes 445
    pharmacological 114, 115, 263–4, 446–7

surgery 165, 456
prognostic markers 99, 452–3, 461–2
QoL 419, 424, 465, 466
radiotherapy 168, 412–19, 462–3
   for liver metastases 463
recurrence 168, 409, 412, 415f, 422, 462
screening 264, 270–1, 446, 465
staging 408, 452
   preoperative 409, 453–4
   restaging after neoadjuvant CRT 410, 418–19
stents 456
stoma care 423, 465
surgery 453
   anal sphincter preservation 411, 417, 418
   audits 169–70, 423
   emergency 456
   endoscopic polypectomy 167, 411, 456–7
   follow-up procedures 170, 422–3, 465–6
   in IBD 456
   laparoscopic 412, 455–6
   liver metastases 68, 431–2, 457
   lung metastases 457
   margins of resection 165, 409
   outcomes 412, 457
   perioperative care 411, 454
   peritoneal metastases 457
   prophylactic 165, 456
   resection technique 411–12, 454–5
   risk-adapted procedures 417–18, 418
   splenic flexure tumours 455
   transanal 167, 411
surveillance 313, 422–3, 465–6
survival rates 457, 466
targeted therapies 52, 418, 427–31, 432, 433, 459–60
in the young 46–55, 288, 451
colorectal cancer profile with unknown
   primary 969, 970
colpectomy 584
colposcopy 272
communication with the patient
   end-of-life discussions 297
   genetic counselling 276, 278, 279–81, 288
   and screening uptake 271
   shared decision-making 170–1
comparative genomic hybridization
   (CGH) 677, 720
computed tomography (CT)
   adrenal tumours 930f, 935, 936, 937f
   brain tumours 871
      lymphoma 882, 883f
   cervical cancer (PET/CT) 581
   colorectal cancer 453
      PET/CT 453, 466
      screening 271
   head and neck cancer 337–40
      nasopharyngeal 343
      PET/CT 338–40
      sinonasal 341
   hepatobiliary cancers 512–13, 522, 523f
   lung cancer (PET/CT) 635
   mesothelioma
      peritoneal 537–8
      pleural 665f, 666f
   myeloma (PET/CT) 789f, 790
   oesophageal cancer 371
   oesophageal cancer (PET/CT) 371, 375
   orbital tumours 906
   pancreatic cancer 499f
   phaeochromocytoma 936, 937f

renal cancer 617
   sarcoma 844
   unknown primary (PET/CT) 968
   urothelial cell carcinoma 614, 615–16
computer-adaptive testing of QoL 305–6
computer modelling
   carcinogenicity 147
   pharmacokinetics 215
condensin 35
confidence intervals 225–6
confocal laser microscopy 677
conformal radiotherapy 178, 180–1, 376
confounding factors in trial design 102
congenital adrenal hyperplasia 933
conization of the cervix 581
conjunctival tumours 904
   lymphoma 911–12, 912f
   melanoma 907–8, 907f, 907f
CONKO-001 trial 491, 494
Conn's syndrome 930–1
consent procedures
   clinical trials 230t, 231
   radiotherapy 182
continual reassessment method (CRM) 224
contrast-enhanced ultrasound (CEUS) 512
controls for biomarker tests 105
conus medullaris tumours 889–90
core binding factor AML 705
corticosteroids
   acute lymphoblastic leukaemia 716, 725, 730
   aldosterone-producing adenoma 929f, 930–1
   brain tumours 872, 882, 891
   chronic lymphocytic leukaemia 768
   for fatigue 296
   hydrocortisone replacement therapy 930, 932
   hypercortisolism see Cushing syndrome
   lymphoma 817–18, 882
   myeloma 793, 794b, 796
   spinal tumours 688, 893
costs of cancer care 241
   biomarker tests 104
   to cancer survivors 319
   controlling 239–41
   cost-effectiveness analysis 238–9
   end-of-life care 241
   ethics 232–3, 240–1
   to individual patients 237–8, 240–1, 319
   in metastatic CRC 424
   to society at large 236–7
   targeted therapies 53, 238
cotinine 128
counselling see genetic counselling
Cowden's syndrome 451
COX2 inhibitors
   colorectal cancer prevention 264, 446–7
   penile cancer 607
   skin cancer prevention 697–8
CpG island methylation 77, 122
   breast cancer 549
   colorectal cancer 448–9, 452
   gastric cancer 390, 391
   inhibition 709
   oesophageal cancer (of p16 gene
      CDKN2A) 367
cranial nerves
   laryngeal nerve 369, 374, 634
   optic nerve 879, 884, 885, 906
   paraganglioma 355–6
   vestibular schwannoma 893–4
craniofacial surgery 341
craniopharyngioma 887, 939

CRC see colorectal cancer
C-reactive protein (CRP) 113
CREBBP gene (CREB-binding protein,
   CBP) 716, 721t, 723, 815
crizotinib 630, 646, 858
CRLF2 gene 719, 721t
Crohn's disease 444, 456
Cronkhite–Canada syndrome 451
CROSS trial 377, 379
CRP (C-reactive protein) 113
CRT see chemoradiotherapy
cryoglobulin 787
cryosurgery 611, 618, 692
CRYSTAL trial 429, 430t, 431
CSCs see cancer stem cells
CT see computed tomography
CTCs (circulating tumour cells) 67, 93–4
   unknown primary 966–7
CTL (cytotoxic T-cells) (CD8+) 6, 111, 112, 114
CTLA4 inhibitors 115, 687
CTNNB1 gene (β-catenin) 29, 393
CUP see cancer of unknown primary
Cushing syndrome
   adrenal adenoma 928–30
   adrenal carcinoma 932
   ectopic ACTHoma 945t, 950, 955t
   pituitary adenoma 939, 942–3
cutaneous T-cell lymphoma 814, 831–2
cyclin-dependent kinase inhibitors (CKI) 28, 33, 34
   CDKN1B 390
   p16 see p16 protein/CDKN2A gene
cyclin-dependent kinases (CDK) 28, 31–3
   CDK4 in melanoma 675t
   in DNA replication control 34
   in G1/S phase transition 34–5, 367
   in mitosis 34–5, 36
cyclins 28
   cyclin-CDK1 complexes 32–3, 34–5
   D1 331, 366, 784
   D3 816, 817
   E 390, 578
   ubiquitination 33, 36
cyclophosphamide 212t
   breast cancer 561
   chronic lymphocytic leukaemia 768, 769
   lymphoma (CHOP) 817–18
   myeloma 794b
cystectomy 615
cystoscopy 614, 616
cytarabine (cytosine arabinoside) 193, 704, 706, 709
   post-remission 709–10
cytochrome P-450 enzymes
   activation of carcinogens 129, 145
   drug metabolism 189, 190, 211, 214
   polymorphisms 190
cytogenetic abnormalities see chromosome
   instability; translocations
cytokines
   and inflammation 8, 110
   linking local and systemic immune
      response 113–14
   pathogenesis of gastric cancer 389
   as therapeutic targets 115
   and T lymphocytes 111
cytosine arabinoside (cytarabine) 193, 704, 706, 709
   post-remission 709–10
cytotoxic T-cells (CTL) (CD8+) 6, 111, 112, 114

D

dabrafenib 686
dacarbazine 858
dairy products 157
Dargent's operation 582
dasatinib
  acute lymphoblastic leukaemia 727
  chronic lymphocytic leukaemia 770
  chronic myeloid leukaemia 757–8, 763, 764
    monitoring response 765
    resistance 764
DASISION trial 757, 760, 761t, 763, 764
databases
  cancer registries 169
  radiotherapy treatment 184
daunorubicin
  acute lymphoblastic leukaemia 725
  acute myeloid leukaemia 702, 706, 708f
DCIS (ductal carcinoma in situ) 269, 552, 554, 559
DDR (DNA damage response) pathway 76–7, 82–4
deafness 893
death-inducing signalling complex (DISC) 44
DECISION trial 921–2
decitabine 709
defensive medicine 240
denosumab 563
depression 296–7, 317–18, 872
dermatofibrosarcoma protuberans (DFSP) 17, 849t, 853–4, 858
derm(at)oscopy 677
dexamethasone
  acute lymphoblastic leukaemia 725, 730
  brain tumours 872, 891
  for fatigue 296
  myeloma 793, 794b, 796
dexamethasone suppression test 928, 943
diabetes insipidus 940
diabetes mellitus 445–6, 497
diarrhoea 375, 948, 950
diclofenac 695
diet
  and breast cancer 319, 546
  and cancer risk 156–8, 365, 388, 445, 465, 546
  and colorectal cancer 157, 445, 465
  drug bioavailability 211
  and pancreatic cancer 497
  supplements and cancer prevention 158, 264, 445
  in survivors 319, 320t, 465
diethylstilbestrol 581
diffuse large B-cell lymphoma (DLBCL)
  chemotherapy 817–20
  classification
    by transcriptional profiles 815–16
    by WHO 813
  epidemiology 808
  genetic profiles 815, 815–16
  PMBL 816, 829
  radiotherapy 828–9
digital rectal examination 408, 610
dihydropyrimidine dehydrogenase (DPD) deficiency 214
diphencyprone 683
direct-to-consumer (DTC) genetic testing 286
DIS3 gene 784
DISC (death-inducing signalling complex) 44
disseminated tumour cells (DTC) 63, 65, 93–4

distribution of drugs 211
DLBCL see diffuse large B-cell lymphoma
DNA damage
  by carcinogens 129, 143, 144
  by ionizing radiation 150, 173–4
  by UV light 674
  double strand breaks (DSBs) 76–7, 82–4, 783
DNA methylation 77, 122
  breast cancer 549
  colorectal cancer 448–9, 452
  gastric cancer 390, 391
  inhibition 709
  myeloma 785
  oesophageal cancer (of p16 gene CDKN2A) 367
DNA repair 7, 72
  BER pathway 75–6, 84, 450
  in the cell cycle 28, 36–7, 84
  in CSCs 89
  DDR pathway 76–7, 82–4
  MMR pathway 74–5, 76, 447–8
  NER pathway 75
DNA replication 31, 34
  disruption by chemotherapy agents 186, 187, 193
DNMT3A gene 701, 702
docetaxel 212t
  breast cancer 561
  gastric cancer 403
  head and neck cancer 342, 348
  lung cancer 643, 644
  sarcoma 858
dopamine 935, 937
dopamine agonists 941, 942
dormancy 64–7
  see also quiescence of CSCs
dose-limiting toxicity 191, 192, 220–1
DOT1L methyltransferase 719
double strand breaks (DSB) 76–7, 82–4, 783
dovitinib 619
Down syndrome 719, 723
doxorubicin 212t
  liver cancer 518, 519, 521
  lymphoma (CHOP) 817–18
  mesothelioma 539
  myeloma 794b
  sarcoma 857, 859
DPC4 gene/SMAD4 protein 451, 479, 480
DPP10 gene 660
driver mutations 3, 7–8
drug-eluting beads 517
DSB (double strand breaks) 76–7, 82–4, 783
DTC (disseminated tumour cells) 63, 65, 93–4
ductal carcinoma in situ (DCIS) 269, 552, 554, 559
dumping syndrome 375
dutasteride 264–5
Dutch Gastric Cancer trial 163, 398–9
DWI magnetic resonance imaging 338
dyskaryosis 272
dysphagia 306, 369, 382

E

E2F transcription factors 33–4, 37, 390
E3 ubiquitin ligases 16
  APC 33, 36
  Cbl 24–5
  in mesothelioma 543
  SOCS 14, 25
early detection of cancer 246

early T-cell precursor ALL (ETP ALL) 722
EATL (enteropathy-associated T-cell lymphoma) 814, 831
EBV see Epstein–Barr virus
ECM (extracellular matrix) 480
  angiogenesis 49–51
  cancer cell invasiveness 61, 65–7, 481
  see also tumour microenvironment
ECOG 2993 trial 726, 727
ECOG E1900 trial 702
ECOG E2906 trial 706
ECOG E5202 trial 461
economics
  biomarker test uptake 104
  costs of cancer care 241
    to cancer survivors 319
    controlling 239–41
    cost-effectiveness analysis 238–9, 309
    end-of-life care 241
    ethics 232–3, 240–1
    to individual patients 237–8, 240–1, 319
    in metastatic CRC 424
    to society at large 236–7
    targeted therapies 53, 238
  multidisciplinary teams 198
  resource availability in cancer control planning 250, 251
  vaccines 257, 258, 259–60
Edmonton Staging System (ESS)/revised (rESS) 296
Edmonton Symptom Assessment Scale (ESAS) 294, 303
effect size in QoL assessments 309
EGF see epidermal growth factor
EGFR see epidermal growth factor receptor
elderly patients
  acute myeloid leukaemia 702–4, 708–9, 710, 711
  colorectal cancer 418, 424, 459, 464
  glioblastoma 876
  lung cancer 643
  multidisciplinary care 205, 464
  myeloma 796
  surgery 164
electrochemotherapy 352
electron-photon therapy 664
embolization therapy see trans-arterial chemoembolization (TACE) of hepatic tumours
employment of cancer survivors 319
EMT see epithelial-mesenchymal transition
endocrine therapy 187, 213t
  breast cancer 187, 562, 970
    in combination with RT 559
    prediction of response 551
    prevention 262–3
  carcinogenic 145t
  endometrial cancer 592
  liver cancer 519
  prostate cancer 187, 264–5, 612
endocytosis 24
end-of-life care 293, 297
  cost of futile treatment 241
endometrial cancer
  case study 595–6
  causes and risk factors 156t, 576, 578
  chemotherapy 592
  endocrine therapy 592
  genetic profiles 578
  histopathology 578–9

imaging 583, 589*f*
incidence 576, 577
lymph node involvement 583, 596
Lynch syndrome 578, 583
molecular biology 578, 583
radiotherapy 589–91, 596
surgery 583–4, 595–6
targeted therapies 592
endorectal ultrasound (ERUS) 409
endoscopic retrograde
    cholangiopancreatography
    (ERCP) 513–14
endoscopic ultrasound (EUS)
  hepatobiliary cancers 513
  oesophageal cancer 371, 372
endoscopy
  bronchoscopy 634
  cholangioscopy 514
  colorectal
    colonoscopy 271, 453, 465
    flexible sigmoidoscopy 270–1, 408
    polypectomy 167, 411, 456–7
    rectoscopy 408
  colposcopy 272
  mediastinoscopy 635
  neuroendocrine tumours 949*f*
  oesophageal
    imaging 369, 371, 372
    resection 372
  unknown primary 968
  urinary tract 614, 616
  see also laparoscopy
endosomes 24
endothelial precursor cells (EPCs) 66
energy metabolism of cancer cells 61, 119–23
  as a hallmark of cancer 6, 119
  regulation by mTOR pathway 26–7, 120
  therapeutic targets 123
ENESTnd trial 761, 761*t*, 764
enhanced recovery after surgery (ERAS) 167,
  454
enteropathy-associated T-cell lymphoma
  (EATL) 814, 831
enzalutamide 612
EORTC 08941 trial 640
EORTC 20981 trial 823
EORTC 22844/22845 trials 880
EORTC 22921 trial 420, 422
EORTC 24891 trial 349
EORTC 24954 trial 349
EORTC 26951 trial 878
EORTC QLQ-C30 questionnaire 303, 304–5,
  308–9
eosinophils 111, 756
EPCAM/EPCAM (epithelial cell adhesion
  molecule)
  catumaxomab (anti-CD3/EPCAM) 91, 115
  as a marker for CSCs 90, 94
  mutations 276, 282, 286*f*
ependymoma 869*t*
  intracranial 880
  spinal 888, 889–90, 889*f*
epidemiology
  acute lymphoblastic leukaemia 715, 723
  acute myeloid leukaemia 131, 702–4, 706
  adrenal tumours 928, 930, 931, 933, 935
  bladder cancer 613
  brain tumours 867
  breast cancer 156*t*, 262, 546–7
    negative risk factors 158, 319, 546

radiotherapy 151, 152
  smoking 131, 132
cancer control planning data 248–9
cancer registries 169
cervical cancer 131, 139, 258, 576, 577
cholangiocarcinoma 509–10, 511
chronic lymphocytic leukaemia 766
chronic myeloid leukaemia 754
colorectal cancer 156, 157, 263, 278*t*, 444–6
cost implications of rising incidence 237
endometrial cancer 156*t*, 576, 577–8
eyelid tumours 904
gallbladder cancer 508–9, 510
gastric cancer 156*t*, 388, 389
geographic differences 342, 365, 388, 444,
  508, 602, 628, 754, 808
hairy cell leukaemia 770
head and neck cancer 157, 329
  laryngeal/hypolaryngeal 130, 347
  nasopharyngeal 342
  oropharyngeal 345–6
  salivary gland 353
  sinonasal 340
hepatitis B 256
liver cancer 131, 140, 508, 510–11
lung cancer 151, 628, 646, 648
  and smoking 127, 128*f*, 130, 132, 628
lymphoma 808–9, 912
melanoma 674–6, 908
mesothelioma 533–4, 659
myeloma 782
oesophageal cancer 156*t*, 157, 365, 367
orbital tumours 906
ovarian cancer 576
pancreatic cancer 156*t*, 478
penile cancer 602
phaeochromocytoma 935
pituitary tumours 938*t*, 939
prostate cancer 157, 264, 609
renal cancer 616–17
sarcoma 844, 855, 856
skin cancer 674–6, 690–1, 696
survivors of cancer 312
thymic tumours 655
thyroid cancer 151, 918–19, 923
unknown primary 966–7
urothelial cell cancer 615
uveal melanoma 908
vaginal cancer 576
vulvar cancer 576
epidermal growth factor (EGF) 14, 24
  TGFα 368, 480
epidermal growth factor receptor (EGFR)
  (ErbB1, HER1) 14–15, 24–5, 188
  inhibitors 15, 188
    basal cell carcinoma 693
    block DSB repair 83–4
    colorectal cancer 418, 429–30, 432, 433,
    453, 459–60
    head and neck cancer 346, 348, 352–3
    liver cancer 520
    lung cancer 629, 643, 643–4, 644–6
    pancreatic cancer 496
    penile cancer 607
    pharmacokinetics 213*t*
  molecular biology
    breast cancer 548
    gastric cancer 389
    head and neck cancer 331
    lung cancer 629

mesothelioma 534
  oesophageal cancer 366, 368
  pancreatic cancer 480
  penile cancer 606–7
  thymic tumours 656
  unknown primary 966
  and viruses 25
epidermolysis bullosa 691
epigenetics
  acute lymphoblastic leukaemia 716
  acute myeloid leukaemia 701, 705
  DNA methylation *see* DNA methylation
  histone methylation/demethylation
    701, 785
  imprinting of IGF2 13
  mesothelioma 659–60
  myeloma 785
epileptic seizures 871, 872
epirubicin 212*t*, 378, 382
epithelial-mesenchymal transition (EMT) 5,
  6, 9
  and CSCs 92–3
  invasion of cancer cells 61
  pancreatic cancer 481
  and TGFβ 29–30
epithelioid sarcoma 854
Epstein–Barr virus (EBV) 136–7
  EBV+ lymphoproliferative disorders 137,
    814
  lymphoma 136, 336, 832
  nasopharyngeal carcinoma 136, 333, 343
equipment, research 104
ErbB1 *see* epidermal growth factor receptor
  (EGFR)
ErbB2 *see* HER2/neu-positive (ErbB2)
  cancers
ErbB3 (HER3) 14, 24, 548–9
ErbB family 14
ERCC1 protein 639
ERCP (endoscopic retrograde
  cholangiopancreatography) 513–14
erectile dysfunction 316, 611
ERG gene 720
eribulin 562
ERK signalling pathway *see* RAS/RAF/MAPK
  signalling pathway
erlotinib 213*t*
  colorectal cancer 433
  liver cancer 520
  lung cancer 643, 644, 645*t*
  pancreatic cancer 496
ER-positive cancer
  breast 547, 548, 552–3
    chemotherapy 561
    endocrine therapy 562
    targeted therapies 563
  liver 519
ERUS (endorectal ultrasound) 409
erythromycin 375
erythroplasia of Queyrat 603
ESAS questionnaire 294, 303
ESPAC1/3/4 trials 491, 494
ethics 229–34
  chemoprevention 263
  clinical trials 221, 229–32
  cost of care 232–3
    moral hazard 240–1
  drug shortages 232, 233*t*, 238
  resources 233–4
ethmoid tumours 340, 341, 342

ethnicity
  lymphoma 808
  melanoma 675–6
  myeloma 782
  nasopharyngeal carcinoma 342
  screening rates for colon cancer 282
etoposide 187, 213t
  as cause of AML 706
  lung cancer 646, 647, 648
  lymphoma
    CHOEP 817–18
    R-CHOEP 818
ETV6-RUNX1 fusion gene 715, 718, 720
EUROCARE registry 169
European Organization for Research and
    Treatment of Cancer Core QoL
    Questionnaire (EORTC QLQ-C30) 303,
    304–5, 308–9
European Registration of Cancer Care
    (EURECCA) 169
EUS see endoscopic ultrasound
everolimus 213t
  breast cancer 563
  liver cancer 521
  neuroendocrine tumours 956t, 957
  renal cancer 619
evidence-based medicine 240, 250
Ewing sarcoma/PNET 844, 847, 855–6
  extraskeletal 855, 860
  genetic profiles 849t, 855
  treatment 856, 857, 860
EWSR1 gene 849t
excretion of drugs 189–90, 214
exemestane 562
exercise
  and cancer prevention in survivors 319,
    320t, 465
  for cancer-related fatigue 296
  and cancer risk 156
EXPERT-C trial 418, 422
exportin 1/XPO1 767
external beam radiotherapy (EBRT) 178–80
  see also radiotherapy
extracellular matrix (ECM) 480
  angiogenesis 49–51
  cancer cell invasiveness 61, 65–7, 481
  see also tumour microenvironment
extramedullary plasmacytoma 787, 801
extrapleural pneumonectomy (EPP) 661, 662,
    663–4, 663f
  in multimodality therapy 665–9
eyelid tumours 904–5
eye tumours
  choroidal lymphoma 913t, 914
  conjunctival lymphoma 911–12, 912f
  conjunctival melanoma 907–8, 907f, 907f
  iridal tumours 908, 910, 913t, 914
  metastasis to 906–7, 907, 914
  orbital tumours 905–7
    invasion from sinonasal tumours 341,
      342, 907
  retinal lymphoma 912–14, 912f
  uveal lymphoma 914
  uveal melanoma 908–11

F
FA (Fanconi anaemia) 76–7, 278t
facial nerve 354, 893–4
FACT-G questionnaire 303, 304, 306–7
faecal incontinence 316, 419

faecal occult blood testing 270
fallopian tubes 579
  bilateral salpingo-oophorectomy 280, 586
false negative (type II) error 224
false positive (type I) error 224, 226
FAM46C gene 784
familial adenomatous polyposis (FAP)
  APC gene mutations 29, 77, 288, 450
  attenuated form 288, 450
  fundic gland polyps 393
  genetic counselling 288
  prophylactic surgery 165, 456
  screening 411
familial atypical multiple mole/melanoma
    syndrome (FAMMM) 166, 675, 908
familial cancer syndromes see hereditary
    cancer syndromes
familial medullary thyroid carcinoma 923, 923t
families
  of cancer survivors 219
  relatives at-risk of hereditary syndromes 278,
    280–1
family history 276, 281
family information service (FIS) 280
FAMMM syndrome 166, 675, 908
Fanconi's anaemia 278t
  FA genes 76–7
FAP see familial adenomatous polyposis
fast track surgery 167
fatigue
  cancer-related 294, 296, 767
  in cancer survivors 313–14
fat tissue see obesity
fatty acid synthesis 123
F-box genes 578, 816
FDG-PET see positron emission tomography
fear
  of a positive genetic test 279
  of recurrence 318
females
  faecal occult blood tests 271
  fertility after treatment 317, 464–5, 810
    gynaecological cancer surgery 582, 584,
      586
  gallbladder cancer 509t
  lung cancer 628
  oestrogen-secreting tumours 933
  pituitary tumours 940, 941
  second cancers after Hodgkin disease 153
  smoking and cancer risk 130
  unknown primary site cancers 969, 970
  virilizing tumours 932, 933
feminizing tumours 933
fertility
  preservation strategies 317
    in colorectal cancer 465
    gynaecological cancer surgery 582, 584,
      586
    in lymphoma 810
    testicular cancer 609
FFCD 9901/9102 trials 379, 380–1
FGF see fibroblast growth factor
FGFR see fibroblast growth factor receptor
fibre, dietary 157, 445
fibroblast growth factor (FGF) 15–16
  gastric cancer 391
  oesophageal cancer 368–9
fibroblast growth factor receptor (FGFR) 15–16
  breast cancer 547
  gastric cancer 391

renal cancer 619
fibronectin 65
filum terminale tumours 888, 889–90
finasteride 264–5
FIRE-3 trial 429
FISH see fluorescence in situ hybridization
5α-reductase inhibitors 187, 264–5
FL see follicular lymphoma
FLAGS trial 402t, 403
flavopiridol (alvocidib) 770
flexible sigmoidoscopy 270–1, 408
flow cytometry
  acute lymphoblastic leukaemia 712–13, 722
  acute myeloid leukaemia 705, 712
  chronic lymphocytic leukaemia 766
  chronic myeloid leukaemia 756
  hairy cell leukaemia 771
  myeloma 789–90
  prolymphocytic leukaemia 772, 773
FLT3-ITD mutations (in AML) 699, 702
  inhibitors 712
fludarabine 768–9
fluorescence in situ hybridization (FISH) 677–8
  chronic myeloid leukaemia 756, 760
  myeloma 790
fluoropyrimidines see 5-fluorouracil;
    capecitabine
5-fluorouracil (5-FU)
  colorectal cancer 418, 419, 420, 424–7,
    458–9
    contraindicated 453, 460
  gastric cancer 401, 402, 403
  gynaecological cancers 592
  head and neck cancer 345, 346, 348
  oesophageal cancer 377, 378, 381, 382
  pancreatic cancer 490, 495–6
  penile carcinoma in situ 603
  pharmacokinetics 212t, 214
  squamous cell carcinoma 694
flushing
  carcinoid syndrome 951
  premature menopause 317t
FNCLCC/FFCD trial 400, 401t
FOLFIRINOX regime 239, 495–6
FOLFIRI regime 426
FOLFOXIRI regime 427
FOLFOX regime 426, 519
folinic acid (leucovorin) 495–6
follicular epithelial thyroid cancer 67, 918–23
follicular lymphoma (FL) 808, 813
  genetic profiles 815
  treatment 823, 825, 828
follow-up care 183, 320–1
  surgical audits 169–70, 423
  see also surveillance
FOXO (forkhead) transcription factors 28, 29
FOXP3+ T-lymphocytes (regulatory
    T-cells) 112, 114
  inhibitors 115, 687
fractional cell kill hypothesis 189
fractionation of radiotherapy 177–8
fractures, in myeloma 786, 797, 798
Framework Convention on Tobacco Control
    (WHO) 133
France 237
fruit and vegetables in the diet 156–7
5-FU see 5-fluorouracil
fulvestrant 213t, 562
Functional Assessment of Cancer Therapy–
    General (FACT–G) 303, 304, 306–7

fundic gland polyps 288, 393
fundoscopy
metastases 914
retinal lymphoma 912
uveal melanoma 909f

G
G1/G2 (gap) phases 31
G1 to S phase transition 33–4, 84, 367
in myeloma 783–4
gallbladder cancer (GBC)
causes and risk factors 508–9, 510
chemotherapy 524, 525
clinical presentation 522
ERCP 513–14
histopathology 511
imaging 522, 523f
incidence 508
lymph node involvement 522, 523, 524
palliative care 513, 524–5
surgery 522–4
survival rates 524
gallstones 508–9
Gardasil®/Gardasil® 9 (HPV vaccines) 258
Gardner's syndrome 450
garlic 156
gastrectomy 396–7, 399–400
laparoscopic 399
gastric anatomy 392
gastric cancer
causes and risk factors 156t, 388, 389
chemoradiotherapy 400
chemotherapy 402–3
adjuvant 400–1
palliative 402–3
perioperative 400
classification 388, 393–4
diffuse-type 388, 391–2, 395, 396
genetic profiles 389–93, 396, 403
genetic syndromes 288, 396
histopathology 370, 388, 392–6
incidence 388
intestinal-type 388, 389–91, 394, 396
lymph node involvement 163, 397–9
station definitions 398
macroscopic appearance 394f
metastatic 395–6
chemotherapy 402–3
laparoscopy 400
molecular biology 389–92, 396, 403
neuroendocrine tumours 953
palliative care 399, 402–3, 404
premalignant lesions 388, 392–3
staging 394b
surgery 396–7
adjuvant/neoadjuvant therapies 400–1
laparoscopic 399, 400
lymphadenectomy 163, 397–9
palliative 399
reduction 399–400
survival rates 400
targeted therapies 396, 402, 403–4
gastric outlet obstruction 375
gastrinoma 945t, 947–50, 954t
gastritis, atrophic 388, 392–3
gastroenteropancreatic neuroendocrine
neoplasms see neuroendocrine tumours
gastrointestinal stromal tumours (GIST) 17, 51
gastrointestinal tract
bleeding 270, 369

melanoma metastases 685
primary cancers see colorectal cancer; gastric
cancer; oesophageal cancer; small bowel
cancer
gastro-oesophageal junction cancer
(GEJ) 369–70
treatment 376, 377–8, 381, 382
see also oesophageal cancer
gastro-oesophageal reflux disease (GORD) 367
gastroparesis, post-operative 374–5, 488
GAVI Alliance 257, 258
gefitinib 213t, 645–6, 645t
GEJ see gastro-oesophageal junction cancer
gemcitabine 212t
cholangiocarcinoma 526
lung cancer 643
pancreatic cancer 490, 494–5
sarcoma 858
gemtuzumab ozogamicin 707
Genansense® (oblimersen) 44
gender see females; males
gene expression analysis 84
breast cancer 99, 548–51, 561
colorectal cancer 461–2
head and neck cancer 331
mesothelioma 660
NSCLC 119
uveal melanoma 911
genetic counselling 276–88
at-risk relatives 278, 280–1
breast cancer 165–6, 280, 282
children and young adults 288
DTC tests 286
family information service 280
identification of mutations 277, 278–9
Lynch syndrome 279, 280–2
screening of all CRC cases 282–6
medullary thyroid cancer 918, 924
melanoma 675
missed in ethnic minorities 282
psychosocial impact 279–80
service provision 278
genetic instability 72–9
acute lymphoblastic leukaemia 715–23
acute myeloid leukaemia 699
chronic lymphocytic leukaemia 767
chronic myeloid leukaemia 754, 755, 756,
759–60
colorectal cancer 282, 444, 447–9, 460–1
in CSCs 91
DLBCL 816
endometrial cancer 578
gastric cancer 390–1
genotoxic carcinogens 143, 144
as a hallmark of cancer 7–8
and inflammation 444
melanoma 677–8
mesothelioma 660
in metastatic cells 65
myeloma 783–4, 784, 786t
sarcoma 849–50t, 850
in sporadic cancers 72, 77–8
unknown primary cancer 966, 968
genetic profiles
acute lymphoblastic leukaemia 713, 715–16
B-cell lineages 716–21
and risk of ALL 723
T-cell lineages 717t, 721–2
acute myeloid leukaemia 699–702, 705,
711, 718

adrenal adenoma 928
brain tumours 122, 868, 870f, 877
breast cancer 99, 165–6, 547–51, 561
cervical cancer 577
chronic lymphocytic leukaemia 767, 814–15
chronic myeloid leukaemia 755, 756
monitoring changes 759–60, 763–4
colorectal cancer 99, 447–9, 460–1
BRAF and KRAS 429, 449, 460
endometrial cancer 578
gastric cancer 389–93, 396, 403
hairy cell leukaemia 770, 814
head and neck cancer 329–31, 355
lung cancer 119, 628–30, 631, 644, 646
lymphoma 809, 814–15
ALCL 813–14
Burkitt 817
DLBCL 815, 815–16
PMBL 816
T-cell 832
melanoma 674, 675t, 677–8, 679–80, 907
mesothelioma
peritoneal 534
pleural 660
myeloma 782, 783–4
at relapse 799
prognostic 783, 791
test methods 790
oesophageal cancer 366–7, 368–9
ovarian cancer 579
pancreatic cancer 478–80
penile cancer 606–7
pituitary tumours 939
prolymphocytic leukaemia 772, 773
sarcoma 849–50
thyroid cancer 919, 921, 923–4
unknown primary cancer 966–7, 968
genetic syndromes see hereditary cancer
syndromes
genital warts 258
genitourinary cancers see penile cancer;
prostate cancer; renal cancer; testicular
cancer; urothelial cell carcinoma
genome-wide association studies (GWAS) 723
germ cell tumours
pineal 881, 882
testicular 306–7, 607–9
germinal centres 783, 784f, 815
GHRHoma (growth hormone-releasing
hormone-secreting tumour) 951
GIST (gastrointestinal stromal tumours) 17, 51
GITSG trials 490, 493
glans penis 603–4
Glasgow Prognostic Score (GPS) 112–13
Gleason score 610
Gleevec® see imatinib
glioblastoma
in the elderly 876
genetic profiles 122, 868, 870f
imaging 874–5, 874f, 875f
spinal 890
treatment 872, 875–6
glioma
classification 869t
high-grade 872, 873–8
low-grade 878–80
management of complications 872
see also astrocytoma; ependymoma;
glioblastoma; oligodendroglioma
glucagonoma 945t, 950, 954t

glucocorticoid-remediable aldosteronism 930, 931
glucose metabolism 6, 61, 119–23
glutamine metabolism 6
glycine metabolism 91
glycogen synthesis 123
glycolysis 6, 61, 119–22
goals of care discussions 295f
GOG-169/179/204 trials 592
goitre 919
Gompertzian growth model 188–9
gonadotrophin-releasing hormone (GnRH)
       analogues 187, 612
gonadotrophins
    hCG as a tumour marker 607, 608, 881
    and pituitary tumours
       deficiency 940
       excess 939
GORD (gastro-oesophageal reflux disease) 367
Gorlin's syndrome 277t, 690, 873, 905
GORTEC trial 349
government policy 245–52
gp130 (glycoprotein receptor 130) 14
GPS (Glasgow Prognostic Score) 112–13
graft-versus-host disease (GVHD) 726, 758
graft-versus-leukaemia (GVL) effect 726, 758
graft-versus-myeloma effect 795
granulocytes 756
grapefruit juice 211
Graves' disease 918
GRB2 (growth factor receptor-bound protein
    2) 11, 15, 24, 25
growth factors 11–18, 23–5
    see also epidermal growth factor (EGF);
       fibroblast growth factor (FGF);
       hepatocyte growth factor (HGF);
       insulin-like growth factor (IGF1/IGF2);
       platelet-derived growth factor (PDGF);
       transforming growth factor β (TGFβ);
       vascular endothelial growth factor
       (VEGF)
growth hormone (GH)
    deficiency 940
    excess 939, 942
growth hormone-releasing hormone-secreting
       tumour (GHRHoma) 951
GTPase activating proteins (GAPs) 25, 26
GTPases (RAS family) 25
    see also KRAS oncogene; NRAS oncogene
guaiac based faecal occult blood testing
       (gFOBT) 270
gynaecological cancers see cervical cancer;
       endometrial cancer; ovarian cancer;
       vaginal cancer; vulvar cancer

H
HAEMACARE Project (Europe) 808
haematogenous metastasis 62–3
haematopoietic stem cell transplantation
    acute lymphoblastic leukaemia 713–14,
       726–7, 727–8
    acute myeloid leukaemia 699, 710–11, 712
    adverse effects 316
    amyloidosis 800–1
    chronic myeloid leukaemia 758, 765
    conditioning 826–7
       reduced-intensity 711, 727, 758, 827
    lymphoma 822, 823, 826–7
    myeloma 795, 796, 799
    POEMS syndrome 800
    prolymphocytic leukaemia 773

haematuria 613
Haemoccult II® test 270
haemodialysis 797
haemorrhage
    acute promyelocytic leukaemia 705
    endometrial cancer 583
    oesophageal cancer 369
    after pancreatic surgery 488
hairy cell leukaemia (HCL) 770–2, 814
hairy cell leukaemia-variant (HCL-v) 774
half-life of a drug 210
halogenated carcinogens 144t
hamartomatous polyposis syndromes 451
hamartomatous polyps 452
Hashimoto's thyroiditis 920, 923
HBV see hepatitis B virus
HCC (hepatocellular carcinoma) see liver cancer
hCG (human chorionic gonadotrophin) 607,
       608, 881
HCL (hairy cell leukaemia) 770–2, 814
HCL-v (hairy cell leukaemia-variant) 774
HCV (hepatitis C virus) 140, 510–11
headache 868, 871, 940
head and neck cancer 329–56
    causes and risk factors 157, 329, 340
    chemoradiotherapy
       laryngeal/hypopharyngeal tumours 348–9
       nasopharyngeal 343
       oropharyngeal 346
       sinonasal lymphoma 829, 832
       unknown primary 350
    chemotherapy
       nasopharyngeal carcinoma 343–4
       oral cavity tumours 345
       palliative 352, 354
       salivary gland tumours 354
       sinonasal tumours 342
    clinical presentation
       laryngeal/hypopharyngeal 347
       nasopharyngeal tumours 343
       oropharyngeal tumours 345
       paraganglioma 355
       salivary gland tumours 353
       sinonasal tumours 340–1
    EBV-associated 136, 333, 336, 343
    eyelid tumours 904–5
    eye tumours see eye tumours
    genetic profiles 329–31, 355
    histopathology 331–6, 353
    HPV-associated 329
       histopathology 333
       molecular biology 84, 329, 330f, 331
       treatment 84, 346
    hypopharyngeal 337, 338, 347–9
    imaging 337–40, 341, 343, 349, 353, 355
    incidence 340, 342, 345, 347, 353
    laryngeal 130, 157, 337, 338, 347–9, 351
    lymph node involvement
       imaging 337, 339
       nasopharyngeal tumours 343
       oropharyngeal tumours 345
       pathology report 334
       salivary gland tumours 354
       unknown primary 349–51
    metastatic
       imaging 337, 339
       treatment 344, 348
    molecular biology 329–31
       CSCs 87t
       subtypes 331

multidisciplinary care 203t, 205
    nasopharyngeal 136, 333, 333f, 342–4
    oral cavity 157, 344–5
    orbital tumours 905–7
    oropharyngeal 84, 157, 329, 333, 333f, 345–7
    paraganglioma 355–6, 935
    photodynamic therapy 344, 352
    premalignant lesions 331, 345
    radiotherapy
       adverse effects 306, 316, 343, 344, 348
       imaging after 338, 340
       laryngeal/hypopharyngeal tumours 348
       nasopharyngeal carcinoma 343, 344
       oral cavity tumours 345
       oropharyngeal tumours 84, 346–7
       paragangliomas 355–6
       QoL issues 306
       recurrent disease 352
       salivary gland tumours 354
       sinonasal tumours 341–2, 829, 832
       unknown primary 350
    recurrence 175f, 351
       imaging 338, 339–40
       treatment 344, 348, 351–3
    salivary gland 336, 353–5
    sinonasal 334, 336t, 340–2
       lymphoma 336, 829, 832
       orbital invasion 341, 342, 907
    skull base tumours 335t, 336t, 893–4
    staging 341, 349–50
    surgery
       intraoperative evaluation 333–4
       laryngeal/hypopharyngeal tumours 347,
          348, 349, 351
       nasopharyngeal carcinoma 344
       oral cavity tumours 344–5
       oropharyngeal tumours 347
       paragangliomas 355–6
       recurrent disease 344, 351–2
       salivary gland tumours 354
       sinonasal tumours 341, 342
       unknown primary 350
    survival rates 342, 355
    targeted therapies
       laryngeal/hypolaryngeal 348
       metastatic disease 352–3
       oropharyngeal 346
       salivary gland tumours 355t
    thyroid cancer 67, 151, 337
    unknown primary 349–51, 968, 969, 970
health behaviour modification 156–7, 319–20,
       465
health economics see economics
hearing loss 893
heart disease
    amyloidosis 800
    carcinoid syndrome 951, 958
    cardiotoxicity of cancer treatment 315, 377,
       559, 560, 730, 823
heated intraoperative chemotherapy
    intraperitoneal (HIPEC) 167, 457, 540
    thoracic 667
hedgehog (Hh) signalling pathway 391
    basal cell carcinoma 691, 693
    pancreatic cancer 481
Hedinger's syndrome (endocardial
       fibrosis) 951, 958
HeLa cells 139
Helicobacter pylori 388, 389, 390, 392
    antibiotic therapy 392

gallbladder cancer 509, 510
helper T-cells (CD4+) 111, 112, 114
hepatic artery 517, 524f
hepatic drug metabolism 189–90, 214
  and hepatic impairment 190
hepatitis B virus (HBV) 139
  liver cancer 140, 256, 510
    reactivation 521–2
  nasopharyngeal carcinoma 343
  vaccines 256–7
hepatitis C virus (HCV) 140, 510–11
hepatocellular carcinoma (HCC) see liver
  cancer
hepatocyte growth factor (HGF) 11–13
  gastric cancer 390, 391
  liver cancer 520
  MET mutations in unknown primary 966
hepatolithiasis 510
HER1 see epidermal growth factor receptor
  (EGFR)
HER2/neu-positive (ErbB2) cancers
  breast 547–8
    chemotherapy 560
    cost of targeted therapy 238
    radiotherapy + trastuzumab 559
    targeted therapies 67, 553, 562–3, 564–5, 892
  gastric 389–90, 396, 402, 403
  oesophageal 378, 382
  unknown primary 966
HER3 (ErbB3) 14, 24, 548–9
Herceptin® see trastuzumab
hereditary cancer syndromes 72, 78, 277–8t
  acute lymphoblastic leukaemia 723
  adrenal tumours 930, 931, 935
  breast/ovarian 165–6, 280, 546–7
  CNS tumours 868t
  colorectal 277t, 278f, 449–51
    see also familial adenomatous polyposis
      (FAP); Lynch syndrome
  DTC genetic tests 286
  gastric cancer 288, 396
  genetic counselling 276, 288
    at-risk relatives 278, 280–1
    children and young adults 288
    family information service 280
    identification of mutations 277, 278–9
    missed in ethnic minorities 282
    psychosocial impact 279–80
    service provision 278
  genetic screening of cancer cases 282–6
  melanoma 166, 674–5, 908
  MEN1 166, 939, 944, 948
  MEN2A/2B 918, 923–4, 926, 926–7, 935
  MUTYH-associated polyposis 75, 450
  oesophageal cancer (tylosis) 365
  pancreatic cancer 478
  phaeochromocytoma 926, 935
  pituitary tumours 939
  prophylactic surgery 165, 280, 456, 554
  renal cancer 616–17
  skin cancer 166, 674–5, 690–1, 905
  thyroid cancer 918, 919, 923–4
  upper urinary tract cancer 615
  uveal melanoma 908
hereditary non-polyposis colorectal cancer
  (HNPCC) see Lynch syndrome
herpesviruses 136
  EBV 136–7
    EBV+ lymphoproliferative disorders
      137, 814

  lymphoma 136, 336, 832
    nasopharyngeal carcinoma 136, 333, 343
  Kaposi's sarcoma-associated 137–9
HGF see hepatocyte growth factor
HIF (hypoxia-inducible transcription factor)
  system 5, 121–2, 122–3
high intensity focused ultrasound (HIFU) 516,
  611
high-precision conformal radiotherapy 178,
  180–1, 376
HIPEC (hyperthermic intraperitoneal
  chemotherapy) 167, 457, 540
Hiroshima A-bomb survivors 150, 706
histone acetyltransferases 815
  see also CREBBP gene
histones
  H3F3A in glioblastoma 868
  methylation/demethylation 701, 785
HIV-associated tumours 137–9, 808
HL see Hodgkin lymphoma
HMG-CoA reductase inhibitors (statins) 115
HNPCC (hereditary non-polyposis colorectal
  cancer) see Lynch syndrome
HNSCC see head and neck cancer
hoarseness (laryngeal nerve damage) 369,
  374, 634
Hodgkin lymphoma (HL/CHL)
  chemotherapy 821–2
  classification 813b
  clinical types 809–10
  EBV infections 136
  paediatric 831
  radiotherapy 829–31
  second cancers in survivors 152, 153
  targeted therapies 816, 822
home care, palliative 294
homologous recombination DNA repair
  82, 84
hormonal therapy see endocrine therapy
hormone replacement therapy 546
hospice care 294f
hot drinks 365
hot flashes see flushing
HOX genes 722
HPV see human papilloma virus
HR-type DLBCL 815
HTLV1 (human T-cell leukaemia virus 1) 139,
  832
human chorionic gonadotrophin (hCG) 607,
  608, 881
human papilloma virus (HPV)
  cervical cancer 139, 258, 577
  and EGFR 25
  head and neck cancer 329
    histopathology 333
    molecular biology 84, 329, 330f, 331
    treatment 84, 346
  penile cancer 606, 607
  radiosensitivity of tumours 84
  screening tests 273
  vaccines 258–9, 272–3, 606
  vaginal cancer 580
  vulvar cancer 581
human T-cell leukaemia virus 1 (HTLV-1)
  139, 832
humoral immune response 111, 113
Hürthle (oncocytic) cell carcinoma 920
hydrocephalus 871, 880–1, 887
hydrocortisone 930, 932
2-hydroxyglutarate (2-HG) 122, 701

5-hydroxyindoleacetic acid (5-HIAA) 951
hydroxyurea 756
hyperaldosteronism 930–1
hypercalcaemia 786, 797
hypercortisolism see Cushing syndrome
hyperdiploidy 716
hyperfractionated radiotherapy 178
hyperleukocytosis 706
hyperlipidaemia 787
hyperparathyroidism 926–7
hyperplastic polyposis syndrome 451
hyperprolactinaemia 938–9, 941
hypertension 936
hyperthermic intraperitoneal chemotherapy
  (HIPEC) 167, 457, 540
hyperuricaemia 706, 787
hyperviscosity/ hypervolaemia syndrome
  787, 797
hypodiploidy 716–17
hypofractionated radiotherapy 178, 416, 556
hypoglycaemia syndrome 945t, 946–7
hypokalaemia 931
hypomethylation agents 709
hyponatraemia 787
hypopharyngeal cancer 337, 338, 347–9
hypopituitarism 940, 941
hypothalamic tumours 938t
hypothyroidism 316, 920
  pituitary 940
  and radio-iodine treatment 921
hypoxia
  hypoxic phenotype in unknown primary
    cancers 966
  metabolic effects 122
  promotion of genetic instability 78
  radiotherapy efficacy 173–4, 178
hypoxia-inducible transcription factor (HIF)
  system 5, 121–2, 122–3
hysterectomy
  in cervical cancer 582
  in endometrial cancer 583–4
  in ovarian cancer 586

I
ibritumomab tiuxetan 824–5
ibrutinib 770, 820
idarubicin 818
IDH1/IDH2 genes (isocitrate
  dehydrogenase)
  acute myeloid leukaemia 700–1, 702
  glioma 122, 868, 875, 877
  T-cell lymphoma 815
IFN-α see interferon alpha
ifosfamide 212t, 857–8, 859, 861
IGF see insulin-like growth factor
  (IGF1/IGF2)
IGFR see insulin-like growth factor receptor
  (IGFR1/IGFR2)
IGRT (image-guided radiotherapy) 182, 183
IKZF1 gene 719, 720, 721t, 723
IL1a (interleukin 1 alpha) 391
IL1b (interleukin 1 beta) 389
IL2 (interleukin 2) 687
IL6 (interleukin 6) 14, 113–14
  anti-IL6 therapy 14, 115
IL8 (interleukin 8) 113–14
IL10 (interleukin 10) 389
image-guided adaptive brachytherapy
  588, 595
image-guided radiotherapy (IGRT) 182, 183

imaging
　　adrenal tumours 930f, 931, 932, 935,
　　　　936, 937f
　　bladder cancer 614
　　bone metastases 610, 949f
　　brain tumours 871–2
　　　　choroid plexus 894
　　　　craniopharyngioma 887
　　　　ependymoma 880
　　　　glioblastoma 874–5, 874f, 875f
　　　　high-grade (anaplastic) glioma 876–7, 877f
　　　　intraoperative 872, 875
　　　　low-grade glioma 878–9, 879f
　　　　lymphoma 882, 883f
　　　　medulloblastoma 880
　　　　meningioma 884–5, 884f
　　　　metastatic disease 891
　　　　pineal tumours 881
　　carcinoids (intestinal) 951, 952f, 953f
　　cervical cancer 581, 594f
　　cholangiocarcinoma 512, 513–14, 525f
　　colorectal cancer 408–11, 453, 466
　　costs 237
　　endometrial cancer 583, 589f
　　eyelid tumours 904
　　gallbladder cancer 522, 523f
　　gastrinoma 948
　　head and neck cancer 337–40
　　　　nasopharyngeal 343
　　　　paraganglioma 355
　　　　salivary glands 353
　　　　sinonasal 341
　　　　unknown primary 349
　　insulinoma 946–7, 948f
　　liver cancer 511–12, 513, 514
　　　　for regional therapies 517
　　lung cancer 635, 638
　　lymphoma 811
　　　　cerebral 882, 883f
　　melanoma 677, 680, 682, 684, 908
　　mesothelioma
　　　　asbestos 661
　　　　peritoneal 537–8
　　　　pleural 661, 663, 665, 666f
　　myeloma 788f, 789f, 790
　　oesophageal cancer 370–1, 375
　　orbital tumours 906
　　pancreatic cancer 485, 498, 499f
　　penile cancer 602, 604f, 605f
　　phaeochromocytoma 936, 937f
　　pituitary tumours 886, 940, 941f
　　prostate cancer 123, 610
　　renal cancer 617
　　sarcoma 844
　　spinal tumours 789f, 790, 888, 889f, 890f
　　testicular cancer 607–8
　　thyroid cancer 337, 920–1, 922, 927
　　unknown primary 349, 968
　　upper urinary tract cancer 614, 615–16
　　vaginal cancer 584
　　VIPoma 950
imatinib (Gleevec®) 213t
　　acute lymphoblastic leukaemia 714, 719,
　　　　720, 727–9
　　adverse effects 757
　　chordoma 861
　　chronic myeloid leukaemia 757
　　　　high-dose 765
　　　　monitoring response 758–63
　　　　resistance 757, 763–4

dermatofibrosarcoma protuberans 17, 858
　　resistance 89, 729, 757, 763–5
imiquimod 693, 695
immortality of cells 5
immune system 109–15
　　hallmarks of cancer 6–7, 110f
　　local response 109–12
　　in progression/metastasis 66, 112
　　and response to chemotherapy 549
　　systemic response 112–14
　　as a therapeutic target 14, 114–15, 549, 687
　　see also inflammation
immunodrug conjugates
　　brentuximab vedotin 822, 825–6, 832
　　gemtuzumab ozogamicin 707
　　inotuzumab ozogamicin 826
　　trastuzumab-emtansine 238, 563, 565
immunoglobulin deficiency in
　　　　myeloma 786–7, 798
immunoglobulin detection in myeloma 787–9
immunoglobulin production 782–3, 815
immunohistochemistry
　　atypical fibroxanthoma 697
　　breast cancer 552–3, 560–1
　　DNA repair proteins 84, 448, 639
　　lung cancer 630, 633, 639
　　melanoma 680, 907
　　mesothelioma 535t, 536, 661–2
　　myeloma 788f
　　neuroendocrine tumours 944–5
　　ovarian cancer 580
　　pancreatic cancer 482
　　pituitary adenoma 938
　　retinal lymphoma 912
　　sarcoma 847–8
　　T-cell infiltrates 112
　　unknown primary site 967–8
immunomodulatory drugs
　　chronic lymphocytic leukaemia 770
　　myeloma 793, 794b, 795–6, 798, 799
immunophenotype
　　acute lymphoblastic leukaemia 713, 722
　　acute myeloid leukaemia 705, 712
　　chronic lymphocytic leukaemia 766
　　hairy cell leukaemia 771
　　myeloma 789–90
　　prolymphocytic leukaemia 772, 773
immunosuppression
　　AIDS-associated tumours 137–9, 808
　　iatrogenic 192, 757, 768, 769, 772, 774
　　lymphoma 808
　　myeloma 786–7, 798
　　PTLD 136–7, 813b, 814
　　skin cancer 690
immunotherapy
　　adoptive 687, 712, 770
　　BCG therapy 615
　　targeting the immune response 14, 115, 687
　　vaccines 259–60
　　　　melanoma 686–7
　　　　myeloma 798
　　　　prostate cancer (Sipuleucel-T) 115, 259, 612
　　see also interferon alpha; monoclonal
　　　　antibody therapies
imprinting of IGF2 13
IMRT see intensity-modulated radiotherapy
incidentalomas, adrenal 933–5
incontinence
　　faecal 316, 419
　　urinary 316, 611

incremental cost effectiveness ratio (ICER) 239
induced pluripotent stem cells (iPS) 89–90
infections
　　H. pylori
　　　　gallbladder cancer 509, 510
　　　　gastric cancer 388, 389, 390, 392
　　in leukaemia
　　　　AML 706
　　　　CLL 766, 768, 769
　　　　HCL 770
　　　　opportunistic infections after
　　　　　　alemtuzumab therapy 769, 774
　　liver flukes 509–10, 511
　　and lymphoma 808
　　in myeloma 786–7, 798
　　see also viruses
infertility see fertility
infiltrating immune cells (IICs) 8
inflammation 8, 66
　　anti-inflammatory drugs 114–15
　　　　colorectal cancer prevention 114, 264,
　　　　　　446–7
　　　　skin cancer prevention 697–8
　　cholangiocarcinoma 509–10
　　colorectal cancer and IBD 444, 456
　　gallbladder cancer 508–9
　　local response 109–12
　　mesothelioma 533–4
　　systemic response 112–14
　　targeted therapies 115
inflammatory bowel disease 444, 456
inflammatory myofibroblastic tumour 849t, 858
information provision 170–1, 798
informed consent
　　clinical trials 230t, 231
　　radiotherapy 182
inotuzumab ozogamicin 826
in silico tests of carcinogenicity 147
insulin 445
insulin-like growth factor (IGF1/IGF2) 13–14,
　　　　23–4
　　colorectal cancer 445
　　GH-secreting tumours 942
insulin-like growth factor receptor (IGF1R/
　　　　IGF2R) 13–14, 23–4
　　breast cancer 547
　　pancreatic cancer 481
insulinoma 943, 945t, 946–7, 954t
insulin receptor (IR) 13, 23
intensity-modulated radiotherapy (IMRT) 180,
　　　　181–2
　　laryngeal/hypopharyngeal tumours 348
　　mesothelioma 664
　　nasopharyngeal tumours 343
　　oesophageal cancer 376
　　oropharyngeal tumours 346–7
　　sinonasal tumours 341–2
intention-to-treat (ITT) principle 226
interferon alpha (IFN-α)
　　adverse effects 756
　　chronic myeloid leukaemia 756
　　hairy cell leukaemia 772
　　hepatitis C 140
　　melanoma 682, 687
　　myeloma 795
　　neuroendocrine tumours 955, 956t, 957
　　renal cell carcinoma 618
Intergroup 0116 trial 381, 400, 401t
Intergroup 0139 trial 640
interleukin 1 alpha (IL1a) 391

interleukin 1 beta (IL1b) 389
interleukin 2 (IL2) 687
interleukin 6 (IL6) 14, 113–14
    anti-IL6 therapy 14, 115
interleukin 8 (IL8) 113–14
interleukin 10 (IL10) 389
International Finance Facility for Immunisation
        (IFFIm) 260
intestinal metaplasia of the oesophagus 375
intestinal metaplasia of the stomach 393
intracranial hypertension 871, 887
intraductal papillary mucinous neoplasm
        (IPMN) 479–80, 484t, 488–9
intraepithelial neoplasia
    cervical 272, 577
    gastric 393
    oesophageal 366
    pancreatic 479, 483f, 484, 489
intrahepatic cholangiocarcinoma (IHCC) see
        cholangiocarcinoma
intraoperative chemotherapy
    intraperitoneal 167, 457, 540
    thoracic 667
intraoperative radiation therapy (IORT)
    breast cancer 556–7
    colorectal cancer 463
    sarcoma 856
intraperitoneal chemotherapy
    HIPEC 167, 457, 540
    for mesothelioma 540–2
    for ovarian cancer 593, 596, 597
invasion 17, 61–2, 481
    as a hallmark of cancer 5–6
in vitro tests of carcinogenicity 147
IORT see intraoperative radiation therapy
ipilimumab 115, 687
IRE (irreversible electroporation) 518, 611
Iressa® (gefitinib) 213t, 645–6, 645t
irinotecan 187
    colorectal cancer 425–7, 459
    gastric cancer 403
    lung cancer 648
    nanoliposomes 496
    neuroendocrine tumours 957t
    pancreatic cancer 495–6
    pharmacokinetics 213t, 214
    thyroid cancer 927
iris
    lymphoma 913t
    melanoma 908, 910
    metastases 914
IRIS trial 757, 761, 763
irreversible electroporation (IRE) 518, 611
IRTA1 epitope 814
isocitrate dehydrogenase see IDH1/IDH2 genes
isolated limb perfusion/infusion (ILP/ILI) 683,
        696, 860
ISS risk stratification for myeloma 791
ixabepilone 562

J
Jagged1 (Notch ligand) 50f, 392
JAK/STAT signalling pathway (Janus
        kinases) 14, 25
    acute lymphoblastic leukaemia 719, 720, 721t
    lymphoma (PMBL) 816
    myeloma 786
Japan
    gastric cancer 397–8, 400
    Hiroshima A-bomb survivors 150, 706

jaundice, obstructive
    hepatobiliary cancer 513–14, 522, 524–5, 526f
    pancreatic cancer 497, 498
JCOG 9501 trial 397–8
JCOG 9912 trial 402t, 403
juvenile polyposis 451

K
Kaposi's sarcoma 137–9
Kausch–Whipple procedure 486
keratoacanthoma 686, 694, 695
Ki67 protein 553, 561, 944
kidney
    allowable radiation dose 377
    cancer see renal cancer (RCC)
    drug excretion 189–90, 214
        and renal impairment 190
    failure (in myeloma) 787, 797
    nephrectomy 617–18
KiSS1 gene 966
KIT oncogene/KIT/RTK 548, 656, 686, 966
KLASS 01 trial 399
KLHL6 gene 767
KRAS oncogene
    colorectal cancer 429, 449, 460
    gastric cancer 389
    lung cancer 629
    ovarian cancer 579
    pancreatic cancer 479, 480
Krukenberg tumour 395
Ku protein (XRCC5/XRCC6 dimer) 76, 84

L
lacrimal gland carcinoma 906
lactate dehydrogenase (LDH) 123, 680, 684f
lactate metabolism 6, 122
lambrolizumab 687
laparoscopy 166
    colorectal cancer 412, 455–6
    gastric cancer 399, 400
    hysterectomy 583–4
    nephrectomy 617, 618
    pancreatic surgery 487
    peritoneal mesothelioma 538
lapatinib 563, 564
    brain metastases 565, 892
LAPTM4B gene 551
large cell carcinoma (LCC) 632
large cell neuroendocrine carcinoma
        (LCNEC) 632, 648, 649
large granular lymphocytic leukaemia (LGL) 774
laryngeal cancer
    clinical presentation 347
    epidemiology 130, 157, 347
    imaging 337, 338
    larynx preservation 349
    treatment 347–9, 351
laryngeal nerve damage 369, 374, 634
laser surgery 167, 348, 603, 611
Lauren classification (gastric cancer) 394–5
LCC (large cell carcinoma) 632
LCIS (lobular carcinoma in situ) 552, 554
LCNEC (large cell neuroendocrine
        carcinoma) 632, 648, 649
LDH (lactate dehydrogenase) 123, 680, 684f
lead time bias 267
leather bottle stomach (linitis plastica) 388,
        393–4, 395
legal issues (defensive medicine) 240
leiomyosarcoma 854, 858

lenalidomide
    chronic lymphocytic leukaemia 770
    myeloma 793, 794b, 795, 796, 799
length bias 267
lentigo maligna melanoma 678, 905
letrozole 562
leucovorin (folinic acid) 495–6
leukaemia
    acute lymphoblastic see acute lymphoblastic
        leukaemia (ALL)
    acute myeloid see acute myeloid leukaemia
        (AML)
    acute promyelocytic 704, 705
    adult T-cell 139, 832
    chronic lymphocytic see chronic
        lymphocytic leukaemia (CLL)
    chronic myeloid see chronic myeloid
        leukaemia (CML)
    hairy cell (HCL) 770–2, 814
    hairy cell-variant (HCL-v) 772
    large granular lymphocytic (LGL) 774
    plasma cell (PCL) 799–800
    prolymphocytic (PLL) 766, 772–3
    radiation-induced 150, 151, 706
levamisole 458
levothyroxine 922, 923, 928
LGL (large granular lymphocytic
        leukaemia) 774
Life Span Study (LLS) 150
lifestyle 155–8
    impact on survival rates 158
    risk factors for cancer 155
        alcohol consumption 157, 320t, 366t, 446, 546
        alcohol plus smoking 130, 329
        body weight 155–6, 237, 320t, 367, 445, 546
        diet 156–8, 365, 388, 445, 465, 546
        physical activity 156
        smoking see smoking
    of survivors 319–20, 465
Li-Fraumeni syndrome 277t
light-chain deposition 787
    amyloidosis 800–1
light-chain detection in myeloma 787–9, 791
linifanib 520
linitis plastica 388, 393–4, 395
liothyronine 921
lipids
    hyperlipidaemia 787
    synthesis 123
liposarcoma 849t, 850
    myxoid/round cell 852f, 853, 857, 858
    pleomorphic 854
    well-differentiated 845, 852–3
liver cancer
    ablation techniques 167, 516–17, 517–18
    assessment of liver function 514
    biopsy 514
    causes and risk factors 131, 140, 157, 508,
        510–11
    chemotherapy 518–19
        chemosaturation technique 517
        in combination with targeted
            therapies 521
        HBV reactivation 521–2
        TACE 516, 517, 521
    cirrhosis 508, 510, 514, 515
    HBV 140, 256, 510
        reactivation 521–2
        vaccination 256–7
    HCV 140, 510–11

liver cancer (*Cont.*)
  histopathology 511
  imaging 511–12, 513, 514
    for regional therapies 517
  intrahepatic cholangiocarcinoma 509, 510
    see also cholangiocarcinoma
  macroscopic appearance 508*f*, 514*f*, 516*f*
  metastatic from other sites 62, 64
    colorectal cancer 67–8, 204, 431–2, 457, 463
    imaging 513
    melanoma 685, 910
    neuroendocrine tumours 948*f*, 950,
      953–4, 953*f*, 958
    unknown primary 972
  molecular biology 520
  radiotherapy (SIRT) 517, 958
  staging 514–15, 516*f*
  surgery
    resection 515
    transplantation 514, 515, 953–4
  surveillance 514
  targeted therapies 51, 54, 519–21
    adjuvant 521
liver flukes 509–10, 511
liver metabolism (of drugs) 189–90, 214
  and hepatic impairment 190
liver stone disease 510
LKB1/LKB1 (liver kinase B1) 121, 451
LNH03-2B trial 819–20
LNH03-6B trial 818
LNH98-5 trial 818
lobular carcinoma in situ (LCIS) 552, 554
low- and middle-income countries (LMICs)
  burden of cancer 245, 256
  cancer control planning 245–52
  HBV vaccination 256–7
  HPV vaccination 258
lumiliximab 770
lung
  adverse effects of systemic therapies 316
  extrapleural pneumonectomy (for
    mesothelioma) 661, 663–4, 663*f*
    in multimodality therapy 665–9
    pre-operative lung function tests 662
  post-operative complications 374, 379
  radiation-induced pneumonitis 177, 316,
    559, 560
  RT dose in oesophageal cancer 377, 379
lung cancer 628–49
  ACTHoma 945*t*, 950, 955*t*
  adenocarcinoma 130, 629–30, 630–31, 644
    acinar pattern 631*f*
    lepidic pattern 630*f*
    micropapillary pattern 631*f*
  biopsy/cytology 633, 634
  carcinoid tumours 632, 648–9
  causes and risk factors
    occupational carcinogens 151, 628
    radon 151, 628
    smoking 127–8, 130, 132, 628
  chemoradiotherapy
    NSCLC 640–41
    SCLC 646–7
  chemotherapy
    carcinoid tumours 648–9
    elderly patients 643
    LCNEC 649
    NSCLC (early stage) 638–9
    NSCLC (first-line therapy) 641–3
    NSCLC (maintenance therapy) 643
    NSCLC (metastatic) 641, 642*t*

NSCLC (second-line therapy) 644
NSCLC (with targeted therapies) 629,
  643–4, 645
SCLC 68, 647–8
clinical presentation 633–4
diagnosis 633, 634
elderly patients 643
genetic profiles 119, 628–30, 631, 644, 646
histopathology 119, 630–33
imaging 635, 638
incidence 628
large cell carcinoma 632
lymph node involvement 631, 635, 637*f*
  carcinoid tumours 648
  neuroendocrine tumours 648–9
  NSCLC 641, 642*t*, 646
  SCLC 647–8
  surgery 635–6, 638
  symptoms 634
metastatic from other sites 62*t*, 64
  colon 457
  melanoma 685
  sarcoma 844, 859, 861
metastatic to other sites 641, 646, 647–8
  prophylactic brain irradiation 647, 648
mixed types 633
molecular biology 119, 628–30, 631
  ALK mutations 629–30, 646
  CSCs 87*t*
  EGFR mutations 629, 644
mortality 128*f*, 628
multidisciplinary care 199, 201*t*, 204
neuroendocrine tumours 631–2, 648–9
non-small cell *see* non-small cell lung cancer
  (NSCLC)
palliative care 307–8, 641
premalignant lesions 630, 631
prevention
  pharmacological 265
  smoking cessation 132–4
radiotherapy
  brain metastases 646, 647, 648
  NSCLC (early-stage) 639
  NSCLC (locally advanced) 640–1
  SCLC 647, 648
sarcomatoid carcinoma 632–3
screening 273
small-cell *see* small cell lung cancer (SCLC)
squamous cell carcinoma 630, 631
staging 635, 636*t*, 637*f*, 638*t*
surgery
  carcinoid tumours 648
  early stage NCSLC 635–8
  locally advanced NSCLC 640
  SCLC 646
survival rates 628, 646, 648
targeted therapies
  with chemotherapy 629, 643–4, 645
  driver mutations present 641, 644–6
  maintenance therapy 643
  metastatic disease 641
  resistance to 629, 646
  second-line therapy 644
lymphatic system
  gastric nodal stations 398*t*
  germinal centres 783, 784*t*, 815
  metastatic spread via 62
lymph node metastases
  breast cancer
    chemo/radiotherapy 68, 558–9

sentinel node surgery 168, 555
cervical cancer 577, 581–2, 595
chronic lymphocytic leukaemia 766
colorectal cancer
  imaging 409–10
  management 415, 419
  prognosis 452
  risk factors in early cancer 457*t*
endometrial cancer 583, 596
eyelid tumours 904
gallbladder cancer 522, 523, 524
gastric cancer 163, 397–9
head and neck cancer
  imaging 338, 339
  nasopharyngeal tumours 343
  oropharyngeal tumours 345
  pathology report 334
  salivary gland tumours 354
  unknown primary 349–51
lung cancer 631, 635, 637*f*
  carcinoid tumours 648
  surgery 635–6, 638
melanoma 168, 679, 680–2, 682–3, 688
mesothelioma
  peritoneal 536
  pleural 661, 663
oesophageal cancer 371, 372–3, 376
ovarian cancer 586, 587
pancreatic cancer 482, 486
penile cancer 602, 604–5, 606
prostate cancer 610, 611
renal cancer 618
sentinel nodes *see* sentinel node procedure
skin cancer, non-melanoma 693, 696, 697
thyroid cancer 921, 924, 926, 927
unknown primary 969, 970
vaginal cancer 584–5
vulvar cancer 585, 591
lymphocytes *see* B cells; T cells
lymphoedema 316
lymphoma 808–32
  AIDS-associated 137, 808
  Burkitt 39, 136, 808, 817
  cerebral 811, 826, 882–4, 914
  chemoradiotherapy 822, 828–9, 831
  chemotherapy 817
    aggressive B-cell 817–20
    CNS disease 882–3
    Hodgkin 821–2
    indolent B-cell 821, 822*t*, 824*t*
    mantle cell 820
    NK/T-cell 832
    pre-transplant conditioning 826–7
    relapsed disease 822–3
    T-cell 832
  classification 809, 812–14, 831–2
  clinical presentation 810, 882, 884, 912
  clinical types 809–10
  diagnosis 810–11, 832
    CNS disease 882
    ocular disease 912
  emergencies 810
  epidemiology 808–9
  genetic profiles 809, 814–15
    ALCL 813–14
    Burkitt 817
    DLBCL 815, 815–16
    PMBL 816
    T-cell lymphoma 832
  historical overview 810*f*

Hodgkin *see* Hodgkin lymphoma
imaging 811
   CNS disease 882, 883*f*
incidence 808, 809*f*, 912
indolent forms 809, 810, 814, 820–1, 824*t*, 828
ocular 913*t*
   choroidal 914
   conjunctival 911–12, 912*f*
   uveal 914
   vitreoretinal 912–14, 912*f*
palliative care 828
prognosis 811–12
   CNS disease 882
   retinal disease 914
radioimmunotherapy 824–5
radiotherapy 820, 822, 827–31
   CNS disease 883–4
   retinal disease 912
   total body irradiation pre-transplant 827
relapsed disease 822–3
   Hodgkin 822
   T-cell lymphomas 832
second cancers in survivors 152, 153
sinonasal 336, 829, 832
stem cell transplantation 822, 823, 826–7
targeted therapies 823–4
   aggressive B-cell 815, 818–20
   Hodgkin 816, 822
   indolent B-cell 821, 824*t*
   Mab-drug conjugates 825–6, 832
   mantle cell 820
   radioimmunotherapy 824–5
   retinal disease 912
thyroid 918, 920, 923
viruses 136, 808, 832
Lynch syndrome (HNPCC) 279, 280–2
   clinical features 281*b*
   endometrial cancer 578, 583
   genetic testing of all CRC cases 282–6
   mutations 75, 277*t*, 282, 450–1
   prophylactic surgery 165, 456
   upper urinary tract cancer 615

M
MACH-NC meta-analysis 346, 348, 351
macrophages, tumour-associated 66, 109, 110–11, 114, 549
MAGIC trial 400, 401*t*
magnetic resonance imaging (MRI)
   brain tumours 871–2
      craniopharyngioma 887
      glioblastoma 874*f*, 875*f*
      high-grade glioma 877*f*
      low-grade glioma 878–9, 879*f*
      meningioma 884*f*
      pituitary adenoma 886
   breast cancer screening 267
   cervical cancer 581, 594*f*
   colorectal cancer 409–11
   endometrial cancer 583
   head and neck cancer 337–8, 341
   hepatobiliary cancers 513, 522
   mesothelioma 666*f*
   myeloma 788*f*, 789*f*, 790
   penile cancer 604*f*, 605*f*
   phaeochromocytoma 936
   pituitary tumours 940, 941*f*
   prostate cancer 610
   sarcoma 844
   spinal ependymoma 889*f*

unknown primary site 968
urothelial cell carcinoma 616
vaginal cancer 584
males
   breast cancer 166, 559
   faecal occult blood tests 271
   feminizing tumours 933
   fertility after treatment 317, 465, 609, 810
   HPV vaccination 606
   lung cancer 628
   pituitary tumours 940, 941
   unknown primary site cancers 969, 970, 971
malignant fibrous histiocytoma 697
malignant peripheral nerve sheath tumour 854
malnutrition 164
MALT lymphoma 828
Mammaprint® 561
mammography 267–70, 968
mantle cell lymphoma (MCL) 809, 813, 814, 820
MAPK signalling pathway (mitogen-activated protein kinase) *see* RAS/RAF/MAPK signalling pathway
marginal zone lymphoma (MZL) 814
Marjolin's ulcer 690
marriage, and cancer survivors 319
Masaoka-Koga staging of thymic tumours 655, 656*t*
masking (blinding) in RCT design 222–3
mast cells 66, 111
mastectomy
   adjuvant RT 557–8
   margins of resection 165
   prophylactic 280, 554
MATE (MDT software) 205
matrix metalloproteinases (MMP) 17, 481
maxillary sinus tumours 340, 341
maximum tolerated dose (MTD) 190
   compared with metronomic dosing 66
   identified in Phase I studies 220–1
MC1R gene (melanocortin-1 receptor) 675
MCL (mantle cell lymphoma) 809, 813, 814, 820
MCPM (multicystic peritoneal mesothelioma) 534, 536, 537–8, 540
MCT1/MCT4 (monocarboxylate transporters) 122
MDACC classification of CML 754
MDACC classification of 755*t*
MDM2 gene/Mdm2 protein 37, 660, 850
MDT *see* multidisciplinary care/teams
meat, in the diet 157, 445
mediastinoscopy 635
Medical Outcomes Study Short-Form Health Survey (SF-36) 303, 308
medico-legal issues (defensive medicine) 240
medroxyprogesterone acetate 308, 592
medullary carcinoma, thyroid (MTC) 918, 923–8
medulloblastoma 880–1
megakaryocytes 756
meibomian glands 905
MEK kinase (MAP2K) 26
   inhibitors 629, 686
   see also RAS/RAF/MAPK signalling pathway
melanocytic tumours of uncertain malignant potential 677
melanoma 674–89
   causes and risk factors 674–5, 676, 905, 908
   chemotherapy 683, 687
   classification 678
   conjunctival 907–8, 907*f*, 907*f*

CSCs 87–8*t*, 91–2, 674
diagnosis 676–7, 907, 908–9
eyelid 905
genetic profiles 674, 675*t*, 677–8, 679–80, 907
genetic syndromes 166, 674–5
histopathology 677, 678*t*, 907, 911
imaging 677, 680, 682, 684, 908
immunotherapy 682, 686–7
incidence 675–6
lymph node involvement 168, 679, 680–2, 682–3, 688
macroscopic appearance 676–7
   uveal 909*f*
metastatic 684–8, 689
   to the brain 685, 688, 689, 892
   from conjunctiva 907
   from uvea 910, 911
   in transit (satellites) 679, 683, 907
molecular biology 674, 678
mucosal 335, 689
multidisciplinary care 689
prognosis 678–9, 679*f*, 681*f*
   ocular melanoma 907, 911
radiotherapy 682–3, 688
   in uveal melanoma 909–10, 911
recurrence 679, 683–4, 907
staging 680
surgery 680, 681*t*, 689
   conjunctival melanoma 907
   limb amputation 683
   lymph nodes 168, 680–2
   stage IV disease 684–5
   uveal melanoma 909, 910
surveillance 683–4
   uveal 910, 911
targeted therapies 115, 682, 685–6, 687, 892
unknown primary site 688, 970, 971
uveal 908–11
see also skin cancers, non-melanoma
MELD score 515*t*
melphalan 683, 794*b*, 795, 796
MEN1 (multiple endocrine neoplasia type 1) 166, 277*t*, 939, 944, 948
MEN2A/2B (multiple endocrine neoplasia type 2A/2B) 277*t*
   phaeochromocytoma 926, 935
   thyroid cancer 918, 923–4, 926
   treatment 926–7
men *see* males
menarche 546
meningeal tumours 869*t*
meningioma 884–6
   spinal 888
menopause
   breast cancer risk 546
   premature 317
MERCURY trial 409
Merkel cell carcinoma (MCC) 140, 696–7, 905
Merkel cell polyomavirus (MCV) 140, 696
mesenchymal-to-epithelial transition (MET) 9
mesorectal fascia (MRF) 409, 410
mesothelioma
   causes and risk factors 533–4, 659
   chemoradiotherapy 669
   chemotherapy
      adjuvant 665–7
      heated intraoperative 540–2, 667
      neoadjuvant 667–9
      systemic 538–40, 664–5

mesothelioma (*Cont.*)
  clinical presentation 536–7
  diagnosis 534, 536–8, 661
  epidemiology 533–4, 659
  genetic profiles 534, 660
  histopathology
    peritoneal 534–6
    pleural 661–2
  imaging
    asbestos 661
    peritoneal 537–8
    pleural 661, 663, 665, 666*f*
  laparoscopy 538
  lymph node involvement
    peritoneal 536
    pleural 661, 663
  macroscopic appearance
    peritoneal 533*f*, 535
    pleural 661
  molecular biology
    peritoneal 534, 542–3, 542*f*
    pleural 659–60
  multicystic peritoneal form 534, 536, 537–8, 540
  multimodality treatment 664, 665–9
  palliative care 538–9, 664
  peritoneal 533–43
  photodynamic therapy 669
  pleural 659–69
  prognosis 538, 660
  radiotherapy 664, 669
  recurrence 663–4
  staging
    peritoneal 538, 539*t*
    pleural 662
  surgery
    peritoneal 540
    pleural 661, 662–4
  survival rates 533, 664
  targeted therapies 542–3
  tumour markers 538
  well-differentiated papillary peritoneal
      form 534, 536
MET (HGF receptor) 11–13
  gastric cancer 390, 391
  liver cancer 520
  unknown primary 966
metabolic syndrome 316
metabolism of cancer cells
  energy production 6, 61, 119–23
    mTOR signalling 26–7, 120
  glycogen synthesis 123
  as a hallmark of cancer 6, 119
  lactate 6, 122
  lipid synthesis 123
  therapeutic targets 123
metabolism of carcinogens 145–7
metabolism of drugs 189–90, 211, 214
  first-pass 189, 211
metals, carcinogenic 145*t*
metanephrines 935, 936
metaphase 35
metaplasia, intestinal 375, 393
metastasis 62–7
  bladder cancer 615
  to bone 62–3, 64
    from breast cancer 560, 563–4
    from melanoma 685, 688
    from neuroendocrine tumours 949*f*
    from prostate cancer 64, 612
    PSA-elevated unknown primary 970, 971

treatment of bone pain 612, 688
  to brain 62–3, 64, 890–1
    from acute lymphoblastic leukaemia 718,
        726, 730
    from breast 565, 892
    from lung 646, 647, 648
    from melanoma 685, 688, 689, 892
    pharmacodynamic resistance 646
    prophylactic irradiation 647, 648
    treatment 565, 891–2
  breast cancer *see* breast cancer, metastatic
  and cause of death 63–4
  cervical cancer 592
  circulating tumour cells 67, 93–4
  colorectal cancer *see* colorectal cancer
      (CRC), metastatic
  and CSCs 93–4
  dormancy and progression 63, 64–7
  to the eye 914
  gastric cancer 395–6, 400, 402–3
  as a hallmark of cancer 5–6
  head and neck cancer 337, 339, 344, 348
  invasion 17, 61–2, 481
  to liver 62, 64
    from colon 67–8, 204, 431–2, 457, 463
    imaging 513
    from melanoma 685, 910
    from neuroendocrine tumours 948*f*, 950,
        953–4, 953*f*, 958
    from unknown primary 972
  to lung 62*t*, 64
    from colon 457
    from melanoma 685
    from primary lung tumours 646
    from sarcoma 844, 859, 861
  from lung cancer 641, 646, 647–8
  to lymph nodes *see* lymph node metastases
  mechanisms of spread 62–3
  melanoma 684–8, 689, 892
    from conjunctiva 907
    from uvea 910, 911
    in transit (satellite lesions) 679, 683, 907
  molecular pathways 64*t*
  neuroendocrine tumours 944, 946*t*, 948*f*,
      949*f*, 950, 953*f*
  to the orbit 906–7, 907
  from ovarian cancer 586–7
  to the ovary 395, 580
  pancreatic cancer 479, 494–6
  peritoneal carcinomatosis 63, 64
    colorectal cancer 167, 457, 534
    gastric cancer 395, 400
    ovarian cancer 586–7
  to the pituitary 939
  prostate cancer 612
  renal cancer 618–19
  sarcoma 844, 852, 853, 854, 857, 859, 861
  site of metastases 62*t*, 64
  site of primary tumour 62–3
  skin cancer
    BCC 693
    melanoma 679, 683, 684–8, 689, 892
    Merkel cell 697
    SCC 696
  to spine 888, 890*f*, 892–3
    from melanoma 685, 688
  testicular cancer 608, 609
  thyroid cancer
    medullary 926, 927
    papillary/follicular 919, 921, 922

treatment 67–8
  upper urinary tract cancer 616
  see also cancer of unknown primary
metastasis-initiating cells (MICs) 93–4
metastasis-suppressor genes 966
metformin 123
methadone 296
methotrexate 187, 212*t*, 211
  cerebral lymphoma 882
  CNS prophylaxis of ALL 726
  head and neck cancer 352
  osteosarcoma 861
methylation of DNA 77, 122
  breast cancer 549
  colorectal cancer 448–9, 452
  gastric cancer 390, 391
  inhibition 709
  oesophageal cancer (of p16 gene
      CDKN2A) 367
methylation of histones 701, 785
methylphenidate 296
METMab® 12
Metorchis conjunctus 511
metyrapone 943
MGMT/MGMT (O-6-methylguanine DNA
      methyltransferase) 449, 876, 877
  in elderly patients 876
MGUS (monoclonal gammopathy of
      undetermined significance) 782, 787
  amyloidosis 800
  diagnosis 790*t*
  management 791–2
  progression risk 790–1
^{123}I-MIBG scintigraphy 936
microarray profiling 660
micropthalmia transcription factor (MITF) 674
microRNAs (miRs) 67, 549
microsatellite instability (MSI) 75
  colorectal cancer 447–8, 460–1
  endometrial cancer 578
  gastric cancer 390–1
microtubules 186–7
milk, in the diet 157
minimally invasive surgery 166–7
  oesophageal 372, 373
  see also laparoscopy; thermal ablation
minor salivary gland (MiSG) cancer 353
  radiotherapy 354
  surgery 354
  survival rates 355
MInT trial 818, 819
mismatch repair (MMR) pathway 74–5, 76
  colorectal cancer 447–8, 449, 460–1
    HNPCC (Lynch syndrome) 75, 277*t*, 282,
        450–1, 578
  endometrial cancer 578
  gastric cancer 391
mitochondria
  and apoptosis 42–3
  tumour suppressor genes 122–3
mitogens 34
mitomycin 615
mitomycin C 187
mitosis 31
  in CAFs 67
  inhibition by chemotherapy agents 186–7
  mitotic rate in melanoma 678–9
  regulation 34–6
mitotane 932, 933, 943
mitotic spindle 35

checkpoint 36
mitoxantrone 519
mixed malignant Müllerian tumours
        (MMMT) 579
mixed polyposis syndrome 451
MLH1 gene (mismatch repair) 74, 75, 76
    colorectal cancer 448, 449, 451
    endometrial cancer 578
    gastric cancer 391
MLL gene fusion/rearrangement 702, 718–19,
        720, 722
MM *see* myeloma
MMP (matrix metalloproteinases) 17, 481
MMR *see* mismatch repair (MMR) pathway
MMSET gene 785
modafenil 296
moderate hypofractionation of RT 178
Mohs' surgery 692, 695–6, 905
monoclonal antibody therapies
    ant-CD33 (gemtuzumab) 707
    anti-angiogenesis *see* bevacizumab;
        ramucirumab
    anti-CD3 (blinatumomab) 730
    anti-CD3/EPCAM (catumaxomab) 91, 115
    anti-CD20 823–5
        see also ofatumumab; rituximab
    anti-CD23 (lumiliximab) 770
    anti-CD30 (brentuximab) 822, 825–6, 832
    anti-CD44 (bevatuzumab) 90
    anti-CD52 (alemtuzumab) 769, 773, 774
    anti-CTL4 (ipilimumab, tremelimumab) 115,
        687
    anti-EGFR *see* cetuximab; necitumumab;
        panitumumab
    anti-HER2 *see* pertuzumab; trastuzumab
    anti-IL6 (siltuximab) 14, 115
    anti-PD-1 (nivolumab, lambrolizumab) 115,
        644, 687, 816
    anti-RANK ligand (denosumab) 563
    anti-VEGF/VEGFR *see* bevacuzumab;
        ramucirumab
    immunodrug conjugates
        brentuximab vedotin 822, 825–6, 832
        gemtuzumab ozogamicin 707
        inotuzumab ozogamicin 826
        trastuzumab-emtansine 238, 563, 565
    radioimmunotherapy 824–5
monoclonal B-cell lymphocytosis (MBL) 813, 814
monoclonal gammopathy of undetermined
        significance *see* MGUS
monocytes 113
moral hazard, in healthcare costs 240–1
morphine 296
MOSAIC trial 459, 460
motesanib 54
mouth, dry 343
mouth cancer 157, 344–5
MPM (malignant pleural mesothelioma) *see*
        pleural mesothelioma
MPOWER Report (WHO) 133
MRC-COIN trial 429, 430*t*
MRC-FOCUS trial 426–7
MRI *see* magnetic resonance imaging
MSH2 gene (mismatch repair) 74, 75, 276, 282, 451
MSH6 gene (mismatch repair) 74, 75, 282, 450*f*
MSI *see* microsatellite instability
MSLT-I trial 681
MSLT-II trial 682
MTC (medullary thyroid carcinoma) 918,
        923–8

MTD *see* maximum tolerated dose
mTOR signalling pathway (mammalian target
        of rapamycin)
    acute lymphoblastic leukaemia 719
    autophagy 27, 47, 120
    breast cancer 563
    endometrial cancer 592
    inhibitors *see* everolimus; temsirolimus
    liver cancer 520, 521
    mesothelioma 534, 542–3
    myeloma 786
    regulation of metabolism 26–7, 120
    renal cancer 619
    sarcoma 858
mucin 392
mucinous adenocarcinoma
    gastric 394
    lung 631
mucinous cystic neoplasm (MCN),
        pancreatic 479–80, 483*f*, 484*t*, 489
mucoepidermoid carcinoma (MEC) 336–7
mucosa-associated lymphatic tissue (MALT)
        lymphoma 828
mucosal melanoma 335, 689
Muir–Torre syndrome 285*f*, 451
multicentric Castleman's disease 139
multicystic peritoneal mesothelioma
        (MCPM) 534, 536, 537–8, 540
multidisciplinary care/teams (MDTs) 169, 182,
        196–206
    benefits and problems 197–9, 205, 464
    brain tumours 872
    breast cancer 199, 200*t*, 564–5
    colorectal cancer 201*t*, 204, 433, 454, 463–6
    future developments 205
    gynaecological cancers 202–3*t*, 204, 593–7
    head and neck cancer 203*t*, 205
    lung cancer 199, 201*t*, 204
    melanoma 689
    myeloma 798
    oesophageal cancer 201*t*, 204
    organization of MDTs 196–7, 198
    palliative care 293, 297–8
    pancreatic cancer 202*t*, 204, 497–9
    prostate cancer 202*t*, 204
    thymic tumours 657
multidrug resistance 89, 191–2
multileaf collimators 180*f*
multiple endocrine neoplasia type 1
        (MEN1) 166, 277*t*, 939, 944, 948
multiple endocrine neoplasia type 2A/2B
        (MEN2A/2B) 277*t*
    phaeochromocytoma 926, 935
    thyroid cancer 918, 923–4, 926
        treatment 926–7
multiple myeloma *see* myeloma
Municon trials 380
muramil tripeptide 861
mutations associated with cancer 7–8, 23, 38–9,
        98, 278–9
    see also genetic instability; genetic profiles
MUTYH-associated polyposis 75, 450
MYC/Myc/c-Myc oncogene 28–9, 121–2
    Burkitt lymphoma 817
    DLBCL 816
    myeloma 786
MYD88 gene 767, 815
myeloblasts
    acute myeloid leukaemia 705
    chronic myeloid leukaemia 756

myelodysplastic syndrome (MDS) 701, 705
myeloid derived suppressor cells (MDSC) 66, 112
myeloid leukaemia *see* acute myeloid
        leukaemia (AML); chronic myeloid
        leukaemia (CML)
myeloma (MM) 782–99
    causes and risk factors 782
    chemotherapy 792–3
        at relapse 799
        consolidation 795
        induction 793–5
        maintenance 793, 795–6
        older patients 796
    clinical presentation 786–7
    complications and emergencies 786–7
        management 792, 797–8
    diagnosis 787–90
    genetic profiles 782, 783–5, 786
        at relapse 799
        prognostic 783, 791
        test methods 790
    imaging 788*f*, 789*f*, 790
    incidence 782
    MGUS 782, 787
        amyloidosis 800
        diagnosis 790*t*
        management 791–2
        progression risk 790–1
    molecular biology 782–6
    monitoring response to treatment 791, 792*t*,
        798
    relapse 798–9
    risk stratification 790–1, 798–9
    smouldering 790*t*, 791, 792
    stem cell transplantation 795, 796, 799
    surveillance 791–2
    survival rates 793
myeloproliferative diseases 25
    see also chronic myeloid leukaemia
myelosuppression, iatrogenic 192, 757, 768,
        769, 772, 774
myofibroblasts 111
    inflammatory myofibroblastic tumour 849*t*, 858
myxofibrosarcoma 854
myxoid liposarcoma 849*t*, 852*f*, 853, 857, 858
MZL (marginal zone lymphoma) 814

N
nab-paclitaxel 496–7, 562
NADPH 122
naevi 674, 677
    choroidal 908, 909*f*
    dysplastic (atypical) 675–6, 677
Nakamura classification (gastric cancer) 395
NAMPT (nicotinamide
        phosphoribosyltransferase) 123
nanoliposomes 496
NAPOLI-1 trial 496
nasal cavity tumours 340–2
nasopharyngeal carcinoma (NPC) 342–4
    and EBV 136, 333, 343
    histopathology 333*f*
national cancer control plans (NCCP) 245–52
National Institute for Health and Clinical
        Excellence (NICE) (UK) 239
natural killer cells
    NK-cell LGL 774
    NK-cell lymphomas 334*f*, 812*b*, 829, 832
natural orifice transluminal endoscopic surgery
        (NOTES) 166

navitoclax 44
NCCP (national cancer control plans) 245–52
NCCTG-N0147 trial 459–60
NCCTG N9831 trial 563
necitumumab 644
neck cancer *see* head and neck cancer
necrosis/necroptosis 4, 44–5, 112
   radiation-induced 174
negative predictive value (NPV) 105
nelarabine 730
NeoALTTO trial 564
NeoSphere trial 564
nephrectomy 617–18
nephroureterectomy 616
NER (nucleotide excision repair) pathway 75, 639
   in XP 690–1
nerve sheath tumours
   malignant peripheral NST 854
   optic meningioma 884, 885
   spinal neurofibroma 888
   vestibular schwannoma 893–4
Netherlands 676t
neuroblastoma, olfactory 335, 342
neuroendocrine tumours 943–59
   ACTHoma 945t, 950, 955t
   carcinoids 944, 945t, 951–2, 954t
      atypical 632, 648, 945t, 955t
      heart disease 951, 958
      lung 632, 648–9
   classification 943–4
   clinical presentation 648, 945–6, 947–8,
      950, 951
   diagnosis 649, 946–7, 948, 950, 951, 952–3
   endoscopy 949f
   gastric 953
   GHRHoma 951
   glucagonoma 945t, 950, 954t
   histopathology 484, 632, 944–5, 947f
   imaging 946–7, 948, 949f, 953, 953f
   insulinoma 943, 945t, 946–7, 954t
   lung 631–2, 648–9, 950
   metastasis 944, 946t
      bone 949f
      liver 948f, 950, 953–4, 953f, 958
   non-functional tumours 945t, 952–3
   pancreatic 484, 945t, 946–50, 954–5t
   phaeochromocytoma 926, 929f, 935–8
   prognosis 946t
   site 944
   somatostatinoma 945t, 950, 955t
   treatment 947, 948–50, 950, 951–2, 953–9, 970
      chemotherapy 648–9, 948, 956–7t, 958
      interferon-α 955, 956t, 957
      of liver metastases 950, 953–4, 958
      of lung tumours 648–9
      radionuclide therapy 649, 958
      somatostatin analogues 649, 946, 947, 952,
         954–5, 956t, 957
      surgery 648, 948, 951, 953–4
      targeted therapies 51, 956t, 957–8
   unknown primary 944, 968, 969, 970
   Verner–Morrison syndrome (VIPoma) 945t,
      950, 955t
   Zollinger–Ellison syndrome 945t, 947–50, 954t
neurofibroma, spinal 888
neurofibromatosis type 1/type 2 (NF1/
   NF2) 277t, 868t, 873, 935
   NF2 mutations in mesothelioma 660
   vestibular schwannoma 894
neuropathic pain 798

neutrophils 111, 113
   neutropaenia 296, 757
New Zealand 675–6
next generation sequencing 548, 660, 702
NF1/NF2 genes *see* neurofibromatosis type
   1/type 2
NFκB signalling pathway 114, 481–2
   leukaemia 90
   myeloma 786
   pancreatic cancer 482
NHEJ (non-homologous end joining) DNA
   repair 76, 82
NHL-B trial 817–18
NHL (non-Hodgkin lymphoma) *see* lymphoma
nicotinamide 698
nicotinamide phosphoribosyltransferase
   (NAMPT) 123
nilotinib 757–8, 761, 764
   monitoring response 765
nintedanib 644
nitric oxide synthase (NOS) 91, 389
N-nitrosamines 128, 144t, 157
nivolumab 644, 687, 816
NK-cell large granular lymphocytic
   leukaemia 774
NK-cell lymphomas 334f, 812b, 829, 832
non-alcoholic steatohepatitis (NASH) 508
non-communicable disease control 246
non-epidermolytic palmoplantar keratoderma
   (tylosis) 365
non-germinoma germ cell tumour (pineal) 882
non-Hodgkin lymphoma (NHL) *see* lymphoma
non-homologous end joining (NHEJ) DNA
   repair 76, 82
non-inferiority design in RCTs 222
non-seminoma germ cell tumour (NSGST)
   (testicular) 607, 608
non-small cell lung cancer (NSCLC)
   chemoradiotherapy 640–1
   chemotherapy
      early stage disease 638–9
      first-line therapy 641–3
      maintenance therapy 643
      metastatic disease 641, 642t
      second-line therapy 644
      with targeted therapies 629, 643–4, 645
   histopathology 119, 630–1, 632–3
   metastatic 640, 641t, 645
   molecular biology 119, 629–30
   radiotherapy
      early stage 639
      locally advanced 640–1
   surgery
      early stage 635–8
      locally advanced 640
   targeted therapies
      with chemotherapy 629, 643–4, 645
      driver mutations present 641, 644–6
      maintenance therapy 643
      metastatic disease 641
      resistance to 629, 646
      second-line therapy 644
non-steroidal anti-inflammatory drugs
   (NSAIDs) 114–15
   colorectal cancer prevention 114, 264,
      446–7
   in myeloma 798
   skin cancer prevention 697–8
noradrenaline 930
Nordic 7 trial 429, 430t

normal tissue complication probability
   (NTCP) 173, 176
Notch signalling pathway 51
   gastric cancer 392
   NOTCH1 mutations in CLL 767, 815
   pancreatic cancer 481
NPC *see* nasopharyngeal carcinoma
NPM1 gene 699, 702
NPV (negative predictive value) 105
NRAS oncogene 679, 686
NSABP C07 trial 459, 460
NSABP C08 trial 52, 459
NSAIDs *see* non-steroidal anti-inflammatory
   drugs
NSCLC *see* non-small cell lung cancer
NT5C2 gene 721t, 723
NTCP (normal tissue complication
   probability) 173, 176
nuclear envelope breakdown during mitosis 35
nuclear medicine *see* positron emission
   tomography; radionuclide scans;
   radionuclide therapy
nucleotide excision repair (NER) pathway 75, 639
   in XP 690–1
null hypothesis 222f
nurses
   clinical nurse specialists 196, 198
   nurse practitioners and colorectal cancer 465
NUT midline carcinoma 334
nutrition *see* diet

O
obesity
   and cancer risk 155–6, 237, 320t, 367, 445, 546
   liver imaging 512
obinutuzumab 824
oblimersen (Genansense®) 44
occupational cancers
   biliary 509, 510
   bladder 613
   lung 151, 628
   sinonasal 340
Octreoscan® 648, 952f, 968
octreotide
   neuroendocrine tumours 649, 947, 952,
      954–5, 956t, 957
   pituitary tumours 942
   thymic tumours 656
ocular tumours *see* eye tumours
oculo(dermal) melanocytosis 908
oesophageal cancer
   adenocarcinoma 365, 367–9
      Siewert classification 369–70
      treatment 376, 377–8, 381, 382
   causes and risk factors 156t, 157, 365, 367
   chemoradiotherapy 372, 377, 378–9
      adjuvant 381
      neoadjuvant 379, 380–1
   chemotherapy 377–8
      adjuvant 381
      neoadjuvant 379–80
      palliative 381–2
   clinical presentation 369
   diagnosis 369–71
   genetic profiles 366–7, 368–9
   genetic syndromes 365
   histopathology 365–6, 367–8
   imaging 370–1, 375
   incidence 365
   lymph node involvement 371, 372–3, 376

molecular biology 366–7, 368–9
multidisciplinary care 201t, 204
palliative care 381–2
premalignant lesions 365–6, 367–8
QoL 375
radiotherapy 375–7, 378
  palliative 382
squamous cell carcinoma 365–7, 377, 382
staging 369, 370–1
surgery 371–4, 378, 379–80
  complications 374–5
  palliative 382
survival rates 373t, 374t, 380
targeted therapies 378, 382
oesophagectomy 371–2, 372–4, 378
adjuvant therapies 381
complications 374–5, 379
neoadjuvant therapies 379–81
oesophagitis, reflux 374
oesophagography 371
oestrogen receptor antagonists 187, 262–3
  see also tamoxifen
oestrogen receptor-positive cancer see
  ER-positive cancer
oestrogen-related receptors (ERRs) 121, 123
oestrogens, feminizing tumours 933
oestrogen therapy in prostate cancer 612
ofatumumab 768, 770, 824
olaparib 563, 593
olfactory neuroblastoma (ONB) 335, 342
oligoastrocytoma 869t, 877
oligodendroglioma 869t
anaplastic 872, 874, 878
low-grade 878–9
oncogene addiction 90, 631
oncogenes 38–9, 38t
cell cycle control 28, 28–9
and cell metabolism 120, 121–2
colorectal cancer 429, 449, 460
gastric cancer 389–90, 396
head and neck cancer 331
lung cancer 629–30
melanoma 675t
myeloma 784
oesophageal cancer 366, 368–9
oncogene-induced DNA replication
  stress 78
ovarian cancer 579
unknown primary 966
  see also BRAF oncogene; epidermal growth
  factor receptor; KIT oncogene/KIT/
  RTK; KRAS oncogene; MYC/Myc/c-Myc
  oncogene; NRAS oncogene
OncotypeDx®
breast cancer 99, 549, 561
colorectal cancer 461
OPC see oropharyngeal cancer
operator effects 102
opioids 296
opisthorchiasis 509–10, 511
optic nerve
glioma 879
meningioma 884, 885
orbital tumours 906
OPUS trial 429, 430t
oral administration of drugs 210
oral cavity cancer 157, 344–5
oral contraceptives 546
orbital exenteration 905, 907
orbital tumours 905–7

invasion from sinonasal tumours 341,
  342, 907
  see also eye
orchiectomy 608
oropharyngeal cancer (OPC)
clinical presentation 345
epidemiology 157, 345–6
HPV-associated 84, 329, 345
  histopathology 333, 333f
treatment 84, 346–7
osteoblastic metastases 64, 612, 970, 971
osteoclastic metastases 64
from breast cancer 560, 563–4
osteolytic lesions in myeloma 786
osteonecrosis, steroid-induced 730
osteoporosis/osteopenia 316, 317
osteosarcoma 844, 846b, 849t, 855, 860–1
outpatient care, palliative 294
ovarian cancer
case study 596–7
causes and risk factors 576
chemotherapy 68, 587, 592–3, 596, 597
genetic profiles 579
hereditary syndromes 165–6, 280
histopathology 579–80
incidence 576
lymph node involvement 586, 587
metastatic from other sites 395, 580
metastatic to other sites 586–7
molecular biology 579, 580
  CSCs 88t
multidisciplinary care 202–3t, 204, 596–7
prevention 280
radiotherapy 591
screening 166, 576
surgery 585–7, 596–7
  prophylactic 280
targeted therapies 53–4, 593
ovarian cancer profile with unknown
  primary 969, 970
ovary
cysts 579
polycystic ovary syndrome 933
transposition before RT for cervical
  cancer 582–3
oxaliplatin 187, 212t
colorectal cancer 418, 419, 425–7, 459, 460
gastric cancer 401, 402, 403
neuroendocrine tumours 957t
oesophageal cancer 377, 378, 382
pancreatic cancer 495–6
oxidative phosphorylation 6
OxPhos-type DLBCL 815

P
p14ARF 480
p16 protein/CDKN2A gene
acute lymphoblastic leukaemia 723
DLBCL 816
FAMMM syndrome 166
head and neck cancer 329–31
melanoma 675, 686
mesothelioma 534, 660
oesophageal cancer 367
p16INK4A 480
pancreatic cancer 479, 480
p53 protein/TP53 gene
acute lymphoblastic leukaemia 717, 721t, 723
cervical cancer 577
endometrial cancer 578

function
apoptosis 5, 28, 61
cell cycle control 3–4, 28
DNA damage response 7, 28, 36–7
glycolysis regulation 122
regulation by Mdm2 37
gastric cancer 390
head and neck cancer 329, 331
lung cancer 630
lymphoma (DLBCL) 816
myeloma 784
oesophageal cancer 366, 369
ovarian cancer 579
pancreatic cancer 480
penile cancer 607
squamous cell carcinoma 693
and SV40-T virus 136
unknown primary cancer 966
vulvar cancer 581
p70S6K1 (S6 kinase 1) 27
p73 protein/TP73 gene 390
p107 (pocket protein) 33
p130 (pocket protein) 33
paclitaxel
breast cancer 562
ovarian cancer 592–3
pancreatic cancer 496–7
pharmacokinetics 212t, 215
sarcoma 858
paediatric cancer
acute lymphoblastic leukaemia 715
adverse effects of treatment 730
genetic profiles 716–21, 722
relapsed 729–30
treatment 724, 725, 727–8
adrenal carcinoma 932
brain tumours 868, 873, 880, 881
Hodgkin lymphoma 831
juvenile polyposis 451
FAP 288, 450
in MEN 2B patients 926
sarcoma 855, 857
second cancers in survivors 152–3
pain
assessment 296
bone pain 612, 688, 786, 798
chronic, in survivors 314–15
control 296
bone pain 612, 688, 798
chronic pain 315
in pancreatic cancer 497
spinal tumours 892
eyelid tumours 904
spinal tumours 887, 892
palliative care 293–9
biliary cancers 513, 524–5, 526f
brain metastases 565, 891
breast cancer 559–60
colorectal cancer 424, 432, 456
depression 296–7
end-of-life discussions 297
fatigue 294, 296
gastric cancer 399, 402–3, 404
head and neck cancer 352, 354
a key element of cancer control planning 246
lung cancer 307–8, 641
lymphoma 828
mesothelioma 538–9, 664
oesophageal cancer 381–2
outcomes 297

palliative care (*Cont.*)
 pain relief 296, 612
 pancreatic cancer 488, 497
 prostate cancer 612
 and QoL 303, 307–8
 referral to 294*t*
 sarcoma 857, 859
 service provision 293–4, 297–8
 for spinal cord compression 688, 892–3
 surgery 168, 382, 488
 symptom assessment and management 294–7, 303
 unknown primary cancer 971*t*
pancreatic cancer
 borderline resectable 485, 492–3, 498–9
 CA19-9 497
 case study 498–9
 causes and risk factors 156*t*, 478
 chemoradiotherapy 489–94
  adjuvant 491, 493–4
  neoadjuvant 492–3, 494, 498
  unresectable disease 490–1
 chemotherapy 494–6, 496–7
  before chemoradiotherapy 490–1
 clinical presentation 478
 cost-effectiveness analysis 239
 genetic profiles 478–80
 hereditary syndromes 478
 histopathology 482–5
 imaging 485, 498, 499*f*
 immunohistochemistry 482
 incidence 478
 locally advanced (unresectable) 482, 485, 490–1, 498–9
 lymph node involvement 482, 486
 macroscopic appearance 482
 metastatic 479, 494–6
 molecular biology 478–82, 496
  CSCs 88*t*, 481
 mortality 478
 multidisciplinary care 202*t*, 204, 497–9
 neuroendocrine tumours 484, 945*t*, 946–50, 954–5*t*
 non-adenocarcinoma 484
 palliative care 488, 497
 premalignant lesions 479–80, 484, 488–9
 prognosis 68, 478, 483
 radiotherapy *see* pancreatic cancer, chemoradiotherapy
 screening 166
 staging 482–3
 surgery 164, 485–9, 487*f*
  complications 488
  after CRT 491
  palliative 488
  premalignant lesions 488–9
 survival time 483, 488
 targeted therapies 51, 496
pancreatic fistula 488
pancreatic intraepithelial neoplasia (PanIN) 479, 483*f*, 484, 489
pancreaticoduodenectomy 486
pancreatitis 482
pancreatoblastoma 484
panitumumab 429
papillary adenocarcinoma, gastric 394, 395*f*
papillary squamous carcinoma 332
papillary thyroid carcinoma 67, 918–23
papillary urothelial neoplasm of low malignant potential 613
para-aortic lymph nodes

gastric cancer 397
 gynaecological cancers 582, 583, 586
paraganglioma
 adrenal 935, 936
 head and neck 355–6, 935
paranasal sinus tumours *see* sinonasal tumours
paraneoplastic syndromes 943–52, 954–5*t*
 in lung cancer 634, 648
 POEMS 800
 see also Conn's syndrome; Cushing syndrome
parapituitary tumours 938*t*
paraprotein 782
 associated symptoms 787, 792
 measurement 787–9, 791
parasitic infestations (liver flukes) 509–10, 511
parathyroid disorders 926–7
parosteal osteosarcoma 855
parotid gland cancer 353
 radiotherapy 354
 surgery 354
 survival rates 355*t*
PARP/PARP-1 (poly(ADP-ribose)polymerase) protein 77, 84
 inhibitors 77
  breast cancer 548, 563
  ovarian cancer 593
PARSPORT trial 347
parthenolide 90
pasireotide 943, 947, 954
passenger mutations 7
passive smoking 127, 132, 628
patched (*PTCH* gene) 277*t*, 481, 690, 693
patient education 170–1, 676, 798
Patient-Reported Outcome Measurement Information System (PROMIS) 305–6
PAX5 gene 720, 721*t*, 723
pazopanib 51, 54
 adverse effects 53
 renal cancer 618, 619
 sarcoma 858
PCA3 test (prostate cancer) 610
PCL (plasma cell leukaemia) 799–800
PCNSL (primary CNS lymphoma) 811, 826, 882–4, 914
PCPT trial 264–5
PCR *see* polymerase chain reaction
PD-1 protein (programmed death 1) 115, 816
 inhibitors 644, 687, 816
PDGF *see* platelet-derived growth factor (PDGF)
PDGFR *see* platelet-derived growth factor receptor (PDGFR)
PDT *see* photodynamic therapy
pegvisomant 942
pegylated interferon 140, 682
pelvic exenteration 582, 587
pelvis, bone sarcoma 855
pemetrexed 212*t*
 lung cancer 643, 644
 mesothelioma 539–40, 541–2, 664–5
penile cancer 602–7
 carcinoma in situ 603
 chemotherapy 603, 606
 diagnosis 602
 genetic profile 606–7
 histopathology 602
 and HPV 606, 607
 imaging 602, 604*f*, 605*f*
 incidence 602
 laser therapy 603
 lymph node involvement 602, 604–5, 606

macroscopic appearance 602, 603*f*
 molecular biology 606–7
 radiotherapy 604
 surgery 602, 603–5
 survival rates 605–6
 targeted therapies 607
pentostatin 772
peptide receptor-mediated radionuclide therapy (PRRT) 958
pericytes 8, 51
peripheral B-cell lymphomas *see* lymphoma
peripheral neuro-ectodermic tumour (PNET) *see* Ewing sarcoma; medulloblastoma
peripheral T-cell lymphomas (PTCL) *see* T-cell lymphomas (TCL)
peritoneal adenocarcinoma, unknown primary 969, 970
peritoneal cancer index (PCI) 538, 539*f*
peritoneal dissemination/carcinomatosis 63, 64
 colorectal cancer 167, 457, 534
 gastric cancer 395, 400
 ovarian cancer 534, 586–7
peritoneal mesothelioma 533–43
 causes and risk factors 533–4
 chemotherapy
  intraperitoneal 540–2
  systemic 538–40
 clinical presentation 536–7
 diagnosis 534, 536–8
 epidemiology 533–4
 genetic profiles 534
 histopathology 534–6
 imaging 537–8
 laparoscopy 538
 lymph node involvement 536
 macroscopic appearance 533*f*, 535
 molecular biology 534, 542–3, 542*f*
 multicystic 534, 536, 537–8, 540
 staging 538, 539*t*
 surgery 540
 targeted therapies 542–3
 tumour markers 538
 well-differentiated papillary 534, 536
peritonectomy 540
per-protocol analysis 226
personal growth in survivors 318–19
personalized medicine 98
 hereditary syndromes 276, 280
 pharmacogenomics 99–100, 190, 216
 radiotherapy 184
pertuzumab 563, 564–5
PET *see* positron emission tomography
Peutz–Jeghers syndrome 277*t*, 451
PGP (P-glycoprotein) 192
pH, intracellular 122
phaeochromocytoma 929*f*, 935–7
 malignant 937–8
 surgery 926, 936
 with thyroid cancer 926
pharmacodynamic resistance 646
pharmacodynamics 209
 biomarkers 100–1, 209–10, 215–16
pharmacogenomics 99–100, 190, 216, 966–7
pharmacokinetics 189–90, 209, 210–15
 intraperitoneal pemetrexed 541
pharyngeal cancer *see* hypopharyngeal cancer; nasopharyngeal cancer; oropharyngeal cancer
PHF6 gene 722
Philadelphia chromosome (Ph)

acute lymphoblastic leukaemia 713, 715, 719, 727–9
  chronic myeloid leukaemia 754, 755
    additional abnormalities 756, 759–60
phospholipase Cγ (PLCγ) 15, 17
photodynamic therapy (PDT)
  actinic keratoses 695
  basal cell carcinoma 693
  head and neck cancer 344, 352
  mesothelioma 669
physical exercise
  and cancer prevention in survivors 319, 320t, 465
  for cancer-related fatigue 296
  and cancer risk 156
phytochemicals 157
PI3K signalling pathway (phosphatidylinositol 3-kinase) 26, 114
  activation by growth factors 11, 13, 16, 17, 24
  acute lymphoblastic leukaemia 717
  breast cancer 547, 548
  Burkitt lymphoma 817
  endometrial cancer 578
  head and neck cancer 331
  liver cancer 520
  melanoma 686
  metabolic reprogramming 120
  myeloma 786
  pancreatic cancer 480, 481
PICALM-MLLT10 (CALM-AF10) fusion gene 722
pilocytic astrocytoma, spinal 888
pineal tumours 869t, 881–2
pipe smoking 131, 628
pituitary apoplexy 886, 940
pituitary tumours 938–43
  adenoma 886–7, 938–9
  carcinoma 938, 939
  clinical presentation 886, 940, 941, 942–3, 942t
  craniopharyngioma 887, 939
  Cushing disease 939, 942–3
  diagnosis 940, 942, 943
  epidemiology 938t, 939
  genetics 939
  gonadotrophin-secreting 939
  growth hormone-secreting 939, 942
  imaging 886, 940, 941f
  metastatic from other sites 939
  non-functioning 939, 940
  pharmacological treatments 941, 942, 943
  prolactinoma 938–9, 941–2
  radiotherapy 886–7, 941, 942, 943
  surgery 886, 940–1, 941, 942, 943
  TSH-secreting 939
pixantrone 823
placebos in clinical trials 231
plasma cell dyscrasias
  amyloidosis 800–1
  extramedullary plasmacytoma 787, 801
  myeloma see myeloma
  plasma cell leukaemia (PCL) 799–800
  POEMS 800
  solitary plasmacytoma of bone 801
plasma cells
  in the diagnosis of myeloma 789–90
  normal development 782–3, 784f
plasmapheresis 797
platelet-derived growth factor (PDGF) 17–18, 481, 534
platelet-derived growth factor receptor (PDGFR) 17–18

acute lymphoblastic leukaemia 720
dermatofibrosarcoma protuberans 17, 858
mesothelioma 534
platelets (in CML) 756
platinum-based agents see carboplatin; cisplatin; oxaliplatin
pleomorphic adenoma 336, 906
pleomorphic liposarcoma/sarcoma 854
pleural hyaline plaques 661
pleural mesothelioma 659–69
  asbestos 659, 661
  chemoradiotherapy 669
  chemotherapy
    adjuvant 665–7
    heated intraoperative (HIOC) 667
    neoadjuvant 667–9
    systemic 664–5
  diagnosis 661
  genetic profiles 660
  histopathology 661–2
  imaging 661, 663, 665, 666f
  lymph node involvement 661, 663
  macroscopic appearance 661
  molecular biology 659–60
  multimodality treatment 664, 665–9
  palliative care 664
  photodynamic therapy 669
  prognosis 660
  radiotherapy 664, 669
  recurrence 663–4
  staging 662
  surgery 661, 662–4
  survival rates 664
pleurectomy/decortication 661, 662, 663–4, 663f
  adjuvant therapies 669
PLL (prolymphocytic leukaemia) 766, 772–4
PMBL (primary mediastinal large B-cell lymphoma) 816, 829
PML-RARA fusion gene 699
PMS2/PMS2 75, 276, 451
PNET (primitive/peripheral neuro-ectodermal tumour) see Ewing sarcoma; medulloblastoma
pneumonectomy 638
  extrapleural 661, 662, 663–4, 663f
  in multimodality therapy 665–9
pneumonitis, iatrogenic 316
  radiation-induced 177, 316, 559, 560
pocket proteins 33
  see also pRb (retinoblastoma protein, RB1)
POEMS syndrome 800
POET trial 380
point mutation instability (PIN) 76
Polo-like kinases 35
polycyclic aromatic hydrocarbons (PAHs) 128, 144t, 157
polycystic ovary syndrome 933
polymerase chain reaction (PCR) 680
  acute lymphoblastic leukaemia 728–9
  chronic myeloid leukaemia 756, 760
polyposis syndromes 451
  FAP see familial adenomatous polyposis
  MUTYH-associated 75, 450
polyps
  endoscopic polypectomy 167, 411, 456–7
  fundic gland 288, 393
  gallbladder 509
  histopathology 452
pomalidomide 794b, 799
ponatinib 758, 764, 765

poorly-differentiated carcinoma with midline distribution 969, 970
population effects 102
positive predictive value (PPV) 105
positron emission tomography (PET) 61
  head and neck cancer 338–40, 349
  hepatobiliary cancers 513, 522
  lymphoma 811
  PET/CT
    cervical cancer 581
    colorectal cancer 453, 466
    head and neck cancer 338–40
    lung cancer 635
    mesothelioma 666f
    myeloma 789f, 790
    oesophageal cancer 371, 375
    unknown primary 968
  prostate cancer 123
  vaginal cancer 584
post-operative complications see surgery, complications
post-translational modification in cell cycle control 33–4
post-transplant lymphoproliferative disorder (PTLD) 136–7, 813b, 814
potassium, hypokalaemia 931
power (1–β) 224
PPV (positive predictive value) 105
pRb (retinoblastoma protein, RB1) 28, 33–4, 39
  cervical cancer 577
  head and neck cancer 331
  oesophageal cancer 367
precision of biomarker tests 105
prednisolone 768, 793, 794b, 796
prednisone 817–18
pregnancy
  thyroid cancer 922–3
  see also fertility
premalignant lesions
  breast 269, 552, 554, 559
  cervical 272, 577
  colorectal 408, 411, 451–2, 456
  gastric 388, 392–3
  head and neck 331, 345
  lung 630, 631
  oesophageal 365–6, 367–8
  pancreatic 479–80, 484, 488–9
  penile 603
prepuce 603
pre-RC (pre-replicative) complex 34
prevention
  of brain metastases in lung cancer 647, 648
  breast cancer 158, 262–3, 280, 554
  colorectal cancer 165, 263–4, 445, 446–7, 456
  a key element of cancer control planning 246
  lifestyle changes 156–7, 158, 319, 445
  lung cancer 132–4, 265
  ovarian cancer 280
  pharmacological 114–15, 262–5, 446–7, 697–8
  prostate cancer 264–5
  of recurrence 313, 319–20, 465–6
  screening see screening
  skin cancers 676, 697–8
  smoking control/cessation 132–4, 320t
  surgery (in hereditary syndromes) 165, 280, 456, 554
  vaccination 256
    against HBV 256–7
    against HPV 258–9, 272–3, 606

primary mediastinal large B-cell lymphoma
(PMBL) 816, 829
primary sclerosing cholangitis (PSC) 509
primitive neuro-ectodermal tumour
(PNET) *see* Ewing sarcoma;
medulloblastoma
processed meat 157, 445
PROCTOR/SCRIPT trial 420
progestins 308, 592
programmed cell death 4–5, 42–7, 112
radiation-induced 174
see also apoptosis; autophagy
prolactinoma 938–9, 941–2
prolymphocytic leukaemia (PLL) 766, 772–4
PROMID trial 649
prophylaxis *see* prevention
proportion of treatment effect (PTE) 223
proptosis 906
prostate cancer 609–12
active surveillance 610–11
biopsy 610
castrate resistant 612
causes and risk factors 157, 609
chemotherapy 612
clinical presentation 610
digital rectal examination 610
endocrine therapy 187, 264–5, 612
histopathology 610
imaging 123, 610
incidence 264, 609
local treatments 611
lymph node involvement 610, 611
metastasis 64, 612
multidisciplinary care 202t, 204
palliative care 612
prevention 264–5
PSA 273, 610, 611, 612
radiotherapy 611, 612
second cancers in survivors 152
risk groups 610, 611t
screening 273, 609
Sipuleucel-T vaccine 115, 259, 612
surgery 316, 611, 611–12
watchful waiting 611
prostate-specific antigen (PSA) 273, 610, 611,
612, 970
proteasome inhibitors (bortezomib)
mantle cell lymphoma 820
myeloma 793, 794b, 795, 796, 798, 799
plasma cell leukaemia 800
protein binding of drugs 211
protein kinase B *see* AKT signalling pathway
protein kinase C (PKCβ) 815
protein synthesis 27
proteinuria 782, 787
proton beam radiotherapy 179–80, 463, 873,
893, 910
proto-oncogenes 38–9
see also oncogenes
PSA (prostate-specific antigen) 273, 610, 611,
612, 970
psoriasis treatment 690
psychological factors
in cancer patients 296–7, 872, 911
in cancer survivors 317–19, 466
effect of MDTs on healthcare workers 205
in genetic counselling 279–80
PTCH (patched) 277t, 481, 690, 693
PTEN gene/PTEN protein 26, 277t, 451,
548, 578

pterygopalatine fossa tumours 341
PTLD (post-transplant lymphoproliferative
disorder) 136–7, 813b, 814
PTPN11 gene 716, 717, 723
public health
cancer control planning 245–52
challenges 251–2
international initiatives 246, 252
key elements 246
the process 246–51
cost of cancer care 236–40
genetic counselling 276–88
prevention of cancer *see* prevention
screening *see* screening
and smoking 132–4
sun exposure education 676
purine analogues 187, 768–9, 772, 773
pyloric dilatation 375
pylorus-preserving pancreaticoduodenectomy
(PPPD) 486
pyrimidine analogues 187, 212t
see also 5-fluorouracil; capecitabine; cytosine
arabinoside; gemcitabine
pyruvate kinase 122

Q

quality-adjusted life years (QALYs) 239
quality assurance/quality control (QA/QC)
biomarker tests 106
mammography 268
in surgery 169–70, 423
quality of life (QoL)
assessment methods 302–10
colorectal cancer 419, 424, 465, 466
ocular cancer 911
after oesophagectomy 375
in survivors of cancer 306–7
physical morbidity 313–17
psychosocial morbidity 317–19, 466
QUASAR trials 420, 421t, 460
questionnaires (QoL) 303–8
quiescence of CSCs 88–9, 91

R

radiation-induced cancers 150–1, 444–5, 706
acute myeloid leukaemia 706
after radiotherapy 151–3, 419, 560, 873, 905,
918–19
radon 151, 628
sarcoma 854–5
skin cancer 690
thyroid cancer 151, 918–19
radiofrequency ablation (RFA) 167, 372,
517–18
radioimmunotherapy 824–5
radionuclide scans
adrenal tumours 931
bone metastases 610, 949f
neuroendocrine tumours 648, 952f, 968
phaeochromocytoma 936
thyroid cancer 920, 922
radionuclide therapy
bone metastases 612
lymphoma (Mab conjugates) 824–5
neuroendocrine tumours 649, 958
selective internal (SIRT) 517, 958
thyroid cancer (^{131}I) 67, 921, 922, 927
radiotherapy (RT) 173–84
3D (conformal with 3D treatment
planning) 178, 180–1, 376

3D (image-guided adaptive
brachytherapy) 588, 595
adverse effects 176–7
in breast cancer 152, 153, 559, 560
cardiotoxicity 315, 377, 559, 560
in colorectal cancer 419
of cranial irradiation 730, 873, 883, 891
of episcleral brachytherapy 910b, 910f
and fractionation schedule 177–8
in gynaecological cancers 590, 591
in head and neck cancer 306, 316, 343,
344, 348
lung damage 177, 316, 559, 560
pain 315
second cancers 151–3, 419, 560, 873, 905,
918–19
spinal irradiation 889
for benign disease 151
bone metastases 685, 688
brachytherapy *see* brachytherapy
brain tumours 872–3
choroid plexus 894
craniopharyngioma 887
in the elderly 876
ependymoma 881
glioblastoma 876
high-grade (anaplastic) glioma 877–8
low-grade glioma 880
lymphoma 883–4
medulloblastoma 881
meningioma 885–6
metastatic disease 565, 646, 647, 648, 685,
688, 891–2
pineal tumours 882
breast cancer 152, 153, 556–60, 565
cervical cancer 587–8, 593–5
surgery to reduce morbidity from 582–3
in children 152–3, 730
colorectal cancer 168, 412–19, 462–3
liver metastases 463
in combination with chemotherapy *see*
chemoradiotherapy
and DNA repair 82–4, 89
dose 175–6
beam composition and strength 178–80,
183–4
fractionation 177–8
emergencies 183
endometrial cancer 589–91, 596
follow-up 183
future developments 183–4
head and neck cancer
adverse effects 306, 316, 343, 344, 348
imaging after treatment 338, 340
laryngeal/hypopharyngeal 348
nasopharyngeal 343, 344
oral cavity 345
oropharyngeal 84, 346–7
paragangliomas 355–6
QoL issues 306
recurrent disease 352
salivary gland tumours 354
sinonasal 341–2
unknown primary 350
image-guided 182, 183
brachytherapy 588, 595
intensity-modulated *see* intensity-modulated
radiotherapy (IMRT)
intraoperative (IORT) 463, 556–7, 856
liver cancer 517

lung cancer
  brain metastases 646, 647, 648
  NSCLC (early stage) 639
  NSCLC (locally advanced) 640–1
  SCLC 647, 648
lymphoma 820, 822, 827–31
  CNS disease 883–4
  retinal 912
  total body irradiation pre-transplant 827
mechanism of action 173–4
melanoma 682–3, 688
  uveal 909–10, 911
mesothelioma 664, 669
methods 181–3
monitoring and verification 183
multidisciplinary care 182
oesophageal cancer 375–7, 378, 382
orbital tumours 906
ovarian cancer 591
pancreatic cancer see chemoradiotherapy
  (CRT), pancreatic cancer
patient set-up 183
penile cancer 604
physics 178–80
pituitary tumours 886–7, 941, 942, 943
POEMS syndrome 800
prostate cancer 611, 612
  second cancers in survivors 152
radiosensitivity 83–4, 184
  of CSCs 176
sarcoma 856, 856–7
skin cancer
  BCC 692–3
  melanoma 682–3, 688
  Merkel cell carcinoma 697
  SCC 696
skull base tumours 893
spinal tumours 889
  astrocytoma 890
  ependymoma 890
  metastatic 688, 893
  re-irradiation 873, 889
stereotactic see stereotactic body/brain
  radiotherapy (SBRT)
targeting 174–5, 178, 375
testicular cancer 608
therapeutic window 173
thymic tumours 656, 657
thyroid cancer 927
timing of pre-operative RT 168
treatment planning 173, 176, 180–1, 182–3
  brain tumours 872
  lymphoma 828, 830–1, 830f
  oesophageal cancer 375–6
  unknown primary 350
  vaginal cancer 584, 590–1
  vestibular schwannoma 894
  vulvar cancer 591
  whole abdomen 463, 540, 591
radon exposure 151, 628
RAF see RAS/RAF/MAPK signalling pathway
RAG (recombinase activating gene)
  enzymes 720
Rai staging of chronic lymphocytic
  leukaemia 767
raloxifene 187, 263t
ramucirumab 54, 188
  colorectal cancer 431
  gastro-oesophageal cancers 382, 404
  lung cancer 644

randomized clinical trials (RCTs)
  analysis 225–6
  design
    Phase II/III combined 224–5
    Phase III 221–3
  ethics
    placebo use 231
    research biopsies 231–2
  for screening tests 267
RANK ligands 482, 563
rapamycin 47
RAS/RAF/MAPK signalling pathway 25–6
  activation by growth factors 11, 15, 17, 24, 25
  acute lymphoblastic leukaemia 716, 717, 723
  cell cycle/CDK activation 28
  colorectal cancer 429
  gastric cancer 389
  inhibitors 682, 685–6, 892, 921–2
  liver cancer 520, 521
  melanoma 674, 682, 685–6, 892
  myeloma 784, 786
  pancreatic cancer 480
  squamous cell carcinoma 686, 693
  thyroid cancer 919, 921–2
  see also BRAF oncogene; KRAS oncogene;
    NRAS oncogene
rationing of care/drugs 232, 233t, 238
RB1 gene see pRb (retinoblastoma protein,
  RB1)
RCC see renal cancer
RCTs see randomized clinical trials
reactive oxygen species (ROS) 44, 89, 122, 145
reagent batch effects 102
REAL-2 trial 382, 402t, 403
receptor tyrosine kinases (RTKs) 14, 23
  see also epidermal growth factor receptor
    (EGFR); fibroblast growth factor
    receptor (FGFR); insulin-like growth
    factor receptor (IGFR1/IGFR2); MET
    (HGF receptor); platelet-derived growth
    factor receptor (PDGFR); vascular
    endothelial growth factor receptor
    (VEGFR)
recombinase activating gene (RAG)
  enzymes 720
RECOURSE trial 431
rectal cancer 408–19
  chemoradiotherapy
    adjuvant 415, 418
    neoadjuvant 168, 416–19
  chemotherapy 419–22
  definition 408, 415
  imaging 408–11
  lymph node involvement 409–10, 415, 419
  neuroendocrine tumours 952
  radiotherapy 168, 412–19
  recurrence 409, 412, 415f
  staging/restaging 408, 409, 410, 418–19
  surgery
    anal sphincter preservation 411, 417, 418
    audits 169–70
    endoscopic polypectomy 167, 411
    follow-up procedures 170, 422–3, 465–6
    margins of resection 165, 409
    outcomes 412
    preoperative preparation 411
    resection technique 411–12
    risk-adapted procedures 417–18, 418
    TEM 167, 411
  see also colorectal cancer

rectal examination 408, 610
rectoscopy 408
red eye 904
REDUCE trial 264–5
reference ranges of biomarker tests 105
referral
  to expert centres 168, 170, 485, 607, 850–1
  to palliative care 294t
reflux disease
  GORD 367
  post-oesophagectomy 374
REGARD trial 382, 404
registries 169
regorafenib 49, 51, 431
regulatory (suppressor) T-lymphocytes
  112, 114
  inhibitors 115, 687
rehabilitation 246
relatives
  at-risk of hereditary syndromes 278, 280–1
  of cancer survivors 219
REMARK criteria 100b
renal allowable radiation dose 377
renal cancer (RCC) 616–19
  causes and risk factors 616–17
  diagnosis 617
  histopathology 616
  surgery 617–18
  targeted therapies 51–2, 618–19
renal excretion of drugs 189–90, 214
  and renal impairment 190
renal failure in myeloma 787, 797
renin 931
research and development
  biomarker tests 101–6
  pharmaceuticals see clinical trials
response rate (RR) 221
RET gene
  genetic screening 924
  thyroid cancer 918, 919, 923–4
retinal lymphoma 912–14, 912f
retinoblastoma protein see pRb (retinoblastoma
  protein, RB1)
retinoic acid 699, 704
retinoids 696, 697
retroperitoneal sarcoma
  radiotherapy 857
  surgery 852, 853f, 853t
RFA (radiofrequency ablation) 167, 372,
  517–18
rhabdomyosarcoma 336
rheumatic disease 774
RICOVER-60 trial 818, 829
RIP 1/RIP3 (receptor-interacting protein
  kinase) 44–5
rituximab 823
  chronic lymphocytic leukaemia 768–9
  lymphoma
    with chemotherapy 818–20, 823, 824t
    maintenance therapy 823
    mantle cell lymphoma 820
    retinal 912
  mechanism of action 823–4
  PTLD 137
robotic surgery 166
  hysterectomy 584
  transoral 347, 348
ROS1 gene 629–30
ROS (reactive oxygen species) 44, 89, 122, 145
round cell liposarcoma 849t, 853, 857, 858

RT *see* radiotherapy
RTOG 0129 trial 346
RTOG 0617 trial 641
RTOG 8501 trial 378–9
RTOG 9111 trial 349
RTOG 9207 trial 377
RTOG 9402 trial 878
RTOG 9405 trial 379
RTOG 9704 trial 491, 493, 494
RTOG 9802 trial 880
RUN3X gene 392
RUNX1 gene 720
   ETV6-RUNX1 fusion gene 715, 718, 720
ruxolitinib 14, 719

S
S-1 (fluoropyrimidine) 382, 401, 403
S6 kinase 1 (p70S6K1) 27
sacrum 855
salinomycin 91
salivary gland tumours 336, 353–5
salivary type lung carcinoma 633
Salmonella spp. 509, 510
salpingo-oophorectomy 280, 586
salt (sodium chloride), dietary 157–8
Sanger sequencing methods 680
sarcoma 844–61
  of bone *see* bone, sarcoma
  chemotherapy
    bone 856, 860–1
     isolated limb perfusion 860
    soft tissue 857–60
  classification 845, 845–6b
  diagnosis 844–5, 846–7, 850
    expert referral 850–1
  genetic profiles 849–50
  grading 848–9
  head and neck 336
  histopathology 846–9
  imaging 844
  incidence 844, 855, 856
  metastasis 844, 852, 853, 854, 857, 859, 861
  palliative care 857, 859
  radiotherapy 856, 856–7
  recurrence 851t, 854
  surgery 851–6, 859
  targeted therapies 54, 850, 858–9, 861
sarcomatoid carcinoma, lung 632–3
sarcomatoid squamous carcinoma 332–3
SBRT *see* stereotactic body/brain radiotherapy
scalp angiosarcoma 854
SCC *see* squamous cell carcinoma
scintigraphy *see* radionuclide scans
SCLC *see* small-cell lung cancer
screening 267–73
  breast cancer 166, 267–70
  cervical cancer 258, 272–3
  colorectal cancer 264, 270–1, 282, 446, 465
  for hereditary syndromes 282
  interval cancers 269, 271
  a key element of cancer control planning 246
  lung cancer 273
  melanoma 166
  ovarian cancer 166, 576
  over-diagnosis/over-treatment 269
  pancreatic cancer 166
  principles 268b
  prostate cancer 273, 609
  and socioeconomic status 271, 282
  in survivors of cancer 313

  see also surveillance
SCRIPT trial 420
SDH (succinate dehydrogenase) 122, 355, 935
sebaceous carcinoma 905
secondhand smoke 127, 132, 628
secretin 948
securin 36
'seed and soil' hypothesis of metastatic
    spread 63
seizures 871, 872
selective internal radionuclide therapy
    (SIRT) 517, 958
sellar region tumours 869t
  craniopharyngioma 887, 939
selumetinib 629
seminoma germ cell tumour (SGST) 607, 608
senescence 78, 480
  radiation-induced 174
sensitivity (analytical) 105
sensitivity (clinical) 105
sentinel node procedure
  breast cancer 168, 555
  cervical cancer 582
  colorectal cancer 169
  endometrial cancer 583
  melanoma 168, 679, 681–2
  Merkel cell carcinoma 697
  penile cancer 605
  squamous cell carcinoma 696
  vaginal cancer 584–5
  vulvar cancer 585
SERMs (selective estrogen receptor
    modulators) 187, 262–3
  see also tamoxifen
serotoninoma *see* carcinoids
serous endometrial intraepithelial carcinoma
    (SEIC) 578
serous papillary adenocarcinoma of the
    peritoneal cavity 969, 970
serous tubal intraepithelial carcinoma
    (STIC) 579
serrated polyps 452
serum free light-chain (SFLC) 787–9, 791
service provision
  for cancer survivors 320–1
  genetic counselling 278
  palliative care 293–4, 297–8
sex steroids
  feminizing tumours 933
  virilizing tumours 932, 933
sexual dysfunction 316–17
  after prostate surgery 316, 611
  after vaginal surgery 584
SF-36 questionnaire 303, 308
SH2/SH3 (Src homology) domain 25
shared decision-making 170–1
  end-of-life discussions 297
  fertility preservation 317
Siewert classification of GEJ cancer 369–70
sigmoidoscopy 270–1, 408
signalling pathways 11–18, 23–30
  see also AKT signalling pathway; JAK/STAT
    signalling pathway; mTOR signalling
    pathway; PI3K signalling pathway; RAS/
    RAF/MAPK signalling pathway; Wnt
    signalling pathway
signet-ring-cell carcinoma
  colorectal 453
  gastric 394, 395f, 396
significance (statistical/clinical) 224, 308

siltuximab 14, 115
Simon's two-stage design 221
Simpson classification (meningioma
    resection) 885
simultaneous integrated boosts (SIB) 181–2
single-strand annealing (SSA) DNA repair 82
sinonasal tumours 334–5, 336t, 340–2
  lymphoma 336, 829, 832
  orbital invasion 341, 342, 907
sinonasal undifferentiated carcinoma
    (SNUC) 334–5
SINS score (spinal instability neoplastic
    score) 892
Sipuleucel-T 115, 259, 612
skin cancers, non-melanoma 690–8
  atypical fibroxanthoma 697
  basal cell carcinoma 690, 691–3, 904–5
  causes and risk factors 690–1, 693, 696,
    904–5
  chemotherapy 693, 694, 696, 697
  cutaneous T-cell lymphoma 814, 831–2
  eyelid tumours 904–5
  genetic syndromes 690–1, 905
  histopathology 692f, 695f, 696, 697
  incidence 690, 696, 904
  lymph node involvement 693, 696, 697, 904
  macroscopic appearance 691, 691f, 694, 694f,
    696, 905
  Merkel cell carcinoma 140, 696–7, 905
  metastasis 693, 696, 697
  molecular biology 691, 693
  prevention 697–8
  prognosis 692, 696
  radiotherapy 692–3, 696, 697
  squamous cell carcinoma 686, 690, 691,
    693–6, 697–8, 905
  surgery 692, 695–6, 905
  surveillance 693, 696
  targeted therapies 693
  topical therapies 693, 694–5
  xeroderma pigmentosum 75, 690–1, 905
  see also melanoma
skull base tumours 335t, 336t, 893
  sinonasal 334, 340–2
Slug (transcription factor) 29–30
SMAC protein 45
SMAD proteins 16, 29
  SMAD4/*DPC4* 451, 479, 480
small bowel cancer
  melanoma metastases 685
  neuroendocrine tumours 951–2
small-cell gynaecological cancers 593
small-cell lung cancer (SCLC)
  chemoradiotherapy in early stage
    disease 646–7
  chemotherapy
    metastatic disease 647–8
    resistance 68
  classification 646
  cranial irradiation 647, 648
  histopathology 631–2
  surgery 647
small round blue cell tumours
  childhood sarcoma 857
  olfactory neuroblastoma 334
smoking 127–34
  and alcohol 130, 329
  carcinogenesis 127–9
  colorectal cancer 446
  control/cessation 132–4, 320t

epidemiology of cancer 127, 129–32, 134
lung cancer 127, 128f, 130, 132, 628
markers of exposure 128
oesophageal cancer 366t
oncologists' role 133–4
oropharyngeal cancer 346
pancreatic cancer 478
passive 127, 132, 628
in survivors 319, 320t
SMO/smoothened 481, 693
smouldering myeloma (SMM) 790t, 791, 792
Snail (transcription factor) 29–30
social functioning in cancer survivors 319
societal costs of cancer care 236–7
socioeconomic status
and delayed diagnosis/missed screening 271, 282
lymphoma 808–9
SOCS (suppressor of cytokine signalling) 14, 25
sodium
dietary 157–8
hyponatraemia 787
soft tissue plasmacytomas 787, 801
soft tissue sarcoma (STS)
chemotherapy 857–60
classification 845, 845–6b
diagnosis 844, 845, 846–7, 850
genetic profiles 849–50
grading 848–9
histopathology 846–7, 848
imaging 844
incidence 844
metastatic disease 844, 852, 853, 854, 857, 859
radiotherapy 856–7
surgery 851–5, 859
targeted therapies 858–9
Sokal risk score (CML) 754
solid-pseudopapillary tumour, pancreatic 483f, 484
solitary fibrous tumour 535
solitary plasmacytoma of bone (SPB) 801
somatic hypermutation 783
somatostatin analogues (SSA)
imaging receptor-bearing tumours 648, 952f, 968
neuroendocrine tumours 649, 947, 952, 954–5, 956t, 957
pituitary tumours 942, 943
thymic tumours 656
somatostatinoma 945t, 950, 955t
somnolence syndrome 873
sonidegib 693
sorafenib 49, 51, 52t
adverse effects 53, 922
liver cancer 51, 519–20
combination therapies 521
with TACE 521
thyroid cancer 921–2
SOS (Son of Sevenless) 25
SPACE trial 521
specificity 105
S phase 31
control of DNA replication 31, 34
G1 to S phase transition 33–4, 84
in myeloma 783–4
spinal cord compression 685, 688, 797, 887–8, 892–3
spinal cord radiotherapy dose 377, 889
spinal tumours 887–90
clinical presentation 887–8, 892

imaging 789f, 790, 888, 889f, 890f
metastatic 888, 890f, 892–3
melanoma 685, 688
myeloma 786, 789f, 790, 797
pain relief 892
radiotherapy 889
astrocytoma 890
ependymoma 890
metastases 688, 893
re-irradiation 873, 889
sarcoma 855, 856
surgery 688, 888–9, 892
astrocytoma 890
ependymoma 889–90
SPIRITS trial 402t, 403
spironolactone 931
Spitz naevi 675, 677
spleen
gastric cancer 397
hairy cell leukaemia 770, 771
melanoma metastases 685
splenectomy 397, 771
splenic flexure tumours 455
squamous cell carcinoma (SCC)
cutaneous 693–6
and BRAF inhibitor treatment for melanoma 686, 693
causes and risk factors 690, 691, 693
prevention 697–8
eyelid 905
lung 630, 631
oesophageal 365–7, 377, 382
penile 603t
in situ (Bowen's disease) 603, 694, 694f, 695, 696
see also cervical cancer; head and neck cancer; vaginal cancer; vulvar cancer
SREBPs (sterol regulatory element binding proteins) 123
SSA see somatostatin analogues
staging 164
adrenal carcinoma 932t
breast cancer 553–4
chronic lymphocytic leukaemia 767
chronic myeloid leukaemia 754, 755t
colorectal cancer 408, 452
preoperative 409, 453–4
restaging after neoadjuvant CRT 410, 418–19
gastric cancer 394b
head and neck cancer 341, 349–50
liver cancer 514–15, 516f
lung cancer 635, 636t, 637f, 638t
melanoma 680
mesothelioma
peritoneal 538, 539t
pleural 662
oesophageal cancer 369, 370–1
pancreatic cancer 482–3
penile cancer 602
renal cancer 617
restaging (after pre-operative therapy) 165, 410, 418–19
testicular cancer 607–8
thymic tumours 655, 656t
thyroid cancer 922, 924
urothelial cell cancer 613, 615
stakeholders in NCCPs 247
STAT3 see JAK/STAT signalling pathway
statins (HMG-CoA reductase inhibitors) 115

stem cells in tumours see cancer stem cells (CSCs)
stem cell transplantation see haematopoietic stem cell transplantation
stents
biliary 497, 525, 526f
colonic 456
oesophageal 382
stereotactic body/brain radiotherapy (SBRT) 179, 182
brain tumours 688, 873, 878, 891
liver metastases 463
lung cancer 639
nasopharyngeal carcinoma 344
STIM trial 758, 763
STK11 gene 451
stomach anatomy 392
stomach cancer see gastric cancer
stomas 316, 423
stoma therapists 465
STORM trial 521
stratification in RCT design 222
streptozocin 956t, 958
stroma
breast cancer 549
CSC niche 8–9, 89
immune/inflammatory response 109–12, 114
myeloma 785–6
pancreatic cancer 480–1
role in metastasis 65–7
STS see soft tissue sarcoma
subependymoma 879
submandibular gland cancer 353
radiotherapy 354
surgery 354
survival rates 355
succinate dehydrogenase (SDH) 122, 355, 935
sunbeds 676, 691
sun exposure
eyelid cancer 904
melanoma 674, 675, 676
other skin cancer 690, 691, 693
sunscreen 694, 697
xeroderma pigmentosum 75, 690–1, 905
sunitinib 49, 52t, 54
adverse effects 53
liver cancer 520
neuroendocrine tumours 51, 956t, 957
renal cancer 51, 618, 619
sarcoma 858
superficial spreading melanoma 678
superiority design in RCTs 222
supportive care see palliative care; survivors of cancer
surgery 163–71
adjuvant or neoadjuvant procedures 168
adrenal tumours 930, 931, 933, 935, 936
audits 169–70, 423
bladder cancer 614, 615
brain tumours 872
choroid plexus 894
craniopharyngioma 887
glioblastoma 875, 876
low-grade glioma 879
medulloblastoma 880–1
meningioma 885
metastatic 891
pineal 881–2

surgery (*Cont.*)
breast cancer 163, 165, 168, 307, 553–6
prophylactic 280, 554
shared decision-making 170–1
cervical cancer 581–3, 593
cholangiocarcinoma 525
colorectal cancer *see* colorectal cancer
(CRC), surgery
complications 315*t*
of cervical cancer surgery 582
of oesophagectomy 374–5
pain 314
of pancreatic surgery 488
of prostatectomy 316, 611
elderly patients 164
endometrial cancer 583–4, 595–6
in expert centres 168, 170, 373–4, 399, 485
eyelid tumours 905
gallbladder cancer 522–4
gastric cancer 396–7
adjuvant/neoadjuvant therapies 400–1
laparoscopic 399, 400
lymphadenectomy 163, 397–9
palliative 399
reduction 399–400
head and neck cancer
intraoperative evaluation 333–4
laryngeal/hypopharyngeal 347, 348, 349,
351
nasopharyngeal 344
oral cavity 344–5
oropharyngeal 347
paragangliomas 355–6
recurrent disease 344, 351–2
salivary gland tumours 354
sinonasal 341, 342
unknown primary 350
history 163–4
liver cancer
resection 515
transplantation 514, 515
lung cancer
carcinoid tumours 648
early stage NCSLC 635–8
locally advanced NCSLC 640
SCLC 647
margins of resection 165, 409, 554
melanoma 680, 681*t*, 689
amputation 683
conjunctival disease 907
lymph nodes 168, 680–2
stage IV disease 684–5
uveal 909, 910
mesothelioma
peritoneal 540
pleural 661, 662–4
minimally invasive 166–7
see also laparoscopy; thermal ablation
neuroendocrine tumours 648, 948, 951, 953–4
oesophageal cancer 371–4, 378, 379–80
complications 374–5
palliative 382
orbital tumours 907
ovarian cancer 585–7, 596–7
palliative 168, 382, 488
pancreatic cancer 164, 485–8, 487*f*
after CRT 491
palliative 488
premalignant lesions 488–9
penile cancer 602, 603–5
perioperative care 167, 411, 454

phaeochromocytoma 926, 936
pituitary tumours 886, 940–1, 941, 942, 943
planning 164–5, 169
prophylactic
for breast/ovarian cancer 280, 554
for colorectal cancer 165, 456
prostate cancer 316, 611, 611–12
registries 169
renal cancer 617–18
resectability 164–5
sarcoma 851–6, 859
sentinel node *see* sentinel node procedure
shared decision-making 170–1
skin cancer
atypical fibroxanthoma 697
BCC 692
eyelid 905
melanoma 680–2, 683, 684–5, 689
SCC 695–6
spinal tumours 688, 888–9, 892
astrocytoma 890
ependymoma 889–90
testicular cancer 608, 609
thymic tumours 655–6, 657
thyroid cancer 921, 926–7
reoperation 927
unknown primary 350, 970
urothelial cell carcinoma 614, 615
vaginal cancer 584–5
vestibular schwannoma 893–4
vulvar cancer 585
surrogate endpoints 223, 494, 497
surveillance 312–13
colorectal cancer 313, 422–3, 465–6
liver cancer 514
melanoma 683–4, 910
myeloma 791–2, 798
prostate cancer 610–11
renal cancer 617
skin cancer 683–4, 693, 696
testicular cancer 608
thyroid cancer 922, 928
uveal melanoma 910
see also screening
survivin 542
survivors of cancer 312–21
care planning 246, 320–1
of colorectal cancer 422–3, 465–6
demographics 312
future developments 321
guidelines 321
physical long-term/late effects 313–17
pregnancy after thyroid cancer 923
prevention of recurrence/new primaries 313,
319–20, 465–6
psychosocial long-term/late effects 317–19,
466, 873
QoL 306–7, 466
second cancers
associated with chemotherapy 706
associated with radiotherapy 151–3, 419,
560, 873, 905, 918–19
surveillance/screening 312–13
swallowing difficulties 306, 369, 382
synovial sarcoma 850*t*, 854
synthetic lethality 77, 84, 123, 548

T

TACE (trans-arterial chemoembolization) of
hepatic tumours 516, 517
with adjuvant sorafenib 521

neuroendocrine tumour metastases 950, 958
TAL1 gene 722
talc granulomata 661
T-ALL (T-lineage ALL)
early T-cell precursor ALL 722
genetic profiles 717*t*, 721–2
metastasis 730
prognosis 713
tamoxifen 187
breast cancer 562
in combination with RT 559
prediction of response 551
prevention 262
liver cancer 519
pharmacokinetics 190, 214
TAM (tumour-associated macrophages) 66,
109, 110–11, 114, 549
tandutinib 54
targeted therapies 9*f*
acute lymphoblastic leukaemia 713, 714, 719
Ph+ ALL 727–9
relapsed disease 730
acute myeloid leukaemia 89, 90, 707, 712
angiogenesis 49, 51–7, 187–8
apoptosis 44
autophagy 47
basal cell carcinoma 693
brain tumours 874, 876, 878
metastatic disease 892
breast cancer 54, 67, 562–3, 564–5, 892
in combination with RT 559
costs 238
resistance 548
chronic lymphocytic leukaemia 768–70
chronic myeloid leukaemia 754, 756–8
monitoring response 758–63, 765
refractory/recurrent disease 764–5
resistance 89, 757, 763–4, 765
therapy may be stopped without
recurrence 765–6
clinical trial designs 224–5
colorectal cancer 52, 418, 427–31, 432, 433,
459–60
CSCs 90–1, 93
endometrial cancer 592
gastric cancer 396, 402, 403–4
growth factors 12–13, 14, 15, 16, 17, 18
head and neck cancer
laryngeal/hypolaryngeal 348
metastatic disease 352–3
oropharyngeal 346
immune system/inflammation 14, 115, 687
liver cancer 51, 54, 519–21
adjuvant 521
lung cancer
with chemotherapy 629, 643–4, 645
driver mutations present 641, 644–6
maintenance therapy 643
metastatic disease 641
resistance 629, 646
second-line therapy 644
lymphomas 823–4
aggressive B-cell 815, 818–20
Hodgkin 816, 822
indolent B-cell 821, 824*t*
Mab-drug conjugates 825–6, 832
mantle cell 820
radioimmunotherapy 824–5
retinal 912
melanoma 115, 682, 685–6, 687, 892
mesothelioma 542–3

metabolism of cancer cells 123
metastatic disease 68*t*
neuroendocrine tumours 51, 956*t*, 957–8
oesophageal cancer 378, 382
ovarian cancer 53–4, 593
pancreatic cancer 51, 496
penile cancer 607
renal cancer 51–2, 618–19
resistance
    to crizotinib 646
    in CSCs 89, 91
    to EGFR inhibitors 548, 629, 646
    to imatinib (BCR-ABL mutations) 89, 757,
        763–4, 765
    to trastuzumab 548
sarcoma 54, 850, 858–9, 861
thymic tumours 656
thyroid cancer 921–2, 927–8
vestibular schwannoma 894
TAS-102 431
TAX 323/TAX 324 trials 348
taxanes
breast cancer 561, 562
gastric cancer 403
head and neck cancer 342, 348
lung cancer 643, 644
mechanism of action 186–7
oesophageal cancer 377, 378, 382
pancreatic cancer 496–7
pharmacokinetics 212*t*, 215
prostate cancer 612
sarcoma 858
T-cell lymphomas (TCL)
ALCL 813–14, 825–6, 832
classification 812–13*b*, 813–14, 831–2
genetic profiles 815
NK/T-cell 334*f*, 812*b*, 829, 832
T cells
adult T-cell leukaemia/lymphoma 139, 832
circulating 114
infiltrating 111–12
T-ALL
    early T-cell precursor ALL 722
    genetic profiles 717*t*, 721–2
    metastasis 730
    prognosis 713
as therapeutic targets 115
T-LGL 774
T-PLL 773–4
TCF3-PBX1 fusion gene 718
TDM1 (trastuzumab-emtansine) 238, 563, 565
teenagers *see* adolescents
tegafur *see* UFT
telomeres/telomerase 5, 7, 77–8
mesothelioma 534
pancreatic cancer 480
temozolomide 858, 872, 873, 876, 878, 956*t*
temsirolimus 213*t*, 592, 820
teratoma 609, 881
testicular cancer 306–7, 607–9
acute lymphoblastic leukaemia 730
testosterone 612, 933
TET2 gene 701, 702, 815
TGFα (transforming growth factor α) 368, 480
TGFβ *see* transforming growth factor β
thalidomide 793, 794*b*, 795, 799
therapeutic misconception 230–1
thermal ablation 167
liver cancer 167, 516, 517–18
melanoma 683
non-melanoma skin cancer 692

penile cancer 603
prostate cancer 611
renal cancer 618
thiopurine methyltransferase (TPMT)
    100, 726
thoracotomy 638
thromboprophylaxis
colorectal surgery 411, 454
glioma 872
myeloma 798
pancreatic cancer 497
pleural mesothelioma surgery 662
thrombospondin-1 (TSP-1) 966
thymus tumours (thymoma/thymic
    carcinoma) 655–7
thyroglobulin 920, 922
thyroid cancer 918–28
anaplastic 918, 919, 920*f*, 922
biopsy 921, 924
causes and risk factors 151, 918–19
chemotherapy 922, 927
classification 918*t*
clinical presentation 918, 919, 923, 924
diagnosis 920–1, 924–6
follicular epithelial 67, 918–23
genetic profiles 919, 921, 923–4
genetic syndromes 918, 919, 923–4
    screening 924
histopathology 919–20, 920*f*, 924
imaging 337, 920–1, 922, 927
incidence 919, 923
lymph node involvement 921, 924, 926, 927
lymphoma 918, 920, 923
medullary 918, 923–8
metastasis
    medullary cancer 926, 927
    papillary/follicular cancer 67, 919, 921,
        922
molecular biology 919, 921
pregnancy 922–3
prognosis 922, 928
radio-iodine therapy 67, 921, 922, 927
radiotherapy 927
staging 922, 924
surgery 921, 926–7
    reoperation 927
surveillance 922, 928
targeted therapies 921–2, 927–8
thyroid function tests 920, 922
thyroxine replacement therapy 922,
    923, 928
tumour markers 924–6, 927, 928
thyroid gland
iatrogenic hypothyroidism 316
thyroidectomy 921, 926–7
thyroid-stimulating hormone (TSH) 918, 920
and pituitary tumours 939, 940
stimulation (pre-^{131}I therapy) 921
suppression (post-treatment) 922, 923
TICs (tumour-initiating cells) *see* cancer stem
    cells (CSCs)
TIDEL-I/TIDEL-II trials 761
TILs (tumour infiltrating lymphocytes) 111,
    687
tissue banks 101–2, 106
tivozanib 54
TKIs *see* tyrosine kinase inhibitors
T-LGL (T-cell large granular lymphocytic
    leukaemia) 774
TLX1/TLX3 genes 722
T lymphocytes *see* T cells

TME *see* tumour microenvironment
TNF (tumour necrosis factor) family 43–4, 44,
    389, 860
TNM staging 164
breast cancer 553–4
colorectal cancer 408, 452
gastric cancer 394*b*
head and neck cancer 341, 349–50
lung cancer 635, 636*t*, 637*f*, 638*t*
mesothelioma (peritoneal) 538, 539*t*
oesophageal cancer 369, 370
penile cancer 602
renal cancer 617
thyroid cancer 924
urothelial cell cancer 613, 615
tobacco industry 132
tobacco use *see* smoking
ToGA trial 382, 402*t*, 403
tongue base 333, 347
tonsils 333, 351
TOPGEAR trial 380
topical chemotherapy
basal cell carcinoma 693
melanoma 683
penile carcinoma in situ 603
squamous cell carcinoma and
    precursors 694–5
topoisomerase inhibitors *see* etoposide;
    irinotecan; topotecan
topotecan 187, 213*t*, 592, 648
tositumomab 824–5
total glans resurfacing (TGR) 603
total mesometrial resection (TMMR) 582
TP53 see p53 protein/*TP53* gene
TP73 gene/p73 protein 390
T-PLL (T-cell prolymphocytic
    leukaemia) 773–4
TPMT (thiopurine methyltransferase)
    100, 726
trabectedin 858
trachelectomy 582
tracheo-bronchial fistula 369
TRAIL receptor 43, 44
trametinib 686
transanal endoscopic microsurgery (TEM)
    167, 411
trans-arterial chemoembolization (TACE) of
    hepatic tumours 516, 517
with adjuvant sorafenib 521
neuroendocrine tumour metastases
    950, 958
transforming growth factor α (TGFα)
    368, 480
transforming growth factor β (TGFβ) 16–17,
    29–30, 90–1
colorectal cancer 451
gastric cancer 392
pancreatic cancer 480
translocations 38–9, 715
in acute lymphoblastic leukaemia 715, 717*t*,
    718–19, 721–2
in acute myeloid leukaemia 699
in DLBCL 816
in myeloma 783–4, 784, 786*t*
in sarcoma 849–50*t*, 850
t(1;19)(p13;q22) (*TCF3-PBX1*) 718
t(9;22)(q34;q11) *see* Philadelphia
    chromosome (Ph)
t(12;21)(p13;q22) (*ETV6-RUNX1*) 715, 718,
    720
transoral robotic surgery 347, 348

transplantation
  haematopoietic stem cells
    acute lymphoblastic leukaemia 713–14,
      726–7, 727–8
    acute myeloid leukaemia 699, 710–11, 712
    adverse effects 316
    amyloidosis 800–1
    chronic myeloid leukaemia 758, 765
    conditioning 826–7
    reduced-intensity 711, 727, 758, 827
    lymphoma 822, 823, 826–7
    myeloma 795, 796, 799
    POEMS syndrome 800
    prolymphocytic leukaemia 773
  liver
    for cholangiocarcinoma 525
    for liver cancer 514, 515
    for neuroendocrine tumour
      metastases 953–4
transrectal ultrasound (TRUS) 610
transurethral resection 614
TRAP (tartrate-resistant acid
  phosphatase) 771
trastuzumab (Herceptin®)
  breast cancer 67, 553, 562–3, 564–5
    in combination with radiotherapy 559
    resistance 548
  cardiotoxicity 315, 559
  cost 238
  gastric cancer 396, 402, 403
  oesophageal cancer 378, 382
trastuzumab-emtansine (TDM1) 238, 563, 565
TRA/TRB/TRD/TRG genes 721
tremelimumab 687
TRUS (transrectal ultrasound) 610
TSC1/TSC2 complex (tuberous sclerosis) 26–7
TSH see thyroid-stimulating hormone
tubular adenocarcinoma, gastric 394, 395f
tumour-associated macrophages (TAM) 66,
  109, 110–11, 114, 549
tumour infiltrating lymphocytes (TILs) 111,
  687
tumour-initiating cells (TICs) see cancer stem
  cells (CSCs)
tumour lysis syndrome 706
tumour markers 98–9
  AFP 881
    liver cancer 514
    testicular cancer 607, 608
  CA19-9 497
  CA-125 538, 969
  calcitonin 924–6, 927, 928
  CEA 466, 926, 928
  hCG 607, 608, 881
  in lymphoma 810
  in mesothelioma 538
  PSA 273, 610, 611, 612, 970
  in unknown primary cancer 968, 969
tumour microenvironment (TME)
  breast cancer 549
  CSC niche 8–9, 89
  immune/inflammatory response 109–12,
    114
  myeloma 785–6
  pancreatic cancer 480–1
  role in metastasis 65–7
tumour necrosis factor (TNF) family 43–4, 44,
  389, 860
tumour suppressor genes (TSGs) 4, 38t, 39
  breast cancer 548

cervical cancer 577
colorectal cancer 449, 451
endometrial cancer 578
gastric cancer 390, 396
head and neck cancer 329–31
lung cancer 630
mesothelioma 534, 660
mitochondrial 122–3
mutations caused by tobacco smoke 129
myeloma 784
oesophageal cancer 366–7, 369
ovarian cancer 579
pancreatic cancer 480
penile cancer 607
repression can lead to self-renewal
  potential 89–90
unknown primary 966
vulvar cancer 581
see also BRCA1/BRCA2 genes; p16
  protein/CDKN2A gene; p53
  protein/TP53 gene; pRb (retinoblastoma
  protein, RB1)
Turcot's syndrome 451
tylosis 365
type I (false positive) error 224, 226
type II (false negative) error 224
tyrosine kinase inhibitors (TKIs)
  anti-ALK 630, 646
  anti-BCR-ABL see bosutinib; dasatinib;
    imatinib
  anti-BRAF 682, 685–6, 892, 921–2
    see also sorafenib
  anti-EGFR see afatinib; erlotinib; gefitinib
  anti-EGFR/HER2 see lapatinib
  anti-FGFR see dovitinib
  anti-JAK 14, 719
  anti-MEK 629, 686
  anti-PDGFR see imatinib
  anti-VEGFR 54
    see also axitinib; pazopanib; sorafenib;
      sunitinib
  in chronic myeloid leukaemia 754, 756–8
    monitoring response 758–63, 765
    refractory/recurrent disease 764–5
    resistance 89, 757, 763–4, 765
    therapy may be stopped without
      recurrence 765–6
  multi-kinase inhibitors see regorafenib;
    sorafenib; vandetanib

U
ubiquitin ligases 16
  APC 33, 36
  Cbl 24–5
  in mesothelioma 543
  SOCS 14, 25
UFT (tegafur + uracil) 425, 519
UGT1A1 gene 214
UK
  breast cancer screening 267–8
  cervical cancer screening 272
  colorectal cancer screening 270
  cost of cancer care 239
  HPV vaccination 272
  melanoma 676t
UKALLXII/US ECOG 2993 trial 726, 727
UKELD score 515t
ulceration, melanoma 678
ulcerative colitis 444, 456
ULK1-4 kinases 27, 47

ultrasmall superparamagnetic particles of iron
  oxide (USPIO) 409
ultrasound
  breast cancer screening 267
  colorectal cancer 409
  endometrial cancer 583
  head and neck cancer 337
  hepatobiliary cancers 511–12, 513, 514, 522
  melanoma 682, 908
  oesophageal cancer 371, 372
  orbital tumours 906
  prostate cancer 610
  testicular cancer 607–8
  therapeutic (HIFU) 516, 611
  thyroid cancer 920–1, 922
  urothelial cell carcinoma 614
UNFOLDER trial 829
United Nations (UN), on cancer control 246
unknown primary see cancer of unknown
  primary (CUP)
UPA/PAI assay 561
upper urinary tract (ureteric) cancer 614,
  615–16
ureterocolic anastomosis 446
ureteroscopy 616
uric acid, hyperuricaemia 706, 787
urinary analysis
  myeloma 782, 787
  urothelial cell carcinoma 613–14, 616
urinary incontinence 316, 611
urothelial cell carcinoma 612–16
  biomarkers 614, 616
  diagnosis 613–14, 615–16
  epidemiology 613, 615
  histopathology 613
  treatment 614–15, 616
USA
  chronic myeloid leukaemia 754
  colorectal cancer 415, 444
  cost of cancer care 236, 237, 238, 240
    'choosing wisely' campaign 240
  defensive medicine 240
  lymphoma 808
  melanoma 676t
  pancreatic cancer 478
  survivors of cancer 312
uterine cancer see cervical cancer; endometrial
  cancer
uveal lymphoma 914
uveal melanoma 908–11
uveitis 882
UV light
  eyelid cancer 904
  melanoma 674, 675, 676
  other skin cancer 690, 691, 693
  xeroderma pigmentosum 75, 690–1, 905

V
V325 trial 402t, 403
vaccines 256–60
  economics 257, 258, 259–60
  HBV 256–7
  HPV 258–9, 272–3, 606
  in melanoma 686–7
  in myeloma 798
  Sipuleucel-T (for prostate cancer) 115, 259, 612
vaginal bleeding 583, 933
vaginal cancer
  chemotherapy 592
  epidemiology 576

histopathology 580–1
HPV-related 580
imaging 584
lymph node involvement 584–5
radiotherapy 584, 590–1
surgery 584–5
vaginal hysterectomy 583
vaginal vault brachytherapy 589–90, 596
validation of biomarker tests 105–6, 216
vandetanib 927
vascular disrupting agents (VDAs) 54, 55t, 56t
vascular endothelial growth factor (VEGF)
inhibitors
adverse effects 53
breast cancer 54, 563
colorectal cancer 52, 427–8, 429–30, 432, 459
liver cancer 519, 520
lung cancer 643
mechanism of action 52–3, 187
oesophageal cancer 382
ovarian cancer 53–4, 593
pancreatic cancer 496
molecular biology 49, 50–1, 66
oesophageal cancer 368
pancreatic cancer 480–1
POEMS syndrome 800
unknown primary 966
vascular endothelial growth factor receptor
(VEGFR) 49, 51–2, 54
inhibitors
adverse effects 53
colorectal cancer 431
gastro-oesophageal cancers 382, 404
liver cancer 51, 519–20, 521
lung cancer 644
mechanism of action 187–8
renal cancer 51–2, 618–19
vascular system
angiogenesis see angiogenesis
metastatic spread via 62–3
vatalanib 54
Vd (volume of distribution) 211
vegetables and fruit in the diet 156–7
VEGF see vascular endothelial growth factor
(VEGF)
VEGFR see vascular endothelial growth factor
receptor (VEGFR)
vemurafenib 682, 685–6, 892
vena cava, renal cancer spread to 618
venous thromboembolism see
thromboprophylaxis
Verner–Morrison syndrome (VIPoma) 945t,
950, 955t

verrucous carcinoma
head and neck 332
penile 603
vaginal/vulvar 581
vertebral collapse in myeloma 786, 789f,
790, 797
vestibular schwannoma 893–4
Vienna classification (gastrointestinal epithelial
neoplasia) 368t
vinca alkaloids 186, 213t
lymphoma (CHOP) 817–18
VIPoma (vasoactive intestinal polypeptide-
secreting) 945t, 950, 955t
virilizing tumours 932, 933
viruses, oncogenic 136–41
and EGFR 25
immune response 6
lymphoma 808, 832
see also hepatitis B virus; hepatitis C virus;
herpesviruses; human papilloma virus
vision, disturbances in
brain tumours 882, 886
orbital tumours 906
pituitary tumours 940
vismodegib 693
vitamins 264, 445, 698
vitreoretinal lymphoma (VRL) 912–14, 912f
vocal cord paralysis 374
volunteer bias 267
von Hippel-Lindau syndrome (VHL) 616–17,
873, 935
vulvar cancer
chemoradiotherapy 591
chemotherapy 592
epidemiology 576
histopathology 581
HPV-related 581
lymph node involvement 585, 591
molecular biology 581
radiotherapy 591
surgery 585

W
warfarin 214
watchful waiting 610–11
weight see body weight
well-differentiated liposarcoma 845, 849t,
852–3
well-differentiated papillary peritoneal
mesothelioma (WDPPM) 534, 536
Well's syndrome 766
Werner syndrome 278t

WHEL (Women's Healthy Eating and Living)
study 319
Whipple procedure 486
Whipple's triad see insulinoma
white blood cell count
acute lymphoblastic leukaemia 712–13
acute myeloid leukaemia 706
chronic lymphocytic leukaemia 766
chronic myeloid leukaemia 756
WHO see World Health Organization
whole abdominal radiation therapy
(WART) 463, 540, 591
whole-body digital photography 677
whole brain radiation therapy (WBRT) 565,
646, 685, 688, 883–4, 891–2
whole-genome sequencing 548, 702
Wilms' tumour 277t
see also WT1 protein
Wnt signalling pathway 29
gastric cancer 390, 393
pancreatic cancer 481
women see females
Women's Intervention Nutrition Study
(WINS) 319
World Health Organization (WHO)
bladder cancer grading 613b, 613t
on cancer control planning 246, 247, 251
on cancer vaccines 257, 258
CNS tumour classification 867, 869t
gastric cancer classification 394
lymphoma classification 809, 812–14, 831–2
neuroendocrine tumour classification 946t
sarcoma classification 845, 845–6b
thymic tumour classification 655, 656t
on tobacco control 133
WT1 protein 580

X
XBP1 (transcription factor) 783
xeroderma pigmentosum (XP) 75, 690–1, 905
xerostomia (dry mouth) 343
XPO1/exportin1 767
X-rays, myeloma 790
XRCC5/XRCC6 dimer (Ku) 76, 84

Y
YWHAZ gene 551

Z
ZAP-70 (zeta-associated protein) 767
zoledronic acid 563, 797
Zollinger–Ellison syndrome 945t, 947–50, 954t